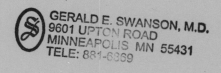
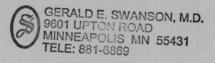
Paid ⟶ # 4656(

Ordered ⟶ 1/19/03
$105 44

Therapy in Nephrology and Hypertension

SECOND EDITION

A Companion to
Brenner and Rector's
THE KIDNEY

Edited by

Hugh R. Brady MD PhD FRCPI
Professor of Medicine and Therapeutics
Department of Medicine and Therapeutics
University College Dublin
Mater Misericordiae University Hospital
Dublin
Ireland

Christopher S. Wilcox MD PhD FRCP FACP
Chief, Division of Nephrology and Hypertension
Vice-Chair, Department of Medicine
Director, Cardiovascular–Kidney Institute
Georgetown University
Washington, DC
USA

SAUNDERS

London • Edinburgh • New York • Philadelphia • St Louis • Sydney • Toronto 2003

WB SAUNDERS
An imprint of Elsevier Science Limited

First edition 1999

ISBN 0721696813

British Library Cataloguing in Publication Data
A catalogue record for this book is available from the British Library

Library of Congress Cataloging in Publication Data
A catalog record for this book is available from the Library of Congress

Notice
Medical knowledge is constantly changing. Standard safety precautions must be followed, but as new research and clinical experience broaden our knowledge, changes in treatment and drug therapy may become necessary or appropriate. Readers are advised to check the most current product information provided by the manufacturer of each drug to be administered to verify the recommended dose, the method and duration of administration, and contraindications. It is the responsibility of the practitioner, relying on experience and knowledge of the patient, to determine dosages and the best treatment for each individual patient. Neither the Publisher nor the editor/contributor assumes any liability for any injury and/or damage to persons or property arising from this publication.
The Publisher

 ELSEVIER SCIENCE   your source for books, journals and multimedia in the health sciences
www.elsevierhealth.com

Printed in Spain by Grafos SA

The Publisher's policy is to use paper manufactured from sustainable forests

Commissioning Editor: *Susan Pioli*
Project Development Manager: *Louise Cook*
Project Managers: *Prepress Projects Ltd and Aoibhe O'Shea*
Illustration Manager: *Mick Ruddy*
Designer: *Andy Chapman*
Illustrator: *Tim Loughhead*

To my parents: Hugh and Carmel Brady.

– HRB

To my wife and children: Linda, Mark, Juliette, Stuart, and Phillip.

– CSW

We also dedicate this second edition to our mentors, who have been a source of inspiration to us:

Faisel S. Nashat, Professor Sir Stanley Peart, Gerhard Giebisch, George E. Schreiner, and Barry M. Brenner.

– HRB and CSW

I demand of my students the patience of poetry and the passion of science.

– Vladimir Nabokov

Contents

Contents

Preface

In the first edition of *Therapy in Nephrology and Hypertension* we used the parent textbook *Brenner and Rector's The Kidney* as a springboard from which to launch an amplified discussion of the rationale, specifics, efficacy, and limitations of current renal and hypertension therapeutics. We challenged our panel of expert contributors to summarize and critique clinical trials and to make treatment recommendations based on the results of these trials. Where clinical trials were too few or flawed to allow consensus, we further challenged our contributors to make recommendations based on a combination of the evidence available and their own personal experience and to suggest trials that would clarify treatment strategies going forward.

It was with some anxiety that we chose to launch a second edition some four years after the first. Had therapy evolved sufficiently to justify a second edition? Had therapy evolved at all? While we appreciate that the final decision in this regard will be made by our readers, it was heartening that our contributors accepted our second invitation with great enthusiasm and that their contributions provide tangible evidence that the explosion in knowledge of the mechanisms of renal disease and the great surge in activity in the world of clinical investigation and clinical trials is advancing renal hypertension and therapeutics in a manner that would have been unimaginable a decade ago. As should be evident from the text, many vexing questions have been answered through improved trial design, and new agents and regimens have emerged on the landscape that offer hope where none existed before.

In keeping with the style of the first edition, the updated text relies on multiple short chapters that have been designed to make the information accessible and comprehensive to the expert in nephrology and hypertension and the general internist, fellow, or student. Clinical features, pathology, pathophysiology, and diagnosis are discussed only briefly to launch a detailed discussion of therapy. For more comprehensive discussion of the former aspects of renal disease and hypertension, readers are referred to the parent text *Brenner and Rector's The Kidney*. In an effort to sustain the energy and vitality embodied in the first edition, we decided to arbitrarily "roll over" approximately one-third of our contributors with each subsequent edition. With regard to hypertension, the sections on the management of essential and secondary hypertension have been expanded significantly, reflecting the impressive volume of new clinical trial activity in these areas. In response to suggestions by our readers and reviewers, we have included a new section on the treatment of renal disease in children. With reference to the field of adult nephrology, new or expanded chapters have been included addressing the cardiovascular complications of endstage renal disease and the management of cardiovascular risk factors such as hypercholesterolemia, hyperhomocysteinemia, and oxidative stress. In the area of anemia management, the introduction of darbopoietin (a novel erythroid stimulating peptide) into clinical practice offers the first alternative to erythropoietin. With an eye on the wider impact of endstage renal disease on the patient and society, new chapters are included on measures to improve quality of life, on palliative and supportive care, and on the health economics of the treatment of endstage renal disease.

Once again, our readers will determine the success of this textbook. Your comments, criticisms, and suggestions following the publication of our first edition were much appreciated and have had a significant impact on our shaping of this new text. We look forward to your feedback over the coming months and years and sincerely hope that the second edition of *Therapy in Nephrology and Hypertension* assists you with the management of your patients and with the design of new therapeutic strategies and regimens that will advance the treatment of renal disease and hypertension going forward.

Hugh R. Brady
Christopher S. Wilcox
2003

Contributors

Marcin Adamczak MD
Department of Internal Medicine
Section Nephrology
University of Heidelberg
Heidelberg
Germany;
Assistant in Department of Nephrology,
Endocrinology and Metabolic Diseases
Silesian University School of Medicine
Katowice
Poland

Gerald B Appel MD
Professor of Clinical Medicine
Director of Clinical Nephrology
Columbia University College of
Physicians and Surgeons
Columbia Presbyterian Center of
New York – Presbyterian Hospital
New York, NY
USA

Shakil Aslam MD
Assistant Professor of Medicine
Division of Nephrology and
Hypertension
Georgetown University
Washington, DC
USA

Robert C Atkins DSc FRACP
Professor, Department of Medicine
Director, Department of Nephrology
Monash Medical Centre
Melbourne, Victoria
Australia

Howard A Austin III MD
Adjunct Professor of Medicine
Uniformed Services University of the
Health Sciences;
Senior Clinical Investigator
National Institute of Diabetes and
Digestive and Kidney Diseases
National Institutes of Health
Bethesda, MD
USA

James E Balow MD
Professor of Medicine
Uniformed Services University of the
Health Sciences;
Clinical Director and Chief
Kidney Disease Section
National Institute of Diabetes and
Digestive and Kidney Diseases
National Institutes of Health
Bethesda, MD
USA

Brendan J Barrett MB MSc FRCPI
FRCPC
Professor of Medicine
Division of Nephrology and Clinical
Epidemiology Unit
Patient Research Centre
Health Sciences Centre
St John's, NF
Canada

Bryan N Becker MD FACP
Associate Professor of Nephrology
Head, Nephrology Section
University of Wisconsin
Madison, WI
USA

Rinaldo Bellomo MD
Professor of Medicine
University of Melbourne;
Director of Intensive Care Research
Staff Specialist in Intensive Care
Department of Intensive Care
Austin & Repatriation Medical Centre
Heidelberg, Victoria
Australia

Tomas Berl MD
Professor of Medicine
University of Colorado
Denver, CO
USA

Peter G Blake MB FRCPC FRCPI
Professor of Medicine
University of Western Ontario
London, ON
Canada

Catherine Blake PhD MMedSc
College Lecturer
University College Dublin
School of Physiotherapy
Mater Misericordiae University Hospital
Dublin
Ireland

Roy D Bloom MD
Assistant Professor of Medicine
Renal Division
University of Pennsylvania
School of Medicine
Philadelphia, PA
USA

Dimitrios T Boumpas MD
Professor and Chairman
Department of Internal Medicine
University of Crete Medical School
Heraklion
Crete
Greece

Joseph V Bonventre MD PhD
Robert H Ebert Professor of
Molecular Medicine
Department of Medicine
Harvard Medical School;
Director, Division of Health Sciences
and Technology
Massachusetts Institute of Technology;
Physician, Medical Services
Massachusetts General Hospital
Boston, MA
USA

Hugh R Brady MD PhD FRCPI
Professor of Medicine and Therapeutics
Department of Medicine and
Therapeutics
University College Dublin
Mater Misericordiae University Hospital
Dublin
Ireland

D Craig Brater MD
Dean
Indiana University School of Medicine
Indianapolis, IN
USA

William E Braun MD
Department of Nephrology and
Hypertension
Consultant, Organ Transplantation
Cleveland Clinic Foundation
Cleveland, OH
USA

Emmanuel L Bravo MD
Consultant
Department of Nephrology
and Hypertension
Cleveland Clinic Foundation
Cleveland, OH
USA

Alessandra Brendolan MD
Nephrologist
Department of Nephrology
St Bortolo Hospital
Vicenza
Italy

Barry M Brenner MD
Director Emeritus, Renal Division
Brigham and Women's Hospital;
Samuel A Levine Professor of Medicine
Harvard Medical School
Boston, MA
USA

David M Briscoe MB MRCP
Associate Professor
Harvard Medical School
Division of Nephrology
Children's Hospital
Boston, MA
USA

Giovambattista Capasso MD
Associate Professor of Nephrology
Second University of Naples
Naples
Italy

Culley C Carson III MD
Rhodes Distinguished Professor and
Chief of Urology
University of North Carolina
at Chapel Hill
School of Medicine
Chapel Hill, NC
USA

Steven J Chadban MD PhD FRACP
Nephrologist and Transplant Physician
Renal Medicine
Royal Prince Alfred Hospital
Camperdown, NSW
Australia

Arlene Chapman MD
Professor of Medicine
Director of Hypertension and Renal
Diseases Research
Emory University School of Medicine
Atlanta, GA
USA

Glenn M Chertow MD MPH
Associate Professor of Medicine
Division of Nephrology and
Department of Medicine
University of California
San Francisco, CA
USA

Russell W Chesney MD
Le Bonheur Professor and Chair
Department of Pediatrics
University of Tennessee Health
Science Center
Le Bonheur Children's Hospital
Memphis, TN
USA

Fredric L Coe MD
Professor of Medicine and Physiology
Nephrology Section
Department of Medicine
University of Chicago
Chicago, IL
USA

Lewis M Cohen MD
Associate Professor of Psychiatry
Tufts University School of Medicine;
Co-director, Psychiatric Consultation
Service
Baystate Medical Center
Springfield, MA
USA

Paul R Conlin MD
Assistant Professor of Medicine
Harvard Medical School;
Director, Endocrinology
Training Program
Division of Endocrinology, Diabetes,
and Hypertension
Brigham and Women's Hospital
Boston, MA
USA

Gary C Curhan MD ScD
Associate Professor of Medicine
and Epidemiology
Harvard Medical School and
Harvard School of Public Health
Channing Laboratory
Boston, MA
USA

John J Curtis MD
Professor of Medicine and
Professor of Surgery
University of Alabama at Birmingham
Division of Nephrology
Birmingham, AL
USA

Bryan M Curtis MD FRCPC
Research Fellow
Division of Nephrology and Clinical
Epidemiology Unit
Patient Research Centre
Health Sciences Centre
St John's, NF
Canada

Giuseppe D'Amico MD
Professor of Medicine
San Carlo Borromeo Hospital
Milan
Italy

Donald C Dafoe MD
Samuel D Gross Professor and
Chairman
Department of Surgery
Jefferson Medical College
Philadelphia, PA
USA

Simon Davies MD FRCP
Reader in Nephrology
Centre for Science and Technology in
Medicine
Keele University
Staffordshire
UK

Raffaele De Caterina MD PhD
Professor of Cardiology
Director, University Cardiology Division
"G D'Annunzio" University – Chieti;
Director, Laboratory for Thrombosis
and Vascular Research
CNR Institute of Clinical Physiology
Pisa
Italy

Laura M Dember MD
Assistant Professor of Medicine
Boston University School of Medicine
Attending Physician, Renal Section
Boston University Medical Center
Boston, MA
USA

Mark Denton BSc PhD MRCP
Specialist Registrar in Renal Medicine
Guy's Hospital
London
UK

J Eric Derkson MD
Chief Resident
University of North Carolina
at Chapel Hill
School of Medicine
Chapel Hill, NC
USA

Hamish Dobbie MB
Clinical Research Fellow
Centre for Nephrology
The Middlesex Hospital
London
UK

Alden M Doyle MD MPH MS
Assistant Professor of Medicine
Renal Division
University of Pennsylvania
School of Medicine
Philadelphia, PA
USA

Tilman B Drüeke MD FRCP
Director of Research and
Associate Professor
Division of Nephrology
Hôpital Necker
Paris Cedex 15
France

Wilfred Druml MD
Professor of Medicine
Klinik für Innere Medizin III
Abteilung für Nephrologie
University of Vienna
Vienna
Austria

Thomas D DuBose Jr MD
Professor and Chair
Department of Internal Medicine
Wake Forest University Health Sciences
Winston-Salem, NC
USA

Lance D Dworkin MD
Professor of Medicine
Brown University Medical School
Rhode Island Hospital
Providence, RI
USA

David H Ellison MD
Head, Division of Nephrology
and Hypertension
Professor of Medicine and Physiology
and Pharmacology
Staff Physician, Department of
Veterans' Affairs
Oregon Health and Science University
Portland, OR
USA

Murray Epstein MD FACP
Professor of Medicine
University of Miami School of Medicine
Miami, FL
USA

Joseph A Eustace MB MRCPI MHS
Assistant Professor
Departments of Medicine and
Epidemiology
Johns Hopkins University School
of Medicine
Baltimore, MD
USA

Ronald J Falk MD
Doc J Thurston Professor of Medicine
Chief, Division of Nephrology and
Hypertension
University of North Carolina
at Chapel Hill
School of Medicine
Chapel Hill, NC
USA

John Feehally MA DM FRCP
Professor of Renal Medicine
Department of Nephrology
Leicester General Hospital
Leicester
UK

M Roy First MD
Professor of Medicine
Director, Section of Transplantation
Division of Nephrology
University of Cincinnati
Cincinnati, OH
USA

Maxwell E Fisher MD
Renal Fellow
Department of Medicine
Vanderbilt University
Nashville, TN
USA

John M Fitzpatrick MCh FRCSI
FCUrol FRCS
Professor and Chairman
and Consultant Urologist
Department of Surgery
University College Dublin
Dublin
Ireland

Robert N Foley MB MSc FRCPI FRCPC
Director
Nephrology Analytical Services
Minneapolis, MN
USA

Alessandro Fornasieri MD
Consultant
Division of Nephrology
San Carlo Hospital
Milan
Italy

John H Galla MD
Professor Emeritus of Medicine
Division of Nephrology and
Hypertension
Department of Medicine
University of Cincinnati
Cincinnati, OH
USA

Marc B Garnick MD
Clinical Professor of Medicine
Harvard Medical School;
Associate in Medicine and
Genitourinary Oncology
Department of Hematology/Oncology
Beth Israel Deaconess Medical Center
Boston, MA
USA

Robert S Gaston MD
Professor of Medicine and Professor
of Surgery
Division of Nephrology
University of Alabama at Birmingham
Birmingham, AL
USA

Michael J Germain MD FACP
Associate Professor of Medicine
Tufts University School of Medicine;
Medical Director
Renal Transplantation Service
Baystate Medical Center
Springfield, MA
USA

David A Goldfarb MD
Head, Section of Renal Transplantation
Urological Institute
Cleveland Clinic Foundation
Cleveland, OH
USA

Eddie L Greene MD
Associate Professor of Medicine
Department of Internal Medicine
Division of Nephrology
Mayo Clinic and Mayo School of
Medicine
Rochester, MN
USA

Todd F Griffith MD
Fellow in Nephrology
Duke Institute for Renal Outcomes
Research and Health Policy
Division of Nephrology
Duke University Medical Center
Durham, NC
USA

Scott M Grundy MD PhD
Professor of Internal Medicine
University of Texas Southwestern
Medical Center
Dallas, TX
USA

Mitchell L Halperin MD
Professor of Medicine
University of Toronto
St Michael's Hospital
Toronto, ON
Canada

Richard K Halterman MD
Clinical Instructor
University of Colorado
Denver, CO
USA

Peter Hewins MRCP
Clinical Research Training Fellow in
Nephrology
Division of Medical Sciences
The Medical School
Birmingham
UK

Norman K Hollenberg MD PhD
Professor
Harvard Medical School
Boston, MA
USA

Enyu Imai MD PhD
Professor of Medicine
Renal Section
Osaka University School of Medicine
Osaka
Japan

Bertrand L Jaber MD
Assistant Professor of Medicine
Tufts University School of Medicine
Tufts New England Medical Center
Boston, MA
USA

Sarbjit V Jassal MB MRCP MSc
FRCPC MD
Assistant Professor
University of Toronto
Staff Physician
University Health Network
Toronto, ON
Canada

Rosy E Joseph MD
Hackenstock University Medical Center
Hackenstock, NJ
USA

Kamel S Kamel MD
Associate Professor of Medicine
University of Toronto
St Michael's Hospital
Toronto, ON
Canada

Norman M Kaplan MD
Clinical Professor of Internal Medicine
University of Texas
Southwestern Medical School
Dallas, TX
USA

Joana E Kist-van Holthe MD
Renal Fellow
Division of Nephrology
Children's Hospital
Harvard Medical School
Boston, MA
USA

Saulo Klahr MD
John E and Adaline Simon Professor
of Medicine
Department of Internal Medicine
Washington University
School of Medicine
Barnes-Jewish Hospital of St Louis
St Louis, MO
USA

Mary E Klotman MD
Murray Rosenberg Professor of
Medicine
Chief, Division of Infectious Diseases
Mount Sinai School of Medicine
New York, NY
USA

Paul E Klotman MD
Murray Rosenberg Professor of Medicine
Chairman, Samuel F Bronfman
Department of Medicine
Mount Sinai School of Medicine
New York, NY
USA

Stephen M Korbet MD
Professor of Medicine
Section of Nephrology
Department of Medicine
Rush-Presbyterian-St Luke's Medical
Center
Chicago, IL
USA

Eugene C Kovalik MD CM FRCPC
FACP
Duke University Medical Center
Durham, NC
USA

Lawrence R Krakoff MD
Professor of Medicine
Mount Sinai School of Medicine
New York, NY
USA

Jerrold S Levine MD
Assistant Professor of Medicine
Section of Nephrology
The University of Chicago
Chicago, IL
USA

Jeremy B Levy MA PhD ILTM MRCP
Consultant Nephrologist
Imperial College School of Medicine
Hammersmith Hospital
London
UK

Francisco Llach MD FACP
Professor of Medicine
Director of Clinical Nephrology
Division of Nephrology and
Hypertension
Georgetown University
Washington, DC
USA

Iain C Macdougall MD BSc FRCP
Consultant Nephrologist and
Honorary Senior Lecturer
King's College Hospital
London
UK

François Madore MD MSc
Assistant Professor of Medicine
Centre de Recherche
Hôpital du Sacré-Coeur de Montréal
Montréal, Québec
Canada

Samuel J Mann MD
Associate Professor of Clinical Medicine
Department of Medicine
Hypertension Division
New York Presbyterian Hospital –
Cornell Medical School
New York, NY
USA

Ziad A Massy MD PhD
Professor of Pharmacology
University of Picardie;
Praticien Hospitalier of Nephrology and
Research Associate
INSERM U507
Necker Hospital
Paris
France

Tahsin Masud MB BS
Assistant Professor of Medicine
Renal Division
Emory University School of Medicine
Atlanta, GA
USA

Michael McKusick MD
Assistant Professor of Radiology
Department of Radiology
Section of Vascular and Interventional
Radiology
Mayo Clinic
Rochester, MN
USA

Ashraf I Mikhail MB BCh MSc MRCP
Clinical Research Fellow
King's College Hospital
London
UK

Luigi Minetti MD
Professor of Nephrology
Clinical Research Center for
Rare Diseases
Bergamo
Italy

William E Mitch MD
Edward Randall Distinguished Professor
of Medicine
Chair, Department of Medicine
University of Texas,
Galveston, TX
USA

Carl Erik Mogensen MD Dr Med Sci
Professor of Medicine
Department of Diabetes and
Endocrinology
Aarhus Kommunehospital
Aarhus
Denmark

Alvin H Moss MD
Professor of Medicine
Section of Nephrology
Director, Center for Health Ethics
and Law
Robert C Byrd Health Sciences Center
West Virginia University
Morgantown, WV
USA

Patrick H Nachman MD
Assistant Professor of Medicine
Division of Nephrology and
Hypertension
University of North Carolina
at Chapel Hill
School of Medicine
Chapel Hill, NC
USA

Eric G Neilson MD FACP
Morgan Professor and Chairman
Department of Medicine
Vanderbilt University
Nashville, TN
USA

Elizabeth H Nora MD PhD
Medical Resident
Department of Internal Medicine
Mayo Clinic
Rochester, MN
USA

Marina Noris Chem Pharm D
Head, Laboratory of Immunology and
Genetics of Rare Diseases and
Transplantation
Mario Negri Institute for
Pharmacological Research
Bergamo
Italy

Andrew C Novick MD
Chairman, Urological Institute
Cleveland Clinic Foundation
Cleveland, OH
USA

Yvonne M O'Meara MD FRCPI
Senior Lecturer in Medicine
University College Dublin
Consultant Physician
Mater Misericordiae University Hospital
Dublin
Ireland

Man S Oh MD
Professor of Medicine
State University of New York
Health Science Center at Brooklyn
Brooklyn, NY
USA

Caitlin Carroll Oppenheimer MPH
Senior Research Scientist
National Organization for Research at
the University of Chicago
Washington, DC
USA

Dimitrios G Oreopoulos MD PhD
FRCPC FACP FRCTS
Professor of Medicine
University of Toronto
Director of Peritoneal Dialysis Program
University Health Network
Toronto, ON
Canada

William F Owen Jr MD
Chief Scientist
Baxter Healthcare – Renal
Waukegan, IL;
Adjunct Professor of Medicine
Duke University School of Medicine
Durham, NC
USA

Vasilios Papademetriou MD FACC
FACP
Professor of Medicine
Georgetown University;
Director Hypertension and
Cardiovascular Research
Department of Veterans' Affairs
Medical Center
Washington, DC
USA

Patrick S Parfrey MD FRCPC
University Research Professor
Division of Nephrology and Clinical
Epidemiology Unit
Patient Research Centre
Health Sciences Centre
St John's, NF
Canada

Joan H Parks MBA
Research Associate and
Assistant Professor
Nephrology Section
Department of Medicine
University of Chicago
Chicago, IL
USA

Manish P Patel MD
Chief Resident
University of North Carolina
at Chapel Hill
School of Medicine
Chapel Hill, NC
USA

V Ram Peddi MD
Associate Professor of Medicine
Division of Nephrology
University of Cincinnati
Cincinnati, OH
USA

Brian JG Pereira MD MBA
Louisa C Endicott Professor of Medicine
Tufts University School of Medicine
Tufts New England Medical Center
Boston, MA
USA

William D Plant BSc MB MRCPI
FRCPE
Consultant Renal Physician
Cork University Hospital
Wilton
Cork
Ireland

Charles D Pusey MSc FRCP FRCPath
Professor of Renal Medicine
Imperial College School of Medicine
Hammersmith Hospital
London
UK

Hamid Rabb MD
Physician Director
Kidney Transplant Program
Associate Professor
Department of Medicine
Johns Hopkins University School of
Medicine
Baltimore, MD
USA

Brian D Radbill MD
Nephrology Fellow
Nephrology Division
Mount Sinai School of Medicine
New York, NY
USA

Donal Reddan MB MHS MRCPI
Associate in Medicine
Duke Institute for Renal Outcomes
Research and Health Policy
and Durham VA Medical Center;
Division of Nephrology
Duke University Medical Center
Durham, NC
USA

Andrew J Rees MSc FRCP
Regius Professor of Medicine
University of Aberdeen;
Consultant Physician
Aberdeen Royal Infirmary
Aberdeen
UK

Giuseppe Remuzzi MD
Professor of Medicine and Director
Mario Negri Institute for
Pharmacological Research;
Director of Division of Nephrology
and Dialysis
Azienda Ospedaliera Ospedali Riuniti
di Bergamo
Bergamo
Italy

Eberhard Ritz MD
Professor of Medicine
Department of Internal Medicine
Section Nephrology
University of Heidelberg
Heidelberg
Germany

Nancy M Rodig MD
Instructor in Pediatrics
Division of Nephrology
Children's Hospital
Harvard Medical School
Boston, MA
USA

Claudio Ronco MD
Director
Department of Nephrology
St Bortolo Hospital
Vicenza
Italy

Robert H Rubin MD FACP FCCP
Osborne Professor of Health Sciences
and Technology and
Professor of Medicine
Harvard Medical School;
Director, Center for Experimental
Pharmacology and Therapeutics
Massachusetts Institute of Technology;
Associate Director, Division of
Infectious Disease
Brigham and Women's Hospital
Boston, MA
USA

Robert J Rubin MD FACP
Clinical Professor of Medicine
Division of Nephrology and
Hypertension
Georgetown University
Washington, DC
USA

Piero Ruggenenti MD
Assistant Professor
Mario Negri Institute for
Pharmacological Research
Division of Nephrology and Dialysis
Azienda Ospedaliera Ospedali Riuniti
di Bergamo
Bergamo
Italy

David J Salant MD
Professor of Medicine
Boston University School of Medicine
Chief, Renal Section
Boston University Medical Center
Boston, MA
USA

Paul W Sanders MD
Professor of Medicine
University of Alabama at Birmingham
Birmingham, AL
USA

Caroline OS Savage PhD FRCP
Professor of Nephrology
Division of Medical Sciences
The Medical School
Birmingham
UK

Mohamed H Sayegh MD
Associate Professor of Medicine
Harvard Medical School
Brigham and Women's Hospital
Boston, MA
USA

Arrigo Schieppati MD
Associate Physician
Nephrology and Dialysis Unit
Azienda Ospedaliera Ospedali Riuniti
di Bergamo
Bergamo
Italy

Gerald Schulman MD
Associate Professor
Vanderbilt University School of
Medicine
Nashville, TN
USA

Steve J Schwab MD
Duke University Medical Center
Durham, NC
USA

Joshua A Schwimmer MD
Clinical Fellow in Nephrology
Columbia University College of
Physicians and Surgeons
Columbia Presbyterian Center of New
York – Presbyterian Hospital
New York, NY
USA

Douglas G Shemin MD
Clinical Associate Professor of Medicine
Brown University Medical School
Renal Division
Rhode Island Hospital
Providence, RI
USA

Alice M Sheridan MD
Instructor in Medicine
Harvard Medical School;
Assistant in Medicine
Massachusetts General Hospital
Boston, MA
USA

Karen V Smirnakis MD PhD
Instructor in Medicine
Harvard Medical School;
Chief Resident and Assistant in
Medicine
Massachusetts General Hospital
Boston, MA
USA

Virend K Somers MD PhD
Professor of Medicine
Division of Cardiovascular Diseases and
Division of Hypertension
Mayo Clinic
Rochester, MN
USA

Michael JG Somers MD
Assistant in Medicine and Assistant
Professor of Pediatrics
Division of Nephrology
Children's Hospital
Harvard Medical School
Boston, MA
USA

Renuka Sothinathan MB BAOBCh
MHS
Senior Fellow
Division of Nephrology
Johns Hopkins University School
of Medicine
Baltimore, MD
USA

Robert O Stuart MD
Assistant Professor of Medicine
Division of Nephrology and
Hypertension, VASDHS;
Director, VASDHS GeneChip
Core Facility;
Co-leader, UCSD Cancer Center
Microarray Shared Resource
La Jolla, CA
USA

Vikas P Sukhatme MD PhD
Professor of Medicine, Renal Section
Beth Israel Deaconess Medical Center
and Harvard Medical School
Boston, MA
USA

Maarten W Taal MB ChB MMed FCP
Consultant Renal Physician
Renal Unit
Derby City General Hospital
Derby
UK

Edward G Tessier PharmD MPH
BCPS
Clinical Associate Professor of Medicine
Springfield College
Springfield, MA
USA

Stephen C Textor MD
Professor of Medicine
Divisions of Hypertension and
Nephrology
Mayo Clinic
Rochester, MN
USA

Joshua M Thurman MD
Clinical Instructor
University of Colorado
Denver, CO
USA

Nina E Tolkoff-Rubin MD FACP
Medical Director of Transplantation
Chief of Hemodialysis and
Peritoneal Dialysis
Director of End Stage Renal
Disease Program
Massachusetts General Hospital;
Associate Professor of Medicine
Harvard Medical School
Boston, MA
USA

Robert Toto MD
Professor of Medicine
University of Texas Southwestern
Medical Center
Dallas, TX
USA

Laurence A Turka MD
C Mahlon Kline Professor of Medicine
Chief, Renal – Electrolyte and
Hypertension Division
University of Pennsylvania
School of Medicine
Philadelphia, PA
USA

A Neil Turner PhD FRCP
Professor of Nephrology
University of Edinburgh
Edinburgh Royal Infirmary
Edinburgh
UK

Jason G Umans MD PhD
Associate Professor of Medicine
Division of Nephrology and
Hypertension
Georgetown University
Washington, DC
USA

Robert Unwin BM PhD FRCP
Professor of Nephrology and
Physiology
Centre for Nephrology and
Department of Physiology
The Middlesex Hospital
London
UK

Joseph A Vassalotti MD
Assistant Professor of Medicine
Nephrology Division
Director, Hemodialysis Services
Mount Sinai School of Medicine
New York, NY
USA

Gloria Lena Vega PhD
Professor of Clinical Nutrition
Center for Human Nutrition
University of Texas Southwestern
Medical Center
Dallas, TX
USA

Francisco Velasquez-Forero MD
Senior Investigator
Bone Metabolic Research Unit
Hospital Infantil de Mexico
Mexico DF

John P Vella MD FRCPI FACP
Assistant Professor of Medicine
Division of Nephrology
University of Vermont
School of Medicine;
Medical Director of Renal
Transplantation
Maine Medical Center
Portland, ME
USA

Sushrut S Waikar MD
Chief Medical Resident
Division of Nephrology and
Department of Medicine
University of San Francisco
San Francisco, CA
USA

David C Wheeler MD FRCP
Senior Lecturer in Nephrology
Centre for Nephrology
Royal Free Campus
Royal Free and University College
Medical School
London
UK

Christopher S Wilcox MD PhD FRCP
FACP
Chief, Division of Nephrology and
Hypertension
Vice-Chair, Department of Medicine
Director, Cardiovascular–Kidney
Institute
Georgetown University
Washington, DC
USA

John D Williams MD FRCP
Professor of Nephrology
University of Wales College of
Medicine
Cardiff
UK

James F Winchester MD FRCP FACP
Chief Medical Officer
RenalTech International
New York, NY
USA

Gunter Wolf MD
Associate Professor of Internal Medicine
Department of Medicine
Division of Nephrology
University Hospital Eppendorf
Hamburg
Germany

Alan SL Yu MB BChir
Assistant Professor of Medicine
University of Southern California Keck
School of Medicine
Los Angeles, CA
USA

Martin Zeier MD
Department of Internal Medicine
Section Nephrology
University of Heidelberg
Heidelberg
Germany

PART I
Acute Renal Failure

HUGH R. BRADY

Crystalloids, Colloids, and Pressors in Prerenal Acute Renal Failure

Sushrut S. Waikar and Glenn M. Chertow

Volume replacement in prerenal renal failure
- Crystalloids
- Colloids
- Albumin
- Hydroxyethyl starch
- Dextrans and gelatin
- Crystalloids versus colloids

Pressors in acute renal failure
- Dopamine
- Norepinephrine
- Epinephrine and phenylephrine
- Dobutamine
- Vasopressin
- Choice of pressor

Prerenal azotemia is the most common cause of acute renal failure (ARF), accounting for 40% of cases in hospitalized patients[1] and 60% of community-acquired cases.[2] The hallmark of prerenal azotemia is inadequate renal perfusion, which may arise from hypovolemia, low cardiac output, low systemic vascular resistance, or renal vasoconstriction. By definition, ARF from prerenal causes is reversible if the inciting cause(s) is removed. The high morbidity and mortality attributable to ARF in hospitalized patients underscores the importance of effectively managing prerenal azotemia, especially before irreversible kidney damage occurs.

Therapies for prerenal azotemia should focus on the presumed cause for inadequate renal perfusion. Offending drugs, such as cyclooxygenase inhibitors, should be discontinued if possible, and cardiac function in cases of low cardiac output should be optimized. This chapter will focus on two common and controversial questions in the management of patients with prerenal azotemia: are crystalloids or colloids the preferred solution for volume replacement? and which vasopressor is the most effective (and least offensive) for patients with ARF and hypotension refractory to fluid therapy?

Volume replacement in prerenal renal failure

Hypovolemia sufficient to cause prerenal ARF is common in a number of clinical settings, including burns, the postoperative period, pancreatitis, gastrointestinal losses, sepsis, dehydration, and hemorrhage. The goal of volume repletion in prerenal ARF is to restore renal perfusion for adequate glomerular filtration. Successful volume resuscitation in hypovolemic patients requires the restoration

of tissue perfusion and avoidance of the untoward effects of volume overload, such as pulmonary edema. The optimal fluid composition for volume resuscitation has been the subject of considerable debate for decades. Crystalloid solutions, consisting of water and electrolytes, with or without dextrose, have been compared with the more expensive colloid solutions, which contain larger molecules that are relatively impermeable to capillary membranes. The crystalloid versus colloid debate continues even after the publication of no fewer than three recent metaanalyses suggesting that colloid administration does not improve survival relative to crystalloids.[3–5] Indeed, practice patterns vary widely around the world. A 1998 survey of intensive care units in Germany[6] showed the most commonly used solution for volume replacement to be hydroxyethyl starch (67%), followed by crystalloids (55%); albumin was rarely used (2%). In the USA, crystalloids were decidedly more popular; among colloids, albumin was by far the most commonly prescribed (83%).[7]

Crystalloids

Isotonic crystalloid solutions distribute throughout the extracellular compartment, of which approximately 25% is intravascular and 75% interstitial in healthy individuals.[8] Therefore, approximately one-fourth of the infused volume of isotonic crystalloid remains within the intravascular compartment (these assumptions may not hold in the critically ill).

Isotonic saline is the initial treatment of choice for most patients with significant hypovolemia leading to prerenal azotemia. Saline is inexpensive, readily available, and without significant deleterious effects in most instances. Large volumes of saline infusion can, however, cause hyperchloremic metabolic acidosis through "hemodilution" as nonbicarbonate-containing solutions are infused while bicarbonate-containing fluids (e.g. urine, stool) may still be excreted. The American College of Surgeons recommends the use of lactated Ringer's solution (LR) over normal saline as the initial fluid of choice in hemorrhagic shock. Lactated Ringer's solution may be expected to expand the extracellular volume slightly less effectively than normal saline, which contains a higher sodium concentration. The lactate in LR is metabolized by the liver to bicarbonate; small clinical trials have shown that infusion of buffered solutions such as LR, Normosol or Plasma-Lyte produces acidosis less frequently than an equivalent volume of isotonic saline.[9–11] No study, however, has linked the type of crystalloid solution to relevant clinical outcomes. Furthermore, patients with prerenal azotemia may exhibit an alkalosis (usually hypochloremic, and occasionally termed a "contraction" alkalosis), making the concern over the hyperchloremic acidosis with normal saline less relevant. Underlying acidosis is more common with pre-existing chronic renal insufficiency (CRI). Choosing among these isotonic solutions has become a matter of preference as no comparative clinical trials of adequate power have been conducted. In the setting of hyperchloremic meta-bolic acidosis, LR, hypotonic saline with added sodium bicarbonate (e.g. 0.45% or 0.225% saline with 50 mEq or 100 mEq of sodium bicarbonate respectively), Plasma-lyte, or Normosol may be used instead of normal (0.9% NaCl) saline. When using solutions containing potassium or magnesium, care must be taken to avoid iatrogenic electrolyte complications, particularly in patients with CRI.

Hypotonic saline solutions are commonly used as maintenance intravenous fluids in hospitalized patients. The excess free water in hypotonic saline distributes throughout the total body water (TBW) space, thereby limiting the restoration of intravascular volume compared with isotonic solutions. Hypotonic saline can be used for volume replacement in the setting of mild volume deficits and in the case of hypernatremia, in which a free water deficit exists. Since insensible losses are low in electrolytes, true "maintenance" fluids should be hypotonic.

Hypertonic saline solutions are often used in trauma settings and for patients following burns. Hypertonic saline is also used for hypotension and cramps in patients undergoing intermittent hemodialysis. By drawing water from the intracellular into the intravascular space, small volumes of hypertonic saline may result in relatively larger increases in circulating volume. Hypertonic saline has been shown to enhance myocardial contractility in animal and human studies and to increase venous return.[12,13] Wade et al[14] performed a metaanalysis of 12 studies that used hypertonic solutions for trauma resuscitation.[15–23] Results from six studies comparing hypertonic saline with isotonic resuscitation showed no difference in survival to discharge at 30 days. Eight studies compared hypertonic saline plus dextran, a colloid, with isotonic saline; a trend toward improved survival with hypertonic saline plus dextran (weighted difference in mortality, 3.5%) was observed but was not statistically significant. To date, trials employing hypertonic saline have been small in size and have not examined clinically relevant endpoints such as risk of ARF or changes in glomerular filtration rate (GFR) or creatinine clearance. Future studies on specific patient subgroups, such as those with myocardial and/or renal dysfunction, may help to define specific indications for hypertonic saline administration.

Colloids

Colloid solutions (albumin, hydroxyethyl starch, gelatins, dextrans) contain oncotically active molecules which should in theory remain within the intravascular compartment and provide an oncotic gradient favoring diffusive entry of water from the interstitium. While often grouped collectively, the individual colloid solutions have distinct pharmacologic profiles and exert different clinical effects when used for volume replacement in prerenal azotemia.

Albumin

Albumin infusion is widely used for volume expansion in multiple clinical conditions, including trauma, shock from multiple causes, and the perioperative period. Human serum albumin is extremely expensive, costing twice as much as hydroxyethyl starch and 30 times as much as sodium chloride on a milliliter per milliliter basis. The frequency of albumin administration in many academic and community-based health centers exceeds contemporary practice guidelines on the appropriate indications for its use.[7] The Cochrane Injuries Group published a systematic review of albumin use in critically ill patients with hypovolemia, burns, and hypoproteinemia.[24] Thirty randomized controlled trials comprising 1419 patients were included. The investigators found increased mortality with albumin administration. The pooled relative risk (RR) of death for patients treated with albumin was 1.68 (95% confidence interval (CI) 1.26–2.23) compared with all crystalloid solutions or no fluid administrations. A subsequent metaanalysis by Wilkes and Navickis[4] refuted the Cochrane investigators' conclusions about the dangers of albumin administration; the RR for mortality in their metaanalysis of 55 trials was 1.11 (95% CI 0.95–1.28). While conflicting quantitatively, these two metaanalyses do agree qualitatively that there is no evidence for the superiority of albumin in these clinical settings.

Only a few trials have investigated the effects of albumin on renal function, or examined its use in patients with, or at risk for, ARF (see Table 1.1). One such study, a disease-specific, randomized controlled trial, contradicts the findings of the two meta-analyses on albumin.[25] Sort et al[25] evaluated the effects of albumin on plasma volume expansion in patients with cirrhosis and spontaneous bacterial peritonitis (SBP). Acute renal failure develops in approximately one-third of patients with SBP and is among the most potent predictors of inhospital mortality.[39] Albumin infusion was remarkably effective in this population: 10% of patients given albumin plus antibiotics developed acute renal failure compared with 33% of patients given antibiotics alone ($P = 0.002$). Inhospital mortality was reduced by more than 60% (10% versus 29%, $P = 0.01$). Importantly, patients with evidence of septic shock or volume depletion were excluded from this study, and the control group received placebo instead of crystalloid.

The generalizability of this study, i.e. should albumin be the intravenous solution of choice for volume repletion in cirrhotic patients, is unclear. Based on metaanalyses of multiple trials, the routine use of albumin in the USA is probably excessive given the absence of data supporting its benefit on survival. However, specific populations may exist in which albumin is preferred. Further studies comparing albumin and crystalloid are needed, particularly in patients with, or at risk for, a variety of forms of liver or kidney disease. For now, specific recommendations on the use of albumin will have to await the completion of well-designed trials examining kidney-specific outcomes as well as mortality.

Table 1.1 Crystalloids and colloids: selected studies

Reference	Setting	No. of patients	Intervention	Study period	Renal outcomes
6	Surgical ICU (trauma and postoperative patients with sepsis)	300	1 10% HES 2 20% albumin	5 days	No differences in SCr
25	Patients with cirrhosis and spontaneous bacterial peritonitis; ~ 40% with ARF at enrollment	126	1 Albumin 20% + antibiotics 2 Antibiotics alone	90 days	ARF (defined as 50% increase in BUN or SCr) developed in only 10% of patients treated with albumin and 33% treated with antibiotics alone
26	Hypovolemia due to multiple medical or surgical causes	50	1 5% Albumin 2 6% HES	24 h	No differences in SCr
27	ICU patients with sepsis; majority with ARF at study inclusion	129	1 6% HES 2 3% Gelatin	28 days	HES treatment increased risk of ARF, defined as twofold increase in SCr or need for RRT
28	Elective major abdominal surgery	60	1 Gelatin 2 HES 70 3 HES 200	3 days	No differences in SCr
29	Elective aortic reconstruction surgery	58	1 LR 2 Hypertonic saline	3 days	No differences in SCr or CrCl
30	Elective abdominal aortic surgery	20	1 Dextran-60 in LR 2 LR	24 h	No differences in SCr
31	Elective abdominal aortic surgery	16	1 25% albumin 2 LR	1 day	No differences in CrCl
32	Hypovolemic trauma patients	52	1 "Standard resuscitation" 2 Above + albumin	Average of 55 h	GFR lower in albumin group (one-time measurement of GFR, not change, compared between groups)
33	Elective abdominal aortic surgery	24	1 Albumin 2 LR 3 0.45% saline	48 h	No differences in BUN, SCr
34	Burn victims resuscitated with LR followed by albumin × 4 h	6	Albumin 25%, 3 mL/kg/h × 4 h	4 h	After albumin administration, ERPF was unchanged and GFR decreased by 32% (PAH and insulin used to measure effect of albumin on GFR and ERPF)
35	Medical/surgical ICU	475	1 Albumin 4.5% 2 Polygeline (gelatin)	30 days	No differences in "ARF" in 112 patients hospitalized > 5 days
36	Elective major abdominal surgery	30	1 20% albumin 2 LR	6 days	No differences in BUN, SCr
37	Elective total hip arthroplasty	41	1 6% HES 2 5% albumin	6 h	No differences in CrCl
38	Vascular leak syndrome from IL-2 therapy	107	1 5% albumin 2 0.9% saline	5 days	No differences in SCr

HES, hydroxyethyl starch; LR, lactated Ringer's; ARF, acute renal failure; SCr, serum creatinine; BUN, blood urea nitrogen; GFR, glomerular filtration rate; RRT, renal replacement therapy; ICU, intensive care unit; CrCl, creatinine clearance; PAH, para-aminohippurate.

Hydroxyethyl starch

Hydroxyethyl starch (HES) is a synthetic polymer derived from the starch amylopectin. In the USA, only one preparation is commercially available, whereas in Europe a wider range of solutions is in use of varying concentrations, mean molecular weight, and molar substitutions. Hydroxyethyl starch effectively restores circulating volume by remaining largely within the intravascular space and increasing colloid oncotic pressure. Several trials have demonstrated HES to be a safe and effective volume expander in critically ill patients.[26,40,41] Although HES can affect coagulation profiles, HES has not generally been associated with bleeding diatheses.[42]

More concerning is the association of HES with ARF. In a randomized study of intravascular volume treatment of 69 brain-dead organ donors, HES treatment resulted in impaired renal function in kidney transplant recipients.[43] Schortgen et al[27] studied 129 patients with severe sepsis and randomized patients to receive gelatin (another class of artificial colloid) or HES. A majority of these patients had moderate renal dysfunction at inclusion, most frequently from prerenal causes. Acute renal failure, defined as a need for renal replacement therapy or a doubling of serum creatinine concentration, developed in 42% of patients treated with HES and 23% of patients treated with gelatin ($P = 0.028$; OR for ARF, 2.32; 95% CI, 1.02–5.34). Mortality did not differ between the two groups, highlighting the importance of examining outcomes other than survival in studies of modest scope. The exact mechanism of HES-induced ARF is unknown, and at least one small study has suggested no adverse effect on renal function in elderly patients.[28] HES may worsen renal function by raising plasma oncotic pressure and thus diminishing glomerular filtration rate.[44] Based on these findings and on the absence of clearly demonstrable clinical benefit, HES should be avoided in patients with renal failure of any cause.

Dextrans and gelatin

The dextrans are mixtures of glucose polymers of various sizes and molecular weights. Two preparations, dextran 70 and dextran 40, are available for use and are both effective in volume expansion. Dextran 70 is the solution used more often for volume resuscitation because of its longer duration of effect. Several potentially severe toxicities may occur with dextran infusion: anaphylaxis, bleeding diatheses, and ARF.[45] As with HES, reduction in glomerular filtration by hyperoncotic plasma is postulated to be the cause of ARF.[44] In patients with cirrhosis and tense ascites undergoing large volume paracentesis – a population at high risk of developing ARF – dextran 70 administration was shown to be as safe and effective as albumin.[46] In patients with established ARF, however, dextrans should not be administered.

Gelatin solutions are modified collagen derivates made from bovine raw material. They are not available commercially in the USA. The intravascular half-life of gelatins is relatively short, making them the least effective of synthetic colloids for volume expansion.

Crystalloids versus colloids

Intravenous fluids are equivalent in principle to drug therapies. The decision to use one class of fluid over another should be subjected to the same critical thought process and reliance on evidence that ideally takes place with conventional drugs. Whereas recent metaanalyses are a useful addition to the body of literature on the choice of intravenous fluids for volume replacement, they have not settled the debate.

Unfortunately, most of the literature on volume repletion has not studied patients with prerenal azotemia. Selected trials that have reported renal outcomes or included patients with renal disease are listed in Table 1.2. Patients with prerenal azotemia represent a high-risk population that might benefit from one or another volume replacement strategy. An otherwise unrecognized treatment benefit from crystalloids or a specific colloid may be more readily demonstrable in this population.

Crystalloids are the preferred therapy for volume repletion for patients with prerenal azotemia. Certain colloids, such as dextrans and hydroxyethylstarch, should be avoided because of the risk of further impairing glomerular filtration. While risk factors have not been clearly identified, prerenal azotemia is thought to be an important contributing cause to the nephrotoxicity of other agents, such as radiocontrast, cis-platinum, aminoglycosides, and amphotericin B. Further studies are warranted on the use of albumin versus crystalloids in patients with or at risk for ARF, especially those with chronic liver disease. Future trials on volume replacement strategies should examine organ-specific outcomes along with survival, length of stay, and costs to help guide clinicians with these important management decisions.

Pressors in acute renal failure

Prerenal azotemia may arise from an imbalance between renal and systemic vascular resistance, even in normovolemic states. The most common clinical scenario in which this occurs is the sepsis syndrome. Renal failure in the setting of sepsis is common and remains a grave prognostic sign. Systemic vasodilation, abnormal intrarenal hemodynamics, and a complex cascade involving endogenous mediators of inflammation and thrombosis contribute to ARF in sepsis.[68–70] In septic shock unresponsive to crystalloid or colloid infusion, vasopressor agents are used to restore mean arterial pressure to a level sufficient for cerebral and coronary perfusion. The kidneys, however, may be unfortunate casualties of the pharmacologic management of shock. Renal blood flow and intrarenal hemodynamics can be impaired in sepsis alone as well as by well-intentioned vasopressor drugs. For patients with ARF and sepsis, the ideal vasopressor agent would increase mean arterial pressure while also improving renal and glomerular hemodynamics. Unfortunately, no such drug has been demonstrated to exist. Vasopressor agents commonly in use include dopamine, dobutamine, norepinephrine, epinephrine, phenylephrine, and vasopressin. Large, well-designed clinical trials comparing the safety and efficacy of these drugs in septic shock are lacking. The existing data on renal outcomes with the use of vasopressor drugs are reviewed below.

Dopamine

Dopamine has emerged as the first-line agent in the management of septic shock unresponsive to aggressive fluid management.[71] In healthy adults and animal models,

Table 1.2   Vasopressors: selected studies

Reference	Setting	No. of patients	Pressor(s) studied	Outcomes
47	Volunteers with normal renal function ($n = 28$) and varying degrees of renal insufficiency ($n = 127$)	165	Dopamine (1.5–2.0 µg/kg/min)	Dopamine increased effective renal plasma flow and GFR. The effect was most pronounced in subjects with normal GFR and absent if GFR < 50 mL/min
48	Medical ICU patients with septic shock. Randomized, short-term intervention trial	20	Dopamine (mean 26 µg/kg/min) and norepinephrine (mean 0.18 µg/kg/min). Study period 3 h	Dopamine increase MAP by increasing cardiac index. Norepinephrine increased MAP by increasing SVRI. Dopamine decreased and norepinephrine increased the gastric intramucosal pH
49	Medical ICU patients with septic shock. Prospective, double-blind randomized trial	32	Dopamine (2.5–25 µg/kg/min) and norepinephrine (0.5–5 µg/kg/min). Study period was time of required vasopressor support	Norepinephrine was more effective than dopamine in restoring mean increased in patients successfully treated with both dopamine and norepinephrine
50	Medical and surgical ICU patients with severe septic shock. Open-label, non-randomized, prospective study	10	Dopamine, dobutamine, and norepinephrine. Study period was duration of ICU stay	Norepinephrine reversed hypotension after dopamine and dobutamine failed. No renal outcomes
51	Medical and surgical ICU patients with septic shock. Open-label, prospective study of norepinephrine in patients not responding to dopamine	12	Dopamine (max. 15 µg/kg/min) and norepinephrine (0.5–1.0 µg/kg/min). Hemodynamic measurements carried out 20 min after starting norepinephrine	Norepinephrine reversed shock in 10 of 12 patients. Urine output increased with norepinephrine treatment
52	Medical ICU patients with shock from bacterial sepsis or severe falciparum malaria. Prospective, controlled, crossover trial employing invasive hemodynamic studies of systemic and renal blood flow	19	Dopamine (2.5–10 µg/kg/min) and epinephrine (0.1–0.5 µg/kg/min). Measurements made every 45 min during stepped infusions; total study period < 12 h	Dopamine increased and epinephrine decreased fractional renal blood flow. Neither drug significantly affected CrCl or urine output
53	Healthy male volunteers. Single blinded, randomized, placebo-controlled trial. Renal plasma flow and GFR measured with [125I]-iothalamte and [131I]-hippurate	7	Dopamine (4 µg/kg/min) or placebo added to norepinephrine (0.04–0.15 µg/kg/min)	Norepinephrine decreased renal plasma flow but did not change GFR. Concomitant dopamine administration prevented the decrease in renal plasma flow and increased sodium excretion
54	Healthy male volunteers. Prospective, single-blind, randomized study	6	Dopamine (3 µg/kg/min) and norepinephrine (0.076–0.164 µg/kg/min). Study period 3 h	Norepinephrine decreased renal blood flow; adding dopamine returned renal blood flow to baseline values. No changes noted in urine output and glomerular filtration rate
55	Medical and surgical ICU patients with two criteria for SIRS and early renal dysfunction. Multicenter, randomized, double-blind, placebo-controlled trial	324	Dopamine (2 µg/kg/min) Infusion of drug or placebo continued until need for RRT, death, adverse event, clinical improvement, or discharge from ICU	No difference in peak SCr, need for renal replacement therapy, duration of ICU or hospital stay, and mortality
56	Cohort study of oliguric patients randomized to the placebo arm of a multicenter intervention trial	395	Dopamine at varying doses, classified as none, ≤ 3 µg/kg/min, and > 3 µg/kg/min	Administration of dopamine was not associated with a difference in incidence of acute renal failure, need for RRT, or 28-day survival

Table 1.2 Vasopressors: selected studies (*cont'd*)

Reference	Setting	No. of patients	Pressor(s) studied	Outcomes
57	Medical and surgical ICU patients with septic shock. Prospective, open-label study	25	Norepinephrine (0.5–1.5 µg/kg/min) and dopamine (mean 14.2 ± 2 µg/kg/min. Study period 24–240 h	Norepinephrine had no deleterious renal effect; urine flow rate, creatinine, and osmolar clearance increased while free water clearance and FE_{Na} decreased
58	Medical ICU patients with septic shock. Prospective, crossover design	10	Dopamine (mean 20.1 µg/kg/min) and norepinephrine (mean 0.32 µg/kg/min). Study period 1 h for each drug	Dopamine increased blood pressure mainly via inotropic effects; norepinephrine by vasoconstriction. Similar effects on right ventricular performance. No significant difference in urine output
59	Medical and surgical ICU patients with septic shock. Retrospective study	15	Norepinephrine (0.05–0.24 µg/kg/min). Measurements made when norepinephrine infusion rate was fixed	In patients with serum lactate < 20 mg/dL, norepinephrine increased urine flow and SVRI and had no effect on CrCl. In patients with serum lactate > 20 mg/dL, norepinephrine did not increase urine flow or SVRI, and decreased CrCl significantly
60	Prospective observational cohort study of consecutive patients with septic shock	97	Norepinephrine, dopamine, epinephrine. Study period was duration of ICU stay	Norepinephrine administration was associated with improved survival compared with other vasopressors; non-randomized, open-label, observational study. No renal outcomes
61	Medical and surgical ICU patients with septic shock. Retrospective analysis of patients treated with norepinephrine (alone and with other pressors)	24	Norepinephrine (0.5–1.1 µg/kg/min). Measurements made 30 min after stable norepinephrine dose was obtained	In 20 of 24 patients, normalization of systemic hemodynamics was followed by increased urine flow and increased CrCl
62	Medical ICU patients with septic shock. Prospective, crossover design	8	Epinephrine (0.13–1.0 µg/kg/min), dobutamine (8.3–18.1 µg/kg/min) and norepinephrine (0.08–0.68 µg/kg/min). Two-hour infusions of epinephrine versus dobutamine plus norepinephrine	Epinephrine had no beneficial hemodynamic effects. Lactate concentration was increased with epinephrine. Splanchnic perfusion was impaired with epinephrine
63	Medical ICU patients with shock from bacterial sepsis or severe falciparum malaria. Open, randomized, crossover study	23	Dopamine (2.5–10 µg/kg/min) and epinephrine (0.1–0.5 µg/kg/min). Measurements made every 45 min during stepped infusions; total study period < 12 h	All patients completed the dopamine portion of the study; study was terminated in 84% of patients receiving epinephrine because of the development of lactic acidosis. No significant difference in hemodynamic effects
64	Critically ill medical and surgical ICU patients with SCr < 3.4 mg/dL. Prospective, randomized, double-blind study	23	Dopamine (200 µg/min) and dobutamine (175 µg/min). Study period 5 h	Dopamine increased urine output but did not change CrCl. Dobutamine increased CrCl and had no effect on urine output
65	Hemodynamically stable surgical and medical ICU patients with CrCl between 30 and 80 mL/min. Prospective, single-blind, randomized study	12	Dopamine (3–12 µg/kg/min) and dobutamine (3–12 µg/kg/min). Study period 4 h	Dopamine increased CrCl, diuresis, and FeNa. Dobutamine had no effect on these parameters

Table 1.2 Vasopressors: selected studies (*cont'd*)

Reference	Setting	No. of patients	Pressor(s) studied	Outcomes
66	Nonoliguric medical and surgical ICU patients with sepsis syndrome not in shock. Double blind, crossover design	16	Dopamine (3 µg/kg/min)	Dopamine infusion increased urine volume but did not affect gastric intramucosal pH, urinary sodium excretion, or CrCl
67	Cohort study of patients with acute renal failure randomized to the placebo arm of a multicenter intervention trial.	256	Dopamine at varying doses, classified as none, ≤ 3 µg/kg/min, and > 3 µg/kg/min	Relative risk of death or dialysis with administration of low-dose dopamine was 0.82, 95% CI 0.42–1.60

CrCl, creatinine clearance; SCr, serum creatinine; GFR, glomerular filtration rate; FE_{Na}, fractional excretion of sodium; SIRS, systemic inflammatory response syndrome; MAP, mean arterial pressure; SVRI, systemic vascular resistance index; RRT, renal replacement therapy; CI, confidence interval; ICU, intensive care unit.

dopamine exerts a dose-dependent pharmacologic effect on peripheral catecholamine receptors. At doses of less than 5 µg/kg/min, dopamine predominantly stimulates DA-1 and DA-2 receptors in coronary, mesenteric, and renal vessels, resulting in vasodilation. Sometimes described as "renal-dose" dopamine, low-dose dopamine infusions are used worldwide for putative but unsubstantiated beneficial effects on renal function. At doses of 5–10 µg/kg/min, dopamine increases the cardiac index through stimulation of cardiac β_1-adrenoreceptors. At higher doses, dopamine exerts vasoconstrictive effects through stimulation of α_1-adrenergic receptors. Importantly, this dose-dependent effect upon different receptor classes may not hold true in critically ill patients, in whom plasma clearance of dopamine is impaired.[72] In addition, low doses of dopamine may not increase renal plasma flow or GFR in patients with renal insufficiency.[47]

In hyperdynamic shock from sepsis, dopamine augments blood pressure principally by α_1-adrenergic receptor-mediated increase in cardiac index.[48] Whether dopamine is renoprotective when used as a first-line agent for septic shock is not clear. Some studies have suggested that dopamine is less effective than norepinephrine in restoring mean arterial pressure[49–51] and that norepinephrine more favorably affects splanchnic circulation.[48] To date, no clinical trials of adequate size have compared dopamine with other vasopressor agents to establish one drug as the safest or most beneficial in terms of renal function or survival.

Day et al[52] studied the effects of dopamine and epinephrine on renal hemodynamics in 14 patients with severe malaria and five with severe sepsis; the investigators used renal vein catheters to directly measure renal hemodynamics and creatinine clearance during stepped infusions of the study drugs over a period of several hours. At a dose of 2.5 µg/kg/min, dopamine increased renal blood flow by 37% (95% CI 13–61%; $P = 0.007$) and renal blood flow (RBF) as a fraction of cardiac output by 35% (95% CI 10–59%; $P = 0.014$). At 10 µg/kg/min, however, RBF and RBF/cardiac output (CO) were not statistically significantly different from baseline. As the dose was reduced

back to 2.5 µg/kg/min, RBF and RBF/CO did not increase and remained unchanged from baseline. Creatinine clearance, calculated using arterial and renal vein creatinine measurements at each point in the study, was not affected by dopamine or epinephrine. These data suggest that any beneficial effect of dopamine on renal hemodynamics in sepsis disappears with increasing doses and may be transient even at low doses.

Dopamine is commonly employed in low doses as an adjunct to vasopressors such as norepinephrine to offset renal vasoconstriction induced by α_1-adrenergic agonists. Intuitively appealing, the administration of low-dose dopamine has been shown to be effective in improving renal blood flow in dogs and healthy volunteers treated with norepinephrine.[53,54,73] In clinical trials of sepsis, however, the addition of low-dose dopamine to other vasopressors has been ineffective in improving renal function or survival. A multicenter, prospective, randomized, placebo-controlled trial involving 328 patients with the systemic inflammatory response syndrome (SIRS) and early renal dysfunction showed no benefit of low-dose dopamine (2 µg/kg/min) on peak serum creatinine, need for renal replacement therapy, duration of ICU stay, or survival.[55] Another observational study involving 395 patients with septic shock and oliguria who were randomized to the placebo arm of a multicenter intervention trial showed no benefit to the use of low-dose dopamine.[56] Low-dose dopamine has not been demonstrated to be effective in the prevention or treatment of ARF in patients with septic shock in the absence of systemic hypotension, or in individuals with established ARF.[55,67]

Norepinephrine

Norepinephrine is a potent vasopressor with predominant α-adrenergic and less pronounced β-adrenergic effects. This agent has traditionally been reserved as a treatment of last resort for refractory hypotension owing to concern over potentially deleterious vasoconstriction of the splanchnic and renal circulations. Newer data have challenged the conventional wisdom that norepinephrine causes excessive vasoconstriction and organ dysfunction (see below).

That norepinephrine is a more potent vasopressor than dopamine was shown in a small, prospective, double-blind, randomized trial involving adults with hyperdynamic septic shock.[49] Only 5 out of 16 patients were successfully treated with dopamine (10–25 µg/kg/min) compared with 15 out of 16 treated with norepinephrine (1.5 ± 1.2 µg/kg/min) ($P < 0.001$). No apparent adverse effect on organ perfusion or urine output was noted. Other retrospective and prospective observational studies have confirmed that norepinephrine is effective in patients with septic shock and not associated with adverse renal outcomes.[51,57–61] In 20 septic patients randomized to dopamine or norepinephrine infusion, Marik and Mohedin[48] showed that splanchnic oxygen utilization – as estimated by indirect calorimetry and gastric pH tonometry – was impaired in patients randomized to dopamine compared with norepinephrine. Despite its reputation for impairing blood flow in the splanchnic bed and renal circulation, norepinephrine may in fact optimize regional circulation. The possibility that norepinephrine may improve glomerular filtration rate by efferent arteriolar vasoconstriction is intriguing and deserves further study in prospective, randomized clinical trials.

Epinephrine and phenylephrine

Epinephrine, an α- and β-adrenergic agonist, is generally used after volume repletion and other vasopressors have failed to restore adequate mean arterial pressure. Epinephrine administration can cause lactic acidosis and may impair splanchnic blood flow,[62,63,74] making it a second-line agent in the treatment of septic shock. Invasive renal hemodynamic monitoring of patients with severe sepsis and severe falciparum malaria[52] showed epinephrine decreased renal blood flow and increased renal vascular resistance both in absolute terms and compared with dopamine; no effect on creatinine clearance, however, was noted with either drug.

Phenylephrine is a selective α-adrenergic agonist that can be used when tachyarrhythmias limit the use of other vasopressor agents with α-agonist properties. Few clinical studies have examined its role in hyperdynamic septic shock,[75–77] and no studies have examined its effects on renal function or its role in patients with renal insufficiency.

Dobutamine

Dobutamine is an inotropic agent with predominant α_1- and α_2-adrenergic agonist effects. The impairment of myocardial function seen in septic shock[78] has led to the investigation of positive inotropes in the resuscitation of septic patients. Dobutamine has been studied as a part of goal-directed therapy of hemodynamics in septic shock with conflicting results. A large, multicenter, prospective randomized study found no improvement in survival or morbidity with dobutamine as part of hemodynamic treatment aimed at achieving supranormal cardiac index.[79] A more recent study employing earlier goal-directed therapy with dobutamine and other interventions showed a reduction of inhospital mortality from 46.5% to 30.5%.[80]

Dobutamine has been compared with dopamine in critically ill patients at risk of ARF. Duke et al[64] studied the effects of sequential infusions of dopamine and dobutamine on urine volume, creatinine clearance, and fractional excretion of sodium in 18 critically ill patients. These authors found that low-dose dopamine increased urine volume but did not increase creatinine clearance; dobutamine at a dose of 175 µg/min, on the other hand, increased creatinine clearance without increasing urine volume. Ichai et al[65] compared the renal effects of low to high doses of dopamine and dobutamine in 12 critically ill patients with mild nonoliguric ARF. These investigators found that dopamine favorably modified all indices of renal function, including urine volume, fractional excretion of sodium and water, and creatinine clearance; in this study, dobutamine administration had no statistically significant effect. A small study of patients with septic shock treated with norepinephrine showed that the addition of dobutamine had no beneficial effect on renal function.[81] Therefore, the available evidence on the effects of dobutamine (and other inotropes with vasodilatory properties) on renal function is mixed.

Vasopressin

Vasopressin, also known as antidiuretic hormone (ADH), is an endogenous peptide hormone secreted by the posterior pituitary gland principally in response to hyperosmolality and hypovolemia. Vasopressin exerts a direct vasoconstrictor effect on the systemic vasculature by binding to V_1 receptors. Osmoregulation is mediated by V_2 receptors located in the renal collecting duct system and endothelial cells. The pharmacologic use of vasopressin has been established in variceal hemorrhage and diabetes insipidus. More recently, interest in the use of nonadrenergic vasoactive substances has led to the study of vasopressin in cardiac arrest[82,83] and septic shock.

Patients with vasodilatory septic shock may have inappropriately low plasma levels of vasopressin, and may be very sensitive to administration of low doses of vasopressin.[84,85] In a randomized, placebo-controlled trial of vasopressin in 10 patients with septic shock ($n = 10$, five in each group), vasopressin treatment at a dose of 0.04 U/min resulted in improved systolic blood pressure and withdrawal of other catecholamine vasopressors compared with placebo.[86] A retrospective study of 50 patients who received vasopressin for septic shock showed improved mean arterial pressure, increased urine output, and decreased pressor requirements.[87]

The renal effects of vasopressin are complex and not well studied in septic shock. At low doses, vasopressin induces diuresis in patients with hepatorenal syndrome, congestive heart failure, and septic shock.[85,86,88] At higher doses, however, animal studies have shown a dose-dependent fall in renal blood flow, GFR, and sodium excretion.[89,90]

Choice of pressor

The available data on patients with septic shock and prerenal ARF do not allow for definitive recommendations on a "one size fits all" choice of a vasopressor agent, both generally and when one considers the kidneys specifically. What has become clear is that dopamine, although widely used to treat or prevent ARF in critically ill patients, has no obvious specific renal protective effect in humans. Whether dopamine is superior to other vasopressor therapies as an empiric first-line agent in septic shock is not clear. Norepinephrine deserves further study in patients with septic shock, particularly to assess its effects on renal outcomes compared with dopamine. Epinephrine should be used after other agents have failed to increase mean arterial pressure. Phenylephrine has a role in the treatment of patients with shock who suffer tachyarrhythmias from α-adrenergic agonists. Dobutamine as a part of early goal-directed hemodynamic therapy may improve outcomes in septic shock. Vasopressin, a nonadrenergic agent, has only recently been studied in clinical trials. Prospective, randomized clinical trials are needed to provide guidance to clinicians choosing among vasoactive substances in the treatment of patients in shock with prerenal renal failure.

References

1. Nolan CR, Anderson RJ: Hospital-acquired acute renal failure. J Am Soc Nephrol 1998;9:710.
2. Liano F, Pascual J: Epidemiology of acute renal failure: a prospective, multicenter, community-based study. Madrid Acute Renal Failure Study Group. Kidney Int 1996;50:811.
3. Alderson P, Schierhout G, Roberts I, et al: Colloids versus crystalloids for fluid resuscitation in critically ill patients. Cochrane Database Syst Rev 2000;2:CD000567.
4. Wilkes MM, Navickis RJ: Patient survival after human albumin administration. A meta-analysis of randomized, controlled trials. Ann Intern Med 2001;135:149.
5. Choi PT, Yip G, Quinonez LG, et al: Crystalloids vs. colloids in fluid resuscitation: a systematic review. Crit Care Med 1999;27:200.
6. Boldt J, Lenz M, Kumle B, et al: Volume replacement strategies on intensive care units: results from a postal survey. Intensive Care Med 1998;24:147.
7. Yim JM, Vermeulen LC, Erstad BL, et al: Albumin and nonprotein colloid solution use in US academic health centers. Arch Intern Med 1995;155:2450.
8. Berne RM, Levy MN: Principles of Physiology, 2nd edn. St. Louis, MO, Mosby, 1996.
9. Scheingraber S, Rehm M, Sehmisch C, et al: Rapid saline infusion produces hyperchloremic acidosis in patients undergoing gynecologic surgery. Anesthesiology 1999;90:1265.
10. McFarlane C, Lee A: A comparison of Plasmalyte 148 and 0.9% saline for intra-operative fluid replacement. Anaesthesia 1994;49:779.
11. Williams EL, Hildebrand KL, McCormick SA, et al: The effect of intravenous lactated Ringer's solution versus 0.9% sodium chloride solution on serum osmolality in human volunteers. Anesth Analg 1999;88:999.
12. Mouren S, Delayance S, Mion G, et al: Mechanisms of increased myocardial contractility with hypertonic saline solutions in isolated blood-perfused rabbit hearts. Anesth Analg 1995;81:777.
13. Goertz AW, Mehl T, Lindner KH, et al: Effect of 7.2% hypertonic saline/6% hetastarch on left ventricular contractility in anesthetized humans. Anesthesiology 1995;82:1389.
14. Wade CE, Kramer GC, Grady JJ, et al: Efficacy of hypertonic 7.5% saline and 6% dextran-70 in treating trauma: a meta-analysis of controlled clinical studies. Surgery 1997;122:609.
15. Younes RN, Aun F, Accioly CQ, et al: Hypertonic solutions in the treatment of hypovolemic shock: a prospective, randomized study in patients admitted to the emergency room. Surgery 1992;111:380.
16. Holcroft JW, Vassar MJ, Turner JE, et al: 3% NaCl and 7.5% NaCl/dextran 70 in the resuscitation of severely injured patients. Ann Surg 1987;206:279.
17. Holcroft JW, Vassar MJ, Perry CA, et al: Perspectives on clinical trials for hypertonic saline/dextran solutions for the treatment of traumatic shock. Braz J Med Biol Res 1989;22:291.
18. Maningas PA, Mattox KL, Pepe PE, et al: Hypertonic saline–dextran solutions for the prehospital management of traumatic hypotension. Am J Surg 1989;157:528.
19. Mattox KL, Maningas PA, Moore EE, et al: Prehospital hypertonic saline/dextran infusion for post-traumatic hypotension. The U.S.A. Multicenter Trial. Ann Surg 1991;213:482.
20. Vassar MJ, Perry CA, Holcroft JW: Analysis of potential risks associated with 7.5% sodium chloride resuscitation of traumatic shock. Arch Surg 1990;125:1309.
21. Vassar MJ, Perry CA, Gannaway WL, et al: 7.5% sodium chloride/dextran for resuscitation of trauma patients undergoing helicopter transport. Arch Surg 1991;126:1065.
22. Vassar MJ, Perry CA, Holcroft JW: Prehospital resuscitation of hypotensive trauma patients with 7.5% NaCl versus 7.5% NaCl with added dextran: a controlled trial. J Trauma 1993;34:622.
23. Vassar MJ, Fischer RP, O'Brien PE, et al: A multicenter trial for resuscitation of injured patients with 7.5% sodium chloride. The effect of added dextran 70. The Multicenter Group for the Study of Hypertonic Saline in Trauma Patients. Arch Surg 1993;128:1003.
24. Human albumin administration in critically ill patients: systematic review of randomised controlled trials. Cochrane Injuries Group Albumin Reviewers. Br Med J 1998;317:235.
25. Sort P, Navasa M, Arroyo V, et al: Effect of intravenous albumin on renal impairment and mortality in patients with cirrhosis and spontaneous bacterial peritonitis. N Engl J Med 1999;341:403.
26. Puri VK, Howard M, Paidipaty BB, et al: Resuscitation in hypovolemia and shock: a prospective study of hydroxyethyl starch and albumin. Crit Care Med 1983;11:518.
27. Schortgen F, Lacherade JC, Bruneel F, et al: Effects of hydroxyethylstarch and gelatin on renal function in severe sepsis: a multicentre randomised study. Lancet 2001;357:911.
28. Kumle B, Boldt J, Piper S, et al: The influence of different intravascular volume replacement regimens on renal function in the elderly. Anesth Analg 1999;89:1124.
29. Shackford SR, Sise MJ, Fridlund PH, et al: Hypertonic sodium lactate versus lactated ringer's solution for intravenous fluid therapy in operations on the abdominal aorta. Surgery 1983;94:41.
30. Dawidson IJ, Willms CD, Sandor ZF, et al: Ringer's lactate with or without 3% dextran-60 as volume expanders during abdominal aortic surgery. Crit Care Med 1991;19:36.
31. Skillman JJ, Restall DS, Salzman EW: Randomized trial of albumin vs. electrolyte solutions during abdominal aortic operations. Surgery 1975;78:291.
32. Lucas CE, Weaver D, Higgins RF, et al: Effects of albumin versus non-albumin resuscitation on plasma volume and renal excretory function. J Trauma 1978;18:564.
33. Boutros AR, Ruess R, Olson L, et al: Comparison of hemodynamic, pulmonary, and renal effects of use of three types of fluids after major surgical procedures on the abdominal aorta. Crit Care Med 1979;7:9.
34. Gore DC, Dalton JM, Gehr TW: Colloid infusions reduce glomerular filtration in resuscitated burn victims. J Trauma 1996;40:356.
35. Stockwell MA, Scott A, Day A, et al: Colloid solutions in the critically ill. A randomised comparison of albumin and polygeline 2. Serum albumin concentration and incidences of pulmonary oedema and acute renal failure. Anaesthesia 1992;47:7.
36. Zetterstrom H, Hedstrand U: Albumin treatment following major surgery. I. Effects on plasma oncotic pressure, renal function and peripheral oedema. Acta Anaesthesiol Scand 1981;25:125.
37. Vogt NH, Bothner U, Lerch G, et al: Large-dose administration of 6% hydroxyethyl starch 200/0.5 total hip arthroplasty: plasma homeostasis, hemostasis, and renal function compared to use of 5% human albumin. Anesth Analg 1996;83:262.
38. Pockaj BA, Yang JC, Lotze MT, et al: A prospective randomized trial evaluating colloid versus crystalloid resuscitation in the treatment of

the vascular leak syndrome associated with interleukin-2 therapy. J Immunother 1994;15:22.

39. Follo A, Llovet JM, Navasa M, et al: Renal impairment after spontaneous bacterial peritonitis in cirrhosis: incidence, clinical course, predictive factors and prognosis. Hepatology 1994;20:1495.

40. Hankeln K, Radel C, Beez M, et al: Comparison of hydroxyethyl starch and lactated Ringer's solution on hemodynamics and oxygen transport of critically ill patients in prospective crossover studies. Crit Care Med 1989;17:133.

41. Rackow EC, Falk JL, Fein IA, et al: Fluid resuscitation in circulatory shock: a comparison of the cardiorespiratory effects of albumin, hetastarch, and saline solutions in patients with hypovolemic and septic shock. Crit Care Med 1983;11:839.

42. Strauss RG: Review of the effects of hydroxyethyl starch on the blood coagulation system. Transfusion 1981;21:299.

43. Cittanova ML, Leblanc I, Legendre C, et al: Effect of hydroxyethylstarch in brain-dead kidney donors on renal function in kidney-transplant recipients. Lancet 1996;348:1620.

44. Moran M, Kapsner C: Acute renal failure associated with elevated plasma oncotic pressure. N Engl J Med 1987;317:150.

45. Griffel MI, Kaufman BS: Pharmacology of colloids and crystalloids. Crit Care Clin 1992;8:235.

46. Fassio E, Terg R, Landeira G, et al: Paracentesis with Dextran 70 vs. paracentesis with albumin in cirrhosis with tense ascites. Results of a randomized study. J Hepatol 1992;14:310.

47. ter Wee PM, Smit AJ, Rosman JB, et al: Effect of intravenous infusion of low-dose dopamine on renal function in normal individuals and in patients with renal disease. Am J Nephrol 1986;6:42.

48. Marik PE, Mohedin M: The contrasting effects of dopamine and norepinephrine on systemic and splanchnic oxygen utilization in hyperdynamic sepsis. JAMA 1994;272:1354.

49. Martin C, Papazian L, Perrin G, et al: Norepinephrine or dopamine for the treatment of hyperdynamic septic shock? Chest 1993;103:1826.

50. Meadows D, Edwards JD, Wilkins RG, et al: Reversal of intractable septic shock with norepinephrine therapy. Crit Care Med 1988;16:663.

51. Desjars P, Pinaud M, Potel G, et al: A reappraisal of norepinephrine therapy in human septic shock. Crit Care Med 1987;15:134.

52. Day NP, Phu NH, Mai NT, et al: Effects of dopamine and epinephrine infusions on renal hemodynamics in severe malaria and severe sepsis. Crit Care Med 2000;28:1353.

53. Hoogenberg K, Smit AJ, Girbes AR: Effects of low-dose dopamine on renal and systemic hemodynamics during incremental norepine-phrine infusion in healthy volunteers. Crit Care Med 1998;26:260.

54. Richer M, Robert S, Lebel M: Renal hemodynamics during norepinephrine and low-dose dopamine infusions in man. Crit Care Med 1996;24:1150.

55. Bellomo R, Chapman M, Finfer S, et al: Low-dose dopamine in patients with early renal dysfunction: a placebo-controlled randomised trial. Australian and New Zealand Intensive Care Society (ANZICS) Clinical Trials Group. Lancet 2000;356:2139.

56. Marik PE, Iglesias J: Low-dose dopamine does not prevent acute renal failure in patients with septic shock and oliguria. NORASEPT II Study Investigators. Am J Med 1999;107:387.

57. Desjars P, Pinaud M, Bugnon D, et al: Norepinephrine therapy has no deleterious renal effects in human septic shock. Crit Care Med 1989;17:426.

58. Schreuder WO, Schneider AJ, Groeneveld AB, et al: Effect of dopamine vs norepinephrine on hemodynamics in septic shock. Emphasis on right ventricular performance. Chest 1989;95:1282.

59. Fukuoka T, Nishimura M, Imanaka H, et al: Effects of norepinephrine on renal function in septic patients with normal and elevated serum lactate levels. Crit Care Med 1989;17:1104.

60. Martin C, Viviand X, Leone M, et al: Effect of norepinephrine on the outcome of septic shock. Crit Care Med 2000;28:2758.

61. Marin C, Eon B, Saux P, et al: Renal effects of norepinephrine used to treat septic shock patients. Crit Care Med 1990;18:282.

62. Meier-Hellmann A, Reinhart K, Bredle DL, et al: Epinephrine impairs splanchnic perfusion in septic shock. Crit Care Med 1997;25:399.

63. Day NP, Phu NH, Bethell DP, et al: The effects of dopamine and adrenaline infusions on acid–base balance and systemic haemodynamics in severe infection. Lancet 1996;348:219.

64. Duke GJ, Briedis JH, Weaver RA: Renal support in critically ill patients: low-dose dopamine or low-dose dobutamine? Crit Care Med 1994;22:1919.

65. Ichai C, Soubielle J, Carles M, et al: Comparison of the renal effects of low to high doses of dopamine and dobutamine in critically ill patients: a single-blind randomized study. Crit Care Med 2000;28:921.

66. Olson D, Pohlman A, Hall JB: Administration of low-dose dopamine to nonoliguric patients with sepsis syndrome does not raise intramucosal gastric pH nor improve creatinine clearance. Am J Resp Crit Care Med 1996;154(6 Pt 1):1664.

67. Chertow GM, Sayegh MH, Allgren RL, et al: Is the administration of dopamine associated with adverse or favorable outcomes in acute renal failure? Auriculin Anaritide Acute Renal Failure Study Group. Am J Med 1996;101:49.

68. Bock HA: Pathophysiology of acute renal failure in septic shock: from prerenal to renal failure. Kidney Int Suppl 1998;64:S15.

69. Thijs A, Thijs LG: Pathogenesis of renal failure in sepsis. Kidney Int Suppl 1998;66:S34.

70. Bone RC: The pathogenesis of sepsis. Ann Intern Med 1991;115:457.

71. Task Force of the American College of Critical Care Medicine, Society of Critical Care Medicine: Practice parameters for hemodynamic support of sepsis in adult patients in sepsis. Crit Care Med 1999;27:639.

72. Juste RN, Moran L, Hooper J, et al: Dopamine clearance in critically ill patients. Intensive Care Med 1998;24:1217.

73. Schaer GL, Fink MP, Parrillo JE: Norepinephrine alone versus norepinephrine plus low-dose dopamine: enhanced renal blood flow with combination pressor therapy. Crit Care Med 1985;13:492.

74. Levy B, Bollaert PE, Charpentier C, et al: Comparison of norepinephrine and dobutamine to epinephrine for hemodynamics, lactate metabolism, and gastric tonometric variables in septic shock: a prospective, randomized study. Intensive Care Med 1997;23:282.

75. Yamazaki T, Shimada Y, Taenaka N, et al: Circulatory responses to afterloading with phenylephrine in hyperdynamic sepsis. Crit Care Med 1982;10:432.

76. Flancbaum L, Dick M, Dasta J, et al: A dose–response study of phenylephrine in critically ill, septic surgical patients. Eur J Clin Pharmacol 1997;51:461.

77. Gregory JS, Bonfiglio MF, Dasta JF, et al: Experience with phenylephrine as a component of the pharmacologic support of septic shock. Crit Care Med 1991;19:1395.

78. Parker MM, Shelhamer JH, Bacharach SL, et al: Profound but reversible myocardial depression in patients with septic shock. Ann Intern Med 1984;100:483.

79. Gattinoni L, Brazzi L, Pelosi P, et al: A trial of goal-oriented hemodynamic therapy in critically ill patients. SvO2 Collaborative Group. N Engl J Med 1995;333:1025.

80. Rivers E, Nguyen B, Havstad S, et al: Early goal-directed therapy in the treatment of severe sepsis and septic shock. N Engl J Med 2001;345:1368.

81. Levy B, Nace L, Bollaert PE, et al: Comparison of systemic and regional effects of dobutamine and dopexamine in norepinephrine-treated septic shock. Intensive Care Med 1999;25:942.

82. Lindner KH, Dirks B, Strohmenger HU, et al: Randomised comparison of epinephrine and vasopressin in patients with out-of-hospital ventricular fibrillation. Lancet 1997;349:535.

83. Stiell IG, Hebert PC, Wells GA, et al: Vasopressin versus epinephrine for inhospital cardiac arrest: a randomised controlled trial. Lancet 2001;358:105.

84. Landry DW, Levin HR, Gallant EM, et al: Vasopressin deficiency contributes to the vasodilation of septic shock. Circulation 1997;95:1122.

85. Landry DW, Levin HR, Gallant EM, et al: Vasopressin pressor hypersensitivity in vasodilatory septic shock. Crit Care Med 1997;25:1279.

86. Malay MB, Ashton RC Jr, Landry DW, et al: Low-dose vasopressin in the treatment of vasodilatory septic shock. J Trauma 1999;47:699.

87. Holmes CL, Walley KR, Chittock DR, et al: The effects of vasopressin on hemodynamics and renal function in severe septic shock: a case series. Intensive Care Med 2001;27:1416.

88. Eisenman A, Armali Z, Enat R, et al: Low-dose vasopressin restores diuresis both in patients with hepatorenal syndrome and in anuric patients with end-stage heart failure. J Intern Med 1999;246:183.

89. Harrison-Bernard LM, Carmines PK: Juxtamedullary microvascular responses to arginine vasopressin in rat kidney. Am J Physiol 1994;267(2 Pt 2):F249.

90. McVicar AJ: Dose–response effects of pressor doses of arginine vasopressin on renal haemodynamics in the rat. J Physiol 1988;404:535.

Overview of the Pathogenesis and Management of Acute Tubular Necrosis

Alice M. Sheridan

Acute tubular necrosis
Nephrotoxic acute renal failure
Therapy
Supportive treatment
Dialysis
Summary

Acute renal failure (ARF) is a syndrome defined by an acute reduction in glomerular filtration rate (GFR).[1] ARF occurs in 1–5% of all hospitalized patients, carries a mortality ranging from 46% to 90%, and is often classified according to its etiology, which can be prerenal, postrenal, or intrinsic renal.[2,3] Prerenal ARF is defined by a reduction in renal perfusion that occurs in the absence of parenchymal disease. Postrenal ARF results from obstruction of the urinary outflow tract. Intrinsic or intrarenal ARF is due to a parenchymal lesion of the tubules, the glomerulus, vessels, or interstitium. The most common cause of intrinsic ARF is acute tubular necrosis (ATN), which may be due to either an ischemic (50%) or toxic (35%) insult to the kidney.[4] Diseases such as interstitial nephritis, acute glomerulonephritis, or vasculitis cause the remainder of cases of intrinsic ARF. Nephrotoxins most often cause either prerenal ARF or ATN but may also cause acute interstitial nephritis or, less commonly, vasculitis. This chapter provides an overview of the pathogenesis of ATN, agents commonly associated with nephrotoxic injury, and the treatment of intrinsic ARF, and particularly of ATN. It is intended to set the stage for more detailed discussions of specific treatment modalities in subsequent chapters.

Acute tubular necrosis

Ischemic ATN results from an abrupt transient decrease in renal blood flow and is often associated with multiple organ failure and sepsis. Prerenal ARF predisposes patients toward the development of ATN, and these syndromes may be considered part of a continuum.[3] Nephrotoxin-induced ATN results from drugs, radiocontrast agents, and hemoglobin- or myoglobin-associated pigment that causes vasoconstriction resulting in ischemia as well as direct injury to tubular epithelial or vascular endothelial cells.

Statistically, isolated ischemic ATN carries a worse prognosis than isolated nephrotoxic ATN.[5] The poor prognosis associated with ischemic compared with nephrotoxic ATN may be due to the higher prevalence of associated comorbidities that adversely affect outcome rather than differences in pathogenesis. Clinically, however, it is often difficult to assign an exclusive etiology to ATN as critically ill patients, who are the most susceptible to ATN, often sustain several renal insults during a hospital course, including hemodynamic compromise, nephrotoxic antibiotics, and diagnostic studies requiring the administration of radiocontrast agents.

Our knowledge of the pathogenesis of ATN derives primarily from animal models of ischemic or mixed ischemic and nephrotoxic injury. Ischemic ATN involves the activation of signaling cascades, which results in preglomerular vasoconstriction, leukocyte accumulation, and direct injury to the tubule epithelial cells.[6]

A number of vasoconstrictor influences have been implicated in abnormal vascular tone during the maintenance phase of ischemic renal injury, including angiotensin II, thromboxane A_2, prostaglandin (PG) H_2, leukotrienes C_4 and D_4, endothelin-1, adenosine, and sympathetic nerve stimulation.[7] Ischemic ATN also involves an inflammatory response that results in leukocyte infiltration, tissue edema, and compromise of microvascular blood flow.[8] The infiltration of leukocytes into tissues is dependent on the enhanced expression of adhesion molecules, including selectins and integrins.[9] Integrins interact with immunoglobulin-like adhesion molecules such as interstitial cell adhesion molecules (ICAM) or vascular cell adhesion molecules (VCAM). Animal studies have implicated ICAM-1 in the pathogenesis of ischemia-induced ATN.[10] Chemokines, which recruit and activate leukocytes, and selectins are upregulated by inflammatory cytokines, such as interleukin 1 (IL-1) and tumor necrosis factor α (TNFα).[11] Reactive oxygen species (ROS) may upregulate chemokine expression,[12] and complement may play a role in potentiation of leukocyte–endothelial interactions.[13]

Ischemic ATN also results in direct injury to proximal tubule cells.[14] Sublethal injury is manifested by changes in cell polarity and paracellular permeability as well as desquamation, resulting in the backleak of glomerular filtrate and intraluminal obstruction contributing to decreased GFR.[15] With more severe or sustained ischemia, the epithelial cell is irreversibly damaged, resulting in necrosis or apoptosis, especially when other toxic influences such as ROS are present.[16] ROS are produced by numerous sources, including mitochondrial electron transport, cyclooxygenases, lipoxygenases, and mixed function oxidases of the endoplasmic reticulum and xanthine oxidase system.[17] ROS injure tubular epithelial cells by causing the peroxidation of lipid membranes, protein denaturation, and DNA strand breaks.[18] Lipid peroxidation by ROS enhances permeability and impairs enzymatic processes and ion pumps. ROS-induced strand breaks in DNA result in the activation of DNA repair mechanisms, including the nuclear enzyme poly(ADP-ribose) synthetase (PARS). PARS transfers ADP-ribose from nicotinamide adenine diphosphate (NAD) to nuclear proteins. With excessive activation of PARS, NAD is depleted thus inhibiting cellular ATP generation and worsening injury. This amplification of injury, called the PARS suicide, may be a major mechanism by which oxygen- and nitrogen-derived ROS cause direct cell toxicity.[19]

Ischemic ATN is characterized by enhanced tissue phospholipase activity, which results in the generation of inflammatory mediators and can directly alter the composition of cell membranes and their barrier functions.[14] Metabolic products of phospholipase activation include eicosanoids, which are vasoactive and chemoattractant for neutrophils, and platelet-activating factor (PAF) which also contributes to ischemia–reperfusion injury.[20] Additionally, arachidonic acid or its metabolites have been implicated in signal transduction pathways that are involved in inflammation, mitogenesis, and cellular differentiation.[21] Arachidonic acid derivatives are ligands for the peroxisomal proliferator activated receptors (PPAR), which are ligand-dependent nuclear transcription factors.[22] In a rat model of ischemia, PPAR activators protect against ischemic injury, possibly by preventing the ischemia-induced reduction of acyl coenzyme A oxidase and cytochrome P450.[23]

Activation of the mitogen-activated protein (MAP) family of kinases, including the extracellular signal-related kinases (ERKs), the stress response protein kinases (SAPKs), and the p38 family of kinases, contributes to cell injury and death from ischemia–reperfusion.[24] Numerous studies have demonstrated that whereas the ERK1/2 cascade is critical to the mitogenic response, to cellular differentiation, and, in some cells, to the induction of hypertrophy, the SAPKs and the p38 family are activated by cellular stress. The SAPKs have been implicated in cell injury and are increased with ischemia–reperfusion in vivo and ATP depletion in vitro.[25] Some argue that the outcome of ATN is predicated by the balance between the SAPKs, which promote apoptosis, and the ERKs, which inhibit apoptosis and commit surviving cells to a proliferative, reparative response.[26]

During recovery from ischemia–reperfusion injury, surviving tubular epithelial cells dedifferentiate and proliferate, eventually replacing the irreversibly injured tubular epithelial cells and restoring tubular integrity.[27] This regeneration parallels kidney organogenesis in the high rate of DNA synthesis and apoptosis[28] and in patterns of gene expression.[29]

Nephrotoxic acute renal failure

The major mechanisms by which nephrotoxic agents cause ARF include decreased perfusion, direct vascular or tubular cell injury (ATN), acute interstitial nephritis (AIN), and damage to the glomerular basement membrane. Less commonly, nephrotoxic agents precipitate in the lumen of renal tubules, causing obstructive ARF.[30] The most common cause of drug-induced ARF is prerenal ARF caused by either nonsteroidal anti-inflammatory agents (NSAIDs) or angiotensin-converting enzyme (ACE) inhibitors. Prerenal ARF is the most common manifestation of NSAID-induced

toxicity and accounts for 16% of all cases of drug-induced ARF.[31] NSAID-induced ARF is caused by the inhibition of prostaglandins that counteract angiotensin-induced vasoconstriction of the afferent arteriole in high renin states such as volume depletion, cirrhosis, and congestive heart failure.[32] NSAIDs also induce hyporenin hypoaldosteronism via the inhibition of PGI_2 and PGE_2 that stimulate renin release. NSAID-induced PGE_2 inhibition enhances sodium reabsorption by the medullary thick ascending limb, which inhibits delivery to the distal tubule worsening hyporenin-induced hyperkalemia.[33] Cyclooxygenase (COX) 1 and 2 are the rate-limiting enzymes for prostaglandin production. Whereas COX-1 is constitutively expressed at constant levels throughout the kidney, COX-2 expression is increased by various stimuli, including the modulation of salt intake.[34] Both non-selective and selective COX-2 inhibitors cause ARF.[33,35] NSAIDs also cause acute and chronic interstitial nephritis, independently of their effect on prostaglandins.[31] AIN occurs within days to weeks after initiation of the NSAID and full or partial recovery may occur up to 1 year after NSAIDs are withdrawn. NSAID-induced AIN may be associated with membranous nephropathy that is histologically indistinguishable from idiopathic membranous nephropathy.[36] ACE inhibitors and angiotensin receptor blockers (ARBs) cause ARF by inhibiting the vasoconstrictive effect of angiotensin on the efferent renal arteriole, which causes a decrease in transglomerular pressure in high renin states.[32] The ACE inhibition-induced reduction in GFR is especially pronounced in patients with bilateral renal artery stenosis or unilateral stenosis of a solitary kidney where transglomerular pressure is renin dependent.

Nephrotoxin-induced ATN results from drugs, such as aminoglycosides, amphotericin B, and cisplatin, that cause direct cellular injury.[32] Aminoglycosides are the most common cause of nephrotoxin-induced ATN. ATN occurs in 5–10% of patients who receive aminoglycosides, and typically presents 7–10 days after initiation of the drug.[37] Aminoglycosides are reabsorbed by proximal tubule cells and accumulate in high intracellular concentrations that are poorly approximated by serum levels. Whereas the half-life of aminoglycosides in serum is only 3 h, the intracellular half-life is markedly prolonged, resulting in a cumulative toxicity that often presents after serum levels are no longer detected. Amphotericin B causes both vasoconstriction and direct toxicity to both distal and proximal tubule cell membranes.[38] ATN occurs in 25–30% of patients who receive amphotericin B.[39] Cell toxicity, mediated by insertion of the polyene agent into the cell membrane, is mitigated by a liposomal amphotericin preparation,[38] although the more costly liposomal amphotericin is best reserved for patients who are at high risk for ATN. Risk factors associated with amphotericin-induced ATN include a higher dose, longer duration of therapy, higher level of care at initiation of treatment, and the concomitant use of cyclosporine.[40] Calcineurin inhibitors cause reversible vasoconstriction of the renal arteriole and are also directly toxic to endothelial and tubular cells. Long-term use of calcineurin inhibitors results in a structural arteriolopathy and tubulopathy that progresses after discontinuation of the drug. Endothelin-1, released from both damaged endothelial and proximal tubule cells, may play a role in both acute and chronic calcineurin inhibitor-induced injury.[41] Nephrotoxic ATN may also result from the release of endogenous heme and myoglobin pigment from hemolysis or rhabdomyolysis caused by trauma or by agents such as ethanol and lovastatin.[32]

Therapy

The treatment of ARF, and particularly of ATN, includes consideration of its prophylaxis and the medical and dialytic support of the patient during its course. Few specific interventions have been conclusively shown to prevent the development or hasten recovery of ATN. Although significant progress has been made in defining the major components of ATN, the interventions that proved effective in animal models of ischemic injury have failed to show any beneficial effect in human trials of established ATN. Therapeutic trials have centered on vasoactive substances, diuretics, the inhibition of ROS, and the stimulation of recovery via growth factors. The rationale for the many trials of vasoactive agents arose from the belief that persistent vasoconstriction was a predominant mechanism during the maintenance phase of ATN.[7] Animal models and various clinical trials have evaluated the effects of dopamine, calcium channel blockers, and atrial natriuretic peptide (ANP) on the prevention and outcome of established ATN. The rationale for the use of dopamine in ATN is based upon its DA_1 receptor-mediated, renal-specific effects that include vasodilation and inhibition of tubular sodium transport resulting in an increase in renal blood flow, diuresis, and natriuresis. Clinical trials, however, have failed to show a beneficial effect of dopamine on the prevention and outcome of ATN, possibly because of dopamine's confounding multiple dose-dependent effects mediated by different receptor types, including DA_2 and α and β adrenergic receptors.[42,43] DA_1-selective agonists, such as fenolodopam, may provide potential prophylaxis or therapy of ATN; however, further studies of this agent are necessary in order to determine its utility.[44] Although ANP had great theoretical appeal based on its mechanism of action and its proven benefit in animal models of ATN,[45] clinical trials showed no benefit in either treatment of established oliguric[46] and nonoliguric ATN[47] or in prophylaxis of radiocontrast-induced ATN.[48] Although endothelin receptor blockade was shown to prevent radiocontrast-induced ATN in animal models, it had no effect on, or was detrimental to, outcome in human clinical trials of ATN.[49] The calcium channel blocker diltiazem has been shown to have a beneficial effect on the outcome of ATN in the transplanted kidney,[50] although this agent has not been well studied in other forms of ATN and may have an adverse hypotensive effect in ATN associated with multiorgan failure.[3]

It was initially believed that diuretics, by increasing urine flow, could relieve the intraluminal obstruction that contributes to the low GFR characteristic of ATN.

However, as discussed in Chapter 5, neither loop diuretics nor mannitol have been shown to either affect the course of established ATN or prevent its onset.[51] Loop diuretics may, however, convert oliguric to nonoliguric ATN, which may facilitate medical management and obviate the need for dialysis.

ROS scavengers, such as superoxide dismutase, glutathione, and vitamin E, and inhibitors of ROS production, such as deferoxamine, protect against renal injury in animal models, suggesting that they may play a role in the treatment of ATN.[52] The result of a preliminary trial suggests that the antioxidant acetylcysteine (600 mg orally twice daily) may provide partial protection from radiocontrast-induced ATN in high-risk patients with underlying chronic renal insufficiency.[53] As discussed in Chapter 5, theophylline (800 mg in divided doses for 2 days prior to the study) also appears to reduce the incidence of contrast nephropathy in high-risk patients. Other potential therapies, including the administration of growth factors to enhance the proliferation of sublethally injured proximal tubule cells,[54] have not proved useful in the prophylaxis or treatment of ATN.

Supportive treatment (Table 2.1)

The careful management of intravascular volume status is the cornerstone of ARF prevention strategy, especially in patients who require diagnostic studies or therapies that expose them to nephrotoxins. Volume depletion is a well-recognized risk factor for nephrotoxin-induced ARF, and its correction with judicious administration of fluids should be performed prior to diagnostic tests requiring radiocontrast. Drugs known to cause prerenal azotemia, such as ACE inhibitors, ARBs, or NSAIDs, should be discontinued, if possible, prior to the administration of radiocontrast to patients at high risk for radiocontrast-induced ATN. Volume management is equally important in patients at risk for ischemia-induced ATN and may require the use of invasive monitoring of either central venous pressure or, in patients with either respiratory or cardiac disease, pulmonary artery occlusion pressure. As ischemia-induced ATN is often part of the multiorgan failure syndrome that occurs as a result of sepsis, the aggressive control of infection with appropriate antibiotics and debridement may be among the most effective measures to prevent ischemic ATN. Medications should be carefully reviewed in all patients who are at risk for ischemic ATN or nephrotoxin-induced ARF. Known nephrotoxins, such as aminoglycosides and amphotericin B, should be used sparingly, and every attempt should be made to avoid their concurrent use.

Volume repletion and alkalinization of urine prevents ARF due to rhabdomyolysis[55] and is recommended whenever rhabdomyolysis is anticipated (such as trauma involving a crush injury) or in any condition in which the serum creatine phosphokinase exceeds 12 000–15 000 U/L. Acute urate nephropathy is caused by the precipitation of uric acid in the distal lumen and is often a manifestation of tumor lysis syndrome resulting from the treatment of

Table 2.1 Management of established ARF

Volume overload	Furosemide bolus (40–100 mg) or infusion (0.1–0.4 mg/kg/h following bolus of 0.1 mg/kg). May be given with thiazide Dialysis or ultrafiltration
Hyperkalemia	Restriction of potassium intake to < 2 g/day. Discontinue K-sparing diuretics Sodium polystyrene sulfonate, orally (20 g given with 100 ml of 20% sorbitol) or rectally (50 g) Intravenous insulin (10 units) with dextrose (50 ml of 50% solution) Intravenous $NaHCO_3$ (50–100 mEq) Intravenous calcium gluconate (10 ml of 10% solution) Dialysis
Hyponatremia	Restriction of dietary free water intake to < 1 L daily Restriction of hypotonic intravenous solutions
Acidosis	Intravenous $NaHCO_3$ Dialysis
Hyperphosphatemia	Restriction of dietary phosphorus intake (< 800 mg/day) Phosphorus binding agents (calcium carbonate 500–1000 mg elemental calcium t.i.d. with meals; calcium acetate 667–1334 mg t.i.d. with meals; sevelamer hydrochloride 800–1600 mg t.i.d. with meals)
Hypermagnesemia	Restriction of magnesium intake (especially antacids)
Hyperuricemia	Allopurinol (dosage adjusted for glomerular filtration rate Alkalinization of urine and forced diuresis or dialysis
Uremic platelet dysfunction	Maintenance of hematocrit > 30% Desmopressin (DDAVP) (0.3 mg/kg i.v.) Cryoprecipitate
Nutrition	Caloric intake: 25–35 kcal/kg daily Protein intake: 0.6–1.5 g/kg daily

Adapted from Brady HR, Singer GG: Acute renal failure. Lancet 1995;346:1533–1540.

lymphomatous or myeloproliferative tumors.[56] The inhibition of xanthine oxidase with allopurinol (600–900 mg daily), volume administration, and the alkalinization of urine to increase the solubility of urate all decrease the incidence of urate nephropathy and are recommended whenever a large tumor lysis is anticipated.

Supportive care of the patient with established ARF from any cause requires careful attention to volume and electrolyte status. Volume overload should be treated with loop diuretics that may be given concurrently with a thiazide. A continuous infusion of the loop diuretic may yield a higher urine output compared with comparable doses given as a bolus.[57] Diuretic nonresponders should be evaluated for early institution of renal replacement therapy. Hyperkalemia and metabolic acidosis may be initially treated with sodium resins, insulin, glucose, and bicarbonate but both conditions commonly necessitate renal replacement therapy. Medications of patients with ARF should be carefully reviewed and dosages adjusted for a reduced GFR. As it is not possible to calculate the GFR based on a rapidly changing serum creatinine, it is often necessary to follow serum drug levels to prevent toxicity of particular agents.

Nutritional status is an important determinant of mortality in all patients with ARF[58] (extensively discussed in Chapter 10). The energy requirement of patients with ARF depends on the associated illness. Oxygen consumption is increased 20–30% by multiorgan failure of sepsis, though not by isolated ARF. Depending on the severity of the associated illness, patients with ARF should receive 25–35 kcal/kg/day. ARF is characterized by a marked increase in protein catabolism caused by insulin resistance, acidosis, and increased circulating levels of TNFα and interleukins. Hyperparathyroidism and the suppression of growth factors may also cause an increase in catabolism.[59] Depending on associated illnesses, patients with ARF require a protein intake of 0.6–1.5 g/kg daily, and a rising blood urea nitrogen should not limit protein intake. Although enteral feeding is preferred, total or partial parenteral feeding may be necessary to meet caloric and protein requirements. Other metabolic abnormalities associated with ARF include hyperglycemia due to insulin resistance, hypertriglyceridemia, and low cholesterol. Hyperglycemia should be treated with exogenous insulin.[59,60]

Patients with ARF are at risk for bleeding secondary to acquired platelet dysfunction that is only partially corrected with dialysis. Patients should be evaluated with skin bleeding times prior to any operative procedures. Patients who have bleeding times greater than 10 min are at high risk for hemorrhage and should have their bleeding time normalized with intensive dialysis or with administration of desmopressin (DDAVP) or estrogen. The transfusion of packed cells to a hematocrit greater than 30% may improve coagulation parameters.[61] Patients with ARF are at greater risk for infection and should be aggressively worked up and treated for suspected infections.

Dialysis

About 85% of patients with oliguric ARF and 30% of patients with nonoliguric ARF will eventually require dialysis.[4] The criteria for dialysis of ARF are the same as those required for the institution of chronic hemodialysis, although an argument may be made to initiate dialysis earlier for the patient with ARF and multiorgan failure. Clearly the patient who remains oliguric or anuric despite a trial of diuretics and who is receiving multiple intravenous infusions, including total parenteral nutrition, is unlikely to escape dialysis. Similarly, patients who present with hyperkalemia and acidosis may be temporized with medical therapy but will likely eventually require dialysis, unless the oliguria can be reversed.[62] A well-dialyzed patient has a more competent immune response and less of a bleeding diathesis, supporting the argument for early intervention with renal replacement therapy. On the other hand, hemodialysis is not risk free. Placement of a hemodialysis catheter carries a significant risk of bleeding, pneumothorax, and line-associated sepsis. Ischemic ATN is characterized by loss of autoregulation that causes an injured kidney to be more sensitive to hypotensive episodes that may occur during dialysis. Dialysis with a bioincompatible membrane may cause additional injury by the activation of complement and neutrophils.[63] In the high-risk, hemodynamically unstable patient, dialysis-associated risks are partially mitigated by the use of continuous replacement modalities, which are less likely than intermittent hemodialysis to cause hypotension, and by use of a biocompatible membrane.

Summary

ARF from all causes is treated by careful modulation of volume and electrolyte status using medical and/or renal replacement therapy. Careful attention to infection, nutrition, and the possibility of bleeding disorders will maximize survival until the recovery of renal function.

References

1. Nissenson AR: Acute renal failure: definition and pathogenesis. Kidney Int 1998;Suppl 66:S7–S10.
2. Chertow GM, Christiansen CL, Cleary PD, Munro C, Lazarus JM: Prognostic stratification in critically ill patients with acute renal failure requiring dialysis. Arch Intern Med 1995;155:1505–1511.
3. Thadhani R, Pascual M, Bonventre JV: Acute renal failure. N Engl J Med 1996;334:1448–1460.
4. Star RA: Treatment of acute renal failure. Kidney Int 1998;54:1817–1831.
5. Weisberg LS, Allgren RL, Genter FC, Kurnik BR: Cause of acute tubular necrosis affects its prognosis. Arch Intern Med 1997;157:1833–1838.
6. Bonventre JV: Mechanisms of ischemic acute renal failure. Kidney Int 1993;43:1160–1178.
7. Conger J: Hemodynamic factors in acute renal failure. Adv Renal Replacement Ther 1997;4:25–37.
8. Linas SL, Shanley PF, Whittenburg D, et al: Neutrophils accentuate ischemia-reperfusion injury in isolated perfused rat kidneys. Am J Physiol 1988;255: F728–F735.
9. Molitoris BA, Marrs J: The role of adhesion molecules in ischemic acute renal failure. Am J Med 1999;106:583–592.
10. Kelly KJ, Williams WWJ, Colvin RB, et al: Antibody to intercellular adhesion molecule-1 protects the kidneys against ischemic injury. Proc Natl Acad Sci USA 1994;91:812–816.
11. Donnahoo KK, Meng X, Ayala A, et al: Early kidney TNFα expression mediates neutrophil infiltration and injury after renal ischemia–reperfusion. Am J Physiol 1999;277:R922–R929.
12. Ishibashi N, Weisbrot-Lefkowitz M, Reuhl K, et al: Modulation of chemokine expression during ischemia/reperfusion in transgenic mice overproducing human glutathione peroxidases. J Immunol 1999;163:5666–5677.
13. Zhou W, Farrar CA, Abe K, et al: Predominant role for C5b-9 in renal ischemia/reperfusion injury. J Clin Invest 2000;105: 1363–1371.
14. Venkatachalam MA, Patel YJ, Kreisberg JI, et al: Energy thresholds that determine membrane integrity and injury in a renal epithelial cell line (LLC-P_{K1}). Relationship to phospholipid degradation and unesterified fatty acid accumulation. J Clin Invest 1988;81:745–758.
15. Molitoris BA: Ischemia-induced loss of epithelial polarity: potential role of the actin cytoskeleton. Am J Physiol 1991;260:F769–F778.
16. Schumer M, Colombel MC, Sawczuk IS, et al: Morphologic, biochemical and molecular evidence of apoptosis during the reperfusion phase and after brief periods of renal ischemia. Am J Pathol 1992;140:831–838.
17. Ueda N, Kaushal GP, Shah SV: Apoptotic mechanisms in acute renal failure. Am J Med 2000;108: 403–415.
18. Chatterjee PK, Cuzzocrea S, Thiemermann C: Inhibitors of poly (ADP-ribose) synthetase protect rat proximal tubules against oxidant stress. Kidney Int 1999;56:973–984.
19. Berger NA: Poly (ADP-ribose) in the cellular response to DNA damage. Radiat Res 1985;101:4–15.
20. Kelly KJ, Tolkoff-Rubin NE, Rubin RH, et al: An oral platelet-activating factor antagonist, R0-24-4736, protects the rat kidney from ischemic injury. Am J Physiol 1996; 271:F1061–F1067.
21. Dennis EA: The growing phospholipase A_2 superfamily of signal transduction enzymes. Trends Biochem Sci 1997;22:1–2.
22. Devchand PR, Keller H, Peters JM, et al: The PPARα-leukotriene B_4 pathway to inflammation control. Nature 1996;384:39–43.
23. Portilla D: Carnitine palmitoyltransferase enzyme inhibition protects proximal tubules during hypoxia. Kidney Int 1997;52:429–437.
24. Bonventre JV, Force T: Mitogen-activated protein kinases and transcriptional responses in renal injury and repair. Curr Opin Nephrol Hypertens 1998;4:425–433.
25. Pombo CM, Bonventre JV, Avruch J, et al: The stress-activated protein kinases are major c-Jun amino-terminal kinases activated by ischemia and reperfusion. J Biol Chem 1994;269:26546–26551.
26. di Mari JF, Davis R, Safirstein RL: MAPK activation determines renal epithelial cell survival during oxidative injury. Am J Physiol 1999;277:F195–F203.
27. Safirstein R: Renal regeneration: reiterating a developmental paradigm. Kidney Int 1999;56:1599–1600.
28. Shimizu A, Yamanaka N: Apoptosis and cell desquamation in repair process of ischemic tubular necrosis. Virchows Arch B Cell Pathol 1993;64:171–180.
29. Bacallao R, Fine LG: Molecular events in the organization of renal tubular epithelium: from nephrogenesis to regeneration. Am J Physiol 1989;257: F913–F924.
30. Hewitt WR, Goldstein RS, Hook JB: Toxic responses of the kidney. In Klasses CD, Doull J, Amdur MO (eds): Casarett and Doull's Toxicology. New York: Macmillan, 1990, pp 354–382.

31. Pugliese F, Cinotti GA: Nonsteroidal anti-inflammatory drugs (NSAIDs) and the kidney. Nephrol Dial Transplant 1997;12:386–388.
32. Choudhury D, Ahmed Z: Drug-induced nephrotoxicity. Med Clin North Am 1997;81:705–717.
33. Brater DC: Effects of nonsteroidal anti-inflammatory drugs on renal function: focus on cyclooxygenase-2-selective inhibition. Am J Med 1999;107(6A):65S–70S; discussion 70S–71S.
34. Harris RC, Breyer MD: Physiological regulation of cyclooxygenase-2 in the kidney. Am J Physiol 2001;281:F1–F11.
35. Komers R, Anderson S, Epstein M: Renal and cardiovascular effects of selective cyclooxygenase-2 inhibitors. Am J Kidney Dis 2001;38:1145–1157.
36. Radford MG Jr, Holley KE, Grande JP, et al: Reversible membranous nephropathy associated with the use of nonsteroidal anti-inflammatory drugs. JAMA 1996;276:466–469.
37. Appel GB: Aminoglycoside nephrotoxicity. Am J Med 1990;88(3C):16S–20S; discussion 38S–42S.
38. Zager RA, Bredl CR, Schimpf BA: Direct amphotericin B-mediated tubular toxicity: assessments of selected cytoprotective agents. Kidney Int 1992;41:1588–1594.
39. Bates DW, Su L, Yu DT, et al: Mortality and costs of acute renal failure associated with amphotericin B therapy. Clin Infect Dis 2001;32:686–693.
40. Bates DW, Su L, Yu DT, et al: Correlates of acute renal failure in patients receiving parenteral amphotericin B. Kidney Int 2001;60:1452–1459.
41. Campistol JM, Sacks SH: Mechanisms of nephrotoxicity. Transplantation 2000;69(Suppl):SS5–SS10.
42. Denton MD, Chertow GM, Brady HR: "Renal-dose" dopamine for the treatment of acute renal failure: scientific rationale, experimental studies and clinical trials. Kidney Int 1996;50:4–14.
43. Kellum JA, Decker JM: Use of dopamine in acute renal failure: a meta-analysis. Crit Care Med 2001;29:1526–1531.
44. Murphy MB, Murray C, Shorten GD: Fenoldopam: a selective peripheral dopamine-receptor agonist for the treatment of severe hypertension. N Engl J Med 2001;345:1548–1558.
45. Nakamoto M, Shapiro JI, Shanley PF, et al: In vitro and in vivo protective effect of atriopeptin III on ischemic acute renal failure. J Clin Invest 1987;80:698–705.
46. Allgren, RL, Marbury TC, Rahman SN, et al: Anaritide in acute tubular necrosis. Auriculin Anaritide Acute Renal Failure Study Group. N Engl J Med 1997;336:828–834.
47. Lewis J, Salem MM, Chertow GM, et al: Atrial natriuretic factor in oliguric acute renal failure. Anaritide Acute Renal Failure Study Group. Am J Kidney Dis 2000;36:767–774.
48. Kurnik BR, Allgren RL, Genter FC, et al: Prospective study of atrial natriuretic peptide for the prevention of radiocontrast-induced nephropathy. Am J Kidney Dis 1998;31:674–680.
49. Wang A, Holcslaw T, Bashore TM, et al: Exacerbation of radiocontrast nephrotoxicity by endothelin receptor antagonism. Kidney Int 2000;57:1675–1680.
50. Wagner K, Albrecht S, Neumayer HH: Prevention of posttransplant acute tubular necrosis by the calcium antagonist diltiazem: a prospective randomized study. Am J Nephrol 1987;7:287–291.
51. Solomon R, Werner C, Mann D, et al: Effects of saline, mannitol, and furosemide to prevent acute decreases in renal function induced by radiocontrast agents. N Engl J Med 1994;331:1416–1420.
52. Paller MS: Renal work, glutathione and susceptibility to free radical-mediated postischemic injury. Kidney Int 1988;33:843–849.
53. Tepel M, van der Giet M, Schwarzfeld C, et al: Prevention of radiographic-contrast-agent-induced reductions in renal function by acetylcysteine. N Engl J Med 2000;343:180–184.
54. Hirschberg R, Brunori G, Kopple JD, et al: Effects of insulin-like growth factor I on renal function in normal men. Kidney Int 1993;43:387–397.
55. Zager RA: Rhabdomyolysis and myohemoglobinuric acute renal failure. Kidney Int 1996;49:314–326.
56. Maesaka JK, Fishbane S: Regulation of renal urate excretion: a critical review. Am J Kidney Dis 1998;32:917–933.
57. Martin SJ, Danziger LH: Continuous infusion of loop diuretics in the critically ill: a review of the literature. Crit Care Med 1994;22:1323–1329.
58. Fiaccadori E, Lombardi M, Leonardi S, et al: Prevalence and clinical outcome associated with preexisting malnutrition in acute renal failure: a prospective cohort study. J Am Soc Nephrol 1999;10:581–593.
59. Druml W: Nutritional management of acute renal failure. Am J Kidney Dis 2001;37(Suppl 2):S89–S94.
60. Leverve X, Barnoud D: Stress metabolism and nutritional support in acute renal failure. Kidney Int 1998;Suppl 66:S62–S66.
61. Paganini EP: Hematologic abnormalities. In Daugirdas JT, Ing TS (eds): Handbook of Dialysis. Boston: Little Brown, 1994, pp 445–468.
62. Bellomo R, Ronco C: Indications and criteria for initiating renal replacement therapy in the intensive care unit. Kidney Int 1998;Suppl 66:S106–S109.
63. Hakim RM, Wingard RL, Parker RA: Effect of the dialysis membrane in the treatment of patients with acute renal failure. N Engl J Med 1994;331:1338–1342.

Dopamine Therapy in Acute Renal Failure

Mark Denton and Hugh R. Brady

Low-dose dopamine (1–3 µg/kg/min) is prescribed worldwide for the prevention and treatment of acute renal failure (ARF), to correct oliguria, and to preserve renal perfusion in patients receiving systemic vasopressors. Its popularity stems from physiological studies performed in the early 1970s that showed that low-dose dopamine infusion caused selective renal vasodilation, increased renal blood flow, and induced a natriuresis and diuresis in animals and healthy humans. As prerenal azotemia and ischemic acute tubular necrosis arising from reduced renal blood flow are major causes of ARF in the hospital setting, it seems logical to use a pharmacologic agent that may selectively enhance renal blood flow. Enthusiasm for dopamine has been further fuelled by multiple small and uncontrolled studies in the literature reporting beneficial effects of low-dose dopamine in patients with renal impairment from a variety of causes. However, larger clinical studies have failed to demonstrate that low-dose dopamine can either prevent the development of ARF in high-risk settings or affect the outcome of patients with established renal failure. Many editorials and reviews have advised against its use, owing to the paucity of supportive evidence and an increasingly recognized side-effect profile.[1–6] Yet, low-dose dopamine continues to be used extensively, particularly in the surgical intensive care unit. Several large good-quality studies examining the effect of low-dose dopamine infusion on renal function in a variety of clinical settings have been published. This chapter reviews the mechanisms of action of intrarenal and infused dopamine and summarizes the data from clinical studies. The effects of selective dopamine receptor agonists and dopamine precursors will also be discussed.

Physiology of intrarenal dopamine

Dopamine is synthesized by the kidney and is a critical regulator of sodium excretion.[7,8] It achieves this by directly inhibiting sodium reabsorption via inhibition of sodium transporters along almost the entire length of the nephron and by interacting with other regulators of sodium excretion, including atrial natriuretic peptide (ANP), catecholamines, vasopressin (AVP), angiotensin, and prostaglandins.[8] This physiologic role of dopamine is important to the understanding of the effects of exogenous dopamine and will therefore be discussed briefly in this section.

Proximal tubule epithelial cells synthesize dopamine from the substrate L-dopa using the enzyme L-amino acid decarboxylase. L-Dopa enters the cell from the tubular lumen by a sodium-coupled transport mechanism. Dietary sodium load is the major factor controlling intrarenal dopamine synthesis; the exact mechanism linking increased salt intake to increased renal dopamine synthesis is not understood. Upon synthesis, intrarenal dopamine may act in an autocrine fashion by binding dopamine receptors on the proximal tubule cell or pass along the urinary space to bind to specific receptors on distal portions of the nephron. Importantly, the natriuretic effect of dopamine is prominent in states of sodium loading and is weak or negligible in salt-depleted states.[9,10]

Dopamine inhibits the activity of the Na/K ATPase in the proximal tubule, the thick ascending limb of Henle, the distal tubule, and the collecting duct. Dopamine also has profound effects on sodium entry into tubule cells via inhibition of the Na/H exchanger and Na/PO$_4$ exchanger in the proximal tubule. Dopamine also inhibits the Na/Cl cotransporter in the thick ascending limb and the AVP-stimulated sodium transporter in the collecting duct.

Intrarenal dopamine interacts with other hormonal regulators of sodium excretion. For example, the natriuretic effect of ANP is dependent on renal dopamine receptors. Conversely, the inhibitory effect of dopamine on the proximal tubule Na/H exchanger is potentiated by ANP. Dopamine and α-adrenergic agonists counteract each other's effect on the basolateral Na/K ATPase. In addition, dopamine inhibits the stimulatory effect of angiotensin on Na/K ATPase in part by inhibition of angiotensin I receptor expression. AVP-dependent sodium and water transport in the cortical collecting duct is inhibited by stimulation of dopamine receptors at these sites. Finally, dopamine enhances the synthesis of other locally acting natriuretic compounds, such as prostaglandin E_2 (PGE_2).

Dopamine (DA) receptors are expressed on the renal vasculature.[11] DA_1 receptors are localized within the vessel wall media, whereas DA_2 receptors are present in the adventitia and are probably localized presynaptically on sympathetic nerve terminals. The vascular effects of dopamine in the kidney are mediated by dopamine released by dopaminergic nerves and circulating dopamine but not dopamine synthesized by the proximal tubules.[8]

Recent studies have examined the activity of renally synthesized dopamine in disease. In patients with both acute and chronic heart failure, proximal tubular uptake of the precursor L-dopa is enhanced perhaps to preserve renal dopamine production.[12] Patients with renal parenchymal disease have reduced activity of their renal dopaminergic system.[13]

Effect of exogenous dopamine on renal function in healthy persons

Dopamine can bind to three major types of receptor: the DA receptor, the β-adrenoreceptor, and the α-adrenoreceptor.[14] There are differences in the affinity of these receptors for dopamine, and this accounts for the dose–response profile observed with infusion. In general, selective dopamine receptor stimulation occurs within an infusion rate range of 0.5–3 μg/kg/min. Further increases in infusion rate between 3 and 10 μg/kg/min result in increasing β-adrenoreceptor stimulation, and increased α-adrenoreceptor stimulation occurs at a rate between 5 and 20 μg/kg/min. These dose ranges are only approximate and must be interpreted with caution because they were derived from small studies using healthy patients.[14] In general, studies have shown a poor correlation between infusion rates and plasma dopamine levels in critically ill patients.[15] There is a high interpatient and intrapatient variability in the effects of any given dopamine infusion rate.[16] Thus, low-dose dopamine should not be referred to as "renal dose" dopamine because at this infusion rate (0.5–3 μg/kg/min) it is possible that all three receptor types are stimulated. Consistent with this, tachycardia is frequently seen in patients receiving low-dose dopamine.[17] Dopamine clearance is reduced in critically ill patients and in patients with renal impairment.[15]

In healthy adults, dopamine infusion increases renal blood flow (RBF); the mechanism for this effect is dependent on the infusion rate.[18–20] At low infusion rates, dopamine induces renal vasodilation and increases RBF and can do this without any change in systemic hemodynamics – an effect mediated by dopaminergic receptors on the intrarenal vasculature.[21,22] This effect can be mimicked by selective DA_1 receptor agonists such as

fenoldapam.[23] Stimulation of presynaptic DA_2 receptors on sympathetic nerve terminals with inhibition of norepinephrine release may further augment renal vasodilation and RBF.[24] With higher infusion rates, RBF is increased as a consequence of increases in cardiac output, mediated by β-adrenoreceptor stimulation.[25] In healthy humans, low-dose dopamine counteracts the reduction in RBF observed with norepinephrine infusion.[26,27]

Knowledge of how low-dose dopamine affects the intrarenal distribution of blood flow is important since specific areas of the kidney are more susceptible to ischemic injury than others. Most animal models have shown a preferential increase in cortical flow with dopamine.[7] This was confirmed in humans by Hollenberg et al[28] using a xenon washout technique. Dopamine-induced PGE_2 production may also enhance inner medullary blood flow.[29] Thus, dopamine may shunt blood away from the outer medulla, which would be detrimental in states of renal hypoperfusion given that the outer medulla contains the pars recta of the proximal tubule and the medullary thick ascending limb – two highly metabolically active portions of the nephron. In a study of patients with severe sepsis, low-dose dopamine increased renal blood flow, but this was accompanied by a reduction in the renal oxygen extraction ratio, which led to no net change in renal oxygen consumption.[30]

Low-dose dopamine has minimal effects on the glomerular filtration rate (GFR) in healthy subjects.[16,20] Most studies report a mild increase in GFR of approximately 10–20%, whereas others report no change as assessed by creatinine clearance or iothalamate clearance. Increases in GFR are mediated by preferential afferent arteriolar vasodilation and an increase in intraglomerular pressure, as demonstrated in single-nephron studies.[31] The ultrafiltration coefficient remains unchanged with dopamine infusion.[7] The selective DA_1 receptor agonist fenoldopam did not change the GFR in healthy adults.[23]

The hemodynamic effects of low-dose dopamine infusion in healthy subjects differ with age, race, extracellular fluid volume status,[32] and duration of infusion.[33] In neonates, activation of α-adrenoreceptors occurs at much lower infusion rates.[34] In general, the selective vasodilatory effects of dopamine are not seen in young children.[6] With increasing age, the effects of dopamine on RBF and GFR are attenuated, perhaps because of impaired renal prostaglandin production.[35,36] African-Americans are more likely to exhibit pressor responses to low-dose dopamine than Caucasians.[37] African-Americans also appear to be more resistant to the natriuretic effects of dopamine.[37]

A natriuresis is the most consistent physiologic response to low-dose dopamine in healthy humans.[20] This effect is rapid in onset and may be profound. It is abrogated by extracellular fluid volume depletion[32] and typically wanes after 24 h of infusion, perhaps as a result of counteractive antinatriuretic factors or perhaps dopamine receptor downregulation.[19,33,38,39] Oral dopamine receptor antagonists commonly used as antiemetic agents or to enhance gastric motility may or may not counteract the hemodynamic and natriuretic effects of dopamine.[40,41] In addition to the direct tubular effects of dopamine, dopamine infusion may induce natriuresis by inhibiting adrenal aldosterone production.[42,43]

Effects of exogenous dopamine on renal function in disease states

The effects of low-dose dopamine observed in healthy individuals cannot necessarily be extrapolated to patients with disease. Many studies have examined the effects of short-term administration of low-dose dopamine to critically ill patients in the intensive care unit or patients with renal or cardiovascular disease. These studies frequently use the patient as their own control and examine cardiovascular and renal parameters before, during, and after a limited infusion period. A number of these studies are summarized in Table 3.1.

In general, the effects of low-dose dopamine infusion on renal hemodynamics and renal function are inconsistent and are frequently attenuated in patients with coexisting disease states. Ter Wee and colleagues[44] reported that patients with renal disease and a baseline GFR of less than 50 mL/min showed no change in RBF or GFR with dopamine infusion. McDonald et al[19] reported that, in contrast to normal subjects, patients with heart failure do not exhibit an increase in RBF or GFR with low-dose dopamine. Similar findings have been reported in hypertensive patients,[45] in patients with septic shock, and in critically ill patients on vasopressor therapy.[17,46] In critically ill patients with nonoliguric renal impairment, low-dose dopamine did increase creatinine clearance (associated with increased cardiac index) and urine sodium excretion, but this effect disappeared after 48 h of infusion.[39] In a group of patients who underwent infrarenal surgery, low-dose dopamine did increase RBF and GFR, but this is reported to be entirely secondary to an increase in cardiac output and not due to selective renal vasodilation.[43] In a prospective crossover study comparing dobutamine (mean dose, 2.5 µg/kg/min) with dopamine (mean dose 2.9 µg/kg/min) in critically ill patients, dopamine acted primarily as a diuretic and had no effect on creatinine clearance, whereas dobutamine, which had a greater effect on cardiac index, increased creatinine clearance.[17] In postcardiac surgery patients, dopamine was no more effective than dobutamine in increasing RBF and GFR.[47] Dopamine, however, was more effective in inducing a diuresis.[47] In general, the most consistent effect of low-dose dopamine in hospitalized patients is natriuresis and diuresis.[48]

There are probably multiple explanations accounting for the reduced efficacy of low-dose dopamine in disease states. Likely causes include abnormal vasculature (atherosclerosis or hypertensive vasculopathy), altered intravascular volume status, counteractive effects of other vasoactive hormones, and intrinsic renal disease. It is well established that intrinsic renal mechanisms act to decrease RBF in patients with acute tubular necrosis, even after renal perfusion pressures are restored. In addition, hypoxia is associated with an attenuated renal hemodynamic response to low-dose dopamine.[49] Finally, plasma dopamine clearance is lower in critically ill patients, and therefore the concept of selective renovasodilation with low-dose dopamine is invalid in this population.[15,50]

Value of low-dose dopamine infusion in patients with severe heart failure

Patients with severe cardiac failure suffer chronic renal hypoperfusion owing to a low cardiac output state and renal vasoconstriction caused by overactivity of the sympathetic nervous system and renin–angiotensin system. Secondary salt and water retention results in massive extracellular volume expansion and further cardiac decompensation because of excessive preload. These patients are frequently given a trial infusion of dobutamine and dopamine; the former for its ability to augment cardiac output and the latter for its purported renal vasodilatory and natriuretic effects. What evidence is there to support the use of low-dose dopamine in this setting?

The evidence is mixed, but in general there are no good trials examining this issue. El Allaf et al[51] reported that in patients with acute myocardial infarction and cardiac failure addition of low-dose dopamine to dobutamine therapy (2.5 µg/kg/min) did not alter cardiac output, heart rate, or blood pressure but did increase urine output by > 60%. In patients with cardiomyopathy, addition of low-dose dopamine to dobutamine did not augment cardiac output, RBF, GFR, or urine output.[52] Dopamine did not augment furosemide-induced diuresis in patients with chronic heart failure.[53]

In 20 patients with congestive heart failure who were being aggressively diuresed with loop diuretics, randomization to low-dose dopamine infusion was associated with improvement of blood urea nitrogen (BUN), creatinine, and creatinine and urine output in contrast to a modest decrease in renal function in the control group.[54] In a similar trial, the combination of low-dose dopamine and low-dose loop diuretic was compared with high-dose loop diuretic in patients with refractory heart failure. In both groups, the drugs induced equal weight loss and improved symptoms, but patients in the dopamine group had greater preservation of renal function.[55] Dopamine analogs have also been used in patients with heart failure. In a small randomized controlled trial, the oral dopamine precursor L-dopa increased urine output and sodium excretion in patients with cardiac failure resistant to the effects of diuretics.[56] In contrast, intravenous fenoldopam did not induce a natriuresis in patients with severe heart failure.[57]

In summary, there is insufficient evidence to support the use of low-dose dopamine in patients with cardiac failure requiring dobutamine infusion for inotropic support. There is some evidence to suggest that low-dose dopamine may enable a reduction in diuretic dosage. Patients with cardiac failure are resistant to the renal hemodynamic effects of dopamine, exhibiting at best a modest diuretic effect of this drug.

Table 3.1 Studies examining the hemodynamic and renal effects of low-dose dopamine in patients with disease

Study	Clinical setting	Dopamine regimen µg/kg/min	Dopamine regimen Duration (h)	Parameter	Response to dopamine Unit	Response to dopamine Pre	Response to dopamine Post	Significant difference?	Comment
Bughi et al[24] (n = 8)	Hypertension subjects	1	3	MAP	mmHg	108	103	No	Similar results with fenoldapam
				RBF	L/min/m²	1098 ± 85	1061 ± 101	No	
				U_{NA}	mmol/3 h	17 ± 3	34 ± 3	Yes	
				UO	L/3 h	0.31 ± 0.1	0.45 ± 0.1	Yes	
McDonald et al[19] (n = 6)	Cardiac failure	1–4	4	RBF	mL/min	217	321	No	In a parallel study dopamine increased RBF and GFR in normal subjects
				GFR	mL/min	61	80	No	
				U_{NA}	mmol/h	4.9	20.1	Yes	
				UO	mL/h	156	314	Yes	
ter Wee et al[44] (n = 42)	Chronic renal impairment (GFR < 50)	2	2	RBF	mL/min per 1.73 m²	129	137	No	
				GFR	mL/min per 1.73 m²	27	28	No	
Lherm et al[46] (n = 15)	Septic shock on norepinephrine	2	2	HR	beats/min	101 ± 18	106 ± 17	No	In same study dopamine did increase CrCl/U_{Na}/UO in sepsis syndrome
				MAP	mmHg	78 ± 10	76 ± 11	No	
				CO	L/min	7.9 ± 2	8.1 ± 2	No	
				CrCl	mL/min	60 ± 35	52 ± 31	No	
				U_{NA}	mmol/2 h	11 ± 5	11 ± 4	No	
				UO	mL/2 h	201 ± 131	184 ± 111	No	
Girbes et al[43] (n = 7)	Postinfrarenal AAA repair	4	1	HR	beats/min	84	88	No	
				CI	L/min/m²	2.77	3.34	Yes	
				RBF	mL/min per 1.73 m²	676	809	Yes	
				GFR	mL/min per 1.73 m²	80	97	Yes	
				U_{NA}	mmol/h	11.9	28	Yes	
				UO	mL/h	115	260	Yes	
Ichai et al[39] (n = 12)	Critically ill nonoliguric renal impairment	3	4	HR	beats/min	95 ± 21	96 ± 23	No	Dobutamine did not exhibit these effects
				MAP	mmHg	79 ± 7	79 ± 10	No	The CrCl and U_{Na} decreased to baseline after 48 h infusion in sister paper
				CI	L/min	3.8 ± 0.9	4.2 ± 1	Yes	
				CrCl	mL/min	61 ± 17	80 ± 20	Yes	
				U_{NA}	mmol/2 h	8	16	Yes	
				UO	mL/h	48 ± 21	79 ± 62	Yes	

Table 3.1 Studies examining the hemodynamic and renal effects of low-dose dopamine in patients with disease (cont'd)

| Study | Clinical setting | Dopamine regimen | | Parameter | Response to dopamine | | | Significant | Comment |
		µg/kg/min	Duration (h)		Unit	Pre	Post	difference?	
Davis et al[113] (n = 15)	Oliguria postcardiac surgery	100 µg/min	4	CrCl	mL/min	70 ± 120	115 ± 13	Yes	
				U_NA	mmol/4 h	1.3	6	Yes	
				UO	mL/h	22 ± 2	54 ± 9	Yes	
Duke et al[17] (n = 18)	Critically ill	200 µg/min	5	HR	beats/min	95 ± 24	102 ± 24	Yes	
				MAP	kPa	11.1 ± 1.7	11.6 ± 2.0	No	
				CI	L/min/m²	3.5 ± 0.8	3.8 ± 1.0	No	
				CrCl	mL/min	79 ± 38	88 ± 42	No	
				UO	mL/h	90 ± 44	145 ± 148	Yes	
Girbes et al[112] (n = 8)	Sepsis/epinephrine (Creat < 180)	4	1	HR	beats/min	124 ± 24	124 ± 24	Yes	
				CO	L/min	7.9 ± 1.7	7.9 ± 1.7	Yes	
				CrCl	mL/min	109(29–126)	134(20–179)	No	
				U_NA	mmol/h	4(0–48)	13(1–55)	Yes	
				UO	mL/h	103(60–240)	133(21–170)	Yes	

Creat, serum creatinine; CO, cardiac output; CI, cardiac index; CrCl, creatinine clearance; GFR, glomerular filtration rate; HR, heart rate; MAP, mean arterial pressure; U_NA, urine sodium excretion; UO, urine output; RBF, renal blood flow.

Low-dose dopamine in conjunction with systemic vasopressors

Low-dose dopamine is commonly administered to patients with septic shock requiring pressor support with systemic vasoconstrictors, with the goal of maximizing renal perfusion in this setting. However, there is very little evidence to support this clinical practice. In healthy humans, pressor doses of norepinephrine lower RBF, and this can be normalized by coadministration of low-dose dopamine.[27] However, in patients with septic shock requiring norepinephrine for pressor support, addition of low-dose dopamine did not improve creatinine clearance or urine output.[46] In a similar study, low-dose dopamine did not improve creatinine clearance, but did increase urine output when coadministered with norepinephrine.[58] Marin and coworkers[59,60] reported that addition of norepinephrine alone is sufficient to restore renal perfusion and urine output in patients with septic shock. Furthermore, norepinephrine was more effective than high-dose dopamine in preserving RBF in this patient population.[61]

Value of low-dose dopamine in preventing acute renal failure in high-risk patients

A limitation in the efficacy of any treatment designed to prevent ARF is the difficulty in predicting its occurrence and hence the correct timing of treatment. However, when patients are about to undergo a high-risk procedure, prophylactic administration of renoprotective agents can be timed appropriately. In these circumstances, judgment is required as to whether it is appropriate to expose all patients to the potential side-effects of a given drug when the potential benefit may be gained by only a few patients. Several well-defined clinical situations are associated with renal hypoperfusion and a high risk of developing ARF. These include cardiac, vascular, and biliary surgery, renal and liver transplantation, and exposure to radiocontrast agents or vasoactive drugs. The prophylactic administration of low-dose dopamine in an attempt to prevent renal hypoperfusion and injury has been evaluated in these settings.

Prevention of acute renal failure during cardiopulmonary bypass and infrarenal cross-clamping

Table 3.2 lists the major prospective controlled trials that have examined the ability of low-dose dopamine to prevent ARF in patients undergoing either cardiopulmonary bypass for cardiac surgery or infrarenal cross-clamping for abdominal aortic surgery. Five studies have examined the efficacy of low-dose dopamine infusion in the prevention of ARF during cardiac surgery.[62–66] Three studies have examined the efficacy of low-dose dopamine infusion in the

prevention of ARF during peripheral vascular surgery.[67–69] All studies failed to demonstrate a beneficial effect of dopamine on renal function, as assessed by BUN, creatinine, or creatinine clearance. However, the incidence of ARF in the control groups of some of these studies was low (perhaps a result of study participation), making it difficult to detect a benefit of dopamine. Three studies examined evidence for more subtle ischemic renal damage by measuring markers of tubule injury such as urinary retinal binding protein and β_2-microglobulin.[64–66] Overall, prophylactic low-dose dopamine infusion appeared to be associated with increased renal tubular injury.

Halpenny et al[70] reported the effects of the selective DA_1 agonist fenoldopam in patients undergoing cardiopulmonary bypass. In a small but randomized and controlled trial, fenoldopam treatment was associated with preservation of creatinine clearance post procedure.[70] In an uncontrolled trial, fenoldopam was associated with a rapid return of renal function to baseline levels after aortic cross-clamping.[71] Prospective controlled trials are needed to assess the true value of fenoldopam infusion in the prevention of ARF during high-risk surgery.

Prevention of acute renal failure in renal transplantation

The renal allograft is subject to ischemic injury during the process of transplantation and from the vasoconstrictive effects of high-dose calcineurin inhibitors. Five studies have examined the role of perioperative low-dose dopamine infusion during renal transplantation, including three prospective studies[72–74] and two retrospective studies[75,76] involving a total of 367 patients. Endpoints measured included incidence of ARF post transplantation, delayed graft function, requirements for dialysis, and allograft GFR at various points after transplantation. Four studies indicated no beneficial effects of perioperative dopamine infusion on allograft function. Indeed, dopamine-induced natriuresis and diuresis were often associated with fluid and electrolyte management problems in these patients. Carmellini and colleagues[73] reported a small but significantly higher GFR in dopamine-treated allografts 1 month post transplantation. Consistent with this apparent lack of efficacy of dopamine in renal transplant patients, Spicer et al[77] demonstrated an insensitivity of recently implanted kidneys to the vasodilatory effects of dopamine, as assessed by Doppler ultrasound of the renal vasculature. In contrast, Hansen et al[78] reported that low-dose dopamine did increase effective renal plasma flow (ERPF) and GFR in transplanted patients on cyclosporine. This variable response may be due to differences in baseline transplant function and/or cyclosporine dosing.

Prevention of acute renal failure in liver transplantation and hepatobiliary surgery

Liver transplantation is associated with a high incidence of renal failure, in part from the chronic renal hypoperfusion

Table 3.2 Prospective randomized controlled trials examining the ability of low-dose dopamine to prevent acute renal failure in patients undergoing cardiovascular surgery

Study	Clinical setting	Dopamine regimen	Parameter	Control Pre-operative	Control Post-operative	Dopamine Pre-operative	Dopamine Post-operative	Significant difference?	Comment
Myles et al[63] (n = 52)	Elective CABG	3 μg/kg/min presurgery and 24 h post	BUN	NR	NR	NR	NR	–	CrCl Creat and UO assessed at day 7 postoperatively. No ARF in control group
			Creat	1.02 ± 0.05	1.03 ± 0.05	1.05 ± 0.05	1.13 ± 0.14	No	
			CrCl	127 ± 12	107 ± 15	104 ± 16	91 ± 16	No	
			UO	NR	342 ± 130	NR	305 ± 160	No	
Tang et al[64] (n = 42)	Cardiac surgery	3 μg/kg/min presurgery and 48 h post	BUN*	5.2 ± 0.4	6.5 ± 1.5	4.5 ± 0.3	6.4 ± 1.0	No	Parameters assessed at day 5. Dopamine use associated with worse tubular injury (assessed by urine retinol-binding protein) (UO = mL/h)
			Creat	120 ± 5	113 ± 4	110 ± 6	1.13 ± 0.14	No	
			UO*	27 ± 7	21 ± 4	28 ± 5	23 ± 4	No	
Lassnigg et al[62] (n = 82)	Cardiac surgery	2 μg/kg/min presurgery and 48 h post	BUN	17.3 ± 5.9	23.7 ± 10.7	16.2 ± 6.1	25.7 ± 8.1	No	ARF defined by increase in Creat > 0.5. Statistically more ARF in third group receiving frusemide alone
			Creat	0.96 ± 0.23	1.1 ± 0.36	0.98 ± 0.23	1.21 ± 0.45	No	
			CrCl	99 ± 47	95 ± 54	101 ± 35	72 ± 35	No	
			ARF	–	1(2.3%)	–	0(0%)	No	
Baldwin et al[67] (n = 37)	Elective abdominal aortic surgery	3 μg/kg/min post surgery for 24 h	BUN	6.8	5.8	6.8	5.8	No	Parameters assessed at day 5. No ARF in control group. Trend toward increased UO in control group
			Creat	1.3	1.2	1.2	1.2	No	
			CrCl	72	83	89	85	No	
			UO	NR	NR	NR	NR	–	
Paul et al[68] (n = 27)	Elective infrarenal aortic clamping	3 μg/kg/min post surgery for 24 h Mannitol	BUN	NR	NR	NR	NR	–	Parameters assessed at day 1 postoperatively. CrCl decreased in both groups by 50% during clamp period (UO = mL/day)
			Creat	NR	NR	NR	NR	–	
			CrCl	96 ± 10	92 ± 7	92 ± 7	92 ± 7	No	
			UO	150 ± 30	115 ± 30	130 ± 30	100 ± 30	No	
de Lasson et al[69] (n = 30)	Elective peripheral vascular surgery	3 μg/kg/min presurgery and 24 h post	REF	380	350	320	373	No	Parameters assessed at day 1 postoperatively. RBF (^{131}I-hippurate) and GFR (^{125}I-thalamate) measured 24 h postoperatively (mL/min per 1.73 m²) (UO = mL/day) (values estimated from figure)
			GFR	91	78	80	86	No	
			UO	–	1163	–	1933	Yes	

ARF, acute renal failure; BUN, blood urea nitrogen; CABG, coronary artery bypass grafting; Creat, serum creatinine; CrCl, creatinine clearance (mL/min); GFR, glomerular filtration rate; NR, not reported; RBF, renal blood flow; U_{Na}, urine sodium excretion; UO, urine output; BUN and Creat expressed as mg/dL unless marked by an asterisk, which indicates SI units.

that complicates liver failure and the nephrotoxicity of hyperbilirubinemia and calcineurin inhibitors. In a prospective controlled trial involving 48 patients, perioperative infusion of dopamine was not associated with improved renal function (creatinine clearance and radionuclide GFR measured at 24 h and 1 month post surgery respectively) compared with control.[79] However, only 4% of control patients developed ARF compared with 40–60% in some series. Two trials have assessed the value of prophylactic low-dose dopamine infusion inpatients with hyperbilirubinemia undergoing surgery.[80,81] In a prospective randomized controlled trial involving 40 patients, Wahbah et al[80] concluded that administration of low-dose dopamine conferred no additional benefit over adequate hydration. Similarly, Parks et al[81] randomized 23 patients to dopamine or saline infusion during surgery for obstructive jaundice and found no benefit of dopamine infusion on renal function. However, in this latter trial, there was no ARF in the control group.

Prevention of radiocontrast-induced nephropathy

Radiocontrast agents are a major cause of hospital-acquired ARF. Diabetics, patients with preexisting renal impairment, and patients with intravascular volume depletion are most at risk of radiocontrast-induced nephropathy (RCIN). In the majority of cases, RCIN is mild and reversible; however, contrast exposure may precipitate the need for permanent dialysis in patients with baseline chronic renal failure. The mechanism for this effect is contrast-induced intrarenal vasoconstriction. The role of prophylactic dopamine therapy, therefore, to prevent RCIN has been an area of much interest. Table 3.3 summarizes the prospective controlled trials that have assessed the value of low-dose dopamine infusion for the prevention of RCIN.

There are six prospective, controlled, randomized trials containing over 340 patients undergoing coronary and aortic angiography.[82–87] Most of these patients would be considered at high risk of RCIN on the basis of having diabetes or chronic renal impairment. The majority of studies compared dopamine with placebo in patients who were receiving saline infusion to ensure adequate hydration. The primary measure of efficacy was peak creatinine post procedure. Five out of the six studies reported no benefit of dopamine infusion. Rather, in some studies, subgroups of patients appeared to do worse on dopamine. This may be secondary to the natriuretic effects of dopamine leading to intravascular volume depletion. Furthermore, Abizaid et al[87] reported that, in those patients who developed RCIN, continuation of dopamine infusion was associated with delayed recovery.

No prospective controlled trials have examined the efficacy of the selective DA_1 agonist fenoldopam for the prevention of radiocontrast-induced ARF.[88] Proponents argue that, unlike dopamine, fenoldopam does not have α-adrenoreceptor activity and may therefore be more vasodilatory. Two large case series (one with 46 patients and the other with 150) reported a favorable outcome in consecutive high-risk patients undergoing angiography with fenoldopam infusion.[89,90] The incidence of ARF,

defined by a greater than 25% increase in baseline serum creatinine, was 13% and 5%, respectively, compared with higher rates (38% and 19%) noted in historical controls.

Prevention of drug-induced nephrotoxicity

A variety of drugs are known to induce renal vasoconstriction and a prerenal state, including nonsteroidal anti-inflammatory agents, amphotericin B, and interleukin 2 (IL-2) therapy. Prospective, randomized, controlled trials have examined the ability of low-dose dopamine infusion to counteract renal vasoconstriction induced by these drugs. Indomethacin therapy for closure of a patent ductus arteriosus in preterm neonates can be associated with renal impairment. In two trials, low-dose dopamine did not attenuate the development of oliguria or mean increase in creatinine observed with indomethacin therapy.[91,92] Prophylactic administration of low-dose dopamine did not affect the renal outcome of patients receiving systemic high-dose IL-2 therapy[93] or amphotericin B treatment in bone marrow transplant and leukemia patients.[94,95] In this latter study, dopamine infusion was associated with a high incidence of adverse reactions. Finally, low-dose dopamine failed to prevent cisplatin-induced ARF in a prospective randomized study.[96]

In summary, the value of low-dose dopamine infusion for the prevention of ARF has been assessed in a variety of high-risk settings. When assessed in prospective controlled trials, studies invariably show a lack of efficacy on major endpoints such as postprocedure creatinine level or GFR, development of ARF, or requirement for dialysis. A possible criticism of these trials is insufficient patients and low rates of renal injury in control groups, making it difficult to demonstrate a potential benefit of dopamine. However, the overriding sense from these trials is a lack of benefit. A meta-analysis of these studies reported no benefit of low-dose dopamine in the prevention of ARF.[97] The lack of efficacy may be due to (1) absent or insufficient renovasodilatory effects of low-dose dopamine in these patients; (2) detrimental effects of dopamine on intrarenal distribution blood flow; (3) increased energy demands on distal segments of the nephron owing to increased delivery of solute; and (4) intravascular volume depletion because of natriuretic effects. Consistent with this last explanation, trials examining the efficacy of loop diuretics in the prevention of ARF have shown a detrimental effect.[62]

Influence of low-dose dopamine on established acute renal failure

Established acute tubular necrosis is associated with a reduced GFR owing to several mechanisms, including: (1) impaired glomerular perfusion secondary to pre-glomerular vasoconstriction; (2) backleakage of glomerular filtrate through injured tubular epithelium; and (3) obstruction of the renal tubules by cellular debris. Proponents of low-dose dopamine infusion argue that

Table 3.3 Prospective randomized controlled trials examining the ability of low-dose dopamine to prevent radiocontrast-induced nephropathy

Study	Study population	Dopamine regimen	Control	Parameter	Renal function				Significant difference	Comment
					Control		Dopamine			
					Pre-operative	Post-operative	Pre-operative	Post-operative		
Stevens et al[85] (n = 77)	"High-risk" patients DM,CRF,PVD Coronary angiography	2 µg/kg/min and saline infusion, furosemide and mannitol	Saline	Creat UO ARF RRT	2.6 ± 0.9 – – –	3.1 ± 1.2 122 ± 54 14.50% 9.10%	2.2 ± 0.4 – – –	2.7 ± 1.2 167 ± 58 13.60% 4.50%	No Yes No No	Parameters assessed at 24 and 48 h ARF defined by increase in Creat > 0.5 mg/dL
Gare et al[82] (n = 66)	Coronary angiography in patients with DM and/or CRF	2 µg/kg/min and saline infusion, for 48 h	Saline	BUN* Creat*	7.3 ± 0.5 100.6 ± 5.2	7.9 ± 0.8 112.3 ± 8.0	6.9 ± 0.5 100.3 ± 5.4	7.6 ± 0.6 117.5 ± 8.8	No No	Peak Creat within 5 days post contrast Subgroup of patients with peripheral vascular disease did worse with dopamine
Hans et al[83] (n = 55)	CRF (Creat 1.4–3.5) Abdominal angiography	2.5 µg/kg/min 1 h pre/12 h post	Saline	ARF	–	44%	–	18%	Yes	ARF defined by increase in Creat > 0.5 mg/dL by day 4 post. No RRT required
Abizaid et al[87] (n = 40)	CRF (Creat > 1.5) Coronary angiography	2.5 µg/kg/min 2 h pre and saline infusion (1 mg/kg/h) 12 h pre	Saline	Creat ARF	2.3 ± 0.8 –	2.8 ± 1.1 6(30%)	1.9 ± 0.3 –	2.5 ± 0.6 10(50%)	No No	Creat is peak value post procedure ARF defined by Creat > 25% above baseline
Weisberg et al[86] (n = 50)	CRF (Creat > 1.8) Coronary angiography	2.5 µg/kg/min during and 2 h post	Saline	RBF Creat ARF	247 ± 55 > 1.8 –	NR NR 40%	171 ± 23 > 1.8 –	NR NR 30%	Yes – No	ARF defined by Creat > 25% above baseline RBF: thermodilution (mL/min per kidney)
Kapoor et al[84] (n = 40)	Coronary angiography	5 µg/kg/min 30 min pre and 6 h post	Saline	BUN Creat ARF	20 ± 13 1.5 ± 7 –	23 ± 8 2.0 ± 1.0 50%	16 ± 8 1.5 ± 0.3 –	15 ± 6 1.4 ± 0.3 0%	No Yes Yes	ARF defined by Creat > 25% above baseline In all cases ARF mild and reversible

ARF, acute renal failure; BUN, blood urea nitrogen; CRF, chronic renal failure; Creat, serum creatinine; DM, diabetes mellitus; NR, not reported; PVD, peripheral vascular disease; RBF, renal blood flow; RRT, renal replacement therapy; UO, urine output; BUN and Creat expressed as mg/dL unless marked by an asterisk, which indicates SI units.

dopamine may improve the outcome of acute tubular necrosis by: (1) improving renal perfusion; (2) inhibiting tubular transport processes and therefore improving the oxygen supply/demand relationship; and (3) "flushing" out renal tubules by inducing a diuresis.

Until recently, there were no prospective controlled trials evaluating the efficacy of low-dose dopamine in patients with established ARF. Several case series had reported variable success with dopamine in established ARF, but because there were no control groups for comparison it was impossible to differentiate response from natural history.

Table 3.4 lists the prospective controlled trials evaluating the efficacy of low-dose dopamine in patients with established ARF. The largest of these studies randomized 328 intensive care unit patients with sepsis syndrome with evidence of early renal dysfunction (either prolonged oliguria or increased serum creatinine) to low-dose dopamine or saline infusion.[98] The majority of patients were receiving catecholamines or phosphodiesterase inhibitors for blood pressure support. Low-dose dopamine had no effect on serum creatinine, on requirements for dialysis, on duration of stay in the intensive care unit, or on patient survival. The incidence of acute renal failure was high in both groups, with approximately 25% of patients requiring dialysis. This study provides the most convincing data for abandoning the use of low-dose dopamine in critically ill oliguric patients.

Chertow et al[99] performed secondary analysis of 165 patients from the placebo arm of the auriculin anaritide acute renal failure study. All patients within the placebo arm were adults with ARF and a clinical history consistent with acute tubular necrosis. Low-dose dopamine had been administered to a proportion of these patients at the discretion of the physician. Low-dose dopamine treatment was not associated with reduced risk of death or dialysis. Marik and Iglesias[100] performed a similar secondary analysis of 168 patients with oliguria within the placebo arm of the NORASEPT II study – a multicenter randomized trial of anti-tumor necrosis factor (TNF)-α monoclonal antibodies in septic shock. The incidence of ARF, requirement for renal replacement therapy, and patient survival were no different in oliguric patients who received low-dose dopamine infusion from those patients who did not. A criticism of both of these reports is that because the original trial was not set up to study the effects of dopamine, treatment was based on physician judgment rather than randomization.

Finally, smaller studies have examined the value of dopamine infusion in the treatment of established ARF from radiocontrast exposure,[87] malarial infection,[30] IL-2 therapy,[101–103] and cyclosporine A with variable results.[104]

To summarize, the bulk of the evidence suggests that low-dose dopamine does not alter the outcome of established ARF from a variety of causes. These disappointing results may be due to several factors: (1) the renal hemodynamic effects of dopamine appear to be attenuated in critically ill patients; (2) dopamine may have a detrimental effect on the intrarenal distribution of blood flow; and (3) inhibition of proximal tubule solute

reabsorption may enhance distal delivery of solute and increase the workload of distal nephron segments. The practice of administering low-dose dopamine in ARF has evolved from the belief that increasing urine output improves outcome in this condition. This opinion is based on the improved prognosis and lower mortality rates observed with nonoliguric ARF compared with patients with oliguric ARF. Nevertheless, there is no evidence that converting oliguric ARF to the nonoliguric state improves prognosis.

Potentially deleterious effects of dopamine

Although proponents advocate the use of low-dose dopamine in ARF on the grounds that it may improve renal function and is unlikely to harm the patient, evidence is accumulating that this is a misconception. The following complications of low-dose dopamine infusion have been reported:

1. Dopamine may cause local extravasation of dopamine, resulting in distal gangrene and skin necrosis.
2. β-Adrenoreceptor agonism can increase myocardial oxygen demand and precipitate tachyarrhythymias and myocardial ischemia.[17]
3. Dopamine may cause a ventilation perfusion mismatch and hypoxemia.[17,105] Furthermore, dopamine can suppress the respiratory drive induced by hypoxemia.[106] Hypoxemia may worsen myocardial ischemia and potentially delay the recovery from ischemic acute tubular necrosis.
4. Although dopamine augments total splanchnic blood flow, it may cause shunting of blood away from the intestinal mucosa.[107–109] Mucosal ischemia promotes bacterial translocation and septicemia.
5. When administered to patients without close monitoring of fluid balance, the natriuretic effects of dopamine may promote intravascular volume depletion.
6. Increased delivery of sodium to the distal nephron causes hypokalemia, hypophosphatemia, and hypomagnesemia.
7. Dopamine infusion inhibits prolactin and growth hormone secretion. Lymphocyte function is suppressed in hypoprolactinemia.[110] Growth hormone deficiency may worsen the catabolic state in critically ill patients.[111]

Conclusion

In summary, low-dose dopamine does promote renal vasodilation, augment RBF, and induce a natriuresis in healthy humans. However, these effects are attenuated in patients with underlying vascular disease, cardiac failure, or chronic renal disease or in patients who are critically ill and/or receiving vasopressors for hemodynamic support in the intensive care unit. When administered prophylactically to patients who are undergoing procedures deemed high risk for the development of ARF, randomized

Table 3.4 Studies examining the effects of low-dose dopamine in established acute renal failure

Study	Study type	Clinical setting	Dopamine regimen	Parameter	Renal function				Significant difference	Comment
					Control		Dopamine			
					Pre-operative	Post-operative	Pre-operative	Post-operative		
ANZICS[98] (n = 328)	Prospective controlled randomized	Critically ill with renal dysfunction (4 h oliguria or increased Creat)	2 μg/kg/min until endpoint	BUN*	14.4 ± 7	23 ± 12	14.3 ± 8	20 ± 10	No	BUN and Creat represent peak levels post start infusion UO after 48 h treatment (UO = mL/h)
				Creat*	182 ± 81	249 ± 147	183 ± 85	245 ± 144	No	
				UO	50 ± 59	109 ± 95	37 ± 40	99 ± 83	No	
				RRT	–	40(25%)	–	35(22%)	No	
				% ICU discharge		67%		64%	No	
Marik and Iglesias[100] (n = 168)	Secondary analysis of prospective controlled trial	Septic shock; oliguria	< 3 μg/kg/min until endpoint	Creat	1.6 ± 0.8	–	1.7 ± 1.0	–	No	Data derived from placebo arm of NORASEPT II study. ARF defined by Creat > 3.5 mg/dL or 2× above baseline
				ARF	–	29%	–	29%	No	
				RRT	–	13%	–	13%	No	
				28-day surveillance	–	66%	–	64%	No	
Chertow et al[99] (n = 165)	Secondary of prospective controlled trial	ARF with clinical characteristics of ATN	3 μg/kg/min until endpoint	Creat	5.3 ± 2.7	–	4.2 ± 1.5	–	No	Data derived from placebo arm of ANP trial. No difference in risk of death or requirement for dialysis
				Oliguria (%)	22	–	15	–	No	
Abizaid et al[87] (n = 72)	Prospective controlled randomized	Radiocontrast ATN	2.5 μg/kg/min up to 4 days	Creat	2.2 ± 0.5	2.7 ± 0.6	2.1 ± 0.9	3.7 ± 1.3	Yes	Dopamine group did worse. Post Creat represents peak value
				RRT	–	0	–	4(11%)	Yes	
Lumlertgul et al[114] (n = 8)	Prospective controlled randomized	Malaria-induced ARF	1 μg/kg/min for 4 days; furosemide	Creat	3.5 ± 0.2	9.9 ± 0.2	3.7 ± 0.4	2.9 ± 0.4	Yes	Parameters assessed at day 6. Mean recovery time was 9 days in dopamine group vs 17 days in control
				CrCl	13 ± 0.8	NR	12.8 ± 0.6	NR	No	

ARF, acute renal failure; ATN, acute tubular necrosis; BUN, blood urea nitrogen; Creat, serum creatinine; CrCl, creatinine clearance (mL/min); NR, not reported; RRT, renal replacement therapy; UO, urine output; BUN and Creat expressed as mg/dL unless marked by an asterisk, which indicates SI units.

controlled trials have universally failed to demonstrate improved renal outcome with low-dose dopamine infusion. Until recently, there were no large trials assessing the efficacy of low-dose dopamine in established ARF. The results of the Australian and New Zealand Intensive Care Society (ANZICS) clinical trial now clearly show that low-dose dopamine given to critically ill patients with early renal dysfunction has no effect on serum creatinine, requirement for renal replacement therapy, duration of stay in the intensive care unit, or mortality. Thus, there is currently no justification for the use of low-dose dopamine for renal protection. These recommendations should not preclude the use of dopamine for its systemic effects in heart failure or septic shock, when dopamine, like other inotropes/vasopressors, may afford a valuable increase in cardiac output and tissue perfusion.

References

1. Thompson BT, Cockrill BA: Renal-dose dopamine: a siren song? Lancet 1994;344:7–8.
2. Denton MD, Chertow GM, Brady HR: "Renal-dose" dopamine for the treatment of acute renal failure: scientific rationale, experimental studies and clinical trials. Kidney Int 1996;50:4–14.
3. Corwin HL, Lisbon A: Renal dose dopamine: long on conjecture, short on fact. Crit Care Med 2000;28:1657–1658.
4. O'Hara JF Jr: Low-dose "renal" dopamine. Anesthesiol Clin North Am 2000;18:835–851.
5. Galley HF: Renal-dose dopamine: will the message now get through? Lancet 2000;356:2112–113.
6. Prins I, Plotz FB, Uiterwaal CS, et al: Low-dose dopamine in neonatal and pediatric intensive care: a systematic review. Intensive Care Med 2001;27:206–210.
7. Lee MR: Dopamine and the kidney: ten years on. Clin Sci (Lond) 1993;84:357–375.
8. Aperia AC: Intrarenal dopamine: a key signal in the interactive regulation of sodium metabolism. Annu Rev Physiol 2000;62:621–647.
9. Hansell P, Fasching A: The effect of dopamine receptor blockade on natriuresis is dependent on the degree of hypervolemia. Kidney Int 1991;39:253–258.
10. Bryan AG, Bolsin SN, Vianna PT, et al: Modification of the diuretic and natriuretic effects of a dopamine infusion by fluid loading in preoperative cardiac surgical patients. J Cardiothorac Vasc Anesth 1995;9:158–163.
11. Carey RM, Siragy HM, Ragsdale NV, et al: Dopamine-1 and dopamine-2 mechanisms in the control of renal function. Am J Hypertens 1990;3:59S–63S.
12. Ferreira A, Bettencourt P, Pestana M, et al: Renal synthesis of dopamine in asymptomatic post-infarction left ventricular systolic dysfunction. Clin Sci (Lond) 2000;99:195–200.
13. Pestana M, Jardim H, Correia F, et al: Renal dopaminergic mechanisms in renal parenchymal diseases and hypertension. Nephrol Dial Transplant 2001;16:53–59.
14. D'Orio V, el Allaf D, Juchmes J, et al: The use of low doses of dopamine in intensive care medicine. Arch Int Physiol Biochim 1984;92:S11–S20.
15. Juste RN, Moran L, Hooper J, et al: Dopamine clearance in critically ill patients. Intensive Care Med 1998;24:1217–1220.
16. MacGregor DA, Butterworth JFT, Zaloga CP, et al: Hemodynamic and renal effects of dopexamine and dobutamine in patients with reduced cardiac output following coronary artery bypass grafting. Chest 1994;106:835–841.
17. Duke GJ, Briedis JH, Weaver RA. Renal support in critically ill patients: low-dose dopamine or low-dose dobutamine? Crit Care Med 1994;22:1919–1925.
18. Goldberg LI. Dopamine: clinical uses of an endogenous catecholamine. N Engl J Med 1974;291:707–710.
19. McDonald R, Goldberg L, McNay J: Effects of dopamine in man: augmentation of sodium excretion, glomerular filtration and renal plasma flow. J Clin Invest 1964;43:1116.
20. Olsen NV: Effects of dopamine on renal haemodynamics tubular function and sodium excretion in normal humans. Danish Med Bull 1998;45:282–297.
21. Hughes JM, Beck TR, Rose CE Jr, et al: The effect of selective dopamine-1 receptor stimulation on renal and adrenal function in man. J Clin Endocrinol Metab 1988;66:518–525.
22. Yura T, Yuasa S, Fukunaga M, et al: Role for Doppler ultrasound in the assessment of renal circulation: effects of dopamine and dobutamine on renal hemodynamics in humans. Nephron 1995;71:168–175.
23. Mathur VS, Swan SK, Lambrecht LJ, et al: The effects of fenoldopam, a selective dopamine receptor agonist, on systemic and renal hemodynamics in normotensive subjects. Crit Care Med 1999;27:1832–1837.
24. Bughi S, Jost-Vu E, Antonipillai I, et al: Effect of dopamine2 blockade on renal function under varied sodium intake. J Clin Endocrinol Metab 1994;78:1079–1084.
25. Olsen NV, Lang-Jensen T, Hansen JM, et al: Effects of acute beta-adrenoceptor blockade with metoprolol on the renal response to dopamine in normal humans. Br J Clin Pharmacol 1994;37:347–353.
26. Hoogenberg K, Smit AJ, Girbes AR: Effects of low-dose dopamine on renal and systemic hemodynamics during incremental norepinephrine infusion in healthy volunteers. Crit Care Med 1998;26:260–265.
27. Richer M, Robert S, Lebel M: Renal hemodynamics during norepinephrine and low-dose dopamine infusions in man. Crit Care Med 1996;24:1150–1156.
28. Hollenberg NK, Adams DF, Mendell P et al: Renal vascular responses to dopamine: haemodynamic and angiographic observations in normal man. Clin Sci Mol Med 1973;45:733–742.
29. Hubbard PC, Henderson IW: Renal dopamine and the tubular handling of sodium. J Mol Endocrinol 1995;14:139–155.
30. Day NP, Phu NH, Mai NT, et al: Effects of dopamine and epinephrine infusions on renal hemodynamics in severe malaria and severe sepsis. Crit Care Med 2000;28:1353–1362.
31. Seri I, Aperia A: Contribution of dopamine 2 receptors to dopamine-induced increase in glomerular filtration rate. Am J Physiol 1988;254:F196–F201.
32. Agnoli GC, Cacciari M, Garutti C, et al: Effects of extracellular fluid volume changes on renal response to low-dose dopamine infusion in normal women. Clin Physiol 1987;7:465–479.
33. Orme ML, Breckenridge A, Dollery CT: The effects of long term administration of dopamine on renal function in hypertensive patients. Eur J Clin Pharmacol 1973;6:150–155.
34. Seri I, Rudas G, Bors Z, et al: Effects of low-dose dopamine infusion on cardiovascular and renal functions, cerebral blood flow, and plasma catecholamine levels in sick preterm neonates. Pediatr Res 1993;34:742–749.
35. Mulkerrin E, Epstein FH, Clark BA: Reduced renal response to low-dose dopamine infusion in the elderly. J Gerontol A Biol Sci Med Sci 1995;50:M271–M275.
36. Fuiano G, Sund S, Mazza G, et al: Renal hemodynamic response to maximal vasodilating stimulus in healthy older subjects. Kidney Int 2001;59:1052–1058.
37. Marinac JS, Willsie SK, Dew M, et al: Pharmacodynamic effects of dopamine stratified by race. Am J Ther 2001;8:27–34.
38. Braun GG, Bahlmann F, Brandl M, Knoll R: Long term administration of dopamine: is there a development of tolerance? Prog Clin Biol Res 1989;308:1097–1099.
39. Ichai C, Passeron C, Carles M, et al: Prolonged low-dose dopamine infusion induces a transient improvement in renal function in hemodynamically stable, critically ill patients: a single-blind, prospective, controlled study. Crit Care Med 2000;28:1329–1335.
40. MacDonald TM: Metoclopramide, domperidone and dopamine in man: actions and interactions. Eur J Clin Pharmacol 1991;40:225–230.
41. Munn J, Tooley M, Bolsin S, et al: Effect of metoclopramide on renal vascular resistance index and renal function in patients receiving a low-dose infusion of dopamine. Br J Anaesth 1993;71:379–382.
42. Smit AJ, Meijer S, Wesseling H, et al: Effect of metoclopramide on dopamine-induced changes in renal function in healthy controls and in patients with renal disease. Clin Sci (Lond) 1988;75:421–428.
43. Girbes AR, Lieverse AG, Smit AJ, et al: Lack of specific renal haemodynamic effects of different doses of dopamine after infrarenal aortic surgery. Br J Anaesth 1996;77:753–757.

44. ter Wee PM, Smit AJ, Rosman JB, et al: Effect of intravenous infusion of low-dose dopamine on renal function in normal individuals and in patients with renal disease. Am J Nephrol 1986;6:42–46.

45. Bughi S, Horton R, Antonipillai I, et al: Comparison of dopamine and fenoldopam effects on renal blood flow and prostacyclin excretion in normal and essential hypertensive subjects. J Clin Endocrinol Metab 1989;69:1116–1121.

46. Lherm T, Troche G, Rossignol M, et al: Renal effects of low-dose dopamine in patients with sepsis syndrome or septic shock treated with catecholamines. Intensive Care Med 1996;22: 213–219.

47. Hilberman M, Maseda J, Stinson EB, et al: The diuretic properties of dopamine in patients after open-heart operation. Anesthesiology 1984;61:489–494.

48. Pavoni V, Verri M, Ferraro L, et al: Plasma dopamine concentration and effects of low dopamine doses on urinary output after major vascular surgery. Kidney Int Suppl 1998;66:S75–S80.

49. Olsen NV, Hansen JM, Kanstrup IL, et al: Renal hemodynamics, tubular function, and response to low-dose dopamine during acute hypoxia in humans. J Appl Physiol 1993;74:2166–2173.

50. Notterman DA, Greenwald BM, Moran F, et al: Dopamine clearance in critically ill infants and children: effect of age and organ system dysfunction. Clin Pharmacol Ther 1990;48:138–147.

51. el Allaf D, Cremers S, D'Orio V, et al: Combined haemodynamic effects of low doses of dopamine and dobutamine in patients with acute infarction and cardiac failure. Arch Int Physiol Biochim 1984;92:S49–S55.

52. Leier CV, Heban PT, Huss P, et al: Comparative systemic and regional hemodynamic effects of dopamine and dobutamine in patients with cardiomyopathic heart failure. Circulation 1978;58:466–475.

53. Good J, Frost G, Oakley CM, et al: The renal effects of dopamine and dobutamine in stable chronic heart failure. Postgrad Med J 1992;68:S7–S11.

54. Varriale P, Mossavi A: The benefit of low-dose dopamine during vigorous diuresis for congestive heart failure associated with renal insufficiency: does it protect renal function? Clin Cardiol 1997;20:627–630.

55. Cotter G, Weissgarten J, Metzkor E, et al: Increased toxicity of high-dose furosemide versus low-dose dopamine in the treatment of refractory congestive heart failure. Clin Pharmacol Ther 1997;62:187–193.

56. Grossman E, Shenkar A, Peleg E, et al: Renal effects of L-DOPA in heart failure. J Cardiovasc Pharmacol 1999;33:922–928.

57. Patel JJ, Mitha AS, Sareli P, et al: Intravenous fenoldopam infusion in severe heart failure. Cardiovasc Drugs Ther 1993;7:97–101.

58. Juste RN, Panikkar K, Soni N: The effects of low-dose dopamine infusions on haemodynamic and renal parameters in patients with septic shock requiring treatment with noradrenaline. Intensive Care Med 1998;24:564–568.

59. Marin C, Eon B, Saux P, et al: Renal effects of norepinephrine used to treat septic shock patients. Crit Care Med 1990;18: 282–285.

60. Redl-Wenzl EM, Armbruster C, Edelmann G, et al: The effects of norepinephrine on hemodynamics and renal function in severe septic shock states. Intensive Care Med 1993;19:151–154.

61. Martin C, Papazian L, Perrin G, et al: Norepinephrine or dopamine for the treatment of hyperdynamic septic shock? Chest 1993;103:1826–1831.

62. Lassnigg A, Donner E, Grubhofer G, et al: Lack of renoprotective effects of dopamine and furosemide during cardiac surgery. J Am Soc Nephrol 2000;11:97–104.

63. Myles PS, Buckland MR, Schenk NJ, et al: Effect of "renal-dose" dopamine on renal function following cardiac surgery. Anaesth Intensive Care 1993;21:56–61.

64. Tang AT, El-Gamel A, Keevil B, et al: The effect of "renal-dose" dopamine on renal tubular function following cardiac surgery: assessed by measuring retinol binding protein (RBP). Eur J Cardiothorac Surg 1999;15:717–721.

65. Sumeray M, Robertson C, Lapsley M, et al: Low dose dopamine infusion reduces renal tubular injury following cardiopulmonary bypass surgery. J Nephrol 2001;14:397–402.

66. Yavuz S, Ayabakan N, Dilek K, et al: Renal dose dopamine in open heart surgery. Does it protect renal tubular function? J Cardiovasc Surg (Torino) 2002;43:25–30.

67. Baldwin L, Henderson A, Hickman P: Effect of postoperative low-dose dopamine on renal function after elective major vascular surgery. Ann Intern Med 1994;120:744–747.

68. Paul MD, Mazer CD, Byrick RJ, et al: Influence of mannitol and dopamine on renal function during elective infrarenal aortic clamping in man. Am J Nephrol 1986;6:427–434.

69. de Lasson L, Hansen HE, Juhl B, et al: A randomised, clinical study of the effect of low-dose dopamine on central and renal haemodynamics in infrarenal aortic surgery. Eur J Vasc Endovasc Surg 1995;10:82–90.

70. Halpenny M, Lakshmi S, O'Donnell A, et al: Fenoldopam: renal and splanchnic effects in patients undergoing coronary artery bypass grafting. Anaesthesia 2001;56:953–960.

71. Gilbert TB, Hasnain JU, Flinn WR, et al: Fenoldopam infusion associated with preserving renal function after aortic cross-clamping for aneurysm repair. J Cardiovasc Pharmacol Ther 2001;6:31–36.

72. Grundmann R, Kindler J, Meider G, et al: Dopamine treatment of human cadaver kidney graft recipients: a prospectively randomized trial. Klin Wochenschr 1982;60:193–197.

73. Carmellini M, Romagnoli J, Giulianotti PC, et al: Dopamine lowers the incidence of delayed graft function in transplanted kidney patients treated with cyclosporine A. Transplant Proc 1994;26:2626–2629.

74. Kadieva VS, Friedman L, Margolius LP, et al: The effect of dopamine on graft function in patients undergoing renal transplantation. Anesth Analg 1993;76:362–365.

75. DeLosAngeles A, Bacquero A, Bannet A, et al: Dopamine and furosemide infusion for the prevention of post-transplant oliguric renal failure. Kidney Int 1985;27:239.

76. Sandberg J, Tyden G, Groth CG, et al: Low-dose dopamine infusion following cadaveric renal transplantation: no effect on the incidence of ATN. Transplant Proc 1992;24:357.

77. Spicer ST, Gruenewald S, O'Connell PJ, et al: Low-dose dopamine after kidney transplantation: assessment by Doppler ultrasound. Clin Transplant 1999;13:479–483.

78. Hansen JM, Olsen NV, Leyssac PP: Renal effects of amino acids and dopamine in renal transplant recipients treated with or without cyclosporin A. Clin Sci (Lond) 1996;91:489–496.

79. Swygert TH, Roberts LC, Valek TR, et al: Effect of intraoperative low-dose dopamine on renal function in liver transplant recipients. Anesthesiology 1991;75:571–576.

80. Wahbah AM, el-Hefny MO, Wafa EM, et al: Perioperative renal protection in patients with obstructive jaundice using drug combinations. Hepatogastroenterology 2000;47: 1691–1694.

81. Parks RW, Diamond T, McCrory DC, et al: Prospective study of postoperative renal function in obstructive jaundice and the effect of perioperative dopamine. Br J Surg 1994;81:437–439.

82. Gare M, Haviv YS, Ben-Yehuda A, et al: The renal effect of low-dose dopamine in high-risk patients undergoing coronary angiography. J Am Coll Cardiol 1999;34:1682–1688.

83. Hans SS, Hans BA, Dhillon R, et al: Effect of dopamine on renal function after arteriography in patients with pre-existing renal insufficiency. Am Surg 1998;64:432–436.

84. Kapoor A, Sinha N, Sharma RK, et al: Use of dopamine in prevention of contrast induced acute renal failure: a randomised study. Int J Cardiol 1996;53:233–236.

85. Stevens MA, McCullough PA, Tobin KJ, et al: A prospective randomized trial of prevention measures in patients at high risk for contrast nephropathy: results of the P.R.I.N.C.E. Study. Prevention of Radiocontrast Induced Nephropathy Clinical Evaluation. J Am Coll Cardiol 1999;33:403–411.

86. Weisberg LS, Kurnik PB, Kurnik BR: Risk of radiocontrast nephropathy in patients with and without diabetes mellitus. Kidney Int 1994;45:259–265.

87. Abizaid AS, Clark CE, Mintz GS, et al: Effects of dopamine and aminophylline on contrast-induced acute renal failure after coronary angioplasty in patients with preexisting renal insufficiency. Am J Cardiol 1999;83:260–263.

88. Chu VL, Cheng JW: Fenoldopam in the prevention of contrast media-induced acute renal failure. Ann Pharmacother 2001;35:1278–1282.

89. Madyoon H, Croushore L, Weaver D, et al: Use of fenoldopam to prevent radiocontrast nephropathy in high-risk patients. Catheter Cardiovasc Intervention 2001;53:341–345.

90. Kini AS, Mitre CA, Kim M, et al: A protocol for prevention of radiographic contrast nephropathy during percutaneous coronary intervention: effect of selective dopamine receptor agonist fenoldopam. Catheter Cardiovasc Intervention 2002;55:169–173.

91. Fajardo CA, Whyte RK, Steele BT: Effect of dopamine on failure of indomethacin to close the patent ductus arteriosus. J Pediatr 1992;121:771–775.

92. Baenziger O, Waldvogel K, Ghelfi D, et al: Can dopamine prevent the renal side effects of indomethacin? A prospective randomized clinical study. Klin Pediatr 1999;211:438–441.

93. Cormier JN, Hurst R, Vasselli J, et al: A prospective randomized evaluation of the prophylactic use of low-dose dopamine in cancer patients receiving interleukin-2. J Immunother 1997;20:292–300.

94. Camp MJ, Wingard JR, Gilmore CE, et al: Efficacy of low-dose dopamine in preventing amphotericin B nephrotoxicity in bone marrow transplant patients and leukemia patients. Antimicrob Agents Chemother 1998;42:3103–3106.

95. Costa S, Nucci M. Can we decrease amphotericin nephrotoxicity? Curr Opin Crit Care 2001;7:379–383.

96. Somlo G, Doroshow JH, Lev-Ran A, et al: Effect of low-dose prophylactic dopamine on high-dose cisplatin-induced electrolyte wasting, ototoxicity, and epidermal growth factor excretion: a randomized, placebo-controlled, double-blind trial. J Clin Oncol 1995;13:1231–1237.

97. Kellum JA, J MD: Use of dopamine in acute renal failure: a meta-analysis. Crit Care Med 2001;29:1526–1531.

98. Bellomo R, Chapman M, Finfer S, et al: Low-dose dopamine in patients with early renal dysfunction: a placebo-controlled randomised trial. Australian and New Zealand Intensive Care Society (ANZICS) Clinical Trials Group. Lancet 2000;356:2139–2143.

99. Chertow GM, Sayegh MH, Allgren RL, et al: Is the administration of dopamine associated with adverse or favorable outcomes in acute renal failure? Auriculin Anaritide Acute Renal Failure Study Group. Am J Med 1996;101:49–53.

100. Marik PE, Iglesias J: Low-dose dopamine does not prevent acute renal failure in patients with septic shock and oliguria. NORASEPT II Study Investigators. Am J Med 1999;107:387–390.

101. Cochat P, Floret D, Bouffet E, et al: Renal effects of continuous infusion of recombinant interleukin-2 in children. Pediatr Nephrol 1991;5:33–37.

102. Palmieri G, Morabito A, Lauria R, et al: Low-dose dopamine induces early recovery of recombinant interleukin-2: impaired renal function. Eur J Cancer 1993;8:1119–1122.

103. Memoli B, De Nicola L, Libetta C, et al: Interleukin-2-induced renal dysfunction in cancer patients is reversed by low-dose dopamine infusion. Am J Kidney Dis 1995;26:27–33.

104. Conte G, Dal Canton A, Sabbatini M, et al: Acute cyclosporine renal dysfunction reversed by dopamine infusion in healthy subjects. Kidney Int 1989;36:1086–1092.

105. Johnson RL Jr: Low-dose dopamine and oxygen transport by the lung. Circulation 1998;98:97–99.

106. van de Borne P, Oren R, Somers VK: Dopamine depresses minute ventilation in patients with heart failure. Circulation 1998;98:126–131.

107. Giraud GD, MacCannell KL: Decreased nutrient blood flow during dopamine- and epinephrine-induced intestinal vasodilation. J Pharmacol Exp Ther 1984;230:214–220.

108. Segal JM, Phang PT, Walley KR: Low-dose dopamine hastens onset of gut ischemia in a porcine model of hemorrhagic shock. J Appl Physiol 1992;73:1159–1164.

109. Marik PE, Mohedin M: The contrasting effects of dopamine and norepinephrine on systemic and splanchnic oxygen utilization in hyperdynamic sepsis. JAMA 1994;272:1354–1357.

110. Clodi M, Kotzmann H, Riedl M, et al: The long-acting dopamine agonist bromocriptine mesylate as additive immunosuppressive drug after kidney transplantation. Nephrol Dial Transplant 1997;12:748–752.

111. Van den Berghe G, de Zegher F: Anterior pituitary function during critical illness and dopamine treatment. Crit Care Med 1996;24:1580–1590.

112. Girbes AR, Patten MT, McCloskey BV, et al: The renal and neurohormonal effects of the addition of low-dose dopamine in septic critically ill patients. Intens Care Med 2000;26:685–689.

113. Davis RF, Lappus DF, Kirklin JK, et al: Acute oliguria after cardiopulmonary bypass: renal functional improvement with low dose dopamine infusion. Crit Care Med 1982;10:852.

114. Lumlertgul D, Keoplung M, Sitprija V, Moolaor P, Shwangool P: Frusemide and dopamine in malarial acute renal failure. Nephron 1989;52:40–44.

Diuretics in Acute Renal Failure

Karen V. Smirnakis and Alan S.L. Yu

Background

Acute renal failure (ARF) is exceedingly common, occurring in 1–5% of all hospitalized patients,[1] but despite advances in supportive care the mortality remains quite high. Diuretics are one of the most commonly used agents in the management of ARF. They have been used to prevent the development of ARF, to reverse early or incipient ARF, to convert oliguric to nonoliguric ARF, and to accelerate recovery of established ARF. However, evidence to support the benefit of diuretic therapy for each of these indications is limited at best. Only mannitol and the loop diuretics have been carefully studied in this setting. We discuss the potential mechanisms of benefit for these agents in ARF and review the clinical data regarding their use in human ARF. Complications of diuretic therapy are considered, and recommendations given for usage and dosing of diuretics.

Multiple pathophysiologic factors contribute to renal injury in ARF, including vasoconstriction, reduced glomerular capillary permeability, tubular obstruction by casts and swollen epithelial cells, and backleak of filtrate through an altered epithelium.[2,3] There is a potential beneficial role for diuretics in several of these steps. Firstly, mannitol increases renal blood flow in both the renal cortex and medulla by reducing renal vascular resistance.[4] Secondly, by increasing urine flow, mannitol could lead to relief of tubular obstruction by casts and cellular debris and to a reduction in the concentration of tubular toxins such as myoglobin or hemoglobin.[5] Finally, mannitol may reduce epithelial cell swelling[6] as well as scavenge harmful free radicals,[7] thereby ameliorating hypoxic reperfusion injury. The loop diuretics also have vasodilatory properties and may act to increase renal blood flow. However, it has been postulated that the increased renal blood flow induced by loop diuretics may be maldistributed and potentially harmful.[8,9] Like mannitol, the loop diuretics increase urine flow and could relieve tubular obstruction and reduce the concentration of tubular toxins.[5] Furthermore, by inhibiting active solute transport, loop diuretics reduce the oxygen and ATP requirements of the tubular epithelium, thereby possibly improving tolerance of hypoxia.[10]

Extensive data from animal studies suggest that diuretics given prophylactically prior to renal injury, or very early in so-called "incipient" ARF, may ameliorate the subsequent course of ARF, while their administration once ARF is established has generally been ineffective (see Conger[11] for review). However, the data supporting a beneficial role for diuretics in human ARF are inconsistent. Evaluation of the available human studies is further complicated by the heterogeneity of ARF. Thus, these studies vary widely in the underlying etiology of renal injury, the severity of disease, and the phase of ARF at which the diuretics were administered. With the exception of a few small randomized controlled trials, most of the data are from retrospective or case–control studies that are confounded by multiple factors. We focus on the recent prospective clinical trials (Table 4.1) and refer the reader to several excellent reviews[12–16] for a summary of the earlier work.

Role of mannitol in the prevention and treatment of acute renal failure

The prophylactic use of mannitol began in the 1960s when it was introduced for use in patients undergoing cardiovascular surgery to maintain intraoperative urine flow.[17] Since that time, prophylactic use of mannitol has been recommended for patients at high risk of ARF in various clinical settings, including cardiac or vascular surgery, radiocontrast administration, obstructive jaundice, rhabdomyolysis, and renal transplantation. However, seven prospective clinical trials examining the use of mannitol for prophylaxis failed to show improvement in renal function or mortality. The first four negative trials have been summarized recently by Conger.[13] Three of the trials examined the use of mannitol to prevent ARF in surgical patients and one examined its use in preventing contrast-induced ARF. In the time since the Conger review, three additional studies have been performed. Nicholson et al[18] performed a randomized controlled study of the effects of preoperative mannitol or saline on the development of postoperative ARF in 28 consecutive patients undergoing elective aortic aneurysm repair. Despite an increase in urine output in the first 24 h after surgery in the group who received mannitol, there was no difference in renal function between the two groups. However, based on an assessment of urinary markers that purportedly indicate early glomerular and tubular injury, the authors suggested that mannitol provides protection against

Table 4.1   Summary of randomized controlled clinical trials of diuretics in acute renal failure (ARF)

Intervention	Control	Mode of therapy	Etiology of ARF	Total no. of patients	Effect of intervention on renal function	Reference
Mannitol	Saline	Prophylaxis	Postoperative	28	None	18
Mannitol and saline	Saline	Prophylaxis	Radiocontrast	78	Worse	8
Mannitol and saline	Saline	Prophylaxis	Radiocontrast	50	None	20
Mannitol, furosemide, dopamine and saline	Saline	Prophylaxis	Radiocontrast	98	None	19
Mannitol and saline	Saline	Prophylaxis	Cadaveric renal transplantation	131	Better	23
Furosemide and saline	Saline	Prophylaxis	Postoperative	126	Worse	29
Furosemide and saline	Saline	Prophylaxis	Radiocontrast	78	Worse	8
Furosemide	Saline	Prophylaxis	Radiocontrast	18	Worse	31
Furosemide bolus and infusion	Furosemide bolus	Established ARF	Trauma or surgery	58	None	33
Furosemide/torsemide, mannitol and dopamine	Mannitol and dopamine	Established ARF	Mixed	92	None	32
Mannitol, furosemide, and dopamine infusion	Loop diuretic intermittent bolus	Established ARF	Cardiac surgery	100	?*	33

*Reduction in requirement for dialysis, but creatinine not reported.

subclinical renal injury. In Solomon et al's study,[8] which randomized patients with mild chronic renal failure undergoing intravenous radiocontrast administration to receive mannitol, furosemide, or saline alone, the mannitol-treated group had no reduction in the incidence of ARF, and actually had an increased serum creatinine at 24 h. Similar results were found in a prospective randomized controlled trial of patients undergoing radiocontrast administration by Stevens et al.[19] Patients were randomized to a split experimental arm, which consisted of mannitol, furosemide, dopamine, and saline for patients with a pulmonary capillary wedge pressure (PCWP) greater than 20 mmHg, or furosemide, dopamine, and saline (without mannitol) for patients with a lower PCWP. Patients in the control arm received saline alone. The authors found no change in the serum creatinine between the experimental and control arms. The lack of benefit found in these two studies confirms that seen in diabetic patients in an earlier study on the effects of mannitol for prevention of radiocontrast-induced ARF.[20]

Forced alkaline diuresis with intravenous fluids and mannitol is widely used in the treatment of patients with rhabdomyolysis.[21] This regimen is believed to prevent intratubular precipitation and obstruction by myoglobin. In this setting, mannitol is theoretically superior to loop diuretics, which tend to acidify the urine, and is safe so long as the patient is not anuric. However, only one clinical trial has examined the use of mannitol independently from fluid resuscitation. In this small retrospective study by Homsi et al,[22] no difference in renal function was found between patients who received prophylactic mannitol, sodium bicarbonate, and saline compared with patients who received saline alone.

Mannitol may have a beneficial role in the prevention of ARF following renal transplantation. Van Valenberg et al[23] demonstrated a beneficial effect in cadaveric renal transplant recipients who received mannitol at the time of transplant. This was supported by the finding that inclusion of mannitol in the donor organ perfusate resulted in a faster decline in the recipient's serum creatinine post transplant.[24] The practice of using mannitol in renal transplantation varies by center, and its potential benefit remains to be confirmed by larger multicenter trials.

There have been no controlled studies of the use of mannitol in early or established ARF. While several uncontrolled studies performed prior to 1970 demonstrate that mannitol can restore urine flow when administered early in the course of oliguric ARF (see later), there is no evidence that it improves outcome in terms of renal function.[25–28]

Role of loop diuretics in the prevention and treatment of acute renal failure

Furosemide is widely used to prevent the development of ARF despite lack of evidence of its efficacy in humans. A survey of the members of the European Workgroup of Cardiothoracic Intensivists reportedly showed 11 of 38 centers using continuous furosemide for renoprotection, and 34 of 38 centers using furosemide bolus injections to maintain urine output greater than 0.5 mL/kg/h.[29] To address the effectiveness of furosemide in this setting, Lassnigg and colleagues[29] recently performed a double-blind randomized controlled trial examining the effectiveness of furosemide and dopamine in preventing ARF following cardiac surgery: 126 patients with normal preoperative renal function were assigned to receive dopamine, furosemide, or normal saline starting at the beginning of surgery and continuing for 48 h after surgery or until discharge from the intensive care unit, whichever came first. The group receiving furosemide had an increase in plasma creatinine that was twice as high as the other two groups. As the increased sodium and water excretion in the furosemide group was not fully replaced, these results could potentially be due to relative hypovolemia, though objective indices such as PCWP were not significantly different between the two groups. Nevertheless the absence of benefit is consistent with the findings of an earlier retrospective controlled study of ARF prophylaxis following open-heart surgery that showed no benefit of furosemide administration.[30]

Three other prospective controlled studies have evaluated the role of furosemide in preventing ARF induced by radiocontrast material and found no benefit.[8,19,31] In two of the studies, administration of furosemide prior to radiocontrast resulted in worsening of the decline in renal function that was associated with net loss of body weight,[8,31] again suggesting that it had caused hypovolemia.

The remainder of the clinical trials examine the role of furosemide in established ARF. Several retrospective studies, reviewed by Conger,[13] found no effect of furosemide on renal function or mortality in patients with ARF of various etiologies. There have been three randomized controlled trials of loop diuretics in established ARF. A prospective controlled study of torsemide or furosemide showed no difference in renal recovery, need for dialysis, or mortality in loop-diuretic treated patients compared with controls that received no loop diuretics.[32] However, all patients enrolled in this study also received dopamine and mannitol. Brown et al[33] randomized 58 patients with established ARF to receive either a one-time bolus of furosemide, or a bolus followed by a continuous infusion. While the continuous infusion was more effective at reversing oliguria, there was no difference in the need for dialysis, duration of renal failure, or mortality between the two groups. Sirivella et al[34] published a randomized trial of intermittent bolus diuretics given "as recommended by the nephrologist" versus a continuous infusion of a solution containing mannitol, furosemide, and dopamine in cardiac surgery patients with established postoperative oliguric or anuric ARF. Significantly more patients in the latter group experienced "diuresis." Notably, 90% of the patients receiving intermittent bolus diuretics required dialysis compared with only 6.7% of the patients receiving the continuous infusion of furosemide, dopamine, and saline. However, this study was flawed because there was no true control group. Thus, it is unclear what treatment the "intermittent bolus" group received. Furthermore, the serum creatinine at initiation of hemodialysis was not reported, so it is unclear if the results reflect differences in renal function or, as seems more likely, in volume management (see later). In summary, we find insufficient evidence to support the use of loop diuretics for prevention or treatment of ARF, and some evidence to suggest that they may be harmful if given intercurrently with an acute renal insult.

Diuretics in the management of complications of acute renal failure

While there is no evidence that diuretics are effective at preventing or altering the course of ARF, they are very useful in the management of oliguria and volume overload in this setting. Several studies have shown that diuretics administered early in the course of oliguric ARF, usually within 24–48 h of onset,[27,28,35] can induce a sustained diuresis in some patients, in some cases even after a single bolus dose. While individuals successfully converted from oliguric to nonoliguric ARF in this manner have a better prognosis than those who are diuretic-resistant,[28] this likely reflects the milder severity of their underlying renal injury and not any effect of the diuretic to alter the natural history of the disease. Thus, diuretic-responsive patients not only had a shorter duration of oliguria but also higher urine output and better urinary concentrating ability than diuretic-resistant patients.[26,28,36] Successful reversal of oliguria, even in the initial absence of overt hypervolemia, might be expected to reduce the subsequent need for dialysis or ultrafiltration. Indeed this has been shown in some studies[34] though not in others.[33] Our approach is to administer a single bolus of a diuretic within 24 h of the onset of oliguria, once established ARF has been confirmed, in an attempt to convert to nonoliguric ARF. We favor loop diuretics over mannitol because they appear to be safer and may also be more effective.[35] If there is no diuretic response to a maximally effective dose (see later), further doses should not be given as there is a significant risk of ototoxicity.[33,35] If there is a diuretic response but it is transient and not sustained, further doses of diuretic, given either as repeated boluses or as a continuous infusion, should be given only if required in a hypervolemic patient to maintain appropriate fluid balance.

Pharmacology and dosage recommendations

Mannitol may be given in boluses of 12.5–25 g, or as a continuous infusion of up to 200 g per 24 h. It is rapidly distributed in the extracellular space, results in the onset of diuresis within 15–30 min, and has a half-life of 70–100 min in the setting of normal renal function. In the setting of renal dysfunction, mannitol may accumulate and cause plasma volume expansion as well as itself causing ARF.[37,38] It should therefore be administered with caution, if at all, to anuric patients. As with all diuretics, caution should be used to avoid inducing hypovolemia from overdiuresis and thereby exacerbating the renal injury.

The effectiveness of loop diuretics in patients with ARF is reduced due to decreased urinary excretion. This may be overcome by using higher doses than usual. Treatment should be initiated with an intravenous bolus dose. Reasonable starting doses are 40 mg furosemide, 1 mg bumetanide, or 25 mg torsemide. If there is no response within 30–60 min, the dose should be increased by repeatedly doubling the dosage until either diuresis is achieved or the maximum safe dose is reached. For furosemide, we consider a maximum single dose of 200–250 mg i.v. with a maximum total daily dose of 1 g to be safe. Higher doses may incur an unacceptable risk of ototoxicity.[33]

If the loop diuretic alone is ineffective, a thiazide diuretic may also be added (e.g. chlorothiazide 250 or 500 mg i.v., given 30 min before a 200 mg i.v. bolus of furosemide). This combination has been studied in chronic renal failure,[39] but can also be effective in ARF. Thiazide diuretics alone are ineffective when the glomerular filtration rate falls below 30 mL/min, but may retain benefit when added to a regimen containing a loop diuretic. If no increase in urine output occurs in response to 200 mg of furosemide given in combination with a thiazide diuretic, further doses should not be administered until recovery of renal function is evident.

In patients with severe hypoalbuminemia, the volume of distribution of furosemide (normally tightly protein-bound in plasma) is markedly increased and urinary concentrations lower, thus limiting its effectiveness as a diuretic. To overcome this, administration of intravenous furosemide premixed with albumin has been proposed,[40] though recent clinical studies have not shown a convincing advantage to this approach.[41]

Increasing the dose of furosemide increases the risks of toxicity. Some advocate maintaining a continuous infusion of intravenous loop diuretics in order to maintain a safe and constant plasma level. An infusion of furosemide may be given at 5–40 mg/h following a bolus dose.[42] The half-life of furosemide is intermediate, with bumetanide having a shorter half-life and torsemide having a longer half-life. Therefore, the benefits of continuous infusion may be greater for bumetanide and furosemide than for torsemide.

References

1. Hou SH, Bushinsky DA, Wish JB, et al: Hospital-acquired renal insufficiency: a prospective study. Am J Med 1983;74:243.
2. Thadhani R, Pascual M, Bonventre JV: Acute renal failure. N Engl J Med 1996;334:1448.
3. Kellum JA: Use of diuretics in the acute care setting. Kidney Int 1998;Suppl 66:S67–S70.
4. Velasquez MT, Notargiacomo AV, Cohn JN: Comparative effects of saline and mannitol on renal cortical blood flow and volume in the dog. Am J Physiol 1973;224:322–327.
5. Star RA: Treatment of acute renal failure. Kidney Int 1998;54:1817.
6. Mason J, Joeris B, Welsch J, et al: Vascular congestion in ischemic renal failure: the role of cell swelling. Miner Electrolyte Metab 1989;15:114–124.
7. Magovern GJ, Bolling SF, Casale AS, et al: The mechanisms of mannitol in reducing ischemic injury: hyperosmolarity or hydroxyl scavenger? Circulation 1984;70(Suppl 1):91–95.
8. Solomon R, Werner C, Mann D, et al: Effects of saline, mannitol, and furosemide to prevent acute decreases in renal function induced by radiocontrast agents. N Engl J Med 1994;331:1416–1420.
9. Brezis M, Rosen S: Hypoxia of the renal medulla: its implications for disease. N Engl J Med 1995;332:647–655.
10. Brezis M, Rosen S, Silva P, et al: Transport activity modified thick ascending limb damage in the isolated perfused kidney. Kidney Int 1984;25:65–72.
11. Conger JD: Drug therapy in acute renal failure. In Lazarus JM, Brenner BM (eds): Acute Renal Failure. New York: Churchill Livingstone, 1993, pp 527–552.
12. Fink M: Are diuretics useful in the treatment or prevention of acute renal failure? South Med J 1982;75:329–334.
13. Conger JD: Interventions in clinical acute renal failure: what are the data? Am J Kidney Dis 1995;26:565–576.
14. Shilliday I, Allison MEM: Diuretics in acute renal failure. Renal Failure 16:3–17, 1994.
15. Better OS, Rubinstein I, Winaver JM, et al: Mannitol therapy revisited (1940–1997). Kidney Int 1997;51:886–894.
16. Lameire AL, Vanholder R: Pathophysiologic features and prevention of human and experimental acute tubular necrosis. J Am Soc Nephrol 2001;12:S20–S32.
17. Barry KC, Cohen A, Knochel JP, et al: Mannitol infusion II. The prevention of acute functional renal failure during resection of an aneursysm of the abdominal aorta. N Engl J Med 1961;264:967–971.
18. Nicholson ML, Baker DM, Hopkinson BR, et al: Randomized controlled trial of the effect of mannitol on renal reperfusion injury during aortic aneurysm surgery. Br J Surg 1996;83:1230–1233.
19. Stevens NA, McCullough PA, Tobin KJ, et al: A prospective randomized trial of prevention measures in patients at high risk for contrast nephropathy: Results of the PRINCE study. J Am Coll Cardiol 1999;33:403–411.
20. Weisberg LS, Kurnik PB, Kurnik BRC: Risk of radiocontrast nephropathy in patients with and without diabetes mellitus. Kidney Int 1994;45:259–265.
21. Better OS, Stein JH: Early management of shock and prophylaxis of acute renal failure in traumatic rhabdomyolysis. N Engl J Med 1990;322:825–829.
22. Homsi E, Barreiro MF, Orlando JM, et al: Prophylaxis of acute renal failure in patients with rhabdomyolysis. Renal Failure 1997;19:283–288.
23. Van Valenberg PLJ, Hoitsma AJ, Tiggeler RGWL: Mannitol as an indispensable constituent of an intraoperative hydration protocol for the prevention of acute renal failure after renal cadaveric transplantation. Transplantation 1987;44:784–788.
24. Grino JM, Miravitlles R, Castelao AM: Flush solution with mannitol in the prevention of post-transplant renal failure. Transplant Proc 1987;19:4140–4142.
25. Barry K, Malloy J: Oliguric renal failure: evaluation and therapy by the intravenous infusion of mannitol. JAMA 1962;179:510–514.
26. Eliahou H: Mannitol therpay in oliguria of acute onset. Br Med J 1964;1:807–811.
27. Luke R, Linton A, Briggs J, et al: Mannitol therapy in acute renal failure. Lancet 1965;i:980–984.
28. Luke R, Briggs J, Allison M, et al: Factors determining response to mannitol in acute renal failure. Am J Med Sci 1970;259:168–173.
29. Lassnigg A, Donner E, Grubhofer G, et al: Lack of renoprotective effects of dopamine and furosemide during cardiac surgery. J Am Soc Nephrol 2000;11:97–104.
30. Nuutinen LS, Kairaluioma M, Tuononen S, et al: The effect of furosemide on renal function in open heart surgery. J Cardiovasc Surg 1978;19:471–477.
31. Weinstein JM, Heyman S, Brezis M: Potential deleterious effect of furosemide in radiocontrast nephropathy. Nephron 1992;62:413–415.
32. Shilliday IR, Quinn KJ, Allison ME: Loop diuretics in the management of acute renal failure: a prospective, double-blind, placebo-controlled, randomized study. Nephrol Dial Transplant 1997;12:2592–2596.
33. Brown CB, Ogg CS, Cameron JS: High dose furosemide in acute renal failure: a controlled trial. Clin Nephrol 1981;15:90–96.
34. Sirivella S, Gielchinsky I, Parsonnet V: Mannitol, furosemide, and dopamine infusion in postoperative renal failure complicating cardiac surgery. Ann Thorac Surg 2000;69:501–506.
35. Kjellstrand C: Ethacrynic acid in acute tubular necrosis. Indications and effect on the natural course. Nephron 1972;9:337–348.

36. Scheer RL: The effects of hypertonic mannitol on oliguric patients. Am J Med Sci 1965;250:35–43.

37. van Hengel P, Nikken JJ, de Jong GM, et al: Mannitol-induced acute renal failure. Neth J Med 50:21–24, 1997.

38. Visweswaran P, Massin EK, Dubose TD: Mannitol-induced acute renal failure. J Am Soc Nephrol 1997;8:1028–1033.

39. Fliser D: Loop diuretics and thiazides: the case for their combination in chronic renal failure. Nephrol Dial Transplant 1996;11:408–423.

40. Inoue M, Okajima K, Itoh K, et al: Mechanism of furosemide resistance in analbuminemic rats and hypoalbuminemic patients. Kidney Int 1987;32:198–203.

41. Chalasani N, Gorski JC, Horlander JC Sr, et al: Effects of albumin/furosemide mixtures on responses to furosemide in hypoalbuminemic patients. J Am Soc Nephrol 2001;12:1010–1016.

42. Martin SJ, Danzinger LH: Continuous infusion of loop diuretics in the critically ill: a review of the literature. Crit Care Med 1994;22:1323–1329.

Contrast Nephropathy and Atheroembolism

Bryan M. Curtis, Brendan J. Barrett, and Patrick S. Parfrey

Diagnostic and therapeutic intravascular interventions are commonly performed invasive procedures. Although less invasive techniques, such as magnetic resonance or ultrasound, have begun to replace some diagnostic angiography, this has been offset by a growth in the use of intravascular therapies such as angioplasty and stenting. The nephrotoxic effects of iodinated radiocontrast materials and atheroembolism may lead to acute deterioration in renal function. Atheroembolism can occur without a precipitating event, but its association with catheter-related trauma to plaque links these distinct renal insults in the context of angiographic procedures. In this chapter these topics are considered separately as they differ in terms of pathogenesis, clinical presentation, therapy, and prevention.

Contrast nephropathy

Epidemiology

Iodinated radiocontrast leads to at least minor, transient changes in renal function in almost all cases.[1] The degree and persistence of renal injury is determined by preexisting renal status, concomitant acute renal insults, and the dose and type of contrast used.[2] Factors associated with an increased risk of contrast nephropathy are shown in Table 5.1. The risk is inversely related to preexisting renal function. While diabetics with advanced nephropathy are among the highest risk cases, diabetics with normal serum creatinine seem to be at low risk.[3] Incidence of renal failure ranges from 1.2% to 100% as the number of risk factors increases from zero to four.[4] Differences in definition and patients studied are largely responsible for conflicting estimates of the importance of contrast nephrotoxicity.[3,5] More severe contrast nephropathy typi-

cally manifests as nonoliguric, typically reversible, acute renal failure of varying severity.[4] Concomitant processes, including atheroembolism, may contribute to long-term renal injury. Contrast nephropathy is also associated with increased mortality.[6] At present management of acute renal failure due to contrast nephropathy is supportive. Existing studies of early dialysis fail to show benefit in reducing renal injury.[7,8] Similarly patients already on dialysis do not routinely need dialysis immediately after contrast.[9]

Pathogenetic basis for prevention

Contrast nephropathy likely results from both ischemic injury and direct tubular cell toxicity.[2] A reduction in medullary perfusion, possibly mediated by increased endothelin and adenosine together with reduced nitric oxide and prostacyclin, has been considered important.[2,10] The nature of the contrast, associated ions, concentration, concomitant hypoxia, and oxygen free radical generation are each related to the degree of cellular damage.[2,11] While controversy remains about the exact pathogenesis in humans and the relevance of animal models,[12] pathogenetic considerations underlie recent efforts to reduce contrast nephrotoxicity.

Minimization of contrast nephropathy

Both general and specific means should be employed as outlined in Fig. 5.1. Advances in imaging modalities may permit avoidance of contrast in high-risk cases.[13] Clinical history and examination will identify most risk factors for contrast nephropathy. Renal impairment may be asymptomatic until advanced, but it is impractical to measure renal function before contrast in all cases. If no other risk factors for nephrotoxicity are apparent, it is probably not

Table 5.1 Risk factors for contrast nephropathy

Preexisting renal impairment
Diabetes (with renal impairment)
Decreased effective arterial blood volume
Volume depletion
Heart failure
Nephrosis
Cirrhosis
Concurrent nephrotoxins (e.g. NSAIDs)
High doses of contrast

NSAIDs, nonsteroidal antiinflammatory drugs.

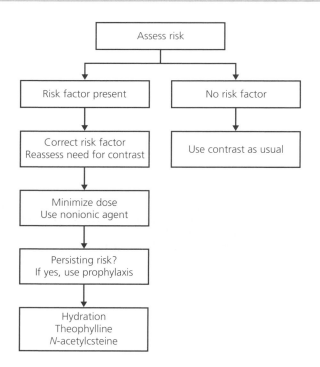

Figure 5.1 Approach to minimizing the risk of contrast nephropathy

with low-dose dopamine, atrial natriuretic peptide (ANP), captopril, calcium channel blockers, prostaglandin (PG) E_1, or endothelin antagonism; and an "antioxidant" approach using theophylline or acetylcysteine. The evidence supporting the use of these measures varies. Studies addressing the use of these therapies are summarized in Tables 5.2–5.4.

Recommended specific prophylactic regimen

Although deliberate hydration has never been tested in a randomized trial versus no therapy, it forms the basis of most prophylactic regimens. The mechanism of protective effect, if any, is not clear but may include correction or prevention of volume depletion, or prevention of protein precipitation in tubules. No single fluid administration protocol has been shown to be better than another. The most important factor may not be the details of the fluid protocol itself, but rather careful assessment and response to patient fluid balance and clinical status, avoiding volume depletion or overload before and after contrast. Many institutions use intravenous 0.45% saline at a rate of 1 mL/kg/h, beginning up to 12 h before contrast and continuing for up to 24 h. This is not practical for ambulatory cases. A small trial suggests that oral pre-hydration, with intravenous fluid as above for 6 h post contrast, may be adequate.[17] Whatever protocol is used, it should be adjusted based on patient tolerance and the degree of diuresis achieved.

In addition to deliberate hydration, theophylline as an antagonist of adenosine action can now be recommended based on consistent benefit in several small trials.[1,34–37] Toxicity has been minor. The trials have included a reasonable proportion of diabetics and patients with renal impairment. In fact the more recent study by Erley et al[36] was limited to patients with preexisting renal impairment. Optimal dosing is unclear. Oral dosing is simplest and 800 mg/day in two divided doses for at least 2 days prior to contrast is our recommendation for now. N-Acetylcysteine 600 mg orally twice a day beginning just prior to contrast is an alternative. This has become widely accepted in many centers because of low cost and toxicity. Efficacy has now been shown in two small trials.[38,39]

necessary to determine renal function.[14] When contrast must be administered in the presence of an uncorrectable or uncorrected risk factor, serum creatinine should be checked before and 48–72 h after contrast. In addition, specific prophylactic measures as discussed later are indicated for high-risk patients. Based on accumulated evidence to date, to minimize contrast nephrotoxicity, nonionic low-osmolality contrast is recommended for patients with renal impairment, especially that due to diabetic nephropathy[15,16].

Specific prophylactic measures

Many specific pathogenetically based prophylactic measures have been tested. These include a "diuretic" approach with deliberate hydration, furosemide, or mannitol, singly or in combination; a "vasodilator" approach

Table 5.2 Trials of specific prophylactic diuretic measures for contrast nephropathy

	Regimen	Evidence	Comments
Fluids	Usual 0.45% saline 1 mL/kg/h i.v. 6 h pre up to 12 h post	No RCT vs. no therapy	Recommended as standard basic therapy. Oral fluids may be adequate[17]
Furosemide	40–80 mg i.v. pre contrast	Several RCTs[18–20]	Trials fail to show benefit or suggest harm. Not recommended
Mannitol	About 25 g i.v. over 1 h pre contrast	Several RCTs[18–20]	Trials fail to show benefit or suggest harm especially in diabetics. Not recommended

RCT, randomized controlled trial.

Table 5.3 Trials of specific prophylactic vasodilator therapies for contrast nephropathy

	Regimen	Evidence	Comments
Dopamine	2–5 µg/kg/min i.v. from pre up to 12 h post	Several RCTs[20–26]	Inconsistent effect, potentially harmful in diabetics. Not recommended
Atrial natriuretic Peptide	50 µg i.v. bolus, 1 µg/min infusion up to 12 h post	Several RCTs[21,27]	Potential for harm in diabetics. Not recommended
Calcium channel blockers	Nifedipine and nitrendipine, single dose p.o. or up to 3 days post	Several RCTs[28–30]	Inadequately powered studies, no convincing benefit. Not recommended
Captopril	25 mg p.o. q8h for 3 days post	1 RCT in diabetics[31]	Small positive study. Needs replication. Not recommended yet
PGE₁	10–40 ng/kg/min i.v. for 6 h	1 RCT[32]	Promising at 20 ng/kg/min. Needs replication. Not recommended yet
Endothelin receptor blockade	SB290670 (nonselective ET receptor blocker)	1 RCT[33]	Deleterious effect. Not recommended

RCT, randomized controlled trial.

Table 5.4 Trials of specific prophylactic antioxidant therapies for contrast nephropathy

	Regimen	Evidence	Comments
Theophylline	4–5 mg/kg i.v. pre contrast ± 0.4 mg/kg/h, or about 800 mg/day in 2 divided doses from 2 days pre up to 3 days post	Several RCTs[1,34–37]	Consistent benefit across studies. Oral regimen is easy to use. Recommended
N-Acetylcysteine	600 mg p.o. q12h × 4 starting 1 day pre	1 RCT[38,39]	Promising and easy to use. Needs replication. Recommended
Allopurinol	4 mg/kg/day p.o. from 1 day pre	1 RCT[11]	Small trial. Benefit limited to hypomagnesemic cases. Not recommended

RCT, randomized controlled trial.

While intravenous infusions of low-dose dopamine and ANP have been associated with benefit in nondiabetics, we feel that these therapies are cumbersome and costly and do not recommend them as routine for prophylaxis. Promising data exist for PGE₁ and captopril, but further trials are warranted to better establish the efficacy of these approaches before they can be strongly recommended.

Atheroembolism

Atheroembolic renal disease is characterized by multifocal occlusions of small arteries by cholesterol emboli. Fragments of atherosclerotic plaques dislodged usually from atheromatous aorta or other major arteries result in a shower of emboli to affected downstream organ(s). A granulomatous inflammatory reaction ensues followed by intimal proliferation and intravascular fibrosis. The subsequent narrowing or occlusion of the vessel lumen can lead to ischemia and infarction.[40] The resultant disease ranges from entirely asymptomatic to a potentially lethal multiorgan clinical syndrome reflecting the underlying organ(s) involved. The kidney is frequently affected because of its vast blood supply and proximity to the aorta. Atheroembolic kidney disease can be difficult to diagnose.[41] Originally reported to occur spontaneously, the following are now known to be predisposing factors: (1) angiographic procedures; (2) anticoagulation; and (3) vascular surgery.[42] The shift in etiology is likely secondary to the increasing use of these therapies.

Epidemiology

Since atheroemboli arise from plaques, risk factors are similar to those for atherosclerosis itself. Each is common in older, hypertensive, male smokers but atheroembolism seems to be rare in blacks.[43] The incidence is difficult to ascertain from the literature because of the diverse clinical spectrum of disease and the lack of prospective studies. Nonetheless, an overall incidence of 0.15–3.4% has been reported after inciting events.[44] After coronary angiography the general incidence is less than 2%.[45] For patients at high risk, however, the incidence may be as much as 24–77%. Finally, atheroembolic kidney disease may account for at least 4% of all inpatient nephrology consultations.[44]

Clinical presentation

Atheroembolism may affect the kidney in a number of ways: (1) asymptomatic atheroembolism; (2) new onset or worsening mild to malignant hypertension; (3) gradual to rapid decline in kidney function; or (4) proteinuria alone.[40,46,47] These effects may be seen immediately after an inciting event, but may also be delayed for months. Kidney dysfunction may range from a mild decrease in glomerular filtration rate to kidney failure requiring dialysis. Atheroembolism in a kidney allograft is a rare complication. It may be of donor vessel origin, presenting as early delayed graft function, or of recipient origin, manifesting like atheroembolism in native kidneys.[48] Overall graft survival is worse if emboli originate from the donor vessel. The frequency of this entity will likely increase given the older population of both donors and recipients.

The diagnosis of atheroembolism is challenging as the spectrum of disease is so variable and nonspecific. Atheroembolism should be included in the differential diagnosis given a clinical outcome following a precipitating event in a patient with multiple risk factors. Contrast nephropathy and acute interstitial nephritis may especially confound the diagnosis or worsen disease course because of the clinical settings in which they occur. Differentiation from other systemic disorders may be difficult. Clinically atheroembolism may mimic vasculitis,[49,50] thrombotic thrombocytopenic purpura,[51] or subacute bacterial endocarditis,[40] and may manifest as a pulmonary–renal syndrome affecting the lungs as an endogenous lipoid pneumonia.[52]

Extrarenal manifestations may help clarify the diagnosis.[46] Cutaneous involvement is common, with acrocyanosis of toes (with preserved pulses) or livedo reticularis. Gastrointestinal involvement is often asymptomatic but nausea, bleeding, or abdominal pain can occur.[53] Abnormal liver function, pancreatitis, and cholecystitis may also occur. Retinal atheroemboli may be visible as Hollenhorst plaques in the retinal vessels. Finally, patients may present with central nervous system involvement.[54,55]

There are no specific laboratory tests to confirm the diagnosis.[41,46] Urinalysis is often abnormal but nonspecific, with mild to moderate proteinuria, microhematuria, and hyaline or granular casts. Urine eosinophils may also be present. Leukocytosis, eosinophilia, thrombocytosis, or anemia can all be seen. Erythrocyte sedimentation rate, C-reactive protein, and fibrin may be elevated. An association with low complement and anti-neutrophil cytoplasmic autoantibodies remains controversial.[56] Other organ involvement may be reflected in the blood work. For example, if the pancreas is affected, serum lipase or amylase may be elevated.

Pathology

Histologic confirmation is required for definitive diagnosis as imaging tests are not specific.[57] Kidney biopsy remains the gold standard, although skin or deep muscle biopsy may suffice in the proper clinical context. These biopsies need to be deep to obtain good-sized dermal or muscle vessels.

The characteristic histology reveals biconvex, needle-shaped clefts in vessels 50–200 μm in diameter (the cholesterol is dissolved during fixation). There is an acute inflammatory response, with hysticocytic multinucleated giant cells, glomerular collapse with basement wrinkling, and tubular atrophy. Some vessels may be completely obliterated with ensuing fibrosis. Focal segmental necrotizing glomerulonephritis, membranoproliferative changes,[58–60] and a cellular variant of focal segmental glomerulerosclerosis[61] have also been described. These pathologic findings may be patchy and thus may be missed.

Outcome

Spontaneous recovery of kidney function has been reported.[62–64] However, with a 1-year mortality rate between 64 and 87%,[42,65,66] the prognosis appears to be dismal. Of survivors, 32% remain on maintenance dialysis. The main causes of death have been recurrent bouts of cholesterol embolism, cardiac failure, and cachexia. Aggressive management targeting these issues had a 1-year survival of 79%.[67]

Management (Fig. 5.2)

Prevention is possible if inciting events, such as angiographies, are avoided in patients at high risk. Aside from identifying clinical risk factors, patients may be imaged by magnetic resonance or transesophageal echo to identify those with extensive atheromatous plaques.[68] It remains controversial whether a brachial versus a femoral approach for angiography reduces embolization.[69]

Management of atheroembolism is predominantly symptomatic and supportive. The focus is on prevention of further embolization and reducing the risk of death. Anticoagulants should be interrupted and angiographic or vascular surgical procedures should be restricted. Cardiac failure should be treated or prevented and cachexia should be minimized by nutritional support.[67] Dialysis therapy should be initiated when indicated. Peritoneal dialysis offers the theoretical advantage of avoiding the need for anticoagulation.[63]

The evidence for specific therapeutic interventions is limited to case reports. These provide limited insight into the effects of therapy as instances of spontaneous remission have been documented.[62–64] There are case reports of improved kidney function following steroid therapy in patients with serum indices reflecting inflammation.[70,71] Additionally, a retrospective study showed no increase in complications with steroid therapy.[67] In theory, statin therapy should help by plaque stabilization. Again, there are case reports of improved kidney function using this class of medications.[72,73] Although there is no clear evidence for their use to treat atheroembolic kidney disease, they may well be indicated in most cases because of concomitant dyslipidemia. The same considerations apply to the use of antiplatelet agents. Surgical interven-

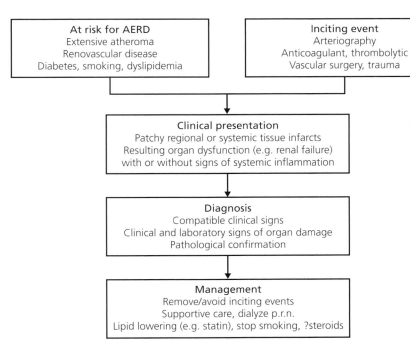

Figure 5.2 Summary of approach to atheroembolic renal disease (AERD).

tion has been tried, but is problematic as the source of the emboli is usually unclear and mortality has been high.[40] It should be limited to life-threatening situations.[67]

References

1. Katholi RE, Taylor GJ, McCann WP, et al: Nephrotoxicity from contrast media: attenuation with theophylline. Radiology 1995;195:17–22.
2. Barrett BJ: Contrast nephrotoxicity. J Am Soc Nephrol 1994;5:125–137.
3. Parfrey PS, Griffiths SM, Barrett BJ, et al: Radiocontrast induced renal failure in diabetes mellitus and in patients with pre-existing renal failure: a prospective controlled study. N Engl J Med 1989;320:143–149.
4. Rich MW, Crecelius CA: Incidence, risk factors, and clinical course of acute renal insufficiency after cardiac catheterization in patients 70 years of age or older. Arch Intern Med 1990;150:1237–1242.
5. Taliercio CP, Vlietstra RE, Fisher LD, et al: Risks for renal dysfunction with cardiac angiography. Ann Intern Med 1986;104:501–504.
6. Levy EM, Viscoli CM, Horwitz RI: The effect of acute renal failure on mortality. A cohort analysis. JAMA 1996;275:1489–1494.
7. Sterner G, Frennby B, Kurkus J, et al: Does post-angiographic hemodialysis reduce the risk of the contrast-medium nephropathy? Scand J Urol Nephrol 2000;34:323–326.
8. Lehnert T, Keller E, Gondolf K, et al: Effect of hemodialysis after contrast medium administration in patients with renal insufficiency. Nephrol Dial Transplant 1998;13:358–362.
9. Younathan CM, Kaude JV, Cook MD, et al: Dialysis is not indicated immediately after administration of nonionic contrast agents in patients with end-stage renal disease treated by maintenance dialysis. Am J Roentgenol 1994;163:969–971.
10. Heyman SN, Brezis M, Epstein FH, et al: Early renal medullary hypoxic injury from radiocontrast and indomethacin. Kidney Int 1991;40:632–642.
11. Katholi RE, Woods WT, Taylor GJ, et al: Oxygen free radicals and contrast nephropathy. Am J Kidney Dis 1998;32:64–71.
12. Oldroyd S, Haylor J, Morcos SK (with reply by Katzberg RW): Endothelin and nephroxicity induced by contrast media. Radiology 1998;207:270–273.
13. Spinosa DJ, Matsumoto AH, Angle JF, et al: Safety of CO_2 and gadodiamide-enhanced angiography for the evaluation and percutaneous treatment of renal artery stenosis in patients with chronic renal insufficiency. Am J Roentgenol 2001; 176:1305–1311.
14. Choyke PL, Cady J, DePollar SL, et al: Determination of serum creatinine prior to iodinated contrast media: is it necessary in all patients? Tech Urol 1998;4:65–69.
15. Barrett BJ, Carlisle EJ: Metaanalysis of the relative nephrotoxicity of high- and low-osmolality iodinated contrast media. Radiology 1993;188:171–178.
16. Rudnick MR, Goldfarb S, Wexler L, et al for the Iohexol Cooperative Study: Nephrotoxicity of ionic and nonionic contrast media in 1196 patients: a randomized trial. Kidney Int 1995;47:254–261.
17. Taylor AJ, Hotchkiss D, Morse RW, et al: PREPARED: PREParation for Angiography in REnal Dysfunction. Chest 1998;114:1570–1574.
18. Solomon R, Werner C, Mann D, et al: Effects of saline, mannitol, and furosemide on acute decreases in renal function induced by radiocontrast agents. N Engl J Med 1994;331:1416–1420.
19. Weinstein J-M, Heyman S, Brezis M: Potential deleterious effect of furosemide in radiocontrast nephropathy. Nephron 1992;62:413–415.
20. Stevens MA, McCullough PA, Tobin KJ, et al: A prospective randomized trial of prevention measures in patients at high risk for contrast nephropathy. J Am Coll Cardiol 1999;33:403–411.
21. Weisberg LS, Kurnik PB, Kurnik BRC: Risk of radiocontrast nephropathy in patients with and without diabetes mellitus. Kidney Int 1994;45:259–265.
22. Hans B, Hans SS, Mittal VK, et al: Renal functional response to dopamine during and after arteriography in patients with chronic renal insufficiency. Radiology 1990;176:651–654.
23. Hall KA, Wong RW, Hunter GC, et al: Contrast-induced nephrotoxicity: the effects of vasodilator therapy. J Surg Res 1992;53:317–320.
24. Weisberg LS, Kurnik PB, Kurnik BRC: Dopamine and renal blood flow in radiocontrast-induced nephropathy in humans. Renal Failure 1993;15:61–68.
25. Gare M, Haviv YS, Ben-Yehuda A, et al: The renal effect of low-dose dopamine in high-risk patients undergoing coronary angiography. J Am Coll Cardiol 1999;34:1682–1688.
26. Kapoor A, Sinha N, Sharma RK, et al: Use of dopamine in prevention of contrast induced acute renal failure: a randomized study. Int J Cardiol 1996;53:233–236.
27. Kurnik BRC, Weisberg LS, Cuttler IM, et al: Effects of atrial natriuretic peptide versus mannitol on renal blood flow during radiocontrast infusion in chronic renal failure. J Lab Clin Med 1990;116:27–35.
28. Neumayer H-H, Junge W, Kufner A, et al: Prevention of radiocontrast-media-induced nephrotoxicity by the calcium channel blocker nitrendipine: a prospective randomised clinical trial. Nephrol Dial Transplant 1989;4:1030–1036.
29. Russo D, Testa A, Volpe LD, et al: Randomized prospective study on renal effects of two different contrast media in humans: protective

role of a calcium channel blocker. Nephron 1990;55:254–257.

30. Khoury Z, Schlicht JR, Como J, et al: The effect of prophylactic nifedipine on renal function in patients administered contrast media. Pharmacotherapy 1995;15:59–65.

31. Gupta RK, Kapoor A, Tewari S, et al: Captopril for prevention of contrast-induced nephropathy in diabetic patients: a randomised study. Indian Heart J 1999;51:521–526.

32. Sketch MH, Whelton A, Schollmayer E, et al and the Prostaglandin E_1 Study Group: Prevention of contrast media-induced renal dysfunction with prostaglandin E_1: a randomized, double-blind, placebo-controlled study. Am J Ther 2001;8:155–162.

33. Wang A, Holcslaw T, Bashore TM, et al: Exacerbation of radiocontrast nephrotoxicity by endothelin receptor antagonism. Kidney Int 2000;57:1675–1680.

34. Erley CM, Duda SH, Schlepckow S, et al: Adenosine antagonist theophylline prevents the reduction of glomerular filtration rate after contrast media application. Kidney Int 1994;45:1425–1431.

35. Abizaid AS, Clark CE, Mintz GS, et al: Effects of dopamine and aminophylline on contrast-induced acute renal failure after coronary angioplasty in patients with pre-existing renal insufficiency. Am J Cardiol 1999;83:260–263.

36. Erley CM, Duda SH, Rehfuss D, et al: Prevention of radiocontrast-media-induced nephropathy in patients with pre-exisintg renal insufficiency by hydration in combination with the adenosine antagonist theophylline. Nephrol Dial Transplant 1999;14:1146–1149.

37. Kolonko A, Wiecek A, Kokot F: The nonselective adenosine antagonist theophylline does prevent renal dysfunction induced by radiographic contrast agents. J Nephrol 1998;11:151–156.

38. Tepel M, van der Giet M, Schwarzfeld C, et al: Prevention of radiographic-contrast-agent-induced reductions in renal function by acetylcysteine. N Engl J Med 2000;343:180–184.

39. Diaz-Sandoval LJ, Kosowsky BD, Losordo DW: Acetylcysteine to prevent angiography-related renal tissue injury (APART trial). Am J Cardiol 2002;89:356–358.

40. Scolari F, Tardanico R, Zani R, et al: Cholesterol crystal embolism: a recognizable cause of renal disease. Am J Kidney Dis 2000;36:1089–1109.

41. Scoble JE, O'Donnell PJ: Renal atheroembolic disease: the Cinderella of nephrology? Nephrol Dial Transplant 1996;11:1516–1517.

42. Fine MJ, Kapoor W, Falanga V: Cholesterol crystal embolization: a review of 221 cases in the English literature. Angiology 1987;38:769–784.

43. Saklayen MG: Atheroembolic renal disease: preferential occurrence in whites only. Am J Nephrol 1989;9:87–88.

44. Mayo RR, Swartz RD: Redefining the incidence of clinically detectable atheroembolism. Am J Med 1996;100:524–529.

45. Saklayen MG, Gupta S, Suryaprasad A, Azmeh W: Incidence of atheroembolic renal failure after coronary angiography: a prospective study. Angiology 1997;48:609–613.

46. Thadhani RI, Camargo CA, Xavier RJ, Fang LS, Bazari H: Atheroembolic renal failure after invasive procedures. Natural history based on 52 histologically proven cases. Medicine 1995;74:350–358.

47. Scolari F, Bracchi M, Valzorio B, et al: Cholesterol atheromatous embolism: an increasing recognized cause of acute renal failure. Nephrol Dial Transplant 1996;11:1607–1612.

48. Ripple MG, Charney D, Nadasdy T: Cholesterol embolization in renal allografts. Transplantation 2000;69:2221–2225.

49. Young DK, Burton MF, Herman JH: Multiple cholesterol emboli syndrome simulating systemic necrotizing vasculitis. J Rheumatol 1986;13:423–426.

50. Peat DS, Mathieson PW: Cholesterol emboli may mimic systemic vasculitis. Br Med J 1996;313:546–547.

51. Sannes MR, Modi KS: Acute renal failure and thrombocytopenia after ticlopidine: not necessarily thrombotic thrombocytopenic purpura. Nephrol Dial Transplant 2000;15:1076–1079.

52. Ducloux D, Schuller V, Ranfaing E, et al: Is atheroembolic disease a new differential diagnosis of pulmonary–renal syndrome? Nephrol Dial Transplant 1998;13:1259–1261.

53. Zanen AL, Rietveld AP, Tjen HS: Cholesterol-embolism: diagnosis by endoscopy. Endoscopy 1994;26:257–259.

54. Desnuelle C, Lanteri-Minet M, Hofman P, Butori C, Bedoucha P, Chatel M: Cholesterol emboli with neurological manifestation in the spinal cord. Rev Neurol (Paris) 1992;148:715–718.

55. Robson MG, Scoble JE: Atheroembolic disease. Br J Hosp Med 1996;55:648–652.

56. Kaplan-Pavlovcic S, Vizjak A, Vene N, Ferluga D: Antineutrophil cytoplasmic autoantibodies in atheroembolic disease. Nephrol Dial Transplant 1998;13:985–987.

57. Peixoto AJ, Reilly RF, Crowley ST: Delayed gallium-67 uptake in renal atheroembolic disease. Am J Kidney Dis 1999;34:161–165.

58. Hannedouche T, Godin M, Courtois H, et al: Necrotizing glomerulonephritis and renal cholesterol embolization. Nephron 1986;42:271–272.

59. Goldman M, Thoua Y, Dhaene M, Toussaint C: Necrotizing glomerulonephritis associated with cholesterol microemboli. Br Med J 1985;290:205–206.

60. Remy P, Jacquot C, Nochy D, d'Auzac C, Yeni P, Bariety J: Cholesterol atheroembolic renal disease with necrotizing glomerulonephritis. Am J Nephrol 1987;7:164–165.

61. Greenberg A, Bastacky SI, Iqbal A, Borochovitz D, Johnson JP: Focal segmental glomerulosclerosis associated with nephrotic syndrome in cholesterol atheroembolism: clinicopathological correlations. Am J Kidney Dis 1997;29:334–344.

62. Rumpf KW, Schult S, Mueller GA: Simvastatin treatment in cholesterol emboli syndrome. Lancet 1998;352:321–322.

63. Smith MC, Ghose MK, Henry AR: The clinical spectrum of renal cholesterol embolization. Am J Med 1981;71:174–180.

64. Siemons L, van den Heuvel P, Parizel G, Buyssens N, DeBroe ME, Cuykens JJ: Peritoneal dialysis in acute renal failure due to cholesterol embolization: two cases of recovery of renal function and extended survival. Clin Nephrol 1987;28:205–208.

65. Lye WC, Cheah JS, Sinniah R: Renal cholesterol embolic disease. Case report and review of the literature Am J Nephrol 1993;13:489–493.

66. Dahlberg PJ, Frecentese DF, Cogbill TH: Cholesterol embolism: experience with 22 histologically proven cases. Surgery 1989;105:737–746.

67. Belenfant X, Meyrier A, Jacquot C: Supportive treatment improves survival in multivisceral cholesterol crystal embolism. Am J Kidney Dis 1999;33:840–850.

68. Orr WP, Banning AP: Aortic atherosclerotic debris detected by trans-oesophageal echocardiography: a risk factor for cholesterol embolization. Q J Med 1999;92:341–346.

69. Johnson LW, Esente P, Giambartolomei A, et al: Peripheral vascular complications of coronary angioplasty by the femoral and brachial techniques. Cathet Cardiovasc Diagn 1994;31:165–172.

70. Graziani G, Santostasi S, Angelini C, Badalamenti S: Corticosteroids in cholesterol emboli. Nephron 2001;87:371–373.

71. Stabellini N, Rizzioli E, Trapassi MR, Fabbian F, Catalano C, Gilli P: Renal cholesterol microembolism: is steroid therapy effective? Nephron 2000;86:239–240.

72. Woolfsen RG, Lachman H: Improvement in renal cholesterol emboli syndrome after simvastatin. Lancet 1998;351:1331–1332.

73. Cabili S, Hochman I, Goor Y: Reversal of gangrenous lesions in the blue toe syndrome with lovastatin: a case report. Angiology 1993;44:821–825.

Hepatorenal Syndrome

Murray Epstein

Several acute azotemic syndromes occur with increased frequency in patients with hepatic and biliary disease. Although acute azotemia often represents classic acute tubular necrosis (ATN), cirrhotic patients may also develop hepatorenal syndrome (HRS), a unique form of renal failure for which a specific cause cannot be elucidated. HRS will be the focus of this chapter.

Background

Progressive oliguric renal failure commonly complicates the course of patients with advanced hepatic disease.[1-4] This condition has been designated by many names, including "functional renal failure" and "the renal failure of cirrhosis," but the most commonly used is HRS, a more appealing, albeit less specific, term. HRS may be defined as unexplained renal failure occurring in patients with liver disease in the absence of clinical, laboratory, or anatomic evidence of other known causes of renal failure.

It should be emphasized that when confronted with a patient who has concomitant renal and hepatic disease, the clinician should consider not only HRS but also a number of potentially treatable disorders that simultaneously involve the liver and the kidney. These disorders, called "pseudo"-HRS, include toxic, hematologic, neoplastic, genetic, hemodynamic, and infectious processes.

The importance of recognizing these disorders lies in the fact that they may be reversible if detected early and treated appropriately.

Clinical features

HRS occurs usually in cirrhotic patients who are alcoholic, although cirrhosis is not a sine qua non for the development of HRS. HRS may complicate other liver diseases, including acute hepatitis, primary biliary cirrhosis, and hepatic malignancy.[1,4-6] Renal failure may develop with great rapidity and often occurs in patients in whom normal serum creatinine levels have been previously documented within a few days of onset of HRS. Papadakis and Arieff[7] have suggested that the serum creatinine level may be a poor index of renal function in patients with chronic liver disease, often masking greatly reduced glomerular filtration rates (GFRs). Implicit in such a formulation is the concept that HRS represents a progression in patients who already have markedly impaired renal function.

Numerous reports have emphasized the development of renal failure following events that reduce effective blood volume, including abdominal paracentesis, vigorous diuretic therapy, gastrointestinal bleeding, sepsis, and surgery, although it can occur in the absence of any apparent precipitating event. In this context, several careful observers have noted that patients with HRS seldom arrive in the hospital with preexisting azotemia; rather, HRS seems to develop in the hospital, suggesting that iatrogenic events might precipitate this syndrome.[1,4]

Almost all patients with HRS have ascites, which is often tense; other clinical stigmata of chronic liver disease and portal hypertension are usually present. Hepatic encephalopathy is a common feature. The degree of jaundice is extremely variable, and occasionally renal failure may develop at a time when the serum bilirubin concentration is decreasing. Thus, although the majority of reports suggest that HRS occurs in patients who manifest evidence of severe hepatocellular disease, it is quite apparent that HRS can occur with minimal jaundice and with little evidence of severe hepatic dysfunction.[1,4] There are no apparent clinical, functional, renal, or hepatic laboratory characteristics that serve to identify patients with cirrhosis who will ultimately develop renal failure.

The overwhelming majority of patients with HRS die, and recovery from HRS is unusual. Most patients die within 3 weeks of the onset of renal failure.[1]

Diagnostic considerations

Although measurement of the serum creatinine concentration is generally the best of the widely available clinical means of assessing the GFR, there is a diagnostic pitfall

Table 6.1 Differential diagnosis of acute azotemia in the patient with liver disease:* important differential urinary findings

Biochemical characteristics	Prerenal azotemia	Hepatorenal syndrome	Acute tubular necrosis (ATN)
Urine sodium concentration (mequiv./L)	< 10	< 10	> 30†
Urine–plasma creatinine ratio	> 30:1	> 30:1	< 20:1
Urine osmolality	At least 200 mosmol/kg > plasma osmolality	At least 200 mosmol/kg plasma osmolality	Relatively similar to plasma osmolality
Urine sediment	Normal	Unremarkable	Casts, cellular debris

*The numbers cited are arbitrary and are meant to highlight the salient differences in these three diagnostic categories; however, the values vary. As an example, U_{Na} may occasionally exceed 10 mequiv./L.

†Radiocontrast agents and sepsis may lower urinary sodium concentration in the patient with acute tubular necrosis. When urinary output is very low, the concentration of sodium may rise.

that may confound diagnosis in the setting of liver disease, i.e. spurious interference with creatinine measurements by a variety of endogenous and exogenous metabolites. Although the interference by bilirubin in the measurement of serum creatinine levels has been recognized in the technical literature for several years,[8] most clinicians are unfamiliar with this phenomenon. The magnitude of the error varies with the autoanalyzer used, but the spurious depression can be as much as 57% with some commonly used instruments.[8] Recognition of this laboratory artifact is important because, depending on the instrument used for bilirubin measurement, an increase in serum creatinine could be masked. Conversely, a decrease in serum creatinine could be interpreted as an improvement in renal function. It has been suggested, however, that the endpoint Jaffe method can overcome the interference of bilirubin.[9] In summary, it is clear that changes in serum creatinine concentrations should be interpreted with caution in the presence of extreme hyperbilirubinemia.

Examination of the urine

Patients with HRS manifest a rather characteristic urine excretory pattern, voiding urine that is practically free of sodium and retaining the capacity to concentrate urine to a modest degree. As seen in Table 6.1, the biochemical characteristics $[U_{Na}]$, $[U_{osm}]$, and $[U_{Cr}]$ (urinary sodium concentration, urinary osmolality, and urinary creatinine concentrations) in such patients are indistinguishable from those seen in the setting of hypovolemia, which emphasizes the importance of considering hypovolemia in any diagnostic evaluation of azotemia in the setting of liver disease. Proteinuria is absent or minimal in HRS.

A clinical setting that may also mimic HRS is myoglobinuric acute renal failure. It is not generally appreciated that, in the setting of renal insufficiency, myoglobin is converted extensively to bilirubin. Furthermore, myoglobinuric ATN is one of the settings of ATN associated with a low $[U_{Na}]$. Thus, the clinician may fall into the trap of falsely diagnosing myoglobinuric ATN as HRS.[1]

Pathogenesis

As detailed in several reviews,[1,4,10] a substantial body of evidence lends strong support to the concept that the renal failure in HRS is functional in nature. Despite the severe derangement of renal function, pathologic abnormalities are minimal and inconsistent.[1,4] Furthermore, tubular functionality integrity is maintained during the renal failure, as manifested by a relatively unimpaired sodium reabsorptive capacity and concentrating ability. Finally, more direct evidence is derived from the demonstration that (1) kidneys transplanted from patients with HRS are capable of resuming normal function in the recipient[11] and (2) renal function returns when the patient with HRS successfully receives a liver transplant.[12]

The factors responsible for the sustained reduction in renal cortical perfusion and suppression of filtration in HRS have not been elucidated. Several major factors have been implicated, including: (1) alterations of the renin-angiotensin system; (2) an increase in sympathetic nervous system activity; (3) alterations in renal eicosanoids, including a relative decrease in renal vasodilatory prostaglandins and an increase in vasoconstrictor thromboxanes; (4) enhanced nitric oxide production with peripheral vasodilatation; (5) elevated plasma endothelin levels; (6) a relative impairment of renal kallikrein production; and (7) endotoxemia (Table 6.2).

Clinical trials and specific recommendations

General considerations

The management of HRS has been discouraging in view of the absence of any reproducible effective treatment modality. Because knowledge about the pathogenesis of HRS is inferential and incomplete, therapy to the present has been supportive. Because iatrogenic events often precipitate this syndrome, and therapy is difficult once the

Table 6.2 Known and postulated mechanisms that may contribute to the renal failure of liver disease

Hormonal
Activation of the renin–angiotensin system
Alterations in renal eicosanoids
    Diminished vasodilatory prostaglandins
    Increased vasoconstrictor thromboxanes
Enhanced nitric oxide production
Elevated plasma endothelin levels
Endotoxemia
Relative impairment of renal kallikrein production
Diminished atrial natriuretic peptides
Vasoactive intestinal peptide
Glomerulopressin deficiency

Neural and hemodynamic
An increase in sympathetic nervous system activity
Alterations in intrarenal blood flow distribution

Table 6.3 Principles of management of the patient with hepatorenal syndrome*

I General measures
   A Try not to make the diagnosis
      1 Attempt to rule out other likely diagnoses
         a Acute renal failure
         b Prerenal azotemia
            Use of CVP or Swan–Ganz catheter
            Volume challenge
   B Primum non nocere
II Specific therapeutic considerations
   A General
      1 Sodium and fluid restriction
      2 Correct acid–base disturbances
      3 Correct severe anemia
      4 Treat encephalopathy
   B Ascites reinfusion
   C Infusion of vasodilators
      1 Acetylcholine
      2 Phentolamine
      3 Prostaglandins A_1 and E
      4 Dopamine
   D Portacaval shunting
   E Dialysis
   F CAVU
   G LeVeen (peritoneovenous) shunt
   H Hepatic transplantation

CVP, central venous pressure; CAVU, continuous arteriovenous ultrafiltration.
*From: Epstein M (ed): The Kidney in Liver Disease, 4th edn. Philadelphia: Hanley & Belfus, 1996.

syndrome is established, prevention constitutes the key to management. Table 6.3 summarizes the principles of management of HRS.

The initial step in management is to not equate decreased renal function with HRS but rather to search diligently for and treat correctable causes of azotemia, such as volume contraction, cardiac decompensation, and urinary tract obstruction. The diagnosis of ATN should clearly be considered because ATN occurs commonly in the cirrhotic patient. Furthermore, cirrhotic patients with ATN may be more likely to recover if supported with dialysis therapy than patients with HRS.

Drugs causing renal failure

Although we commonly invoke the caveat of primum non nocere (first do no harm), it takes on greater meaning than it had in earlier times. Our increasing knowledge of the effects of numerous drugs in the setting of liver disease has now amplified the myriad ways whereby such agents may actually induce acute renal failure in the cirrhotic patient (Table 6.4). Thus, it is well established that nonsteroidal anti-inflammatory drugs that inhibit prostaglandin synthetase activity are capable of inducing detrimental effects on renal function in the patient with liver disease and ascites.[13-16] Similarly, the broad-spectrum antibiotic demeclocylcine has been shown to be capable of inducing acute azotemia in the patient with cirrhosis and ascites.[17,18] Finally, we should be cognizant of the fact that drugs that may be indicated for the management of complications of liver disease (e.g. lactulose for the treatment of hepatic encephalopathy) are capable of inducing profound hypovolemia with resultant azotemia. Clearly, we are encountering ever-increasing "diseases of medical progress" in the management of the patient with advanced liver disease.

β-Blockers have currently achieved widespread acceptance as effective agents in the prophylaxis of recurrent

Table 6.4 Drugs and procedures that impair renal function in the patient with liver disease and ascites

Drugs
Nonsteroidal anti-inflammatory drugs
Demeclocycline
Lactulose
Neomycin
Aminoglycosides

Procedures
Overly vigorous or inordinately rapid diuresis
Nonjudicious abdominal paracentesis

variceal bleeding.[19] Because, on average, propranolol reduces both effective renal plasma flow (ERPF) and GFR by 10–20% in patients with essential hypertension,[20] one might be concerned that these agents might also contribute to renal functional impairment in cirrhosis. In other words, it is conceivable that the administration of some β-blockers might increase the risk of ATN or HRS in patients with advanced liver disease. However, recent information indicates that, in contrast to the situation that occurs in patients with essential hypertension, β-blockers (at least nadolol and propranolol) may not adversely affect renal function in patients with cirrhosis.[21]

Neomycin may cause renal toxicity, especially in the setting of renal dysfunction. Aminoglycosides should be avoided because 30% of cirrhotic patients develop renal failure in the setting of therapeutic nontoxic blood levels.[22,23]

Rule out reversible prerenal azotemia

The next step in management is to exclude reversible prerenal azotemia (see Table 6.3). Diarrhea, vomiting, or vigorous diuresis can cause reversible prerenal azotemia. Diuretics and lactulose should be discontinued if clinically permissible. Because HRS and prerenal azotemia have similar urinary diagnostic indices, one must often use a functional maneuver, i.e. administration of volume expanders, to differentiate between these two entities. In this regard, it should be emphasized that our frame of reference for the cirrhotic patient may be quite different from that of other disease states. The degree of volume expansion necessary to replete the cirrhotic patient may sometimes be marked; occasionally, the patient may require an infusion of massive amounts of colloids.

It should be emphasized that there is no defined regimen that allows one to approximate the amount of volume expanders necessary to replete the cirrhotic patient suspected of being hypovolemic. Rather, I believe that the expanders should be infused in a setting in which alteration of clinical status (blood pressure, urine flow rate, creatinine clearance) as well as central hemodynamics (central venous pressure (CVP), Swan–Ganz catheter) can be monitored. Furthermore, it should be emphasized that the changes in CVP are often more important than the absolute level; that is, a CVP reading may not necessarily be extremely low yet may not change (increase) until large amounts of expanders are administered. Such guidelines do not presuppose that there is a correlation between central hemodynamics and volume deficit. Rather, we use such manometric determinations as a safety guideline to assist us in determining when to discontinue volume expansion in order to avoid overt fluid overload. Expansion should be accomplished by infusion of colloids or packed red blood cells, depending on the severity of the patient's anemia.

Once the correctable causes of renal functional impairment are excluded, the mainstay of therapy is careful restriction of sodium and fluid intake. A number of specific therapeutic measures have been attempted, but none has proved to be of practical value. Attempts at volume expansion with different exogenous expanders have resulted in only transient improvement in renal hemodynamics and function without significant improvement in the outcome.[1] Similarly, attempts at reinfusion of ascites using peritoneal fluid that has been concentrated have not provided any lasting improvement.

Paracentesis

The role of paracentesis in the treatment of HRS, with or without simultaneous plasma volume expansion, remains controversial.[24] The potential renal benefit of a reduction of ascitic fluid volume includes diminished intra-abdominal pressure with possible relief of inferior vena cava obstruction and augmentation of cardiac output. Improvement in renal function, when it occurs, is transient, and because the abnormal hydraulic pressures that sustain ascites formation are not altered by paracentesis, continued fluid removal is necessary and may result in progressive depletion of intravascular volume with subsequent deterioration in cardiac function and renal perfusion. Nevertheless, a subsequent report by Gines and associates suggests that paracentesis may induce a more favorable response than was previously thought.[25]

Renal vasodilators and other pharmacologic approaches

In view of the prominent role assigned to renal cortical ischemia in the pathogenesis of HRS, it is not surprising that there have been numerous attempts to treat HRS with vasodilators.[1] Intrarenal infusion of nonspecific vasodilators such as acetylcholine and papaverine improve renal blood flow but do not augment GFR. Similarly, blockade of vasoconstrictor α-adrenergic nerves by intrarenal infusion of phentolamine or phenoxybenzamine, or by stimulation of vasodilator β-adrenergic nerves with isoproterenol, has no significant effect on GFR.

Direct stimulation of renal dopaminergic receptors by infusion of nonpressor doses of dopamine produces renal vasodilation; however, GFR and urine flow are virtually unaffected despite infusions for as long as 24 h.[26] A report suggests that dopamine infusion for longer periods provides some increase in urine flow and sodium excretion, but these effects are modest and the studies were uncontrolled.[27] Infusion of vasodilator prostaglandins to correct a possible renal prostaglandin deficiency has been unrewarding.[28] In summary, although such therapeutic manipulations with vasodilators have occasionally resulted in salutary effects on renal function, the benefits have not been sustained.

Thromboxane inhibitors

As detailed in a recent review,[14] several investigators have proposed that alterations of thromboxane (Tx) may contribute to the development of renal dysfunction.[29,30] Consequently, there have been attempts to modify the course of HRS by the administration of selective inhibitors of Tx synthesis.[29,31] Whereas nonspecific cyclooxygenase inhibitors, such as indomethacin and aspirin, reduce both Tx and prostaglandin synthesis to varying degrees in different biologic systems, selective inhibitors of Tx synthesis preserve or possibly increase the production of other metabolites of arachidonic acid, such as the potent vasodilator prostacyclin.

Unfortunately, the administration of Tx synthase inhibitors is associated with a number of confounding factors that render the results difficult to interpret.[29,31] Indeed, these drugs may lead to the accumulation of the prostaglandin endoperoxides PGG_2 and PGH_2, which mimic the renal effects of TxA_2 by interacting with the same receptors. As an example, arachidonic acid-induced vasoconstriction in the rat kidney is only partially reduced by pretreatment with a Tx synthase inhibitor, whereas it is completely abolished by the administration of a Tx receptor antagonist.[32]

In an attempt to obviate these problems, Laffi and associates[30] conducted a randomized, double-blind, cross-over trial to characterize the effects of the Tx receptor antagonist ONO-3708 on renal hemodynamics and excretory function in 15 nonazotemic cirrhotic patients with ascites. Urinary TxB_2 excretion was threefold higher than in healthy subjects. The administration of ONO-3708 significantly blocked TxA_2 receptors; bleeding time showed a twofold increase, and platelet aggregation to the Tx receptor agonist U-46619 was abolished in all patients studied. ONO-3708 induced an 86% increase in free water clearance compared with placebo ($P < 0.001$) that was associated with a significant diuresis. Renal plasma flow, as measured by p-aminohippurate (PAH) clearance, increased 14% during Tx receptor blockade ($P < 0.05$), whereas the GFR, as assessed by inulin, was unchanged. Additional studies with Tx receptor antagonists in patients with widely varying degrees of acute renal insufficiency will be required to further define the possible utility of these agents in the treatment of HRS.

Other pharmacologic modalities

In view of the prominent role assigned to renal cortical ischemia in the pathogenesis of HRS, it is not altogether surprising that there have been numerous attempts to treat HRS with vasodilators. The intrarenal infusion of nonspecific vasodilators such as acetylcholine and papaverine improves renal blood flow but does not augment the GFR.[10,33] Similarly, the blockade of vasoconstrictor α-adrenergic nerves by the intrarenal infusion of phentolamine or phenoxybenzamine or the stimulation of vasodilator β-adrenergic nerves with isoproterenol has no significant effect on the GFR.[10,12]

The direct stimulation of renal dopaminergic receptors by the infusion of nonpressor doses of dopamine produces renal vasodilation, but, again, the GFR and urine flow are virtually unaffected despite infusions for as long as 24 h.[34] The recent availability of direct agonists that specifically activate the peripheral dopaminergic system (e.g. fenoldopam) has facilitated future investigations to further delineate the role of dopaminergic activation in treating HRS.[35]

Finally, a variety of other treatment modalities have been proposed, including prednisone, exchange transfusion, charcoal hemoperfusion, xenobiotic cross-circulation, and ex vivo baboon liver perfusion.[1,36] None is of demonstrated benefit, and the actual and potential complications are of sufficient magnitude to dictate great hesitation in their clinical use.

Treatment of hepatorenal syndrome with invasive procedures

Dialytic techniques

Although dialysis has previously been reported to be ineffective in the management of HRS,[37] it is apparent that it may be helpful and is warranted in certain patients (see below).[38]

Peritoneal dialysis

Peritoneal dialysis is not a practical approach for treating patients with HRS. Included among the difficulties in instituting peritoneal dialysis in HRS are (1) coagulopathy requiring surgical rather than percutaneous placement of the catheter, (2) ascites rendering the exchanges less efficient and augmenting protein losses, and (3) insufficient rates of solute clearance.

Hemodialysis and ultrafiltration

Several investigators have reported that hemodialysis is ineffective in the management of HRS.[37-42] Our own recent experience, however, suggests that such a condemnation should be qualified.[38] Although most of the published literature indeed suggests a dismal prognosis for patients who are dialyzed, such reports have dealt almost exclusively with patients with chronic endstage liver disease. Our experience and that of others suggests that in carefully selected patients – i.e. patients with acute hepatic dysfunction, in whom there is reason to believe that the underlying liver disease may reverse (making long-term survival and even spontaneous recovery of renal function possible) – dialytic therapy is indicated.[38] Thus, sporadic case reports describe prolonged survival and improvement in renal function in selected patients with acute, or acute superimposed on chronic, liver disease treated by dialysis alone[38-43] or combined with other modalities.[44]

Dialysis has a pivotal role in the treatment of acute renal failure in patients with severe endstage liver disease who are awaiting hepatic transplantation.[42] Aside from complicating the medical management, the development of acute renal failure in this setting is associated with considerable morbidity and mortality that is not improved by dialysis. Nevertheless, in one study, dialytic therapy was helpful in the life support of patients awaiting liver transplantation, and four of seven patients with HRS experienced recovery of renal function 1–5 weeks after successful hepatic replacement.[42]

In addition to stabilizing renal function, it is often necessary to mobilize fluid either to prevent life-threatening emergencies, such as acute pulmonary edema, or to facilitate administration of requisite fluids such as bicarbonate solutions or hyperalimentation. Although hemodialysis often constitutes the therapeutic modality of choice in effecting such interventions, it is not feasible in many patients with severe liver disease who have associated hemodynamic instability.[38,45] Unfortunately, patients with decompensated cirrhosis frequently become hypotensive in response to the institution of hemodialysis. To circumvent this problem, we have used continuous arteriovenous ultrafiltration (CAVU) as an alternative maneuver in a few patients with HRS and have been successful in mobilizing fluid without concomitant hemodynamic instability.[38,45] Additional experience will be required to clarify the role of this approach in managing patients with HRS.

Peritoneovenous shunts

In 1974, LeVeen and associates[46] introduced the peritoneovenous shunt (PVS) for the treatment of refractory ascites. Subsequently, these authors reported five long-term survivals in nine patients with HRS treated with the PVS. Other reports that followed claimed long-term survival rates approaching 40%.[47–49] Nevertheless, careful scrutiny of the reported cases reveals that diagnosis of HRS was frequently inadequately documented.[50,51]

Only two prospective randomized studies of the role of the PVS in the treatment of HRS have been performed.[52,53] Both studies demonstrated that survival was not prolonged; rather, in reality, patients died with somewhat improved renal function.

On the basis of the available data, it is apparent that a beneficial role for the PVS in the treatment of HRS has not been established. Although some patients exhibit an improvement in renal function, the PVS has not been shown to improve long-term survival or quality of life.[47]

Hepatic transplantation

Hepatic transplantation is the ultimate modality of therapy that results in correction not only of HRS but also of many of the metabolic complications of advanced liver disease.[11,54–56] Of interest, many of these patients are admitted with varying degrees of concomitant renal dysfunction, including HRS. Orthotopic liver transplantation (OLTX) has been reported to reverse HRS acutely.[11,57,58] In 1991, Gonwa and associates[55] reviewed the extensive experience of the Baylor University transplant group and reported good long-term survival with return of acceptable renal function for prolonged periods. They retrospectively reviewed the first 308 patients undergoing OLTX. The incidence of HRS was 10.5%. Patients with HRS manifested an increase in GFR from a baseline of 20 ± 4 mL/min to a mean of 33 ± 3 mL/min at 6 weeks, with a further increase to 46 ± 6 mL/min at 1 year. GFR remained stable at 2 years postoperatively (38 ± 6 mL/min). There was no difference in perioperative (90 day) mortality between HRS and non-HRS patients, despite a worse preoperative status and a more unstable postoperative course. The actuarial 1- and 2-year survival rate for patients with HRS was 77% and did not differ from that of non-HRS patients. These investigators concluded that with aggressive pretransplant and post-transplant management, one can anticipate good results after OLTX in patients with HRS. Gonwa and Wilkinson[56] have since updated the extensive Baylor experience and have confirmed and extended their earlier results.

Seu and associates[59] reviewed retrospectively their experience of 130 adult patients who underwent OLTX. Nineteen patients had HRS for an incidence of 15.1%. The rate of survival was similar for patients with HRS and nonhepatorenal patients. In some patients, renal function improved slowly after OLTX.

Transjugular intrahepatic portosystemic shunt

A few anecdotal reports have appeared describing improvement in renal function in patients with HRS after the insertion of a transjugular intrahepatic portosystemic shunt (TIPS).[60–62] The rationale for this procedure is similar to that for the establishment of a side-to-side portacaval shunt, thus creating a portal to systemic vascular pathway that serves to decompress the portacaval system.[63] Although TIPS obviates the need for performing major vascular surgery, it is not nearly so simple and innocuous a procedure as some of its adherents would propose. It should also be noted that the reported experience is preliminary, and the available data consist mainly of a few preliminary and anecdotal reports. Somberg[64] has written an in-depth review of the rationale and experience with TIPS, as well as considerations regarding its potential future niche in the therapeutic armamentarium. In addition to its potential beneficial effects on renal function in HRS, TIPS may also assist with the management of ascites in patients with advanced liver disease and refractory ascites.

Summary and future directions

In summary, I recommend the following algorithm for the evaluation and management of acute renal failure in cirrhosis (Fig. 6.1). The three important diagnostic considerations are prerenal azotemia, ATN, and HRS. The fractional excretion of sodium (FE_{Na}) or the urinary sodium concentration in a spot urine, and the pulmonary capillary wedge pressure (PCWP) or the CVP, may help to distinguish among these diagnostic possibilities. There is, however, considerable overlap between the three categories, and patients often present with more than one diagnosis. For example, patients with HRS often exhibit ATN, and HRS and prerenal failure often coexist. In fact, the response to colloid infusion is the only feature that helps to differentiate the last two conditions. Of note, because of the low peripheral resistance associated with cirrhosis, volume expansion frequently does not result in a marked increase in CVP or PCWP. Hemodialysis or hemoperfusion is indicated for the management of HRS, complicating acute (reversible) liver injury. In patients with chronic cirrhosis, dialysis may maintain the patient until a suitable liver donor is found. The potential role of TIPS in managing HRS remains to be established by prospective, randomized, clinical trials.

Acknowledgment

I am indebted to Mrs Elsa V. Reina for her expert preparation of the manuscript. Portions of this review have been adapted with permission from an earlier review by the author: Epstein M: Hepatorenal syndrome. *In* Epstein M (ed): The Kidney in Liver Disease, 4th edn. Philadelphia: Hanley & Belfus, 1996, pp 75–108.

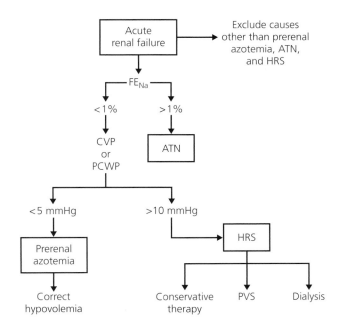

Figure 6.1 Algorithm for the evaluation and management of a cirrhotic patient with acute renal failure. ATN, acute tubular necrosis; CVP, central venous pressure; HRS, hepatorenal syndrome; PCWP, pulmonary capillary wedge pressure; PVS, peritoneovenous shunt; FE$_{Na}$, fractional excretion of sodium. (From Epstein M: Hepatorenal syndrome. In The Kidney in Liver Disease, 4th edn. Philadelphia: Hanley & Belfus, 1996, pp 75–108.)

References

1. Epstein M: Hepatorenal syndrome. In Epstein M (ed): The Kidney in Liver Disease, 4th edn. Philadelphia, Hanley & Belfus, 1996, pp 75–108.
2. Epstein M: Renal functional abnormalities in cirrhosis: pathophysiology and management. In Zakim D, Boyer TD (eds): Hepatology: A Textbook of Liver Disease, 2nd edn. Philadelphia: WB Saunders, 1990, pp 493–512.
3. Epstein M: Liver disease. In Massry SG, Glassock R Jr (eds): Textbook of Nephrology, Vol 2, 3rd edn. Baltimore: Williams & Wilkins, 1995, pp 1105–1117.
4. Epstein M: The hepatorenal syndrome: emerging perspectives of pathophysiology and therapy. J Am Soc Nephrol 1994;4:1735–1753.
5. Ritt DJ, Whelan G, Werner DJ, et al: Acute hepatic necrosis with stupor or coma. Medicine 1969;48:151–172.
6. Vesin P, Roberti A, Vuigie R: Defaillance renale fonctionnelle terminale chez des maladies atteints de cancer du foie, primitif ou secondaire. Semin Hop Paris 1965;26:1216–1220.
7. Papadakis M, Arieff AJ: Unpredictability of clinical evaluation of renal function in cirrhosis: a prospective study. Am J Med 1987;82:945–952.
8. Halstead AC, Nanji AA: Artifactual lowering of serum creatinine in the presence of hyperbilirubinemia – a method dependent artifact. JAMA 1984;251:38–39.
9. Daugherty NA, Hammond KB, Osberg IM: Bilirubin interference with the kinetic Jaffe method for serum creatinine. Clin Chem 1978;24:392–393.
10. Epstein M, Berk DP, Hollenberg NK, et al: Renal failure in the patient with cirrhosis: the role of active vasoconstriction. Am J Med 1970;49:175–185.
11. Koppel MH, Coburn JW, Mims MM, et al: Transplantation of cadaveric kidneys from patients with hepatorenal syndrome: evidence for the functional nature of renal failure in advanced liver disease. N Engl J Med 1969;280:1367–1371.
12. Iwatsuki S, Popovtzer MM, Corman JL, et al: Recovery from hepatorenal syndrome after orthotopic liver transplantation. N Engl J Med 1973;289:1155–1159.
13. Epstein M: Renal prostaglandins and the control of renal function in liver disease. Am J Med 1986;80 (Suppl 1A):46–55.
14. Laffi G, La Villa G, Penzani M, et al: Lipid-derived autacoids and renal function in liver cirrhosis. In Epstein M (ed): The Kidney in Liver Disease. 4th edn. Philadelphia: Hanley & Belfus, 1996, pp 307–337.
15. Epstein M, Lifschitz MD: Renal eicosanoids as determinants of renal function in liver disease. Hepatology 1987;7:1359–1367.
16. Boyer TD, Zia P, Reynolds TB: Effect of indomethacin and prostaglandins AI on renal function and plasma renin activity in alcoholic liver disease. Gastroenterology 1979;77:215–222.
17. Oster JR, Epstein M, Ulano HB: Deterioration of renal function with demeclocycline administration. Curr Ther Res 1976;20:794–801.
18. Carrilho F, Bosch J, Arroyo V, et al: Renal failure associated with demeclocycline in cirrhosis. Ann Intern Med 1977;87:195–197.
19. Lebrec D, Poynard T, Hillon P, et al: Propranolol for prevention of recurrent gastrointestinal bleeding in patients with cirrhosis: a controlled study. N Engl J Med 1981;305:1371–1374.
20. Epstein M, Oster JR: Beta blockers and renal function: a reappraisal. J Clin Hypertens 1985;1:85–99.
21. Bataille C, Bercoff E, Pariente EA, et al: Effects of propranolol on renal blood flow and renal function in patients with cirrhosis. Gastroenterology 1984;86:129–133.
22. Cabrera J, Arroyo V, Ballesta AM, et al: Aminoglycoside nephrotoxicity in cirrhosis. Gastroenterology 1982;82:97–105.
23. Moore RD, Smith CR, Lietman PS: Increased risk of renal dysfunction due to the interaction of liver disease and aminoglycosides. Am J Med 1986;80:1093–1097.
24. Planas R, Gines P, Gines A, Arroyo V: Paracentesis in the management of cirrhotics with ascites. In Epstein M (ed): The Kidney in Liver Disease, 4th edn. Philadelphia: Hanley & Belfus, 1996, pp 479–490.
25. Gines P, Arroyo V, Quintero E, et al: Comparison of paracentesis and diuretics in the treatment of cirrhotics with tense ascites: results of a randomised study. Gastroenterology 1987;93:234–241.
26. Bennett WM, Keeffe E, Melnyk C, et al: Response to dopamine hydrochloride in the hepatorenal syndrome. Arch Intern Med 1975;135:964–971.
27. Wilson JR: Dopamine in the hepatorenal syndrome. JAMA 1977;238:2719–2720.
28. Zusman RM, Axelrod L, Tolkoff-Rubin N: The treatment of the hepatorenal syndrome (HRS) with intrarenal administration of prostaglandin E. Prostaglandins 1977;13:819–830.
29. Zipser RD, Kronborg I, Rector W, et al: Therapeutic trial of thromboxane synthase inhibition in the hepatorenal syndrome. Gastroenterology 1984;87:1228–1232.
30. Laffi G, Marra F, Carloni V, et al: Thromboxane-receptor blockade increases water diuresis in cirrhotic patients with ascites. Gastroenterology 1992;103:1017–1021.
31. Gentilini P, Laffi G, Meacci E, et al: Effects of OKY 046, a thromboxane-synthase inhibitor, on renal function in non-azotemic cirrhotic patients with ascites. Gastroenterology 1988;94:1470–1477.
32. Quilley J, McGiff JC, Nasjletti A: Role of endoperoxides in arachidonic acid-induced vasoconstriction in the isolated perfused kidney of the rat. Br J Pharmacol 1989;96:111–116.
33. Cohn JN, Tristani FE, Khatri M: Renal vasodilator therapy in the hepatorenal syndrome. Med Ann DC 1970;39:1–7.
34. Bennett WM, Keefe E, Melnyk C, et al: Response to dopamine hydrochloride in the hepatorenal syndrome. Arch Intern Med 1975;135:964–971.
35. Singer I, Epstein M: Potential of dopamine A-1 agonists in the management of acute renal failure. Am J Kidney Dis 1998;31:743–755.
36. Horisawa M, Reynolds TB: Exchange transfusion in hepatorenal syndrome with liver disease. Arch Intern Med 1976;136:1135–1137.
37. Perez GO, Oster JR: A critical review of the role of dialysis in the treatment of liver disease. In Epstein M (ed): The Kidney in Liver Disease. New York: Elsevier, 1978, pp 325–336.
38. Perez GO, Golper T, Epstein M, et al: Dialysis, hemofiltration, and other extracorporeal techniques in the treatment of the renal complication of liver disease. In Epstein M (ed): The Kidney in Liver Disease, 4th edn. Philadelphia: Hanley & Belfus, 1996, pp 517–528.
39. Ring-Larsen H, Clausen E, Ranek L: Peritoneal dialysis in hyponatremia due to liver failure. Scand J Gastroenterol 1973;8:33–40.

40. Wilkinson SP, Weston MJ, Parsons V, et al: Dialysis in the treatment of renal failure in patients with liver disease. Clin Nephrol 1977;8:287–292.

41. Coratelli P, Passavanti G, Munn I, et al: New trends in hepatorenal syndrome. Kidney Int 1985;17:S143–S147.

42. Ellis D, Avner ED: Renal failure and dialysis therapy in children with hepatic failure in the perioperative period of orthotopic liver transplantation. Clin Nephrol 1986;25:295–303.

43. Keller F, Wagner K, Lenz T, et al: Hemodialysis in "hepatorenal syndrome:" report on two cases. Gut 1985;26:208–211.

44. Kearns PJ, Polhemus RJ, Oakes D, et al: Hepatorenal syndrome managed with hemodialysis then reversed by peritoneovenous shunting. J Clin Gastroenterol 1985;7:341–343.

45. Epstein M, Perez GO, Bedoya LA, et al: Continuous arteriovenous ultrafiltration in cirrhotic patients with ascites or renal failure. Int J Artific Organs 1986;9:253–256.

46. LeVeen HH, Christoudias G, Luft R, et al: Peritoneovenous shunting for ascites. Ann Surg 1974;180:580–590.

47. Epstein M: Role of the peritoneovenous shunt in the management of ascites and the hepatorenal syndrome. In Epstein M (ed): The Kidney in Liver Disease, 4th edn. Philadelphia: Hanley & Belfus, 1996, pp 491–506.

48. Schroeder ET, Anderson GH, Smulyan H: Effects of a portacaval or peritoneovenous shunt on renin in the hepatorenal syndrome. Kidney Int 1979;15:54–61.

49. Greig PD, Blendis LM, Langer B: Renal and hemodynamic effects of the peritoneovenous shunt. II. Long-term effects. Gastroenterology 1981;80:119–125.

50. Epstein M: The peritoneovenous shunt in the management of ascites and the hepatorenal syndrome. Gastroenterology 1982;82:790–799.

51. Epstein M: The LeVeen shunt for ascites and hepatorenal syndrome. N Engl J Med 1980;302:628–630.

52. Linas SL, Schaffer JW, Moore EE, et al: Peritoneovenous shunt in the management of the hepatorenal syndrome. Kidney Int 1986;30:736–740.

53. Stanley MM, Ochi S, Lee KK, et al: Peritoneovenous shunting as compared with medical treatment in patients with alcoholic cirrhosis and massive ascites. N Engl J Med 1989;321:1632–1638.

54. Starzl TE, VanThiel D, Tzakis AG, et al: Orthotopic liver transplantation for alcoholic cirrhosis. JAMA 1988;260:2542–2544.

55. Gonwa TA, Morris CA, Goldstein RM, et al: Long-term survival and renal function following liver transplantation in patients with and without hepatorenal syndrome – experience in 300 patients. Transplantation 1991;51:428–430.

56. Gonwa TA, Wilkinson AH: Liver transplantation and renal function: results in patients with and without hepatorenal syndrome. In Epstein M (ed): The Kidney in Liver Disease, 4th edn. Philadelphia: Hanley & Belfus, 1996, pp 529–542.

57. Wood RP, Ellis D, Starzl TE: The reversal of the hepatorenal syndrome in four pediatric patients following successful orthotopic liver transplantation. Ann Surg 1987;205:415–419.

58. Gunning TC, Brown MR, Swygert TH, et al: Perioperative renal function in patients undergoing orthotopic liver transplantation. Transplantation 1991;51:422–427.

59. Seu P, Wilkinson A, Shaked A, et al: The hepatorenal syndrome in liver transplant recipients. Am Surg 1991;12:806–809.

60. Conn H: Transjugular intrahepatic portal-systemic shunts: the state of the art. Hepatology 1993;17:148–158.

61. Somberg KA, Lake JR, Tomlanovich SJ, et al: Transjugular intrahepatic portosystemic shunt for refractory ascites: assessment of clinical and humoral response and renal function. Hepatology 1995;21:709–716.

62. Lake J, Ring E, LaBerge J, et al: Transjugular intrahepatic portacaval stent shunt in patients with renal insufficiency. Transplant Proc 1992;25:1766–1767.

63. Orloff MJ: Effect of side-to-side portacaval shunt in intractable ascites, sodium excretion, and aldosterone metabolism in man. Am J Surg 1966;112:287–298.

64. Somberg K: The transjugular intrahepatic portosystemic shunt (TIPS) in the treatment of refractory ascites and hepatorenal syndrome. In Epstein M (ed): The Kidney in Liver Disease, 4th edn. Philadelphia: Hanley & Belfus, 1996, pp 507–516.

CHAPTER 7

Acute Hemodialysis and Acute Peritoneal Dialysis

Renuka Sothinathan and Joseph A. Eustace

Epidemiology

Acute renal failure (ARF) is a protean syndrome of varied severity. Owing to the lack of representative registry data, the proportion of patients with ARF who actually require dialysis is uncertain, but is calculated to be between 5.7 and 13 cases/100 000 population per year.[1,2] Much of the currently available information regarding acute dialysis relates to the intensive care unit (ICU) population, among whom between 3% and 7% of all admissions require renal replacement therapy.[3,4] The mortality rate of such patients often exceeds 50%. This rate has shown at best only moderate improvement over the last three decades, as progress in technologic innovation and improved medical management has been largely equaled by increases in the severity and extent of patient comorbidities.[5] While survival is undeniably influenced by the severity of underlying illness, there is increasing evidence that factors related to the renal failure and/or to the dialysis procedure per se may also affect outcome,[6–8] thus contradicting the once common assertion that, with the availability of dialysis, patients died with renal failure and not from it. In those who do survive, the renal prognosis is usually good, with the majority (82–84%) of survivors regaining independent renal function.[9,10]

Renal replacement modalities

A wide and increasing variety of dialytic strategies are now available to manage ARF. These may be extracorporeal, using an external circuit and an artificial membrane, or instead utilize the abdominal cavity and the peritoneal membrane. The actual technique used may be predominantly diffusion-based (hemodialysis and peritoneal dialysis), convection-based (hemofiltration), or a combination of both processes (hemodiafiltration). While technically the term "dialysis" refers to a pure diffusion-based technique, it is commonly used as the collective term for all forms of renal replacement therapy. We follow this convention, and use the term "hemodialysis" to distinguish the specific diffusion-based extracorporeal modality.

Intermittent hemodialysis (initially daily, then often alternate-day), relatively short duration (3–4 h) treatments remains the commonest dialysis regimen for the management of ARF. In a survey of 831 US nephrologists 70% used intermittent hemodialysis in over 75% of cases requiring acute dialysis.[11] The presence of hemodynamic instability or the need to achieve large-scale volume removal mitigates against standard intermittent dialysis and usually leads to one of the above techniques being prescribed on a near-continuous basis. These continuous modalities require specialized equipment and are discussed and compared with intermittent dialysis in Chapter 8.

Extended duration dialysis

A more recent development has been a hybrid form of extended duration, frequent dialysis. This is performed using standard intermittent hemodialysis equipment but with much slower dialysate and blood flow rates than usual, thus improving hemodynamic tolerance, while requiring less intensive nurse supervision. Two similar approaches to this have been recently explored: extended daily dialysis (EDD) and sustained low-efficiency dialysis (SLED). EDD uses 6–8 h treatment periods, with prescribed blood flows of 200 mL/min and dialysate flows of 300 mL/min. This low-intensity intervention enables one nephrology nurse to monitor two patients undergoing treatment at a given time, reviewing them routinely every 15–30 min. Treatments were well tolerated with median (range) ultrafiltration rates of 3 (1.8–4.4) L/day.[12] In SLED therapy, dialysis is prescribed for 12 h with blood flows of 200 mL/min and dialysate flow rates of 100 mL/min. In a report of 145 treatments in 37 patients with ARF, a mean (± standard deviation) ultra-filtration rate was 2.8 ± 1.5 L per treatment, with an average phosphate removal of 1.5 g per session. Once the program was established the therapy was successfully used pre-dominantly at night-time, thus minimizing scheduling conflicts. Treatment was stopped prematurely in 34% of cases, most commonly due to the circuit clotting or due to intractable hypotension.[13] A rigorous comparison of these several different dialytic strategies is not available, and the techniques used in a given situation usually depend more on available equipment, nursing resources, and local expertise than on evidence-based considerations.

Elective initiation of dialysis

The absolute indications for hemodialysis are well established and represent the presence of uncontrolled uremic toxicity that is refractory to conservative management. Such complications include life-threatening hyper-kalemia, acidosis, fluid overload, or the development of uremic pericarditis or encephalopathy. However, in patients with progressive azotemia the optimal time-point at which to electively start dialysis is unestablished. Many physicians use a blood urea nitrogen (BUN) of 100 as a relative indication for starting dialysis; however, the sensitivity and specificity of this empiric cutoff is unknown.

Prophylactic dialysis

Several studies in the early 1960s attempted to examine the benefit of starting dialysis at a standard predetermined BUN, rather than waiting for the development of the usual absolute or relative indications.[14] Methodologic limita-tions in the design of these studies together with sub-sequent technologic advances limit the relevance of these important early studies to current clinical practice. Based on the available data, we believe that there is no com-pelling evidence supporting prophylactic dialysis using the same universal cutoff level for all patients.

Medical management

Conservative measures may be used to delay dialysis, either in the hope of a spontaneous renal recovery, or to allow the clinical situation to stabilize. However, these measures are of only limited effectiveness and subject the patient to the risk of progressive uremia, as well as to adverse effects of the conservative interventions. Thus, the use of exchange resins may predispose to subacute intestinal obstruction, especially in postsurgical patients,[15,16] the infusion of sodium bicarbonate may precipitate pulmonary edema, while prolonged high-dose diuretics may induce ototoxicity. Although alkali therapy has been traditionally used in the treatment of hyperkalemia, it is usually ineffective for this purpose in the setting of established renal failure.[17]

Renal replacement versus renal support

A major influence on whether to pursue conservative measures or instead electively initiate dialysis is whether renal failure develops as an isolated problem or occurs in the presence of severe comorbidities or multiorgan dysfunction. In the former situation, the essential goal is to palliate the uremic syndrome, while waiting for a spontaneous renal recovery. This usually leads, at least initially, to a more conservative approach and to the aggressive use of nondialytic strategies, together with close sequential monitoring of the biochemical profile and the clinical status of the patient. Alternatively, in the case of multiorgan dysfunction, the overall goals of renal replacement therapy are much broader. Its purpose becomes one of renal support, through the careful use of dialysis to support the critically ill patient and so attenuate both extrarenal, as well as renal, complications.[18]

The decision to initiate dialysis should be based on an assessment of the relevant risks and benefits of renal replacement therapy as individualized to a given patient's clinical circumstances. The decision to delay initiation needs to be reevaluated on a frequent basis and the success of this process is much enhanced if the nephrologist is involved early on in the management of the high-risk patient.[19] As it becomes increasingly evident that an immediate renal recovery is unlikely and that dialysis will eventually be necessary, there is usually little benefit in subjecting the patient to the increasing risks of uncontrolled uremia by the protracted use of conservative measures.

Dialysis dose

Measurement of acute dialysis adequacy

Insufficient evidence is currently available to determine what is either the minimally adequate or the optimal dose of acute intermittent dialysis. Part of this difficulty lies with the lack of consensus regarding how to validly and reliably quantitate the provided dialysis dose in this setting. Several studies have examined the Kt/V, as is widely used in maintenance dialysis, but the marked catabolism associated with ARF and the lack of an underlying steady state contravenes the basic assumption of the formal urea kinetic model. In ARF the protein catabolic rate may rise as high as 1.7 g/kg/day and may vary on a daily basis by as much as 0.8 g/kg.[20] Furthermore, ARF patients are typically volume overloaded, making it difficult to estimate accurately the volume of distribution of urea; they may also demonstrate increased compartment disequilibrium effects.[21] As a result there are substantial challenges to using the Kt/V to quantitate acute dialysis. A preferable option is to use dialysate-based methods, such as the solute removal index (SRI).[22] This method is free of the requirement for a neutral nitrogen balance and is not influenced by intercompartmental effects or the specific dialysis modality, though an equilibrated postdialysis BUN is required to accurately estimate the urea volume of distribution; it also requires specialized equipment to allow either fractional dialysate sampling or the collection of the entire spent dialysate. In a study of 46 intermittent hemodialysis treatments in 28 consecutive patients, Evanson et al[23] found that both the traditional single-pool, variable-volume Kt/V, as well as the equilibrated Kt/V, significantly overestimated the SRI (expressed as a Kt/V equivalent), with means (± standard deviations) of 0.96 ± 0.33, 0.84 ± 0.28, and 0.56 ± 0.27 respectively.

Effect of dose on outcome

The effect of dialysis dose on outcome has been controversial. Gillum et al[24] found no influence of intensive versus nonintensive dialysis on patient survival, although there was a decreased risk of gastrointestinal bleeding. Paganini and colleagues[25] retrospectively reviewed the records of 844 patients and assessed comorbidity using the Cleveland Clinic Comorbidity Scale and dialysis dose using Kt/V. They failed to find a dose–survival effect in patients who had either a very high or a near-normal degree of comorbidity, but a significant association between dose and survival was evident for patients with intermediate degrees

of comorbidities. More recently a dose–outcome association has been shown in a randomized trial of continuous hemofiltration,[7] as well as in a trial of intermittent hemodialysis[8] (Table 7.1). These data support the contention that the more intensive provision of dialysis may improve patient outcomes at least for some patients with ARF.

Prescribed versus delivered dose

While the optimal acute dialysis dose is unknown, it is clear that the provided dose is frequently significantly less than that prescribed.[8,14] Evanson et al[26] found that, although 49% of ARF patients were prescribed a Kt/V of less than 1.2, 70% had a delivered Kt/V that was below this level. The various factors contributing to this discrepancy are outlined in Table 7.2.

Hemodialysis technique

Angioaccess
Access site

The National Kidney Foundation–Kidney Disease Outcomes Quality Initiative (NKF-K/DOQI) practice guidelines recommend that acute hemodialysis access be initially obtained by direct percutaneous placement of either a cuffed or a noncuffed, double-lumen catheter into the femoral, internal jugular, or subclavian vein.[27] The femoral vein is technically the easiest to cannulate, and is associated with the least risk of serious complication. In addition, bleeding from inadvertent arterial puncture can be readily controlled by direct pressure, making it especially suitable in coagulopathic patients. It is essential that an appropriate length femoral catheter is used so that

Table 7.1 Effect of dose of dialysis on outcome of acute renal failure

Reference	Randomized	Subjects enrolled (analyzed)	Interventions	Severity	Oliguria (%)	Age (years)	Patient survival (%)	Renal survival (%)	Duration of dialysis
Schiffl et al[8]	No	160 (146)	*Intermittent HD*	*AP III*					
			Alternate day	85	31	61	28**	NA	16
			Daily	89	36	59	46	NA	9***
Ronco et al[7]	Yes	425 (425)	*CVVH*	*AP II*				*Survivors*	
			20 ml/h/kg	22	100	61	41 ref	95	NA
			35 ml/h/kg	24	100	59	57***	92	NA
			45 ml/h/kg	22	100	63	58***	90	NA
Gillum et al[24]	No	36 (36)	*Pre dialysis*						
			BUN < 100 mg/dL	NA	61	56	48	NA	22
			BUN < 60 mg/dL	NA	72	56	59	NA	23

AP II, APACHE II score; AP III, APACHE III score; BUN, blood urea nitrogen; CVVH, continuous venovenous hemofiltration; HD, hemodialysis; NA, not available; ref, reference category.
Outcomes were not significantly different unless otherwise indicated: **$P < 0.01$; ***$P < 0.001$.

Table 7.2 Factors contributing to underdialysis in acute renal failure

Inadequate prescribed dialysis dose
Dialysis prescription inadequate for patient's needs
Insufficient staff/equipment

Catheter dysfunction
Positional
Fibrin sheath
Vascular stenosis
Access thrombosis

Excess recirculation
Use of inappropriate length catheters
Use of catheter with the lines reversed
Central or local vascular stenosis

Decreased dialyzer function
Inadequate anticoagulation

Failure to allow for down time
Time spent changing the system
Failure to restart after late treatment thrombosis

Early discontinuation
Cardiovascular instability
Scheduling conflicts

the tip reaches the inferior vena cava. At blood flows of 230 mL/min, the mean percentage recirculation using a femoral catheter of less than 20 cm was 26.3% compared with 8.3% using catheters longer than 20 cm ($P = 0.007$).[28] Thoracic catheters should extend at least into the superior vena cava, and typically have significantly less mean recirculation than femoral catheters (0.4% vs. 13.1%, $P < 0.001$).[28] Attempted cannulation of the subclavian vein is associated with higher risk of both immediate (pneumothorax, vessel trauma, hemorrhage) and long-term complications. Subclavian vein stenosis may develop in up to 50% of patients following temporary catheterization,[29] though half of these cases may show spontaneous recannulization within 3 months of catheter removal.[30] The stenosis rate associated with tunneled internal jugular catheters is much lower, 10% in one study.[31] The use of a curved extension with internal jugular catheters, so that the catheter sits over the anterior chest wall, increases patient comfort and decreases catheter mobility and thereby possibly attenuates the complication rate. In view of the above, our personal preference for acute dialysis access is to use the right internal jugular or either femoral vein, the latter especially in high-risk patients, followed by the left internal jugular vein, and to avoid using a subclavian access whenever possible. Patients with femoral catheters should remain on bed rest, and even then we prefer to use the catheter for no more than 48 to 72 h, except in immobilized and closely monitored ICU patients. If dialysis is likely to extend beyond several days, early placement of a tunneled internal jugular catheter should be considered, unless the patient is bacteremic.[27]

The use of portable ultrasound machines, either to identify aberrant anatomy before the procedure or to insert the catheter under direct vision, increases both the first-pass and overall cannulation success rates, while decreasing both the procedure time and the immediate complication rate.[32] Its benefits are supported by a metaanalysis of trials examining nontunneled catheter placement in intensive care.[33]

Catheter outcomes

Temporary hemodialysis catheters have been shown to be an independent risk factor for the development of septicemia.[34] In a study of 168 temporary dialysis catheters, used for a mean of 17.8 days, the cumulative incidence of catheter infection was 21.4%;[35] in another study of 105 noncuffed thoracic catheters (75% subclavian), the bacteremia rate was 6.5 infections per 1000 catheter days, with a linear increase in risk with increased duration of catheterization.[36] In a prospective study of 318 new catheter insertions, Oliver et al[37] found a cumulative incidence of bacteremia of 5.4% after 3 weeks for internal jugular catheters compared with 10.7% after only 1 week with femoral catheters. The relative risk (95% confidence interval) for bacteremia associated with femoral versus internal jugular catheter infection was 3.1 (1.8–5.2). The presence of an exit site infection is a major risk factor for the development of bacteremia, the incidence of which increased from 1.9% on the first day to 13.4% on the second day of the exit site infection.[37]

Empiric antibiotic treatment of catheter-related infections should cover both Gram-positive and Gram-negative bacteria and must take into account local patterns of antimicrobial resistance. Therapy should be adjusted as necessary when sensitivities become available and vancomycin avoided where possible. Tunneled catheters may be initially treated by antibiotics and subsequently exchanged over a wire, but infection of a noncuffed catheter should be treated by catheter removal.[27] Prospective studies support the use of aqueous chlorhexidine at the time of catheter insertion,[38] the use of povidone-iodine at the time of dressing change,[39] and the use of a nonocclusive dressing.[40] The potential benefits of particular catheter materials, and use of antibiotic-impregnated catheters or antimicrobial intraluminal packing protocols are currently under investigation.

Anticoagulation

Anticoagulation is usually necessary in extracorporeal dialysis to prevent dialyzer thrombosis. Progressive clotting leads to increased blood loss, decreased dialyzer efficiency, and additional costs if replacing the dialysis circuit and/or dialyzer becomes necessary. In ARF, the risk for generalized and localized bleeding often precludes the use of systemic anticoagulation. Several alternative strategies to systemic heparinization are available that try to limit dialyzer thrombosis while minimizing the associated risk of hemorrhage (Table 7.3).[41,42] The decision as to which to use depends on physician experience, available

Table 7.3 Anticoagulation strategies in intermittent hemodialysis

Anticoagulation modality	Complexity	Monitoring	Advantages	Disadvantages
Predialysis heparin Dialyzer prerinsed with 20 000 units heparin in 2 L, then flushed with 2 L normal saline	+	None	Easy to use	Increased preparation time
Low-dose systemic heparin Initial bolus 10–25 units/kg, then 5–10 units/kg/h adjusted to ACT of 125–150%	++	ACT	Short duration of effect	Persistent bleeding risk HIT
Regional heparinization Full-dose heparin infused pre dialyzer, neutralized post dialyzer by protamine	+++	ACT	Decreased systemic anticoagulation	Rebound anticoagulation Protamine allergy
Low molecular weight heparin Single bolus pre dialysis (e.g. Dalteparin 5000 units for a 70 kg man)	+	Factor Xa		HIT
Low mocular weight heparinoids Single dose pre dialysis (e.g. Danaproid 34.4 anti-Xa units/kg)	+	Factor Xa	Can use with heparin allergy	Long half-life (~ 24 h)
Regional citrate anticoagulation Infuse trisodium citrate or citrate dextrose A pre dialyzer, with calcium-free dialysate Separate calcium infusion	+++	ACT Ca^{2+}	Highly effective Can use with heparin allergy	Metabolic alkalosis Hypocalcemia
Prostacyclin Constant infusion of 4–5 ng/kg/min	++	None	Can use with heparin allergy Short half-life	Dose-related hypotension Flushing/GI symptoms
Anticoagulation-free dialysis Use high blood flows Regular saline flushes	++	None	Suitable for high-risk patients	Requires close monitoring Blood transfusion difficult Increased dialyzer clotting

ACT, activated clotting time; GI, gastrointestinal; HIT, heparin-induced thrombocytopenia.

resources, and an assessment of the individual patient's risk of bleeding (e.g. recent surgery or preexisting coagulopathy) and the potential consequences of such hemorrhage (e.g. the presence of pericarditis). Several novel additional anticoagulant strategies have been described but are not in widespread use for dialysis, such as serine protease inhibitors, recombinant hirudin, and dermatan sulfate.

Dialysate

Acetate-based dialysate should be avoided in acute dialysis because its several disadvantages (hypoxemia, hypotension, initial exacerbation of acidosis) outweigh the modest benefits of being relatively inexpensive and easy to administer. The need for large volumes of dialysate with standard intermittent hemodialysis, often 120 L or more per treatment, can be greatly reduced by regenerating the dialysate, as in the Sorbent® system.[43] However, this technique is complicated to use and achieves lower clearance rates than standard hemodialysis. Alternatively, the requirement for large volumes of substitution fluid with filtration-based modalities can be avoided by the online generation of replacement fluid and dialysate.[44]

Dialysis membranes

A large and ever-increasing range of dialyzers are currently available for dialysis; these differ in their surface area, composition, behavior, and cost. The initial dialyzers developed were made from cellulose, the structure of which resembles the bacterial cell wall and which activates complement via the alternative pathway. Progressive substitution of the hydroxy groups on the surface of the cellulose membrane (substituted cellulose) greatly attenuates this capability. Alternatively, an entirely synthetic noncellulose-based material may be used. Such membranes are typically more permeable to water (high flux) and show much less activation of complement compared with either of the other two membrane types, but they are substantially more expensive to manufacture. Synthetic low-flux membranes and substituted cellulose high-flux membranes have now been developed, and thus the type of membrane material used no longer indicates the degree of solute or water flux.[45]

The nature and consequences of blood–membrane (bioincompatiblity) interactions have been extensively studied.[46] These interactions are implicated in several of the common complications of acute dialysis, including hypoxemia, hypotension, dialyzer reactions, delayed renal recovery, malnutrition, and immune dysregulation. In addition to complement activation, several other blood–membrane interactions may contribute to the development of these complications, including adsorption of proteins on to the dialyzer surface, altered cytokine transcription by macrophages and neutrophils, and activation of coagulation and contact pathways. While the term "biocompatibility" is usually used in reference to complement activation and release of C3a and C5a, this convention is purely arbitrary and the nature and relative severity of blood–membrane interactions depends on both membrane composition and the particular humoral or cellular system examined. Thus the highly "biocompatible" AN69 membrane is a potent activator of the contact pathway, which predisposes to dialyzer reactions;[47] and although the polymethylmethacrylate (PMMA) membrane shows significantly greater degrees of complement activation than cellulose acetate membranes, the degree of neutrophil activation for both membranes is similar.[48]

Hemodialysis complications

Disequilibrium syndrome

The dialysis disequilibrium syndrome is a constellation of symptoms that occur when patients with severe, often longstanding, azotemia are initially dialyzed in an overly intensive fashion. Symptoms start during or soon after dialysis and may include muscle cramps, restlessness, headaches, nausea, vomiting, and blurred vision. In early reports, pre 1970, generalized seizures and coma were attributed to the syndrome but these are distinctly rare in current clinical practice. Risk factors for developing disequilibrium include extremes of age (pediatric and geriatric populations), intracranial pathology, hepatic

encephalopathy, and recent brain surgery or trauma.[49] While typically complicating the initiation of dialysis, low-grade symptoms may occur in maintenance dialysis patients. The etiology of disequilibrium is believed to relate to cerebral edema, though the exact pathophysiology remains controversial.[50] There is no diagnostic test and the diagnosis is thus one of exclusion. The syndrome is prevented by gradually escalating the intensity of the initial dialysis treatments; one approach to this end is outlined in Table 7.4. Sodium modeling, by dialyzing against a relatively high sodium concentration at the start of dialysis, when the rate of urea removal is highest, helps prevent a sudden decrease in plasma osmolality and resulting cellular edema. Mannitol infusions have been used with a similar rationale, in both the prevention and treatment of severe cases. In high-risk patients an alternative option is to use a low-intensity, continuous dialysis modality. Disequilibrium symptoms, especially when mild, are usually self-limiting and only require symptomatic treatment.

Dialysis reactions
IgE-mediated reactions

Type I hypersensitivity dialyzer reactions are increasingly uncommon, possibly due to improved dialyzer degassing by manufacturers and prerinsing of the membrane immediately before use. A reaction against residual ethylene oxide is suggested by the finding of moderate to high levels of circulating ethylene oxide antibodies in up to 65% of cases.[47] Management consists of discontinuation of dialysis, without rinsing back the blood within it, and the treatment of anaphylaxis with epinephrine and/or steroids as appropriate. Further exposure to ethylene oxide-sterilized membranes should be avoided.

Angiotensin-converting enzyme inhibitor reactions

Negatively charged dialysis membranes, such as AN69, cause contact pathway activation and increase circulating bradykinin levels; if used in conjunction with angiotensin-converting enzyme inhibitors (which decrease bradykinin breakdown), a rapid elevation in serum bradykinin and an anaphylactic-type reaction may develop.[47] For this reason, the aforementioned combination is best avoided in clinical practice.[51]

Table 7.4 Guidelines for the gradual initiation of dialysis in adult patients

Treatment	Day 1	Day 2	Day 3	Subsequent
Membrane size	Small	Small	Large	Large
Duration (h)	2	2.5	3	3–4
Blood flow rate (mL/min)	200	250	300	300+
Dialysate flow rate (mL/min)	500	500	800	800
Sodium modeling	Yes	Yes	Yes	Optional

Hypoxia

Intermittent hemodialysis is associated with hypoxemia by a variety of mechanisms (Table 7.5), although the relative contribution of these mechanisms remains controversial.[52] In a randomized crossover study of six patients with mild to moderate chronic obstructive airways disease, the use of cuprophane as compared to polysulfone was associated with significantly more apneic episodes (17 ± 6 vs. 10 ± 5, $P = 0.05$) and with decrements in Po_2 at 60 min of 17 ± 7 mmHg vs. 4 ± 5 mmHg ($P = 0.10$).[53] This exacerbation of hypoxemia may be reduced by the use of a low bicarbonate dialysate (29 mmol/L) as distinct from either a high bicarbonate dialysate (36 mmol/L) or an acetate dialysate.[54] A prospective randomized crossover study evaluated 10 patients who were dialyzed alternately with either a polysulfone or a cuprophane membrane and with either acetate (36 mequiv./L) or bicarbonate (33 mequiv./L) buffered dialysate.[55] All four dialyzer–dialysate combinations were associated with a decrease in arterial oxygenation but the cuprophane membrane–acetate dialysate combination, compared with the polysulfone membrane–bicarbonate dialysate combination, resulted in significantly more hypoxic episodes (53 vs. 32 events per treatment) and longer duration of desaturation episodes. The use of bicarbonate reduced the total number of desaturations by 70% ($P < 0.05$).[55]

Hypotension

Hemodynamic instability is the commonest complication of acute intermittent hemodialysis. Its etiology is complex and in the setting of uncontrolled azotemia the possibility of cardiac tamponade should always be considered. Dialysis-related hypotension is the principal reason for the use of an extended or continuous dialysis modality. Furthermore, hypotension results in patient discomfort and inefficient solute clearance, the latter due to both reduced solute clearance from underperfused tissues as well as the early discontinuation of dialysis. Hypotension also subjects the patient to the risk of ischemic complications and of recurrent renal ischemia.[56] Most of the objective evidence concerning the pathogenesis and management of dialysis-related hypotension is based on studies of maintenance dialysis patients. The relative efficacy and potential adverse effects of these management strategies may be quite different in a short self-limiting course of acute dialysis as compared to their long-term use in maintenance dialysis.

The pathogenesis of dialysis hypotension is multifactorial and depends on both dialytic and patient-specific influences (Table 7.6). It primarily depends on the rate of ultrafiltration relative to the rate of fluid movement from the intercellular space back into the vasculature (capillary refilling). Unfortunately the simultaneous removal of solute by dialysis decreases the serum osmolality and thus reduces capillary refilling. In addition, the dialysis procedure itself may impair the normal cardiac and neurohumoral compensatory responses to a drop in blood pressure and thus may further exacerbate the severity of the hypotensive episode.

Assessing intravascular volume

Estimation of volume status is particularly challenging in the acutely ill patient. The presence of hypoalbuminemia, multiorgan failure, and the accumulation of third-space fluids may all suggest the presence of severe fluid overload,

Table 7.6 Prevention of dialysis-related hypotension

Procedure related

Ultrafiltration goal too high
Reassess clinical volume status
Hemodynamic monitoring

Ultrafiltration/solute removal rate too high
Reduce ultrafiltration rate/prolong treatment
Online blood volume monitoring
Sodium profiling
Ultrafiltration profiling
Increase capillary refilling (hypertonics)
Change dialysis modality

Impaired vasoconstriction
Avoid acetate dialysate
Decrease dialysate temperature
Midodrine
Nitric oxide inhibitors (methylene blue)
Switch to biocompatible membranes

Patient related

Impaired cardiac function
Drainage of pericardial tamponade
Inotropes
High calcium dialysate

Impaired neurohumoral reflexes
Hold blood pressure medications before dialysis
Avoid food before/during dialysis

Table 7.5 Etiology of dialysis-related hypoxemia

Etiology	Mechanism
Bicarbonate-free dialysate	CO_2 unloading causing decreased Pco_2 and decreased spontaneous ventilation
Complement activation	Pulmonary leukostasis and increased arteriolar–alveolar oxygen gradient
High dialysate bicarbonate	Temporary metabolic alkalosis and respiratory depression

while masking actual intravascular volume contraction. The intravascular volume may be assessed by invasive central venous pressure monitoring or noninvasively by the sonographic measurement of the inferior vena cava diameter,[57] though the latter may be misleading in patients with severe heart failure.[58] Real-time assessment of changes in blood volume can also be measured by a variety of techniques including the online optical measurement of hematocrit.[59] Using these techniques, some though not all investigators have reported changes in blood volume that predict the subsequent development of hypotension.[60] The increasing sophistication of dialyzer monitoring capabilities and associated software offer the possibility of developing closed-loop biofeedback control systems. These would respond automatically to a change in blood pressure or blood volume by adjusting the dialysate sodium or temperature composition.[57] Indeed, one nonrandomized study where the ultrafiltration profile

and infusion of hypertonic saline were automatically adjusted in response to changes in blood pressure supports the potential benefit of such an approach.[61]

Dialysate profiling

The decrease in plasma osmolality and consequent decrease in capillary refilling may be attenuated by use of a high dialysate sodium concentration, which helps to maintain plasma osmolality. The resulting positive sodium balance can be minimized by the use of sodium profiling, where the dialysate sodium concentration is varied over the course of the dialysis treatment.[62] While the hemodynamic benefits of sodium modeling may be offset by the positive sodium balance, increased interdialytic fluid gains, and hypertension, these adverse effects are easier to control in the acute dialysis setting. In randomized controlled trials both high sodium and profiled sodium dialysate were associated with better

Table 7.7 Recent studies in treatment/prevention of dialysis-related hypotension

Reference	No. of patients	Randomized	Crossover	Washout	Interventions	Results	
Oliver et al[63]	33	Yes	Yes	No		*Symptoms*	*Time to event*
					2 weeks: [Na] 142	30.6%	182 min
					2 weeks: profiled UF and [Na] 152 to 142	20.4%*	147 min**
Dheenan et al[64]	10	Yes	Yes	No		*BP*	*Nadir SBP*
					1 week: [Na] 138	Ref	64 ref
					1 week: [Na] 144	Fewer*	72*
					1 week: [Na] 152 to 140	Fewer*	80*
					1 week: sequential UF†	Fewer NS	66 NS
					1 week: dialysate temperature 35°C and [Na] 140	Fewer*	76*
Van der Sande[67]	9	Yes	Yes	No		*SBP‡*	*DBP‡*
					3 sessions: 33 mL 3% NaCl	−8.7 NS	−5.7 NS
					3 sessions:100 mL 20% albumin	+8.7 NS	+2.9 NS
					3 treatments: 100 mL 10% HES	+16.1*	+7.6*
Cruz et al[69]	11 of 18	No	Yes	No		*Nadir SBP*	*Nadir DBP*
					3 weeks: dialysate temperature 37°C	90.6 ref	54.9 ref
					3 weeks: midodrine	103.9**	62.3**
					3 weeks: dialysate temperature 35.5°C	102.6**	61.7**
					3 weeks: midodrine 10 mg and dialysate temperature 35.5°C	103.7**	62.6**

BP, blood pressure; DBP, diastolic blood pressure; HES, hydroxyethylstarch; [Na], dialysate sodium concentration (mequiv./L); SBP, systolic blood pressure; UF, ultrafiltration.
†Sequential UF: half ultrafiltration goal removed as isolated ultrafiltration in first hour, followed by 3 h of regular combined hemodialysis and ultrafiltration.
‡End of treatment vs. time of intervention.
*$P < 0.05$; **$P < 0.01$; ref, reference group; NS, not significant.

hemodynamic stability compared with standard dialysate (Table 7.7).[63,64] The odds ratio (95% confidence interval) for a hypotensive event with combined sodium and ultrafiltration profiling compared with use of standard dialysate was 0.61 (0.39–0.96) ($P < 0.05$).[63]

Hyperoncotic agents

Albumin is often used as a hyperoncotic agent in order to increase intravascular tonicity and promote capillary refilling. However, it is expensive and in a recent meta-analysis of its general use in patients with volume depletion, it was associated with an increased mortality.[65] An uncontrolled study of in-hospital acute dialysis used a stepwise protocol of normal saline, mannitol and, if necessary, albumin to manage hypotension and was able to significantly reduce the use of albumin.[66] A relatively inexpensive and well-tolerated colloid solution is 10% hydroxyethyl-starch, which results in at least equal efficacy in blood pressure support as albumin and which has significantly better efficacy compared with hypertonic saline.[67]

Sequential ultrafiltration

The use of sequential ultrafiltration (an initial separate period of isolated ultrafiltration followed by regular hemodialysis) may result in better tolerance of fluid removal. However, unless the dialysis time is further extended it will lead to a reduction in the already, frequently marginal, total solute clearance, while if a high ultrafiltration rate is applied it may still lead to symptomatic hypotension. In one study, in which half of the total planned fluid removal was achieved with 1 h of isolated ultrafiltration followed by 3 h of regular combined dialysis and ultrafiltration, this sequential approach was no better than standard dialysis.[64]

Impaired vasoconstriction

Several methodologically limited, small, nonrandomized studies have compared hemodynamic stability in intermittent hemodialysis, hemofiltration or hemodiafiltration, with inconclusive results.[68] These dialytic modalities differ in many aspects other than their being based on convective or diffusive processes; in particular the decrease in intravascular volume in patients on dialysis is associated with a subnormal peripheral vasoconstrictive response, thus increasing susceptibility to hypotension. This decrease is not seen with the use of convective-based therapies (isolated ultrafiltration or hemofiltration),[68] and may partially explain the potential hemodynamic superiority attributed to these modalities. Core body temperature and peripheral vasodilation increase significantly with standard hemodialysis but not with the dialysate-free modalities (isolated ultrafiltration or hemofiltration). The effect of hemodiafiltration is more variable and depends on the exact technique used. This increase in core temperature can be avoided by decreasing the dialysate temperature to 35°C (95°F) with significantly better hemodynamic stability.[64,69] The use of cooled dialysate may be limited by development of shivering, cramping, and a sensation of intolerable cold.[64] In some studies,[70] though not all,[69] its efficacy may vary depending on the patient's predialysis core temperature. Patients who are intolerant of cool dialysate may benefit from the predialysis administration of midodrine, a peripherally active α_2-receptor agonist. Midodrine is as effective as cool dialysate but conferred no additional benefits over cool dialysate alone.[69]

Nitric oxide

Beasley and Brenner[71] have suggested that the inappropriate vasodilation seen during dialysis may be mediated by the increased generation or activity of nitric oxide. The use of methylene oxide in one nonrandomized trial of hypotension-prone dialysis patients, without history of cardiac ischemia, resulted in decreased production of plasma and platelet NO_2 and NO_3 (stable breakdown products of nitric oxide) and was associated with significantly improved hemodynamic stability.[72] Interestingly in 18 patients with refractory intradialytic hypotension the use of cool dialysate was associated with both decreased NO_2 and NO_3 levels and improved mean arterial pressure, suggesting a possible role for nitric oxide modulation in the mechanism of action of cool dialysate.[73]

Inotropes

In cases of persistent hypotension, the use of cardiac inotropes and vasoactive agents, in an appropriately monitored environment, may allow treatment with intermittent hemodialysis; however, adequate volume control in this setting is usually only feasible, when there are low-level fluid requirements. A cardiac inotropic effect can also be obtained by use of high-calcium dialysate (1.75 mmol/L).[74] While use of high-calcium dialysate in chronic dialysis is limited by concerns regarding long-term consequences of a positive calcium balance, as with sodium profiling, these concerns may be less of an issue with short-term use in acute dialysis.

Change in modality

If the above corrective measures are ineffective, it remains to either reduce the net ultrafiltration goal and accept a short-term positive fluid balance, a compromise that should be of strictly limited duration, or extend the duration of the intermittent treatment thus allowing for a lower hourly ultrafiltration rate. In cases of severe volume overload, high volume intakes, and marginal hemodynamics, it is frequently necessary to change from intermittent to either a continuous or extended duration therapy.

Delayed renal recovery
Renal hypoperfusion

Dialysis, by precipitating hypotension, may induce recurrent renal ischemia and thus delay renal recovery. The kidney in established or resolving renal failure is especially susceptible to this effect due to the impaired autoregulation of renal blood flow.[56,75]

Bioincompatibility reactions

Considerable evidence suggests that the development of dialyzer–blood bioincompatiblity reactions may also

Table 7.8 Studies of membrane compatibility on recovery of renal function

Reference	No. of sites	Randomized	Patients enrolled	Patients analyzed (total)	Dialyzer†	Flux	AP II	Oliguria‡ (%)	Age (years)	Patient survival (%)	Renal survival§ (%)	Dialysis sessions	Dialysis duration (days)
Native kidney acute renal failure													
Schiffl et al[80]	1	Yes	52	26 / 26 (52)	Cuprophane / PAN	Low / High	24 / 24	31 / 31	65 / 64	35 / 62**	100 / 100	12 / 9	22 / 15
Hakim et al[81]	1	No	83	35 / 37 (72)	Cuprophane / PMMA	Low / Low	29 / 29	43 / 46	50 / 52	37 / 57*	37 / 62*	5 / 17**	11 / 33**
Himmelfarb et al[82]	4	No	NA	81 / 72 (153)	Cuprophane / PS or PMMA	Low / Low	26.4 / 28.1	43 / 46	58.0 / 57.3	46 / 57***	43 / 64***	NA / NA	NA / NA
Kurtal et al[83]	1	No	57	32 / 25 (57)	Cuprophane / Polyflux	Low / High	23 / 23	NA / NA	64 / 65	72 / 64	65 / 66	6.0 / 6.4	NA / NA
Jorres et al[84]	5	Yes	180	76 / 84 (160)	Cuprophane / PMMA	Low / Low	23.3 / 24.4	39 / 33	56.3 / 61.7	58 / 60	57 / 57	5.1 / 5.1	8.9 / 8.5
Albright et al[85]	1	No	66	33 / 33 (66)	CA / PS	Low / High	>25 36 / 30	79 / 73	>70 45% / 30%	30-day 76 / 73	30-day 58 / 39	Per week 3.2 / 3.5	NA / NA
Gastaldello et al[86]	1	Yes	162	53 / 53 / 53 (159)	PS / PS / CA	High / Low / Low	23.2 / 24.8 / 23.1	60 / 60 / 49	60.3 / 60.2 / 59.9	43 / 36 / 45	52.8 / 45.3 / 45.3	6.7 / 5.9 / 6.6	10.7 / 9.9 / 9.1

Table 7.8 Studies of membrane compatibility on recovery of renal function (cont'd)

Reference	No. of sites	Randomized	Patients enrolled	Patients analyzed (total)	Dialyzer†	Flux	AP II	Oliguria‡ (%)	Age (years)	Patient survival (%)	Renal survival§ (%)	Dialysis sessions	Dialysis duration (days)
Ponikvar et al[87]	1	Yes	75	38 34 (72)	PS PAN	Low High	21.7 22.6	40 41	61.3 62.2	18 21	26 24	8.5 7.2	11.2 10.8
Posttransplant acute renal failure													
Valeri et al[88]	1	Yes	53	18 18 (36)	Cuprophane PMMA	Low Low	NA NA	89 89	42.9 42.4	100 100	NA NA	3.6 3.6	8.9 9.5
Ramao et al[106]	1	Yes	53	24 20 (44)	Cuprophane PS	Low Low	NA NA	79 70	44.8 34.8	100 100	100 95	6.7 6.1	14.3 12.3
Woo et al[90]	1	Yes	45	23 18 (41)	PS Cuprophane	Low Low	NA	<1 L/day 100 100	39 50	100 100	91.3 83.3	7 5**	14 11

AP II, APACHE II score; NA, not available.
†Dialyzer type: CA, cellulose acetate; PAN, polyacrylonitrile; PMMA, polymethylmethacrylate; PS, polysulfone.
‡Oliguria < 400 mL/day unless otherwise stated.
§Percent renal recovery among patients who survived.
Outcomes are not significant unless otherwise indicated: *P < 0.1; **P < 0.05; ***P < 0.001.

contribute to delayed renal recovery. There was a significant delay in renal recovery, associated with increased neutrophil infiltration of the glomeruli and vasa recta, in rats that were exposed daily to blood from a cuprophane membrane compared with that from a synthetic polyacrylonitrile membrane.[76] Neutrophil activation has also been shown to prolong ARF in an isolated rat perfusion model of renal ischemia.[77] However, there was no demonstrable effect on renal outcome attributable to bioincompatible membrane exposure in rats dialyzed on the third and seventh day following bilateral renal artery ligation.[78] These disparate results may possibly be explained by differences in the timing of the exposure to the dialysis membrane relative to the induction of renal injury. In a more recent crossover study of 24 dialysis patients, there was no significant difference in the peripheral blood mononuclear cell cytokine release, neutrophil superoxide production, or cellular apoptosis with a low-flux substituted cellulose compared with a low-flux polysulfone dialyzer.[79]

To date, 11 prospective trials have investigated the effect of dialyzer biocompatibility on the recovery of renal function in patients requiring acute intermittent dialysis (Table 7.8).[80-90] Most of these studies are subject to substantial methodologic limitations including an absence of masking, nonrandomized designs, failure to conduct analysis on an intention-to-treat basis, or to adjust for sequential analyses. In addition, none of the studies have adequately controlled for the wide range of potential confounders, especially in achieved dialysis dose, while their limited sample sizes, relative to great heterogeneity of events that may influence outcome in ARF, make it unlikely that such influences were evenly distributed across groups on a purely random basis. These limitations notwithstanding, the early studies,[80-82] but not the later ones,[83,84] comparing unsubstituted cellulose with synthetic membranes found a significant benefit with the synthetic membranes, although in the work of Hakim and Himmelfarb[81,82] this benefit was limited to patients with nonoliguric renal failure. Alternatively the studies that have compared modified cellulose with synthetic membranes have uniformly failed to demonstrate any such benefit.[85-87] This last observation may relate to the larger sample size required to detect a smaller effect size or the lack of any such effect. In view of the available in vitro, animal, and human studies we do not use unsubstituted cellulose dialyzers in acute dialysis and would especially recommend avoiding them in nonoliguric patients. In our opinion there is no convincing evidence from the currently available clinical trial data of improved outcomes in ARF with the use of synthetic as compared with semisynthetic membranes, and therefore the choice as to which to use depends largely on financial considerations.

Peritoneal dialysis

Peritoneal dialysis (PD) remains an effective therapeutic tool in the management of ARF,[91] especially in patients who are not severely catabolic. Its popularity in the treatment of ARF in Europe and the USA has declined, in large part due to the ready availability of hemodialysis. It has been the traditionally used modality in pediatric populations, but with improvements in angioaccess this is no longer the case, at least in specialist centers.[92] Nevertheless, on a global basis, PD remains a widely used and effective treatment strategy for all age groups.[93,94] The potential advantages and disadvantages of PD compared with hemodialysis are shown in Table 7.9.

Acute peritoneal dialysis technique
Peritoneal access

Placement of an acute PD catheter may be done at the bedside with reasonable safety. These stiff, noncuffed stylet catheters are placed directly into the peritoneum by the Seldinger technique under local anesthesia. The risk of bowel perforation is increased in uncooperative patients or with extensive peritoneal adhesions, and may be reduced by placing the catheter under direct vision.[91] Additional complications include catheter infection, occlusion or dislodgement, and the risk of peritonitis. Though it is substantially more complicated, PD has been successfully

Table 7.9 Advantages and disadvantages of peritoneal dialysis

Advantages	Disadvantages
No angioaccess	Risk of bowel perforation at catheter insertion
Technically simple	Difficult post abdominal surgery
No anticoagulation	Less predictable ultrafiltration/solute control
Reduced risk of disequilibrium	Risk of peritonitis
Hemodynamic stability	Hyperglycemia
Biocompatible	Slow rate of solute removal
Peritoneal lavage	Diaphragmatic splinting
Central core warming in hypothermia	Dialysate amino acid/protein losses

performed on patients immediately after abdominal surgery.[95]

Peritoneal dialysate

The availability of standardized peritoneal dialysate solutions has greatly simplified the technique of standard PD. The degree of ultrafiltration is controlled by the osmotic strength of the dialysate. Standard dialysate uses dextrose as the hypertonic agent and lactate as the buffer. The glucose load may exacerbate hyperglycemia, but with adequate insulin coverage it provides a route for substantial caloric supplementation. Lactate should be avoided in fulminant liver failure and severe septic shock and an alternative bicarbonate-buffered dialysate should be used instead.[96] In addition, an amino acid-based dialysate is available which may decrease amino acid loss and improve nitrogen balance.[97]

Prescription

The commonest form of PD practiced in acute dialysis is continuous equilibrium peritoneal dialysis (CEPD), in which 2–3 L of dialysate is placed in the peritoneum, typically on a 4- to 6-hourly exchange schedule so that the composition of dialysate and blood approaches equilibrium prior to the next exchange. Typically this method provides less intense control of azotemia than is achieved with intermittent hemodialysis. The rate of solute clearance and ultrafiltration can be improved by using larger fill volumes, as tolerated, or by increasing the number of exchanges. The use of a cycler greatly facilitates more frequent exchanges and helps decrease the nursing burden associated with frequent exchanges. Several strategies have been suggested to increase efficiency of PD including tidal dialysis, where a proportion of the dwelling dialysate is continuously replaced with fresh dialysate, and continuous-flow PD, in which dialysate is constantly circulated through the abdomen for several hours a day. In a recent crossover study of mild to moderately hypercatabolic patients, the achieved Kt/V with tidal PD (2.43 ± 0.87) was significantly better than with standard CEPD (1.8 ± 0.32). Continuous-flow PD was originally described in the 1960s but was limited by the need and associated expense of using very large volumes of dialysate. In the modern form, this is avoided by recycling the dialysate after it leaves the peritoneum and then reinfusing it into the abdomen. The dialysate is recycled by dialyzing it, in turn, in an extracorporeal dialysis circuit. This technique has all the advantages of PD with greatly increased urea clearance rates;[98] however there are no currently available studies of this modality in the treatment of ARF.

Outcome prediction

The outcome for patients with ARF is influenced by the patient's background state of health, current underlying illness, the etiology of the renal dysfunction, as well as the intensity of dialysis management. Multiple prediction systems have been used to estimate the outcome of acute renal replacement therapy. These may usefully guide patient stratification for research purposes and/or assist in quality control assessments in clinical practice. These systems include either general ICU prognostic indices or ARF-specific instruments. The APACHE II has been the most widely used of the former, although its predictive value when measured on ICU admission in one study was only 58%.[3] Improved results may be obtained by using the APACHE II at the time of onset of renal failure or at the initiation of dialysis,[99] or with the use of the revised APACHE III scoring system. Several renal failure-specific scoring systems have been developed, but are based on small sample sizes, do not have split sample validation, and have poor reproducibility when used outside the institution in which they were developed. In our opinion, the most useful ARF-specific instruments to date are the Cleveland Clinic Foundation (CCF) score[100] and the Individual Severity Index (ISI) score.[101] Using a receiver–operator curve analysis the ISI has similar performance characteristics to the APACHE III.[102]

Suitability for dialysis

The question of whether to advise withholding or withdrawing renal replacement therapy is extremely difficult, raising as it does multiple, often conflicting, medical, economic, lifestyle, and ethical issues, many of which are difficult to accurately quantitate.[103] It is most problematic in a patient who is unable to express their own wishes with regard to future therapy. While none of the above prediction models are able to predict individual prognosis with sufficient reliability, except in extreme cases, they do provide a reasonable framework in which to discuss the clinically likely outcomes. In cases where the outlook appears poor but is not yet hopeless, a trial of dialysis may be useful. In such an approach, the limitations and goals of dialysis should be carefully explained and regular review dates established. To succeed and to allow the elective discontinuation of dialysis, where appropriate, the "trial of dialysis" must be viewed not as a single intervention of predetermined duration, but rather as a process where the patient, their family, and/or legal guardians are guided toward an understanding of the clinical realities and the limitations of the currently available medical technologies. Without this focused dialogue it is often impossible to achieve consensus regarding the discontinuation of dialysis.

In keeping with the increasing proportion of elderly patients in the population, the percentage of patients with ARF who are elderly has dramatically increased. The effect of age on the outcome of ARF remains controversial. Pascual and Liano[104] found that, although the incidence of ARF increased above age 80 years, disease severity and mortality rates were similar to those of patients under age 65, while the mean survival post hospitalization was 19 months in one study of patients aged over 80 years.[105] We believe that "physiologic age" strongly influences patient outcomes and needs to be carefully considered in determining optimal patient management; we equally contend that chronologic age per se should not preclude the active treatment of uremia. Instead, the decision to recommend renal replacement therapy should be based on the expectation of a clinically meaningful recovery, with the restoration of an acceptable quality of life. In the absence of this potential, regardless of the patient's age, we see no role for prolonged dialytic support.

References

1. Cole L, Bellomo R, Silvester W, et al: A prospective, multicenter study of the epidemiology, management, and outcome of severe acute renal failure in a "closed" ICU system. Am J Respir Crit Care Med 2000;162:191–196.
2. Liano F, Pascual J, the Madrid Acute Renal Failure Study Group: Epidemiology of acute renal failure: a prospective multicenter community-based study. Kidney Int 1996;50:811–818.
3. Schaefer JH, Jochimsen F, Keller F, et al: Outcome prediction of acute renal failure in medical intensive care. Intensive Care Med 1991;17:19–24.
4. Brivet FG, Kleinknecht DJ, Loirat P, et al: Acute renal failure in intensive care units. Causes, outcome, and prognostic factors of hospital mortality: a prospective, multicenter study. French Study Group on Acute Renal Failure. Crit Care Med 1996;24:192–198.
5. McCarthy JT: Prognosis of patients with acute renal failure in the intensive care unit: a tale of two eras. Mayo Clin Proc 1996;71:117–126.
6. Levy EM, Viscoli CM, Horwitz RI: The effect of acute renal failure on mortality. JAMA 1996;275:1489–1494.
7. Ronco C, Bellomo R, Homel P, et al: Effects of different doses in continuous veno-venous haemofiltration on outcomes of acute renal failure: a prospective randomized trial. Lancet 2000;355:26–30.
8. Schiffl H, Lang SM, Fischer R: Daily hemodialysis and outcome of acute renal failure. N Engl J Med 2002;346:305–310.
9. Bhandari S, Turney JH: Survivors of acute renal failure who do not recover renal function. Q J Med 1996;89:415–421.
10. Korkeila M, Ruokonen E, Takala J: Costs of care, long term prognosis and quality of life in patients requiring renal replacement therapy during intensive care. Intensive Care Med 2000;26:1824–1831.
11. Mehta RL, Letteri JM: Current status of renal replacement therapy for acute renal failure. Am J Nephrol 1999;19:377–382.
12. Kumar VA, Ceraig M, Depner TA, et al: Extended daily dialysis: a new approach to renal replacement for acute renal failure in the intensive care unit. Am J Kidney Dis 2000;36:294–300.
13. Marshall MR, Golper TA, Shaver MJ, et al: Sustained low-efficiency dialysis for critically ill patients requiring renal replacement therapy. Kidney Int 2001;60:777–785.
14. Chertow GM, Lazarus JM: Intensity of dialysis in established acute renal failure. Semin Dial 1996;9:476–480.
15. Pirenne J, Lledo-Garcia E, Benedetti E, et al: Colon perforation after renal transplantation: a single-institution review. Clin Transplant 1997;11:88–93.
16. Rashid A, Hamilton SR: Necrosis of the gastrointestinal tract in uremic patients as a result of sodium polystyrene sulfonate (Kayexalate) in sorbitol: an underrecognized condition. Am J Surg Pathol 1997;21:60–69.
17. Ahmed J, Weisberg LS: Hyperkalemia in dialysis patients. Semin Dial 2001;14:348–356.
18. Mehta RL: Indications for daily dialysis in the ICU: renal replacement vs. renal support. Blood Purif 2001;19:227–232.
19. Mehta RL, Farkas A, Pascual M: Effect of delayed consultation on outcome from acute renal failure in the ICU. J Am Soc Nephrol 1995;6:471–474.
20. Chima CS, Meyer L, Hummell AC, et al: Protein catabolic rate in patients with acute renal failure on continuous arteriovenous hemofiltration and total parenteral nutrition. J Am Soc Nephrol 1993;3:1516–1521.
21. Paganini EP: Dialysis is not dialysis! Acute dialysis is different and needs help! Am J Kidney Dis 1998;32:832–833.
22. Keshaviah P, Star RA: A new approach to dialysis quantification: an adequacy index based on solute removal. Semin Dial 1994;7:85–90.
23. Evanson JA, Ikizler TA, Wingard R, et al: Measurement of the delivery of dialysis in acute renal failure. Kidney Int 1999;55:1501–1508.
24. Gillum DM, Dixon BS, Yanover MJ, et al: The role of intensive dialysis in acute renal failure. Clin Nephrol 1986;25:249–253.
25. Paganini EP, Tapolyai M, Goormastic M, et al: Establishing a dialysis therapy/patient outcome link in intensive care unit acute dialysis for patients with acute renal failure. Am J Kidney Dis 1996;28(Suppl 3):S81–S89.
26. Evanson JA, Himmelfarb J, Wingard R, et al: Prescribed versus delivered dialysis in acute renal failure patients. Am J Kidney Dis 1998;32:731–738.
27. NKF-K/DOQI III: Clinical practice guidelines for vascular access: update 2000. Am J Kidney Dis 2001;37(Suppl 1):S137–S181.
28. Little MA, Conlon PJ, Walshe JJ: Access recirculation in temporary hemodialysis catheters as measured by the saline dilution technique. Am J Kidney Dis 2000;36:1135–1139.
29. Cimochowski GE, Worley E, Rutherford WE, et al: Superiority of the internal jugular over the subclavian access for temporary dialysis. Nephron 1990;54:154–161.
30. Hernandez D, Diaz F, Rufino M, et al: Subclavian vascular access stenosis in dialysis patients: natural history and risk factors. J Am Soc Nephrol 1998;9:1507–1510.
31. Trerotola SO, Johnson MS, Harris VJ, et al: Outcome of tunneled hemodialysis catheters placed via the right internal jugular vein by interventional radiologists. Radiology 1997;203:489–495.
32. Aslam N, Palevsky PM: Real time ultrasound for placement of dialysis catheters: a new standard of care. Semin Dial 1999;12:1–4.
33. Randolph AG, Cook DJ, Gonzales CA, et al: Ultrasound guidance for placement of central venous catheters: a meta-analysis of the literature. Crit Care Med 1996;24:2053–2058.
34. Powe NR, Jaar B, Furth SL, et al: Septicemia in dialysis patients: incidence, risk factors, and prognosis. Kidney Int 1999;55:1081–1090.
35. Hung KY, Tsai TJ, Yen CJ, et al: Infection associated with double lumen catheterization for temporary haemodialysis: experience of 168 cases. Nephrol Dial Transplant 1995;10:247–251.
36. Kairaitis LK, Gottlieb T: Outcome and complications of temporary haemodialysis catheters. Nephrol Dial Transplant 1999;14:1710–1714.
37. Oliver MJ, Callery SM, Thorpe KE, et al: Risk of bacteremia from temporary hemodialysis catheters by site of insertion and duration of use: a prospective study. Kidney Int 2000;58:2543–2545.
38. Maki DG, Ringer M, Alvarado CJ: Prospective randomised trial of povidone-iodine, alcohol, and chlorhexidine for prevention of infection associated with central venous and arterial catheters. Lancet 1991;338:339–343.
39. Levin A, Mason AJ, Jindal KK, et al: Prevention of hemodialysis subclavian vein catheter infections by topical povidone-iodine. Kidney Int 1991;40:934–938.
40. Conly JM, Grieves K, Peters B: A prospective, randomized study comparing transparent and dry gauze dressings for central venous catheters. J Infect Dis 1989;159:310–319.
41. Ouseph R, Ward RA: Anticoagulation for intermittent hemodialysis. Semin Dial 2000;13:181–187.
42. Chuang P, Parikh C, Reilly RF: A case review: anticoagulation in hemodialysis patients with heparin induced thrombocytopenia. Am J Nephrol 2001;21:226–231.
43. Shapiro WB: The current state of Sorbent hemodialysis. Semin Dial 1990;3:40–45.
44. Canaud B, Bosc JY, Leray H, et al: On-line haemodiafiltration: state of the art. Nephrol Dial Transplant 1998;13(Suppl 5):3–11.
45. Clark WC, Hamburger RJ, Lysaght MJ: Effect of membrane composition and structure on solute removal and biocompatibility in hemodialysis. Kidney Int 1999;56:2005–2015.
46. Hakim RM: Clinical implications of biocompatibility in blood purification membranes. Nephrol Dial Transplant 2000;15(Suppl 2):16–20.
47. Salem MM, Brennan JF: Anaphylactoid reactions in dialysis patients: pathogenesis and management. Semin Dial 1995;8:212–219.
48. Star RA, Kimmel PL: Biocompatibility and acute renal failure. Lancet 2000;355:314.
49. Davenport A: Renal replacement therapy in the patient with acute brain injury. Am J Kidney Dis 2001;37:457–468.
50. Arieff AI: Dialysis disequilibrium syndrome: current concepts on pathogenesis and prevention. Kidney Int 1994;45:629–635.

51. Kammerl MC, Schaefer RM, Schweda F, et al: Extracorporal therapy with AN69 membranes in combination with ACE inhibitors causing severe anaphylactoid reactions: still a current problem. Clin Nephrol 2000;53:486–488.

52. De Broe ME, De Backer WA: Pathophysiology of hemodialysis-associated hypoxemia. Adv Nephrol Necker Hosp 1989;18:297–315.

53. Navarro J, Serrano C, Donna E, et al: Disordered breathing patterns during bicarbonate hemodialysis in COPD. Effect of cuprophane versus polysulfone membranes. ASAIO Trans 1992;38:811–814.

54. Ganss R, Aarseth HP, Nordby G: Prevention of hemodialysis associated hypoxemia by use of low-concentration bicarbonate dialysate. ASAIO Trans 1992;38:820–822.

55. Munger MA, Ateshkadi A, Cheung AK, et al: Cardiopulmonary events during hemodialysis: effects of dialysis membranes and dialysate buffers. Am J Kidney Dis 2000;36:130–139.

56. Conger JD: Does hemodialysis delay recovery from acute renal failure? Semin Dial 1990;3:146–148.

57. Van der Sande FM, Kooman JP, Leunissen KM: Strategies for improving hemodynamic stability in cardiac-compromised dialysis patients. Am J Kidney Dis 2000;35:E19.

58. Mandelbaum A, Ritz E: Vena cava diameter measurement for estimation of dry weight in haemodialysis patients. Nephrol Dial Transplant 1996;11(Suppl 2):24–27.

59. Leypoldt JK, Lindsay RM: Hemodynamic monitoring during hemodialysis. Adv Renal Replacement Ther 1999;6:233–242.

60. Passauer J, Bussemaker E, Gross P: Dialysis hypotension: do we see light at the end of the tunnel? Nephrol Dial Transplant 1998;13:3024–3029.

61. Schmidt R, Roeher O, Hickstein H, et al: Prevention of haemodialysis-induced hypotension by biofeedback control of ultrafiltration and infusion. Nephrol Dial Transplant 2001;16:595–603.

62. Stiller S, Bonnie-Schorn E, Grassmann A, et al: A critical review of sodium profiling for hemodialysis. Semin Dial 2001;14:337–347.

63. Oliver MJ, Edwards LJ, Churchill DN: Impact of sodium and ultrafiltration profiling on hemodialysis-related symptoms. J Am Soc Nephrol 2001;12:151–156.

64. Dheenan S, Henrich WL: Preventing dialysis hypotension: a comparison of usual protective maneuvers. Kidney Int 2001;59:1175–1181.

65. Cochrane Injuries Group Albumin Reviewers: Human albumin administration in critically ill patients. Systematic review of randomized controlled trials. Br Med J 1998;317:235–240.

66. Emili S, Black NA, Paul RV, et al: A protocol-based treatment for intradialytic hypotension in hospitalized hemodialysis patients. Am J Kidney Dis 1999;33:1107–1114.

67. Van der Sande FM, Luik AJ, Kooman JP, et al: Effect of intravenous fluids on blood pressure course during hemodialysis in hypotensive-prone patients. J Am Soc Nephrol 2000;11:550–555.

68. Maggiore Q, Pizzarelli P, Dattolo P, et al: Cardiovascular stability during haemodialysis, haemofiltration and haemodiafiltration. Nephrol Dial Transplant 2000;15(Suppl 1):68–73.

69. Cruz DN, Mahnensmith RL, Brickel HM, et al: Midodrine and cool dialysate are effective therapies for symptomatic intradialytic hypotension. Am J Kidney Dis 1999;33:920–926.

70. Fine A, Penner B: The protective effect of cool dialysate is dependent on patients' predialysis temperature. Am J Kidney Dis 1996;28:262–265.

71. Beasley D, Brenner BM: Role of nitric oxide in hemodialysis hypotension. Kidney Int 1992;38(Suppl 38):s96–s100.

72. Peer G, Itzhakov E, Wollman Y, et al: Methylene blue, a nitric oxide inhibitor, prevents haemodialysis hypotension. Nephrol Dial Transplant 2001;16:1436–1441.

73. Jamil K, Yokoyama K, Takemoto F, et al: Low temperature hemodialysis prevents hypotensive episodes by reducing nitric oxide synthesis. Nephron 2000;84:284–286.

74. Van Der Sande FM, Cheriex EC, van Kuijk WH, et al: Effect of dialysate calcium concentrations on intradialytic blood pressure course in cardiac-compromised patients. Am J Kidney Dis 1998;32:125–131.

75. Solez K, Morel-Maroger L, Sraer JD: The morphology of "acute tubular necrosis" in man: analysis of 57 renal biopsies and a comparison with the glycerol model. Medicine (Baltimore) 1979;58:362–376.

76. Schulman G, Fogo A, Gung A, et al: Complement activation retards resolution of acute ischemic renal failure in the rat. Kidney Int 1991;40:1069–1074.

77. Linas S, Whittenburg D, Parsons PE, et al: Mild renal ischemia activates primed neutrophils to cause acute renal failure. Kidney Int 1992;42:610–616.

78. Kranzlin B, Reuss A, Gretz N, et al: Recovery from ischemic acute renal failure: independence from dialysis membrane type. Nephron 1996;73:644–651.

79. Jaber BL, Cendoroglo M, Balakrishnan VS, et al: Impact of dialyzer membrane selection on cellular responses in acute renal failure: a crossover study. Kidney Int 2000;57:2107–2116.

80. Schiffl H, Lang SM, Konig A, et al: Biocompatible membranes in acute renal failure: prospective case-controlled study. Lancet 1994;344:570–572.

81. Hakim RM, Wingard RL, Parker RA: Effect of the dialysis membrane in the treatment of patients with acute renal failure. N Engl J Med 1994;331:1338–1342.

82. Himmelfarb J, Rubin NT, Chandran P, et al: A multicenter comparison of dialysis membranes in the treatment of acute renal failure requiring dialysis. J Am Soc Nephrol 1998;9:257–266.

83. Kurtal H, von Herrath D, Schaefer K: Is the choice of membrane important for patients with acute renal failure requiring hemodialysis? Artif Organs 1995;19:391–394.

84. Jorres A, Gahl GM, Dobis C, et al: Hemodialysis-membrane biocompatibility and mortality of patients with dialysis-dependent acute renal failure: a prospective randomised multicentre trial. Lancet 1999;354:1337–1341.

85. Albright RC, Smelser JM, McCarthy JT, et al: Patient survival and renal recovery in acute renal failure: randomized comparison of cellulose acetate and polysulfone membrane dialyzers. Mayo Clin Proc 2000;75:1141–1147.

86. Gastaldello K, Melot C, Kahn R, et al: Comparison of cellulose diacetate and polysulfone membranes in the outcome of acute renal failure. A prospective randomized study. Nephrol Dial Transplant 2000;15:224–230.

87. Ponikvar JB, Rus RR, Bren AJ, et al: Low-flux versus high flux synthetic dialysis membrane in acute renal failure: prospective randomized study. Artif Organs 2001;25:946–950.

88. Valeri A, Radhakrishnan J, Ryan R, et al: Biocompatible dialysis membranes and acute renal failure: a study in post operative acute tubular necrosis in cadaveric renal transplant recipients. Clin Nephrol 1996;46:402–409.

89. Romao JE, Jr., Fadil MA, Sabbaga E, et al: Haemodialysis without anticoagulant: haemostasis parameters, fibrinogen kinetic, and dialysis efficiency. Nephrol Dial Transplant 1997;12:106–110.

90. Woo YM, Craig A, King BB, et al: Biocompatible membranes do not promote graft recovery following cadaveric renal transplantation. Clin Nephrol 2002;57:38–44.

91. Ash SR: Peritoneal dialysis in acute renal failure of adults: the safe, effective, and low-cost modality. Contrib Nephrol 2001;132:210–221.

92. Gong W, Tan T, Foong P, et al: Eighteen years experience in pediatric acute dialysis: analysis of predictors of outcome. Pediatr Nephrol 2001;16:212–215.

93. Chitalia VC, Almeida AF, Rai H, et al: Is peritoneal dialysis adequate for hypercatabolic acute renal failure in developing countries? Kidney Int 2002;61:747–757.

94. Chugh KS, Jha V, Chuhg S: Economics of dialysis and transplantation in the developing world. Transplant Proc 1999;31:3275–3277.

95. Hajarizadeh H, Rohrer MJ, Herriman JB, et al: Acute peritoneal dialysis following ruptured abdominal aortic aneurysms. Am J Surg Pathol 1995;170:223–226.

96. Thongboonkerd V, Lumlertgul D, Supajatura V: Better correction of metabolic acidosis, blood pressure control, and phagocytosis with bicarbonate compared to lactate solution in acute peritoneal dialysis. Artif Organs 2001;25:99–108.

97. Kopple JD, Bernard D, Messana J, et al: Treatment of malnourished CAPD patients with an amino acid based dialysate. Kidney Int 1995;47:1148–1157.

98. Ronco C: Continuous flow peritoneal dialysis: is there a need for it? Semin Dial 2001;14:395–400.

99. Parker RA, Himmelfarb J, Tolkoff-Rubin N, et al: Prognosis of patients with acute renal failure requiring dialysis: results of a multicenter study. Am J Kidney Dis 1998;32:432–443.

100. Chertow GM, Lazarus JM, Paganini EP, et al: Predictors of mortality and the provision of dialysis in patients with acute tubular necrosis. J Am Soc Nephrol 1998;9:692–698.

101. Liano F, Gallego A, Pascual J, et al: Prognosis of acute tubular necrosis: an extended prospectively contrasted study. Nephron 1993;63:21–31.

102. Douma CE, Redekop WK, van der Meulen J, et al: Predicting mortality in intensive care patients with acute renal failure treated with dialysis. J Am Soc Nephrol 1997;8:111–117.

103. MacKay K, Moss AH: To dialyze or not to dialyze: an ethical and evidence-based approach to the patients with acute renal failure in the intensive care unit. Adv Renal Replacement Ther 1997;4:288–296.

104. Pascual J, Liano F: Causes and prognosis of acute renal failure in the very old. Madrid Acute Renal Failure Study Group. J Am Geriatr Soc 1998;46:721–725.

105. Akposso K, Hertig A, Couprie R, et al: Acute renal failure in patients over 80 years old: 25-years' experience. Intensive Care Med 2000;26:400–406.

106. Ramao JE, Abensur H, de Castro MC, et al: Effect of dialyser biocompatibility on recovery from acute renal failure after cadaveric renal transplantation. Nephrol Dial Transplant 1999;14:709–712.

Continuous Dialysis Treatments

Claudio Ronco, Alessandra Brendolan, and Rinaldo Bellomo

1. excellent clinical tolerance;
2. excellent capacity for blood purification of different molecules;
3. optimal correction of electrolyte disorders;
4. optimal correction of acid–base disorders;
5. excellent biocompatibility with minimal or no proinflammatory effects;
6. minimal or absent adverse effects, including a negative impact on recovery of the native organ function;
7. possibly improved outcomes;
8. easy institution and easy monitoring of treatment.

Most of these targets have been achieved with the use of continuous therapies. This is especially true of the most recent techniques in which the treatment dose and the applied technology have been optimized.

In order to appreciate the state of the art in the field of CRRT, a short historical review may be useful and appropriate. Since the original description of the different techniques, new modifications have been successfully applied. However we feel that it is important to understand the basic concepts underlying each single technique to better interpret the possible advantages and to better target the prescription of the selected therapy.

Acute renal failure and the need for renal replacement

Acute renal failure is often complicated by multiorgan dysfunction, especially in intensive care patients. Thus the clinical scenario is different from the syndrome typically observed in renal wards. Patients are critically ill and several organ systems are involved in the syndrome. Frequently sepsis and a multiorgan dysfunction syndrome complicate the clinical picture. Under such circumstances, adequate renal replacement therapy must be instituted to provide effective blood purification and correction of the various homeostatic disorders.[1] Standard hemodialysis or peritoneal dialysis have displayed significant limitations in these patients, while continuous renal replacement therapies (CRRT) are rapidly gaining consensus and displaying interesting clinical advantages. The critically ill patient presents with severe hemodynamic instability, sepsis, and septic shock; he or she may require mechanical ventilation, cardiac mechanical support, and other types of vital supports. In these conditions, intermittent hemodialysis appears to produce further hemodynamic instability and only partial correction of the uremic syndrome.[2] Peritoneal dialysis on the other hand may cause mechanical and infectious complications and is limited by the low clearances and ultrafiltration rates. Under these circumstances the logical approach is one of providing a therapy with the following characteristics.

Historical review

In 1977, Peter Kramer described a new technique he called continuous arteriovenous hemofiltration (CAVH).[3] The system originated from an accidental puncture of the femoral artery instead of the femoral vein. Kramer's insight was to connect a highly permeable filter to the arterial access and to return the blood to another venous access thus creating an arteriovenous circuit without the need of a pump. The arteriovenous pressure gradient was adequate to move the blood throughout the circuit and to create sufficient hydrostatic pressure in the filter to produce a certain amount of ultrafiltration. The transmembrane pressure gradient was further increased by lowering the position of the ultrafiltrate collection bag, thus creating a negative pressure in the ultrafiltrate compartment. Blood purification was obtained exclusively by convection and the ultrafiltrate produced was totally or partially replaced with fresh solutions. Anticoagulation was achieved by infusion of heparin in the arterial line. Since that time, several modifications and new techniques have been developed and classified as CRRT.[4]

The low efficiency of CAVH stimulated the use of countercurrent dialysate flow in low-permeable dialyzers (continuous arteriovenous hemodialysis) or highly permeable hemodiafilters (continuous arteriovenous hemodiafiltration).[5,6] The newer membranes allowed the combination of diffusion and convection to remove molecules with a wider spectrum of molecular weights. The arteriovenous circulation was progressively substituted with a veno-venous circulation thanks to the application of peristaltic pumps. Special techniques to reduce the risk of bleeding were developed, including the use of predilution, or the utilization of alternative agents such as citrate, low molecular weight heparin, and prostacyclin.[7] Special filters were designed for particular patients such as neonates or small infants,[8] and heparin-coated membranes were made available for special treatment conditions. The same technology was applied to catheters and lines in order to achieve a completely antithrombogenic surface throughout the whole circuit. finally, a series of machines specifically designed to perform CRRT have been developed and the new technology spurred new interest in the use of CRRT, not only as blood purification techniques but also as possible treatments for multiorgan dysfunction syndromes and septic shock.[9,10]

Mechanisms of solute and water transport

The most important mechanisms of solute and water transport across a semipermeable membrane are diffusion, convection, and ultrafiltration.[10]

Diffusion is a process that occurs in a solution containing solute and solvent molecules. When a semipermeable membrane is placed in this solution, solute molecules that can cross the membrane move from the region where they are in high concentration to the region where they are in low concentration (Fig. 8.1). In reality, molecules move randomly. However, as they tend to reach the same concentration in the space occupied by the solvent, the number of particles crossing the membrane toward the region of lower concentration will be statistically higher. This is therefore a transport mechanism that occurs in presence of a concentration gradient for solutes whose diffusion is not restricted by the porosity of the membrane. Besides the concentration gradient (dc), the diffusion flux is influenced by the characteristics of the membrane including surface area (A) and thickness (dx), the temperature of the solution (T), and the diffusion coefficient of the solute (D). The diffusion flux of a given solute (Jx) is therefore given by equation 8.1:

$$Jx = DTA(dc/dx) \tag{8.1}$$

Using these concepts, one can estimate to a good approximation the clearance value in the presence of given solute, solvent, membrane, and operational conditions. However several factors may influence the final clearance value, leading to certain discrepancies between the theoretically expected value and the empirically obtained valure. As an example, protein binding or electrical charges on the solute may negatively affect the final clearance value. Conversely, an increased amount of convection may contribute to a greater transport of solutes especially in the higher molecular weight range.

Convection is a form of transport that requires movement of fluid across the membrane as a consequence of a transmembrane pressure (TMP) gradient. In conjunction with this fluid transport, the crystalloids present in the solution (but not the cells or colloids retained by the membrane) are transported to the other side of the membrane with a mechanism-defined solvent drag. The fluid transport is defined as ultrafiltration (Fig. 8.2) and it is described by equation 8.2:

$$Jf = Kf \times TMP \tag{8.2}$$

where Kf is the coefficient of hydraulic permeability of the membrane, and TMP = $P_b - P_{uf} - \pi$, where P_b is the hydrostatic pressure of blood, P_{uf} the hydrostatic pressure of ultrafiltrate or dialysate, and π the oncotic pressure generated by plasma proteins in the blood.

The convective flux of a given solute x therefore depends on the amount of ultrafiltration (Jf), the concentration of the solute in plasma water (C_b), and the sieving characteristics of the membrane for the solute (S).

$$Jx = Jf\ C_b\ (1 - s) = Jf\ S \tag{8.3}$$

Under theoretical conditions, the sieving coefficient (S) is regulated by Stavermann's reflection coefficient of the membrane (σ) according to equation 8.4:

$$S = 1 - \sigma \tag{8.4}$$

In the clinical practice, however, as plasma proteins and other factors tend to interfere with the original reflection

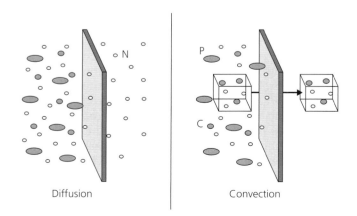

Figure 8.1 Mechanisms of solute removal in different blood purification techniques.

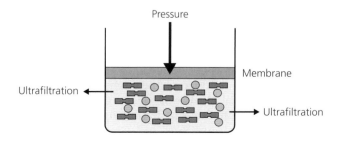

Figure 8.2 Mechanism of ultrafiltration in response to a transmembrane pressure gradient.

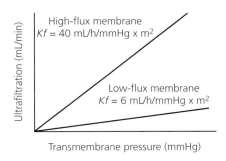 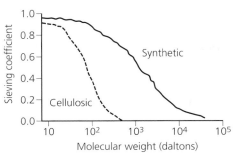

Figure 8.3 Characteristics of dialysis membranes.

coefficient of the membrane, the final observed sieving coefficient always tends to be smaller than that expected from a simple theoretical calculation. Dialysis membranes are classified according to their ultrafiltration coefficient and solute sieving profile in high flux and low flux (Fig. 8.3).

In clinical practice, membranes are mounted on specific devices designed to optimize the performance of the membrane itself. These devices may be designed as either dialyzers, which work generally by diffusion with a countercurrent flux of blood and dialysate, or hemofilters, which work generally by convection. Thanks to the most recent design of membranes, diffusion and convection can be conveniently combined leading to therapies defined as high-flux dialysis or hemodiafiltration where the advantages of both mechanisms are significantly enhanced.

CRRT techniques

Several CRRT techniques are available. These may differ in terms of vascular access and extracorporeal circuit design, frequency and intensity of treatment, mechanism of transport utilized, and type of membrane.[11]

The following descriptions are mostly based on the type of equipment utilized, the operational parameters normally employed, and the target efficiency as far as solute and fluid control are concerned. Most techniques can be performed in either arteriovenous or venovenous mode. The schematic representations presented in the Figures are simple reconstructions of all the components of each technique. The machines illustrated are just examples of an entire family of dedicated equipment available on the market. Finally, a brief description of the most common clinical indications completes the review of the available CRRT techniques.

Arteriovenous or venovenous slow continuous ultrafiltration

Slow continuous ultrafiltration is a treatment typically employed continuously or for only a few hours a day with an arteriovenous or venovenous access (with pump) (Fig. 8.4). The treatment is carried out with high-flux membranes and the objective is to achieve volume control in fluid-overloaded patients. The operational parameters

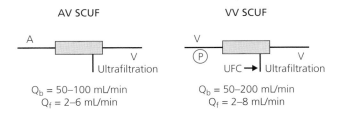

Figure 8.4 Arteriovenous (AV) and venovenous (VV) slow continuous ultrafiltration (SCUF). A, artery; V, vein; P, pump; UFC, ultrafiltrate control provided by a pump or a simple clamp; Q_b, blood flow; Q_f, ultrafiltration rate.

are generally those described in Fig. 8.4. As low filtration rates are required, filters with small surface area are generally employed. When the system is utilized in arteriovenous mode, ultrafiltration is somehow self-limited. When a blood pump is utilized, an ultrafiltration control system should be applied in order to prevent excessive ultrafiltration. Because of the low filtration rates, the treatment is suitable for volume control but not blood purification.

Arteriovenous or venovenous continuous hemofiltration

Continuous hemofiltration is normally applied for an extended period of time up to several weeks. The treatment can be performed in arteriovenous or venovenous mode (Fig. 8.5).

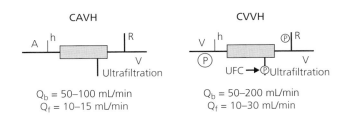

Figure 8.5 Continuous arteriovenous hemofiltration (CAVH) and continuous venovenous hemofiltration (CVVH). A, artery; V, vein; h, heparin; R, reinfusion; P, pump; Uf, ultrafiltrate; UFC, ultrafiltrate control; Q_b, blood flow; Q_f, ultrafiltration rate.

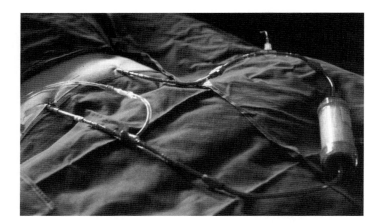

Figure 8.6 Representation of a typical CAVH extracorporeal circuit.

The technique utilizes high-flux membranes and the principal mechanism of solute transport is convection. The operational conditions are described in Fig. 8.5. Ultrafiltration in excess of the amount required for volume control is produced and it is partially or totally replaced by fresh substitution fluid. In CAVH (Fig. 8.6), blood flow is regulated by the arteriovenous pressure gradient and the circuit must be designed to prevent any unnecessary resistance to the circulation. Under these circumstances the rate of ultrafiltration may vary and may be increased by lowering the position of the ultrafiltrate collecting bag. In continuous venovenous hemofiltration (CVVH), the flow is regulated by a pump and the rate of ultrafiltration can significantly increase. In the presence of high filtration rates, systems for ultrafiltration and reinfusion control are generally utilized. Different machines use either volumetric control systems or volumetric pumps regulated by one or multiple scales. Heparin is infused in the arterial line to prevent clotting of the circuit. The replacement solution can be infused either before the filter (pre dilution) or after the filter (post dilution). In the former case, ultrafiltration must be relatively increased to maintain the same efficiency observed in postdilution mode.

Since the ultrafiltrate is replaced by the toxin-free substitution fluid, the treatment is used for blood purification and volume control. A typical machine for CVVH is equipped with an ultrafiltration pump and a scale-controlled reinfusion pump. Once blood flow is set,

average ultrafiltration should not exceed 20% of the overall blood flow rate.

Arteriovenous or venovenous continuous hemodialysis

Continuous hemodialysis is a treatment carried out over an extended period of time using either an arteriovenous access or a venovenous pump-driven circuit. The treatment originally utilized a low-flux membrane such as cuprophane and a countercurrent dialysate flow of 15–20 mL/min.[5] Because of the nature of the membrane and the gradient provided by the dialysate, the principal mechanism of solute transport in this technique is diffusion (Fig. 8.7). Ultrafiltration is obtained exactly in the range of values adequate to maintain the patient's fluid control without the requirement for fluid reinfusion. Recently, with the use of blood pumps, blood flows could be increased and so could be done with dialysate flows. For this reason, dialyzers with higher surface area and modified cellulose membranes, such as triacetate, could be used effectively.[12] When dialysate is run at low flow rates, fluid saturation is almost complete. When dialysate flow is increased despite progressive desaturation of the spent dialysate, there is an increase in small molecular weight solute clearances. In most cases, designated machines, for example the Prisma or Diapact machine, must be used to control inlet

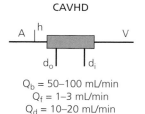

CAVHD

Q_b = 50–100 mL/min
Q_f = 1–3 mL/min
Q_d = 10–20 mL/min

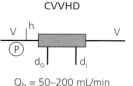

CVVHD

Q_b = 50–200 mL/min
Q_f = 1–5 mL/min
Q_d = 15–30 mL/min

CHFD

Q_b = 50–100 mL/min
Q_f = 1–5 mL/min
Q_d = 50–200 mL/min

Figure 8.7 Continuous arteriovenous hemodialysis (CAVHD), continuous venovenous hemodialysis (CVVHD) and continuous high-flux dialysis (CHFD). A, artery; V, vein; h, heparin; d_o, dialysate outlet; d_i, dialysate inlet; P, pump; Q_b, blood flow; Q_d, dialysate flow; Q_f, ultrafiltration rate.

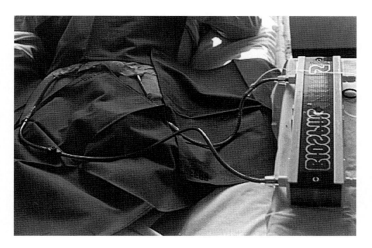

Figure 8.8 Continuous arteriovenous hemodialysis.

and outlet dialysate flows and to achieve the desired volume of ultrafiltration. Figure 8.8 illustrates continuous arteriovenous hemodialysis.

A further modification of these techniques is called continuous high-flux dialysis (CHFD).[9–13] In this technique high-flux dialyzers are utilized in a continuous hemodialysis circuit with continuous ultrafiltration volume control. Since the spontaneous filtration occurring in the hollow fiber dialyzer would be much greater than the desired fluid loss, a positive pressure is automatically applied to the dialysate compartment and the TMP gradient is reduced significantly. This in turn results in a very special pressure profile inside the dialyzer. Large amounts of filtration and consequently of convective transport are maintained in the proximal part of the hemodialyzer despite moderate net filtration. The net fluid balance is obtained thanks to a significant amount of backfiltration of fresh dialysate in the distal portion of the dialyzer. In this technique, diffusion and convection are conveniently combined.

The system can be run in either single-pass or recirculation mode and clearance of middle to high molecular weight solutes can reach values as high as 60% of those observed for small molecules like urea.

Arteriovenous or venovenous continuous hemodiafiltration

Continuous hemodiafiltration (Fig. 8.9) is carried out over an extended period of time in arteriovenous or venovenous mode. The system requires a high-flux hemodiafilter and combines the principles of hemodialysis and hemofiltration. Dialysate is circulated in countercurrent mode to blood and at the same time ultrafiltration is obtained in excess of the desired fluid loss from the patient. This is totally or partially replaced with substitution fluid, in either predilution or postdilution mode. Recent machines (Fig. 8.10) allow a combination of pre and post dilution aiming at combining the advantages of both modalities.

Since this therapy is supposed to combine the advantages of diffusion and convection, optimal clearances are expected for both small and large molecular weight solutes.

Technical aspects

The evolution of CRRT has been accompanied by a parallel evolution in the related technology. A series of double-lumen catheters has been developed in order to achieve higher blood flows with lower flow resistance and reduced risk of recirculation.[9] In some cases double-lumen catheters are substituted by twin separate catheters in order to maximize blood flow and prevent unwanted recirculation. Several machines have incorporated the heparin pump or other systems for regional heparinization and citrate anticoagulation. The most common anticoagulant remains heparin, although high blood flows and predilution techniques allow for smooth operation of CRRT without any anticoagulant in patients at risk. Regional heparinization and the use of citrate is mostly reserved for special cases, as is low molecular weight

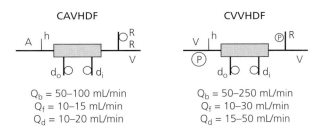

Q_b = 50–100 mL/min
Q_f = 10–15 mL/min
Q_d = 10–20 mL/min

Q_b = 50–250 mL/min
Q_f = 10–30 mL/min
Q_d = 15–50 mL/min

Figure 8.9 Continuous arteriovenous hemodiafiltration (CAVHDF) and continuous venovenous hemodiafiltration (CVVHDF) and the typical operational parameters used for these techniques. A, artery; V, vein; h, heparin; R, reinfusion; d_o, dialysate outlet; d_i, dialysate inlet; P, pump; Q_b, blood flow; Q_d, dialysate flow; Q_f, ultrafiltration rate.

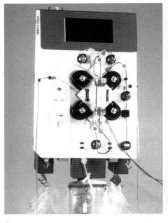
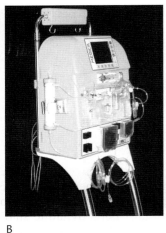
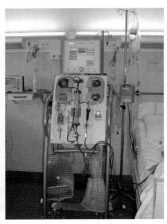

A   B   C

Figure 8.10 (A) Prisma, (B) Equasmart, and (C) Aquarius machines. The easy interface makes them suitable for most of the CRRT techniques available today.

heparin and prostacyclin. In recent years, catheters, blood lines, and filters with heparin bound on the inner surface have been developed. However their use is still experimental and requires further evaluation. Dialyzers with different membranes have been created, making it possible to choose among a variety of membrane materials. Membranes with different porosity and ultrafiltration coefficients are available.[14] There is a tendency to increase the filter surface area since the pumped circulation can operate at higher blood flows compared with arteriovenous circuits. A series of online monitoring techniques are under evaluation, including blood volume monitoring and blood temperature monitoring.[15,16] Finally, a great deal of development has taken place in the operator interface of CRRT machines. Most of these machines are equipped with large color screens and step-by-step guidelines to prime the circuit and run the treatment smoothly and effectively.

Clinical indications

The different techniques described in this chapter have been used in different settings and different clinical conditions. In those departments in which dialysis machines or CRRT equipment are not available, arteriovenous treatments still represent an important resource. In most cases, however, one or more machines, or simply different types or adapted technologies, are available and venovenous pump-driven therapies can be carried out. In this case, the indication for one technique over another is based on the knowledge of the capabilities of each technique and the clinical objectives that the clinician is seeking to achieve. If small molecule clearance is the main target, there is no point in using expensive high-flux membranes. On the other hand, if a wider spectrum of molecules is to be removed, convective therapies or combined diffusive–convective therapies should be implemented. Combination therapies are utilized more and more, especially in the setting of multiorgan failure and acute renal failure complicated by sepsis,[17] and we refer to them in the New horizons section of this chapter.

When blood purification is the main target, the efficiency of CRRT seems to be unparalleled. While inter-mittent hemodialysis displays the typical limitations imposed by the double-pool kinetics of most molecules, CRRT, despite a lower clearance, displays improved removal due to the continuous action and the steady concentration of the solutes in blood. Recent studies have demonstrated that CRRT can improve survival in acute renal failure patients if the dose of treatment is increased up to 35 mL/h/mmHg.[18] This observation has been elaborated by Gotch[19] who described this level of efficiency as the only one approaching the function of the native kidney. Comparing the efficiency of different therapies is complicated and requires special parameters of calculation, such as the standard Kt/V.[20] When comparing hemodialysis and peritoneal dialysis, weekly standard Kt/V as high as 2–2.5 can be obtained. In CRRT, standard Kt/V can be four or five times higher, displaying the enormous superiority of continuous therapies. The same concept can be described for the correction of acid–base and electrolyte derangement. By performing a continuous correction, electrolyte pools can be normalized at the same time as serum concentrations, leading to stable maintenance of an optimal homeostatic equilibrium.[2] The effect of slow and continuous water removal is the other important advantage of these therapies, since continuous refilling from the interstitial space can be obtained. Under such circumstances, overhydrated patients or patients with congestive heart failure can be treated in order to normalize or improve cardiac filling pressures, preload, and afterload, in the absence of dangerous reductions of circulating blood volume.[15]

New horizons

In the clinical scenario of acute renal failure and the application of CRRT, it is worth emphasizing that not only techniques but also the possible clinical indications are continuously evolving. As an example, there is increasing evidence that a beneficial hemodynamic effect can be obtained by CRRT in patients with multiorgan failure and septic shock. Since the explanation for some of the possible benefits seems to be the capacity of these therapies to remove chemical mediators from the patient's circulation, new studies and research have been directed toward the mechanism of humoral response to sepsis and the possibility of attenuating the immunologic disequilibrium that seems to characterize the septic patient.[21] Since some effects induced by CRRT could be related to the removal of proinflammatory mediators, this hypothesis has spurred new interest in the application of therapies with increased convection, such as high-volume hemofiltration, or with membranes characterized by increased sieving coefficients.[22]

High-volume hemofiltration

High-volume hemofiltration is a pure convective therapy that can be performed using two basic schedules.

1. Continuous hemofiltration with a fluid exchange rate > 3 L/h. In this case, if the therapy is performed for 24 h, clearances in the range of 80 L/day can be obtained. The special technical requirements of this technique are the increased blood flow rates and the availability of large volumes of substitution fluid.
2. High-volume hemofiltration can be performed for some hours (3–6) during the day exchanging 6–8 L/h while the patient continues standard CVVH for the rest of the day.

These therapies have been shown to produce a beneficial effect on the patient's hemodynamics, with a significant reduction in the requirement for vasopressor drugs.[22] The technology involved is in most cases borrowed from the chronic hemodialysis setting, although new machines can be suitable for this purpose. The large volumes of fluid exchanged may render the treatment somewhat impractical. However, new methods for online production of substitution fluid may contribute to a reduction in costs and in problems of fluid supply in the near future.

Continuous plasmapheresis–plasma exchange

Continuous plasmapheresis–plasma exchange are techniques basically derived from the classic plasma therapies of the same name, but are performed with lower flow rates and for an extended period of time. The rationale for these therapies is based on the attempt to remove plasma proteins and immunocomplexes considered to be the pathophysiologic source of the patient's disease. Since plasma is filtered across highly porous membranes, large quantities of plasma substitutes, such as fresh frozen plasma, are required for these procedures. Single or repeated sessions can be performed isolated or in conjunction with other blood purification techniques.[23]

Continuous plasmafiltration

Continuous plasmafiltration coupled with adsorption is a special technique that has been recently introduced in an attempt to combine the advantages of CRRT and continuous plasmapheresis without requiring large amounts of plasma substitutes.[24]

The technique consists of two steps. First, blood is circulated through a plasma filter and plasma filtrate is pushed by a pump through a cartridge containing a mixture of hydrophobic resin and uncoated charcoal. Second, the regenerated plasma is returned to the main circuit where blood is reconstituted and eventually dialyzed (Fig. 8.11). Because the patient's own plasma is used for reinfusion, there is no need for substitution fluids and unwanted protein losses are avoided. The technique has been effective in reducing the circulating levels of various cytokines and at the same time has allowed a significant reduction of the pharmacologic requirement to maintain hemodynamic stability.[25] The technique seems to be especially indicated in the early stages of the septic syndrome[25] (Fig. 8.12).

Continuous hemoperfusion–hemodialysis

Continuous hemoperfusion–hemodialysis is another combination therapy that has been mostly used in the past for acute intoxications[26] The technique is based on the placement of a sorbent cartridge in series with the dialyzer in an attempt to remove those toxins not removed by classic blood purification techniques.

One of the major limitations imposed by this technique was the poor biocompatibility of the sorbent. However,

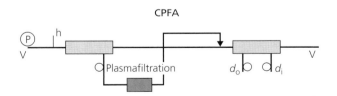

Figure 8.11 Continuous plasmafiltration. V, vein; P, pump; h, heparin; d_o, dialysate outlet; d_i, dialysate inlet.

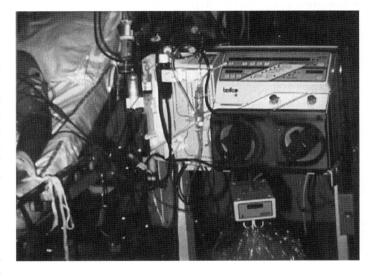

Figure 8.12 Practical application of continuous plasmafiltration.

the most recent sorbent materials are coated with biocompatible surfaces that prevent platelet trapping and clotting activation. Among the sorbent techniques, the attempt to remove circulating endotoxin with antibiotic-coated fibers should be mentioned. The cartridge contains fibers that are coated with an antibiotic (polymyxin B) with high affinity for lipopolysaccharide (LPS).[27] Critical to the success of this therapy seems to be its early application, when high levels of circulating endotoxin can be detected in plasma and the systemic effects of the humoral response to LPS have not yet occurred.

Considerations on treatment dose

Different techniques are today available for the therapy of acute renal failure in the critically ill patient. Continuous therapies seem to display important advantages in terms of clinical tolerance and blood purification capacity.[28] CRRT ensure a steady control of body weight and body hydration. Electrolyte homeostasis together with acid–base balance are well controlled due to the adjustment of the composition of the replacement solution and dialysate. Uremic intoxication is adequately controlled due to the continuous clearance. In particular, 35 mL/h per kg body weight seems to the "renal dose" at which maximal impact on outcomes can be obtained.[18] This limit, beyond which no further effects are observed in the general population, may not be the effective limit for the septic patient. In sepsis in fact, further benefits might be observed at even higher doses of treatment. Whether this is due to removal of proinflammatory mediators or to improved metabolic control is still controversial. However, this latter aspect seems to suggest that a "sepsis dose" could be different from the "renal dose" of CRRT and further studies will be devoted to clarify such a question.

The field is in continuous evolution and prospective randomized controlled trials will soon prove if there is any significant rationale for the application of CRRT and derived techniques in patients with sepsis and multiorgan dysfunction syndromes, beyond the simple indication of acute renal failure.

References

1. Bellomo R, Ronco C: Acute renal failure in the ICU: adequacy of dialysis and the case for continuous therapies. Nephrol Dial Transplant 1996;11:424–428.
2. Bellomo R, Ronco C: Continuous versus intermittent renal replacement therapy in the intensive care unit. Kidney Int 1998;53(Suppl 66):S125–S128.
3. Kramer P, Wigger W, Rieger J, Matthaei D, Scheler F: Arteriovenous hemofiltration: a new and simple method for treatment of over hydrated patients resistant to diuretics. Klin Wochenschr 1977;55:1121–1122.
4. Ronco C, Bellomo R: Continuous renal replacement therapy: evolution in technology and current nomenclature. Kidney Int 1998;53(Suppl 66):S160–S164.
5. Geronemus R, Schneider N: Continuous arterio-venous hemodialysis: a new modality for treatment of acute renal failure. ASAIO Trans 1984;30:610–613.
6. Ronco C: Arterio-venous hemodiafiltration (AVHDF): a possible way to increase urea removal during CAVH. Int J Artif Organs 1985;8:61–62.
7. Mehta RL, Dobos GJ, Ward DM: Anticoagulation in continuous renal replacement therapies. Semin Dial 1992;5:61–68.
8. Ronco C, Bellomo R: Acute renal failure in infancy: treatment by continuous renal replacement therapy. In Ronco C, Bellomo R (eds): Critical Care Nephrology. Dordrecht: Kluwer Academic Publishers, 1998, pp 1335–1350.
9. Ronco C, Bellomo R (eds): Critical Care Nephrology. Dordrecht: Kluwer Academic Publishers, 1998.
10. Ronco C, Ghezzi P, Bellomo R: New perspective in the treatment of acute renal failure. Blood Purif 1999;17:166–172.
11. Ronco C: Continuous renal replacement therapies in the treatment of acute renal failure in intensive care patients. Part 1: Theoretical aspects and techniques. Nephrol Dial Transplant 1994;9(Suppl 4):191–200.
12. Clark WR, Ronco C: Renal replacement therapy in acute renal failure: solute removal mechanism and dose quantification. Kidney Int 1998;53(Suppl 66):S133–S137.
13. Ronco C: Continuous renal replacement therapies for the treatment of acute renal failure in intensive care patients. Clin Nephrol 1993;4:187–198.
14. Ronco C, Ghezzi PM, Hoenich N, Delfino PG: Membranes and filters for hemodialysis. Contrib Nephrol 2000;137:146–157.
15. Ronco C, Brendolan A, Bellomo R: On-line monitoring in continuous renal replacement therapies. Kidney Int 1999;56(Suppl 72):S8–S14.
16. Rahmati S, Ronco F, Spittle M, et al: Validation of the blood temperature monitor for extracorporeal thermal energy balance during in vitro continuous hemodialysis. Renal Research Institute Seminars. In Levin NW, Ronco C (eds): Advances in Endstage Renal Diseases, 2001, pp 245–250.
17. Ronco C, Brendolan A, Bellomo R: Current technology for continuous renal replacement therapies. In Ronco C, Bellomo R (eds): Critical Care Nephrology. Dordrecht: Kluwer Academic Publishers, 1998, pp 1269–1308.
18. Ronco C, Bellomo R, Homel P, et al: Effects of different doses in continuous veno-venous haemofiltration on outcomes of acute renal failure. A prospective randomised trial. Lancet 2000;356:26–30.
19. Gotch FA: Daily hemodialysis is a complex therapy with unproven benefits. Blood Purif 2001;19:211–216.
20. Gotch F: The current place of urea kinetic modeling with respect to different dialysis schedules. Nephrol Dial Transplant 1998;13(Suppl 6):10–14.
21. Tetta C, Mariano F, Ronco C, Bellomo R: Removal and generation of inflammatory mediators during continuous renal replacement therapies. In Ronco C, Bellomo R (eds): Critical Care Nephrology. Dordrecht: Kluwer Academic Publishers, 1998, pp 1239–1248.
22. Bellomo R, Baldwin I, Cole L, Ronco C: Preliminary experience with high volume hemofiltration in human septic shock. Kidney Int 1998;53(Suppl 66):S182–S185.
23. Tetta C, Cavaillon JM, Schulze M, et al: Removal of cytokines and activated complement components in an experimental model of continuous plasma filtration coupled with sorbent adsorption. Nephrol Dial Transplant 1998;13:1458–1464.
24. Berlot G, Tomasini A, Silvestri L, Gullo A: Plasmapheresis in the critically ill patient. Kidney Int 1998;53(Suppl 66):S178–S181.
25. Tetta C, Bellomo R, Brendolan A, et al: Use of adsorptive mechanisms in continuous renal replacement therapies in the critically ill. Kidney Int 1999;56(Suppl 72):S15–S19.
26. La Greca G, Brendolan A, Ghezzi PM, et al: The concept of sorbent in hemodialysis. Int J Artif Organs 1998;21:303–308.
27. Malchesky PS, Zborowski M, Hou KC: Extracorporeal techniques of endotoxin removal: a review of the art and science. Adv Renal Replacement Ther 1995;2:60–69.
28. Ronco C, Bellomo R: Continuous versus intermittent renal replacement therapy in the treatment of acute renal failure. Nephrol Dial Transplant 1998;13:79–85.

Nutritional Management of Acute Renal Failure

Wilfred Druml and William E. Mitch

The objectives for initiating nutritional support in patients with catabolic conditions are to maintain protein stores and correct preexisting or disease-related deficits in lean body mass. These are the same objectives for treating patients with acute renal failure (ARF). However, the specific metabolic alterations and demands created by ARF, the consequences of impaired excretory renal function, and the modifications in nutrient balances induced by renal replacement therapy all have to be taken into consideration.[1] These conditions change the way in which nutritional support is implemented for ARF patients.

The principles of nutritional support for ARF patients also differ from those used to treat patients with chronic renal failure (CRF) because diets or infusions that satisfy the minimal requirements in CRF may not be sufficient for ARF patients. In ARF, it is the degree of hypercatabolism associated with the diseases or disorders linked with ARF and the type and frequency of dialysis, rather than the degree of renal dysfunction, that determine the nutrient requirements of ARF patients.

Despite the well-known difficulties of demonstrating an obviously improved survival of critically ill patients if parenteral nutrition is introduced, there is widespread agreement among clinicians that nutritional therapy is a cornerstone of modern critical care medicine (including the care of patients with ARF). In large part, this agreement is the result of the finding that preexisting and/or hospital-acquired malnutrition are important factors in the high mortality rate of acutely ill patients with ARF.[1-3] Another factor is the recognition that enteral nutrition should be the primary route of nutritional support for patients with ARF, as well as for those patients with catabolic illness but normal renal function.

Metabolic alterations and nutrient requirements in acute renal failure

ARF causes a broad range of disturbed physiological and metabolic functions that contributes to the high rates of morbidity and mortality.[4] However, it is not just ARF that causes these problems: acute damage to the kidney is often a complication of sepsis, trauma, or multiorgan failure, and these disorders also change many of the steps in intermediary metabolism. Finally, there is the impact of the type and intensity of renal replacement therapy. In short, the acute loss of renal excretory function has a profound effect on the "milieu interieur," with specific alterations in the metabolism of proteins, amino acids, carbohydrates, and lipids in addition to the abrupt loss of the ability to precisely control the balance of water, electrolytes, and acid–base.[4] For these reasons, patients with ARF present as a heterogeneous group with different nutrient requirements. The nephrologist must also recognize that nutrient requirements for an individual patient can vary widely during the course of disease (just as the requirements for electrolytes and water change during the development and recovery from ARF).

Energy metabolism and energy requirements

In contrast to the results obtained from experimental models of ARF that indicate a decrease in oxygen consumption (i.e. "uremic hypometabolism"), energy expenditure in patients with uncomplicated ARF is within the normal range. However, disorders which frequently accompany ARF (e.g. sepsis or multiple organ failure) increase oxygen consumption by as much as 30%.[5] Thus, energy requirements for patients with uncomplicated ARF are the same as for normal age-matched controls, whereas energy requirements for ARF patients with other complicating diseases are determined more by the underlying disease process than by a response to ARF.

There are well-defined complications arising from administering excessive quantities of energy substrates (e.g. increased CO_2 production, hyperlipidemia; see below), therefore the prescription for supplying energy should cover, but not exceed, the rate of energy expenditure. In fact, the prescription error should be towards slight underfeeding rather than overfeeding because the former causes fewer complications than the latter. The problem is that the basal energy expenditure (BEE) cannot be measured easily and so is estimated from the Harris–Benedict equation. The energy prescription is based on this calculation plus a "correction" factor for any degree of hypermetabolism (i.e. a "stress factor;" Table 9.1). It is very rare for energy requirements to exceed 130% of BEE.

Amino acid metabolism

A hallmark of ARF is excessive protein catabolism and sustained negative nitrogen balance. Unfortunately, this catabolic response cannot be blocked by strategies solely based on nutritional intervention. The hypercatabolic state causes excessive release of amino acids from skeletal muscle and there is defective utilization of amino acids for protein synthesis in muscle.[6,7] The liver responds by increasing gluconeogenesis (and ureagenesis) and there is a shift to hepatic synthesis of acute-phase reactant proteins. ARF also leads to an imbalance in amino acid pools in plasma and in the intracellular compartment of muscle. Together, these factors lead to defective utilization of amino acids during their intravenous infusion.[8]

Metabolic acidosis and endocrine abnormalities (e.g. release of catabolic hormones, hyperparathyroidism) along with circulating proteases, the release of inflammatory mediators (tumor necrosis factor α (TNFα), inter-leukins, etc.), and increased catabolism stimulated by dialysis all contribute to the accelerated breakdown of protein in ARF (Table 9.2). Metabolic acidosis is a well-recognized factor that stimulates catabolism of essential amino acids and protein, and acidosis causes insulin resistance.[9] This is relevant because a low level of insulin and, presumably, insulin resistance can stimulate catabolism in muscle; in experimental models of ARF, both insulin-mediated stimulation of protein synthesis and inhibition of protein degradation are depressed.[6,10] Besides these catabolic factors, the negative nitrogen balance and loss of lean body mass in ARF patients are augmented when stress factors such as inadequate nutrition, infection, trauma, sepsis, or thermal injury are present.[11,12]

Finally, loss of kidney tissue per se affects protein and amino acid metabolism because the kidney degrades hormones (e.g. insulin, parathyroid hormone) and could contribute to the abnormal responses to these. In addition, several amino acids are synthesized and/or metabolized by the kidney. The loss of kidney function and its synthetic and metabolic functions can make several amino acids (e.g. tyrosine, arginine, serine, and cysteine) indispensable, so they must be included in the diet to provide the substrates for protein synthesis.[1]

Anticatabolic strategies in acute renal failure

The above discussion indicates that nutritional support (including branched chain amino acid infusions) can only minimize the catabolic effects of ARF, but will not eliminate them. It also remains to be shown that specific nutrients such as glutamine or structured lipids will exert a more pronounced beneficial effect on protein balance.[1]

There was support for taking advantage of the anabolic potential of growth factors such as recombinant human growth hormone (rHGH) or insulin-like growth factor 1 (IGF-1) to block catabolism in patients with ARF. In sharp

---

Table 9.1 Estimation of energy requirements

a Calculation of BEE (Harris–Benedict equation)
Males: 66.47 + (13.75 × BW) + (5 × height) – (6.76 × age)
Females:
655.1 + (9.56 × BW) + (1.85 × height) – (4.67 × age)
The average BEE is approximately 25 kcal/kgBW/day

b Stress factor to correct calculated energy requirement for hypermetabolism

Postoperative (no complications)	1.0
Long bone fracture	1.15–1.30
Cancer	1.10–1.30
Peritonitis/sepsis	1.20–1.30
Severe infection/multiple trauma	1.20–1.40
Burns	1.20–2.00 (≈ BEE + % burned body surface area)
Corrected energy requirements (kcal/day) = BEE × stress factor	

BEE, basic energy expenditure; BW, body weight.

Table 9.2 Protein catabolism in acute renal failure: contributing factors

Impairment of metabolic functions by uremic toxins

Endocrine factors
  Insulin resistance
  Increased secretion of catabolic hormones (catecholamines, glucagons, glucocorticoids)
  Hyperparathyroidism
  Suppression of release/resistance to growth factors

Acidosis

Acute-phase reaction: systemic inflammatory response syndrome (activation of cytokine network)

Release of proteases

Inadequate supply of nutritional substrates

Loss of nutritional substrates (renal replacement therapy)

contrast to results obtained from animal experiments, clinical benefits have been disappointing: a multicenter study using recombinant IGF-1 (rIGF-1) in patients with ARF had to be terminated prematurely because of a lack of beneficial effect.[13] Administration of rHGH to critically ill patients (some of whom had ARF) was associated with a higher death rate in a large trial; this therapy was also discontinued.[14]

Cytokines such as interleukins and TNFα can elicit a catabolic response in experimental animals.[11] In patients with various acute diseases and ARF, these factors could cause excessive release of amino acids from skeletal muscle and activation of hepatic amino acid extraction. Anticytokine therapies designed to limit the overwhelming release or action of inflammatory mediators on protein breakdown have been evaluated in animal experiments.

Protein and amino acid requirements

The critical concept for prescribing protein intake is that providing an excess of protein or infusing an excess of amino acids does not force synthesis of protein. For this reason, the recommended level of protein for patients with catabolic illnesses should not exceed 1.5 g/kg/day.[15,16] For patients with uncomplicated ARF, it is suspected that the daily protein or amino acid requirement is nearer the recommended allowance of 0.8 g/kg/day for normal adults rather than the minimum protein level of 0.6 g/kg/day recommended for CRF patients.[1] Unfortunately, there have been only a few attempts to define the optimal intake for protein or amino acids in ARF: in ARF patients without significant catabolic illnesses who were in the polyuric recovery phase of ARF, an amino acid intake of 1 g/kg/day was necessary to achieve a neutral nitrogen balance.[1] There are a few studies of the protein and amino acid requirements of critically ill patients with ARF treated with continuous renal replacement therapy (CRRT). In these catabolic patients, the protein catabolic rate (PCR) calculated from urea kinetics was 1.4–1.7 g/kg/day.[17] There was also an inverse relationship between the amounts of protein and energy provided and the protein catabolic rate – the nitrogen deficit was less in those patients receiving nutritional support. Even so, a protein intake of about 1.5 g/kg/day has been recommended, as for nondialysis critically ill patients.

Unless renal insufficiency will be brief, and there is no associated catabolic illness, the intake of protein or amino acids should be at least 0.8 g/kg/day. It should be emphasized again that hypercatabolism cannot be overcome by increasing protein or protein/amino acid intake above the maximum rate of 1.5 g/kg/day, and that higher intakes or infusions of protein or amino acids will simply stimulate the formation of urea and other nitrogenous waste products and aggravate uremic complications.

For patients treated by hemodialysis or continuous hemofiltration or peritoneal dialysis, an extra protein/amino acid intake of 0.2 g/kg/day should be added to the 0.8 g/kg/day recommended allowance (again to a maximum of 1.5 g/kg/day). This amount should compensate for losses occurring during dialysis therapy.

Carbohydrate metabolism in acute renal failure

ARF is characterized by insulin resistance: the maximum insulin-stimulated glucose uptake by skeletal muscle is lower than normal whereas the insulin concentration causing half maximum uptake is normal, indicating the presence of a postreceptor defect rather than impaired sensitivity.[18] A second feature of abnormal glucose metabolism in ARF is accelerated hepatic gluconeogenesis from amino acids released during protein breakdown. Hepatic extraction of amino acids, the conversion of amino acids to glucose, and urea production are all increased by ARF, and protein breakdown is not suppressed by glucose infusion.[19]

Metabolism of insulin is grossly abnormal in ARF: endogenous insulin secretion is reduced in the basal state and during glucose infusion, and there is blunted catabolism of insulin by the damaged kidney and, surprisingly, also by the liver. The resulting elevation in plasma insulin concentration can contribute to the normal blood glucose levels in several patients with ARF.[4]

Lipid metabolism in acute renal failure

Profound alterations in lipid metabolism occur in patients with ARF: the triglyceride content of plasma lipoproteins is increased, whereas total cholesterol and high-density lipoprotein (HDL) cholesterol are decreased.[1] The major cause of lipid abnormalities is impaired lipolysis as the activities of both lipolytic systems – lipoprotein lipase and hepatic triglyceride lipase – are decreased by > 50% compared with normal values.[20] Whether or not increased hepatic synthesis contributes to hypertriglyceridemia in ARF remains undetermined, but carnitine deficiency does not participate in the development of lipid abnormalities in ARF. Plasma carnitine levels are increased because of increased release from muscle tissue and increased hepatic synthesis.

The nutritional relevance of abnormal lipid metabolism is that the lipid fractions in artificial fat emulsions are metabolized in the same way as the lipids in very low-density lipoprotein (VLDL) particles and, consequently, their elimination is delayed in ARF.[21] The delay in lipolysis in ARF contrasts with findings in other acute illnesses, such as surgery, trauma, or sepsis, in which fat elimination and utilization are enhanced and the oxidation of free fatty acids can help "cover" the increase in energy requirements.

Micronutrients

ARF patients' requirements for water-soluble vitamins are increased by renal replacement therapies. Caution should be used in prescribing vitamin C to ARF patients because it is a precursor of oxalic acid and excess amounts (> 250 mg/day) can result in secondary oxalosis. In contrast to patients with CRF, the requirements of vitamins A, E, and D (but not vitamin K) are increased in patients with ARF and a daily supplement should be provided.[22] Most multivitamin preparations for parenteral infusions contain the recommended daily allowance (RDA) of all necessary vitamins.

Requirements of trace elements have to be defined for ARF patients. This is relevant because hyperalimentation solutions containing trace element supplements carry the risk of inducing toxic effects since the regulation of trace element homeostasis, including both gastrointestinal absorption and renal excretion, is impaired. An exception is selenium because its concentration in plasma and erythrocytes is consistently decreased in patients with ARF and CRF.[23]

Several micronutrients act as part of the organism's defense mechanisms against oxygen free radical-induced injury to cellular components. A profound depression in antioxidant status has been documented in patients with ARF, and although the clinical importance of this effect has not been defined it seems likely to be important in ARF patients as well as in patients with arteriosclerosis.[23]

Metabolic impact of extracorporeal therapy

The metabolic and nutritional changes induced by renal replacement therapies are clinically important. It has been documented that the dialysis procedure (using modern membranes and techniques) stimulates protein catabolism in the body and, specifically, in muscle.[24] This catabolic response persists for at least 2 h after dialysis and contributes to the loss of muscle mass. The mechanism for this response has not been worked out, but protein catabolism could be stimulated by substrate losses or by activation of leukocyte-derived proteases and/or inflammatory mediators of catabolism. Dialysis has less of an inhibitory effect on protein synthesis in muscle.[24] Finally, several water-soluble substances (e.g. vitamins and carnitine) are lost during hemodialysis, and it has been suggested that reactive oxygen species are generated during treatment.

Recently, CRRT (continuous hemofiltration and/or hemodialysis) has been widely used to manage critically ill patients with ARF. The metabolic consequences of these modalities (Table 9.3) could be especially relevant since

Table 9.3 Metabolic effects of continuous renal replacement therapy

Amelioration of uremic intoxication ("renal replacement") *plus*
1 Heat loss
2 Excessive load of substrates (lactate, glucose, etc.)
3 Loss of nutrients (amino acids, vitamins, etc.)
4 Loss of electrolytes (phosphate, magnesium)
5 Elimination of short-chain proteins (hormones, mediators?)
6 Metabolic consequences of bioincompatibility (induction/activation of mediator cascades, stimulation of protein catabolism?)

the treatment is continuous and is associated with high fluid turnover.[25] For all of these reasons and the fact that the provision of large amounts of amino acids and proteins will not force the body to synthesize proteins, the practice of increasing the frequency of dialysis in order to remove the nitrogen-containing waste products and fluids generated by prescribing large amounts of parenteral hyperalimentation should be discarded.

Clinical experiences with nutritional support in acute renal failure

The number of controlled trials examining how nutritional support changes the course and outcome of patients with ARF are few. Some are prospective and fulfill minimal requirements of study design with respect to patient numbers, definition of endpoints, stratification of groups, etc., but most have defects in these requirements.[1] Early reports compared nutritional support with amino acids plus glucose and with glucose alone. Pooled results of the four studies revealed a 64% mortality with glucose infusion compared with a 42% mortality when a more complete parenteral nutrition solution was used. Combining this result with other retrospective investigations leads to the tentative conclusion that nutritional support is beneficial and that critically ill patients with more complications may derive more benefit from nutritional therapy than those patients who are not critically ill.[1]

Regarding the optimal type of amino acid solution and the quantity of amino acids used for patients with ARF, the results are inconclusive in terms of improving the survival rate or the nitrogen balance; however, the numbers of patients studied were small or the control groups were not treated concurrently or were not hypercatabolic.[1] There have been no studies conducted recently, and there have been no systematic evaluations of the potential of enteral nutritional support in patients with ARF.

The ongoing controversy over the beneficial influence of nutritional support in ARF reflects a basic misunderstanding of the objectives of this therapy.[2] Survival will be determined principally by the underlying illness and by the degree of hypercatabolism of associated illnesses; ARF has only a minor influence on this factor. After all, many patients with no renal function are successfully managed by dialysis. Nutrition is just one element of a complex pattern of therapeutic interventions, and patient survival cannot serve as the sole endpoint of an evaluation.

Impact of nutritional interventions on renal function and/or recovery from acute renal failure

In the kidney, starvation will accelerate protein breakdown and impair protein synthesis, whereas refeeding exerts the opposite effects. This is relevant because provision of amino acids or total parenteral nutrition accelerated tissue repair and the recovery of renal function in animals with experimental ARF. This benefit has been more difficult to establish in humans, but results from one study led to the conclusion that nutritional supplements hastened the resolution of ARF.[1] On the other hand, amino acids given in high doses can induce toxic tubular damage in both ischemic and nephrotoxic animal models of ARF. During the "insult phase" of ARF (similar to the "ebb" phase occurring after trauma, major operations, etc.), excessive intake of nutrients can aggravate tissue injury and should be avoided. In part, this "therapeutic paradox" in ARF is related to the increase in metabolic work stimulated by the uptake and metabolism of glucose and amino acids when oxygen is limited. In contrast, several amino acids have a renoprotective influence, namely glycine and, to a lesser degree, alanine. These amino acids can limit tubular injury in ischemic and nephritic experimental models of ARF. Arginine (possibly by producing nitric oxide) reportedly acts to preserve renal function in experimental ARF, although, again, this is an unsettled issue as it could augment tubular injury. Overall, both parenteral and enteral administration of amino acids and protein can augment renal perfusion and renal function; whether this effect can be used to promote tubular repair in ARF remains to be shown.

Various endocrine–metabolic interventions (e.g. administration of thyroxine, growth hormone, epidermal growth factor, IGF-1) have been shown to accelerate regeneration in experimental models of ARF. In the rat, IGF-1 accelerates recovery from ischemic ARF and improves nitrogen balance. Unfortunately, strategies directed at promoting tubular repair and limiting hypercatabolism have not been effective in clinical studies in ARF patients (see above).

Patient classification

Ideally, a specific nutritional program should be designed for each ARF patient. In practice, however, we suggest that there are three strategies which differ according to the extent of protein catabolism associated with the underlying disease (Table 9.4). The reason for this classification is that it addresses the central problem, namely that the degree of hypercatabolism more directly affects outcome than other categories that are based on the cause or degree of renal insufficiency.

The first strategy is for patients who do not exhibit excess catabolism, as estimated from urea appearance rate, i.e. < 5 g nitrogen more than nitrogen intake. In this group, ARF is usually caused by nephrotoxins (e.g. aminoglycosides, contrast media, or mismatched blood transfusions). Generally, these patients can be fed orally and the prognosis for recovery of renal function and for survival is excellent. The second strategy is for patients who exhibit moderate hypercatabolism and have a urea appearance rate exceeding nitrogen intake by 5–10 g/day. These patients frequently suffer from complicating infections, peritonitis, or moderate injury, and generally they require both nutritional support and dialysis. The

Table 9.4 Patient classification and nutrient requirements in patients with acute renal failure

	Extent of catabolism		
	Mild	Moderate	Severe
Excess urea appearance (above N intake)	> 5 g	5–10 g	> 10 g
Clinical setting (examples)	Drug toxicity	Elective surgery ± infection	Severe injury or sepsis
Mortality	20%	60%	> 80%
Dialysis/hemofiltration (frequency)	Rare	As needed	Frequent
Route of nutrient administration	Oral	Enteral and/or parenteral	Enteral and/or parenteral
Energy recommendations (kcal/kg/day)	25	25–30	25–35
Energy substrates	Glucose	Glucose + fat	Glucose + fat
Glucose (g/kg/day)	3.0–5.0	3.0–5.0	3.0–5.0
Fat (g/kg/day)		0.5–1.0	0.8–1.2
Amino acids/protein (g/kg/day)	0.6–1.0 EAA (+ NEAA)	0.8–1.2 EAA + NEAA	1.0–1.5 EAA + NEAA
Nutrients used			
Oral/enteral	Food	Enteral formulas	Enteral formulas
Parenteral		Glucose 50–70% + fat emulsions 10% or 20%	Glucose 50–70% + fat emulsions 10% or 20%
	EAA + specific NEAA solutions (general or "nephro") multivitamin and multitrace element preparations		

EAA, essential amino acids; NEAA, nonessential amino acids.

third strategy is for patients who have ARF in association with severe trauma, burns, or overwhelming sepsis. Their urea appearance rate is markedly elevated (> 10 g/day above nitrogen intake) and treatment strategies, which include enteral or parenteral nutrition and blood pressure or ventilatory support, are complex (Table 9.4). It is of utmost importance to maintain blood glucose concentrations within acceptable levels in critically ill patients and, generally, insulin is required.[26] Dialysis or continuous hemofiltration is used to maintain fluid balance and a blood urea nitrogen (BUN) level below 80–100 mg/dL. Mortality in this group exceeds 60–80%. Again, the key point is that it is not the loss of renal function that accounts for the poor prognosis but rather superimposed hypercatabolism.

Nutrient administration

There are two important questions to be addressed in designing the nutritional regimen: which patients require nutritional support and when should it be initiated? Both decisions are influenced by the nutritional status of the patient as well as the type and degree of hypercatabolism associated with the underlying illness.

During the acute phase of ARF, i.e. within the first 24 h after trauma, surgery, etc., nutritional support should be avoided. Infusion of large quantities of amino acids or glucose during this "ebb phase" will increase oxygen requirements and may well aggravate tubular injury and the degree of functional loss. If the nutritional status of the patient is viewed as normal (e.g. normal plasma protein concentrations, anthropometric measurements, and, importantly, clinical judgment), and if the patient will resume a normal diet within 5 days, no specific nutritional support is necessary. However, if there is evidence of malnourishment, nutritional therapy should be initiated regardless of whether the patient is likely to eat within 5 days. For all patients, an estimate of the type and severity of diseases complicating ARF is required. For patients with evidence of accelerated protein catabolism (Table 9.4, groups moderate and severe), nutritional support should be instituted early and dialysis used to keep the BUN below 80–100 mg/dL (this level is emphasized because the frequency of "uremic" complications arises at a BUN above this value). Finally, metabolic abnormalities from loss of renal function generally occur when creatinine clearance falls below 30 mL/min and nutritional regimens should be designed to counteract specific metabolic abnormalities. The guiding principle is to devise methods that will both prevent the loss of lean body mass (i.e. hospital-acquired malnutrition) and support the patient through the acute illness.

Oral feedings

Oral feedings should be encouraged in every patient who can tolerate them. Initially, 40 g/day of high-quality protein (e.g. egg protein) is given to provide the mean daily protein requirement of about 0.6 g/kg body weight per day. Protein intake should be increased to 0.8 g/kg/day if the BUN remains below 100 mg/dL. For patients requiring dialysis, the protein intake must be raised to 1–1.2 g/kg/day (for the peritoneal dialysis patient, it should be raised to 1.4 g/kg/day to counteract losses of both amino acids and protein). A water-soluble vitamin supplement is recommended because there are losses and a restricted diet may not contain adequate amounts of the vitamins.

Enteral nutrition

Even small amounts of enteral nutrients serve to maintain normal intestinal structure and function and to limit bacterial translocation from the gut; enteral feeding may help to prevent the development of sepsis from intestinal bacteria.[27] Enteral nutrition might also exert a beneficial effect on kidney function, as it does in animal models of ARF: enteral nutrition improved renal function and survival compared with parenteral nutritional strategies.[28] However, there have been no systematic evaluations of the benefits of enteral nutrition in patients with ARF.

Enteral diets are given by mouth or through a small (8–10 Fr), soft, feeding tube positioned with the tip in the stomach or jejunum; nutrients are administered by pump either intermittently or continuously. Gastric contents should be aspirated initially every 2–3 h until there is adequate gastric emptying and intestinal peristalsis to prevent vomiting or bronchopulmonary aspiration. This is important because ARF is associated with impaired gastric and intestinal motility. Nutrients given by feeding tube should be diluted initially, and the amount and concentration of the solution gradually increased over several days until nutritional requirements are satisfied. Potentially treatable side-effects of this strategy include nausea, vomiting, diarrhea, abdominal distention, and cramping.

Enteral feeding formulas

No commercially available enteral mixture has been specifically developed for patients with ARF. Conventional tube-feeding formulas (Table 9.5) designed for subjects with normal renal function are used, but, occasionally, the fixed composition of nutrients and high content of protein and electrolytes (especially potassium and phosphate) can limit their use. Recently, specialized ready-to-use liquid diets have been developed for patients with CRF or for hemodialysis patients; they can also be used for ARF patients (Table 9.5). In patients not requiring extracorporeal therapy, mixtures that consist of a reduced protein content and low electrolyte concentrations are effective if high-quality proteins (in parts as oligopeptides or free amino acids) are used. For ARF patients with excessive catabolism who require dialysis therapy, we recommend preparations with a moderately high protein content and a reduced electrolyte concentration. Whether enteral diets that contain specific nutrients such as glutamine, arginine, ω3 fatty acids, and nucleotides (i.e. "immunonutrition") will exert additional advantages for patients with ARF remains to be shown.

Table 9.5 Enteral diets for patients with renal failure

	Travasorb renal[1]	Salvipeptide nephro[2]	Survimed renal[3]	Replena[4] (Suplena)	Renalcal[5]	Nepro[6]	Nova Source renal[7]	Magnacal renal[8]
	(Clintec)	(Clintec)	(Fresenius)	(Ross)	(Nestle)	(Ross)	(Novartis)	(Mead Johnson)
Volume (mL)	1000	1000	1000	1000	1000	1000	1000	1000
Calories (kcal)	1333.3	2000	1320	2000	2000	2000	2000	2000
(cal/mL)	1.35	2	1.32	2	2	2	2	2
Ratio protein–fat–carbohydrates	7:12:81	8:22:70	6:10:84	6:43:51	6.9:35:58.1	14:43:43	15:45:40	15.3:45:40
Nitrogen (g)	3.42	6.4	3.32	4.8	5.9	11.2	12.2	11.8
kcal/gN	389:1	313:1	398:1	417:1	360:1	179:1	164:1	169:1
Nonprotein (kcal/gN)	363:1	288:1	374:1	393:1	340:1	154:1	140:1	144:1
Osmolality (mosmol/kg)	590	507	600	600	600	635	700	570
Protein (g)	22.9	40	20.8	30	34.4	69.9	74	75
EAA (%)	60	23			67			
NEAA (%)	30	20			33			
Hydrolysate (%)		23	100					
Total protein (%)		34		100		100		100
Carbohydrate (g)	270.5	350	276	256	290.4	215.78	200	200
Monosaccharide–disaccharide (%)	100	3		10		12		
Oligosaccharide (%)		8						
Polysaccharide (%)		69	100	90		88		
Fat (g)	17.7	48	15.2	95.7	82.4	95.6	100	101
LCT (%)	30	50	70	100	30	100	86	80
Essential FA (%)	18	31	52	22		20		
MCT (%)	70	50	30		70		14	20
Sodium (mmol/L)	NA	7.2	15.2	34	NA	36.1	43.5	35
Potassium (mmol/L)	NA	1.5	8	29	NA	27	20.8	32
Phosphorus (mg/L)	NA			728	NA	695	650	800
Vitamins	a	a	a	a	a	a	a	a
Trace elements	b	a	a	a	a	a	a	a

Form/how supplied:
1   Powder diet: 3 bags + 810 mL water = 1050 mL.
2   Power diet: 1 × component I + 1 × component II + 350 mL water × 2 = 1000 mL.
3   Powder diet: 4 bags + 800 mL water = 1000 mL.
4   Ready-to-use liquid diet: taurine + carnitine – supplement, 8 fl oz cans (237 ml).
5   Ready-to-use liquid diet: 250-mL cans.
6   Ready-to-use liquid diet: taurine + carnitine – supplement, 8 fl oz cans (237 ml).
7   Ready-to-use liquid diet: 8 fl oz Tetra Brik Paks (237 ml); 1000-mL ready to hang.
8   Ready-to-use liquid diet: 8 fl oz cans (237 ml).

a, 2000 kcal/day for recommended daily allowance (RDA) of vitamins and trace elements; b, have to be supplied; EAA, essential amino acid; NEAA, nonessential amino acids; FA, fatty acids; LCT, long-chain triglycerides; MCT, medium-chain triglycerides; NA, information not available; RDI, reference daily intake for vitamins and minerals.

Parenteral nutrition (TPN)

Another key concept is that parenteral nutrition should not be viewed as an alternative but rather as a complementary method of providing nutritional support. For many ARF patients, it is often not possible to meet nutritional requirements by the enteral route alone. Moreover, ARF frequently occurs in patients with gastrointestinal dysfunction or pancreatitis or in patients with hypercatabolism and multiple organ dysfunction. In such patients, a total or supplementary amount of parenteral nutrition may become necessary.

Substrates for parenteral nutrition in acute renal failure

Amino acid solutions

There is ongoing controversy about whether parenteral nutrition for patients with ARF should consist of essential amino acids (EAA) exclusively, of a mixture of EAA plus nonessential amino acids (NEAA), or of specifically designed "nephro" solutions containing EAA in modified proportions plus certain NEAA that might become "conditionally essential" (Table 9.6). The use of solutions of EAA alone was based on principles established for treating CRF patients with a low protein diet and an EAA supplement. But there are fundamental differences in the goals of nutritional therapy for the two groups of patients and, therefore, this concept may be inappropriate. Moreover, the use of large amounts of EAA (i.e. > 0.6 g/kg/day) can create an amino acid imbalance that would impair protein conservation. For these reasons, available solutions of EAA for parenteral infusion may be suboptimal, and if the requirement exceeds 0.6 g protein equivalent/kg/day, a solution containing both EAA and NEAA in standard proportions or in special proportions designed to counteract the metabolic changes of renal failure (i.e. "nephro" solutions) is preferred (Table 9.6). As noted, there is no persuasive evidence that infusion mixtures enriched with branched chain amino acids or glutamine will exert a significant anticatabolic effect, but this strategy may complement other treatment regimens and should not be forgotten.

Table 9.6 Amino acid solutions for the treatment of acute renal failure

	Dose requirements	RenAmin® (Clintec)	Aminess® (Clintec)	Aminosyn RF® (Abbott)	Nephr-Amine® (McGaw)	Nephrotect® (Fresenius)
Amino acids (g/L) (g/%)	65 (6.5)	52 (5.2)	52 (5.2)	54 (5.4)	100 (10)	
Volume (mL)	500	400	1000	1000	500	
mosmol/L	600	416	475	435	908	
Nitrogen (g/L)	10	8.3	8.3	6.5	16.3	
Essential amino acids (g/L)						
Isoleucine	1.40	5.00	5.25	4.62	5.60	5.80
Leucine	2.20	6.00	8.25	7.26	8.80	12.80
Lysine acetate/HCl	1.60	4.50	6.00	5.35	6.40	12.00
Methionine	2.20	5.00	8.25	7.26	8.80	2.00
Phenylalanine	2.20	4.90	8.25	7.26	8.80	3.50
Threonine	1.00	3.80	3.75	3.30	4.00	8.20
Trypotophan	0.50	1.60	1.88	1.60	2.00	3.00
Valine	1.60	8.20	6.00	5.20	6.40	8.70
Nonessential amino acids (g/L)						
Alanine		5.60				6.20
Arginine		6.30		6.00		8.20
Glycine		3.00				6.30*
Histidine		4.20	4.12	4.29	2.50	9.80
Proline		3.50				3.00
Serine		3.00				7.60
Tyrosine		0.40				3.00†
Cysteine	–				0.20	0.40
Electrolytes (mEq/L)						
Acetate		60	50	105	44	71
Sodium					5	
Potassium				5.4		
Chloride		31			3	

*Tyrosine is included as dipeptide (glycyl-L-tyrosine).
†Glycine in part is a component of the dipeptide.

Energy substrates

For carbohydrates, glucose is the principal energy substrate when parenteral nutrition is used, but if > 5 g glucose/kg/day is given the extra glucose will not be oxidized for energy but will be used in lipogenesis and stored as fat. This is undesirable and can induce fatty infiltration of the liver. In addition, the excessive carbon dioxide produced when large amounts of glucose are oxidized leads to hypercarbia and increased respiratory demands. Another problem is that the amount of glucose that can be infused is limited by the degree of impairment of glucose utilization that is characteristic of ARF. To reiterate, because of the serious consequences of hyperglycemia, it is necessary to maintain normal glucose levels.[26] Often, excessive quantities of insulin are required and can cause electrolyte disturbances such as hypokalemia or hypophosphatemia. For such patients, some of the energy requirement should be covered by lipid emulsions. Our recommendation is that the most suitable means of providing energy substrates to critically ill patients is not glucose or lipids but glucose plus lipids. Other carbohydrates, including fructose, sorbitol, or xylitol, that are available in some countries but not in the USA should not be used in patients with ARF because of adverse metabolic effects.[1]

Fat emulsions

Advantages of using intravenous lipids to augment energy intake include a high specific energy content, a low osmolality, provision of essential fatty acids, a lower frequency of hepatic side-effects (fatty infiltration of the liver, hyperbilirubinemia), and reduced carbon dioxide production (especially in patients with compromised respiratory function). Even though lipid metabolism is altered by ARF, this should not prevent the use of lipid emulsions, but the amount infused must be adjusted to the patient's capacity to utilize lipids. Usually, 1 g fat/kg/day will not increase plasma triglycerides substantially, and about 20–30% of energy requirements can be met by lipids. Note that lipid emulsions are not hyperosmolar and can be infused into a peripheral vein. Lipids should be avoided in patients who have hyperlipidemia (i.e. plasma triglycerides > 350 mg/dL), in patients with evidence of intravascular coagulation, acidosis (pH < 7.3), or impaired circulation. Lipid emulsions usually contain long-chain triglycerides (LCT), but recently developed emulsions contain a mixture of LCT and medium-chain triglycerides (MCT). These have the potential advantages of undergoing more rapid elimination of fatty acids from plasma, more complete and carnitine-independent metabolism, and a triglyceride-lowering effect. Unfortunately, the defect in lipolysis that is characteristic of ARF cannot be circumvented by using MCT.

Parenteral solutions

There are commercially available solutions containing amino acids, glucose, and lipids with vitamins, trace elements, and electrolytes added as required (insulin can be added or administered separately; Table 9.7). These "all-in-one" solutions containing all the necessary nutrients in a single bag have proven efficacious and are widely accepted. The stability of added fat emulsions should be tested to ensure that the supply of energy is adequate.

To ensure optimal nutrient utilization and to avoid creating metabolic derangements (such as hyperglycemia, hypertriglyceridemia, an excessive rise in BUN, or mineral imbalance), the infusion should be started at a low rate (providing about 50% of requirements) and gradually increased over several days. Optimally, nutrients should be infused continuously over 24 h to avoid marked changes in substrate concentrations and to achieve their maximal utilization in anabolic processes. Because fluids are usually restricted in ARF patients, the parenteral nutrition solutions are hyperosmolar and must be infused through a central venous catheter to avoid damage to veins. Special venous catheters are available both as infusion ports and for temporary dialysis access, but they carry a significant risk of infection.

Table 9.7 "Renal failure fluid" ("all-in-one-solution")

Component	Quantity	Remarks
Glucose (40–70%)	500 mL	In the presence of severe insulin resistance, switch to D30W
Fat emulsion (10–20%)	500 mL	Start with 10%, switch to 20% if TG are < 350 mg/dL
Amino acids (6.5–10%)	500 mL	General or special "nephro" amino acid solutions containing EAA and NEAA
Water-soluble vitamins*	Daily	Limit vitamin C intake < 250 mg/day
Fat-soluble vitamins*	Daily	
Trace elements*	2–4 times weekly	Cave: toxic effects
Electrolytes	As required	Cave: hypophosphatemia or hypokalemia after initiation of TPN
Insulin	As required	Added directly to the solution or given separately

For the "all-in-one solution" with all the components contained in a single bag, the infusion rate is initially 50% of requirements, and is to be increased over a period of 3 days to satisfy requirements.
*Combination products containing the recommended daily allowances.
TG, triglycerides; EAA, essential amino acids; NEAA, nonessential amino acids; TPN, parenteral nutrition.

Complications and monitoring of nutritional support

Complications and side-effects of nutritional support in patients with ARF do not differ fundamentally from those observed when this therapy is used for other patient groups. The major concern is that hypervolemia and electrolyte imbalances can develop rapidly, and that an excessive intake will result in metabolic derangements and waste product accumulation because of the alterations in metabolism caused by ARF. In fact, most complications of parenteral nutrition are related to excessive intake of substrates (e.g. hyperglycemia, hypertriglyceridemia, hyperkalemia, an accelerated increase in BUN or in CO_2 production). It is less likely that deficiencies of minerals, vitamins, or essential fatty acids will develop. Thus, nutritional therapy in ARF patients requires more frequent monitoring than the same treatments used in other patient groups.

Summary

The acute loss of renal function causes complex metabolic abnormalities affecting not only water, electrolyte, and acid–base balance but also amino acid, carbohydrate, and lipid metabolism. Knowledge about the pathophysiology of these metabolic changes, better definitions of nutritional requirements, and advances in nutritional administration techniques have improved the success of this type of therapy for ARF patients. Dietary restrictions based on the principles of treating CRF patients have been largely abandoned in favor of an approach directed at meeting nutrient requirements. Despite the extensive experience with parenteral nutritional support, there is no doubt that enteral nutrition is the preferred type of nutrition; even small amounts of a diet provided into the gastrointestinal tract can help to support intestinal function and, potentially, renal function.

Although nutritional support has not convincingly reduced morbidity and mortality in ARF patients, it should not be abandoned because the poor prognosis for these patients is mainly related to the severity of the underlying illness and associated hypercatabolism. Nutritional therapy, like renal replacement therapy, should be viewed as a means of supporting the patient until the underlying illness is controlled. For future advances, nutritional therapy must leave a quantitatively oriented approach in covering nitrogen and energy requirements and move toward a more qualitative type of metabolic support, taking advantage of the specific pharmacologic effects of nutrients.

References

1. Druml W: Nutritional support in acute renal failure. *In* Mitch WE, Klahr S (eds): Handbook of Nutrition and the Kidney. Philadelphia: Lippincott Raven, 2001.
2. Heyland DK, MacDonald S, Keefe L, Drover JW: Total parenteral nutrition in the critically ill patient: a meta-analysis. JAMA 1998;280:2013–2019.
3. Fiaccadori E, Lombardi M, Leonardi S, Rotelli CF, Tortorella G, Borghetti A: Prevalence and clinical outcome of malnutrition in acute renal failure. JASN 1999;10:581–593.
4. Druml W, Mitch WE: Metabolic abnormalities in acute renal failure. Semin Dial 1996;9:484–490.
5. Schneeweiss B, Stockenhuber F, Druml W, et al: Energy metabolism in acute and chronic renal failure. Am J Clin Nutr 1990;52:596–601.
6. Druml W: Protein metabolism in acute renal failure. Miner Electrolyte Metab 1998;24:47–54.
7. Price SR, Reaich D, Marinovic AC, et al: Mechanisms contributing to muscle wasting in acute uremia: activation of amino acid catabolism. JASN 1998;9:438–443.
8. Druml W, Fischer M, Liebisch B, Lenz K, Roth E: Elimination of amino acids in renal failure. Am J Clin Nutr 1994;60:418–423.
9. Mitch WE, May RC, Maroni BJ, Druml W: Protein and amino acid metabolism in uremia: influence of metabolic acidosis. Kidney Int 1989; 36 (Suppl 27):S205–S207.
10. Mitch WE, Bailey JL, Wang X, Jurkovitz C, Newby D, Price SR: Evaluation of signals activating ubiquitin–proteasome proteolysis in a model of muscle wasting. Am J Physiol 1999;276:C1132–C1138.
11. Mitch WE, Price SR: Transcription factors and muscle cachexia: have we defined a therapeutic target? Lancet 2001;357:734–735.
12. Mitch WE, Goldberg AL: Mechanisms of muscle wasting: the role of the ubiquitin–proteasome system. N Engl J Med 1996;335:1897–1905.
13. Hirschberg R, Kopple J, Lipsett P, et al: Multicenter clinical trial of recombinant human insulin-like growth factor I in patients with acute renal failure. Kidney Int 1999;55:2423–2432.
14. Takala J, Ruokonen E, Webster NR, et al: Increased mortality associated with growth hormone treatment in critically ill adults. N Engl J Med 1999;341:785–792.
15. Wolfe RR, Goodenough RD, Burke JF, Wolfe MH: Response of protein and urea kinetics in burn patients to different levels of protein intake. Ann Surg 1983;197:163–171.
16. Shaw JHF, Wildbore M, Wolfe RR: Whole body protein kinetics in severely septic patients. Ann Surg 1987;205:288–294.
17. Chima CS, Meyer L, Hummell AC, et al: Protein catabolic rate in patients with acute renal failure on continuous arteriovenous hemofiltration and total parenteral nutrition. JASN 1993;3:1516–1521.
18. May RC, Clark AS, Goheer MA, Mitch WE: Specific defects in insulin-mediated muscle metabolism in acute renal failure. Kidney Int 1985;28:490–497.
19. Cianciaruso B, Bellizzi V, Napoli R, Sacca L, Kopple JD: Hepatic uptake and release of glucose, lactate and amino acids in acutely uremic dogs. Metabolism 1991;40:261–290.
20. Druml W, Zechner R, Magometschnigg D, et al: Postheparin lipolytic activity in acute renal failure. Clin Nephrol 1985;23:289–293.
21. Druml W, Fischer M, Sertl S, Schneeweiss B, Lenz K, Widhalm K: Fat elimination in acute renal failure: long-chain vs. medium-chain triglycerides. Am J Clin Nutr 1992;55:468–472.
22. Druml W, Schwarzenhofer M, Apsner R, Hörl WH: Fat soluble vitamins in acute renal failure. Miner Electrolyte Metab 1998;24:220–226.
23. Metnitz PGH, Fischer M, Bartnes S, Steltzer H, Lang TH, Druml W: Impact of acute renal failure on antioxidant status in patients with multiple organ failure. Acta Anaesthesiol Scand 2000;44:236–240.
24. Ikizler TA, Pupim LB, Brouillette JR, et al: Hemodialysis stimulates muscle and whole body protein loss and alters substrate oxidation. Am J Physiol 2002;Endocrinology and Metabolism 282:E107–116.
25. Druml W: Metabolic aspects of continuous renal replacement therapies. Kidney Int 1999;56 (Suppl 72):S56–S61.
26. Van den Berghe G, Wouters P, Weekers F, et al: Intensive insulin therapy in critically ill patients. N Engl J Med 2001;345:1359–1367.
27. Druml W, Mitch WE: Enteral nutrition in renal disease. *In* Rombeau JL, Rolandelli RD (eds): Enteral and Tube Feeding. Philadelphia: WB Saunders, 1997, pp 439–461.
28. Roberts PR, Black KW, Zaloga GP: Enteral feeding improves outcome and protects against glycerol-induced acute renal failure in the rat. Am J Resp Crit Care Med 1997;156:1265–1269.

Experimental Strategies for Acute Renal Failure: the Future

Hamid Rabb and Joseph V. Bonventre

Pathophysiologic mechanisms underlying acute renal failure
Experimental models of acute renal failure
Novel experimental strategies in acute renal failure

Acute renal failure (ARF) related to intrinsic renal causes remains a disease of high prevalence and unacceptably high mortality, despite improvements in critical care and the development of various forms of dialytic therapy. Despite efforts over 40 years to identify interventions to prevent the development of ARF or hasten its recovery once established, the clinician currently has little to offer the patient once ARF has developed except for close monitoring and dialysis.

Effective approaches to prevent and treat ARF will emanate from fundamental understanding of the pathophysiologic processes responsible for the loss of the kidney's ability to function, and the restorative actions that come into play in those patients who recover renal function. Furthermore, effective therapies will be found more efficiently when sensitive and early markers of tubular injury are reliable and easily obtained. This chapter is divided into three sections. In the first we review major pathways that are believed to be important for the pathophysiology of ARF. In the second section we discuss the advantages and limitations of experimental models currently employed to elucidate the pathogenesis of ARF. The third section introduces novel experimental approaches. Owing to limitations on space, we have omitted many experimental approaches and studies. We refer the reader to prior comprehensive reviews on this topic for broader scope and depth.[1–4]

Pathophysiologic mechanisms underlying acute renal failure

While total renal blood flow after ischemia may be close to normal, the distribution of renal blood flow may be markedly abnormal.[3] Due to the unique anatomic features of normal medullary blood flow needed to efficiently concentrate urine, the outer medulla is hypoxic under normal conditions and is particularly sensitive to further decrements in blood flow.[5] After an ischemic episode the outer medulla remains disproportionately hypoxic even after oxygenation to cortex and papilla improves. There is vascular congestion in the outer medulla after ischemia. This is likely related to impaired blood flow through small vessels due to enhanced leukocyte–endothelial interactions, possibly added to by an imbalance between vasoconstrictive and vasodilatory factors affecting the arterioles proximal to these small vessels. There have been a number of studies exploring the balance between renal vasodilatory and constrictive influences in ARF and many therapeutic attempts to increase renal blood flow. Nitric oxide (NO), endothelin (ET), atrial natriuretic peptides, angiotensin II, dopamine, eicosanoids, and platelet-activating factor are candidate mediators of the intrarenal balance between vasoconstriction and vasodilation in the postischemic kidney.[1] Atrial natriuretic peptide (ANP), with its substantial effects on glomerular filtration rate, renal blood flow, and salt and water balance, has been reported to have a protective effect in ARF in several models.[6] However in randomized prospective human trials of ANP, beneficial effects were not observed.[7] Other drugs such as dopamine and calcium channel blockers have been postulated to have protective effects during ARF, but clinical studies have not demonstrated convincing protection. Prostaglandins are known to counteract the vasoconstrictive effects of angiotensin II.[6] The family of phospholipase A_2 enzymes, which act on phospholipids to generate free arachadonic acid, increase in activity with ischemia–reperfusion and have been implicated in the pathophysiology of ARF.[8] The role(s) of these enzymes in human ARF remains unknown, however. After releasing arachidonic acid, this product is metabolized to a variety of eicosanoids. Potential roles for eicosanoids in ARF remain to be elucidated. Future work in this area will be facilitated by the advent of cyclooxygenase subtype-specific inhibitors and the known effects of nonsteroidal anti-inflammatory agents to decrease medullary oxygenation.[9]

The flow of leukocytes through capillaries and small venules can be adversely affected by blood cell–cell interactions, such as platelet plugging, or blood cell–endothelial interactions resulting in leukocyte adhesion and transmigration through the endothelial layer. Platelet plugs and activated leukocytes can enhance vascular permeability and obstruction of microvessels. If this happens in the small vessels of the outer medulla, then the energetically demanding S_3 segment of the proximal tubule will be particularly vulnerable to ischemic injury. A number of experimental studies in rodents have demonstrated an important role for leukocyte–endothelial adhesion molecules, particularly CD11/CD18 and intercellular adhesion molecule (ICAM)-1 in experimental ARF.[10–14] Small clinical trials have suggested that CD11a/CD18 or ICAM-1 could reduce transplant ARF.[15,16] However, larger prospective studies with a CD11a/CD18 or ICAM-1 monoclonal antibody did not reveal a protective effect.[17,18] A major limitation was the experimental design of these clinical trials: the antiadhesive agent was administered after the original insult. In experimental studies the major protective effect was seen when the protective agent was given prior to, or shortly after, the ischemic insult.

Growth factors play a vital role in regulation of embryologic development of the tubule and potentially regulate recovery from ARF. A number of growth factors have enhanced recovery from ARF in experimental models. These include insulin-like growth factor (IGF-1), epidermal growth factor (EGF), and hepatocyte growth factor (HGF), each of which has been shown to hasten recovery in rat models of ARF.[19] The engagement of these growth factors during repair after ARF recapitulates many aspects of renal embryogenesis.[20] Unfortunately clinical trials of IGF-1 have been disappointing, although in both of the published trials the design suffered from, in one case,[21] small numbers of patients with a low incidence of ARF and, in the other,[22] entry criteria for admission into the study that were arguably too broad.

Experimental models of acute renal failure

A number of agents have shown promising results in ameliorating ischemia–reperfusion injury in animal models but failed to display efficacy in human trials.[7,18,22] Thus it is important to evaluate the appropriateness of the available experimental models to disease pathogenesis in humans. Even though experimental approaches to simulate human ARF have specific limitations, they have allowed investigators to elucidate important concepts and further the understanding of the pathogenesis of renal disease. There is a surprising lack of clarity regarding the pathologic features of ARF in humans. Some argue that the disease affects distal tubules with as much regularity as it does proximal tubules.[23,24] This is in contrast to most, but not all,[25] of the animal models, where the damage occurs primarily in the proximal nephron. Others argue that proximal injury predominates in humans also.[3] In humans, focal necrotic changes have been reported in both proximal and distal tubules on biopsy.[26–29] The data on pathologic changes in ARF are limited, however, owing to the absence of outer medullary tissue, which is generally not obtained on biopsy.

The investigator has to choose between a simpler more controlled model such as cell culture versus a more complex and realistic model in animals.[30] There are advantages and limitations of each model system. For example, the effects of glomerular filtrate leaking back across damaged epithelium into the renal interstitium were first observed in animal epithelial cell lines in culture, and were later proven to be a factor in the human manifestations of disease as well.[31,32] Animal models involving occlusion of the major renal vessels or intramuscular injections of glycerol are inherently more complex than isolated tubules, tubular cells, or cell cultures, which become dedifferentiated and change their metabolic characteristics to become less dependent on oxygenation. However, animal models are closer to the human condition, and new interventions should be tested in animals prior to clinical trials.

In the commonly used renal artery clamp model, the animal is subjected to clamping of the renal artery or renal pedicle for 30–60 min with subsequent release and reperfusion. Investigators have realized that in order to produce reliable changes in serum creatinine and blood urea nitrogen they had to pay close attention to a number of important variables. These include the temperature of the animal during the surgery, proper hydration, as well as complete occlusion of the renal artery. Rat models of renal artery occlusion (RAO) are often associated with significant alterations in renal hemodynamics, together with medullary congestion. Many mediators that affect the renal vasculature may improve renal function and ameliorate ischemia–reperfusion injury in rat models by improving renal blood flow and preventing occlusion of vessels in the outer medulla.[33,34] RAO in rats is associated with extensive necrosis of the proximal tubule, with mild damage to the loop of Henle and the distal nephron segment.[35,36]

Mice are being increasingly used to study the pathogenesis of ARF. The use of populations with specific gene alterations remains a fertile field with great scientific potential. Knockout animals with specific deficiencies in cytokines, surface molecules, or cell populations allow the researcher to test molecular pathways in relation to the complexities of the entire organism. In dealing with mice, however, it is important to recognize that different common background strains have strain-specific responses to ARF, highlighting the importance of using appropriate strain controls.[37]

Larger animals such as dog,[38,39] monkey, and pig have also been used in RAO models of ARF. The pig kidney has many similarities to the human kidney both anatomically and physiologically,[40] and may be well suited to simulate the hemodynamic changes encountered during ARF. However, the high costs involved in developing and maintaining such a pig model has limited its use to one of confirmation, where significant findings on rat and murine models can be verified.

Cell culture experiments have yielded significant information on cell regulatory and second messenger systems. The loss of polarity of renal cells secondary to a dysfunction in the Na^+/K^+ ATPase found in ARF was first elucidated in a model in vitro[41] and then translated to humans.[42] Understanding of cytoskeletal structures and their relationship to cell–cell interactions have been important discoveries. However, because of the significant metabolic changes and alterations in differentiation state brought about by placing cells in culture, the models do not truly reflect the conditions experienced by the epithelial cell in vivo. Furthermore ischemia, with its acidosis, substrate limitations, and metabolic waste product accumulation, is not generally modeled in tissue culture or freshly isolated tubules, where the very low cell to media volume ratio does not model the high cell to interstitial volume ratio present in vivo. Thus most experiments in vitro are conducted under metabolic and pH conditions that do not resemble the renal milieu encountered in ARF.

To reduce the metabolic changes observed in cell culture and to preserve the differentiated phenotype of the epithelial cell, investigators have isolated proximal tubule segments and studied them in vitro. During procurement, however, the proximal tubule is subjected to a great physical insult, which may induce sublethal changes. Using proximal tubules it has been found that glycine can exert a protective effect via various mediators in ARF.[43] Despite its limitations the isolation of proximal tubules will remain an important tool to study epithelial cell injury. Even though cell culture experiments will continue to add important information regarding epithelial cell injury and repair, attention to maintenance of a close correlation between in vitro and in vivo studies will likely be most productive in unraveling the pathophysiology of ARF.

In summary, while we can learn much from the animal models of ischemia, we do not know enough about the pathologic features of the human disease to transfer an intervention that works well in animals to humans with a high degree of confidence that it will be effective. We need better information about human ARF and likely will benefit from development of better models of the disease in animals.

Novel experimental strategies in acute renal failure

There are many areas under investigation in ARF and we introduce a selection of these. Preconditioning of the kidney, by prior ischemia, toxic damage, or obstruction, confers a relative resistance to subsequent ARF. Upregulation of heat shock proteins (HSP), particularly HSP 25, as well as activation of stress kinases such as MAPK and JNK may be important in this process.[44] NO has also been invoked as a potential mediator in the preconditioning response.[45] However, there may be some species and stimulus specificity to this, as ischemic preconditioning in a pig ARF model did not appear to have a protective effect on subsequent ischemia.[46]

Recent evidence has indicated an important role for T lymphocytes in ARF.[47–49] This finding was somewhat counterintuitive, given the low numbers of T cells seen in the kidney during ARF, as well as the classic paradigms of T-cell functions. The CD4+ T-cell subset is likely the important T cell in this process, acting in part through CD28 and γ-interferon.[50] In addition to a potentially deleterious role for T cells in ARF, a protective CD4+ of the Th2 subtype has been identified.[51] The utility of therapy directed toward T cells in ARF remains to be tested.

Another way by which to modulate renal hemodynamics as well as reduce inflammation in ARF is by selective activation of A_{2A} adenosine receptors.[52] The exact mechanisms by which these compounds prevent ARF are unclear, but may well involve prevention of circulating leukocytes from attaching to endothelium of the kidney.

Apoptosis is present in some tubular cells during ARF.[53] The regulation of apoptosis during ARF is an exciting area of study.[54] Apoptosis may be linked with inflammation,[55]

caspases,[56] as well as heme oxygenase,[57] which are also potential experimental targets in ARF.

Though most previous work on leukocyte adhesion in ARF has focused on CD11/CD18 and ICAM-1, selectins are also potential targets. Recent work has demonstrated an important role in ARF for specific selectins[58,59] and the selectin ligands.[60,61] Clinical trials in renal transplant ARF are now underway with selectin ligand blockade.

Many new technologies are being developed that provide us with new tools to study ARF. Such powerful tools include representational difference analysis, subtraction hybridization, and gene-chip/micro-array approaches.[62] With these techniques researchers are able to survey the expression patterns of a wide variety of genes and proteins and their activation in tissues. These data have not only characterized the pattern of known gene expression during ARF but also hold the promise to identify novel genes potentially important for the injury or recovery phase of ARF.[63,64] One of the limitations of studying whole-kidney gene expression is that mechanistically one cannot ascertain changes in individual cell types. This problem is being investigated by laser capture microdissection, where groups of cells are selected and their gene expression changes evaluated.[65]

Humes and colleagues have created a bioartificial kidney consisting of a hemofilter in a continuous venovenous hemofiltration circuit containing a cartridge with fibers lined with renal proximal tubule cells. They have called

Table 10.1 Therapeutic targets for human acute renal failure

Some targets/strategies previously evaluated
Insulin-like growth factor 1
Intercellular adhesion molecule 1
CD11a/CD18 (LFA-1)
Atrial natriuretic peptide
Dopamine
Acetylcysteine (successfully applied)

Some agents in current evaluation
Fenoldapam
Selectin ligand inhibitor
Melanocyte-stimulating hormone

Potential targets of future human trials
A_{2A} adenosine receptor
CD4+ T cell
Proteases
Apoptosis
Glycine
Caspase inhibitors
Heme oxygenase
Iron chelators
Endonuclease inhibitors
Growth factors
Poly(ADP-ribose) polymerase
New molecules identified by subtraction/array/proteomic techniques

Combination approaches

this a renal tubule assist device. Using this device in an animal model of endotoxin shock and renal failure, they have recently reported that treatment with a bioartificial kidney resulted in higher circulating levels of the anti-inflammatory cytokine interleukin-10 and better hemodynamic stability in treated animals.[66]

In summary the information explosion that is characterizing biology and medicine in the early part of the twenty-first century, together with high-throughput drug discovery efforts and advances in research technologies and quantitative bioassays, will ultimately lead to a better understanding of and effective therapies for ARF (Table 10.1). These are exciting times for the experimental study of ARF, and hopefully we are at the brink of clinical translation of these basic findings into effective therapies for the prevention and treatment of ARF.

Acknowledgments

H.R. was supported by NIH DK54770 and an NKF Clinical Scientist Award. J.V.B. was supported by NIH MERIT Award DK 39773, DK 38452, and DK 46269.

References

1. Rabb H, Bonventre J: Experimental strategies for acute renal failure – the future. In Brady HR, Wilcox CS (eds): Therapy in Nephrology and Hypertension: a Companion to Brenner and Rector's The Kidney. Philadelphia: WB Saunders, 1999, pp 72–80.
2. Star RA: Treatment of acute renal failure. Kidney Int 1998;54:1817–1831.
3. Thadhani R, Pascual M, Bonventre JV: Acute renal failure. N Engl J Med 1996;334:1448–1460.
4. Molitoris W, Finn W (eds): Acute Renal Failure. A Companion to Brenner and Rector's The Kidney. Philadelphia: WB Saunders, 2001.
5. Brezis M, Rosen S: Hypoxia of the renal medulla: its implications for disease. N Engl J Med 1995;332:647–655.
6. Conger JD: Interventions in clinical acute renal failure: what are the data? Am J Kidney Dis 1995;26:565–576.
7. Allgren RL, Marbury TC, Rahman SN, et al: Anaritide in acute tubular necrosis. Auriculin Anaritide Acute Renal Failure Study Group. N Engl J Med 1997;336:828–834.
8. Bonventre JV: Phospholipase A2 and signal transduction. J Am Soc Nephrol 1992;3:128–150.
9. Burke TJ, Malhotra D, Shapiro JI: Effects of enhanced oxygen release from hemoglobin by rsr13 in acute renal failure model. Kidney Int 2001;60:1407–1414.
10. Kelly KJ, Williams WW, Colvin RB, Bonventre JV: Antibody to intercellular adhesion molecule 1 protects the kidney against ischemic injury. Proc Natl Acad Sci USA 1994;91:812–816.
11. Rabb H, Mendiola CC, Dietz J, et al: Role of CD11a and CD11b in ischemic acute renal failure in rats. Am J Physiol 1994;267:F1052–F1058.
12. Rabb H, Mendiola CC, Saba SR, et al: Antibodies to ICAM-1 protect kidneys in severe ischemic reperfusion injury. Biochem Biophys Res Commun 1995;211:67–73.
13. Kelly KJ, Williams WW, Colvin RB, et al: Intercellular adhesion molecule-1-deficient mice are protected against ischemic renal injury. J Clin Invest 1996;97:1056–1063.
14. Haller H, Dragun D, Miethke A, et al: Antisense oligonucleotides for ICAM-1 attenuate reperfusion injury and renal failure in the rat. Kidney Int 1996;50:473–480.
15. Hourmant M, Bedrossian J, Durand D, et al: A randomized multicenter trial comparing leukocyte function-associated antigen-1 monoclonal antibody with rabbit antithymocyte globulin as induction treatment in first kidney transplantations. Transplantation 1996;62:1565–1570.
16. Haug CE, Colvin RB, Delmonico FL, et al: A phase I trial of immunosuppression with anti-ICAM-1 (CD54) mAb in renal allograft recipients. Transplantation 1993;55:766–772,.
17. LFA 1 delayed graft function trial, Pasteur Marieux, unpublished data.
18. Salmela K, Wramner L, Ekberg H, et al: A randomized multicenter trial of the anti-ICAM-1 monoclonal antibody (enlimomab) for the prevention of acute rejection and delayed onset of graft function in cadaveric renal transplantation: a report of the European Anti-ICAM-1 Renal Transplant Study Group. Transplantation 1999;67:729–736.
19. Hammerman MR, Miller SB: Effects of growth hormone and insulin-like growth factor I on renal growth and function. J Pediatr 1997;131:S17–S19.
20. Bush KT, Keller SH, Nigam SK: Genesis and reversal of the ischemic phenotype in epithelial cells. J Clin Invest 2000;106:621–626.
21. Franklin SC, Moulton M, Sicard GA, et al: Insulin-like growth factor I preserves renal function postoperatively. Am J Physiol 1997;272:F257–F259.
22. Hirschberg R, Kopple J, Lipsett P, et al: Multicenter clinical trial of recombinant human insulin-like growth factor I in patients with acute renal failure. Kidney Int 1999;55:2423–2432.
23. Olsen TS, Hansen HE, Olsen HS: Tubular ultrastructure in acute renal failure: alterations of cellular surfaces (brush-border and basolateral infoldings). Virchows Arch Pathol Anat Histopathol 1985;406:97–104.
24. Solez K, Morel-Maroger L, Sraer JD: The morphology of "acute tubular necrosis" in man: analysis of 57 renal biopsies and a comparison with the glycerol model. Medicine (Baltimore) 1979;58:362–376.
25. Rosen S, Heyman SN: Difficulties in understanding human "acute tubular necrosis": limited data and flawed animal models. Kidney Int 2001;60:1220–1224.
26. Oliver J, MacDowell M, Tracy A: The pathogenesis of acute renal failure associated with traumatic and toxic injury. Renal ischemia, nephrotoxic damage and the ischemic episode. J Clin Invest 1951;30:1307–1351.
27. Jones DB: Ultrastructure of human acute renal failure. Lab Invest 1982;46:254–264.
28. Olsen TS, Hansen HE: Ultrastructure of medullary tubules in ischemic acute tubular necrosis and acute interstitial nephritis in man. APMIS 1990;98:1139–1148.
29. Racusen LC: Pathology of acute renal failure: structure/function correlations. Adv Renal Replacement Ther 1997;4:3–16.
30. Lieberthal W, Nigam SK: Acute renal failure. II. Experimental models of acute renal failure: imperfect but indispensable. Am J Physiol 2000;278:F1–F12.
31. Donohoe JF, Venkatachalam MA, Bernard DB, et al: Tubular leakage and obstruction after renal ischemia: structural–functional correlations. Kidney Int 1978;13:208–222.
32. Moran SM, Myers BD: Pathophysiology of protracted acute renal failure in man. J Clin Invest 1985;76:1140–1148.
33. Conger JD, Falk SA, Yuan BH, et al: Atrial natriuretic peptide and dopamine in a rat model of ischemic acute renal failure. Kidney Int 1989;35:1126–1132.
34. Kelly KJ, Tolkoff-Rubin NE, Rubin RH, et al: An oral platelet-activating factor antagonist, Ro-24-4736, protects the rat kidney from ischemic injury. Am J Physiol 1996;271:F1061–F1067.
35. Glaumann B, Glaumann H, Trump BF: Studies of cellular recovery from injury. III. Ultrastructural studies on the recovery of the pars recta of the proximal tubule (P3 segment) of the rat kidney from temporary ischemia. Virchows Arch B Cell Pathol 1977;25:281–308.
36. Finn WF, Chevalier RL: Recovery from postischemic acute renal failure in the rat. Kidney Int 1979;16:113–123.
37. Burne MJ, Haq M, Matsuse H, et al: Genetic susceptibility to renal ischemia reperfusion injury revealed in a murine model. Transplantation 2000;69:1023–1025.
38. Lewis RM, Rice JH Patton MK, et al: Renal ischemic injury in the dog: characterization and effect of various pharmacologic agents. J Lab Clin Med 1984;104:470–479.
39. Riley AL, Alexander EA, Migdal S, et al: The effect of ischemia on renal blood flow in the dog. Kidney Int 1975;7:27–34.
40. Killion D, Canfield C, Norman J, Rosenthal JT: Exogenous epidermal growth factor fails to accelerate functional recovery in the autotransplanted ischemic pig kidney. J Urol 1993;150:1551–1556.
41. Spiegel DM, Wilson PD, Molitoris BA: Epithelial polarity following ischemia: a requirement for normal cell function. Am J Physiol 1989;256:F430–F436.
42. Alejandro V, Scandling JD Jr, Sibley RK, et al: Mechanisms of filtration failure during postischemic injury of the human kidney. A

study of the reperfused renal allograft. J Clin Invest 1995;95:820–831.

43. Weinberg JM, Venkatachalam MA, Roeser NF, et al: Energetic determinants of tyrosine phosphorylation of focal adhesion proteins during hypoxia/reoxygenation of kidney proximal tubules. Am J Pathol 2001;158:2153–2164.

44. Park KM, Chen A, Bonventre JV: Prevention of kidney ischemia/reperfusion-induced functional injury, MAPK and MAPK kinase activation, and inflammation by remote transient ureteral obstruction. J Biol Chem 2001;276:11870–11876.

45. Bolli R: Cardioprotective function of inducible nitric oxide synthase and role of nitric oxide in myocardial ischemia and preconditioning: an overview of a decade of research. J Mol Cell Cardiol 2001;33:1897–1918.

46. Behrends M, Walz MK, Kribben A, et al: No protection of the porcine kidney by ischaemic preconditioning. Exp Physiol 2000;85:819–827.

47. Takada M, Chandraker A, Nadeau KC, et al: The role of the B7 costimulatory pathway in experimental cold ischemia/reperfusion injury. J Clin Invest 1997;100:1199–1203.

48. Rabb H, Daniels F, O'Donnell M, et al: Pathophysiological role of T lymphocytes in renal ischemia–reperfusion injury in mice. Am J Physiol 2000;279:F525–F531.

49. De Greef KE, Ysebaert DK, Dauwe S, et al: Anti-B7-1 improves kidney function and blocks mononuclear cell adherence in vasa recta after acute renal ischemic injury. Kidney Int 2001;60:1415–1427.

50. Burne M, Daniels F, Elgandour A, et al: Identification of the CD4+ T cell as a major modulator of renal ischemia reperfusion injury. J Clin Invest 2001;108:1283–1290.

51. Yokota N, Daniels F, Rabb H: A protective population of T cells in renal ischemia revealed in the STAT-6 deficient mouse. J Am Soc Nephrol 2001;11:795a.

52. Okusa MD: A2A adenosine receptor: a novel therapeutic target in renal disease. Am J Physiol 2002;282:F10–F18.

53. Beeri R, Symon Z, Brezis M, et al: Rapid DNA fragmentation from hypoxia along the thick ascending limb of rat kidneys. Kidney Int 1995;47:1806–1810.

54. Ueda N, Kasushal GP, Shah SV: Apoptotic mechanisms in acute renal failure. Am J Med 2000;108:403–415.

55. Daeman MA, van't Veer C, Denecker G, et al: Inhibition of apoptosis induced by ischemia–reperfusion prevents inflammation. J Clin Invest 1999;104:541–549.

56. Melnikov VY, Ecder T, Fantuzzi G, et al: Impaired IL-18 processing protects caspase-1-deficient mice from ischemic acute renal failure. J Clin Invest 2001;107:1145–1152.

57. Hill-Kapturezak N, Thamilselvan V, Liu F, et al: Mechanism of heme oxygenase-1 induction by curcumin in human renal proximal tubule cells. Am J Physiol 2001;281:F851–F859.

58. Rabb H, Ramirez G, Xu J, et al: Renal ischemic reperfusion injury in L-selectin deficient mice. Am J Physiol 1996;271:F408–F413.

59. Singbartl K, Ley K: Protection from ischemia–reperfusion induced severe acute renal failure by blocking E-selectin. Crit Care Med 2000;28:2507–2514.

60. Takada M, Nadeau KC, Shaw GD, et al: The cytokine–adhesion molecule cascade in ischemia/reperfusion injury of the rat kidney. Inhibition by a soluble P-selectin ligand. J Clin Invest 1997;99:2682–2690.

61. Nemoto T, Burne MJ, Daniels F, et al: Small molecule selectin ligand inhibition improves outcome in ischemic acute renal failure. Kidney Int 2001;60:2205–2214.

62. Iyer VR, Eisen MB, Ross DT, et al: The transcriptional program in the response of human fibroblasts to serum. Science 1999;283:83–87.

63. Burnham C, Rabb H, Wang Z, Soleimani M: Gene array analysis of rat kidney during renal ischemia reperfusion injury. J Am Soc Nephrol 2000;10:586a.

64. Ichimura T, Bonventre JV, Bailly V, et al: Kidney injury molecule-1 (KIM-1), a putative epithelial cell adhesion molecule containing a novel immunoglobulin domain, is up-regulated in renal cells after injury. J Biol Chem 1998;273:4135–4142.

65. Murakami H, Liotta L, Star RA: IF-LCM: laser capture microdissection of immunofluorescently defined cells for mRNA analysis. Kidney Int 2000;58:1346–1353.

66. Fissell WH, Dyke DB, Weitzel WF, et al: Bioartificial kidney alters cytokine response and hemodynamics in endotoxin-challenged uremic animals. Blood Purif 2002;20:55–60.

PART II
Diseases of Glomeruli, Microvasculature, and Tubulointerstitium

HUGH R. BRADY

Indications for Renal Biopsy

Eberhard Ritz, Marcin Adamczak, and Martin Zeier

How should renal biopsy be done and what requirements must be met?

What is the diagnostic information obtained by renal biopsy?
- What kind of information is provided by the renal biopsy?

What are the potential indications for renal biopsy?
- Microhematuria
- Isolated acute nephritic syndrome
- Rapidly progressive glomerulonephritis
- Nephrotic syndrome
- Focal segmental glomerulosclerosis
- Diabetes mellitus
- Chronic renal failure
- Acute renal failure
- Renal allograft

Renal histology is the gold standard for the diagnosis of renal disease. It has been stated that the nephrologist who does not look at the kidney resembles the hematologist who does not analyze the blood smear. Nephrologists have a number of diagnostic procedures at their disposal, including family history, the patient's history, serologic investigations such as complement, antinuclear antibody (ANA), antineutrophil cytoplasmic antibody (ANCA), antiglomerular basement membrane antibody, hepatitis B virus (HBV) and hepatitis C virus (HCV) serology, cryoglobins, proteinuria, and microscopic analysis of the urinary sediment to mention only a few. If phase-contrast microscopy is used for the analysis of the urinary sediment, the differential diagnosis can be substantially narrowed down. The finding of dysmorphic erythrocytes (acanthocytes), and granular casts, cellular casts or erythrocyte casts is virtually diagnostic of glomerular disease. It has been stated that the analysis of the urinary sediment is a downstream analysis of upstream events. Nevertheless, renal biopsy is very often indispensable for arriving at a definite diagnosis and establishing the indications for treatment.

How should renal biopsy be done and what requirements must be met?

The indication for renal biopsy must consider the relation between diagnostic benefit and potential adverse effects. The technique of renal biopsy has been much improved since the 1950s, when Brun introduced the procedure.[1]

Major advances have been ultrasonographic control of the procedure and reduction of the bore of the needle with controlled spring-loaded advancement of the needle under sterile conditions. Using the ultrasound-guided Biopty T technique (Biopty Radioplast AB, Uppsala, Sweden) we had a single case of macrohematuria requiring interventional radiology (placement of a coil) and three patients who required blood transfusion among 1090 patients. Only 2.2.% had hematoma formation greater than 2×2 cm and macrohematuria was seen in only 8% of patients. Histopathologic diagnosis could be made in 1077 of 1090 biopsies (98.8%). The median number of glomeruli was nine (range 1–37) per biopsy.[2]

In order to minimize the risk of biopsy, a number of preconditions must be met that are summarized in Table 11.1. Conventional renal biopsy is absolutely contraindicated in patients with hemorrhagic diathesis and uncontrolled hypertension. (There have recently been suggestions that in such cases transjugular biopsy may be an alternative.[3]) The risk is definitely higher if the patient has a single kidney, contracted kidneys (i.e. parenchymal width < 9 mm, in which case the yield of tissue is also usually unsatisfactory), anatomically abnormal kidneys (because of the risk of abnormal vascular supply; Duplex sonography suggested), urinary tract infection, or urinary tract obstruction.

A frequent problem is the patient who has inadvertently taken aspirin or nonsteroidal anti-inflammatory drugs (NSAIDs) for a planned biopsy. It is our policy to withdraw these drugs for 5 days, which is usually sufficient to normalize bleeding time. If this is not the case and the indication is urgent, we usually administer DDAVP (1-deamino-8-D-arginine vasopressin, Minirin) at a dose of 0.4 µg/kg body weight. A less recommended alternative is

Table 11.1 Examinations before renal biopsy

Renal ultrasonography
Single kidney?
Orthotopic position?
Normal parenchymal width?
Aberrant vessels (Duplex sonography)
Blood pressure < 140/90 mmHg
Normal prothrombin time, partial thromboplastin time, factor VIII, thrombocyte count, bleeding time
No recent ingestion of aspirin or nonsteroidal anti-inflammatory drugs
Sterile urine culture

the administration of estrogens; we use a total dose of 3 mg/kg divided over 5 days (5 × 0.6 mg/kg conjugated estrogens).[4]

There has been much discussion about whether renal biopsy can be done on an outpatient basis, which offers substantial financial savings.[5] Personally we feel that while this is feasible in many patients there is a small but definite risk of hemorrhage, so we perform renal biopsy on an inpatient basis only.

Late complications of renal biopsy comprise arteriovenous fistulae (which usually close spontaneously but may require invasive angiologic procedures, e.g. coil placement) and Page kidney after perirenal hematoma, i.e. renal compression by perirenal scar tissue with renin-dependent hypertension.

What is the diagnostic information obtained by renal biopsy?

Apart from providing a diagnosis,[6,7] renal biopsy may be helpful in evaluating the course of renal disease. It is by no means exceptional, particularly in renal diseases with flares and remissions such as vasculitis or lupus nephritis, that sequential biopsies are required.[8] This is important in two situations. First, one will be reluctant to administer aggressive immunosuppression in the patient in whom the biopsy shows substantial scarring so that reversibility of the lesion is not very likely. It is often more prudent to let the patient go into endstage renal failure and then perform transplantation, particularly since in lupus nephritis (and less so in vasculitis) recurrence of the disease into the graft is rare. Second, a nephritic urinary sediment in the patient with vasculitis may not always be due to relapse of the disease but to de novo IgA glomerulonephritis, for which aggressive immunosuppressive therapy of vasculitis is of course not indicated.[9]

It goes without saying that optimal information can be obtained from a renal biopsy only if sufficient material is obtained.[10] We try to obtain at least two cores (one for light microscopy and one for immunohistology), and if possible three cores (an additional one for electron microscopy or molecular studies). The advantage of electron microscopy is very often undervalued. Electron microscopy permits recognition of thin basement membrane disease (not an infrequent cause of dysmorphic microhematuria) and is extremely helpful in the diagnosis of Alport syndrome. Beyond this, the exact topographic location of deposits and the evaluation of subcellular details is extremely valuable in arriving at the correct diagnosis.

What kind of information is provided by the renal biopsy?

The type and extent of renal involvement provides prognostic information (more adverse in patients with tubular atrophy, interstitial fibrosis, vascular sclerosis, and focal segmental glomerulosclerosis); it also provides informa-

tion on the potential reversibility of the lesions, e.g. in lupus marked signs of activity (which justify aggressive intervention) vs. marked signs of chronicity, e.g. scarring (which justifies a cautious approach or no intervention at all). Renal biopsy also permits the nephrologist to recognize the coexistence of different renal diseases, e.g. Wegener disease plus IgA glomerulonephritis,[9,11] IgA glomerulonephritis plus minimal-change glomerulonephritis,[12] antiglomerular basement membrane antibody glomerulonephritis plus vasculitis,[13] membranous glomerulonephritis plus rapidly progressive glomerulonephritis (RPGN),[14] or hemolytic–uremic syndrome (HUS) plus glomerulonephritis.[15]

Renal biopsy is often the only procedure which permits an early diagnosis of rare conditions that are difficult or impossible to diagnose noninvasively, such as primary amyloidosis, light-chain deposit disease, lecithin cholesterol acyltransferase deficiency, fibrillary glomerulopathy, sarcoidosis (occasionally renal limited), and infiltration of the kidney, e.g. by B-cell lymphoma restricted to the kidney.

Particularly intriguing is the fact that today the diagnosis of several rare metabolic disorders has consequences for therapeutic intervention, e.g. Fabry disease (for which recombinant enzymatic therapy has become available[16]), oxalosis, cystinosis, and Refsum disease. This list is impressive and should convince the reader that renal biopsy is more than an innocent academic exercise without practical consequences.

What are the potential indications for renal biopsy?

Table 11.2 summarizes the major renal syndromes in which renal biopsy should be considered.[17]

Microhematuria

In our view, microhematuria per se does not justify renal biopsy unless phase-contrast microscopy shows dysmorphic erythrocytes in the urinary sediment, with granular, cellular, or erythrocyte casts. The indication is even stronger if the patient has concomitant proteinuria and/or

---

Table 11.2 Nephrologic syndromes in which renal biopsy should be considered

Asymptomatic hematuria (dysmorphic erythrocytes, erythrocyte casts) ± proteinuria

Acute nephritic syndrome

Rapidly progressive glomerulonephritis

Nephrotic syndrome

Chronic renal failure

Acute renal failure

Renal allograft dysfunction

Table 11.3 Differential diagnosis of asymptomatic hematuria/proteinuria

IgA glomerulonephritis
Alport disease
Thin basement membrane disease
Systemic lupus erythematosus
Initially isolated renal involvement in systemic disease
Membranoproliferative glomerulonephritis

hypertension. (Obviously blood pressure has then to be normalized before renal biopsy.) The major causes of asymptomatic hematuria/proteinuria to consider are summarized in Table 11.3.

Isolated acute nephritic syndrome

An isolated acute nephritic syndrome with acute-onset microhematuria/macrohematuria, proteinuria, edema, and hypertension can be due to postinfectious glomerulonephritis, IgA glomerulonephritis, Henoch–Schönlein purpura, renal-limited Wegener's granulomatosis/microscopic polyarteritis (presumably early stage of RPGN), and rarely systemic lupus erythematosus.

Rapidly progressive glomerulonephritis

RPGN is a nephrologic emergency that requires urgent confirmation by renal biopsy unless there are serious contraindications. Table 11.4 lists the major forms of glomerulonephritis to consider. The biopsy is important for assessing the extent of renal inflammation, activity

Table 11.4 Differential diagnosis of rapidly progressive glomerulonephritis (RPGN)

Immune complex glomerulonephritis
Postinfectious glomerulonephritis
Henoch–Schönlein purpura
Systemic lupus erythematosus
Antiglomerular basement membrane antibody glomerulonephritis
Isolated glomerulonephritis
Goodpasture syndrome (with hemoptysis)
Pauci-immune RPGN
Wegener disease
Microscopic polyangiitis
Renal-limited crescentic glomerulonephritis
Differential diagnosis
Hemolytic–uremic syndrome (enterohemorrhagic *Escherichia coli*, idiopathic) and malignant hypertension including scleroderma kidney. Consider hemolytic–uremic syndrome plus glomerulonephritis!

vs. chronicity of the lesions (reflecting reversibility vs. irreversibility of the lesion), superimposition of diseases such as combination of antiglomerular basement membrane antibody glomerulonephritis and Wegener disease,[13,18] or superimposition of de novo IgA glomerulonephritis mimicking the urinary findings of a relapse of Wegener disease.[9,11]

Nephrotic syndrome

The presence of a nephrotic syndrome, i.e. proteinuria > 3.5 g/1.73 m^2 per 24 h, is a classic indication for renal biopsy.[19] The exception to this rule is the pediatric case where steroid-sensitive minimal-change glomerulonephritis is by far the most frequent condition. There is consensus that in children renal biopsy should be considered only after the response to steroids has been evaluated.[20] The types of renal lesions found are somewhat different in children compared with adults (Table 11.5). Table 11.6 lists the most common glomerular diseases to consider. Rare causes of renal disease identified by renal biopsy include fibrillary glomerulopathy (immunotactoid glomerulonephritis), amyloidosis (AL, AA, transthyretin), light-chain deposit disease, collapsing glomerulopathy, infection-associated glomerulonephritis (e.g. endocarditis, syphilis,

Table 11.5 Nephrotic syndrome in children and adults

	Children (%)	Adults (%)
Minimal-change glomerulonephritis	76	20
Focal segmental glomerulosclerosis	8	15
Membranous glomerulonephritis	7	40
Membranoproliferative glomerulonephritis	4	7
Other	5	18

Table 11.6 Differential diagnosis of nephrotic syndrome

Minimal-change glomerulopathy, focal segmental glomerulosclerosis
Glomerulonephritis
Membranous glomerulonephritis
Membranoproliferative glomerulonephritis
Nephrotic syndrome in systemic diseases
Diabetes (type 1 and type 2)
Amyloidosis (AL, AA, transthyretin)
Heredofamilial disease
Alport disease
Nail patella syndrome
Protein deposit disease
Amyloidosis (AA, AL)
Light-chain deposit disease

HBV, HCV, HIV), protozoan disease (malaria quartana, toxoplasmosis, schistosomiasis, filiariasis), heredofamilial syndromes (Alport disease, nail patella syndrome), immune reactions to medication (gold, penicillamine, NSAIDs, interferon α), illicit drugs (heroin, cocaine), or environmental toxins (poison ivy, bee sting, snake bite).

Focal segmental glomerulosclerosis

The diagnosis of focal segmental glomerulosclerosis (FSGS) requires specific comment (Table 11.7). The diagnosis describes a histologic finding that may have quite different causes with different prognostic implications. Primary FSGS is thought to be due to a circulating factor, because evidence from the first voided urine shows that the condition may recur immediately after transplantation.[21] Primary FSGS responds to steroids more frequently than reported in the past (total remission in 47%, partial remission in 8%[22]), but overall has a very poor prognosis.

The secondary forms of FSGS are thought to be the consequence of glomerular hypertension/hyperfiltration. The associated proteinuria responds particularly well to angiotensin-converting enzyme inhibitors and angiotensin receptor blockers (in contrast to idiopathic FSGS) but does not respond to steroids.[23] Thus, behind a similar glomerular picture there may be a different pathogenesis. It is with this caveat in mind that one must interpret the diagnosis of FSGS and select the respective therapies.

A unique form, frequently but not always associated with HIV, is characterized by a unique glomerular pathology (collapsing glomerulonephritis). It has very poor prognosis.[24]

Diabetes mellitus

A particular bone of contention is the indication for renal biopsy in patients with diabetes mellitus. There is consensus that if the clinical presentation fits into the pattern expected in type 1 diabetic patients, the chances that renal biopsy yields information that alters therapy is very slim indeed, since Kimmelstiel–Wilson glomerulosclerosis will virtually always be found. The issue is more difficult in type 2 diabetic patients, because the temporal pattern between onset of diabetes and development of diabetic nephropathy is somewhat different. While in type 1 diabetic patients it is very unusual that proteinuria occurs before the tenth year of diabetes, this is quite common in type 2 diabetes, presumably because of more and prolonged periods of unrecognized diabetic hyperglycemia before the diagnosis has been made. Table 11.8 summarizes the main indications when biopsy should be considered.

Chronic renal failure

In chronic renal failure, renal biopsy usually shows nonspecific scarring and does not yield further diagnostic information. The biopsy is not without risk if the parenchyma is shrunken and the parenchymal width is < 9 mm. Biopsy should only be considered if transplantation is an option and if recurrent disease in the graft is thought to be a possibility.

Acute renal failure

In the patient with acute renal failure, renal biopsy is usually not indicated. Very often the cause of acute renal failure can be established based on the patient's history.[25] Acute renal dysfunction caused by primary renal disease should be suspected when the patient has a nephritic sediment or when there is clinical or serologic evidence of systemic disease (ANCA, ANA, antiglomerular basement membrane antibodies, thrombocytopenia, and other presentations suggesting HUS). A particular situation necessitating renal biopsy is acute renal failure in the nephrotic patient with minimal-change glomerulonephritis. Renal biopsy may show almost completely normal tissue. The condition is usually, but not always, reversible. Renal biopsy may also be useful for recognizing acute glomerulonephritis and acute interstitial nephritis; the latter is usually a consequence of drug allergy or is idiopathic (e.g. tubulointerstitial nephritis with uveitis) or the result of viral infection (particularly Hanta virus). The biopsy in the patient with acute renal failure may also show acute tubular blockade due to drugs (methotrexate, dextran), acute oxalosis (e.g. after exposure to glycol),

Table 11.7 Focal segmental glomerulosclerosis: potential causes
Primary (idiopathic) focal segmental glomerulosclerosis
HIV or heroin-associated focal segmental glomerulosclerosis
Secondary focal segmental glomerulosclerosis

With reduced renal mass, e.g.
    Oligomeganephronia
    Unilateral renal agenesis
    Renal dysplasia
    Reflux nephropathy
    Massive surgical ablation
    Renal allograft failure

With initially normal renal mass, e.g.
    Diabetes mellitus
    Obesity
    Cyanotic congenital heart failure

Table 11.8 Potential indications for renal biopsy in diabetic patients with nephropathy
Biopsy not indicated when: Typical evolution of renal disease Concomitant retinopathy
Biopsy should be considered when: Renal manifestations atypically early (< 10 years) in type 1 diabetes Dysmorphic erythrocytes/casts Rapid deterioration of renal function Elevated serum creatinine without urine abnormalities

Table 11.9 Indications for renal biopsy in patients with acute renal failure

Progressive loss of renal function

Persisting oliguria

Absence of recognizable cause of acute renal failure

Marked proteinuria or dysmorphic hematuria

Exclusion of systemic disorders

Marked hypertension (exclude hemolytic–uremic syndrome)

Preexisting glomerular disease

Suspected drug allergy

calcium phosphate precipitates (tumor lysis syndrome), or atheroembolism. The indications for renal biopsy are summarized in Table 11.9.

Renal allograft

Biopsy of the graft is superior to aspiration cytology, because it provides more complete assessment of renal structures.

In selected cases, graft biopsy may be performed at the time of transplantation. Particularly in elderly and borderline donors, poor long-term graft function is correlated to renal pathology, specifically to vascular and interstitial lesions, but not to glomerular lesions.

Classically, the most important indication for renal allograft biopsy in the early postoperative period has been suspicion of acute rejection or exclusion of calcineurin inhibitor toxicity. In cases with prolonged postoperative oliguria or anuria, biopsies are necessary because superimposed rejection may not cause any signs and symptoms.

With the recognition that clinically concealed rejection may not be reflected by changes in serum creatinine concentration, protocol biopsies have become increasingly popular and permit early intervention with immunosuppressive treatment. Initial studies show that this improves long-term graft outcome. Protocol renal biopsies may be performed for instance at 8 weeks and 6 months after renal transplantation.

A further indication is chronically deteriorating renal function. Renal biopsy gives useful information whether there is rejection or another abnormality, particularly calcineurin toxicity or recurrent disease, whether the lesion is chronically sclerosing (in which case the chances of reversal by aggressive immune therapy are limited), or

Table 11.10 Simplified Banff schema

Biopsy findings	Banff classification	Possible clinical approach
Normal minor changes or infiltrates, *without* tubular invasion	Normal or "other" nonspecific changes	No treatment, or treat other entity
Mild lymphocytic invasion of tubules (tubulitis)	Borderline changes	No treatment, or treat other entity
Widespread interstitial infiltrate with moderate invasion of tubules	Mild acute rejection (Grade I)*	Treat for rejection if there are clinical signs
(A) Widespread interstitial infiltrate with severe invasion of tubules and/or (B) mild or moderate intimal arteritis	Moderate acute rejection (Grade II)	Treat for rejection, consider antilymphocyte globulin/OKT3 if refractory to steroids
Severe intimal arteritis and/or "transmural" arteritis, fibrinoid change, and medial smooth muscle cell necrosis often with patchy infarction and interstitial hemorrhage	Severe acute rejection (Grade III)	Treat for rejection unless clinical course suggests rejection which cannot be reversed, in which case consider abandoning the graft
Hyaline arteriolar thickening (new onset, not present in implantation biopsy) and/or extensive isomeric vacuolization of tubules, smooth muscle degeneration, thrombotic microangiopathy	Cyclosporine toxicity	Reduce cyclosporine therapy
Tubular cell loss and necrosis, regenerative changes	Acute tubular necrosis	Await recovery
Interstitial fibrosis, tubular atrophy (new-onset arterial fibrous intimal thickening suggests chronic rejection)	Chronic transplant nephropathy	Temporize

Examination should attempt to obtain biopsies with at least two cores containing in aggregate at least one to six glomeruli with arteries. A minimum of seven sections should be cut; three stained with H & E, three with PAS, and one with trichrome.
*In grade I or mild acute rejection, moderate tubulitis is defined as the presence of foci with more than four mononuclear cells in at least one tubular cross-section or group of 10 tubular cells.

whether there is acute rejection (which is often due to patient noncompliance).

Table 11.10 summarizes the features important for the diagnosis of rejection according to the Banff classification.[26] Tables 11.11 and 11.12 give incomplete lists of potential causes of acute (Table 11.11) and chronic (Table 11.12) allograft dysfunction. Apart from light microscopy, further useful information can be obtained by immunohistologic analysis, which differentiates the type of infiltrating cells, shows deposition of complement, and activation of tubuloepithelial cells. A completely new perspective may be provided soon by molecular methods currently under development.

Table 11.11 Differential diagnosis of posttransplantation oliguria

Prerenal cause (salt–volume depletion)

Hyperacute or acute rejection*

Acute renal failure (acute tubular necrosis)*

Calcineurin inhibitor toxicity (cyclosporine, tacrolimus)*

Arterial or venous thrombosis (± graft necrosis)

Graft damage following hydroxyethyl starch administration to the donor*

Viral infection

Nephrotoxic antibiotics

Lymphocele

Recurrent primary disease, particularly focal segmental glomerulosclerosis and oxalosis*

*Conditions in which renal biopsy is diagnostic.

Table 11.12 Differential diagnosis of chronic graft dysfunction

Chronic allograft nephropathy*

Calcineurin inhibitor toxicity*

Recurrent renal disease*

De novo glomerulonephritis*

Diabetic nephropathy (persisting or de novo diabetes)*

Hemolytic–uremic syndrome (recurrent or calcineurin inhibitor triggered)*

Viral disease (cytomegalovirus, polyoma virus, etc.)*

Graft artery stenosis or iliac artery stenosis

Atheroembolism*

Hypercalcemia, oxalosis, oxypurinol nephropathy*

Urinary tract obstruction or infection

*Conditions in which renal biopsy is diagnostic.

The recent trend toward performing more frequent allograft biopsies and even protocol biopsies is justified, because the graft in superficial location can be easily identified by ultrasonography so that the biopsy technique is simple to perform with few complications.

References

1. Iverson P, Brun C: Aspiration biopsy of kidney. Am J Med 1951;11:324–330.
2. Hergesell O, Felten H, Andrassy K, Kuhn K, Ritz E: Safety of ultrasound-guided percutaneous renal biopsy: retrospective analysis of 1090 consecutive cases. Nephrol Dial Transplant 1998;13:975–977.
3. Cluzel P, Martinez F, Bellin MF, et al: Transjugular versus percutaneus renal biopsy for the diagnosis of parenchymal disease: comparison of sampling effectiveness and complications. Radiology 2000;215:689–693.
4. Stiles KP, Yuan CM, Chung EM, Lyon RD, Lane JD, Abbot KC: Renal biopsy in high risk patients with medical diseases of the kidney. Am J Kidney Dis 2000;36:419–433.
5. Fraser IR, Fairley KF: Renal biopsy as an outpatient procedure. Am J Kidney Dis 1995;25:876–878.
6. Turner MW, Hutchinson TA, Barre PE, Prichard S, Jothy S: A prospective study on the impact of the renal biopsy in clinical management. Clin Nephrol 1986;26:217–221.
7. Monteseny J, Kleinknecht D, Meyrier A, et al: Long-term outcome according to renal histological lesions in 118 patients with monoclonal gammopathies. Nephrol Dial Transplant 1998;13:1438–1445.
8. Moroni G, Pasquali S, Quglini S, et al: Clinical and prognostic value of serial renal biopsies in lupus nephritis. Am J Kidney Dis 1999;34:530–539.
9. Andrassy K, Waldherr R, Erb A, Ritz E: De novo glomerulonephritis in patients during remission from Wegener's granulomatosis. Clin Nephrol 1992;38:295–298.
10. Furness PN: ACP Best Practice No 160. Renal biopsy specimens. J Clin Pathol 2000;53:433–438.
11. Vrtovsnik F, Queffeulou G, Skhiri H, et al: Simultaneous IgA nephropathy and Wegener's granulomatosis: overlap or coincidence (the role of renal biopsy). Nephrol Dial Transplant 1999;14:1266–1267.
12. Monga G, Mazzuco G, Barbiano di Belgiojoso G, Confalonieri R, Sacchi G, Bertani T: Pattern of double glomerulopathies. A clinicopathologic study in nine nondiabetic patients. Nephron 1990;56:73–80.
13. Wu MJ, Rajaram R, Shelp WD, Beirne GJ, Burkholder PM: Vasculitis in Goodpasture's syndrome. Arch Pathol Lab Med 1980;104:300–302.
14. Kurki P, Helve T, von Bondorff M, et al: Transformation of membranous glomerulonephritis into crescentic glomerulonephritis with glomerular basement membrane antibodies. Serial determination of anti-GBM before the transplantation. Nephron 1984;38:134–137.
15. Morita S, Sakai T, Okamoto N, et al: Hemolytic uremic syndrome associated with immunoglobin A nephropathy: a case report and review of cases of hemolytic syndrome with glomerular disease. Intern Med 1999;38:495–499.
16. Schiffmann R, Murray GJ, Treco D, et al: Infusion of α-galactosidase A reduces tissue globotriaosylceramide storage in patients with Fabry disease. Proc Natl Acad Sci USA 2000;97:365–370.
17. Fuianno G, Mazza G, Comi N, et al: Current indications for renal biopsy: a questionnaire-based survey. Am J Kidney Dis 2000;35:448–457.
18. Kalluri R, Meyers K, Mogyrosi A, Madaio MP, Neilson EG: Goodpasture syndrome involving overlap with Wegener's granulomatosis and anti-glomerular basement membrane disease. J Am Soc Nephrol 1997;8:1795–1800.
19. Orth SR, Ritz E: The nephrotic syndrome. N Engl J Med 1998;338:1202–1211.
20. Webb NJ, Lewis MA, Iqbal J, Smart PJ, Lendon M, Postlethwaite RJ: Childhood steroid-sensitive nephritic syndrome: does the histology matter? Am J Kidney Dis 1996;27:484–488.
21. Dantal J, Bigot E, Bogers W, et al: Effect of plasma protein adsorption on protein excretion in kidney-transplant recipients with recurrent nephrotic syndrome. N Engl J Med 1994;330:7–14.

22. Meyrier A: Treatment of primary focal segmental glomerulosclerosis. Nephrol Dial Transplant 1999;14:74–78.
23. Schmidt A, Mayer G: The diagnostic trash bin of focal and segmental glomerulosclerosis: an effort to provide rational clinical guidelines. Nephrol Dial Transplant 1999;14:550–552.
24. Barisoni L, Kriz W, Mundel P, D'Agati V: The dysregulated podocyte phenotype: a novel concept in the pathogenesis of collapsing idiopathic focal segmental glomerulosclerosis and HIV associated nephropathy. J Am Soc Nephrol 1999;10:51–61.
25. Haas M, Spargo BH, Wit EJ, Meehan SM: Etiologies and outcome of acute renal insufficiency in older adults: a renal biopsy study of 250 cases. Am J Kidney Dis 2000;35:433–447.
26. Gaber LW, Moore LW, Gaber AO, et al: Utility of standardized histological classification in the management of acute rejections. 1995 Efficacy Endpoints Conference. Transplantation 1998;65:376–380.

Immunosuppressive Therapy in Immunologic Renal Disease and Transplantation

Alden M. Doyle, Laurence A. Turka, and Roy D. Bloom

Outline of the immune response
- Induction phase
- Effector phase

General principles of immunosuppression

Specific immunosuppressive agents (Table 12.1)
- Glucocorticosteroids
  - Mechanism of action
  - Adverse effects
- Azathioprine
  - Mechanism of action
  - Adverse effects
- Mycophenolate mofetil
  - Mechanism of action
  - Adverse effects
- Calcineurin inhibitors (cyclosporine and tacrolimus)
  - Mechanism of action
  - Adverse effects
- TOR inhibitors (sirolimus and everolimus)
  - Mechanism of action
  - Adverse effects
- Cyclophosphamide
  - Mechanism of action
  - Adverse effects
- Polyclonal antilymphocyte preparations
  - Mechanism of action
  - Adverse effects
- Muromonab-CD3 (OKT3)
  - Mechanism of action
  - Adverse effects
- IL-2 receptor antibodies
  - Mechanism of action
  - Adverse effects
- Plasmapheresis/plasma exchange
  - Mechanism of action
  - Adverse effects

The ability to specifically modulate the immune system is a relatively recent advance in medicine, but it has had a profound impact on clinical practice. Specifically, this ability has had dramatic consequences on our capacity to alter the course of autoimmune disease and, perhaps most dramatic, has made the modern era of solid organ transplantation possible.

The goal of this chapter is to provide an overview of the immunosuppressive agents used in transplantation and other immunologically mediated renal diseases. We begin with a general overview of immune responses, focusing on those aspects that are important in understanding the logic behind the clinical use of immunosuppressive drugs.

Next, we outline clinically relevant characteristics of individual immunosuppressive agents, focusing on mechanisms of action, interactions, and toxicities of individual medications. This is meant as a general guide to their use and not as an exhaustive review of individual drugs.

Outline of the immune response

The human immune system can respond to a nearly infinite range of foreign antigens by generating and maintaining immune responses that are rapid, antigen specific, and protective. The cardinal features of this system are (1) specificity to antigenic diversity, (2) memory, and (3) tolerance for self. The vital importance of this system is demonstrated by the rapid demise of infants born with prominent defects in immunity (e.g. severe combined immunodeficiency, or SCID, syndrome) when exposed to the environment. Nonetheless, there are circumstances when the immune system results in untoward clinical effects on its host, as is the case with autoimmunity and transplantation.

There are multiple cell types that play a role in immunity. The majority of cellular components of the immune system are derived from the bone marrow and include T lymphocytes, B lymphocytes, natural killer (NK) cells, macrophages, and dendritic cells. Lymphocytes and NK cells play a central role in most immune responses because they provide specificity through their specialized antigen receptors. Also important are those cells that directly interact with lymphocytes. Some of the interactive cells serve as antigen presenters, and supply the co-stimulatory ligands that are required in conjunction with the appropriate antigens to initiate and sustain the immune response, while others serve as additional effector arms of the immune system, with the ability to kill or neutralize specific targets. Additional nonmarrow-derived cells, such as specialized stromal cells and endothelial cells, provide an appropriate microenvironment in which the other immune cells can function.

The majority of immune responses begin by encounter with an antigen that is recognized as nonself. Under the appropriate conditions, this results in the expansion of antigen-specific T-cell populations, which then provide "help" for the expansion and differentiation of B cells and their production of antigen-specific antibodies. In most cases, this process requires presentation of the antigens by professional antigen-presenting cells (APCs) such as dendritic cells, B-cells, and macrophages that take up the antigenic proteins, process them, and present them to the responding cells in the context of specific accessory molecules. In this way, there are multiple steps required to generate and maintain an immune response, which allows for a high level of control and feedback.

T cells are derived from the thymus and play a central role in *cellular immunity*. As the name implies, cellular immunity requires effector cells to either directly contact target cells or elaborate substances (cytokines) that act over short distances. Cellular immunity accounts for *delayed-type hypersensitivity*, which directs cellular lysis, graft vs. host disease, and the majority of solid organ transplant rejection.

T-cell responses occur when the T-cell receptor (TCR) engages an antigenic peptide presented in the antigen-binding groove of a major histocompatibility complex (MHC) molecule.[1] T cells do not respond to antigen alone, but rather require "antigen presentation" by an MHC molecule in the setting of appropriate costimulation. MHC molecules are broadly divided into class I proteins, which are expressed on all nucleated cells, and class II proteins, which are found predominantly on specialized APCs such as macrophages, dendritic cells, and B cells.[2] MHC class I molecules usually present endogenous (i.e. cytosolic) antigens, thus serving as a means by which the cell displays all of the proteins it is manufacturing. Viral infection or malignant transformation can lead to the expression of neoantigens, which are detected by surveillance of MHC class I molecules. MHC class II molecules present exogenous antigens, which are taken up through phagocytosis (in the case of macrophages and dendritic cells) or immuno-globulin-mediated internalization (in the case of B cells). T lymphocytes themselves are subdivided by the expression of either of two glycoproteins, CD4 or CD8. CD4+ lymphocytes recognize antigen presented by MHC class II molecules, and CD8+ lymphocytes recognize antigen presented by MHC class I molecules.

B cells are produced in the bone marrow and make up the humoral arm of the immune system. B cells express a highly specialized form of antigen receptor, surface immunoglobulin, and are the precursors of plasma cells, which can secrete a soluble form of the immunoglobulin, the antibody. Immunoglobulins belong to four principal classes (IgA, IgE, IgG, IgM), all of which share a common structure that relies on a highly-specific antigen-binding structure.

Induction phase

One can think of immune responses as being divided into distinct induction and effector phases. Most often, antigens that provoke an immune response are encountered in nonlymphoid tissues, where they are picked up and processed by specialized APCs such as dendritic cells. These cells undergo a maturation process that involves expression of cell surface proteins that promote interactions and signaling, then migrate to regional draining lymph nodes where they can present the antigens to T lymphocytes.

When T cells see the presented antigen in the context of the appropriate secondary signals, their populations begin to expand and secrete cytokines, which completes the induction phase of the immune response (Fig. 12.1). Most of the cytokines are derived from CD4+ cells (so-called T helper or Th cells). These cytokines can act on the CD4+ cells themselves in an autocrine fashion, and on other cells in the local microenvironment (CD8+ T cells, macrophages, B cells, etc.) in a paracrine fashion. These cytokines are critically important for the induction of an immune response. Thus, immunosuppressants that act to prevent T-cell activation, inhibit T-cell cytokine production, or block the effects of cytokines are very potent.

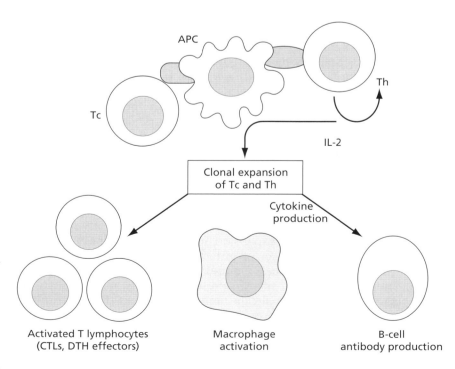

Figure 12.1 Inductive phase of T-cell-mediated immune responses. Most T-cell-mediated immune responses are initiated when CD4+ T cells encounter antigen presented by MHC class II on an antigen-presenting cell (APC). CD4+ cells, often referred to as T helper (Th) cells, are the primary source for cytokines which drive the immune response. These cytokines serve as growth and differentiation factors for CD4+ cells as well as other immune effector cells. For T cells, both CD4+ helper cells and CD8+ cytotoxic T lymphocytes (CTLs), interleukin 2 (IL-2) is the primary growth factor. B cells depend most on IL-4, while interferon-γ is of primary importance in activating macrophages. DTH, delayed-type hypersensitivity; Tc, cytotoxic T cell.

APC

Tc

Th

IL-2

Clonal expansion of Tc and Th

Cytokine production

Activated T lymphocytes (CTLs, DTH effectors)

Macrophage activation

B-cell antibody production

One of the most important cytokines is interleukin 2 (IL-2). This cytokine is a potent growth and survival factor for T and B lymphocytes. Blockade of IL-2 in vitro strongly inhibits both proliferation and survival of T cells. In vivo blockade of IL-2 is slightly less effective, due perhaps to overlapping functions of IL-2 with other important cytokines including interferon (IFN)-γ, IL-4, and IL-15, a cytokine with closely related functions to IL-2.[3] In addition to its effects on T cells, IL-4 is also a potent growth and maturation promoter for B cells (see later), driving their differentiation into antibody-secreting plasma cells. IFN-γ, which is also primarily produced by T cells and NK cells, promotes the activation of macrophages, an integral component of many cellular immune responses.[4]

Effector phase

In this phase of the immune response, activated effector cells including T cells, B cells, NK cells, and macrophages, migrate to the site of original antigen encounter. Once in situ, these activated cells utilize a combination of mechanisms to kill and/or neutralize their targets. In the case of cellular immune responses, the primary mediators are cytotoxic T lymphocytes (CTLs), macrophages, and

selected cytokines produced in the local microenvironment (Fig. 12.2).

CTLs, primarily MHC class I-restricted CD8+ T cells, kill their targets through direct cell–cell contact by either of two means. The first method utilizes proteins such as perforin and granzyme B, which are contained in secretory granules of the CTL.[5] These proteins can create pores in the membranes of the target cells and actuate a cascade that results in cell lysis. The second method of CTL killing is through the Fas–Fas-ligand pathway,[6] in which engagement of Fas by its ligand results in programmed cell death. In each case, CTLs are antigen specific, meaning that they only kill select targets following recognition of antigen and activation of the CTL through its TCR.

Macrophages can kill their target cells in a number of ways. These include phagocytosis of the target cell, or killing by soluble factors such as reactive oxygen intermediates, proteases, and tumor necrosis factor (TNF). Unlike CTLs, which kill their targets in an antigen-specific manner, activated macrophages are antigen nonspecific and will attempt to kill all cells in their local environment. The one exception to this is phagocytosis of antibody-coated cells, which has some degree of specificity conferred upon it by the antibody molecule itself.

Cytokines themselves can directly affect target cells. While some cytokines are growth and differentiation factors, others can cause tissue destruction, particularly TNF and lymphotoxin. These related cytokines are released by activated macrophages, but are also produced by T cells. Thus even in the absence of macrophages, TNF-induced killing is a potent part of cell-mediated immunity.

Humoral immunity is, by definition, antibody mediated (see Fig. 12.2). The initial B-cell response to an antigen is IgM antibody production. As the immune response progresses, B cells receive "help" from T cells in the form of cytokines (such as IL-4) and other signals, the net result of which is proliferation, differentiation to plasma cells, and isotype switching from IgM to other classes of antibodies such as IgG, IgE, or IgA.[7] Antibodies themselves act through several mechanisms, the relative importance of which depends upon the isotype of the antibody, and the nature and anatomic site of the antigen.

1. Antibodies can act by stearic mechanisms, blocking access to and neutralizing an entire molecule or an epitope of the molecule critical for its function.
2. Antibodies can target cells for phagocytosis by macrophages and other cells with Fc receptors (Fc referring to the nonantigen-binding portion of the antibody molecule).
3. Antibodies can fix complement, resulting in both lysis of the cell and in activation of the complement cascade with resultant fibrin deposition, neutrophil recruitment, increase in vascular permeability, etc.

The degree to which cellular and humoral mechanisms are activated in response to an immune stimulus is controlled largely by the type of APC that presents antigen to the T cells (macrophage, B cell, dendritic cell), the cytokines present in the initiating microenvironment, and antigen concentration. The degree to which cellular or

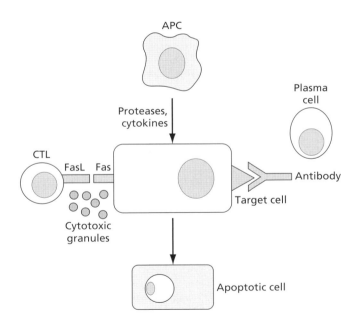

Figure 12.2 Effector phase of T-cell-mediated immune responses. Each type of cell shown in Fig. 12.1 can contribute to immune-mediated damage of target tissues. Cytotoxic T lymphocytes (CTLs) kill their targets via cell–cell contact using either of two mechanisms: perforins or Fas–Fas-ligand (FasL) (see text for details). Activated macrophages secrete soluble substances such as proteases, reactive oxygen intermediates, and tumor necrosis factor, any of which can kill a target cell. B cells act by secretion of antibodies. Once they bind to a target cell, antibodies can act by opsonizing the cell for phagocytosis (by a macrophage or other "scavenger cell"), by priming a cell for antibody-dependent cell-mediated cytotoxicity, or by activating complement leading to direct lysis of the target.

humoral mechanisms are responsible for tissue pathology will vary with the strength and site of the response. For example, organ transplant rejection in previously unsensitized recipients is almost always a cellular response. In contrast, immune complex-mediated glomerulonephritis is a humoral response. The remainder of this chapter focuses on the mechanism of actions and toxicities of immunosuppressive drugs. The choice of drugs for given diseases will vary based on: (1) the type of immune response causing the disease; (2) the relative effects of the drugs on cellular vs. humoral responses; and (3) the safety profiles and toxicities of the drugs in relation to the severity of the disease itself.

General principles of immunosuppression

A general axiom of immunosuppression is that toxicity due to immunodeficiency is inextricably linked to the immunosuppressive efficacy of the drug. As a consequence, the more a patient is immunosuppressed, the more their

chances of untoward effects from deficient immune surveillance. Patients who have immunodeficiencies, whether acquired or congenital, have an increased risk of both infections and neoplasia. With increased understanding of immunology, it may be possible to more specifically modulate immune function and avoid the consequences of broad-based immunosuppression. The Holy Grail of transplantation and the treatment of autoimmunity is to be able to achieve specific tolerance, a state characterized as the absence of a pathogenic immune response without a need for ongoing therapy.

Specific immunosuppressive agents (Table 12.1)

Glucocorticosteroids

Glucocorticoids are potent antiinflammatory and immunosuppressive agents and have been used for these purposes for several decades.

Table 12.1 Immunosuppressive drugs: their mechanisms of action and adverse effects

Drug	Mechanism of action	Adverse effects	Dosing guidelines
Corticosteroids	Inhibition of expression of genes encoding proinflammatory cytokines	Infections; glucose intolerance, hypercholesterolemia; hypertension; impaired wound healing, skin fragility, growth retardation, osteoporosis; central obesity; suppression of pituitary–hypothalamic axis; cataracts, glaucoma; psychosis	Varies according to disease process. Patients on chronic maintenance regimens should undergo biannual bone densitometry and be considered for prophylaxis with antiresorptive therapy and supplementation with calcium and vitamin D
Azathioprine	Competitive inhibitor of purine synthesis	Leukopenia, thrombocytopenia, anemia, hepatotoxicity, increased malignancies	Usually used in combination with calcineurin inhibitors and corticosteroids 1 mg/kg/day. Reduce/discontinue dose if WBC < 4000/mm^3, for chronic anemia, or in presence of severe infection or new malignancy
Mycophenolate mofetil	Noncompetitive inhibitor of inosine monophosphate dehydrogenase; inhibits purine synthesis	Nausea, vomiting, diarrhea, dyspepsia, leukopenia, anemia	Usually used in combination with calcineurin inhibitors and corticosteroids 2 g/day in divided doses with cyclosporine 1–1.5 g/day with tacrolimus. Reduce/discontinue dose if WBC < 4000/mm^3, for chronic anemia, or in presence of severe infection or new malignancy
Cyclosporine	Cyclosporine–cyclophilin complex prevents T-cell activation by inhibition of calcineurin; enhanced TGF-β expression leads to decreased T-cell proliferation	Infections, increased neoplasia; nephrotoxicity; hypertension; hyperlipidemia, glucose intolerance; hyperkalemia, hyperuricemia, and gout, hypomagnesemia; tremor, paresthesias, seizures, encephalopathy; thrombotic microangiopathy, hirsutism, gingival hyperplasia, hepatotoxicity	Usually given in combination with antimetabolite/steroid or steroid alone, rarely as monotherapy. Initial dosage is 3–4 mg/kg/day in divided doses. Target levels depend on use of concomitantly administered drugs and organs transplanted. By immunoassay, target 12-h trough levels are 200–300 ng/ml for first 3–6 months post transplant; 80–200 ng/ml beyond 6 months. Following dosage adjustment, levels can be rechecked 2–3 days later

Table 12.1 Immunosuppressive drugs: their mechanisms of action and adverse effects (*cont'd*)

Drug	Mechanism of action	Adverse effects	Dosing guidelines
Tacrolimus	Tacrolimus–FKBP complex inhibits calcineurin, leading to impaired T-cell activation	Infections, increased neoplasia, hyperglycemia, neurotoxicity including tremor and encephalopathy, hepatoxicity, nephrotoxicity, hyperkalemia, hypomagnesemia, alopecia, hyperlipidemia, diarrhea	Usually given in combination with antimetabolite/steroid or steroid alone, rarely as monotherapy. Initial dosage is 0.1 mg/kg/day in divided doses. Target levels depend on use of concomitantly administered drugs and organs transplanted. By immunoassay, target 12-h trough levels are 8–15 ng/ml for first 3–6 months post transplant; 5–10 ng/ml beyond 6 months. Following dosage adjustment, levels can be rechecked 2–3 days later
Sirolimus	Blocks growth factor-mediated cell proliferation	Infections, increased neoplasia, thrombocytopenia, anemia, leukopenia, hyperlipidemia, edema, lymphocele (renal transplant patients), diarrhea, headaches, interstitial pneumonitis, impaired wound healing	Generally used in combination with calcineurin inhibitors, starting dose 2–4 mg every morning, dosed to target 24-h trough level 4–8 ng/ml. Following dosage adjustment, should wait 5–7 days before rechecking level. Most patients require concomitant use of statin for hyperlipidemia
Cyclophosphamide	Alkylating agent, interferes with T and B cell proliferation and function	Leukopenia, hemorrhagic cystitis, bladder cancer, gonadal toxicity, syndrome of inappropriate ADH secretion	Dosing is usually protocol-based depending on disease process being treated. Blood counts need to be monitored and patients with evidence of bone marrow suppression may require dosage reductions
Polyclonal antilymphocyte antibodies	Cause lymphopenia and impair T-cell responses	Serum sickness, anaphylaxis, hemolysis, leukopenia, thrombocytopenia, fever, volume overload, thrombophlebitis, infections, increased neoplasia	Given as intravenous infusion over 4 h, via central venous catheter, for 3–7 days when used as induction agent, 7–10 days when used to treat acute allograft rejection. Dosage depends on which antibody preparation is used, and should be titrated according to WBC and platelet counts
Anti-CD25 antibodies	Specifically target CD25 on activated lymphocytes	Generally uncommon. Infections may occur; hypersensitivity may occur with basiliximab	These agents have only been used as induction therapy in transplantation in combination with other standard immunosuppressive drugs. Basiliximab is given as two 20 mg doses, the first on day 0 (within 2 h prior to transplantation) and the second on day 4 post transplant. The recommended dose of daclizumab is 1 mg/kg i.v. infusion within 24 h before transplantation (day 0), then every 14 days for four doses, though protocols may vary between centers
OKT3	Specifically targets CD3+ T cells and impairs function	"Cytokine release syndrome": fever, chills, pulmonary edema, hypotension, myalgias, increased clotting, aseptic meningitis, increased neoplasia	5 mg i.v. for 7–10 days for acute allograft rejection

ADH, antidiuretic hormone; TGF-β, transforming growth factor β; WBC, white blood cell.

Mechanism of action

Glucocorticoids affect the transcription of a large number of genes encoding mediators of inflammatory and immune responses. Numerous genes contain DNA regulatory sequences called glucocorticoid-responsive elements (GRE), to which the heterodimeric complex of the glucocorticoid and its cytosolic receptor can bind with resultant stimulation or suppression of transcription of that gene.[8] Corticosteroids decrease the transcription of key cytokines like IL-1α, IL-2, IL-4, IL-6, IL-10, TNFα, and IFN-γ.[9] Corticosteroids may also affect the transcription of genes that do not contain GREs.[10] As evidenced by the large number of target genes for glucocorticoids, their effects are exerted on a variety of cells, including lymphocytes and macrophages. Despite our understanding of the molecular mechanisms of these drugs, it is not certain which mechanisms predominate in vivo, and this may depend on the drug dose used. It appears likely that in the low doses used for daily maintenance therapy for prophylaxis of rejection or the treatment of glomerulonephritis, the antiinflammatory effects mediated through blockade of macrophage products such as IL-1α and TNFα are most important. At high doses, glucocorticoids are directly lympholytic, i.e. they kill T and B cells, and this action may explain the potent immunosuppressive effects of "pulse steroids."

Adverse effects

Given their multiple actions, it is no surprise that glucocorticoids have multiple adverse effects. These depend on the dosage and duration of use, with the majority of effects becoming a serious problem only after prolonged use. As with all immunosuppressive drugs, there is an increased risk of infection (viral, bacterial, and opportunistic). Corticosteroids lead to multiple metabolic abnormalities, including impaired glucose tolerance and hyperlipidemia. Together with the hypertension and volume overload caused by sodium retention, these adverse effects can significantly enhance progression of atherosclerosis and the attendant cardiovascular morbidity and mortality. Corticosteroids have devastating effects on connective tissues, causing poor wound healing, skin fragility, growth retardation in children, accelerated bone loss leading to osteoporosis, avascular necrosis of bones, and proximal myopathy. There may be an increase in the risk of peptic ulceration, although this remains controversial. Redistribution of fat centrally leads to the Cushingoid appearance and central obesity. Posterior subcapsular cataracts are also a problem. Neuropsychiatric manifestations include depression and psychosis. Suppression of the endogenous pituitary–hypothalamic axis may lead to significant adrenal insufficiency in periods of stress or on rapid withdrawal of the drugs. Other, less common adverse effects include pancreatitis, colonic perforation, and cardiac arrhythmias.

Strategies to reduce the adverse effects of corticosteroids rely on utilizing the minimal possible dosage for the correct indication and only for the shortest duration possible. However, premature or abrupt withdrawal of therapy should be avoided to prevent relapse of disease. Dosing of steroids on alternate days may decrease adverse effects, provided this can be done safely. Recent data suggest that corticosteroid-induced osteoporosis may be diminished by the use of calcium and vitamin D supplements as well as the use of agents to decrease bone resorption, including bisphosphonates and calcitonin.[11] The use of combination regimens in which other immunosuppressive agents act as steroid-sparing or steroid-avoiding therapy have also been of great utility in decreasing the incidence of steroid-induced iatrogenic diseases.

Azathioprine

Azathioprine is used for the prevention of transplant rejection, the treatment of a variety of autoimmune diseases, and for the maintenance of remission in certain types of vasculitis.

Mechanism of action

Azathioprine interferes with the synthesis of purines. Purine nucleotides form key elements of DNA and RNA and thus have an important role to play at several levels of the immune response, including DNA synthesis, required for cell proliferation, and RNA transcription, required for protein synthesis. In addition, purines are needed for the glycosylation of adhesion molecules and the activation of lymphocytes and macrophages. Azathioprine is a prodrug, whose active metabolite, 6-mercaptopurine, competitively inhibits the formation of phosphoribosyl pyrophosphate, a key intermediate in purine synthesis. Clearly, the central role of purines in nucleotide metabolism means that all cell types require them. However, lymphocytes are relatively unique in their dependence on de novo purine synthesis. Other cells are able to use a "salvage pathway" for recycling of purines. Thus azathioprine and related compounds (see later) are relatively selective for lymphocytes. Azathioprine use leads to mild lymphopenia without significant changes in subset ratios. There appears to be a dose-dependent depression of antibody production, T-cell proliferation, and NK cell activity.[12]

Adverse effects

Myelosuppression is the major adverse effect of azathioprine use and leads to leukopenia, megaloblastic anemia, and thrombocytopenia in that order of frequency. The dose can be adjusted to the white blood cell (WBC) count, which is usually maintained at levels above 3500/mm^3. Nausea, vomiting, and diarrhea may occur acutely. Hepatotoxicity with elevated liver enzymes may be seen. An increased incidence of hematologic and skin malignancies is reported. There is no significant gonadal dysfunction or teratogenicity due to azathioprine.[12] The use of lower doses in combination regimens has decreased the incidence of adverse effects. It is important to be aware of a significant drug interaction between azathioprine and allopurinol. The latter drug impairs the degradation of the active metabolites of azathioprine, thus greatly potentiating its in vivo effect. Profound and long-lasting neutropenia can occur with concomitant use of both drugs and death from sepsis has been reported. It is wise to consider azathioprine therapy a contraindication to the use of allopurinol. If absolutely necessary, allopurinol should be used with great caution, reducing the dose of azathioprine by at least 70% and monitoring neutrophil counts frequently (i.e. one to two times per week).

Mycophenolate mofetil

Mycophenolate mofetil was developed as an alternative to azathioprine for maintenance immunosuppression in transplant patients, as a steroid-sparing agent, and as a treatment for episodes of acute rejection. Like azathioprine, the use of mycophenolate mofetil has expanded to treatment of a wide variety of autoimmune disorders.

Mechanism of action

Mycophenolate mofetil is metabolized to mycophenolic acid, which causes noncompetitive inhibition of inosine monophosphate dehydrogenase (IMPDH), a key enzyme in the de novo synthesis of guanine nucleotides.[13] Due to their significant dependence on this pathway, in addition to salvage mechanisms for purine synthesis (see section on azathioprine), proliferating lymphocytes are especially susceptible to inhibition of IMPDH. Consequently, exposure to mycophenolic acid impairs T-cell proliferation in response to antigen stimulation, decreases B-cell activity and antibody production, and also decreases adhesion molecule function due to impaired glycosylation.[14]

Adverse effects

Mycophenolate mofetil causes significant gastrointestinal adverse effects that may manifest as severe nausea, vomiting, and diarrhea. Endoscopic evaluation may reveal severe esophagitis and gastritis. It may be necessary to decrease the administered dose or even discontinue the drug because of these adverse reactions. In the clinical trials of mycophenolate mofetil, leukopenia was found to occur at a frequency similar to that seen with the use of azathioprine.[15] An increased incidence of opportunistic infections has been shown, especially tissue-invasive cytomegalovirus disease.

Calcineurin inhibitors (cyclosporine and tacrolimus)

Together, cyclosporine and tacrolimus constitute the calcineurin inhibitor class of drugs. Calcineurin inhibitors are primarily used in combination with other agents for prevention of rejection in solid organ transplantation. With the advent of the first preparations of cyclosporine by Calne, 1-year graft survival rapidly improved, ushering in the modern era of transplantation. More recently, the use of calcineurin inhibitors has expanded to the treatment of a growing variety of autoimmune disorders.

Mechanism of action

Cyclosporine and tacrolimus inhibit the expression of multiple genes involved in T-cell activation and pro-liferation, including IL-2 and other lymphokines.[16] Cyclosporine and tacrolimus bind respectively to cytoplasmic immunophilins called cyclophilin and FK-binding protein (FKBP), thereby producing a complex that inhibits the calcium-sensitive phosphatase calcineurin.[17] Calcineurin normally dephosphorylates transcription factors including NF-AT (nuclear factor of activated T cells), allowing their translocation into the nucleus where they are responsible for induction of gene transcription.[18,19] T lymphocytes are specifically susceptible to calcineurin inhibition due to the limited amount of calcineurin present in these cells.

Adverse effects

Both cyclosporine and tacrolimus are associated with numerous adverse effects, and although there are minor differences in the incidence of individual adverse effects, the spectrum is essentially similar for both agents.

Cyclosporine causes both acute and chronic renal insufficiency. Acute renal insufficiency may be related to renal vasoconstriction as well as tubular toxicity. The vasoconstriction can be marked, involves both the afferent and efferent glomerular arterioles, and persists with time. Long-term use of cyclosporine leads to renal insufficiency due to chronic interstitial disease that is characterized by "striped" interstitial fibrosis. Detailed description of cyclosporine nephrotoxicity is beyond the scope of this chapter and the reader is referred to excellent reviews on the subject.[20,21] Tacrolimus also causes renal insufficiency in a pattern similar to cyclosporine, and while the exact incidence compared with cyclosporine may be controversial there does not appear to be a significant difference.

Cyclosporine is associated with hypertension that appears to be salt-sensitive and associated with low renin levels.[22] It also causes hyperlipidemia and glucose intolerance.[23,24] Tacrolimus causes the same problems but there appears to be a greater tendency to diabetogenicity with a slightly lower incidence of hypertension and hyperlipidemia. The mechanisms underlying the development of these adverse defects are not yet fully clear and strategies to avoid them basically hinge on using the lowest possible doses.

Hyperkalemia is seen with both agents, and may be related to decreased effect of aldosterone as well as decreased delivery of sodium to the distal tubule secondary to renal vasoconstriction. Hyperuricemia with resultant tophaceous gout is more common with cyclosporine. Both drugs lead to magnesium wasting and hypomagnesemia.

Neurotoxicity may occur with both agents and manifests as paresthesias, tremors, convulsions, and encephalopathy. Although it was initially felt that tacrolimus might be more neurotoxic, it appears that both drugs are similar in this regard and that previous results may have been due to inappropriately high tacrolimus levels. Hemolytic–uremic syndrome (HUS) with microangiopathic anemia and thrombocytopenia has been described with cyclosporine and requires discontinuation of the drug. Case reports of the same syndrome with tacrolimus have been published, while other investigators have shown that tacrolimus can be used as a salvage regimen for cyclosporine-induced HUS and thrombotic thrombocytopenic purpura.[25] At high drug levels, hepato-toxicity manifested by hyperbilirubinemia and elevated transaminases may occur with both agents. Hirsutism, coarse facies, and gingival hyperplasia are troubling adverse effects that appear to occur only with cyclosporine and not tacrolimus.

Cyclosporine and tacrolimus are metabolized in the liver using the P450 3A enzymes, and several commonly used drugs including diltiazem, verapamil, erythromycin, clarithromycin, ketoconazole, and other agents metab-olized by the same pathway may cause elevations in drug levels with acute adverse effects.

TOR inhibitors (sirolimus and everolimus)

Sirolimus (rapamycin) has been available for use in renal transplantation since 1999, while everolimus (RAD) is in late stages of phase III clinical studies. Initial trials in humans have used these drugs as maintenance therapy in combination with cyclosporine and steroids. However, since the approval of sirolimus by the Food and Drug Administration (FDA), there have been preliminary reports of use of this drug in combination with steroids alone, with tacrolimus and steroids, with mycophenolate mofetil and steroids, as well as triple therapy strategies that after the first few months call for elimination of the calcineurin inhibitor or steroids.

Mechanism of action

Although TOR inhibitors bind to the immunophilin FKBP just as FK506 does, they act through an entirely different mechanism.[26] The resulting TOR inhibitor–FKBP complex does not bind to calcineurin phosphatase, but rather to cytosolic protein kinases known as "targets of rapamycin" (TOR) that are centrally involved in the regulation of cell proliferation and differentiation. Binding of sirolimus and everolimus to their target site results in inhibition of signal transduction through several growth factor receptors (such as the IL-2 receptor), thus preventing cell cycle progression and immune activation.[27] The net result of these actions is potent antiproliferative activity against T cells and smooth muscle cells, as well as inhibition of antibody production by B cells. Due to actions at a later stage in the immune response, TOR inhibitors can prevent cell proliferation even after immune stimulation and may function syner-gistically with calcineurin inhibitors. While tacrolimus and TOR inhibitors both bind to FKBP and may theoretically antagonize each other if used in com-bination, this does not occur within the pharmacologic spectrum of dosing of these drugs in clinical practice.

Adverse effects

The adverse effect profile of sirolimus is better established than that of everolimus, although preliminary data sug-gest that they are similar. The major adverse effects of sirolimus appear to be related to higher concentrations of drug in the blood. In the early post-transplant period,

impaired wound healing and an increased tendency to lymphoceles has been noted, as well as myelosuppression, with thrombocytopenia, leukopenia, and anemia. Hyper-lipidemia, particularly with hypertriglyceridemia, is a complication of TOR inhibitors that is commonly observed in stable renal transplant recipients. This appears to be worse when sirolimus is used in combination with cyclosporine rather than tacrolimus.[28] There is good evidence that sirolimus augments the blood concen-trations of cyclosporine and vice versa. Of particular importance, while pharmacologic dosing of sirolimus ad-ministered without cyclosporine does not appear to adversely affect renal function, increasing blood levels of sirolimus appear to potentiate the nephrotoxicity of the calcineurin inhibitor when these two drugs are used in combination. Currently, information regarding the clinicopharmacologic interactions between tacrolimus and sirolimus is limited.

Cyclophosphamide

From a renal perspective, this drug is used for the treat-ment of glomerulonephritides that are usually associated with proliferative and crescent histologic lesions and are typically part of a systemic disease process. Examples of such diseases include Wegener granulomatosis, systemic lupus erythematosus, and Goodpasture disease.

Mechanism of action

Cyclophosphamide is a prodrug that is metabolized by the liver to 4-hydroxy-cyclophosphamide and phosphoramide mustard, both highly reactive compounds. These alkyl-ating agents bind and cross-link several important molecules including DNA and thereby interfere with cell proliferation and function. Cyclophosphamide has variable dose-dependent effects on the immune system. The effects vary somewhat based on the route of adminis-tration as well. Cyclophosphamide has been shown to cause dose-dependent lymphopenia, with decreases in both T and B cells, and is a particularly potent inhibitor of antibody formation.

Adverse effects

Cyclophosphamide causes dose-dependent bone marrow suppression, with effects on leukocytes being most pro-minent. In fact, the dose of cyclophosphamide may be adjusted based solely on WBC count, with the goal being avoidance of WBC counts $< 3500/mm^3$. The nadir of leukocyte count typically occurs 2 weeks after intravenous dosing and recovery is usually seen within a week. Anemia and thrombocytopenia occur less frequently.

Hemorrhagic cystitis and increased incidence of transitional cell carcinoma occur more commonly with prolonged oral dosage, but are reportedly rare with intermittent intravenous use. Aggressive hydration as well as the concomitant use of the reducing agent mesna may decrease the risk of this complication.

Gonadal toxicity occurs in every patient, with reduced fertility while on the drug in all patients. Permanent sterility occurs with higher cumulative doses and in the older patient, particularly older women.[29] Men appear to be more susceptible to permanent effects on reproductive function than women.

Nausea, hair loss, and hyponatremia due to increased antidiuretic hormone secretion may also be seen. The latter can be acute and require prompt attention.

Polyclonal antilymphocyte preparations

Antilymphocyte preparations work by binding to peripheral lymphocytes, blocking their function and targeting them for destruction. These agents provide a powerful mechanism for attenuating lymphocyte function, and can be used both as induction therapy and as treatment when rejection has been identified.

Mechanism of action

Polyclonal antibody preparations are IgG fractions isolated from serum of animals (goats, rabbits, or horses) immunized against human lymphocytes. The antigenic preparation used may be cultured lymphoblasts, human thymocytes, or lymphocytes and the antibodies are directed primarily against a variety of surface proteins on T cells, but also on other bone-marrow-derived cells such as B cells, macrophages, and platelets. After administration, antilymphocyte antibody preparations lead to lymphocyte depletion via complement-mediated lysis, removal by the reticuloendothelial system, and antibody-mediated cell-dependent cytotoxicity.[30] In addition lymphocytes that return to the circulation after cessation of therapy show blunted proliferative responses. The variability in the potency of these preparations from batch to batch remains a problematic issue.

Adverse effects

Polyclonal antibody preparations are foreign proteins and may cause a variety of adverse effects, including anaphylaxis, serum sickness, fever, and rash. In addition, cross-reactive antibodies may lead to thrombocytopenia and hemolysis. The high incidence of thrombophlebitis associated with these preparations necessitates the placement of central venous catheters for their administration.[30]

Muromonab-CD3 (OKT3)

Monoclonal antibodies, similar to polyclonal antibodies, are used both as induction therapy and to treat episodes of acute rejection.

Mechanism of action

OKT3 was the first monoclonal antibody approved for human use by the FDA. It is a murine IgG2 antibody directed against the ε chain of the human CD3 complex, which is a protein linked to the TCR. OKT3 is a potent immunosuppressive agent and has several potential mechanisms of action that are similar to that of any antibody (see above). Within minutes after administration of this antibody, CD3+ lymphocytes disappear from the

circulation, returning only after several days. This is a result of complement-mediated lysis and opsonization for clearance by phagocytic cells. OKT3 can also modulate the TCR–CD3 complex off the T-cell surface, thereby rendering T cells, even if present, incapable of antigen recognition.[30] Finally, OKT3, by steric hindrance, may block the binding of the TCR to the antigen–MHC complex. Unlike pharmacologic agents, transient treatment with OKT3, or with polyclonal antilymphocyte preparations, can have longstanding immunosuppressive effects. The reasons are not yet known but probably include the induction of natural immunoregulatory mechanisms.

Adverse effects

The most dangerous adverse effect of OKT3 administration is a "cytokine release syndrome" usually seen during the first few doses and characterized by high fever, chills, headache, arthralgias, nausea, and diarrhea. When severe, aseptic meningitis, hypotension, and pulmonary edema can be seen. These reactions are secondary to transient activation of T cells by OKT3 (due to the antibody binding to proteins in the TCR complex, the normal means of T-cell activation), with release of various cytokines including TNFα.[30] The severity of these reactions may be decreased by premedication with high doses of corticosteroids and antihistamines.[31] It is also important to ensure that the patient is euvolemic prior to administration of OKT3 so as to avoid the occurrence of life-threatening pulmonary edema.

OKT3 in combination with triple-drug immunosuppressive therapy has been shown to cause an increased incidence of lymphomas in cardiac transplant recipients.[32] Some authors contend that the increase in lymphoproliferative disorders is related to the overall degree of cumulative immunosuppression rather than specific agents.[33]

IL-2 receptor antibodies

Two monoclonal antibodies that target the IL-2 receptor were recently approved: the humanized antibody daclizumab and the chimeric antibody basiliximab. These agents have been primarily used as induction therapy in renal transplantation, but like other immunosuppressive agents their use may expand as clinical experience with this class of medications grows.

Mechanism of action

IL-2 receptor antibodies target the α chain of the IL-2 receptor (CD25), blocking the autocrine and paracrine survival and growth effects of IL-2. Because of the central role that IL-2 plays in the antigen-induced proliferation of T cells, use of these drugs results in diminished T-cell responses for at least 4–6 weeks. These agents have been shown clinically to result in a lower incidence of acute rejection compared with standard three-drug therapy in renal transplantation and may allow for steroid-sparing. The exact role for this class of agents has not been well defined.

Adverse effects

IL-2 receptor antibodies are chimeric and have generally been associated with few serious adverse effects, but have still occasionally resulted in hypersensitivity reactions. As with all immunosuppression, the risk of infections increases.

Plasmapheresis/plasma exchange

Plasmapheresis, involving removal and replacement of plasma proteins, is an effective therapy that has been used in a variety of renal diseases and rarely in renal transplantation. Generally, plasmapheresis is administered as an adjunctive therapy together with other immunosuppressive drugs, for greatest efficacy.

Mechanism of action

Plasmapheresis involves the rapid depletion from the circulation of specific factors implicated in the pathogenesis of several different disease processes. Such factors may include autoantibodies or alloantibodies, antigens, immune complexes, light chains, and proteins involved in platelet aggregation or coagulation.

Adverse effects

Besides the potential for excessive immunosuppression, most of the risk associated with plasmapheresis is related to vascular access placement and complications of anticoagulation. Angiotensin-converting enzyme inhibitors should be avoided with patients in whom polyacrylonitrile membranes are being used for plasmapheresis, because of the potential for profound bradykinin activation and the development of angioedema. A similar reaction has been reported with use of this membrane with patients taking angiotensin receptor blockers.

References

1. Matis LA: The molecular basis of T-cell specificity. Annu Rev Immunol 1990;8:65–82.
2. Turka LA: Normal immune responses. *In* Neilson EG, Couser WG (eds): Immunologic Renal Disease, 1st edn. Philadelphia: Lippincott-Raven Publishers, 1997, pp 65–94.
3. Waldmann TA, Dubois S, Sand Tagaya Y: Contrasting roles of IL-2 and IL-15 in the life and death of lymphocytes: implications for immunotherapy. Immunity 2001;14:105–110.
4. Perussia B, Kobayashi M, Rossi ME, et al: Immune interferon enhances functional properties of human granulocytes: role of Fc receptors and effect of lymphotoxin, tumor necrosis factor, and granulocyte-macrophage colony-stimulating factor. J Immunol 1987;138:765–774.
v5. Apasov S, Redegeld F, Sitdovsky M: Cell-mediated cytotoxicity: contact and secreted factors. Curr Opin Immunol 1993;5:404–410.
6. Rouvier E, Luciani M-F, Golstein P: Fas involvement in Ca^{2+} independent T cell-mediated cytotoxicity. J Exp Med 1993;177:195–200.
7. MacLennan IC, Liu YJ, Johnson GD: Maturation and dispersal of B-cell clones during T cell-dependent antibody responses. Immunol Rev 1992;126:143–161.
8. Beato M: Gene regulation by steroid hormones. Cell 1989;56:335–344.
9. Hricik DE, Almawi WY, Strom TB: Trends in the use of glucocorticoids in renal transplantation. Transplantation 1994;57:979–989.
10. Auphan N, DiDonato JA, Rosette C, et al: Immunosuppression by glucocorticoids: inhibition of NF-kappa B activity through induction of I kappa B synthesis. Science 1995;270:286–290.
11. Sambrook P, Birmingham J, Kelly P, et al: Prevention of corticosteroid osteoporosis. A comparison of calcium, calcitriol, and calcitonin. N Engl J Med 1993;328:1747–1752.
12. Lu CY, Sicher SC, Vazquez MA: Prevention and treatment of renal allograft rejection: new therapeutic approaches and new insights into established therapies. J Am Soc Nephrol 1993;4:1239–1256.
13. Sollinger HW: Mycophenolate mofetil for the prevention of acute rejection in primary cadaveric renal allograft recipients. U.S. Renal Transplant Mycophenolate Mofetil Study Group. Transplantation 1995;60:225–232.
14. Allison AC, Eugui EM: Immunosuppressive and other effects of mycophenolic acid and an ester prodrug, mycophenolate mofetil. Immunol Rev 1993;136:5–28.
15. European Mycophenolate Mofetil Cooperative Study Group: Placebo-controlled study of mycophenolate mofetil combined with cyclosporin and corticosteroids for prevention of acute rejection. Lancet 1995;345:1321–1325.
16. Sharma VK, Li B, Khanna A, et al: Which way for drug-mediated immunosuppression? Curr Opin Immunol 1994;6:784–790.
17. O'Keefe SJ, Tamura J, Kincaid RL, et al: FK-506- and CsA-sensitive activation of the interleukin-2 promoter by calcineurin. Nature 1992;357:692–694.
18. Clipstone NA, Crabtree GR: Identification of calcineurin as a key signalling enzyme in T-lymphocyte activation. Nature 1992;357:695–697.
19. Liu J, Farmer JD Jr, Lane WS, et al: Calcineurin is a common target of cyclophilin–cyclosporin A and FKBP–FK506 complexes. Cell 1991;66:807–815.
20. Remuzzi G, Perico N: Cyclosporine-induced renal dysfunction in experimental animals and humans. Kidney Int 1995;52:S70–S74.
21. Porayko MK, Textor SC, Krom RA, et al: Nephrotoxicity of FK 506 and cyclosporine when used as primary immunosuppression in liver transplant recipients. Transplant Proc 1993;25:665–668.
22. Curtis JJ: Hypertension following kidney transplantation. Am J Kidney Dis 1994;23:471–475.
23. Kasiske BL, Tortorice KL, Heim-Duthoy KL, et al: The adverse impact of cyclosporine on serum lipids in renal transplant recipients. Am J Kidney Dis 1991;17:700–707.
24. Roth D, Milgrom M, Esquenazi V, et al: Posttransplant hyperglycemia. Increased incidence in cyclosporine-treated renal allograft recipients. Transplantation 1989;47:278–281.
25. Zarifian A, Meleg-Smith S, O'Donovan R, Tesi RJ, Batuman V: Cyclosporine-associated thrombotic microangiopathy in renal allografts. Kidney Int 1999;55:2457–2466.
26. Morris RE: Rapamycin: FK506's fraternal twin or distant cousin? Immunol Today 1991;12:137–140.
27. Chung J, Kuo CJ, Crabtree GR, et al: Rapamycin–FKBP specifically blocks growth-dependent activation of and signaling by the 70 kd S6 protein kinases. Cell 1992;69:1227–1236.
28. Murgia MG, Jordan S, Kahan BD: The side effect profile of Sirolimus: a phase I study in quiescent cyclosporine–prednisone-treated transplant patients. Kidney Int 1996;49:209–216.
29. Klippel JH: Cyclophosphamide: ovarian and other toxicities. Lupus 1995;4:1–2.
30. Norman DJ: Antilymphocyte antibodies in the treatment of allograft rejection: targets, mechanisms of action, monitoring, and efficacy. Semin Nephrol 1992;12:315–324.
31. Chatenoud L, Ferran C, Legendre C, et al: In vivo cell activation following OKT3 administration. Systemic cytokine release and modulation by corticosteroids. Transplantation 1990;49:697–702.
32. Swinnen LJ, Costanzo-Nordin MR, Fisher SG, et al: Increased incidence of lymphoproliferative disorder after immunosuppression with the monoclonal antibody OKT3 in cardiac-transplant recipients. N Engl J Med 1990;323:1723–1728.
33. Penn I: Cancers complicating organ transplantation. N Engl J Med 1990;323:1767–1769.

Dietary Modulation of the Inflammatory Response

Raffaele De Caterina

The inflammatory reaction and points of attack for its modulation

Inflammation, defined as the reaction of a living vascularized tissue to localized damage,[1] plays a role in both normal repair reactions and the pathogenesis of disease. Inflammatory reactions are usually defined as acute or chronic on the basis of both their temporal duration and the prevailing phenomena occurring. The main features of acute inflammation, lasting minutes to hours, are fluid and plasma protein exudation (edema) and leukocyte (mainly neutrophil) migration.[2] Chronic inflammation lasts longer, is less stereotyped, and is associated histologically with the presence of lymphocytes and macrophages, as well as with the proliferation of small blood vessels and connective tissue.[3] Inflammatory phenomena are the basis of a number of systemic and organ-specific disease processes, ranging from classical rheumatic diseases to bronchial airway hyper-responsiveness, inflammatory bowel disease, kidney diseases, psoriasis, and atopic eczema. Tissue phenomena occurring in inflammation include modification of blood flow and vessel diameter, changes in vascular permeability, leukocyte exudation and phagocytosis, remodeling of the extracellular matrix, and cell proliferation. Each phase of the inflammatory reaction is sustained by the local production of mediators, including vasoactive amines, plasma and tissue proteases, arachidonic acid metabolites, cytokines, chemokines and growth factors, lysosomal components, and reactive oxygen species, each of which may be a theoretical target for drugs or therapeutic interventions. It has recently been appreciated that many of these phases may be modulated by diet. Dietary modulation of the inflammatory reaction is thus now achievable as a therapeutic option in the treatment of a variety of human diseases. Selected dietary components can also be supplemented in amounts not easily achieved through the diet, thus forming truly "pharmacologic" modalities based on dietary components. This chapter reviews the main options presently available for these interventions, their proposed rationale and mechanism of action, clinical results, and some current therapeutic recommendations. Most of these are presently based on manipulation of fatty acid intake, and constitute by far the main topic of this chapter.

Highly unsaturated n-3 fatty acids

Present mainly in seafood, and therefore better known as "fish oils," highly unsaturated fatty acids of the n-3 series (ω-3 fatty acids) are probably the best example of how diet may affect inflammation. These compounds exert a remarkable variety of biologic effects;[4,5] because of this they are currently being tested in a variety of clinical situations as disparate as coronary artery disease,[6,7] hypertension,[8–10] hyperlipidemia,[11] cancer,[12] diabetes,[13] renal diseases,[14] and a number of inflammatory states. The reader is referred to the quoted reviews covering their use in these conditions, while this section focuses on their use in inflammatory states and renal disease.

Biologic properties and effects of n-3 fatty acids and their potential relevance to inflammation

Current medical interest in n-3 fatty acids stems from observations of the different prevalence of some chronic diseases in the Greenland (Eskimo) population relative to Western populations.[15] Diseases with lower prevalence in Eskimos as compared to control Danes include myocardial infarction (the main source of interest for these compounds as preventive agents in coronary artery disease) but also conditions such as psoriasis, bronchial asthma, diabetes mellitus, and thyrotoxicosis,[15] which share a background of inflammation or a derangement of immunity. Increased nutritional intake of fish and marine mammals, which provides an increased supply of n-3 fatty acids, was highlighted as the main factor responsible for such differences.[16,17] Mammals in general cannot synthesize fatty acids with double bonds distal to the ninth carbon atom (numbered from the methyl end of the carbon chain), although they are able, to some extent, to elongate (increase carbon chain length) and further desaturate (increase the number of double bonds) the aliphatic chain. Two main families of long-chain poly-unsaturated fatty acids exist, both derived from linoleic acid (C18:2, n-6) and α-linolenic acid (C18:3), the shortest precursors that cannot be synthesized (Fig. 13.1). Linoleic acid is abundant in oils from most vegetable seeds such as corn and safflower; α-linolenic acid is found in the chloroplasts of green leafy vegetables. Humans can desaturate and elongate α-linolenic acid to eicosapentaenoic acid (EPA) and further to docosahexaenoic acid (DHA). However the elongation and desaturation processes are likely to be slow and possibly further limited with aging[18] and disease conditions.[19] For these reasons, EPA and DHA are considered, to a large extent, nutritionally essential and are nearly exclusively derived from fish. Fish increase their membrane content by eating the phytoplankton, rich in either the precursor α-linolenic acid or the more elongated compounds EPA and DHA. Particularly fatty fish living in cold seas (e.g. mackerel, salmon, and herring) are rich in these compounds, which may give them a selective advantage in preventing low temperature-related loss of membrane fluidity in cell membranes.[18] Concentrated formulations of EPA and DHA are now available from industrial processing of the body fat from fish, and are undergoing clinical trials as dietary supplements or pharmacologic agents.

The n-3 fatty acids exert a remarkable variety of biologic effects, many of which may affect inflammation and clinical conditions related to its presence (Fig. 13.2). The most important of these are now discussed in greater detail.

Production of eicosanoids and related lipid mediators

Until recently, the prevailing hypothesis to explain the variety of effects of n-3 fatty acids was that their action could be related to the different profile of activities of neo-synthesized soluble lipid mediators derived from EPA as

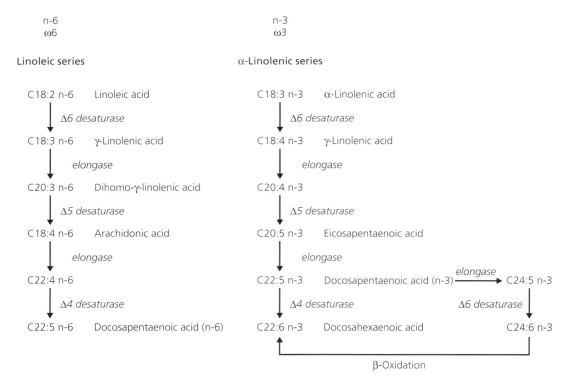

Figure 13.1 Metabolism and nomenclature of the main polyunsaturated fatty acids of the linoleic series (left) and the α-linolenic series (right). The two metabolic pathways, although largely using the same enzymes without appreciable substrate specificity, are entirely distinct and not interconvertible in animals and humans. Regulation of elongase and desaturases is largely unknown. Both pathways use the same enzymes for chain elongation and desaturation. Recent findings, however, have indicated that formation of docosahexaenoic acid (DHA) from 22:5 n-3 occurs through an initial chain elongation to 24:5 n-3 (in either mitochondria or peroxisomes), which is in turn desaturated in microsomes at position 6 to yield 24:6 n-3. The chain is then shortened via β-oxidation to yield DHA. This novel biosynthetic pathway is commonly referred to as "Sprecher's shunt."[122] Dihomo-γ-linolenic acid is the precursor of prostaglandins of the 1 series. Arachidonic acid is the most common eicosanoid precursor; eicosapentaenoic acid (EPA) is the most common precursor of the 3 series prostaglandins and the 5 series leukotrienes, and is the most abundant polyunsaturated fatty acid present in fish oil concentrates; DHA is the most abundant n-3 fatty acid accumulated in tissues (especially the central nervous system) and in fish, and can exert its effects partly by retroconversion to EPA and partly by itself. See text for further details. (Modified from De Caterina R, Endres S, Kristensen S, Schmidt E: n-3 Fatty acids and renal diseases. Am J Kidney Dis 1994;24:397–415, with permission.)

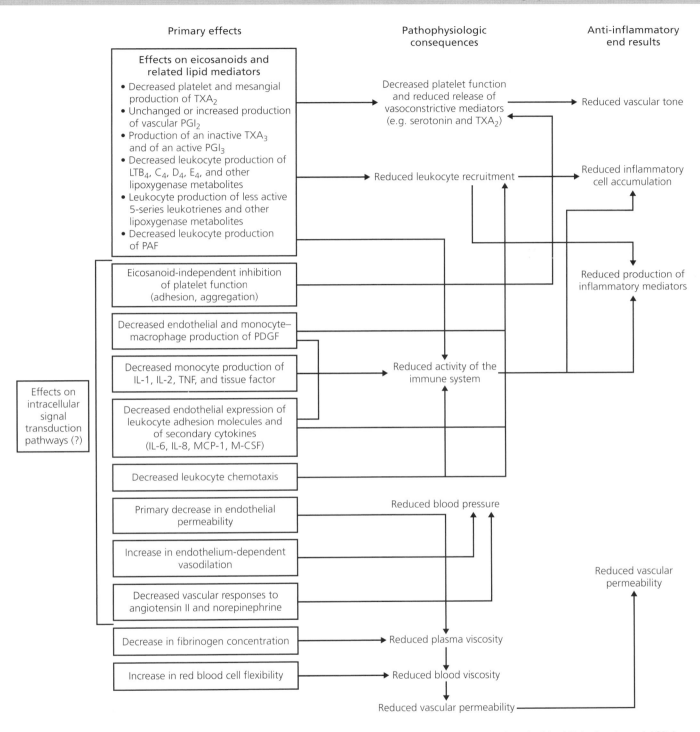

Figure 13.2 Biologic effects of n-3 fatty acids and the rationale for their anti-inflammatory use. IL, interleukin; LT, leukotriene; MCP-1, monocyte chemotactic protein 1; M-CSF, macrophage colony-stimulating factor; PAF, platelet-activating factor; PDGF, platelet-derived growth factor; PG, prostaglandin; TNF, tumor necrosis factor; TX, thromboxane. See text for details and references.

opposed to those derived from the normally more abundant arachidonic acid (AA) (Fig. 13.3). Both AA and EPA are fatty acids with 20 (Greek *eicosa*) carbon atoms and four or five *cis* double bonds, each one inducing a bending of the otherwise linear aliphatic chain. These bendings allow the occurrence of a "hairpin" configuration and the subsequent enzymatic transformation of the fatty acid

precursor in a variety of compounds commonly designated "eicosanoids." This term now encompasses a number of classes of related compounds, named prostaglandins (PG), thromboxanes (TX), leukotrienes (LT), hydroxy and epoxy fatty acids, lipoxins (LX), and isoprostanes. The initial step in the biosynthesis of these compounds is thought to be a receptor- or physical perturbation-mediated influx of Ca^{2+} ions, causing translocation of a cytoplasmic phospholipase A_2 to the cell membrane.[20,21] The enzyme then catalyzes the hydrolysis of the esterified AA in the sn-2 position.[22,23] A variety of phospholipase A_2 enzymes have now been identified, differing in molecular weight, calcium sensitivity, and specificity for AA.[22,23] The activity of these enzymes appears to be increased by a phospholipase A_2-activating protein, which is activated by cytokines such as interleukin 1 (IL-1) and tumor necrosis factor (TNF).[24] A secretory phospholipase A_2 present on the surface of mast cells and other cells may also be involved in the liberation of AA.[25]

Physical or agonist-induced activation of cytoplasmic phospholipase A_2 leads to a liberation of free AA. When EPA partially replaces AA as the polyunsaturated fatty acid in the sn-2 position of glycerophospholipids, free EPA is produced. AA or EPA then becomes available for a variety of enzymes able to drive their further metabolism in directions depending on the cell type where such activation processes occur (see Fig. 13.1). Thus, in platelets and a few other tissues (including the kidney), AA is metabolized to TXA_2, a powerful vasoconstrictor and inducer of platelet activation. The replacement of EPA leads to the production of the much weaker TXA_3. On the other hand, in endothelia, products of AA and EPA are the almost equiactive PGI_2 and PGI_3, both vasodilators and inhibitors of platelet activation. In leukocytes, which are pivotal cells in inflammation, the main metabolism of AA is toward the production of leukotrienes, which are endowed with a variety of properties: LTB_4 causes chemotaxis; LTC_4, LTD_4, and LTE_4 cause vasoconstriction, bronchoconstriction, and endothelial permeabilization. EPA also acts as a poor substrate for AA-metabolizing enzymes, leading to decreased net production of derived compounds (reviewed in references 4, 5, and 26). Lipoxygenase products of EPA are the weaker corresponding leukotrienes of the 5-series (LTB_5, LTC_5, LTD_5, LTE_5) (see Fig. 13.3), although in this regard the most relevant property of n-3 fatty acid incorporation in membrane phospholipids appears to be the reduced production of such mediators.[27] As a result, a shift in the relative abundance of AA and EPA leads to a new balance of eicosanoids, favoring vasodilating, antiplatelet, and less proinflammatory compounds. Elevated TXA_2 (by urinary assays of metabolites of its hydrolytic product TXB_2) has been found in patients with systemic lupus erythematosus[28] and in a variety of renal diseases, including chronic glomerular disease,[29] diabetic nephropathy,[30] renal damage caused by cyclosporine,[31] renal transplant rejection,[32] and proteinuric syndromes.[33–36] Substitution of EPA for AA reduces platelet[8,37–40] as well as renal production of thromboxanes.[36] These changes may be a partial explanation for some of the anti-inflammatory, antihypertensive, and renal effects of n-3 fatty acids.

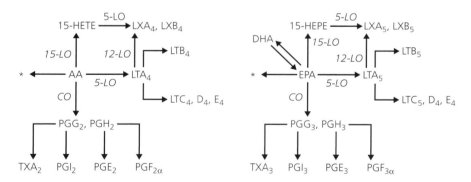

Figure 13.3   An updated schema for the origin of the main eicosanoids derived from the linoleic series (metabolites of arachidonic acid, AA) and the α-linolenic series (metabolites of eicosapentaenoic acid, EPA) with relevance to inflammation physiology and pathophysiology. The best-characterized metabolic pathway, catalyzed by the enzyme prostaglandin (PG)H synthase (cyclooxygenase, CO, of which a constitutive and an inducible form are now known), leads to the formation of prostanoids (prostaglandins and thromboxanes, TX) of the 2 series from AA and of the 3 series from EPA. AA and EPA can also be metabolized in leukocytes and some connective tissue cells via the enzyme 5-lipoxygenase (5-LO) to leukotriene (LT)A_4 and LTA_5 respectively. These labile intermediates can be converted to the more stable LTB (endowed with potent chemotactic properties) or, by the addition of a peptide residue, to the sulfido-peptide leukotrienes (LTC, LTD, LTE), which are powerful vasoconstrictors and able to increase vascular permeability. The schema also outlines the possible complex metabolism of both AA and EPA toward lipoxins (LX), which are also endowed with vasoactive properties. Lipoxins arise through the combined action of 5-LO and other lipoxygenases (15-LO and 12-LO) (15-HETE, 15-hydroxytetraenoic acid; 15-HEPE, 15-hydroxypentaenoic acid). Cell–cell interactions, including exchanges of substrates and of intermediate metabolites, are thought to be particularly relevant to the generation of LO metabolites. On average, metabolites derived from EPA are less active than the corresponding species derived from AA, potentially explaining the reduction in many cellular responses occurring when n-3 fatty acids are added to the diet. More importantly, EPA is a worse substrate for the metabolizing enzymes than AA, leading to a net absolute reduction in the amount of metabolites generated. The schema also outlines the bidirectional relationship of EPA and docosahexaenoic acid (DHA), by which this last compound may serve as a storage compartment for EPA. The asterisk denotes other potential metabolic pathways of AA and EPA to bioactive compounds that have been recently appreciated in particular organ systems. These include the generation of isoprostanes, ω-3 hydroxylation, epioxygenase, and cytochrome P450/allylic oxidation products. (From De Caterina R, Endres S, Kristensen S, Schmidt E: n-3 Fatty acids and renal diseases. Am J Kidney Dis 1994;24:397–415, with permission.)

Modulation of cell activation and cytokine production

In addition to changes in eicosanoid metabolism, increased attention is now being paid to n-3 fatty acids as possible modulators of cytokine production. When administered to healthy volunteers, n-3 fatty acids decrease bacterial lipopolysaccharide (LPS)-induced production of the proinflammatory cytokines IL-1 and TNF from peripheral blood lymphomonocytes.[41,42] In a different setting (cultured human endothelial cells), membrane enrichment of n-3 fatty acids by supplementation of culture medium with DHA reduces the ability of endothelial cells to respond to stimulation with LPS, IL-1, IL-4, or TNF in terms of surface expression of the leukocyte adhesion molecules vascular cell adhesion molecule (VCAM)-1, intercellular adhesion molecule (ICAM)-1, and E-selectin, as well as expression of soluble mediators of "endothelial activation," such as IL-6 and IL-8, able to provide positive feedback for the amplification of the inflammatory response.[43–46] This provides a basis for reduced responsiveness of cells to inflammatory stimuli, probably due to the ability of n-3 fatty acids to modulate the activation of transcription factors (nuclear factor-κB)[43–46] which can coordinate the concerted activation of a variety of genes involved in acute inflammation, atherosclerosis, and modulation of the immune response.[46–48] Other reported properties of n-3 fatty acids, including the ability to modulate the expression of tissue factor by stimulated monocytes[49,50] or the expression of platelet-derived growth factor-like proteins in endothelial cells[51] or monocytes,[52] could be due to the same or similar underlying mechanism of action.

Other biologic properties of n-3 fatty acids related to modulation of inflammation

These include (1) reduction of monocyte and neutrophil chemotaxis[53–56] and leukocyte inflammatory potential,[57] the mechanisms of which have not yet been investigated in detail (possibly cytokine and chemokine production); (2) reduction in total blood viscosity,[58–60] most probably through a combined effect on red blood cell deformability,[18] and plasma viscosity, the main determinant of which, the concentration of fibrinogen, is favorably reduced by these compounds;[61–63] and (3) an increase in endothelium-dependent vasodilation[64,65] and a decrease in vasoconstrictive responses to angiotensin II.[66,67] At least some of these effects may be due to modulation of intracellular signal transduction pathways, partly due to the function of fatty acids as intracellular second messengers themselves in cell activation[68] (see Fig. 13.2). In general, n-3 fatty acids have been found to reduce the increase in intracellular calcium in response to agonists. In particular, the enrichment of cellular phospholipids with DHA inhibits calcium transients.[69–71] In cardiac myocytes this may occur through a modulation of the L-type calcium channel.[72] Alternatively, changes in agonist-induced increase in intracellular calcium may occur through an alteration of the agonist–receptor affinity[73] or cell membrane physicochemical characteristics.[74,75] Postreceptor signaling pathways and the formation of second messengers involved in the mobilization of intracellular calcium may be inhibited by reductions in inositol tris-phosphate production[76,77] or by conversion of fatty acids to cytochrome P450 epoxygenase metabolites.[78,79]

Essential fatty acid deficiency

Over 20 years ago it was established that essential fatty acid (EFA) deficiency was able to prevent the lethal glomerulonephritis that occurs in the New Zealand Black (NZB) × New Zealand White (NZW) model of murine lupus.[80] The original report was followed by others showing similar results for supplementation with n-3 fatty acids in both the NZB × NZW and MRL1pr models of murine lupus.[81–83] A proximal step in the pathogenesis of the glomerulonephritis in murine lupus is the formation of autoantibodies. Suppression of such an event did not appear to be involved in these protective effects. Dietary polyunsaturated fatty acid manipulation was found to be effective even when started late in the disease, after a full expression of the auto-antibody response.[82] Also, investigations on the mechanism of action of EFA deficiency were not able to show clear results on suppression of lymphocyte responses.[84] Therefore it was reasoned that fatty acids had to act distal to the deposition of immune complexes in glomeruli. The original hypothesis entertained at that time was that the efficacy of dietary polyunsaturated fatty acid manipulation was through diminished levels of active cyclooxygenase metabolites.[83] However, several lines of evidence subsequently argued against such a simplistic explanation. These were mainly that (1) pharmacologic inhibition of cyclooxygenase in murine lupus did not reproduce the beneficial effects of fatty acid manipulation[85] and (2) EFA deprivation was not inevitably accompanied by a decrease in tissue AA or the production of cyclooxygenase metabolites.[86] Subsequent studies in normal glomeruli showed that EFA deficiency has the unique ability to modulate macrophage migration, dramatically depleting the resident population of glomerular and renal interstitial macrophages.[87] The specific deficiency of n-6 fatty acids was responsible for these effects, since the administration of linoleic acid (18:2 n-6) but not α-linolenic acid (18:3 n-3) reversed the decrease in macrophage population.[87] These changes were interpreted as due to an attenuated ability of glomeruli from EFA-deficient animals to generate LTB$_4$.[88] More recently, it was observed that EFA deficiency attenuates the immunologic, metabolic, and functional alterations accompanying nephrotoxic nephritis, a model of immune-mediated glomerulonephritis.[89,90] In this model, multiple mechanisms appear operative in different phases, including an early role for neutrophil–platelet interactions, causing increased glomerular LTB$_4$ and thromboxane synthesis and consequent proteinuria, and involving complement and possibly fibrinogen, P-selectin, and eicosanoids.[91] EFA deficiency does not alter neutrophil influx in the glomeruli but affects the acute rise in glomerular LTB$_4$ and thromboxanes,[89] and other neutrophil functions, such as the generation of superoxide anion,[92] similar to what occurs with n-3 fatty acid supplementation.[53] A role for the generation of platelet activating factor (PAF), the production of which is also impaired by EFA deficiency[93] as well as by n-3 fatty acid supplementation,[94] has been postulated.[95] In later phases of nephrotoxic nephritis, the critical cellular effector system is the monocyte macrophage, which appears to mediate the increase in glomerular thromboxane production, proteinuria, and the decline in renal function.[96,97] EFA deficiency dramatically inhibits the elicitation of monocyte macrophages into the glomerulus in this model of renal inflammatory disease, and this effect is not attributable to either PAF or LTB_5 since it is not inhibited by PAF receptor blockade or 5-lipoxygenase inhibition.[98] Also, since no defect in in-vitro sensitivity to chemotactic agents in monocyte/macrophages from EFA-deficient animals is demonstrable,[89] it is likely that glomerular production of a monocyte-specific chemoattractant or monocyte adherence is impaired, similar to results demonstrated with n-3 fatty acid supplementation.[43,45] Fatty acid manipulation with EFA deficiency has also been shown effective in decreasing the late glomerulosclerosis[99,100] that is a consequence of glomerular injury and inflammation regardless of the initiating insult.[101]

Studies in humans with dietary manipulation of fatty acid intake

Along with the elucidation of their many biologic properties, studies have been performed to explore the potential usefulness of dietary supplementation with n-3 fatty acids in a number of pathologic conditions in which inflammation is either the most prominent or an essential component. Such conditions include rhematoid arthritis,[102] systemic lupus erythematosus[103] and other rheumatic diseases,[104] ulcerative colitis,[105–107] Crohn's disease,[108–110] and bronchial asthma.[111] Results of the vast majority of these trials have been critically reviewed.[112] Several well-controlled double-blind trials of the effects of n-3 fatty acids in rheumatoid arthritis have reported statistically significant beneficial effects, which were however of small magnitude and modest clinical impact. Such studies were conducted with doses in the range 5–6 g/day, with minimal adverse effects, justifying the hypothesis that larger doses might possibly have greater clinical efficacy. Inconsistent results, possibly for similar reasons, have also been reported in inflammatory respiratory diseases (namely allergic asthma)[113,114] and inflammatory skin diseases.[115–117] Promising, yet not definitive studies have been reported in systemic lupus erythematosus.[118] A recent double-blind, placebo-controlled clinical trial in patients with Crohn's disease at high risk of relapse has shown that 59% of patients kept on 2.7 g/day of n-3 fatty acids remained in remission compared with 26% in the placebo group.[110] This is certainly the most promising result so far obtained in this disease category. Compared with previous less favorable results obtained by others,[108,109] the authors hypothesize a better compliance in the last study due to a special coating that enhances protection of the n-3 fatty acid capsules against gastric acidity and the consequent occurrence of gastric adverse effects.[110] Also, four double-blind, placebo-controlled trials in ulcerative colitis, with

doses of n-3 fatty acids between 2.7 and 5.4 g/day, have documented moderate clinical improvements, mostly in remission induction.[105–108] The variable results obtained by dietary supplementation with n-3 fatty acids in different inflammatory conditions can possibly be explained by the variable nature of inflammation in these conditions. A unitary explanation of these discrepancies is however lacking at the present time.

Studies with supplementation of n-3 fatty acids in renal disease

Against a background of older literature indicating promising effects in slowing down the progression of glomerular sclerosis and reducing proteinuria in various forms of renal diseases (reviewed in reference 14), more recent human studies fall into the following two main categories.

1. Studies with intermediate mechanistic endpoints show that, in patients on hemodialysis, n-3 fatty acids may ameliorate lipid profile by reducing plasma levels of triglycerides, remnant lipoproteins and, contrary to common expectations, lipid peroxidation;[119] increase high-density lipoprotein cholesterol;[120] synergize the lipid-lowering effects of statins;[121] reduce leukotriene formation;[122] and increase heart rate variability, a prognostic marker of arrhythmic death in these patients.[123] In patients after renal transplantation, n-3 fatty acids may, as in other clinical conditions,[8,10] have favorable effects on blood pressure,[124] and improve cyclosporine absorption and metabolism.[125]

2. Studies with clinical endpoints are mostly confined to the setting of IgA nephropathy (Table 13.1).[126] In this disease, a prospective-double blind trial had originally shown beneficial effects of n-3 fatty acids.[127] This has been confirmed in a follow-up of longer than 6 years of the original cohort.[128]

Vitamins and other nutrients

There are scanty and occasional reports in the literature of other nutrients able to modulate selected examples of inflammation. Thus, plasma levels of pyridoxal-5′-phosphate (vitamin B_6) have been found to be reduced in patients with rheumatoid arthritis, and this reduction is somehow correlated with increased production of the inflammatory mediator TNFα by peripheral blood monocytes.[129] Antioxidant vitamins, mostly vitamin E[130] and β-carotene (vitamin A),[131] have occasionally been reported to modulate the inflammatory response in a variety of experimental and some clinical models. Their effects, although with a clear biologic rationale in interfering with redox-mediated intracellular signal transduction pathways activated by cytokines, are weak at best and their clinical impact appears to be minor.

Conclusions

Modulation of long-chain polyunsaturated fatty acid intake, mostly by increasing the relative proportions of

Table 13.1 Human studies of n-3 fatty acids in IgA nephropathy

Reference	Geographic location	EPA/DHA (g/day)	Duration of treatment (years)	Renal function outcome
Hamazaki et al[132]	Japan (n = 20)	1.6/1.0	1	Stabilized
Pettersson et al[133]	Australia (n = 37)	1.8/1.2	2	Declined
Bennett et al[134]	Sweden (n = 32)	3.3/1.8	0.5	Declined
Donadio[126]	North America (n = 106)	1.8/1.2	2	Stabilized
Donadio et al[127]	North America (n = 73)	3.8/2.9 vs. 1.9/1.5	2	No difference between low dose and high dose

DHA, docosahexaenoic acid; EPA, eicosapentaenoic acid.

n-3 versus n-6 fatty acids, is the clearest example of how diet may modulate the inflammatory process. It is possible that many of the epidemiologic differences in the incidence of inflammatory diseases among different populations can be tracked back to different nutritional intake of selected, quantitatively minor, nutritional components such as n-3 fatty acids. The clarification of the mechanisms of action of these as well as of other dietary components, and a better documentation of the spectrum of clinical possibilities offered by dietary manipulation in the intake of such compounds, linking together classical nutritional science, molecular biology, epidemiology, and clinical medicine, are a frontier for nutritional research in the years to come, and are likely to gain a place for these compounds in the therapy of some inflammatory disorders.

References

1. Robbins S, Cotran R, Kumar V (eds): Inflammation and Repair Processes: Pathologic Basis of Disease, 3rd edn. Philadelphia: WB Saunders, 1984.
2. McIntyre TM, Modur V, Prescott SM, Zimmerman GA: Molecular mechanisms of early inflammation. Thromb Haemost 1997;78:302–305.
3. Majno G: Chronic inflammation: links with angiogenesis and wound healing. Am J Pathol 1998;153:1035–1039.
4. Simopoulos A: Omega-3 fatty acids in health and disease and in growth and development. Am J Clin Nutr 1991;54:438–463.
5. Kristensen S, Schmidt E, De Caterina R, Endres S: n-3 Fatty Acids: Prevention and Treatment in Vascular Disease. Berlin: Springer-Verlag, 1995.
6. Kristensen S, De Caterina R, Schmidt E, Endres S: Fish oil and ischaemic heart disease. Br Heart J 1993;70:212–214.
7. GISSI-Prevenzione Investigators: Dietary supplementation with n-3 polyunsaturated fatty acids and vitamin E after myocardial infarction: results of the GISSI-Prevenzione trial. Lancet 1999;354:447–455.
8. Knapp H, FitzGerald G: Anti-hypertensive effects of fish oil. A controlled study of polyunsaturated fatty acid supplementation in essential hypertension. N Engl J Med 1989;320:1037–1043.
9. Appel L, Miller E, Seidler A, Whelton P: Does supplementation of diet with fish oil reduce blood pressure: a meta-analysis of controlled clinical trials. Arch Intern Med 1993;153:1429–1438.
10. Holm T, Andreassen AK, Aukrust P, et al: Omega-3 fatty acids improve blood pressure control and preserve renal function in hypertensive heart transplant recipients. Eur Heart J 2001;22:428–436.
11. Schmidt E, Kristensen S, De Caterina R, Endres S: The effects of n-3 fatty acids on plasma lipids and lipoproteins and other cardiovascular risk factors in patients with hyperlipidemia. Atherosclerosis 1993;103:107–121.
12. Galli C, Butrum R: Dietary ω3 fatty acids and cancer: an overview. World Rev Nutr Diet 1991;66:446–461.
13. Malasanos T, Stacpoole P: Biological effects of ω3 fatty acids in diabetes mellitus. Diabetes Care 1991;14:1160–1179.
14. De Caterina R, Endres S, Kristensen S, Schmidt E: n-3 Fatty acids and renal diseases. Am J Kidney Dis 1994;24:397–415.
15. Kromann N, Green A: Epidemiological studies in the Upernavik District, Greenland. Acta Med Scand 1980;208:401–406.
16. Dyerberg J, Bang H, Hjorne N: Fatty acid composition of the plasma lipids in Greenland Eskimos. Am J Clin Nutr 1975;28:958–966.
17. Bang H, Dyerberg J, Hjorne N: The composition of food consumed by Greenland Eskimos. Acta Med Scand 1976;200:69–73.
18. Popp-Snijders C, Schouten J, van der Meer J, van der Veen E: Fatty-fish induced changes in membrane lipid composition and viscosity of human erythrocyte suspensions. Scand J Clin Invest 1986;46:253–258.
19. Singer P, Jaeger W, Voigt S, Thiel H: Defective desaturation and elongation of n-6 and n-3 fatty acids in hypertensive patients. Prostaglandins Leukot Med 1984;15:159–165.
20. Sharp J, White D, Chious X, et al: Molecular cloning and expression of human Ca(2+)-sensitive cytosolic phospholipase A2. J Biol Chem 1991;266:14850–14853.
21. Clark J, Lin L, Kriz R, et al: A novel arachidonic acid-selective cytosolic PLA2 contains a Ca(2+)-dependent translocation domain with homology to PKC and GAP. Cell 1991;65:1043–1051.
22. Mayer R, Marshall L: New insights on mammalian phospholipase A2(s): comparison of arachidonoyl-selective and -non selective enzymes. FASEB J 1993;7:339–348.
23. Glaser K, Mobilio D, Chang J, Senko N: Phospholipase A2 enzymes: regulation and inhibition. Trends Pharmacol Sci 1993;14:92–98.
24. Clark M, Ögü L, Conway T, Dispoto J, Crooke S, Bomalaski J: Cloning of a phospholipase A2-activating protein. Proc Natl Acad Sci USA 1991;88:5418–5422.
25. Kramer R, Hession C, Johansen B, et al: Structure and properties of a human non-pancreatic phospholipase A2. J Biol Chem 1989;264:5768–5775.
26. Leaf A, Weber P: Cardiovascular effects of n-3 fatty acids. N Engl J Med 1988;318:549–557.
27. Knapp H: Omega-3 fatty acids in respiratory diseases: a review. J Am Coll Nutr 1995;14:18–23.
28. Patrono C, Ciabattoni G, Remuzzi G, et al: Functional significance of renal prostacyclin and thromboxane A2 production in patients with systemic lupus erythematosus. J Clin Invest 1985;76:1011–1018.
29. Ciabattoni G, Cinotti G, Pierucci A, et al: Effect of sulindac and ibuprofen in patients with chronic glomerular disease. Evidence for the dependence of renal function on prostacyclin. N Engl J Med 1984;310:279–283.
30. Craven P, Melhem M, DeRubertis F: Thromboxane in the pathogenesis of glomerular injury in diabetes. Kidney Int 1992;42:937–946.
31. Perico N, Benigni A, Zoja C, Delaini F, Remuzzi G: Functional significance of exaggerated renal thromboxane A2 synthesis induced by cyclosporin A. Am J Physiol 1986;251:F581–F587.
32. Foegh M, Lim K, Alijani M, Helfrich G, Ramwell P: Thromboxane and inflammatory cell infiltration in the allograft of renal transplant patients. Transplant Proc 1987;19:3633–3636.
33. Remuzzi G, Imberti L, Rossini M, et al: Increased glomerular thromboxane synthesis as a possible cause of proteinuria in experimental nephrosis. J Clin Invest 1985;75:94–101.

34. Stahl R: Die Bedeutung von Eicosanoiden bei glomerulären Erkrankungen. Klin Wochenschr 1986;64:813–823.
35. Remuzzi G, FitzGerald G, Patrono C: Thromboxane synthesis and action within the kidney. Kidney Int 1992;41:1483–1493.
36. De Caterina R, Caprioli R, Giannessi D, et al: n-3 Polyunsaturated fatty acids reduce proteinuria in patients with chronic glomerular disease. Kidney Int 1993;44:843–850.
37. Dyerberg J, Bang H, Stofferson E, Moncada S, Vane J: Eicosapentaenoic acid and prevention of thrombosis and atherosclerosis. Lancet 1978;ii:117–119.
38. von Schacky C, Fischer S, Weber P: Long-term effects of dietary marine w-3 fatty acids upon plasma and cellular lipids, platelet function, and eicosanoids formation in humans. J Clin Invest 1985;76:1626–1631.
39. von Schacky C, Weber P: Metabolism and effects on platelet function of the purified eicosapentaenoic and docosahexaenoic acids in humans. J Clin Invest 1985;76:2446–2450.
40. De Caterina R, Giannessi D, Mazzone A, et al: Vascular prostacyclin is increased in patients ingesting omega-3 polyunsaturated fatty acids before coronary artery bypass graft surgery. Circulation 1990;82:428–438.
41. Endres S, Ghorbany R, Kelley V, et al: The effect of dietary supplementation with n-3 polyunsaturated fatty acids on the synthesis of interleukin-1 and tumor necrosis factor by mononuclear cells. N Engl J Med 1989;320:265–271.
42. Meydani S, Endres S, Wood M, et al: Oral n-3 fatty acid supplementation suppresses cytokine production and lymphocyte proliferation: comparison in young and older women. J Nutr 1991;121:547–555.
43. De Caterina R, Cybulsky MI, Clinton SK, Gimbrone MA Jr, Libby P: The omega-3 fatty acid docosahexaenoate reduces cytokine-induced expression of pro-atherogenic and pro-inflammatory proteins in human endothelial cells. Arterioscler Thromb 1994;14:1829–1836.
44. De Caterina R, Libby P: Control of endothelial leukocyte adhesion molecules by fatty acids. Lipids 1996;31(Suppl 1):557–563.
45. De Caterina R, Liao JK, Libby P: Fatty acid modulation of endothelial activation. Am J Clin Nutr 2000;71:213S–223S.
46. De Caterina R: Endothelial dysfunctions: common denominators in vascular disease. Curr Opin Lipidol 2000;11:9–23.
47. Bauerle P: The inducible transcription activator NF-kB: regulation by distinct protein subunits. Biochim Biophys Acta 1991;1072:63–80.
48. Collins T, Cybuslsky MI: NF-kB: pivotal mediator or innocent bystander in atherogenesis? J Clin Invest 2001;107:255–264.
49. Hansen J, Olsen J, Wilsgard L, Østerud B: Effects of dietary supplementation with cod liver oil on monocyte thromboplastin synthesis, coagulation and fibrinolysis. J Intern Med Suppl 1989;225:133–139.
50. Tremoli E, Eligini S, Colli S, et al: Effects of omega 3 fatty acid ethyl esters on monocyte tissue factor expression. World Rev Nutr Diet 1994;76:55–59.
51. Fox P, DiCorleto P: Fish oils inhibit endothelial cell production of platelet-derived growth factor-like protein. Science 1988;241:453–456.
52. Kaminski W, Jendraschak E, Kiefl R, von Schacky C: Dietary omega-3 fatty acids lower levels of platelet-derived growth factor mRNA in human mononuclear cells. Blood 1993;71:1871–1879.
53. Lee T, Hoover R, Williams J, et al: Effect of dietary enrichment with eicosapentaenoic and docosahexaenoic acids on in vitro neutrophil and monocyte leukotriene generation and neutrophil function. N Engl J Med 1985;312:1217–1224.
54. Schmidt EB, Dyerberg J: n-3 Fatty acids and leucocytes. J Intern Med 1989;225(Suppl 731):151–158.
55. Schmidt E, Pedersen J, Ekelund S, Grunnet N, Jersild C, Dyerberg J: Cod liver oil inhibits neutrophil and monocyte chemotaxis in healthy males. Atherosclerosis 1989;77:53–57.
56. Schmidt E, Pedersen J, Varming K, et al: n-3 Fatty acids and leukocyte chemotaxis. Effects in hyperlipidemia and dose–response studies in healthy men. Arterioscler Thromb 1991;11:429–435,.
57. Fisher M, Upchurch K, Levine P, et al: Effects of dietary fish oil supplementation on polymorphonuclear leucocyte inflammatory potential. Inflammation 1986;10:387–392.
58. Terano T, Hirai A, Hamazaki T, et al: Effect of oral administration of highly purified eicosapentaenoic acid on platelet function, blood viscosity and red cell deformability in healthy human subjects. Atherosclerosis 1983;46:321–331.
59. Cartwright I, Pockley A, Galloway J, Greaves M, Preston F: The effects of dietary w3 polyunsaturated fatty acids on erythrocyte membrane phospholipids, erythrocyte deformability and blood viscosity in healthy volunteers. Atherosclerosis 1985;55:267–281.
60. Ernst E: Effects of n-3 fatty acids on blood rheology. J Intern Med 1989;225(Suppl 731):129–132.
61. Hostmark A, Bjerkedal T, Kierulf P, Flaten H, Ulshagen K: Fish oil and plasma fibrinogen. Br Med J 1988;297:180–181.
62. Radak K, Deck C, Huster G: Dietary supplementation with low-dose fish oils lowers fibrinogen levels: a randomized, double-blind controlled study. Ann Intern Med 1989;111:757–758.
63. Flaten H, Hostmark A, Kierulf P, et al: Fish-oil concentrate: effects on variables related to cardiovascular disease. Am J Clin Nutr 1990;52:300–306.
64. Boulanger C, Schini V, Hendrickson H, Vanhoutte P: Chronic exposure of cultured endothelial cells to eicosapentaenoic acid potentiates the release of endothelium-dependent relaxing factor(s). Br J Pharmacol 1990;99:176–180.
65. Vanhoutte P, Shimokawa H, Boulanger C: Fish oil and the platelet–blood vessel wall interaction. World Rev Nutr Diet 1991;66:233–244.
66. Coddee J, Croft E, Barden A, Mathews E, Vandongen R, Beilin L: An inhibitory effect of dietary polyunsaturated fatty acids on renin secretion in the isolated perfused rat kidney. J Hypertens 1984;2:265–270.
67. Goodfriend T, Ball D: Fatty acids effects on angiotensin receptors. J Cardiovasc Pharmacol 1986;8:1276–1283.
68. Sellmayer A, Obermeier H, Weber C, Weber P: Modulation of cell activation by n-3 fatty acids In De Caterina R, Endres S, Kristensen S, Schmidt E (eds): n-3 Fatty Acids and Vascular Disease. Berlin: Springer-Verlag, 1993, pp 21–30.
69. Hallaq H, Smith T, Leaf A: Protective effect of eicosapentaenoic acid on ouabain toxicity in neonatal rat cardiac myocytes. Proc Natl Acad Sci USA 1990;87:7834–7838.
70. Weber C, Aepfelbacher M, Lux I, Zimmer B, Weber P: Docosahexaenoic acid inhibits PAF and LTD4-stimulated [Ca++]i increase in differentiated monocytic U937 cells. Biochim Biophys Acta 1991;1133:38–45.
71. Locher R, Sachinidis A, Brunner C, Vetter W: Intracellular free calcium concentration and thromboxane A2 formation of vascular smooth muscle cells are influenced by fish oil and n-3 eicosapentaenoic acid. Scand J Lab Invest 1991;51:541–547.
72. Hallaq H, Smith T, Leaf A: Modulation of dihydropyridine-sensitive calcium channels in heart cells by fish oil fatty acids. Proc Natl Acad Sci USA 1992;89:1760–1764.
73. Swann P, Parent C, Croset M, et al: Enrichment of platelet phospholipids with eicosapentaenoic acid and docosahexaenoic acid inhibits thromboxane A2/prostaglandin H2 receptor binding and function. J Biol Chem 1990;265:21692–21697.
74. Salem N, Kim H, Yergey J: Docosahexaenoic acid: membrane function and metabolism. In Simopoulos A, Kifer R, Martin R (eds): Health Effects of Polyunsaturated Fatty Acids in Seafoods. Orlando, FL: Academic Press, 1986, pp 263–318.
75. Ehringer W, Belcher D, Wassal S, Stillwell W: A comparison of the effects of linolenic (18:3 w3) and docosahexaenoic (22:6 w3) acids on phospholipid bilayers. Chem Phys Lipids 1990;54:79–88.
76. Locher R, Sachinidis A, Steiner A, Vogt E, Vetter W: Fish oil affects phosphoinositide turnover and thromboxane A metabolism in cultured vascular smooth cells. Biochim Biophys Acta 1989;1012:279–283.
77. Medini L, Colli S, Mosconi C, Tremoli E, Galli C: Diets rich in n-9, n-6 and n-3 fatty acids differentially affect the generation of inositol phosphates and of thromboxane by stimulated platelets in the rabbit. Biochem Pharmacol 1990;39:129–133.
78. Force T, Hyman G, Hajjar R, Sellmayer A, Bonventre J: Non cyclo-oxygenase metabolites of arachidonic acid amplify the vasopressin-induced Ca2+ signal in glomerular mesangial cells by releasing Ca2+ from intracellular stores. J Biol Chem 1991;266:4295–4302.
79. Oliw E, Sprecher H: Metabolism of polyunsaturated (n-3) fatty acids by monkey seminal vesicles: isolation and biosynthesis of w3 epoxides. Biochim Biophys Acta 1991;1086:287–294.
80. Hurd E, Johnston J, Okita J, MacDonald P, Ziff M, Gilliam J: Prevention of glomerulonephritis and prolonged survival in New Zealand Black/New Zealand White F1 hybrid mice fed an essential fatty acid-deficient diet. J Clin Invest 1981;67:476–485.
81. Prickett J, Robinson D, Steinberg A: Dietary enrichment with the

polyunsaturated fatty acid eicosapentaenoic acid prevents proteinuria and prolongs survival in NZB × NZW F1 mice. J Clin Invest 1981;68:556–559.

82. Robinson D, Prickett J, Polisson R, Steniberg A, Levine L: The protective effect of dietary fish oil in murine lupus. Prostaglandins 1985;30:51–75.

83. Kelley V, Ferretti A, Izui S, Strom T: A fish oil diet rich in eicosapentaenoic acid reduces cyclooxygenase metabolites, and suppresses lupus in MRL-1pr mice. J Immunol 1985;134:1914–1919.

84. Yamanaka W, Clemans G, Hutchinson M: Essential fatty acid deficiency in humans. Prog Lipid Res 1981;19:187–215.

85. Kelley V, Iaui S, Halushka P: Effect of ibuprofen, a fatty acid cyclooxygenase inhibitor on murine lupus. Clin Immunol Immunopathol 1982;25:223–231.

86. Lefkowith J, Filippo B, Sprecher H, Needleman P: Paradoxical conservation of cardiac and renal arachidonate content in essential fatty acid deficiency. J Biol Chem 1985;260:15736–15744.

87. Lefkowith J, Schreiner G: Essential fatty acid deficiency depletes rat glomeruli of resident mesangial macrophages and inhibits angiotensin II-stimulated eicosanoid synthesis. J Clin Invest 1987;80:947–956.

88. Lefkowith J, Morrison A, Schreiner G: Glomerular leukotriene B4 synthesis: manipulation by (n-6) fatty acid deprivation and cellular origin. J Clin Invest 1988;82:1655–1660.

89. Schreiner G, Rovin B, Lefkowith J: The anti-inflammatory effects of essential fatty acid deficiency in experimental glomerulonephritis: the modulation of macrophage migration and eicosanoid metabolism. J Immunol 1989;143:3192–3199.

90. Takahashi K, Kato T, Schreiner G, Ebert J, Badr K: Essential fatty acid deficiency normalizes function and histology in rat nephrotoxic nephritis. Kidney Int 1992;41:1245–1253.

91. Wu X, Pippin J, Lefkowith JB: Neutrophils are critical to the enhanced glomerular arachidonate metabolism in acute nephrotoxic nephritis in rats. J Clin Invest 1993;91:766–773.

92. Gyllenhammar H, Palmblad J: Linoleic acid-deficient rat neutrophils show decreased bactericidal capacity, superoxide formation and membrane depolarization. Immunology 1989;66:616–620.

93. Ramesha C, Pickett W: Platelet-activating factor and leukotriene biosynthesis is inhibited in polymorphonuclear leukocytes depleted of arachidonic acid. J Biol Chem 1986;261:7592–7599.

94. Sperling R, Robin J, Kylander K, Lee T, Lewis R, Austen K: The effects of n-3 polyunsaturated fatty acids on the generation of platelet-activating factor-acether by human monocytes. J Immunol 1987;139:4186–4191.

95. Baldi E, Emancipator S, Hassan M, Dunn M: Platelet activating factor receptor blockade ameliorates murine systemic lupus erythematosus. Kidney Int 1990;38:1030–1038.

96. Takahashi K, Schreiner G, Yamashita K, Christman B, Blair I, Badr K: Predominant functional roles for thromboxane A2 and prostaglandin E2 during late nephrotoxic serum glomerulonephritis in the rat. J Clin Invest 1990;85:1974–1982.

97. Lefkowith J, Nagamatsu T, Pippin J, Schreiner G: Role of leukocytes in metabolic and functional derangements of experimental glomerulonephritis. Am J Physiol 1991;261:F213–F220.

98. Rovin B, Lefkowith J, Schreiner G: Mechanisms underlying the anti-inflammatory effects of essential fatty acid deficiency in experimental glomerulonephritis: inhibited release of a glomerular chemoattractant. J Immunol 1990;145:1238–1245.

99. Diamond J, Pesek I, Ruggieri S, Karnowsky M: Essential fatty acid deficiency during acute puromycin nephrosis ameliorates late renal injury. Am J Physiol 1989;257:F798–F807.

100. Diamond J, Ding G, Frye J, Diamond I: Glomerular macrophages and the mesangial proliferative response in the experimental nephrotic syndrome. Am J Pathol 1992;141:887–894.

101. El Nahas A: Growth factors and glomerular sclerosis. Kidney Int 1992;41:S15–S20.

102. Kremer J, Jubiz W, Michalek A, et al: Fish-oil fatty acid supplementation in active rheumatoid arthritis: a double-blinded, controlled, crossover study. Ann Intern Med 1987;106:497–503.

103. Westberg G, Tarkowski A: Effect of MaxEPA in patients with systemic lupus erythematosus. Scand J Rheumatol 1990;19:137–143.

104. Allen B: Fish oil in combination with other therapies in the treatment of psoriasis. World Rev Nutr Diet 1991;66:436–445.

105. Hawthorne A, Daneshmend T, Hawkey C, et al: Treatment of ulcerative colitis with fish oil supplementation. Gut 1992;33:922–928.

106. Stenson W, Cort D, Rodgers J, et al: Dietary supplementation with fish oil in ulcerative colitis. Ann Intern Med 1992;116:606–614.

107. Aslan A, Triadafilopoulos G: Fish oil fatty acid supplementation in active ulcerative colitis: a double-blind, placebo-controlled, crossover study. Am J Gastroenterol 1992;87:432–437.

108. Lorenz R, Weber P, Szinmau P, Heldwein W, Strasser T, Loeschke K: Supplementation with n-3 fatty acids from fish oil in chronic inflammatory bowel disease: a randomized, placebo-controlled, double-blind cross-over trial. J Intern Med 1989;Suppl 225:225–232.

109. Matè J, Castaños R, Garcia-Samaniego J, Pajares J: Does dietary fish oil maintain the remission of Crohn's disease (CD): a study case control. Gastroenterology 1991;100(Suppl):A228.

110. Belluzzi A, Brignola C, Campieri M, Pera A, Boschi S, Miglioli M: Effect of an enteric-coated fish-oil preparation on relapses in Crohn's disease. N Engl J Med 1996;334:1557–1560.

111. Arm J, Horton C, Mencia-Huerta J, Lee T: The effects of dietary supplementation with fish oil lipids on the airway response to inhaled allergen in bronchial asthma. Am Rev Respir Dis 1989;139:1395–1402.

112. De Caterina R: Summary statement: clinical trials with w3 fatty acids. World Rev Nutr Diet 1994;76:130–132.

113. Dry J, Vincent D: Effect of a fish oil diet on asthma: results of a 1-year double-blind study. Int Arch Allergy Appl Immunol 1991;95:156–157.

114. Thien F, Mencia-Huerta J, Lee T: Dietary fish oil effects on seasonal hay fever and asthma in pollen-sensitive subjects. Am Rev Respir Dis 1993;147:1138–1143.

115. Gupta A, Ellis C, Tellner D, Anderson T, Voorhees J: Double-blind, placebo-controlled study to evaluate the efficacy of fish oil and low-dose UVB in the treatment of psoriasis. Br J Dermatol 1989;120:801–807.

116. Henneicke-von Zepelin H, Mrowietz U, Farber L, et al: Highly purified omega-3-polyunsaturated fatty acids for topical treatment of psoriasis. Results of a double-blind, placebo-controlled multicentre study. Br J Dermatol 1993;129:713–717.

117. Soyland E, Funk J, Rajka G, et al: Effect of dietary supplementation with very-long-chain n-3 fatty acids in patients with psoriasis. N Engl J Med 1993;328:1812–1816.

118. Leiba A, Amital H, Gershwin ME, Shoenfeld Y: Diet and lupus. Lupus 2001;10:246–248.

119. Ando M, Sanaka T, Nihei H: Eicosapentaenoic acid reduces plasma levels of remnant lipoproteins and prevents in vivo peroxidation of LDL in dialysis patients. J Am Soc Nephrol 1999;10:2177–2184.

120. Khajehdehi P: Lipid-lowering effect of polyunsaturated fatty acids in hemodialysis patients. J Renal Nutr 2000;10:191–195.

121. Grekas D, Kassimatis E, Makedou A, Bacharaki D, Bamichas G, Tourkantonis A: Combined treatment with low-dose pravastatin and fish oil in post-renal transplantation dislipidemia. Nephron 2000;88:329–333.

122. Løssl K, Skou HA, Christensen JH, Schmidt EB: The effect of n-3 fatty acids on leukotriene formation from neutrophils in patients on hemodialysis. Lipids 1999;34:S185.

123. Christensen JH, Aarøe J, Knudsen N, et al: Heart rate variability and n-3 fatty acids in patients with chronic renal failure: a pilot study. Clin Nephrol 1998;49:102–106.

124. Santos J, Queirós J, Silva F, et al: Effects of fish oil in cyclosporine-treated renal transplant recipients. Transplant Proc 2000;32:2605–2608.

125. Busnach G, Stragliotto E, Minetti E, et al: Effect of n-3 polyunsaturated fatty acids on cyclosporine pharmacokinetics in kidney graft recipients: a randomized placebo-controlled study. J Nephrol 1998;11:87–93.

126. Donadio JV: The emerging role of omega-3 polyunsaturated fatty acids in the management of patients with IgA nephropathy. J Renal Nutr 2001;11:122–128.

127. Donadio JV, Bergstralh EJ, Offord KP, Spencer DC, Holley KE, for the Mayo Nephrology Collaborative Group: A controlled trial of fish oil in IgA nephropathy. N Engl J Med 1994;331:1194–1199.

128. Donadio JVJ, Grande JP, Bergstralh EJ, Dart RA, Larson TS, Spencer DC, for the Mayo Nephrology Collaborative Group: The long-term outcome of patients with IgA nephropathy treated with fish oil in a controlled trial. J Am Soc Nephrol 1999;10:1772–1777.

129. Roubenoff R, Roubenoff R, Selhub J, et al: Abnormal vitamin B6 status in rheumatoid cachexia. Association with spontaneous tumor necrosis factor alpha production and markers of inflammation. Arthritis Rheum 1995;38:105–109.

130. Pringle K: Modulation of the inflammatory response by antioxidants. Diss Abstr Int 1995;56:690.

131. Driscoll H, Chertow B, Jelic T, et al: Vitamin A status affects the development of diabetes and insulitis in BB rats. Metabolism 1996;45:248–253.

132. Hamazaki T, Tateno S, Shishido H: Eicosapentaenoic acid and IgA nephropathy. Lancet 1984;i:1017–1018.

133. Pettersson EE, Rekola S, Berglund L: Treatment of IgA nephropathy with omega-3 polyunsaturated fatty acids: a prospective, double-blind, randomized study. Clin Nephrol 1994;41:183–190.

134. Bennett WM, Walker RG, Kincaid-Smith P: Treatment of IgA nephropathy with eicosapentaenoic acid (EPA): a two-year prospective trial. Clin Nephrol 1989;41:128–131.

CHAPTER
14

Plasmapheresis in Renal Diseases

François Madore and Hugh R. Brady

Plasma exchange is the removal of plasma from a patient and replacement by fresh-frozen or stored plasma. The procedure is frequently termed "plasmapheresis" when solutions other than plasma (e.g. isotonic saline) are used as replacement fluid. The terms "plasma exchange" and "plasmapheresis" are often used interchangeably, and many authors in the literature do not make the distinction between the two. Plasmapheresis has been applied widely over the several last decades as primary or adjunctive treatment for a number of conditions in which "circulating factors" were believed to contribute to disease pathophysiology. Initially based on anecdotal or uncontrolled studies, indications for plasmapheresis have changed over the years reflecting the availability of evidence largely obtained from controlled prospective studies.

Mechanism of action

Table 14.1 summarizes some potentially beneficial actions of plasmapheresis. Plasmapheresis is often employed to rapidly lower circulating titers of autoantibodies (e.g. antiglomerular basement membrane disease) or immune complexes (e.g. lupus nephritis).[1] Plasmapheresis has also been proposed as a useful adjunct to chemotherapy for removing circulating immunoglobulins or immunoglobulin components in multiple myeloma and other dysproteinemias.[2] Other potential indications include the removal of components other than immunoglobulins. The removal of thrombotic factors has been suggested as an explanation of the effect of plasmapheresis in thrombotic thrombocytopenic purpura (TTP).[3] Infusion of normal plasma may itself have beneficial effects. Indeed, there is evidence that replacement of a deficient plasma component may be the principal mechanism of action of plasmapheresis in TTP.[4] Other theoretical beneficial effects on immune function include depletion of complement products, fibrinogen, and some cytokines, alterations in idiotypic/anti-idiotypic antibody balance, and improvement in reticuloendothelial system function.[5–7]

Table 14.1 Possible mechanisms of action of plasmapheresis*

Mechanism	Example of disease
Removal of circulating pathologic factors	
Antibodies	Antiglomerular basement membrane disease
Immune complexes	Lupus nephritis
Cryoglobulin	Cryoglobulinemia
Myeloma protein	Myeloma cast nephropathy
Prothrombotic factor	Hemolytic–uremic syndrome/thrombotic thrombocytopenic purpura
Replacement of deficient plasma factors	
Antithrombotic or fibrinolytic factor	Hemolytic–uremic syndrome/thrombotic thrombocytopenic purpura
Effects on the immune system	
Removal of complement products	Lupus nephritis
Effect on immune regulation	Transplantation
Improvement in reticuloendothelial system function	Cryoglobulinemia

*Adapted from Madore F, Lazarus M, Brady H: Plasma exchange in renal diseases. J Am Soc Nephrol 1996;7:367–386, with permission.

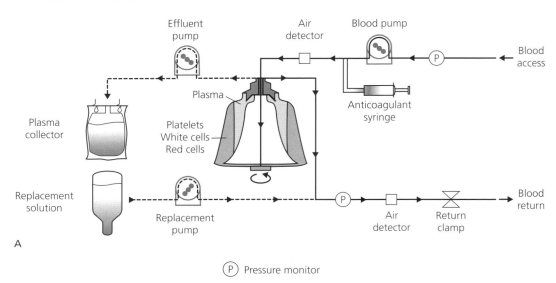

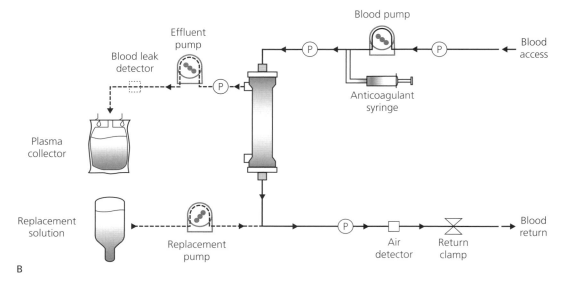

Figure 14.1 Centrifugal separator (A) and membrane filtration (B) systems for plasma exchange. (A) Blood is pumped into the separator container. As the centrifuge revolves, different blood components are separated into discrete layers, which can be harvested separately. Plasma is pumped out of the centrifuge into a collection chamber. Red cells, leukocytes, and platelets are returned to the patient, along with replacement fluid. (B) Blood is pumped into a biocompatible membrane that allows the filtration of plasma while retaining cellular elements.

Technical considerations

Plasmapheresis involves withdrawal of venous blood, separation of plasma from blood cells, and reinfusion of cells plus autologous plasma or another replacement solution. Plasma and blood cells are separated by centrifugation or membrane filtration (Fig. 14.1).

Centrifugation technique

The use of centrifugal force causes whole blood to separate into various components according to their specific gravity. Centrifugation can be intermittent or continuous. With intermittent centrifugation, blood is drawn in successive batches and separated. The cycle is repeated as often as necessary to remove the desired volume of plasma (usually, the equivalent of 1–1.5 plasma volumes or 2.5–4.0 L during a session). Advantages of intermittent centrifugation include relative simplicity of operation, portability of the machines, and adequacy of a single-needle peripheral venipuncture. The disadvantages are slowness (typically > 4 h) and the relatively large extra-corporeal blood volume required (> 225 mL). With continuous-flow equipment, blood is fed continuously into a rapidly rotating bowl in which red cells, leukocytes, platelets, and plasma separate into layers. Any layer or layers can be removed, and the remainder is returned to the patient with replacement fluid (Fig. 14.1A). Continuous-flow centrifugation is faster and most operations (anticoagulation, collection procedures, fluid replacement) are automated. Disadvantages include higher cost, relative immobility of the equipment, and the requirement for either two venipunctures or insertion of a dual-lumen catheter.

Membrane filtration technique

Membrane filtration technology provides an alternative to centrifugation. The patient's blood is pumped through a parallel-plate or hollow-fiber filter at a continuous flow rate, typically 50–200 mL/min (Fig. 14.1B). The membranes usually have pores of 0.2–0.6 µm diameter, sufficient to allow passage of plasma while retaining cells. Several membrane plasma separators are commercially available (e.g. Plasmaflo from Asahi Medical Co. Ltd., Japan; Plasmax from Toray Industries, Japan; CPS-10 from Baxter, USA; Plasmaflux from Fresenius Medical Care AG, Germany; Prisma TPE 2000 from Hospal, France). Plasma is collected and weighed regularly and the infusion rate of replacement fluid is adjusted manually or automatically to maintain intravascular volume. Equipment requirements are relatively minimal, and membrane filtration can be performed using either conventional or continuous hemodialysis equipment. Patients with acute renal failure can receive hemodialysis and plasmapheresis sequentially, using the same machine. In general, plasma can be removed at a rate of 30–50 mL/min (at a blood flow rate of 100 mL/min), and the average time required for a typical membrane filtration is less than 3 h. Potential disadvantages of membrane filtration include activation of complement and leukocytes on the artificial membrane, and the need for a large vein catheter to obtain adequate blood flow rates.

Membrane filtration is as safe and efficient as centrifugal plasmapheresis.[8] The main difference between the techniques is cost of equipment. An automated continuous-flow centrifugal device costs approximately $40 000. Membrane filtration, on the other hand, requires only a blood pump with pressure monitors, available on every standard conventional or continuous hemodialysis machine. Both techniques, however, are roughly comparable in terms of cost per treatment (approximately $400/treatment for nursing time, blood lines, and other basic supplies, plus $300–600/treatment for blood products).

Selective plasmapheresis techniques

More sophisticated approaches achieve more selective removal of immunoglobulins and other specific molecules. Examples include treatment of plasma by cooling (e.g. cryofiltration to remove cryoglobulins), membranes with different pore diameters and filtration/adsorption characteristics (cascade filtration), or perfusion through adsorbent columns (hemadsorption). The use of hemadsorption has been reported for treatment of sepsis, among other indications, to remove endotoxins and other bacterial toxins using absorbent materials with different binding properties.[9]

Anticoagulation

Both centrifugation and membrane plasmapheresis require anticoagulation to prevent activation of the clotting mechanisms within the extracorporeal circuit. The most frequently used anticoagulant for centrifugation procedures is citrate. A continuous infusion of acid-citrate dextrose is given intravenously. The infusion rate is adjusted according to the blood flow rate. Standard unfractionated heparin is the most frequently used anticoagulant for membrane plasmapheresis. The required

dose of heparin is approximately twice that needed for hemodialysis, because a substantial amount of the infused heparin is removed along with the plasma.

Replacement fluids

The typical replacement fluids are fresh-frozen plasma, 5% albumin or other plasma derivatives (e.g. cryosupernatant), and crystalloids (e.g. 0.9% saline, Ringer's lactate). The choice of fluid has implications for the efficacy of the procedure, oncotic pressure, coagulation, and spectrum of adverse effects. Albumin is usually preferred to plasma because of the risk of hypersensitivity reactions and transmission of viral infections with the latter. Albumin (5%) is generally combined with 0.9% saline on a 50:50 (vol%) basis. The exact composition of replacement fluids is tailored to the needs of the patient. For example, plasma is the replacement fluid of choice in patients with hemolytic–uremic syndrome (HUS)–TTP because the infusion of normal plasma may contribute to the replacement of a deficient plasma factor. Plasma may also be preferable in patients at risk of bleeding (e.g. those with liver disease or disseminated intravascular coagulation) or requiring intensive therapy (e.g. daily exchanges for several weeks).

Efficacy of plasmapheresis in specific renal diseases

General comments

Clinical application of plasmapheresis was based initially on anecdotal or uncontrolled studies. The last decade has witnessed a more rigorous reexamination of the efficacy of therapeutic plasma exchange.[10–13] However, for many disorders, there are few prospective controlled clinical trials with adequate statistical power to allow definitive conclusions to be reached regarding the efficacy of plasmapheresis. In addition, other factors complicate the interpretation of published literature. First, the natural history of many diseases under investigation (e.g. lupus) is characterized by spontaneous exacerbations and remissions, making it difficult to evaluate whether any improvement is attributable to plasmapheresis. Second, treatment protocols vary widely between centers, making the comparison between published studies hazardous. Finally, negative studies are inevitably less likely to be published, thereby biasing the literature in favor of plasmapheresis. In the following section, the therapeutic use of plasmapheresis in specific acute renal conditions is reviewed. Consensus plasma exchange regimens are presented for diseases in which there is evidence to support its use.

Antiglomerular basement membrane antibody disease

Antiglomerular basement membrane (anti-GBM) antibody disease typically presents as rapidly progressive glomerulonephritis (RPGN) without or with pulmonary hemorrhage

(Goodpasture syndrome). Circulating anti-GBM antibodies are detected in greater than 90% of patients and, in general, disease activity correlates with the titer of circulating antibodies. Prior to 1975, anti-GBM-induced nephritis had a very poor prognosis,[14,15] and more than 85% of patients treated with steroids and cytotoxic drugs progressed to endstage renal disease (ESRD). Against this background, the results of more than 20 uncontrolled studies including close to 250 patients, published over the past 20 years, suggest that survival rates of greater than 80% and renal preservation rates of greater than 45% may be obtained with therapeutic regimens combining plasmapheresis with immunosuppressive drugs (reviewed in references 16 and 17). These results compare favorably with historical data suggesting patient survival of 45% and progression to ESRD in 85%. The largest published series involves more than 56 patients treated with plasmapheresis and immunosuppression at the Hammersmith Hospital (Table 14.2).[15,18] Of patients undergoing daily 4-L plasmapheresis for at least 14 days, 85% were alive after 2 months, 44% had retained independent renal function, and 41% had progressed to ESRD. Significant recovery of renal function was infrequent in patients who were oliguric, or had a serum creatinine above 600 µmol/L (6.8 mg/dL), or who required dialysis at presentation, even though anti-GBM antibody titers were reduced effectively. Similarly, several different centers have also reported that patients with a serum creatinine above 600 µmol/L are unlikely to respond to therapy and regain renal function.[18]

The specific role of plasmapheresis in therapeutic regimens for anti-GBM disease has never been properly assessed by prospective randomized controlled trials. Only two controlled studies have evaluated the efficacy of plasmapheresis as an adjunct to conventional immunosuppressive therapy in this disease (Table 14.2).[19,20] Although small (17 and 20 patients), both studies suggested a benefit as evidenced by faster decline in anti-GBM antibody titers, lower serum creatinine after therapy, and fewer patients progressing to renal failure. However, the authors were cautious about accepting that plasmapheresis had been responsible for the improved outcome, as the groups receiving plasmapheresis had milder disease than the control groups.

Thus, there is evidence, although largely based on uncontrolled or retrospective studies with historical comparison, that plasmapheresis is a useful adjunct to immunosuppressive drugs (Table 14.2). Plasmapheresis can accelerate disappearance of anti-GBM antibody and improve renal function if instituted promptly. In patients with severe disease (oliguria, dialysis, or serum creatinine > 600 µmol/L (6.8 mg/dL)), plasmapheresis should probably be reserved for treatment of lung hemorrhage because patients are unlikely to regain renal function. As an initial regimen, most experts recommend daily plasmapheresis for 14 days, with 4-L exchanges and albumin solution as replacement fluid. Response to therapy should be monitored by repeated assessments of urine output, serum creatinine, and plasma anti-GBM levels.

Table 14.2 Major clinical trials evaluating the efficacy of plasmapheresis in treatment of antiglomerular basement membrane antibody disease*

| | | | | | | Benefit of plasma exchange | | | |
| | | | | | | Renal outcome[‡] | | Mortality | |
References	Study design	No. of patients	Patients on dialysis at presentation	Number of plasma-phereses	Concomitant therapy[†]	Pheresis (%)	Controls (%)	Pheresis (%)	Controls (%)
Johnson et al[19]	Randomized controlled trial	17	2 of 17	4–17	Steroids Cyclophosphamide	25[§]	67[§]	25	11
Simpson et al[20]	Nonrandomized controlled study	20	7 of 20	10–25	Steroids Cyclophosphamide Azathioprine	38[§]	50[§]	13	25
Hammersmith Group[18]	Uncontrolled case series	59	30 of 59	> 14	Steroids Cyclophosphamide Azathioprine	41[¶]	87[¶]	15[¶]	47[¶]

*Adapted from Madore F, Lazarus M, Brady H: Plasma exchange in renal diseases. J Am Soc Nephrol 1996;7:367–386, with permission.
[†]All concomitant methods of therapy were administered by mouth.
[‡]Expressed as incidence of endstage renal disease.
[§]Significant benefit, but patients receiving plasmapheresis had milder disease.
[¶]Benefit when patients treated with plasmapheresis are compared to historical controls.

Pauci-immune rapidly progressive glomerulonephritis

Approximately 40% of patients with RPGN have pauci-immune crescentic glomerulonephritis due to Wegener granulomatosis, polyarteritis nodosa, or "renal-limited" pauci-immune glomerulonephritis. The majority of these patients have antineutrophil cytoplasmic antibodies (ANCA), which may contribute to the pathophysiology of RPGN. The prognosis of pauci-immune RPGN in general has been poor. The limited available prognostic data indicate that 80% of such patients progress to ESRD without therapy with cytotoxic drugs (see review by Couser[16]).

Five randomized controlled trials have evaluated the efficacy of plasmapheresis as an adjunct to immunosuppressive therapy in patients with pauci-immune RPGN (Table 14.3).[21–25] Two studies randomly assigned patients to receive immunosuppressive agents with or without plasmapheresis, and found no statistically significant difference between the two groups as judged by serum creatinine or dialysis dependency.[21,22] Three other studies provided evidence of benefit in subgroups of patients with severe disease.[23–25] Specifically, patients on dialysis or with a serum creatinine above 800 µmol/L were more likely to respond to plasmapheresis than patients with milder disease. None of the randomized controlled trials reported improvement in patient survival.

In aggregate, these results argue against a role for plasmapheresis in milder forms of RPGN, but suggest a benefit when the technique is used as an adjunct to immunosuppressive therapy in patients with severe disease. The latter conclusions are further supported by the combined results of 12 uncontrolled case series (reviewed in reference 16), which suggest a response rate of 70% for patients with RPGN treated with plasmapheresis, similar to that for patients treated with conventional therapy (response rate 60%). Given the paucity of convincing data, it is impossible to give firm recommendations regarding the specifics of therapy for patients with pauci-immune RPGN. It would seem prudent to reserve plasmapheresis for severe cases and to perform at least four plasmapheresis sessions during the first week of immunosuppressive therapy, using 4-L exchanges and albumin solution as replacement fluid. Response to therapy should be monitored with repeated assessments of urine output, serum creatinine, and possibly ANCA titers.

Immune complex crescentic glomerulonephritis

Most patients with immune complex RPGN have clinical or pathologic evidence of a systemic immune complex disease (e.g. systemic lupus erythematosus) or have a specific category of primary glomerulonephritis (e.g. IgA nephropathy). Plasmapheresis has been advocated mainly in the treatment of lupus, cryoglobulinemia, and IgA nephropathy/Henoch–Schönlein purpura.

Lupus nephritis

Overt nephritis complicates 38–90% of cases of systemic lupus erythematosus. Circulating autoantibodies and immune complexes within glomeruli appear to play a key role in the pathophysiology of lupus nephritis. Case reports and uncontrolled case series have suggested a benefit of plasmapheresis in severe lupus nephritis. However, a large multicenter prospective randomized controlled trial provided strong evidence against its use (Table 14.4).[26] The Lupus Nephritis Collaborative Study Group assessed the value of plasmapheresis as an adjunct to prednisone and cyclophosphamide in 86 patients with severe lupus nephritis (serum creatinine > 2.0 mg/dL or 180 µmol/L). Patients underwent plasmapheresis three times weekly for 4 weeks and were followed for an average of 136 weeks. Plasmapheresis caused a rapid reduction of serum anti-dsDNA antibodies and cryoglobulins, but did not influence renal function or mortality. Importantly, patients receiving plasmapheresis tended to have a worse outcome, which ultimately led the external data monitoring board to recommend early termination of the trial.

Four smaller randomized controlled trials of plasmapheresis have been reported, although some patients included in these trials had mild disease (Table 14.4).[27–30] Plasmapheresis produced significant reduction in circulating immune complexes and anti-DNA antibodies, but the frequency and degree of partial or complete remission was the same in both plasmapheresis and control groups.

Given the failure of standard plasmapheresis protocols to demonstrate a generalized benefit, intensified treatment protocols that combine plasmapheresis with subsequent pulse cyclophosphamide have been suggested.[31,32] Despite initial encouraging studies, the results of a recent randomized controlled trial suggest that plasmapheresis does not provide additional benefit when compared with pulse cyclophosphamide.[33]

In summary, the results of multiple prospective randomized controlled trials do not support a role for plasmapheresis in the treatment of lupus nephritis (Table 14.4). There is experimental and clinical evidence that plasmapheresis induces rapid removal of circulating immune complexes and anti-DNA antibodies, but does not appear to influence renal function, remission rate, or mortality.

Cryoglobulinemia

Precipitation of cryoglobulins within the glomerular capillary lumen can induce a proliferative or membrano-proliferative glomerulonephritis with a variable but sometimes rapidly progressive course. Plasmapheresis has been used to treat cryoglobulinemia for over 20 years without being subjected to a prospective randomized controlled clinical trial.[34] Uncontrolled studies in which greater than five patients were evaluated (reviewed in reference 13) showed that plasmapheresis induced rapid reduction in the cryocrit, improved renal function in 55–87% of patients, and improved survival (~25% mortality rate) compared with historical data (~55% mortality rate). Plasmapheresis is claimed to be most effective in

Table 14.3 Randomized controlled trials evaluating the efficacy of plasmapheresis in treatment of pauci-immune rapidly progressive glomerulonephritis*

References	Study design	No. of patients	Presentation	Initial renal function	ANCA	Number of plasmaphereses	Concomitant therapy	Benefit of plasmapheresis	
								Renal outcome	Mortality§
Glöckner et al[19†]	Randomized controlled trial	26	RPGN: systemic diseases included	46% dialysis dependent	NR	11.3 (mean)	Steroids (p.q.) Aza (p.q.) Cyclo (p.q.)	Improved creatinine clearance:‡§ Pheresis 69% Controls 73%	Pheresis 7% Controls 8%
Cole et al[22†]	Randomized controlled trial	32	RPGN: systemic diseases excluded	34% dialysis dependent	(+) in 71%	>10	Steroids (i.v. + p.q.) Aza (p.q.)	Dialysis requirement:§ Pheresis 75% Controls 71%	Pheresis 13% Controls 0%
Pusey et al[23]	Randomized controlled trial	48	RPGN: systemic diseases included	39% dialysis dependent	NR	9 (mean)	Steroids (p.o.) Aza (p.o.) Cyclo (p.o.)	No benefit for entire group. For dialysis patients, of dialysis:¶ Pheresis 91% Controls 37%	Pheresis 48% Controls 35%
Rifle et al[24†]	Randomized controlled trial	14	RPGN: systemic diseases included	79% dialysis dependent	NR	9 (mean)	Steroids (i.v. + p.o.) Cyclo (p.o.) Hep (s.c.)	Benefit for entire group. For dialysis patients, of dialysis:¶ Pheresis 75% Controls 0%	NR
Mauri et al[25]	Randomized controlled trial	22	RPGN: systemic diseases included	50% with serum creatinine >800 μmol/L	NR	>6 (mean)	Steroids (p.o.) Cyclo (p.o.)	No benefit for entire group. For patients with initial serum creatinine >800 μmol/L, mean serum creatinine:¶ Pheresis 728 μmol/L Controls 1163 μmol/L	NR

ANCA, antineutrophil cytoplasmic antibodies; Aza, azathioprine; Cyclo, cyclophosphamide; Hep, calcium heparinate; NR, not reported; RPGN, rapidly progressive glomerulonephritis.
*Adapted from Madore F, Lazarus M, Brady H: Plasma exchange in renal diseases. J Am Soc Nephrol 1996;7:367–386, with permission.
†Studies included patients with immune complex deposits.
‡Defined as an increase of > 20 mL/min in creatinine clearance compared with pretreatment values or a clearance > 10 mL/min for patients who required dialysis at presentation.
§No statistically significant difference between plasmapheresis group and control group.
¶Added benefit of plasmapheresis versus control group ($P < 0.05$).

Table 14.4 Randomized controlled trials evaluating the efficacy of plasmapheresis in treatment of lupus nephritis*

References	Study design	No. of patients	Disease severity	Initial renal function	Number of plasmaphereses	Concomitant therapy[†]	Benefit of plasmapheresis		Mortality[‡]
							Clinical outcome		
Lewis et al[26]	Randomized controlled trial	86	Severe disease	Mean serum creatinine 180 μmol/L	12	Steroids Cyclo	ESRD:[‡] Pheresis 25% Controls 17%		Pheresis 20% Controls 13%
Wei et al[27]	Randomized controlled trial	20	Mild disease	Creatinine clearance > 20 mL/min	6	Steroids Antimalarias	Activity index (> 50% improvement):[‡] Pheresis 55% Controls 33%		NR
Derksen et al[23]	Randomized controlled trial	20	Unresponsive to conventional	Mean creatinine 30 mL/min	9	Steroids	Remission rate:[‡] Pheresis 33% Controls 18%		NR
French Group[29§]	Randomized controlled trial	12	Active disease	Patients with < 50% crescents[¶]	23	Steroids	Activity score:[‡] Pheresis 34% Controls 39%		NR
Clark et al[25]	Randomized controlled trial	39	Mild disease	Creatinine clearance > 30 mL/min	NR	Steroids Aza	Serum creatinine:[‡] Pheresis 97 μmol/L Controls 124 μmol/L		Pheresis 5% Controls 0%

Aza, azathioprine; Cyclo, cyclophosphamide; ESRD, endstage renal disease; NR, not reported; NSAID, nonsteroidal antiinflammatory drug.
*Adapted from Madore F, Lazarus M, Brady H: Plasma exchange in renal diseases. J Am Soc Nephrol 1996;7:367–386, with permission.
[†]All concomitant methods of therapy were administered by mouth.
[‡]No statistically significant difference between plasmapheresis group and control group.
[§]French Cooperative Study Group on Systemic Lupus Erythematosus.
[¶]Patients with rapidly progressive glomerulonephritis or > 50% crescents on renal biopsy were excluded.

patients with early active inflammation. Because of the uncontrolled nature of all reported studies, it is impossible to determine whether the improvement in renal outcome or survival was due to plasmapheresis or other factors such as patient selection, earlier diagnosis, or concurrent immunosuppressive therapy. In addition, all studies were published before the recognition that hepatitis C is the etiologic agent in most cases of mixed essential cryoglobulinemia and that interferon-α alone or in combination with ribavirin can induce remission. Therefore, the use of plasmapheresis, if any, should be limited to patients with acute active and severe disease. Most investigators advocate combining plasmapheresis with conventional immunosuppression, performing the procedure thrice weekly for the first 2 weeks using 4-L exchanges and albumin solution as replacement fluid.

IgA nephropathy and Henoch–Schönlein purpura

IgA nephropathy and Henoch–Schönlein purpura probably represent a spectrum of manifestations of the same disease and are characterized by mesangial deposition of IgA. Although serum total IgA concentration is elevated in 33–55% of patients, circulating IgA levels do not correlate with severity or activity of disease. The published worldwide experience of plasmapheresis in IgA nephropathy and Henoch–Schönlein purpura is limited to approximately 60 patients, and consists of case reports and small uncontrolled series.[35,36] Plasmapheresis is reported to be beneficial in patients with a rapidly progressive course compared with patients with a more slowly evolving course.[36] Roccatello et al[37] reported on their experience in treating six patients with crescentic IgA disease using plasmapheresis in addition to steroids and cyclophosphamide. All patients improved in the short term but subsequent deterioration in renal function was observed in more than half of these patients.

In summary, no firm conclusions can be drawn regarding the efficacy of plasmapheresis in IgA nephropathy or Henoch–Schönlein purpura because of lack of adequate concurrent controls, small number of subjects, and marked variability in the plasmapheresis regimens. Given the encouraging preliminary results, however, the role of plasmapheresis deserves further study.

Hemolytic–uremic syndrome and thrombotic thrombocytopenic purpura

HUS–TTP probably represent a spectrum of manifestations of the same disease and are characterized by thrombotic microangiopathy with consumptive thrombocytopenia, microangiopathic hemolytic anemia, and renal failure. Therapeutic plasma exchange has been suggested mainly for adult HUS–TTP, although some studies have also included cases with childhood diarrhea-associated HUS. Therapeutic plasma exchange has been proposed to benefit patients with HUS–TTP by (1) replacing a deficient plasma factor with antithrombotic or fibrinolytic activity and/or (2) removing circulating toxins that cause endo-thelial injury and/or platelet aggregation and promote formation of microthrombi. Recent evidence suggests that a deficiency in von Willebrand factor-cleaving protease caused by autoantibodies is responsible for some cases of HUS–TTP.[38,39] In such patients, plasma exchange with fresh-frozen plasma presumably removes the inhibitory antibody and the accumulating von Willebrand multimers in addition to supplying the missing enzyme.

Most of the evidence in favor of the role of plasmapheresis in HUS–TTP originates from uncontrolled or retrospective studies (reviewed in reference 40) and from comparison with historical data. Prior to the introduction of plasma infusion and plasmapheresis, the disease typically progressed rapidly and was almost uniformly fatal (93% fatality rate; 79% within 90 days).[41] With plasmapheresis using fresh-frozen plasma, remission rates of greater than 75% and survival rates greater than 85% have been consistently reported.

There has been no controlled, prospective, randomized, appropriately blinded study comparing plasma exchange with placebo or drug therapy. However, two randomized controlled trials compared plasma exchange to plasma infusion (Table 14.5).[42,43] Rock et al[42] randomized patients with TTP to either plasma exchange or plasma infusion with fresh-frozen plasma and observed that patients receiving plasma exchange had a better response rate and superior survival. Although the authors concluded that plasma exchange is superior to plasma infusion, interpretation should be guarded as patients undergoing plasma exchange received three times as much plasma as patients undergoing plasma infusion. Indeed, a smaller multicenter controlled trial did not observe a difference in outcome when patients were randomized to receive either daily infusions of 15 mL/kg of fresh-frozen plasma or plasma exchange with a mixture of 15 mL/kg of fresh-frozen plasma and 45 mL/kg of 5% albumin as replacement fluid (Table 14.5).[43] Thus, the exact role of plasma removal and plasma infusion in the beneficial effect of plasma exchange remains controversial.

In summary, there is evidence, largely based on studies using historical controls, that plasma exchange improves renal outcome and mortality in adult patients with HUS–TTP. It is unclear whether this benefit is due to plasma infusion alone and replacement of a deficient plasma factor or to plasma exchange and removal of a circulating toxic. In practice, this distinction is rather semantic since it is often necessary to perform plasma exchange in order to administer the desired amount of plasma, given that these patients are often oliguric or anuric and at risk for hypervolemia and pulmonary edema. The most widely recognized plasma exchange protocol involves daily plasma exchange for 7–14 days, using 4-L exchanges and fresh-frozen plasma as replacement fluid. Cryosupernatant may also be used as replacement fluid. Results of earlier reports suggested that the cryosupernatant portion of plasma, in which von Willebrand factor is largely removed, might be more effective than whole plasma.[44,45] However, a recent randomized controlled trial found no difference in efficacy between whole plasma and cryosupernatant plasma.[46]

Table 14.5 Controlled studies comparing the efficacy of plasma exchange versus plasma in treatment of thrombotic thrombocytopenic purpura and hemolytic–uremic syndrome*

References	Study design	No. of patients	Diagnosis	Renal function at presentation	Number of exchange	Other therapies	Benefit of plasma exchange		
							Remission rate[†]	Renal outcome	Mortality
Rock et al[42]	Randomized controlled trial	102	TTP (adults)	Mean serum creatinine 138 μmol/L	3–36	ASA (p.o.) Dipyridamole (p.o.)	PE 78%[‡] Controls 49%	NR	PE 22%[‡] Controls 37%
Henon et al[43]	Randomized controlled trial	40	TTP (adults)	Mean serum creatinine 278 μmol/L	3–35	ASA (p.o.) Dipyridamole (i.v.)	PE 80%[§] Controls 52%	NR	PE 15%[§] Controls 3%

ASA, aspirin; NR, not reported; PE, plasma exchange; TTP, thrombotic thrombocytopenic purpura.
*Adapted from Madore F, Lazarus M, Brady H: Plasma exchange in renal diseases. J Am Soc Nephrol 1996;7:367–386, with permission.
[†]Remission defined as > 150 000 platelets.
[‡]Statistically significant benefit of plasmapheresis versus control group ($P < 0.05$).
[§]No statistically significant difference between plasmapheresis group and control group.

Renal failure associated with multiple myeloma

Renal failure complicates 3–9% of cases of multiple myeloma and portends a poor prognosis. Renal impairment can be caused by a variety of factors, including precipitation of myeloma light chains within renal tubules and direct toxicity to tubule epithelium. Other factors frequently implicated include hypercalcemia, hyperuricemia, amyloidosis, hyperviscosity, infections, and chemotherapeutic agents. Plasmapheresis has been suggested specifically to prevent the renal toxicity associated with myeloma proteins by rapidly reducing their plasma concentration. Two randomized controlled trials of plasmapheresis in multiple myeloma have been reported (Table 14.6).[47,48] Johnson et al[47] randomized

patients to either chemotherapy and forced diuresis with or without plasmapheresis, and could detect only a small and nonsignificant benefit on renal function despite lowering of plasma concentration of myeloma protein. There was no difference in survival between the two groups. In contrast, Zucchelli et al[48] randomized patients to receive steroids and cyclophosphamide with or without plasmapheresis, and observed significant improvements in renal outcome and patient survival. A similar trend was noted in at least three other nonrandomized studies and case series.[2,49,50]

Thus whereas the role of plasmapheresis in multiple myeloma remains controversial, there are sufficient data to justify the use of plasmapheresis as adjunctive therapy in some patients with myeloma cast nephropathy. Given the paucity of data, however, it is impossible to give firm

Table 14.6 Randomized controlled trials evaluating the efficacy of plasmapheresis in treatment of acute renal failure associated with multiple myeloma*

References	Study design	No. of patients	Patients on dialysis at presentation	Number of plasmaphereses	Concomitant therapy	Benefit of plasma exchange	
						Renal outcome[‡]	Mortality[§]
Johnson et al[47]	Randomized controlled trial	21	12 of 21	3–12	Forced diuresis Steroids (p.o.) Melphalan (p.o.)	Discontinuation of dialysis:[¶] Pheresis 43% Controls 0%	Pheresis 25%[¶] Controls 25%
Zucchelli et al[48]	Randomized controlled study	29	24 of 29	5	Forced diuresis Steroids (p.o.) Cyclophosphamide (p.o.)	Discontinuation of dialysis:[‖] Pheresis 48% Controls 18%	Pheresis 34%[‖] Controls 72%

*Adapted from Madore F, Lazarus M, Brady H: Plasma exchange in renal diseases. J Am Soc Nephrol 1996;7:367–386, with permission.
[†]All studies focused on acute or progressive renal failure associated with multiple myeloma and excluded patients with chronic renal impairment.
[‡]Expressed as percentage of patients on dialysis at presentation.
[§]Expressed as percentage of patients from the entire group.
[¶]No statistically significant difference between plasmapheresis group and control group.
[‖]Statistically significant benefit of plasmapheresis versus control group ($P < 0.05$).

recommendations regarding its use. A large multicenter randomized controlled trial currently ongoing should allow more definitive recommendations to be made. Meanwhile, it would seem reasonable to attempt plasmapheresis in myeloma patients with rapidly evolving renal failure. At least five plasmapheresis sessions should be performed initially, using 4-L exchanges and albumin solution as replacement fluid.

Renal transplantation

Plasmapheresis has been used in experimental protocols to prevent or treat renal allograft rejection by removing cytotoxic antibodies and other inflammatory mediators, or to prevent and treat recurrence of primary renal disease in allografts.

Approximately 20% of patients waiting for cadaveric transplantation have high titers of preformed cytotoxic antibodies that render them at high risk for hyperacute and acute allograft rejection. In an attempt to solve this problem, plasmapheresis and immunoadsorption have been advocated as a means of removing cytotoxic antibodies prior to transplantation. In uncontrolled studies, plasmapheresis significantly reduced the titers of antibodies;[51-53] however, this benefit is usually transient and no firm conclusions can be drawn concerning the efficacy of this practice. Prophylactic plasmapheresis has also been studied in highly sensitized patients in the immediate postoperative period, again in an effort to prevent early humoral rejection. Overall, the results did not show a major benefit over conventional antirejection prophylaxis.[13,51,54]

Four randomized controlled trials have been conducted on the efficacy of plasmapheresis in the treatment of established, biopsy-proven acute allograft rejection (Table 14.7).[55-58] Blake et al[55] randomized 85 patients to receive conventional antirejection therapy with or without plasmapheresis for treatment of all episodes of acute rejection occurring within the first 3 months after transplantation. There was no statistically significant difference in 5-year actuarial graft survival, although there was a trend toward superior graft survival in patients undergoing plasmapheresis. Three smaller trials focused on the value of plasmapheresis for treatment of acute rejection with prominent vascular injury on the basis that this clinicopathologic entity is likely mediated in large part by circulating anti-endothelial cell antibodies.[56-58] Two of these studies[56,57] did not observe a significant difference in graft survival, whereas the third study[58] suggested a benefit. Thus, the sum of data published to date do not support the use of therapeutic plasmapheresis for the prevention or treatment of acute rejection.

The literature on therapeutic plasmapheresis in chronic rejection is limited to a few uncontrolled series and the results in general have been disappointing, with improvement in graft function being, at best, modest and usually transient.[13,51] A few uncontrolled studies have suggested a role for plasmapheresis in the prevention and treatment of recurrent glomerular disease, particularly primary focal segmental glomerulosclerosis, after transplantation. In a representative study by Dantal et al[59] patients with recurrent nephrotic syndrome were treated with plasma immunoadsorption using protein A. This technique induced a fall in urinary protein excretion in all

Table 14.7 Randomized controlled trials evaluating the efficacy of plasmapheresis in treatment of established acute allograft rejection*

References	Study design	No. of patients	Features at presentation Diagnosis	Features at presentation Graft biopsy	Number of plasma-phereses	Concomitant therapy	Benefit of plasmapheresis Graft survival	Benefit of plasmapheresis Patients' survival
Blake et al[55]	Randomized controlled trial	85	Acute rejection	Vascular or cellular rejection	5	Steroids (i.v.)	Pheresis 64%[†] Controls 51%	NR
Allen et al[56]	Randomized controlled trial	27	Acute rejection (unresponsive[‡])	Vascular rejection	6	Steroids (i.v.) Heparin (s.c.)	Pheresis 18%[†] Controls 38%	NR
Kirubakaran et al[57]	Randomized controlled trial	24	Acute rejection (severe)	Vascular rejection	8	Steroids (i.v.)	Pheresis 33%[†] Controls 75%	NR
Bonomini et al[58]	Randomized controlled trial	44	Acute rejection (unresponsive[‡])	Vascular rejection	3–7	Steroids (i.v.) Cyclo (p.o.)	Pheresis 70%[§] Controls 19 %	NR

Cyclo, cyclophosphamide; NR, not reported.
*Adapted from Madore F, Lazarus M, Brady H: Plasma exchange in renal diseases. J Am Soc Nephrol 1996;7:367–386, with permission.
[†]No statistically significant difference between plasmapheresis group and control group.
[‡]Acute rejection uunresponsive to conventional therapy with i.v. steroids.
[§]Statistically significant benefit of plasmapheresis versus control group (P < 0.05).

patients by an average of 82%; however, the effect of therapy was transient in all but one patient. Thus there are insufficient data, as yet, to recommend routine use of plasmapheresis in recurrent glomerular disease.

Complications of plasmapheresis

The perception that plasmapheresis is a benign procedure has undoubtedly contributed to its widespread use for unproven indications. The overall incidence of adverse reactions reported in the literature ranges from 1.6 to 25%, with severe reactions occurring in 0.5–3.1% (cf. review in reference 60). The most frequent complications are related to either vascular access or the composition of replacement fluids. Hematomas, pneumothorax, and catheter infections are the most frequent complications of vascular access, complicating 0.02–4% of treatments. Complications related to the replacement fluids include anaphylactoid reactions to fresh-frozen plasma, coagulopathies induced by inadequate replacement of clotting factors, and transmission of viral hepatitis and other infections. Symptomatic hypocalcemia resulting from infusion of citrate (either as the treatment's anticoagulant or in fresh-frozen plasma) complicates 1.5–9% of treatments. Hypotensive episodes occur in 0.4–4% of patients and can be triggered by vasovagal episodes, delayed or inadequate volume replacement, hypo-oncotic fluid replacement, or anaphylaxis. Repeated plasmapheresis has been postulated to be immunosuppressive and to increase the risk of infections in patients receiving immunosuppressive agents. However, infection rates reported from randomized trials in the treatment of lupus nephritis and pauci-immune RPGN do not support this contention.[21–23,61] Infection rates were the same in patients treated with plasmapheresis and those treated conventionally.

Conclusions

Use of plasmapheresis has changed in recent years reflecting the availability of evidence largely obtained from controlled prospective studies. However, the clinical efficacy of plasmapheresis for many renal conditions is still controversial. Plasmapheresis appears to be a useful adjunct to conventional therapy in the treatment of anti-GBM nephritis, severe dialysis-dependent forms of pauci-immune RPGN, and HUS–TTP. Reported data also suggest a possible benefit of plasmapheresis in patients with myeloma cast nephropathy and cryoglobulinemia, but the case for plasmapheresis in these disorders is largely unproven and the reported evidence insufficient to recommend its use outside research settings. In contrast, data from controlled trials do not support a role for plasmapheresis in immune complex-mediated RPGN, such as lupus nephritis, and acute allograft rejection. The more widespread application of prospective, randomized, controlled clinical trials should help to better define the value of plasmapheresis for treatment of renal diseases.

References

1. Shumak KH, Rock GA: Therapeutic plasma exchange. N Engl J Med 1984;310:762–771.
2. Wahlin A, Lofvenberg E, Holm J: Improved survival in multiple myeloma with renal failure. Acta Med Scand 1987;221:205–209.
3. Kelton JG, Neame PB, Walker I, et al: Thrombotic thrombocytopenic purpura: mechanism for effectiveness of plasmapheresis. Clin Res 1979;27:299A.
4. Byrnes JJ, Khurana M: Treatment of thrombotic thrombocytopenic purpura with plasma. N Engl J Med 1977;297:1386–1389.
5. Lockwood CM, Worlledge S, Nicholas A, Cotton C, Peters DK: Reversal of impaired splenic function in patients with nephritis or vasculitis (or both) by plasma exchange. N Engl J Med 1979;300:524–530.
6. Low A, Hotze A, Krapf F, et al: The non specific clearance function of the reticuloendothelial system in patients with immune complex mediated diseases before and after therapeutic plasmapheresis. Rheumatol Int 1985;5:69–72.
7. Bystryn JC, Graf MW, Uhr JW: Regulation of antibody formation by serum antibody. Removal of specific antibody by means of exchange transfusion. J Exp Med 1970;132:1279–1287.
8. Gurland HJ, Lysaght MJ, Samtleben W, Schmidt B: A comparison of centrifugal and membrane-based apheresis formats. Int J Artif Organs 1984;7:35–38.
9. Jaber BL, Pereira BJ: Extracorporeal adsorbent-based strategies in sepsis. Am J Kidney Dis 1997;30:S44–S56.
10. Guillevin L, Bussel A: Indications of plasma exchanges in 2000. Ann Med Interne (Paris) 2000;151:123–135.
11. Winters JL, Pineda AA, McLeod BC, Grima KM: Therapeutic apheresis in renal and metabolic diseases. J Clin Apheresis 2000;15:53–73.
12. Harada T, Miyazaki M, Ozono Y, et al: Therapeutic apheresis for renal diseases. Ther Apheresis 1998;2:193–198.
13. Madore F, Lazarus M, Brady H: Plasma exchange in renal diseases. J Am Soc Nephrol 1996;7:367–386.
14. Wilson CD, Dixon FJ: Anti-glomerular basement membrane antibody-induced glomerulonephritis. Kidney Int 1973;3:74.
15. Rees AJ: Goodpasture's syndrome. In Glassock RJ (ed): Current Therapy in Nephrology and Hypertension. St Louis: Mosby-Year Book, 1992, pp 173–178.
16. Couser WG: Rapidly progressive glomerulonephritis: classification, pathogenetic mechanisms, and therapy. Am J Kidney Dis 1988;11:449–464.
17. Kluth DC, Rees AJ: Anti-glomerular basement membrane disease. J Am Soc Nephrol 1999;10:2446–2453.
18. Turner AN, Rees AJ: Antiglomerular basement membrane disease. In Davison AM, Cameron JS, Grunfeld J-P, Kerr DNS, Ritz E, Winearls CG (eds): Oxford Textbook of Nephrology, 2nd edn. New York: Oxford University Press, 1998, pp 645–666.
19. Johnson JP, Moore JJ, Austin HD, Balow JE, Antonovych TT, Wilson CB: Therapy of anti-glomerular basement membrane antibody disease: analysis of prognostic significance of clinical, pathologic and treatment factors. Medicine (Baltimore) 1985;64:219–227.
20. Simpson IJ, Doak PB, Williams LC, et al: Plasma exchange in Goodpasture's syndrome. Am J Nephrol 1982;2:301–311.
21. Glockner WM, Sieberth HG, Wichmann HE, et al: Plasma exchange and immunosuppression in rapidly progressive glomerulonephritis: a controlled, multi-center study. Clin Nephrol 1988;29:1–8.
22. Cole E, Cattran D, Magil A, et al: A prospective randomized trial of plasma exchange as additive therapy in idiopathic crescentic glomerulonephritis. The Canadian Apheresis Study Group. Am J Kidney Dis 1992;20:261–269.
23. Pusey CD, Rees AJ, Evans DJ, Peters DK, Lockwood CM: Plasma exchange in focal necrotizing glomerulonephritis without anti-GBM antibodies. Kidney Int 1991;40:757–763.
24. Rifle G, Dechelette E: Treatment of rapidly progressive glomerulonephritis by plasma exchange and methylprednisolone pulses. A prospective randomized trial of cyclophosphamide. Interim analysis. The French Cooperative Group. Prog Clin Biol Res 1990;337:263–267.
25. Mauri JM, Gonzales MT, Poveda R, et al: Therapeutic plasma exchange in the treatment of rapidly progressive glomerulonephritis. Plasma Ther Transfus Technol 1985;6:587–591.
26. Lewis EJ, Hunsicker LG, Lan SP, Rohde RD, Lachin JM: A controlled trial of plasmapheresis therapy in severe lupus nephritis. The Lupus Nephritis Collaborative Study Group. N Engl J Med 1992;326:1373–1379.

27. Wei N, Klippel JH, Huston DP, et al: Randomised trial of plasma exchange in mild systemic lupus erythematosus. Lancet 1983;i:17–22.
28. Derksen RH, Hene RJ, Kallenberg CG, Valentijn RM, Kater L: Prospective multicentre trial on the short-term effects of plasma exchange versus cytotoxic drugs in steroid-resistant lupus nephritis. Neth J Med 1988;33:168–177.
29. French Cooperative Group: A randomized trial of plasma exchange in severe acute systemic lupus erythematosous: methodology and interim analysis. Plasm Ther Transfus Technol 1985;6:535–539.
30. Clark WF, Cattran DC, Balfe JW, Williams W, Lindsay RM, Linton AL: Chronic plasma exchange in systemic lupus erythematosus nephritis. Proc Eur Dial Transplant Assoc 1983;20:629–635.
31. Schroeder JO, Euler HH, Löffler H: Synchronization of plasmapheresis and pulse cyclophosphamide in systemic lupus erythematosus. Ann Intern Med 1987;107:344–346.
32. Barr WG, Hubbel EA, Robinson JA: Plasmapheresis and pulse cyclophosphamide in systemic lupus erythematosus. Ann Intern Med 1988;108:152–153.
33. Wallace DJ, Goldfinger D, Pepkowitz SH, et al: Randomized controlled trial of pulse/synchronization cyclophosphamide/apheresis for proliferative lupus nephritis. J Clin Apheresis 1998;13:163–166.
34. Berkman EM, Orlin JB: Use of plasmapheresis and partial plasma exchange in the management of patients with cryoglobulinemia. Transfusion 1980;20:171–178.
35. Nicholls K, Becker G, Walker R, Wright C, Kincaid SP: Plasma exchange in progressive IgA nephropathy. J Clin Apheresis 1990;5:128–132.
36. Coppo R, Basolo B, Roccatello D, et al: Plasma exchange in progressive primary IgA nephropathy. Int J Artif Organs 1985;2:55–58.
37. Roccatello D, Ferro M, Coppo R, Mazzucco G, Quattrocchio G, Piccoli G: Treatment of rapidly progressive IgA nephropathy. Contrib Nephrol 1995;111:177–182.
38. Furlan M, Robles R, Galbusera M, et al: von Willebrand factor-cleaving protease in thrombotic thrombocytopenic purpura and the hemolytic–uremic syndrome. N Engl J Med 1998;339:1578–1584.
39. Tsai HM, Lian EC: Antibodies to von Willebrand factor-cleaving protease in acute thrombotic thrombocytopenic purpura. N Engl J Med 1998;339:1585–1594.
40. Onundarson PT, Rowe JM, Heal JM, Francis CW: Response to plasma exchange and splenectomy in thrombotic thrombocytopenic purpura. A 10-year experience at a single institution. Arch Intern Med 1992;152:791–796.
41. Amorosi EL, Ultmann JE: Thrombotic thrombocytopenic purpura: report of 16 cases and review of the literature. Medicine (Baltimore) 1966;45:139–159.
42. Rock GA, Shumak KH, Buskard NA, et al: Comparison of plasma exchange with plasma infusion in the treatment of thrombotic thrombocytopenic purpura. Canadian Apheresis Study Group. N Engl J Med 1991;325:393–397.
43. Henon P: Treatment of thrombotic thrombopenic purpura. Results of a multicenter randomized clinical study. Presse Med 1991;20:1761–1767.
44. Rock G, Shumak KH, Sutton DM, Buskard NA, Nair RC: Cryosupernatant as replacement fluid for plasma exchange in thrombotic thrombocytopenic purpura. Members of the Canadian Apheresis Group. Br J Haematol 1996;94:383–386.
45. Byrnes JJ, Moake JL, Klug P, Periman P: Effectiveness of the cryosupernatant fraction of plasma in the treatment of refractory thrombotic thrombocytopenic purpura. Am J Hematol 1990;34:169–174.
46. Zeigler ZR, Gryn JF, Rintels PB: Cryopoor plasma does not improve early response in primary adult thrombotic thrombocytopenic purpura. Blood 1998;92:707a.
47. Johnson WJ, Kyle RA, Pineda AA, O'Brien PC, Holley KE: Treatment of renal failure associated with multiple myeloma. Plasmapheresis, hemodialysis, and chemotherapy. Arch Intern Med 1990;150:863–869.
48. Zucchelli P, Pasquali S, Cagnoli L, Rovinetti C: Plasma exchange therapy in acute renal failure due to light chain myeloma. Trans Am Soc Artif Intern Organs 1984;30:36–39.
49. Misiani R, Tiraboschi G, Mingardi G, Mecca G: Management of myeloma kidney: an anti-light-chain approach. Am J Kidney Dis 1987;10:28–33.
50. Pozzi C, Pasquali S, Donini U, et al: Prognostic factors and effectiveness of treatment in acute renal failure due to multiple myeloma: a review of 50 cases. Report of the Italian Renal Immunopathology Group. Clin Nephrol 1987;28:1–9.
51. Frasca GM, Martella D, Vangelista A, Bonomini V: Ten years experience with plasma exchange in renal transplantation. Int J Artif Organs 1991;14:51–55.
52. Hakim RM, Milford E, Himmelfarb J, Wingard R, Lazarus JM, Watt RM: Extracorporeal removal of anti-HLA antibodies in transplant candidates. Am J Kidney Dis 1990;16:423–431.
53. Palmer A, Taube D, Welsh K, Bewick M, Gjorstrup P, Thick M: Removal of anti-HLA antibodies by extracorporeal immunoadsorption to enable renal transplantation. Lancet 1989;i:10–12.
54. Reisaeter AV, Fauchald P, Leivestad T, et al: Plasma exchange in highly sensitized patients as induction therapy after renal transplantation. Transplant Proc 1994;26:1758.
55. Blake P, Sutton D, Cardella CJ: Plasma exchange in acute renal transplant rejection. Prog Clin Biol Res 1990;337:249–252.
56. Allen NH, Dyer P, Geoghegan T, Harris K, Lee HA, Slapak M: Plasma exchange in acute renal allograft rejection. A controlled trial. Transplantation 1983;35:425–428.
57. Kirubakaran MG, Disney AP, Norman J, Pugsley DJ, Mathew TH: A controlled trial of plasmapheresis in the treatment of renal allograft rejection. Transplantation 1981;32:164–165.
58. Bonomini V, Vangelista A, Frasca GM, Di FA, Liviano DAG: Effects of plasmapheresis in renal transplant rejection. A controlled study. Trans Am Soc Artif Intern Organs 1985;31:698–703.
59. Dantal J, Bigot E, Bogers W, et al: Effect of plasma protein adsorption on protein excretion in kidney-transplant recipients with recurrent nephrotic syndrome. N Engl J Med 1994;330:7–14.
60. Mokrzycki MH, Kaplan AA: Therapeutic plasma exchange: complications and management. Am J Kidney Dis 1994;23:817–827.
61. Pohl MA, Lan SP, Berl T: Plasmapheresis does not increase the risk for infection in immunosuppressed patients with severe lupus nephritis. The Lupus Nephritis Collaborative Study Group. Ann Intern Med 1991;114:924–929.

Management of Infection-associated Glomerulonephritis

Steven J. Chadban and Robert C. Atkins

An association between glomerulonephritis and infectious disease has long been recognized. Glomerular damage occurs in infection-associated glomerulonephritis as a result of three pathogenic pathways: the direct renal effects of the invading microorganism, the sepsis-induced dysregulation of systemic circulation and homeostasis, and most importantly the host immune response to microbial antigens. Current clinical therapies actively target the invading organism and provide support for host homeostasis, while the aberrant host immune response is not directly addressed.

The epidemiology of infectious disease and the problems in producing reliable and accurate animal models make infection-associated glomerulonephritis a difficult condition to study. Despite some advances in our understanding of the immunopathogenesis, little impact has been made on specific immunotherapy, and the treatment of infection-associated glomerulonephritis remains largely empirical rather than evidence based. With these limitations in mind, this chapter briefly reviews recent conceptual advances in the understanding of this form of glomerulonephritis, and then discusses current theraputic strategies associated with specific organisms and sites of infection. Approaches to management are provided and avenues amenable to future research highlighted. The renal disease caused by infections with HIV and hepatitis C are covered elsewhere in Part III of this book. Drug dosages, including correction factors for renal dysfunction, are listed in the Appendix to this volume.

Recent developments in infection-associated glomerulonephritis

The epidemiology of infection-associated glomerulonephritis has changed. Classical poststreptococcal glomerulonephritis (PSGN) remains the most common cause of the nephritic syndrome in some communities.[1,2] Staphylococcal infection has, however, become a far more frequent precipitant of glomerulonephritis in developed countries.[3] Infective endocarditis is now the bacterial infection most frequently associated with glomerulonephritis in developed countries, and is predominantly caused by staphylococci introduced via needles or surgery.[3,4] In Europe and North America, hepatitis C is now recognized as a common cause of cryoglobulinemia and mesangiocapillary glomerulonephritis, while on a worldwide scale hepatitis B and malaria persist as dominant causes of the nephrotic syndrome.[5]

As the epidemiology has evolved, the classification of glomerulonephritis resulting from infection has broadened. As the incidence of PSGN in developed countries has declined, infection with an increasing number of other microorganisms has been associated with glomerular disease. The glomerular lesions induced include classical postinfectious "exudative endocapillary" changes, but also mesangioproliferative, mesangiocapillary, crescentic, and membranous lesions. The time-course varies such that clinical glomerulonephritis may become apparent during the acute or chronic infective phase, or during convalescence. Accordingly, the term "postinfectious glomerulonephritis" is best used with specific reference to poststreptococcal disease, while the broader term "infection-associated glomerulonephritis" is the more appropriate nomenclature to apply to the entire spectrum of glomerulonephritis that results from infection.

The importance of host immune status is increasingly recognized as being central to the development of infection-associated glomerulonephritis and to the patient's prognosis. Alcoholism is prevalent throughout the world and is now well recognized as conferring both an increased susceptibility to infection-associated glomerulonephritis and a poor prognosis from this condition.[3,6] Additionally, the immune dysregulation induced by chronic viral infections may enhance patient susceptibility to glomerulonephritis, particularly in the case of infections with hepatitis B, hepatitis C and HIV (see *Brenner and Rector's The Kidney*, Chapter 27).

Progress in molecular biologic technology has facilitated new insights into the pathogenesis of infection-associated glomerulonephritis. Infectious organisms may produce glomerular damage via several mechanisms.

1. direct cytopathic effects, e.g. staphylococcal antigens may induce glomerular damage in the absence of immunoglobulin;[7]
2. host cell-mediated damage due to the presence of the organism within renal cells, with subsequent cell surface antigen expression serving to attract cytotoxic T cells;
3. deposition of circulating immune complexes or cryoglobulins within the glomerulus;
4. formation of in-situ immune complexes to planted infective antigens;
5. induction of autoimmunity via the development of cross-reactive antibodies;
6. indirect effects of infection via cytokine and growth factor induction.[8]

Various infections have been shown to induce glomerular damage via the above-mentioned mechanisms, although one major discrepancy exists. Humans incur infection many times a year during every year of their life, yet only a minority develop clinical nephritis. The reason why only some individuals develop glomerulonephritis in response to infection with particular organisms remains an enigma. Certainly some strains of organism are more nephritogenic than others (e.g. nephritogenic versus non-nephritogenic streptococci). Patient susceptibility factors have also been identified, such as complement deficiency, while others remain unidentified but inferred, such as familial susceptibility to PSGN (see *Brenner and Rector's The Kidney*, Chapter 26). It appears likely that several infection-dependent and host-dependent factors must interact to produce infection-associated glomerulonephritis.

The diagnosis of infection-associated glomerulonephritis should be considered in three broad clinical settings. First, the patient who develops renal dysfunction or an abnormal urinary sediment in the context of an infectious illness may have infection-associated glomerulonephritis. This should be differentiated from renal tract infection, interstitial nephritis (due to infection or therapy), preexisting or concurrent renal disease, and the indirect effects of fever on urinary protein and red cell content (see *Brenner and Rector's The Kidney*, Chapter 26). Second, infection-associated glomerulonephritis remains underdiagnosed as a cause of glomerulonephritis in the general community and should therefore be considered in all patients presenting with glomerular abnormalities.[9] Risk factors for infection with potentially nephritogenic organisms should be sought for on history. Examination for signs of infection should be performed, such as skin rash, needle tracks, and stigmata of endocarditis. Specific serologic investigations, tailored to the epidemiology of infectious disease relevant to the patient, should be undertaken. Percutaneous renal biopsy should be performed in all cases in the absence of significant contraindications.[9] Finally, an infection-related exacerbation should be considered in patients with preexisting glomerulonephritis who develop an unexplained flare of their disease.[10]

The prognosis for recovery from infection-associated glomerulonephritis remains linked to the interaction between host factors and the infecting organism. Recent therapeutic developments have made little impact, with the exceptions of antibiotic prophylaxis for at-risk populations during epidemics of "nephritogenic" streptococcal infection[2] and the use of α-interferon (α-IFN) or lamivudine for the treatment of glomerulonephritis associated with hepatitis B and C viruses. Thus, the prognosis has changed in line with the epidemiology. In areas where infection-associated glomerulonephritis remains primarily streptococcal, the prognosis remains generally favorable, at least in the short to medium term.[1,11] However, in communities where the majority of cases of infection-associated glomerulonephritis are due to staphylococcal infection occurring in alcoholics or intravenous drug abusers, the prognosis is relatively poor for both patient and renal survival.[3,12]

Is resolution of the clinical episode of acute infection-associated glomerulonephritis all that matters? Long-term follow-up studies of survivors of PSGN have revealed clinical (hypertension, proteinuria) and subclinical (reduced glomerular filtration rate, impaired renal functional reserve, fibrosis and glomerulosclerosis on biopsy) renal abnormalities in a significant proportion, and renal failure in a minority.[11,13] Whether these findings are applicable to all forms of infection-associated glomerulonephritis is unknown. Also unknown is whether such asymptomatic abnormalities indicate a significant increase in the lifetime risk of renal failure, cardiovascular disease, or overall mortality for these patients. This information is required in order to provide accurate prognostic information for both the patient and caring physician, and to facilitate the development and utilization of renoprotective strategies during the acute and "recovery" phases of infection-associated glomerulonephritis (see Part XII, Chapter 66 of this book).

Bacterial infections

Streptococcus
Poststreptococcal glomerulonephritis

The management of classical PSGN involves three phases: (1) the prompt treatment of streptococcal infections in the community; (2) the management of the patient with nephritis; and (3) the prevention or detection of strepto-coccal disease and PSGN among the patient's contacts.

Animal data have demonstrated that penicillin given within 3 days of the onset of streptococcal infection is able to prevent the development of nephritis.[14] Although there is no conclusive evidence that antibiotic treatment of pharyngitis or impetigo in humans is effective in preventing the development of PSGN, such treatment seems logical to reduce the streptococcal antigenic load. Additionally, antibiotics may prevent the development of suppurative complications in the individual and hopefully reduce the prevalence of pathogenic streptococci in the community. Thus, as the cost and adverse-effect profile of penicillin is favorable, it should be given to patients with clinically probable and/or culture-positive streptococcal pharyngitis or impetigo. The appropriate dosage for adults is 1.2 million units of benzathine benzylpenicillin as a single intramuscular injection, or 250 mg of phenoxy-methyl penicillin every 6 h orally for 10 days. Children should receive half doses, and erythromycin should be given to individuals who are allergic to penicillin.

The diagnosis of PSGN is made in a patient who has historical and/or laboratory evidence of antecedent streptococcal infection, which was followed by a latent period prior to the development of nephritis. The laboratory finding of decreased C3 is a sensitive but not specific supporting feature. Renal biopsy is often required for the diagnosis in endemic cases, though less so in the epidemic situation, to differentiate PSGN from other causes of the nephritic syndrome (see *Brenner and Rector's The Kidney*, Chapter 26).

Once the diagnosis is made, patient management involves three phases. First, penicillin is given in a bid to eliminate streptococcal antigenemia. Second, features of the nephritic syndrome are treated supportively. If hyper-tension or signs of volume overload are present, sodium intake should be minimized and fluid intake restricted to 1000 mL/day in mild cases and 500 mL/day in moderate to severe cases. In addition, loop diuretics should be used to restore urine volume. Therapy should be guided by the maintenance of strict fluid balance records including daily weights. In cases of severe volume overload with immi-nent or actual hypertensive encephalopathy or pulmonary edema, morphine, oxygen, sedation, ventilation, intra-venous nitrates, and hydralazine may be required. In this setting, urgent hemodialysis including ultrafiltration is often the most effective and physiologic therapeutic maneuver. With good supportive care as above, attention to nutrition, and the treatment of intercurrent iatrogenic infection, an acute mortality of less than 1% can be expected.[11] Resolution is spontaneous and generally complete within several months. Patients with an adult-onset, nephrotic-range or persistent proteinuria, extensive crescent formation, and heavy capillary IgG/C3 deposition on biopsy are an exception to this rule, and commonly exhibit an incomplete renal recovery. A minority will progress to endstage renal failure.[11,13]

Combined immunosuppressive and anticoagulant therapy has been trialed in severe PSGN in children and was not found to be of benefit.[15] Persisting hypertension should be treated, probably with an angiotensin-converting enzyme inhibitor. Acute PSGN recurs only rarely, due to the development of type-specific, long-lasting and protective immunity to streptococcal M protein.

Management of the patient in the long term is the third and most controversial aspect of treatment. Studies of patients up to 20 years after an episode of acute PSGN reveal conflicting results but clear trends in terms of renal outcome. The vast majority of patients recover acutely, but 5–60% will show features of subclinical renal dysfunction (proteinuria or reduced creatinine clearance, fibrosis and glomerulosclerosis on biopsy) or hypertension during the next 10–20 years[11,13] and almost all patients with "resolved" PSGN can be shown to have a reduced renal functional reserve. Asymptomatic abnormalities are a more common sequelae of PSGN in the adult rather than in the child. Whether such abnormalities indicate a significant increase in the lifetime risk of the development of progressive renal failure remains to be determined. At this stage it would seem prudent to monitor all patients who recover from PSGN with annual assessment of blood pressure, 24-h urinary protein excretion, and creatinine clearance. Hypertension should be treated aggressively, and the development of proteinuria or reduced creatinine clearance should prompt the adoption of general measures for the preservation of renal function (see Part XII, Chapter 66 of this book).

Epidemics of PSGN continue to occur in communities that have relatively poor hygiene and overcrowding. The administration of penicillin (2.4 million units i.m. for adults, half dose for children) to all community members during such outbreaks appears to be of benefit.[2]

Other streptococcal infections

Viridans streptococci have classically been implicated as the major cause of subacute bacterial endocarditis, while *Streptococcus faecalis* (enterococcus) is an increasingly recognized cause of acute endocarditis. These and other groups of streptococci have been documented as causes of proliferative glomerulonephritis, both focal and diffuse, in the setting of infectious endocarditis and other visceral infections. Principles of diagnosis and management are similar to those detailed below for staphylococcal endo-carditis. Antibiotic resistance is becoming problematic. The emergence of penicillin-resistant streptococci requires the usage of penicillin plus an aminoglycoside, until bacterial sensitivities are defined. Enterococci are generally penicillin insensitive and require combination therapy with gentamicin and ampicillin, which act synergistically. Vancomycin is indicated if enterococci with high-level penicillin resistance are isolated; however, the develop-ment of vancomycin-resistant enterococci is a major concern.[16] Vigilant monitoring of aminoglycoside and vancomycin levels are required to avoid toxicity.

Staphylococcus
Staphylococcal endocarditis

Staphylococcal endocarditis may occur on normal, damaged, or prosthetic valves on either the left or right side of the heart. Infection of a previously normal tricuspid valve is particularly commonly seen in intravenous drug abusers. The presentation may be acute, particularly in the case of *Staphylococcus aureus* infection, or chronic, as is typically seen with coagulase-negative staphylococcal endocarditis.

Glomerulonephritis occurs in 20–80% of cases of infective endocarditis and may be recognized at any stage of the illness.[4] In cases of infective endocarditis complicated by glomerulonephritis, circulating immune complexes (90% of cases), rheumatoid factors (10–70%), and cryoglobulins (84–95%) are present, while C3 is frequently reduced in serum. No serologic marker has consistently been shown to have predictive value in identifying the presence or absence of glomerulonephritis in patients with endocarditis. Serology may be more useful for monitoring therapy, as the persistence of circulating immune complexes and C3 depletion, despite antibiotic treatment, has been shown to indicate the failure of therapy and a high probability of persistent glomerulo-nephritis.[4] Microbiologic identification, including the determination of antibiotic sensitivities, is crucial in establishing a therapeutic plan. Renal biopsy is also crucial to both confirm the diagnosis and provide prognostic information. Biopsy may reveal either focal or diffuse proliferative changes, often accompanied by an exudate of neutrophils. Crescents are less commonly seen. Immuno-fluorescence reveals granular staining for C3, which is often but not always accompanied by IgG or IgM. Staphylococcal antigens have frequently been reported within damaged glomeruli in the absence of immuno-globulin and rarely in the absence of C3, suggesting that staphylococci may induce either direct or complement-mediated renal injury, independent of immunoglobulin.[7]

Treatment involves the intravenous administration of bactericidal antibiotics at dosages appropriate for renal function (see Appendix). The role of surgery is to restore valve function and remove foci of infection where necessary. This requires an ongoing evaluation of the patient, in consultation with the involved infectious disease and cardiac teams. The persistence of glomerulo-nephritis, despite the apparent resolution of infection, is an additional indication to reassess the affected heart valve with a view to surgery, as the surgical removal of a sterile vegetation has been associated with improvement in renal function.[17] Supportive measures for renal and cardiac function and the optimization of host nutrition and immune status are important components of therapy. Drug and alcohol withdrawal, malnutrition, immuno-suppression, and infection (both preexisting and hospital acquired) are major contributors to the high rates of morbidity (50%) and mortality (11%) seen in patients with infection-associated glomerulonephritis.[3] Additionally, screening tests for concurrent disease, such as HIV and viral hepatitis, should be undertaken to avoid diagnostic confusion and to optimize management.

The likelihood of renal and patient recovery depend on host status, control of infection, and the degree of renal damage as assessed by both clinical and biopsy parameters. Cases in which severe crescentic disease has been present on renal biopsy, or where renal dysfunction has persisted or evolved despite clinical eradication of infection, have prompted the use of immunosuppressive therapy: 35 cases of infection-associated glomerulonephritis (including 11 cases of classical PSGN) treated with immunosuppressants have been reported[3,15,17–24] (Table 15.1). Endocarditis was the most frequently associated infection. One controlled trial of prednisolone, cyclophosphamide, dipyridamole, and azathioprine in children with crescentic PSGN showed no benefit over placebo.[15] All other reports involved uncontrolled therapeutic trials of corticosteroids (100%), cyclophosphamide (44%), azathioprine (4%), heparin (4%), dipyridamole (8%), and plasmapheresis (20%), used either singly or in various combinations and always in conjunction with antibiotics. Indices of renal function improved in 52% of cases. No specific reports of therapy-related morbidity or mortality were made; however, 12% of patients progressed to terminal renal failure and 8% of patients died of "multiple complications" including renal failure. Thus, on the basis of this uncontrolled data, the role of immunosuppressive therapy for infection-associated glomerulonephritis is difficult to determine. Bearing in mind the potential for positive publication bias, these results clearly highlight the need to mount a prospective controlled clinical trial of immunosuppressive therapy for selected cases of infection-associated glomerulonephritis. Without such a trial to examine the safety and efficacy of immunosuppression in this setting, this form of treatment cannot be broadly recommended, except for consideration in cases with severe renal failure unresponsive to documented clearance of infection.[22]

Staphylococcal septicemia

Proliferative glomerulonephritis was documented in 35% of cases of fatal staphylococcal septicemia at autopsy.[25] Treatment is similar to that for infectious endocarditis, in addition to a rigorous search for primary (e.g. skin, bone, joint) and secondary (e.g. heart, lung) sites of infection.

Visceral abscess

Abscesses within abdominal viscera, bone, joint, lung, and other tissues have been associated with infection-asso-ciated glomerulonephritis. *Staphylococcus aureus*, and less commonly other organisms, has been cultured from the abscess fluid. Although blood cultures have frequently been negative in reported cases, bacterial antigens have been identified within glomerular deposits, accompanied by immunoglobulin and complement components. Thus, an immune-mediated infection-associated glomerulo-nephritis occurs that produces a proliferative renal lesion associated with a nephritic clinical presentation, frequently accompanied by severe acute renal failure.[26]

Table 15.1 Immunosuppressive treatment of glomerulonephritis associated with bacterial infection: published reports and trials

Reference	Infection	Patients	Histology	Treatment	Outcome
Montseny et al[3]	Various, unspecified	17	Crescents (12) Endo (5)	Prednisone (17) Cyclophosphamide (8)	5 resolved, 8 CRF, 2 ESRD, 2 deceased
Vanwalleghem et al[23]	S. aureus prosthesis	1	Crescents 27%	Prednisone	Improved
Yamashita et al[24]	S. aureus pneumonia	1	?	Plasmapheresis Prednisone	Improved, late ESRD
Rovzar et al[19]	S. viridans endocarditis	1	Crescents > 50%	Plasmapheresis Prednisone Azathioprine	Improved
McKenzie et al[18]	Endocarditis	1	Crescents 60%	Plasmapheresis Prednisone	Improved
Ayres et al[20]	Streptococcal endocarditis	1	Crescents 80%	Prednisone Cyclophosphamide Heparin Dipyridamole	Improved
McKinsey et al[21]	S. aureus septicemia	1	Some crescents	Prednisone	Improved
Kupari et al[22]	Dental abscess	1	Crescents 80%	Plasmapheresis Prednisone Cyclophosphamide	Resolved
Roy et al[16]	PSGN	5 treated 5 control	Crescents 70% Crescents 65%	Prednisone Azathioprine Cyclophosphamide Dipyridamole	Resolved*
Fairley et al[25]	PSGN	1	Crescents 83%	Plasmapheresis Prednisone Cyclophosphamide Dipyridamole	Resolved

CRF, chronic renal failure; Endo, endoproliferative glomerulonephritis; ESRD, endstage renal disease; PSGN, poststreptococcal glomerulonephritis.
*All patients showed resolution of clinical indicators of renal damage; however, two patients died of causes thought to be unrelated to therapy.[16]

Successful eradication of the antigen, via surgical evacuation and appropriate antibiotic therapy, has resulted in clinical resolution of nephritis in the majority of reported cases.

Shunt nephritis

Ventriculoatrial shunts, inserted for the treatment of hydrocephalus, may rarely become colonized by coagulase-negative staphylococci, or other organisms of low virulence such as *Propionibacterium acnes*.[27] Such colonization is associated with the development of mesangiocapillary glomerulonephritis, manifest by heavy proteinuria, hematuria, and renal impairment. The diagnosis may be confirmed by positive culture of blood, cerebrospinal fluid, or the shunt itself. Removal of the shunt, combined with appropriate antibiotic therapy, leads to an improvement in renal function in the majority of cases. Given the potential morbidity associated with shunt removal and replacement, treatment of the infection with antibiotics alone has been attempted, with clearance of infection and restoration of renal function reported.[28]

Pneumococcus

Pneumococcal pneumonia, endocarditis, and other infections have been associated with glomerulonephritis. Immune-mediated renal disease is induced via mechanisms similar to those described for staphylococcal infection, though pneumococcal capsular antigen has additionally been detected within a cryoprecipitate obtained from one patient with infection-associated glomerulonephritis. Treatment involves the same principles as discussed for staphylococcal infections. Penicillin is the antibiotic of choice, except in areas of drug-resistant pneumococci, where initial treatment with vancomycin plus penicillin is advisable pending antibiotic sensitivity determination.[29]

Gram-negative bacteria

Typhoid fever

Although uncommon in typhoid fever, a diffuse proliferative infection-associated glomerulonephritis may occur and is generally associated with a relatively mild nephritic clinical presentation. Glomerulonephritis must be differentiated from cystitis, pyelonephritis, and acute tubular necrosis, all of which may occur in the context of this illness. In contrast, acute infection with various species of *Salmonella* has been associated with the onset of the nephrotic syndrome in patients with coexistent hepatosplenic schistosomiasis. Nephrosis has been found to resolve on the eradication of salmonella carriage by treatment with cotrimoxazole or ampicillin.[30]

Other bacterial infections

Glomerulonephritis has been reported following enteritis caused by *Yersinia entercolitica*. Pneumonia or lung abscess due to *Klebsiella pneumoniae*, *Haemophilus influenzae*, *Mycoplasma pneumoniae*, *Pseudomonas aeruginosa*, *Chlamydia psittaci*, and *Legionella pneumophila* have rarely been reported to cause glomerulonephritis. *Escherichia coli*, meningococci and other Gram-negative, Gram-positive, and anaerobic bacteria causing septicemia, peritonitis, subphrenic abscess, osteomyelitis, meningitis, and septic abortion have also been linked to infection-associated glomerulonephritis. As a generalization, this rare complication of infection has been found to resolve following the eradication of infection with antibiotic treatment and/or surgery.

Mycobacteria

Leprosy

Approximately 10 million people worldwide have leprosy; of these, 6–8% can be expected to have glomerulonephritis.[31] Most commonly a mesangioproliferative lesion has been found on biopsy, with evidence of IgG and C3 deposition on immunofluorescence microscopy; mycobacterial antigens within glomeruli have been documented. Nephritis is generally clinically mild, with low-grade proteinuria and minimal impairment of renal function. Cases of rapidly progressive glomerulonephritis have been reported, generally in the context of an episode of erythema nodosum leprae, where spontaneous or treatment-associated systemic immune-complex disease occurs, superimposed on the course of previously indolent lepromatous leprosy. Standard treatment for erythema nodosum leprae, consisting of prednisone 1 mg/kg/day orally, was reported to produce a rapid resolution.[31] In general, glomerulonephritis due to leprosy responds clinically to bacteriologic cure, though drug treatment may be complicated by the development erythema nodosum leprae or drug adverse effects.[32] Interstitial nephritis and renal amyloidosis are also documented in patients with leprosy. As opposed to glomerulonephritis, amyloid produces more severe proteinuria and renal impairment and consequently carries a poor prognosis.

Tuberculosis

Tuberculosis may produce direct renal infection and cavitation, or glomerular involvement through the development of amyloidosis, but has only rarely been reported as a cause of glomerulonephritis. Treatment involves antituberculous chemotherapy (see Part VI).

Spirochetes

Syphilis

The prevalence of syphilis is increasing worldwide. As congenital, secondary, and tertiary syphilis have been associated with various forms of glomerulonephritis, renal gumma formation, and amyloidosis, the incidence of renal presentations of syphilis may also be anticipated to rise. Congenital syphilis may result in membranous nephropathy. Acquired secondary and tertiary syphilis in adults may also produce a nephrotic presentation in association with minimal change or membranous features on biopsy. A nephritic presentation may also occur, with typical proliferative glomerular changes of infection-associated glomerulonephritis seen on biopsy. Granular deposition of IgG and C3 is generally demonstrable by immunofluorescence, suggesting an immune-complex basis. Treatment of syphilis with penicillin, 2.4 million units by weekly intramuscular injection for 3 weeks, has led to the resolution of proteinuria in the majority of cases.[33]

Leptospirosis

Leptospirosis has been associated with a mesangioproliferative glomerulonephritis, but far more commonly induces acute interstitial nephritis or acute tubular necrosis in the setting of Weil syndrome. Regardless of the renal lesion produced, treatment involves intensive supportive care and antibiotic treatment, which is of proven benefit if started within the first 5 days of infection. Doxycycline 200 mg/day orally is effective in mild cases. Penicillin, 1.5 million units every 6 h for 7 days, is preferred for severe disease. Exchange transfusion may have a role in reducing hyperbilirubinemia, which may contribute to the renal toxicity in Weil syndrome. The renal lesion is entirely reversible upon resolution of the infection.[34]

Viral infections

Viruses in general

Viral infection is almost ubiquitous in humans. However, clinically relevant infection-associated glomerulonephritis due to viral infection is rare. Circulating immune complexes may be found in the serum of patients at some stage in the course of nearly all acute viral infections. Indeed, glomerulonephritis in the setting of viral infection is associated with the glomerular deposition of immune complexes. This is accompanied by endothelial and/or mesangial cell proliferation and rarely by extracapillary crescent formation. Why only a minority of people develop glomerulonephritis upon infection with virus is unknown. The probable explanation is that multiple virus-dependent factors (nephritogenicity, virulence, capacity for immunomodulation and chronicity) and host-dependent factors (immune competence, cytokine response, glomerular response) interact to determine the glomerular consequences of infection.[35] The management of acute virus-associated glomerulonephritis is directed at clearance of the viral infection, which generally occurs spontaneously, and the provision of supportive care when required. The management of chronic virus-associated glomerulonephritis additionally involves the use of specific antiviral or immunomodulatory therapies, discussed later in the case of hepatitis B virus and in Chapter 27 for hepatitis C virus and HIV.

Viral hepatitis
Hepatitis B

Hepatitis B virus (HBV) has been linked with many glomerular pathologies. In patients with membranous, mesangiocapillary, mesangioproliferative, and polyarteritis nodosa-associated glomerulonephritis, the repeated demonstration of viral antigens (HBsAg, HBcAg, and HBeAg) and specific antibody within glomerular deposits, and the clearly increased incidence of these types of glomerulonephritis in HBsAg-positive patients, provides strong evidence for the etiologic role of HBV.[36] Other forms of glomerulonephritis, including focal glomerulosclerosis, minimal change disease, and lupus nephropathy, have been inconclusively linked to HBV infection.[37]

The vast majority of cases of HBV-associated glomerulonephritis are seen in chronic carriers (HBsAg positive). Membranous nephropathy is the commonest form and is seen predominantly in areas where HBV infection is endemic and infection is acquired during infancy. Males are more commonly affected, a past history of hepatitis is rare, and physical and biochemical evidence of liver disease is generally lacking. Nephrotic syndrome is the most common manifestation of renal involvement and this may remit spontaneously in 30–60% of cases in children or with seroconversion to anti-HBe antibody-positive status. Progression to renal failure is uncommon in children, but has been reported to occur in 29% of adults followed for 5 years.[36,37]

The management of HBV-associated membranous nephropathy involves both supportive care and selective use of antiviral agents. Symptomatic management of features of the nephrotic syndrome, treatment of hypertension, and long-term follow-up should be employed in all cases. Specific therapy for membranous nephropathy related to HBV infection has been attempted using recombinant human α-IFN.[36–41] Treatment of Taiwanese children in an open controlled trial resulted in remission of proteinuria in 100% of children receiving 5–8 million units of α-IFN daily for 3 months compared with 50% of controls.[38] However, seroconversion was incomplete and adverse effects, particularly psychiatric, were common. The treatment of adults from areas of endemic HBV

appears to be relatively unrewarding.[37] In contrast, case reports and one uncontrolled trial from nonendemic areas have described high response rates to α-IFN, in terms of loss of HBV DNA and antigens from the circulation, improvement in indices of liver damage, and reduction in proteinuria and symptoms of the nephrotic syndrome.[39–41] The long-term impacts on renal function and patient morbidity in this setting appear beneficial. A paper from the National Institutes of Health that reported the follow-up (for up to 7 years) of all patients with HBV-associated membranous nephropathy (11) treated with α-IFN demonstrated sustained reductions in proteinuria and stabilization of renal function in 73% of cases. Improvement was associated with the clearance of HBV DNA from serum and an improvement in liver histology and function.[41] Thus, given the progressive nature of HBV-associated membranous nephropathy in adults, a trial of therapy with α-IFN appears justified. Dosage and duration are arbitrary: 5 million units three times weekly for 4 months appears to be appropriate.[41] The dosage should be halved if serious or intolerable adverse effects occur, as was the case in 53% of patients reported by Conjeevaram et al.[41] Progress should be assessed by the evaluation of serologic markers of viral persistence, including HBV DNA and HBsAg/Ab, and by parameters of renal function, including 24-h protein excretion and creatinine clearance.

Immunosuppressive treatment with steroids has been trialed in HBV-related membranous nephropathy.[36] Treatment was associated with serologic evidence of enhanced viral replication. A follow-up biopsy performed on one patient demonstrated histologic progression and the presence of virus-like particles within glomeruli. Thus, steroids should be avoided for patients with membranous nephropathy who are HBsAg seropositive.

Mesangioproliferative and mesangiocapillary glomerulonephritis are less common forms of HBV-associated glomerulonephritis. The clinical presentation and clinical courses are similar to those of the primary diseases and the risk of progression to renal failure is high. As in the case of HBV-associated membranous nephropathy, antiviral therapy with α-IFN has been reported to induce renal remission in association with seroconversion (loss of HBsAg and HBeAg and appearance of anti-HBe).[41–43] Given the variable course of these diseases and the cost, adverse effects, and lack of controlled trial evidence, the use of interferon therapy should probably be limited to those with progressive disease and/or progressive liver disease. The use of lamivudine and other newer antiviral agents has not been reported. The use of immunosuppressant drugs has not been studied and should probably be avoided given the high risk of promoting viral replication.[36]

HBV-related polyarteritis is an uncommon condition seen in areas where HBV infection occurs via blood transfusion, needle sharing, or sexual transmission and is therefore largely a disease of young adults. A mild and often asymptomatic hepatitis is followed within 6 months by a systemic vasculitis producing fever, arthralgias, and rash. Renal damage may present with hypertension, nephritic syndrome, or renal failure, and involvement of the myocardium, gut, lung, and nervous system may also be seen in a clinical presentation similar to classical polyarteritis nodosa. Patients typically have a mild elevation of liver enzymes, are seropositive for HBs and HBe antigens, and may have IgM anti-HBs antibodies in serum, consistent with recent infection. Antineutrophil cytoplasmic antibody titers are typically negative. The diagnosis may be established by renal biopsy or by angiography revealing medium-calibre vessel changes including aneurysms. Controlled data on the treatment of this rare condition are absent; however, successful combination therapy with lamivudine, steroids, cyclophosphamide, and plasma exchange has been reported.[44,45]

Clearance of virus from the circulation with α-IFN therapy followed by orthotopic liver transplantation may lead to resolution of glomerular disease. Resolution of mesangiocapillary glomerulonephritis has been reported following liver transplantation, despite the persistence of HBsAg positivity in one case.[46] In contrast, the use of α-IFN in patients with functioning kidney and liver transplants has been associated with an increase in the incidence of rejection, and therefore should not be used in these patients.[47]

Other hepatitis viruses

Hepatitis A has been reported to cause immune-complex mesangioproliferative glomerulonephritis. The management of this uncommon complication of hepatitis A virus infection is supportive, and nephritis resolves with recovery from the infection. Glomerulonephritis associated with hepatitis C virus is discussed later in Part III of this book (see Part II Chapter 27).

Hantaan virus

Hantaan and related viruses induce an illness known as "nephropathia epidemica" or "haemorrhagic fever with renal syndrome," which is endemic in areas of Southeast Asia and southern Europe and appears in epidemics worldwide.[48] Spread by the inhalation of aerosolized virus containing particles formed from the excreta of infected mice, these viruses induce a spectrum of disease that ranges from a mild febrile illness to a life-threatening disorder. Severe disease is characterized by several phases. Initially high fever and myalgias dominate, while facial and truncal flushing and petechiae develop in association with thrombocytopenia. Fever suddenly subsides after several days, but profound hypotension develops associated with oliguric acute renal failure. Systemic hypotension, derangements of intrarenal vasomotor tone, coagulation, and associated interstitial nephritis contribute to renal injury. Mesangiocapillary glomerulonephritis has been reported; however, glomerular involvement is generally minor.

The diagnosis is confirmed by a rise in titer of specific antibody to Hantaan virus between serum samples taken 1 week apart. Leptospirosis and scrub typhus should be excluded, also on serologic grounds, as these agents may produce a similar illness but are amenable to treatment with tetracyclines. Treatment of hemorrhagic fever with renal syndrome is supportive only.[48] A specific vaccine is currently under trial in Korea.

Herpes-type viruses

Generally mild and spontaneously resolving acute nephritis has been reported as a rare complication of various infections, including infectious mononucleosis, pneumonitis, encephalitis, and congenital infection with Epstein–Barr virus, cytomegalovirus, varicella, and herpes simplex virus. Specific antiviral therapy is indicated for critical organ infection rather than for glomerulonephritis, which tends to resolve on control of the infection.

Other viruses

Smith et al[49] reported a 3.8% incidence of glomerulonephritis following nonstreptococcal upper respiratory tract infection in American army recruits. Presumably, the majority of these infections were viral in etiology. Recovery was spontaneous and clinically complete (except in one patient with a past history of PSGN) but took up to 12 months in some cases. In nephrologic practice, virus-associated glomerulonephritis is a far less frequently encountered cause of glomerulonephritis than these figures would indicate. This is probably due to underdetection. Given the apparently benign clinical course of infection-associated glomerulonephritis following "viral" upper respiratory tract infection, biopsy does not appear to be indicated except in cases of diagnostic uncertainty. However, the degree of renal functional impairment, as documented above, does indicate a need for follow-up of blood pressure and renal function in such patients. Whether the long-term prognosis of patients with virus-associated glomerulonephritis is similar to that for patients with PSGN is unknown.

Human parvovirus B19 has recently been identified as a cause of collapsing glomerulopathy, a variant of focal and segmental glomerulosclerosis. This virus is common and typically causes a mild nonspecific illness, but has been associated with red cell aplasia in a minority of patients. Parvovirus B19 DNA was identified within glomeruli in the majority of cases of supposedly idiopathic collapsing glomerulopathy in one study.[50] HIV infection has also been associated with collapsing glomerulopathy. The clinical presentation is similar to primary focal and segmental glomerulosclerosis and progression to renal failure is frequent.

Cases of glomerulonephritis have been reported in association with mumps, measles, and enteroviral infections (Coxsackie B5 virus and echovirus). Generally, these have produced only a mild nephritic illness that resolved spontaneously.

Rickettsial infections

Rocky Mountain spotted fever

Rocky Mountain spotted fever, in severe cases, results in a multiorgan vasculitis involving the central nervous system, myocardium, and kidney. Renal involvement is predominantly tubulointerstitial, as prerenal factors (vasculitis and myocardial depression) combine with a perivascular interstitial nephritis to produce acute renal failure. Glomerular involvement has been described but is overshadowed by the interstitial lesions. One case of infection-associated glomerulonephritis has been reported in which a nephritic illness, associated with typical postinfectious changes on biopsy, occurred 2 weeks after an acute episode of Rocky Mountain spotted fever. Spontaneous resolution occurred.[51]

Q fever

Immune complex mesangioproliferative glomerulonephritis has been reported in cases of both endocarditis and sepsis due to *Coxiella burnetii*. Antiphospholipid and anti-DNA autoantibodies have been detected in the sera of these patients, suggesting that the development of antibodies to *Coxiella* antigens cross-reactive to host antigens may have a role in the pathogenesis of Q fever. The diagnosis is based on clinical features and confirmed by serology. Treatment is with doxycycline 100 mg/day orally for 1 week for sepsis, or longer for endocarditis, where surgical removal of the vegetation, with or without valve replacement, is often required. Renal manifestations have been reported to resolve with cure of the infection.[52]

Scrub typhus

Rickettsia tsutsugamushi, like other rickettsias, has a predilection for the endothelium. Glomerulonephritis has been reported as a rare sequelae of scrub typhus. The clinical illness produced is similar to that seen in infections with leptospirosis and Hantaan virus, and should be distinguished on epidemiologic and serologic grounds. Treatment with doxycycline 100 mg/day orally for 1 week is beneficial at any stage of the illness.

Fungal infections

Mucocutaneous candidiasis has been reported as a cause of immune complex-mediated mesangiocapillary glomerulonephritis. Proteinuria and renal function improved on clearance of the infection.[53]

Clinical renal involvement may occur in disseminated histoplasmosis. Proliferative glomerulonephritis, associated with the presence of circulating immune complexes, has been reported in a case of acute primary disseminated histoplasmosis. Renal manifestations resolved following spontaneous recovery from the infection.[54] However, disseminated infection in immunocompromised or nonresolving patients does require therapy with antifungal agents.

Parasitic infections

Malaria

Falciparum malaria

Transient glomerulonephritis may be a common sequelae of infection with *Plasmodium falciparum*, but it is generally mild and undetected. Glomerulonephritis has been demonstrated in 18% of patients with fatal falciparum malaria.[55] Renal failure is a significant contributor to the mortality of severe falciparum infection; however, acute renal failure in this setting is usually due to acute tubular necrosis, which results from shock, renal vasoconstriction, intravascular coagulation, direct tubular toxicity, and hyperbilirubinemia.[8] Treatment with intravenous quinine and supportive care including hemodialysis is beneficial. Exchange transfusion, designed to reduce parasite load and hyperbilirubinemia, has been reported to be beneficial in selected situations. Elimination of the parasite is accompanied by the resolution of renal abnormalities in surviving patients.[56]

Quartan malaria

The incidence of childhood nephrotic syndrome is 20–60 times more frequent in areas where infection with *P. malariae* is endemic, in comparison with nonendemic areas. A small percentage of patients, mainly children, with quartan malaria develop an immune complex glomerulonephritis. Histologically, this is characterized initially by glomerular capillary wall thickening, due to subendothelial immune complex deposition, which evolves to produce capillary collapse and diffuse mesangial sclerosis. The characteristic clinical presentation is with the nephrotic syndrome. Disease progression is the rule, with the development of hypertension and progressive renal failure leading to death in 3–5 years. Neither antimalarial treatment nor immunosuppressive therapies have been shown to improve the renal outcome in this condition. Thus the main therapeutic hope for the future is prevention, either through the development of a vaccine for *P. malariae* or by reducing the prevalence of the organism.[5]

Schistosomiasis

Chronic hepatosplenic schistosomiasis due to infestation with *Schistosoma haematobium* (endemic in Africa and the Middle East), *S. mansoni* (Africa, South America, and the Middle East), and *S. japonicum* (Middle East and Asia) has been associated with immune complex glomerulonephritis.[57] Glomerulopathy has rarely been reported in the setting of infestation with *S. japonicum* and an etiologic role has been disputed.

Hepatosplenic schistosomiasis due to *S. haematobium* has been associated with two cases of mesangiocapillary glomerulonephritis and one of minimal change disease, all of which responded clinically to antischistosomal treatment.[58,59] However, the vast majority of cases of renal disease seen in association with *S. haematobium* are due to coinfection with *Salmonella* species, as indicated by the presence of fever and isolation of the organism from blood cultures. In this setting, proteinuria and renal impairment have been shown to respond to treatment of the salmonellosis, with or without antischistosomal treatment.[30] Antischistosomal treatment is indicated because persistence of the schistosomiasis renders these patients susceptible to recurrences of renal disease on reexposure to salmonella.

In contrast, glomerular involvement in *S. mansoni* infection is relatively common. Though rarely reported in the earlier hepatointestinal phase, glomerulopathy is seen in 12–15% of patients who develop hepatosplenic disease. Glomerulonephritis is due to immune complex disease. A mesangioproliferative or mesangiocapillary lesion may be seen on biopsy and may evolve to focal glomerulo-sclerosis. Patients are frequently nephrotic. Hypertension and progressive renal failure may develop. Treatment with prednisone, with or without cyclophosphamide, has induced occasional remissions, whereas treatment with antischistosomal drugs has been unsuccessful in altering the course of the renal disease. Amyloidosis may also occur as a complication of chronic schistosomiasis.[57]

Other parasites

Toxoplasmosis has rarely been associated with glomerulonephritis. Whether nephritis will be increasingly recognized in the setting of toxoplasmosis associated with AIDS and other immunocompromised states remains to be seen.

Visceral leishmaniasis has been reported in association with a mild nephritic illness due to mesangioproliferative glomerulonephritis; however, this occurrence is rare and a direct causal link has not been firmly established.

Filariasis due to *Wuchereria bancrofti* has been shown to produce glomerulonephritis with antigen and specific antibody demonstrable within glomeruli. Filariasis caused by *Onchocerca volvulus* and *Loa loa* has also been linked to various types of glomerulonephritis, largely by way of immune complex deposition. Additionally, microfilariae have been demonstrated within glomerular capillaries in association with an eosinophilic tubulointerstitial nephritis. The presentation of acute filarial nephropathy is generally nephritic and is responsive to treatment with diethylcarbamazine. Chronic filarial nephropathy more commonly produces a nephrotic presentation and responds poorly to antifilarial drugs.[5]

Summary and future directions

Infection with various microbes can cause glomerulonephritis in humans. The percentage of infectious illnesses that result in a clinically apparent episode of infection-associated glomerulonephritis is, however, very small. While the underdiagnosis of infection-associated glomerulonephritis[9] may account for a fraction of this discrepancy, it is clear that a complex interaction of host- and microbe-related factors are involved in determining whether or not an individual develops glomerulonephritis as a consequence of infection with a particular organism. Such factors remain to be elucidated.

Fortunately the vast majority of cases of infection-associated glomerulonephritis resolve following either spontaneous or treatment-induced clearance of the underlying infection. A few patients incur progressive renal disease. In some cases this is caused by a failure of, or a delay in, the clearance of infection. In others, progression may occur despite microbiologic cure. The mechanisms behind progressive disease also remain unclear. As a consequence, therapeutic approaches have been limited to the provision of supportive care and the use of un-controlled empirical trials of therapy, based on regimens that have been successful in the treatment of other forms of glomerulonephritis. Advances in specific therapy for infection-associated glomerulonephritis will require a better understanding of the pathogenetic mechanisms involved. In the interim, if empirical therapies are to be used then surely it is time for a coordinated effort in mounting a controlled trial of, for example, immunosuppression in infection-associated glomerulonephritis.

Little is known of the long-term consequences of infection-associated glomerulonephritis, with the exception of the follow-up studies of patients after PSGN by Baldwin[13] and Rodriguez-Iturbe[11] and more recently of patients with infection-associated glomerulonephritis of various etiologies by Montseny et al.[3] The diligent work of these teams has clearly indicated that a significant proportion of patients manifest hypertension, proteinuria, and progressive renal failure as long-term sequelae of infection-associated glomerulonephritis. The risk of development of these late sequelae for patients with mild or subclinical infection-associated glomerulonephritis is unknown. What is clear is that patients with infection-associated glomerulonephritis should be followed long term in order to screen for the development of late sequelae amenable to management by conventional renoprotective measures (see Part XII, Chapter 66 of this book). Whether treatment following the acute episode of infection-associated glomerulonephritis with, for example, angiotensin-converting enzyme inhibitors would retard the development of late sequelae is unknown.

In conclusion, several general principles are applicable to the treatment of infection-associated glomerulonephritis, and these are depicted as a treatment algorithm in Fig. 15.1. First, prevention should be attempted. This can be accomplished by reducing the prevalence of infection with nephritogenic organisms in the community, as has been partially achieved in the case of PSGN in developed countries. Prevention remains a difficult issue for many other infections such as neonatal hepatitis B and malaria. Attention to host-dependent risk factors for the development of infection-associated glomerulonephritis, such as alcoholism and intravenous drug abuse, are difficult but potentially modifiable problems of public health. Second, the treatment of cases of infection-associated glomerulonephritis should involve the identification and elimination of the infecting organism, combined with supportive care of the patient. Contacts who may be at risk of infection with the same organism should be identified, screened, and given prophylactic treatment if indicated. Long-term follow-up of the patient is indicated. Finally, coordinated investigation into the pathogenesis, natural history, and therapy of this heterogeneous group of disorders is to be supported.

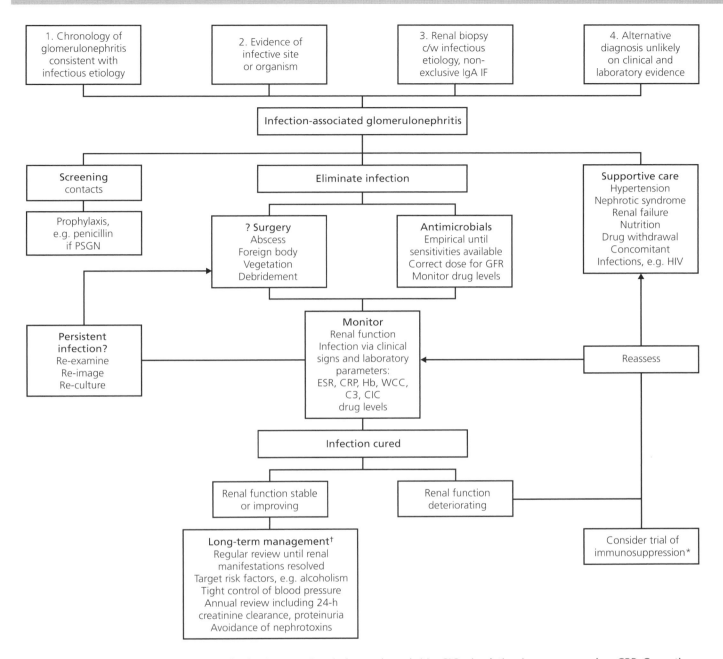

Figure 15.1 Diagnosis and mangement of infection-associated glomerulonephritis. CIC, circulating immune complex; CRP, C-reactive protein; ESR, erythrocyte sedimentation rate; GFR, glomerular filtration rate; Hb, hemoglobin; HIV, human immunodeficiency virus; PSGN, poststreptococcal glomerulonephritis; WCC, white cell count. *Anecdotal evidence only, see text. †See Part XII of this book.

References

1. Tapaneya-Olarn W, Osatakul S, Chatasingh S, et al: Acute glomerulonephritis in children: a prospective study. J Med Assoc Thai 1989;72(Suppl 1):35.
2. Streeton CL, Hanna JN, Messer RD, et al: An epidemic of acute post-streptococcal glomerulonephritis among aboriginal children. J Paediatr Child Health 1995;31:245.
3. Montseny J, Meyrier A, Kleinkeecht D, et al: The current spectrum of infectious glomerulonephritis. Medicine 1995;74:63.
4. Neugarten J, Baldwin DS: Glomerulonephritis in bacterial endocarditis. Am J Med 1984;77:297.
5. Chugh KS, Sakhuja V: Glomerular diseases in the tropics. Am J Nephrol 1990;10:437.
6. Keller CK, Andrassy K, Waldherr R, et al: Postinfectious glomerulonephritis: is there a link to alcoholism? Q J Med 1994;87:97.
7. Angangco R, Thiru S, Oliveira DBG: Pauci-immune glomerulonephritis associated with bacterial infection. Nephrol Dial Transplant 1993;8:754.
8. Eiam-Ong S, Sitprija V: Falciparum malaria and the kidney: a model of inflammation. Am J Kidney Dis 1998;32:361–375.
9. Jones JM, Davison AM: Persistent infection as a cause of renal disease in patients submitted to renal biopsy: a report from the Glomerulonephritis Registry of the United Kingdom MRC. Q J Med 1986;58:123.
10. Rees AJ, Lockwood CM, Peters DK: Enhanced allergic tissue injury in Goodpasture's syndrome by intercurrent bacterial infection. Br Med J 1977;2:723.
11. Rodriguez-Iturbe B: Epidemic poststreptococcal glomerulonephritis. Kidney Int 1984;25:129.

12. Zent R, Van Zyl Smit R, Duffield M, et al: Crescentic nephritis at Groote Schuur Hospital, Cape Town, South Africa: not a benign disease. Clin Nephrol 1994;42:22.

13. Baldwin DS: Post-streptococcal glomerulonephritis: a progressive disease? Am J Med 1977;62:1.

14. Bergholm AM, Holm SE: Effect of early penicillin treatment on the development of experimental poststreptococcal glomerulonephritis. Acta Pathol Microbiol Immunol Scand 1983;91:271.

15. Roy S III, Murphy WM, Arant BS Jr: Poststreptococcal crescenteric glomerulonephritis in children: comparison of quintuple therapy versus supportive care. J Pediatr 1981;98:403.

16. Frieden TR, Munsiff SS, Low DE, et al: Emergence of vancomycin-resistant enterococci in New York city. Lancet 1993;342:76.

17. McKenzie PE, Taylor AE, Woodroffe AJ, et al: Plasmapheresis in glomerulonephritis. Clin Nephrol 1979;12:97.

18. Rovzar MA, Logan JL, Ogden DA, et al: Immunosuppressive therapy and plasmapheresis in rapidly progressive glomerulonephritis associated with bacterial endocarditis. Am J Kidney Dis 1986;7:428.

19. Ayres BF, Bastian PD, Haines D, et al: Renal and cardiac complications of drug abuse. Med J Aust 1976;2:489.

20. McKinsey DS, McMurray TI, Flynn JM: Immune complex glomerulonephritis associated with *Staphylococcus aureus* bacteremia: response to corticosteroid therapy. Rev Infect Dis 1990;12:125.

21. Kupari M, Teerenhovi L: Plasma exchanges in the treatment of rapidly progressive glomerulonephritis associated with chronic dental infection. Acta Med Scand 1981;210:511.

22. Vanwalleghem J, Maes B, Van Damme B, Verberckmoes R, Vanrenterghem Y: Steroids for deep-infection-associated glomerulonephritis: a two-edged sword. Nephrol Dial Transplant 1998;13:773–775.

23. Yamashita Y, Tanase T, Terada Y, et al: Glomerulonephritis after methicillin-resistant *Staphylococcus aureus* infection resulting in end-stage renal failure. Intern Med 2001;40:424–427.

24. Fairley C, Mathews DC, Becker GJ: Rapid development of diffuse crescents in post-streptococcal glomerulonephritis. Clin Nephrol 1987;28:256–260.

25. Powell DEB: Non-suppurative lesions in staphylococcal septicaemia. J Pathol Bacteriol 1961;82:141.

26. Beaufils M, Morel-Maroger L, Sraer JD, et al: Acute renal failure of glomerular origin during visceral abscesses. N Engl J Med 1976;295:185.

27. Beeler BA, Crowder JG, Smith JW: *Propionibacterium acnes*: pathogen in central nervous system shunt infection. Report of three cases including immune complex glomerulonephritis. Am J Med 1976;61:935.

28. Saiz Garcia F, Zubimendi Herranz A, Silva Gonzalez C: Nephritis caused by a shunt. Cure of the nephropathy without the need of a surgical replacement of the ventriculo-atrial valve. Rev Clin Esp 1982;164:123.

29. Tomasz A: The pneumococcus at the gates. N Engl J Med 1995;333:514.

30. Abdul-Fattah MM, Yossef SM, Ebraheem ME, et al: Schistosomal glomerulopathy: a putative role for commonly associated *Salmonella* infection. J Egypt Soc Parasitol 1995;25:165.

31. Ahsan BF, Wheeler D, Palmer BF: Leprosy-associated renal disease: case report and review of the literature. J Am Soc Nephrol 1995;5:1546.

32. Jakeman P: Risk of relapse in multibacillary leprosy. Lancet 1995;345:4.

33. Hunte W, Al-Ghraoui F, Cohen R: Secondary syphilis and the nephrotic syndrome. J Am Soc Nephrol 1993;3:1351.

34. Kim MJ: Recent advances in leptospirosis research based on molecular biology. Infection 1994;26:109.

35. Glassock RJ: Immune complex-induced glomerular injury in viral diseases: an overview. Kidney Int 1991;40(Suppl 35):S5.

36. Lai KN, Mac-Moune F: Clinical features and the natural course of hepatitis B related glomerulopathy in adults. Kidney Int 1991;40(Suppl 35):S40–S45.

37. Lai KN, Li PKT, Lui SF, et al: Membranous nephropathy related to hepatitis B virus in adults. N Engl J Med 1991;324:1457.

38. Lai CL, Lok AS, Lin HJ, et al: Placebo-controlled trial of recombinant alpha2-interferon in chinese HbsAg carrier children. Lancet 1987;ii:877–880.

39. Shapiro RJ, Steinbrecher UP, Magil A: Remission of nephrotic syndrome of HBV-associated membranous glomerulopathy following treatment with interferon. Am J Nephrol 1995;15:343.

40. Lisker-Melman M, Webb D, Di Bisceglie AM: Glomerulonephritis caused by chronic hepatitis B virus infection: treatment with recombinant human alpha-interferon. Ann Intern Med 1989;111:479.

41. Conjeevaram HS, Hoofnagle JH, Austin HA, et al: Long-term outcome of hepatitis B virus-related glomerulonephritis after therapy with interferon alfa. Gastroenterology 1995;109:540.

42. Abbas NA, Pitt MA, Green AT, Solomon LR: Successful treatment of hepatitis B virus (HBV)-associated membranoproliferative glomerulonephritis (MPGN) with alpha interferon. Nephrol Dial Transplant 1999;14:1272–1275.

43. Dhiman RK, Kohli HS, Das G, Joshi K, Chawla Y, Sakhuja V: Remission of HBV-related mesangioproliferative glomerulonephritis after interferon therapy. Nephrol Dial Transplant 1999;14:176–178.

44. Erhardt A, Sagir A, Guillevin L, Neuen-Jacob E, Haussinger D: Successful treatment of hepatitis B virus associated polyarteritis nodosa with a combination of prednisolone, alpha-interferon and lamivudine. J Hepatol 2000;33:677–683.

45. Gupta S, Piraka C, Jaffe M: Lamivudine in the treatment of polyarteritis nodosa associated with acute hepatitis B. N Engl J Med 2001;344:1645–1646.

46. Quan A, Portale A, Foster S, et al: Resolution of hepatitis B virus-related membranoproliferative glomerulonephritis after orthotopic liver transplantation. Pediatr Nephrol 1995;9:599.

47. Feray C, Samuel C, Gigou M, et al: An open trial of interferon alpha recombinant for hepatitis C after liver transplantation: anti-viral effects and risk of rejection. Hepatology 1995;22:1084.

48. Bruno P, Hassell LH, Brown J, Tanner W, Lau A: The protean manifestations of haemorrhagic fever with renal syndrome. A retrospective view of 26 cases from Korea. Ann Intern Med 1990;113:385–391.

49. Smith MC, Cooke JH, Zimmerman DM, et al: Asymptomatic glomerulonephritis after non-streptococcal upper respiratory infections. Ann Intern Med 1979;91:697.

50. Moudgil A, Nast CC, Bagga A, et al: Association of parvovirus B19 infection with idiopathic collapsing glomerulopathy. Kidney Int 2001;59:2126–2133.

51. Quigg RJ, Gaines R, Wakely PE Jr, et al: Acute glomerulonephritis in a patient with Rocky Mountain spotted fever. Am J Kidney Dis 1991;17:339.

52. Tolosa-Vilella C, Rodriguez-Jornet A, Font-Rocabanyera A, et al: Mesangioproliferative glomerulonephritis and antibodies to phospholipids in a patient with acute Q fever: a case report. Clin Infect Dis 1995;21:196.

53. Chesney RW, O'Regan S, Guyda HJ, et al: *Candida* endocrinopathy syndrome with membranoproliferative glomerulonephritis: demonstration of glomerular *Candida* antigen. Clin Nephrol 1976;5:232.

54. Bullock WE, Artz RP, Bhathena D, et al: Histoplasmosis. Association with circulating immune complexes, eosinophilia, and mesangiopathic glomerulonephritis. Arch Intern Med 1979;139:700.

55. Spitz S: The pathology of acute falciparum malaria. Milit Surg 1946;99:555.

56. Sitprija V: Nephropathy in falciparum malaria. Kidney Int 1988;34:867.

57. Barsoum R: Schistosomal glomerulopathies. Kidney Int 1993;44:1.

58. Greenham R, Cameron AH: *Schistosoma haematobium* and the nephrotic syndrome. Trans R Soc Trop Med Hyg 1980;74:609.

59. Turner I, Ibels LS, Alexander JH, et al: Minimal change glomerulonephritis associated with *Schistosoma hematobium* infection: resolution with praziquantel treatment. Aust NZ J Med 1987;17:596.

Cryoglobulinemia

Giuseppe D'Amico and Alessandro Fornasieri

Clinical features, pathology, and pathophysiology
Treatment
- Antiviral therapy of HCV infection
- Antiviral therapy in HCV infection associated with mixed cryoglobulinemia
- Treatment of renal complications associated with mixed cryoglobulinemia and HCV infection
    - Treatment of the chronic stages of the renal disease
    - Therapy of acute exacerbations of cryoglobulinemic glomerulonephritis and renal vasculitis
- Treatment of renal complications associated with mixed cryoglobulinemia in the absence of HCV infection

Clinical features, pathology, and pathophysiology

Cryoglobulinemia is a pathologic condition in which the blood contains immunoglobulins that precipitate reversibly in the cold. Two types of mixed cryoglobulinemia (MC), which are composed of at least two immunoglobulins, have been described. In both types, a polyclonal IgG is bound to another immunoglobulin that is an antiglobulin (i.e. it acts as an anti-IgG rheumatoid factor). The important difference between these two types of MC is that in type II MC the antiglobulin component, which is usually of the IgM class, is monoclonal, while in type III MC it is polyclonal.

It has been demonstrated only recently that hepatitis C virus (HCV) infection can be associated with the clinical syndrome, which was first described by Meltzer[1] in 1966 and which is characterized by purpura, weakness, arthralgia, and, in some cases, glomerular lesions. This had previously been defined as "essential" mixed cryoglobulinemia, since underlying or associated disease had not been found. Probably through the infection of B lymphocytes, HCV induces their dysregulation toward the production of polyclonal (type III MC) or monoclonal (type II MC) rheumatoid factors with cryoprecipitable properties. It has been found that a peculiar type of membranoproliferative glomerulonephritis called "cryoglobulinemic glomerulonephritis" can occur only when type II MC with an IgMκ monoclonal rheumatoid factor is induced by HCV infection. This is characterized by intense monocyte infiltration and subendothelial or interluminal deposition of the cryoglobulins (reviewed in references 2 and 3).

An acute nephritic syndrome, with usually macroscopic hematuria, severe proteinuria, hypertension, and a sudden increase in blood urea nitrogen, is present at the onset of the renal disease in approximately 25% of patients, sometimes complicated by acute oliguric renal failure. Renal and extrarenal vasculitis are frequently present. Isolated proteinuria with microscopic hematuria is the most frequent presenting renal syndrome and is sometimes associated with signs of moderate chronic renal insufficiency or, less frequently, proteinuria in the nephrotic range. The corresponding histologic picture is of a membranoproliferative glomerulonephritis with less conspicuous intraluminal deposits and monocyte infiltration, sometimes with a lobular pattern, while immunofluorescence shows subendothelial deposits of IgM, IgG, and C3, sometimes segmental.

A minority of patients present with isolated urinary abnormalities and may have a rather nonspecific picture of mild segmental mesangial proliferation, without significant monocyte infiltration and capillary wall alterations. Arterial hypertension is frequently found at the time of the apparent onset of renal disease, even in patients without nephritic syndrome.

In nearly one-third of patients, even in those who present with an acute nephritis syndrome or severe nephrotic syndrome, remission of renal symptoms occurs. Remission after an acute nephritic syndrome may occur even before any treatment is started. In one-third of patients, the renal disease has a rather indolent course and, despite the persistence of urinary abnormalities, does not progress to renal failure for several years. In as many as 20% of patients, reversible clinical exacerbations such as nephritic syndrome or nephrotic syndrome occur during the course of the disease and are sometimes associated with flare-ups of systemic signs of the disease.

If a moderate degree of renal insufficiency is not already present at clinical onset, it is frequently found during later stages of the disease. However, progression to endstage renal failure is less common than was believed in the past, even in patients with multiple relapses. Chronic uremia developed in only 10% of patients reported in the literature, usually several years after the onset of renal symptoms. The most frequent causes of death in patients with essential MC are systemic vasculitis, infection, and cardiovascular and cerebrovascular accidents.[4]

Treatment

Antiviral therapy of HCV infection

The most extensively used antiviral agent has been interferon-α (IFN-α). A large number of studies, some of which were controlled, and some recent metaanalyses are now available on the effect of this drug in the control of the infection and its hepatic consequences in patients without associated cryoglobulinemia.[5–11] The conclusions can be summarized as follows.

1. Sustained virologic response (defined as undetectable serum HCV RNA levels 6 months after completion of treatment) is obtained in no more than 15–20% of patients after an initial 12-month course of IFN-α at the standard dose of 3 million units three times a week.
2. More intense treatment courses of IFN-α (6–10 million units three times a week, or each day for the first 4–6 weeks) give only marginally more favorable results.
3. A high baseline viral load (pretreatment HCV RNA > 2 million copies/mL), the persistence of viremia 4–12 weeks after the start of treatment and the viral genotype 1b are the strongest predictors of lack of long-term response to therapy with this drug.
4. Sustained virologic response to IFN-α interrupts the progression of hepatic damage.
5. Even in patients with persisting positivity of HCV RNA, maintenance therapy for 2 years may prevent histologic progression of hepatic damage.[10]

More recently another antiviral agent, ribavirin, a guanidine analog with a broad spectrum of activity against RNA and DNA viruses, has been administered with IFN-α to better control viral infection. The majority of investigators agree that combined treatment of IFN-α (at the above-mentioned doses) and ribavirin (1000–1200 mg/day orally for at least 6 months) increases the sustained virologic response in 40–45% of patients. When viral genotype 1b is present, 12 months of treatment with both drugs can give better results.[12–16] Contraindications to such combined therapy include the existence of severe psychiatric illness, seizure disorders, severe cardiovascular disease, autoimmune diseases, poorly controlled diabetes mellitus, severe anemia, leukopenia or thrombocytopenia, and decompensated cirrhosis.[16]

Combined treatment can produce adverse effects that in about 10% of patients necessitate discontinuation: the more frequent and severe are hemolytic anemia, leukopenia, thrombocytopenia, neuropsychiatric symptoms (depression, insomnia, anxiety, irritability), gastrointestinal disorders (anorexia, nausea, vomiting), and skin disorders (pruritus, rash, alopecia).

Finally, a very recent randomized trial[17] used the combination of ribavirin with a new biologically active molecule obtained by addition of polyethyleneglycol to interferon (peginterferon alfa-2b). This can be administered subcutaneously once a week and further increases the sustained virologic response in > 50% of patients.

Antiviral therapy in HCV infection associated with mixed cryoglobulinemia

Infection of B lymphocytes by HCV in MC has been documented by many investigators (reviewed in reference 2), and it is probable that eradication of the viral infection with antiviral agents can influence the production of new cryoglobulins and therefore the systemic and renal damage they may induce.

In 1993–1994, three controlled trials on the effect of IFN-α in HCV infection complicated by MC were reported (Table 16.1). The trial of Ferri et al[18] was a crossover-controlled trial in 26 patients with documented HCV infection and clinically active MC (purpura, liver, and/or neurologic involvement) but without evident signs of renal involvement. The trial alternated 6 months with and 6 months without IFN-α therapy (2 million units daily for a month, then every other day for 5 months). The majority of patients were on low-dose steroid treatment before the trial and this medication was continued during the trial. A significant improvement of purpura, together with a reduction of cryoglobulins and transaminases, was reported during IFN-α treatment compared to the periods without treatment. A rebound phenomenon was commonly observed during these drug-free intervals. In three patients, signs of renal involvement appeared during the treatment period.

In the randomized controlled trial of Misiani et al,[19] 53 patients with HCV-associated type II MC, three-fourths of whom had some mild renal involvement, were assigned to receive either symptomatic therapy or IFN-α for 6 months (1.5 million units daily for 1 week, then 3 million units thrice weekly for the following 23 weeks). Even in this trial many patients in both subgroups were receiving low-dose steroid treatment before the start of the trial and continued to take it. IFN-α eradicated the viremia in 60% of patients, improved the systemic signs of the disease, and reduced the cryocrit, although no beneficial effects on liver damage were documented. With regard to the renal disease, only a small but constant reduction in serum creatinine was reported, without significant change in proteinuria. Despite these beneficial effects in 60% of treated patients, none became completely free of the abnormalities that characterize MC and all patients relapsed after IFN-α was discontinued.

In the randomized controlled trial by Dammacco et al,[20] 65 patients with type II MC due to HCV infection were assigned to four groups:

Group A: 3 millions units of natural IFN-α three times a week for 1 year
Group B: IFN-α as in group A plus 16 mg oral 6-methylprednisolone (6MP) on "non-IFN-α" days
Group C: 16 mg/day of 6MP only
Group D: no treatment.

A good response, arbitrarily defined as reduction of cryocrit to less than 50%, associated with improvement of systemic signs, was obtained in approximately half the patients given IFN-α alone or IFN-α plus 6MP, but in only 17% of those given the steroid alone. As in the previous trials, the favorable effect was limited to patients in whom HCV RNA became negative (42% and 50%, respectively, in groups A and B). In patients treated with 6MP only, despite the demonstration of clinical and biochemical remission in a minority of patients, a significant increase of HCV RNA levels was demonstrated at the end of the treatment in 5 of 13 patients. After discontinuation of the trial, recurrence of signs of MC was a frequent phenomenon, but clinical relapse was delayed in patients receiving the

Table 16.1 Results of three controlled trials of treatment with interferon-α in patients with mixed cryoglobulinemia associated with hepatitis C virus infection

Reference	Type of Cryo	No. of patients	Type of trial	Disappearance of viraemia	Cryocrit	Systemic signs	Signs of liver damage	Signs of renal damage
				Effects of treatment				
Ferri et al[18]	Types II and III MC	26	Crossover 6 months IFN-α, 6 months no treatment*	13%	Reduced[†]	Improved[†]	Reduction of SGPT	None at start; in three patients signs appeared during the treatment
Misian et al[19]	Type II MC	53	Randomized controlled 6 months IFN-α vs. no treatment*	60%[‡]	Reduced[†§]	Improved[†§]	No effect	Present at start in 75%; small but consistent reduction in serum creatinine[§]
Dammacco et al[20]	Type II MC	65	Randomized controlled (A) IFN-α alone (B) IFN-α + 6MP (C) 6MP alone (D) No treatment	(A) 42% (B) 50% (C) increase in some cases	Good response in 52% of patients in groups A and B, and in 17% of patients in group C			Present at start in 43%; improved in 1 of 3 patients in group A and in 2 of five patients in group B. No improvement in group C

HCV, hepatitis C virus; IFN-α, interferon-α; MC, mixed cryoglobulinemia; 6MP, 6-methylprednisolone; SGPT, serum glutamate pyruvate transaminase.
*Low-dose steroids, already administered before the trial, were maintained during the trial.
[†]Rebound occurred after discontinuation of treatment.
[‡]Recurrence after 6 months in 13 of 15 patients.
[§]Only in patients with disappearance of HCV RNA.

combined treatment (IFN-α plus 6MP) compared with those treated with IFN-α alone.

Many subsequent studies[21–26] have confirmed the efficacy of antiviral therapy (IFN-α with or without ribavirin) in controlling the extrarenal clinical manifestations of cryoglobulinemia, suggested that improvement in cryoglobulinemia-related symptoms can be achieved even without complete biochemical or virologic responses,[24] and that the presence of cryoglobulins does not affect the response to antiviral treatment in patients with HCV infection.[22,23]

Treatment of renal complications associated with mixed cryoglobulinemia and HCV infection

Unfortunately, the data on the effect of antiviral therapy in glomerulonephritis associated with HCV infection, usually with concomitant cryoglobulinemia, are still controversial. A uncontrolled study[27] of the effect of IFN-α in 14 patients reported a 60% reduction of proteinuria. Many anecdotal case reports in the last few years have indicated a favorable effect of IFN-α alone, or in combination with ribavirin, in individual patients with membranoproliferative glomerulonephritis but no controlled trials

have been performed. However, most nephrologists treat acute flare-ups of the renal disease with anti-inflammatory (steroids) and immunosuppressive (cyclophosphamide) therapy, in addition to antiviral treatment, as was used extensively in the 1990s before the viral etiology of cryoglobulinemic glomerulonephritis was appreciated.

We therefore recommend a different therapeutic approach to the renal complications of HCV-associated cryoglobulinemia in chronic and acute stages.

Treatment of the chronic stages of the renal disease

In the absence of signs of acute glomerular disease and/or vasculitis, the antiviral therapy indicated in Table 16.2 is the only treatment. The available data do not completely support the policy, still widely utilized by nephrologists, of giving maintenance treatment with low-dose oral steroids, with IFN-α or after its discontinuation. Some favorable systemic effects can be obtained, but the natural history of cryoglobulinemic glomerulonephritis seems to be scarcely influenced, while some evidence exists of possible negative effects of steroids on the viremia.

Therapy of acute exacerbations of cryoglobulinemic glomerulonephritis and renal vasculitis

Acute flare-ups of the renal disease, characterized by an acute nephritic syndrome or a nephrotic syndrome with

Table 16.2 Treatment of mixed cryoglobulinemia associated with HCV infection in the absence of severe signs of renal involvement

Interferon-α: 3 million units twice weekly for 1 year (the drug can be discontinued after 6 months if HCV RNA does not disappear from the blood)
or
Interferon-α plus ribavirin: 3 million units of interferon-α three times weekly plus 1.0–1.2 g/day orally of ribavirin, both for 6–12 months

Low-dose maintenance oral steroids: to control some systemic and renal signs of mixed cryoglobulinemia (?)

less rapid functional deterioration, usually associated with recurrence of the systemic signs of MC (purpura, arthralgia, visceral vasculitis), still occur despite the widespread use of IFN-α. In our opinion they deserve the same aggressive therapy that was used before the viral etiology of the disease became evident. Although these acute manifestations of cryoglobulinemic glomerulonephritis and vasculitis are in some cases spontaneously reversible, in past years nephrologists who did not treat this clinical condition aggressively observed that irreversible complete loss of renal function can occur. Before the viral origin of "essential" MC was shown, such misfortunes prompted investigators to use the same anti-inflammatory and cytotoxic drugs that successfully treated other types of rapidly progressive glomerulonephritis as well as antineutrophil cytoplasmic antibody-positive renal vasculitis. Although data from uncontrolled trials using oral steroids and/or cyclophosphamide were initially discouraging, subsequent experience with a regimen based on intravenous high-dose methylprednisolone pulses at the beginning of the steroid treatment,[28] eventually administered with cyclophosphamide, led nephrologists to consider this regimen probably more efficacious since it frequently induced a rapid improvement in the systemic signs of the disease, a progressive regression of the impaired renal function (often with normalization of glomerular filtration rate or serum creatinine), and a reduction of proteinuria.[3] Plasma exchange or cryofiltration apheresis has been added in more severe cases. Indeed, although a precise relationship between the level of circulating cryoglobulins and severity of renal damage induced by their intraglomerular deposition has not been confirmed by many investigators, the rationale for sharply reducing their level in the blood with such methods appears convincing. Significant amounts of cryoproteins can be removed with this technique; this prevents local cryoprecipitation in small renal vessels, restores reticuloendothelial system functions that have been saturated by the chronic overload of circulating cryoglobulins, and removes from the blood potentially toxic mediators of inflammation. Many uncontrolled studies have reported rapid improvement in serum creatinine, proteinuria, and cryocrit after plasmapheresis or cryofiltration.[29–32] However, in most trials

this treatment was combined with corticosteroids and cyclophosphamide (to avoid rebound production of cryoglobulins by B cells), so that it is difficult to assess whether the beneficial effects were attributable to the plasmapheresis per se, to the concomitant immunosuppression, or to the combination of the two treatments.

Over the last 15 years in two renal units in Milano, we have routinely used a therapeutic regimen that includes steroids (short courses of intravenous methylprednisolone pulses, followed by oral prednisone), cyclophosphamide (especially when signs of renal and/or systemic vasculitis were present), and, in the most acute cases, plasmapheresis.[3] No evident signs of worsening of the liver involvement, as indicated by the level of hepatic enzymes, were found in more than 50 patients treated as indicated above, nor did increased incidences of serious infectious complications occur.

Is this intensive anti-inflammatory and cytotoxic treatment still necessary, despite the availability of antiviral drugs? Our personal experience is that, in the presence of the acute signs of renal involvement in MC, IFN-α is unable to control the clinical situation, and in order to avoid progression of the renal damage we therefore think it is essential to administer IFN-α in combination with the anti-inflammatory and cytotoxic drugs (and eventually also plasma exchange according to the protocol in Table 16.3). Obviously a controlled trial is now mandatory to investigate the effect of IFN-α or other antiviral drugs given alone compared with the same antiviral drugs combined with anti-iflammatory and cytotoxic drugs plus plasmapheresis. Such a trial must establish, by scientifically rigorous procedures, the superiority of the combination treatment, but at the same time must seek to identify the possible adverse effects on the course of the viral disease and its organ complications (especially liver and nervous system), monitoring also the serum level of viremia by measurement of HCV RNA.

Table 16.3 Treatment of mixed cryoglobulinemia associated with HCV infection in the presence of severe acute signs of renal involvement (glomerulonephritis and vasculitis)

Interferon-α (eventually plus other antiviral agents): schedule as in Table 16.2
plus
Steroids: 0.75–1 g/day of methylprednisolone i.v. for three consecutive days, followed by oral prednisone for 6 months (0.5 mg/kg body weight daily, tapered over a few weeks until small maintenance doses are achieved)
plus
Cyclophosphamide: 2 mg/kg for 3–6 months, especially when signs of severe renal and systemic vasculitis are present
plus
Plasmapheresis: exchanges of 3 L of plasma three times weekly for 2 or 3 weeks, in the most severe cases

Treatment of renal complications associated with mixed cryoglobulinemia in the absence of HCV infection

In 5–10% of patients with type II MC and cryoglobulinemic glomerulonephritis, the concomitant presence of HCV infection can be excluded even with accurate repeated analyses, and the etiology remains obscure. We could not find any consistent difference in the clinical presentation, clinical course, and/or histologic features of these patients compared with those in whom HCV infection was responsible for the cryoglobulinemia.[3]

The treatment of these cases is therefore similar to that used in all cases of cryoglobulinemic glomerulonephritis before the 1990s. In the chronic stages, low doses of steroids may be prescribed when some systemic signs of MC appear, even though, as we have said, the natural history of cryoglobulinemic glomerulonephritis seems to be scarcely influenced. Acute exacerbations of the renal disease should be treated with the same strategy described for glomerulonephritis associated with HCV infection, with the exception of the antiviral therapy. In our experience, the results have been similar.

References

1. Meltzer J, Clauvel JP, Danon F, et al: Biological and clinical significance of cryoglobulins. A report of 86 cases. Am J Med 1974;57:775–778.
2. D'Amico G, Fornasieri A: Cryoglobulinemic glomerulonephritis: a membranoproliferative glomerulonephritis induced by hepatitis C virus. Am J Kidney Dis 1995;25:361–369.
3. D'Amico G: Renal involvement in hepatitis C infection: cryoglobulinemic glomerulonephritis. Kidney Int 1998;54:650–671.
4. Tarantino G, Campise M, Banfi G, et al: Long term predictors of survival in essential mixed cryoglobulinemic glomerulonephritis. Kidney Int 1995;47:618–623.
5. Di Bisceglie AM, Martin P, Kassianides C, et al: Recombinant interferon alfa therapy for chronic hepatitis C: a randomized, double-blind, placebo-controlled trial. N Engl J Med 1989;321:1506–1510.
6. Davis GL, Balart LA, Schiff ER, et al: Treatment of chronic hepatitis C with recombinant interferon alfa: a multicenter randomized, controlled trial. N Engl J Med 1989;321:1501–1506.
7. Nishiguchi S, Kuroki T, Nakatani S, et al: Randomised trial of effects of interferon-alpha on incidence of hepatocellular carcinoma in chronic active hepatitis C with cirrhosis. Lancet 1995;346:1051–1055.
8. Hoofnagle JH, Di Bisceglie AM: The treatment of chronic viral hepatitis. Drug Therapy 1997;336:347–356.
9. Reichard O, Glaumann H, Fryden A, et al: Long-term follow-up of chronic hepatitis C patients with sustained virological response to alpha-interferon. J Hepatol 1999;30:783–787.
10. Shiffman ML, Hofmann CM, Contos MS, et al: A randomized controlled trial of maintenance interferon therapy for patients with chronic hepatitis C virus and persistent viremia. Gastroenterology 1999;117:1164–1172.
11. Lauer GM, Walker BD: Hepatitis C virus infection. N Engl J Med 2001;345:41–52.
12. Poynard T, Marcellin P, Lee SS, et al: Randomised trial of interferon alpha2b plus ribavirin for 48 weeks or for 24 weeks versus interferon alpha2b plus placebo for 48 weeks for treatment of chronic infection with hepatitis C virus. Lancet 1998;352:1426–1432.
13. McHutchison JG, Gordon SC, Schiff ET, et al: Interferon alfa-2b alone or in combination with ribavirin as initial treatment for chronic hepatitis C. N Engl J Med 1998;339:1485–1492.
14. Davis GL, Esteban-Mur R, Rustgi V, et al: Interferon alfa-2b alone or in combination with ribavirin for the treatment of relpase of chronic hepatitis C. N Engl J Med 1998;339:1493–1499.
15. Reichard O, Norkran G, Frydén A, et al: Randomised, double-blind, placebo-controlled trial of interferon α-2b with and without ribavirin for chronic hepatitis C. Lancet 1998;351:83–87.
16. Lin OS, Keeffe EB: Current treatment strategies for chronic hepatitis B and C. Annu Rev Med 2001;52:29–49.
17. Manns MP, McHutchison JG, Gordon SC, et al: Peginterferon alfa-2b plus ribavirin compared with interferon alfa-2b plus ribavirin for initial treatment of chronic hepatitis C. a randomised trial. Lancet 2001;358:958–965.
18. Ferri C, Marzo E, Longobardo, G et al: Interferon-α in mixed cryoglobulinemia patients: a randomized, crossover-controlled trial. Blood 1993;81:1132–1136.
19. Misiani R, Bellavita P, Fenili D, et al: Interferon alfa-2a therapy in cryoglobulinemia associated with hepatitis C virus. N Engl J Med 1994;330:751–756.
20. Dammacco F, Sansonno D, Han JH, et al: Natural interferon-α versus its combination with 6-methyl-prednisolone in the therapy of type II mixed cryoglobulinemia: a long-term, randomized, controlled study. Blood 1994;84:3336–3343.
21. Dispenzieri A, Gorevic PD: Cryoglobulinemia. Hematol Oncol Clin North Am 1999;13:1315–1349.
22. Pellicano R, Marietti G, Leone N, et al: Mixed cryoglobulinaemia associated with hepatitis C virus infection: a predictor factor for treatment with interferon? J Gastroenterol Hepatol 1999;14:1108–1111.
23. Calleja JL, Albillos A, Moreno-Otero R, et al: Sustained response to interferon-alpha plus ribavirin in hepatitis C virus-associated symptomatic mixed cryoglobulinaemia. Aliment Pharmacol Ther 1999;13:1179–1186.
24. Zuckerman E, Keren D, Slobodin G, et al: Treatment of refractory, symptomatic, hepatitis C virus related mixed cryoglobulinemia with ribavirin and interferon-alpha. J Rheumatol 2000;27:2172–2178.
25. Lunel F, Cacoub P: Treatment of autoimmune and extra-hepatic manifestations of HCV infection. Ann Med Interne (Paris) 2000;151:58–64.
26. Agnello V: Therapy for cryoglobulinemia secondary to hepatitis C virus: the need for tailored protocols and multiclinic studies. J Rheumatol 2000;27:2065–2067.
27. Johnson RJ, Gretch DR, Couser WG, et al: Hepatitis C virus-associated glomerulonephritis. Effect of α-interferon therapy. Kidney Int 1994;46:1700–1704.
28. De Vecchi A, Montagnino G, Pozzi C, et al: Intravenous methylprednisolone pulse therapy in essential mixed cryoglobulinemia nephropathy. Clin Nephrol 1983;19:221–227.
29. Berkman EM, Orlin JB: Use of plasmapheresis and partial plasma exchange in the management of patients with cryoglobulinemia. Transfusion 1980;20:171–178.
30. Sinico RA, Fornasieri A, Fiorini G, et al: Plasma exchange in the treatment of essential mixed cryoglobulinemia nephropathy. Long-term follow up. Int J Artif Organs 1985;2:15–18.
31. Siami GA, Siami FS, Ferguson P, et al: Cryofiltration apheresis for treatment of cryoglobulinemia associated with hepatitis C. ASAIO Trans 1995;41:315–318.
32. Kiyomoto H, Hitomi H, Hosotani Y, et al: The effect of combination therapy with interferon and cryofiltration on mesangial proliferative glomerulonephritis originating from mixed cryoglobulinemia in chronic hepatitis C virus infection. Ther Apheresis 1999;3:329–333.

CHAPTER

17

Lupus Nephritis

James E. Balow, Dimitrios T. Boumpas, and Howard A. Austin III

Review of clinical trials
- Animal studies
- Human studies
  - Corticosteroids
  - Azathioprine
  - Cyclophosphamide
  - Mycophenolate mofetil (MMF)
  - Plasma exchange
Specific recommendations
- Assessment of prognosis and selection of patients for treatment
- Treatment options
- Relapses of lupus nephritis
- SLE and endstage renal failure
Future directions
- Experimental therapies
- Unanswered questions

Systemic lupus erythematosus (SLE) is a complex systemic disease which develops from a massive overproduction of polyclonal antibodies and impaired clearance of immune complexes.[1,2] Many of the antibodies are autoreactive, either from loss of self-tolerance or from antigenic cross-reactivity, and are used as criteria for the diagnosis of SLE.[3] Renal disease results from deposition of pathogenic immune complexes and infiltration of lymphoid cells within glomeruli, interstitium, and extraglomerular vessels.[4–6] These humoral and cellular components, along with a host of soluble mediators, evoke a cascade of inflammation, cell death or proliferation, vasculopathy, and fibrogenesis.[7,8] Cumulative evidence indicates that complex interactions between environmental factors and disease susceptibility genes contribute to the pathogenesis of SLE and lupus nephritis.[1,2]

It is well recognized that renal involvement adversely affects the prognosis of SLE. Indeed, patients often consider kidney disease to be one of the most dreaded complications of SLE. The empathic physician can help the patient to realize that the prognosis of lupus nephritis is not uniformly grave and that effective therapies are available for many forms of the disease.[9–14] Patients should know that prognosis varies greatly among the many clinical and pathologic forms of lupus renal disease.[12–14]

Delineation of the specific type of renal involvement is critical to effective clinical management. This process depends on diligent surveillance of patients for hypertension and other clinical and serological evidence of lupus activity, as well as periodic screening by appropriate renal function tests. Urinalysis is clearly one of the most

cost-effective methods of detecting renal involvement, but special efforts on the part of the clinician are usually needed to verify routine clinical laboratory assessment of urine sediment.[15] Proteinuria is conveniently assessed by measures of protein-to-creatinine ratios on random urine specimens. Renal biopsies are usually indicated to help delineate the exact type and severity of pathologic lesions early in the course of lupus nephritis.[16–18] A particularly noteworthy study has shown that deferral of renal biopsy is commonly associated with a delay in implementation of cytotoxic drug therapy.[19] Thus, information from early renal biopsy has a substantive impact on development of a comprehensive treatment plan for patients with lupus nephritis. Management of hypertension and the secondary complications of lupus nephritis are addressed elsewhere in this volume. The present chapter will focus on immuno-suppressive drug treatment of the various pathologically defined forms of lupus nephritis. An excellent review of the pharmacodynamics of several of these immuno-suppressive agents has recently been published.[20]

Review of clinical trials

Animal studies

Important insights into the pathogenesis and treatment of lupus nephritis have emerged from studies of murine models of SLE (e.g. NZB/W, SWR/NZB, MRL/lpr, BXSB). The different strains of lupus-prone mice appear to have distinct immunological defects which may have counterparts in the diversity of mechanisms underlying human SLE.[1,2,21] Several strains of lupus mice succumb within a relatively narrow window of time from complications of lupus nephritis; the strain-specific predictable natural history has made them apt subjects for testing new therapies.

Table 17.1 presents a highly simplified overview of experimental therapies which have been tested in the murine models of lupus nephritis. The therapies have been ranked according to their impact on survival (mostly representing amelioration of lupus nephritis). As noted, many therapeutic interventions have a favorable effect on the course of these models. Cyclophosphamide has one of the highest therapeutic indices, for which there is parallel evidence in human SLE. Particularly intriguing is a recent study showing that a combination of cyclophosphamide and the costimulation inhibitor CTLA4-Ig had a dramatic effect on the advanced stages of murine lupus nephritis.[22] Bone marrow transplantation and gene therapy are more complex processes which, hopefully, will offer future prospects for definitive treatment and perhaps "cure" of SLE and lupus nephritis.

Table 17.1 Overview of experimental treatments on survival in murine lupus nephritis

Major benefit
Cyclophosphamide
T-/B-cell costimulation inhibitors (anti-CD154, CTLA4-Ig, and other B7 inhibitors)
Total lymphoid irradiation
Bone marrow transplantation
Gene therapy

Moderate benefit
Sex hormones (in females): castration, androgens, estrogen antagonists, bromocriptine
Chemical immunosuppression: glucocorticoids, azathioprine, mycophenolate mofetil, methotrexate, cyclosporine A, tacrilimus, sirolimus, deoxyspergualin, ornithine decarboxylase inhibitors, dimethylthiourea, 5-azacytidine
Inflammation modulators: prostaglandin E analogs, free radical scavengers, platelet activating factor receptor antagonists, thromboxane synthase and receptor antagonists, nitric oxide synthase inhibitors, endothelin A receptor antagonists
Cytokine antagonists against: IFN-α, soluble IFN-α receptors, IL-2 receptors, IL-6, IL-6 receptors, IL-10, TNF, TGF-β, CSF-1, soluble IL-4 receptors
Monoclonal antibodies against: Ia, nephritogenic idiotypes, T cells, B cells, C5b-9 complement
Anticoagulants: heparin, heparinoids
Fibrinolytic agents: ancrod
DNA-related agents: recombinant murine DNase; bacterial DNA immunization; synthetic oligonucleotide conjugate (LJP-394 DNA toleragen in BXSB mice)
Dietary manipulation: protein, calorie, and fat restriction; fish oil and flax seed supplements

IFN, interferon; IL, interleukin; TNF, tumor necrosis factor; TGF, transforming growth factor; CSF, colony stimulating factor.

Human studies

While there is general consensus that the outlook for patients with lupus nephritis has improved greatly over the past half century, there remains substantial controversy about which factors are principally responsible for this improvement in prognosis.[23–25] A particularly confounding issue is the tremendous diversity in prognosis among patients in different geographic centers. Descriptions of natural history of lupus nephritis range from dismal odds of renal survival despite aggressive immunosuppressive treatment in some populations[26–29] to excellent long-term survivals with only modest immunosuppressive therapy in other populations.[12,13,25,30] Thus, studies must be extended in order to understand important differences in the biology of SLE and their impact on the natural history of lupus nephritis among different demographic populations.[31,32] In the mean time, reliable attributions of treatment efficacy must be based on the results of prospective, randomized, controlled clinical trials in patients with lupus nephritis.[33]

Table 17.2 presents a synopsis of the controlled therapeutic trials which constitute the foundation for our current recommendations for treatment of proliferative lupus nephritis.[34–54] The reader may be surprised to observe that fewer than 1000 patients have been enrolled in these various clinical trials to date. The format of Table 17.2 permits a ready comparison of the diverse treatment regimens tested in these trials. Table 17.3 includes expanded descriptions of the controlled trials in lupus nephritis. Results of the common treatment regimens (drug, route of administration, duration) are grouped together in this table. The criteria for renal disease, the specific treatment regimens, and the conclusions suggested by these major therapeutic trials are presented for each study.

Corticosteroids

The merit of high-dose corticosteroids in patients with various forms of lupus nephritis has never been rigorously proven by modern clinical trial methodology. There have been no controlled clinical trials proving the benefit of corticosteroids over supportive therapy in lupus nephritis, nor have there been any studies directly comparing conventional prednisone with methylprednisolone pulse therapy. Indeed, it is unlikely that prospective clinical trials comparing placebo, low-dose, and high-dose corticosteroids for lupus nephritis will ever be performed owing to the potentially confounding effects of the standard clinical practice of using high-dose corticosteroids as first-line treatment for the myriad of extrarenal manifestations and complications of SLE. The best advice for the practitioner is not to withhold corticosteroids for fear of complications, but rather to test regularly the feasibility of reducing doses (preferably to alternate day) and to be willing to substitute alternative immunosuppressive drug strategies if clinical response is delayed. Physicians treating patients with SLE and lupus nephritis should always be inclined to reduce dosages of corticosteroids to the lowest necessary for disease control in order to minimize the risk of their insidious complications.

Azathioprine

The majority of studies indicate that azathioprine adds marginally to the efficacy of prednisone alone. Thus, at the present time, azathioprine is used as primary therapy mainly in milder forms of lupus nephritis and in patients strongly opposed to receiving cyclophosphamide. Direct comparison of azathioprine with cyclophosphamide for induction therapy has only been tested in National Institutes of Health (NIH) studies.[38,39,41,42] These studies showed that azathioprine was not as efficacious as cyclophosphamide, measured by improvement of urine sediment, proteinuria, lupus activity, and serologies.

Early results (after 8 months) of an ongoing controlled trial in the Netherlands have suggested that a regimen of pulse methylprednisolone and azathioprine is similar to a regimen of pulse cyclophosphamide.[55] Azathioprine continues to be used in many centers around the world as maintenance therapy – often after patients have had substantial improvement or achieved remission of lupus

Table 17.2 Tabulation of controlled immunosuppressive drug trials in lupus nephritis

Year	Reference	No. patients	Pred only	MP short	MP long	AZ	CY p.o. short	CY p.o. long	AZ + CY	CY i.v. short	CY i.v. long	CY i.v. mini	MP i.v. + CY i.v.	PE + CY	Ig i.v.	MMF
1971	34	35	C			E										
1972	35	19	C			E										
1973	37	50	C			E										
1974	38	38	C			E		E								
1975	40	24	C			E										
1978	43	50	C				E									
1986	41	107	C			E		E	E	E						
1992	45	56		C						E	E					
1994	46	29		C						E						
1999	49	14								C					E	
2000	50	42					C									E
2001	48	82			C					E			E			
2002	52	90									C	E				
Plasmapheresis studies																
1992	53	86					C							E		
1998	54	18								C				E		

AZ, azathioprine; CY, cyclophosphamide; MP, methylprednisolone; PE, plasma exchange; Pred, prednisone; Ig, immunoglobulin; MMF, mycophenolate mofetil; short, treatment for up to 6 months; long, treatment for more than 6 months; i.v., intravenous; p.o., oral; mini, low dose; C, comparison (main control) group; E, experimental group.

Table 17.3 Synopsis of controlled immunosuppressive drug and plasma exchange trials in lupus nephritis

Azathioprine: extended oral therapy

Sztejnbok et al[34]
Renal disease: creatinine clearance < 75 mL/min or proteinuria > 0.5 g/day. *Treatment*: prednisone vs. prednisone plus azathioprine for 1–4 years. *Conclusions*: azathioprine decreased morbidity and mortality, reduced steroid requirements, reduced exacerbations, maintained better renal function

Donadio et al[35,36]
Renal disease: active proliferative glomerulonephritis on biopsy. *Treatment*: prednisone vs. prednisone plus azathioprine for 1–3 years. *Conclusions*: no clinical or pathologic (repeat biopsy) benefit of azathioprine over prednisone alone at 6 months; no difference in disease activity or rate of renal flares at 30 months

Cade et al[37]
Renal disease: proliferative lupus nephritis on biopsy. *Treatment*: prednisone vs. prednisone and azathioprine vs. azathioprine alone vs. azathioprine and heparin. *Conclusions*: all regimens containing azathioprine were superior to prednisone alone in maintaining adequate kidney function and in survival

Steinberg and Decker;[38] Decker et al[39]
Renal disease: active urinary sediment with diffuse (mostly proliferative) lupus nephritis on biopsy. *Treatment*: prednisone vs. prednisone plus azathioprine for up to 44 months. *Conclusions*: no significant benefit of azathioprine over prednisone on lupus disease activity, serologies, or renal outcomes

Hahn et al[40]
Renal disease: proteinuria, active sediment, decreased GFR (nephritis on biopsy in 20/24 patients). *Treatment*: prednisone vs. prednisone plus azathioprine for 18–24 months. *Conclusions*: no renal or extrarenal disease benefits of azathioprine

Austin et al;[41] Steinberg and Steinberg[42]
Renal disease: active urinary sediment with lupus nephritis (mostly proliferative) on biopsy. *Treatment*: prednisone vs. prednisone plus azathioprine until major drug toxicity, renal failure or sustained remission of nephritis. *Conclusions*: azathioprine did not reduce risk of ESRD compared with prednisone alone during 10 or more years of observation

Azathioprine plus cyclophosphamide combination: extended oral therapy

Austin et al;[41] Steinberg and Steinberg[42]
Renal disease: active urinary sediment with lupus nephritis (mostly proliferative) on biopsy. *Treatment*: prednisone vs. prednisone plus

Table 17.3 Synopsis of controlled immunosuppressive drug and plasma exchange trials in lupus nephritis (*cont'd*)

azathioprine and cyclophosphamide combination until major drug toxicity, renal failure or sustained remission of nephritis. *Conclusions*: after 5 years of observation, azathioprine plus cyclophosphamide significantly reduced risk of ESRD compared with prednisone alone

Cyclophosphamide: 6 months of oral therapy
Donadio et al[43,44]
Renal disease: severe proliferative lupus nephritis on biopsy with clinical evidence of progression. *Treatment*: prednisone vs. prednisone plus oral cyclophosphamide for 6 months. *Conclusions*: the short course of cyclophosphamide significantly improved the probability of a stable renal course over the first 4 years of observation, but there was no difference in late risk of renal failure

Cyclophosphamide: oral therapy extended until complete remission
Steinberg and Decker;[38] **Decker et al**[39]
Renal disease: active urinary sediment with diffuse (mostly proliferative) lupus nephritis on biopsy. *Treatment*: prednisone vs. prednisone plus cyclophosphamide for up to 44 months. *Conclusions*: cyclophosphamide associated with reduced disease activity, serologies, urinary abnormalities, and a trend toward reduced rates of unfavorable major outcomes (death or ESRD) at 28 months

Austin et al;[41] **Steinberg and Steinberg**[42]
Renal disease: active urinary sediment with lupus nephritis (mostly proliferative) on biopsy. *Treatment*: prednisone vs. prednisone plus cyclophosphamide until major drug toxicity, renal failure or sustained remission of nephritis. *Conclusions*: after 5 years of observation, cyclophosphamide significantly reduced risk of ESRD compared with prednisone alone

Cyclophosphamide: extended quarterly intravenous pulse therapy
Austin et al;[41] **Steinberg and Steinberg**[42]
Renal disease: active urinary sediment with lupus nephritis (mostly proliferative) on biopsy. *Treatment*: prednisone vs. prednisone plus pulse cyclophosphamide until major drug toxicity, renal failure, or sustained remission of nephritis. *Conclusions*: after 5 years of observation, cyclophosphamide significantly reduced risk of ESRD compared with prednisone alone and was less toxic than regimens containing daily cyclophosphamide

Cyclophosphamide: monthly and quarterly pulse therapies
Boumpas et al[45]
Renal disease: active urinary sediment, reduced renal function, or severely active lupus nephritis on biopsy. *Treatment*: monthly pulse methylprednisolone for 6 months vs. monthly pulse cyclophosphamide for 6 months vs. monthly pulse cyclophosphamide for 6 months followed by quarterly pulse cyclophosphamide for 2 years. *Conclusions*: treatment with the extended course of pulse cyclophosphamide significantly reduced the probability of doubling serum creatinine compared with pulse methylprednisolone; relapse after initial improvement of nephritis was increased after the short course compared with the extended course of pulse cyclophosphamide

Sesso et al[46]
Renal disease: severe lupus nephritis. *Treatment*: pulse methylprednisolone vs. pulse cyclophosphamide each given monthly for 4 months followed by two quarterly pulse treatments. *Conclusions*: at 18 months, no difference in probability of doubling creatinine or developing ESRD

Combination pulse methylprednisolone and cyclophosphamide
Gourley et al;[47] **Illei et al**[48]
Renal disease: active urinary sediment, proteinuria, proliferative lupus nephritis on biopsy. *Treatment*: pulse methylprednisolone monthly for at least 1 year vs. pulse cyclophosphamide monthly for 6 months then quarterly vs. combination pulse methylprednisolone and cyclophosphamide therapy. *Conclusions*: renal remission was least likely with pulse methylprednisolone therapy; remissions tended to be established more rapidly with combination pulse methylprednisolone and cyclophosphamide therapy

Cyclophosphamide: low- vs. high-dose pulse therapy with azathioprine maintenance
Houssiau et al[52]
Renal disease: proliferative lupus nephritis. *Treatment*: high doses (≤ 1.5 g) pulse cyclophosphamide monthly for 6 months followed by two quarterly doses vs. low doses (0.5 g fixed dose) of pulse cyclophosphamide fortnightly for six doses. *Conclusions*: after median follow-up of 3.5 years, there were no substantive differences in the proportions of favorable and unfavorable renal outcomes

Mycophenolate mofetil: with azathioprine maintenance
Chan et al[50,51]
Renal disease: proliferative lupus nephritis with > 1 g/day proteinuria. *Treatment*: mycophenolate with switch to azathioprine at 12 months vs. daily oral cyclophosphamide with switch to azathioprine at 6 months. *Conclusions*: at 12 months, there were no differences in favorable or unfavorable renal outcomes between the two treatment arms; however, after an additional year of follow-up into the azathioprine maintenance phase of treatment, patients who initially received mycophenolate had significantly more relapses than patients receiving cyclophosphamide induction therapy

Table 17.3 Synopsis of controlled immunosuppressive drug and plasma exchange trials in lupus nephritis (*cont'd*)

Plasma exchange: with short-course oral cyclophosphamide
Lewis et al[53]
Renal disease: proliferative or mixed membranous and proliferative lupus nephritis on biopsy. *Treatment*: prednisone and daily oral cyclophosphamide (8 weeks) only vs. prednisone and cyclophosphamide combined with thrice weekly plasmapheresis for 4 weeks. *Conclusions*: plasmapheresis does not improve the clinical outcome in severe lupus nephritis compared with that achieved with prednisone and cyclophosphamide alone

Plasma exchange: with synchronized intravenous pulse cyclophosphamide
Wallace et al[54]
Renal disease: active proliferative lupus nephritis. *Treatment*: prednisone and six cycles of monthly high-dose pulse cyclophosphamide vs. prednisone and 6-monthly cycles of synchronized plasma exchanges (3 consecutive days) followed by high-dose pulse cyclophosphamide. *Conclusions*: changes in SLE activity and renal outcomes were similar in both treatment groups; addition of plasma exchange to a regimen of corticosteroids and pulse cyclophosphamide is not indicated in severe SLE

ESRD, endstage renal disease; SLE, systemic lupus erythematosus.

nephritis with cyclophosphamide therapy. Preliminary results of an ongoing controlled clinical trial in the USA have recently suggested that azathioprine may be as effective as quarterly pulse cyclophosphamide for maintenance therapy.[56]

Cyclophosphamide

Daily oral cyclophosphamide has been used as part of several regimens for treatment of lupus nephritis. Conclusions about efficacy and toxicity have differed dramatically, depending mostly on the duration of cyclophosphamide administration and on the measure of renal outcome. Short-term cyclophosphamide therapy (2–6 months) has been shown to be more efficacious than prednisone alone in decreasing activity and stabilizing lupus nephritis.[38,43] However, the short course of cyclophosphamide did not eliminate the subsequent risk of renal failure.[44] On the other hand, continuation of cyclophosphamide until the patients achieved sustained remission was shown to decrease the risk of late renal failure.[41]

The cumulative toxicity of extended courses of daily cyclophosphamide provides a substantial argument against the use of protracted daily cyclophosphamide therapy for lupus nephritis[57] – a conclusion which emerges from studies of systemic vasculitis.[58] Intermittent pulse therapy has become the preferred method for administering cyclophosphamide, including treatment of children with lupus nephritis.[59,60] This approach is based mostly on experience in oncology, where it has long been practice to use high, intermittent dosing as a method of maximizing the therapeutic index of cyclophosphamide as well as other chemotherapeutic drugs. Pulse cyclophosphamide was tested extensively in murine and human lupus nephritis during the 1970s. The prolongation of survival in lupus mice was dramatic.[3] Demonstration of comparable benefit of cyclophosphamide in a human cohort with moderately severe lupus nephritis required a protracted period of observation and analysis of multiple endpoints, including urinary findings, stabilization of renal pathology,[61] and ultimately reduction in risk of renal failure as measures of favorable outcome.[41,42]

After demonstration of the efficacy of prolonged courses of quarterly pulse cyclophosphamide, a subsequent trial was designed to evaluate shorter (6 months), more intense regimens of monthly pulse cyclophosphamide and monthly pulse methylprednisolone for patients with severe proliferative lupus nephritis (presence of renal insufficiency, necrosis, and/or cellular crescents). Neither of these regimens was as effective in preserving renal function or in preventing lupus relapses over a 5-year period as monthly pulse cyclophosphamide followed by 2 years of quarterly maintenance pulse therapy.[45] Neither this study nor the study by Sesso et al[46] showed any short-term (i.e. 18 months) differences in renal function outcomes among patients treated with 4–6 months of pulse methylprednisolone versus pulse cyclophosphamide.

The most recent NIH clinical trial comparing extended courses of pulse methylprednisolone alone, pulse cyclophosphamide alone, and the combination of pulse therapies showed that renal remission was achieved somewhat more rapidly with combination pulse therapy and was least likely with pulse methylprednisolone alone.[47,48]

In short, neither pulse methylprednisolone (in either short or extended courses) nor short courses of pulse cyclophosphamide is as efficacious as extended courses of pulse cyclophosphamide in reducing the risk of renal progression or in achieving sustained remission of lupus nephritis. Nonetheless, pulse cyclophosphamide is not universally effective in controlling lupus nephritis; administration of cyclophosphamide is moderately burdensome for the patient; and cumulative doses of cyclophosphamide pose substantial risk of permanent gonadal toxicity. All of these concerns have prompted continued search for more effective, simple, and safe induction and maintenance immunosuppressive drug regimens for lupus nephritis.

Mycophenolate mofetil (MMF)

Based principally on studies showing greater efficacy of mycophenolate over azathioprine in reducing transplant rejection, several investigators began exploring the use of mycophenolate in lupus nephritis (particularly for patients adverse or refractory to cyclophosphamide).[62–65]

There are several issues impinging on the decision to use mycophenolate. Among the most attractive attributes of mycophenolate is its lack of gonadal and urinary bladder toxicity (compared with cyclophosphamide). A recent controlled trial showed that induction therapy with mycophenolate was similar to daily oral cyclophosphamide for achieving remission.[50] In a preliminary follow-up report, these investigators found that relapses following conversion to maintenance azathioprine therapy were more common in patients initially treated with mycophenolate than with cyclophosphamide.[51] These results suggest that cyclophosphamide induction confers a longer period of stability than does mycophenolate. Sustained treatment with mycophenolate, or a more effective alternative than azathioprine, may be necessary to reduce the tendency to early relapse. If long-term maintenance is necessary, the extremely high cost of mycophenolate could become a practical limitation. Prospective studies in progress should address the effectiveness of lower cost azathioprine as maintenance therapy following induction of remission by either cyclophosphamide or mycophenolate. It is noteworthy that a prospective, multicentered clinical trial is in progress comparing mycophenolate with standard pulse cyclophosphamide as induction therapy for proliferative lupus nephritis.[66]

Plasma exchange

Plasma exchange and immunosuppressive drug therapy has had theoretical appeal as a method to rapidly eliminate pathogenic immune complexes and to inhibit production of autoantibodies.[67,68] Early uncontrolled studies claimed remarkable effectiveness of this dual approach, but this has not been confirmed by controlled therapeutic trials. Neither plasma exchange combined with conventional prednisone and cyclophosphamide[53] nor plasma exchange synchronized with high-dose pulse cyclophosphamide has been found to be superior to immunosuppressive drug therapy alone.[54]

Specific recommendations

Assessment of prognosis and selection of patients for treatment

Lupus nephritis is extremely heterogeneous, both clinically and pathologically. Many variables affect renal prognosis and a composite of risk factors can be used in justifying treatment strategies. Table 17.4 contains a selected list of factors associated with adverse prognosis and high risk of renal progression in lupus nephritis.[12,25,69,70] Some of these factors may be evident at presentation and remain static; others change substantially during the course of lupus nephritis. While the impact of each factor is different and not easily compared, in general, the greater the number of factors present at any one time, the more unfavorable the renal prognosis and the stronger the indications for aggressive immunosuppressive therapy.

Some comments regarding the impact of race on prognosis seem timely. Black race and Hispanic ethnicity

Table 17.4 Factors associated with adverse prognosis and high risk of renal progression in lupus nephritis

Demographic: black race; male gender;* extremes of age at onset of SLE;* limited access to health care

Clinical: hypertension; severe extrarenal (especially neuropsychiatric) lupus activity; failure to achieve or marked delay to renal remission; multiple relapses of lupus nephritis; pregnancy

Laboratory: nephritic urinary sediment; azotemia; anemia; thrombocytopenia; thrombotic microangiopathy (with or without antiphospholipid antibodies); hypocomplementemia (especially falling levels); high anti-DNA (especially rising titers); persistent severe nephrotic syndrome (atherosclerotic and thrombotic diathesis)

Renal pathology: contracted kidney size;† proliferative glomerulonephritis (WHO class III, IV); mixed membranous (V) and proliferative (III–IV) glomerulonephritis; cellular crescents; fibrinoid necrosis; very high activity index; moderate-to-high chronicity index;† combinations of active (e.g. cellular crescents) and chronic histologic features (e.g. interstitial fibrosis); subendothelial deposits

*There is controversy regarding the level of impact of these prognostic factors.
†These prognostic factors per se are not indications for treatment.
SLE, systemic lupus erythematosus.

have been shown to be associated with poor prognosis of lupus nephritis.[27–29,70] Some studies suggest that black patients with proliferative lupus nephritis respond much less favorably than other racial groups to pulse cyclophosphamide[29] and other interventions.[71] While this issue clearly warrants continued study, the reader should be mindful that diverse racial mixes may contribute to reported differences in course, prognosis, and treatment responses among studies from different centers around the world.

Treatment options

Presentation of the various treatment options and practical recommendations for management of lupus nephritis will be concentrated in table format. Nearly all of the commonly available immunosuppressive drugs have been used in management of lupus nephritis and, as described above, only some have been subjected to scientifically rigorous comparisons.[72–85] Table 17.5 contains general comments on various choices of immunosuppressive agents, adjunctive therapies for secondary complications of lupus nephritis, and a selective overview of experimental therapies for proliferative and membranous lupus nephropathies.

Table 17.6 provides practical advice for administration of pulse cyclophosphamide therapy. Pulse cyclophosphamide was initially administered during an overnight hospital stay with the intent of ensuring bladder protection through brisk diuresis and control of nausea

Table 17.5 Therapeutic options for management of lupus nephritis

Immunosuppressive drug therapy

Prednisone
Initiate at 1.0 mg/kg/day; continue for no more than 8 weeks (except when extreme clinical conditions mandate); taper to alternate day therapy in doses of 0.25 mg/kg every other day; use alternative immunosuppressive drugs rather than continued daily prednisone therapy, whenever possible; maintain assiduous surveillance and protection against steroid-induced osteoporosis (i.e. exercise, calcium, bisphosphonates)

Methylprednisolone pulse therapy
Initiate at 1.0 g/m^2 daily for 3 days for severe activity (rapidly progressive renal failure, crescentic glomerulonephritis); option to repeat pulse doses at monthly intervals; may combine with pulse cyclophosphamide in severe or refractory cases

Cyclophosphamide
Intermittent pulse therapy has highest therapeutic index; conventional daily cyclophosphamide therapy (2 mg/kg/day) mostly avoided, or used for < 3 months; see Table 17.6 for details on administration of pulse cyclophosphamide

Azathioprine
Alternative agent in SLE; mostly used for extrarenal disease, in mild lupus nephritis, as maintenance after period of improvement induced by cyclophosphamide, or as a steroid-sparing agent in patients who require sustained high doses of prednisone or in those unwilling to accept/tolerate cyclophosphamide treatment

Mycophenolate mofetil
Preliminary results are encouraging for use of this drug as an alternative to cyclophosphamide, both for induction and maintenance therapy; expense may limit use as an alternative drug

Cyclosporine
Alternative immunosuppressive drug with limited, if any, role in proliferative lupus nephritis; more favorable evidence for use in lupus membranous nephropathy; generally used in low doses (e.g. < 5 mg/kg/day); tends to aggravate hypertension and worsen renal function; expense may limit use as alternative drug

Intravenous immunoglobulins
Expensive, short-term therapy; mostly used in lupus for immune-mediated thrombocytopenia or refractory CNS disease; immunosuppressive properties (e.g. suppression of pathogenic anti-DNA idiotypes) under study

Plasma exchange
Controlled trials have not demonstrated benefit of plasmapheresis in lupus nephritis; mostly used for microangiopathic complications of lupus, such as vasculopathy of superimposed thrombotic thrombocytopenic purpura

Methotrexate
Mostly used as adjunct or alternative anti-inflammatory therapy for extrarenal manifestations of SLE; use in lupus nephritis very limited and mostly anecdotal

Adjunctive therapies for secondary complications of renal disease
Angiotensin antagonists (converting enzyme inhibitors and receptor antagonists)
Glomerular proteinuria persisting after control of active nephritis may be decreased by these agents (this must be balanced against their potential adverse effects on GFR and serum potassium)

Antihypertensives
Treatment of hypertension and drug choices follow standard guidelines; use blood pressure goals appropriate for age of patient (see Chapters 52–57)

Lipid-lowering drugs
For control of hyperlipidemia of nephrotic syndrome; usually start HMG-CoA-reductase inhibitors (statins) and/or fibric acid derivatives if nephrotic syndrome persists for more than 2–3 months (see Chapter 28)

SLE, systemic lupus erythematosus; CNS, central nervous system.

and vomiting. The newer serotonin receptor antagonists (e.g. ondansetron, granisetron) have revolutionized nausea control and have allowed the safe administration of pulse cyclophosphamide in the outpatient setting. Some risk of complications of pulse cyclophosphamide remains even with careful dose adjustment and meticulous monitoring. Herpes zoster in this patient population is aggravating but rarely life-threatening. The risk of gonadal toxicity is dependent on age and total dose.[86–88] Encouraging preliminary data suggest that gonadal toxicity may be reduced by suppressing ovarian function by an analog of gonadotropin-releasing hormone.[88]

Table 17.6 Recommendations for administration and monitoring of pulse cyclophosphamide therapy

- Estimate GFR by standard methods

- Calculate BSA (m²): $\text{BSA} = \sqrt{\dfrac{\text{Height (cm)} \times \text{Weight (kg)}}{3600}}$

- Cyclophosphamide (Cytoxan) dosing and administration:
  - Initial dose CY is 0.75 g/m² (*important note*: start with 0.5 g/m² of CY if glomerular filtration rate is less than one-third of that expected)
  - Administer CY in 150 mL normal saline i.v. over 30–60 min (*alternative*: equivalent dose of pulse CY may be taken orally in highly motivated and compliant patients)[56]

- Obtain WBC at days 10 and 14 after each CY treatment (*note*: advise patient to delay prednisone until after blood tests drawn to avoid transient steroid-induced leukocytosis)

- Adjust subsequent doses of CY to keep nadir WBC above 1500/µL (escalate CY to maximum dose of 1.0 g/m² unless WBC nadir falls below 1500/µL)

- Repeat CY doses monthly (every 3 weeks in patients with extremely aggressive disease) for 6 months, then quarterly for 1 year *after* remission achieved (defined by: inactive urine sediment, proteinuria < 1 g/day, normalization of complement (and ideally anti-DNA), and a state of minimal or no activity of extrarenal lupus)

- Protect bladder against CY-induced hemorrhagic cystitis:
  - Induce diuresis with 5% dextrose and 0.45% saline (e.g. 2 L at 250 mL/h) and encourage frequent voiding; continue high-dose oral fluids for 24 h; counsel patients to return to clinic if they cannot sustain ingestion of enteral fluids
  - Give mesna (Mesnex) (each dose 20% of total CY dose) intravenously or orally at 0, 2, 4 and 6 h after CY dosing (*note*: use of mesna strongly urged whenever sustained diuresis may be difficult to achieve, or if pulse CY is given in outpatient setting)
  - If patients anticipated to have difficulty with sustaining diuresis (e.g. severe nephrotic syndrome) or with voiding, insert a three-way Foley catheter with continuous bladder flushing with standard antibiotic irrigating solution (e.g. 3 L) for 24 h to minimize risk of hemorrhagic cystitis

- Antiemetics (usually administered orally):
  - Dexamethasone (Decadron) 10 mg single dose *plus*:
  - Serotonin receptor antagonists: granisetron (Kytril) 1–2 mg with CY dose (usually repeat dose in 12 h); ondansetron (Zofran) 8 mg t.i.d. for 1–2 days (more costly)

- Monitor fluid balance during diuresis: if patient develops progressive fluid accumulation, use diuretics to reestablish fluid balance

- Complications of pulse CY:
  - *Expected*: nausea and vomiting (central effect of CY) mostly controlled by serotonin receptor antagonists; transient hair thinning (rarely severe at CY doses ≤ 1 g/m²)
  - *Common*: significant infection diathesis only if leukopenia not carefully controlled; modest increase in herpes zoster (very low risk dissemination); infertility (male and female); amenorrhea proportional to age of the patient during treatment and to the cumulative dose of CY[57,58]
  - *Rare*: syndrome inappropriate antidiuretic hormone (SIADH) (occasionally produces severe hyponatremia during the 24 h following CY administration in the context of positive fluid balance); transient hepatocellular injury with severe elevations in bilirubin and transaminases (very rare)

GFR, glomerular filtration rate; BSA, body surface area; CY, cyclophosphamide; WBC, whole blood count

Unfortunately, no consensus has been reached on approaches to gonadal protection during cytotoxic drug therapy. While fertility status is normally a supercharged issue, the high-risk patient should be thoughtfully counseled not to risk compromise of both future health and fertility (owing to renal failure) by rejecting effective therapy for lupus nephritis. Malignancy in SLE has been exaggerated in the past; indeed, cancer diathesis is quite low for both SLE and its treatment with immunosuppressive drugs.[89,90]

Table 17.7 provides a set of practical guidelines for treatment of proliferative lupus nephritis. The recommendations are organized by severity of disease, induction therapies, and maintenance regimens, as well as alternative approaches to treatment. Table 17.8 contains guidelines and recommendations for treatment of lupus membranous nephropathy.[82,91]

Relapses of lupus nephritis

One of the most perplexing aspects of the natural history of SLE is its remitting and relapsing course. Modern treatment neither cures lupus nor completely prevents exacerbations. Furthermore, each major exacerbation is expected to leave residual and cumulative irreversible (often subclinical) damage. Approximately one-third to one-half of patients have a relapse of nephritis after achieving partial or complete remission of proliferative lupus nephritis.[43,45,92–100] Nephritic exacerbations clearly have adverse effects on renal prognosis, while proteinuric exacerbations have much less prognostic importance.[98] These observations argue in support of strategies to minimize probabilities of flares of nephritis. One controlled trial has suggested that rises of anti-DNA activity predict impending flares, which could be averted

Table 17.7 Treatment of diffuse (and severe focal) proliferative lupus nephritis

I. Recommended initial treatment
  A. Moderate disease: defined by limited number and severity of risk factors (Table 17.4)
    1. Prednisone (1.0 mg/kg/day): limited trial (up to 8 weeks)
      a. If *complete* response occurs, including clearing of cellular casts and proteinuria, normalization of complement, and minimal lupus activity, simply taper prednisone to alternate day (~ 0.25 mg/kg) and monitor for flares of nephritis
      b. If no or incomplete response to prednisone, or nephritis worsens, start monthly pulse cyclophosphamide (follow protocol below for severe disease)
    NB Do not delay this therapeutic decision beyond 8 weeks because of a partial response to prednisone.
  B. Severe disease: defined by presence of a constellation of high-risk factors (Table 17.4)
    1. Prednisone (1.0 mg/kg/day tapered) plus:
    2. Monthly pulse cyclophosphamide (0.75 g/m^2) (0.5 g/m^2 if GFR is less than one-third normal) for 6 months; increase dose of cyclophosphamide by up to 0.25 g/m^2 increments, to maximum of 1.0 g/m^2 unless total leukocytes fall below 1500/μL at the 10- to 14-day nadir point

II. Recommended transition to maintenance immunosuppressive drug therapy or early discontinuance of induction therapy (at 6 months)
  A. In selected patients, pulse cyclophosphamide may be stopped and treatment continued with alternate day prednisone (0.25 mg/kg) alone. Such patients have exquisitely responsive nephritis (defined by complete clearing of cellular casts and proteinuria, normal complement, and minimal lupus activity within the first 6 months). Limited duration of cyclophosphamide therapy is also important for patients giving high priority to maintaining fertility while accepting the risk of low-grade activity of lupus nephritis
  B. The majority of patients with proliferative lupus nephritis will not be in full remission at 6 months. Convert this group to maintenance pulse cyclophosphamide every 3 months (doses adjusted by same guidelines used during the induction therapy phase)
  NB Microscopic hematuria often does not clear for several months, even when most other clinical parameters have remitted; by itself, microscopic hematuria is usually not a sufficient reason to abandon a particular therapeutic program

III. Alternative induction and maintenance treatment regimens
  A. Induction therapy: prednisone (1.0 mg/kg/day tapered) plus:
    1. Pulse methylprednisolone 1.0 g/m^2 daily for three doses; may repeat pulses at 4-week intervals and continue for 6–12 months if there is steady progress toward remission
    2. Mycophenolate mofetil, 0.5–2.0 g/day; titrate dose as tolerated (GI side-effects mostly dose limiting; low to moderate risk of bone marrow suppression)
    3. Daily oral cyclophosphamide, 2 mg/kg/day for 2–6 months (risks greater gonadal and urinary bladder toxicities)
    4. Daily oral chlorambucil, 3–6 mg/m^2/day for 2–6 months (uncommonly used)
    5. Oral pulse cyclophosphamide, ranging from 0.5 g weekly to 1.0 g/m^2 monthly (used only in highly motivated, fastidiously compliant patients)
  B. Maintenance therapy: alternate day prednisone (~ 0.25 mg/kg) plus:
    1. Azathioprine, 2 mg/kg/day
    2. Mycophenolate mofetil, 0.5–2.0 g/day

IV. Duration of therapy
  A. Cyclophosphamide: continue quarterly maintenance cyclophosphamide treatments for 1 year *after* remission of lupus nephritis is achieved (defined by: inactive urine sediment, proteinuria < 1 g/day, normalization of complement (and ideally anti-DNA), and a state of minimal or no activity of extrarenal lupus). Patients with isolated fixed proteinuria or persistently elevated anti-DNA (i.e. without other supportive signs of active lupus nephritis) may be considered in remission. If uncertainty persists, findings on repeat renal biopsy may be extremely useful in defining status of renal disease and indications for ongoing therapy
  B. Alternate day prednisone: tapered in very small increments to discontinuance if the patient has been in sustained complete remission for > 3 years

GFR, glomerular filtration rate; GI, gastrointestinal.

by preemptive boosts in corticosteroid therapy.[93] While many agree with the general value of monitoring anti-DNA (or other serologic) activity, most clinicians would use this information as motivation to intensify clinical screening for supportive signs of lupus activity prior to boosting therapy. Several studies have shown that cyclophosphamide is more effective than steroids, and perhaps mycophenolate, in preventing renal flares. However, the risk–benefit of prolonged maintenance courses of cyclophosphamide remains controversial. Studies to define the optimally safe and effective maintenance therapies should continue to be a major clinical research

Table 17.8 Treatment of lupus membranous nephropathy*

I. Mixed membranous and proliferative nephropathies: treat as proliferative lupus nephritis (Table 17.7)

II. Membranous nephropathy with nephrotic-range proteinuria:
 A. First-line treatment is usually high-dose alternate day prednisone (e.g. 1–2 mg/kg) for 2 months; taper to ~0.25 mg/kg alternate days within 3–4 months
 B. Optional adjuncts to prednisone therapy
  1. Cyclosporine, ≤5 mg/kg/day
  2. Pulse cyclophosphamide, ≤1 g/m² every 1–3 months
  3. Pulse methylprednisolone alternating with cyclophosphamide (or chlorambucil): pulse methylprednisolone, 1.0 g/day for 3 days followed by 27 days of prednisone (0.5 mg/kg/day) alternating with 30 days of cyclophosphamide 2 mg/kg/day (or chlorambucil 3–6 mg/m²/day); three cycles of each therapy over a 6-month period
  4. Oral cyclophosphamide, 2 mg/kg/day

III. Membranous nephropathy with non-nephrotic proteinuria: treat according to extrarenal disease activity; consider angiotensin antagonists to minimize proteinuria and statins for hyperlipidemia; monitor patients carefully for evidence of progression to nephrotic syndrome or to mixed membranous and proliferative nephropathy

*See also Chapter 24.

focus. At the present time, it appears that one can justifiably choose among several options of maintenance therapy aimed at reducing the risk of relapse, including quarterly pulse cyclophosphamide, azathioprine, or mycophenolate.

SLE and endstage renal failure

None of the current regimens for treatment of lupus nephritis is fully effective in preventing renal failure. However, severe glomerulonephritis with uremia is not synonymous with irreversible, endstage renal failure in lupus nephritis. The rate of evolution of renal failure has very important implications for treatment. Rapidly progressive renal failure, usually due to necrotizing and crescentic glomerulonephritis, is often reversible with effective treatment. Patients with evidence of active nephritis (specifically, nephritic urine sediment), even if oliguric and in advanced renal failure, warrant treatment with pulse methylprednisolone, prednisone, and pulse cyclophosphamide for approximately 3 months into maintenance dialysis therapy.

This disease profile can be contrasted with that of patients who progress slowly and insidiously to irreversible endstage renal failure. In the latter case, one should avoid the desperate and injudicious use of aggressive immunosuppressive drug therapy in the setting of "burned out" lupus (e.g. renal failure in the context of contracted kidneys and urine sediment showing predominantly broad, waxy casts). On the other hand, a

substantial proportion of patients on maintenance hemodialysis continue to manifest or experience flares of lupus activity which are clearly indications for continued treatment.[25,101,102] A cautious, incremental prescription of prednisone and immunosuppressive drug therapy in such patients is warranted in order not to increase susceptibility to major infections in the uremic host.

Kidney transplantation is a viable alternative for patients with endstage renal disease caused by lupus nephritis. Clinically active lupus is rare, but evidence of recurrence of lupus nephritis in the allograft is increasingly recognized, although it is a rare cause of allograft loss.[103–105]

Future directions

Experimental therapies

There are a number of novel therapies which are candidates for further testing in lupus mice (Table 17.1) and eventual application to human SLE and lupus nephritis. Translational work has begun employing different methods aimed at overhauling the disordered immune system of patients with severe and conventional treatment-refractory SLE. Recent availability of therapeutic granulocyte colony-stimulating factor (G-CSF) has allowed immunoablative regimens involving extreme doses of cyclophosphamide (e.g. 200 mg/kg) with or without adjunctive fludarabine, total body irradiation, and antithymocyte globulin to be tested.[106–111] Results to date are encouraging, but these immunoablative and reconstituting regimens are associated with substantial morbidity, high costs, and not insignificant risk of failure, relapse, and death.[112]

Unanswered questions

Several issues remain to be addressed in future clinical trials. These include, among others: (1) studies of the comparative benefits of recycling short-term, intense immunosuppressive drug treatment for relapses versus long-term, low-intensity maintenance therapies to avert relapses and minimize cumulative renal damage in lupus nephritis, (2) identification of maintenance therapy with the best therapeutic index, (3) assessment of risks and benefits of early treatment of mesangial disease, and (4) studies to define optimal treatment of lupus membranous nephropathy.

References

1. Lahita RG (ed): Systemic Lupus Erythematosus, 3rd edn. San Diego: Academic Press, 1999.
2. Wallace DJ, Hahn BH (eds): Dubois' Lupus Erythematosus, 6th edn. Philadelphia: Lippincott Williams & Wilkins, 2002.
3. Hahn BH: Antibodies to DNA. N Engl J Med 1998;338:1359.
4. Balow JE, Boumpas DT, Austin HA: Renal Disease. In Schur P (ed): The Clinical Management of Systemic Lupus Erythematosus, 2nd edn. Philadelphia: Lippincott-Raven, 1996, p 109.
5. Appel GB, Radhakrishnan J, D'Agati V: Secondary glomerular diseases. In Brenner BM (ed): Brenner & Rector's The Kidney, 6th edn. Philadelphia: WB Saunders, 2000, p 1350.

6. Lewis EJ, Schwartz MM, Korbet SM (eds): Lupus Nephritis. Oxford: Oxford University Press, 1999.

7. Oates JC, Gilkeson GS: Mediators of injury in lupus nephritis. Curr Opin Rheumatol 2002;14:498.

8. Kewalramani R, Singh AK: Immunopathogenesis of lupus and lupus nephritis: recent insights. Curr Opin Nephrol Hypertens 2002;11:273.

9. Balow JE, Austin HA: Progress in the treatment of proliferative lupus nephritis. Curr Opin Nephrol Hypertens 2000;9:107.

10. Esdaile JM: How to manage patients with lupus nephritis. Best Pract Res Clin Rheumatol 2002;16:195.

11. Ponticelli C: Treatment of lupus nephritis – the advantages of a flexible approach. Nephrol Dial Transplant 1997;12:2057.

12. Cameron JS: Lupus nephritis. J Am Soc Nephrol 1999;10:413.

13. Donadio JV Jr, Hart GM, Bergstralh EJ, et al: Prognostic determinants in lupus nephritis: a long-term clinicopathologic study. Lupus 1995;4:109.

14. Huong DL, Papo T, Beaufils H, et al: Renal involvement in systemic lupus erythematosus. A study of 180 patients from a single center. Medicine (Baltimore) 1999;78:148.

15. Rasoulpour M, Banco L, Laut JM, et al: Inability of community-based laboratories to identify pathological casts in urine samples. Arch Pediatr Adolesc Med 1996;150:1201.

16. Grande JP, Balow JE: Renal biopsy in lupus nephritis. Lupus 1998;7:611.

17. Esdaile JM: Current role of renal biopsy in patients with SLE. Baillieres Clin Rheumatol 1998;12:433.

18. Churg J, Bernstein J, Glassock RJ: Lupus nephritis. In Renal Disease: Classification and Atlas of Glomerular Diseases, 2nd edn. New York, Igaku-Shoin, 1995, p 151.

19. Esdaile JM, MacKenzie T, Kashgarian M, et al: The benefit of early treatment with immunosuppressive agents in lupus nephritis. J Rheumatol 1994;21:2046.

20. Dambrin C, Klupp J, Morris RE: Pharmacodynamics of immunosuppressive drugs. Curr Opin Nephrol Hypertens 2000;15:557.

21. Hahn BH: Lessons in lupus: the mighty mouse. Lupus 2001;10:589.

22. Daikh DI, Wofsy D: Reversal of murine lupus nephritis with CTLA4Ig and cyclophosphamide. J Immunol 2001;166:2913.

23. Lewis EJ: The treatment of lupus nephritis: revisiting Galen (editorial). Ann Intern Med 2001;135:296.

24. Donadio JV Jr, Glassock RJ: Immunosuppressive drug therapy in lupus nephritis. Am J Kidney Dis 1993;21:239.

25. Berden JH. Lupus nephritis (Nephrology Forum). Kidney Int 1997;52:538.

26. Bakir AA, Levy PS, Dunea G: The prognosis of lupus nephritis in African-Americans: a retrospective analysis. Am J Kidney Dis 1994;24:159.

27. Baqi N, Moazami S, Singh A, et al: Lupus nephritis in children: a longitudinal study of prognostic factors and therapy. J Am Soc Nephrol 1996;7:924.

28. Conlon PJ, Fischer CA, Levesque MC, et al: Clinical, biochemical and pathological predictors of poor response to intravenous cyclophosphamide in patients with proliferative lupus nephritis. Clin Nephrol 1996;46:170.

29. Dooley MA, Hogan S, Jennette JC, et al: Cyclophosphamide therapy for lupus nephritis: poor renal survival in black Americans. Kidney Int 1997;51:1188.

30. Gruppo Italiano per lo Studio della Nefrite Lupica (GISNEL): Lupus nephritis: prognostic factors and probability of maintaining life-supporting renal function 10 years after the diagnosis. Am J Kidney Dis 1992;19:473.

31. Bastian HM, Roseman JM, McGwin G, et al: Systemic lupus erythematosus in three ethnic groups. XII. Risk factors for lupus nephritis after diagnosis. Lupus 2002;11:152.

32. Seligman VA, Lum RF, Olson JL, et al: Demographic differences in the development of lupus nephritis: a retrospective analysis. Am J Med 2002;112:729.

33. Balow JE: Choosing treatment for proliferative lupus nephritis (editorial). Arthritis Rheum 2002;46:1981.

34. Sztejnbok M, Stewart A, Diamond H, et al: Azathioprine in the treatment of systemic lupus erythematosus: a controlled study. Arthritis Rheum 1971;14:639.

35. Donadio JV Jr, Holley KE, Wagoner RD, et al: Treatment of lupus nephritis with prednisone and combined prednisone and azathioprine. Ann Intern Med 1972;77:829.

36. Donadio JV Jr, Holley KE, Wagoner RD, et al: Further observations on the treatment of lupus nephritis with prednisone and combined prednisone and azathioprine. Arthritis Rheum 1974;17:573.

37. Cade R, Spooner G, Schlein E, et al: Comparison of azathioprine, prednisone, and heparin alone or combined in treating lupus nephritis. Nephron 1973;10:37.

38. Steinberg AD, Decker JL: A double-blind controlled trial comparing cyclophosphamide, azathioprine and placebo in the treatment of lupus glomerulonephritis. Arthritis Rheum 1974;17:923.

39. Decker JL, Klippel JH, Plotz PH, et al: Cyclophosphamide or azathioprine in lupus glomerulonephritis. Ann Intern Med 1975;83:606.

40. Hahn BH, Kantor OS, Osterland CK: Azathioprine plus prednisone compared with prednisone alone in the treatment of systemic lupus erythematosus. Ann Intern Med 1975;83:597.

41. Austin HA, Klippel JH, Balow JE, et al: Therapy of lupus nephritis: controlled trial of prednisone and cytotoxic drugs. N Engl J Med 1986;314:614.

42. Steinberg AD, Steinberg SC: Long-term preservation of renal function in patient with lupus nephritis receiving treatment that includes cyclophosphamide versus those treated with prednisone only. Arthritis Rheum 1991;34:945.

43. Donadio JV Jr, Holley KE, Ferguson RH, et al: Treatment of diffuse proliferative lupus nephritis with prednisone and combined prednisone and cyclophosphamide. N Engl J Med 1978;299:1151.

44. Donadio JV Jr, Holley KE, Ilstrup DM: Cytotoxic drug treatment of lupus nephritis. Am J Kidney Dis 1982;2(Suppl):178.

45. Boumpas DT, Austin HA, Vaughan EM, et al: Severe lupus nephritis: controlled trial of pulse methylprednisolone versus two different regimens of pulse cyclophosphamide. Lancet 1992;340:741.

46. Sesso R, Monteiro M, Sato E, et al: A controlled trial of pulse cyclophosphamide versus pulse methylprednisolone in severe lupus nephritis. Lupus 1994;3:107.

47. Gourley MF, Austin HA, Scott D, et al: Methylprednisolone and cyclophosphamide, alone or in combination, in patients with lupus nephritis: a randomized, controlled trial. Ann Intern Med 1996;125:549.

48. Illei GG, Austin HA, Crane M, et al: Combination therapy with pulse cyclophosphamide plus pulse methylprednisolone improves long-term renal outcome without adding toxicity in patients with lupus nephritis. Ann Intern Med 2001;135:248.

49. Boletis JN, Ioannidis JP, Boki KA, et al: Intravenous immunoglobulin compared with cyclophosphamide for proliferative lupus nephritis. Lancet 1999;354:569.

50. Chan TM, Li FK, Tang CS, et al: Efficacy of mycophenolate mofetil in patients with diffuse proliferative lupus nephritis. N Engl J Med 2000;343:1156.

51. Chan TM, Wong WS, Lau CS, et al: Prolonged follow-up of patients with diffuse proliferative lupus nephritis (DPLN) treated with prednisolone and mycophenolate mofetil (MMF). J Am Soc Nephrol 2001;12:195A.

52. Houssiau FA, Vasconcelos C, D'Cruz DD, et al: Immunosuppressive therapy in lupus nephritis: the Euro-Lupus Nephritis Trial, a randomized trial of low-dose versus high-dose intravenous cyclophosphamide. Arthritis Rheum 2002;46:2121.

53. Lewis EJ, Hunsicker LG, Lan SP, et al: A controlled trial of plasmapheresis therapy in severe lupus nephritis. N Engl J Med 1992;326:1373.

54. Wallace DJ, Goldfinger D, Pepkowitz SH, et al: Randomized controlled trial of pulse/synchronization cyclophosphamide/apheresis for proliferative lupus nephritis. J Clin Apheresis 1998;13:163.

55. Ligtenberg G, Grootscholten CM, Derkson RH, Berden JH: Cyclophosphamide pulse therapy versus azathioprine and methylprednisolone pulses in proliferative lupus nephritis: first results of a randomized, prospective multicenter study (abstract). J Am Soc Nephrol 2002;13:14A.

56. Contreras G, Pardo V, Leclercq B, et al: Maintenance therapy for proliferative forms of lupus nephritis: a randomized clinical trial comparing quarterly intravenous cyclophosphamide (IVCY) versus oral mycophenolate mofetil (MMF) or azathioprine (AZA) (abstract). J Am Soc Nephrol 2002;13:15A.

57. Mok CC, Ho CT, Siu YP, et al: Treatment of diffuse proliferative lupus glomerulonephritis: a comparison of two cyclophosphamide-containing regimens. Am J Kidney Dis 2001;38:256.

58. Haubitz M, Schellong S, Gobel U, et al: Intravenous pulse

administration of cyclophosphamide versus daily oral treatment in patients with antineutrophil cytoplasmic antibody-associated vasculitis and renal involvement: a prospective, randomized study. Arthritis Rheum 1998;41:1835.

59. Lehman TJ, Onel K: Intermittent intravenous cyclophosphamide arrests progression of the renal chronicity index in childhood systemic lupus erythematosus. J Pediatr 2000;136:243.

60. Barbano G, Gusmano R, Damasio B, et al: Childhood-onset lupus nephritis: a single-center experience of pulse intravenous cyclophosphamide therapy. J Nephrol 2002;15:123.

61. Balow JE, Austin HA, Muenz LR, et al: Effect of treatment on the evolution of renal abnormalities in lupus nephritis. N Engl J Med 1984;311:491.

62. Choi MJ, Eustace JA, Gimenez LF, et al: Mycophenolate mofetil treatment for primary glomerular diseases. Kidney Int 2002;61:1098.

63. Dooley MA, Cosio FG, Nachman PH, et al: Mycophenolate mofetil therapy in lupus nephritis: clinical observations. J Am Soc Nephrol 1999;10:833.

64. Karim MY, Alba P, Cuadrado MJ, et al: Mycophenolate mofetil for systemic lupus erythematosus refractory to other immunosuppressive agents. Rheumatology 2002;41:876.

65. Mok CC, Lai KN: Mycophenolate mofetil in lupus glomerulonephritis. Am J Kidney Dis 2002;40:447.

66. Ginzler EM: Clinical trials in lupus nephritis. Curr Rheumatol Rep 2001;3:199.

67. Madore F, Lazarus JM, Brady HR: Therapeutic plasma exchange in renal diseases. J Am Soc Nephrol 1996;7:367.

68. Wallace DJ: Apheresis for lupus erythematosus. Lupus 1999;8:174.

69. Austin HA, Boumpas DT, Vaughan EM, et al: Predicting renal outcomes in severe lupus nephritis: contributions of clinical and histologic data. Kidney Int 1994;45:544.

70. Austin HA, Boumpas DT, Vaughan EM, et al: High-risk features of lupus nephritis: importance of race and clinical and histological factors in 166 patients. Nephrol Dial Transplant 1995;10:1620.

71. Lea JP: Lupus nephritis in African Americans. Am J Med Sci 2002;323:85.

72. Dawisha SM, Yarboro CH, Vaughan EM, et al: Outpatient monthly oral bolus cyclophosphamide therapy in systemic lupus erythematosus. J Rheumatol 1996;23:273.

73. Mok CC, Ho CT, Siu YP, et al: Treatment of diffuse proliferative lupus glomerulonephritis: a comparison of two cyclophosphamide-containing regimens. Am J Kidney Dis 2001;38:256.

74. Davis JC, Austin HA, Boumpas DT, et al: A pilot study of 2-chloro-2′-deoxyadenosine in the treatment of systemic lupus erythematosus-associated glomerulonephritis. Arthritis Rheum 1998;41:335.

75. Davis JC, Manzi S, Yarboro C, et al: Recombinant human DNase I (rhDNase) in patients with lupus nephritis. Lupus 1999;8:68.

76. Huang W, Sinha J, Newman J, et al: The effect of anti-CD40 ligand antibody on B cells in human systemic lupus erythematosus. Arthritis Rheum 2002;46:1554.

77. Miescher PA, Favre H, Lemoine R, et al: Drug combination therapy of systemic lupus erythematosus. Semin Immunopathol 1994;16:295.

78. Remer CF, Weisman MH, Wallace DJ: Benefits of leflunomide in systemic lupus erythematosus: a pilot observational study. Lupus 2001;10:480.

79. Tam LS, Li EK, Leung CB, et al: Long-term treatment of lupus nephritis with cyclosporin A. Q J Med 1998;91:573.

80. Radhakrishnan J, Kunis CL, D'Agati V, et al: Cyclosporine treatment of lupus membranous nephropathy. Clin Nephrol 1994;42:147.

81. Austin HA, Vaughan EM, Balow JE: Lupus membranous nephropathy: randomized controlled trial of prednisone, cyclosporine, and cyclophosphamide (Abstract). J Am Soc Nephrol 2000;11:81A.

82. Moroni G, Maccario M, Banfi G, et al: Treatment of membranous lupus nephritis. Am J Kidney Dis 1998;31:681.

83. Hallegua D, Wallace DJ, Metzger AL, et al: Cyclosporine for lupus membranous nephritis: experience with ten patients and review of the literature. Lupus 2000;9:241.

84. Chan TM, Li FK, Hao WK, et al: Treatment of membranous lupus nephritis with nephrotic syndrome by sequential immunosuppression. Lupus 1999;8:545.

85. Silvestris F, D'Amore O, Cafforio P, et al: Intravenous immune globulin therapy of lupus nephritis: use of pathogenic anti-DNA reactive IgG. Clin Exp Immunol 1996;104(Suppl 1):91.

86. Boumpas DT, Austin HA, Vaughan EM, et al: Risk for sustained amenorrhea in patients with systemic lupus erythematosus

receiving intermittent pulse cyclophosphamide therapy. Ann Intern Med 1993;119:366.

87. McDermott EM, Powell RJ: Incidence of ovarian failure in systemic lupus after treatment with pulse cyclophosphamide. Ann Rheum Dis 1996;55:224.

88. Blumenfeld Z, Shapiro D, Shteinberg M, et al: Preservation of fertility and ovarian function and minimizing gonadotoxicity in young women with systemic lupus erythematosus treated by chemotherapy. Lupus 2000;9:401.

89. Abu-Shakra M, Ehrenfeld M, Shoenfeld Y: Systemic lupus erythematosus and cancer: associated or not? Lupus 2002;11:137.

90. Cibere J, Sibley J, Haga M: Systemic lupus erythematosus and the risk of malignancy. Lupus 2001;10:394.

91. Sloan RP, Schwartz MM, Korbet SM, et al: Long-term outcome in systemic lupus erythematosus membranous glomerulonephritis. J Am Soc Nephrol 1996;7:299.

92. Bootsma H, Spronk P, Derksen R, et al: Prevention of relapses in systemic lupus erythematosus. Lancet 1995;345:1595.

93. Ciruelo E, de la Cruz J, Lopez I, et al: Cumulative rate of relapse of lupus nephritis after successful treatment with cyclophosphamide. Arthritis Rheum 1996;39:2028.

94. Hill GS, Delahousse M, Nochy D, et al: Outcome of relapse in lupus nephritis: roles of reversal of renal fibrosis and response of inflammation to therapy. Kidney Int 2002;61:2176.

95. Illei GG, Takada K, Parkin D, et al: Renal flares are common in patients with severe proliferative lupus nephritis treated with pulse immunosuppressive therapy. Arthritis Rheum 2002;46:995.

96. Ioannides JP, Boki KA, Katsorida ME, et al: Remission, relapse, and re-remission of proliferative lupus nephritis treated with cyclophosphamide. Kidney Int 2000;57:258.

97. Korbet SM, Lewis EJ, Schwartz MM, et al: Factors predictive of outcome in severe lupus nephritis. Lupus Nephritis Collaborative Study Group. Am J Kidney Dis 2000;35:904.

98. Moroni G, Quaglini S, Maccario M, et al: "Nephritic flares" are predictors of bad long-term renal outcome in lupus nephritis. Kidney Int 1996;50:2047.

99. Ponticelli C, Moroni G: Flares in lupus nephritis: incidence, impact on renal survival and management. Lupus 1998;7:635.

100. Swaak AJG, van den Brink HG, Smeenk RJT, et al: Systemic lupus erythematosus. Disease outcome in patients with a disease duration of at least 10 years: second evaluation. Lupus 2001;10:51.

101. Krane NK, Burjak K, Archie M, et al: Persistent disease activity in end-stage renal disease. Am J Kidney Dis 1999;33:872.

102. Ward MM: Cardiovascular and cerebrovascular morbidity and mortality among women with end-stage renal disease attributable to lupus nephritis. Am J Kidney Dis 2000;36:516.

103. Lochhead KM, Pirsch JD, D'Alessandro AM, et al: Risk factors for renal allograft loss in patients with systemic lupus erythematosus. Kidney Int 1996;49:512.

104. Stone JH, Millward CL, Olson JL, et al: Frequency of recurrent lupus nephritis among ninety-seven renal transplant patients during the cyclosporine era. Arthritis Rheum 1998;41:678.

105. Ward MM: Outcomes of renal transplantation among patients with end-stage renal disease caused by lupus nephritis. Kidney Int 2000;57:2136.

106. Brodsky RA, Petri M, Smith BD, et al: Immunoablative high-dose cyclophosphamide without stem cell rescue for refractory, severe autoimmune disease. Ann Intern Med 1998;129:1031.

107. Brodsky RA: High-dose cyclophosphamide for aplastic anemia and autoimmune diseases. Curr Opin Oncol 2002;14:143.

108. Traynor AE, Schroeder J, Rosa RM, et al: Treatment of severe systemic lupus erythematosus with high-dose chemotherapy and haematopoietic stem-cell transplantation: a phase 1 study. Lancet 2000;356:701.

109. Brunner M, Greinix HT, Redlich K, et al: Autologous blood stem cell transplantation in refractory systemic lupus erythematosus with severe pulmonary impairment. Arthritis Rheum 2002;46:1580.

110. Furst DE: Stem cell transplantation for autoimmune disease: progress and problems. Curr Opin Rheumatol 2002;14:220.

111. Marmont AM: Lupus: tinkering with haematopoietic stem cells. Lupus 2001;10:769.

112. Shaughnessy PJ, Ririe DW, Ornstein DL, et al: Graft failure in a patient with systemic lupus erythematosus (SLE) treated with high-dose immunosuppression and autologous stem cell rescue. Bone Marrow Transplantation 2001;27:221.

IgA Nephropathy and Henoch–Schönlein Purpura

John Feehally

Background

IgA nephropathy

IgA nephropathy (IgAN) is a common pattern of glomerulonephritis defined by mesangial IgA deposition.[1] Recurrent macroscopic hematuria is the most frequent clinical presentation, and typically occurs in the second and third decades of life. Other patients present with microscopic hematuria, proteinuria, and slowly progressive renal failure. Clinical features at the time of diagnosis indicating a poor prognosis include proteinuria > 1 g per 24 h and arterial hypertension.[2] Adverse histopathologic features include glomerular sclerosis, tubular atrophy, and interstitial fibrosis.[2] Rapidly progressive renal failure is unusual; it may result from acute tubular necrosis as a consequence of macroscopic hematuria or superimposed crescentic nephritis. Recurrent IgA deposition after transplantation is common, and may be associated with slowly progressive graft failure.[3]

Henoch–Schönlein nephritis

Henoch–Schönlein purpura (HSP) is a systemic vasculitis with characteristic rash, abdominal pain, and arthralgia; it is particularly common in childhood but may occur at any age. Tissue IgA deposition is a hallmark of HSP. The nephritis that accompanies HSP (HS nephritis) may be histologically indistinguishable from IgAN,[4] although a nephritic/nephrotic presentation with relatively rapid progression to renal failure is more common than in IgAN. It is probable that IgAN is a monosymptomatic form of HSP.[4,5]

Disease mechanisms in IgA nephropathy and Henoch–Schönlein nephritis

IgAN and HSP share many abnormalities of the IgA immune system.[5] Exaggerated polymeric IgA1 (pIgA1) responses are typical, although increases in circulating IgA1 are modest. Most evidence suggests that the increased pIgA1 originates from the bone marrow rather than the mucosa.[6] The mechanism of mesangial IgA deposition is not understood, although IgAN and HS nephritis are often regarded as immune complex diseases. Altered glycosylation of IgA1 may promote mesangial IgA deposition.[7] Mechanisms of ongoing inflammation and scarring are probably common to other forms of chronic glomerulonephritis without IgA deposition. There is increasing evidence for genetic susceptibility to IgAN and HSP, for example the high prevalence of urinary abnormalities in first- and second-degree relatives of those with IgAN, and the substantial number of multiplex families, in some of which both HSP and IgAN occur.[8,9]

Treatment approaches

Therapeutic strategies

With this background, the following approaches to treatment in IgAN could be considered.

- Reduce production of nephritogenic IgA.
- Prevent glomerular IgA deposition or promote its removal.
- Alter early immune and inflammatory events that follow IgA deposition.
- Alter later nonspecific events that promote progressive renal failure.
- Prevent recurrent disease after transplant.

Therapeutic endpoints

It is also important to consider how the success of any therapeutic intervention might be judged.

Hematuria

Reduction of episodes of macroscopic hematuria is a clear-cut goal but should not be taken to represent the loss of all disease activity. Properly controlled studies are needed since the natural history of IgAN is that macroscopic hematuria becomes less common with time without intervention.

Proteinuria

Reduction in proteinuria is an attractive short- and long-term goal. If patients are nephrotic, the clinical benefits of reducing proteinuria and correcting serum albumin are unequivocal. However, treatment trial strategy often selects patients using nonnephrotic proteinuria as a marker of poor prognosis. The benefit of modest reductions in proteinuria, even if statistically significant, is uncertain unless accompanied by preservation of renal function.

Prevention of renal failure

Prevention of endstage renal disease (ESRD) is the ultimate goal. However, IgAN is usually so slowly progressive that surrogate markers are required to provide data within an acceptable time frame. Doubling of serum creatinine or reduction in glomerular filtration rate (GFR) can be complemented by histologic data from serial renal biopsy.

Problems of study design

Study group heterogeneity

It cannot be certain that patients with mesangial IgA deposition always share a common disease process but at present it remains the defining criterion for these studies. Renal histology can be useful in study recruitment to minimize heterogeneity but this will be less useful if the interval between biopsy and recruitment is prolonged. Furthermore, the choice of histologic criteria remains controversial. Patients with HSP have been excluded from most available studies; it is therefore still uncertain whether any strategies developed for IgAN are indeed applicable to HS nephritis.

Risk versus benefit

In slowly progressive disease the balance of risk versus benefit if prolonged treatment is considered is often unfavorable. Acute immune interventions are also not easy to plan. If there is crescentic nephritis with renal failure, intensive treatment is justifiable; more often, visible hematuria is clinically striking but transient and produces no functional renal impairment, weakening the justification for therapy. In any case, clinically apparent hematuria is likely to represent the tip of an iceberg of ongoing injury, so that shaping and timing the intensity of therapy, even if rational treatments were available, is difficult.

The good prognosis for many patients, particularly those with isolated hematuria, argues against their involvement in prolonged studies of therapies with potential adverse effects. On the other hand, the selection of patients by proteinuria can introduce heterogeneity because proteinuria may reflect both active immune injury and fixed chronic damage. Any study using proteinuria as an entry criterion will provide therapeutic guidance for only a minority of patients with IgAN.

Randomized controlled trials

The need for randomized controlled trials (RCTs) of adequate power to answer questions about the prevention of chronic renal failure in IgAN is pressing. The use of historical controls is of limited value since earlier cohorts of patients may not be comparable, for example because of changing attitudes over recent years in accepted blood pressure targets and in the use of medications that interrupt the renin–angiotensin system. It is disappointing, despite the prevalence of IgAN and consensus about its definition and natural history, that there are so few published RCTs. Available studies are clearly defined in this chapter as RCTs and are shown in the tables. Those available in 1998 have been critically reviewed.[10] There have been no RCTs in HS nephritis.

Age of subjects

There is no specific evidence that IgAN is a distinctive disease process when onset is in childhood rather than adult life; nevertheless, the application to adult practice of trial findings in children remains uncertain.[11]

Defining early and late disease

The distinction between early inflammatory processes in IgAN and later nonspecific processes leading to renal failure is not easily made and is somewhat artificial. In a disease as indolent as IgAN such processes will inevitably be concurrent. Diagnosis, defined by the time of renal biopsy, may be many years after the onset of the disease. RCTs of corticosteroids and immunosuppressive regimens have mostly recruited patients with proteinuria and preserved renal function, while studies of fish oil have in general recruited those with proteinuria and impaired excretory function. However one study, recently completed and not yet reported, makes a direct comparison of fish oils and corticosteroids.[12]

Treatment of IgA nephropathy

Reduction of IgA production
Reduce mucosal antigen challenge

Attempts have been made in uncontrolled studies to modify food antigen intake or alter mucosal permeability pharmacologically. These have been of little benefit.[13] There is no role for prophylactic antibiotics.

Tonsillectomy

Tonsillectomy has been shown to reduce the frequency of episodic hematuria when tonsillitis is the provoking infection.[14] However, in retrospective studies there is no evidence that tonsillectomy reduces the incidence of progressive renal failure.[15] The lack of RCTs to resolve this question is particularly important because the natural history of IgAN is that episodes of macroscopic hematuria become less frequent with time independent of any specific treatment.

Phenytoin

Phenytoin reduces serum IgA levels and was given in an RCT for 2 years, but it produced no benefit to renal function or proteinuria nor in renal histology in repeat biopsies after treatment.[16]

Other approaches for reducing IgA production

There are no other known strategies for reducing relevant IgA production. There is no evidence that any immunosuppressive treatment used in IgAN alters circulating IgA levels, although the possibility cannot be excluded that a number of immune manipulations may reduce a specific subset of nephritogenic pIgA1 molecules. However, no intervention is known to modify the abnormal IgA1 glycosylation found in IgAN.

Prevention and removal of IgA deposits

The ideal treatment for IgAN would remove IgA from the glomerulus and prevent further IgA deposition. This remains a remote prospect while IgA deposition is so poorly understood. Such a treatment would also need to be extremely safe because it would require application to large numbers of patients with benign disease unless reliable early markers of progression risk were available. The high prevalence of recurrent IgA deposition after transplantation suggests that conventional immuno-

suppression does not prevent IgA deposition even if it may alter subsequent inflammatory events.

Alteration of immune and inflammatory events that follow IgA deposition
Rapidly progressive renal failure associated with crescentic IgA nephritis

In this uncommon situation, the risk–benefit balance is most strongly placed in favor of intensive immunosuppressive therapy, since if crescentic IgA nephritis is not treated there will almost inevitably be rapid progression to ESRD. Unfortunately there are no available RCTs.

There are a number of case reports, of which nine have been reviewed by Lai.[17] The largest single-center experiences in adults are nine cases reported by Macintyre et al,[18] 12 reported by Roccatello et al,[19] and 16 reported by Harper et al.[20] Reports in 19 children have been reviewed.[11] Treatment in the majority of cases has included prednisolone and cyclophosphamide, often combined with plasma exchange. It is not possible to make firm conclusions from these data. The decision to treat is usually made on histologic evidence of aggressive glomerular injury, and most reports include some patients with preserved renal function at the time treatment is initiated as well as those with rapidly progressive renal failure. Early clinical response is favorable as in other crescentic nephritis but medium-term results may be disappointing: 60% of treated patients reached ESRD by 12 months in one series[21] and 25% reached ESRD over longer follow-up in another.[20] However a subset of patients has been reported with circulating IgG–antineutrophil cytoplasmic antibody (ANCA) who have a more favorable response to immunosuppressive therapy, similar to that seen in other types of ANCA-positive crescentic nephritis.[22]

An RCT of immunosuppressive treatments in crescentic IgAN would be particularly valuable, but this is an uncommon condition and such a trial may never be achieved. On the available evidence the use of corticosteroids and cyclophosphamide is justified, but there is insufficient information to recommend the addition of plasma exchange.

Early treatment with immunosuppressive/ anti-inflammatory regimens

Interventions have been made in IgAN soon after diagnosis in those with active disease, even when renal function is still preserved. Treatments have included corticosteroids, cyclophosphamide, azathioprine, and pooled human immunoglobulin. In some studies they have been combined with antiplatelet agents and warfarin. The great majority of such studies are restricted to those with proteinuria > 1 g per 24 h, an arbitrary threshold known to be associated with significant risk of progression. The minority with nephrotic syndrome have been excluded from most studies.

Corticosteroids There has been interest in the potential role of corticosteroids for many years, supported mostly by evidence from uncontrolled trials. In adults with heavy proteinuria,[23] corticosteroids appeared to preserve renal function if initial creatinine clearance was > 70 mL/min, and the same group reported 10-year follow-up in moderate proteinuria that suggests reduced risk of ESRD with corticosteroids.[24]

However there have been only four RCTs of corticosteroids (Table 18.1). Three months of treatment in children with low-grade proteinuria showed no benefit.[25] Four months of treatment in nephrotic adults showed no overall benefit,[26] although there was a minority with very minor histologic changes who responded rapidly to treatment (see section Nephrotic syndrome and IgAN).

A recent RCT evaluated 12 months of corticosteroids with antiplatelet agents in nonnephrotic proteinuria with preserved renal function;[27] the control group also received antiplatelet agents. There was a reduction in proteinuria and improvement in histology, but the design and power of the study prevented investigation of any possible protection of renal function.

A larger RCT of 6 months' treatment with corticosteroids showed not only a reduction in proteinuria but also a significant reduction in the risk of a twofold rise in serum creatinine or ESRD.[28] Further analysis shows that the benefit is sustained for up to 6 years of follow-up.[29] Angiotensin-converting enzyme (ACE) inhibitors were not used in all patients in this study but were used in equal proportions in both corticosteroid-treated patients and control subjects. The authors also report a lack of steroid adverse effects despite the substantial dosage over 6 months.

This study remains the only evidence from an RCT that corticosteroids prevent renal failure in IgAN with proteinuria > 1 g per 24 h. However the benefit must be viewed in context; analysis shows that the protection was no greater than that afforded by female gender,[29] emphasizing the need to understand better the many factors that contribute to the highly variable natural history of IgAN. A further study is underway to assess the additional benefit of azathioprine with corticosteroids in similar patients, although unfortunately this study will not contain a control group not receiving corticosteroids.[30] Another study is currently investigating the additional benefits of 6 months of treatment with corticosteroids in patients with IgAN with proteinuria > 1 g per 24 h receiving long-term ACE inhibitor therapy.[31]

Cyclophosphamide (see Table 18.2) Cyclophosphamide has been used in combination with warfarin and dipyridamole in two RCTs that are not consistent. Two studies of very similar design both showed modest reduction in proteinuria,[32,33] but the preservation of renal function in one study[32] could not be confirmed.[31] Cyclophosphamide has not been used alone in IgAN. In any case, many physicians regard the risk of cyclophosphamide as unacceptable in young adults with IgAN. Further studies

Table 18.1 Randomized controlled trials of corticosteroid treatment in IgA nephropathy

Reference	Entry criteria	Number on active treatment	Treatment period (months)	Follow-up (months)	Proteinuria before treatment (mean, g/24h)	Proteinuria after treatment (mean, g/24h)	Other benefits	Comment
Lai et al[26]	Nephrotic Serum creatinine < 3 mg/dL	17 (adults)	4	12–106	6.5	2.3	Remission of nephrotic syndrome in 6 of 7 with minor histologic change	40% had steroid-related adverse effects
Welch et al[25]	Serum creatinine < 1.6 mg/dL	20 (children)	3	6	0.7	0.6	None	
Pozzi et al[28,29]	Urine protein 1–3.5 g/24 h Serum creatinine < 1.5 mg/dL	43 (adults)	6	60–120	2.0	0.67	Risk of ESRD reduced	No major adverse effects reported
Shoji et al[27]	Urine protein < 1.5 g/24 h Serum creatinine < 1.5 mg/dL	11 (adults)	12	13	0.8	0.3	Histologic improvement	All received dipyridamole None received ACE inhibitors

ACE, angiotensin-converting enzyme; ESRD, endstage renal disease.

Table 18.2 Randomized controlled trials of immunosuppressive treatment in IgA nephropathy*

Reference	Entry criteria	Agents	Number on active treatment	Duration of treatment (months)	Follow-up (months)	Benefit	Comment
Woo et al[32]	Serum creatinine <1.5 mg/dL Urine protein < 5 g/24 h	Cyclophosphamide +dipyridamole/warfarin	27	6	60	Proteinuria reduced (mean 2.4 to 0.8 g/24 h) Glomerulosclerosis prevented	Cyclophosphamide for 6 months Dipyridamole/warfarin for 24 months
Walker et al[33]	Serum creatinine 1.1–1.8 mg/dL Urine protein > 1 g/24 h	Cyclophosphamide +dipyridamole/warfarin	25	6	24	Proteinuria reduced (mean 1.7 to 1.2 g/24 h) Renal function unchanged	Cyclophosphamide for 6 months Dipyridamole/warfarin for 36 months
Yoshikawa et al[37]	Active biopsy CC normal Not nephrotic	Azathioprine + prednisolone + dipyridamole + low-dose warfarin	39 (children)	24	24	Proteinuria reduced (mean 1.3 to 0.2 g/24 h) Glomerulosclerosis prevented Intensity of IgA deposits reduced	Control group received dipyridamole/warfarin Renal function normal and unchanged in both groups
Lai et al[38]	Urine protein > 1.5 g/24 h	Cyclosporine	9	3	6	Transient reduction in proteinuria (mean 4.2 to 1.3 g/24 h)	Parallel fall in renal function reversed when cyclosporine was withdrawn

CC, creatinine clearance.
*There are no randomized controlled trials of immunosuppressive agents in crescentic/vasculitic IgA nephropathy; available data are discussed in the text.

have therefore assessed the combination of warfarin and dipyridamole without cyclophosphamide (see section Antiplatelet agents).

Azathioprine (see Table 18.2) In an open study of children with aggressive disease, azathioprine with prednisolone appeared to preserve renal function.[34] In a long-term retrospective study,[35] azathioprine with prednisolone preserved renal function but unfortunately the control group is not comparable. A nonrandomized trial of azathioprine or chlorambucil in adults showed no benefit for either agent.[36] An RCT in children of 2 years of treatment with prednisolone and azathioprine (combined with antiplatelet agents) showed a reduction in proteinuria and lessening of active glomerular injury on repeat renal biopsy.[37] However, all subjects had preserved renal function at recruitment and the rather short duration of follow-up precluded any investigation of an effect on preservation of renal function.

Cyclosporine (see Table 18.2) Cyclosporine has been used in one RCT.[36] There was a reversible fall in proteinuria but this occurred in parallel with a fall in creatinine clearance, suggesting the changes were a hemodynamic effect of cyclosporine rather than an immune-modulating effect.

Pooled human immunoglobulin The immunomodulatory and anti-inflammatory effects of pooled human immunoglobulin are poorly defined but they have some benefit in uncontrolled studies in systemic vasculitis and lupus. They have little short-term toxicity, although long-term effects have not yet been well documented. Open studies of immunoglobulin have been reported in both "severe" IgAN (heavy proteinuria with falling GFR)[39] and "moderate" IgAN (persistent proteinuria with GFR > 70 mL/min).[40] Proteinuria diminished, deterioration in GFR slowed in the severe group, and histologic activity scores lessened where repeat renal biopsies were available. No prospective controlled trial is yet available for this promising approach.

Nephrotic syndrome in IgA nephropathy

Nephrotic syndrome occurs in only 10% of IgAN. In many of these patients the heavy proteinuria is a manifestation of significant structural glomerular damage and progressive renal dysfunction. However a small minority, both adults and children, have nephrosis with minimal glomerular change on renal biopsy, although there are IgA deposits with hematuria; proteinuria remits promptly in response to corticosteroids.[26] In these patients, two common glomerular diseases may coincide: minimal-change nephrotic syndrome and IgAN.[41,42] This observation justifies a trial of high-dose corticosteroids, using a regimen appropriate for minimal change disease, in IgAN with nephrotic syndrome and preserved renal function when light microscopy shows minimal glomerular injury. However, there is no evidence to support prolonged exposure to corticosteroids if there is not a prompt response, nor their use in nephrotic syndrome in the presence of significant glomerular inflammation. Unfortunately all recent RCTs of corticosteroids in IgAN have excluded those with nephrotic-range proteinuria, so there is little evidence to inform treatment choices for nephrotic IgAN with significant histologic glomerular injury.

Treatment of slowly progressive IgA nephropathy

There is little to suggest that the events of progressive glomerular injury are unique to IgAN. The growing experimental evidence on mesangial injury and its resolution under the influence of growth factors and cytokines seems to be applicable to mesangial glomerulonephritis whether or not there are IgA deposits. The adverse influence of hypertension and the likely role of proteinuria in progression likewise are common to all glomerular disease.

Treatments available are nonspecific. They are reported as treatments for IgAN but it is more precise to regard them as treatments for chronic glomerular disease, of which IgAN is the commonest and most easily defined. (The immunosuppressive strategems reviewed above may equally be nonspecific in their efficacy.) The main approaches include treatment of hypertension and the use of antiplatelet agents, anticoagulants, fish oil, and HMG-CoA reductase inhibitors.

Predicting risk of progression

At diagnosis conventional clinical and histologic criteria predict cohorts of patients with a poor prognosis.[2] Attempts continue to refine such analyses further in order to improve prediction of outcome early in follow-up for the individual patient. In particular it would be valuable to predict those who will do badly even if they show none of the known adverse features at diagnosis, in order to identify those who require more intensive therapy.[43] Genetic markers for risk of progression have been studied, in particular I/D polymorphisms of the ACE gene.[44] However, the association between the ACE DD genotype and risk of progression is not reliable enough to influence treatment strategies for the individual patient, nor to inform stratification in design of treatment trials.

Antiplatelet agents

The main studies are summarized in Table 18.3. Two studies of dipyridamole/warfarin in combination with cyclophosphamide produced conflicting results (see Table 18.2). In the study in children given azathioprine and corticosteroids, all subjects received dipyridamole/warfarin[37] so no effect of these agents can be inferred. Two RCTs of dipyridamole/warfarin alone are inconsistent: there was no benefit in one,[45] but some reduction in proteinuria and protection from renal impairment in the other.[46]

Hypertension and the role of ACE inhibitors

There is compelling evidence for the benefit of lowering blood pressure in the treatment of chronic progressive glomerular disease. In IgAN, evidence is accumulating that casual clinic blood pressure measurements may under-

Table 18.3 Randomized controlled trials of antiplatelet/anticoagulant treatment in IgA nephropathy

Reference	Entry criteria	Agents	Number on active treatment	Duration of treatment (months)	Follow-up (months)	Benefit	Comment
Woo et al[32]	Serum creatinine < 1.5 mg/dL Urine protein < 5 g/24 h	Dipyridamole/warfarin (+ cyclophosphamide)	27	36	60	Urine protein reduced (mean 2.4 to 0.8 g/24 h) Glomerulosclerosis prevented	Cyclophosphamide for 6 months
Walker et al[33]	Serum creatinine 1.1–1.8 mg/dL Urine protein > 1 g/24 h	Dipyridamole/warfarin (+ cyclophosphamide)	25	24	24	Urine protein reduced (mean 1.7 to 1.2 g/24 h) Renal function unchanged	Cyclophosphamide for 6 months
Chan et al[45]	Serum creatinine < 1.5 mg/dL Urine protein < 2 g/24 h	Dipyridamole/warfarin	19	33	33	None	
Lee et al[46]	Serum creatinine 1.6–3 mg/dL	Dipyridamole/warfarin	11	36	60	Proteinuria reduced (mean 1.4 to 0.6 g/24 h) Renal function maintained	

Table 18.4 Randomized controlled trials of angiotensin-converting enzyme (ACE) inhibitor treatment in IgA nephropathy

Reference	Type of study	Entry criteria	Number on ACE treatment	Follow-up (months)	Outcome	Comment
Maschio et al[49]	Placebo controlled crossover	Urine protein 1–2.5 g/24 h Normotensive	8	8	Proteinuria reduced (mean 1.8 to 1.4 g/24 h)	Short-term study: ? functional importance of minor reduction in proteinuria
Perico et al[50]	RCT Enalapril vs. irbesartan ± indomethacin	Urine protein 0.5–4 g/24 h Serum creatinine < 2.5 mg/dL	10	1	Proteinuria reduced by 55–61% Effect of enalapril = irbesartan Potentiated by indomethacin	Short-term study
Banniste et al[52]	RCT Enalapril vs. nifedipine	Hypertensive GFR 30–90 mL/min	12	12	Proteinuria reduced (mean 2.0 to 1.2 g/24 h) Renal function not different	
Cheng et al[53]	RCT Captopril vs. nadolol/ticlopidine	Urine protein > 1 g/24 h Serum creatinine 1.3–4.4 mg/dL Hypertensive Sclerosis on biopsy	31	> 36	No difference in proteinuria, blood pressure, or renal impairment between ACE inhibitor and nadolol	Advanced disease at time of study

GFR, glomerular filtration rate; RCT, randomized clinical trial.

estimate the early impact of hypertension as judged by ambulatory blood pressure monitoring and echocardiographic evidence of increased left ventricular mass.[47] The impact of the early active management of blood pressure on the long-term cardiovascular morbidity and mortality of these patients will be considerable, independent of any effect on the preservation of renal function. There is also powerful evidence for the primary role of ACE inhibitors in chronic proteinuric renal disease in view of their additional benefits in lowering proteinuria and preserving renal function.[48] However, specific evidence on the role of ACE inhibitors in IgAN is scant (Table 18.4). Short-term randomized studies in normotensive proteinuric IgAN confirm that an ACE inhibitor reduces proteinuria to the same degree as an angiotensin receptor antagonist (ATRA), an effect potentiated by indomethacin.[49,50] Furthermore, the combination of ACE inhibitor and ATRA produces a significant additional fall in proteinuria.[51] The only two RCTs of ACE inhibitors in hypertensive IgAN showed no benefit, although this may be attributable to the relatively short follow-up in one study[52] and the inclusion of patients with advanced disease in the other.[53] However, two retrospective studies in IgAN demonstrated the benefit of using ACE inhibitors for hypertension compared with β-blockers[54] and a wide range of other agents.[55] A placebo-controlled RCT of ACE inhibitors in IgAN with proteinuria > 1 g per 24 h is under way.[56] Despite the relative dearth of specific information in IgAN, ACE inhibitors are recommended as preferred treatment for hypertensive IgAN and should also be considered for normotensive IgAN with significant proteinuria (> 1 g per 24 h).

Fish oil

The available studies are summarized in Table 18.5. The favorable effects of supplementing the diet with ω-3 fatty acids in the form of fish oil include reductions in eicosanoid and cytokine production, changes in membrane fluidity and rheology, and reduced platelet aggregability. These features should significantly reduce the adverse influence of many mechanisms thought to impact on progression of chronic glomerular disease. Fish oil treatment does not have the drawbacks associated with immunosuppressive treatment. It is safe apart from a decrease in blood coaguability, which is not usually a practical problem, and an unpleasant taste with flatulence, which may make compliance difficult.

The study of Donadio et al[61] provides convincing evidence of protection with 6 months of treatment with fish oil (12 g daily). However, an unexpected finding was that fish oil did not significantly reduce proteinuria, which is a major risk factor for progression and which has been reduced in all other studies of agents that are renoprotective in IgAN. The benefit was sustained in a longer follow-up of the same cohort, although treatment allocations were not always sustained after the original trial period was completed.[62] A further study showed no difference in outcome between a high (24 g daily) and low (12 g daily) dose of fish oil; once again, proteinuria did not lessen during follow-up.[63] However, these studies conflict with the smaller study of Bennett et al,[58] which showed no benefit of fish oil. Pettersson et al[60] may have failed to show benefit because of the short follow-up period of 6 months. A metaanalysis of these studies suggests that the available evidence does not yet give unequivocal support for the use of fish oil.[64] A further confirmatory study of fish oil would be of great value. An RCT of fish oil compared with corticosteroids has completed recruitment but no interim analysis is yet available.[12]

HMG-CoA reductase inhibitors

One small RCT showed that 6 months of treatment with the HMG-CoA reductase inhibitor fluvastatin gave a 41% reduction in proteinuria with no effect on GFR.[65] Further prolonged studies are needed to confirm this effect.

Posttransplant recurrence

Mesangial IgA deposition after transplantation is common, occurring in up to 50% of patients whose primary renal disease was IgAN.[66] Graft survival is no worse in registry

Table 18.5 Fish oil treatment in IgA nephropathy

Reference	Entry criteria	Number on active treatment	Duration of treatment (months)	Outcome	Comment
Hamazaki et al[57]	No details	10	12	Renal function stabilized	Randomization not described
Bennett et al[58]	**Proteinuria**	**17**	**24**	**No benefit**	
Cheng et al[59]	Creatinine 3.6 (2–6) mg/dL	11	10 (8–12)	No benefit	Advanced renal impairment at recruitment
Petterson et al[60]	Proteinuria > 0.5 g/24 h Creatinine < 2.8 mg/dL	15	6	No benefit	
Donadio et al[61,62]	**Proteinuria > 1 g/24 h Creatinine < 3 mg/dL**	**55**	**24**	**Fish oils lessened deterioration in renal function**	**Proteinuria unchanged Poor prognosis in control group**
Donadio et al[63]	**Proteinuria 1.7–3.6 g/24 h Serum creatinine 1.5–4.9 mg/dL**	**73 (high vs. low dose)**	**24**	**No difference between high- and low-dose fish oils**	**No control group not receiving fish oils Proteinuria unchanged**

Randomized controlled trials in **bold**.

data than for other primary renal disease; however, recent data indicate that IgA deposition is accompanied by the slow onset of glomerular injury, indistinguishable histologically from disease in native kidneys and often at the same tempo.[3] There is no substantial evidence that any particular immunosuppressive regimen reduces the risk of recurrent IgA deposits or prevents any subsequent glomerular injury. One recent study in Chinese patients suggests that the risk of recurrence may be higher in live related donor transplant than in live unrelated or cadaveric donation,[67] but numerous other studies do not support this. On present evidence there is no need to recommend any restriction in the use of live as opposed to cadaveric donors.

Treatment of Henoch–Schönlein nephritis

There are no prospective RCTs to guide the treatment of HS nephritis. Most available data are in children. Most therapeutic studies of IgAN exclude those with HSP so it is uncertain whether a number of potential treatments have a role in HS nephritis. Available studies usually include children whose renal abnormalities have been severe or persistent enough to warrant referral to a nephrologist.

Many patients have transient nephritis during the early phase of HSP, which spontaneously remits and requires no treatment. It is has been proposed that early use of corticosteroids in HSP may prevent nephritis[68] but this has not been confirmed in other nonrandomized studies.[11]

Rapidly progressive renal failure due to crescentic nephritis

Crescentic nephritis is more common than in IgAN, particularly early in the course of HSP. There is little information on treatment in adults; five studies report experience in 81 children.[11] Regimens are variable and include corticosteroids and cyclophosphamide, with the addition of pulse methylprednisolone in some cases; two studies used plasma exchange alone. Precise entry criteria varied in the extent of proteinuria, renal impairment, and histologic injury. Short-term outcomes are encouraging, for example Oner et al[69] report that 11 of 12 children had normal GFR at 3 months despite a GFR < 40 mL/min and > 60% crescents at presentation. However, in the middle term, 20% of reported cases had an adverse outcome including ESRD.[11]

Active Henoch–Schönlein nephritis without renal failure

In less aggressive HS nephritis there is little information. Corticosteroids alone have never been shown to be beneficial.[11] Apparently promising findings with combination therapy of corticosteroids, cyclophosphamide, and antiplatelet agents have only been reported in small nonrandomized studies.[11] A recent nonrandomized study reported that prednisolone/azathioprine preserved renal function and improved histologic appearances, but relied on comparison with historical controls.[70] There are only five patients with HS nephritis included in the promising studies of immunoglobulin.[39,40]

Slowly progressive renal failure

While the renal histology and clinical course of slowly progressive HS nephritis and IgAN may be indistinguishable, patients with HS nephritis have not been included in the RCTs of corticosteroids, fish oil, or antiplatelet agents.

Transplant recurrence

Graft recurrence of HS nephritis is common. There is some evidence that it is more common and more likely to cause graft loss in children receiving live related donor kidneys than cadaver kidneys,[71] although this is not confirmed in adults.[72] No treatment is known to reduce risk of recurrence.

Treatment recommendations

On the evidence reviewed above, specific treatment recommendations are described in Tables 18.6 and 18.7 for the different clinical patterns of IgAN and HS nephritis.

The most controversial issue remains the treatment of IgAN with proteinuria > 1 g per 24 h. Physicians are increasingly using corticosteroids when there is preserved renal function (serum creatinine < 1.5 mg/dL) and fish oils when there is more renal impairment (serum creatinine > 1.5 mg/dL). However, in my opinion the case is not yet made for either of these therapies. Tight control of blood pressure and reduction of proteinuria with ACE inhibitors should be the first line of treatment. If physicians wish to consider additional therapy with fish oil or corticosteroids, this should only be contemplated if proteinuria persists at > 1 g per 24 h on maximal ACE inhibitor with blood pressure < 130/80.

Future directions

Specific treatment to prevent mesangial IgA deposition is the ideal goal but remains a remote prospect until the fundamentals of the disease mechanism are understood. It seems unlikely that controlled trials of crescentic IgAN or crescentic HS nephritis will ever be mounted. Prevention of slowly progressive renal failure remains the most promising field, particularly as this may inform the management of chronic glomerular disease other than that associated with IgA deposition. Further studies confirming the value of fish oil and corticosteroids are required. The value of combining ACE inhibitors and ATRAs requires formal confirmation in prospective studies, as does the potential role for HMG-CoA reductase inhibitors. Other low-risk strategies need to be developed from an understanding of the mechanisms of progressive renal scarring.

Table 18.6 Treatment recommendations for IgA nephropathy

Recurrent macroscopic hematuria (preserved renal function)
No specific treatment (no role for antibiotics or tonsillectomy)

Macroscopic hematuria with acute renal failure (renal biopsy mandatory)
Acute tubular necrosis
Supportive measures only
Crescentic nephritis
Induction
    Prednisolone 0.5–1 mg/kg/day for up to 8 weeks
    Cyclophosphamide 2 mg/kg/day for up to 8 weeks
    No evidence favoring oral or intravenous route: follow local practice
Maintenance
    Prednisolone in reducing dosage
    Azathioprine 2.5 mg/kg/day

Proteinuria < 1 g/24 h (± microscopic hematuria)
No specific treatment

Nephrotic syndrome (with minimal change on light microscopy)
Prednisolone 0.5–1 mg/kg/day (children 60 mg/m^2/day) for up to 8 weeks

Proteinuria > 1 g/24 h (± microscopic hematuria)
ACE inhibitor

If proteinuria still > 1 g/24 h on maximal ACE inhibitor, serum creatinine < 1.5 mg/dL
Consider corticosteroids: 0.5 mg/kg on alternate days for 6 months

If proteinuria still > 1 g/24 h on maximal ACE inhibitor, serum creatinine > 1.5 mg/dL
Consider fish oil 12 g daily for 6 months

Hypertension
ACE inhibitors are agents of first choice
Target blood pressure 130/80

Transplantation
No special measures required

ACE, angiotensin-converting enzyme.

Table 18.7 Treatment recommendations for Henoch–Schönlein nephritis

Crescentic nephritis
Regimen as above for crescentic IgA nephropathy

All other Henoch–Schönlein nephritis (including nephrotic syndrome)
No specific treatment; supportive measures only

Hypertension
ACE inhibitor agent of first choice

Transplantation
Cadaveric donor may be preferable to live related donor in children

ACE, angiotensin-converting enzyme.

References

1. Falk RJ, Jennette JC, Nachman PJ: IgA nephropathy. *In* Brenner BM (ed): The Kidney, Vol II, 6th edn. Philadelphia: WB Saunders, 2000, pp 1302–1310.
2. D'Amico G: Natural history of idiopathic IgA nephropathy: role of clinical and histological prognostic factors. Am J Kidney Dis 2000;36:227–237.
3. Floege J, Burg M, Kliem V: Recurrent IgA nephropathy after kidney transplantation: not a benign condition. Nephrol Dial Transplant 1998;13:1933–1935.
4. Appell GB, Radhakrishnan J, D'Agati V: Schönlein–Henoch purpura. *In* Brenner BM (ed): The Kidney, Vol II, 6th edn. Philadelphia: WB Saunders, 2000, pp 1379–1382.
5. Davin JC, ten Berge IJ, Weening J: What is the difference between IgA nephropathy and Henoch–Schönlein purpura nephritis? Kidney Int 2001;59:823–834.
6. Feehally J, Allen AC: Pathogenesis of IgA nephropathy. Ann Med Interne (Paris) 1999;150:91–98.
7. Allen AC, Bailey EM, Brenchley PEC, et al: Mesangial IgA1 in IgA nephropathy exhibits aberrant O-glycosylation: observations in three patients. Kidney Int 2001;60:969–973.
8. Schena FP Scivittaro V, Ranieri E, et al: Abnormalities of the IgA immune system in members of unrelated pedigrees from patients with IgA nephropathy. Clin Exp Immunol 1993;92:139–144.

9. Levy M: Familial cases of Berger's disease and anaphylactoid purpura: more frequent than previously thought. Am J Med 1989;87:246–248.

10. Nolin L, Courteau M: Management of IgA nephropathy: evidence-based recommendations. Kidney Int 1999;Suppl 70:S56–S62.

11. Wyatt RJ, Hogg RJ: Evidence-based assessment of treatment options for children with IgA nephropathies. Pediatr Nephrol 2001;16;156–167.

12. Hogg RJ: A randomised placebo-controlled multicenter trial evaluating alternate-day prednisone and fish oil supplements in young patients with immunoglobulin A nephropathy. Am J Kidney Dis 1995;26:792–796.

13. Feehally J: Strategies for the management of IgA nephropathy. In Andreucci ,VE (ed): Annual Yearbook of Nephrology, Dialysis and Transplantation. Oxford: Oxford University Press, 1996, pp 23–29.

14. Clarkson AR , Woodroffe AJ: Therapeutic perspectives in mesangial IgA nephropathy. Contrib Nephrol 1984;40:187–194.

15. Rasche FM, Schwarz A, Keller F: Tonsillectomy does not prevent a progressive course in IgA nephropathy. Clin Nephrol 1999;51:147–152.

16. Clarkson AR, Seymour AE, Woodroffe AJ, et al: Controlled trial of phenytoin therapy in IgA nephropathy. Clin Nephrol 1980;13:215–218.

17. Lai KN, MacMoune Lai F, Leung ACT et al. Plasma exchange in patients with rapidly progressive idiopathic IgA nephropathy: a report of two cases and review of the literature. Am J Kidney Dis 1987;10:66–70.

18. Macintyre CW, Fluck RJ, Lambie SH: Steoid and cyclophosphamide therapy for crescentic IgA nephropathy associated with crescentic change: an effective treatment. Clin Nephrol 2001;56:193–198.

19. Roccatello D, Ferro G, Cesano D, et al: Steroid and cyclophosphamide in IgA nephropathy. Nephrol Dial Transplant 2000;15:833–835.

20. Harper L, Ferreira M, Howie AJ, et al: Treatment of vasculitic IgA nephropathy. J Nephrol 2000;13:360–366.

21. Roccatello D, Ferro M, Coppo R, et al: Report on intensive treatment of extracapillary glomerulonephritis with focus on crescentic IgA nephropathy. Nephrol Dial Transplant 1995;10:2054–2059.

22. Haas M, Jafri J, Bartosh SM, et al: ANCA-associated crescentic glomerulonephritis with mesangial IgA deposits. Am J Kidney Dis 2000;36:709–718.

23. Kobayashi Y, Fujii K, Hiki Y, et al: Steroid therapy in IgA nephropathy: a retrospective study in heavy proteinuric cases. Nephron 1988;48:12–17.

24. Kobayashi Y, Hiki Y, Kokubo T, et al: Steroid therapy during the early stage of progressive IgA nephropathy. Nephron 1996;72:237–242.

25. Welch TR, Fryer C, Shely E, et al: Double blind controlled trial of short term prednisone therapy in immunoglobulin A glomerulonephritis. J Pediatr 1992;121:474–477.

26. Lai KN, Lai FM, Ho CP, et al: Corticosteroid therapy in IgA nephropathy with nephrotic syndrome: a long-term controlled trial. Clin Nephrol 1986;26:174–180.

27. Shoji T, Nakanashi I, Suzuki A, et al: Early treatment with corticosteroids ameliorates proteinuria, proliferative lesions, and mesangial phenotypic modulation in adult diffuse proliferative IgA nephropathy. Am J Kidney Dis 2000;35:194–201.

28. Pozzi C, Bolasco PG, Fogazzi GB, et al: Corticosteroids in IgA nephropathy: a randomised controlled trial. Lancet 1999;353:883–887.

29. Locatelli F, Pozzi C, Del Vecchio L, et al: Role of proteinuria reduction in the progression of IgA nephropathy. Ren Fail 2001;23:495–505.

30. Locatelli F, Pozzi C, Del Vecchio L, et al: Combined treatment with steroids and azathioprine in IgA nephropathy: design of a prospective randomised multicentre trial. J Nephrol 1999;12:308–311.

31. Manno C, Gesualdo L, D'Altri C, Rossini M, Grandaliano G, Schena FP: Prospective randomised controlled multicenter trial on steroids plus ramipril in proteinuric IgA nephropathy. J Nephrol 2001;14:248–252.

32. Woo KT, Lee GSL, Lau YK, et al: Effects of triple therapy in IgA nephritis: a follow-up study 5 years later. Clin Nephrol 1991;36:60–66.

33. Walker RG, Yu SH, Owen JE, et al: The treatment of mesangial IgA nephropathy with cyclophosphamide, dipyridamole amd warfarin:a two-year prospective trial. Clin Nephrol 1990;34:103–107.

34. Andreoli SP, Bergstein JM: Treatment of severe IgA nephropathy in children. Pediatr Nephrol 1989;3:248–253.

35. Goumenos D, Ahuja M, Shortland JR, et al: Can immunosuppressive drugs slow the progression of IgA nephropathy? Nephrol Dial Transplant 1995;10:1173–1181.

36. Lagrue G, Bernard D, Bariety J, et al: Traitment par la chlorambucil et azathioprine dans les glomerulonephrites primitives. Resultats d'une etude "controlee". J Urol Nephrol 1975;9:655–672.

37. Yoshikawa N, Ito H, Sakai Y, et al: A controlled trial of combined therapy for newly diagnoses severe childhood IgA nephropathy. J Am Soc Nephrol 1999;10:101–109.

38. Lai KN, MacMoune Lai F, Li PKT, et al: Cyclosporin treatment of IgA nephropathy: a short term controlled trial. Br Med J 1987;295:1165–1168.

39. Rostoker G, Desvaux-Belghiti D, Pilatte Y, et al: High-dose immunoglobulin therapy for severe IgA nephropathy and Henoch–Schönlein purpura. Ann Intern Med 1994;120:476–484.

40. Rostoker G, Desvaux-Belghiti D, Pilatte Y, et al: Immunomodulation with low-dose immunoglobulins for moderate IgA nephropathy and Henoch–Schönlein purpura. Preliminary results of a prospective uncontrolled trial. Nephron 1995;69:327–334.

41. Furuse A, Hiramatsu M, Adachi N, et al: Dramatic response to corticosteroid therapy of nephrotic syndrome associated with IgA nephropathy. Int J Pediatr Nephrol 1985;6:205–206.

42. Clive DM, Galvanek DG, Silva FG: Mesangial immunoglobulin A deposits in minimal change nephrotic syndrome: a report of an older patient and a review of the literature. Am J Nephrol 1990;10:31–36.

43. Feehally J: Predicting prognosis in IgA nephropathy. Am J Kidney Dis 2001;38:881–883.

44. Hsu SI, Ramirez B, Winn MP, Bonventre JV, Owen WF: Evidence for genetic factors in the development and progression of IgA nephropathy. Kidney Int 2000;57:1818–1835.

45. Chan MK, Kwan SYL, Chan KW, et al: Controlled trial of antiplatelet agents in mesangial IgA glomerulonephritis. Am J Kidney Dis 1987;9:417–421.

46. Lee GSL, Choong HL, Chang GSC, Woo KT: Three-year randomised controlled trial of dipyridamole and low-dose warfarin in patients with IgA nephropathy and renal impairment. Nephrology 1997;3:117–121.

47. Stefanski A, Schmidt KG, Waldherr R, Ritz E: Early increase in blood pressure and diastolic left ventricular malfunction in patients with glomerulonephritis. Kidney Int 1995;54:926–931.

48. The GISEN Group: Randomised placebo-controlled trial of effect of ramipril on decline in glomerular filtration rate and risk of terminal renal failure in proteinuric, non-diabetic nephropathy. Lancet 1997;349:1857–1863.

49. Maschio G, Cagnoli L, Claroni F, et al: ACE inhibition reduces proteinuria in normotensive patients with IgA nephropathy: a multicentre, randomised placebo-controlled trial. Nephrol Dial Transplant 1994;9:265–269.

50. Perico N, Remuzzi A, Sangalli F, et al: The antiproteinuric effect of angiotensin antagonism in human IgA nephropathy is potentiated by indomethacin. J Am Soc Nephrol 1998;9:2308–2317.

51. Russo D, Minutolo R, Pisani R, et al: Additive antiproteinuric effect of converting enzyme inhibitor and losartan in normotensive patients with IgA nephropathy. Am J Kidney Dis 2001;33:851–856.

52. Bannister KM, Weaver A, Clarkson AR, Woodroffe AJ: Effect of angiotensin-converting enzyme and calcium channel inhibition on progression of IgA nephropathy. Contrib Nephrol 1995; 111:184–193.

53. Cheng IKP, Fang GX, Wong MC, Ji YL, Chan KW, Yeung HWD: A randomised prospective comparison of nadolol, captopril with or without ticlopidine on disease progression in IgA nephropathy. Nephrology 1998;4:19–26.

54. Rekola S, Bergstrand A, Bucht H, et al: Deterioration rate in hypertensive IgA nephropathy: comparison of a converting enzyme inhibitor and β-blocking agents. Nephron 1991;57:57–60.

55. Cattran D, Greenwood C, Ritchie S: Long-term benefits of angiotensin-converting enzyme inhibitor therapy in patients with severe immunoglobulin A therapy: a comparison to patients receiving treatment with other antihypertensive agents and to those receiving no therapy. Am J Kidney Dis 1994;23:247–254.

56. Coppo R: Angiotensin-converting enzyme inhibitors in young patients with IgA nephropathy. Nephrol Dial Transplant 1999;14:840–841.

57. Hamazaki T, Tateno S, Shishido H: Eicosapentanoic acid and IgA nephropathy. Lancet 1984;i:1017–1018.

58. Bennett WM, Walker RG, Kincaid-Smith P: Treatment of IgA nephropathy with eicosapentaenoic acid (EPA): a two-year prospective trial. Clin Nephrol 1989;31:128–129.

59. Cheng IKP, Chan PCK, Chan MK: The effects of fish-oil dietary supplementation on the progression of mesangial IgA glomerulonephritis. Nephrol Dial Transplant 1990;5:241–246.

60. Pettersson EE, Rekola S, Berglund L, et al: Treatment of IgA nephropathy with omega-3-polyunsaturated fatty acids: a prospective, double-blind, randomised study. Clin Nephrol 1994;41:183–190.

61. Donadio JV, Bergstalh EJ, Offord KP, et al: A controlled trial of fish oil in IgA nephropathy. N Engl J Med 1994;331:1194–1199.

62. Donadio JV, Grande JP, Bergstralh EJ, et al: The long-term outcome of patients with IgA nephropathy treated with fish oil in a controlled trial. J Am Soc Nephrol 1999;10:1772–1777.

63. Donadio JV, Larson TS, Bergstralh EJ, Grande JP: A randomised trial of high-dose compared with low-dose omega-3 fatty acids in severe IgA nephropathy. J Am Soc Nephrol 2001;12:791–799.

64. Dillon JJ: Fish oil therapy for IgA nephropathy: efficacy and interstudy variability. J Am Soc Nephrol 1997;8:1739–1744.

65. Buemi M, Allegra A, Corica F, et al: Effect of fluvistatin on proteinuria in patients with immunoglobulin A nephropathy. Clin Pharmacol Ther 2000;67:427–431.

66. Odum J, Peh CA, Clarkson AR, et al: Recurrent mesangial IgA nephritis following renal transplantation. Nephrol Dial Transplant 1994;9:309–312.

67. Wang AYM, Lai FM, Yu AW-Y, et al: Recurrent IgA nephropathy in renal transplant allografts. J Am Soc Nephrol 2001;38:588–596.

68. Mollica F, LiVolti S, Garozzo R, et al: Effectiveness of early prednisone treatment in preventing the development of nephropathy in anaphylactoid purpura. Eur J Pediatr 1992;151:140–144.

69. Oner A, Tinaztepe K, Erdogan O: The effect of triple therapy on rapidly progressive type of Henoch–Schönlein nephritis. Pediatr Nephrol 1995;9:6–10.

70. Foster BJ, Bernard C, Drummond KN, Sharma AK: Effective therapy for Henoch–Schönlein purpura nephritis with prednisone and azathioprine: a clinical and histopathologic study. J Pediatr 2000;136:370–375.

71. Hasegawa A: Fate of renal grafts with recurrent Henoch–Schönlein purpura nephritis in children. Transplant Proc 1989;21:2130.

72. Meulders Q, Pirson Y, Cosyns J-P, et al: Course of Henoch–Schonlein nephritis after renal transplantation. Transplantation 1994;48:1179–1186.

Crescentic Glomerulonephritis

Jeremy B. Levy and Charles D. Pusey

Background

The term "crescentic glomerulonephritis" as a diagnostic label should now have sunk into oblivion. Certainly the presence of extracapillary cellular proliferation within Bowman's space should still be referred to as a crescent, as part of a descriptive analysis of the light microscopic changes of a renal biopsy. However, it should now be possible, in most cases, to provide a precise diagnostic label as to the underlying cause for this pathologic change.

Crescentic proliferation and its clinical corollary, rapidly progressive glomerulonephritis (RPGN), are found in a number of different diseases and appear to represent a final common pathway of intraglomerular inflammation.[1,2] The best classification of crescentic nephritis has divided patients into three groups on the basis of the underlying immunopathology:[1] (1) those with antiglomerular basement membrane (anti-GBM) disease; (2) those with immune deposits and cellular proliferation within the glomerular tuft; and (3) those without immune deposits. Up to 50% of patients have either anti-GBM disease (Goodpasture disease) or a clearly identifiable primary or secondary underlying glomerulonephritis that has undergone crescentic transformation, for example systemic lupus erythematosus (SLE), infectious endocarditis, postinfectious glomerulonephritis, IgA nephropathy, membranoproliferative glomerulonephritis, etc. However, 50–70% of all cases of crescentic glomerulonephritis have no apparent underlying primary glomerulonephritis and no, or few, immune deposits on immunomicroscopy, and these have been described as "pauci-immune" (Table 19.1).[1,3,4] It has become increasingly clear that the majority of pauci-immune crescentic nephritides are associated with the presence of antineutrophil cytoplasmic antibodies (ANCA).[5,6] A review of all the crescentic biopsies from our own unit over the last decade showed that of 145 biopsies 37% were pauci-immune with an ANCA-associated vasculitis as the cause, 23% were caused by SLE,

12% by IgA nephropathy, and 12% by anti-GBM disease (Table 19.1). Specific clinical features, together with characteristic biopsy findings, may enable the condition to be labeled as either Wegener granulomatosis (WG) or microscopic polyangiitis (MP),[7] leaving a small group of patients with isolated pauci-immune glomerulonephritis in the absence of any systemic manifestations. The identification of ANCA[8–10] has led to the recognition that most of these cases are not truly idiopathic, since patients have detectable circulating ANCA and their condition should thus be labeled as "renal-limited vasculitis."[5,6,11] There remains a group of ANCA-negative patients whose underlying pathophysiology is still undefined, although clinically their condition resembles ANCA-positive RPGN.[12] An alternative classification of crescentic nephritis separates primary glomerulonephritis (including renal-limited anti-GBM disease, pauci-immune glomerulonephritis, immune complex glomerulonephritis, and idiopathic crescentic glomerulonephritis) from crescentic nephritis associated with infectious diseases (endocarditis, hepatitis B and C viruses, etc.), with multisystem diseases (SLE, Goodpasture disease, Henoch–Schönlein purpura, systemic vasculitis), or with drugs (penicillamine, rifampicin, allopurinol, etc.).[2] Finally, most studies of RPGN have shown that the percentage of crescents in a renal biopsy specimen is not in itself a predictive factor for recovery of renal function or response to treatment, although it does frequently correlate with initial serum creatinine. The degree of tubulointerstitial damage and the percentage of normal glomeruli are both more useful prognostic factors.[13,14]

Angangco and colleagues[5] reanalyzed all patients presenting with crescentic nephritis over a 10-year period; 7% of all their renal biopsies showed crescentic proliferation. Of these 82 cases, 10 had anti-GBM disease and 35 were secondary to a variety of nephritic processes, including rheumatoid arthritis, mixed connective tissue disease, SLE, cryoglobulinemia, IgA nephropathy, membranoproliferative glomerulonephritis, and accelerated hypertension; 36 patients had ANCA-associated disease (two WG, 25 small-vessel vasculitis, either WG or MP, and nine idiopathic crescentic nephritis in the presence of ANCA). Only 1 of 82 crescentic biopsies was truly idiopathic, without circulating antibody or systemic features. However, even in this patient, ANCA with myeloperoxidase specificity had been positive on one occasion at low titer.

Ferrario et al[6] also retrospectively evaluated their previously labeled idiopathic crescentic glomerulonephritides, having first excluded those with anti-GBM disease or an identifiable primary glomerulonephritis. All patients could be divided into two groups on the basis of the presence of intraglomerular segmental necrosis. Of 41

Table 19.1   Diseases causing crescentic and rapidly progressive glomerulonephritis

	Heilmann et al (1987)[77] (n = 64)	Keller et al (1989)[78] (n = 46)	Ritz et al (1991)[79] (n = 38)	Levy & Winearls (1994)[4] (n = 48)	Angangco et al (1994)[5] (v = 82)	Hammersmith data (2001)* (n = 145)
ANCA-associated vasculitis	—	—	—		—	37
Microscopic polyarteritis	16	—	18	25	30	—
Wegener granulomatosis	9	4	34	23	2	—
Anti-GBM disease	20	20	8	15	12	6
Idiopathic crescentic glomerulonephritis	23	61	—	8	1	6
Kidney-limited vasculitis	—	—	—	—	11	—
Systemic lupus erythematosus	—	7	8	6	2	23
Henoch–Schönlein purpura	3	2	13	8	17	1
Postinfectious glomerulonephritis	—	—	13	2	4	3
Polyarteritis nodosa	—	4	—	4	—	—
Churg–Strauss syndrome	—	—	—	2	—	1
Cryoglobulinemia	2	—	—	2	1	1
Mixed connective tissue disease	—	—	—	4	1	—
Rheumatoid arthritis	—	—	—	—	5	—
Systemic vasculitis	20	—	—	—	—	—
Primary glomerulonephritis (IgA, membranous, MCGN)	6	2	5	—	12	22

ANCA, antineutrophil cytoplasmic antibody; GBM, glomerular basement membrane; MCGN, mesangiocapillary glomerulonephritis.
Figures given are percentages.
*Hammersmith data are unpublished results.

patients identified over a 20-year period with idiopathic crescentic nephritis, 25 had variable degrees of intraglomerular segmental necrosis, while 16 had no necrosis in any capillary loops. This latter nonnecrotic group had less acute interstitial inflammation but more mesangial proliferation within the biopsy than patients with segmental necrosis. The nonnecrotic biopsies also had substantially more deposition of complement C3 and immunoglobulin in the capillary walls and mesangium than those with necrosis. In the necrotic group 12 of 13 patients tested were ANCA positive compared with none of the eight tested in the proliferative nonnecrotic group. On the basis of these pathologic and serologic findings, Ferrario et al suggested that all patients with segmental tuft necrosis and crescentic glomerulonephritis actually have renal-limited vasculitis.[6] The ANCA-negative patients without segmental necrosis but with more pronounced mesangial proliferation and increased immune deposits have a true but unidentified primary glomerulonephritis that has developed into rapidly progressive disease with segmental disruption of the GBM, escape of cells and fibrin through these gaps, and the formation of a crescent.

The crescent causes compression of the glomerular tuft, making recognition of the underlying primary nephritis difficult because of the distortion involved. These authors, therefore, also suggest that truly idiopathic crescentic glomerulonephritis does not exist. In contrast, Hedger et al[12] retrospectively reviewed all patients with pauci-immune RPGN presenting to a single unit in the UK from 1986 to 1996. Over this period 128 patients were seen (giving an incidence of 3.9 per million population per year), of whom 93 (73%) were ANCA positive but 35 (27%) repeatedly ANCA negative. The ANCA-negative cohort presented earlier but otherwise had very similar clinical characteristics as the ANCA-positive patients. In our experience, almost all patients with crescentic nephritis and segmental necrosis in whom other diagnoses have been excluded have a positive ANCA assay. Thus we believe that truly idiopathic crescentic glomerulonephritis is extremely rare. It should not be forgotten, however, that pauci-immune RPGN is generally common, for example making up 31% of all cases of acute renal insufficiency in adults aged over 60 in Chicago – the commonest single diagnosis.[15]

Diagnosis

Making an accurate diagnosis in patients with RPGN is critically important, as both the nature of the therapy and the response to treatment will be very different depending on the precise diagnosis (see following chapters). All patients presenting clinically with RPGN or evidence of vasculitis should have a renal biopsy and appropriate serologic investigations[7,16] performed as a matter of urgency.[17] Assays for anti-GBM antibodies, ANCA, lupus serology, and complement are particularly important, as well as measures of an acute-phase response. ANCA should be assessed by indirect immunofluorescence on ethanol-fixed neutrophils with confirmation of the antigen specificity by enzyme-linked immunosorbent assay (ELISA) against purified proteinase 3 and myeloperoxidase. The renal biopsy should be carefully analyzed for the presence of segmental necrosis and for any immune deposits. Patients with pauci-immune glomerulonephritis usually do have some deposition of complement C3 and immunoglobulin within the mesangium and along the capillary loops, and it is important to try to localize and quantitate the immune deposits to distinguish those patients with truly pauci-immune disease from those who may have underlying primary glomerulonephritis.[18] Increasing numbers of patients with crescentic nephritis are being recognized as having both ANCA and anti-GBM antibodies, so-called "double-positive" patients.[19] The outcome in these patients is unclear but in our experience may be poor and more like that seen with anti-GBM disease. Thus all anti-GBM antibody-positive patients, or those with linear immunoglobulin deposited along the GBM on renal biopsy, should have ANCA assays performed, since this might influence subsequent management.

Clinical trials

The heterogeneity of crescentic glomerulonephritis has confounded many clinical trials of therapy. Early studies included patients with diseases as diverse as postinfectious nephritis, SLE, WG, and renal-limited vasculitis, and very few studies have clearly separated patients into appropriate diagnostic groups.[20,21] It has become clear that the immunopathologic classification of crescentic nephritis is critically important for deciding the precise nature of the treatment to be used and in predicting response to therapy. Subsequent chapters discuss precise treatment regimens for anti-GBM disease, the ANCA-associated glomerulonephritides, and primary glomerulonephritis in crescentic phase, so we just give a brief overview of the therapeutic interventions that have been used in crescentic nephritis in general. However, the evidence base for many of the interventions discussed below is poor. There are very few prospective randomized controlled trials in any of the glomerulonephritides and most reports are based on cohorts of patients treated in a single center.

Patients with anti-GBM disease respond well to therapy if they present before they require dialysis, with patient survival rates in excess of 90% and renal survival rates of 72%.[22–24] Patients already dependent on dialysis do substantially less well, with very few of these coming off dialysis (at most around 10%). This is in contrast to dialysis-dependent patients with ANCA-associated vasculitides, either WG or MP, in whom a good response to therapy has been shown if treated aggressively (see later).[4,22,25] Patients with primary glomerulonephritis in a crescentic phase generally have a poor response to therapy.[2] In Ferrario's reevaluation of their cases of idiopathic crescentic glomerulonephritis,[6] patients without focal necrosis, who were ANCA negative and thought to have a primary but unidentifiable chronic glomerulonephritis complicated by crescent formation, responded poorly to immunosuppression, with almost 60% requiring renal support at follow-up. In contrast, no patients with segmental necrosis and a positive ANCA required renal replacement therapy. Some patients with crescentic IgA nephropathy have been reported to respond to aggressive immunosuppression with plasma exchange (PE), steroids, and cytotoxic drugs; however, treatment seems simply to delay the onset of endstage renal disease rather than prevent renal failure.[26,27]

Treatment for crescentic glomerulonephritis is usually divided into two phases: the induction period and maintenance treatment. Historically, the outcome of patients with crescentic nephritis was dramatically improved with the introduction of oral immunosuppression as induction therapy, particularly the addition of cyclophosphamide to corticosteroids as described by Fauci at the National Institutes of Health for patients with WG.[28–31] A similar regimen was subsequently applied to patients with MP.[25,31] In Goodpasture disease, the introduction of combined immunosuppression, steroids, and PE in the mid-1970s led to a dramatic improvement in patient and renal survival.[32–34] Treatments used for induction therapy in crescentic glomerulonephritis have included oral and intravenous steroids, oral and intravenous cyclophosphamide, and PE.

Induction treatments
Plasma exchange

The rationale for the use of PE in Goodpasture disease is based on the known pathogenicity of the autoantibodies and the ability of PE, when combined with immunosuppression, to remove circulating antibodies rapidly and suppress their further production. However, only one small controlled trial has been performed,[35] in which nine patients were randomized to receive oral steroids and cyclophosphamide and eight patients to receive additional PE: 2 of 8 patients receiving PE developed endstage renal failure compared with six of nine receiving drugs alone. This beneficial effect, though not dramatic, occurred despite a low intensity of treatment, with plasma exchanges only every 3 days. The outcome of patients treated since 1980 has been dramatically better than historic controls. The largest experience of PE in anti-GBM disease was reported by Levy et al[24] in 71 patients all treated intensively with PE, prednisolone, and cyclophosphamide. Patients with an initial creatinine < 500 μmol/L had a good outcome, with 74% retaining independent renal function in the long term. Similar results were achieved in patients with severe renal failure (creatinine > 500 μmol/L) but who did not require immediate dialysis: 69% had independent renal function at last follow-up. Dialysis-dependent patients rarely, but occasionally, recovered renal function (8%).

The rationale for the use of PE in MP, WG, and "idiopathic" crescentic nephritis was initially based on the similarity of the renal pathology to Goodpasture disease, namely severe focal necrotizing crescentic nephritis and the presumed "immune complex etiology." The identification of ANCA in these conditions strengthens the rationale for the use of PE, although the precise role of the autoantibodies in the pathogenesis of these diseases is not yet clearly defined (see later chapters). Five controlled trials of the value of PE in non-anti-GBM RPGN have been performed.[21,36–39] Glockner et al[21] could not demonstrate any additional benefit of twice-weekly PE in 14 patients with crescentic RPGN compared with 12 controls treated with oral prednisolone, cyclophosphamide, and azathioprine. However, the patients included in this study were a heterogeneous group, including those with WG, polyarteritis nodosa, SLE, scleroderma, and idiopathic RPGN. Furthermore, patients with oliguria were excluded and three patients in the control group were subsequently successfully treated with PE.

The Hammersmith Hospital controlled trial of PE only treated patients with WG, MP, or idiopathic RPGN, and randomized 48 patients to conventional treatment with oral steroids, cyclophosphamide and azathioprine, either with or without intensive PE (at least five exchanges in the first 7 days).[36] In this study, PE was of no additional benefit in patients with moderate or severe renal disease who were not dialysis-dependent at presentation. However, 10 of 11 dialysis-dependent patients receiving PE discontinued dialysis compared with only 3 of 8 receiving oral immunosuppression alone. Although ANCA were not routinely measured at that time, these patients fell into diagnostic categories now associated with ANCA. Rifle and Dechelette[38] also showed a benefit of PE in dialysis-dependent patients: 6 of 8 patients receiving PE recovered renal function but none of six treated with drugs alone.

The Canadian apheresis study group[32] added PE to induction therapy of intravenous methylprednisolone followed by oral prednisolone and azathioprine. This study excluded patients with systemic disease and included one patient with postinfectious RPGN in the PE group. There was no demonstrable benefit of PE in the nondialysis-dependent patients. However, in dialysis-dependent patients, a nonsignificant trend in benefit was evident: three of four patients receiving PE discontinued dialysis compared with two of seven in the control group.

Most recently, Zauner et al[39] prospectively randomized 39 patients with non-anti-GBM crescentic nephritis to receive PE in addition to standard immunosuppression (pulsed methylprednisolone, oral steroids, and oral cyclophosphamide): 6 of 11 dialysis-dependent patients recovered renal function overall but with no difference in outcome between the two groups. Combining the results

from the controlled trials clearly demonstrates a significant benefit of PE only in dialysis-dependent patients. In total, 25 of 31 dialysis-dependent patients (81%) treated with PE had independent renal function at follow-up compared with 8 of 25 (32%) treated with immunosuppressive drugs alone.

Guillevin et al[40] reported no benefit of PE in vasculitis in two prospective randomized controlled trials, although very few patients in these studies had severe renal disease. Stegmayr et al[41] conducted a randomized controlled trial of PE versus protein A immunoadsorption in 44 patients with RPGN and > 50% crescents: 7 of 10 dialysis-dependent patients discontinued dialysis, with no difference between the two antibody removal strategies. Frasca et al[42,43] reported their uncontrolled experience with PE in ANCA-associated RPGN (either WG or MP). Patients were treated with oral steroids, oral cyclophosphamide, defibritide (an antithrombotic agent), and daily PE for 3–10 sessions. All 10 dialysis-dependent patients came off renal support with this treatment regimen, although in the long term one patient required renal replacement therapy. Levy and Winearls[4] retrospectively analyzed the response to treatment of all the patients with crescentic glomerulonephritis presenting to a single renal unit. Only patients with MP, WG, or idiopathic crescentic glomerulonephritis were studied in detail. Patients received either PE or intravenous methylprednisolone together with oral steroids and oral cyclophosphamide. Some patients received both intravenous steroids and PE, and separating the effects of the two treatment modalities was difficult. Patient survival at 1 and 3 years was 86%, with a renal survival rate of 78%. In this study, 9 of 11 dialysis-dependent patients who received PE recovered renal function compared with five of nine patients who were not plasmapheresed. Finally, Gaskin and Pusey[25] reported that 74% of patients with ANCA-associated vasculitis could recover renal function from dependency on dialysis if treated with intensive PE in addition to oral immunosuppression.

Combining the outcome of treatment of dialysis-dependent patients with crescentic nephritis receiving conventional treatment with or without PE from published data over the last 10 years, 104 of 139 patients (75%) came off dialysis with PE as opposed to only 87 of 157 patients (55%) treated with oral or intravenous steroids and cyclophosphamide (Table 19.2). A prospective randomized controlled trial of PE versus intravenous methylprednisolone in the treatment of patients with ANCA-associated vasculitis and severe renal failure has been completed and confirms the benefit of PE over methylprednisolone. Around 70% of patients treated with PE survived with independent renal function compared with less than 50% of those treated with methylprednisolone. PE has also been used in patients with crescentic IgA disease and other primary glomerulonephritides. There are no controlled trials and results have been variable.

Intravenous methylprednisolone

Intravenous methylprednisolone has also been advocated for the treatment of crescentic glomerulonephritis, usually

Table 19.2 Outcome of patients who present with severe renal failure (dialysis dependent or creatinine > 600 μmol/L) with rapidly progessive glomerulonephritis caused by renal vasculitis according to induction therapy, with or without plasma exchange

Reference	Patients recovering renal function with PE and immunosuppression	Patients recovering renal function with oral or i.v. immunosuppression only	Comments
Glockner et al[21]	6/8	3/4	Randomized controlled trial; oral drugs
Keller et al[78]	6/11	5/12	Oral and i.v. steroids
Bolton & Sturgill[45]	—	14/19	All received i.v. MP
Falk et al[53]	—	6/12	i.v. MP 7 mg/kg added to oral drugs
Rifle & Dechelette[38]	6/8	0/6	Randomized controlled trial
Andrassy et al[46]	—	11/12	All received i.v. MP
Pusey et al[36]	10/11	3/8	Randomized controlled trial; oral drugs
Cole et al[37]	3/4	2/7	Randomized controlled trial; i.v. MP
Frasca et al[43]	10/10	—	Oral drugs
Garrett et al[10]	—	7/17	All received i.v. MP
Bindi et al[80]	0/3	0/5	Received oral or i.v. steroids
Levy & Winearls[4]	9/11	5/9	Some received i.v. MP
Pettersson et al[47]	—	31/46	Oral drugs predominantly
Gaskin & Pusey[25]	54/73	—	All received intensive PE
Zauner et al[39]			6/11 came off dialysis; no difference with or without PE
Total	104/139 (75%)	87/157 (55%)	

PE, plasma exchange; MP, methylprednisolone.

in place of PE. There has now been one controlled study comparing the two treatment modalities, a European trial of intravenous methylprednisolone versus PE as induction therapy in crescentic nephritis, in which steroids were significantly less effective than PE[44] (see above). There have been no controlled trials of oral versus intravenous steroids. Intravenous methylprednisolone is certainly cheaper and easier to administer than PE but there is a suggestion of an increased incidence of infection complicating its use, as well as an increased risk of osteoporosis in older patients. Stevens et al[20] compared PE with intravenous methylprednisolone in 15 patients with dialysis-dependent crescentic nephritis and reported that both treatments were equally effective. Patients in this study had a variety of underlying diseases, including anti-GBM disease, Henoch–Schönlein purpura, WG, and polyarteritis nodosa. Bolton and Sturgill[45] reported good results in dialysis-dependent patients with pauci-immune RPGN or vasculitis (excluding WG), with 14 of 19 dialysis-dependent patients treated with intravenous methylprednisolone coming off dialysis. However, this study used very large doses of methylprednisolone (30 mg/kg/day for 3 days, maximum 3 g/day). Andrassy et al[46] also used intravenous methylprednisolone successfully at much lower doses (250 mg/day for 3 days) enabling 11 of 12 dialysis-

dependent patients with WG to recover renal function. In contrast, Garrett et al[10] reported improved renal function in only 7 of 17 (41%) patients with ANCA-associated RPGN treated with high-dose intravenous steroids. One of the more recent studies[47] simply used oral prednisolone (1 mg/kg/day) and oral cyclophosphamide (2 mg/kg/day) in 46 patients with pauci-immune necrotizing crescentic ANCA-associated glomerulonephritis (either WG, MP, or renal-limited vasculitis). After 33 months of follow-up, 31 of 46 (67%) had independent renal function with a median creatinine value of 179 μmol/L. However, only 14 of these patients were initially dialysis dependent, and eight (17%) had died within 1 year.

Other treatments

Intravenous cyclophosphamide has also been used in patients with crescentic glomerulonephritis, in view of the successful use of this treatment modality in patients with severe SLE.[48–50] Results from these studies are conflicting (see subsequent chapters). However, in most studies the incidence of adverse effects is reduced with pulsed intravenous cyclophosphamide, probably because of the reduction in total dose administered and the concomitant use of mesna to prevent bladder toxicity.[50] However, intravenous cyclophosphamide seems less efficacious in successfully limiting renal inflammation.[25,50,51] Guillevin and Haubitz both reported an inferior rate of recovery from dialysis dependence in patients treated with intravenous cyclophosphamide compared with the response to oral therapy,[50,51] and Aaserod demonstrated an increased relapse rate in over 108 patients treated with intravenous compared with oral cyclophosphamide.[13,52] However, Falk and Haubitz both showed equivalence of the two treatment regimens in small numbers of patients.[53,54] A recent metaanalysis of all published data confirmed a significant reduction in leukopenia and infectious complications of pulsed intravenous cyclophosphamide, and a trend to more relapses but equal numbers of patients reaching endstage renal disease or death.[55]

Methotrexate has been used successfully in place of cyclophosphamide in a number of patients with WG but without severe crescentic nephritis, since it should be avoided in renal failure (see subsequent chapters).[56,57] A handful of cases of severe crescentic nephritis responding to cyclosporine have also been reported.[58,59] The use of intravenous immunoglobulin (IVIG) appears to be more successful. Jayne and Lockwood[60] treated 26 patients with WG, MP, and rheumatoid vasculitis in whom disease was refractory to conventional therapy with steroids and cytotoxic drugs. IVIG was given as Sandoglobulin at a total dose of 2 g/kg over 5 days. By 2 months, 50% of the patients had achieved a full remission, while the remainder had a partial remission of their disease. After 1 year of follow-up, 19 of 26 patients were still in remission and one patient had died from overwhelming sepsis. However, most of these patients were still on oral cyclophosphamide or azathioprine and oral prednisolone. A subsequent randomized controlled trial of IVIG (2 g/kg total dose) in 34 patients with ANCA-associated vasculitis demonstrated modest treatment responses (14 of 17 patients improved compared with 6 of 17 placebo treated).[61] Benefit was not maintained in the long term, and a reversible rise in serum creatinine was a common complication. Richter et al[62] reported much less promising results in nine patients with ANCA-associated vasculitis who had responded incompletely to conventional therapy. No patient achieved a complete remission with IVIG. The major concern regarding the use of IVIG has been the frequent (usually reversible) deterioration in renal function in patients with an initial creatinine > 200 μmol/L.[63] Such nephrotoxicity makes it difficult to justify the use of IVIG as preferred treatment in patients with severe crescentic nephritis.

Mycophenolate has been used to treat patients with a variety of immune-mediated nephritides, usually for chronic disease. Stegeman et al[64] used mycophenolate for induction of remission in patients with active WG who were intolerant of cyclophosphamide. Most achieved complete remission but over 20% relapsed subsequently. Adverse effects included leukopenia, anemia, abdominal pain, and diarrhea, and were usually dose related.

Maintenance therapy

Long-term maintenance therapy is usually required for crescentic nephritis associated with ANCA. Up to 50% of

patients will relapse with systemic or local disease.[25] In the Hammersmith series, use of long-term maintenance therapy and tailoring treatment according to ANCA status has reduced the relapse rate at 5 years from 53% to 22%.[25] The majority of patients in this series were still taking a cytotoxic agent in the third year, usually azathioprine. The choice of drug has been clarified by the recent CYCAZAREM trial results, although the duration of maintenance therapy remains controversial. The long-term use of cyclophosphamide has been associated with significant adverse effects,[65] while azathioprine is usually well tolerated with reduced risk of hematologic or urothelial malignancy. The CYCAZAREM randomized controlled trial clearly demonstrated that 3 months of cyclophosphamide followed by a switch to oral azathioprine was equally efficacious as continued cyclophosphamide after induction of remission. Relapse rates, mortality, and endstage renal disease were identical in both arms of the study, and there was a trend to less severe complications in patients receiving azathioprine as long-term maintenance therapy.[66] There should no longer be a place for the routine use of cyclophosphamide as maintenance therapy in ANCA-associated RPGN. In patients who relapse on azathioprine, or who are intolerant of it, the use of methotrexate or mycophenolate mofetil as maintenance therapy may be considered. Cyclosporine, pulsed intravenous cyclophosphamide and deoxyspergualin are also agents which could, in theory, provide useful immunosuppression; however, data are limited to small uncontrolled case series. In contrast, patients with anti-GBM disease rarely relapse and do not require long-term maintenance therapy.[24,67] Their immunosuppression should generally be withdrawn within 6 months of diagnosis.

Refractory disease has also been treated with anti-T-lymphocyte antibodies. Lockwood et al[68] used a combination of two humanized monoclonal antibodies, Campath 1H directed against CDw52 and an anti-CD4 antibody, in four patients and achieved a sustained remission in three. Antithymocyte globulin has also achieved a favorable response in a few patients with refractory WG, but again relapses were common. In view of the probable importance of ANCA in the pathogenesis of vasculitis, semi-specific removal of these antibodies has been attempted using L-tryptophan immunoadsorption[69] and more specifically with myeloperoxidase-bound immunosorbent columns to remove antimyeloperoxidase ANCA antibodies.[70] Therapy against tumor necrosis factor (TNF) using either blocking antibodies or soluble TNF receptors is showing promise in the treatment of acute and chronic disease, and trials are in progress. Finally, at least two patients with severe disease have received immunoablation with autologous bone marrow stem cell transplant, both of whom were apparently well 6 months after the procedure.

Outcome

Crescentic ANCA-positive RPGN should be controlled with conventional therapy in more than 70% of patients.[25] Levy and Winearls[4] reported patient-survival rates at 1 and 3 years of 86.3% in 31 patients with crescentic glomerulonephritis (of various etiologies) and an overall renal survival rate of 78%. Of these 31 patients, 20 were dialysis dependent at presentation. In the Hammersmith series of 73 patients with WG or MP and an initial creatinine value > 500 μmol/L who were treated with oral steroids, cyclophosphamide, and PE, 73% were alive with improved renal function 2 months after presentation.[25] Stegmayr et al[41] treated patients with severe renal failure and RPGN in a similar fashion (with PE or immunoadsorption) and were able to show that 70% came off dialysis. Gordon et al[71] reported 82% survival at 3 months in 150 patients with small-vessel vasculitis treated with steroids and oral or intravenous cyclophosphamide, while Aaserod et al[52] showed 74% and 75% patient and renal survival at 5 years, with 55% patients coming off dialysis. The outcome in recent studies, including patients with severe crescentic nephritis, is shown in Table 19.3. Renal recovery usually occurs within 1 month but can be delayed substantially after the initiation of therapy (up to 4 months in our experience). Patients with extensive interstitial damage on their initial renal biopsy, marked glomerulosclerosis, or a long history of untreated disease often respond to initial induction therapy but subsequently have declining renal function and ultimately require renal replacement therapy.[13,39,72] Increasing age has also been associated with a worse outcome. Patients who achieve a serum creatinine of < 200 μmol/L are subsequently much less likely to require renal support. Patients who suffer relapses of disease with further renal damage are at risk of long term renal failure; hence the need to prevent relapses and maintain prolonged remission.

The severity of the renal insult is particularly important in determining the outcome of patients with anti-GBM antibody-mediated crescentic nephritis, very few of whom come off dialysis despite aggressive treatment.[24] Overall less than 10% of patients with anti-GBM disease who present with a creatinine value > 500–600 μmol/L recover independent renal function, although we have found that as long as patients do not require dialysis at presentation, even those with severe renal failure, can recover renal function.[24] In those patients presenting with a serum creatinine < 600 μmol/L the outcome is good, with more than 70% retaining independent renal function at 1 year.[24] The poor outlook in patients with anti-GBM disease and advanced renal failure is in marked contrast to the outcome of patients with ANCA-associated crescentic nephritis or renal-limited vasculitis, in whom a substantial number dependent on dialysis at presentation show improved renal function with adequate immuno-suppression.[25,39,41] The long-term outcome in patients with anti-GBM disease who recover renal function is good, particularly as the disease does not relapse. Most patients will have sustained independent renal function, unless the initial renal biopsy demonstrated significant interstitial scarring. The prognosis in other crescentic nephritides is variable. Sumekthul et al[73] examined patients with SLE and crescentic RPGN and found that 38% required long-term renal replacement therapy despite aggressive treatment. In IgA disease, the importance of crescents remains somewhat controversial, with studies reporting both positive and negative predictive value for long-term renal failure,[74,75] although most of these patients did not have true RPGN.

Specific recommendations for treatment

It is critically important that a specific diagnosis is made in all patients with light microscopic changes of crescentic glomerulonephritis and clinical presentation with RPGN. For example, the recommended treatment regimen will vary considerably between a patient with anti-GBM disease presenting on dialysis and a patient with MP presenting similarly (Fig. 19.1). Subsequent chapters detail appropriate treatment protocols for individual disease entities. Patients with ANCA-negative renal-limited vasculitis should be treated in the same way as those with ANCA-positive systemic vasculitis, since the renal prognosis is otherwise poor. We recommend that ANCA-positive patients presenting with a creatinine value < 500 μmol/L should be treated with oral prednisolone (1 mg/kg/day), oral cyclophosphamide (2 mg/kg/day, with dose reduction in the elderly), and prophylactic cotrimoxazole, anti-fungals, and histamine H_2 antagonists or proton-pump inhibitors. Patients who present with a creatinine value > 500 μmol/L or who are dialysis dependent should receive urgent PE using human albumin solution supplemented with calcium. Fresh-frozen plasma should be added to the replacement fluids within 3 days of renal biopsy or in the presence of bleeding. PE should be repeated frequently and regularly to provide at least seven 4-L exchanges within the first 2 weeks. If PE is unavailable, intravenous methylprednisolone (~15 mg/kg/day, maximum 1 g/day) should be given for three consecutive days. The definitive trial comparing these two strategies in patients with severe renal failure showed significant benefit of PE over methylprednisolone. One week after initiation of therapy oral prednisolone should be slowly reduced, so that patients are receiving 20 mg by 6 weeks and 10 mg by 6 months after the initial diagnosis. Cyclophosphamide should only be used for 3 months and subsequently changed to oral azathioprine (2 mg/kg/day) (as shown by the Cycazarem trial[66]). Renal function, urine deposit, and white blood cell count should be closely monitored, as should inflammatory markers and ANCA. Treatment should be continued for at least 2 years, and longer if there has been any evidence of disease relapse.

Patients presenting with anti-GBM disease and a serum creatinine value < 500 μmol/L are treated with oral cyclophosphamide (2 mg/kg/day), oral prednisolone (initially 1 mg/kg/day), and PE (at least seven exchanges, continued until autoantibodies are undetectable). Despite the lack of evidence, if PE is unavailable intravenous methylprednisolone (~15 mg/kg/day) should be given for three days, particularly in the presence of pulmonary hemorrhage. However, no long-term maintenance therapy is required and all drugs are withdrawn within 6–9 months. Close monitoring of renal function, urine deposit, white cell

Table 19.3 Outcome in severe crescentic glomerulonephritis

Reference	Diagnoses	Treatment	Alive with independent renal function (%)
Coward et al[81] (n = 18)	WG, MP	IVMP, P, Cyc, Aza, PE	50
Fuiano et al[82] (n = 5)	WG, MP	IVMP, P, Cyc, Aza, PE	60
Glockner et al[21] (n = 12)	WG, RLV, MP	P, Cyc, Aza, PE	67
Bolton & Sturgill[45] (n = 19)	MP, RLV	IVMP, P	74
Falk et al[53] (n = 12)	ANCA + GN	IVMP, P, Cyc	50
Rifle & Dechelette[38] (n = 14)	MP, WG, RLV	PE, IVMP, P, Cyc	43
Pusey et al[36] (n = 31)	MP, WG, RLV	P, Cyc, Aza PE, P, Cyc, Aza	60 69
Andrassy et al[46] (n = 14)	WG	IVMP, P, Cyc, PE in 2	93
Garrett et al[10] (n = 19)	ANCA + GN	IVMP, P, Cyc, Aza, PE	41
Cole et al[37] (n = 11)	RLV	IVMP, P, Aza PE, IVMP, P, Aza	29 75
Frasca et al[43] (n = 10)	ANCA + GN	PE, IVMP, P, Aza	80
Bindi et al[80] (n = 17)	ANCA + GN	IVMP, P, Cyc, PE in 6	47
Levy & Winearls[4] (n = 20)	WG, MP, RLV	P, Cyc, PE, IVMP	70
Haubitz et al[51] (n = 15)	WG, MP	IVMP, P, oral Cyc IVMP, P, i.v. Cyc	66 14
Pettersson et al[47] (n = 46)	WG, MP, RLV	P, Cyc, Aza	67
Higgins et al[83] (n = 7) (all > 70 years)	WG, MP	P, Cyc, Aza	29
Gaskin & Pusey[25] (n = 80)	WG, MP, RLV	PE, P, Cyc	73
McLaughlin et al[84] (n = 47)	WG, MP, RLV	P, Cyc, Aza, IVMP, PE in 3	61
Westman et al[76] (n = 123)	WG, MP	P, Cyc, Aza, IVMP, PE	78
Stegmayr et al[41] (n = 44)	WG, MP	PE, IA, P, Cyc	70
Aaserod et al[52] (n = 108)	WG	IVMP, P, Cyc, PE	86
Cohen & Clark[72] (n = 94)	WG, MP, RLV	IVMP, P, Cyc, PE	57
Zauner et al[39] (n = 39)	WG, MP	IVMP, P, Cyc PE, P, Cyc	85 70

ANCA + GN, antineutrophil cytoplasmic antibody-positive glomerulonephritis; Aza, azathioprine; Cyc, cyclophosphamide; IA, immunoadsorption; IVMP, intravenous methylprednisolone; MP, microscopic polyangiitis; P, oral prednisolone; PE, plasma exchange; RLV, renal-limited vasculitis; WG, Wegener granulomatosis.

count, and anti-GBM antibodies are important, particularly in the early stages of treatment when sepsis, fluid overload, and smoking can induce disease relapses. Patients presenting with oliguria or severe renal failure are treated similarly if pulmonary hemorrhage is a significant feature or if the renal biopsy suggests recent injury. However, if the biopsy of dialysis-dependent patients (without pulmonary hemorrhage) shows a high percentage of fibrous crescents, interstitial scarring, and chronic changes, without any reversible features (such as tubular necrosis), it may be reasonable to withhold aggressive immunosuppression and simply institute dialysis and monitor the natural decline in anti-GBM antibodies. A number of

insults can precipitate pulmonary hemorrhage in the presence of anti-GBM antibodies, so care should be taken to treat infections early and to warn the patient to avoid smoking.

Crescentic primary glomerulonephritis rarely responds to immunosuppression. However, we would use the biopsy as a guide to therapy, based on the degree of interstitial damage, the cellularity of the crescents, and number of obsolescent glomeruli. If treatment is considered, it would usually comprise cyclophosphamide and oral steroids as above. In contrast, crescentic secondary glomerulonephritis more often responds to immunosuppressive therapy. Patients with SLE who present with crescentic

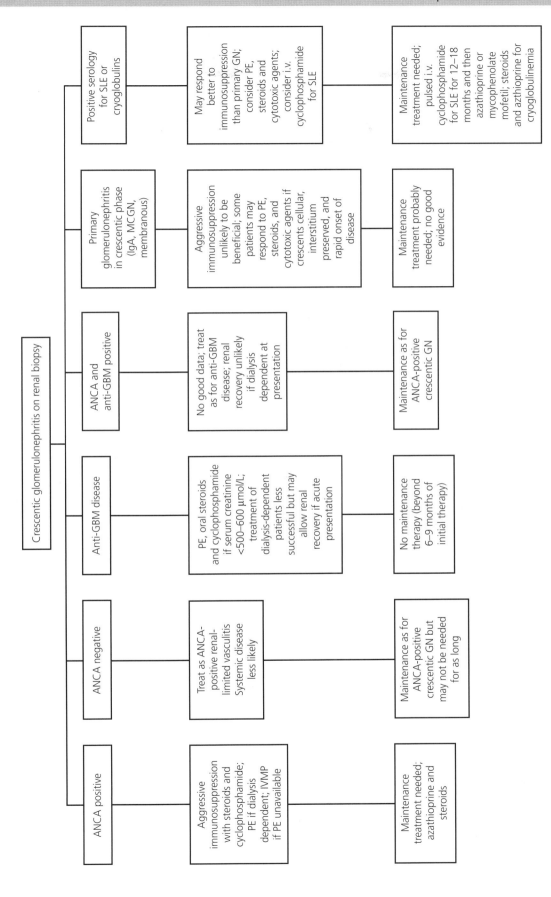

Figure 19.1 Management of crescentic glomerulonephritis. ANCA, antineutrophil cytoplasmic antibody; GN, glomerulonephritis; IVMP, intravenous methylprednisolone; MCGN, mesangiocapillary glomerulonephritis; PE, plasma exchange; SLE, systemic lupus erythematosus.

glomerulonephritis may benefit from pulsed intravenous cyclophosphamide in addition to oral or intravenous steroids (see later chapters). Recent trials of PE (in addition to immunosuppression) in patients with lupus nephritis have failed to show any benefit. However, the patients included in these studies had a wide range of renal impairment, so the potential benefit of PE in those with crescentic glomerulonephritis presenting with oliguria and dialysis dependence has not been addressed. Patients with crescentic glomerulonephritis secondary to cryo-globulinemia usually respond to PE in conjunction with cytotoxic agents and steroids, and may show a marked improvement in renal function (see later chapters).

Future directions

The detailed analysis of the pan-European trials of PE versus intravenous methylprednisolone in the induction phase of treatment for MP, WG, or renal-limited vasculitis and severe renal failure are eagerly awaited.[44] The use of methotrexate in limited disease is also under investigation. Other planned trials include a comparison of intravenous and oral cyclophosphamide, the use of myco-phenolate mofetil in maintaining remission, and anti-TNF therapies. In our limited experience, IVIG appears to offers hope for some patients resistant to, or intolerant of, conventional therapy. Monoclonal antibody therapy, or appropriate fusion proteins, will probably contribute to future treatment regimens, using agents directed against T-cell antigens, endothelial cell antigens, and proinflam-matory cytokines (including TNF), as reported in various experimental models of glomerulonephritis. Trials of anti-CD4 and anti-CDw52 monoclonal antibodies as rescue therapy in systemic vasculitis are already underway. As the molecular mechanisms involved in crescentic glomerulo-nephritis are dissected, it will be possible to design more specific forms of immunotherapy, such as analogue peptides involved in the MHC–T-cell receptor trimolecular complex.

References

1. Rees AJ, Cameron JS: Crescentic glomerulonephritis. *In* Cameron JS, Davison AM, Grunfeld JP, Kerr D, Ritz E (eds): Oxford Textbook of Clinical Nephrology. Oxford: Oxford University Press, 1992, pp 418–438.
2. Glassock RJ, Cohen EH, Adler SG: Primary glomerular disease. *In* Brenner BM (ed): The Kidney, 5th edn. Philadelphia: WB Saunders, 1996, pp 1392–1497.
3. Neild GH, Cameron JS, Ogg CS, et al: Rapidly progressive glomerulonephritis with extensive glomerular crescent formation. Q J Med 1983;52:395–416.
4. Levy JB, Winearls CG: Rapidly progressive glomerulonephritis: what should be first-line therapy? Nephron 1994;67:402–407.
5. Angangco R, Thiru S, Esnault VL, Short AK, Lockwood CM, Oliveira DB: Does truly "idiopathic" crescentic glomerulonephritis exist? Nephrol Dial Transplant 1994;9:630–636.
6. Ferrario F, Tadros MT, Napodano P, Sinico RA, Fellin G, D'Amico G: Critical re-evaluation of 41 cases of "idiopathic" crescentic glomerulonephritis. Clin Nephrol 1994;41:1–9.
7. Adler SG, Cohen AH, Glassock RJ: Secondary glomerular diseases. *In* Brenner BM (ed): The Kidney, 5th edn. Philadelphia: WB Saunders, 1996, pp 1498–1596.
8. Jennette JC, Wilkman AS, Falk RJ: Anti-neutrophil cytoplasmic autoantibody-associated glomerulonephritis and vasculitis. Am J Pathol 1989;135:921–930.
9. Cohen Tervaert JW, Goldschmeding R, Elema JD, et al: Autoantibodies against myeloid lysosomal enzymes in crescentic glomerulonephritis. Kidney Int 1990;37:799–806.
10. Garrett PJ, Dewhurst AG, Morgan LS, Mason JC, Dathan JR: Renal disease associated with circulating antineutrophil cytoplasmic activity. Q J Med 1992;85:731–749.
11. Ferrario F, Tadros M, Napodano P, et al: Rapidly progressive glomerulonephritis: is there still an "idiopathic" subgroup? Adv Exp Med Biol 1993;336:431–434.
12. Hedger N, Stevens J, Drey N, Walker S, Roderick P: Incidence and outcome of pauci-immune rapidly progressive glomerulonephritis in Wessex, UK: a 10 year retrospective study. Nephrol Dial Transplant 2000;15:1593–1599.
13. Aaserod K, Bostad L, Hammerstrom J, Jorstad S, Iversen BM: Renal histopathology and clinical course in 94 patients with Wegener's granulomatosis. Nephrol Dial Transplant 2001;16:953–966.
14. Sasatomi Y, Kiyoshi Y, Takabeyashi S: A clinical and pathological study on the characteristics and factors influencing the prognosis of crescentic glomerulonephritis using a cluster analysis. Pathol Int 1999;49:781–785.
15. Haas M, Spargo BH, Wit EJ, Meehan SM: Etiologies and outcome of acute renal insufficiency in older adults: a renal biopsy study of 259 cases. Am J Kidney Dis 2000;35:433–447.
16. Pusey CD, Rees AJ: Rapidly progressive glomerulonephritis and anti-glomerular basement membrane disease. *In* Weatherall DJ, Ledingham JGG, Warrell DA (eds): Oxford Textbook of Medicine, 3rd edn. Oxford: Oxford University Press, 1996, pp 3162–3166.
17. Ferrario F, Rastaldi MP, D'Amico G: The crucial role of renal biopsy in the management of ANCA-associated renal vasculitis. Nephrol Dial Transplant 1996;11:726–728.
18. Jennette JC, Falk RJ: Clinical and pathological classification of ANCA-associated vasculitis: what are the controversies? Clin Exp Immunol 1995;101(Suppl 1):18–22.
19. Levy JB, Hammad T, Coulthart A, Dougan T, Pusey CD: Features and outcome of patients with both anti-glomerular basement membrane (anti-GBM) antibodies and anti-neutrophil cytoplasm antibodies (ANCA). J Am Soc Nephrol 2001;12:113A.
20. Stevens ME, McConnell M, Bone JM: Aggressive treatment with pulse methylprednisolone or plasma exchange is justified in rapidly progressive glomerulonephritis. Proc Eur Dial Transplant Assoc 1982;19:724–731.
21. Glockner WM, Sieberth HG, Wichmann HE, et al: Plasma exchange and immunosuppression in rapidly progressive glomerulonephritis: a controlled multi-center study. Clin Nephrol 1988;29:1–8.
22. Levy JB, Pusey CD: Still a role for plasma exchange in rapidly progressive glomerulonephritis? J Nephrol 1997;10:7–13.
23. Levy JB, Pusey CD: Anti-GBM antibody mediated disease. *In* Wilkinson R, Jamison R (eds): Nephrology. London: Chapman & Hall, 1997, pp 599–615.
24. Levy JB, Turner AN, Rees AJ, Pusey CD: Long term outcome of anti-glomerular basement membrane antibody disease treated with plasma exchange and immunosuppression. Ann Intern Med 2001;134:1033–1042.
25. Gaskin G, Pusey CD: Systemic vasculitis. *In* Davison A, Cameron JS, Grunfeld JP, Kerr DNS, Ritz E, Winearls CG (eds): Oxford Textbook of Clinical Nephrology, 2nd edn. Oxford: Oxford University Press, 1997, pp 877–911.
26. Lai KN, Lai FN, Leung ACT, Ho CP, Vallance-Owen J: Plasma exchange in patients with rapidly progressive idiopathic IgA nephropathy: a report of two cases and review of the literature. Am J Kidney Dis 1987;10:66–70.
27. Roccatello D, Ferro M, Coppo R, Giraudo G, Quattrocchio G, Piccoli G: Report on intensive treatment of extracapillary glomerulonephritis with focus on crescentic IgA nephropathy. Nephrol Dial Transplant 1995;10:2054–2059.
28. Fauci AS, Wolff SM: Wegener's granulomatosis: studies in eighteen patients and a review of the literature. Medicine (Baltimore) 1973;52:535–561.
29. Fauci AS, Haynes BF, Katz P, Wolff SM: Wegener's granulomatosis: prospective clinical and therapeutic experience with 85 patients for 21 years. Ann Intern Med 1983;98:76–85.
30. Hind CRK, Paraskevakou H, Lockwood CM, Evans DJ, Peters DK, Rees AJ: Prognosis after immunouppression of patients with crescentic nephritis requiring dialysis. Lancet 1983;i:263–265.

31. Fuiano G, Cameron JS, Raftery M, Hartley BH, Williams DG, Ogg CS: Improved prognosis of renal microscopic polyarteritis in recent years. Nephrol Dial Transplant 1988;3:383–391.

32. Lockwood CM, Boulton-Jones JM, Lowenthal RM, Simpson IJ, Peters DK: Recovery from Goodpasture's syndrome after immunosuppressive treatment and plasmapheresis. Br Med J 1975;2:252–254.

33. Lockwood CM, Rees AJ, Pearson TA, Evans DJ, Peters DK, Wilson CB: Immunosuppression and plasma-exchange in the treatment of Goodpasture's syndrome. Lancet 1976;i:711–715.

34. Lockwood CM, Pinching AJ, Sweny P, et al: Plasma exchange and immunosuppression in the treatment of fulminating immune complex crescentic nephritis. Lancet 1977;i:63–67.

35. Johnson JP, Moore JJ, Austin HJ, Blalow JE, Antonovych TT, Wilson CB: Therapy of anti-glomerular basement membrane antibody disease: analysis of prognostic significance of clinical, pathological and treatment factors. Medicine (Baltimore) 1985;64:219–227.

36. Pusey CD, Rees AJ, Evans DJ, Peters DK, Lockwood CM: Plasma exchange in focal necrotizing glomerulonephritis without anti-GBM antibodies. Kidney Int 1991;40:757–763.

37. Cole E, Cattran D, Magil A, et al: A prospective randomised trial of plasma exchange as additive therapy in idiopathic crescentic glomerulonephritis. Am J Kidney Dis 1992;20:261–269.

38. Rifle G, Dechelette E: Treatment of rapidly progressive glomerulonephritis by plasma exchange and methylprednisolone pulses. A prospective randomised trial of cyclophosphamide. Interim analysis. Prog Clin Biol Res 1990;337:263–267.

39. Zauner I, Bach D, Kramer BK, et al: Predictive value of initial histology and effect of plasmapheresis on long term prognosis of rapidly progressive glomerulonephritis. Am J Kidney Dis 2002;39:28–35.

40. Guillevin L, Lhote F, Cohen P, et al: Lack of superiority of corticosteroids plus pulse cyclophosphamide and plasma exchanges to corticosteroids plus pulse cyclophosphamide alone in the treatment of polyarteritis nodosa and Churg Strauss syndrome patients with poor prognostic factors. A prospective randomised trial in 62 patients. Arthritis Rheum 1995;38:1638–1645.

41. Stegmayr BG, Almroth G, Berlin G, et al: Plasma exchange or immunoadsorption in patients with rapidly progressive crescentic glomerulonephritis. A Swedish multi-center study. Int J Artif Organs 1999;22:81–87.

42. Frasca GM, Zoumparidis NG, Borgnino LC, Neri L, Neri L, Vangelista A: Combined treatment in Wegener's granulomatosis with crescentic glomerulonephritis: clinical course and long-term oucome. Int J Artif Organs 1993;16:11–19.

43. Frasca GM, Zoumparidis LG, Borgnino LC, Neri L, Vangelista A, Bonomini V: Plasma exchange treatment in rapidly progressive glomerulonephritis associated with anti-neutrophil cytoplasmic antibodies. Int J Artif Organs 1992;15:181–184.

44. Rasmussen N, Jayne DRW, Abramowicz D, et al: European therapeutic trials in ANCA associated systemic vasculitis: disease scoring, consensus regimens and proposed clinical trials. Clin Exp Immunol 1995;101(Suppl 1):29–34.

45. Bolton WK, Sturgill BC: Methylprednisolone therapy for acute crescentic rapidly progressive glomerulonephritis. Am J Nephrol 1989;9:368–375.

46. Andrassy K, Erb A, Koderisch J, Waldherr R, Ritz E: Wegener's granulomatosis with renal involvement: patient survival and correlations between initial renal function, renal histology, therapy and renal outcome. Clin Nephrol 1991;35:139–147.

47. Pettersson EE, Sundelin B, Heigel Z: Incidence and outcome of pauci-immune necrotizing and crescentic glomerulonephritis in adults. Clin Nephrol 1995;43:141–149.

48. Austin HA, Klippel JH, Balow JE, et al: Therapy of lupus nephritis. Controlled trial of prednisone and cytotoxic drugs. N Engl J Med 1986;314:614–619.

49. Reinhold-Keller E, Kekow J, Schnabel A, et al: Influence of disease manifestations and antineutrophil cytoplasmic antibody titer on the response to pulse cyclophosphamide therapy in patients with Wegener's granulomatosis. Arthritis Rheum 1994;39:919–924.

50. Guillevin L, Lhote F, Jarrousse B, et al: Treatment of severe Wegener's granulomatosis: a prospective trial comparing prednisone, pulse cyclophosphamide versus prednisone and oral cyclophosphamide. Clin Exp Immunol 1995;101(Suppl 1):43 (abstract).

51. Haubitz M, Brunkhorst R, Schellong S, Gobel U, Schwek HJ, Koch KM: A prospective randomised study comparing daily oral versus monthly intravenous cyclophosphamide in patients with ANCA associated vasculitis and renal involvement (preliminary results) (abstract). Clin Exp Immunol 1995;101(Suppl 1):43.

52. Aaserod K, Iversen B, Hammerstrom J, et al: Wegener's granulomatosis: clinical course in 108 patients with renal involvement. Nephrol Dial Transplant 2000;15:611–618.

53. Falk RJ, Hogan S, Carey TS, Jennette JC: Clinical course of anti-neutrophil cytoplasmic autoantibody-associated glomerulonephritis and vasculitis. Ann Intern Med 1990;113:656–663.

54. Haubitz M, Frei U, Rother U, Brunkhorst R, Koch KM: Cyclophosphamide pulse therapy in Wegeners granulomatosis. Nephrol Dial Transplant 1991;6:531–535.

55. de Groot K, Adu D, Savage COS: The value of pulse cyclophosphamide in ANCA associated vasculitis: meta-analysis and critical review. Nephrol Dial Transplant 2001;16:2018–2027.

56. Hoffman GS, Leavitt RY, Kerr GS, et al: The treatment of Wegeners granulomatosis with glucocorticoids and methotrexate. Arthritis Rheum 1992;35:1322–1329.

57. Sneller MC, Hoffman GS, Talar-Williams C, Kerr GS, Hallahan CW, Fauci AS: An analysis of 42 Wegeners granulomatosis patients treated with methotrexate and prednisone. Arthritis Rheum 1995;18:608–613.

58. Borleffs JCC, Derksen RHWM, Hene RJ: Treatment of Wegeners granulomatosis with cyclosporin. Ann Rheum Dis 1987;46:175.

59. Gremmell F, Druml W, Schmidt, et al: Cyclosporin in Wegeners granulomatosis. Ann Intern Med 1988;108:491–492.

60. Jayne DRW, Lockwood CM: Pooled intravenous immunoglobulin in the management of systemic vasculitis. Adv Exp Med Biol 1993;336:469–472.

61. Jayne DRW, Chapel H, Adu D, et al: Intravenous immunoglobulin for ANCA associated systemic vasculitis with persistent disease activity. Q J Med 2000;93:433–439.

62. Richter C, Schnabel A, Csernok E, De Groot K, Reinhold-Keller E, Gross WL: Treatment of anti-neutrophil cytoplasmic antibody (ANCA)-associated systemic vasculitis with high-dose intravenous immunoglobulin. Clin Exp Immunol 1995;101:2–7.

63. Levy JB, Pusey CD: Renal failure and intravenous immunoglobulin. Q J Med 2000;93:751–755.

64. Stegeman CA, Cohen Tervaert JW: Mycophenolate mofetil for remission induction in patients with active Wegener's granulomatosis intolerant of cyclophosphamide. J Am Soc Nephrol 2000;11:98A.

65. Hoffman GS, Leavitt RY, Fleisher TA, Minor JR, Fauci AS: Treatment of Wegener's granulomatosis with intermittent high dose intravenous cyclophosphamide. Am J Med 1990;89:403–410.

66. Jayne D, Rasmussen N. European collaborative trials in vasculitis: EUVAS update and latest results. Clin Exp Immunol 2000;120(Suppl 1):13–15.

67. Levy JB, Lachmann RH, Pusey CD: Recurrent Goodpasture's disease. Am J Kidney Dis 1996;27:573–578.

68. Lockwood CM, Thiru S, Isaacs JD, Hale G, Waldmann H: Long term remission of intractable systemic vasculitis with monoclonal antibody therapy. Lancet 1993;341:1620–1622.

69. Elliott JD, Lockwood CM, Hale G, Waldmann H: Semi-specific immuno-absorption and monoclonal antibody therapy in ANCA positive vasculitis: experience in four cases. Autoimmunity 1998;28:163–171.

70. Alexandre S, Moguilevsky N, Paindavoine P, et al: Specific MPO immunoabsorption for the treatment of vasculitis. Clin Exp Immunol 2000;120(Suppl 1):43.

71. Gordon M, Luqmani RA, Adu D, et al: Relapses in patients with systemic vasculitis. Q J Med 1993;86:779–789.

72. Cohen BA, Clark WF: Pauci-immune renal vasculitis: natural history, prognostic factors and impact of therapy. Am J Kidney Dis 2000;36:914–924.

73. Sumekthul V, Chalermsanyakorn P, Changsirikulchai S, Radinahamed P: Lupus nephritis: a challenging cause of rapidly progressive crescentic glomerulonephritis. Lupus 2000;9:424–428.

74. Haas M: Histologic subclassification of IgA nephropathy: a clinicopathologic study of 244 cases. Am J Kidney Dis 1997;29:829–842.

75. D'Amico G: Natural history of idiopathic IgA nephropathy: role of clinical and histological prognostic factors. Am J Kidney Dis 2000;36:227–237.

76. Westman KWA, Bygren PG, Olsson H, Ranstam J, Wieslander J: Relapse rate, renal survival and cancer morbidity in patients with

Wegener's granulomatosis or microscopic polyangiitis with renal involvement. J Am Soc Nephrol 1998;9:842–852.

77. Heilman JL, Offord KP, Holley KE, Velosa JA: Analysis of risk factors for patient and renal survival in crescentic glomerulonephritis. Am J Kidney Dis 1987;9:98–107.

78. Keller F, Oehlenberg B, Kunzendorf U, Schwarz A, Offermann G: Long-term treatment and prognosis of rapidly progressive glomerulonephritis. Clin Nephol 1989;31:190–197.

79. Ritz E, Andrassy K, Kuster S, Waldherr R: Wegener's granulomatosis, microscopic polyarteritis and pauciimmune crescentic glomerulonephritis. An overview. Contrib Nephrol 1991;94:1–12.

80. Bindi P, Mougenot B, Mentre F, et al: Necrotizing crescentic glomerulonephritis without significant immune deposits: a clinical and serological study. Q J Med 1993;86:55–68.

81. Coward RA, Hamdy NA, Shortland JS, Brown CB: Renal micropolyarteritis: a treatable condition. Nephrol Dial Transplant 1986;1:31–37.

82. Fuiano G, Cameron JS, Raftery M, Hartley BH, Williams DG, Ogg CS: Improved prognosis of renal microscopic polyarteritis in recent years. Nephrol Dial Transplant 1988;3:383–391.

83. Higgins RM, Goldsmith DJ, Connolly J, et al: Vasculitis and rapidly progressive glomerulonephritis in the elderly. Postgrad Med J 1996;72:41–44.

84. McLaughlin K, Jerimiah P, Fox JG, Mactier RA, Simpson K, Boulton-Jones JM: Has the prognosis for patients with pauci-immune necrotizing glomerulonephritis improved? Nephrol Dial Transplant 1998:13;1696–1701.

Antiglomerular Basement Membrane Antibody Disease

A. Neil Turner and Andrew J. Rees

Background

Goodpasture, or antiglomerular basement membrane (anti-GBM), disease is an uncommon but usually severe disease caused by autoimmunity to a component of certain basement membranes.[1] Autoantibodies to this component, the "Goodpasture antigen", define the disorder. Anti-GBM antibodies had been used for nearly 100 years to induce experimental nephritis before the human disease was identified, and Goodpasture disease remains one of the few types of human nephritis in which there is considerable understanding of the mechanisms leading to renal injury. It was also the first type of inflammatory glomerulonephritis for which effective treatment was developed. This was a landmark because similar therapy was then applied to other types of rapidly progressive glomerulonephritis (RPGN), in which it was often even more effective.

Clinical and pathologic features

Ernest Goodpasture reported a single patient with lung hemorrhage and RPGN in 1919. Although Goodpasture's name is now firmly associated with anti-GBM disease, it is now clear that this syndrome occurs more commonly in small-vessel vasculitis (see Chapter 21). Accordingly, it is important to determine the underlying disorder as there are prognostic and therapeutic differences.

Typical patients present with fulminant disease of short duration, although minor symptoms, particularly of lung disease, may have been present for weeks or occasionally much longer. The phenomenon of a sudden crescendo in disease intensity is common, and it is often only when this occurs that the disease is diagnosed. In such patients the time window in which treatment can salvage renal function, or even life, is short, and rapid diagnosis and treatment are essential if this is to be achieved.[1,2]

Patients may also present with renal disease alone or with pulmonary disease alone. As the symptoms of minor renal disease are nonspecific, it is common for presentation with isolated renal disease to be late. Lung hemorrhage, on the other hand, often causes hemoptysis relatively early, and patients often seek medical attention at a time when signs of renal involvement may be minimal. Usually at least microscopic hematuria is present. Patients occasionally present with subacute renal disease, leading to nephrotic syndrome with hematuria and variable renal impairment, although mild or rapidly progressive renal disease is much more common.

Even where the diagnosis appears to be obvious, renal biopsy is important for prognostic reasons and thus in guiding therapy.

Diagnosis

Diagnosis rests on the demonstration of anti-GBM antibodies, either fixed to basement membranes of affected organs or in the circulation. As systemic vasculitis may cause a similar clinical picture and even overlap with Goodpasture disease, measurement of antineutrophil cytoplasmic antibodies (ANCA) is essential whenever the diagnosis is contemplated. The most sensitive technique for detection of antibodies is direct immunohistologic examination of a renal biopsy. Linear fixation of immunoglobulin is described in several other circumstances, but the concurrence of linear antibody fixation and crescentic nephritis occurs only in Goodpasture disease or in systemic vasculitis associated with Goodpasture autoantibodies.[2] Direct immunohistology of lung biopsies is less reliable because antibody binding may be patchy. Indirect immunohistology using patients' sera (demonstrating binding of antibodies to GBM on sections of normal kidney) is an unreliable technique that will only identify high-titer anti-GBM sera. Immunoassays for circulating anti-GBM antibodies are valuable but their reliability varies.[3] High titers of antibodies are usually found in patients with fulminant or rapidly progressive disease, and false-negative results should in these circumstances be very uncommon. False positives are occasionally found, according to the quality of the antigen used as the ligand. False-negative results are most likely in patients with relatively low antibody titers, typically associated with isolated lung disease or minor or slowly progressive renal disease. False-negative results may also be encountered in the post-transplant anti-GBM disease that occurs in some patients with Alport syndrome, even in the presence of quite florid disease, because the target of anti-GBM antibodies may be different (described below).

Basis of lung hemorrhage

Lung hemorrhage occurs in about 50% of patients at some stage but, unlike renal injury, its severity and incidence correlate poorly with antibody titers. There is clear evidence from epidemiologic and anecdotal observations, and from animal models, that local injury to the lung influences the occurrence of pulmonary hemorrhage and is likely to account for these observations. In patients, several surveys have confirmed a close association of lung hemorrhage with cigarette smoking. Anecdotally, other inhaled substances, notably gasoline and other volatile organic compounds, have also precipitated pulmonary hemorrhage. Pulmonary or other infection and volume overload have also been associated with lung hemorrhage.

Alport post-transplant anti-GBM disease

While renal transplantation in Alport syndrome is generally successful and overall graft survival rate is at least as good as for other patients, up to 5% of patients may develop crescentic nephritis in the allograft with linear binding of immunoglobulin to the GBM.[4] In the majority of cases the graft is lost and retransplantation has been unsuccessful. Typically the disease develops some months after a first or second allograft, and is recognized at a stage when the glomeruli have already been destroyed. In subsequent allografts the disease develops within weeks or even days and progresses much more rapidly. A few patients have shown less aggressive disease and retained their allografts in these circumstances. Disease is limited to the donor organ.

Most patients with Alport syndrome lack the network of tissue-specific type IV collagen chains ($\alpha3/\alpha4/\alpha5$) that make up the collagen framework of normal GBM. They are replaced by $\alpha1/\alpha2$ chains of type IV collagen, the isoforms that form the collagen component of most basement membranes in the body. This seems to be inadequate for long-term structural stability in the GBM, or the cochlea, although Alport lungs do not seem to suffer from the absence of $\alpha3/\alpha4/\alpha5$ in the alveolar basement membrane. Antibodies in Alport anti-GBM disease are therefore directed toward components of the donor GBM missing from their own basement membranes, and are therefore *allo*antibodies rather than *auto*antibodies.[5] Most cases of Alport syndrome can be attributed to mutations of the gene encoding the $\alpha5$ chain of type IV collagen, which is located on the X chromosome; the usual target of allo-antibodies in Alport anti-GBM disease is the NC1 domain of $\alpha5$(IV) collagen.[5] This is distinct from the Goodpasture antigen, which is carried on the 70% homologous NC1 domain of the $\alpha3$ chain of type IV collagen, and explains

why immunoassays optimized to detect the autoantibodies of spontaneous Goodpasture disease may fail to detect the alloantibodies of Alport anti-GBM disease.

Clinical trials
Development of current regimens

Before the 1970s, a variety of treatments had been suggested for Goodpasture disease, ranging from the use of corticosteroids and azathioprine to bilateral nephrectomy, the latter a last resort for intractable pulmonary hemorrhage.[2] None had been consistently successful. Wilson and Dixon's observation that 12.5% of patients survived 1 year or more with functioning kidneys after an episode of Goodpasture disease affecting lungs and kidneys was in keeping with other series of the era.[2,6] At that time, based on the demonstration that circulating autoantibodies in the disease were directly pathogenic, a potentially highly toxic combination treatment was devised and tested in several patients.[7] The combination had three elements:

- intensive plasma exchange to remove autoantibodies;
- cytotoxic therapy, based on cyclophosphamide,[8] to prevent their resynthesis;
- corticosteroids as adjunctive anti-inflammatory agents.

The initial results were spectacularly good in a group of patients who otherwise would have been expected to have an extremely bad prognosis. Lung hemorrhage was arrested, usually within days, and recovery or preservation of renal function was reported. The initial studies were extended, and similar regimens applied elsewhere met with equally impressive results.[9–13] Plasma exchange combined with cyclophosphamide and corticosteroids has become the standard treatment for Goodpasture disease. None of the early studies was controlled, but the improvement in renal function was dramatically different from previous experience and was temporally related to the start of treatment.

Effectiveness and outcome

In subsequent years, the limits of the effectiveness of this therapy and its potential hazards have been delineated. The major cause of morbidity has been infection, often related to neutropenia. The cytotoxic therapy employed in the first series comprised both cyclophosphamide and azathioprine. This almost always led to leukopenia, and in recent years most have used cyclophosphamide alone without any obvious loss of effectiveness. Some have used significantly less intensive regimens, with less cyclophosphamide and/or less plasma exchange. It has been our impression, supported to some extent by published results, that this has been less effective, although fair comparison of series from different centers and countries is extremely difficult (Table 20.1).[9,12–16]

The mortality of Goodpasture disease is now much improved, although renal survival remains poor. The reason

Table 20.1 Results of treatment in series using immunosuppression and plasma exchange*

| Reference | Number of patients in study | Percentage with independent renal function at 1 year according to initial creatinine level[†] | | Notes on treatment given |
		≥ 600 µmol/L	< 600 µmol/L	
Briggs et al[9]	15	36% (4/11)	0% (0/4)	Only 4/15 received plasma exchange
Simpson et al[12]	12	70% (7/10)	0% (0/2)	8/12 received plasma exchange
Johnson et al[14]	17	69% (7/13)	0% (0/4)	Less cyclophosphamide than in Table 20.2. Half received plasma exchange, but only every third day, and using frozen plasma
Walker et al[13]	22	82% (9/11)	18% (2/11)	Slightly less cyclophosphamide and plasma exchange than in Table 20.2
Herody et al[15]	22	93% (13/14)	0% (0/15)	Variable amounts of plasma exchange and different immunosuppressive regimens were used
Hammersmith, 1975–99	71	95% (18/19)	15% (8/52)	As Table 20.2, except early patients also received azathioprine 1 mg/kg/day

Untreated patients have been excluded. Treated patients are divided into two groups according to their creatinine at the time treatment commenced, or at presentation if this is not available.
*Modified from Turner AN, Rees AJ: Antiglomerular basement membrane antibody disease. In Cameron JS, Davison AM, Grunfeld JP, Kerr DNS, Ritz E (eds): Oxford Textbook of Clinical Nephrology. Oxford: Oxford University Press, 1998, pp 647–666. By permission of Oxford University Press.
[†]The percentage of patients who were alive and not requiring dialysis at 1 year is shown (number and total number in that group at presentation are shown in parentheses). 600 µmol/L is equivalent to 6.8 mg/dL.

for this is the late stage at which treatment is instituted in most patients. Early treatment is of course difficult in a disease that evolves rapidly and normally is only diagnosed when that evolution occurs, but there is a very clear relationship between the severity of renal disease at presentation and the outcome (Table 20.1). Those who require dialysis or who present with oliguria or a serum creatinine > 500–600 µmol/L (~ 6–7 mg/dL) have a low probability of regaining useful renal function even with the most aggressive therapy. It has therefore been argued that they should not be subjected to the risks of such treatment, unless they have pulmonary hemorrhage. This is discussed further in the section Specific recommendations.

If ANCA are found as well as anti-GBM antibodies, the renal prognosis may be better. Some of these patients have evidence of vasculitic disease in other organs, but in some the disease is limited to kidneys or to lungs and kidneys. Several authors have reported that such patients are more likely to recover renal function from dependence on dialysis than patients with anti-GBM antibodies alone.[17–19] This may be because in most the anti-GBM response is a secondary phenomenon, a response to GBM damage caused by small-vessel vasculitis. The similarity of the response to treatment to that seen in pauci-immune RPGN is part of the evidence for this, although anti-GBM titers also tend to be lower and to fall rapidly with treatment. Some patients have clear evidence of vasculitis outside the kidneys and lungs. ANCA are most commonly directed against the neutrophil granule enzyme myeloperoxidase.

Autoantibody levels are usually rapidly suppressed by these treatments, and usually remain so after only a short period of therapy. Thereafter, recurrences are uncommon. Interestingly they seem to be particularly likely in patients with lung disease but only minor renal disease.[20] In untreated patients (those with endstage renal disease but no lung disease) antibodies may persist for 1 or 2 years or even longer. Ultimately, the immune response is therefore usually self-limiting, although treatment speeds the inhibition of autoantibody synthesis.[21]

Role of individual treatment components

Historical evidence suggests that corticosteroids alone, or azathioprine alone or in combination with corticosteroids, are not effective treatments.[2] Plasma exchange given alone leads to rapid resynthesis of autoantibodies.[22] The only randomized controlled trial in Goodpasture disease addressed the role of plasma exchange.[14] Although the results showed a better outcome in those receiving plasma exchange, the plasma exchange group had less severe renal disease than the drugs-only group, and the authors were justifiably cautious about making firm conclusions from these results. Both the plasma exchange and cyclophosphamide regimen used in this work were less intensive than recommended here, and this may be reflected in the slightly disappointing results (only 69% of patients with creatinine < 6.8 mg/dL recovered renal function) (see Table 20.1). Nevertheless the study did usefully show that patients with mild renal disease could do well with oral cyclophosphamide and prednisolone alone.

Pulsed intravenous methylprednisolone has been widely used in RPGN of other types, and in Goodpasture disease has sometimes been used in place of plasma exchange following an initial encouraging report.[23] Bolton and Sturgill's nonrandomized study of the use of pulses of methylprednisolone in crescentic nephritis of various types included 17 patients with Goodpasture disease, although most of these had advanced disease requiring dialysis.[24] The report only discusses effects on renal function, and methylprednisolone was given without other immuno-suppression. Of the four nonoliguric patients who were treated, only two retained renal function. Williams et al[25] reported failures of pulsed corticosteroid therapy in arresting pulmonary hemorrhage; Johnson et al[14] felt that it might stop pulmonary hemorrhage but had no impact on renal disease. Of major concern with the use of large doses of corticosteroids is the increased risk of secondary infection, sometimes opportunistic but usually a common bacterial infection. There is clear evidence in Goodpasture disease[26] and in animal models[27] that infections may precipitate or exacerbate lung hemorrhage and aggravate renal injury. We do not believe that the safety and efficiency of high-dose steroids have been established as an alternative to plasma exchange in this disease, in which there is a clear basis for removing autoantibodies.

Other effects of current regimens

While the original rationale for current treatment regimens was to control autoantibody levels, it is clear that therapy does substantially more than this. Plasma exchange depletes clotting factors, complement components, and other known and unknown mediators of renal damage, as well as circulating antibodies. While protein A immunoadsorption removes immunoglobulins much more specifically and appears to be equally effective clinically, it has been undertaken in only a few patients and no real comparison has been made. Similarly, cyclophosphamide suppresses antibody resynthesis but also has profound effects on cell-mediated immunity. It is effective in other autoimmune diseases where there is no evidence of a role for autoantibodies. It is not possible to disentangle these effects of the treatments from those originally intended.

Other agents for Goodpasture disease

Isolated reports describe the use of cyclosporine but give conflicting impressions of effectiveness.[28,29] Cyclosporine, deoxyspergualin, and anti-T-lymphocyte antibodies have been effective in animal models of Goodpasture disease, but usually these treatments have been given from the onset of the disease and it is not clear how closely these models mimic the human immune response.

Post-transplant anti-GBM disease

Renal transplantation undertaken in the presence of anti-GBM antibodies has been associated with recurrence of the disease in the allograft, although this has not occurred in all instances. Now that immunoassays for anti-GBM antibodies are widely available, recurrence seems to have become rare. More frequent is the development of post-transplant anti-GBM disease in patients in whom the original renal diagnosis was Alport syndrome.[4] In a proportion of patients this diagnosis may not have been made beforehand, because of lack of knowledge of family background, new mutations, or autosomal disease. Typically, patients are deaf and have developed endstage renal failure at a relatively young age. They are more likely to have a large gene deletion as the causative mutation. Once the disease has developed, the graft is almost always lost despite treatment, although often the disease is recognized late and initial treatments have often been those used to reverse graft rejection. Thus, many failures of high-dose corticosteroids are recorded, as are some for antilymphocyte antibodies. In those very few reported instances in which the graft has been retained, the treatments used were not particularly unusual.

Children, pregnancy, and the elderly

Goodpasture disease is very rare in childhood but has been reported in children as young as 2 years old. Lung hemorrhage is unusual in childhood examples. The reported numbers are very small, although there is evidence that response to treatment can be at least as good as that of adults.

Three case reports suggest that the fetus may not be directly harmed by maternal anti-GBM disease, although placental transfer of the predominantly IgG1 autoantibodies is to be expected. However, the fetus will clearly be harmed by maternal pulmonary hemorrhage and renal failure, and the prevention of these is usually the main concern. Anti-GBM disease in the elderly is less likely to be accompanied by lung hemorrhage, but anti-GBM antibodies are more likely to be associated with ANCA in this age group, which may be a relatively good prognostic feature. Elderly patients are more susceptible to leukopenia and infection, as well as to other complications of therapy. Doses of cyclophosphamide should be reduced. The risks of commencing or continuing aggressive treatment need to be balanced with these risks.

Specific recommendations

Drug treatment and antibody removal

None of the components of currently accepted therapy for Goodpasture disease has been subjected to analysis by rigorous controlled trial, nor are they now likely to be. The recommendations made here are therefore based on theoretical considerations, including the observation that the autoantibodies are directly pathogenic and that this is therefore at least in part an antibody-mediated disease, and on analysis of the effects of this and similar treatments. Our regimen for acute severe disease is shown in Table 20.2. The protocol is more intensive than that used by some, but an intensive regimen is required to suppress

Table 20.2 Treatment recommendations for acute Goodpasture disease

Prednisolone
1 mg/kg per 24 h orally. Reduce at weekly intervals to achieve one-sixth of this dose by 8 weeks. (For a starting daily dose of 60 mg, weekly reductions to 45 mg, 30 mg, 25 mg, 20 mg, 15 mg, 12.5 mg, 10 mg.) Maintain this dose to 3 months, stop by 4 months

Cyclophosphamide
3 mg/kg per 24 h orally, rounded down to the nearest 50 mg. Patients over 55 years should receive a reduced dose, 2–2.5 mg/kg. Administer by daily intravenous injection if unable to take orally

Plasma exchange
Daily exchange of 4 L of plasma for 5% human albumin for 14 days or until the circulating antibody is suppressed. In the presence of pulmonary hemorrhage, or within 48 h of an invasive procedure, 300–400 mL of fresh-frozen plasma is given at the end of each treatment. If white blood cell count $< 3.5 \times 10^9$ L, stop cyclophosphamide until it recovers. Resume at lower dose if cessation has been necessary

Monitoring
Daily blood count during plasma exchange and while antibody titer still elevated. At least twice weekly during first month, and weekly thereafter. Baseline Kco, with further measurements as indicated. Daily coagulation tests during plasma exchange to monitor for significant depletion of clotting factors. Initially, daily checks of renal and hepatic function, glucose

Prophylaxis against complications of treatment
Oral nystatin or similar for 1 month. Histamine H_2 antagonist during corticosteroid therapy. Prophylaxis against *Pneumocystis* infection during cyclophosphamide therapy. Avoid other antibiotics unless indicated. Close monitoring for signs of infection with full investigation of any fever

autoantibody levels as rapidly as possible. Some patients may not require such aggressive therapy, perhaps those with slight lung hemorrhage and minimal, if any, non-progressive renal disease. It is our practice to use full treatment for all patients with severe lung hemorrhage or with significant but recoverable renal disease. The risk of very rapid acceleration of disease is real, and it can be devastating.

A separate question is whether some patients with severe renal damage but no lung hemorrhage should not be given immunosuppressive treatment or plasma exchange. Given that most dialysis-dependent patients, or even those with creatinine values > 600 μmol/L (6.8 mg/dL), do not recover renal function, there is a strong case for withholding treatment in these circumstance.[30,31] There are several important caveats associated with this policy.

- Some patients in these circumstances have recoverable disease, as shown in several series and case reports (Fig. 20.1). Some have been shown on renal biopsy to have acute tubular necrosis, so that the nephritis was not as severe as perceived clinically. Others had very acute and recent onset of severe disease, and the biopsy appearances were notable for the very cellular (and uniform) crescents affecting most or all glomeruli. Renal biopsy is therefore an essential part of the assessment of such patients; if there is any doubt, it is safer to commence treatment until further information is available. There is little hazard from a few days of treatment but much to lose by delaying.
- Patients with ANCA as well as anti-GBM antibodies may have a better renal prognosis with treatment than those with anti-GBM antibodies alone, unless the renal biopsy shows advanced scarring. They may also be at risk of extrarenal vasculitis.

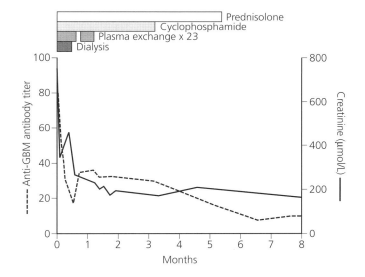

Figure 20.1 Response to treatment of a dialysis-requiring patient with Goodpasture disease (renal disease only, no lung hemorrhage). This patient had 85% crescents but very acute disease. Such a response is unusually good but many instances have been reported (see text).

- Lung hemorrhage may occur as a late development in response to infection, toxic exposure, or other stimuli, and should be guarded against and looked for. This is uncommon but a significant risk.
- Withholding treatment extends the interval before renal transplantation is possible, sometimes to years, because antibody levels subside much more slowly.

The specific contribution of plasma exchange to disease that is not immediately life-threatening or rapidly progressive is uncertain, but it does allow more rapid control of anti-GBM antibody levels and reduces the risk of an acceleration of disease activity. Protein A immunoadsorption may permit even more rapid control of autoantibody levels[32] and apparent effectiveness at arresting pulmonary hemorrhage has been reported;[33] however it does not remove other factors that may contribute to renal injury and is labor intensive and technically demanding. When it is available, the fact that it reduces the need for blood components may make the overall cost similar to that of plasma exchange.

Whether treatment with cyclophosphamide and prednisolone (but not plasma exchange) accelerates the disappearance of anti-GBM antibodies in comparison with no treatment has not been clearly shown.

Because the risks of pulsed methylprednisolone therapy may outweigh potential benefits, we believe that it is not an adequate substitute for intensive plasma exchange in severe disease. The use of other therapeutic agents must be regarded as experimental in the absence of adequate reported data.

Supportive treatment

As in other severe illnesses, it is likely that attention to details other than the primary therapy may be critical in determining outcome. These include details of respiratory, renal, and other supportive care.

Lung hemorrhage is precipitated or exacerbated by fluid overload, pulmonary or remote infections, and by pulmonary irritants and toxins. Experimentally, this includes oxygen toxicity, so in the intensive care setting fractional inspired oxygen concentration should be kept as low as is compatible with adequate tissue oxygenation. On recovery, patients should be prohibited from smoking.

The major cause of morbidity and mortality after the first few days is infection. These can be minimized by avoidance of nonessential intravascular lines and by adhering rigorously to protocols for the care of those that are in place. Neutrophil counts should be monitored carefully and cyclophosphamide dose adjusted accordingly. Prophylactic agents should be given as indicated (see Table 20.2). Granulocyte colony-stimulating factor (filgrastim) can be useful for severe neutropenia.

Post-transplant anti-GBM disease

Avoidance of transplantation in the presence of circulating antibodies should reduce the risk of disease recurrence, and an additional delay of 12 months has been recommended. We have reduced this to 6 months in some instances without evidence of disease recurrence. Recurrences of spontaneous Goodpasture disease should respond to similar treatments to those used for the disorder in native kidneys.

Alport post-transplant anti-GBM disease is different, in that the response is to a "foreign" antigen (alloantigen) not an autoantigen, and there are very few examples of effective therapy on which to base recommendations. It is

important to appreciate the low sensitivity of standard assays for anti-GBM antibodies in these circumstances, particularly as it seems very likely that, as in spontaneous Goodpasture diesease, early recognition and aggressive treatment aimed at suppressing the antibody response are critical to success. Renal biopsy, including immunofluorescence examination to identify GBM-fixed immunoglobulin, is usually the quickest way to make the diagnosis, and antibody titers can be followed subsequently by using an assay based on crude antigen or by sending samples to a center with access to recombinant or hightly purified antigens. Intensive plasma exchange appears to be a critical part of management. Anti-T-cell therapies do not appear to be powerfully effective when used alone. There are obvious problems in using antilymphocyte antibodies in combination with plasma exchange. By analogy with spontaneous anti-GBM disease, cyclophosphamide is likely to be substantially better at suppressing disease than azathioprine. We are aware of one notable success using mycophenolate mofetil after cyclophosphamide had to be stopped because of bone marrow toxicity.

Future directions

Familiarity with treatment regimens and improvements in intensive care have improved death rates, but there has been little further improvement in renal outcome since combination therapy was first described. Indeed, in the UK, physicians' familiarity with immunosuppressive regimens and the much wider availability of plasma exchange has reduced the rate of referral of patients with this and similar diseases to centers where there is more accumulated experience. This may not be in patients' best interests.

At present, improved outcomes are heavily dependent on more rapid recognition and diagnosis, and earlier institution of currently available therapies. It is interesting to speculate why treatment at apparently similar stages of disease is less effective in Goodpasture disease than in other types of RPGN. It may be that while they appear histologically similar, the underlying structural damage is more severe in Goodpasture disease. Alternatively, other factors may have to be understood that could be controlled by additional therapies. Specific immunoadsorption may become a way to remove anti-GBM antibodies without rendering the patient hypogammaglobulinemic,[34] although there is no reason to think it should be any more effective or technically simpler than protein A immunoadsorption, which removes most IgG.

Research models of anti-GBM disease have suggested ways in which the inflammatory response may be down-regulated by agents that interfere with the localization of leukocytes to the inflamed glomerulus or by decreasing their activation state once there. Examples include inhibition of lymphocyte costimulation with molecules directed against CD80/CD86 or CD40; therapies designed to inhibit proinflammatory cytokines (tumor necrosis factor and interleukin 1); or infusion of anti-inflammatory cytokines (interleukin 10). Models of anti-GBM disease have been used extensively to determine the efficiency of such approaches and to assess the newer immunosuppressive agents. Many of these agents are being used in phase I clinical trials[35,36] and several could be applicable to human disease.[36] Because of the rarity of Goodpasture disease it is unlikely that randomized clinical trials of this disease alone could be viable, even between multiple centers. However, from work in human and model systems, information about the immune and inflammatory responses in Goodpasture disease is so much more extensive than in other types of nephritis that further therapies are likely to spring from it.

References

1. Falk RJ, Jenelte JC, Nachman PH: Primary Glomerular Diseases. *In* Brenner BM (ed): Benner and Rector's The Kidney, 6th edn. Philadelphia: WB Saunders, 2000, pp 1317–1347.

2. Turner AN, Rees AJ: Antiglomerular basement membrane disease. *In* Davison AM, Cameron JS, Grunfeld J-P, Kerr DNS, Ritz E, Winearls CG (eds): Oxford Textbook of Clinical Nephrology, 3rd edn. Oxford: Oxford University Press, 2002, in press.

3. Litwin CM, Mouritsen CL, Wilfahrt PA, Schroder MC, Hill HR: Anti-glomerular basement membrane disease: role of enzyme-linked immunosorbent assays in diagnosis. Biochem Mol Med 1996;59:52–56.

4. Kashtan CE, Michael AF: Alport syndrome. Kidney Int 1996;50:1445–1463.

5. Brainwood D, Kashtan C, Gubler MC, Turner AN: Targets of alloantibodies in Alport anti-glomerular basement membrane disease after renal transplantation. Kidney Int 1998;53:762–766.

6. Wilson CB, Dixon FJ: Anti-glomerular basement membrane antibody-induced glomerulonephritis. Kidney Int 1973;3:74–89.

7. Lockwood CM, Rees AJ, Pearson TA, Evans DJ, Peters DK, Wilson CB: Immunosuppression and plasma-exchange in the treatment of Goodpasture's syndrome. Lancet 1976;i:711–715.

8. Couser WG: Goodpasture's syndrome: a response to nitrogen mustard. Am J Med Sci 1974;268:175–179.

9. Briggs WA, Johnson JP, Teichman S, Yeager HC, Wilson CB: Antiglomerular basement membrane antibody-mediated glomerulonephritis and Goodpasture's syndrome. Medicine (Baltimore) 1979;58:348–361.

10. Finch RA, Rutsky EA, McGowan E, Wilson CB: Treatment of Goodpasture's syndrome with immunosuppression and plasmapheresis. South Med J 1979;72:1288–1290.

11. Johnson JP, Whitman W, Briggs WA, Wilson CB: Plasmapheresis and immunosuppressive agents in antibasement membrane antibody-induced Goodpasture's syndrome. Am J Med 1978;64:354–359.

12. Simpson IJ, Doak PB, Williams LC, et al: Plasma exchange in Goodpasture's syndrome. Am J Nephrol 1982;2:301–311.

13. Walker RG, Scheinkestel C, Becker GJ, Owen JE, Dowling JP, Kincaid Smith P: Clinical and morphological aspects of the management of crescentic anti-glomerular basement membrane antibody (anti-GBM) nephritis/Goodpasture's syndrome. Q J Med 1985;54:75–89.

14. Johnson JP, Moore JJ, Austin HA, Balow JE, Antonovych TT, Wilson CB: Therapy of anti-glomerular basement membrane antibody disease: analysis of prognostic significance of clinical, pathologic and treatment factors. Medicine (Baltimore) 1985;64:219–227.

15. Herody M, Bobrie G, Gouarin C, Grunfeld JP, Noel LH: Anti-GBM disease: predictive value of clinical, histological and serological data. Clin Nephrol 1993;40:249–255.

16. Levy JB, Turner AN, Rees AJ, Pusey CD: Long-term outcome of anti-glomerular basement membrane antibody disease treated with plasma exchange and immunosuppression. Ann Intern Med 2001;134:1033–1042.

17. Bosch X, Mirapeix E, Font J, et al: Prognostic implication of anti-neutrophil cytoplasmic autoantibodies with myeloperoxidase specificity in anti-glomerular basement membrane disease. Clin Nephrol 1991;36:107–113.

18. Jayne DRW, Marshall PD, Jones SJ, Lockwood CM: Autoantibodies to glomerular basement membrane and neutrophil cytoplasm in rapidly progressive glomerulonephritis. Kidney Int 1990;37:965–970.

19. Saxena R, Bygren P, Rasmussen N, Wieslander J: Circulating autoantibodies in patients with extracapillary glomerulonephritis. Nephrol Dial Transplant 1991;6:389–397.

20. Levy JB, Lachmann RH, Pusey CD: Recurrent Goodpasture's disease. Am J Kidney Dis 1996;27:573–578.

21. Lockwood CM, Pusey CD, Rees AJ, Peters DK: Plasma exchange in the treatment of immune complex disease. Clin Immunol Allergy 1981;1:433–455.

22. Proskey AJ, Weatherbee L, Easterling RE, Greene JAJ, Weller JM: Goodpasture's syndrome. A report of five cases and review of the literature. Am J Med 1970;48:162–173.

23. de Torrente A, Popovtzer M, Guggenheim SJ, et al: Serious pulmonary hemorrhage, glomerulonephritis and massive steroid therapy. Ann Intern Med 1975;83:218–219.

24. Bolton WK, Sturgill BC: Methylprednisolone therapy for acute crescentic rapidly progressive glomerulonephritis. Am J Nephrol 1989;9:368–375.

25. Williams PS, Davenport A, McDicken I, Ashby D, Bone JM: Increased incidence of anti-glomerular basement membrane antibody (anti-GBM) nephritis in the Mersey region, September 1984–October 1985. Q J Med 1988;68:727–733.

26. Rees AJ, Lockwood CM, Peters DK: Enhanced allergic tissue injury in Goodpasture's syndrome by intercurrent bacterial infection. Br Med J 1977;2:723–726.

27. Tomosugi NI, Cashman SJ, Hay H, et al: Modulation of antibody-mediated glomerular injury in vivo by bacterial lipopolysaccharide, tumor necrosis factor, and IL-1. J Immunol 1989;142:3083–3090.

28. Querin S, Schurch W, Beaulieu R: Ciclosporin in Goodpasture's syndrome. Nephron 1992;60:355–359.

29. Pepys EO, Rees AJ, Pepys MB: Enumeration of lymphocyte populations in whole peripheral blood of patients with antibody-mediated nephritis during treatment with cyclosporin A. Immunol Lett 1982;4:211–214.

30. Hind CRK, Paraskevakou H, Lockwood CM, Evans DJ, Peters DK, Rees AJ: Prognosis after immunosuppression of patients with crescentic nephritis requiring dialysis. Lancet 1983;i:263–265.

31. Flores JC, Taube D, Savage COS, Cameron JS, Lockwood CM, Ogg CS: Clinical and immunological evolution of oliguric anti-GBM nephritis treated by haemodialysis. Lancet 1986;i:5–8.

32. Bygren P, Freiburghaus C, Lindholm T, Simonsen O, Thysell H, Wieslander J: Goodpasture's syndrome treated with staphylococcal protein A immunoadsorption (letter). Lancet 1985;ii:1295–1296.

33. Moreso F, Poveda R, Gil-Vernet S, et al: Therapeutic immunoadsorption in Goodpasture disease. Med Clin (Barc) 1995;105:59–61.

34. Boutaud AA, Kalluri R, Kahsai TZ, Noelken ME, Hudson BG: Goodpasture syndrome: selective removal of anti-α3 (IV) collagen autoantibodies. A potential therapeutic alternative to plasmapheresis. Exp Nephrol 1996;4:205–212.

35. Atkins RC, Nikolic-Paterson DJ, Song Q, Lan HY: Modulators of crescentic glomerulonephritis. J Am Soc Nephrol 1996;7:2271–2278.

36. Kunzendorf U, Pohl T, Bulfone-Paus S, et al: Immunomodulation in experimental and clinical nephrology using chimeric proteins. Kidney Blood Press Res 1997;19:201–204.

Treatment of ANCA-associated Small-vessel Vasculitis

Patrick H. Nachman and Ronald J. Falk

Various forms of vasculitis may affect the kidney. The classification of vasculitides was agreed upon at the 1993 Chapel Hill Consensus Conference for the Nomenclature of Systemic Vasculitis[1] and is based on the predilection for injury of the different vascular beds (Table 21.1). Conceptually, vasculitides may be organized based on three different mechanisms of injury: (1) immune complex-mediated vasculitis; (2) direct antibody-mediated attack; or (3) pauci-immune necrotizing vasculitides. Immune complex-mediated vasculitis includes Henoch–Schönlein purpura, cryoglobulinemic vasculitis, rheumatoid vasculitis, and lupus vasculitis. Direct antibody-mediated disease includes antiglomerular basement membrane (anti-GBM) disease, Goodpasture syndrome, and Kawasaki disease (antiendothelial cell antibodies). Pauci-immune small-vessel vasculitis (SVV) includes microscopic polyangiitis, Wegener granulomatosis, and Churg–Strauss syndrome. The pauci-immune vasculitides are associated with antineutrophil cytoplasmic autoantibodies (ANCA) and are the focus of this chapter.

Microscopic polyangiitis is a necrotizing angiitis involving capillaries, venules, and arterioles. The vascular beds of one or more organs may be involved simultaneously or at different times, including the kidneys, lungs, skin, spleen, liver, heart, and muscle. Alternatively, the disease may be limited to the kidneys alone, causing a necrotizing and crescentic glomerulonephritis. Damaged vessels have focal fibrinoid necrosis with perivascular infiltrates of neutrophils or mononuclear leukocytes. Wegener granulomatosis is characterized by necrotizing granulomatous inflammation found in the upper or lower respiratory tract and may occur without overt vasculitis. Churg–Strauss syndrome is defined by the presence of eosinophil-rich granulomatous inflammation and vasculitis in patients with a history of eosinophilia and asthma. The necrotizing glomerulonephritis and vasculitis found in Wegener granulomatosis and Churg–Strauss syndrome can be pathologically identical to that found in microscopic polyangiitis. It is characterized by segmental fibrinoid necrosis, crescent formation,[2] and the absence of immune reactants.

ANCA react with constituents of neutrophils and monocytes. By indirect immunofluorescence microscopy on alcohol-fixed neutrophils, two patterns of ANCA staining can be distinguished: a cytoplasmic pattern (C-ANCA) and a perinuclear pattern (P-ANCA). The majority of C-ANCA react with proteinase 3 (PR3-ANCA). In necrotizing SVV, P-ANCA react with myeloperoxidase (MPO-ANCA).[3,4] Wegener granulomatosis is usually associated with circulating PR3-ANCA, but as many as 20% of patients may have MPO-ANCA.[5] Conversely, PR3-ANCA can be found in patients with microscopic polyangiitis and necrotizing glomerulonephritis without evidence of Wegener granulomatosis. MPO-ANCA are more commonly found in patients with microscopic polyangiitis and those with necrotizing and crescentic glomerulonephritis without evidence of extrarenal SVV. MPO-ANCA is the most common ANCA subtype in Churg–Strauss syndrome. Thus, despite a predominance of antigenic specificity for each of the diseases, neither ANCA subtype allows differentiation between the three phenotypes of necrotizing vasculitis.

Clinical features of the disease

ANCA SVV is more common in Caucasians than African-Americans, with a ratio of 7–8:1. Females and males are equally affected, and while patients are typically 55 years or older, patients of any age may have this disease.[6–9] Clinical features of the renal disease are usually that of hematuria, with dysmorphic red blood cells and red blood cell casts. Proteinuria tends to be in the subnephrotic range with a mean of 2–3 g/day, although some patients have as much as 20 g/day. ANCA-associated glomerulonephritis frequently presents as a rapidly progressive glomerulonephritis, although the syndromes of asymptomatic hematuria with minimal amounts of proteinuria or acute nephritis are common as well.

At least 50% of patients with ANCA necrotizing glomerulonephritis have pulmonary disease spanning the spectrum from severe life-threatening pulmonary hemorrhage

Table 21.1 Names and definitions adopted by the Chapel Hill Consensus Conference on the Nomenclature of Systemic Vasculitis*

Large vessel vasculitis	
Giant cell (temporal) arteritis	Granulomatous arteritis of the aorta and its major branches, with a predilection for the extracranial branches of the carotid artery. Often associated with polymyalgia rheumatica
Takayasu arteritis	Granulomatous inflammation of the aorta and its major branches
Medium-sized vessel vasculitis	
Polyarteritis nodosa	Necrotizing inflammation of medium-sized or small arteries without glomerulonephritis or vasculitis in arterioles, capillaries, or venules
Kawasaki disease	Arteritis involving large, medium-sized, and small arteries, and associated with mucocutaneous lymph node syndrome. Coronary arteries are often involved. Aorta and veins may be involved. Usually occurs in children
Small-vessel vasculitis	
Wegener granulomatosis[†]	Granulomatous inflammation involving the respiratory tract and necrotizing vasculitis affecting small to medium-sized vessels, e.g. capillaries, venules, arterioles, and arteries. Necrotizing glomerulonephritis is common
Churg–Strauss syndrome[†]	Eosinophil-rich and granulomatous inflammation involving the respiratory tract and necrotizing vasculitis affecting small to medium-sized vessels, and associated with asthma and blood eosinophilia
Microscopic polyangiitis[†]	Necrotizing vasculitis with few or no immune deposits affecting small vessels, i.e. capillaries, venules, or arterioles. Necrotizing glomerulonephritis is very common. Pulmonary capillaritis often occurs
Henoch–Schönlein purpura	Vasculitis with IgA-dominant immune deposits affecting small vessels, i.e. capillaries, venules, or arterioles. Typically involves skin, gut, and glomeruli, and is associated with arthralgias or arthritis
Essential cryoglobulinemic vasculitis	Vasculitis with cryoglobulin immune deposits affecting small vessels, i.e. capillaries, venules, or arterioles, and associated with cryoglobulins in serum. Skin and glomeruli are often involved
Cutaneous leukocytoclastic angiitis	Isolated cutaneous leukocytoclastic angiitis without systemic vasculitis or glomerulonephritis

* Modified with permission from Jennette JC, Falk RJ, Andrassy K, et al: Nomenclature of systemic vasculitides. Proposal of an international consensus conference. Arthritis Rheum 1994;37:187–192.
[†]The ANCA-associated vasculitides.

to fleeting alveolar infiltrates.[6,10,11] Massive pulmonary hemorrhage affects about 10% of patients with ANCA glomerulonephritis, and is associated with a mortality rate of 50%.

In the evaluation of pulmonary disease in the setting of a glomerulonephritis, it is imperative to exclude the possibility of an infectious etiology, especially when pulmonary infiltrates with or without hemoptysis develop in the setting of prior or ongoing immunosuppressive treatment. Recurrent vasculitis must be differentiated from infection, with special attention to *Pneumocystis carinii*, *Mycobacterium tuberculosis*, or fungal pathogens. Bronchoscopy, including bronchoalveolar lavage, may differentiate infection from alveolar hemorrhage. Similarly, infections of the upper respiratory tract mimic vasculitic lesions in the nose, sinus, and ear. Fiberoptic translumination of the upper airways with biopsy allows differentiation of vascular inflammation from infections.

Common dermal vasculitic findings are palpable purpura (usually in the lower extremities), petechia, ulcers, nodules, ecchymoses, and bullae. Urticaria is a much more common manifestation of SVV in the skin than previously considered.

The neurologic manifestations of ANCA SVV are peripheral neuropathies typically of mononeuritis multiplex. Occasionally, patients have central nervous system inflammation, specifically granulomatous meningeal inflammation observed on magnetic resonance imaging. Capillary inflammation is not seen on routine magnetic resonance scanning, yet seizure activity, presumably secondary to vasculitis, responds to immunosuppressive treatment.

Several other organ systems are involved. Gastrointestinal disease, found in one-third of patients with ANCA SVV, may present with gastric or duodenal ulcers detected by endoscopic examination. Vasculitis of the small and large intestine results in gastrointestinal bleeding or, if severe, perforation of the viscus as a consequence of transmural infarction. Iritis, uveitis, and episcleritis result in painful red eyes. These lesions are frequently present in a "subclinical" fashion and require slit-lamp ophthalmologic evaluation. Almost all patients have a prodrome of a "flu-like" illness with malaise, myalgias, and arthralgias. Many patients have arthropathy that migrates from joint to joint.

Diagnosis

The differential diagnosis of ANCA necrotizing glomerulonephritis includes lupus nephritis, anti-GBM disease, and other aggressive forms of glomerulonephritis. Patients with thrombotic microangiopathies may present a picture that mimics necrotizing glomerulonephritis. However, these patients do not have MPO- or PR3-ANCA and have features typical of a microangiopathic hemolytic disease. ANCA can be found in 20% of patients with anti-GBM disease, concomitant with anti-GBM antibodies. Patients with immune complex forms of glomerulonephritis, including membranous nephropathy with crescent transformation, may have positive MPO- or PR3-ANCA. In these individuals, a search for extrarenal SVV is warranted.

The decision as to whether a renal biopsy is essential for the management of ANCA glomerulonephritis rests on three factors: the accuracy of the ANCA methodology, the risks associated with therapy, and the "pretest probability" based on the features of the patient's clinical syndrome.

In a study of 1000 patients with proliferative and/or necrotizing glomerulonephritis with or without crescentic disease and a serologic test for either PR3- or MPO-ANCA,[12] the sensitivity of ANCA for pauci-immune glomerulonephritis was only 80% with a specificity of 89%. Considering the prevalence of pauci-immune glomerulonephritis in this patient cohort is 45%, the positive predictive value of ANCA was 86%, the false-positive rate 14% and the "false"-negative rate 16%. These results preclude the use of ANCA testing alone as the determinant for treatment, especially if one considers the serious risks inherent in the treatment of SVV with potent antiinflammatory and immunosuppressive drugs. The distribution of ANCA reactivity in patients with aggressive glomerular diseases is shown in Table 21.2.

On the other hand, if the prevalence of disease in the selected patient population (based on the clinical picture) is relatively high (> 50%), then the positive predictive value for the spectrum of pauci-immune necrotizing glomerulonephritis is > 99%.[13] In such a setting, expert ANCA testing may obviate the need for pathologic confirmation of necrotizing vasculitis in some emergency situations.

Based on these data, it is our contention that a renal biopsy is mandatory for the definitive diagnosis of pauci-immune SVV, whether associated with circulating ANCA or not (ANCA negative, about 10% of cases). Serologic data, the clinical spectrum of disease, and a pathologic diagnosis should be considered together in order to provide maximal information for meaningful patient-informed consent. However, in the setting of a rapidly progressive glomerulonephriti, or a pulmonary–renal vasculitic syndrome, we would not delay the initiation of treatment with pulse methylprednisolone until a biopsy

result is obtained, because prompt initiation of treatment is an essential determinant of outcome.

Prognostic factors

Several studies have examined the question of prognostic factors in ANCA SVV.[8,14–16] These studies point to the entry serum creatinine, the presence of pulmonary disease, severity of renal disease, and even the entry white blood cell count as important predictors of outcomes. In our experience,[8] the presence of pulmonary hemorrhage was the most important determinant of patient survival, whereas other pulmonary findings (e.g. infiltrates, nodules, or cavities) did not increase the risk of death.

The risk of endstage renal disease was largely attributable to the entry serum creatinine, even when such variables as the presence of extrarenal disease or pulmonary findings were incorporated into the model.[8] The findings on renal biopsy were predictive of outcome only to the extent that interstitial fibrosis was an independent risk factor only in individuals with an entry serum creatinine of < 3 mg/dL. In a more recent study, the percentage of normal glomeruli was the histologic feature that correlated most significantly with renal outcome.[17]

Although the entry serum creatinine is the single most important prognostic marker for the development of endstage renal disease, there was no concentration beyond which the chance of recovery was too small to justify treatment. However, patients with ANCA SVV who require dialysis at the time of presentation have a decreased chance of recovery compared with patients who are not dialysis dependent (50% vs. > 70%).

Treatment

Induction therapy

To date, the cornerstone of treatment of SVV remains the use of a combination of corticosteroids and cyclophosphamide as initially suggested by Fauci et al.[18]

Since renal prognosis appears to be determined by early treatment, it is reasonable to minimize inflammation with prompt, aggressive therapy. Typically, patients are given methylprednisolone 7 mg/kg/day for 3 days followed by daily oral prednisone. Prednisone is then started at a dose of 1 mg/kg for the first month, tapered to an alternate-day

Table 21.2 Distribution of ANCA in patients with pauci-immune, anti-GBM, and immune complex-mediated glomerulonephritis

	Pauci-immune glomerulonephritis (%)	Anti-GBM glomerulonephritis (%)	Immune complex glomerulonephritis (%)
ANCA positive	36	1	5
ANCA negative	9	2	47

ANCA, antineutrophil cytoplasmic antibodies; GBM, glomerular basement membrane.

regimen during the second month, and discontinued by the end of the third to fourth month. Cyclophosphamide is administered either intravenously or orally. Intravenous cyclophosphamide is administered on a monthly basis beginning at a dose of 0.5 g/m^2, adjusting the dose upward to 1 g/m^2 based on 2-week leukocyte counts.[7,9] Oral cyclophosphamide should begin at a dose of 2 mg/kg/day.[18] All forms of cyclophosphamide dosage should be titrated to keep the nadir leukocyte count > 3000/μL. The leukocyte count may decrease significantly with decreasing doses of prednisone, and the dosage of cyclophosphamide may need lowering accordingly.

The optimum length of therapy with cyclophosphamide has not been determined. An indefinite use of cyclophosphamide is prohibited by its associated risks, including a 15% incidence of transitional cell carcinoma in the bladder seen in patients treated with long-term oral cyclophosphamide.[19] In patients achieving complete remission within 6 months of therapy, treatment can be stopped with the institution of close patient follow-up. In those individuals with persistently active disease at 6 months, it is reasonable to continue cyclophosphamide therapy for a full 12 months. Another protocol consists of 3 months only of cyclophosphamide followed by azathioprine (2 mg/kg/day) for the duration of therapy.[20] Most patients may stop this form of therapy at 6–12 months.

In a randomized controlled study, the oral and intravenous cyclophosphamide regimen resulted in comparable remission rates. Whereas the oral regimen afforded a lower rate of relapse (13% vs. 59%) than the intravenous regimen, it was also associated with a significantly higher rate of serious infections. The overall outcome at the end of the study was similar in both groups.[21] In our experience (based on the retrospective review of 142 patients) the two modalities result in equivalent rates of remission and relapse. The intravenous regimen allows for a total dose of cyclophosphamide that is two to three times smaller than the oral regimen. As a consequence, there is a substantial decrease in neutropenia and both minor and major infections. However, the most concerning feature of cyclophosphamide therapy is its long-term mutagenic risk, especially transitional cell carcinoma of the bladder.[19] That risk is commensurate to the cumulative dose received. Although there are currently no data comparing the carcinogenic risk of monthly intravenous pulses of cyclophosphamide and daily oral dosing, it is hoped that the risk of malignancy would be reduced with the smaller doses used in the intravenous regimen.

That cyclophosphamide is a necessary adjunct to prednisone has been appreciated for years.[18] In our experience, we have learned that treatment with prednisone alone resulted in a fivefold increase in the risk of death and a threefold increase in the risk of relapse compared with treatment with cyclophosphamide.[8,9]

Treatment of dialysis-dependent patients

At least 20% of patients with ANCA SVV will require dialysis at the time of diagnosis. Half of these patients may come off dialysis within 8–12 weeks of therapy. It is currently impossible to predict at the initiation of treatment which patient will recover sufficient renal function to discontinue dialysis. For patients who do respond to treatment, the dialysis-free interval may last from as little as a few weeks to 3–4 years.[9] The degree of immunosuppression warranted during the first 12 weeks of dialysis depends on the risk–benefit ratio. It is our practice to treat dialysis-dependent patients for at least 8–12 weeks with pulse methylprednisolone followed by oral prednisone as described above. If patients have return or improvement of renal function, we add cyclophosphamide to the corticosteroid regimen. The addition to plasmapheresis may increase the chance of renal recovery in this subset of patients.[22] Because of the risk of severe bone marrow suppression and immunosuppression in patients on dialysis, the use of cyclophosphamide in patients on dialysis should only be undertaken with extreme caution. The latter drug is definitely indicated for patients with life- or organ-threatening disease (e.g. alveolar hemorrhage).

Transplantation

Recurrence after transplantation of ANCA glomerulonephritis and SVV has been reported on numerous occasions.[23–26] Time to recurrence varies widely, from 5 days after transplantation to more than 4 years.[25,27] The very early recurrences were not in patients with active disease at the time of transplantation.

The rate of recurrence is difficult to assess with confidence from the literature, because most of the reports are anecdotal case reports. Based on a pooled analysis of published data, added to the experience at the universities of North Carolina and Lund, Sweden, the rate of recurrence appears to be about 20%. Patients with Wegener granulomatosis were more likely to relapse than patients with microscopic polyangiitis or necrotizing crescentic glomerulonephritis alone. There were no statistically significant differences in relapse rates between patients treated and those not treated with cyclosporine, or between those with or without circulating ANCA at the time of transplant.[28] If the patient is clinically in remission, it is probably not necessary to delay transplantation until a negative ANCA serology is attained. It is our opinion that transplantation should be delayed in patients with active disease and in patients with rising ANCA titers after a period with undetectable titers.

Recurrence is not confined to the transplanted kidney but can occur throughout the upper and lower respiratory tract and can affect other organs.[26,29,30] In the majority of reported cases, recurrent disease after transplantation responded well to treatment with cyclophosphamide and pulse corticosteroids.

Relationship of serial ANCA titers and disease

The relationship of ANCA titers as a disease-monitoring test has been the subject of several investigations. ANCA titers rise during relapse in 23–77% of cases.[31,32] ANCA titers may increase without overt clinical relapse and, in some patients, persistently high ANCA titers are found in conjunction with clinical remission. In contrast, some patients have a clinical relapse that is not associated with any rise in ANCA titers. In general, a rise in ANCA titer should raise questions about the possibility of a clinical relapse, and it is reasonable to presume that the disappearance of ANCA is associated with absence of clinical activity.

In a prospective randomized trial of immunosuppression in response to a fourfold increase in ANCA titer, Cohen Tervaert et al[33] were able to demonstrate a reduction in the rate of relapses in the treated group. In this study, however, 30% of patients who had a rise in titer but received no "prophylactic" treatment did not suffer a clinical relapse, and a few patients who did relapse did so more than a year later. This approach, therefore, has the disadvantage of unnecessarily exposing a significant number of patients to the dangers of cyclophosphamide and high-dose corticosteroids.

Serial ANCA testing may be of greater importance with regard to treatment decisions in some patients than others. It has been argued that the serial measurement of ANCA of specific isotypes (e.g. IgG3) could better predict the occurrence of a relapse. This contention is not substantiated by a retrospective analysis of 169 consecutive sera obtained over a median of 21 months from 18 patients with ANCA SVV.[34] For these reasons, our approach to initiating a second course of treatment is based not on ANCA titers but on the constellation of findings on clinical course, physical examination, and serologies. As of now, ANCA titers should not be used as the sole determinant in beginning or altering immunosuppressive therapy.

Response to treatment

The terms "remission" and "relapse" are defined in Table 21.3.[8] Treatment with cyclophosphamide is beneficial over the use of corticosteroids alone for achieving a remission as well as for patient survival.[8,9] Patients treated with either intravenous or oral cyclophosphamide have a long-term remission rate of 60–85%. We found no difference in the rate of response to treatment between patients with microscopic polyangiitis and those with necrotizing crescentic glomerulonephritis alone (77% vs. 78%). Patients with Wegener granulomatosis may have a better chance of remission than patients with microscopic polyangiitis or necrotizing crescentic glomerulonephritis.

Relapse

The risk of relapse after an initial response to treatment is of the order of 30–45%.[9,35,36] Based on the retrospective review of 142 patients with ANCA SVV treated with corticosteroids and cyclophosphamide, we found that patients with C-ANCA were twice as likely to suffer a relapse than patients with P-ANCA.[37] Among patients with P-ANCA, sinus involvement is associated with a fourfold increased risk of relapse.

In our patients with ANCA-associated microscopic polyangiitis and necrotizing crescentic glomerulonephritis, 80% of relapses occurred within the first 18

Table 21.3 Criteria for treatment response*

Remission

Stabilization or improvement of renal function (as measured by serum creatinine), resolution of hematuria, and resolution of extrarenal manifestations of systemic vasculitis. Persistence of proteinuria was not considered indicative of persistence of disease activity

Remission on therapy

Achievement of remission while still receiving immunosuppressive medication or corticosteroids at a dose > 7.5 mg/day of prednisone or its equivalent

Treatment resistance

Progressive decline in renal function with persistence of an active urine sediment, *or*

Persistence or new appearance of any extrarenal manifestation of vasculitis despite immunosuppressive therapy

Relapse

Occurrence of at least one of the following.

1. Rapid rise in serum creatinine accompanied by an active urine sediment
2. Renal biopsy demonstrating active necrosis or crescent formation
3. Hemoptysis, pulmonary hemorrhage, or new or expanding nodules without evidence for infection
4. Active vasculitis of the respiratory or gastrointestinal tracts as demonstrated by endoscopy with biopsy
5. Iritis or uveitis
6. New mononeuritis multiplex
7. Necrotizing vasculitis identified by biopsy in any tissue

*Modified from Nachman PH, Hogan SL, Jennette JC, Falk RJ: Treatment response and relapse in antineutrophil cytoplasmic autoantibody-associated microscopic polyangiitis and glomerulonephritis. J Am Soc Nephrol 1996;7:33–39.

months after cessation of therapy, although a few continued to occur with prolonged follow-up. This clustering of relapse within the first years after treatment was not observed in the retrospective study by Gordon et al,[35] which may be a result of maintenance therapy with corticosteroids or azathioprine. Both studies suggest the need for close follow-up for at least 2 years after the end of treatment. We found that treatment with cyclophosphamide confers a threefold decrease in the risk of relapse compared with treatment with corticosteroids alone. When compared with pulsed intravenous cyclophosphamide, treatment with a daily oral regimen may be associated with a lower risk of relapse,[21] although this potential benefit should be weighed against the higher risk of serious infections associated with this treatment modality.

Relapse typically occurs in the same organ system initially affected by the disease, although new organ system involvement occurs as well. Relapses in the kidney are heralded by the recurrence of microscopic hematuria, red blood cell casts, and worsening renal function. Fluctuations in the amount of proteinuria are not good indicators of active disease, and are related to glomerulosclerosis. Many patients' relapses are heralded by recurrence of a migratory polyarthropathy or recurrence of occult disease.

Fortunately, a similar rate of response is achieved in the treatment of relapse and initial disease.[9] Retreatment is therefore an important and beneficial option. Full-blown vasculitic relapse should be treated with a repeat course of prednisone and cyclophosphamide. In general, these patients require maintenance on long-term immunosuppression with azathioprine, methotrexate, mycophenolate mofetil, or cyclophosphamide. How to best treat milder relapses is a matter of substantial investigation. It is in an effort to limit the exposure of relapsing patients to repetitive cycles of cytotoxic drugs and their associated risks[12,38,39] that alternative or adjunctive less toxic therapies are sought and being evaluated.

Adjunctive and alternative treatment strategies

Trimethoprim–sulfamethoxazole

Trimethoprim–sulfamethoxazole is suggested as the initial treatment of selected patients with Wegener granulomatosis limited to the upper respiratory tract, reserving corticosteroid therapy for patients who fail antibiotic therapy.[40,41] The rationale for this approach is largely based on empiric data, but is supported by the fact that chronic nasal carriage of *Staphylococcus aureus* is a risk factor for relapse in Wegener granulomatosis.[42]

In assessing the role of trimethoprim–sulfamethoxazole in the prevention of relapse in patients already treated with cyclophosphamide and/or prednisone, a prospective placebo-controlled trial with trimethoprim–sulfamethoxazole was performed in 81 patients with Wegener granulomatosis.[42] In 20% of these patients, therapy was stopped

due to adverse effects. The number of relapses was significantly reduced in the groups assigned to trimethoprim–sulfamethoxazole, although the benefit was limited to relapse involving the upper respiratory tract not the lower respiratory tract or the kidney. In contrast, Reinhold-Keller et al[41] found that "maintenance" therapy with trimethoprim–sulfamethoxazole (after cyclophosphamide treatment) was associated with an increased rate of relapses compared with no maintenance treatment (42% vs. 29% respectively). Similarly, in a randomized trial of 65 patients with Wegener granulomatosis comparing methotrexate and trimethoprim–sulfamethoxazole,[43] methotrexate therapy was more effective in maintaining remission than trimethoprim–sulfamethoxazole used alone or in combination with prednisone. Thus the use of trimethoprim–sulfamethoxazole in patients with Wegener granulomatosis remains a matter of controversy, and its beneficial effects seem to be limited to the respiratory tract.

Methotrexate

In an open-label pilot study, Hoffman et al[44] treated 29 patients with Wegener granulomatosis who did not have immediately life-threatening disease with weekly oral methotrexate and daily corticosteroids. This study revealed a response rate of 76% and a remission rate of 69%. These results, as well as the incidence of severe life-threatening infections, were comparable to those achieved with the cyclophosphamide-based regimen. In an extension of this study (total 40 patients),[45] the continued use of methotrexate for 1 year after clinical remission failed to prevent relapses from occurring, because 64% of recurrences occurred while patients were taking methotrexate. In contrast, in a randomized study of 65 patients, those who received maintenance weekly intravenous methotrexate suffered significantly fewer relapses than patients treated with trimethoprim–sulfamethoxazole. This beneficial effect came at a cost of a twofold increase in adverse effects in patients receiving methotrexate. Methotrexate is thus a useful form of therapy for SVV, especially in individuals with normal or near-normal renal function and predominantly extrarenal manifestations of vasculitis.[44] Methotrexate should not be used if the serum creatinine is > 2 mg/dL or creatinine clearance is < 60 mL/min. Whether methotrexate offers an effective, safe, and practical approach to maintenance therapy remains to be determined, and this treatment is not convincingly supported by the data currently available.

Plasmapheresis

A number of noncontrolled reports of beneficial effects of plasmapheresis in the treatment of ANCA-associated SVV and glomerulonephritis are available in the literature.[46,47] To date, several randomized controlled trials have addressed the issue of plasmapheresis.[48–53] Although these studies differ with respect to patient selection and the concurrent immunosuppressive treatment regimen, none found a beneficial effect of plasmapheresis over immunosuppressive treatment alone in patients with limited disease or in patients with mild or moderate renal dysfunction. In a subgroup analysis of patients who required dialysis, Pusey et al[48] reported that a greater number of dialysis-dependent patients treated with plasmapheresis recovered renal function. This beneficial effect is further suggested by a pooled analysis of dialysis-requiring patients from the published randomized controlled trials.[22]

The routine use of plasmapheresis in patients with ANCA SVV is therefore not supported by the current data, with the exception of patients with pulmonary hemorrhage. The addition of plasmapheresis to conventional treatment with cyclophosphamide and corticosteroids appears to be of benefit in reversing diffuse alveolar hemorrhage and improving the mortality of patients with this life-threatening manifestation of ANCA vasculitis.[54,55] Whether dialysis-dependent patients would benefit from the addition of plasmapheresis awaits confirmation in a larger randomized trial.

Intravenous immunoglobulin

High-dose pooled immunoglobulin has been used in the treatment of various autoimmune diseases. Several possible Fc and F(ab)-mediated mechanisms by which intravenous immunoglobulin (IVIG) exerts its immuno-modulatory effect have been suggested,[56,57] including providing the patients with anti-idiotype antibodies that inhibit the action of the offending autoantibodies (in this case ANCA).[58,59] IVIG therapy is used in the treatment of patients with ANCA-associated glomerulonephritis and vasculitis and results in variable degrees of benefit. To date, the published reports on the use of IVIG in the treatment of ANCA SVV consist mostly of case reports or series including a small number of patients. Almost all patients described received treatment with other immuno-suppressive regimens and were "poor responders."[58,60-63] Recently, a randomized controlled trial assessed the effect of a single course of IVIG (0.4 g/kg/day for 5 days, total 2 g/kg) when added to conventional therapy with high-dose corticosteroids and cyclophosphamide. The addition of IVIG resulted in a more rapid decrease in disease activity and C-reactive protein levels when measured 2 and 4 weeks later but had no effect on these outcome measures after 3 months, nor did it affect the ANCA levels or the cumulative exposure to immunosuppressive drugs.[64] Although the effects of a single course were not long-lasting, this study suggests a beneficial role for IVIG in the management of patients with persistent or frequently relapsing disease.

Mycophenolate mofetil

Mycophenolate mofetil (MMF) is a reversible inhibitor of the enzyme inosine monophosphate dehydrogenase, a critical rate-limiting enzyme in the de novo synthesis of purines. As lymphocytes require a fully functioning de novo pathway for purine synthesis and proliferation, MMF functions as a relatively lymphocyte-selective antimeta-bolite. In vitro, MMF blocks proliferation of both B and T cells, inhibits antibody formation and the generation of cytotoxic T cells, and decreases the expression of adhesion molecules on lymphocytes that impairs their ability to bind to endothelial cells. Preliminary small-scale pilot studies suggest that MMF may have a role in the treatment of mild or moderate ANCA SVV[65] or as "maintenance" therapy to prevent relapse.[66] There are currently no sufficient data to support its use in the treatment of life- or organ-threatening disease or as a preferred drug.

Cyclosporine

There are a few reports of beneficial response to treatment with cyclosporine, including frequently relapsing patients.[67,68] However, experience with the use of cyclosporine is limited to case reports or small series of patients. This drug does not seem to be able to prevent relapses, as evidenced by the significant rate of relapses in the post-transplant population.[28]

Novel therapies

The last few years have witnessed the development of a number of "biologic" immunomodulatory products such as humanized monoclonal antibodies and fusion proteins designed to block various inflammatory pathways. Because of their selective effect on specific mechanisms of inflammation, these products hold the promise of efficacy in the treatment of patients with ANCA SVV, while decreasing the severity of adverse effects. Unfortunately, none has been sufficiently investigated yet in the treatment of ANCA SVV. Of these, the tumor necrosis factor receptor–Fc fusion protein etanercept[69] is the subject of a current phase II controlled trial comparing its efficacy and safety with that of the traditional regimen of daily oral cyclophosphamide or methotrexate and corticosteroids in the treatment of patients with ANCA-associated vasculitis. In an open-label study of 20 patients with persistently active Wegener granulomatosis, the addition of etanercept to baseline immunosuppressive drugs resulted in a reduction of disease activity, although the rate of relapses was high (75%).[70]

Supportive therapy

As aggressive corticosteroids and cyclophosphamide remain the cornerstone of therapy of ANCA SVV, special effort must be exercised to minimize the short- and long-term complications of treatment. The most prominent adverse effects of this form of therapy are infection, ovarian failure (especially with a prolonged course of cyclophosphamide), bone disease, and cataract formation. In addition, the use of cyclophosphamide is associated with an increased risk of skin, hematopoietic, and transitional cell carcinoma of the urinary tract,[19] whereas the use of azathioprine is associated with skin cancer.[36]

Whenever corticosteroids are used, measures must be taken to minimize the development of osteoporosis,[71] with the early institution of calcium and vitamin D supplementation and, in selected patients with established osteoporosis, calcitonin or bisphosphonates (if not contra-indicated by azotemia or esophagitis). Rigorous control of blood pressure with sodium restriction and antihyperten-sive therapy is essential to minimize the additive effect of hypertension in loss of renal function following active nephritis. Hormonal manipulation during cytotoxic therapy may allow the preservation of gonadal function. In men, the use of testosterone during cyclophosphamide treatment appears to prevent irreversible azoospermia,[72] whereas the gonadotropin-releasing hormone agonist leuprolide may help prevent premature ovarian failure in women.[73]

Conclusion

The last few years have brought a substantial improvement in our understanding of the spectrum of small-vessel vasculitis, and especially its association with ANCA. A better definition of the effects of various therapies on specific aspects of these syndromes is now emerging. While our knowledge base remains inadequate in formulating more specific novel therapies, our immuno-suppressive armamentarium is expanding and promises to do so even further in the next few years. It is evident that no one strategy is uniformly applicable to all patients with SVV. The choice of a particular drug regimen must be tailored to the individual needs of each patient, taking into account the spectrum of organ involvement, the level of disease activity, and the degree of exposure to prior immunosuppression. From the clinical perspective, the most important progress lies perhaps in the better recognition of the many faces of SVV, and a better understanding of its long-term course of relapsing disease. One can hope that an improved ability to prospectively use of available therapies thus minimizing their toxic effects. This improved knowledge is of particular value as one keeps in mind that the single most important predictor of outcome remains an early diagnosis and the prompt initiation of therapy.

References

1. Jennette JC, Falk RJ, Andrassy K, et al: Nomenclature of systemic vasculitides. Proposal of an international consensus conference. Arthritis Rheum 1994;37:187–192.
2. Jennette JC, Wilkman AS, Falk RJ: Anti-neutrophil cytoplasmic autoantibody-associated glomerulonephritis and vasculitis. Am J Pathol 1989;135:921–930.
3. Falk RJ, Jennette JC: Anti-neutrophil cytoplasmic autoantibodies with specificity for myeloperoxidase in patients with systemic vasculitis and idiopathic necrotizing and crescentic glomerulonephritis. N Engl J Med 1988;318:1651–1657.
4. Hagen EC, Ballieux BE, van Es LA, Daha MR, Van Der Woude FJ: Antineutrophil cytoplasmic autoantibodies: a review of the antigens involved, the assays, and the clinical and possible pathogenetic consequences. Blood 1993;81:1996–2002.
5. Hagen EC, Daha MR, Hermans J, et al: Diagnostic value of standardized assays for anti-neutrophil cytoplasmic antibodies in idiopathic systemic vasculitis. EC/BCR Project for ANCA Assay Standardization. Kidney Int 1998;53:743–753.
6. Fienberg R, Mark EJ, Goodman M, McCluskey RT, Niles JL: Correlation of antineutrophil cytoplasmic antibodies with the extrarenal histopathology of Wegener's (pathergic) granulomatosis and related forms of vasculitis. Hum Pathol 1993;24:160–168.
7. Falk RJ, Hogan S, Carey TS, Jennette JC: Clinical course of anti-neutrophil cytoplasmic autoantibody-associated glomerulonephritis and systemic vasculitis. The Glomerular Disease Collaborative Network. Ann Intern Med 1990;113:656–663.
8. Hogan SL, Nachman PH, Wilkman AS, Jennette JC, Falk RJ: Prognostic markers in patients with antineutrophil cytoplasmic autoantibody-associated microscopic polyangiitis and glomerulonephritis. J Am Soc Nephrol 1996;7:23–32.
9. Nachman PH, Hogan SL, Jennette JC, Falk RJ: Treatment response and relapse in antineutrophil cytoplasmic autoantibody-associated microscopic polyangiitis and glomerulonephritis. J Am Soc Nephrol 1996;7:33–39.
10. Lotze MT, Matory YL, Rayner AA, et al: Clinical effects and toxicity of interleukin-2 in patients with cancer. Cancer 1986;58:2764–2772.
11. Sarna GP, Figlin RA, Pertcheck M, Altrock B, Kradjian SA: Systemic administration of recombinant methionyl human interleukin-2 (Ala 125) to cancer patients: clinical results. J Biol Response Mod 1989;8:16–24.
12. Falk RJ, Moore DT, Hogan SL, Jennette JC: A renal biopsy is essential for the management of ANCA-positive patients with glomerulonephritis. Sarcoidosis Vasc Diffuse Lung Dis 1996;13:230–231.
13. Niles JL, Pan GL, Collins AB, et al: Antigen-specific radioimmunoassays for anti-neutrophil cytoplasmic antibodies in the diagnosis of rapidly progressive glomerulonephritis. J Am Soc Nephrol 1991;2:27–36.
14. Savage CO, Winearls CG, Evans DJ, Rees AJ, Lockwood CM: Microscopic polyarteritis: presentation, pathology and prognosis. Q J Med 1985;56:467–483.
15. Dupre-Goudable C, Keriven O, Modesto A, Ton TH, Durand D, Suc JM: In Wegener's granulomatosis initial renal biopsy predicts response to treatment better than peak plasma creatinine. Contrib Nephrol 1991;94:181–185.
16. Briedigkeit L, Kettritz R, Gobel U, Natusch R: Prognostic factors in Wegener's granulomatosis. Postgrad Med J 1993;69:856–861.
17. Bajema IM, Hagen EC, Hermans J, et al: Kidney biopsy as a predictor for renal outcome in ANCA-associated necrotizing glomerulonephritis. Kidney Int 1999;56:1751–1758.
18. Fauci AS, Katz P, Haynes BF, Wolff SM: Cyclophosphamide therapy of severe systemic necrotizing vasculitis. N Engl J Med 1979;301:235–238.
19. Tarlar-Williams C, Hijazi Y, Walther M: Cyclophosphamide-induced cystitis and bladder cancer in patients with Wegener's granulomatosis. Ann Intern Med 1996;124:477–484.
20. Gaskin G, Savage CO, Ryan JJ, et al: Anti-neutrophil cytoplasmic antibodies and disease activity during long-term follow-up of 70 patients with systemic vasculitis. Nephrol Dial Transplant 1991;6:689–694.
21. Guillevin L, Cordier JF, Lhote F, et al: A prospective, multicenter, randomized trial comparing steroids and pulse cyclophosphamide versus steroids and oral cyclophosphamide in the treatment of generalized Wegener's granulomatosis. Arthritis Rheum 1997;40:2187–2198.
22. Gaskin G, Pusey CD: Plasmapheresis in antineutrophil cytoplasmic antibody-associated systemic vasculitis. Ther Apheresis 2001;5:176–181.
23. Frasca GM, Neri L, Martello M, Sestigiani E, Borgnino LC, Bonomini V: Renal transplantation in patients with microscopic polyarteritis and antimyeloperoxidase antibodies: report of three cases. Nephron 1996;72:82–85.
24. Clarke AE, Bitton A, Eappen R, Danoff DS, Esdaile JM: Treatment of Wegener's granulomatosis after renal transplantation: is cyclosporine the preferred treatment? Transplantation 1990;50:1047–1051.
25. Haubitz M, Olbricht CJ, Maschek H, Frei U, Koch KM: Lethal relapse of Wegener's disease 4 years after successful kidney transplantation (letter). Nephron 1995;71:118–120.
26. Rosenstein ED, Ribot S, Ventresca E, Kramer N: Recurrence of Wegener's granulomatosis following renal transplantation. Br J Rheumatol 1994;33:869–871.
27. Reaich D, Cooper N, Main J: Rapid catastrophic onset of Wegener's granulomatosis in a renal transplant. Nephron 1994;67:354–357.
28. Nachman PH, Segelmark M, Westman K, et al: Recurrent ANCA-associated small vessel vasculitis after transplantation: a pooled analysis. Kidney Int 1999;56:1544–1550.
29. Rich LM, Piering WF: Ureteral stenosis due to recurrent Wegener's granulomatosis after kidney transplantation. J Am Soc Nephrol 1994;4:1516–1521.
30. Boubenider SA, Akhtar M, Alfurayh O, Algazlan S, Taibah K, Qunibi W: Late recurrence of Wegener's granulomatosis presenting as tracheal stenosis in a renal transplant patient. Clin Transplant 1994;8:5–9.
31. Cohen Tervaert JW, Stegeman CA, Kallenberg CGM: Serial ANCA testing is useful in monitoring disease activity of patients with ANCA-associated vasculitis. Sarcoidosis Vasc Diffuse Lung Dis 1996;13:241–245.

32. De'Oliviera J, Gaskin G, Dash A, Rees AJ, Pusey CD: Relationship between disease activity and anti-neutrophil cytoplasmic antibody concentration in long-term management of systemic vasculitis. Am J Kidney Dis 1995;25:380–389.

33. Cohen Tervaert JW, Huitema MG, Hene RJ, et al: Prevention of relapses in Wegener's granulomatosis by treatment based on antineutrophil cytoplasmic antibody titre. Lancet 1990;336:709–711.

34. Nowack R, Grab I, Flores S, Schnulle P, Yard B, van der Waude F: ANCA titres, even of IgG subclasses, and soluble CD14 fail to predict relapses in patients with ANCA-associated vasculitis. Nephrol Dial Transplant 2001;16:1631–1637.

35. Gordon M, Luqmani RA, Adu D, et al: Relapses in patients with a systemic vasculitis. Q J Med 1993;86:779–789.

36. Westman KW, Bygren PG, Olsson H, Ranstam J, Wieslander J: Relapse rate, renal survival, and cancer morbidity in patients with Wegener's granulomatosis or microscopic polyangiitis with renal involvement. J Am Soc Nephrol 1998;9:842–852.

37. Hogan SL, Nachman PH, Jennette JC, Falk RJ: The role of ANCA pattern and diagnosis in clinical presentation and outcomes in ANCA-associated small vessel vasculitis (ANCA-SVV). J Am Soc Nephrol 1999;10:104A.

38. Niles JL: A renal biopsy is essential for the management of ANCA-positive patients with glomerulonephritis: the contra-view. Sarcoidosis Vasc Diffuse Lung Dis 1996;13:232–234.

39. Bosch X, Lopez-Soto A, Mirapeix E, Font J, Ingelmo M, Urbano-Marquez A: Antineutrophil cytoplasmic autoantibody-associated alveolar capillaritis in patients presenting with pulmonary hemorrhage. Arch Pathol Lab Med 1994;118:517–522.

40. DeRemee RA, McDonald TJ, Weiland LH: Wegener's granulomatosis: observations on treatment with antimicrobial agents. Mayo Clin Proc 1985;60:27–32.

41. Reinhold-Keller E, DeGroot K, Rudert H, Nolle B, Heller M, Gross WL: Response to trimethoprim/sulfamethoxazole in Wegener's granulomatosis depends on the phase of disease. Q J Med 1996;89:15–23.

42. Stegeman CA, Cohen Tervaert JW, De Jong PE, Kallenberg CG: Trimethoprim–sulfamethoxazole (co-trimoxazole) for the prevention of relapses of Wegener's granulomatosis. Dutch Co-Trimoxazole Wegener Study Group. N Engl J Med 1996;335:16–20.

43. DeGroot K, Reinhold-Keller E, Taub NA, Paulsen J, Heller M, Nolle B: Maintenance of remission therapy in 65 patients with generalized Wegener's granulomatosis: methotrexate versus trimethoprim–sulfamethoxazole. Sarcoidosis Vasc Diffuse Lung Dis 1996;13:276.

44. Hoffman GS, Leavitt RY, Kerr GS, Fauci AS: The treatment of Wegener's granulomatosis with glucocorticoids and methotrexate. Arthritis Rheum 1992;35:1322–1329.

45. Sneller MC, Hoffman GS, Talar-Williams C, Kerr GS, Hallahan CW, Fauci AS: An analysis of forty-two Wegener's granulomatosis patients treated with methotrexate and prednisone. Arthritis Rheum 1995;38:608–613.

46. Frasca GM, Zoumparidis NG, Borgnino LC, Neri L, Vangelista A, Bonomini V: Plasma exchange treatment in rapidly progressive glomerulonephritis associated with anti-neutrophil cytoplasmic autoantibodies. Int J Artif Organs 1992;15:181–184.

47. Frasca GM, Zoumparidis NG, Borgnino LC, et al: Combined treatment in Wegener's granulomatosis with crescentic glomerulonephritis: clinical course and long-term outcome. Int J Artif Organs 1993;16:11–19.

48. Pusey CD, Rees AJ, Evans DJ, Peters DK, Lockwood CM: Plasma exchange in focal necrotizing glomerulonephritis without anti-GBM antibodies. Kidney Int 1991;40:757–763.

49. Guillevin L, Lhote F, Cohen P, et al: Corticosteroids plus pulse cyclophosphamide and plasma exchanges versus corticosteroids plus pulse cyclophosphamide alone in the treatment of polyarteritis nodosa and Churg–Strauss syndrome patients with factors predicting poor prognosis. A prospective, randomized trial in sixty-two patients. Arthritis Rheum 1995;38:1638–1645.

50. Guillevin L, Fain O, Lhote F, et al: Lack of superiority of steroids plus plasma exchange to steroids alone in the treatment of polyarteritis nodosa and Churg–Strauss syndrome. A prospective, randomized trial in 78 patients. Arthritis Rheum 1992;35:208–215.

51. Guillevin L, Cevallos R, Durand G, Lhote F, Jarrousse B, Callard P: Treatment of glomerulonephritis in microscopic polyangiitis and Churg–Strauss syndrome. Indications of plasma exchanges, meta-analysis of 2 randomized studies on 140 patients, 32 with glomerulonephritis. Ann Med Interne (Paris) 1997;148:198–204.

52. Cole E, Cattran D, Magil A, et al: A prospective randomized trial of plasma exchange as additive therapy in idiopathic crescentic glomerulonephritis. The Canadian Apheresis Study Group. Am J Kidney Dis 1992;20:261–269.

53. Zauner I, Bach D, Braun N, et al: Predictive value of initial histology and effect of plasmapheresis on long-term prognosis of rapidly progressive glomerulonephritis. Am J Kidney Dis 2002;39:28–35.

54. Klemmer PJ, Chalermskulrat W, Reif MS, Hogan SL, Henke DC, Falk RJ: Treatment with plasmaphersis in diffuse alveolar hemorrhage in ANCA-SVV. Clin Exp Immunol 2000;120(Suppl 1):73.

55. Gallagher H, Kwan JT, Jayne DR: Pulmonary renal syndrome: a 4-year, single-center experience. Am J Kidney Dis 2002;39:42–47.

56. Jordan SC: Treatment of systemic and renal-limited vasculitic disorders with pooled human intravenous immune globulin. J Clin Immunol 1995;15(Suppl):76S–85S.

57. Bussel A, Boulechfar H, Naim R: Immunoglobulins or plasma exchange? Synchronization of plasma exchange and intravenous polyvalent immunoglobulins. A consecutive study of 11 patients. Ann Med Interne (Paris) 1993;144:532–538.

58. Jayne DR, Esnault VL, Lockwood CM: Anti-idiotype antibodies to anti-myeloperoxidase autoantibodies in patients with systemic vasculitis. J Autoimmun 1993;6:221–226.

59. Rossi F, Jayne DR, Lockwood CM, Kazatchkine MD: Anti-idiotypes against anti-neutrophil cytoplasmic antigen autoantibodies in normal human polyspecific IgG for therapeutic use and in the remission sera of patients with systemic vasculitis. Clin Exp Immunol 1991;83:298–303.

60. Jayne DR, Davies MJ, Fox CJ, Black CM, Lockwood CM: Treatment of systemic vasculitis with pooled intravenous immunoglobulin. Lancet 1991;337:1137–1139.

61. Tuso P, Moudgil A, Hay J, et al: Treatment of antineutrophil cytoplasmic autoantibody-positive systemic vasculitis and glomerulonephritis with pooled intravenous gammaglobulin. Am J Kidney Dis 1992;20:504–508.

62. Richter C, Schnabel A, Csernok E, De G, Reinhold K, Gross WL: Treatment of anti-neutrophil cytoplasmic antibody (ANCA)-associated systemic vasculitis with high-dose intravenous immunoglobulin. Clin Exp Immunol 1995;101:2–7.

63. Richter C, Schnabel A, Csernok E, Reinhold-Keller E, Gross WL: Treatment of Wegener's granulomatosis with intravenous immunoglobulin. Adv Exp Med Biol 1993;336:487–489.

64. Jayne DR, Chapel H, Adu D, et al: Intravenous immunoglobulin for ANCA-associated systemic vasculitis with persistent disease activity. Q J Med 2000;93:433–439.

65. Nachman PH, Joy MS, Hogan SL, Jennette JC, Falk RJ: Preliminary results of a pilot study on the use of mycophenolate mofetil (MMF) in relapsing ANCA small vessel vasculitis (ANCA-SVV). J Am Soc Nephrol 2000;11:158.

66. Nowack R, Gobel U, Klooker P, Hergesell O, Andrassy K, Van Der Woude FJ: Mycophenolate mofetil for maintenance therapy of Wegener's granulomatosis and microscopic polyangiitis: a pilot study in 11 patients with renal involvement. J Am Soc Nephrol 1999;10:1965–1971.

67. Allen NB, Caldwell DS, Rice JR, McCallum RM: Cyclosporin A therapy for Wegener's granulomatosis. Adv Exp Med Biol 1993;336:473–476.

68. Georganas C, Ioakimidis D, Iatrou C, et al: Relapsing Wegener's granulomatosis: successful treatment with cyclosporin-A. Clin Rheumatol 1996;15:189–192.

69. Etanercept. Soluble tumour necrosis factor receptor, TNF receptor fusion protein,TNFR-Fc, TNR 001, Enbrel. Drugs R D 2000;1:75–77.

70. Stone JH, Uhlfelder ML, Hellmann DB, Crook S, Bedocs NM, Hoffman GS: Etanercept combined with conventional treatment in Wegener's granulomatosis: a six-month open-label trial to evaluate safety. Arthritis Rheum 2001;44:1149–1154.

71. Recommendations for the prevention and treatment of glucocorticoid-induced osteoporosis. American College of Rheumatology Task Force on Osteoporosis Guidelines. Arthritis Rheum 1996;39:1791–1801.

72. Masala A, Faedda R, Alagna S, et al: Use of testosterone to prevent cyclophosphamide-induced azoospermia. Ann Intern Med 1997;126:292–295.

73. Dooley MA, Patterson CC, Hogan SL, et al: Preservation of ovarian function using depot leuprolide acetate during cyclophosphamide therapy for severe lupus nephritis. Arthritis Rheum 2000;43:2858.

Minimal Change Disease

Laura M. Dember and David J. Salant

Background

Minimal change disease (MCD) is an idiopathic glomerular disease that accounts for 70–90% of cases of idiopathic nephrotic syndrome in children and 10–15% of cases in adults.[1] The name MCD has largely superseded the older terms "lipoid nephrosis," "nil disease," and "idiopathic nephrotic syndrome." The disorder is characterized by the rapid onset of severe, symptomatic nephrotic syndrome with well-preserved renal function, almost normal glomerular histology except for generalized podocyte effacement, and a remarkable sensitivity to treatment with glucocorticoids. Because relapse is common and repeated courses of glucocorticoids are associated with significant toxicities, MCD remains one of the major therapeutic challenges in clinical nephrology.

Clinical features, pathology, and pathogenesis

Clinical features

The clinical presentation of MCD is that of a pure nephrotic syndrome with heavy proteinuria, hypoalbuminemia, hyperlipidemia, and edema formation. Albumin is the predominant urine protein, although moderately selective or nonselective proteinuria has been observed in a significant proportion of adults with MCD.[2] Urinalysis reveals lipiduria, and mild microscopic hematuria may occur, especially in adults. Macroscopic hematuria is rare, and red blood cell casts are not present. Renal tubular cells and granular casts may be seen in the acute renal failure that occurs occasionally in association with MCD. Moderate hypertension is present in 13–30% of cases and is more frequent in adults.[1,2] Serum creatinine may be slightly elevated at the time of presentation.[1–3] The elevation in blood pressure and creatinine typically resolves with remission of the nephrotic syndrome. Adults are more likely to develop acute renal failure than children.[3–5] The renal failure is usually reversible and is often preceded by severe edema formation. Histologic evidence of ischemic tubular injury has been observed in many cases, but the mechanism of the acute renal failure is not known.[6]

The course of MCD is characterized by multiple remissions and relapses of the nephrotic syndrome and a marked sensitivity to glucocorticoid therapy. In children, the frequency of relapses tends to decrease with age, and in most cases the episodes cease after several years. The long-term renal outcome of MCD is good and fewer than 5% of patients develop endstage renal disease.[7] In general, the course of the disease is similar in children and adults. Age-related differences in the response to treatment and the frequency of relapses are discussed in detail in subsequent sections of this chapter.

Pathology

Because the diagnosis of MCD is in many respects a diagnosis of exclusion, the challenge for the clinician is to avoid misclassifying lesions of focal segmental glomerulosclerosis (FSGS) as MCD. Such misclassification has obvious implications for interpreting clinical studies. Those histologic features that should raise suspicion for FSGS are noted in the discussion that follows.

By light microscopy the glomeruli in MCD usually appear normal. There may be a slight increase in mesangial cellularity, and the visceral epithelial cells may be swollen. The capillaries are patent and the walls are not thickened. Dilatation of the glomerular capillaries is common and may be due to loss of compliance of the capillary wall resulting from epithelial cell alterations. Glomerular size is usually normal. Enlarged but otherwise normal-appearing glomeruli may be predictive of steroid unresponsiveness or subsequent development of FSGS.[8] Doubly refractile lipid droplets and periodic acid–Schiff-positive protein droplets may be seen in the cells of the proximal tubule. Focal tubular atrophy and mild segmental interstitial fibrosis are accepted by some authorities as features of MCD; however, if tubulointerstitial changes are diffuse or severe it is likely that FSGS is present. In adults, particularly in elderly patients, vascular changes may be present but are thought to be due to associated conditions such as hypertension rather than MCD.

The results of immunofluorescence studies are negative for immunoglobulin or complement deposition in most cases of MCD. Mesangial IgM, IgG, or C3 deposits have been reported in up to 20% of cases of MCD in some series and are felt by most investigators to be the result of nonspecific trapping of circulating immunoglobulins.[6] It has been suggested that heavy mesangial IgM deposition, especially in conjunction with some degree of mesangial hypercellularity, may be a marker of glucocorticoid unresponsiveness and/or subsequent development of FSGS. However, this idea remains controversial.[6]

Electron microscopy reveals the major morphologic features of MCD: effacement of the glomerular visceral epithelial cell (podocyte) foot processes and obliteration of the slit pore complex. These abnormalities are not specific for MCD and occur in other conditions associated with heavy proteinuria. The extent of the foot process effacement and obliteration of the slit pore complex does not correlate with the amount of proteinuria but has been shown to correlate with the decrement in glomerular filtration rate (GFR).[9] Other electron microscopic features of the podocytes include hypertrophy, increased numbers of pinocytic vesicles and intracytoplasmic lipid and protein droplets, and microvillous transformation of their free surfaces. The endothelial cells lining the capillary loop show normal fenestration, and the glomerular basement membrane is usually of normal thickness.[6]

Pathogenesis

The etiology of MCD is unknown. Experimental animal models developed to analyze the mechanisms underlying proteinuria and clearance studies in human patients suggest that there is a loss of both charge selectivity and size selectivity of the glomerular filter.[6,10] Changes in the anionic composition of the glomerular capillary wall are thought to underlie the impairment in charge selectivity and may, in fact, produce defects in size selectivity as well.[11] Whether the primary abnormality occurs in the glomerular basement membrane or in the visceral epithelial cells is not clear. Epithelial cell injury, which is the predominant histologic feature of MCD, may be either the cause or the result of loss of the anionic constituents of the glomerular capillary wall. An immunologic basis of MCD, more specifically a disorder of T-lymphocyte function, is suggested by the response to immunosuppressive agents, by the association of minimal change lesions with Hodgkin disease, and by multiple alterations in the in vitro function of T cells from MCD patients.[1] The observation that supernatants of cultured lymphocytes from patients with MCD can increase capillary wall permeability and induce loss of glomerular polyanions has led to a search for vascular permeability factors secreted by the T cells of these patients.[12,13]

An unresolved question is whether MCD and FSGS represent two distinct clinicopathologic entities or whether they are variants of a single disease process.[6] The differences in responsiveness to glucocorticoids and in long-term renal outcome support the former view. The demonstration of FSGS lesions in subsequent biopsies from patients with an initial histologic diagnosis of MCD has been offered as evidence that MCD can "progress" to FSGS. However, the possibility of histologic misclassification due to sampling error limits the conclusions that can be drawn from such observations.

Clinical trials

The impetus for treating MCD arises mainly from the consequences of the nephrotic state, which include malaise from anasarca, as well as a predisposition to infection, thrombosis, malnutrition, and possibly atherogenesis. Prior to the availability of antibiotics and glucocorticoids, the mortality of nephrotic syndrome was greater than 50% with the majority of the deaths during this period resulting from infection.[14] It has been argued that proteinuria itself may be nephrotoxic and contribute to progressive renal injury. Indeed, in MCD, as in other glomerulopathies, the attainment of remission of nephrotic syndrome is associated with good long-term renal outcome.[7,15] Although it is not known whether remission of nephrotic syndrome serves as a favorable prognostic indicator or whether it actually affects the outcome, the latter possibility has been offered as an additional reason to treat MCD.[16]

Because persistent nephrotic syndrome is considered especially harmful in children, most pediatric nephrologists promptly treat the first episode and relapses.[17] The decision to begin treatment in adults is somewhat more complicated because the consequences of the nephrotic syndrome may be less significant and the therapy is generally less well tolerated.

Terminology

The course of MCD is often described in terms of the response to glucocorticoid treatment. The classification scheme outlined in Table 22.1 evolved out of experience with children with idiopathic nephrotic syndrome but is used in the adult literature as well. However, as will become clear later in this chapter, the definition of steroid-resistant disease should probably differ for children and adults. The criteria for complete remission and relapse shown in Table 22.1 were established by the International Study of Kidney Disease in Children (ISKDC).[18] Although the definitions of these outcomes are relatively uniform in subsequent studies, some variation does exist. Consequently, the ability to generalize from the findings is somewhat limited. Interpretation of the literature is also complicated by the inclusion of patients with primary glomerulopathies other than MCD.

Table 22.1 Classification of minimal change disease based on response to glucocorticoid treatment

Steroid-responsive	Complete remission of proteinuria within 8 weeks of initiating glucocorticoid treatment
Frequently relapsing	Initially steroid-responsive but relapses at rate of two per 6 months or six per 18 months
Steroid-dependent	Initially steroid-responsive but relapse during tapering of glucocorticoids or within 2 weeks of discontinuing glucocorticoids
Steroid-resistant	No remission within 8 weeks of initiating glucocorticoid treatment
Complete remission	Reduction in urinary protein excretion to < 4 mg/h/m^2 or 0–trace by urine dipstick for three consecutive days
Relapse	Reappearance of proteinuria ≥ 4 mg/h/m^2 for three consecutive days

Natural history of untreated minimal change disease

A clear understanding of the natural history of a disease facilitates both the interpretation of uncontrolled treatment trials and clinical decisions regarding the use of therapies with potential toxicities. Unfortunately, the natural history of untreated MCD has been difficult to establish because the use of glucocorticoids is extremely widespread, and data from the era before glucocorticoids are limited by infrequent histologic classification. Spontaneous remissions do occur in MCD and have been reported in 10–75% of patients who received only supportive therapy.[19–23] The accuracy of these estimates is limited by the small numbers of untreated patients and, in many cases, the lack of randomization. Although the occurrence of spontaneous remissions has led some investigators to recommend a period of observation before starting treatment, this is impractical because such a remission may not happen until months or years after the onset of disease.

Treatment with glucocorticoids
Results in children

Table 22.2 summarizes selected studies that evaluate glucocorticoid therapy for childhood MCD.[18,24–28] Although there are no controlled trials directly comparing glucocorticoid therapy with supportive therapy as initial treatment of childhood MCD, the overwhelming consensus is that both the likelihood and the rapidity of remission are increased with glucocorticoids. In the ISKDC, a multicenter, prospective, uncontrolled trial, 93% of children achieved complete remission with an 8-week

course of prednisone.[18] The dose of prednisone used in this study was arbitrarily set at 60 mg/m^2/day (up to 80 mg/day) for 4 weeks followed by 4 weeks of "intermittent" prednisone at 40 mg/m^2 for three consecutive days out of seven. Subsequently, the Arbeitsgemeinschaft für Pädiatrische Nephrologie (APN), a large multicenter study from Germany, and a single-center study in Japan both showed that a prolonged course of alternate-day prednis(ol)one, given after an initial course of daily prednis(ol)one, resulted in fewer relapses than a short alternate-day course[26] or the intermittent regimen used in the ISKDC trial.[27] The prolonged regimens were not associated with an increase in the cumulative dose or toxicity of glucocorticoids. Bagga et al[28] found a trend toward a longer duration of first remission with an initial 16-week course of prednisolone daily for 8 weeks and alternate days for 8 weeks compared with an initial 8-week course. However, the total number of relapses during a 2-year follow-up period did not differ between the two groups, and the cumulative glucocorticoid dose was greater in the prolonged therapy group than in the standard therapy group.

Even with more intensive initial treatment protocols, as many as 60% of children will have a relapse within 12 months,[28] and approximately 40% will have a frequently relapsing course[29] (see Table 22.1). Thus, the major challenge is managing frequently relapsing MCD. Using individual polyrelapsing children as their own controls, the APN compared alternate-day prednisolone with intermittent prednisolone (in both cases following 4 weeks of daily therapy) in frequent relapsers and found a lower relapse rate with alternate-day therapy.[24] However, neither treatment was completely satisfactory: 43% of the alternate-day group suffered at least one relapse during the 6-month treatment period (compared with 72% in the intermittent group) and almost all patients relapsed during the subsequent 6 months. The use of intravenous methylprednisolone pulse therapy followed by "low-dose" oral prednisone produced a similar remission rate and relapse rate as the "standard therapy" (60 mg/m^2/day) but was associated with fewer glucocorticoid-induced adverse effects.[25] This study included both children and adults. While the efficacy data were analyzed separately for adults and children, the adverse effect data were analyzed together. Given age-related differences in glucocorticoid toxicities, the conclusions that can be drawn from such an analysis are somewhat limited. Induction therapy with alternate-day glucocorticoids has not been studied in children.

Results in adults

Table 22.3 summarizes the results of studies evaluating glucocorticoid treatment of MCD in adults.[2–5,22,30] All except one of these studies are retrospective analyses. It should be noted that there was marked variation in the treatment regimens used, particularly with regard to duration and tapering schemes. Remission of nephrotic syndrome was achieved in 81–90% of adults treated with glucocorticoids in these studies, a remission rate similar to that of children. However, the time to remit after starting

Table 22.2 Studies of glucocorticoid treatment of minimal change disease in children

Reference	Design	Clinical setting[1]	Mean follow-up	Treatment	Control	Complete remission (%)		Relapse (%)[2]		Comments
						Treatment	Control	Treatment	Control	
ISKDC[18] (n = 363)	Prospective Uncontrolled	Initial episode	8 weeks	Prednisone, daily then intermittent				NA		
APN[24] (n = 48)	Prospective Controlled Randomized	Frequently relapsing	12 months	Prednisone, daily then alternate day[4]	Prednisone, daily then intermittent[5]	NA	NA	43 $P < 0.05$	72	Relapse rates shown are for treatment period. No significant difference during subsequent 6 months
Imbasciati et al[25] (n = 67)	Prospective Controlled Randomized	Initial episode or relapse	18 months	i.v. pulse then prednisone, low dose[6]	Prednisone, high dose[7]	94	97	68	64	Time to response shorter in methylprednisolone group
APN[26] (n = 61)	Prospective Controlled Randomized	Initial episode	8 months	Prednisone, short duration[8]	Prednisone, standard duration[9]			81 $P = 0.001$	59	
Ueda et al[27] (n = 46)	Prospective Controlled Randomized	Initial episode	3.8 years	Prednisolone, daily, then long taper[10]	Prednisolone, daily then short intermittent[11]	100	100	29	62	Relapse rate significantly lower in long duration group within first 6 months after treatment
Bagga et al[28] (n = 51)	Prospective Controlled Randomized	Initial episode	28 months	Prednisolone, prolonged daily then alternate day[12]	Prednisolone, standard daily, then alternate day[13]	100	100	73	91	Only patients with remission by 4 weeks included. Cumulative steroid dose significantly greater in prolonged daily group

APN, Arbeitsgemeinschaft für Pädiatrische Nephrologie; ISKDC, International Study of Kidney Diseases in Children; NA, not available.

[1] See Table 22.1 for general definition of frequently relapsing disease. Criteria in studies may vary somewhat from those in Table 22.1.
[2] P-value is shown if difference is significant ($P < 0.05$).
[3] Prednisone 60 mg/m²/day in divided doses for 4 weeks, then 40 mg/m²/day in divided doses 3 consecutive days out of 7 for 4 weeks.
[4] Prednisone 60 mg/m²/day in divided doses until remission, then prednisone 35 mg/m² on alternate days for 6 months.
[5] Prednisone 60 mg/m²/day in divided doses until remission, then prednisone 40 mg/m²/day in divided doses 3 consecutive days out of 7 for 6 months.
[6] Methylprednisolone 20 mg/kg/day i.v. for 3 days, prednisone 20 mg/m²/day for 4 weeks, then 20 mg/m² on alternate days and and taper off over 4 months.
[7] Prednisone 60 mg/m²/day for 4 weeks, then 40 mg/m² on alternate days and taper off over 4 months.
[8] Prednisone 60 mg/m²/day until remission, then prednisone 40 mg/m²/day on alternate days for 4 weeks. Relapse: 60 mg/m²/day until remission, then 40 mg/m² on alternate days for 4 weeks.
[9] Prednisone 60 mg/m²/day for 4 weeks, then prednisone 40 mg/m² on alternate days for 4 weeks, then taper off over 5 months.
[10] Prednisolone 60 mg/m²/day for 4 weeks, then prednisolone 60 mg/m² on alternate days for 4 weeks, then taper off over 5 months.
[11] Prednisolone 60 mg/m²/day for 4 weeks, then prednisolone 40 mg/m²/day for 3 consecutive days out of 7 for 4 weeks.
[12] Prednisolone 2 mg/kg/day for 4 weeks, then 1.5 mg/kg/day on alternate days for 4 weeks, then 1.0 mg/kg on alternate days for 4 weeks.
[13] Prednisolone 2 mg/kg/day for 4 weeks, then 1.5 mg/kg on alternate days for 4 weeks.

Table 22.3 Studies of glucocorticoid treatment of minimal change disease in adults

Reference[1]	Design	Clinical setting	Mean follow-up	Treatment	Complete remission (%)	Complete remission (%)			Relapse (%)[2]	Comments
						Week 8	Week 16	Week 28		
Black et al[22] (n = 31)	Prospective Controlled	Initial episode	> 2 years	Prednisone daily[3]	80	NA	NA	NA	NA	Low doses of prednisone used. Complete remission rate estimated (refers to treated patients only)
Wang et al[5] (n = 109)	Retrospective Uncontrolled	Initial episode or relapse	2.0 years	Prednisolone, alternate day[4]	83		NA	NA	NA	Young patients (82% had onset of disease before age 30 years)
Nolasco et al[2] (n = 75)	Retrospective Uncontrolled	Initial episode	7.5 years	Prednisone daily[6]	77	60	73	77	76	Significantly higher relapse rate in younger patients (age < 45 years)
Nair et al[30] (n = 58)	Retrospective Uncontrolled	Initial episode	3.0 years	Prednisolone, alternate day[7]	93	82	93	NA	31	Mean age of patients low (27.7 years)
Korbet et al[3] (n = 34)	Retrospective Uncontrolled	Initial episode	5.3 years	Prednisone daily[8]	91	51	77	85	65	Significantly greater time to achieve remission in older patients (age > 40 years)
Fujimoto et al[4] (n = 33)	Retrospective Uncontrolled	Initial episode	3.9 years	Prednisolone daily[9]	97	76	97	NA	34	Mean age of patients low (27.7 years)

NA, not available.

[1] Only patients treated with glucocorticoids alone are included.

[2] Study compared prednisone with supportive treatment in variety of glomerular diseases. Only MCD patients included in table. Unable to determine spontaneous remission rate from data because some control group patients received prednisone during follow-up.

[3] Prednisone dose varied (mean initial dose 26 mg/day). Treatment duration 6–48 months.

[4] Prednisolone 60 mg/day for 1 week, then 120 mg on alternate days until remission, and tapered off over 10–16 months.

[5] Extension of Cameron et al.[31]

[6] Prednisone 60 mg/day for 1 week, then 45 mg/day for 4 weeks and taper off over 3–15 weeks. Mean duration of treatment 13 weeks.

[7] Prednisolone 2 mg/kg (maximum 120 mg) on alternate days for 6–12 weeks, then tapered off over 12 weeks.

[8] Prednisone ≥ 60 mg/day for 1–3 months and tapered off over 1–40 months. Mean duration of treatment 8.1 months.

[9] Prednisolone 1 mg/kg/day for 4–8 weeks, then tapered off over approximately 9 months.

treatment was greater in the adults. In the study by Nolasco et al,[2] 60% of adults were in remission within 8 weeks of starting treatment and 73% in remission within 16 weeks. Similar results were reported by Korbet et al.[3] The experience of Fujimoto et al[4] differed somewhat in that a higher percentage (76%) were in remission within 8 weeks, and by 16 weeks 90% of adults achieved remission. The reason for the more rapid response to glucocorticoid treatment in the study by Fujimoto et al may be due to the younger age of the patients (mean 27.7 years in Fujimoto et al's study vs. 40.7 and 42 years in the research by Korbet et al and Nolasco et al, respectively). The analysis by Korbet et al does, in fact, suggest that the time to remission after initiation of glucocorticoids is shorter in younger adults than in older adults. It is also possible that genetic and environmental factors may influence the outcome. Meyrier and Simon[19] pooled all the published cases of adults treated with glucocorticoids between 1961 and 1987 and found that of 302 patients, 74.8% had complete remission, 7% had partial remission, and 18.2% had no response. The lower rate of complete remission in this pooled data may be due to shorter duration of treatment and inclusion of patients treated for relapses as well as initial disease.

The results of these studies suggest that similar proportions (70–80%) of adults and children have at least one relapse. However, adults appear to be less likely than children to have frequently relapsing or steroid-dependent disease (21% in Nolasco et al[2] compared with 40% in the ISKDC[29]).

Initial treatment of MCD with alternate-day glucocorticoids has been evaluated in adults.[5,23,30] Nair et al[30] retrospectively analyzed the outcomes of 58 adults treated with prednisolone at 2 mg/kg (with maximum of 120 mg) as a single dose every 48 h. Tapering began once remission was achieved. In contrast to the experience described earlier with daily prednisone, 82% of patients in this study were in remission within 6 weeks, 93% were in remission within 12 weeks, and only 31% of patients relapsed during the follow-up period. The low relapse rate has been attributed to the more gradual tapering regimen used for many of the patients in this study. The experience of Wang et al[5] using alternate-day prednisolone in Malaysian adults with MCD was less impressive. Remission occurred in 78% of 109 patients but, in many cases, was not achieved until 6 months or more of treatment. The rationale for alternate-day treatment is to decrease the adverse effects of the glucocorticoids. Although the authors of both these studies commented that the adverse effects were low using an alternate-day regimen, this claim has not been substantiated by a prospective comparison with daily dosing.

Treatment with alkylating agents
Results in children
The use of therapies other than glucocorticoids has generally been reserved for those patients with frequently relapsing, steroid-dependent, or steroid-resistant MCD. Table 22.4 summarizes selected studies evaluating the efficacy of cyclophosphamide and chlorambucil in such patients.[2,31–38] In a prospective controlled study, the ISKDC compared cyclophosphamide with "intermittent" prednisone in children with frequently relapsing nephrotic syndrome and found a lower relapse rate in the cyclophosphamide group compared with the prednisone group (48% vs. 88%).[32] While this result is consistent with the findings of earlier studies[39,40] and supports the use of alkylating agents in frequently relapsing disease, separate analyses were not performed for the patients with MCD and FSGS, thus preventing firm conclusions regarding MCD per se. Furthermore, the "intermittent" prednisone regimen used in this study has been shown to be less effective than alternate-day therapy in preventing relapse.[24]

Alkylating agents appear to be less effective in steroid-dependent disease than in frequently relapsing disease. In one of the APN studies, frequently relapsing and steroid-dependent children were treated with either cyclophosphamide and prednisone or chlorambucil and prednisone.[36] Such treatment produced a remission rate of 72% in the frequent relapsers but only 28% in the steroid-dependent patients. There is controversy as to whether or not an increase in the duration of the alkylating agent improves the response in steroid-dependent disease. In a separate study of steroid-dependent children with MCD, the APN found that a 12-week course of cyclophosphamide was associated with a higher 2-year relapse-free rate (67%) than was an 8-week course (22%).[37] However, Ueda et al[38] found no difference in the 5-year relapse-free rates in steroid-dependent MCD patients treated for 8 or 12 weeks (24% and 25%, respectively).

There are fewer studies of alkylating agents for steroid-resistant MCD. This probably reflects the relative rarity of steroid resistance in true MCD. Uncontrolled studies suggest that steroid-resistant patients with MCD may respond to cyclophosphamide;[41,42] however, in the ISKDC, the early nonresponsive patients (i.e., those who had not remitted after 8 weeks of prednisone) treated with cyclophosphamide plus prednisone did not show a greater remission rate than those treated with prednisone alone.[32] It should be noted, however, that among those who did respond, the remission occurred earlier in the cyclophosphamide group than in the prednisone group (mean interval between beginning of treatment and remission 38.4 days and 95.5 days, respectively). In the one study in which they were directly compared, chlorambucil and cyclophosphamide appeared to be equally effective in frequently relapsing MCD and equally ineffective in steroid-dependent disease.[36]

Results in adults
In comparison with children, fewer data are available in adults with regard to the response of MCD to alkylating agents. The retrospective analysis by Nolasco et al[2] showed that 69% of adults treated with cyclophosphamide achieved remission. Moreover, 58% of those who remitted did so within 8 weeks of the initiation of therapy. The duration of remission was longer after treatment with cyclophosphamide than with prednisone in this series.

Table 22.4 Studies of alkylating agents in minimal change disease

Reference	Design	Clinical setting[1]	Mean follow-up	Treatment	Control	Complete remission (%) Treatment	Complete remission (%) Control	Relapse (%)[2] Treatment	Relapse (%)[2] Control	Comments
Cameron et al[31] (n = 58)	Retrospective Uncontrolled	Children FR MCD	5.8 years	Cyclophosphamide		98		66		Relapse-free half-life: 2.8 years. Duration of treatment variable (2–30 weeks)
ISKDC[32] (n = 96)	Prospective Controlled Randomized	Children FR, SR NS	NA	Cyclophosphamide ± prednisone, intermittent	Prednisone, intermittent	SR: 56	40	FR: 48 $P < 0.001$	88	Treatment for FR patients: cylophosphamide alone Treatment for SR patients: cyclophosphamide + intermittent prednisone
Grupe et al[33] (n = 21)	Prospective Controlled Randomized	Children FR, SD NS	1.7 years	Chlorambucil + prednisone	Prednisone			0 $P < 0.005$	100	Mean dose of chlorambucil (16.9 mg/kg) above gonadal toxicity limit
Al-Khader et al[34] (n = 14)	Prospective Controlled Randomized	Adults MCD	6 years	Cyclophosphamide	Supportive therapy	87	25	0	0	Statistical significance of difference in remission rates not provided in publication
Williams et al[35] (n = 59)	Retrospective Uncontrolled	Children FR, SD, SR NS	5 years	Chlorambucil + prednisone				15		Duration of remission same with high (> 0.3 mg/kg/day) or low (< 0.3 mg/kg/day) dose of chlorambucil
APN[36] (n = 50)	Prospective Controlled Randomized	Children FR, SD MCD	2.5 years	Cyclophosphamide + prednisone taper	Chlorambucil + prednisone taper			FR: 37 SD: 72	12 69	Significantly higher relapse rate in SD patients than in FR patients (cyclophosphamide and chlorambucil patients combined)
Nolasco et al[2] (n = 36)	Retrospective Uncontrolled	Adults Initial episode FR, SD, SR MCD	> 4 years	Cyclophosphamide ± prednisone		69		41		
APN[37] (n = 36)	Prospective Historically controlled	Children SD MCD	2 years	Cyclophosphamide + prednisone taper 12 weeks	Cyclophosphamide + prednisone taper 8 weeks			33 $P = 0.018$	78	Control group comprised the treatment group from APN[31]
Ueda et al[38] (n = 73)	Prospective Controlled Randomized	Children SD MCD	5.3 years	Cyclophosphamide + prednisolone 12 weeks	Cyclophosphamide +prednisolone 8 weeks			76	75	As with relapse rate, there was was no significant difference in time to relapse between groups

APN, Arbeitsgemeinschaft für Pädiatrische Nephrologie; FR, frequently relapsing; ISKDC, International Study of Kidney Diseases in Children; MCD, minimal change disease; NA, not available; NS, idiopathic nephrotic syndrome; SD, steroid dependent; SR, steroid resistant. Criteria in studies may vary somewhat from those in Table 22.1. NS indicates that patient group includes those with idiopathic nephrotic syndrome, not necessarily only patients with MCD.

[1]See Table 22.1 for general definitions of frequently relapsing, steroid-dependent, and steroid-resistant.

[2]P-value is shown if difference is significant ($P < 0.05$).

Two-thirds of those who responded to cyclophosphamide were still in remission 4 years after treatment. In a small prospective controlled study, Al-Khader et al[34] treated eight adult MCD patients with cyclophosphamide and compared the outcome to that in eight patients treated with supportive therapy (diuretics). Seven of those treated with cyclophosphamide attained remission, whereas two of the control patients remitted spontaneously. None of the patients in either group who achieved remission had a relapse during a mean follow-up period of 6 years. Although this appears to be an impressive outcome, six patients required treatment for longer than 1 month to achieve remission and it is possible that an equally good result would have been obtained with glucocorticoids.

Toxicity of alkylating agents

The bulk of the data in children and adults suggest that cyclophosphamide or chlorambucil therapy, in conjunction with glucocorticoids, will induce remissions of longer duration than those resulting from glucocorticoids alone in frequently relapsing patients, and that these drugs may decrease glucocorticoid requirements in steroid-dependent patients. The major toxicities of these agents include reversible alopecia, susceptibility to viral and fungal infections, gonadal failure, and late development of malignancy. Cyclophosphamide can cause hemorrhagic cystitis and chlorambucil has been associated with the development of seizures. The risk of irreversible gonadal failure increases with patient age (particularly for women) and cumulative dose. Gonadal failure is usually reversible if the total cumulative dose of cyclophosphamide or chlorambucil is less than 200 mg/kg or 10 mg/kg, respectively. Most cases of late malignancy following treatment with these agents have occurred in patients treated for at least 1 year. The risk of malignancy with short-term therapy with chlorambucil or cyclophosphamide is not known. The "steroid-sparing" effect of alkylating agents has been considered a justification for their use in frequently relapsing and steroid-dependent cases. Although patients who enter prolonged remission after such therapy will be spared further steroid toxicity, there is a risk of additive toxicity in those who relapse or fail to respond. Therefore alkylating agents should be limited to those patients suffering severe steroid toxicity or uncontrolled disease.

Treatment with cyclosporine

Multiple small uncontrolled studies suggesting beneficial effects of cyclosporine in patients with frequently relapsing or steroid-dependent MCD provided the rationale for the larger trials summarized in Table 22.5.[43–47] All but one of these studies included patients with FSGS as well as MCD, and in most cases separate analyses of the patients with MCD were not performed. Two multicenter, randomized, controlled studies by Ponticelli et al[43,44] showed that cyclosporine, at doses of 5 mg/kg/day in adults and 6 mg/kg/day in children, is highly effective in maintaining remission in steroid-dependent or frequently relapsing nephrotic syndrome (88% with cyclosporine vs. 68% with cyclophosphamide), and is capable of producing at least a partial remission in 60% of steroid-resistant cases. In the steroid-responsive patients, the relapse rate and glucocorticoid requirement were reduced during treatment with cyclosporine. However, in both of these studies, relapse occurred in approximately 70% of patients after cyclosporine was discontinued.

The need for prolonged courses of treatment with cyclosporine, owing to the high relapse rate following its discontinuation, has raised concern about chronic cyclosporine nephrotoxicity. Somewhat to the surprise of those involved in the early trials of cyclosporine treatment in MCD, the drug appeared to be well tolerated in the short term, with no discernible alteration in serum creatinine or GFR measurements.[48] On the other hand, histologic changes have been documented in the absence of changes in the serum creatinine level. Habib and Niaudet[49] reviewed serial renal biopsies in 42 children with nephrotic syndrome (35 with MCD and seven with FSGS) treated with cyclosporine for 4–63 months. Tubulointerstitial lesions developed in 24 patients, and none of the nine patients with "extensive lesions" had a reduction in GFR.

Although the high relapse rate and potential nephrotoxicity of cyclosporine have relegated it to third-line therapy behind glucocorticoids and alkylating agents for steroid-dependent or steroid-resistant disease, the results of a long-term study by Meyrier et al[46] in adults with MCD and FSGS give cause to reconsider this position. The essential findings in this study are that adults with MCD (confirmed on repeat biopsy) can be treated with cyclosporine for an extended period (up to 78 months) without loss of renal function and with scant histologic evidence of cyclosporine nephrotoxicity as long as the dose does not exceed 5.5 mg/kg/day. Not only did this cyclosporine therapy produce complete remission in 86% (19 of 22) of these steroid-dependent or steroid-resistant patients, but remission was also sustained (for 5 months to 6 years) in 10 patients in whom cyclosporine was discontinued after 1–5 years. In this study, the factors that were most predictive of histologic cyclosporine nephrotoxicity included dosage greater than 5.5 mg/kg/day, the presence of renal insufficiency prior to treatment, and the percentage of glomeruli with lesions of FSGS on pretreatment biopsy. A similar paucity of cyclosporine nephrotoxicity in adult MCD was reported by Ittel et al.[47] Although these authors did not observe permanent remission in their patients, they were able to maintain partial or complete remission in 15 steroid-dependent or steroid-resistant MCD patients for 7–91 months. Only one patient showed mild interstitial fibrosis suggestive of cyclosporine toxicity. Cyclosporine trough whole-blood levels were kept at 50–150 ng/mL at a mean dose of approximately 4.5 mg/kg/day.

Evaluations of the nephrotoxicity of long-term cyclosporine treatment in children with MCD have included small numbers of patients and have had varied results. Inoue et al[50] found histologic evidence of cyclosporine toxicity in 7 of 13 children following a 2-year course of treatment for steroid-dependent MCD. The changes

Table 22.5 Studies of cyclosporine in minimal change disease

Reference	Design	Clinical setting[1]	Mean follow-up	Treatment	Control	Complete remission (%)		Relapse (%)[2]		Comments
						Treatment	Control	Treatment	Control	
Ponticelli et al[43] (n = 41)	Prospective Controlled Randomized	Children Adults SR MCD, FSGS	1.5 years (median)	Cyclosporine 6 months, then taper	Supportive therapy	32 $P < 0.05$	0	69[3]	NA	Complete or partial remission in 60% of cyclosporine group vs. 16% of control group
Ponticelli et al[44] (n = 66)	Prospective Controlled Randomized	Children Adults FR, SD MCD, FSGS	1.7 years	Cyclosporine 9 months	Cyclophosphamide 8 weeks			75	37	P value for % relapse not provided in publication
Hulton et al[45] (n = 40)	Prospective Uncontrolled	Children SD MCD	2 years	Cyclosporine 12–63 months				72		All relapsed after cyclosporine withdrawal
Meyrier et al[46] (n = 36)	Prospective Uncontrolled	Adults SD, SR MCD, FSGS	1.6 years	Cyclosporine 6–78 months (mean 19.6 months)		86[4]				Serial biopsy study. Sustained remission in 10 MCD patients after cyclosporine withdrawal
Ittel et al[47] (n = 40)	Prospective Uncontrolled	Adults FR, SD, SR MCD, FSGS	2.7 years (median)	Cyclosporine 6–91 months (median 32 months)		60[5]				Serial biopsy study. All relapsed after cyclosporine withdrawal

FSGS, focal segmental glomerulosclerosis; FR, frequently relapsing; MCD, minimal change disease; NA, not available; SD, steroid dependent; SR, steroid resistant.

[1]See Table 22.1 for definitions of frequently relapsing, steroid dependent, and steroid resistant. Criteria in studies may vary somewhat from those in Table 22.1.
[2]P-value is shown if difference is significant ($P < 0.05$).
[3]Relapse rate for patients who had complete or partial remission.
[4]Refers to MCD patients only (n = 22).
[5]Refers to MCD patients only (n = 15).

were considered moderate or severe in five of the patients. Much lower rates of cyclosporine toxicity have been reported by others. Gregory et al[51] biopsied 12 of 22 children with steroid-dependent or steroid-resistant nephrotic syndrome after 12–41 months of cyclosporine treatment. Two patients, both with IgM nephropathy, had progression of interstitial fibrosis and tubular atrophy present on biopsies before cyclosporine administaration. None of the other patients had histologic evidence of nephrotoxicity. Hino et al[52] found mild tubular atrophy with striped interstitial fibrosis in 2 of 13 children biopsied after 12–43 months of cyclosporine treatment, while Kano et al[53] found such changes in only 1 of 14 children treated with low-dose cyclosporine (1.6–3.1 mg/kg/day) for 2 years. In both of these studies there was no apparent correlation between either the cyclosporine dose or mean trough level and the development of histologic changes, and the serum creatinine did not increase following cyclosporine treatment in those patients with biopsy evidence of nephrotoxicity. The stability of the serum creatinine was particularly noteworthy in the study by Hino et al because creatinine values were available at 2–10.5 years following completion of the cyclosporine treatment.

Thus although it has yet to be determined whether prolonged treatment with cyclosporine is "curative" or simply sustains remission until the disease "burns out," it is worth considering maintenance cyclosporine as an alternative to cyclophosphamide in severe steroid-dependent, steroid-resistant, or even frequently relapsing adults, especially those in their reproductive years. Indeed, some authorities argue that short-term, low-dose cyclosporine might even be preferable to glucocorticoids as preferred therapy, although no prospective data are currently available to support this position.

Treatment with azathioprine, mizoribine, and levamisole

Most of the data on the use of azathioprine in MCD comes from anecdotal reports, and the general view is that this drug has limited value in the treatment of this disease. In the only controlled study examining its use in MCD, Abramowicz et al[54] found that azathioprine was ineffective in 31 children with steroid-resistant nephrotic syndrome (only five of the patients had MCD). More promising results were reported by Cade et al[55] who treated 13 adults (eight with MCD) with prolonged courses (4 years) of azathiaprine and found that all the patients had a progressive reduction in proteinuria and ultimately achieved complete remission. The results of this study, and the reduced toxicity profile of azathiaprine compared with the alkylating agents, have led some investigators to argue for further evaluation of its efficacy in MCD.[19]

Mizoribine, like azathioprine, interferes with purine biosynthesis and thereby inhibits lymphocyte proliferation. This agent is not available in the USA but has been studied in Japan in children with frequently relapsing nephrotic syndrome.[56] In this multicenter, double-blind, placebo-controlled trial involving 197 children, there was no difference in the relapse rate between mizoribine-treated patients and controls; however, subset analysis showed a reduction in the relapse rate in the subset of mizoribine-treated patients who were 10 years of age or younger. The lack of a demonstrable benefit of the drug in the entire study population was attributed to a relatively low relapse rate in the older children. Renal biopsies were performed in 76% of patients and approximately 40% of patients in each treatment arm had MCD. However, information is not provided to enable correlation between histologic diagnosis and outcome. Comparisons of mizoribine with either cytotoxic agents or cyclosporine have not been reported.

Mycophenolate mofetil, an inhibitor of purine synthesis that is more effective than azathioprine in preventing acute rejection of renal allografts, was studied in a small series of patients with a variety of glomerular diseases.[57] Glucocorticoid discontinuation was possible following initiation of mycophenolate mofetil in the two patients with relapsing MCD. Other than this report, there are no data regarding the use of this drug in MCD.

Levamisole, an immunopotentiating drug, has been used as a steroid-sparing agent in children with frequently relapsing disease. The British Association for Paediatric Nephrology[58] performed a controlled study of 61 children treated with levamisole or placebo after a steroid-induced remission. Of 31 patients treated with levamisole, 14 were in remission at the end of a 3–4 month treatment period compared with 3 of 30 patients treated with a placebo. However, discontinuation of the drug was associated with a rapid relapse, and only four of the reponders were still in remission at the end of the study. The one other prospective controlled trial of levamisole found that treatment with this drug resulted in a statistically nonsignificant increase in the proportion of patients with a sustained glucocorticoid-induced remission.[59]

Specific recommendations

Although maintaining MCD patients free of urine protein could probably be accomplished in more than 90% of cases using prednisone, cyclophosphamide, or cyclosporine, such regimens are associated with significant toxicity. Thus the therapeutic challenge of this disease is to identify the treatment with the highest probability of producing a sustained remission with the lowest risk of toxicity. The literature reviewed earlier is helpful in this regard but is not conclusive. Individual patient variation remains a major factor in choosing among treatment options. Therefore, the recommendations that follow (summarized in Figs 22.1 and 22.2) should be viewed as flexible guidelines rather than definitive treatment protocols.

Regardless of the specific therapy used, symptomatic management of nephrotic patients should include dietary sodium and fluid restriction to prevent further edema formation. Diuretics may be necessary before specific therapy takes effect, and high doses are often required because of the marked sodium avidity that accompanies nephrotic syndrome. Angiotensin-converting enzyme

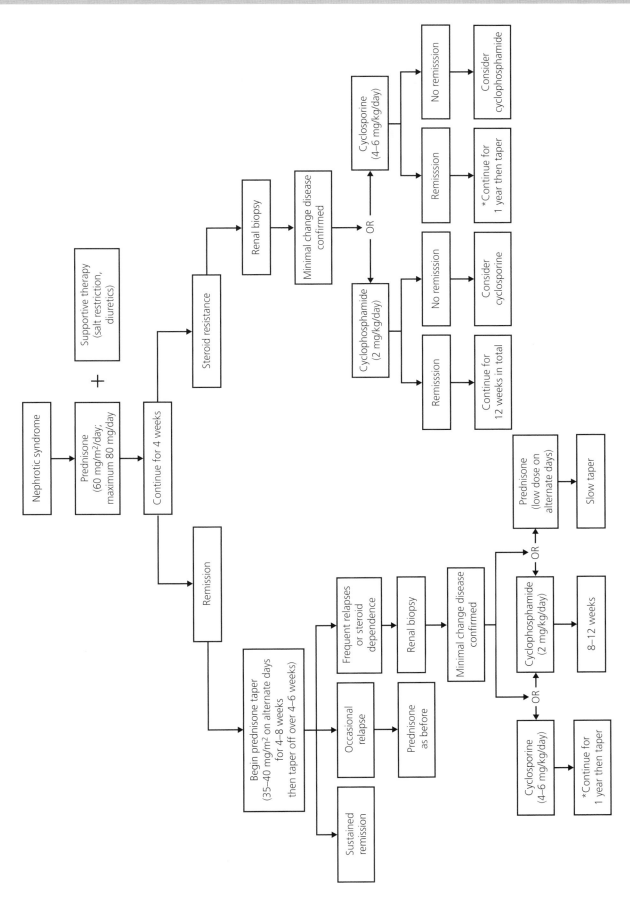

Figure 22.1 Treatment algorithm for children with minimal change disease. *Renal biopsy should be performed to evaluate for cyclosporine toxicity before continuing cyclosporine treatment beyond 1 year.

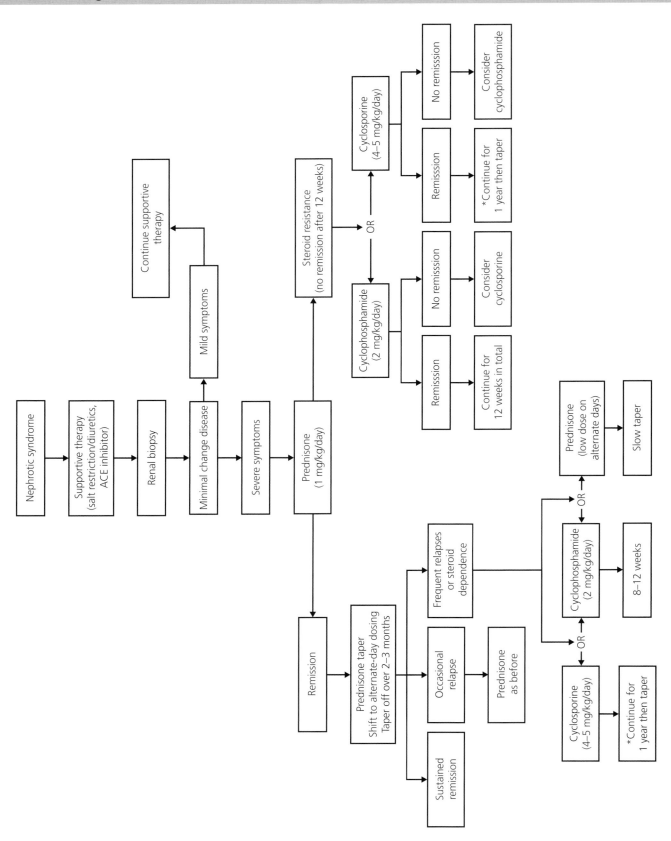

Figure 22.2 Treatment algorithm for adults with minimal change disease. ACE, angiotensin-converting enzyme. *Renal biopsy should be performed to evaluate for cyclosporine toxicity before continuing cyclosporine treatment beyond 1 year.

inhibitors may decrease proteinuria in nephrotic patients and thus may have a role during initial management or in steroid-resistant patients; however, one should be alert to the possibility of an acute reduction in GFR from alterations in intrarenal hemodynamics. To prevent glucocorticoid-induced osteoporosis, we recommend a daily intake (either through diet or supplements) of 1500 mg of calcium and 400–800 international units of vitamin D (with age-appropriate reductions in children) for all patients during glucocorticoid therapy. Additionally, for adult patients receiving long-term glucocorticoid treatment, it may be appropriate to obtain a baseline bone mineral density measurement and to consider further prophylactic treatment with bisphosphonates, hormone replacement therapy, or calcitonin.[60] Although the risk of accelerated atherogenesis in patients with MCD is debated, the use of lipid-lowering agents (preferably 3-hydroxy-3-methyl-glutaryl coenzyme A reductase inhibitors) should be considered in hyperlipidemic patients with sustained proteinuria. Nephrotic patients are also at risk for thromboembolic disease; however, routine anticoagulation is not recommended for patients with MCD.

Almost all children with idiopathic nephrotic syndrome should be treated empirically with glucocorticoids because of the high probability that they have MCD. A typical regimen for a first attack is prednisone 60 mg/m^2/day with a maximum of 80 mg/day, given as a single daily dose for 4 weeks. The dose is reduced to 35–40 mg/m^2 every other day for the subsequent 4 weeks and then tapered off over an additional 4 weeks. A more gradual tapering scheme, preferred by some, consists of alternate-day dosing at 60 mg/m^2 for 8 weeks after the initial 4 weeks of daily therapy, with tapering over an additional 4–6 weeks, such that the total duration of therapy is approximately 4–5 months. A reduction in proteinuria will occur in most children after 2 weeks of treatment. If proteinuria persists in a child after 4 weeks of treatment, a renal biopsy should be performed.

Since MCD accounts for only 10–15% of cases of nephrotic syndrome in adults, a renal biopsy should be performed prior to initiating therapy. If secondary causes of MCD have been eliminated, we recommend treatment with prednisone at 1 mg/kg as a single daily dose. As the response to glucocorticoids occurs less rapidly in adults than in children, the prednisone therapy should be continued for 12 weeks before the disease is considered to be steroid resistant. A progressive shift to alternate-day dosing beginning at 1 mg/kg should be started 1 week after proteinuria remits and tapered off over 2–3 months. Initial treatment with alternate-day prednisone at 2 mg/kg, with a maximum dose of 120 mg every other day, may also be effective and have fewer adverse effects, but there is less published experience with such a regimen.

Treatment of MCD relapses must take into account their frequency and the severity of glucocorticoid-related toxicities. A first relapse in either a child or adult can usually be treated with a second course of prednisone, with tapering beginning as soon as remission occurs. We recommend gradual, rather than rapid, tapering of the second course of prednisone therapy because available data

suggest that this results in a lower probability of a subsequent relapse. However, this approach may not necessarily result in a lower cumulative glucocorticoid dose.

If a relapse occurs during prednisone tapering, the prednisone dose should be increased immediately to the level at which remission occurred. In most cases, remission will result and a relatively rapid taper can begin. As the dose at which the relapse occurred is approached, the rate of tapering should be made more gradual in order to decrease the likelihood of a second relapse. We recommend that the patient or parent monitor the urine for protein by using a dipstick during the taper to facilitate early detection of relapse.

In some cases of frequently relapsing or steroid-dependent MCD, remission can be sustained with long-term, low-dose, alternate-day prednisone therapy. However, the doses required to maintain remission may be intolerably high, in which case alkylating agents should be considered. Indeed, elderly patients may tolerate cyclophosphamide better than glucocorticoids. Although cyclophosphamide and chlorambucil appear to be similarly effective, we prefer cyclophosphamide 2 mg/kg/day for 8–12 weeks in frequently relapsing disease and for 12 weeks in steroid-dependent disease. Prednisone is usually administered with the cyclophosphamide, although this may not necessarily improve efficacy. Patients are often already taking glucocorticoids when the decision is made to start therapy with an alkylating agent. A potential benefit of inducing a remission with glucocorticoids before starting cyclophosphamide therapy is that it may allow the high fluid intake required for protection against cystitis. The usual dose of chlorambucil is 0.1–0.2 mg/kg/day. The cumulative doses of cyclophosphamide and chlorambucil should be kept to less than 200 mg/kg and 10 mg/kg, respectively, in order to avoid gonadal toxicity. The leukocyte count should be monitored during treatment with alkylating agents, with dose adjustments as needed to maintain the count between 2000 and 5000 cells/mm^3.

Cyclosporine is a reasonable option for patients who have a relapse after one or two courses of cyclophosphamide therapy and may even be a good alternative to an alkylating agent in young adults. The dose of cyclosporine should be initiated at 4–5 mg/kg/day in adults and 4–6 mg/kg/day in children, and adjusted to maintain a whole-blood trough level by monoclonal antibody assay of 100–150 ng/mL. Treatment should be continued for 1 year and then tapered off. If a relapse occurs, cyclosporine should be restarted at the dose that maintained remission but in adults should not exceed 5.5 mg/kg/day. If a response to cyclosporine has not occurred within 3–4 months, the drug should be discontinued. It is important to note that the optimal dose for long-term cyclosporine therapy in children has not been established. In the studies describing outcomes with cyclosporine treatment for greater than 1 year, many of the children had mean trough levels that were less than 100 ng/mL. Steroid-dependent patients may require low doses of prednisone together with cyclosporine to stay in remission and are more likely than frequent relapsers to relapse after discontinuation of cyclosporine therapy. Serum creatinine and creatinine clearance should be monitored periodically during administration of cyclosporine; however, early cyclosporine nephrotoxicity may not be accompanied by changes in these measurements. Therefore, repeat renal biopsy to look for nephrotoxicity is advisable in patients requiring treatment with cyclosporine for more than 1 year.

Steroid-resistant MCD is rare. Children who have nephrotic syndrome that does not remit with prednisone should undergo renal biopsy because it is likely that they actually have FSGS. Adults who have presumed MCD based on a biopsy performed prior to treatment may actually have had FSGS that was not apparent on the initial biopsy. Steroid-resistant MCD can be treated with alkylating agents or with cyclosporine using the regimens described for frequently relapsing or steroid-dependent disease, although such patients are less likely to respond.

In conclusion, despite many years of accumulated experience with immunosuppressive agents, the treatment of polyrelapsing MCD remains a challenge. The approach we have outlined favors a shift from repeated courses of high-dose glucocorticoids or alkylating agents to a maintenance type of treatment with longer courses of low-dose, alternate-day glucocorticoids or cyclosporine. In the final analysis, however, treatment must be customized according to the clinical and demographic features of each patient.

References

1. Falk RJ, Jennette JC, Nachman PH: Primary glomerular diseases. *In* Brenner BM (ed): Brenner and Rector's The Kidney, Vol 2, 6th edn. Philadelphia: WB Saunders, 2000, pp 1263–1349.
2. Nolasco F, Cameron JS, Heywood EF, Hicks J, Ogg C, Williams DG: Adult-onset minimal change nephrotic syndrome: a long-term follow-up. Kidney Int 1986;29:1215–1223.
3. Korbet SM, Schwartz MM, Lewis EJ: Minimal change glomerulopathy of adulthood. Am J Nephrol 1988;8:291–297.
4. Fujimoto S, Yamamoto Y, Hisanaga S, Morita S, Eto T, Tanaka K: Minimal change nephrotic syndrome in adults: response to corticosteroid therapy and frequency of relapse. Am J Kidney Dis 1991;17:687–692.
5. Wang F, Looi LM, Chua CT: Minimal change glomerular disease in Malaysian adults and use of alternate day steroid therapy. Q J Med 1982;51:312.
6. Nadasdy T, Silva FG, Hogg RJ: Minimal change nephrotic syndrome–focal sclerosis complex (including IgM nephropathy and diffuse mesangial hypercellularity). *In* Tisher CC, Brenner BM (eds): Renal Pathology: With Clinical and Functional Correlations, Vol 1, 2nd edn. Philadelphia: JB Lippincott, 1994, pp 330–389.
7. Tarshish P, Tobin JN, Bernstein J, Edelmann CM Jr: Prognostic significance of the early course of minimal change nephrotic syndrome: report of the International Study of Kidney Disease in Children. J Am Soc Nephrol 1997;8:769–776.
8. Fogo A, Hawkins EP, Berry PL, et al: Glomerular hypertrophy in minimal change disease predicts subsequent progression to focal glomerular sclerosis. Kidney Int 1990;38:115–123.
9. Guasch A, Myers BD: Determinants of glomerular hypofiltration in nephrotic patients with minimal change nephropathy. J Am Soc Nephrol 1994;4:1571–1581.
10. Guasch A, Deen WM, Myers BD: Charge selectivity of the glomerular filtration barrier in healthy and nephrotic humans. J Clin Invest 1993;92:2274–2282.
11. Bertolatus JA, Hunsicker LG: Glomerular sieving of anionic and neutral bovine albumins in proteinuric rats. Kidney Int 1985;28:467–476.
12. Koyama A, Fujisaki M, Kobayashi M, Igarashi M, Narita M: A glomerular permeability factor produced by human T cell hybridomas. Kidney Int 1991;40:453–460.
13. Maruyama K, Tomizawa S, Seki Y, Arai H, Kuroume T: Inhibition of vascular permeability factor production by ciclosporin in minimal change nephrotic syndrome. Nephron 1992;62:27–30.
14. Cameron JS: The long-term outcome of glomerular diseases. *In* Schrier RN, Gottschalk CW (eds): Diseases of the Kidney, Vol 2, 5th edn. Boston: Little, Brown, 1992, pp 1919–1981.
15. Idelson BA, Smithline N, Smith GW, Harrington JT: Prognosis in steroid-treated idiopathic nephrotic syndrome in adults. Analysis of major predictive factors after ten-year follow-up. Arch Intern Med 1977;137:891–896.
16. Glassock RJ: Therapy of idiopathic nephrotic syndrome in adults. A conservative or aggressive therapeutic approach? Am J Nephrol 1993;13:422–428.
17. Brodehl J: Conventional therapy for idiopathic nephrotic syndrome in children. Clin Nephrol 1991;35:S8–S15.
18. Report of the International Study of Kidney Disease in Children: The primary nephrotic syndrome in children. Identification of patients with minimal change nephrotic syndrome from initial response to prednisone. J Pediatr 1981;98:561–564.
19. Meyrier A, Simon P: Treatment of corticoresistant idiopathic nephrotic syndrome in the adult: minimal change disease and focal segmental glomerulosclerosis. Adv Nephrol Necker Hosp 1988;17:127–150.
20. Wingen AM, Muller-Wiefel DE, Scharer K: Spontaneous remissions in frequently relapsing and steroid dependent idiopathic nephrotic syndrome. Clin Nephrol 1985;23:35–40.
21. Schena FP, Cameron JS: Treatment of proteinuric idiopathic glomerulonephritides in adults: a retrospective survey. Am J Med 1988;85:315–326.
22. Black DAK, Rose G, Brewer DB: Controlled trial of prednisone in adult patients with the nephrotic syndrome. Br Med J 1970;3:421–426.
23. Coggins CH: Minimal change nephrosis in adults. *In* Zurukzoglu W (ed): Proceedings of the 8th International Congress of Nephrology. Basel: Karger, 1981, pp 336–344.
24. Report of Arbeitsgemeinschaft für Pädiatrische Nephrologie: Alternate-day prednisone is more effective than intermittent prednisone in frequently relapsing nephrotic syndrome. Eur J Pediatr 1981;135:229–237.
25. Imbasciati E, Gusmano R, Edefonti A, et al: Controlled trial of methylprednisolone pulses and low dose oral prednisone for the minimal change nephrotic syndrome. Br Med J 1985;291:1305–1308.
26. Arbeitsgemeinschaft für Pädiatrische Nephrologie: Short versus standard prednisone therapy for initial treatment of idiopathic nephrotic syndrome in children. Lancet 1988;i:380–383.
27. Ueda N, Chihara M, Kawaguchi S, et al: Intermittent versus long-term tapering prednisolone for initial therapy in children with idiopathic nephrotic syndrome. J Pediatr 1988;112:122–126.
28. Bagga A, Hari P, Srivastava RN: Prolonged versus standard prednisolone therapy for initial episode of nephrotic syndrome. Pediatr Nephrol 1999;13:824–827.
29. Report of the International Study of Kidney Disease in Children: Nephrotic syndrome in children: a randomized trial comparing two prednisone regimens in steroid-responsive patients who relapse early. J Pediatr 1979;95:239–243.
30. Nair RB, Date A, Kirubakaran MG, Shastry JC: Minimal change nephrotic syndrome in adults treated with alternate-day steroids. Nephron 1987;47:209–210.
31. Cameron JS, Chantler C, Ogg CS, White RH: Long-term stability of remission in nephrotic syndrome after treatment with cyclophosphamide. Br Med J 1974;4:7–11.
32. Report of the International Study of Kidney Disease in Children: Prospective, controlled trial of cylcophosphamide therapy in children with the nephrotic syndrome after treatment with cyclophosphamide. Lancet 1974;ii:423–427.
33. Grupe WE, Makker SP, Ingelfinger JR: Chlorambucil treatment of frequently relapsing nephrotic syndrome. N Engl J Med 1976;295:746–749.
34. Al-Khader AA, Lien JW, Aber GM: Cyclophosphamide alone in the treatment of adult patients with minimal change glomerulonephritis. Clin Nephrol 1979;11:26–30.
35. Williams SA, Makker SP, Ingelfinger JR, Grupe WE: Long-term evaluation of chlorambucil plus prednisone in the idiopathic nephrotic syndrome of childhood. N Engl J Med 1980;302:929–933.

36. Arbeitsgemeinschaft fur Pädiatrische Nephrologie: Effect of cytotoxic drugs in frequently relapsing nephrotic syndrome with and without steroid dependence. N Engl J Med 1982;306:451–454.
37. Report of Arbeitsgemeinschaft fur Pädiatrische Nephrologie: Cyclophosphamide treatment of steroid dependent nephrotic syndrome: comparison of eight week with 12 week course. Arch Dis Child 1987;62:1102–1106.
38. Ueda N, Kuno K, Ito S: Eight and 12 week courses of cyclophosphamide in nephrotic syndrome. Arch Dis Child 1990;65:1147–1150.
39. Barratt TM, Soothill JF: Controlled trial of cyclophosphamide in steroid-sensitive relapsing nephrotic syndrome of childhood. Lancet 1970;ii:479–482.
40. Chiu J, McLaine PN, Drummond KN: A controlled prospective study of cyclophosphamide in relapsing, corticosteroid-responsive, minimal-lesion nephrotic syndrome in childhood. J Pediatr 1973;82:607–613.
41. Bergstrand A, Bollgren I, Samuelsson A, Tornroth T, Wasserman J, Winberg J: Idiopathic nephrotic syndrome of childhood: cyclophosphamide induced conversion from steroid refractory to highly steroid sensitive disease. Clin Nephrol 1973;1:302–306.
42. Ponticelli C, Passerini P: Treatment of the nephrotic syndrome associated with primary glomerulonephritis. Kidney Int 1994;46:595–604.
43. Ponticelli C, Rizzoni G, Edefonti A, et al: A randomized trial of cyclosporine in steroid-resistant idiopathic nephrotic syndrome. Kidney Int 1993;43:1377–1384.
44. Ponticelli C, Edefonti A, Ghio L, et al: Cyclosporin versus cyclophosphamide for patients with steroid-dependent and frequently relapsing idiopathic nephrotic syndrome: a multicentre randomized controlled trial. Nephrol Dial Transplant 1993;8:1326–1332.
45. Hulton SA, Neuhaus TJ, Dillon MJ, Barratt TM: Long-term cyclosporin A treatment of minimal change nephrotic syndrome of childhood. Pediatr Nephrol 1994;8:401–403.
46. Meyrier A, Noel LH, Auriche P, Callard P: Long-term renal tolerance of cyclosporin A treatment in adult idiopathic nephrotic syndrome. Collaborative Group of the Societe de Nephrologie. Kidney Int 1994;45:1446–1456.
47. Ittel TH, Clasen W, Fuhs M, Kindler J, Mihatsch MJ, Sieberth HG: Long-term ciclosporine A treatment in adults with minimal change nephrotic syndrome or focal segmental glomerulosclerosis. Clin Nephrol 1995;44:156–162.
48. Collaborative Study Group of Sandimmun® in Nephrotic Syndrome: Safety and tolerability of cyclosporin A (Sandimmun®) in idiopathic nephrotic syndrome. Clin Nephrol 1991;35:S48–S60.
49. Habib R, Niaudet P: Comparison between pre- and posttreatment renal biopsies in children receiving ciclosporine for idiopathic nephrosis. Clin Nephrol 1994;42:141–146.
50. Inoue Y, Iijima K, Nakamura H, Yoshikawa N: Two-year cyclosporin treatment in children with steroid-dependent nephrotic syndrome. Pediatr Nephrol 1999;13:33–38.
51. Gregory MJ, Smoyer WE, Sedman A, et al: Long-term cyclosporine therapy for pediatric nephrotic syndrome: a clinical and histologic analysis. J Am Soc Nephrol 1996;7:543–549.
52. Hino S, Takemura T, Okada M, et al: Follow-up study of children with nephrotic syndrome treated with a long-term moderate dose of cyclosporine. Am J Kidney Dis 1998;31:932–939.
53. Kano K, Kyo K, Yamada Y, Ito S, Ando T, Arisaka O: Comparison between pre- and posttreatment clinical and renal biopsies in children receiving low dose cyclosporine-A for steroid-dependent nephrotic syndrome. Clin Nephrol 1999;52:19–24.
54. Abramowicz M, Barnett HL, Edelmann CM Jr, et al: Controlled trial of azathioprine in children with nephrotic syndrome. A report for the International Study of Kidney Disease in children. Lancet 1970;i:959–961.
55. Cade R, Mars D, Privette M, et al: Effect of long-term azathioprine administration in adults with minimal change glomerulonephritis and nephrotic syndrome resistant to corticosteroids. Arch Intern Med 1986;146:737–741.
56. Yoshioka K, Ohashi Y, Sakai T, et al: A multicenter trial of mizoribine compared with placebo in children with frequently relapsing nephrotic syndrome. Kidney Int 2000;58:317–324.
57. Briggs WA, Choi MJ, Scheel PJ: Successful mycophenolate mofetil treatment of glomerular disease. Am J Kidney Dis 1998;31:213–217.
58. British Association for Paediatric Nephrology: Levamisole for corticosteroid-dependent nephrotic syndrome in childhood. Lancet 1991;337:1555–1557.
59. Dayal U, Dayal AK, Shastry JC, Raghupathy P: Use of levamisole in maintaining remission in steroid-sensitive nephrotic syndrome in children. Nephron 1994;66:408–412.
60. American College of Rheumatology Task Force on Osteoporosis Guidelines: Recommendations for the prevention and treatment of glucocorticoid-induced osteoporosis. Arthritis Rheum 1996;39:1791–1801.

Primary Focal Segmental Glomerulosclerosis

Stephen M. Korbet

Primary focal segmental glomerulosclerosis (FSGS) is a clinicopathologic entity defined by the presence of proteinuria and by segmental glomerular scars involving some but not all glomeruli. In contrast to minimal change disease, nephrotic patients with FSGS often present with hematuria, hypertension, and renal insufficiency, are significantly less responsive to steroid therapy, and have a progressive course to endstage renal disease (ESRD).[1-3]

Primary FSGS accounts for 7–35% of glomerular lesions in children and adults presenting with the nephrotic syndrome.[4-12] Over the last 20 years there has been a twofold to threefold increase in the incidence of this lesion in both adults and children.[9,11-15] The reason for this observation is unknown but some have attributed it in part to an increase in the identification of histologic variants of FSGS.[9,13,16-18] Additionally, it is now recognized that the prevalence of primary FSGS in nephrotic black patients is two to four times that in white patients (50–60% vs. 20–25%).[8,10,11,19-21] The progressive nature of this lesion and the high recurrence rate in transplanted kidneys[22] has made the treatment of primary FSGS a serious concern to nephrologists.

Pathogenesis

The pathogenesis of primary FSGS, although not well understood, appears to be the result of a circulating factor(s), possibly a lymphokine or cytokine.[23,24] This leads to glomerular epithelial cell injury that results in segmental scar formation and ultimately glomerular obsolescence, resulting in alterations in intraglomerular hemodynamics that along with local mediators of renal injury (i.e. angiotensin II, transforming growth factor β, plasminogen activator inhibitor 1) leads to progressive renal disease.[25,26] The best evidence supporting the presence of a circulating factor stems from the frequent recurrence of primary FSGS in allografts and subsequent resolution of disease with plasmapheresis.[24,27,28]

It is well recognized that a morphologically similar lesion to FSGS may result in a number of settings, with a clinical presentation indistinguishable from primary FSGS.[17,29,30] Since the pathogenesis and treatment of these disorders may differ significantly, familial forms of FSGS and secondary conditions associated with FSGS (e.g. morbid obesity, HIV infection, states leading to reduced nephron mass such as reflux and sickle-cell nephropathies) must be excluded before making the diagnosis of primary FSGS.

Pathology

The glomerular lesion of "classic FSGS" is characterized by a focal segmental scar. The involved glomerular capillaries are obliterated by a collagenized scar and collapsed wrinkled basement membranes; the endothelium is lost or replaced by foam cells (macrophages); the overlying epithelial cells may be prominent but they do not appear increased in number; and there may be a dense fibrous scar formed between the involved segment and Bowman's capsule. In many cases the scar contains areas of hyalinosis. The uninvolved portions of the glomeruli with segmental scars and the remaining glomeruli in the biopsy are essentially normal. Although FSGS is not an immunoglobulin-mediated disease, deposits of IgM and the C3 component of complement are frequently seen within the segmental scars and concentrated in the hyalinosis lesions. Ultrastructurally, there is foot process effacement, seen in both involved and uninvolved glomeruli. The degree of foot process effacement is variable.[31]

A number of histologic features may be seen in association with the diagnosis of FSGS, including mesangial hypercellularity, foam cells, mesangial deposits of IgM, the location of the segmental scar in the glomerulus, hyalinosis, and pathologic changes in the podocytes. Several of these are referred to as "variants" of primary FSGS.[16-18] The cellular or collapsing lesion (variant) of FSGS has gained much interest recently.[16,17,32-37] This lesion is defined by segmental or global collapse of glomerular capillaries, which often contain foam cells that are associated with hypertrophy and hyperplasia of the surrounding visceral glomerular epithelial cells. When the cellular lesion is isolated to the take-off of the proximal tubule it has been called the "tip lesion."

Clinical presentation

The presenting feature in all patients with primary FSGS is proteinuria, frequently resulting in the nephrotic syndrome, although a nonnephrotic presentation (proteinuria < 3.0 g per 24 h without hypoalbuminemia) is not

Table 23.1 Presenting features*

	Children	Adults
Number	506	786
Nephrotic	88%	76%
Male	54%	62%
Hypertensive	26%	43%
Hematuria	50%	40%
Renal insufficiency	19%	34%

*Data derived from references 1, 4, 6, 7, 37–39, 43, 46, 51, 55, 59, 65, 66, 69, 70, 72, 90, 113–123.

unusual, particularly in adults (Table 23.1). In addition, microscopic hematuria, hypertension, and renal insufficiency are common presenting features. Although Newman et al[38] found that adults were more likely to have hypertension and renal insufficiency at presentation than children, Pei et al[39] found that the occurrence of hematuria, hypertension, and level of renal function did not significantly differ between these two groups. However, both studies found that adults presented with the nephrotic syndrome less frequently than children (41–55% vs. 75–76% respectively).[38,39]

However, the presentation for patients with primary FSGS may differ among the histologic variants. In contrast with classic FSGS, the cellular lesion has a black racial predominance and these patients are more likely to be nephrotic at presentation.[33–35,37] Massive proteinuria (> 10 g/day) at presentation is much more common among patients with the cellular lesion (44–67% of patients) compared with patients with classic FSGS (4–11% of patients). Furthermore, while the time from presentation to biopsy is significantly shorter, patients with the cellular lesion present with more advanced renal insufficiency. In one series, over 60% of patients with the cellular lesion presented with a serum creatinine ≥ 2.0 mg/dL compared with less than 10% of patients with classic FSGS.[33]

Clinical course

The degree of proteinuria at presentation has consistently been of prognostic significance.[7,40–44] The presence of nephrotic-range proteinuria (> 3–3.5 g per 24 h) predicts outcome in primary FSGS, with 50% of patients reaching ESRD over 5–10 years.[7,41–44] Patients with massive proteinuria (> 10 g per 24 h) have an even more malignant course, with essentially all patients progressing to ESRD within 5 years.[41,45] This is in contrast to the more favorable prognosis in patients with nonnephrotic proteinuria, in which renal survival of over 80% is observed after 10 years.[7,41–44] An additional clinical feature of prognostic significance is the presenting serum creatinine. The serum creatinine exhibits an inverse relationship with progression to ESRD: patients with a serum creatinine > 1.3 mg/dL

have a significantly poorer renal survival than those with a serum creatinine ≤ 1.3 mg/dL.[10,40,42,44,46]

It has been suggested that racial differences in the course of primary FSGS may exist. In nephrotic children with FSGS, Ingulli and Tejani[10] found that 78% of black patients progressed to ESRD over an 8.5-year follow-up compared with only 33% of white patients. This experience has been confirmed by some[47,48] but not all studies in children with FSGS.[49,50] In our own experience with adults, black patients tend to present less often with nonnephrotic-range proteinuria than white patients (14% vs. 52%) and in this respect may have a poorer prognosis.[42,44] However, when evaluating nephrotic patients, we found no significant racial difference in the rate of decline of renal function or the number of patients reaching ESRD.[42,44]

Given the above, it is interesting to note that multivariate analyses of baseline clinical features have often demonstrated that only the level of serum creatinine, rather than proteinuria, is predictive of progression to ESRD.[37,40,41,44] This may be explained by the unusually high rate of remission, and the associated improvement in long-term renal survival, in the nephrotic patients reported in these studies.[37,39,44] When patients entering a remission are eliminated from analysis, both proteinuria and serum creatinine become predictive.[44]

When the prognostic importance of various pathologic features have been studied, neither the proportion of glomeruli with segmental scars nor the proportion of glomeruli with global sclerosis are predictive of outcome. The histologic feature that has been predictive of a poor prognosis most consistently is the presence of advanced (> 20%) interstitial fibrosis.[16,37,44,51] Recent studies have now shown that the presence of the cellular lesion also portends a significantly poorer prognosis than that of classic FSGS.[9,33,34,37,52–54] Initial studies suggested that patients with the "tip lesion" had a better response to therapy and a more benign clinical course than patients with classic FSGS lesions.[55,56] However, a number of investigators were unable to reproduce these observations, concluding that the response to treatment and renal survival (30–50% at 10 years) was not significantly different from that in FSGS patients without the tip lesion.[16,17,57]

Remission

Of all the clinical and histologic characteristics evaluated in primary FSGS, only remission of proteinuria predicts a favorable outcome in nephrotic patients with primary FSGS.[37,39,44,51,58] In nephrotic adults and children alike, less than 15% of patients entering a complete remission (defined as proteinuria < 0.3 g per 24 h) progress to ESRD, whereas up to 50% of persistently nephrotic patients progress to ESRD over 5 years (Table 23.2). Even a partial remission (variably defined as a proteinuria of less than 2–3 g per 24 h but more than 0.3–0.5 g per 24 h, or as a 50% or greater decrease in proteinuria) is associated with a less rapid decline in renal function compared with patients in whom the nephrotic syndrome persists.[40,59,60] Unfortunately, spontaneous remissions are rare, occurring

Table 23.2 Prognosis according to response to treatment*

	Follow-up (years)	Patients progressing to ESRD		
		Complete remission	Partial remission	No response
Adults	5.5	2/119 (1.7%)	9/67 (13%)	94/175 (54%)
Children	7.0	10/70 (14%)	0/12 (0%)	60/161 (37%)
Total		12/189 (6%)	9/79 (11%)	154/336 (46%)

ESRD, endstage renal disease.
*Data derived from references 4, 7, 37–39, 43, 46, 55, 58, 59, 65, 66, 69, 70, 90, 113, 115, 117, 118, 122, 123.

in less than 5% of nephrotic patients with primary FSGS.[37,58] However, patients receiving a course of treatment with steroids are four to ten times more likely to enter a remission than untreated patients.[37,51] Since no clinical or histologic feature at presentation allows one to predict which patients will enter a remission, the response to a course of "treatment" becomes the best clinical indicator of outcome.[37,39,61]

Initial therapy and response

The initial treatment for primary FSGS in children has followed the regimen outlined for the treatment of primary nephrotic syndrome by the International Study of Kidney Disease in Children (ISKDC). This consists of prednisone 60 mg/m^2/day (up to 80 mg/day) given in

divided doses for 4 weeks, followed by 40 mg/m^2/day (up to 60 mg/day) given in divided doses, three consecutive days out of seven, for 4 weeks and then discontinued.[5,55] Although this protocol has been found to be satisfactory for the treatment of children with the highly steroid-sensitive lesion of minimal-change glomerulopathy, the data suggest that it may be inadequate for those with primary FSGS. The complete remission rate for children with primary FSGS using this treatment protocol has been as high as 51%, although in over 80% of studies it has not exceeded 30% (Table 23.3).

Evidence supporting the concept that children with FSGS may be undertreated has been provided by Pei and colleagues,[39,58] who reported a complete remission in 44% of children with primary FSGS using a more prolonged initial course of prednisone therapy. The median cumulative dose of prednisone per treatment course (median

Table 23.3 Response to treatment in children

Reference	Year	No.	Complete remission	Partial remission	No response	Follow-up (years)
White et al[1]	1970	12	2 (17%)	0	10 (83%)	7
Habib & Kleinknecht[4]	1971	46	9 (20%)	6 (13%)	31 (67%)	5
Hyman & Burkholder[115]	1974	13	0	0	13 (100%)	5.1
Nash et al[121]	1976	20	2 (10%)	0	18 (90%)	3.3
Newman et al[38]	1976	16	3 (19%)	6 (38%)	7 (43%)	7
Mongeau et al[72]	1981	23	6 (26%)	1 (4%)	16 (70%)	8
ISKDC[5]	1981	37	11 (30%)	0	26 (70%)	0.2
Arbus et al[70]	1982	51	26 (51%)	0	25 (49%)	10.6
SWPNG[6]	1985	38	9 (24%)	0	29 (76%)	4.8
Yoshikawa et al[55]	1986	45	8 (18%)	0	37 (82%)	5.5
Pei et al[39]	1987	34	15 (44%)	0	19 (56%)	4.5
Morita et al[120]	1990	43	5 (12%)	0	38 (88%)	9.3
Cattran & Rao[58]	1998	32	15 (47%)	0	17 (53%)	12.5
Frishberg et al[114]	1998	47	14 (30%)	0	33 (70%)	6

ISKDC, International Study of Kidney Disease in Children; SWPNG, Southwest Pediatric Nephrology Group.

6 months) was 120 mg/kg (0.3–2.0 mg/kg). The median time to remission was 3 months, with patients entering a remission doing so within 6 months of initiating therapy. In half the patients, cytotoxic drugs (cyclophosphamide or azathioprine) were used in addition to prednisone, with a median dose per treatment course of 90 mg/kg for a median duration of 2 months. The renal survival for those patients with a complete remission was 100% at 15 years compared with 73%, 58%, and 51% at 5, 10, and 15 years in patients who failed to respond.[39,58,62] Half of the unresponsive patients had doubled their serum creatinine by 4 years. Based on these findings, these authors recommended that nephrotic patients with primary FSGS be treated with a course of steroids for up to 6 months. While it appears that improved response rates are attainable with a more prolonged initial course of steroids in children with primary FSGS, the optimal dose and duration of therapy needs to be defined.

The early experience with the response to steroid therapy in nephrotic adults with primary FSGS was quite disappointing. Complete remission rates of less than 20% were observed in virtually every study published prior to 1980 (Tables 23.4 and 23.5). In 50% of these reports no patient attained a complete remission. Based on this experience, it is not surprising that nephrologists became less than enthusiastic or even reluctant to subject their adult patients with primary FSGS to a course of steroids or immunosuppressive therapy.[63] This is evident in the study of Pei et al,[39] who found that only 42% of nephrotic adults with primary FSGS received treatment compared with 95% of children.

Since 1980, however, a different experience in the response to treatment of adult FSGS has evolved (Tables 23.4 and 23.5). In over 80% of studies, complete remission rates in excess of 30% have been reported, with the majority being 40% or more. Insight into the marked dichotomy in remission rates may be gained by evaluating and comparing the treatment protocols used in those studies attaining complete remission rates of less than 30% with those attaining complete remission rates of 30% or more (Table 23.6). In making this comparison, the most obvious difference was the duration of therapy, since the initial dose of prednisone utilized has been similar (0.5–2 mg/kg/day). The total duration of therapy in those

Table 23.4 Response to treatment in adults

Reference	Year	No.	Complete remission	Partial remission	No response	Follow-up (years)
Lim et al[118]	1974	10	0	1 (10%)	9 (90%)	3.9
Jenis et al[117]	1974	6	0	2 (33%)	4(67%)	2.8
Velsoa et al[123]	1975	34	4 (12%)	10 (29%)	20 (59%)	6.5
Saint-Hillier et al[69]	1975	23	16 (70%)	0	7 (30%)	5.5
Newman et al[38]	1976	8	0	4 (50%)	4 (50%)	3.8
Boltonet al[65]	1977	10	0	4 (40%)	6 (60%)	3.4
Cameron et al[43]	1978	20	2 (10%)	0	18 (90%)	9.5
Beaufils et al7	1978	26	5 (19%)	8 (31%)	13 (50%)	5.5
Korbet et al[42]	1986	16	5 (31%)	3 (19%)	8 (50%)	5
Miyata et al[119]	1986	32	14 (44%)	4 (12%)	14 (44%)	6
Pei et al[39]	1987	18	7 (39%)	0	11 (61%)	5
Chan et al[46]	1991	13	3 (23%)	4 (31%)	6 (46%)	6.8
Banfi et al[59]	1991	59	36 (61%)	0	23 (39%)	6.3
Agarwal et al[113]	1993	38	12 (32%)	10 (26%)	16 (42%)	2.8
Nagai et al[66]	1994	9	4 (44%)	1 (11%)	4 (44%)	2.5
Rydel et al[44]	1995	30	10 (33%)	5 (17%)	15 (50%)	5.2
Shiiki et al[122]	1996	35	12 (34%)	11 (31%)	12 (34%)	5
Cattran & Rao[58]	1998	17	8 (47%)	0	9 (53%)	11.25
Ponticelli et al[51]	1999	80	29 (36%)	13 (16%)	38 (48%)	7
Schwartz et al[37]	1999	42	14 (33%)	8 (19%)	20 (48%)	6.25
Alexopoulos et al[90]	2000	11	3 (28%)	4 (36%)	4 (36%)	4.75

Table 23.5 Initial treatment in adults*

Treatment	No.	Complete remission	Partial remission	No response
Steroids	405	141 (35%)	79 (20%)	185 (46%)
Before 1980	103	19 (18%)	23 (22%)	61 (59%)
After 1980	302	122 (40%)	56 (19%)	124 (41%)
Cytotoxics + steroids	115	35 (30%)	13 (11%)	67 (58%)
Before 1980	34	8 (23%)	6 (18%)	20 (59%)
After 1980	81	27 (33%)	7 (9%)	47 (58%)

*Data derived from references 7, 37–39, 42–44, 46, 51, 59, 65, 66, 69, 90, 113, 117–119, 122, 123.

Table 23.6 Initial steroid treatment in adults with focal segmental glomerulosclerosis

Reference	Dose (mg/kg/day)	High-dose duration (months)	Total duration (months)
≥ 30% Complete remissions			
Saint-Hillier et al[69]	0.5–1.5	3	6–12
Korbet et al[37,42,44]	0.5–1.0	2–3	6–8
Pei et al[39,58]	0.3–2.0		8
Banfi et al[51,59]	0.5–1.0	2	6–9
Agarwal et al[113]	1.0	2–3	6
Shiiki et al[122]	0.5–1.0	1–2	36
Alexopoulos et al[90]	1.0	> 1	24
< 30% Complete remissions			
Lim et al[118]	0.5–1.5		2
Velosa et al[123]	0.5–1.0	1	2
Beaufils et al[7]	1.0–1.5	1	3

studies with a poor response rate was 2 months or less compared with an average of 5–9 months in studies achieving high remission rates (Table 23.6). Ponticelli et al[51] reported a complete remission in only 15% of patients treated with steroids for less than 4 months, while 61% of patients treated for 4 months or more entered a complete remission. The initial period of daily high-dose steroids may also be an important factor. In most studies achieving 30% or more complete remission rates, a period of "high-dose" steroids was maintained for 2–3 months before tapering. Rydel et al[44] found that those patients achieving a remission had received an initial period of high-dose prednisone (≥ 60 mg/day) for a significantly longer duration than nonresponders (median 3 vs. 1 month respectively), even though both groups had a similar total duration of treatment (median 4 vs. 5 months respectively).

Less than one-third of adults who ultimately achieve a complete remission do so by 8 weeks of therapy. The median time to complete remission is 3–4 months, with the majority of patients reaching a complete remission by 5–9 months from the beginning of treatment.[39,42,44,58,59] Based on this experience, it has now been proposed that steroid resistance in adults be defined as the persistence of the nephrotic syndrome after a 4-month trial of therapy with prednisone at a dose of 1 mg/kg/day.[64]

While the presence of the cellular lesion has generally been associated with poor therapeutic response, with remissions in less than 20% of treated patients,[33,34,52,53] we have observed no difference in the remission rate for patients with cellular FSGS compared with patients with classic FSGS. We found that remission was achieved in 52% of patients with cellular FSGS (complete, 32%; partial, 20%) and 53% of patients with classic FSGS (complete, 35%; partial, 18%).[37] However, the remission rate was lower (only 23%) in those patients whose biopsies demonstrated more than 20% involvement of glomeruli with cellular lesions.[37] The reason for the different response rates among studies is not clear but may relate to differences in therapeutic approach or the presence of more advanced renal disease at biopsy (serum creatinine at biopsy > 3.5 mg/dL) in those studies experiencing a poor response.[33–35,54]

The use of alternate-day steroid therapy has been considered to minimize the potential for complications associated with daily steroid use, particularly in older adults. To date, however, the response to alternate-day steroids has been disappointing in young adults.[65] Of 10 patients (average age 29 years) treated by Bolton et al[65] with 60–120 mg of prednisone every other day for 9–12 months, none sustained a complete remission. However,

Nagai et al[66] attained a complete remission in 44% (5/9) of their elderly (> 60 years of age) nephrotic patients with primary FSGS using 1.0–1.6 mg/kg (up to 100 mg) every other day for 3–5 months. Over 37 months of follow-up, no relapses occurred and no patient with a complete remission progressed to ESRD compared with 47% of untreated or nonresponsive patients. Furthermore, the therapy was well tolerated without obvious complication. The excellent response rate with alternate-day steroid therapy in the elderly (comparable to that in younger adults on daily steroid therapy) may be due to the significant decrease in clearance of steroids observed in the elderly, leading to a higher relative serum concentration of steroid and/or a more sustained steroid effect.[67,68]

Approximately 20% of adults have received cytotoxic agents along with steroids as initial therapy (Table 23.5), although this appears to confer no added benefit in attaining a complete remission compared with steroids alone.[51,59] However, their use may induce a more stable remission than steroids alone.[51,59,69] Banfi and colleagues[51,59] found a lower relapse rate (18%) in patients initially receiving cytotoxic agents (cyclophosphamide 2 mg/kg/day, chlorambucil 0.1–0.2 mg/kg/day, or azathioprine 2 mg/kg/day for a median of 5–19 months) in addition to steroids compared with patients treated with steroid alone (55% relapsed). Ultimately, the proportion of patients in complete remission (47% vs. 59% respectively) was not significantly different between the two groups.

Treatment of relapsing patients

The improved outcome incurred by a remission in primary FSGS is dependent on that remission being sustained, since recurrence of the nephrotic syndrome portends a prognosis similar to primary nonresponders.[41,70] The duration of the initial remission is longer and overall relapse rate less in adults compared with children (25% vs. 80%).[39,58] Fortunately, for those patients who relapse, the majority (> 75%) are able to achieve another remission with retreatment.[39,58,59] Patients who remain in remission for 10 years or more have an excellent prognosis and are unlikely to subsequently relapse.[71]

The therapeutic approach to the patient who relapses depends on the frequency with which relapses occur. In the patient who relapses after a prolonged period off steroids (6 months or more), a second course of steroid therapy could be sufficient. For patients who are frequent relapsers (two or more relapses within 6 months, or three or four or more within 12 months) or dependent on steroids (two relapses occurring with steroid taper or a relapse within 1 month of ending treatment), or those patients in whom a more steroid conservative approach may be desired, the use of cytotoxic agents or cyclosporine has been beneficial.

A course of cytotoxic therapy (cyclophosphamide 2 mg/kg/day or chlorambucil 0.1–0.2 mg/kg/day for 2–3 months), often in combination with prednisone, leads to the reestablishment of a remission in over 70% of children and adults (Table 23.7). Response to these agents is associated with a reduction in the rate of relapse resulting in more prolonged remissions, eliminating the need for additional courses of steroids.[51,59,71,72]

Cyclosporine (5–6 mg/kg/day) is also highly successful in reestablishing a remission in steroid-responsive patients with primary FSGS who have gone on to relapse (Table 23.8). Response is seen within the first month of treatment in the majority of patients. However, the remission is generally maintained only with continuous cyclosporine therapy because most patients (≥ 75%) relapse, often within 2 months of taper or discontinuation of the drug.[73–77] In these patients cyclosporine dependency becomes the trade-off for the treatment of steroid-dependent patients with FSGS.

In a prospective randomized trial, Ponticelli et al[78] compared a 2-month course of cyclophosphamide (2.5 mg/kg/day) with 9 months of cyclosporine (5–6 mg/kg/day) in a group of frequently relapsing or steroid-dependent patients with idiopathic nephrotic syndrome after reestablishing a complete remission on prednisone. The prednisone was tapered after 5 weeks of randomization. After 9 months of follow-up from randomization, 25% of cyclosporine-treated patients and 33% of cyclophosphamide-treated patients had relapsed. By 24 months of follow-up, 75% of cyclosporine-treated patients had relapsed compared with only 37% of patients who

Table 23.7 Response to cytotoxic therapy*

Initial response to steroids	No.	Complete remission	Partial remission	No response
Steroid-responsive				
Children	25	13 (52%)	5 (20%)	7 (28%)
Adults	18	9 (50%)	5 (28%)	4 (22%)
Total	43	22 (51%)	10 (23%)	11 (26%)
Steroid-resistant				
Children	140	28 (20%)	22 (16%)	90 (64%)
Adults	45	3 (7%)	5 (11%)	37 (82%)
Total	185	31 (17%)	27 (15%)	127 (69%)

*Data derived from references 4, 43, 51, 55, 59, 69, 70, 72, 80, 81, 92, 118.

Table 23.8 Response to cyclosporine therapy*

Initial response to steroids	No.	Complete remission	Partial remission	No response
Steroid-responsive				
Children	7	6 (86%)	1 (14%)	0
Adults	8	5 (63%)	0	3 (38%)
Total	15	11 (73%)	1 (7%)	3 (20%)
Steroid-resistant				
Children	151	65 (43%)	18 (12%)	68 (45%)
Adults	130	17 (13%)	43 (33%)	70 (54%)
Total	281	82 (29%)	61 (22%)	138 (49%)

*Data derived from references 51, 62, 75–77, 85, 87, 124–136.

Table 23.9 Methylprednisolone protocol for children with focal segmental glomerulosclerosis*

Week	Methylprednisolone[†]	Prednisone[‡]	Cytotoxic therapy
1–2	30 mg/kg, thrice weekly	None	None
3–10	30 mg/kg, q 1 week	2 mg/kg q.o.d.	None
11–18	30 mg/kg, q 2 weeks	2 mg/kg q.o.d.	§
19–52	30 mg/kg, q 4 weeks	2 mg/kg q.o.d.	None
53–78	30 mg/kg, q 8 weeks	2 mg/kg q.o.d.	None

*From Mendoza SA, Reznik VM, Griswold WR, Krensky AM, Yorgin PD, Tune BM: Treatment of steroid-resistant focal segmental glomerulosclerosis with methylprednisone and alkylating agents. Pediatr Nephrol 1990;4:303–307; Tune BM, Kirpekar R, Sibley RK, Reznik VM, Griswold WR, Mendoza SA: Intravenous methylprednisolone and oral alkylating agent therapy of prednisone-resistant pediatric focal segmental glomerulosclerosis: a long-term follow-up. Clin Nephrol 1995;43:84–88.
[†]Up to 1000 mg per dose.
[‡]Up to 60 mg.
§At week 11, treatment failures are given either cyclophosphamide 2 mg/kg/day or chlorambucil 0.2 mg/kg/day for 8–12 weeks.

received cyclophosphamide. Thus, for the frequently relapsing or steroid-dependent patient with FSGS, a course of therapy with a cytotoxic agent would appear to offer the greatest overall benefit.

Treatment of steroid-resistant patients

One approach taken by some pediatric nephrologists in children initially resistant to the standard course of steroid therapy is a more intense course of treatment with pulse methylprednisolone and alkylating agents (Table 23.9). In uncontrolled trials using this aggressive protocol, Tune and colleagues[48,79] have reported remission rates of more than 60% in steroid-resistant children with FSGS. However, the same degree of success with pulse methylprednisolone therapy has not been experienced by others (Table 23.10). The differences in remission rates noted among studies have been attributed to variations in methylprednisolone protocol and the proportion of patients treated with alkylating agents (Table 23.10).[49,50]

Alternate therapeutic approaches in steroid-resistant FSGS are the same as in steroid-responsive patients (i.e. cyclophosphamide or chlorambucil, and cyclosporine). Unfortunately, the response to these agents in steroid-resistant FSGS has been disappointing in adults and children compared with that of steroid-responsive patients (see Tables 23.7 and 23.8). In the only prospective randomized trial evaluating the benefit of cyclophosphamide in steroid-resistant children with FSGS, the addition of a 90-day course of cyclophosphamide (2.5 mg/kg/day) to alternate-day prednisone (40 mg/m² for 12 months) achieved no better response than the prolonged course of alternate-day prednisone alone (complete remission 25% vs. 28% respectively).[80,81] It was therefore concluded that cyclophosphamide offered no additional benefit to a prolonged course of steroids alone and should not be used in children.[80,81]

Recently, mycophenolate mofetil has been tried in a small number of adults with steroid-resistant FSGS and has resulted in improvement in proteinuria and stabilization of renal function, although it has not resulted in complete remissions.[82–84] Furthermore, frequent gastrointestinal

Table 23.10 Response to pulse methylprednisolone and cytotoxic therapy

Reference	No.	Complete remission	Partial remission	No response	Cytotoxic therapy (%)*
Tune et al[49]	11	7 (64%)	2 (18%)	2 (18%)	100
Tune et al[48]	32	21 (66%)	3 (9%)	8 (25%)	78
Aviles et al[137]	5	3 (60%)	0	2 (40%)	60
Guillot & Kim[91]	15	4 (27%)	4 (27%)	7 (46%)	53
Waldo et al[47]	10	0	0	10 (100%)	20

*Proportion of patients treated with cytotoxic therapy.

symptoms have resulted in discontinuation of therapy in 15% of patients in one study.[83]

The overall results with the use of cyclosporine in steroid-resistant FSGS have been more favorable in children than adults, in whom less than 15% attain a complete remission (see Table 23.8). The combined use of a low dose of prednisone with cyclosporine may enhance the likelihood of remission.[85] However, if a response to cyclosporine is not observed by 4–6 months, it is unlikely to occur.[75,86]

Several prospective, randomized, controlled trials of cyclosporine (4–6 mg/kg/day, in two divided doses, for 6 months) have been conducted in adults[62,76] and children[76,87] with steroid-resistant FSGS (Table 23.11). Cyclosporine was adjusted to maintain a 10–12 h whole-blood trough level of 125–225 ng/mL by monoclonal radioimmunoassay[62] or 250–600 ng/mL by polyclonal radioimmunoassay.[76,87] In the two studies evaluating primarily adults,[62,76] the complete remission rate was only 13% and 21%, although none of the patients in the control group achieved a complete remission. In every study patients treated with cyclosporine had a significantly higher remission rate (complete and partial) than patients in the control group. After discontinuation of cyclosporine, 60% of patients followed by Cattran et al[62] and 75% of patients followed by Ponticelli et al[76] had

relapsed by 12 months. Nonetheless, at 50 months of follow-up Cattran et al[62] found that a 50% reduction in creatinine clearance occurred in only 25% of cyclosporine-treated patients compared with 52% of patients on placebo, and that the renal survival at 4 years was 72% in the cyclosporine-treated group compared with 49% in the placebo group. Thus, continuation of cyclosporine therapy is required to maintain the remission in proteinuria; however, even with relapse, a beneficial effect resulting in the preservation of renal function may be observed in some patients. Whether prolonged use of low-dose cyclosporine (required to maintain a remission in some patients) results in the same degree of nephrotoxicity as that associated with patients maintained on doses of 4–8 mg/kg/day is not known and needs to be evaluated. Recent evidence suggests that patients remaining in remission on cyclosporine for over 12 months may be slowly tapered off cyclosporine without subsequent relapse.[64] Thus an attempt at tapering cyclosporine in patients with a prolonged remission should be made in order to minimize the potential for nephrotoxicity.

The results of a pilot trial using FK 506 in seven patients with steroid-resistant nephrotic syndrome (five with FSGS) was recently reported.[88] A remission was seen in four patients, two complete and two partial, after 3 months of therapy; however, all patients had a 50% reduction

Table 23.11 Randomized controlled trials of cyclosporine in steroid-resistant focal segmental glomerulosclerosis

	No.	Complete remission	Partial remission	P value
Ponticelli et al[76]				
Cyclosporine	14	21%	36%	< 0.001
Control	19	0	16%	
Cattran et al[62]				
Cyclosporine	26	12%	57%	< 0.001
Placebo	23	0	4%	
Lieberman et al[87]				
Cyclosporine	12	33%	66%	< 0.05
Placebo	12	0	17%	

in proteinuria at some point during treatment. As with cyclosporine, discontinuation of FK 506 resulted in relapses of proteinuria to the pretreatment level and nephrotoxicity was the most common adverse effect. Whether FK 506 offers any added benefit over cyclosporine in steroid-resistant patients requires further study. While none of the present therapeutic options generates much cause for optimism in treating steroid-resistant FSGS, cyclosporine appears to have a risk–benefit advantage over that of cytotoxic agents.

Complications of steroid or immunosuppressive therapy

The use of prolonged courses of steroids and immuno-suppressive agents raises concern regarding potential adverse effects in children and adults alike. While significant adverse effects from high-dose and prolonged courses of steroid therapy have not been routinely encountered, even in studies with average treatment durations of up to 9 months, one must be cautious because the retrospective nature of most studies makes it difficult to track and assess adverse effects accurately.[5,37,39,42,44,51,59,66,69,89,90] A cushingoid appearance is the most common complication reported, seen in up to 33% of cases, while proximal myopathy (16%), hypertension (5%), gastric discomfort (5%), and diabetes mellitus (2–5%) occur less frequently.[51,90] Although severe adverse effects are observed infrequently, they have usually been encountered in the setting of combined treatment with cytotoxic agents or cyclosporine.[51,58]

In children, prolonged courses of high-dose intravenous methylprednisolone have not been without a cost. The development of cataracts (22%), hypertension (17%), slowed growth (17%), leukopenia (19%), and infectious complications (17%) were not infrequent in patients treated by Mendoza et al.[79] In another study, the use of pulse steroid therapy led to sepsis in 20% (3/15) of children treated, leading to the death of one patient.[91]

Similarly, reports of adverse events (infections, malignancy, infertility) from the use of cytotoxic agents are rare.[39,51,58,59,72,80,92] Even though the duration of treatment has been as long as 19 months,[59] the majority of patients receive cytotoxic therapy for 2–3 months.[39,80,92] Nonetheless, concern regarding the development of gonadal dysfunction or malignancy is appropriate when alkylating agents are used for a prolonged period. The cumulative dose received by a patient during a 2–3 month course of cyclophosphamide at 2 mg/kg/day is 120–180 mg/kg (or 8.4–12.6 g in a 70-kg patient). This is below the dose generally associated with gonadal dysfunction (> 300 mg/kg; > 10 mg/kg for chlorambucil) or the development of acute leukemia (> 10–25 g; > 1 g for chlorambucil).[93,94] However, a 6- or 9-month course of cyclophosphamide (total dose 360–540 mg/kg or 25–39 g), as used in some studies, does put patients at a greatly increased risk of these complications (gonadal dysfunction in 50% of women and 80–100% of men[94]) and should be avoided. Furthermore, it must be recognized that the

development of malignancy (i.e. acute leukemia or bladder cancer) may not be apparent until years after receiving the therapy.[93] Ponticelli et al[51] reported malignancies in three (3.7%) patients (two with lung cancer, one of whom had received a total of 42 g of cyclophosphamide and the other 0.9 g of chlorambucil, and one with Kaposi sarcoma after 2 months of cyclophosphamide and 11 weeks of cyclosporine). Thus, the course of cytotoxic treatment should be limited and the patients monitored closely. In children or young adults on cyclophosphamide it is recommended that the cumulative dose delivered be no greater than 250 mg/kg in order to prevent gonadal toxicity.[93]

The extrarenal adverse effects of cyclosporine therapy are reportedly few, although it is the potential renal toxicity of long-term cyclosporine therapy that is of greatest concern. It has been clearly shown that continuous cyclosporine use over 12–38 months is associated with nephrotoxicity as determined by significant increases in tubulointerstitial fibrosis.[64,77,95] The development of nephrotoxicity may not be apparent clinically as there is a lack of correlation between the structural damage and renal function. Thus in those patients requiring cyclosporine therapy for more than 12 months, it has been suggested that a repeat biopsy be obtained to assess the extent of cyclosporine nephrotoxicity.[64]

An additional cause for concern is the recent observation that cyclosporine may actually accelerate the course of FSGS to ESRD. Meyrier et al[64] found that renal function continued to deteriorate in FSGS patients who had received cyclosporine for an average of 12 months. A significant increase in glomeruli with segmental scars, obsolescent glomeruli, and interstitial fibrosis/infiltrates compared with biopsies before cyclosporine administration was demonstrated. These findings were observed even in FSGS patients who were otherwise in remission. The severity of tubulointerstitial lesions/fibrosis in follow-up biopsies of patients on cyclosporine correlated positively and significantly with the percentage of glomeruli with segmental scars on the initial biopsy, the serum creatinine at the time of initial renal biopsy, and the cyclosporine dosage (> 5.5 mg/kg/day). Thus, the use of cyclosporine could be problematic in patients with FSGS, particularly those with preexisting renal insufficiency and tubulointerstitial disease, and should be used cautiously in this setting.

Other treatment considerations

Control of blood pressure (mean arterial pressure of ≤ 92 mmHg or ≤ 125/75 mmHg) and the use of angiotensin-converting enzyme (ACE) inhibitors have been shown to reduce proteinuria and the rate of decline in glomerular filtration rate (GFR) by as much as 50% in patients with primary glomerulopathies, including FSGS.[96–100] Whether angiotensin II receptor blockers (ARBs) will have the same beneficial effect as ACE inhibitors in patients with primary glomerulopathies is unknown. The only study to date that has compared the use of ACE inhibitors with ARBs in proteinuric patients with IgA nephropathy demonstrated a similar reduction in proteinuria from baseline for ACE inhibitors (61%) and ARBs (55%) after 4 weeks of therapy.[101,102] While blood pressure control and ACE inhibitors are beneficial in reducing proteinuria and progression of renal disease, they rarely lead to remission of nephrotic syndrome.[98] Irrespective, the treatment for both nephrotic and nonnephrotic patients with primary FSGS must include good blood pressure control and the use of ACE inhibitors (and/or ARBs).

Nonsteroidal antiinflammatory drugs (NSAIDs) have been used in severely nephrotic patients unresponsive to the more conventional therapies. In an uncontrolled study, Velosa et al[103] treated 30 patients with steroid-resistant nephrotic syndrome (16 with FSGS) with a 2-month course of meclofenamate. Slightly over 50% of patients responded with a reduction in proteinuria of greater than 40%, with the average proteinuria decreasing from 13 to 4 g per 24 h at follow-up 12 months later. This was associated with stable renal function as determined by serum creatinine. In contrast, 75% of patients not responding to the NSAID had progressive renal failure, with 50% reaching ESRD. In a few case reports, complete remissions have been attained in patients with steroid-resistant FSGS using NSAIDs.[28,104]

While the combined use of NSAIDs and ACE inhibitors in patients with primary glomerulopathies have an additive effect on the reduction in proteinuria,[101,105] this can be associated with a marked decline in GFR and rise in serum potassium levels.[105] In one study using combined therapy, an increase in potassium of more than 1.0 mEq/L was observed in 60% of patients; in 30% of patients this therapy resulted in levels greater than 6.0 mEq/L.[105] If this combination is used, close monitoring of electrolytes and renal function is required due to its life-threatening potential.

The use of plasmapheresis or immunoadsorption in the treatment of FSGS has been proposed based on the premise that the circulating factor(s) responsible for FSGS will be removed.[23,27,106] Recent trials of this approach in transplant patients with recurrent FSGS have resulted in intriguing findings. In two independent trials, one using plasmapheresis[27] and the other immunoadsorption,[106] patients treated for recurrent nephrotic syndrome had significant reductions in proteinuria of 58–82%. This has resulted in lasting remissions in some patients associated with marked histologic improvement in glomerular abnormalities. The success in these patients has been attributed to the early detection and treatment of the recurrent disease (within 1 week after onset of proteinuria). The use of plasmapheresis in primary FSGS has been limited but, in general, has not met with the same beneficial results seen in recurrent FSGS.[107–111] However, in a study by Mitwalli[110] that used a combination of steroids, cyclophosphamide, and plasmapheresis (17 sessions over 6 months), a remission was attained in 73% (8/11) of steroid-resistant adults with primary FSGS.[110] Additionally, Franke et al[111] achieved a remission with pulse methylprednisolone, cyclo-

sporine, and plasma exchange in 57% (4/7) of children with previously steroid- and cyclosporine-resistant primary FSGS. The variability in success of plasmapheresis in primary FSGS suggests that factors other than the "permeability factor" may dominate in patients who have had their disease for a more prolonged period. A therapeutic protocol for prospectively testing the value of apheresis in resistant primary and recurrent FSGS has been proposed.[112]

Specific recommendations

The use of ACE inhibitors (or ARBs) along with good blood pressure control should be part of the therapeutic approach for all patients with primary glomerulopathies, nephrotic or nonnephrotic, and particularly FSGS. In nephrotic patients with primary FSGS, recent experience has provided a note of optimism in the use of immunosuppressive agents for treating this otherwise progressive glomerulopathy. As a result, a course of steroid therapy in primary FSGS is warranted in nephrotic patients with reasonably well-preserved renal function (serum creatinine ≤ 3 mg/dL) in whom it is not otherwise contraindicated. As an initial approach to treatment in adults, prednisone is given at a dose of 1 mg/kg/day (up to 80 mg) for 3–4 months (Table 23.12). In the elderly (≥ 60 years of age), an initial alternate-day regimen of prednisone (1–2 mg/kg up to 120 mg) for 4–5 months may be prudent. In patients showing a response to treatment (i.e. a remission or ≥ 50% reduction in proteinuria), the dose can be slowly tapered over an additional 3 months. For patients unresponsive to the initial course of therapy, a more rapid taper, over 4 weeks, could be utilized in order to minimize further steroid exposure.

In patients who relapse or become steroid-dependent, the use of cytotoxic agents appears most beneficial in achieving a more sustained remission. In order to minimize the toxicity of this therapy, the course of treatment should ideally be limited to 2–3 months. The use of cyclosporine in this setting is also effective but risks the likelihood of nephrotoxicity from long-term cyclosporine dependency.

Of greatest concern are those patients who are steroid resistant as they are resilient to most forms of therapy presently available and ultimately progress to ESRD. Unfortunately, complete remission rates in nephrotic adults with FSGS have been unimpressive with either cytotoxic agents or cyclosporine. However, cyclosporine appears to have a better overall response rate than cytotoxic agents. Patients responding to cyclosporine therapy will usually do so by 4–6 months. Since relapse is common after cyclosporine is discontinued, responders to cyclosporine therapy may require a more prolonged course to maintain the remission. Ideally, this should be done with the lowest dose capable of maintaining a remission in order to minimize the possible nephrotoxicity. Patients in remission for more than 12 months on cyclosporine may be successfully tapered without relapse.

Table 23.12 Treatment recommendations for nephrotic adults with primary focal segmental glomerulosclerosis

Initial therapy
A. Prednisone 1 mg/kg/day (up to 80 mg) for 3–4 months
B. In the elderly (≥ 60 years of age), alternate-day prednisone (1–2 mg/kg up to 120 mg) for 4–5 months
   1. In patients showing a response to treatment, slowly taper prednisone over 3 months
   2. In steroid-resistant patients taper prednisone over 4 weeks and consider cyclosporine therapy

Therapy for relapsing or steroid-dependent patients
A. Cyclophosphamide 2 mg/kg/day or chlorambucil 0.1–0.2 mg/kg/day for 2–3 months
or
B. Cyclosporine 5–6 mg/kg/day for 6 months
   1. Adjusted to maintain a trough level of 125–225 ng/mL
   2. If response is attained, continue for a total of 1 year and then try to slowly taper off
   3. High rate of relapse/cyclosporine dependence
   4. If no response by 6 months, discontinue cyclosporine
C. In patients who relapse after a prolonged remission off prednisone (> 6 months), consider a second course of prednisone therapy alone

Therapy for steroid-resistant patients
A. Cyclosporine 5–6 mg/kg/day for 6 months
   1. Adjusted to maintain a trough level of 125–225 ng/mL
   2. If response is attained, continue for a total of 1 year and then try to slowly taper off
   3. High rate of relapse/cyclosporine dependence
   4. If no response by 6 months, discontinue cyclosporine
B. Low-dose prednisone (15 mg/day) may enhance response to cyclosporine
   1. Continue for 6 months then taper off over 4–8 weeks

References

1. White RHR, Glasgow EF, Mills RJ: Clinicopathologic study of nephrotic syndrome in childhood. Lancet 1970;i:1353–1359.
2. Abramowicz M, Barnett HL, Edelmann CM Jr, et al: Controlled trial of azathioprine in children with nephrotic syndrome: A report of the international study of kidney disease in children. Lancet 1970;ii:959–961.
3. Habib R: Focal glomerular sclerosis. Kidney Int 1973;4:355–361.
4. Habib R, Kleinknecht C: The primary nephrotic syndrome of childhood: classification and clinicopathologic study of 406 cases. *In* Sommers S (ed): Pathology Annual. New York: Appelton-Century Crofts, 1971, pp 427–434.
5. International Study of Kidney Disease in Children: The primary nephrotic syndrome in children. Identification of patients with minimal change nephrotic syndrome from initial response to prednisone. J Pediatr 1981;98:561–564.
6. A Report of the Southwest Pediatric Nephrology Study Group: Focal segmental glomerulosclerosis in children with idiopathic nephrotic syndrome. Kidney Int 1985;27:442–449.
7. Beaufils H, Alphonse JC, Guedon J, Legrain M: Focal glomerulosclerosis: natural history and treatment. Nephron 1978;21:75–85.
8. Korbet SM, Genchi R, Borok RZ, Schwartz MM: The racial prevalence of glomerular lesions in nephrotic adults. Am J Kidney Dis 1996;27:647–651.
9. Haas M, Spargo BH, Coventry S: Increasing incidence of focal-segmental glomerulosclerosis among adult nephropathies: a 20-year renal biopsy study. Am J Kidney Dis 1995;26:740–750.
10. Ingulli E, Tejani A: Racial differences in the incidence and renal outcome of idiopathic focal segmental glomerulosclerosis in children. Pediatr Nephrol 1991;5:393–397.
11. Bonilla-Felix M, Parra C, Dajani T, et al: Changing patterns in the histopathology of idiopathic nephrotic syndrome in children. Kidney Int 1999;55:1885–1890.
12. Braden GL, Mulhern JG, O'Shea MH, Nash SV, Ucci AA Jr, Germain MJ: Changing incidence of glomerular diseases in adults. Am J Kidney Dis 2000;35:878–883.
13. Barisoni L, Valeri A, Radhakrishnan J, Nash M, Appel G, D'Agati V: Focal segmental glomerulosclerosis: a 20-year epidemiological perspective. J Am Soc Nephrol 1994;5:347.
14. Gulati S, Sharma AP, Sharma RK, Gupta A: Changing trends of histopathology in childhood nephrotic syndrome. Am J Kidney Dis 1999;34:646–650.
15. Haas M, Meehan SM, Karrison TG, Spargo BH: Changing etiologies of unexplained adult nephrotic syndrome: a comparison of renal biopsy findings from 1976–1979 and 1995–1997. Am J Kidney Dis 1997;30:621–631.
16. Schwartz MM, Korbet SM, Rydel JJ, Borok RZ, Genchi R: Primary focal segmental glomerular sclerosis in adults: Prognostic value of histologic variants. Am J Kidney Dis 1995;25:845–852.
17. Schwartz MM, Korbet SM: Primary focal segmental glomerulosclerosis: pathology, histologic variants, and pathogenesis. Am J Kidney Dis 1993;22:874–883.
18. D'Agati V: The many masks of focal segmental glomerulosclerosis. Kidney Int 1994;46:1223–1241.
19. Bakir AA, Bazilinski NG, Rhee HL, Ainis H, Dunea G: Focal segmental glomerulosclerosis. A common entity in nephrotic black adults. Arch Intern Med 1989;149:1802–1804.
20. Pontier PJ, Patel TG: Racial differences in the prevalence and presentation of glomerular disease in adults. Clin Nephrol 1994;42:79–84.
21. Pinn-Wiggins VW: Nephrotic syndrome in blacks: histopathologic perspectives. Transplant Proc 1987;19:49–55.
22. Lewis EJ: Recurrent focal sclerosis after renal transplantation. Kidney Int 1982;22:315–323.
23. Ritz E: Pathogenesis of "idiopathic" nephrotic syndrome. N Engl J Med 1994;330:61–62.
24. Savin VJ, Sharma R, Sharma M, et al: Circulating factor associated with increased glomerular permeability to albumin in recurrent focal segmental glomerulosclerosis. N Engl J Med 1996;334:878–883.
25. Neuringer JR, Brenner BM: Hemodynamic theory of progressive renal disease. Am J Kidney Dis 1993;22:98–104.
26. Fogo AB: Progression and potential regression of glomerulosclerosis. Kidney Int 2001;59:804–819.
27. Artero ML, Sharma R, Savin V, Vincenti F: Plasmapheresis reduces proteinuria and serum capacity to injure glomeruli in patients with recurrent focal glomerulosclerosis. Am J Kidney Dis 1994;23:574–581.

28. Korbet SM, Schwartz MM, Lewis EJ: Recurrent nephrotic syndrome in renal allografts. Am J Kidney Dis 1988;11:270–276.

29. Rennke HG, Klein PS: Pathogenesis and significance of nonprimary focal and segmental glomerulosclerosis. Am J Kidney Dis 1989;13:443–456.

30. Conlon PJ, Lynn K, Winn MP, et al: Spectrum of disease in familial focal and segmental glomerulosclerosis. Kidney Int 1999;56:1863–1871.

31. Olson JL, Schwartz MM: The nephrotic syndrome: minimal change disease, focal segmental glomerulosclerosis and miscellaneous causes. In Jennette JC, Olson JL, Schwartz MM, et al (eds): Heptinstall's Pathology of the Kidney, 5th edn. New York: Lippincott-Raven, 1998, pp 212–221.

32. Schwartz MM, Lewis EJ: Focal segmental glomerular sclerosis: the cellular lesion. Kidney Int 1985;28:968–974.

33. Detwiler RK, Falk RJ, Hogan SL, Jennette JC: Collapsing gloemerulopathy: a clinically and pathologically distinct variant of focal segmental glomerulosclerosis. Kidney Int 1994;45:1416–1424.

34. Valeri A, Barisoni L, Appel G, Seigle R, D'Agati V: Idiopathic collapsing focal segmental glomerulosclerosis: a clinicopathologic study. Kidney Int 1996;50:1734–1746.

35. Weiss MA, Daquioag E, Margolin EG, Pollak VE: Nephrotic syndrome, progressive irreversible renal failure and glomerular "collapse": a new clinicopathologic entity? Am J Med 1986;7:20–28.

36. Meyrier AY: Collapsing glomerulopathy: expanding interest in a shrinking tuft. Am J Kidney Dis 1999;33:801–803.

37. Schwartz MM, Evans J, Bain R, Korbet SM: Focal segmental glomerulosclerosis: prognostic implications of the cellular lesion. J Am Soc Nephrol 1999;10:1900–1907.

38. Newman WJ, Tisher CC, McCoy RC, et al: Focal glomerular sclerosis: contrasting clinical patterns in children and adults. Medicine 1976;55:67–87.

39. Pei Y, Cattran D, Delmore T, Katz A, Lang A, Rance P: Evidence suggesting under-treatment in adults with idiopathic focal segmental glomerulosclerosis. Am J Med 1987;82:938–944.

40. Wehrmann M, Bohle A, Held H, Schumm G, Kendziorra H, Pressler H: Long-term prognosis of focal sclerosing glomerulonephritis: an analysis of 250 cases with particular regard to tubulointerstitial changes. Clin Nephrol 1990;33:115–122.

41. Velosa JA, Holley KE, Torres VE, Offord KP: Significance of proteinuria on the outcome of renal function in patients with focal segmental glomerulosclerosis. Mayo Clin Proc 1983;58:568–577.

42. Korbet SM, Schwartz MM, Lewis EJ: The prognosis of focal segmental glomerular sclerosis of adulthood. Medicine 1986;65:304–311.

43. Cameron JS, Turner DR, Ogg CS, Chantler C, Williams DG: The long-term prognosis of patients with focal segmental glomerulosclerosis. Clin Nephrol 1978;10:213–218.

44. Rydel JJ, Korbet SM, Borok RZ, Schwartz MM: Focal segmental glomerular sclerosis in adults: presentation, course and response to treatment. Am J Kidney Dis 1995;25:534–542.

45. Brown CB, Cameron JS, Turner DR, et al: Focal segmental glomerulosclerosis with rapid decline in renal function ("malignant FSGS"). Clin Nephrol 1978;10:51–61.

46. Chan PCK, Chan KW, Cheng IKP, Chan MK: Focal sclerosing glomerulopathy: risk factors of progression and optimal mode of treatment. Int Urol Nephrol 1991;239:619–629.

47. Waldo FB, Benfield MR, Kohaut EC: Methylprednisolone treatment of patients with steroid-resistant nephrotic syndrome. Pediatr Nephrol 1992;6:503–505.

48. Tune BM, Kirpekar R, Sibley RK, Reznik VM, Griswold WR, Mendoza SA: Intravenous methylprednisolone and oral alkylating agent therapy of prednisone-resistant pediatric focal segmental glomerulosclerosis: a long-term follow-up. Clin Nephrol 1995;43:84–88.

49. Tune BM, Lieberman E, Mendoza SA: Steroid-resistant nephrotic focal segmental glomerulosclerosis: a treatable disease. Pediatr Nephrol 1996;10:772–778.

50. Tune BM, Mendoza SA: Treatment of the idiopathic nephrotic syndrome: regimens and outcomes in children and adults. J Am Soc Nephrol 1997;8:824–832.

51. Ponticelli C, Villa M, Banfi G, et al: Can prolonged treatment improve the prognosis in adults with focal segmental glomerulosclerosis? Am J Kidney Dis 1999;34:618–625.

52. Laurinavicius A, Hurwitz S, Rennke HG: Collapsing glomerulopathy in HIV and non-HIV patients: a clinicopathological and follow-up study. Kidney Int 1999;56:2203–2213.

53. Singh HK, Baldree LA, McKenney DW, Hogan SL, Jennette JC: Idiopathic collapsing glomerulopathy in children. Pediatr Nephrol 2000;14:132–137.

54. Korbet SM, Schwartz MM: Primary focal segmental glomerulosclerosis: a treatable lesion with variable outcomes. Nephrology 2001;6:47–56.

55. Yoshikawa N, Ito H, Akamatsu R, et al: Focal segmental glomerulosclerosis with and without nephrotic syndrome in children. J Pediatr 1986;109:65–70.

56. Howie AJ, Brewer DB: Further studies on the glomerular tip lesion: early and late stages and life table analysis. J Pathol 1985;147:245–255.

57. Cameron JS: The enigma of focal segmental glomerulosclerosis. Kidney Int 1996;50(Suppl 57):S119–S131.

58. Cattran DC, Rao P: Long-term outcome in children and adults with classic focal segmental glomerulosclerosis. Am J Kidney Dis 1998;32:72–79.

59. Banfi G, Moriggi M, Sabadini E, Fellin G, D'Amico G, Ponticelli C: The impact of prolonged immunosuppression on the outcome of idiopathic focal–segmental glomerulosclerosis with nephrotic syndrome in adults. A collaborative retrospective study. Clin Nephrol 1991;36:53–59.

60. Korbet SM, Schwartz MM, Lewis EJ: Primary focal segmental glomerulosclerosis: clinical course and response to therapy. Am J Kidney Dis 1994;23:773–783.

61. Cattran DC: Are all patients with idiopathic focal segmental glomerulosclerosis (FSGS) created equal? Nephrol Dial Transplant 1998;13:1107–1109.

62. Cattran DC, Appel GB, Hebert LA, et al: A randomized trial of cyclosporine in patients with steroid-resistant focal segmental glomerulosclerosis. Kidney Int 1999;56:2220–2226.

63. Korbet SM: The treatment of focal segmental glomerulosclerosis: steroid-resistance or steroid-reluctance? Kidney 1992;1:1–2.

64. Meyrier A, Noel LH, Auriche P, et al: Long-term renal tolerance of cyclosporin A treatment in adult idiopathic nephrotic syndrome. Kidney Int 1994;45:1446–1456.

65. Bolton WK, Atuk NO, Sturgil BC, Westervelt FB Jr: Therapy of the idiopathic nephrotic syndrome with alternate day steroids. Am J Med 1977;62:60–70.

66. Nagai R, Cattran DC, Pei Y: Steroid therapy and prognosis of focal segmental glomerulosclerosis in the elderly. Clin Nephrol 1994;42:18–21.

67. Tornatore KM, Logue G, Venuto RC, Davis PJ: Pharmacokinetics of methylprednisolone in elderly and young healthy adult males. J Am Geriatr Soc 1994;42:1118–1122.

68. Stuck AE, Frey BM, Frey FJ: Kinetics of prednisolone and endogenous cortisol suppression in the elderly. Clin Pharmacol Ther 1988;43:354–362.

69. Saint-Hillier Y, Morel-Maroger L, Woodrow D, Richet G: Focal and segmental hyalinosis. Adv Nephrol 1975;5:67–88.

70. Arbus GS, Poucell S, Bacheyie GS, Baumal R: Focal segmental glomerulosclerosis with idiopathic nephrotic syndrome: three types of clinical response. J Pediatr 1982;101:40–45.

71. Mongeau JG, Robitaille PO, Clermont MJ, Merouani A, Russo P: Focal segmental glomerulosclerosis (FSG) 20 years later. From toddler to grown up. Clin Nephrol 1993;40:1–6.

72. Mongeau JG, Corneille L, Robitaille PO, O'Regan S, Pelletier M: Primary nephrosis in childhood associated with focal glomerular sclerosis: is long-term prognosis that severe? Kidney Int 1981;20:743–746.

73. Meyrier A, Simon P: Treatment of corticoresistant idiopathic nephrotic syndrome in the adult: minimal change disease and focal segmental glomerulosclerosis. Adv Nephrol 1988;17:127–150.

74. Meyrier A, Collaborative Group of the Société de Néphrologie: Cyclosporin in the treatment of nephrosis. Am J Nephrol 1989;9(Suppl 1):65–71.

75. Meyrier A, Condamin MC, Broneer D, Collaborative Group of the Société de Néphrologie: Treatment of adult idiopathic nephrotic syndrome with cyclosporin A: minimal-change disease and focal–segmental glomerulosclerosis. Clin Nephrol 1991;35(Suppl 1):37–42.

76. Ponticelli C, Rizzoni G, Edefonti A, et al: A randomized trial of cyclosporine in steroid resistant idiopathic nephrotic syndrome. Kidney Int 1993;43:1377–1384.

77. Melocoton TL, Kamil ES, Cohen AH, Fine RN: Long-term cyclosporine A treatment of steroid-resistant and steroid-dependent nephrotic syndrome. Am J Kidney Dis 1991;18:583–588.

78. Ponticelli C, Edefonti A, Ghio L, et al: Cyclosporin versus cyclophosphamide for patients with steroid dependent and frequently relapsing idiopathic nephrotic syndrome: a multicenter randomized controlled trial. Nephrol Dial Transplant 1993;8:1326–1332.

79. Mendoza SA, Reznik VM, Griswold WR, Krensky AM, Yorgin PD, Tune BM: Treatment of steroid-resistant focal segmental glomerulosclerosis with methylprednisone and alkylating agents. Pediatr Nephrol 1990;4:303–307.

80. Tarshish P, Tobin JN, Bernstein J, Edelmann CM Jr: Cyclophosphamide does not benefit patients with focal segmental glomerulosclerosis: a report of the International Study of Kidney Disease in Children. Pediatr Nephrol 1996;10:590–593.

81. International Study of Kidney Disease in Children: Cyclophosphamide therapy in focal segmental glomerular sclerosis: a controlled clinical trial. Pediatr Res 1982;16:320.

82. Briggs WA, Choi MJ, Scheel PJ Jr: Successful mycophenolate mofetil treatment of glomerular disease. Am J Kidney Dis 1998;31:213–217.

83. Briggs WA, Choi MJ, Gimenez LF, Scheel PJ Jr: Treatment of primary glomerulopathies with mycophenolate mofetil. J Am Soc Nephrol 1998;9:84A.

84. Radhakrishnan J, Wang MM, Matalon A, Cattran DC, Appel GB: Mycophenolate mofetil treatment of idiopathic focal segmental glomerular sclerosis. J Am Soc Nephrol 1999;10:114A.

85. Niaudet P, French Society of Pediatric Nephrology: Treatment of childhood steroid-resistant idiopathic nephrosis with a combination of cyclosporine and prednisone. J Pediatr 1994;125:981–986.

86. Meyrier A: Treatment of nephrotic syndrome with cyclosporin A. What remains in 1994? Nephrol Dial Transplant 1994;9:596–598.

87. Lieberman KV, Tejani A for the New York–New Jersey Pediatric Nephrology Study Group: A randomized double-blind placebo-controlled trial of cyclosporine in steroid-resistant idiopathic focal segmental glomerulosclerosis in children. J Am Soc Nephrol 1996;7:56–63.

88. McCauley J, Shapiro R, Ellis D, Igdal H, Tzakis A, Starzl T: Pilot trial of FK 506 in the management of steroid-resistant nephrotic syndrome. Nephrol Dial Transplant 1993;8:1286–1290.

89. Splendiani G, Costanzi S, Sturniolo A, et al: Treatment of idiopathic glomerulonepritis in the elderly. Contrib Nephrol 1993;105:139–143.

90. Alexopoulos E, Stangou M, Papagianni A, Pantzaki A, Papadimitriou M: Factors influencing the course and the response to treatment in primary focal segmental glomerulosclerosis. Nephrol Dial Transplant 2000;15:1348–1356.

91. Guillot AP, Kim MS: Pulse steroid therapy does not alter the course of focal segmental glomerulosclerosis. J Am Soc Nephrol 1993;4:276.

92. Geary DF, Farine M, Thorner P, Baumal R: Response to cyclophosphamide in steroid-resistant focal segmental glomerulosclerosis: a reappraisal. Clin Nephrol 1984;22:109–113.

93. Lewis EJ: Management of the nephrotic syndrome in adults. *In* Cameron JS, Glassock RJ (eds): The Nephrotic Syndrome. New York: Marcel Dekker, 1988, pp 461–521.

94. Rivkees SA, Crawford JD: The relationship of gonadal activity and chemotherapy-induced gonadal damage. JAMA 1988;259:2123–2125.

95. Habib R, Niaudet P: Comparison between pre- and posttreatment renal biopsies in children receiving cyclosporine for idiopathic nephrosis. Clin Nephrol 1994;42:141–146.

96. Maschio G, Alberti D, Janin G, et al: Effect of the angiotensin-converting-enzyme inhibitor benazepril on the progression of chronic renal insufficiency. N Engl J Med 1996;334:939–945.

97. Peterson JC, Adler S, Burkart JM, et al: Blood pressure control, proteinuria, and the progression of renal disease. The Modification of Diet in Renal Disease Study. Ann Intern Med 1995;123:754–762.

98. Praga M, Hernández E, Montoyo C, Andrés A, Ruilope LM, Rodicio JL: Long-term beneficial effects of angiotensin-converting enzyme inhibition in patients with nephrotic proteinuria. Am J Kidney Dis 1992;20:240–248.

99. Ruggenenti P, Perna A, Gherardi G, Benini R, Remuzzi G: Chronic proteinuric nephropathies: outcomes and response to treatment in a prospective cohort of 352 patients with different patterns of renal injury. Am J Kidney Dis 2000;35:1155–1165.

100. The GISEN Group: Randomized placebo-controlled trial of effect of ramipril on decline in glomerular filtration rate and risk of terminal renal failure in proteinuric, nondiabetic nephropathy. Lancet 1997;349:1857–1863.

101. Perico N, Remuzzi A, Sangalli F, et al: The antiproteinuric effect of angiotensin antagonism in human IgA nephropathy is potentiated by indomethacin. J Am Soc Nephrol 1998;9:2308–2317.

102. Taal MW, Brenner BM: Renoprotective benefits of RAS inhibition: from ACEI to angiotensin II antagonists. Kidney Int 2000;57:1803–1817.

103. Velosa JA, Torres VE, Donadio JV, Wagoner RD, Holley KE, Offord KP: Treatment of severe nephrotic syndrome with meclofenamate: an uncontrolled pilot study. Mayo Clin Proc 1985;60:586–592.

104. Torres VE, Velosa JA, Holley KE, Frohnert PP, Zincke H, Sterioff S: Meclofenamate treatment of recurrent idiopathic nephrotic syndrome with focal segmental glomerulosclerosis after renal transplantation. Mayo Clin Proc 1984;59:146–152.

105. Heeg JE, de-Jong PE, Vriesendorp R, de-Zeeuw D: Additive antiproteinuric effect of the NSAID indomethacin and the ACE inhibitor lisinopril. Am J Nephrol 1990;10(Suppl 1):94–97.

106. Dantal J, Bigot E, Bogers W, et al: Effect of plasma protein adsorption on protein excretion in kidney-transplant recipients with recurrent nephrotic syndrome. N Engl J Med 1994;330:7–14.

107. Feld SM, Figueroa P, Savin V, et al: Plasmapheresis in the treatment of steroid-resistant focal segmental glomerulosclerosis in native kidneys. Am J Kidney Dis 1998;32:230–237.

108. Haas M, Godfrin Y, Oberbauer R, et al: Plasma immunadsorption treatment in patients with primary focal and segmental glomerulosclerosis. Nephrol Dial Transplant 1998;13:2013–2016.

109. Ginsburg DS, Dau P: Plasmapheresis in the treatment of steroid-resistant focal segmental glomerulosclerosis. Clin Nephrol 1997;48:282–287.

110. Mitwalli AH: Adding plasmapheresis to corticosteroids and alkylating agents: does it benefit patients with focal segmental glomerulosclerosis? Nephrol Dial Transplant 1998;13:1524–1528.

111. Franke D, Zimmering M, Wolfish N, Ehrich JH, Filler G: Treatment of FSGS with plasma exchange and immunadsorption. Pediatr Nephrol 2000;14:965–969.

112. Moriconi L, Passalacqua S, Pretagostini R, et al: Apheresis in primary focal segmental glomerulosclerosis of native and transplanted kidneys: a therapeutic protocol. J Nephrol 2000;13:347–351.

113. Agarwal SK, Dash SC, Tiwari SC, Bhuyan UN: Idiopathic adult focal segmental glomerulosclerosis: a clinicopathological study and response to steroid. Nephron 1993;63:168–171.

114. Frishberg Y, Becker-Cohen R, Halle D, et al: Genetic polymorphisms of the renin–angiotensin system and the outcome of focal segmental glomerulosclerosis in children. Kidney Int 1998;54:1843–1849.

115. Hyman LR, Burkholder PM: Focal sclerosing glomerulonephropathy with hylanosis. J Pediatr 1974;84:217–225.

116. International Study of Kidney Disease in Children: Nephrotic syndrome in children: prediction of histopathology from clinical and laboratory characteristics at time of diagnosis. Kidney Int 1978;13:159–165.

117. Jenis EH, Teichman S, Briggs WA, et al: Focal segmental glomerulosclerosis. Am J Med 1974;57:695–705.

118. Lim VS, Sibley R, Spargo B: Adult lipoid nephrosis: clinicopathological correlations. Ann Intern Med 1974;81:314–320.

119. Miyata J, Takebayashi S, Taguchi T, Harada T: Evaluation and correlation of clinical and histological features of focal segmental glomerulosclerosis. Nephron 1986;44:115–120.

120. Morita M, White RHR, Coad NAG, Raafat F: The clinical significance of the glomerular location of segmental lesion in focal segmental glomerulosclerosis. Clin Nephrol 1990;33:211–219.

121. Nash MA, Greifer I, Olbing H, Bennett B, Spitzer A: The significance of focal sclerotic lesions of glomeruli in children. J Pediatr 1976;88:806–813.

122. Shiiki H, Nishino T, Uyama H, et al: Clinical and morphological predictors of renal outcome in adult patients with focal and segmental glomerulosclerosis (FSGS). Clin Nephrol 1996;46:362–368.

123. Velosa JA, Donadio JV, Holley KE: Focal sclerosing glomerulonephropathy: a clinicopathologic study. Mayo Clin Proc 1975;50:121–133.

124. Brandis M, Burghard R, Leititis J, Zimmerhackl B, Hildebrandt F, Helmchen U: Cyclosporine A for treatment of nephrotic syndromes. Transplant Proc 1988;20(Suppl 4):275–279.

125. Brodehl J, Hoyer PF: Cyclosporin in idiopathic nephrotic syndrome of children. Am J Nephrol 1989;9(Suppl 1):61–64.

235

126. Delaney MP, Dukes DC, Edmunds ME: Cyclosporin A in refactory idiopathic nephrotic syndrome: 5 years clinical experience. Postgrad Med J 1994;70:891–894.

127. Garin EH, Orak JK, Hiott KL, Sutherland SE: Cyclosporine therapy for steroid-resistant nephrotic syndrome. Am J Dis Child 1988;142:985–988.

128. Ingulli E, Singh A, Baqui N, Ahmad H, Moazami S, Tejani A: Aggressive, long-term cyclosporine therapy for steroid-resistant focal segmental glomerulosclerosis. J Am Soc Nephrol 1995;5:1820–1825.

129. Ittel TH, Clasen W, Fuhs M, Kindler J, Mihatsch MJ, Sieberth H-G: Long-term ciclosporine A treatment in adults with minimal change nephrotic syndrome or focal segmental glomerulosclerosis. Clin Nephrol 1995;44:156–162.

130. Maher ER, Sweny P, Chappel M, Varghese Z, Moorhead JF: Cyclosporin in the treatment of steroid-responsive and steroid-resistant nephrotic syndrome in adults. Nephrol Dial Transplant 1988;3:728–732.

131. Ponticelli C, Rivolta E: Cyclosporine in nephrotic syndrome. Transplant Proc 1988;20:253–258.

132. Singh A, Tejani C, Tejani A: One-center experience with cyclosporine in refractory nephrotic syndrome in children. Pediatr Nephrol 1999;13:26–32.

133. Tejani A, Butt K, Trachtman H, Suthanthiran M, Rosenthal CJ, Khawar MR: Cyclosporine A induced remission of relapsing nephrotic syndrome in children. Kidney Int† 1988;33:729–734.

134. Waldo FB, Benfield MR, Kohaut EC: Therapy of focal and segmental glomerulosclerosis with methylprednisolone, cyclosporine A, and prednisone. Pediatr Nephrol 1998;12:397–400.

135. Waldo FB, Kohaut EC: Therapy of focal–segmental glomerulosclerosis with cyclosporine A. Pediatr Nephrol 1987;1:180–182.

136. Walker RG, Kincaid-Smith P: The effects of treatment of corticosteroid-resistant idiopathic (primary) focal segmental hyalinosis and sclerosis (focal glomerulosclerosis) with cyclosporin. Nephron 1990;54:117–121.

137. Aviles DH, Irwin KC, Dublin LS, Vehaskari VM: Aggressive treatment of severe idiopathic focal segmental glomerulosclerosis. Pediatr Nephrol 1999;13:298–300.

Idiopathic Membranous Nephropathy

Howard A. Austin III

Membranous nephropathy is a common cause of adult-onset nephrotic syndrome, accounting for about 20% of cases.[1] Characteristic renal biopsy changes include diffuse glomerular capillary wall thickening and subepithelial and/or intramembranous electron-dense deposits (described further in reference 2). Various medications and toxins as well as certain rheumatologic, neoplastic, and infectious diseases account for approximately 20% of membranous nephropathy from developed countries.[3] The underlying cause (e.g. neoplasia or systemic lupus erythematosus) may not be evident at presentation in some patients, requiring an ongoing evaluation to ferret out a specific, and it is hoped treatable, disorder.[3] Treatment of secondary membranous nephropathy is beyond the scope of this chapter.

Natural history

Despite evidence that immunologic mechanisms induce glomerular injury in membranous nephropathy, immunosuppressive drug treatments are not justified for all patients with this disorder. The clinical course of idiopathic membranous nephropathy is highly variable. Approximately 20% of adult patients progress to endstage renal disease within 10 years,[4] while another 25% typically experience complete spontaneous remissions of proteinuria.[5] Since spontaneous remissions may occur after several months (or even years) of follow-up, a period of observation may be required to fully evaluate the prognosis of some individuals. Patients with persistent proteinuria and hyperlipidemia are at increased risk for cardiovascular and thromboembolic complications of the nephrotic syndrome. Ordonez et al[6] found that patients with the nephrotic syndrome had a fivefold increased risk of myocardial infarction (after statistical adjustment for hypertension and cigarette smoking) compared with age- and sex-matched control subjects who participated in the same health plan. Thus nephrotic syndrome is an independent risk factor for accelerated coronary artery disease.

The nephrotic syndrome due to membranous nephropathy is also associated with an increased risk for thromboembolic complications. Epidemiologic data are highly variable; estimates for the prevalence of renal vein thrombosis among patients with membranous nephropathy range from 5% to 63%. The prevalence of other deep vein thrombosis in this population of patients appears to be comparable, ranging from 9% to 44%. Concern for the morbidity and mortality associated with pulmonary embolism has led to interest in the possible role of prophylactic anticoagulation for patients with severe nephrotic syndrome due to membranous nephropathy. By decision analysis, the risks of life-threatening complications of pulmonary embolism appear to outweigh those associated with anticoagulation.[7] However, data from prospective randomized clinical trials are not available to support this approach.

Survival data compiled by Hogan et al[8] illustrate the potential morbidity and mortality attributed to idiopathic membranous nephropathy. A pooled analysis of outcomes in clinical studies of this disorder was conducted to estimate "renal" survival, defined as the probability of not progressing to endstage renal failure and not succumbing to death from kidney disease or from cardiovascular events associated with persistent nephrotic syndrome. Employing this approach, the probability of renal survival was 86% at 5 years, 65% at 10 years, and 59% at 15 years.

Prognostic indicators

Generalizations about the prognosis of patients with idiopathic membranous nephropathy are of limited value because the natural history of this disorder is highly variable. To refine estimates of prognosis and to derive relatively objective criteria for instituting therapeutic interventions, investigators have sought to identify high-risk subgroups of patients. Several potentially important prognostic factors have been examined (Table 24.1). In a chronic disorder subject to spontaneous remissions, clinical observations acquired during a period of time are likely to be stronger predictors of long-term renal function outcome than those obtained at a single time-point. Thus, patients observed to have declining renal function due to membranous nephropathy are at particularly high risk for progressive deterioration in renal function.[9] Furthermore,

Table 24.1 Idiopathic membranous nephropathy: indications for immunosuppressive treatment in patients with nephrotic proteinuria

Very strong indicators
Declining renal function
Persistent severe proteinuria, e.g.
　≥ 8 g/day for ≥ 6 months
　≥ 6 g/day for ≥ 6–9 months
Superimposed crescents

Strong indicators
Persistent moderate nephrotic proteinuria, e.g. ≥ 4 g/day for
　≥ 6–18 months
Very severe proteinuria when first evaluated, e.g. ≥ 10 g/day
　(sequential observations not available)
Impaired renal function at presentation (longitudinal data not
　available)
Chronic tubulointerstitial changes
　Interstitial fibrosis
　Tubular atrophy
Atherosclerotic or thromboembolic complications of the
　nephrotic syndrome

Moderately strong indicators
Male gender
Older age (> 50 years)
Hypertension
Focal segmental glomerulosclerosis
Stage 3 glomerular lesions
Interstitial mononuclear infiltrates
Hyaline vascular lesions

persistent high-grade proteinuria is more predictive than a comparable degree of proteinuria at a single point in time. Pei et al[10] observed that persistent severe proteinuria (≥ 8 g/day for ≥ 6 months) was associated with a 66% probability of progression to chronic renal insufficiency (defined as creatinine clearance < 60 mL/min per 1.73 m^2 for ≥ 12 months). This observation is important because once patients with membranous nephropathy manifest deteriorating renal function, they are at high risk for further progression to endstage renal disease. Pei et al also recommended that patients be reviewed to determine whether they have had less severe proteinuria for longer periods. Thus they observed that patients with proteinuria of at least 6 g/day for 9 months or more had a 55% probability of developing chronic renal insufficiency. A moderate level of persistent nephrotic proteinuria (≥ 4 g/day) for a longer time (≥ 18 months) was also associated with an increased risk of chronic renal insufficiency. In these cases, the predictive value of persistent proteinuria was enhanced substantially by considering additional prognostic factors, namely the creatinine clearance at the start of persistent proteinuria and the rate of change of creatinine clearance during the period of persistent proteinuria.

Concern that prolonged observation might delay therapy excessively in some patients has prompted Cattran et al[11] to reassess the predictive models by employing a 6-month period of observation for all levels of persistent proteinuria. A mathematical model was derived and validated by employing data from two additional distinct populations of patients. The algorithm uses the highest level of proteinuria that persisted for a 6-month interval as well as the initial value and the rate of change of creatinine clearance during the period of persistent proteinuria. The equation and examples of how to calculate the probability of progression to chronic renal insufficiency are described in reference 11.

Observation of patients for the evolution of time-dependent prognostic factors is recommended for some, but not all, cases of idiopathic membranous nephropathy. Patients that present with combinations of ominous time-independent features (see Table 24.1) should be considered for treatment without prolonged observation in an effort to reduce the risks of irreversible renal parenchymal injury as well as cardiovascular and thromboembolic complications of the nephrotic syndrome.

Clinical trials and specific recommendations

Nephrotic-range proteinuria

Patients who present with moderate degrees of nephrotic (or subnephrotic)-range proteinuria without other compelling indications of a poor prognosis are frequently treated, at least initially, without immunosuppression. These patients may benefit from angiotensin-converting enzyme (ACE) inhibitors, angiotensin II receptor antagonists, and lipid-lowering agents. Whereas the response to ACE inhibitors is not consistent in this population, modulation of intrarenal hemodynamic parameters may reduce proteinuria by as much as 50%[12-14] and may reduce the risk for progressive glomerular sclerosis as well. The beneficial effect of ACE inhibition on slowing the progression of renal insufficiency is most pronounced among patients with proteinuria (> 1 g/day); a relatively low blood pressure target (< 125/75 mmHg) has been recommended for these individuals.[15,16] Studies in other populations of nephrotic patients suggest that a low-protein diet may augment the hemodynamic effect of ACE inhibitors.[17]

It is important to address coronary risk factors in patients with the nephrotic syndrome.[18] Whereas ACE inhibitors may reduce proteinuria and partially correct hyperlipidemia, specific lipid-lowering agents are often indicated as well. 3-Hydroxy-3-methylglutaryl coenzyme A (HMG-CoA) reductase inhibitors are widely used for this purpose and typically lead to 30–45% decrements in low-density lipoprotein (LDL) cholesterol.[19-21]

The role of alternate-day oral glucocorticoids (similar to that employed in the US Collaborative Study[22]) has been debated. There is widespread appropriate skepticism regarding the efficacy of oral prednisone regimens for membranous nephropathy based on the negative results of the Toronto[23] and the British Medical Research Council[24] collaborative trials (Table 24.2). It could be

Table 24.2 Selected studies of immunosuppressive drug regimens

Reference	Design	Baseline	Treatment	Outcome
Short-term corticosteroid therapy				
CSAINS[22]	RCT	Creatinine clearance > 42 mL/min/1.73 m² Proteinuria ≥ 3.5 g/day per 1.73 m²	Prednisone (n = 34) vs. placebo (n = 38) for at least 8 weeks	Corticosteroids decreased proteinuria transiently and reduced the risk of renal insufficiency compared with controls, some of whom deteriorated unusually rapidly
Cattran et al[23]	RCT	Creatinine clearance ≥ 15 mL/min/1.73 m² Proteinuria ≥ 0.3 g/day	Prednisone (n = 81) vs. no specific treatment (n = 77) for 6 months	Six-month course of alternate-day prednisone was of no benefit
Cameron et al[24]	RCT	Creatinine clearance ≥ 30 mL/min Proteinuria > 3.5 g/day.	Prednisolone (n = 52) vs. placebo (n = 51) for 8 weeks	No sustained benefit of corticosteroids on renal function or proteinuria
Alternate-month corticosteroid and cytotoxic drug therapy				
Ponticelli et al[26,25,28]	RCT	Plasma creatinine ≤ 150 µmol/L Proteinuria > 3.5 g/day	Methylprednisolone alternating monthly with chlorambucil (n = 42) vs.control (n = 39) for 6 months	Treatment favored remission of nephrotic syndrome and preservation of renal function
Ponticelli et al[27]	RCT	Plasma creatinine ≤ 150 µmol/L Proteinuria > 3.5 g/day	Methylprednisolone alternating monthly with chlorambucil (n = 45) vs. methylprednisolone alone (n = 47) for 6 months	Combination drug regimen associated with earlier remission of the nephrotic syndrome
Reichert et al[46]	RCT	Nephrotic syndrome and deteriorating renal function	Methylprednisolone alternating monthly with chlorambucil (n = 9) vs. monthly pulse cyclophosphamide and pulse methylprednisolone every 2 months (n = 9) for 6 months	Renal function improved on chlorambucil regimen but not on pulse cyclophosphamide
Ponticelli et al[29]	RCT	Plasma creatinine ≤ 150 µmol/L Proteinuria > 3.5 g/day	Methylprednisolone alternating monthly with either chlorambucil (n = 50) or cyclophosphamide (n = 45) for 6 months	Regimens were equally effective in inducing remission of the nephrotic syndrome and preserving renal function
Intermittent monthly pulses of cyclophosphamide				
Falk et al[56]	RCT	Deteriorating renal function or persistent nephrotic syndrome with morbid complications	Pulse methylprednisolone, oral corticosteroids, and 6 months of i.v. cyclophosphamide (n = 13) vs alternate-day prednisone alone (n = 13)	Combination treatment did not improve renal outcomes

239

Table 24.2 Selected studies of immunosuppressive drug regimens (cont'd)

Reference	Design	Baseline	Treatment	Outcome
Intermittent monthly pulses of cyclophosphamide				
Reichert et al[46]	RCT	Nephrotic syndrome and deteriorating renal function	Methylprednisolone alternating monthly with chlorambucil (n = 9) vs. monthly pulse cyclophosphamide and pulse methylprednisolone every 2 months (n = 9) for 6 months	Renal function improved on chlorambucil regimen but not on pulse cyclophosphamide
Daily oral cyclophosphamide				
Donadio et al[68]	RCT	GFR 33–117 mL/min/1.73 m² Proteinuria 2–17 g/day	Cyclophosphamide (n = 11) vs no drug (n = 11) for 1 year	No difference in proteinuria, renal function or morphology between groups after treatment
West et al[51] and Jindal et al[52]	Nonrandomized concurrent controls	Impaired renal function and nephrotic proteinuria	Cyclophosphamide for 8–54 months (n = 9) vs control (n = 17)	Treatment favored remission of nephrotic syndrome and preservation of renal function
Bruns et al[53]	Case series	Progressive renal dysfunction Proteinuria > 3.5 g/day	Cyclophosphamide (n = 11) and prednisone for up to 1 year	Plasma creatinine and proteinuria decreased significantly
Murphy et al[69]	RCT	Plasma creatinine 50–280 µmol/L Proteinuria 0.5–13 g/day (13 patients in each group were nephrotic)	Cyclophosphamide for 6 months plus dipyridamole and warfarin for 2 years (n = 19) vs no treatment (n = 21)	Greater reduction in proteinuria observed in the treatment group
Branten et al[54]	Randomized and nonrandomized treatment assignments	Nephrotic syndrome and deteriorating renal function	Methylprednisolone alternating monthly with chlorambucil for 6 months (n = 15) vs. cyclophosphamide for 1 year plus corticosteroids (n = 17)	Cyclophosphamide regimen was associated with more sustained improvement in renal function, more frequent remissions of proteinuria, and fewer adverse effects that interrupted treatment.
Cyclosporine				
Cattran et al[57]	RCT	Declining renal function Persistent proteinuria ≥ 3.5 g/day	Cyclosporine (n = 9) vs. placebo (n = 8)	Average proteinuria and rate of renal function deterioration were reduced in the cyclosporine group, but not the placebo group
Cattran et al[30]	RCT	Creatinine clearance ≥ 42 mL/min/1.73 m² Nephrotic-range proteinuria despite at least 8 weeks of prednisone ≥ 1 mg/kg/day	Cyclosporine plus low-dose prednisone (n = 28) vs. placebo (n = 23) plus low-dose prednisone	Complete or partial remissions of proteinuria in 75% of the cyclosporine group and 22% of the placebo group; 50% of remissions relapsed in both groups

CSAINS, Collaborative Study of the Adult Idiopathic Nephrotic Syndrome; GFR, glomerular filtration rate; RCT, randomized controlled trial.

argued that differences in criteria for selection of patients and in treatment regimens may have contributed to differences in outcomes observed in these three clinical trials. Admission to the US Collaborative Study was limited to patients with somewhat better renal function than permitted at entry into the other two trials. The US Collaborative Study employed a higher dose of prednisone than used in the Toronto Glomerulonephritis Study and permitted a longer course of prednisone (that included a tapering schedule and retreatment for relapses) than was used in the British Medical Research Council Trial. These considerations raise the possibility that a course of alternate-day prednisone, modeled after the regimen used in the US Collaborative Study, may be effective for some patients without excessive toxicity. However, relapses of proteinuria occurred in a substantial number of prednisone-treated patients in the US Collaborative Study. Consequently, corticosteroids alone failed to increase the rate of long-term remissions of proteinuria in each of these controlled trials. Furthermore, corticosteroids appeared to prevent deterioration in renal function only in the US Collaborative Trial; the apparent efficacy of corticosteroid therapy in this study may reflect the unusually high incidence of adverse outcomes in the control group. The aggregate impression is that corticosteroid therapy offers only marginal benefits, if any. Consequently, investigators have sought to identify combination immunosuppressive drug regimens that might be more beneficial (Table 24.2).

Nephrotic syndrome complicated by high-risk features (glomerular filtration rate ≥ 50 mL/min)

Several studies support the value of cytotoxic drug regimens that combine corticosteroids with either chlorambucil or cyclophosphamide for the treatment of patients with idiopathic membranous nephropathy, nephrotic syndrome, and well-preserved renal function (see Table 24.2).

Chlorambucil

The most convincing evidence has emerged from the multicenter, prospective, randomized clinical trials of Ponticelli and colleagues. They have shown that a 6-month regimen of alternate-month corticosteroids and chlorambucil reduces the risk of deterioration in renal function as well as the duration of the nephrotic syndrome.[25-28] The recommendation to employ chlorambucil and methylprednisolone for this subset of patients is supported by well-controlled clinical observations. However, a substantial number of patients are unable to tolerate the regimen. Ponticelli et al[28] reported that 4 of 42 patients in one study had to discontinue this therapy because of adverse effects (two because of peptic ulcers that developed while on methylprednisolone, one because of pneumonia, and one because of gastric intolerance to chlorambucil). The potential advantage of this approach must be balanced against the risks of malignancy, gonadal toxicity, reversible myelosuppression, infection, gastro-

intestinal intolerance, and hepatotoxicity associated with chlorambucil. Furthermore, patients should be informed that the long-term toxicities of this and other cytotoxic drug regimens for membranous nephropathy have not been fully defined.

Cyclophosphamide

Since most nephrologists are more familiar with cyclophosphamide than chlorambucil, Ponticelli et al[29] conducted a multicenter controlled clinical trial to compare the efficacy and toxicity of these two alkylating agents when alternated with corticosteroids for the treatment of idiopathic membranous nephropathy. The two regimens appeared to be equally effective, and both are recommended for the treatment of this subset of patients (Table 24.3). The authors observed a complete or partial remission of the nephrotic syndrome in 82% of patients in the chlorambucil group and 93% of patients in the cyclophosphamide group. Approximately 30% of patients in each group experienced a relapse between 6 and 30 months after stopping treatment. Renal function tended to improve and then stabilize in both treatment groups. Notably, fewer patients stopped therapy prematurely because of adverse events in the cyclophosphamide group (4.5%) than in the chlorambucil group (12%).

Cyclosporine

A randomized clinical trial reported by Cattran et al[30] compared a 6-month course of cyclosporine to placebo in 51 patients with steroid-resistant idiopathic membranous nephropathy, nephrotic-range proteinuria, and a creatinine clearance ≥ 42 mL/min per 1.73 m^2. Adverse effects of cyclosporine included reversible decrements in renal

---

Table 24.3 Idiopathic membranous nephropathy: proposed treatment for patients with strong indications for immunosuppression (GFR ≥ 50 mL/min)

*Recommended approaches**
Alternate-month corticosteroids and chlorambucil for 6 months
   Months 1, 3, and 5: methylprednisolone 1 g i.v. daily for 3 days followed by 0.4 mg/kg/day orally for 27 days
   Months 2, 4, and 6: chlorambucil 0.2 mg/kg/day orally for 30 days
Alternate-month corticosteroids and cyclophosphamide for 6 months
   Months 1, 3, and 5: methylprednisolone (as above)
   Months 2, 4, and 6: cyclophosphamide 2.5 mg/kg/day (initial dose) orally for 30 days

*Alternative approaches**
Cyclosporine 3.5 mg/kg/day (initial dose) and low-dose prednisone for 6–12 months.
No immunosuppression

GFR, glomerular filtration rate.
*Treatment includes angiotensin-converting enzyme inhibition, angiotensin II receptor antagonists, hydroxymethylglutaryl coenzyme A reductase inhibitors, and diuretics as needed.

function, an increased occurrence and severity of hypertension, and nausea. Two patients in each group progressed to renal insufficiency, defined as a doubling of serum creatinine. A complete or partial remission of proteinuria evolved by week 26 in 75% of the cyclosporine group and 22% of the control group (P < 0.001). By week 72, relapse occurred in approximately 50% of patients in each group. The authors questioned whether the high relapse rate observed in this study was related to the dose (3.5 mg/kg/day) or the duration of treatment (6 months rather than 1 year).

Fritsche et al[31] analyzed data from the German Cyclosporine in Nephrotic Syndrome Study Group in an effort to estimate the optimal duration of cyclosporine therapy for idiopathic membranous nephropathy. They observed that complete remissions occurred up to 20 months after starting cyclosporine; the median treatment period prior to a complete remission was 225 days in this study. Presently, there is insufficient information to determine the optimal duration of cyclosporine therapy for idiopathic membranous nephropathy. The high-risk characteristics of these patients justify a 6–12 month course of cyclosporine if the patient can be followed very closely (initially weekly, then biweekly). The hazard of chronic cyclosporine nephrotoxicity can be minimized by initiating treatment at 3.5 mg/kg/day or less and by frequent dose adjustments in order to avoid an increase of 30% or more in serum creatinine over baseline levels. Unfortunately, relapse of nephrotic syndrome has been observed in approximately one-third of patients even after extended courses of cyclosporine for idiopathic membranous nephropathy.[32]

Mycophenolate mofetil

A small number of patients have received mycophenolate mofetil (MMF) for relapsing or resistant idiopathic membranous nephropathy. Briggs et al[33] observed substantial reductions in proteinuria in three patients treated with MMF monotherapy or in combination with low-dose corticosteroids; MMF doses less than 0.75 g twice daily appeared to be ineffective. Miller et al[34] treated 16 nephrotic patients who had failed to achieve a satisfactory response on corticosteroids, cytotoxic drugs, and/or cyclosporine. MMF (initial dose 500–2000 mg/day) was associated with a 50% reduction in proteinuria in six patients and a sustained partial remission in two patients. MMF was discontinued due to adverse events in two patients (one had persistent diarrhea and the other had varicella-zoster infection). Additional study is needed to determine the role of MMF for the treatment of idiopathic membranous nephropathy.

Nephrotic syndrome in elderly patients

Attention has been focused on the challenge of treating idiopathic membranous nephropathy in elderly patients. Considering that there is no evidence that corticosteroids alone improve clinical outcomes for this subgroup[35–37] and that these patients are at increased risk for complications associated with corticosteroid therapy, prednisone alone is

not recommended for elderly patients with idiopathic membranous nephropathy. Although there is preliminary evidence that alternate-month methylprednisolone and chlorambucil are more effective for this subgroup than corticosteroids alone, elderly patients appear to be particularly susceptible to the potential toxicities of methylprednisolone and chlorambucil.[35,36,38,39] Consequently, the initial dose of chlorambucil should be reduced to 0.1 mg/kg/day and pulse methylprednisolone should be eliminated or infused over at least an hour to reduce the risk of cardiac arrhythmias.[35,36]

Bizzarri et al[40] evaluated a regimen in which corticosteroids were alternated monthly with cyclophosphamide for 6 months or more. They observed a comparable number of complete or partial remissions of the nephrotic syndrome in 17 elderly (> 65 years) and 27 younger (< 65 years) patients. On average, renal function declined at approximately the same rate in the two age groups.

Zent et al[37] reported a retrospective study in which 74 elderly patients with idiopathic membranous nephropathy were compared with 249 younger patients with the same diagnosis. One-third of the elderly patients received corticosteroids alone and approximately 10% received other immunosuppressive drugs. These authors found no evidence that prednisone therapy improved outcomes in elderly patients. Comparable numbers of elderly and younger patients achieved a complete remission of proteinuria. Although more elderly patients developed chronic renal insufficiency (creatinine clearance < 50 mL/min), this appears to reflect an age-related loss of renal function reserve prior to disease onset rather than a difference in the rate of renal function deterioration after the disease became manifest. The study concludes that steroid and cytotoxic drug treatments for the elderly should be limited to those at high risk for deterioration of renal function because of the increased incidence of treatment-associated adverse events in this population of patients.

To more fully evaluate the impact of immunosuppressive drug treatments for idiopathic membranous nephropathy, Piccoli et al[41] estimated quality-adjusted life expectancy in years (QALY) associated with various regimens. For a 60-year-old nephrotic patient, the advantage of alternate-month methylprednisolone and chlorambucil therapy was approximately 3.3 QALY more than supportive therapy and 1.2 QALY more than a regimen of intravenous pulse and alternate-day oral methylprednisolone alone. Concern has been expressed that the advantage of alternate-month methylprednisolone and chlorambucil, estimated as QALY, is modest for elderly patients. On the other hand, some elderly patients with severe symptomatic nephrotic syndrome may prefer this approach.

Nephrotic syndrome complicated by high-risk features (glomerular filtration rate < 50 mL/min)

Several immunosuppressive drug regimens have been proposed for the treatment of nephrotic patients with impaired and declining renal function (Table 24.4); none is clearly superior. Pulse methylprednisolone regimens have yielded favorable short-term outcomes in some patients, but long-term outcomes have been less satisfactory.[42] Combining corticosteroids and azathioprine has led to inconsistent results in this population of patients.[43–45] Studies of MMF have not focused on patients with impaired renal function.

Chlorambucil

Although there is considerable experience using alternate-month corticosteroids and chlorambucil for patients with well-preserved renal function, efforts to apply this regimen to patients with reduced glomerular filtration rate (GFR) have met with discordant results and a relatively high incidence of adverse events. To address this issue, modified dosage schedules have been studied for azotemic patients.[46–49] A reduced dose of chlorambucil (~ 0.12 mg/kg/day) appears to ameliorate toxicity in patients with impaired renal function.[50] Concerns regarding the toxicity of corticosteroids in these patients has led several investigators to omit pulse methylprednisolone or to use alternate-day rather than daily oral prednisolone. Because the aggregate experience suggests that intravenous pulse methylprednisolone may contribute to favorable short-term outcomes in patients with declining renal function,[42,48,49] 0.5–1 g doses of pulse methylprednisolone are recommended, rather than omitting this component of the therapy (Table 24.4).

Table 24.4 Idiopathic membranous nephropathy: treatment for patients with strong indications for immunosuppression (GFR < 50 mL/min)

Recommended approaches*
Cyclosporine 3.5 mg/kg/day (initial dose) for 12 months
Cyclophosphamide 1.5 mg/kg/day (initial dose) for 1 year plus prednisone 1 mg/kg every other day for 8 weeks; then taper to 0.25 mg/kg every other day for the duration of therapy
Alternate-month corticosteroids and chlorambucil for 6 months
    Months 1, 3, and 5: methylprednisolone 0.5–1.0 g i.v. daily for 3 days followed by 0.4 mg/kg/day (or 1 mg/kg every other day) orally for 27 days
    Months 2, 4, and 6: chlorambucil 0.12 mg/kg/day (initial dose) orally for 30 days
Alternate-month corticosteroids and cyclophosphamide for 6 months
    Months 1, 3, and 5: methylprednisolone (as above)
    Months 2, 4, and 6: cyclophosphamide 1.5–2.0 mg/kg/day orally for 30 days

Alternative approaches*
Methylprednisolone 1.0 g i.v. daily for 3 days plus prednisone 1 mg/kg every other day for 4 weeks followed by gradual tapering; combined with azathioprine (1–2 mg/kg/day)
No immunosuppression

GFR, glomerular filtration rate.
*Treatment includes angiotensin-converting enzyme inhibition, angiotensin II receptor antagonists, hydroxymethylglutaryl coenzyme A reductase inhibitors, and diuretics as needed.

Cyclophosphamide

Several regimens that combine corticosteroids and cyclophosphamide may be considered for the treatment of nephrotic patients with impaired renal function (see Table 24.2). There is evidence that cyclophosphamide can be substituted for chlorambucil in the Ponticelli regimen for patients with well-preserved renal function, but this approach has not been rigorously evaluated for patients with impaired and declining renal function. Intuitively, this appears to be a reasonable (but unproven) approach given the extensive experience employing cyclophosphamide for the treatment of severe glomerular diseases and the relatively brief (3-month) exposure to a cytotoxic drug in the Ponticelli regimen.

Alternatively, several groups[51–54] have studied daily oral cyclophosphamide and corticosteroids for a year or more in patients with declining renal function. Renal function stabilized or improved and partial remissions of nephrotic proteinuria were observed in most patients treated by investigators in Toronto[51,52] and Pittsburgh.[53] These results were superior to those observed among concurrent (non-randomized) control subjects,[51,52] but serious complications of treatment were observed including leukopenia, infections, amenorrhea, and cancer. Extended oral cyclophosphamide regimens for the treatment of Wegener granulomatosis have been associated an 11-fold increase in the incidence of lymphomas and a 33-fold increase in bladder cancers.[55]

In an effort to reduce the toxicity of cytotoxic drug regimens, several investigators have evaluated intermittent pulse regimens of cyclophosphamide and methylprednisolone for high-risk patients with progressive disease. Falk et al[56] observed that an intensive regimen of monthly pulse cyclophosphamide (for 6 months), pulse methylprednisolone (for 3 days), and alternate-day prednisone (starting at 1 mg/kg) was not superior to alternate-day prednisone alone (starting at 2 mg/kg) for patients with deteriorating renal function or persistent proteinuria associated with morbid complications.

A few prospective studies have compared cytotoxic drug regimens for the treatment of patients with nephrotic syndrome and declining renal function. Reichert et al[46] showed that a 6-month regimen of alternate-month methylprednisolone and chlorambucil was more effective than a 6-month regimen of monthly pulse cyclophosphamide and alternate-month pulse methylprednisolone. Branten et al[54] reported that daily oral cyclophosphamide and corticosteroids for a year was more effective than alternate-month methylprednisolone and chlorambucil for 6 months. Stable renal function and remissions of proteinuria were observed more frequently after cyclophosphamide treatment for 1 year. Treatment was modified, interrupted, or terminated prematurely because of adverse effects significantly more frequently in the chlorambucil group than in the cyclophosphamide group. Although 60% of the patients were randomly assigned to their treatment groups, this was a complex study in which treatment strategies evolved over time. Initially, patients were randomized to alternate-month chlorambucil and corticosteroids (*n* = 9) versus intravenous pulses of cyclophosphamide and methylprednisolone. When the latter regimen proved to be ineffective, seven patients were treated in a pilot study of daily oral cyclophosphamide and corticosteroids for a year. Subsequently, patients were randomly assigned to alternate-month chlorambucil and corticosteroids for 6 months (n = 5) versus daily oral cyclophosphamide and corticosteroids (n = 5) for 1 year. Five patients unwilling to participate in the study received the cyclophosphamide regimen. Consequently, the treatment comparison included some patients who were not randomized concurrently and others who were not randomized at all. Additional studies are needed to compare the risks and benefits of various cytotoxic drug regimens for nephrotic patients with declining renal function.

Cyclosporine

Future studies should include comparisons of the long-term efficacy and toxicity of cyclosporine and cytotoxic drug regimens. There has been interest in cyclosporine for patients with idiopathic membranous nephropathy, persistent nephrotic-range proteinuria, and declining renal function since Cattran et al[57] reported the results of a controlled clinical trial in which 17 patients with these characteristics were randomized to receive either cyclosporine (initially 3.5 mg/kg/day in two divided doses) or placebo for 12 months. Proteinuria and the rate of decline in creatinine clearance decreased significantly in the cyclosporine group (but not in the placebo group). Improvement in renal function and proteinuria was sustained in 75% of patients for a mean follow-up period of 21 months after cyclosporine was discontinued. Six of the nine cyclosporine-treated patients experienced elevations in serum creatinine (≥ 30%) that reversed in five after dose reduction. Cyclosporine-treated patients also tended to require additional antihypertensive medication to maintain adequate blood pressure control. Geddes and Cattran[58] have recommended cyclosporine as preferred immunosuppressive therapy for patients with high-grade proteinuria and renal insufficiency. On the other hand, Ponticelli and Villa[59] have underscored the nephrotoxic potential of cyclosporine and have suggested that patients with impaired renal function (creatinine clearance < 60 mL/min), severe hypertension, or severe interstitial fibrosis and tubular atrophy should not receive cyclosporine.

Summary

Clearly, the optimal immunosuppressive therapy for patients with persistent high-grade proteinuria and renal insufficiency has not been determined. Table 24.4 depicts several recommended treatments. While the recommendation to offer cyclosporine to patients with impaired renal function has been debated,[58,59] evidence supporting this approach includes a small, randomized, controlled clinical trial.[57] Toxicities are largely reversible if the cyclosporine dose is adjusted in response to early signs of toxicity detected by very close follow-up of these patients. Studies supporting the use of alternate-month corticosteroid and cytotoxic drug therapy in patients with renal dysfunction include a small, randomized, controlled clinical trial[46] and several uncontrolled case series.[47–50]

Renal function has tended to improve or stabilize at least transiently and toxicity has been modulated by dose reduction. Alternative cytotoxic drug regimens have been studied as well (see Table 24.2). Intermittent pulse cyclophosphamide has not proven to be effective.[46,56] Daily oral cyclophosphamide and corticosteroids for 1 year or more has been employed as salvage therapy for patients with progressive renal failure. Evidence supporting this approach includes a nonrandomized trial with concurrent controls,[51,52] a clinical study that included randomized and nonrandomized patients,[54] and uncontrolled case series.[53] Although Branten et al[54] noted fewer short-term adverse effects among patients receiving daily oral cyclophosphamide and corticosteroids for 1 year than among those treated with alternate-month chlorambucil and corticosteroids for 6 months, it is the long-term toxicities of extended courses of daily oral cytotoxic drug therapy that prompt the greatest concern. Thus, daily oral cyclophosphamide and corticosteroids should be reserved for patients manifesting progressive renal insufficiency who understand and accept the potential long-term toxicities of this approach. Studies of experimental approaches offer the hope that less toxic interventions may be available in the future.[60–67]

At present, the choice of cyclosporine, cytotoxic drug therapy, or no immunosuppression should reflect the priorities of the individual patient as well as comorbid conditions that might affect the risk profile of each approach. Furthermore, attention should be focused on the comprehensive management of cardiovascular risk factors that are frequently observed in this population of patients. Modulation of nonimmunologic factors that influence the rate of progression of chronic renal disease are likely to contribute to quality of life and to extend survival by delaying the need for dialysis. Thus, dietary modifications, diuretics, ACE inhibitors, angiotensin II receptor antagonists, and lipid-lowering agents are important therapeutic interventions that should be considered in all patients with membranous nephropathy in order to reduce the morbidity and mortality associated with nephrotic syndrome.

References

1. Cameron JS, Glassock RJ: The natural history and outcome of the nephrotic syndrome. In Cameron JS, Glassock RJ (eds): The Nephrotic Syndrome. New York: Marcel Dekker, 1987, pp 999–1033.
2. Falk RJ, Jennette JC, Nachman PH: Primary glomerular diseases. In Brenner BM (ed): The Kidney, 6th edn. Philadelphia: WB Saunders, 2000, pp 1263–1349.
3. Glassock RJ: Secondary membranous glomerulonephritis. Nephrol Dial Transplant 1992;7(Suppl 1):64–71.
4. Cattran DC, Pei Y, Greenwood C: Predicting progression in membranous glomerulonephritis. Nephrol Dial Transplant 1992;7(Suppl 1):48–52.
5. Noel LH, Zanetti M, Droz D, et al: Long-term prognosis of idiopathic membranous glomerulonephritis: study of 116 untreated patients. Am J Med 1979;66:82–90.
6. Ordonez JD, Hiatt RA, Killebrew EJ, et al: The increased risk of coronary heart disease associated with nephrotic syndrome. Kidney Int 1993;44:638–642.
7. Sarasin FP, Schifferli JA: Prophylactic oral anticoagulation in nephrotic patients with idiopathic membranous nephropathy. Kidney Int 1994;45:578–585.

8. Hogan SL, Muller KE, Jennette JC, et al: A review of therapeutic studies of idiopathic membranous glomerulopathy. Am J Kidney Dis 1995;25:862–875.
9. Davison AM, Cameron JS, Kerr DNS, et al: The natural history of renal function in untreated idiopathic membranous glomerulonephritis in adults. Clin Nephrol 1984;22:61–67.
10. Pei Y, Cattran D, Greenwood C: Predicting chronic renal insufficiency in idiopathic membranous glomerulonephritis. Kidney Int 1992;42:960–966.
11. Cattran DC, Pei Y, Greenwood CMT, et al: Validation of a predictive model of idiopathic membranous nephropathy: its clinical and research implications. Kidney Int 1997;51:901–907.
12. Thomas DM, Hillis AN, Coles GA, et al: Enalapril can treat the proteinuria of membranous glomerulonephritis without detriment to systemic or renal hemodynamics. Am J Kidney Dis 1991;18:38–43.
13. Gansevoort RT, Heeg JE, Vriesendorp R, et al: Antiproteinuric drugs in patients with idiopathic membranous glomerulopathy. Nephrol Dial Transplant 1992;7(Suppl 1):91–96.
14. Ruggenenti P, Mosconi L, Vendramin G, et al: ACE inhibition improves glomerular size selectivity in patients with idiopathic membranous nephropathy and persistent nephrotic syndrome. Am J Kidney Dis 2000;35:381–391.
15. Joint National Committee on Prevention, Detection, Evaluation, and Treatment of High Blood Pressure: The Sixth Report of the Joint National Committee on Prevention, Detection, Evaluation, and Treatment of High Blood Pressure. Arch Intern Med 1997;157:2413–2446.
16. Marcantoni C, Jafar TH, Oldrizzi L, et al: The role of systemic hypertension in the progression of nondiabetic renal disease. Kidney Int 2000;57(Suppl 75):44–48.
17. Ruilope LM, Casal MC, Praga M, et al: Additive antiproteinuric effect of converting enzyme inhibition and a low dose protein intake. J Am Soc Nephrol 1992;3:1307–1311.
18. Radhakrishnan J, Appel AS, Valeri A, et al: The nephrotic syndrome, lipids, and risk factors for cardiovascular disease. Am J Kidney Dis 1993;22:135–142.
19. Golper TA, Illingworth DR, Morris CD, et al: Lovastatin in the treatment of multifactorial hyperlipidemia associated with proteinuria. Am J Kidney Dis 1989;13:312–320.
20. Spitalewitz S, Porush JG, Cattran D, et al: Treatment of hyperlipidemia in the nephrotic syndrome: the effects of pravastatin therapy. Am J Kidney Dis 1993;22:143–150.
21. Thomas ME, Harris KPG, Ramaswamy C, et al: Simvastatin therapy for hypercholesterolemic patients with nephrotic syndrome or significant proteinuria. Kidney Int 1993;44:1124–1129.
22. Collaborative Study of the Adult Idiopathic Nephrotic Syndrome: A controlled study of short-term prednisone treatment in adults with membranous nephropathy. N Engl J Med 1979;301:1301–1306.
23. Cattran DC, Delmore T, Roscoe J, et al: A randomized controlled trial of prednisone in patients with idiopathic membranous nephropathy. N Engl J Med 1989;320:210–215.
24. Cameron JS, Healy MJR, Adu D: The Medical Research Council Trial of short-term high-dose alternate day prednisolone in idiopathic membranous nephropathy with nephrotic syndrome in adults. Q J Med 1990;74:133–156.
25. Ponticelli C, Zucchelli P, Passerini P, et al: A randomized trial of methylprednisolone and chlorambucil in idiopathic membranous nephropathy. N Engl J Med 1989;320:8–13.
26. Ponticelli C, Zucchelli P, Imbasciati E, et al: Controlled trial of methylprednisolone and chlorambucil in idiopathic membranous nephropathy. N Engl J Med 1984;310:946–950.
27. Ponticelli C, Zucchelli P, Passerini P, et al: Methylprednisolone plus chlorambucil as compared with methylprednisolone alone for the treatment of idiopathic membranous nephropathy. N Engl J Med 1992;327:599–603.
28. Ponticelli C, Zucchelli P, Passerini P, et al: A 10-year follow-up of a randomized study with methylprednisolone and chlorambucil in membranous nephropathy. Kidney Int 1995;48:1600–1604.
29. Ponticelli C, Altieri P, Scolar F, et al: A randomized study comparing methylprednisolone plus chlorambucil versus methylprednisolone plus cyclophosphamide in idiopathic membranous nephropathy. J Am Soc Nephrol 1998;9:444–450.
30. Cattran DC, Appel GB, Hebert LA, et al: Cyclosporine in patients with steroid-resistant membranous nephropathy: a randomized trial. Kidney Int 2001;59:1484–1490.
31. Fritsche L, Budde K, Farber L, et al: Treatment of membranous glomerulopathy with cyclosporin A: how much patience is required? Nephrol Dial Transplant 1999;14:1036–1038.
32. Rostoker G, Belghiti D, Ben Maadi A, et al: Long-term cyclosporin A therapy for severe idiopathic membranous nephropathy. Nephron 1993;63:335–341.
33. Briggs WA, Choi MJ, Scheel PJ: Successful mycophenolate mofetil treatment of glomerular disease. Am J Kidney Dis 1998;31:213–217.
34. Miller G, Zimmerman R, Radhakrishnan J, et al: Use of mycophenolate mofetil in resistant membranous nephropathy. Am J Kidney Dis 2000;36:250–256.
35. Ponticelli C, Passerini P, Cresseri D: Primary glomerular diseases in the elderly. Glomerulonephritis in the elderly. Geriatr Nephrol Urol 1996;6:105–112.
36. Cameron JS: Nephrotic syndrome in the elderly. Semin Nephrol 1996;16:319–329.
37. Zent R, Nagai R, Cattran DC: Idiopathic membranous nephropathy in the elderly: a comparative study. Am J Kidney Dis 1997;29:200–206.
38. Passerini P, Como G, Vigano E, et al: Idiopathic membranous nephropathy in the elderly. Nephrol Dial Transplant 1993;8:1321–1325.
39. Rollino C, Roccatello D, Vallero A: Membranous glomerulonephritis in the elderly. Is therapy still worthwhile? Geriatr Nephrol Urol 1995;5:97–104.
40. Bizzarri D, Imperiali P, Duranti E, et al: Idiopathic membranous glomerulonephritis in the elderly. Contrib Nephrol 1993;105:65–70.
41. Piccoli A, Pillon L, Passerini P, et al: Therapy for idiopathic membranous nephropathy: tailoring the choice by decision analysis. Kidney Int 1994;45:1193–1202.
42. Short CD, Solomon LR, Gokal R, et al: Methylprednisolone in patients with membranous nephropathy and declining renal function. Q J Med 1987;65:929–940.
43. Bone JM, Rostom R, Williams PS: "Progressive" versus "indolent" idiopathic membranous glomerulonephritis. Q J Med 1997;90:699–706.
44. Ahuja M, Goumenos D, Shortland JR, et al: Does immunosuppression with prednisolone and azathioprine alter the progression of idiopathic membranous nephropathy? Am J Kidney Dis 1999;34:521–529.
45. Brown JH, Douglas AF, Murphy BG, et al: Treatment of renal failure in idiopathic membranous nephropathy with azathioprine and prednisolone. Nephrol Dial Transplant 1998;13:443–448.
46. Reichert LJM, Huysmans FTM, Assmann K, et al: Preserving renal function in patients with membranous nephropathy: daily oral chlorambucil compared with intermittent monthly pulses of cyclophosphamide. Ann Intern Med 1994;121:328–333.
47. Mathieson PW, Turner AN, Maidment CGH, et al: Prednisolone and chlorambucil treatment in idiopathic membranous nephropathy with deteriorating renal function. Lancet 1988;ii:869–872.
48. Warwick GL, Geddes CC, Jones Boulton JM: Prednisolone and chlorambucil therapy for idiopathic membranous nephropathy with progressive renal failure. Q J Med 1994;87:223–229.
49. Brunkhorst R, Wrenger E, Koch KM: Low-dose prednisolone/chlorambucil therapy in patients with severe membranous glomerulonephritis. Clin Invest 1994;72:277–282.
50. Mathieson P: Treating progressive and indolent MGN. Q J Med 1998;91:167.
51. West ML, Jindal KK, Bear RA, et al: A controlled trial of cyclophosphamide in patients with membranous glomerulonephritis. Kidney Int 1987;32:579–584.
52. Jindal K, West M, Bear R, et al: Long-term benefits of therapy with cyclophosphamide and prednisone in patients with membranous glomerulonephritis and impaired renal function. Am J Kidney Dis 1992;19:61–67.
53. Bruns FJ, Adler S, Fraley DS, et al: Sustained remission of membranous glomerulonephritis after cyclophosphamide and prednisone. Ann Intern Med 1991;114:725–730.
54. Branten AJW, Reichert LJM, Koene RAP, et al: Oral cyclophosphamide versus chlorambucil in the treatment of patients with membranous nephropathy and renal insufficiency. Q J Med 1998;91:359–366.
55. Hoffman GS, Kerr GS, Leavitt RY, et al: Wegener granulomatosis: an analysis of 158 patients. Ann Intern Med 1992;116:488–498.
56. Falk RJ, Hogan SL, Muller KE, et al: Treatment of progressive membranous glomerulopathy. A randomized trial comparing cyclophosphamide and corticosteroids with corticosteroids alone. Ann Intern Med 1992;116:438–445.

57. Cattran DC, Greenwood C, Ritchie S, et al: A controlled trial of cyclosporine in patients with progressive membranous nephropathy. Kidney Int 1995;47:1130–1135.

58. Geddes CC, Cattran DC: The treatment of idiopathic membranous nephropathy. Semin Nephrol 2000;20:299–308.

59. Ponticelli C, Villa M: Does cyclosporin have a role in the treatment of membranous nephropathy? Nephrol Dial Transplant 1999;14:23–25.

60. Palla R, Cirami C, Panichi V, et al: Intravenous immunoglobulin therapy of membranous nephropathy. Efficacy and safety. Clin Nephrol 1991;35:98–104.

61. Nangaku M, Pippin J, Richardson CA, et al: Beneficial effects of systemic immunoglobulin in experimental membranous nephropathy. Kidney Int 1996;50:2054–2062.

62. Yokoyama H, Goshima S, Wada T, et al: The short- and long-term outcomes of membranous nephropathy treated with intravenous immune globulin therapy. Nephrol Dial Transplant 1999;14:2379–2386.

63. Ducloux D, Bresson-Vautrin C, Chalopin J-M: Use of pentoxifyllin in membranous nephropathy. Lancet 2001;357:1672–1673.

64. Wang Y, Hu Q, Madri JA, et al: Amelioration of lupus-like autoimmune disease in NZB/W F1 mice after treatment with a blocking monoclonal antibody specific for complement component C5. Proc Natl Acad Sci USA 1996;93:8563–8568.

65. Esnault VLM, Besnier D, Testa A, et al: Effect of protein A immunoadsorption in nephrotic syndrome of various etiologies. J Am Soc Nephrol 1999;10:2014–2017.

66. Al-Wakeel J, Mitwalli A, Tarif N, et al: Role of interferon-α in the treatment of primary glomerulonephritis. Am J Kidney Dis 1999;33:1142–1146.

67. Braun N, Frank J, Biesalski HK, et al: Antioxidative treatment retards progression of idiopathic membranous nephropathy. Nephron 2000;86:208–209.

68. Donadio JV, Holley KE, Anderson CF, Taylor WF: Controlled trial of cyclophosphamide in patients with membranous nephropathy. Kidney Int 1974;6:431–439.

69. Murphy BF, McDonald I, Fairley KF, Kincaid-Smith PS: Randomized controlled trial of cyclophosphamide, warfarin and dipyridamole in idiopathic membranous glomerulonephritis. Clin Nephrol 1992;37:229–234.

Idiopathic Membranoproliferative Glomerulonephritis

Peter Hewins and Caroline O.S. Savage

When is treatment of membranoproliferative glomerunephritis necessary?
General measures to retard the progression of glomerular disease
Corticosterroid therapy
Cytotoxic therapies
Antiplatelet agents and anticoagulants
Plasma exchange
Renal transplantation
Novel therapeutic possibilities

Membranoproliferative glomerulonephritis (MPGN) is an uncommon disease, present in 5–10% of renal biopsies. Hypocomplementemia is frequent and serum nephritic factors may be detected. Subdivision into types 1, 2, and 3 on the basis of electron microscopy likely still disguises considerable etiologic heterogeneity. These factors have frustrated efforts to determine best treatment strategies. Many cases are secondary to systemic disease, particularly infection or autoimmune disease. Most recently, the association with hepatitis C virus (HCV) infection was recognized. The extent of HCV infection among previously reported series of "idiopathic" MPGN probably varies geographically. Secondary cases must be systematically excluded, particularly before considering immunosuppression. Efforts to dissect pathogenic mechanisms in MPGN continue and the armamentarium of potential therapies available to treat glomerular disease grows. Although only limited recommendations are feasible at present, there is room for optimism with regard to their refinement.

When is treatment of membranoproliferative glomerulonephritis necessary?

The natural history of MPGN is widely regarded as aggressive, with 40–60% renal survival at 10 years, justifying treatment in a significant proportion of patients. Approximately 5% of cases spontaneously remit, most often those presenting as an acute postinfectious nephritis. Childhood MPGN initially progresses more slowly but beyond 10 years has a similar outcome to adult MPGN. Heavy proteinuria, renal impairment, hypertension, longer disease duration, glomerular sclerosis and crescents, and tubulointerstitial damage have been reported as adverse predictors, although not all studies have concurred.[1,2] The influence of tubulointerstitial damage on MPGN

progression was recently contested in a small study comparing MPGN with IgA nephropathy, possibly reflecting differences in the mechanisms of interstitial leukocyte infiltration.[3] Some studies suggest that type 2 MPGN has a worse outcome, although it is the least common type and patient numbers are consequently small. Much of the data on the natural history of MPGN relates to cohorts recruited from the 1960s onwards, and applicability to patients diagnosed today cannot necessarily be assumed. General measures employed in managing glomerular disease (see later) may affect progression and caution is essential when using historical data to justify potentially toxic treatments for MPGN, particularly because it is predominantly a disease of childhood and young adults.

General measures to retard the progression of glomerular disease (Fig. 25.1)

Data are now available that demonstrate the importance of aggressive blood pressure control and reducing proteinuria in all glomerular diseases. Although such measures cannot influence the causes of MPGN, they are achievable without major adverse effects and will very likely impact upon its progression. Angiotensin-converting enzyme (ACE) inhibitors and angiotensin II antagonists are agents of first choice, improving renal survival by altering renal hemodynamics and possibly also limiting leukocyte recruitment into the kidney. Statin therapy may also retard glomerular disease progression. Dietary salt restriction and cessation of smoking should not be overlooked. These measures should form the basis of therapy for all patients with MPGN. In the absence of progressive renal impairment or nephrotic proteinuria, no other treatment is warranted.

Corticosteroid therapy (Table 25.1)

West and colleagues have examined the effects of prolonged uncontrolled corticosteroid treatment in childhood MPGN. Most patients received alternate-day prednisolone (ADP) and some also received other immunosuppressants. In 71 patients, 10- and 20-year renal survival were calculated at 82 and 56% respectively from disease onset.[4] Survival from treatment initiation was not significantly different. Treatment was reportedly well tolerated. The outcome was favorable compared with that of a historical untreated group; however, it has been claimed that when disease onset and treatment initiation do not coincide, a spurious treatment benefit may arise by virtue

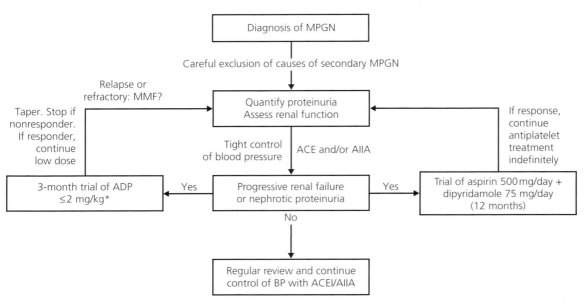

Figure 25.1 Flow diagram for suggested treatment of idiopathic membranoproliferative glomerulonephritis (MPGN). ACE, angiotensin-converting enzyme; ADP, alternate-day prednisolone; AIIA, angiotensin II antagonists; MMF, mycophenolate mofetil. *Use antiosteoporotic measures in adults and avoid alternate-day prednisolone at puberty due to growth delay.

Table 25.1 Trials of steroid therapy in childhood membranoproliferative glomerulonephritis

Reference	No. of patients	Type of trial	Treatment time*	Follow-up*	Regimen	Outcome
McEnery[4]	71 (only 50 ADP)	Uncontrolled	7.7 years	10.6 years	ADP 2–2.5 mg/kg tapered	10-year renal survival: 75% (cf. 50% historically)
Tarshish[7]	80 (47 ADP, 33 placebo)	Controlled	41 months	Unspecified, maximum 170 months	ADP 40 mg/m² vs. placebo	130-months renal survival: 61% ADP vs. 12% placebo ($P = 0.07$)
Ford et al[8]	19	Uncontrolled	38 months	6.5 years	DP or ADP 2 mg/kg tapered ± MP	GFR increased from 80 to 126 mL/min/1.73 m² and none nephrotic
Bergstein & Andreoli[9]	16 (all T1)	Uncontrolled	37 months	52 months	MP + ADP 2 mg/kg	GFR increased from 97 to 127 mL/min/1.73 m². Proteinuria decreased from 5.3 to 1.1 g/24 h
Braun et al[6†]	21 (T1) 25 (T3)	Uncontrolled	93 months (T1) 96 months (T3)	107 months (T1) 106 months (T3)	ADP 2 mg/kg tapered	Change in GFR: +6.3 mL/min (T1) +34.8 mL/min (T3)

ADP, alternate-day prednisolone; DP, daily prednisolone; GFR, glomerular filtration rate; MP, methylprednisolone; T1, type 1 membranoproliferative glomerulonephritis; T3, type 3 membranoproliferative glomerulonephritis.
*Mean treatment and follow-up duration.
†Patients in this trial were also included in the trial by McEnery (1990).[4]

of the survival of treated patients up until enrolment.[5] West has also suggested that type 3 MPGN is less responsive to ADP than type 1.[6] Final mean glomerular filtration rate (GFR) and renal survival were similar but mean GFR at entry was significantly lower in type 1 and stabilized while it fell in type 3. It is possible that type 1 MPGN simply progressed more rapidly, with a larger subset of patients already having lost renal function before enrolment. Subcapsular cataracts and growth failure occurred in 11 and 17% respectively. The International Study of Kidney Disease in Children failed to convincingly establish the benefits of extended ADP in proteinuric MPGN with preserved renal function in a randomized trial ($n = 80$).[7] The significance of improved renal survival in the treatment group at 130 months was marginal (62% vs. 12%, $P = 0.07$) and prior to this time-point the survival curves were much closer together. Furthermore, mean disease duration prior to entry was 9 months longer in the placebo arm, which would bias outcome if longer duration is a poor prognostic marker. Six ADP-treated children withdrew due to steroid-related adverse effects, including three with hypertensive encephalopathy (two placebo-treated children became encephalopathic). Renal function deteriorated in 7 of 12 children who withdrew from ADP. Hypertension was readily treatable in two uncontrolled studies of ADP plus methylprednisolone therapy ($n = 16$ and $n = 19$).[8,9] Indeed, the improved mean GFR in one trial probably resulted in part from antihypertensive therapy (89% received ACE inhibitors).[8] In the second trial, GFR and proteinuria improved after only 3 months of treatment, although mean duration of therapy was 37 months.[9] Data on the treatment of adult MPGN with steroids are extremely limited. In summary, corticosteroids may arrest disease progression in at least some patients but the cumulative doses used will be unacceptable to many nephrologists. It remains to be determined whether lower doses can be combined with other agents with safer effect.

Cytotoxic therapies (Table 25.2)

Many, largely uncontrolled, trials have combined cyclophosphamide with anticoagulant or antiplatelet treatments since the 1970s. None has demonstrated a convincing advantage in adults[10] and serious adverse effects were not uncommon. More recently, an uncontrolled study of steroids plus cyclophosphamide in a mixed population of children and adults reported complete remission in 15 of 19 patients and progression in only one after the first treatment cycle, although there were eight relapses.[11] Mean cyclophosphamide dose was 35 g per cycle and 40% experienced gonadal failure. In a separate study, pulsed cyclophosphamide (6 g total) plus prednisolone produced transient reductions in nephrotic proteinuria in six patients but all subsequently developed severe renal impairment.[12] A study of 10 children with aggressive MPGN suggested that azathioprine combined with prednisolone and antiplatelets/anticoagulants was effective.[13] Six remitted but follow-up was limited to 5 years.

Newer agents may be worth examining in MPGN. Mycophenolate mofetil (MMF) has been used in various refractory nephritides with encouraging results. One report has claimed efficacy of MMF combined with interferon-α in HCV-associated MPGN.[14] In addition to specifically inhibiting lymphocyte proliferation, MMF has been shown to limit mesangial and smooth muscle proliferation. A nephrotic patient with idiopathic MPGN exhibited a significant reduction in proteinuria in response to deoxspergualin.[15] However, the effect was transient and associated with significant leukopenia. It was suggested that improvement correlated with the disappearance of $CD16^+$ monocytes.

Table 25.2 Cytotoxic, antiplatelet, and anticoagulant trials in membranoproliferative glomerulonephritis (mainly adults)

Reference	No. of patients	Type of trial	Treatment time*	Follow-up*	Regimen	Outcome
Zimmerman et al[16]	18	Crossover	12 months	12–24 months	D + W vs. untreated	↓ reciprocal serum creatinine and ↓ proteinuria in treatment arm (unpaired analysis only)
Donadio et al[17,5]	40	Controlled	12 months	Up to 7 years[17] Up to > 10 years[5]	Aspirin + D vs. untreated	10-year renal survival: 49% treatment vs. 41% untreated (NS)
Schena & Cameron[10]	222 treated 79 untreated	Retrospective survey*	Variable	Variable 1–7.8 years	Variable: 188 had cytotoxics	Improved/stable renal function: 59.4% treatment vs. 51.9% untreated (NS)
Faedda et al[11]	19	Uncontrolled	10 months per cycle 21% ESRD	7.4 years	MP + CP + ADP	Proteinuria: ↓ from 3.9 to 0.9 g/24 h
Zauner et al[18]	18 (T1)	Controlled	36 months	36 months	Aspirin + D vs. untreated	Proteinuria: ↓ from 8.3 to 1.6 g/24 h ($P < 0.02$ treatment vs. untreated Change in creatinine: NS
Toz et al[12]	6	Uncontrolled	6 months	60 months	Pulse CP + DP	Proteinuria: ↓ at 6 months 100% ESRD at 60 months

ADP, alternate-day prednisolone; CP, cyclophosphamide; D, dipyridamole; DP, daily prednisolone; ESRD, endstage renal disease; MP, methylprednisolone; NS, not significant; T1, type 1 membranoproliferative glomerulonephritis; W, warfarin.
*Retrospective survey of trials in adult membranoproliferative glomerulonephritis up to 1988.

Antiplatelet agents and anticoagulants (Table 25.2)

Leukocyte infiltration, immune complex deposition, and complement derangement, although variable, provide a rationale for immunosuppressive therapy in MPGN. Antiplatelet therapies are employed on the basis of platelet activation and reduced half-life in MPGN. There is little evidence that platelets contribute to the glomerular immune deposits, although perturbations of platelet-activating factor release might direct leukocyte recruitment. Aspirin and dipyridamole could also act via inhibition of intrarenal prostaglandin synthesis or by altering the balance between thromboxane production and endothelial cell prostacyclin release. In a crossover trial ($n = 18$), unpaired analysis of warfarin plus dipyridamole vs. placebo showed stable creatinine in the treatment group but a significant increase in serum creatinine in the placebo group.[16] Proteinuria also fell significantly with treatment. However, analysis of patients completing crossover failed to support an overall benefit of treatment and there were significant bleeding risks, with one death from intracranial hemorrhage. Encouraging results from a randomized trial ($n = 40$) of aspirin plus dipyridamole vs. placebo were not confirmed by life-table analysis from initiation of treatment.[5,17] No effect on proteinuria was demonstrated in that trial but another study comparing aspirin and dipyridamole with placebo ($n = 18$ adults) reported significant reduction in heavy proteinuria with treatment and no excess bleeding.[18] Sizeable but comparable reductions in blood pressure were achieved in the two groups and more patients in the placebo arm received ACE inhibitors, suggesting that the treatment regimen had additional benefit. Aspirin may affect glomerular hemodynamics and leukocyte function in addition to platelet function. The prothrombotic nature of nephrosis also makes antiplatelet therapy attractive. Larger, prolonged, and controlled trials of antiplatelet agents using full-dose ACE inhibitors or angiotensin II antagonists and optimized blood pressure are warranted.

Plasma exchange

The benefits of plasma exchange in MPGN are unclear and the need for long-term treatment may limit its potential utility. A small number of patients have been treated, mainly late in the course of the disease and without added immunosuppression. Isolated cases have shown temporary improvement.[19] There is no evidence to suggest that patients with circulating nephritic factors respond more readily to plasma exchange.

Renal transplantation

Young patients with endstage renal disease are often compelling candidates for transplantation. MPGN types 1 and 2 recur in 20–30% and ≥ 50% of allograft recipients respectively.[20,21] No clear predictors of recurrence have been identified. Significant proteinuria is typically detected. The risk of graft loss has been calculated as 11.6% (range 3–26.7% in 164 cases) in recurrent type 1 MPGN and is probably similar in type 2 MPGN, although 50% loss has been reported.[21,22] Exclusion of cases where other factors contributed to graft loss may have underestimated the impact of disease recurrence. The influence of calcineurin inhibitor therapy on MPGN is uncertain but probably limited. MPGN recurrence may be more common with living related donation and in a second graft when it recurred in a first kidney.[20]

Novel therapeutic possibilities

New treatments for MPGN will require a clearer knowledge of its etiopathogenesis. The pathogenic significance of deranged complement regulation is made more intriguing by the development of type 2 MPGN in humans and animals with inherited deficiencies of factor H, the physiologic regulator of C3 convertase. Therapeutic manipulation of this system would be an attractive option. However, the relationship between complement and MPGN is likely a complex one and may not be a potential therapeutic target in all cases. Novel treatments to limit leukocyte-mediated damage to the kidney without exposing patients to dangerous adverse effects will be applicable in many glomerulonephritides including MPGN. At present, the patient with MPGN associated with significant proteinuria or renal impairment presents a challenge to the nephrologist.

References

1. D'Amico G, Ferrario F: Mesangiocapillary glomerulonephritis. J Am Soc Nephrol 1992;2:S159–S166.
2. Bennett WM, Fassett RG, Walker RG, et al: Mesangiocapillary glomerulonephritis type II: clinical features of progressive disease. Am J Kidney Dis 1989;13:469–476.
3. Soma J, Ootaka T, Sato H, et al: Tubulointerstitial changes are less important in membranoproliferative glomerulonephritis than in IgA nephropathy. Nephron 2000;86:230–231.
4. McEnery PT: Membranoproliferative glomerulonephritis: the Cincinnati experience. Cumulative renal survival from 1957 to 1989. J Paediatr 1990;116:S109–S114.
5. Donadio JV, Offord KP: Reassessment of treatment results in membranoproliferative glomerulonephritis, with emphasis on life-table analysis. Am J Kidney Disease 1989;14:445–451.
6. Braun MC, West CD, Strife F: Differences between membranoproliferative glomerulonephritis types I and III in long term response to an alternate day prednisolone regimen. Am J Kidney Dis 1999;34:1022–1032.
7. Tarshish P, Bernstein J, Tobin JN, Eldermann CM: Treatment of mesangiocapillary glomerulonephritis with alternate day prednisolone: a report of the International Study of Kidney Disease in Children. Pediatr Nephrol 1992;6:123–130.
8. Ford DM, Brisco DM, Shanley PF, Lum GM: Childhood membranoproliferative glomerulonephritis type 1: limited steroid therapy. Kidney Int 1992;41:1606–1612.
9. Bergstein JM, Andreoli SP: Response of type I membranoproliferative glomerulonephritis to pulse methylprednisolone and alternate day prednisolone. Pediatr Nephrol 1995;9:268–271.
10. Schena FP, Cameron JS: Treatment of proteinuric idiopathic glomerulonephritides in adults: a retrospective survey. Am J Med 1988;85:315–326.
11. Faedda R, Satta A, Tanda F, et al: Immunosuppressive treatment of membranoproliferative glomerulonephritis. Nephron 1994;67:59–65.
12. Toz H, Ok E, Unsal A, et al: Effectiveness of pulse cyclophosphamide

plus oral steroid therapy in idiopathic membranoproliferative glomerulonephritis. Nephrol Dial Transplant 1997;12:1081–1082.

13. Chapman SJ, Cameron JS, Chantler C, Turner D: Treatment of mesangiocapillary glomerulonephritis in children with combined immunosuppression and anticoagulation. Arch Dis Child 1980;55:446–451.

14. Reed MJ, Alexander GJM, Thiru S, Smith KGC: Hepatitis C associated glomerulonephritis: a novel therapeutic approach. Nephrol Dial Transplant 2001;16:869–871.

15. Hotta O, Furuta T, Chiba S, et al: Immunosuppressive effects of deoxyspergualin in proliferative glomerulonephritis. Am J Kidney Dis 1999;34:894–901.

16. Zimmerman SW, Moorthy AV, Dreher WH, et al: Prospective trial of warfarin and dipyridamole in patients with membranoproliferative glomerulonephritis. Am J Kidney Dis 1983;75:920–927.

17. Donadio JV, Anderson CF, Mitchell JC, et al: Membranoproliferative glomerulonephritis: a prospective clinical trial of platelet inhibitor therapy. N Engl J Med 1984;310:1421–1426.

18. Zauner I, Bohler J, Braun N, et al: Effect of aspirn and dipyridamole on proteinuria in idiopathic membranoproliferative glomerulonephritis: a multicentre prospective clinical trial. Nephrol Dial Transplant 1994;9:619–622.

19. McGinley E, Watkins R, McLay A, Boulton-Jones JM: Plasma exchange in the treatment of mesangiocapillary glomerulonephritis. Nephron 1985;40:385–390.

20. Andresdottir M, Assman KJM, Hoitsma AJ, et al: Recurrence of type 1 membranoproliferative glomerulonephritis after renal transplantation. Transplantation 1997;63:1628–1633.

21. Andresdottir M, Assman KJM, Hoitsma AJ, et al: Renal transplantation in patients with dense deposit disease: morphological characteristics of recurrent disease and clinical outcome. Nephrol Dial Transplant 1999;14:1723–1731.

22. Shimizu T, Tanabe K, Oshima T, et al: Recurrence of membranoproliferative glomerulonephritis in renal allografts. Transplant Proc 1998;30:3910–3913.

Amyloid, Fibrillary, and Other Glomerular Deposition Diseases

Joshua A. Schwimmer, Rosy E. Joseph, and Gerald B. Appel

Amyloidosis

Background

Amyloidosis comprises a group of chronic infiltrative diseases characterized by the extracellular deposition of insoluble protein fibrils in various organs.[1–3] The characteristic feature of all amyloid proteins is their ability to form a β-pleated sheet configuration on x-ray diffraction, which lends them unique staining properties. Moreover, all types of amyloid contain serum amyloid P (SAP) component, a 25-kDa glycoprotein constituting 15% of the amyloid. Amyloid fibrils are composed of different proteins, which determine the type of amyloid deposition. In primary (AL) amyloidosis the fibrils consist of part of the variable portion of immunoglobulin light chains. The most common form of secondary amyloidosis involving the kidneys is due to the deposition of serum amyloid A (SAA) protein in association with chronic inflammatory states. Other forms of amyloid are rarely associated with kidney disease.

The diagnosis of amyloidosis is made on the basis of clinical features and biopsy confirmation (Fig. 26.1). AL amyloid should be suspected when any patient has circulating serum monoclonal M proteins, especially in conjunction with cardiac disease, peripheral neuropathy, gastrointestinal symptoms, or the nephrotic syndrome. Likewise, nephrotic patients with evidence of chronic infections or inflammatory conditions may have secondary amyloidosis. SAP scintigraphy after injection of radiolabeled SAP may allow noninvasive diagnosis of amyloidosis, quantification of the extent of organ system involvement, and noninvasive assessment of the response to treatment.[4] However, this technique is available in only a few centers. Fat pad aspirates from both AL and AA amyloidosis patients have been found to be diagnostic in 70–80% of cases, bone marrow aspirates in only 50%, and rectal biopsies in as many as 73%. In patients with clinical renal disease and adequate tissue sampling the sensitivity of

renal biopsy approaches 100%. Renal biopsy can also be helpful in ruling out involvement by other renal disease in patients with known amyloidosis of other organ systems.

Under light microscopy, amyloid appears as an amorphous material that stains pink with hematoxylin–eosin and metachromatically with crystal or methyl violet. With Congo red it produces an apple-green birefringence under polarized light. Amyloid deposition may be confined to the glomeruli or may also be seen in tubular basement membranes, interstitium, and blood vessels. Under electron microscopy, typical nonbranching, 8–10 nm wide fibrils are seen. Immunohistochemical analysis with antisera to λ and κ light chains and SAA protein can differentiate between the types of renal amyloid.

Clinical trials and specific recommendations

Primary amyloidosis (Table 26.1)

In AL amyloidosis the deposited fibrils are composed of the N-terminal amino acid residues of the variable region of an immunoglobulin light chain. It is not clear what factors allow the proteins of some patients to aggregate

Table 26.1 Treatment of glomerular deposition diseases

Disease	Typical treatment regimens
AL amyloid	High-dose melphalan (200 mg/m^2) and stem cell transplantation *or* Melphalan (0.15–0.25 mg/kg/day) and prednisone (0.8–1.5 mg/kg/day) in 4–7 day cycles every 6 weeks with or without colchicine (0.6 mg b.i.d.)
AA amyloid	Treat underlying inflammatory disease Colchicine 1.2–2 mg/day Consider pulse cyclophosphamide (1 g per month for 6 months followed by 1 g per 3 months) or chlorambucil (4 mg/day for 1 week followed by 6 mg/day for 3 weeks)
Familial Mediterranean fever	Colchicine 2 mg/day if tolerated
Fibrillary glomerulopathy	Consider treatment of pattern on light microscopy
Monoclonal immunoglobulin deposition disease	Consider melphalan or other cytotoxic agents, prednisone, and/or plasmapheresis

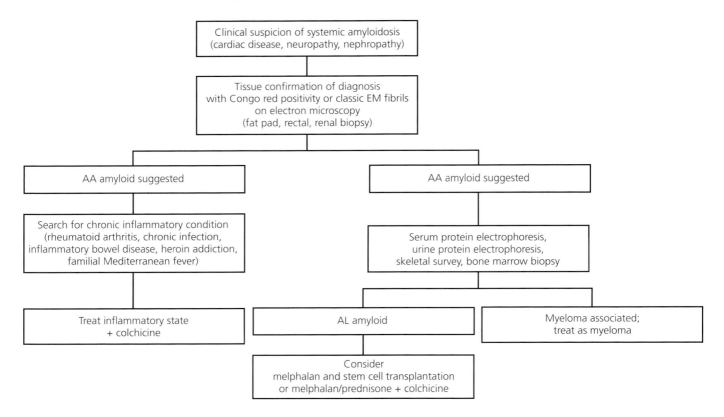

Figure 26.1 Evaluation and treatment of systemic amyloidosis.

into amyloid fibrils. One such property may be the ability to be taken up by macrophages, where proteins are metabolized to preamyloid fragments that have chemical properties that allow aggregation. In AL amyloidosis, λ light chains predominate over κ chains and there is an increased incidence of monoclonal λ type VI. The median age at diagnosis in AL amyloidosis is almost 65 years and only 1% of patients are younger than 40 years. AL amyloidosis occurs twice as often in men as in women. Patients usually present with weight loss, weakness, and other nonspecific complaints including shortness of breath, peripheral edema, pain due to peripheral neuropathy, purpura, and gross bleeding. They may have an enlarged liver, spleen, or rarely lymph node enlargement or macroglossia. Usually there is multiple organ involvement: kidneys are affected in 50%, heart in 40%, and peripheral nerves in 26%. Approximately 25% of patients have nephrotic syndrome on diagnosis, whereas others have lesser degrees of proteinuria or azotemia. Urinalysis is typically bland, although microhematuria and cellular casts have been reported.

Prognosis is poor in many patients with AL amyloidosis: median survival in some series in the past was only 20 months.[1] Survival is shortened if there is evidence of congestive heart failure (to 6–9 months), λ (vs. κ) monoclonal light chains in the urine, elevated serum creatinine, or evidence of interstitial fibrosis on kidney biopsy. Most deaths result from cardiac involvement, followed in frequency by renal disease. Before treatment is instituted, assessment of the extent of organ system involvement is

important and may include electrocardiography, echocardiography, Holter monitoring, CT of the abdomen, gastric emptying scans and malabsorption work-up, nerve conduction studies, bone marrow biopsy and skeletal survey to rule out lytic bone lesions.

Treatment strategies for AL amyloidosis should be focused on the risks and benefits of therapy in the individual patient. Since the disease is associated with a proliferation of a single clone of plasma cells, most therapies concentrate on strategies to decrease the production of monoclonal light chains akin to therapy for multiple myeloma. A variety of chemotherapeutic drugs, including melphalan and prednisone, chlorambucil, azathioprine, cyclophosphamide, and others, have been used. Recent major clinical trials have centered on the use of melphalan and prednisone. Steroids alone do not seem to work, and the benefit of melphalan and prednisone over melphalan alone in amyloidosis has not been addressed. An early placebo-controlled study in 1978 involving 55 patients randomized to receive either melphalan and prednisone or placebo could show no overall survival benefit from chemotherapy, although some of the patients in the treatment group appeared to do particularly well.[5]

The Mayo Clinic group retrospectively reviewed data on 153 AL amyloidosis patients treated with melphalan and prednisone between 1969 and 1982.[6] Melphalan had been initiated at 0.15 mg/kg/day in two divided doses and prednisone at 0.8 mg/kg/day for 7 days with cycles repeated every 6 weeks and melphalan dose adjusted until a 50% reduction in white blood cells or platelets was achieved.

Response to therapy was defined as regression of organ manifestations of amyloidosis. Only 27 of the 153 patients (18%) fulfilled the response criteria. The median survival time for responders was 89.4 months vs. 14.7 months for those who did not respond. Of the responders, 78% survived 5 years; of the nonresponders, only 7%. However, 7 of 27 patients who responded eventually developed a myelodysplatic syndrome or acute leukemia, perhaps due to prolonged exposure to melphalan. Patients with renal amyloidosis as their major organ involvement did better than other groups (overall response rate of 25%). A response to therapy in these patients was defined as 50% reduction in nephrotic-range proteinuria in the absence of a rise in serum creatinine and a return to normal creatinine in those with azotemia at initiation of therapy. An elevated serum creatinine decreased the likelihood of response (< 10% if abnormal and 0% response if > 3 mg/dL). For those with nephrotic-range proteinuria, normal creatinine, and no cardiac involvement, the overall response rate was 39%. The median time for full response was 1 year, although beneficial effects were noted earlier. The authors concluded that in view of the increased survival of those who responded to therapy, a trial of melphalan and prednisone was warranted. In view of its leukemogenic effects, however, total dose of melphalan should not exceed 600 mg nor should treatment period exceed 1 year.

As a result of its benefit in secondary amyloidosis, treatment with colchicine has also been attempted for primary amyloidosis (see later).[7-9] Cohen et al[10] in 1987 treated 53 patients with colchicine 0.5 mg, one or two tablets per day, and compared the results with retrospective ones from controls. An equal number of patients in both groups (22%) received additional chemotherapy. Relative risk of death associated with the colchicine-treated group was 0.35 (P < 0.001) compared with the control group. Median survival for controls was 6 months and for treated patients 17 months. In a regression analysis, variables found to have a significant beneficial effect on survival were treatment with colchicine, female sex, and longer interval from diagnosis to referral or treatment (the latter may indicate disease severity). The reason for better survival of females in both groups is unclear.

A more recent trial by Kyle et al[7] confirmed the superiority of melphalan and prednisone, with or without colchicine, over colchicine alone: 220 patients with AL amyloidosis were randomly assigned to either colchicine alone (0.6 mg twice daily), melphalan (0.15 mg/kg/day) and prednisone (0.8 mg/kg/day), or melphalan plus prednisone and colchicine. Therapy was continued for 7 days in 6-week cycles. The dose of melphalan was increased until leukopenia or thrombocytopenia developed, and the dose of colchicine was increased until limited by gastrointestinal adverse effects. The median duration of survival was 8.5 months in the colchicine group, 18 months in the group treated with melphalan and prednisone, and 17 months in the group treated with melphalan, prednisone, and colchicine (P < 0.001). Of patients treated with regimens containing melphalan and prednisone, 28% showed a positive response in serum or urine protein values compared with only 3% of patients treated with colchicine alone (P < 0.001). However, there was no significant difference in urine protein excretion or renal insufficiency in the groups treated with melphalan and prednisone vs. those treated with colchicine alone: 18% of patients treated with melphalan and prednisone had a 50% reduction in proteinuria compared with 6% of patients treated with colchicine (P = 0.23). Renal failure requiring dialysis developed in 21% of patients treated with colchicine, 21% of patients treated with melphalan and prednisone, and 14% of patients treated with combined therapy (P = 0.64). Recently, a trial compared treatment with melphalan and prednisone to treatment with a five-drug regimen containing vincristine, carmustine, melphalan, cyclophosphamide, and prednisone. There was no difference in response rate or patient survival.[11]

Dimethyl sulfoxide has been shown to induce disappearance of amyloid deposits in casein-treated mice, and a number of isolated case reports have been published that show benefit from its use in a few patients, including one who remained well after 4 years of treatment.[12] It has also been shown to be of benefit when instilled locally for amyloidosis of the bladder and in a case of secondary gastrointestinal amyloidosis related to adult-onset Still disease.[13,14] In our own experience it has not favorably influenced the course of systemic amyloidosis.

One report noted the rapid clinical improvement in a patient with AL amyloidosis associated with multiple myeloma when treated with 4-iodo-4-dexoydoxorubicin. In a follow-up study of eight patients with AL amyloidosis, five demonstrated clinical benefit.[15] Evidence of reduction of interventricular septum thickness was attributed to amyloid resorption in two patients (including one in whom massive urinary excretion of amyloid fragments was seen) and a large reduction in size of an amyloidoma as well as the spleen and liver in another. The main toxicity was found to be reversible granulocytopenia. No large-scale studies of treatment with 4-iodo-4-dexoydoxorubicin have been published at this time.

High-dose dexamethasone has been evaluated as an alternate treatment for AL amyloidosis.[16,17] In a phase II trial, Gertz et al[16] treated 25 patients with AL amyloidosis with high-dose dexamethasone. Only 12% of patients responded, and the median group survival was 13.8 months. While high-dose dexamethasone may occasionally be of benefit, it does not appear to be superior to treatment with melphalan and prednisone.

The most promising results for treatment of AL amyloidosis have come from studies using high-dose chemotherapy followed by peripheral blood stem-cell transplantation.[18-21] In selected case reports, there has been resolution of the nephrotic syndrome and significant improvement of organ amyloid infiltration.[22,23] In an early study, Comenzo et al[24] reported treatment of 25 patients with dose-intensive intravenous melphalan (200 mg/m²) followed by autologous peripheral blood stem-cell transplantation. Early mortality (< 3 months) associated with the therapy was 20%. Of surviving patients, 60% had a complete hematologic response. At a median follow-up of 24 months, 68% of patients were alive and the median survival had not yet been reached. Significant predictors of improved survival included involvement of two or fewer major organ systems (87% vs. 40%, P < 0.05) and lack of predominant cardiac involvement (82% vs. 38%, P < 0.05); 14 patients had renal involvement (defined as proteinuria > 500 mg/day) and all survived to follow-up. Of patients with renal involvement, 64% responded to therapy with at least a 50% decrease in proteinuria without worsening azotemia. The mean daily proteinuria decreased from 6030 mg before treatment to 1573 mg after treatment (P < 0.1). None of the patients had progressive renal insufficiency requiring dialysis. The most common toxicities included mucositis (21%), nausea and vomiting (19%), diarrhea (15%), peripheral edema (11%), pulmonary edema (8%), and worsening renal failure (8%).

A recent study by Dember et al[18] specifically investigated the effect of this treatment on patients with renal amyloidosis. Patients were eligible if they were at least 18 years of age, had a Southwest Oncology Group performance status score of 0–3, had a left ventricular ejection fraction greater than 40%, and had a supine systolic blood pressure greater than 85 mmHg. In total, 65 patients with AL amyloidosis and renal involvement (urine protein excretion > 1 g/day) were treated with dose-intensive melphalan followed by autologous blood stem-cell transplantation, of whom 77% survived to 1 year. A renal response, defined as a 50% reduction in proteinuria without a 25% reduction in creatinine clearance, occurred in 34% of patients, although in the majority the response was delayed for more than 3 months. Analyzing only patients surviving at least 1 year, 36% of patients had a renal response at 12 months and 52% patients responded at 24 months. A complete hematologic response was obtained in 42% of patients alive at 1 year, and patients with a hematologic response were significantly more likely to have a renal response (71% vs. 11%, P < 0.001). Progressive renal insufficiency requiring dialysis developed in 8% of patients. Toxicities of therapy were significant. In 23% of patients, the serum creatinine doubled or increased by 1 mg/dL during the 100 days after treatment, while 3% of patients required temporary dialysis. Other toxicities included mucositis (53%), peripheral edema (23%), bacteremia (19%), pulmonary edema (18%), elevated liver function tests (13%), gastrointestinal bleeding (10%), and nongastrointestinal bleeding (10%).

At present, for younger AL amyloid patients with isolated renal involvement and little evidence of other organ involvement, we recommend dose-intensive intravenous melphalan (200 mg/m^2) and autologous blood stem-cell transplantation. However, only a minority of patients are good candidates, and this therapy is also associated with significant toxicity and is still currently limited to a few medical centers.[25] An alternative to be considered is melphalan (0.15–0.25 mg/kg/day) and prednisone (0.8–1.5 mg/kg/day) in 4- to 7-day cycles repeated every 6 weeks in an attempt to decrease production of the abnormal plasma cell clone that produces the AL light chain that leads to fibril deposition. In addition, 0.6 mg of colchicine twice daily may be given. Medication doses should be increased as tolerated and must be adjusted for leukopenia,

thrombocytopenia, and gastrointestinal adverse effects. Supportive care measures important for ongoing symptomatic relief include diuretics and salt restriction for those with edema related to the nephrotic syndrome. Intravenous albumin infusions provide only transient benefit. Those with orthostatic hypotension may also benefit from compression stockings and should be instructed to rise slowly from supine or seated positions. Fludrocortisone may be of use but has the limiting adverse effect of fluid retention in these patients. Recent isolated cases have shown benefit from midodrine, an oral α-adrenergic agonist that can raise blood pressure in some amyloid patients who have orthostatic hypotension.[26] Gastric atony can be improved with small frequent meals and metoclopramide hydrochloride. Jejunostomy feeds or total parenteral nutrition may become necessary. Peripheral nervous system involvement may be ameliorated with physical therapy or with amitriptyline or carbamazepine.

Secondary amyloidosis (see Table 26.1)

Secondary (AA) amyloidosis occurs in patients with chronic inflammatory diseases such as rheumatoid arthritis, bronchiectasis, osteomyelitis, inflammatory bowel disease, some neoplasms, familial Mediterranean fever (FMF), and in chronic heroin addicts who inject drugs subcutaneously. Currently, longstanding rheumatoid arthritis accounts for the majority of cases, although geography and numbers of chronically addicted patients affect local distribution of cases as well. A major component of these amyloid deposits is AA protein, which comprises the N-terminal end of the larger acute-phase reactant SAA produced by hepatocytes. More than 90% of SAA circulates in association with high-density lipoprotein (HDL). A major role of SAA may be to direct HDL to areas of inflammation, where it can remove cholesterol accumulations after cellular injury. Among patients with chronic inflammatory states, increased levels of SAA occur equally in patients with and without amyloid deposition. Thus, some additional unknown stimulus is required to induce amyloid fibrils to form and precipitate. Approximately 25% of patients with amyloidosis related to AA protein have glomerular involvement, and they often present with proteinuria or the nephrotic syndrome and progressive renal insufficiency.

Treatment of most cases of AA amyloidosis focuses on aggressive treatment of the underlying inflammatory disease, which can lead to stabilization of renal function, reduction of proteinuria, and partial resolution of amyloid deposits. Surgical debridement or removal of an infectious focus appears to be of benefit. Antiinflammatory medications and immunosuppressive agents may be helpful for rheumatoid arthritis and inflammatory bowel disease. Prognosis is usually good if the underlying disease can be controlled and systemic deposition is not already extensive.

In 1987 and 1993 Berglund et al[27,28] reported on the use of alkylating agents to treat AA amyloidosis secondary to rheumatic diseases. They describe a total of 16 patients treated with cyclophosphamide, and subsequently chlorambucil, who demonstrated evidence of increased glomerular filtration rate and decreased proteinuria, with a renal survival rate of 75% at 10 years. The initial dosage of chlorambucil was 4 mg/day for the first week and 6 mg/day for the subsequent 3 weeks. The dose is increased every third week, as necessary to achieve the treatment goals of lymphopenia, normalization of C-reactive protein/SAA levels, and remission of the underlying arthritis. The major adverse effects of alkylating agents are increased risks of infection and malignancies, the risk being related to the total dose received. Another study of 51 patients with juvenile rheumatoid arthritis and AA amyloidosis treated with chlorambucil demonstrated a decrease in proteinuria of 64% after 3 years of continuous treatment. Of the treated patients, 68% were alive at 15-year follow-up compared with 0% survival among historical controls.[29] A small retrospective study of 15 patients with renal AA amyloidosis in association with rheumatoid arthritis showed that patients treated with pulse cyclophosphamide (1 g per month for 6 months followed by 1 g every 3 months) had a lower rate of renal function loss ($P < 0.02$) and higher median survival (165 months vs. 46 months, $P < 0.03$) compared with untreated patients. Several other small studies have documented benefit for patients treated with either cyclosporine or azathioprine, including improvement in proteinuria, prolonged survival compared with controls, and in two cases regression of amyloid deposits on repeat biopsy.[30] A recent retrospective study showed that patients with AA amyloidosis associated with rheumatoid arthritis, who were treated with pulse cyclophosphamide, had a lower rate of renal function loss (follow-up creatinine 268 mmol/L vs. 435 mmol/L, $P = 0.012$) and higher median survival (165 months vs. 46 months, $P = 0.026$) compared with untreated patients.[31] Further prospective studies are needed to clarify the appropriate use of these agents in the treatment of AA amyloidosis.

FMF is an autosomal recessive trait carried on the short arm of chromosome 16 that is seen primarily in Sephardic Jews, Turks, Armenians, and Arabs. The disease manifests as recurrent attacks of fever and serositis and is associated with the development of amyloidosis in as many as 90% of untreated patients. Colchicine has been successfully used to prevent febrile attacks in FMF since the early 1970s. Its mechanism of action is not known, although colchicine has been shown to decrease both suppressor T-cell activity and chemotaxis, which may be involved in the pathogenesis of the disease.

A 1986 study evaluated more than 1000 patients with FMF who were treated with colchicine 1–2 mg/day and who were followed for 4–11 years.[32] Among 906 compliant patients, proteinuria developed in only four (1.7%), whereas in the noncompliant the rate was 48.9% ($P < 0.0001$); 110 patients (11%) had renal involvement at the initiation of the study. Among 86 patients with proteinuria but not the nephrotic syndrome, proteinuria resolved in five and stabilized in 68. Renal function deteriorated in all 24 patients with the nephrotic syndrome at presentation and in 13 with nonnephrotic proteinuria. A retrospective analysis was published in 1994 of 68 FMF patients who presented with at least 0.5 g of proteinuria daily and serum

creatinine of < 2.5 mg/dL and who were treated with colchicine and followed for a minimum of 5 years.[33] Renal function worsened in 46% of patients. Patients whose renal function worsened were more likely to have a creatinine ≥ 1.5 mg/dL at baseline ($P < 0.01$) and were more likely to have been treated with ≤ 1.5 mg/day of colchicine ($P < 0.001$). These data suggest that in FMF the daily dose of colchicine should be 2 mg/day. Major gastrointestinal adverse effects, including diarrhea and nausea, must be treated if this dose of colchicine is to be continued. Additionally, colchicine should be continued even when it appears to have no effect in controlling febrile attacks. At this dosage, colchicine does not appear to prevent progression once the creatinine is elevated but does appear to delay the onset of endstage renal disease (ESRD). Of note, patients with renal failure may be predisposed to drug toxicity and gastrointestinal symptoms that require dose reduction. However, whatever dose is tolerated should be continued on the assumption that it may prevent amyloid deposition in other tissues.

Secondary amyloidosis is also seen in drug abusers with suppurative skin lesions secondary to subcutaneous injection of drugs ("skin-popping"). In an autopsy study of 150 addicts, 14% of those who had subcutaneous infections and 26% of those who had chronic suppurative infections had renal amyloidosis.[34] In a study at our center, nearly all of these patients were African-Americans and most were males. In comparison with those with heroin-induced focal sclerosis, patients with amyloidosis were almost 10 years older (mean age 41 years) and had a longer history of substance abuse, suggesting that they had exhausted sites of intravenous access and had resorted to skin-popping.[35] Sporadic case reports have described responses to colchicine therapy in addicts with secondary amyloidosis, but the key to improvement, or at least halting of disease progression, appears to be treatment of the underlying infections and cessation of skin-popping.

At present, we recommend that treatment of AA amyloidosis be centered on a thorough search for the inflammatory source that stimulates SAA production. We attempt to correct the basic inflammatory disease (e.g. control active inflammatory bowel disease or rheumatoid arthritis) and use colchicine 1.2–2 mg/day in these patients. Supportive measures are similar to those for AL amyloidosis.

Treatment of the amyloid patient with endstage renal disease

Patients with amyloidosis have a median survival of 8.2 months from the start of dialysis.[36] The cause of death in two-thirds has been a complication related to cardiac amyloid. There appears to be no survival advantage to the use of a specific dialysis modality such as peritoneal dialysis or hemodialysis.

An Italian study describes the course of patients diagnosed with both AA and AL amyloidosis who received dialysis.[37] Of 61 patients, 18 died within 1 month of the initiation of therapy. For the remaining patients they found the survival rate to be approximately 55% at 2 years and 30% at 5 years, approximately 20% lower than that observed in an age-matched general population with ESRD. The median survival time was 25 months from the initiation of dialysis, longer than that found by other authors, and four patients survived over 10 years. Cardiovascular complications were common, including arrhythmias, heart block, heart failure, and orthostatic hypotension. In this study a major problem was intradialytic hypotension. For the patients on chronic ambulatory peritoneal dialysis, the incidence of hypotension and the cause of death did not differ significantly from that found in patients on hemodialysis. However, there did seem to be an increased incidence of peritonitis in patients with amyloidosis, with worse outcomes as compared with the general peritoneal dialysis population.

There has not been extensive experience with renal transplantation in AL amyloidosis. Most reported transplant recipients have had AA amyloidosis. A reported series of transplant recipients included 45 patients, three with AL amyloidosis and 42 with AA amyloidosis (33 due to rheumatoid arthritis and nine to other inflammatory diseases).[38] When compared to controls with similar HLA matching and treatment regimens, the study found an overall low patient survival in amyloidosis patients, particular in the early post-transplant period among those over 40 years of age. Graft survival, however, was somewhat better than in patients transplanted for glomerulonephritis; more amyloidosis patients died with a functioning graft, a fact that has been noted elsewhere. There also appears to be a tendency toward fewer episodes of rejection, which, when they occur, are better tolerated by these patients. The rate of recurrence of amyloidosis in the allograft is unclear but may be as high as 20%, depending on duration of survival and pattern of amyloidosis. At present renal transplantation is a reasonable treatment for patients with ESRD related to amyloidosis whose systemic disease is well controlled and who do not have extensive or life-threatening extrarenal involvement.

Fibrillary and immunotactoid glomerulopathy (see Table 26.1)

Recent studies have documented a pattern of glomerular disease related to precipitation of fibrils larger than those found in amyloidosis. Patients have been divided into two groups depending on fibril size: fibrillary glomerulopathy (fibrils ~ 20 nm in diameter) and immunotactoid glomerulopathy (fibrils 30–50 nm in diameter). Similar cases had previously been reported as amyloid-like glomerulopathy, Congo red-negative amyloid-like glomerulonephritis, and nonamyloidotic fibrillary glomerulopathy. The diagnosis of these diseases is made solely on renal biopsy. Light microscopic findings are not diagnostic and are very pleomorphic, including mesangial proliferation as well as membranous, membranoproliferative, and crescentic glomerulonephritis. The pathognomonic findings are visible on electron microscopy, with nonbranching fibrils of 20–50 nm diameter arranged randomly in the mesangial

matrix and basement membranes. Immunofluorescence in these patients is often positive for immunoglobulin G (especially IgG4), C3, and both κ and λ chains.[39]

Fibrillary glomerulopathy accounts for over 90% of cases. In comparison to patients with fibrillary glomerulopathy, Fogo et al[40] found that those patients with immunotactoid glomerulopathy tended to be older, to have a less rapidly progressive course, and to be more likely to have an associated lymphoproliferative disease. Fibrillary glomerulopathy is usually an isolated renal entity not associated with a systemic disease, although a few cases associated with chronic lymphocytic leukemia or B-cell lymphoma have been described.

Most patients are adults, all have proteinuria (70% nephrotic range), and the majority have hypertension and hematuria. Renal insufficiency is often found on presentation and progression to ESRD is frequent. Timecourse to development of ESRD appears to be more rapid than in patients with renal amyloidosis, particularly in patients who are older and have elevated serum creatinine values at presentation. No effective therapy is known. Some clinicians choose to treat the light microscopic pattern (e.g. crescentic, membranous, or membranoproliferative glomerulonephritis) and ignore the presence of the precipitated fibrils. Prednisone and cyclophosphamide have been tried without benefit in most patients;[41] however, in some patients with crescentic glomerulonephritis associated with classic fibrillary deposits on electron microscopy this therapy has led to a dramatic reduction in serum creatinine and proteinuria, and some patients were able to discontinue dialysis support. We have tried daily colchicine therapy, although this has not been demonstrated to be of benefit. In patients with fibrillary glomerulopathy associated with chronic lymphocytic leukemia, treatment of the underlying disease with chemotherapy has been associated with improved renal function and decreased proteinuria. Experience with transplantation is limited. Several patients have undergone transplantation with prolonged graft function, but fibrillary glomerulopathy recurs in approximately 50%.[42,43] Supportive measures and treatment of associated manifestations of the nephrotic syndrome (e.g. edema, hyperlipidemia, thrombotic tendency) should be initiated when necessary.

Monoclonal immunoglobulin deposition disease (see Table 26.1)

Monoclonal immunoglobulin deposition disease (MIDD) is characterized by the deposition of monoclonal light-and/or heavy-chain deposits in basement membranes.[44–48] In contrast to amyloidosis, these proteins do not bind Congo red stain, do not form fibrils or β-pleated sheets, and are not associated with amyloid P protein. Light microscopy reveals a nodular sclerosing glomerulopathy, which may be accompanied by tubular casts if there is coexisting myeloma cast nephropathy. Immunoflorescence reveals a single class of immunoglobulin light-and/or heavy-chain staining along the glomerular and tubular basement membranes. The deposits appear granular (and not fibrillar) on electron microscopy.

MIDD is classified into three types: light-chain deposition disease (LCDD), light- and heavy-chain deposition disease (LHCDD), and heavy-chain deposition disease (HCDD).[46–48] LCDD accounts for the majority of cases of MIDD. In 80% of cases, κ light chains are present and are usually derived from the constant region of the immunoglobulin light chain. Most patients are over 40 years old, and there is a high incidence of multiple myeloma and lymphoplasmacytic B-cell disorders. Approximately one-third of patients with MIDD have coexisting multiple myeloma and myeloma cast nephropathy. Patients with MIDD may have involvement of myocardium, peripheral nerves, liver, and glomerulus, with clinical manifestations similar to those found in patients with amyloidosis. Most patients with MIDD involving the kidneys have renal insufficiency, proteinuria (nephrotic range in half of patients), and hypertension. Patients with LCDD and myeloma cast nephropathy have significantly lower creatinine clearances at presentation compared with patients with MIDD alone. Most patients with HCDD will have low complement levels and are positive for hepatitis C virus antibody but polymerase chain reaction (PCR) negative.[48]

The optimal therapy for LCDD is unclear.[48–50] Patients are often treated with melphalan or other cytotoxic agents, prednisone, and occasionally with plasmapheresis. Treatment of LCDD has led to stabilization or improvement of renal function in some cases. However, therapies are unsuccessful in patients with a serum creatinine above 4 mg/dL at presentation, and a higher initial serum creatinine is significantly associated with worse renal and patient survival. With therapy, patient survival is 90% at 1 year and 50–70% at 5 years. Renal survival is 67% at 1 year and 20–35% at 5 years.[48,50] Patients with LCDD and myeloma cast nephropathy have a significantly worse prognosis, with a mean time to ESRD of 4 months and mean time to death of 22 months.[48] Cases of HCDD are rare, and most patients have progressive renal failure despite treatment with steroids or cytotoxic agents.[47,48] Some patients with MIDD have been successfully transplanted, but recurrence of MIDD in the allograft has been reported.[51–54]

References

1. Appel GB, Radhakrishnan J, D'Agati V: Secondary glomerular disease. In Brenner B (ed): Brenner and Rector's The Kidney, 6th edn. Philadelphia: WB Saunders, 2000, pp 1386.
2. Gertz MA, Lacy MQ, Dispenzieri A: Immunoglobulin light chain amyloidosis and the kidney. Kidney Int 2002;61:1–9.
3. Korbet SM, Schwartz MM, Lewis EJ: The fibrillary glomerulopathies. Am J Kidney Dis 1994;23:751–765.
4. Tan SY, Pepys MB, Hawkins PN: Treatment of amyloidosis. Am J Kidney Dis 1995;26:267–285.
5. Kyle RA, Greipp PR: Primary systemic amyloidosis: comparison of melphalan and prednisone versus placebo. Blood 1978;52:818–827.
6. Gertz MA, Kyle RA, Greipp PR: Response rates and survival in primary systemic amyloidosis. Blood 1991;77:257–262.
7. Kyle RA, Gertz MA, Greipp PR, et al: A trial of three regimens for primary amyloidosis: colchicine alone, melphalan and prednisone, and melphalan, prednisone, and colchicine. N Engl J Med 1997;336:1202–1207.
8. Kyle RA, Greipp PR, Garton JP, et al: Primary systemic amyloidosis. Comparison of melphalan/prednisone versus colchicine. Am J Med 1985;79:708–716.
9. Skinner M, Anderson J, Simms R, et al: Treatment of 100 patients with primary amyloidosis: a randomized trial of melphalan, prednisone, and colchicine versus colchicine only. Am J Med 1996;100:290–298.
10. Cohen AS, Rubinow A, Anderson JJ, et al: Survival of patients with primary (AL) amyloidosis. Colchicine-treated cases from 1976 to 1983 compared with cases seen in previous years (1961 to 1973). Am J Med 1987;82:1182–1190.
11. Gertz MA, Lacy MQ, Lust JA, et al: Prospective randomized trial of melphalan and prednisone versus vincristine, carmustine, melphalan, cyclophosphamide, and prednisone in the treatment of primary systemic amyloidosis. J Clin Oncol 1999;17:262–267.
12. Wang WJ, Lin CS, Wong CK: Response of systemic amyloidosis to dimethyl sulfoxide. J Am Acad Dermatol 1986;15:402–405.
13. Takahashi A, Matsumoto J, Nishimura S, et al: Improvement of endoscopic and histologic findings of AA-type gastrointestinal amyloidosis by treatment with dimethyl sulfoxide and prednisolone. Gastroenterol Jpn 1985;20:143–147.
14. Tokunaka S, Osanai H, Morikawa M, et al: Experience with dimethyl sulfoxide treatment for primary localized amyloidosis of the bladder. J Urol 1986;135:580–582.
15. Gianni L, Bellotti V, Gianni AM, et al: New drug therapy of amyloidoses: resorption of AL-type deposits with 4'-iodo-4'-deoxydoxorubicin. Blood 1995;86:855–861.
16. Gertz MA, Lacy MQ, Lust JA, et al: Phase II trial of high-dose dexamethasone for untreated patients with primary systemic amyloidosis. Med Oncol 1999;16:104–109.
17. Gertz MA, Lacy MQ, Lust JA, et al: Phase II trial of high-dose dexamethasone for previously treated immunoglobulin light-chain amyloidosis. Am J Hematol 1999;61:115–119.
18. Dember LM, Sanchorawala V, Seldin DC, et al: Effect of dose-intensive intravenous melphalan and autologous blood stem-cell transplantation on AL amyloidosis-associated renal disease. Ann Intern Med 2001;134:746–753.
19. Comenzo RL: Hematopoietic cell transplantation for primary systemic amyloidosis: what have we learned? Leuk Lymphoma 2000;37:245–258.
20. Gertz MA, Lacy MQ, Gastineau DA, et al: Blood stem cell transplantation as therapy for primary systemic amyloidosis (AL). Bone Marrow Transplant 2000;26:963–969.
21. Moreau P, Leblond V, Bourquelot P, et al: Prognostic factors for survival and response after high-dose therapy and autologous stem cell transplantation in systemic AL amyloidosis: a report on 21 patients. Br J Haematol 1998;101:766–769.
22. Patriarca F, Geromin A, Fanin R, et al: Improvement of amyloid-related symptoms after autologous stem cell transplantation in a patient with hepatomegaly, macroglossia and purpura. Bone Marrow Transplant 1999;24:433–435.
23. Sezer O, Schmid P, Shweigert M, et al: Rapid reversal of nephrotic syndrome due to primary systemic AL amyloidosis after VAD and subsequent high-dose chemotherapy with autologous stem cell support. Bone Marrow Transplant 1999;23:967–969.
24. Comenzo RL, Vosburgh E, Falk RH, et al: Dose-intensive melphalan with blood stem-cell support for the treatment of AL (amyloid light-chain) amyloidosis: survival and responses in 25 patients. Blood 1998;91:3662–3670.
25. Gertz MA, Lacy MQ, Dispenzieri A: Myeloablative chemotherapy with stem cell rescue for the treatment of primary systemic amyloidosis: a status report. Bone Marrow Transplant 2000;25:465–470.
26. Blowey DL, Balfe JW, Gupta I, et al: Midodrine efficacy and pharmacokinetics in a patient with recurrent intradialytic hypotension. Am J Kidney Dis 1996;28:132–136.
27. Berglund K, Thysell H, Keller C: Results, principles and pitfalls in the management of renal AA-amyloidosis: a 10–21 year followup of 16 patients with rheumatic disease treated with alkylating cytostatics. J Rheumatol 1993;20:2051–2057.
28. Berglund K, Keller C, Thysell H: Alkylating cytostatic treatment in renal amyloidosis secondary to rheumatic disease. Ann Rheum Dis 1987;46:757–762.
29. Schnitzer TJ, Ansell BM: Amyloidosis in juvenile chronic polyarthritis. Arthritis Rheum 1977;20(Suppl):245–252.

30. Falck HM, Skrifvars BOW: Treatment of rheumatoid arthritis with cyclophosphamide. *In* Glenner GG, Costa PD, de Freitas F (eds): Amyloid and Amyloidosis. Amsterdam: Excerpta Medica, 1980, pp 590.

31. Chevrel G, Jenvrin C, McGregor B, et al: Renal type AA amyloidosis associated with rheumatoid arthritis: a cohort study showing improved survival on treatment with pulse cyclophosphamide. Rheumatology (Oxford) 2001;40:821–825.

32. Zemer D, Pras M, Sohar E, et al: Colchicine in the prevention and treatment of the amyloidosis of familial Mediterranean fever. N Engl J Med 1986;314:1001–1005.

33. Livneh A, Zemer D, Langevitz P, et al: Colchicine treatment of AA amyloidosis of familial Mediterranean fever. An analysis of factors affecting outcome. Arthritis Rheum 1994;37:1804–1811.

34. Menchel S, Cohen D, Gross E, et al: AA protein-related renal amyloidosis in drug addicts. Am J Pathol 1983;112:195–199.

35. Kunis CLK, Ward H, Appel GB: Renal disease associated with drugs of abuse. *In* Debroe M, Porter G, Bennett WM, Verpooten GA (eds): Clinical Nephrotoxins: Renal Injury from Drugs and Chemicals, 2nd edn. Dordrecht: Kluwer Academic Publishers, 1998, pp 397–411.

36. Gertz MA, Kyle RA, O'Fallon WM: Dialysis support of patients with primary systemic amyloidosis. A study of 211 patients. Arch Intern Med 1992;152:2245–2250.

37. Moroni G, Banfi G, Montoli A, et al: Chronic dialysis in patients with systemic amyloidosis: the experience in northern Italy. Clin Nephrol 1992;38:81–85.

38. Pasternack A, Ahonen J, Kuhlback B: Renal transplantation in 45 patients with amyloidosis. Transplantation 1986;42:598–601.

39. Iskandar SS, Falk RJ, Jennette JC: Clinical and pathologic features of fibrillary glomerulonephritis. Kidney Int 1992;42:1401–1407.

40. Fogo A, Qureshi N, Horn RG: Morphologic and clinical features of fibrillary glomerulonephritis versus immunotactoid glomerulopathy. Am J Kidney Dis 1993;22:367–377.

41. D'Agati V, Sacchi G, Truong L: Fibrillary glomerulopathy: defining the disease spectrum (abstract). J Am Soc Nephrol 1991;2:590.

42. Pronovost PH, Brady HR, Gunning ME, et al: Clinical features, predictors of disease progression and results of renal transplantation in fibrillary/immunotactoid glomerulopathy. Nephrol Dial Transplant 1996;11:837–842.

43. Samaniego M, Nadasdy GM, Laszik Z, et al: Outcome of renal transplantation in fibrillary glomerulonephritis. Clin Nephrol 2001; 55:159–166.

44. Sanders PW, Herrera GA: Monoclonal immunoglobulin light chain-related renal diseases. Semin Nephrol 1993;13:324–341.

45. Buxbaum J, Gallo G: Nonamyloidotic monoclonal immunoglobulin deposition disease. Light-chain, heavy-chain, and light- and heavy-chain deposition diseases. Hematol Oncol Clin North Am 1999;13:1235–1248.

46. Alpers CE: Glomerulopathies of dysproteinemias, abnormal immunoglobulin deposition, and lymphoproliferative disorders. Curr Opin Nephrol Hypertens 1994;3:349–355.

47. Kambham N, Markowitz GS, Appel GB, et al: Heavy chain deposition disease: the disease spectrum. Am J Kidney Dis 1999;33:954–962.

48. Lin J, Markowitz GS, Valeri AM, et al: Renal monoclonal immunoglobulin deposition disease: the disease spectrum. J Am Soc Nephrol 2001;12:1482–1492.

49. Pozzi C, Fogazzi GB, Banfi G, et al: Renal disease and patient survival in light chain deposition disease. Clin Nephrol 1995;43:281–287.

50. Heilman RL, Velosa JA, Holley KE, et al: Long-term follow-up and response to chemotherapy in patients with light-chain deposition disease. Am J Kidney Dis 1992;20:34–41.

51. Short AK, O'Donoghue DJ, Riad HN, et al: Recurrence of light chain nephropathy in a renal allograft. A case report and review of the literature. Am J Nephrol 2001;21:237–240.

52. Herzenberg AM, Kiaii M, Magil AB: Heavy chain deposition disease: recurrence in a renal transplant and report of IgG(2) subtype. Am J Kidney Dis 2000;35:E25.

53. Lin JJ, Miller F, Waltzer W, et al: Recurrence of immunoglobulin A-kappa crystalline deposition disease after kidney transplantation. Am J Kidney Dis 1995;25:75–78.

54. Gerlag PG, Koene RA, Berden JH: Renal transplantation in light chain nephropathy: case report and review of the literature. Clin Nephrol 1986;25:101–104.

Hepatitis- and HIV-related Renal Diseases

Joseph A. Vassalotti, Brian D. Radbill, Mary E. Klotman, and Paul E. Klotman

Hepatitis B virus and renal disease

Background

Hepatitis B virus (HBV) is a major cause of acute and chronic hepatitis, cirrhosis, and hepatocellular carcinoma, and is associated with renal disease. This partially double-stranded circular DNA virus was discovered in 1966.[1] It remains endemic in Southeast Asia, China, and Africa, whereas the USA has low levels of infection with less than 0.5% or approximately 1 million chronic carriers. The universal vaccination of the general population in Western Europe and the USA should ultimately eliminate HBV infection in those populations.

HBV-associated renal disease

Renal diseases associated with HBV include membranous nephropathy (MN), membranoproliferative colleagues (MPGN) without cryoglobulinemia, and macroscopic polyarteritis nodosa (PAN) (Table 27.1).

Membranous nephropathy

Children in HBV endemic areas are most likely to have membranous nephropathy.[2] Patients present with hematuria and proteinuria or nephritic syndrome. Serologic studies in the majority of patients reveal HBs and HBe antigenemia. Complement levels are usually normal. The etiologic role of HBV in renal disease is supported by the detection of HBe antigen in glomerular deposits[3] and the remission of proteinuria that typically occurs within 6 months of clearing the HBe antigen.[4] Spontaneous remission has been reported in 84% of children after 10 years.[4] One series of 21 adult-onset HBV MN revealed a poorer prognosis with progressive renal failure in 29% and endstage renal disease (ESRD) in 10% after 60 months' mean observation.[5]

Membranoproliferative glomerulonephritis

The MPGN lesion is the most common HBV glomerular disease in adults.[2] It usually occurs in the absence of cryoglobulins. Most reported cases of HBV associated with cryoglobulinemia involve patients coinfected with the hepatitis C virus (HCV) or those who presented before HCV testing was available.[6] Since spontaneous improvement is rare, prognosis with this lesion is poorer than HBV MN.

Polyarteritis nodosa

Patients with this complication of HBV infection present with hematuria, renal failure, new onset or severe hypertension, which may be malignant, and abdominal pain. Mononeuritis multiplex and orchiepididymitis are common. The characteristic lesions are aneurysms of

Table 27.1 Estimated frequency of glomerular diseases associated with viral hepatitis and HIV

	HBV	HCV	HIV
Minimal change disease	+/–	+/–	+
IgA nephropathy	+/–	+/–	++
Membranous nephropathy	+++	+	+
MPGN	++	++	+
MPGN plus cryoglobulinemia	+/–	+++	+/–
Focal and segmental glomerulosclerosis	+/–	+/–	+++
Polyarteritis nodosa	+++	+	+
Thrombotic microangiopathy	–	+/–	+++

MPGN, membranoproliferative glomerulonephritis; +/–, case reports without clear association; +, isolated case reports; ++, occasional reports; +++, common association.

medium-sized arteries of the kidney and mesentery. Diagnosis utilizing clinical features coupled with magnetic resonance angiography has the advantages of a lower morbidity than renal biopsy and absence of radiocontrast nephrotoxicity associated with conventional angiography. Serologic studies typically reveal high levels of HBV DNA and the absence of antineutrophil cytoplasmic antibody. The HBe antigen (Ag) is the most likely candidate for inducing immune complexes.[7] Proteinuria, elevated serum creatinine, and gastrointestinal involvement confer the highest mortality, with death usually following gastrointestinal hemorrhage, infarct, or perforation.[8]

Treatment
Corticosteroids

Use of corticosteroids in HBV-infected patients can enhance viral replication. HBV MN responds poorly to steroid therapy[3] and should be avoided.[9] Few published data are available regarding corticosteroid use in HBV MPGN. To control the life-threatening manifestations of HBV PAN, however, a 1- to 2-week course of steroids (daily prednisone 1 mg/kg) in combination with plasma exchange (PE) and antiviral therapy is important. The duration of immunosuppressive therapy should be tailored to the severity of the PAN manifestations.

Interferon

A US retrospective series of 10 HBV MN, four HBV MPGN, and one unsuccessful biopsy patient treated with 16 weeks of daily or alternate-day 5 million units subcutaneous (s.c.) interferon α_{2b} (IFN-α_{2b}) demonstrated resolution of hepatitis B e antigen (HBeAg) and improvement in proteinuria in eight patients (53%).[10] Seven of eight responders had HBV MN, whereas four of the seven non-responders had HBV MPGN.[10] Results were also promising in a Chinese open trial of steroid-resistant HBV MN in children randomized to 5–8 million units IFN-α_{2b} s.c. three

times weekly or supportive treatment alone.[11] After 1 year of therapy, proteinuria resolved in all 20 treated patients and in only 7 of 20 (35%) who were untreated. HBeAg cleared in 16 (80%) IFN-α patients compared with none in the control group. A series of six HBV PAN patients treated with this agent in addition to a short course of steroids and PE resulted in excellent overall outcome.[12]

Lamivudine (3TC)

There are few data in the literature regarding lamivudine in MN or MPGN associated with HBV. Using lamivudine 100 mg daily as part of the HBV PAN regimen, 9 of 10 patients recovered and HBeAg cleared in seven.[7] Given the direct role of the virus in these renal entities, it is reasonable to assume that 3TC as well as some of the newer hepatitis B antivirals, including adefovir and tenofovir, will play a role in treatment. In higher doses, adefovir is associated with renal toxicity; however, this complication has not been reported in the lower doses proposed for HBV.

Plasma exchange

Alternate-day plasma exchange is used to clear immune complexes in HBV PAN during the initial treatment when the disease is most active.

HBV and renal replacement
Management of HBV in ESRD

The prevalence of HBs antigenemia in US hemodialysis (HD) patients has remarkably decreased from 7.8% in 1976 to 0.9% by 1999,[13] as a result of vaccination, segregation of infected patients and their dialysis equipment from susceptible ones, and improved adherence to infection-control protocol. Testing HBsAg monthly in all susceptible hemodialysis patients is recommended to detect seroconverters.[13]

Effects of HBV on renal transplant recipients

Cirrhosis and reduced graft survival complicate renal transplantation in HBV-infected dialysis patients in the absence of antiviral therapy, but published series are conflicting regarding mortality rates.[14,15] Antilymphocyte globulin use is more frequent in HBV-infected renal transplant recipients who develop hepatic failure.[16] Both preoperative[17] and post-transplant[18] lamivudine therapy has been used with reports of frequent elimination of HBV DNA. One nonrandomized study showed a recurrence of HBV DNA in 10% and 42% of patients treated before and after renal transplantation respectively.[17] The optimal timing and duration of pretransplant lamivudine therapy require further study.

Hepatitis C virus and renal disease

Background

The single-stranded RNA hepatitis C virus (HCV) identified in 1989 as the causative agent for non-A/non-B hepatitis[19] is a major cause of chronic hepatitis, cirrhosis, and hepatocellular carcinoma. The prevalence of antibody to HCV (anti-HCV) in the USA is 1.8%, or an estimated 3.9 million people nationwide.[20] Because HCV is transmitted mainly via parenteral routes, intravenous drug users and recipients of blood transfusions prior to 1987 are high-risk populations, with estimated prevalence rates of 79% and 87% respectively.[21] Sexual and vertical transmission are uncommon, and the source of HCV infection is unknown in approximately 10% of patients.[21]

HCV-associated renal disease
(See also Chapter 16)

Glomerulonephritis

The prevalence of glomerulonephritis in HCV-infected patients is unknown. Investigators have reported an increased prevalence of anti-HCV in patients with membranous nephropathy (MN), but the evidence supporting a direct relationship between HCV and MN is questionable. HCV MN closely resembles idiopathic MN with normal complements, absent rheumatoid factor and cryoglobulins, and similar pathology.[22] Although a few cases of HCV PAN exist in the literature,[23] HBV PAN is much more common. The renal disease most clearly associated with HCV is membranoproliferative glomerulonephritis (MPGN), with[24-26] and without cryoglobulinemia (Table 27.1).[22,27-29] The association between cryoglobulinemic glomerulonephritis (CGN) and HCV is especially striking, with studies reporting 100% anti-HCV positivity in patients with biopsy-proven CGN.[29,30]

Essential mixed cryoglobulinemia

Cryoglobulins or immunoglobulins that reversibly precipitate in the cold cause renal disease via immune complex deposition in small- and medium-sized arteries. Three types of cryoglobulinemias are recognized based on the components of the cryoprecipitate.[31] Type I cryoglobulins are composed of an isolated monoclonal immunoglobulin, whereas types II and III are mixed cryoglobulins. Mixed cryoglobulinemias make up two-thirds of cases and are composed of a polyclonal immunoglobulin G (IgG) bound to another immunoglobulin (usually of the IgM class) that has rheumatoid factor (RF) activity. The IgM component is monoclonal in type II and polyclonal in type III. Prior to the discovery of hepatitis C, approximately 30% of mixed cryoglobulinemias had no clear etiology and were classified as essential mixed cryoglobulinemia (EMC).[32] However, recent studies have shown that up to 90% of patients with EMC have evidence of HCV infection.[33]

Clinical and pathologic presentation of HCV-associated CGN

The most frequent clinical presentation of cryoglobulinemic glomerulonephritis is proteinuria, microscopic hematuria, moderate chronic renal insufficiency, and hypertension, whereas 25% present with acute nephritis and 20% develop nephrotic syndrome.[33,34] Skin purpura is common and hypocomplementemia is universal. The

course of CGN is characterized by exacerbations and remissions, with rare progression to endstage renal disease. Long-term follow-up of patients with CGN demonstrates significant mortality from cardiovascular disease, infection, and cirrhosis before renal replacement therapy is required.[35] Histologically, CGN may be differentiated from idiopathic MPGN on light microscopic examination by a number of distinguishing features. These include increased number of infiltrating leukocytes (typically monocytes), milder mesangial involvement, vasculitis of small- and medium-sized arteries, and the presence of intraluminal hyaline thrombi.[33,36,37] Cylindrical, fibrillar structures, characteristic of cryoglobulins, are found in intraluminal and subendothelial deposits on electron microscopy.[38,39]

Pathogenesis of HCV-associated CGN

Although the pathogenesis of HCV CGN is unknown, D'Amico and Fornasieri[37] proposed that HCV infection progresses from type III to type II mixed cryoglobulinemia, which ultimately results in a membranoproliferative glomerulonephritis. An initial step in this process is thought to be HCV infection of B lymphocytes. Ferri and colleagues[40] reported finding HCV RNA in peripheral blood mononuclear cells of 81% of patients with type II mixed cryoglobulinemia. The HCV-infected B cells are stimulated to overproduce polyclonal immunoglobulins and thereby generate IgM with anti-IgG (RF) activity (type III). There is subsequently a shift from polyclonal to monoclonal (type II) immunoglobulin production. This results in the creation of monoclonal IgMk RF, which deposits within the glomerular matrix and leads to the proliferative inflammatory changes seen in CGN. The pathogenic role of cryoglobulins is supported by the work of Fornasieri and colleagues[41] in which mice injected with solubilized mixed cryoglobulins (type II) collected from humans with HCV CGN developed a similar cryoglobulinemic MPGN.

Treatment

Corticosteroids, immunosuppressives, and plasma exchange

Case reports demonstrate variable success in the treatment of HCV CGN with cyclophosphamide[42] and cryofiltration in combination with corticosteroids.[43] Retrospective studies of patients with CGN prior to the discovery of HCV have shown improvements in serum creatinine levels and proteinuria using pulse steroids[44] and plasma exchange, the latter used in combination with steroids or cytotoxic agents.[45]

IFN-α and ribavirin

Since the discovery of HCV, the management of HCV CGN has focused on antiviral therapy. The standard treatment of HCV in patients with normal renal function is a combination of IFN-α_{2b} (3 million units s.c. three times per week) and ribavirin (1000–1200 mg daily) for 24–48 weeks.[46,47] Although there are case reports regarding the use of IFN-α alone[48] or in combination with the nucleoside analog ribavirin[49,50] for the treatment of HCV-associated glomerulonephritis, it is still unclear whether treatment with IFN-α, a therapy demonstrated to lower viral load in

HCV-infected patients with normal renal function, can attenuate or improve the course of renal disease.

In a prospective, randomized, controlled trial, Misiani and colleagues[51] studied 53 patients with HCV CGN. Half of the patients were treated with IFN-α_{2a} 3 million units s.c. three times weekly for 24 weeks, while the other half were controls. The average serum creatinine was 1.2 and 1.3 mg/dL in the IFN-α and control groups respectively. Approximately 75% of the patients in both groups were characterized as having renal disease at entry into the study, defined by the presence of one of the following: microscopic hematuria, proteinuria, hypertension, or mild-to-moderate renal failure (peak serum creatinine 3.5 mg/dL in both groups). Renal biopsies were not documented. Fifteen of 25 IFN-α-treated patients displayed a small decrease in the mean serum creatinine (from 1.3 to 1.15 mg/dL) and no detectable HCV RNA, whereas untreated patients had a small average serum creatinine increase (from 1.55 to 1.65 mg/dL) and evidence of ongoing viral infection. Unfortunately, after IFN-α therapy was discontinued, HCV RNA and cryoglobulinemia recurred in all 15 patients.

In another prospective trial, Dammacco et al[52] randomized 65 patients with mixed cryoglobulinemia into the following four treatment arms: IFN-α, 3 million units intramuscularly three times per week for 48 weeks (n = 15); 6-methyl-prednisolone (6MP) 16 mg/day orally for 48 weeks (n = 18); IFN-α plus 6MP as above on non-IFN-α days for 48 weeks (n =17); and supportive treatment (n = 15). An average of 43% of the patients in each of the four treatment arms was characterized as having renal involvement, and approximately 80% of the patients were anti-HCV positive. Renal involvement was determined as in the previous study without renal biopsy sampling. A 50% cryocrit decrement was achieved in 53% of patients in both IFN-α arms, and in 17% of 6MP subjects. Proteinuria and renal function improved in one of three patients in the IFN-α arm and in two of the five patients in the IFN-α plus 6MP arm.

In a prospective uncontrolled trial of 34 anti-HCV-positive patients with proteinuria (approximately 60–80% in the nephrotic range), Johnson and colleagues[53] treated 19 patients with IFN-α 3 million units s.c. three times per week for 6–12 months. Although proteinuria was significantly reduced, no significant improvement was observed in mean serum creatinine levels – from 2.0 to 1.5 mg/dL. HCV was undetectable in six patients after IFN-α therapy, but recurred in all patients 3 months after completion of a course of IFN-α. Although IFN-α therapy is an important consideration to prevent liver disease progression, IFN-α monotherapy in HCV CGN is of limited efficacy and has significant side-effects. The role of longer acting pegylated interferon in CGN should be explored in prospective trials.

HCV and renal replacement
Management of HCV in ESRD

Patients undergoing HD have a higher prevalence of anti-HCV than the general population,[54] the average ranging from 5% to 44% in US dialysis units[55,56] depending on the sensitivity of the antibody employed and the prevalence of risk factors in the ESRD population. The likelihood of HCV infection while on HD is directly related to the number of blood transfusions a patient has received and the duration of HD therapy,[57] with an estimated 10% per year cumulative risk.[58] Chronic liver disease is often clinically and biochemically silent in ESRD. There is often no history of jaundice and only one-third of HD patients with biopsy-proven chronic hepatitis have elevated alanine aminotransferase (ALT) levels.[57] Furthermore, anti-HCV-positive dialysis patients awaiting renal transplantation are at increased risk of death from all causes (including liver failure) compared with anti-HCV-negative dialysis patients.[59] Several documented outbreaks of patient-to-patient HCV transmission have occurred in hemodialysis units almost certainly as a result of breaches in infection-control protocol.[13,56] Recent Centers for Disease Control and Prevention (CDC) screening recommendations for hemodialysis patients include monitoring ALT levels monthly, HCV antibody testing for all new patients, and HCV antibody testing at 6-month intervals for all anti-HCV-negative patients.[13] Unlike HBV, there are no recommendations regarding HCV-infected patient treatment with dedicated machines, or prohibition of dialyzer reprocessing. The results of HCV screening should be used to evaluate individual patients as well as contribute to an infection-control program, with emphasis on detection of HCV transmission and proper implementation of infection-control measures.

Unfortunately, optimal therapy for the dialysis patient with HCV infection is complicated by antiviral side-effects. Ribavirin and its metabolites, normally cleared by the kidney, accumulate in ESRD, resulting in a severe hemolytic anemia which would be poorly tolerated in this population with a high prevalence of anemia and coronary artery disease. Monotherapy with IFN-α_{2b} for HCV infection in HD patients has been advocated instead, but intolerance to adverse effects may limit its efficacy.[60] Clinical trials of pegylated interferon are ongoing in patients treated with HD.

Effects of HCV on renal transplant recipients

Anti-HCV-positive renal transplant recipients have higher mortality rates and shorter long-term graft survival than anti-HCV-negative recipients.[61,62] However, HCV-infected renal transplant recipients appear to have better survival rates than their HCV-infected counterparts maintained on chronic hemodialysis.[59,63] Because of a shortage of cadaveric kidneys, outcomes in anti-HCV-positive renal transplant recipients were studied by Morales and colleagues[64] who found no differences in liver disease, graft survival, or mortality when either anti-HCV-positive or anti-HCV-negative donor kidneys were transplanted. Therefore, donor kidneys of patients infected with HCV can be reasonably allocated to HCV-infected recipients with informed consent. One study supports the practice of antiviral therapy preoperatively in anti-HCV-positive dialysis patients, regardless of donor status, to avoid enhanced viral replication after transplantation.[65] Most authors do not recommend IFN-α therapy after renal transplantation because this agent is both only partially effective[66] and frequently associated with acute rejection.[66,67]

Human immunodeficiency virus and renal disease

Background

The human retrovirus, HIV-1, was discovered in 1983,[68] 2 years after the first series of AIDS cases was published.[69] HIV infection prevalence varies widely from significantly less than 1% in industrialized nations to over 20% in parts of the African continent, although studies documenting the renal complications have primarily come from the former.[70]

HIV-associated renal disease

Spectrums of renal syndromes are associated with HIV, including acute renal failure, hyponatremia, adrenal insufficiency, and glomerular disease. The focus of this section is the glomerular diseases associated with HIV infection, dominantly HIV-associated nephropathy (HIVAN), HIV-associated immune complex disease (HIV ICD), and HIV-associated thrombotic microangiopathy (HIV TM) (see Table 27.1).

Pathogenesis

The pathogenesis of HIVAN is poorly characterized, but mounting evidence supports a role for direct infection of renal tissue. HIV-1 mRNA and DNA are detected in renal tubular epithelial cells and podocytes of HIVAN patients.[71,72] The mechanism of viral podocyte entry and the relationship between infection and HIVAN pathogenesis are unknown.

Indications for renal biopsy

Renal biopsy is usually required for precise diagnosis of HIV-infected patients with significant proteinuria or renal failure of unknown etiology, since one retrospective review of 136 renal biopsies revealed only 65% had HIVAN.[73] HIV TM may be underrepresented in biopsy series (1 of 136 in the retrospective review) because this entity usually requires a peripheral blood smear and clinical characteristics to establish a diagnosis.

HIV-associated nephropathy

Heavy proteinuria, and hypoalbuminemia, accompanied by renal failure that progresses to ESRD in 8–16 weeks is the typical course. Hypertension, hyerlipidemia, hematuria, and edema are variably identified. Renal sonogram reveals normal or increased kidney sizes even in advanced renal failure. Although presentation can occur at any time, HIVAN generally is a complication of advanced HIV infection.[74] Epidemiology is remarkable for male and Black race predominance.[74] Classic renal pathology includes focal and segmental glomerulosclerosis with capillary collapse, tubular atrophy, tubular microcystic dilatation, interstitial infiltrate, and, on electron microscopy, endo-

Table 27.2 Classic pathology in HIV-associated nephropathy (HIVAN)

Focal and segmental glomerulosclerosis with capillary collapse
Tubular atrophy
Tubular microcystic dilatation
Interstitial infiltrate
Endothelial tubuloreticular structures

thelial tubular reticular structures (Table 27.2).[73] None of these five findings is absolutely specific as they are less frequently found in idiopathic focal and segmental glomerulosclerosis;[73] however, when found in aggregate, the diagnosis of HIVAN is highly likely. Voluntary HIV testing should be offered to patients with heavy proteinuria and suggestive biopsy findings.

HIV-associated renal disease in children

Biopsies in HIV-infected children with renal disease reveal mesangial hyperplasia, the most common lesion, in 50% and HIVAN in approximately one-third.[75] There is a high incidence of mesangial hyperplasia in African-Americans, but in contrast to HIVAN, 30–60% of cases are female. Clinical onset follows 1–5 years after vertical transmission. Progression to ESRD usually requires 1–3 years.

HIV-associated immune complex disease

A variety of glomerular diseases are described in HIV-infected patients, including minimal change disease, IgA nephropathy or other mesangial proliferative glomerulonephritis, MN, MPGN, and crescentic glomerulonephritis. In contrast to HIVAN, HIV ICD patients more likely have hematuria, hypocomplementemia, mild-to-moderate proteinuria, and gradual progressive renal disease. Although Blacks predominate in most series, patients of non-African heritage are well represented. One review of 26 renal biopsies in HIV-infected Italians, 19 of whom were intravenous drug abusers, revealed HIV ICD in all 26 and no patients with HIVAN.[76] An interesting French series of 60 renal biopsies in HIV-infected subjects showed HIVAN in 23 of 29 Blacks and 3 of 31 Caucasians ($P < 0.001$), and HIV ICD in six Blacks and 16 Caucasians.[77] HIV ICD resembles idiopathic lesions, except for the variable presence of tubuloreticular structures. The latter are a general marker for interferon activity, and thus do not imply retroviral infection. Although a few HIV ICD cases demonstrate evidence supporting HIV-mediated immune complex disease,[78] the relationship between infection and ICD is not established in the majority of published cases.

HIV thrombotic microangiopathy

Like idiopathic TM, the original pentad of microangiopathic hemolytic anemia, thrombocytopenia, renal dysfunction, neurological signs, and noninfectious fever is found in a minority of HIV TM patients at presentation.[79] Microangiopathic hemolytic anemia, thrombocytopenia, and elevated serum lactate dehydrogenase (LDH) are required to establish the diagnosis of HIV TM,[79] which includes hemolytic uremic syndrome and thrombotic thrombocytopenic purpura. HIV infection is commonly associated with TM in urban areas – 12% in Miami[80] and 14% in San Francisco.[79] HIV TM is distinguished from the idiopathic form by high 1-year mortality, approaching 100% even with treatment in AIDS patients.[79-81] High serum LDH levels (> 2500 U/L) at presentation carry a poor prognosis.[82]

Antiretroviral therapy

A primary principle of secondary glomerular disease therapy is to treat the underlying process. Accordingly, improvement in HIVAN and HIV TM has been reported using azidothymidine (AZT), and more recently highly active antiretroviral therapy (HAART) (see Table 27.3). Pre- and post-HAART renal biopsies in two HIVAN cases in two reports demonstrated dramatic improvement in kidney pathology and reversal of dialysis requirement with HAART.[71,83] In one instance, the importance of the kidney as a long-term reservoir was underscored by persistent evidence of retroviral RNA in renal epithelium after such recovery.[71] Proteinuria in one child with HIV-associated nephrotic syndrome in the absence of renal biopsy resolved after HAART.[84] One case of HIV ICD (membranous nephropathy) revealed improvement in proteinuria from 20 g daily to trace after HAART.[85] A retrospective cohort study of HIVAN in 19 patients revealed attenuation of renal disease progression in the eight protease-inhibitor-treated subjects.[86] Major flaws of the study included biopsy documentation in only six individuals and frequent concomitant angiotensin-converting enzyme inhibitor (ACEI) and glucocorticoid use. Despite the absence of prospective trials, HAART is the first-line therapy of HIV-related renal disorders. It clearly improves survival, decreases opportunistic infection, delays progression to AIDS, and has the potential to reverse renal disease. Medication expense, compliance, and drug toxicities are the major limitations to therapy. Prospective trials of HAART controlled for concomitant ACEI and glucocorticoid use are needed to further define the role of these interventions.

Angiotensin-converting enzyme inhibitors

Two nonrandomized studies of adult HIVAN patients showed improvements in proteinuria and attenuation of renal failure progression using ACEI therapy (Table 27.4).[87,88] Burns and colleagues used 10 mg fosinopril daily in 12 of 20 normotensive patients with biopsy-proven HIVAN. Only four treated and three untreated patients received antiviral drugs, and no patient was treated with steroids or HAART.[87] After 12 weeks, the mean serum creatinine and daily proteinuria levels in ACEI-treated and control nephrotic subjects were 2.0 versus 9.2 mg/dL ($P = 0.02$), respectively, and in untreated nephrotic patients were 2.8 versus 10.5 g ($P = 0.008$) respectively. After 24 weeks, ACEI-treated nonnephrotic subjects also significantly benefited from fosinopril therapy compared with controls, with a mean serum creatinine level of 1.5 versus 4.9 mg/dL ($P = 0.006$), respectively, as well as a daily proteinuria level of 1.25 versus 8.5 g ($P = 0.006$) respectively. A major weakness of the study was that controls refused ACEI treatment. Kimmel and colleagues[88] used captopril 6.25–25 mg three times daily, as tolerated, in 9 of 18 biopsy-documented African-American patients with HIVAN showing significantly improved renal survival: 156 versus 37 days in the nine controls matched by age, race, sex, CD4 cell count, and serum creatinine

Table 27.3 Antiretroviral therapy and renal dysfunction

	Normal	CrCl 10–50	CrCl < 10
Nucleoside analogs			
Abacavir	300 mg b.i.d.	Same	Same
Didianosine	200 mg b.i.d.	150 mg q.d.	100 mg q.d.
Lamivudine	150 mg b.i.d.	100 mg q.d.	50 mg q.d.
Stavudine	40 mg b.i.d.	20 mg b.i.d.	20 mg q.d.
Zalcitabine	0.75 mg t.i.d.	0.75 mg q.d.	Avoid
Zidovudine	200 mg t.i.d.	100 mg t.i.d.	100 mg t.i.d.
Nonnucleoside reverse transcriptase inhibitors			
Delavirdine	400 mg t.i.d.	Same	Same
Efavirenz	600 mg q.d.	Same	Same
Nevirapine	200 mg q.d. for 14 days, then b.i.d.	Same	Same
Protease inhibitors			
Amprenavir	1200 mg b.i.d.	Same	Same
Indinavir	800 mg t.i.d.	Same	Same
Nelfinavir	750 mg t.i.d.	Same	Same
Ritonavir	600 mg b.i.d.	Same	Same
Saquinavir	600 mg t.i.d.	Same	Same

CrCl, creatinine clearance.

Table 27.4 Summary of intervention trials

Design	Treated (n)	Control (n)	Therapy	Outcome	Comment	Reference: disease
Retrospective	15	NA	IFN-α	53% HBeAg cleared long term	Better response with MN than MPGN	10: HBV MN and MPGN
Prospective, randomized	20	20	IFN-α	100% proteinuria resolution, 80% HBeAg cleared	All subjects were steroid resistant	11: HBV MN
Retrospective	10	NA	3TC 100 mg q.d.	70% HBeAg cleared	Concomitant PE and steroids	7: HBV PAN
Prospective, randomized	26	26	IFN-α	60% HCV RNA cleared	HCV RNA and cryoglobulins recurred in all	51: HCV CGN
Prospective, randomized	50 (A, 15; B, 17; C, 18)	15	A, IFN-α alone; B, IFN-α + 6MP; C, 6MP alone	↓ Cryocrit (A, 53%; B, 53%; C, 17%)	Relapse (A, 75%; B, 60%; C, 100%)	52: HCV CGN
Prospective, uncontrolled	19	NA	IFN-α	HCV RNA cleared (6), proteinuria reduced	HCV RNA recurred in all	53: HCV MPGN and CGN
Retrospective cohort	8	11	Protease inhibitor	Slower decline in CrCl	Biopsy (6), ACEI (5), prednisone (5)	86: HIVAN
Prospective, nonrandomized	12	8	Fosinopril 10 mg q.d.	SCr 2.0 mg/dL vs. 9.2 mg/dL, proteinuria 2.8 g vs. 10.5 g daily	Controls refused ACEI	87: HIVAN
Retrospective cohort	9	9	Captopril 6.25–25 mg t.i.d.	Renal survival, 156 vs. 37 days	One suicide ACEI group	88: HIVAN
Retrospective	20	NA	Prednisone 60 mg q.d.	SCr 8.1 to 3.0 mg/dL in 17	Infectious complications common	90: HIVAN
Retrospective cohort	15	87	Prednisone 1 mg/kg q.d.	Renal survival improved	No significant proteinuria attenuation	91: HIVAN
Retrospective cohort	13	8	Prednisone 60 mg q.d.	Renal survival improved	No mortality benefit, steroid group, increased hospital days	92: HIVAN

NA, not available; IFN-α, interferon α; HBeAg, hepatitis B e antigen; MN, membranous nephropathy; MPGN, membranoproliferative glomerulonephritis; HBV, hepatitis B virus; 3TC, lamivudine; PE, plasma exchange; PAN, polyarteritis nodosa; HCV, hepatitis C virus; CGN, cryoglobulinemic glomerulonephritis; 6MP, 6-methylprednisolone; CrCl, creatinine clearance; ACEI, angiotensin-converting enzyme inhibitor; HIVAN, HIV-associated nephropathy; SCr, serum creatinine.

levels. Antiviral therapy was administered in six captopril-treated and in seven untreated patients, whereas no patient received HAART or steroid therapy. The precise mechanism of ACEI in HIVAN is unknown, but antiviral protease properties have been proposed.[89]

Corticosteroids

A number of case reports and retrospective series have shown improvement in renal function and proteinuria with oral prednisone therapy in adult patients with HIVAN, although studies in children with HIV and renal disease have been disappointing. The adult studies have employed a steroid taper over months. Smith and colleagues[90] treated 20 patients with HIVAN, 17 of whom were biopsy proven, with 60 mg prednisone daily for 2–11 weeks (mean 4 weeks). All 20 patients had AIDS, 19 of whom were treated with antiviral therapy, but none was treated with HAART or ACEI. Initial response to gluco-

corticoid therapy was impressive, with a mean decrease in creatinine from 8.1 to 3.0 mg/dL (P < 0.001) in 17 cases. After 44 weeks' median follow-up, eight patients required dialysis therapy and 11 died of complications of AIDS. Steroid complications in this study are difficult to evaluate in the absence of a control group. A French retrospective review of 102 patients with biopsy-proven HIVAN revealed improved dialysis-free survival but no significant difference in mortality in 15 patients treated for 2–6 weeks with 1 mg/kg daily prednisone or prednisolone.[91]

In a retrospective cohort study of 21 patients with biopsy-documented HIVAN, Eustace and colleagues[92] found 6-month independent renal function in 7 of 13 subjects treated for 1 month with 60 mg daily prednisone compared with one of eight controls (P = 0.06). Only 1 of 21 patients was treated with ACEI. Importantly, four patients in each group did not receive any antiviral therapy, and no patient received HAART. Although the

Table 27.5 Typical treatment regimen for the glomerular diseases indicated

	HBV MN	HBV MPGN	HBV PAN	HCV CGN	HIVAN	HIV ICD	HIV TM
First line	IFN-α	IFN-α	PE, steroids, and 3TC	IFN-α	HAART + ACEI	HAART + ACEI	PE and HAART
Second line	3TC	3TC	PE, steroids, and IFN-α	Pegylated IFN-α?	HAART	HAART	PE and steroids
Third line	Adefovir or tenofovir?	Adefovir or tenofovir?	PE, steroids, adefovir, or tenofovir?	?	Steroids	?	PE and ACEI

HBV, hepatitis B virus; MN, membranous nephropathy; MPGN, membranoproliferative glomerulonephritis; PAN, polyarteritis nodosa; HCV, hepatitis C virus; CGN, cryoglobulinemic glomerulonephritis; HIVAN, HIV-associated nephropathy; ICD, HIV-associated immune complex disease; HIV TM, HIV-associated thrombotic microangiopathy; IFN-α, interferon α; PE, plasma exchange; 3TC, lamivudine; HAART, highly active antiretroviral therapy; ACEI, angiotensin-converting enzyme inhibitor.

follow-up period was inconsistent, the rate of infection and hospitalization was similar in both groups. However, the steroid-treated patients had significantly more inhospital days, and again no mortality benefit was shown. The presumed role of corticosteroids in HIVAN is improvement in interstitial inflammation, as one case report documented pre- and posttherapy biopsies with significantly improved interstitial infiltrate as well as similar glomerular morphology.[93] Retrospective studies have shown only modest improvement in proteinuria (typically nephrotic to approximately 2 g/day) or no significant proteinuria attenuation.[91] The potential risks of therapy and unknown long-term effects make steroids a third-line agent in selected HIVAN cases (Table 27.5).

Plasmapheresis

Daily plasma exchange using fresh–frozen plasma is the standard treatment of HIV TM until LDH and platelet counts improve.[80,82] The use of HAART as part of this regimen should be evaluated.

HIV and renal replacement
Management of HIV in ESRD

HIVAN is now the third leading cause of ESRD in young US Black adults.[94]

The prevalence of HIV infection in dialysis patients varies by center location and by demographics of the local ESRD population. Twenty percent of dialysis patients in urban centers are HIV-positive compared with few or no infected patients in dialysis centers in suburban communities or those with a much lower percentage of African-Americans. Voluntary confidential HIV testing should be considered in all dialysis patients as improved mortality and potential to reversal of dialysis dependence may be associated with HAART.[89] Both peritoneal and hemodialysis should be considered in such patients.

Effects of HIV on renal transplant recipients

Case reports published before HAART was available suggest that patients with asymptomatic HIV infection who have undergone renal transplantation have increased morbidity and mortality compared with uninfected ESRD patients.[95] In 1998, given the shortage of organs and uncertain prognosis, the majority of US renal transplant program directors would not transplant kidneys to asymptomatic HIV-infected patients with endstage renal disease.[96] However, recent advances in therapy may make renal transplantation a reasonable option for patients with an undetectable viral burden.

References

1. Purcell RH: The discovery of the hepatitis viruses. Gastroenterology 1993;104:955–963.
2. Lee HS, Choi Y, Yu SH, et al: A renal biopsy study of hepatitis B virus-associated nephropathy in Korea. Kidney Int 1988;34:537–543.
3. Lin CY: Clinical features and natural course of HBV-related glomerulopathy in children. Kidney Int 1991;35 (Suppl):S46–S53.
4. Gilbert RD, Wiggelinkhuizen J: The clinical course of hepatitis B virus-associated nephropathy. Pediatr Nephrol 1994;8:11–14.
5. Lai KN, Li PK, Lui SF, et al: Membranous nephropathy related to hepatitis B virus in adults. N Engl J Med 1991;324:1457–1463.
6. Gower RG, Sausker WF, Kohler PF, et al: Small vessel vasculitis caused by hepatitis B virus immune complexes: small vessel vasculitis and HBsAG. J Allergy Clin Immunol 1978;62:222–228.
7. Trepo C, Guillevin L: Polyarteritis nodosa and extrahepatic manifestations of HBV infection: the case against autoimmune intervention in pathogenesis. J Autoimmun 2001;16:269–274.
8. Guillevin L, Lhote F, Gayraud M, et al: Prognostic factors in polyarteritis nodosa and Churg–Strauss syndrome: a prospective study in 342 patients. Medicine 1996;75:17–28.
9. Lai KN, Tam JS, Lin HJ, et al: The therapeutic dilemma of the usage of corticosteroid in patients with membranous nephropathy and persistent hepatitis B virus surface antigenaemia. Nephron 1990;54:12–17.
10. Conjeevaram HS, Hoofnagle JH, Austin HA, et al: Long-term outcome of hepatitis B virus-related glomerulonephritis after therapy with interferon alfa. Gastroenterology 1995;109:540–546.
11. Lin CY: Treatment of hepatitis B virus-associated membranous nephropathy with recombinant alpha-interferon. Kidney Int 1995;47:225–230.
12. Guillevin L, Lhote F, Cohen P, et al: Polyarteritis nodosa related to hepatitis B virus: a prospective study with long-term observation of 41 patients. Medicine 1995;74:238–253.
13. Centers for Disease Control and Prevention. Recommendations for preventing transmission of infections among chronic hemodialysis patients. MMWR 2001;50(RR-5):20–24.
14. Fornairon S, Pol S, Legendre C, et al: The long-term virologic and pathologic impact of renal transplantation on chronic hepatitis B virus infection. Transplantation 1996;62:297–299.
15. Harnett JD, Zeldis JB, Parfrey PS, et al: Hepatitis B disease in dialysis and transplant patients: further epidemiologic and serologic studies. Transplantation 1987;44:369–376.
16. Lee WC, Wu MJ, Cheng CH, et al: Lamivudine is effective for the treatment of reactivation of hepatitis B virus and fulminant hepatic failure in renal transplant recipients. Am J Kidney Dis 2001;38:1074–1081.

17. Han DJ, Kim TH, Park SK, et al: Results on preemptive or prophylactic treatment of lamivudine in HBsAg (+) renal allograft recipients: comparison with salvage treatment after hepatic dysfunction with HBV recurrence. Transplantation 2001;71:387–394.

18. Kletzmayr J, Watschinger B, Muller C, et al: Twelve months of lamivudine treatment for chronic hepatitis B virus infection in renal transplant recipients. Transplantation 2000;70:1404–1407.

19. Choo Q-L, Kuo G, Weiner AJ, et al: Isolation of a cDNA clone derived from a blood-borne non-A, non-B viral hepatitis genome. Science 1989;244:359–362.

20. Alter MJ, Kruszon-Moran D, Nainan OV, et al: The prevalence of hepatitis C virus infection in the United States, 1988 through 1994. N Engl J Med 1999;341:556–562.

21. Alter MJ: Hepatitis C virus infection in the United States. J Hepatol 1999;31 (Suppl 1):88–91.

22. Pouteil-Noble C, Maiza H, Dijoud F, et al: Glomerular disease associated with hepatitis C virus infection in native kidneys. Nephrol Dial Transplant 2000;15 (Suppl 8):28–33.

23. Cacoub P, Lunel-Fabiani, F, Huong Du LT: Polyarteritis and hepatitis C infection. Ann Intern Med 1992;116:605.

24. Agnello V, Chung RT, Kaplan LM: A role for hepatitis C virus infection in type II cryglobulinemia. N Engl J Med 1992;327:1490–1495.

25. Wong VS, Egner W, Elsey T, et al: Incidence, character and clinical relevance of mixed cryoglobulinemia in patients with chronic hepatitis C virus infection. Clin Exp Immunol 1996;104:25–31.

26. Harle JR, Disdier P, Dussol B, et al: Membranoproliferative glomerulonephritis and hepatitis C infection. Lancet 1993;341:904.

27. Yamabe H, Fukushi K, Ohsawa H, et al: Hepatitis C virus (HCV) infection may be an important cause of membranoproliferative glomerulonephritis in Japan (abstract). J Am Soc Nephrol 1993;4:291.

28. Johnson RJ, Gretch DR, Yamabe H, et al: Membranoproliferative glomerulonephritis associated with hepatitis C virus infection. N Engl J Med 1993;328:465–470.

29. Fabrizi F, Pozzi C, Farina M, et al: Hepatitis C virus infection and acute or chronic glomerulonephritis: an epidemiological and clinical appraisal. Nephrol Dial Transplant 1998;13:1991–1997.

30. Pasquariello A, Ferri C, Moriconi L, et al: Cryoglobulinemic membranoproliferative glomerulonephritis associated with hepatitis C virus. Am J Nephrol 1993;13:300–304.

31. Brouet JC, Clauvel JP, Danon F, et al: Biological and clinical significance of cryoglobulins: a report of 86 cases. Am J Med 1974;57:775–778.

32. D'Amico G, Colasanti G, Ferrario F, et al: Renal involvement in essential mixed cryoglobulinemia. Kidney Int 1989;35:1004–1014.

33. D'Amico G: Renal involvement in hepatitis C infection: cryoglobulinemic glomerulonephritis. Kidney Int 1998;54:650–671.

34. Tarantino A, De Vecchi A, Montagnino G, et al: Renal disease in essential mixed cryoglobulinemia: longterm follow-up of 44 patients. Q J Med 1981;50:1–30.

35. Tarantino A, Campise M, Banfi G, et al: Long-term predictors of survival in essential mixed cryoglobulinemic glomerulonephritis. Kidney Int 1995;47:618–623.

36. Falk RJ, Jennette JC, Nachman PH: Primary glomerular disease. In Brenner BM (ed): Brenner & Rector's The Kidney. Philadelphia: WB Saunders, 2000, pp 1292–1297.

37. D'Amico G, Fornasieri A: Cryoglobulinemic glomerulonephritis: a membranoproliferative glomerulonephritis induced by hepatitis C virus. Am J Kidney Dis 1995;25:361–369.

38. Cordonnier D, Martin H, Groslambert P, et al: Mixed IgG–IgM cryoglobulinemia with glomerulonephritis: immunochemical, fluorescent and ultrastructural study of kidney and in vitro cryoprecipitate. Am J Med 1975;59:867–872.

39. Feiner H, Gallo G: Ultrastructure in glomerulonephritis associated with cryoglobulinemia: a report of six cases and review of the literature. Am J Pathol 1977;88:145–155.

40. Ferri C, Monti M, La Civita, L, et al: Infection of peripheral blood mononuclear cells by hepatitis C virus in mixed cryoglobulinemia. Blood 1993;82:3701–3704.

41. Fornasieri A, Li M, Armelloni S, et al: Glomerulonephritis induced by human IgMk–IgG cryoglobulins in mice. Lab Invest 1993;69:531–540.

42. Quigg RJ, Brathwaite M, Gardner DF, et al: Successful cyclophosphamide treatment of cryoglobulinemic membranoproliferative glomerulonephritis associated with hepatitis C infection. Am J Kidney Dis 1995;25:798–800.

43. Mori Y, Kishimoto N, Imai Y, et al: Cryofiltration and oral corticosteroids provide successful treatment for an elderly patient with cryoglobulinemic glomerulonephritis associated with hepatitis C infection. Intern Med 2000;39:564–569.

44. De Vecchi A, Montagnino G, Pozzi C, et al: Intravenous methylprednisolone pulse therapy in essential mixed cryoglobulinemic nephropathy. Clin Nephrol 1983;19:221–227.

45. Sinico RA, Fornasieri A, Fiorini G, et al: Plasma exchange in the treatment of essential mixed cryoglobulinemic nephropathy: long-term follow-up. Int J Artif Organs 1984;8 (Suppl 2):15–18.

46. McHutchison JG, Gordon SC, Schiff ER, et al: Interferon alpha-2b alone or in combination with ribavirin as initial treatment for chronic hepatitis C. N Engl J Med 1998;339:1485–1492.

47. Reichard O, Norkrans G, Frydén A, et al: Randomised, double-blind, placebo-controlled trial of interferon alpha-2b with and without ribavirin for chronic hepatitis C. Lancet 1998;351:83–87.

48. Willson RA: The benefit of long-term interferon alfa therapy for symptomatic mixed cryoglobulinemia (cutaneous vasculitis/membranoproliferative glomerulonephritis) associated with chronic hepatitis C infection. J Clin Gastroenterol 2001;33:137–140.

49. Misiani R, Bellavita P, Baio P, et al: Successful treatment of HCV-associated cryoglobulinemic glomerulonephritis with a combination of interferon-alpha and ribavirin. Nephrol Dial Transplant 1999;14:1558–1560.

50. Garini G, Allegri L, Carnevali L, et al: Interferon-alpha in combination with ribavirin as initial treatment for hepatitis C virus-associated cryoglobulinemic membranoproliferative glomerulonephritis. Am J Kidney Dis 2001;38(6):1–5.

51. Misiani R, Bellavita P, Fenili D, et al: Interferon alfa-2a therapy in cryoglobulinemia associated with hepatitis C virus. N Engl J Med 1994;330:751–756.

52. Dammacco F, Sansonno D, Han JH, et al: Natural interferon-alpha versus its combination with 6-methyl-prednisolone in the therapy of type II mixed cryoglobulinemia: a long-term, randomized, controlled study. Blood 1994;84:3336–3343.

53. Johnson RJ, Gretch DR, Couser WG, et al: Hepatitis C virus-associated glomerulonephritis: effect of alpha-interferon therapy. Kidney Int 1994;46:1700–1704

54. Zeldis JB, Depner TA, Kuramoto IK, et al: The prevalence of hepatitis C virus antibodies among hemodialysis patients. Ann Intern Med 1990;112:958–960.

55. Moyer LA, Alter MJ: Hepatitis C virus in the hemodialysis setting: a review with recommendations for control. Semin Dial 1994;7:124–127.

56. Wreghitt TG: Blood-borne virus infections in dialysis units – a review. Rev Med Virol 1999;9:101–109.

57. Pereira BJG, Levey AS: Hepatitis C virus infection in dialysis and renal transplantation. Kidney Int 1997;51:981–999.

58. Hardy NM, Sandroni S, Danielson S, et al: Antibody to hepatitis C virus increases with time on dialysis. Clin Nephrol 1992;38:44–48.

59. Pereira BJG, Svetlozar NN, Bouthot BA, et al: Effect of hepatitis C infection and renal transplantation on survival in end-stage renal disease. Kidney Int 1998;53:1374–1381.

60. Degos F, Pol S, Laffite V, et al: Multicentric prospective assessment of the tolerance and efficacy of alpha-2b in hemodialysis patients. Hepatology 1999;30:365A.

61. Pereira BJG, Wright TL, Schmid CH, et al: The impact of pretransplantation hepatitis C infection on the outcome of renal transplantation. Transplantation 1995;60:799–805.

62. Legendre C, Garrigue V, Le Bihan C, et al: Harmful long-term impact of hepatitis C virus infection in kidney transplant recipients. Transplantation 1998;65:667–670.

63. Knoll GA, Tankersley MR, Lee JY, et al: The impact of renal transplantation on survival in hepatitis C-positive end-stage renal disease patients. Am J Kidney Dis 1997;29:608–614.

64. Morales JM, Campistol JM, Castellano G, et al: Transplantation of kidneys from donors with hepatitis C antibody into recipients with pre-transplant anti-HCV. Kidney Int 1995;47:236–240.

65. Casanovas-Taltavull T, Baliellas C, Benasco C, et al: Efficacy of interferon for chronic hepatitis C virus-related hepatitis in kidney transplant candidates on hemodialysis: results after transplantation. Am J Gastroenterol 2001;96:1170–1177.

66. Hanafusa T, Ichikawa Y, Kishikawa H, et al: Retrospective study on the impact of hepatitis C virus infection on kidney transplant patients over 20 years. Transplantation 1998;66:471–476.

67. Magnone M, Holley JL, Shapiro R, et al: Interferon-alpha-induced acute renal allograft rejection. Transplantation 1995;59:1068–1070.
68. Barre-Sinoussi F, Chermann JC, Rey F, et al: Isolation of a T-lymphotropic retrovirus from a patient at risk for acquired immune deficiency syndrome (AIDS). Science 1983;220:868–871.
69. Siegal FP, Lopez C, Hammer GS, et al: Severe acquired immunodeficiency in male homosexuals, manifested by chronic perianal ulcerative herpes simplex lesions. N Engl J Med 1981;305:1439–1444.
70. Walker N, Garcia-Calleja JM, Heaton L, et al: Epidemiological analysis of the quality of HIV sero-surveillance in the world: how well do we track the epidemic? AIDS 2001;15:1545–1554.
71. Winston JA, Bruggeman LA, Ross MD, et al: Nephropathy and establishment of a renal reservoir of HIV type 1 during primary infection. N Engl J Med 2001;344:1979–1984.
72. Bruggeman LA, Ross MD, Tanji N, et al: Renal epithelium is a previously unrecognized site of HIV-1 infection. J Am Soc Nephrol 2000;11:2079–2087.
73. D'Agati V, Appel GB: Renal pathology of human immunodeficiency virus infection. Semin Nephrol 1998;18:406–421.
74. Winston JA, Klotman ME, Klotman PE: HIV-associated nephropathy is a late, not early, manifestation of HIV-1 infection. Kidney Int 1999;55:1036–1040.
75. Ray PE, Rakusan T, Loechelt BJ, et al: Human immunodeficiency virus (HIV)-associated nephropathy in children from the Washington, D.C. area: 12 years' experience. Semin Nephrol 1998;18:396–405.
76. Casanova S, Mazzucco G, Barbiano di Belgiojoso G, et al: Pattern of glomerular involvement in human immunodeficiency virus-infected patients: an Italian study. Am J Kidney Dis 1995;26:446–453.
77. Nochy D, Glotz D, Dosquet P, et al: Renal disease associated with HIV infection: a multicentric study of 60 patients from Paris hospitals. Nephrol Dial Transplant 1993;8:11–19.
78. Kimmel PL, Phillips TM, Ferreira-Centeno A, et al: Brief report: idiotypic IgA nephropathy in patients with human immunodeficiency virus infection. N Engl J Med 1992;327:702–706.
79. Thompson CE, Damon LE, Ries CA, et al: Thrombotic microangiopathies in the 1980s: clinical features, response to treatment, and the impact of the human immunodeficiency virus epidemic. Blood 1992;80:1890–1895.
80. Ucar A, Fernandez HF, Byrnes JJ, et al: Thrombotic microangiopathy and retroviral infections: a 13-year experience. Am J Hematol 1994;45:304–309.
81. Gadallah MF, el-Shahawy MA, Campese VM, et al: Disparate prognosis of thrombotic microangiopathy in HIV-infected patients with and without AIDS. Am J Nephrol 1996;16:446–450.
82. Abraham B, Baud O, Bonnet E, et al: Thrombotic microangiopathy during HIV infection. Presse Med 2001;30:581–585.
83. Wali RK, Drachenberg CI, Papadimitriou JC, et al: HIV-1-associated nephropathy and response to highly-active antiretroviral therapy. Lancet 1998;352:783–784.
84. Viani RM, Dankner WM, Muelenaer PA, et al: Resolution of HIV-associated nephrotic syndrome with highly active antiretroviral therapy delivered by gastrostomy tube. Pediatrics 1999;104:1394–1396.
85. Dellow E, Unwin R, Miller R, et al: Protease inhibitor therapy for HIV infection: the effect on HIV-associated nephrotic syndrome. Nephrol Dial Transplant 1999;14:744–777.
86. Szczech LA, Edwards LJ, Sanders LL, et al: Protease inhibitors are associated with a slowed progression of HIV-related renal diseases. Clin Nephrol 2002;57:336–341.
87. Burns GC, Paul SK, Toth IR, et al: Effect of angiotensin-converting enzyme inhibition in HIV-associated nephropathy. J Am Soc Nephrol 1997;8:1140–1146.
88. Kimmel PL, Mishkin GJ, Umana WO: Captopril and renal survival in patients with human immunodeficiency virus nephropathy. Am J Kidney Dis 1996;28:202–208.
89. Kimmel PL, Bosch JP, Vassalotti JA: Treatment of human immunodeficiency virus (HIV)-associated nephropathy. Semin Nephrol 1998;18:446–458.
90. Smith MC, Austen JL, Carey JT, et al: Prednisone improves renal function and proteinuria in human immunodeficiency virus-associated nephropathy. Am J Med 1996;101:41–48.
91. Laradi A, Mallet A, Beaufils H, et al: HIV-associated nephropathy: outcome and prognosis factors. Groupe d'Etudes Nephrologiques d'Ile de France. J Am Soc Nephrol 1998;9:2327–2335.
92. Eustace JA, Nuermberger E, Choi M, et al: Cohort study of the treatment of severe HIV-associated nephropathy with corticosteroids. Kidney Int 2000;58:1253–1260.
93. Briggs WA, Tanawattanacharoen S, Choi MJ, et al: Clinicopathologic correlates of prednisone treatment of human immunodeficiency virus-associated nephropathy. Am J Kidney Dis 1996;28:618–621.
94. Winston JA, Burns GC, Klotman PE: The human immunodeficiency virus (HIV) epidemic and HIV-associated nephropathy. Semin Nephrol 1998;18:373–377.
95. Lang P, Niaudet P: Update and outcome of renal transplant patients with human immunodeficiency virus. The Groupe Cooperatif de Transplantation de l'Ile de France. Transplant Proc 1991;23(1 Pt 2):1352–1353.
96. Spital A: Should all human immunodeficiency virus-infected patients with end-stage renal disease be excluded from transplantation? The views of U.S. transplant centers. Transplantation 1998;65:1187–1191.

Management of Complications of Nephrotic Syndrome

Yvonne M. O'Meara and Jerrold S. Levine

Background

The nephrotic syndrome (NS) is a clinical complex characterized by proteinuria of more than 3.5 g/1.73 m^2 per 24 h (in practice > 3.0–3.5 g per 24 h), hypoalbuminemia, edema, hyperlipidemia, and lipiduria.[1-4] The key component is proteinuria, which results from altered permeability of the glomerular filtration barrier, namely the glomerular basement membrane and podocytes with their slit diaphragms. Proteinuria sets in motion a series of homeostatic and compensatory mechanisms that result in the clinical features of NS.[1,2] These features can occur with lesser degrees of proteinuria or may be absent even in patients with massive proteinuria. While the diseases and pathogenic mechanisms underlying NS are diverse, the result is alteration in the charge- and/or size-selective properties of the glomerular capillary wall such that permeability to albumin and other intermediate-sized macromolecules is enhanced.[3,4]

Management of NS focuses on (1) treatment of the causative disease where possible, generally with a combination of immunosuppressive drugs such as corticosteroids, cytotoxic agents, and calcineurin inhibitors, and (2) treatment of the complications that are responsible for much of the morbidity associated with this condition. In this chapter we discuss management of the complications of NS. Specifically, we address the treatment of hypoalbuminemia, edema, hyperlipidemia, abnormalities of calcium homeostasis, thromboembolic phenomena, and

increased susceptibility to infection. It must be stressed that in many areas there is a dearth of prospective controlled clinical trials, so that recommendations on treatment remain somewhat empiric. Where there is controversy or inadequate data regarding the management of a particular problem, the authors' view is presented.

Hypoalbuminemia/proteinuria

It is becoming increasingly clear that proteinuria per se may be deleterious to the kidney and play a role in the progression of renal disease.[5] The rate of progression is increased in patients with heavy proteinuria, and interventions that reduce urinary protein excretion have been demonstrated to slow the rate of decline of glomerular filtration rate (GFR) in both diabetic and nondiabetic renal disease.[6,7] The sequelae of hypoalbuminemia include an increased risk of acute renal failure (from renal hypoperfusion and filtration failure), systemic and renal drug toxicity (because of alterations in free and protein-bound drug levels), enhanced platelet aggregability, hyperlipidemia, and edema formation.[1] Protein malnutrition is an important complication, particularly in children, in whom normal growth and development may become stunted. Although outside the scope of this chapter, drug dosing needs to be approached with care in patients with nephrotic syndrome, especially those with hypoalbuminemia and impaired renal function.[8] Not only will hepatic and renal clearances be affected but the range of therapeutic levels will need to be lowered for drugs having a high degree of protein binding, since therapeutic ranges are typically based on total drug concentration rather than the bioactive free portion.

In general, the greater the magnitude of the proteinuria, the lower the serum albumin concentration. However, this relationship is not constant, and many patients do not develop hypoalbuminemia even in the presence of persistent heavy proteinuria. Other factors that may contribute to reduced serum albumin levels in patients with nephrotic-range proteinuria include an inappropriately low rate of hepatic albumin synthesis and, although controversial, an increased rate of renal albumin catabolism.[1]

Management

Therapeutic strategies employed to reduce proteinuria and increase serum albumin levels include manipulations of dietary protein intake and treatment with a combination of angiotensin-converting enzyme (ACE) inhibitors, angiotensin receptor antagonists (ATRA), or nonsteroidal anti-inflammatory drugs (NSAIDs). The antiproteinuric mechanism(s) are thought to involve both hemodynamic and local factors affecting glomerular permselectivity characteristics. These measures may confer substantial benefit in patients with severe NS, for whom much of the morbidity derives from persistent heavy proteinuria. Furthermore, a reduction in proteinuria may be associated with slowing of the rate of progression of the underlying renal disease (see later).

Manipulation of dietary protein intake

Although early reports advocated the use of high-protein diets to treat hypoalbuminemia, more recent work has called into question the rationale and efficacy of such an approach. In general, it appears that a high-protein diet results in increases in the rates of both hepatic albumin synthesis and urinary protein loss such that the plasma albumin level fails to increase and may actually decrease.[1,9,10] Furthermore, a high protein intake, by increasing glomerular capillary pressures, has been implicated in the progression of a variety of renal diseases.[11]

Early studies suggested that ingestion of a low-protein diet may reduce urinary protein loss, although this effect was offset by a concomitant decline in hepatic albumin synthesis, so that serum albumin concentrations were not consistently increased.[9,12,13] Recent studies have failed to show a consistent effect of dietary protein restriction on proteinuria. In a randomized crossover trial, Remuzzi et al[14] found that protein restriction (0.6 mg/kg/day) had no effect on renal hemodynamics or proteinuria in nephrotic patients with membranous nephropathy. D'Amico et al[15] reported similarly disappointing results with a protein-restricted diet that was supplemented with essential amino acids and contained a high ratio of polyunsaturated to saturated fats. At variance with these results, Giordano et al[16] reported a significant reduction in proteinuria (38%) and a small but significant increase in serum albumin in seven patients with NS ingesting a low-protein diet for 4 weeks (0.55 g/kg/day plus 1 g of dietary protein per gram of daily protein excretion). Walser et al[17] studied 16 nephrotic patients fed a very low protein diet (0.33 g/kg/day) supplemented with 10–20 g/day of essential amino acids for an average of 10 months. All patients had a reduction in proteinuria and an increase in serum albumin. Indeed, for the five patients with an initial GFR > 30 mL/min the response was especially dramatic, with the serum albumin increasing from 2.5 to 3.8 g/dL and proteinuria declining from 9.1 to 1.9 g/day.

Debate also continues about the potential risk of increasing protein malnutrition by restriction of dietary protein intake in patients who are already severely hypoalbuminemic.[13,18,19] Lack of patient tolerability and the need for close nutritional monitoring are additional factors that may dissuade prescription of such regimens.

Until the benefits and potential risks of dietary protein manipulation are further clarified, it would appear reasonable to advise a moderate dietary protein intake of 0.8–1.0 g/kg/day in adults, although in children an intake of about 1.2 g/kg/day may be preferable to avoid the hazards of growth retardation. Indeed, Lim et al[20] showed that nephrotic patients ingesting 0.84 g/kg/day protein maintained a positive nitrogen balance of 0.5 g/day.

Similarly, Maroni et al[21] demonstrated positive nitrogen balance in a group of patients consuming 0.8 g/kg/day protein plus 1 g protein per gram of urine protein. Finally, to achieve optimal nutrition, an adequate energy intake (≥ 146 kJ/kg/day) must also be assured.

Angiotensin-converting enzyme inhibitors

ACE inhibitors can reduce proteinuria by as much as 50% in a variety of proteinuric states without decreasing GFR or effective renal plasma flow (ERPF).[22,23] The mechanism of this effect is still debated but appears to entail both hemodynamic and structural factors. Structural factors may predominate, since the maximum antiproteinuric effect takes 4–8 weeks to develop. This would also explain why short-term infusion of angiotensin reversed the renal and systemic hemodynamic effects of ACE inhibitors without affecting the reduction in proteinuria.[24] Moreover, ACE inhibitors have been shown to reduce selectively the fractional clearance of large molecular weight dextrans, suggesting a direct improvement in the size-selective properties of the filtration barrier.[25,26] Whether this effect is mediated via inhibition of angiotensin or other angiotensin-independent effects of ACE inhibitors is not yet clear.

The antiproteinuric effect of ACE inhibitors is dose dependent and apparently independent of changes in systemic blood pressure. Agents that lower blood pressure to a comparable degree do not affect proteinuria. The degree of reduction in proteinuria varies considerably among patients, and some may not respond at all. Importantly, the antiproteinuric effect of ACE inhibitors appears to depend on sodium restriction. Heeg et al[22] showed that a high sodium intake (200 mmol/day) abrogated the reduction in proteinuria mediated by lisinopril during a period of low salt intake (50 mmol/day). Buter et al[27] demonstrated that addition of a thiazide diuretic to patients ingesting a high-sodium diet can reverse the blunting effect of high sodium intake on reduction of proteinuria. Finally, the effects of ACE inhibitors tend to be greater in patients with higher baseline proteinuria, probably because of the greater room for a measurable reduction.[28]

It is now well established that ACE inhibitors slow progression of both diabetic and nondiabetic renal disease.[6,7,29–33] In the REIN trial of ACE inhibitors in proteinuric renal disease, the renoprotective effect of ramipril correlated with the observed reduction in proteinuria.[6] A recent metaanalysis of 11 randomized controlled trials involving 1860 patients demonstrated a clear beneficial effect of ACE inhibitors in nondiabetic proteinuric renal disease, an effect that again was more pronounced in patients with higher levels of baseline proteinuria.[33]

Debate continues as to whether ATRA have equivalent antiproteinuric and renoprotective effects as ACE inhibitors.[34,35] In short-term studies involving small numbers of patients, similar reductions in proteinuria have been observed with both agents.[36–39] Because ACE inhibitors and ATRA antagonize the effects of angiotensin through different mechanisms, a rationale exists for using both drugs in combination. Several small studies have demonstrated an additive antiproteinuric effect with the combination of ACE inhibitors and ATRA without adverse effects on renal function.[39–41] Definitive data on the long-term renoprotective benefits of ATRA in nondiabetic renal disease are still pending. However, two recent studies in type 2 diabetes mellitus demonstrated a slowing of progression of diabetic nephropathy in patients treated with losartan or irbesartan.[42,43] Unfortunately, neither of these studies included an ACE inhibitor limb, and hence it is not possible to compare the protection conferred by ATRA with that of ACE inhibitors. Such reservations aside, the data thus far suggest an equivalent benefit for the two classes of drugs. We recommend ACE inhibitors as preferred therapy to reduce proteinuria in most patients, reserving the addition of ATRA for patients who are intolerant of ACE inhibitors or in whom ACE inhibitors fail to achieve the desired response. In light of recent data, ATRA are also a reasonable choice in patients with nephropathy secondary to type 2 diabetes mellitus. The combination of an ACE inhibitor with ATRA is a reasonable therapeutic option in patients who have an inadequate response to either agent alone. ACE inhibitors and ATRA have a number of important adverse effects in patients with renal disease, including reduction of GFR and hyperkalemia. Patients must therefore be monitored carefully following introduction of either agent.

Nonsteroidal anti-inflammatory drugs

NSAIDs reduce proteinuria to a comparable degree as ACE inhibitors.[44,45] The mechanism of action is not known, although there is evidence to suggest that reduced proteinuria depends on inhibition of renal prostaglandin synthesis. In a small study of seven nephrotic patients, a significant correlation was observed between the fall in proteinuria and decreased renal PGE_2 excretion.[46] Indomethacin improves the profile of fractional dextran clearance and reduces flux through the shunt pathway, a major source of abnormal proteinuria in NS.[47]

The beneficial effect of NSAIDs occurs more rapidly than that of ACE inhibitors (1–3 days), and in some studies is associated with reductions in both GFR and ERPF.[45] Sodium depletion enhances both the antiproteinuric effect and the observed decline in GFR.[44] While lisinopril and indomethacin had an additive effect in lowering proteinuria, the combination produced a pronounced fall in GFR and significant hyperkalemia.[45] In another study, indomethacin had an additive antiproteinuric effect in combination with either the ACE inhibitor enalapril or the ATRA irbesartan.[38] No adverse effect on renal hemodynamics was seen with short-term administration.[38] NSAIDs have a number of adverse renal effects, including hyperkalemia, acute renal failure, and salt and water retention. In general, we recommend that ACE inhibitors be used as preferred antiproteinuric agents and that NSAIDs be reserved for patients who are refractory to other measures.

Measures to ablate renal function in refractory nephrotic syndrome

Therapeutic ablation of renal function may be considered in occasional patients with refractory complications of NS, particularly when renal function is already depressed. A variety of measures have been used, including medical nephrectomy with NSAIDs, percutaneous transfemoral embolization using artificial agents or autologous blood clot, balloon occlusion of the renal arteries, and surgical nephrectomy.[48–51] Bilateral renal arterial embolization with autologous blood clot is probably the safest of the methods but should be considered only as a last resort in intractable cases.[51]

Edema

Edema is one of the most common symptoms of NS and frequently the reason patients come to medical attention. Fluid accumulates predominantly in areas of dependency or low tissue pressure. Hence, periorbital edema is common in the morning and leg edema at the end of the day. Pleural effusions and ascites occur frequently, but pulmonary edema does not occur in the presence of normal cardiac function. In patients with very low plasma oncotic pressure (< 8 mmHg), minor elevations in left atrial filling pressure may lead to pulmonary edema despite the normally protective low-pressure features of the pulmonary circuit.[3]

The classic theory of edema formation in NS postulates that hypoalbuminemia leads to decreased intravascular oncotic pressure with leakage of extracellular fluid from the blood to the interstitium and a fall in blood volume. Hypovolemia then leads to activation of both the renin–angiotensin–aldosterone axis and sympathetic nervous system, as well as release of antidiuretic hormone and suppression of atrial natriuretic peptide, thereby signaling the kidney to retain salt and water.[52] However, it is now clear that this classic theory applies to only a minority of patients, since the majority of patients with established NS have normal or even elevated blood volumes and stimulation of the renin–angiotensin–aldosterone axis is not consistently present.[53] Hence, primary renal sodium retention must also contribute to edema formation, although the factors responsible for this sodium avidity, and the role of hypoalbuminemia in its genesis, remain unclear.[54] Given the heterogeneity of NS in terms of patient age, underlying pathophysiologic process, and level of renal function, it is likely that different mechanisms of sodium retention exist in different patients.[55]

Management (See also Chapter 95)

Treatment of edema involves restriction of dietary sodium and the judicious use of diuretics. Considerable improvement should be possible for nearly all patients. For many patients, however, complete resolution of edema is not only unattainable but also undesirable because of the risk of volume contraction. In the case of mild edema, dietary sodium restriction to 100–150 mequiv./day may be sufficient by itself. Restriction to less than 100 mequiv. is indicated in patients with more severe edema. Compliance with sodium restriction can be ascertained by measuring 24-h urinary excretion of sodium. Institution of diuretic therapy is indicated in patients with symptomatic edema unresponsive to sodium restriction.

Furosemide pharmacokinetics and pharmacodynamics are often abnormal in patients with NS, many of whom show a degree of diuretic resistance. Although the following discussion focuses on the loop diuretic furosemide, similar principles apply to the loop diuretic bumetanide, thiazide diuretics, and the potassium-sparing diuretics amiloride and triamterene. The diuretic effect of furosemide depends on binding to, and inhibition of, a specific transporter located in the luminal membrane of the loop of Henle. Since furosemide is highly protein bound (> 90%), it cannot enter the urine by glomerular filtration. Entry into the urine occurs instead via secretion by the proximal tubule. Binding of furosemide to albumin aids secretion in two ways: (1) because of its tight association with albumin, furosemide is restricted to the vascular space and therefore has a higher rate of delivery to the kidney; and (2) optimal secretion of furosemide seems to depend on the presence of albumin.

Thus, several mechanisms may account for diuretic resistance observed in patients with NS and hypoalbuminemia.[56,57]

1. Oral bioavailability may be reduced because of bowel wall edema and impaired absorption.
2. In the presence of hypoalbuminemia, furosemide will be incompletely bound to albumin and therefore diffuse from the vascular space, thereby decreasing delivery of furosemide to the kidney.[58]
3. Given the dependence of proximal secretion on albumin, transport of delivered furosemide into the tubular lumen may be suboptimal.
4. Even that fraction of furosemide entering the urinary space may be limited in efficacy, since the furosemide may bind to filtered albumin, thereby limiting the availability of free drug to interact with its receptor on the tubular brush border.[59]
5. There may be a degree of tubular resistance to the natriuretic effect of furosemide, as suggested by studies showing a lesser response to a given dose of drug in nephrotic patients compared with normal controls.[60] However, in some instances, this may merely reflect the coexistence of renal impairment in nephrotic subjects.[61]
6. A continued high dietary sodium intake and the ingestion of NSAIDs may also cause an inadequate diuretic response.

A recent study casts doubt on the contribution of urinary protein binding of loop diuretics to diuretic resistance in NS.[62] In this study, coadministration of sulfisoxazole with furosemide was used to displace furosemide from binding to urinary albumin but failed to enhance the natriuretic effect. Moreover, despite an observed increase in the volume of distribution of furosemide, there was no reduction in the rate of diuretic excretion, thereby questioning the pharmacodynamic role of hypoalbuminemia per se. These results suggest that diminished tubular responsiveness and/or increased sodium avidity may be more important mechanisms of diuretic resistance in NS.

Dosing recommendations for diuretics in NS are empirically derived and will vary according to the degree of diuretic resistance.[57,63] In normal subjects, the doses of furosemide and bumetanide required to produce a maximal diuresis are 40 mg and 1 mg respectively. In patients with nephrotic edema, for the reasons discussed above, higher doses may be necessary to achieve an adequate diuretic response. Higher doses will also be necessary in patients with reduced GFR. For patients with normal renal function, therapy is usually commenced with furosemide 40 mg i.v. or 80 mg p.o. or bumetanide 1 mg i.v. or p.o.[57,63] In patients with severe edema, initial therapy should be given intravenously in case intestinal absorption of the diuretic is impaired. For patients with renal impairment, these doses should be doubled. If a satisfactory response is not achieved, the initial dose should be titrated upwards, with a ceiling of three times the starting dose. Doses of furosemide as high as 160–240 mg p.o. may be necessary in patients with moderate renal impairment (GFR 20–50 mL/min), and as high as 360–400 mg when the GFR is less than 20 mL/min.[63] Once an effective dose is found, there is no advantage to increasing this dose. If the response to once-daily dosing is inadequate, the diuretic can be given twice daily. The duration of action of furosemide is 3–6 h so that giving the drug twice daily will limit the period of postdiuretic compensatory sodium retention.

Some authors advocate intravenous coadministration of furosemide and albumin for patients with severe refractory edema. The use of such a regimen presumes that pharmacokinetic factors contribute importantly to diuretic resistance. In the most successful study, an equimolar infusion of salt-poor albumin (40 mg furosemide premixed with 6 g salt-poor albumin) increased recovery of furosemide from the urine and led to an enhanced diuretic response.[58] More recent studies have provided less encouraging results. Fliser et al[64] infused 60 mg of furosemide plus 200 ml of 20% human albumin to a group of nephrotic patients. The rate of urinary furosemide excretion was unchanged, suggesting that the observed modest increase in sodium excretion and urine volume was secondary to alterations in renal hemodynamics. Other workers failed to find any potentiation of furosemide by intravenous albumin.[65–67] Some of this lack of effect may be due to the fact that the albumin and furosemide were not admixed prior to infusion or that furosemide was administered at submaximal doses. In addition, in some studies the natriuretic response to furosemide alone was substantial, suggesting that the patients studied may not have been truly diuretic resistant. Taken together, these studies are consistent with a critical role for primary sodium retention in the pathophysiology of the edema of NS. Based on current evidence we recommend that the combination of furosemide and albumin should be reserved for patients with refractory edema. When used in combination, the drugs should be admixed before intravenous administration.

If the response to furosemide alone is inadequate, a thiazide diuretic can be added, since the combination of two drugs acting at different sites may yield a synergistic response with enhanced natriuresis.[68] Thiazide diuretics may be adequate therapy for patients with mild edema and normal renal function. However, they are generally ineffective in the presence of renal impairment (GFR < 20 to 30 mL/min). It is important to note that some patients show an exaggerated response to the combination of a thiazide and loop diuretic, and severe volume contraction and dangerous hypokalemia can result. Careful monitoring for the first few days is therefore essential. Metolazone may also be useful in the treatment of nephrotic edema, either alone or combined with a loop diuretic.[69]

As discussed above, stimulation of the renin–angiotensin–aldosterone system is highly variable in patients with NS, so that the response to aldosterone antagonists is highly inconsistent.[52] Aldosterone antagonists may be most useful in conjunction with loop diuretics to prevent hypokalemia. On the other hand, hyperkalemia is always a risk with this class of diuretics, particularly in patients with diminished renal function.

Intravenous infusion of salt-poor albumin is sometimes employed for the treatment of intractable nephrotic edema and in some patients appears to restore diuretic responsiveness (300 mL of 15% albumin infused over 45 min, followed by furosemide bolus to establish a diuresis, given on alternate days).[70] This treatment is expensive and any benefit is short-lived because of rapid excretion of the injected albumin in the urine as well as redistribution to the tissue spaces. Despite these considerations, some authors recommend that a therapeutic trial of 50–75 g albumin for 2–3 days be undertaken in patients in whom diuretics have effected no improvement in their edema or in whom complications of diuretic therapy preclude further increases in drug dose.[2] Infusion of hyperoncotic albumin can precipitate pulmonary edema in patients with severe hypoproteinemia so they should be monitored closely during therapy. The use of ultrafiltration for the treatment of edema resistant to standard therapy has also been described but should only rarely be necessary.[71]

All patients must be carefully monitored for adverse effects of diuretics. Particular attention must be paid to intravascular volume status because of the risk of precipitating prerenal failure. Changes in orthostatic blood pressure, neck vein distension, and the ratio of blood urea nitrogen to serum creatinine are helpful in assessing intravascular volume. In patients who have evidence of volume depletion and in whom diuretics exacerbate a prerenal state, bed rest and the use of support stockings may help mobilize edema.

Hyperlipidemia

A host of abnormalities of lipid metabolism exist in patients with NS.[72,73] These include elevations in all of the following: total plasma cholesterol, very low density lipoprotein (VLDL), intermediate-density lipoprotein (IDL), low-density lipoprotein (LDL), and lipoprotein (a) (Lp(a)). Triglyceride levels may also be elevated, particularly in patients with very heavy proteinuria. While levels of high-density lipoprotein (HDL) are variable, the distribution

among subclasses is altered such that HDL2 is decreased and HDL3 is increased. Elevated levels of apoproteins B, C, and E have also been shown, while the levels of apoproteins AI and AII, the major apoproteins in HDL, have been reported as normal. Qualitative abnormalities in lipoprotein composition are also described.[72]

The mechanisms of hyperlipoproteinemia in NS have not been fully elucidated. Increased hepatic synthesis of apoprotein B-containing lipoproteins, stimulated by decreased plasma oncotic pressure, may be an important factor.[72] In general, however, decreased lipid catabolism is thought to play a more important role than hepatic overproduction of lipoproteins.[74–76] Depletion of endothelial-bound lipoprotein lipase (LPL) and alterations in the binding capacity of VLDL are thought to contribute importantly to decreased catabolism.[76] Lowered plasma viscosity, reduced oncotic pressure, reduced plasma tonicity, urinary loss of liporegulatory substances, and decreased LPL activity may all play a role in the genesis of hyperlipidemia.[2]

Although the same lipid abnormalities in nonnephrotic populations have been associated with an increased incidence of cardiovascular disease, there is controversy as to whether these findings can be extrapolated to NS. Most reports on cardiovascular disease in NS are small, retrospective, and lack appropriate control groups, perhaps accounting for their conflicting results.[77,78] A more recent retrospective study of 142 patients with NS documented a 5.5-fold increased risk of myocardial infarction after controlling for other risk factors such as hypertension and smoking.[79] Until the results of prospective controlled trials dictate otherwise, it seems prudent to treat severe and prolonged hyperlipidemia, particularly in patients with other cardiovascular risk factors.[74,80]

Hyperlipidemia has also been implicated in accelerating glomerular injury.[72,81] Indeed, similar pathophysiologic mechanisms are thought to contribute to progression of both glomerulosclerosis and atherosclerosis.[82] Such considerations provide an additional rationale for treatment of nephrotic hyperlipidemia. While treatment of hyperlipidemia retards progression of glomerular disease in some animal models, conclusive data in human studies are lacking. However, in a recent metaanalysis of 12 trials in which lipid-lowering agents were administered to patients with proteinuric renal diseases, a significant reduction in the rate of decline of GFR was observed that correlated with study duration.[83] A nonsignificant trend toward reduction in proteinuria was also found.

Management

The approach to management of nephrotic hyperlipidemia is similar to that for nonnephrotic patients and consists of dietary measures, oral lipid-lowering agents, and modification of associated risk factors such as smoking and hypertension.[73,80,84] Available studies are small, mostly uncontrolled, and of short duration. Most studies were designed to test short-term efficacy and safety of specific therapeutic interventions, rather than long-term benefits on cardiac or progressive renal disease. Thus recommendations regarding treatment are based on limited data, much of which awaits confirmation in long-term, prospective, controlled studies.

Dietary manipulations

Given the magnitude of hyperlipidemia seen in association with NS, dietary measures alone, unless highly restrictive, are usually ineffective as sole therapy.[15,84–86] Institution of a moderately restricted diet low in cholesterol (< 300 mg) and fat, with a high ratio of polyunsaturated to saturated fats, during the run-in phase of small trials of lipid-lowering agents failed to effect any significant improvement in lipid parameters.[87–89] More impressive results have been reported with more restricted diets. After 6 months on a diet low in cholesterol (< 200 mg), low in fat (< 30% total calories), and rich in polyunsaturated fatty acids, total and LDL cholesterol decreased by 24% and 27% respectively.[15] A vegetarian soy-based diet low in fat and protein, and essentially cholesterol free, decreased total cholesterol by 28% and LDL by 33% in 20 nephrotic patients over an 8-week period.[90] It is doubtful if such strict diets would be tolerated by most patients with NS. Moreover, the long-term safety of such diets has not been assessed. Uncontrolled human studies have suggested that a diet high in long-chain ω3 polyunsaturated fatty acids (e.g. enriched in fish oil) may decrease total plasma triglycerides and cholesterol as well as reduce proteinuria.[91,92] As other studies have failed to confirm this effect,[85] further evaluation is needed before the routine use of fish oil supplementation can be recommended.

Pharmacologic therapy

A variety of agents have been used in the treatment of nephrotic hyperlipidemia, including bile acid sequestrants, fibric acid derivatives, probucol, and hydroxymethylglutaryl coenzyme A (HMG-CoA) reductase inhibitors. The bile acid sequestrants, cholestyramine and colestipol, lowered LDL cholesterol by 19–32% and total cholesterol by 8–20%.[93,94] However, these drugs are not ideal first-line agents because of a high incidence of gastrointestinal adverse effects and a tendency to increase triglyceride levels. The fibric acid derivative gemfibrozil reduced triglycerides by 51%, total cholesterol by 15%, and LDL by 12.5%, while increasing HDL by 18%, in a 6-week randomized, double-blinded, placebo-controlled trial in 11 patients.[95] Addition of the resin colestipol led to further improvements in lipid parameters but the combination was poorly tolerated. Gemfibrozil alone was well tolerated, though one patient developed a markedly elevated creatine phosphokinase (CPK) following vigorous exercise. Clofibrate, an older fibric acid derivative, has been associated with severe adverse effects in patients with renal impairment and should be avoided.[96] The use of probucol effected a moderate reduction in total and LDL cholesterol in two studies, but reductions also occurred in HDL cholesterol.[94,97]

HMG-CoA reductase inhibitors decrease hepatic cholesterol production by inhibiting the rate-limiting enzyme involved in cholesterol synthesis. These agents reduce total cholesterol, LDL cholesterol, and VLDL triglycerides, and in some studies also increase HDL cholesterol.[86–89,93,98–110] Lp(a) levels were reduced in one study in patients with high baseline levels[107] but they were unchanged in two other studies.[89,106] The results of treatment with HMG-CoA reductase inhibitors are summarized in Table 28.1. In a 2-year follow-up of the patients reported by Rabelink et al,[108] there was a significant reduction in proteinuria and an increase in serum albumin. Similarly, in the patients reported by Rayner et al[86] there was a reduction in proteinuria and an increase in serum albumin that became manifest after 12 months of treatment with simvastatin. The effect did not reach statistical significance, probably because of small numbers. This effect has not been found in other studies.[100,102] In general, HMG-CoA reductase inhibitors are well tolerated and appear to be safe in studies up to 2 years in duration. Occasional patients have developed mild asymptomatic increases in aspartate aminotransferase[87,99] or CPK,[86,88,102,103,106,109] but in most instances these did not necessitate withdrawal of the drug. In the cited studies, only one instance of rhabdomyolysis occurred and this was after severe exercise.[102] A posterior lens opacity developed in one patient in the study of Warwick et al.[103] In a recent metaanalysis of studies on treatment of nephrotic hyperlipidemia, HMG-CoA reductase inhibitors were found to be the most effective therapy.[111]

Finally, there is some evidence to suggest that antiproteinuric treatment with ACE inhjibitors may be accompanied by an improvement in lipid parameters. Keilani et al[112] reported 13% and 15% reductions in total and LDL cholesterol, respectively, in a group of patients with moderate proteinuria without NS. A reduction in Lp(a) also occurred, but only three patients had frankly elevated levels at the start of the trial. The combination of an ACE inhibitor and NSAID effected reductions in total cholesterol, LDL cholesterol, and Lp(a) in nine patients with nephrotic-range proteinuria.[113] These alterations in lipid parameters correlated with reductions in proteinuria.

A reasonable approach to the management of nephrotic hyperlipidemia is to institute therapy with an HMG-CoA reductase inhibitor in conjunction with a low-cholesterol diet. Modification of other risk factors, such as smoking and obesity, is also important. If this regimen is inadequate, a bile acid sequestrant may be added if triglyceride levels are not excessive. If triglycerides are very high and/or HDL levels are low, a fibric acid analog such as gemfibrozil could be added. The long-term safety of these treatments in NS and the benefits of such strategies in lowering the incidence of cardiovascular disease or delaying the progression of glomerulosclerosis await confirmation in long-term studies.

Abnormalities of calcium homeostasis

Hypocalcemia (both total and ionized) and secondary hyperparathyroidism have been variably described in NS.

Table 28.1 HMG-CoA reductase inhibitors in the treatment of nephrotic hyperlipidemia

Reference	Drug (maximum dose)	No. of patients	Duration	Alterations in lipid parameters (%)				
				TC	LDL	HDL	TRIG	Lp(a)
Elisaf et al[100]	Lovastatin (20 mg/day)	16	1 year	−47	−55	−4	−37	NA
Biesenbach & Zazgornik[88]	Lovastatin (20 mg/day)	10	12 weeks	−25	−35	+11	−13	NA
Vega & Grundy[98]	Lovastatin (40 mg/day)	3	8 weeks	−31	−30	+35	−40	NA
Martins Prata et al[105]	Lovastatin (40 mg/day)	7	2 years	−44	−49	+21	−46	NA
Kasiske et al[87]	Lovastatin (40 mg/day)	12	6 weeks	−27	−27	−2	−30	NA
Golper et al[99]	Lovastatin (80 mg/day)	10	24 weeks	−33	−45	+1	−23	NA
Chan et al[102]	Lovastatin (80 mg/day)	12	24 weeks	−31	−43	+17	−18	NA
Brown et al[107]	Lovastatin (80 mg/day)	12 (group1)[†]	8 weeks	−36	−43	+19	−57	−32*
		8 (group2)[†]	8 weeks	−31	−42	0	−6	−8*
Rabelink et al[93]	Simvastatin (40 mg/day)	10	6 weeks	−36	−39	+21	−39	NA
Bazzato et al[101]	Simvastatin (40 mg/day)	20	18 weeks	−44	−52	+37	−49	NA
Warwick et al[103]	Simvastatin (40 mg/day)	16	12 weeks	−37*	−44*	+10*	−25*	NA
Thomas et al[104]‡	Simvastatin (40 mg/day)	11	24 weeks	−33	−31	−2	−25*	NA
Wanner et al[106]	Simvastatin (40 mg/day)	10 (Gp1)§	12 weeks	−31	−35	0	−21	0
		8 (Gp2)§	12 weeks	−43	−54	−13	−24	+1
Rayner et al[86]	Simvastatin (40 mg/day)	9	19 weeks	−50	−55	nc	nc	NA
Olbricht et al[109]	Simvastatin (40 mg/day)	20	2 years	−39	−47	+1	−30	nc
Spitalewitz et al[89]‡	Pravastatin (40 mg/day)	13	24 weeks	−22	−28	+8	−19	nc (n=4)
Matzkies et al[110]	Fluvastatin (40 mg/day)	9	1 year	−31	−29	nc	−19	nc

HDL, HDL cholesterol; LDL, LDL cholesterol; Lp(a), lipoprotein (a); NA, not assessed; nc, no change; TC, total cholesterol; TRIG, triglycerides.
*Median percentage change; all other results are mean percentage change.
†Group 1 Lp(a) < 30 mg/dL; group 2 Lp(a) > 30 mg/dL.
‡Randomized controlled trial.
§Group 1, primary renal disease; group 2, diabetic nephropathy.

Potential mechanisms include reduced intestinal absorption of calcium and a blunted calcemic response to parathyroid hormone.[1] Moreover, levels of 25-hydroxycholecalciferol (25-OH-D), the precursor of the active vitamin, are reduced in most patients with NS, probably because of loss of this metabolite in the urine bound to its vitamin D carrier protein.[114,115] Levels of the physiologically active 1,25-dihydroxycholecalciferol (1,25-$(OH)_2$-D) are more variable, being normal in some studies and low in others.[1]

Despite these alterations in calcium and vitamin D metabolism, studies have yielded conflicting data regarding the incidence of bone disease in patients with NS.[115,116] In one study, bone structure was largely normal among patients with normal renal function. Severe demineralization and bone resorption occurred only in association with deterioration of renal function.[117] Nevertheless, bone abnormalities were more pronounced in patients with NS than in a control group with comparable azotemia but lacking proteinuria. Others have reported evidence of osteomalacia and secondary hyperparathyroidism even in patients with normal renal function.[118] A more recent study of 30 adults with NS and normal renal function documented normal bone histology in one-third of patients and osteomalacia in 57% of the group.[115] The presence of osteomalacia correlated with the degree of proteinuria and the duration of NS.[115] It seems clear that the potential for osteomalacia exists in these patients, and may increase as renal failure supervenes.

Management

Treatment with oral vitamin D therapy should be prescribed for patients with evidence of osteomalacia or secondary hyperparathyroidism, patients with persistently low serum ionized calcium levels, patients in whom progressive renal insufficiency is anticipated, and patients who have unremitting or frequently relapsing NS.[119]

Unfortunately, there is little information available on the optimal formulation or dose for vitamin D replacement in NS. In one study, vitamin D_3 (25 µg) was administered daily for a period of 4–52 weeks to nine nephrotic patients with documented low levels of 25-OH-D and 1,25-$(OH)_2$-D.[120] Normalization of 25-OH-D levels occurred in 8 of 9 patients, and normalization of 1,25-$(OH)_2$-D levels in five patients in whom the baseline serum creatinine was normal. Serum calcium levels should be monitored closely in patients on vitamin D replacement therapy. Measurement of bone mineral density should be considered in patients with persistent nephrotic syndrome, particulary if they have received high doses of corticosteroids or have additional risk factors for osteoporosis.

Hypercoagulability and thromboembolism

Numerous defects in coagulation factors, clotting inhibitors, the fibrinolytic system, and platelet function have been invoked to explain the hypercoagulable state that exists in patients with NS.[121-123] There is a distinct lack of uniformity among the various studies. In general, levels of fibrinogen, factor V, factor VII, and α_2-antiplasmin are increased, whereas those of factor IX, factor XI, factor XII, antithrombin III, plasminogen, and α_1-antitrypsin are reduced. Disturbances in platelet physiology that could promote clotting include increased aggregability, increased levels of β-thromboglobulin (a protein released at the time of platelet aggregation), and increased levels of von Willebrand factor. The cause of enhanced platelet aggregability is most likely multifactorial, with hypoalbuminemia, hyperlipidemia, and hyperfibrinogenemia all playing a role.[124] Despite these multiple abnormalities, a direct relationship has yet to be established between any specific defect and the occurrence of thromboembolic complications.[125]

About 20% (range 8–44%) of adult NS patients develop thromboembolic complications other than renal vein thrombosis (RVT). As many as 50% of these episodes are clinically silent.[121] Arterial thromboses occur much less frequently than venous thromboses and have been described in the pulmonary, femoral, mesenteric, and coronary arteries. The incidence of RVT varies in different series from 2 to 60%, with an average of 35%. RVT is most common in membranous nephropathy.[126] Chronic RVT is usually asymptomatic and can only be diagnosed with certainty by renal venography. Long-term follow-up of established cases indicates that chronic RVT is generally benign, with a low incidence of thromboembolic episodes in patients who are anticoagulated.[126,127] Moreover, there appear to be no adverse effects on renal function or the degree of proteinuria.[2] Acute RVT is less frequent. Patients usually present with flank pain and tenderness, macroscopic hematuria, and deterioration in renal function. Routine venography is not recommended in NS patients, with the possible exception of patients with membranous glomerulopathy, who have a higher incidence of thromboembolic complications, particularly if the serum albumin is less than 2 g/dL. Venography should be reserved for patients with features suggestive of acute RVT, an unexplained rapid deterioration in renal function, or symptoms suggestive of an acute thromboembolic event such as pulmonary embolus.

Management

Management of the thrombotic tendency in NS involves preventative measures such as avoiding immobilization or volume depletion, both of which increase the risk of clotting. Patients with a history of thromboembolism prior to the onset of NS should receive prophylactic anticoagulation if they are immobilized or have other major risk factors for clotting. In patients who experience an episode of thrombus or embolus, anticoagulants should be continued for as long as the nephrotic state persists.[122] Intravenous heparin followed by warfarin is the standard treatment for acute RVT.[122,126,127] The international normalized ratio (INR) must be carefully monitored in nephrotic patients as warfarin kinetics are affected by NS, and dose adjustment may be necessary with changes in serum albumin level.[128] Although fibrinolytic therapy has been successfully used in isolated patients,[129-132] it does not appear to be superior to standard anticoagulant therapy.

The issue of prophylactic anticoagulation in NS is controversial. Prophylaxis with the low-molecular-weight heparin enoxaparin was recently studied in 55 adult patients for periods of 2–48 months.[133] No thrombotic episodes occurred during therapy, as evidenced by renal vein Doppler ultrasonography, lower leg Doppler ultrasonography, and lung ventilation–perfusion scintigriphy. There were no documented adverse effects, and patients found self-administration of the once-daily dose to be tolerable. Some authors advocate the use of prophylaxis in patients with membranous nephropathy on the grounds that these are the patients at highest risk of thrombotic complications.[4,134,135] A recent study using a decision analysis model concluded that the benefits of prophylactic anticoagulation begun at the time of diagnosis of NS due to membranous nephropathy outweighed the risks of bleeding.[134] Despite the arguments in favor of prophylactic anticoagulation, its routine use in all nephrotic patients cannot be recommended. Further prospective controlled studies are indicated to determine both the necessity and optimal prophylactic anticoagulant regimens for patients with NS.

Increased susceptibility to infection

A number of immunologic abnormalities have been documented in patients with NS. These include depressed immunoglobulin levels due to urinary loss, impaired antibody generation, defective opsonization due to depressed levels of complement factor B, and abnormalities of cell-mediated immunity.[1] In many patients, nonspecific depression of immune responses may occur because of malnutrition, vitamin D deficiency, or immuno-suppressive therapy. These abnormalities may result in an increased susceptibility to infection, with the peritoneum and lungs being the sites most frequently involved.

Before the introduction of antibiotics, pulmonary, meningeal, or peritoneal infection with encapsulated organisms, such as *Streptococcus*, *Hemophilus*, or *Klebsiella* species, was a common cause of death, particularly in children. In recent years, the incidence of infection with these agents has fallen, although adult patients continue to display an increased incidence of infection with Gram-negative bacteria.[136]

Management

Aggressive antibiotic therapy should be instituted at the first suspicion of infection. Prophylactic use of antibiotics, pneumococcal vaccine, or intravenous administration of hyperimmune globulin should be considered in high-risk cases. Vaccination should be given whenever possible during periods of remission, as NS may impair the antibody response to vaccination.[137] In one study, despite an adequate initial response to vaccination, 50% of vaccinated patients after 1 year failed to maintain adequate antibody concentrations against several pneumococcal capsular antigens.[138] Nonetheless, pneumococcal vaccination is still recommended for children over 2 years of age and for adults with severely depressed immunoglobulins, particularly if NS is likely to be persistent or if renal failure supervenes.[1,2] Although intravenous immunoglobulin has been used in NS,[136] insufficient data preclude specific recommendations.

References

1. Bernard DB: Extra-renal manifestations of nephrotic syndrome. Kidney Int 1988;33:1184–1202.
2. Harris RC, Ismail N: Extrarenal complications of the nephrotic syndrome. Am J Kidney Dis 1994;23:447–497.
3. Falk RJ, Jennette JC, Nachman PH: Primary glomerular disease. *In* Brenner BM (ed): The Kidney, 6th edn. Philadelphia: WB Saunders, 2000, pp 1263–1349.
4. Orth SR, Ritz E: The nephrotic syndrome. N Engl J Med 1998;338:1202–1211.
5. Ruggenenti P, Remuzzi G: The role of protein traffic in the progression of renal diseases. Annu Rev Med 2000;51:315–327.
6. The GISEN Group (Gruppo Italiano di Studi Epidemiologici in Nefrologia): Randomised placebo-controlled trial of effect of ramipril on decline in glomerular filtration rate and risk of terminal renal failure in proteinuric, non-diabetic nephropathy. Lancet 1997;349:1857–1863.
7. Lewis EJ, Hunsicker LG, Bain RP, et al: The effect of angiotensin-converting enzyme inhibition in diabetic nephropathy. N Engl J Med 1993;329:1456–1462.
8. Gugler R, Shoeman DW, Huffman DH, et al: Pharmacokinetics of drugs in patients with the nephrotic syndrome. J Clin Invest 1975;55:1182–1189.
9. Kaysen GA, Kirkpatrick WG, Couser WG: Albumin homeostasis in the nephrotic rat: nutritional considerations. Am J Physiol 1984;247:F192–F202.
10. Kaysen GA, Gambertoglio J, Jiminez I, et al: Effect of dietary protein intake on albumin homeostasis in nephrotic patients. Kidney Int 1986;29:572–577.
11. Brenner BM, Meyer TW, Hostetter TH: Dietary protein intake and the progressive nature of kidney disease: the role of hemodynamically mediated glomerular injury in the pathogenesis of progressive glomerulosclerosis in aging, renal ablation, and intrinsic renal disease. N Engl J Med 1982;307:652–659.
12. Aparicio M, Bouchet JL, Gin H, et al: Effect of a low-protein diet on urinary albumin excretion in uremic patients. Nephron 1988;50:288–291.
13. Don BR, Kaysen GA, Hutchinson FN, et al: The effect of angiotensin-converting enzyme inhibition and dietary protein restriction in the treatment of proteinuria. Am J Kidney Dis 1991;17:10–17.
14. Remuzzi A, Perticucci E, Battaglia C, et al: Low-protein diet and glomerular size-selective function in membranous glomerulopathy. Am J Kidney Dis 1991;17:317–322.
15. D'Amico G, Remuzzi G, Maschio G, et al: Effect of dietary proteins and lipids in patients with membranous nephropathy and nephrotic syndrome. Clin Nephrol 1991;35:237–242.
16. Giordano M, de Feo P, Lucidi P, et al: Effects of dietary protein restriction on fibrinogen and albumin metabolism in nephrotic patients. Kidney Int 2001;60:235–242.
17. Walser M, Hill S, Tomalis EA: Treatment of nephrotic adults with a supplemented, very low-protein diet. Am J Kidney Dis 1996;28:354–364.
18. Feehally J, Baker F, Walls J: Dietary protein manipulation in experimental nephrotic syndrome. Nephron 1988;50:247–252.
19. Aparicio M, Chauveau P, Combe C: Are supplemented low-protein diets nutritionally safe? Am J Kidney Dis 2001;37(Suppl 2):S71–S76.
20. Lim VS, Wolfson M, Yarasheski KE, et al: Leucine turnover in patients with nephrotic syndrome: evidence suggesting body protein conservation. J Am Soc Nephrol 1998;9:1067–1073.
21. Maroni BJ, Staffeld C, Young VR, et al: Mechanisms permitting nephrotic patients to achieve nitrogen equilibrium with a protein-restricted diet. J Clin Invest 1997;99:2479–2487.
22. Heeg JE, De Jong PE, van der Hem GK, et al: Efficacy and variability of the antiproteinuric effect of ACE inhibition by lisinopril. Kidney Int 1989;36:272–279.
23. Brunner HR: ACE inhibitors in renal disease. Kidney Int 1992;42:463–479.
24. Heeg JE, de Jong PE, van der Hem GK, et al: Angiotensin II does not acutely reverse the reduction of proteinuria by long-term ACE inhibition. Kidney Int 1991;40:734–741.
25. Meyer TW, Morelli E, Loon N, et al: Converting enzyme inhibition and glomerular size selectivity in diabetic nephropathy. J Am Soc Nephrol 1990;1:S64–S68.
26. Thomas DM, Hillis AN, Coles GA, et al: Enalapril can treat the proteinuria of membranous glomerulonephritis without detriment to systemic or renal hemodynamics. Am J Kidney Dis 1991;18:38–43.
27. Buter H, Hemmelder MH, Navis G, et al: The blunting of the antiproteinuric effect of ACE inhibition by high sodium intake can be restored by hydrochlorothiazide. Nephrol Dial Transplant 1998;13:1682–1685.
28. Jafar TH, Stark PC, Schmid CH, et al: Proteinuria as a modifiable risk factor for the progression of non-diabetic renal disease. Kidney Int 2001;60:1131–1140.
29. Maschio G, Alberti D, Janin G, et al: Effect of the angiotensin-converting-enzyme inhibitor benazepril on the progression of chronic renal insufficiency. N Engl J Med 1996;334:939–945.
30. Ruggenenti P, Perna A, Gherardi G, et al: Renal function and requirement for dialysis in chronic nephropathy patients on long-term ramipril: REIN follow-up trial. Lancet 1998;352:1252–1256.
31. Ruggenenti P, Perna A, Gherardi G, et al: Renoprotective properties of ACE-inhibition in non-diabetic nephropathies with non-nephrotic proteinuria. Lancet 1999;354:359–364.
32. Ruggenenti P, Perna A, Gherardi G, et al: Chronic proteinuric nephropathies: outcomes and response to treatment in a prospective cohort of 352 patients with different patterns of renal injury. Am J Kidney Dis 2000;35:1155–1165.
33. Jafar TH, Schmid CH, Landa M, et al: Angiotensin-converting enzyme inhibitors and progression of nondiabetic renal disease. A meta-analysis of patient-level data. Ann Intern Med 2001;135:73–87.
34. Ichikawa I: Will angiotensin II receptor antagonists be renoprotective in humans? Kidney Int 1996;50:684–692.
35. Taal MW, Brenner BM: Renoprotective benefits of RAS inhibition: from ACEI to angiotensin II antagonists. Kidney Int 2000;57:1803–1817.
36. Gansevoort RT, de Zeeuw D, Shahinfar S, et al: Effects of the angiotensin II antagonist losartan in hypertensive patients with renal disease. J Hypertens 1994;12:S37–S42.

37. Plum J, Bunten B, Nemeth R, et al: Effects of the angiotensin II antagonist valsartan on blood pressure, proteinuria, and renal hemodynamics in patients with chronic renal failure and hypertension. J Am Soc Nephrol 1998;9:2223–2234.

38. Perico N, Remuzzi A, Sangalli F, et al: The antiproteinuric effect of angiotensin antagonism in human IgA nephropathy is potentiated by indomethacin. J Am Soc Nephrol 1998;9:2308–2317.

39. Zoccali C, Valvo E, Russo D, et al: Antiproteinuric effect of losartan in patients with chronic renal diseases. Nephrol Dial Transplant 1997;12:234–235.

40. Russo D, Pisani A, Balletta MM, et al: Additive antiproteinuric effect of converting enzyme inhibitor and losartan in normotensive patients with IgA nephropathy. Am J Kidney Dis 1999;33:851–856.

41. Ruilope LM, Aldigier JC, Ponticelli C, et al: Safety of the combination of valsartan and benazepril in patients with chronic renal disease. European Group for the Investigation of Valsartan in Chronic Renal Disease. J Hypertens 2000;18:89–95.

42. Brenner BM, Cooper ME, de Zeeuw D, et al: Effects of losartan on renal and cardiovascular outcomes in patients with type 2 diabetes and nephropathy. N Engl J Med 2001;345:861–869.

43. Lewis EJ, Hunsicker LJ, Clarke WR, et al: Renoprotective effect of the angiotensin-receptor antagonist irbesartan in patients with nephropathy due to type 2 diabetes. N Engl J Med 2001;345:851–860.

44. Donker AJM, Brentjens JRH, van der Hem GK, et al: Treatment of the nephrotic syndrome with indomethacin. Nephron 1978;22:374–381.

45. Heeg JE, de Jong PE, Vriesendorp R, et al: Additive antiproteinuric effect of the NSAID indomethacin and the ACE inhibitor lisinopril. Am J Nephrol 1990;10(Suppl 1):94–97.

46. Vriesendorp R, de Zeeuw D, de Jong PE, et al: Reduction of urinary protein and prostaglandin E2 excretion in the nephrotic syndrome by non-steroidal anti-inflammatory drugs. Clin Nephrol 1986;25:105–110.

47. Golbetz H, Black V, Shemesh O, et al: Mechanism of the antiproteinuric effect of indomethacin in nephrotic humans. Am J Physiol 1989;256:F44–F51.

48. Avram MM, Lepner HI, Gan AC: Medical nephrectomy. The use of metallic salts for the control of massive proteinuria in the nephrotic syndrome. Proc Am Soc Artif Intern Organs 1976;22:431–438.

49. McCarron DA, Rubin RJ, Barnes BA, et al: Therapeutic bilateral renal infarction in end-stage renal disease. N Engl J Med 1976;294:652.

50. Baumelou A, Legrain M: Medical nephrectomy with anti-inflammatory non-steroidal drugs. Br Med J 1982;284:234.

51. Olivero JL, Pedro Frommer J, Gonzalez JM: Medical nephrectomy: the last resort for intractable complications of the nephrotic syndrome. Am J Kidney Dis 1993;21:260–263.

52. Abraham WT, Schrier RW: Edematous disorders: pathophysiology of renal sodium and water retention and treatment with diuretics. Curr Opin Nephrol Hypertens 1993;2:798–805.

53. Palmer BF, Alpern RJ: Pathogenesis of edema formation in the nephrotic syndrome. Kidney Int 1997;51(Suppl 59):S21–S27.

54. Dorhout Mees EJ, Koomans HA: Understanding the nephrotic syndrome: what's new in a decade? Nephron 1995;70:1–10.

55. Vande Walle JGJ, Donckerwolcke RA, Koomans HA: Pathophysiology of edema formation in children with nephrotic syndrome not due to minimal change disease. J Am Soc Nephrol 1999;10:323–331.

56. Wilcox CS: Diuretics. In Brenner BM (ed): The Kidney, 5th edn. Philadelphia: WB Saunders, 2000, pp 2219–2252.

57. Brater DC: Diuretic therapy. N Engl J Med 1998;339:387–395.

58. Inoue M, Okajima K, Itoh K, et al: Mechanism of furosemide resistance in analbuminemic rats and hypoalbuminemic patients. Kidney Int 1987;32:198–203.

59. Kirchner KA, Voelker JR, Brater DC: Binding inhibitors restore furosemide potency in tubule fluid containing albumin. Kidney Int 1991;41:418–424.

60. Sjostrom PA, Odlind BG, Beermann BA, et al: Pharmacokinetics and effects of furosemide in patients with the nephrotic syndrome. Eur J Clin Pharmacol 1989;37:173–180.

61. Danielsen H, Pedersen EB, Madsen M, et al: Abnormal renal sodium excretion in the nephrotic syndrome after furosemide: relation to glomerular filtration rate. Acta Med Scand 1985;217:513–518.

62. Agarwal R, Gorski JC, Sundblad K, et al: Urinary protein binding does not affect response to furosemide in patients with nephrotic syndrome. J Am Soc Nephrol 2000;11:1100–1105.

63. Rose BD: Diuretics. Kidney Int 1991;39:336–352.

64. Fliser D, Zurbruggen I, Mutschler E, et al: Coadministration of albumin and furosemide in patients with the nephrotic syndrome. Kidney Int 1999;55:629–634.

65. Akcicek F, Yalniz T, Basci A, et al: Diuretic effect of frusemide in patients with nephrotic syndrome: is it potentiated by intravenous albumin? Br Med J 1995;310:162–163.

66. Sjostrom PA, Odlind BG: Effect of albumin on diuretic treatment in the nephrotic syndrome. Br Med J 1995;310:1537.

67. Chalasani N, Gorski JC, Horlander JC, et al: Effects of albumin/furosemide mixtures on responses to furosemide in hypoalbuminemic patients. J Am Soc Nephrol 2001;12:1010–1016.

68. Nakahama H, Orita Y, Yamazaki M, et al: Pharmacokinetic and pharmacodynamic interactions between furosemide and hydrochlorothiazide in nephrotic patients. Nephron 1988;49:223–227.

69. Dargie HJ, Allison MEM, Kennedy AC, et al: Efficacy of metolazone in patients with renal edema. Clin Nephrol 1974;2:157–160.

70. Davison AM, Lambie AT, Verth AH, et al: Salt-poor human albumin in management of nephrotic syndrome. Br Med J 1974;1:481–484.

71. Fauchald P, Noddeland H, Norseth J: An evaluation of ultrafiltration as treatment of diuretic-resistant oedema in nephrotic syndrome. Acta Med Scand 1985;217:127–131.

72. Wheeler DC, Bernard DB: Lipid abnormalities in the nephrotic syndrome: causes, consequences and treatment. Am J Kidney Dis 1994;23:331–346.

73. Warwick GL, Packard CJ: Pathogenesis of lipid abnormalities in patients with nephrotic syndrome/proteinuria: clinical implications. Miner Electrolyte Metab 1993;19:115–126.

74. Keane WF, St Peter JV, Kasiske BL: Is the aggressive management of hyperlipidemia in nephrotic syndrome mandatory? Kidney Int 1992;42(Suppl 38):134–141.

75. Kaysen GA, de Sain-van der Velden MGM: New insights into lipid metabolism in the nephrotic syndrome. Kidney Int 1999;55(Suppl 71):S18–S21.

76. Shearer GC, Stevenson FT, Atkinson DN, et al: Hypoalbuminemia and proteinuria contribute separately to reduced lipoprotein catabolism in the nephrotic syndrome. Kidney Int 2001;59:179–189.

77. Wass V, Cameron JS: Cardiovascular disease and the nephrotic syndrome: the other side of the coin. Nephron 1981;27:58–61.

78. Mallick NP, Short CD: The nephrotic syndrome and ischaemic heart disease. Nephron 1981;27:54–57.

79. Ordonez JD, Hiatt RA, Killebrew EJ, et al: The increased risk of coronary heart disease associated with nephrotic syndrome. Kidney Int 1993;44:638–642.

80. Olbricht CJ, Koch KM: Treatment of hyperlipidemia in nephrotic syndrome: time for a change? Nephron 1992;62:125–129.

81. Keane WF, Kasiske BL, O'Donnell MP, et al: The role of altered lipid metabolism in the progression of renal disease: experimental evidence. Am J Kidney Dis 1991;17(Suppl 1):38–42.

82. Diamond JR, Karnovsky MJ: Focal and segmental glomerulosclerosis: analogies to atherosclerosis. Kidney Int 1988;33:917–924.

83. Fried LF, Orchard TJ, Kasiske BL, et al: Effect of lipid reduction on the progression of renal disease: a meta-analysis. Kidney Int 2001;59:260–269.

84. Grundy SM: Management of hyperlipidemia of kidney disease. Kidney Int 1990;37:847–853.

85. D'Amico G, Gentile MG. Influence of diet on lipid abnormalities in human renal disease. Am J Kidney Dis 1993;22:151–157.

86. Rayner BL, Byrne MJ, van Zyl Smit R: A prospective clinical trial comparing the treatment of idiopathic membranous nephropathy and nephrotic syndrome with simvastatin and diet, versus diet alone. Clin Nephrol 1996;46:219–224.

87. Kasiske BL, Velosa JA, Halstenson CE, et al: The effects of lovastatin in hyperlipidemic patients with nephrotic syndrome. Am J Kidney Dis 1990;15:8–15.

88. Biesenbach G, Zazgornik J: Lovastatin in the treatment of hypercholesterolemia in nephrotic syndrome due to diabetic nephropathy stage IV–V. Clin Nephrol 1992;37:274–279.

89. Spitalewitz S, Porush JG, Cattran D, et al: Treatment of hyperlipidemia in the nephrotic syndrome: the effects of pravastatin therapy. Am J Kidney Dis 1993;22:143–150.

90. D'Amico G, Gentile MG, Manna G, et al: Effect of vegetarian soy diet on hyperlipidemia in nephrotic syndrome. Lancet 1992;339:1131–1134.

91. Hall AV, Parbtani A, Clark WF, et al: Omega-3 fatty acid supplementation in primary nephrotic syndrome: effects on plasma lipids and coagulopathy. J Am Soc Nephrol 1992;2:1321–1329.

92. De Caterina R, Caprioli R, Giannessi D, et al: n-3 Fatty acids reduce proteinuria in patients with chronic glomerular disease. Kidney Int 1993;44:843–850.

93. Rabelink AJ, Hene RJ, Erkelens DW, et al: Effects of simvastatin and cholestyramine on lipoprotein profile in hyperlipidemia of nephrotic syndrome. Lancet 1988;ii:1335–1338.

94. Valeri A, Gelfand J, Blum C, et al: Treatment of the hyperlipidemia of the nephrotic syndrome: a controlled trial. Am J Kidney Dis 1986;8:388–396.

95. Groggel GC, Cheung AK, Ellis-Benigni K, et al: Treatment of nephrotic hyperlipoproteinemia with gemfibrozil. Kidney Int 1989;36:266–271.

96. Bridgman JF, Rosen SM, Thorp JM: Complications during clofibrate treatment of nephrotic-syndrome hyperlipoproteinemia. Lancet 1972;ii:506–509.

97. Iida H, Izumino K, Asaka M, et al: Effect of probucol on hyperlipidemia in patients with nephrotic syndrome. Nephron 1987;47:280–283.

98. Vega GL, Grundy SM: Lovastatin therapy in nephrotic hyperlipidemia: effects on lipoprotein metabolism. Kidney Int 1988;33:1160–1168.

99. Golper TA, Illingworth RD, Morris CD, et al: Lovastatin in the treatment of multifactorial hyperlipidemia associated with proteinuria. Am J Kidney Dis 1989;13:312–320.

100. Elisaf M, Dardamanis M, Pappas M, et al: Treatment of nephrotic hyperlipidemia with lovastatin. Clin Nephrol 1991;36:50–51.

101. Bazzato G, Landini S, Fracasso A, et al: Treatment of nephrotic syndrome hyperlipidemia with simvastatin. Curr Ther Res 1991;50:744–752.

102. Chan PC, Robinson JD, Yeung WC, et al: Lovastatin in glomerulonephritis patients with hyperlipidaemia and heavy proteinuria. Nephrol Dial Transplant 1992;7:93–99.

103. Warwick GL, Packard CJ, Murray L, et al: Effect of simvastatin on plasma lipid and lipoprotein concentrations and low-density lipoprotein metabolism in the nephrotic syndrome. Clin Sci 1992;82:701–708.

104. Thomas ME, Harris KPG, Ramaswamy C, et al: Simvastatin therapy for hypercholesterolemic patients with nephrotic syndrome or significant proteinuria. Kidney Int 1993;44:1124–1129.

105. Martins Prata M, Nogueira AC, Reimao Pinto J, et al: Long-term effect of lovastatin on lipoprotein profile in patients with primary nephrotic syndrome. Clin Nephrol 1994;41:277–283.

106. Wanner C, Bohler J, Eckardt HG: Effects of simvastatin on lipoprotein (a) and lipoprotein composition in patients with nephrotic syndrome. Clin Nephrol 1994;41:138–143.

107. Brown CD, Azrolan N, Thomas L, et al: Reduction of lipoprotein (a) following treatment with lovastatin in patients with unremitting nephrotic syndrome. Am J Kidney Dis 1995;26:170–177.

108. Rabelink AJ, Hene RJ, Erkelens DW, et al: Partial remission of nephrotic syndrome in patients on long-term simvastatin. Lancet 1990;335:1045–1046.

109. Olbricht CJ, Wanner C, Thiery J, et al: Simvastatin in nephrotic syndrome. Kidney Int 1999;56:(Suppl 71):S113–S116.

110. Matzkies FK, Bahner U, Teschner M, et al: Efficiency of 1-year treatment with fluvastatin in hyperlipidemic patients with nephrotic syndrome. Am J Nephrol 1999;19:492–494.

111. Massy ZA, Ma JZ, Louis TA, et al: Lipid-lowering therapy in patients with renal disease. Kidney Int 1995;48:188–198.

112. Keilani T, Schlueter WA, Levin ML, et al: Improvement of lipid abnormalities associated with proteinuria using fosinopril, an angiotensin-converting enzyme inhibitor. Ann Intern Med 1993;118:246–254.

113. Gansevoort RT, Heeg JE, Dikkeschei FD, et al: Symptomatic anti-proteinuric treatment decreases serum lipoprotein (a) concentration in patients with glomerular proteinuria. Nephrol Dial Transplant 1994;9:244–250.

114. Sato KA, Gary RW, Lemann J: Urinary excretion of 25-hydroxyvitamin D in health and nephrotic syndrome. J Lab Clin Med 1980;69:325–330.

115. Mittal SK, Dash SC, Tiwari SC, et al: Bone histology in patients with nephrotic syndrome and normal renal function. Kidney Int 1999;55:1912–1919.

116. Korkor A, Schwartz J, Bergfeld M, et al: Absence of metabolic bone disease in adult patients with the nephrotic syndrome and normal renal function. J Clin Endocrinol Metab 1983;56:496–500.

117. Tessitore N, Bonucci E, D'Angelo A, et al: Bone histology and calcium metabolism in patients with nephrotic syndrome and normal or reduced renal function. Nephron 1984;37:153–159.

118. Malluche HH, Goldstein DA, Massry SG: Osteomalacia and hyperparathyroid bone disease in patients with nephrotic syndrome. J Clin Invest 1979;63:494–500.

119. Alon U, Chan JCM: Calcium and vitamin D homeostasis in the nephrotic syndrome: current status. Nephron 1984;36:1–4.

120. Haldimann B, Trechsel U: Vitamin D replacement therapy in patients with nephrotic syndrome. Mineral Electrolyte Metab 1983;9:154–156.

121. Llach F: Hypercoagulability, renal vein thrombosis and other thrombotic complications of nephrotic syndrome. Kidney Int 1985;28:429–439.

122. Cameron JS: Coagulation and thromboembolic complications in the nephrotic syndrome. Adv Nephrol 1984;13:75–114.

123. Rabelink TJ, Zwaginga JJ, Koomans HA, et al: Thrombosis and hemostasis in renal disease. Kidney Int 1994;46:287–296.

124. Machleidt C, Mettang T, Starz E, et al: Multifactorial genesis of enhanced platelet aggregability in patients with nephrotic syndrome. Kidney Int 1989;36:1119–1124.

125. Robert A, Olmer M, Sampol J, et al: Clinical correlation between hypercoagulability and thromboembolic phenomena. Kidney Int 1987;31:830–835.

126. Llach F, Papper S, Massry SG: The clinical spectrum of renal vein thrombosis: acute and chronic. Am J Med 1980;69:819–827.

127. Wagoner RD, Stanson AW, Holley KE, et al: Renal vein thrombosis in idiopathic membranous glomerulopathy and nephrotic syndrome: incidence and significance. Kidney Int 1983;23:368–374.

128. Ganeval D, Fischer AM, Barre J, et al: Pharmacokinetics of warfarin in the nephrotic syndrome and effect on vitamin K-dependent clotting factors. Clin Nephrol 1986;25:75–80.

129. Burrow CR, Walker G, Bell WR, et al: Streptokinase salvage of renal function after renal vein thrombosis. Ann Intern Med 1984;100:237–238.

130. Crowley JP, Matarese RA, Quevedo SF, et al: Fibrinolytic therapy for bilateral renal vein thrombosis. Arch Intern Med 1984;144:159–160.

131. Morrisey EC, McDonald BR, Rabetoy GM: Resolution of proteinuria secondary to bilateral renal vein thrombosis after treatment with systemic thrombolytic therapy. Am J Kidney Dis 1997;29:615–619.

132. Lam K-K, Lui C-C: Successful treatment of acute inferior vena cava and unilateral renal vein thrombosis by local infusion of recombinant tissue plasminogen activator. Am J Kidney Dis 1998;32:1075–1079.

133. Rostoker G, Durand-Zaleski I, Petit-Phar M, et al: Prevention of thrombotic complications of the nephrotic syndrome by the low-molecular-weight heparin enoxaparin. Nephron 1995;69:20–28.

134. Sarasin FP, Schifferli JA: Prophylactic oral anticoagulation in nephrotic patients with idiopathic membranous nephropathy. Kidney Int 1994;45:578–585.

135. Bellomo R, Atkins RC: Membranous nephropathy and thromboembolism: Is prophylactic anticoagulation warranted? Nephron 1993;63:249–254.

136. Ogi M, Yokoyama H, Tomosugi N, et al: Risk factors for infection and immunoglobulin replacement therapy in adult nephrotic syndrome. Am J Kidney Dis 1994;24:427–436.

137. Garin EH, Sausville PJ, Richard GA: Impaired primary antibody response in experimental nephrotic syndrome. Clin Exp Immunol 1983;52:595–598.

138. Spika JS, Halsey NA, Le CT, et al: Decline of vaccine-induced antipneumococcal antibody in children with nephrotic syndrome. Am J Kidney Dis 1986;7:466–470.

Thrombotic Microangiopathies

Piero Ruggenenti, Marina Noris, and Giuseppe Remuzzi

Background

The term "thrombotic microangiopathy" (TMA) defines a lesion of vessel wall thickening (mainly arterioles or capillaries), intraluminal platelet thrombosis, and partial or complete obstruction of the vessel lumina. Depending on whether renal or brain lesions prevail, two pathologically indistinguishable but clinically different entities have been described: hemolytic–uremic syndrome (HUS) and thrombotic thrombocytopenic purpura (TTP). Injury to the endothelial cell is most likely central in provoking the sequence of events leading to TMA. Loss of physiologic thromboresistance, leukocyte adhesion to damaged endothelium, complement consumption, abnormal von Willebrand factor (vWF) release and fragmentation, and increased vascular shear stress may then sustain and amplify the microangiopathic process. Intrinsic abnormalities of the complement system and the vWF pathway may account for a genetic predisposition to the disease that may play a paramount role in familial and recurrent forms. Due to their poor outcome and response to treatment these congenital (genetic) forms are considered separately from acquired forms, whose outcome depends strongly on whether the underlying etiology can be treated or removed. The pathogenesis of acquired forms is only briefly reviewed in order to provide background to the different specific treatments. The mechanisms of genetic forms are discussed in more detail since they have been clarified only recently and will certainly have major relevance in identifying specific treatment modalities in the next few years. Forms without a recognized genetic predisposition or precipitating agent are referred to as idiopathic forms and are discussed separately from acquired and genetic forms (Table 29.1).

Acquired

These are by far the most common forms of TMA. Toxins, autoantibodies, pregnancy, systemic diseases, and drugs have been associated with TMA that may present with the clinical features of HUS or TTP. In most of these cases early recognition and removal or treatment of the underlying condition is therefore of paramount importance in achieving remission.

Shigatoxin-associated thrombotic microangiopathy

Shigatoxin (Stx)-associated HUS, the most frequent form of TMA, is associated with infection by certain strains of *Escherichia coli or Shigella dysenteriae* that produce a

Table 29.1 Classification of thrombotic microangiopathies

	Clinical features
Acquired forms	
Shigatoxin-associated	HUS
Neuraminidase-associated	HUS
vWF protease deficiency-associated	TTP (often recurrent)
Pregnancy-associated	HUS, TTP, HELLP syndrome
Systemic disease-associated	HUS, TTP
Drug-associated	HUS, TTP
Transplantation-associated	HUS (de novo or recurrent), TTP
Genetic forms	
Factor H abnormalities	HUS (often recurrent and familial)
vWF protease deficiency	HUS, TTP (often recurrent and familial)
Others	HUS, TTP (often recurrent and familial)
Idiopathic	HUS, TTP

HELLP, hemolysis, elevated liver enzymes and low platelet count; HUS, hemolytic–uremic syndrome; TTP, thrombotic thrombocytopenic purpura; vWF, von Willebrand factor.

powerful exotoxin (Stx).[1] The term "shigatoxin" was initially used to describe the exotoxin produced by *Sh. dysenteriae* type 1. Later, some strains of *E. coli* (mostly serotype 0157:H7) isolated from human cases with diarrhea were found to produce a toxin similar to that produced by *Sh. dysenteriae*. This toxin was subsequently given different names, such as "shiga-like toxin" due to its similarities with shigatoxin, or "verotoxin" because of its cytopathic effect on Vero cells (i.e. African green monkey kidney cells). However, the terms "shiga-like toxin" or "verotoxin" should now be abandoned and only "shigatoxin" used to describe the exotoxins produced by *Sh. dysenteriae* and *E. coli*. After food contaminated by Stx-producing *E. coli* or *Sh. dysenteriae* is injested, the toxin is released in the gut and causes watery or, more often, bloody diarrhea because of its direct effect on the intestinal mucosa. If Stx moves through the intestinal mucosa to reach the systemic circulation, full-blown HUS may develop. Stx-associated HUS is usually considered to have a good outcome, with complete recovery in about 90% of cases. However, 3–5% of patients die during the acute phase, up to 5% are left with severe renal and extrarenal sequelae, and about 40% will still have low glomerular filtration rate (GFR) at 10-year follow-up. Age under 2 years, severe gastrointestinal prodromes, elevated white cell count, and anuria early in the course of the disease are predictors of the severity of HUS. Anuria for more than 10 days or need for dialysis in the acute phase, as well as proteinuria at 12 months follow-up, have been associated with an increased risk of chronic renal failure in the long term. Patched cortical necrosis or involvement of more than 50% of glomeruli are further predictors of poor outcome.

Diagnosis rests on detection of *E. coli* 0157:H7 in stool cultures. Serologic tests for antibodies to Stx and 0157 lipopolysaccharide can be performed in research laboratories. Tests are being developed for rapid detection of *E. coli* 0157:H7 and shigatoxin in stools.

Undercooked ground beef is the commonest source of infection, although ham, turkey, cheese, unpasteurized milk, and water have also been implicated. Secondary person-to-person contact is an important route of transmission in institutional centers, particularly daycare centers and nursing homes. Infected patients should be excluded from daycare centers until two consecutive stool cultures are negative for *E. coli* 0157:H7 in order to prevent further transmission. However, the most important preventive measure in childcare centers is supervised hand washing.

Supportive therapy

In typical Stx-associated HUS of children the mortality rate has significantly decreased over the last 40 years, probably as the result of better supportive management of anemia, renal failure, hypertension, and electrolyte and water imbalance. Bowel rest is important for the enterohemorrhagic colitis linked with Stx-associated HUS. Antibiotics given to treat infection due to Stx-producing *E. coli* 0157:H7 have been found to increase 17-fold[2] the risk of overt HUS. Indeed, antibiotic-induced injury to the bacterial membrane might favor the acute release of large amounts of preformed toxin. Alternatively, antibiotic therapy might give *E. coli* 0157:H7 a selective advantage if these organisms are not as readily eliminated from the bowel as the normal intestinal flora. Moreover, several antimicrobial drugs, particularly the quinolones, trimethoprim, and furazolidone, are potent inducers of the expression of the Stx 2 gene and may increase the level of toxin in the intestine. However, the above considerations do not necessarily apply to many cases of bloody diarrhea, particularly in South America and India, precipitated by *E. coli* strains other than 0157:H7 or by other bacteria, such as *Sh. dysenteriae* type 1. For instance, when hemorrhagic colitis is caused by *Sh. dysenteriae* type 1, early and empiric antibiotic treatment shortens the duration of diarrhea, decreases the incidence of complications, and reduces the risk of transmission by shortening the duration of bacterial shedding. Thus, in developing countries where *Shigella* is the most frequent cause of hemorrhagic colitis, antibiotic therapy should be started early and even before the involved pathogen is identified.

Plasma manipulation and other specific treatments

No specific therapy aimed at preventing or limiting the microangiopathic process has been proved to affect the course of Stx-associated HUS in children. Two prospective controlled trials found that plasma therapy may limit short-term renal lesions but does not affect long-term renal outcome and patient survival[3,4] (Table 29.2). Heparin and antithrombotic agents may increase the risk of bleeding and should be avoided. Whether tissue-type plasminogen activator, which discriminates between fibrin and fibrin-bound plasminogen, gives a better risk–benefit profile in the treatment of HUS is worth investigating.

Table 29.2 Controlled studies of specific treatments of different forms of thrombotic microangiopathy

Reference	Design	Clinical features	No. of patients	Treatment Cases	Controls	Outcome
Childhood series						
Loirat et al[36]	Prospective Randomized Multicenter	HUS	33	Heparin Urokinase	Supportive	Comparable survival, clinical outcomes, and histology changes in cases and controls
Vandamme-Lombaerts et al[37]	Prospective Randomized Monocenter	HUS	58	Heparin Dipyridamole	Supportive	Comparable survival, clinical outcomes, and histology changes in cases and controls
Loirat et al[38]	Prospective Randomized Monocenter	HUS	79	FFP (10 mL/kg/day)	Supportive	Lower serum creatinine at 6 months (63 ± 21 vs. 48 ± 13 µmol/L, $P < 0.005$) and less cases of cortical necrosis (0 vs. 7, $P < 0.02$) in cases than in controls
Rizzoni et al[3]	Prospective Randomized Multicenter	HUS	32	FFP (10–30 mL/kg/day)	Supportive	Comparable survival, clinical outcomes, and histology changes in cases and controls
Gianviti et al[39]	Retrospective Multicenter	HUS (with ARF)	33	PE (3–10 exchanges)	Supportive	Less residual renal insufficiency (GFR < 80 mL/min) in cases than in controls (18% vs. 43%)
Adult series						
Italian Group[40]	Retrospective Multicenter	TTP	29	PE (3–15 exchanges)	Steroids Antiplatelets	Less mortality (18% vs. 43%) and more remissions (86% vs. 57%) in cases than in controls
French Group[41]	Retrospective Multicenter	HUS	53	PE (2–21 exchanges)	Supportive	Less mortality (0% vs. 23%) and less ESRD (26% vs. 64%) in cases than in controls
Henon[42]	Prospective Randomized Multicenter	TTP (with ARF)	40	PE (3–35 exchanges)	FFP, ASA Dipyridamole	Less mortality (15% vs. 43%) and more remissions (80% vs. 52%) in cases than in control
Rock et al[15]	Prospective Randomized Multicenter	TTP	102	PE (3–36 exchanges)	FFP, ASA Dipyridamole	Less mortality (22% vs. 37%) and more remissions (78% vs. 49%) in cases than in controls

ARF, acute renal failure; ASA, acetylsalicylic acid; ESRD, endstage renal disease; FFP, fresh-frozen plasma; GFR, glomerular filtration rate; HUS, hemolytic–uremic syndrome; PE, plasma exchange; TTP, thrombotic thrombocytopenic purpura.

Efficacy of specific treatments in adult patients is difficult to evaluate, since most information is derived by uncontrolled series that may also include cases of HUS not caused by Stx (Table 29.2). In particular, no prospective randomized trials are available to establish definitively whether plasma infusion or exchange may offer some specific benefit as compared to supportive treatment alone. However, comparative analyses of two large series of patients treated with[5] or without[6] plasma suggest that plasma therapy may dramatically decrease overall mortality of *E. coli* 0157:H7-associated HUS. These findings lead us and others to consider plasma infusion or exchange suitable for adult patients, particularly in those with severe renal insufficiency and central nervous system involvement.

Rescue treatment

In occasional patients, increased shear stress and platelet activation in the damaged renal microvasculature may sustain the microangiopathic process even after the precipitating factor has been exhausted.[1] In these rare cases, persistent thrombocytopenia associated with severe refractory hypertension and signs of hypertensive encephalopathy may put the patient in imminent danger of death. In such dramatic cases bilateral nephrectomy was followed within 2 weeks by complete hematologic and clinical remission.[7]

The rationale of the procedure rests on evidence that removing the kidneys eliminates a major site of vWF fragmentation; this limits platelet activation and protects patients from the further spreading of microvascular lesions.[7] However, bilateral nephrectomy is irreversible and should be considered only for patients in whom all other approaches have failed. Potential candidates are patients who are plasma resistant (defined as more than 20 days of exchange or infusion with no improvement in clinical and laboratory findings) or plasma dependent (patients who have to be continuously infused with plasma to remain in remission, and in whom the platelet count invariably drops, with signs of hemolysis, within a few days after plasma is discontinued).

Nephrectomy should not be considered unless a renal biopsy (taken as soon as the platelet count rises, even transiently, with plasma to a level where the procedure is safe) shows chronic diffuse lesions associated with signs of the disease, i.e. arteriolar thrombosis and myointimal proliferation. Finally, nephrectomy should be considered only in the presence of life-threatening signs such as major neurologic dysfunction or coma, or uncontrolled bleeding as a consequence of refractory thrombocytopenia.

Neuraminidase-associated thrombotic microangiopathy

This is a rare but potentially fatal disease that may complicate pneumonia or, less frequently, meningitis caused by Streptococcus pneumoniae. By removing sialic acid from cell membranes, the neuraminidase produced by Strep. pneumoniae exposes the Thomsen–Friedenreich antigen to preformed circulating IgM antibodies.[8] Binding of circulating preformed IgM antibodies to this cryptic antigen exposed on platelet and endothelial cell surfaces causes platelet aggregation and endothelial damage. Binding of IgM antibodies to the antigen expressed on circulating erythrocytes may also explain why Coombs-positive hemolytic anemia is so frequently reported in patients with neuraminidase-induced HUS. The clinical picture is usually severe, with respiratory distress, neurologic involvement, and coma.

Therapy

The outcome is strongly dependent on the effectiveness of antibiotic therapy. In theory, plasma, either infused or exchanged, is contraindicated because adult plasma contains antibodies against the Thomsen–Friedenreich antigen that may accelerate polyagglutination and hemolysis.[8] Thus patients should be treated only with antibiotics and washed red cells. However, in some cases, plasma therapy, occasionally in combination with steroids, has been associated with recovery.

Thrombotic microangiopathy associated with acquired deficiency of von Willebrand factor-cleaving protease

This is a recently categorized form of TMA that most likely accounts for the majority of cases so far reported as acute idiopathic or sporadic TTP. Recent studies have found that in 70–90% of patients with a clinical diagnosis of acute TTP there is a severe deficiency of a plasma metallo-

protease that in normal individuals cleaves ultralarge vWF multimers as soon as they are secreted.[9] The finding that in most patients a circulating IgG autoantibody blocks the vWF-cleaving protease suggests an autoimmune pathogenesis for the disease.[10–12] Further evidence for the pathogenetic role of this autoantibody is demonstrated by the observations that it usually disappears from the circulation when effective treatment achieves remission and that this occurs in parallel with the normalization of plasma vWF-cleaving protease activity. Although TTP associated with vWF-cleaving protease inhibitors is usually sporadic, recurrent episodes have also been reported due to reappearance of the inhibitor in the circulation several weeks or even months after the resolution of the presenting episode. Notably, autoantibodies against the vWF-cleaving protease have also been observed in patients developing TTP during treatment with antiplatelet drugs such as ticlopidine (see section Drug-associated thrombotic microangiopathy).

The clinical picture is usually severe, with an abrupt onset of neurologic signs, purpura, and fever.[13] Neurologic symptoms usually dominate the clinical picture and may be fleeting and fluctuating, probably because of continuous thrombi formation and dispersion in the brain microcirculation.

Supportive therapy, plasma manipulation, and other specific treatments

In the early 1960s, TTP was almost invariably fatal but now, thanks to earlier diagnosis, improved intensive care facilities, and new techniques such as plasma therapy, survival may reach 90%.[14,15]

Plasma manipulation is the cornerstone of therapy of the acute episode. Plasma may serve to induce remission of the disease by replacing defective protease activity. In theory, compared with infusion, exchange may offer the advantage of rapidly removing antibodies to the vWF-cleaving protease. However, this needs to be proven in controlled trials. In addition, corticosteroids might inhibit the synthesis of antiprotease autoantibodies. Of 108 patients with either TTP or HUS, 30 were recently reported to have recovered after treatment with corticosteroids alone.[14] All of them, however, had mild forms and none of them were tested for vWF-cleaving protease activity. Again, the potential therapeutic benefit of these drugs needs to be tested in ad hoc studies in which response to treatment is evaluated selectively in patients with circulating antibodies to the vWF-cleaving protease.

Rescue treatments

Plasma cryosupernatant Cryosupernatant fraction (i.e. plasma from which a cryoprecipitate containing the largest plasma vWF multimers, fibrinogen, and fibronectin have been removed) instead of fresh-frozen plasma has been successful in treating a small number of patients who did not respond to repeated exchanges or infusions with fresh-frozen plasma.[16] The rationale for this approach is that plasma cryosupernatant may provide the same beneficial factor(s) found in whole plasma (in this case, the defective/inhibited vWF protease activity) but does not contain those factors (including large vWF multimers) that may actually sustain the microangiopathic process until remission is achieved. On this basis, the use of plasma cryosupernatant has been suggested as preferred therapy. However, results of a few small randomized studies failed to find differences between the two products.[17]

Splenectomy Deterioration in clinical status, with a decrease in hematocrit and platelet count and high serum lactate dehydrogenase, was reported in six patients undergoing splenectomy because of refractoriness to corticosteroids and plasma exchange: four patients became comatose and one died abruptly.[14] The five surviving patients progressively recovered after the reinstitution of plasma exchange. Another study showed a higher mortality rate and longer disease duration in 13 patients undergoing splenectomy compared with 39 patients continuing on plasma therapy.[18] Splenectomy was therefore not considered an effective treatment for TTP refractory to plasma therapy.

The above studies, however, were far from conclusive because of their retrospective design and because they included unselected series of patients. Splenectomy may have a specific role in the subset of patients with autoantibodies against vWF-cleaving protease that persist in the circulation despite immunosuppressive therapy.[10] In this setting splenectomy might achieve persistent remission by removing a major site of antibody synthesis. Three patients with TTP and high levels of autoantibodies against vWF-cleaving protease entered remission after splenectomy. In all three patients, splenectomy was followed by disappearance of the inhibitor and normalization of protease activity.[10] In another patient, prolonged treatment by plasma exchange and plasma infusion and corticosteroid therapy resulted in transient disappearance of the vWF-cleaving protease inhibitor.[19] Later in the course of the disease the patient's platelet count again gradually decreased with concomitant reappearance of the inhibitor, leading to several relapses of acute TTP. Splenectomy, performed 1 year after the first episode of TTP, resulted in disappearance of the autoantibody and normalization of protease activity and stable and complete remission of the disease. However, these reports are far from conclusive and further studies with a larger number of patients are needed to prove the therapeutic value of this irreversible procedure.

Platelet transfusion The severe thrombocytopenia in TTP has led many physicians to administer platelet transfusions, with the aim of preventing severe bleeding complications. However, reports of sudden death, decreased survival, and delayed recovery after platelet transfusion dramatically document the danger of giving platelets to patients with TTP. Thus platelet transfusions are contraindicated in acute TTP, except in cases of life-threatening bleeding.

Pregnancy-associated thrombotic microangiopathy

TMA associated with pregnancy includes TTP (usually in the early phases of pregnancy), the HELLP syndrome (usually near term), and HUS (usually post partum).[20]

Thrombotic thrombocytopenic purpura

TTP develops during the antepartum period in 89% of cases, usually within 24 weeks. Later in the course of pregnancy, clinical features of TTP and preeclampsia may overlap. Despite limited experience, available series show that the maternal mortality rate has fallen from 68% to almost zero with the institution of plasma therapy.[20] Delivery is recommended only for those patients who do not respond to plasma therapy. However, delivery is by no means the treatment of choice for preeclampsia/HELLP syndrome.

Measurement of plasma antithrombin (AT) III activity has been suggested as a useful tool for differentiating TTP and preeclampsia. TTP is most likely before gestational week 28 and when AT III plasma activity is normal. Plasma therapy could be tried and, if effective, should be continued until term and/or complete remission of the disease. Delivery can be considered as "rescue" after failure of plasma therapy. The role of other treatments often employed in idiopathic TTP remains elusive.

After week 34 of gestation, preeclampsia is more likely and is usually associated with decreased plasma AT III activity. Delivery is the treatment of choice and is usually followed by complete recovery within 24–48 h. Persistent disease may be an indication to attempt a course of plasma therapy. Between 28 and 34 weeks, the optimal treatment is controversial. Some hold that delivery should always be considered preferred therapy, whereas others believe that if there is no evidence of fetal distress and plasma AT III activity is normal, a course of plasma therapy can be reasonably attempted before inducing delivery.[21]

HELLP syndrome

The HELLP (*h*emolysis, *e*levated *l*iver enzymes and *l*ow *p*latelet count) syndrome is simply a form of severe preeclampsia in which, besides hypertension and renal dysfunction, there is evidence of microangiopathic hemolysis and liver involvement. The syndrome is most common in white multiparous women with a history of poor pregnancy outcome. It arises in the antepartum period in 70% of cases. Symptoms usually arise within 24–48 h post partum, occasionally after an uncomplicated pregnancy.[20]

Diagnosis is based on:

1. hemolysis (defined as fragmented erythrocytes in the circulation and lactate dehydrogenase (LDH) ≥ 600 U/L);
2. elevated liver enzymes (serum glutamate oxaloacetate transaminase > 70 U/L);
3. low platelet count (< 100 000/μL).[19]

Overt disseminated intravascular coagulation is reported in 25% of cases. Intrahepatic hemorrhage, subcapsular liver hematoma, and liver rupture are rare life-threatening complications. The maternal and perinatal mortality rates are 0–24% and 7.7–60% respectively. Most of the perinatal deaths are related to abruptio placentae, intrauterine asphyxia, and extreme prematurity. As many as 44% of the infants are growth retarded.

Termination of pregnancy is the only definitive therapy. Hydralazine or dihydralazine are the preferred drugs for controlling pregnancy-induced hypertension, with magnesium sulfate to prevent and treat convulsions. Both peritoneal dialysis and hemodialysis have been used to treat acute renal failure. Platelet transfusions are needed for clinical bleeding or severe thrombocytopenia (platelet count < 20 000/μL).

In approximately 5% of patients with HELLP syndrome, symptoms and laboratory abnormalities do not improve after delivery. These are cases with central nervous system abnormalities, associated with renal and cardiopulmonary dysfunction and activation of coagulation. Uncontrolled studies suggest that plasma exchange may help recovery in patients with persistent evidence of disease 72 h or more after delivery. However, plasma therapy is ineffective during pregnancy and may increase fetal and maternal risk when used to delay delivery. Preliminary evidence suggests that after birth corticosteroids may speed up disease recovery, and before birth may postpone delivery of previable fetuses and reduce the mother's need for blood products.

Postpartum hemolytic–uremic syndrome

By definition, postpartum HUS follows a normal delivery by no more than 6 months.[1] The clinical course is usually fulminant. Supportive care including dialysis, transfusions, and careful fluid management remains the most important form of treatment. Whether plasma therapy improves survival or limits renal sequelae has not been established. Antiplatelet agents, heparin, and antithrombotic therapy may enhance the risk of bleeding and have no proven efficacy.

Thrombotic microangiopathy associated with systemic disease

Prevention and treatment of TMA associated with systemic diseases largely rests on specific treatment of the underlying conditions.

Antiphospholipid syndrome, systemic lupus erythematosus, scleroderma, malignant hypertension

Plasma therapy should always be attempted in TMA associated with systemic diseases even if its efficacy in this setting is poorly defined. In the antiphospholipid syndrome, the relationships between the various antiphospholipid antibodies and the clinical manifestations of the disease are not clarified. Thus, oral anticoagulation remains the only treatment of proven efficacy for preventing and treating microvascular and macrovascular thrombosis, even if concomitant thrombocytopenia may increase the risk of hemorrhagic complications. Control of blood pressure is the cornerstone of treatment of TMA associated with scleroderma crisis and malignant hypertension.

Human immunodeficiency virus

HUS and TTP are both among the complications of AIDS, which may account for as much as 30% of hospitalized HUS/TTP cases. Plasma manipulation appears the only feasible approach. Uncontrolled series provide evidence that the survival rate in HIV patients without AIDS is comparable to that of idiopathic TTP. In contrast, patients with AIDS-associated TTP almost invariably have a poor outcome and do not appear to benefit from plasma therapy.[21]

Cancer

TMA complicates almost 6% of cases of metastatic carcinoma. The prognosis is extremely poor and most patients die within a few weeks. Therapy is minimally effective. Administration of blood products to correct symptomatic anemia often results in exacerbation of the syndrome, with rapid worsening of hemolysis, deterioration of renal function, and pulmonary edema.

Drug-associated thrombotic microangiopathy
Mitomycin and anticancer drugs

A form of TMA resembling HUS has been described in cancer patients treated with mitomycin C. Disease manifestation is dose related, renal dysfunction being reported in less than 2% of patients given a cumulative dose < 50 mg/m^2 and in more than 28% of those given > 50 mg/m^2 or receiving more than one course of therapy. Platinum- and bleomycin-containing combinations have also been reported to induce HUS. The fatality rate is close to 79% and median time to death is about 4 weeks. Patients surviving the acute phase often remain on chronic dialysis, or die later of recurrence of the tumor or metastases. It has been suggested that the syndrome may be prevented by giving steroids during mitomycin treatment but this needs to be confirmed in prospective controlled trials. Plasma exchange is usually attempted but its effectiveness is unproved.

Antiplatelet drugs

TMA has been reported in 1 in 1600–5000 patients treated with ticlopidine. Neurologic abnormalities occur within 1 month of treatment in 80% of cases. The overall survival rate is 67% and is improved by early treatment withdrawal and plasma therapy. Generation of an autoantibody against vWF-cleaving protease may be involved in the pathogenesis of ticlopidine-associated TTP. Seven patients who developed TTP 2–7 weeks after initiation of ticlopidine therapy had severely decreased levels of vWF-cleaving protease, with the appearance of IgG molecules in their blood that inhibited the vWF-cleaving protease activity.[22] The deficiency resolved after ticlopidine therapy was discontinued and plasmapheresis was instituted. Eleven cases have been reported during treatment with clopidogrel, a new antiaggregating agent that has achieved widespread clinical use because of its safety profile. All patients had neurologic involvement and were treated with plasma exchange: eight fully recovered, two had relapses that rapidly recovered after retreatment with plasma exchange, and one died. Half the patients were concomitantly treated with cholesterol-lowering drugs;

conceivably, these drugs should be avoided in clopidogrel-treated patients.

Quinine

Quinine-induced TMA is a rare, recently defined condition characterized by predominant renal impairment. It typically occurs in patients presensitized by prior exposure to quinine and rapidly follows reingestion of the drug. Quinine is generally used to treat muscle cramps but is also contained in beverages (tonic water and bitter lemon drinks). Quinine-dependent antiplatelet, antierythrocyte, and antigranulocyte antibodies have been involved in the pathogenesis of the disease. Despite the dramatic presenting symptoms and severe renal failure, the outcome is usually good if cessation of quinine and institution of plasma exchange are carried out early enough. Recovery of renal function is described in most cases. Avoidance of quinine is necessary to prevent recurrence.

Thrombotic microangiopathy associated with bone marrow and solid organ transplantation

Among acquired forms of HUS, post-transplant HUS is being reported with increasing frequency and may be affecting a progressively larger number of patients worldwide. Although poorly defined, the incidence of the disease is remarkably higher in the transplant than in the general population, most likely because of the clustering of several risk factors in this particular setting. In renal transplant recipients, HUS may occur for the first time in patients who have never suffered the disease (de novo post-transplant HUS) or may affect patients whose primary cause of endstage renal disease (ESRD) is HUS (recurrent post-transplant HUS). Treatment of post-transplant HUS rests on removal of the inciting factor(s), relief of symptoms, and plasma infusion or exchange. No other approach has proven effective.[23]

De novo post-transplant hemolytic–uremic syndrome

This form occurs in renal and extrarenal transplant recipients and is usually triggered by immunosuppressive drugs such as calcineurin inhibitors or, less frequently, by virus infections and acute vascular rejection (specifically renal transplant recipients). A peculiar form of de novo post-transplant HUS may affect bone marrow transplant recipients, usually in the setting of graft-versus-host disease (GVHD) or intensive GVHD prophylaxis, including total body irradiation.

Therapy Drug withdrawal or dose reduction is the preferred therapy for de novo cyclosporine- or tacrolimus-associated forms, but by itself is effective in less than 50% of cases.[23] A remarkably higher success rate (84%) has been reported with adjunctive plasma infusion or exchange. A similar response rate has been reported, but in much smaller series, with intravenous IgG infusion, the rationale being to neutralize hypothetical circulating cytotoxic or platelet agglutinating factors. Once remission is achieved,

anecdotal reports suggest that patient rechallenge with decreased doses of cyclosporine or tacrolimus, switching from one drug to the other, or replacement of both drugs with mycophenolate mofetil maintains adequate immunosuppression without further disease recurrence. Very recently, compassionate treatment with rapamycin has been associated with a remarkably good outcome in 15 patients with cyclosporine- or tacrolimus-associated post-transplant HUS, with no patient requiring rapamicin withdrawal because of disease recurrence.[23] Monoclonal antibodies to the IL-2 receptor may also be a valid option for maintaining adequate immunosuppression, thus avoiding the toxic effects of calcineurin inhibitors. The outcome of de novo forms that occur in the setting of viral infection parallels the response to treatment of the underlying disease. Despite intensive plasma therapy or rescue treatment with plasma cryosupernatant or protein A immunoadsorption, the outcome of de novo forms that complicate bone marrow transplantation is still dramatically poor, with a mortality rate close to 90%. In addition to the severity of the microangiopathic process (quantified on the basis of serum LDH levels and percentage circulating fragmented erythrocytes), infection, progressive GVHD, or relapse of the underlying disease may account for this discouraging figure.

Recurrent post-transplant hemolytic–uremic syndrome

This is most frequently reported in patients who progress to ESRD because of HUS due to causes other than Stx and particularly in those with genetic forms. Whether the precipitating factors associated with de novo HUS also contribute to disease recurrence in the renal graft is still debatable. This is consistent, albeit not proven, with evidence that a precipitating factor is often observed or suspected in patients with recurrent disease.

Therapy Recurrent forms usually do not respond to any type of therapy and are associated with a graft loss close to 100%. On this basis, renal transplantation should be considered an effective and safe treatment of ESRD only for patients with Stx-associated HUS. In patients with HUS due to other causes, particularly the genetic forms, renal transplantation should be considered extremely carefully. In particular, until new strategies to effectively limit or prevent recurrence become available, renal transplantation is contraindicated in familial/relapsing forms and in all cases with a well-characterized genetic abnormality predisposing to the disease.[23]

Genetic (thrombotic microangiopathy associated with congenital defects)

These forms are rare, often occur in families (mainly but not exclusively children), and frequently relapse even after complete recovery of the presenting episode. Depending on the defect involved and the age of disease onset, these forms may present with the clinical features of HUS or

TTP or both in different members of the same family or in different episodes in the same patient. ESRD, permanent neurologic sequelae, and death are the final outcomes in the majority of cases.[1] Therapy seldom achieves persistent remission of the disease. Genetic counseling is therefore of paramount importance. In cases with recognized genetic mutations, antenatal diagnosis by amniocentesis or chorionic villus biopsy is possible and the carrier state can be identified.

Factor H abnormalities

Intrinsic abnormalities of the complement system due to deficiency of factor H, a plasma protein that inhibits the activation of the alternative pathway of complement, have been found in a number of TMA cases that almost invariably present with the clinical features of HUS.[24,25] Genetic studies in large families have found that an area on chromosome 1q32, where factor H is located, segregates with the disease.[26] Subsequently, about 20 mutations of the factor H gene have been found.[24,27] All described cases had heterozygous mutations, with the exception of members of a Bedouin family with very early-onset disease, who displayed a 24-bp homozygous deletion in the last exon of the factor H gene that resulted in less than 10% of the normal factor H plasma concentration.[24,27] Heterozygous nonsense mutations may also result in reduced (50%) factor H protein concentrations.[25] However, the majority of heterozygous point mutations are missense mutations leading to a single amino acid change in short consensus repeat 20 (SCR20), the most C-terminal individually folded domain of factor H.[24,27] The resulting mutant proteins are functionally inactive, since they have lost the ability to bind either sialic acid molecules on endothelial cells or C3 or both,[24] but are normally translated and secreted, which accounts for the normal plasma concentrations of factor H as measured by commonly used laboratory assays. This point is important for clinicians. Since not all patients with heterozygous mutations have a persistent reduction in complement C3, the diagnosis of factor H-related HUS cannot be dismissed just because concentrations of C3 and factor H are normal.

Heterozygous mutations are associated with incomplete penetrance of the disease as documented by a number of healthy carriers described within families.[24,26,27] Heterozygous factor H mutations have also been reported in patients with sporadic or recurrent HUS with no familial history; in some of these patients, DNA analysis of parental samples revealed that the mutation had been inherited from an unaffected parent.[24,26,27] Thus, in a proportion of patients who present with sporadic or recurrent HUS, there is an underlying genetic predisposition and this may have implications for other family members. It is possible that the genetic change is a predisposing factor and that an environmental insult then precipitates the disorder, although it is also possible that polymorphisms in other genes may combine to determine the HUS phenotype.

Supporting a role for factor H deficiency in the pathogenesis of HUS is the complement dependence of some models of glomerular thrombosis, e.g. the generalized Shwartzman reaction in rabbits, and various immune-mediated models accelerated by lipopolysaccharide. However, the observation that factor H-deficient individuals occasionally have long remissions or do not present until late in life suggests that a "second hit" is needed, at least in the heterozygous form. Preceding infection is commonly reported but specific trigger factors remain unknown.[25] When the insult occurs (e.g. during infection and/or inflammation), the release of inflammatory mediators causes endothelial damage and promotes the activation and tissue deposition of the C3 convertase of the alternative pathway of complement. Whereas in healthy individuals such activation would be contained by the immediate binding of factor H to damaged endothelium and subendothelium, in patients carrying factor H mutations suboptimal factor H function is unable to efficiently restrict the activation of the alternative pathway of complement, allowing the propagation of vascular injury and expression of the disease.

Irrespective of the pattern of inheritance, the clinical course of factor H-related genetic HUS is characterized by persistent severe hypertension, a high rate of relapse, and progression to ESRD.[1,23]

Therapy

Treatment is based on plasma exchange or infusion. There is anecdotal evidence that infusion of normal plasma can provide enough factor H to induce remission of the disease. However, there is concern that the benefit of plasma therapy seems to reduce over time.

Renal transplantation has been attempted in patients with ESRD, although the frequency of disease recurrence in the graft is around 100%. In most patients the disease manifested on the transplanted kidney within 30 days after surgery. Thus in patients with ESRD caused by HUS, screening for factor H mutations should be mandatory before their inclusion in a transplant list. We have recently provided evidence that in a 2-year-old child who had progressed to ESRD because of HUS associated with a heterozygous mutation in SCR20 of the factor H gene, split liver transplantation protected the simultaneously transplanted kidney from recurrence of the disease by restoring the production of normal factor H and preventing uncontrolled complement activation.[28] In this setting, therefore, combined liver and renal transplantation may be an effective way to gain independence from chronic dialysis, and may be life-saving in those infants who have a poor life expectancy on dialysis.

Deficiency of von Willebrand factor protease activity

This rare form of TMA is associated with a congenital defect of a plasma metalloprotease that cleaves ultralarge vWF multimers into smaller multimers. The defect was originally described in TTP;[9,10] however, emerging data indicate that patients with HUS[29] may also have a complete lack of vWF-cleaving protease activity, albeit less frequently. Thus on clinical grounds a possible congenital defect of vWF-cleaving protease cannot be excluded only on the basis of predominant renal localization of disease manifestation. TMA associated with congenital vWF-cleaving protease deficiency presented either in families or in patients with no familial history of the disease.[9,10,29,30] In both cases, the disease is inherited as an autosomal recessive trait, as documented by vWF-cleaving protease levels in healthy relatives of patients that fell into a bimodal distribution with a group with half-normal values (consistent with carriers) and another with normal values.[29]

Recurrences are very frequent and may occur even after symptom-free periods of months or years. Although they are more frequent in adults, relapsing forms of TMA have also been reported in children with congenital deficiency of vWF-cleaving protease in whom renal symptoms are predominant.[30]

The gene encoding the protease (ADAMTS13) has been recently identified and cloned.[30,32] In families with a history of TTP, sequence analysis of patients' DNA identified 12 mutations in the ADAMTS13 gene.[30] Affected individuals within families were either homozygous for the same mutation or compound heterozygous for two different mutations, confirming that the disease is inherited as a recessive trait.

Therapy

Therapy of ADAMTS13-associated TMA involves plasma infusion or exchange to replenish the active protease. In fact, providing just 5% normal enzymatic activity may be sufficient to degrade large vWF multimers, which may be relevant for inducing remission of the microangiopathic process; this effect is sustained over time due to the relatively long half-life (2–4 days) of the protease. In two brothers with complete deficiency of the protease and relapsing TTP, disease remission was achieved by plasmapheresis and was concurrent with an almost full recovery of vWF-cleaving protease activity. Both patients achieved a long-lasting remission, although protease activity decreased to less than 20% over 20 days after withdrawal of plasma therapy.[33] One patient of ours with relapsing TTP due to congenital deficiency of vWF-cleaving protease and who had more than 100 relapses over 7 years was given different forms of treatment on different occasions: exchange, plasma infusion alone, or plasma removed and replaced with albumin and saline.[31] Clinical remission and normalization of platelet count within a few days was invariably obtained with plasma exchange or infusion, but plasma removal never raised the platelet count. Thus plasma infusion is likely the preferred treatment for HUS or TTP associated with congenital deficiency of vWF-cleaving protease. Although individual attacks usually respond to treatment, long-term prognosis is invariably poor if therapy fails to achieve lasting remission.

Other genetic forms

It is possible that the mutations described earlier account for just a minority of genetic forms. Patients with decreased C3 but no evidence of factor H abnormalities have been described. In these rare cases, uncontrolled activation of the alternative complement pathway may be due to genetic defects in other complement regulatory proteins, including DAF, CR1, CR2, C4-binding protein. Other cases may be associated with still unrecognized genetic defects. Among these are familial forms transmitted with a dominant or recessive pattern of inheritance that may manifest with the features of HUS or TTP in different members of the same family or in different recurrences in the same patient.

Therapy

Plasma infusion or exchange is the only therapy that may have some effect. Regardless of treatment, however, disease outcome is usually poor.

Idiopathic

These are forms of unknown etiology with progressive deterioration of renal function and neurologic involvement that may resemble TTP. They may follow a progressive course to ESRD or death and very likely constitute a disease closer to TTP that requires more specific therapies to halt the progression of the microangiopathic process. These cases recur more often after renal transplantation.[23]

Therapy

Plasma infusion and exchange have been retrospectively found to limit residual renal insufficiency or the risk of ESRD in children. Uncontrolled studies suggest that plasma infusion or exchange may markedly lower the mortality rate and risk of ESRD in adults.[1,34] Intravenous immunoglobulins have been suggested in order to limit neurologic involvement, but their effectiveness is still unproved. Bilateral nephrectomy (see earlier) may be attempted as rescue therapy in patients with severe renal involvement, refractory hypertension/thrombocytopenia, and hypertensive encephalopathy.

Specific recommendations

In addition to symptomatic treatment, various specific therapies have been suggested for the different forms of TMA (Tables 29.2–29.4). However, no clear-cut guidelines are available to identify which patients should be treated, which therapies should be chosen, and how these should be given.

A general consensus has been agreed that therapies aimed at halting the microangiopathic process (i.e. plasma exchange or infusion) should always be tried in genetic forms of HUS, adult forms of HUS, and TTP in order to minimize the risk of death or long-term sequelae. In contrast, this approach is not risk effective in childhood Stx-associated HUS, which usually recovers spontaneously.

The role of specific therapies in all other forms of TMA is still unclear. Whenever indicated, specific therapy should be started as soon as diagnosis is established in order to speed up disease recovery and minimize

Table 29.3 Specific therapies commonly used in thrombotic microangiopathy: dose and route of administration

	Dose	Route
Antiplatelet agents		
Aspirin	325–1300 mg/day	Oral
Dipyridamole	400–600 mg/day	Oral
Dextran 70	500 mg twice daily	i.v. injection
Prostacyclin	4–20 mg/kg/min	Continuous i.v. infusion
Antithrombotic agents		
Heparin	5000 units	Bolus i.v. injection
	750–1000 units/h	Continuous i.v. infusion
Streptokinase	250 000 units	Bolus i.v. injection
	100 000 units/h	Continuous i.v. infusion
Antioxidants		
Vitamin E	1000 mg/m^2/day	Oral
Immunosuppressive agents		
Prednisone	200 mg tapered to 60 mg/day	Oral during active disease
	then 5 mg reduction per week	Oral after remission
Prednisolone	200 mg tapered to 60 mg/day	i.v. if hepatic dysfunction
Immunoglobulins	400 mg/kg/day	i.v. infusion
Vincristine	1.4 mg/m^2 on day 1	i.v. injection
	1 mg every 4 days	i.v. injection up to four doses
Fresh-frozen plasma		
Infusion	20–30 mL/kg on day 1	i.v. infusion
	10–20 mL/kg/day	i.v. infusion up to remission
Exchange	1–2 plasma volumes/day	i.v. up to remission
Cryosupernatant	See plasma infusion/exchange	See plasma infusion/exchange
Sodium detergent treated	See plasma infusion/exchange	See plasma infusion/exchange

Table 29.4 Indications for plasma infusion/exchange in the different forms of thrombotic microangiopathy

Disease	Comment
Acquired	
Shigatoxin-associated	
Childhood forms	No (usually complete spontaneous recovery)
Adult forms	Probably yes (to minimize the risk of sequelae)
Neuraminidase-associated	Probably yes (combined with steroids)
vWF protease deficiency	Yes (life-saving, probably combined with steroids)
Pregnancy-associated	
TTP	Yes (life-saving)
HELLP syndrome	Probably yes (in selected cases and after delivery)
Postpartum HUS	Probably yes (but often ineffective)
Systemic disease-associated	Probably yes (combined with treatment of underlying disease)
Drug-associated	Probably yes (combined with drug withdrawal)
Transplant-associated	Probably yes (but often ineffective)
Genetic	
Factor H abnormalities	Yes (but often ineffective)
vWF protease deficiency	Yes (life-saving)
Others	Yes (but often ineffective)
Idiopathic	Probably yes

HELLP, hemolysis, elevated liver enzymes and low platelet count; HUS, hemolytic–uremic syndrome; TTP, thrombotic thrombocytopenic purpura; vWF, von Willebrand factor.

morbidity and mortality. Treatment should be continued until complete disease remission is achieved.

Platelet count and serum LDH are the most sensitive markers for monitoring the response to therapy. In conditions associated with decreased platelet production (cancer- or AIDS-associated TMA), serum LDH concentration is a more reliable indicator of disease activity than platelet count. In pregnancy-associated TMA, monitoring serum transaminases may be helpful.

Plasma manipulation

The infusion is intended to deliver the equivalent of one plasma volume (~ 30 mL/kg body weight) over the first 24 h and about 20 mL/kg daily thereafter. To avoid fluid overload, diuretics or ultrafiltration may be employed. The exchange procedure is usually intended to replace one to two plasma volumes every day.

Two procedures are available for plasma separation in the setting of plasma exchange: filtration and centrifugation. The total extracorporeal volume of the plasma circuit affects the choice of procedure. It is estimated that the total extracorporeal volume should not exceed 8–10% of total blood volume of the patient (taken as 100 mL/kg in infants < 10 kg, and 80 mL/kg in children > 10 kg). Thus, the filtration system, which has an extracorporeal volume of less than 100 mL, is preferred for small children and patients with cardiovascular instability. Plasma centrifugation is the standard procedure for all other cases.

Other specific treatments

In a large series of TTP patients,[15] 200 mg/day of oral prednisone (or 200 mg/day of intravenous prednisolone in patients with evidence of hepatic dysfunction) were given until complete normalization of the markers of hemolysis, when corticosteroids were rapidly tapered to 60 mg/day and then more slowly by 5 mg/week. In the HELLP syndrome, dexamethasone 10 mg i.v. was given every 12 h until delivery and for 36 h thereafter.

The recommended initial dose of vincristine is 1.4 mg/m^2 i.v. (not to exceed 2 mg), followed by 1 mg i.v. every 4 days until complete remission is achieved. On account of its severe neurotoxicity, the drug should be used with caution.

Antiplatelet agents have been given by a variety of schedules. Dipyridamole (400 mg/day) and aspirin (325 mg/day) are usually given for at least 2 weeks and up to disease remission.[14]

PGI$_2$ (epoprostenol), infused at the recommended doses of 10–20 ng/kg/min, may cause hypotension, headache, facial flushing, and diarrhea. Stable analogs have recently been developed but their effectiveness remains to be investigated in controlled trials.

The suggested doses of antithrombotic agents used in HUS are given in Table 29.3. Oral vitamin E 1000 mg/m^2/day is usually given until complete remission of the disease. Other antioxidants available for trial include allopurinol, deferoxamine, and superoxide dismutase.

Rescue treatments

When cryosupernatant fraction (i.e. plasma from which the cryoprecipitate containing the largest plasma vWF multimers, fibrinogen, and fibronectin has been removed) is used, during the infusion or exchange procedure patients should be given the same volumes as reported earlier for whole plasma (see Table 29.2).

Bilateral nephrectomy and splenectomy are irreversible procedures and should be considered only for patients at imminent risk of death or with disabling disease. In patients at increased risk of bleeding because of severe refractory thrombocytopenia, platelet transfusion may be indicated before surgery.

Future directions

Acquired forms

Research efforts are aimed at identifying more specific approaches that may interfere with the causes of endothelial injury (e.g. Stx) and the sequence of events triggered by endothelial damage. New agents targeted to prevent organ exposure to Stx are currently under evaluation.[35] The most promising are Synsorb-Pk, a resin composed of repeated synthetic carbohydrate determinants linked to colloidal silica that binds Stx; recombinant modified E. coli that displays a Stx receptor mimic on its surface that adsorbs and neutralizes Stx with very high efficiency; and "STARFISH", an oligovalent, water-soluble carbohydrate ligand that can simultaneously engage all five B subunits of two toxin molecules. These approaches offer potent new weapons against hemorrhagic diarrhea and HUS caused by Stx-producing E. coli. Oral administration of Synsorb-Pk or recombinant modified E. coli could efficiently clear toxin from the gut, whereas intravenous administration of "STARFISH" might help to prevent toxin already in the circulation from destroying kidney microvessels. Preliminary analyses of an ongoing trial in Canada found that early treatment (within 2 days after onset of diarrhea) with Synsorb-Pk decreased the risk of HUS from 17% to 7%. Toxin-neutralizing antibodies might be a future possible prevention for E. coli infection. In fact, natural infection with E. coli 0157 does not confer immunity and no human vaccine is currently available. Nevertheless, Stx vaccines have been shown effective in preventing related diseases in animals. Generalized pasteurization of ground beef through irradiation will further help to limit/prevent E. coli 0157 and other foodborne pathogen infection.

Agents to prevent shear-induced, vWF-mediated platelet aggregation in vitro may hold promise in the therapy of TMA, in which high shear stress forces in damaged microvessels may sustain vWF-mediated intravascular platelet thrombosis. These agents include aurin tricarboxylic acid, a potent inhibitor of large vWF multimer binding to the platelet surface glycoprotein Ib receptor, now under investigation as an arterial antithrombotic agent; recombinant fragments of the vWF monomer, which competitively block the binding of vWF multimers to glycoprotein Ib; and monoclonal antibodies to the Arg-Gly-Asp binding region for glycoprotein IIb/IIIa on monomeric subunits of vWF multimers.

An alternative approach is aimed at identifying the plasma component(s) that might induce remission of HUS and TTP (one of these might be the vWF protease found to be defective in some forms of TMA). A plasma fraction that substantially retains the beneficial activity of whole plasma would reduce the total amount of plasma proteins infused, limiting the risk of allergic reactions and fluid overload. The active plasma fraction in lyophilized form could be made available to centers that lack facilities for plasma exchange: it would allow prompt treatment of the disease at considerably lower cost and would limit the risk of viral infection. Novel techniques such as solvent–detergent virus inactivation, whereby viruses are inactivated by a lipid solvent and detergent that disrupt the lipid envelope, are being evaluated for their ability to limit viral contamination of plasma without lowering its effectiveness.

However, clinical trials to assess the effectiveness of the above treatments are difficult to design properly. In view of the good outcome of childhood HUS, trials invariably require several hundreds of patients to ensure they have the power to demonstrate an additional beneficial effect of the treatment under evaluation compared with supportive therapy alone. On the other hand, adult HUS and TTP patients are often so ill that treatments are usually attempted in combination, thus confounding data interpretation. This may explain why the majority of information on treatment of TMA comes from retrospective and often uncontrolled reports rather than from prospective randomized trials.

Genetic forms

New information derived from recent genetic studies will hopefully broaden the perspective of new specific treatments for patients with genetic forms of HUS and TTP. Specific replacement therapies with recombinant factor H and vWF cleaving protease could become a viable alternative to plasma treatment. This is reasonably feasible for patients with ADAMTS13 gene mutations, since even a small (5% of normal) vWF-cleaving protease activity may be sufficient to degrade large vWF multimers. Finally, when sequencing of the factor H and ADAMTS13 genes is completed, gene therapy will become a realistic option for patients with inherited HUS or TTP.

References

1. Ruggenenti P, Noris M, Remuzzi G: Thrombotic microangiopathy, hemolytic uremic syndrome, and thrombotic thrombocytopenic purpura. Kidney Int 2001;60:831–846.
2. Wong CS, Jelacic S, Habeeb RL, Watkins SL, Tarr PI: The risk of the hemolytic–uremic syndrome after antibiotic treatment of Escherichia coli 0157:H7 infections. N Engl J Med 2000;342:1930–1936.
3. Rizzoni G, Claris-Appiani A, Edefonti A: Plasma infusion for hemolytic uremic syndrome in children: results of a multicenter controlled trial. J Pediatr 1988;112:284–290.
4. Loirat C, Veyradier A, Foulard M, et al: von Willebrand factor (vWF)-cleaving protease activity in pediatric hemolytic uremic syndrome (HUS) (abstract). Pediatr Nephrol 2001;16:617A.
5. Dundas S, Murphy J, Soutar RL, Jones GA, Hutchinson SJ, Todd WTA: Effectiveness of therapeutic plasma exchange in the 1996 Lanarkshire Escherichia coli 0157:H7 outbreak. Lancet 1999;354:1327–1330.
6. Carter AO, Borczyk AA, Carlson JA, Harvey B, Hockin JC, Karmali MA: A severe outbreak of Escherichia coli 0157:H7-associated hemorrhagic colitis in a nursing home. N Engl J Med 1987;317:1496–1500.
7. Remuzzi G, Galbusera M, Salvadori M, Rizzoni G, Paris S, Ruggenenti P: Bilateral nephrectomy stopped disease progression in plasma-resistant hemolytic uremic syndrome with neurological signs and coma. Kidney Int 1996;49:282–286.
8. McGraw ME, Lendon M, Stevens RF, Postlethwaite RJ, Taylor CM: Hemolytic uremic syndrome and the Thomsen Friedenreich antigen. Pediatr Nephrol 1989;3:135–139.
9. Furlan M, Robles R, Lammle B: Partial purification and characterization of a protease from human plasma cleaving von Willebrand factor to fragments produced by in vivo proteolysis. Blood 1996;87:4223–4234.
10. Furlan M, Robles R, Galbusera M, et al: von Willebrand factor-cleaving protease in thrombotic thrombocytopenic purpura and the hemolytic–uremic syndrome. N Engl J Med 1998;339:1578–1584.
11. Tsai HM, Lia ECY: Antibodies to von Willebrand factor-cleaving protease in acute thrombotic thrombocytopenic purpura. N Engl J Med 1998;339:1585–1594.
12. Veyradier A, Obert B, Houllier A, Meyer D, Girma JP: Specific von Willebrand factor-cleaving protease in thrombotic microangiopathies: a study of 111 cases. Blood 2001;98:1765–1772.
13. Caletti MG, Gallo G, Gianantonio CA: Development of focal segmental sclerosis and hyalinosis in hemolytic uremic syndrome. Pediatr Nephrol 1996;10:687–692.
14. Bell WR, Braine HG, Ness PM, Kickler TS: Improved survival in thrombotic thrombocytopenic purpura–hemolytic uremic syndrome. Clinical experience in 108 patients. N Engl J Med 1991;325:398–403.
15. Rock GA, Shumak KH, Buskard NA, et al: Comparison of plasma exchange with plasma infusion in the treatment of thrombotic thrombocytopenic purpura. N Engl J Med 1991;325:393–397.
16. Byrnes JJ, Moake JL, Klug P, Periman P: Effectiveness of the cryosupernatant fraction of plasma in the treatment of refractory thrombotic thrombocytopenic purpura. Am J Hematol 1990;34:169–174.
17. Rock G, Shumak KH, Sutton DM, Buskard NA, Nair RC: Cryosupernatant as replacement fluid for plasma exchange in thrombotic thrombocytopenic purpura. Members of the Canadian Apheresis Group. Br J Haematol 1996;94:383–386.
18. Hayward CP, Sutton DM, Carter WH Jr, et al: Treatment outcomes in patients with adult thrombotic thrombocytopenic purpura–hemolytic uremic syndrome. Arch Intern Med 1994;154:982–987.
19. Furlan M, Robles R, Solenthaler M, Lammle B: Acquired deficiency of von Willebrand factor-cleaving protease in a patient with thrombotic thrombocytopenic purpura. Blood 1998;91:2839–2846.
20. Weiner CP: Thrombotic microangiopathy in pregnancy and the postpartum period. Semin Hematol 1987;24:119–129.
21. Ruggenenti P, Remuzzi G: The pathophysiology and management of thrombotic thrombocytopenic purpura. Eur J Haematol 1996;56:191–207.
22. Tsai H-M, Rice L, Sarode R, Chow TW, Moake JL: Antibody inhibitors to von Willebrand factor metalloproteinase and increased binding of von Willebrand factor to platelets in ticlopidine-associated thrombotic thrombocytopenic purpura. Ann Intern Med 2000;132:794–799.
23. Ruggenenti P: Post-transplant hemolytic-uremic syndrome. Kidney Int 2002;62:1093–1104.
24. Taylor CM: Complement factor H and the haemolytic uraemic syndrome. Lancet 2001;358:1200–1202.
25. Noris M, Ruggenenti P, Perna A, et al: Hypocomplementemia discloses genetic predisposition to hemolytic uremic syndrome and thrombotic thrombocytopenic purpura: role of factor H abnormalities. Italian Registry of Familial and Recurrent Hemolytic Uremic Syndrome/Thrombotic Thrombocytopenic Purpura. J Am Soc Nephrol 1999;10:281–293.
26. Warwicker P, Goodship THJ, Donne RL, et al: Genetic studies into

inherited and sporadic hemolytic uremic syndrome. Kidney Int 1998;53:836–844.

27. Caprioli J, Bettinaglio P, Zipfel PF, et al: The molecular basis of familial hemolytic uremic syndrome: mutation analysis of factor H gene reveals a hot spot in short consensus repeat 20. J Am Soc Nephrol 2001;12:297–307.

28. Remuzzi G, Ruggenenti P, Codazzi D, et al: Combined split liver and kidney transplant to cure familial and recurrent HUS. Lancet 2001;359:1671–1672.

29. Veyradier A, Obert B, Houllier A, Meyer D, Girma JP: Specific von Willebrand factor-cleaving protease in thrombotic microangiopathies: a study of 111 cases. Blood 2001;98:1765–1772.

30. Levy GG, Nichols WC, Lian EC: Mutations in a member of the ADAMTS gene family cause thrombotic thrombocytopenic purpura. Nature 2001;413:488–494.

31. Ruggenenti P, Galbusera M, Plata Cornejo R, Bellavita P, Remuzzi G: Thrombotic thrombocytopenic purpura: evidence that infusion rather than removal of plasma induces remission of the disease. Am J Kidney Dis 1993;21:314–318.

32. Fujikawa K, Suzuki H, McMullen B, Chung D: Purification of human von Willebrand factor-cleaving protease and its identification as a new member of the metalloproteinase family. Blood 2001;98:1662–1666.

33. Furlan M, Robles R, Morselli B, Sandoz P, Lammle B: Recovery and half-life of von Willebrand factor-cleaving protease after plasma therapy in patients with thrombotic thrombocytopenic purpura. Thromb Hemost 1999;81:8–13.

34. George JN: How I treat patients with thrombotic thrombocytopenic purpura–hemolytic uremic syndrome. Blood 2000;96:1223–1229.

35. Trachtman H, Christen E: Pathogenesis, treatment, and therapeutic trials in hemolytic uremic syndrome. Curr Opin Pediatr 1999;11:162–168.

36. Loirat C, Beaufils F, Sonsino E, et al: Treatment of childhood hemolytic-uremic syndrome with urokinase. Cooperative controlled trial. Arch Fr Pédiatr 1984;41:15–19.

37. Vandamme-Lombaerts R, Proesmans W, Van Damme B, et al: Heparin plus dipyridamole in chlildhood hemolytic uremic syndrome: a prospective, randomized study. J Pediatr 1988;113:913–918.

38. Loirat C, Sonsino E, Hinglais N, et al: Treatment of the childhood haemolytic uraemic syndrome with plasma: a multicenter randomized controlled trial. Pediatr Nephrol 1988;2:279–285.

39. Gianviti A, Perna A, Caringella A, et al. Plasma exchange in children with hemolytic–uremic syndrome at risk of poor outcome. Am J Kidney Dis 1993;22:264–266.

40. Italian Cooperative Group for the Study of Thrombotic Thrombocytopenic Purpura. Thrombotic thrombocytopenic purpura (TTP) treatment: Italian cooperative retrospective study on 29 cases. Haematologica 1986;71:39–43.

41. French Cooperative Study Group for Adult HUS. Adult hemolytic uremic syndrome with renal microangiopathy. Outcome according to therapeutic protocol in 53 cases. Ann Med Interne 1992;143:27–32.

42. Henon Ph pour le Group Francais d'Etude Multicentrique sur le PTT (GFEM). Traitement du purpura thrombotique thrombopénique. Résultats d'une étude clinique multicentrique randomisée. Press Méd 1991;20:1761–1767.

Treatment of Acute Interstitial Nephritis

Maxwell E. Fisher and Eric G. Neilson

Background

Allergic interstitial nephritis, also known as acute interstitial nephritis (AIN), is characterized by acute renal failure resulting from immune-mediated tubulointerstitial injury. The reported incidence of this disorder varies from 1–3% of all cases of acute renal failure to 8–15% of patients who underwent a renal biopsy for the diagnosis of acute renal failure. All advanced cases of chronic renal failure show evidence of secondary tubulointerstitial disease, and almost 25% of patients with endstage renal disease may have suffered from primary tubulointerstitial injury.[1]

AIN is characterized by infiltration of the interstitium by mononuclear cells, with relatively normal glomeruli and vascular structures initially. There is usually evidence of tubular injury as manifested by disruption of the tubular basement membrane and interstitial edema, with distortion of the normal architecture. Eosinophils and neutrophils may also be seen in the cellular infiltrate and predominate in certain varieties of interstitial nephritis.[1] Eventually, there is conversion of epithelial units to fibroblasts for fibrogenesis.[2,3]

While some forms of interstitial nephritis may be idiopathic in origin, all forms are likely to have an immunologic basis. Most cases are due to a known etiologic factor. The causes of AIN may be divided into one of three major categories: drug induced, infectious, and systemic immune disorders. Comprehensive reviews of the various causes of AIN are available.[1] A large number of drugs have been implicated in the causation of interstitial nephritis but some, such as β-lactam antibiotics, nonsteroidal anti-inflammatory drugs (NSAIDs), sulfonamides, anticonvulsants, allopurinol, rifampin, cimetidine, and thiazides, are incriminated more frequently.[4,5] AIN may occur in various infectious diseases, particularly in children, but is characteristically seen in viral infections, leptospirosis, legionella, and diphtheria.[1] Finally, interstitial nephritis may occur in association with uveitis in the tubulo-interstitial nephritis–uveitis (TINU) syndrome or may be a manifestation of a systemic autoimmune disorder such as systemic lupus erythematosus, Sjögren syndrome, or sarcoidosis.[1]

AIN results in a sudden decrement in renal function in association with other clinical features that may vary depending on etiology. Infectious and systemic autoimmune disorders may provide specific clues that point toward their existence. In the most common clinical scenario, that of drug-induced allergic interstitial nephritis, a patient who has defervesced in response to antibiotic therapy for an infectious illness develops a recrudescence of fever associated with a decline in renal function and a skin rash. It is important to note, however, that the classic triad of fever, skin rash, and eosinophilia is found in few patients with interstitial nephritis.[6,7] Individual components of the triad may occur more frequently. Urinalysis typically reveals leukocyturia with eosinophiluria, microscopic hematuria, and nonnephrotic-range proteinuria. Eosinophiluria (defined as > 1% of urinary white blood cells being eosinophils) is best detected using Hansel stain but is neither sensitive nor specific enough to diagnose interstitial nephritis with certainty.[8] Interstitial nephritis caused by NSAIDs is often characterized by the absence of features of hypersensitivity and by the occurrence of nephrotic-range proteinuria.[9] The diagnosis of AIN is typically made on the basis of clinical suspicion and the absence of features to support alternative causes, such as acute tubular necrosis or obstruction resulting in acute renal failure.

A renal biopsy is extremely valuable when establishing the diagnosis of AIN. In a patient who can tolerate the procedure and possible immunosuppressive therapy without excessive risk, we strongly recommend that a renal biopsy be obtained.[10] Pathologic examination of the renal tissue helps not only to establish the diagnosis with certainty but may also provide important prognostic information that may have an impact on the choice of therapy.

AIN is characterized by a mononuclear interstitial infiltrate consisting of lymphocytes, plasma cells, and occasionally eosinophils. Neutrophils may predominate in AIN of infectious origin. Tubulitis, characterized by disruption of the tubular basement membrane and lymphocytic invasion of the tubules, may be seen. Interstitial edema and hemorrhage may be present.[11,12] Fibrosis may be seen as early as 10 days after the onset of illness, and when extensive portends a poor prognosis. Granuloma formation is seen in more severe cases of drug-induced AIN[13] and may also occur in sarcoidosis and TINU syndrome.[14] Diffuse infiltrates, granulomas, and extensive fibrosis suggest severe disease with poorer outcomes.[10,15] Immunofluorescence studies typically reveal no immune deposits, but linear staining due to antitubular basement membrane antibody deposition as well as deposition of immune complexes with complement are seen in a few cases.[12]

Overall, drug-induced AIN is more frequently related to permanent renal injury than disease secondary to infection or idiopathic etiologies. Of all medications causing AIN, NSAIDs seem to correlate with the highest risk of permanent renal insufficiency.[15] Furthermore, a recent evaluation of all renal biopsies done at one large institution demonstrated AIN is becoming more frequent as a cause of acute renal failure, implicated as etiology in 18.6% of cases of acute renal failure in patients older than 60 years.[16]

Although AIN is often considered a benign disease, in aging populations a significant number of patients will develop acute renal failure requiring dialysis. Renal dysfunction is occasionally reversible in the long term, but a meaningful proportion of patients may be left with residual renal damage. A poorer outcome with development of endstage renal disease may occur with continued exposure to an offending agent.[17] Therefore, it is extremely important that the diagnosis of AIN be established early and confirmed if necessary by biopsy, so that appropriate therapeutic measures can be instituted.

Clinical approach

The literature pertaining to AIN is characterized by elegant experimental data from animal models that provide key insights into the pathogenic mechanisms of the disease and a solid framework on which a rational approach to therapy can be based. Clinical data regarding appropriate therapeutic interventions are unfortunately limited to anecdotal experience, case reports, and retrospective, uncontrolled, nonrandomized descriptions often involving small numbers of patients. This is not surprising given that primary AIN results from numerous causes, is relatively uncommon, and represents a highly heterogeneous group of patients.

A detailed discussion of the pathogenic mechanisms is beyond the scope of this chapter, and the reader is referred to some excellent reviews elsewhere.[1,11,18] Most forms of interstitial nephritis are the result of immune-mediated injury, with cellular mechanisms playing a key role in the initiation and perpetuation of inflammation. This assessment is well supported by studies in several experimental animal models. Rodents genetically predisposed to the development of interstitial nephritis show a spontaneous loss of tolerance to tubular antigens and a resultant immune response.[19,20] Drugs and infectious agents may induce an immune response by serving as a hapten bridge to the tubulointerstitium that renders it immunogenic, or they may cause tubulointerstitial damage thus creating nephritogenic neoantigens.[21,22] In addition the tubulointerstitium may be damaged as an innocent bystander, through cross-reactivity of an immune response against an infectious agent[23,24] or from a local cytokine bath provided by metabolic or hemodymanic alterations.[25] Once antigen recognition has occurred, several endogenous regulatory networks are brought into play. T cells appear to be central to this response and are responsible for the release of various cytokines and chemokines that mediate amplification of injury and recruitment of other cell types including B cells.[1] Furthermore, these inflammatory cells, including macrophages, lymphocytes, and activated tubular cells, produce many cytokines that serve to modulate a fibrogenic response. The most important inflammatory molecules in vivo include transforming growth factor β (TGFβ), epidermal growth factor, fibroblast growth factor 2, endothelin 1, and platelet-derived growth factor ββ, which stimulate the destruction of basement membrane, induce epithelial–mesenchymal transition (EMT) forming new fibroblasts, and generate the abundant extracellular matrix associated with renal interstitial fibrosis.[3] Of these cytokines, TGF-β is probably the most important yet identified.[26] It acts to induce EMT, chemotaxis, and extracellular matrix in fibroblasts as well as inhibition of the production and action of metalloproteinases.[4] It is not surprising therefore that therapy in the clinic has attempted to modulate the nephritogenic immune response.

The use of immunosuppressive drugs in the treatment of AIN remains controversial because there are no randomized, controlled, prospective trials that address this issue. However, there are numerous clinical reports and several small, nonrandomized, and retrospective series demonstrating the occasional benefit of corticosteroids in the treatment of interstitial nephritis casued by immune disorders, like sarcoidosis, TINU, or drugs (Table 30.1). Given the seemingly heterogeneous nature of this group of patients, the relative scarcity of clinical cases, and the fact that there may be ethical dilemmas involved in withholding therapy from a patient who does not improve with observation, it seems unlikely that any such trials will be forthcoming. In fact, the first retrospective study that comes closest to a reasonable trial was published almost

Table 30.1 Clinical treatments for acute interstitial nephritis

Reference	Year	Type of trial	No. of patients	Results/conclusion
Chazan et al[27]	1972	Retrospective	5	3 patients treated with prednisone, 2 were not. Lower baseline creatinine and decreased time in reaching baseline creatinine in treated group
Galpin et al[28]	1978	Retrospective	14	Serum creatinine normalized in 6/8 patients in treated group (oral prednisone) vs. 2/6 in control group. All patients had methicillin-induced AIN

Continued

Table 30.1 Clinical treatments for acute interstitial nephritis (*cont'd*)

Reference	Year	Type of trial	No. of patients	Results/conclusion
Linton et al[29]	1980	Retrospective	9	Prednisone 60 mg/day for 6–12 days was given to all patients not showing recovery (7/9). Renal function returned to baseline in all patients within 10 days
Laberke[17]	1980	Retrospective	27	7 patients treated with prednisone, 20 without. Lower baseline serum creatinine in steroid-treated patients
Pusey et al[30]	1983	Retrospective	7	High dose i.v. steroids given in seven episodes to 5 patients; 2 patients received no steroids. Rapid normalization of renal function in all patients treated with i.v. steroids 500–1000 mg/day for 1–2 days
Handa[31]	1986	Retrospective	10	4 patients treated with prednisone, 6 without. More rapid improvement in renal function in patients receiving steroids
Buysen et al[32]	1990	Retrospective	27	10 patients showing worsening renal function despite withdrawal of offending medication were given steroids. All 10 patients demonstrated a positive response, with 6/10 returning to baseline renal function
Joh et al[33]	1990	Retrospective	10	7 patients treated with steroids (some received i.v., some p.o.). Failure of 2 patients in steroid-treated group to recover renal function leading to chronic dialysis
Porile et al[34]	1990	Retrospective	43	43 cases were reviewed from the literature. All patients had AIN secondary to NSAIDs. 24 patients received steroids, 19 did not. No alteration in clinical course could be attributed to steroids
Shibasaki et al[35]	1991	Retrospective	14	6 patients treated with pulse steroids. Unable to conclude whether steroid pulse therapy has beneficial effect
Koselj et al[36]	1993	Retrospective	23	All patients received i.v. pulse steroids or oral prednisone. No strong association could be observed between corticosteroids and outcome
Bhaumik et al[37]	1996	Retrospective	19	6 patients received prednisone, 13 did not. No effect of steroids on extent of renal recovery or time required could be demonstrated
Vanherweghem et al[38]	1996	Retrospective	35	12 patients received steroids, 23 did not. 2/12 patients in steroid group progressed to hemodialysis in 1 year compared with 16/23 patients in control group on hemodialysis by end of 1 year. All patients had interstitial fibrosis secondary to herb-associated nephropathy
O'Riordan et al[39]	2001	Retrospective	5	All patients had sarcoid granulomatous interstitial nephritis. All patients received oral prednisolone. 4/5 patients showed marked improvement in creatinine clearance within 10 days of therapy
Gion et al[40]	2000	Retrospective	6	All patients had tubulointerstitial nephritis and uveitis (TINU) syndrome. All patients received oral steroids with normalization of renal function. All 6 patients developed recurrence of uveitis, which failed to respond to topical or oral steroids. 5/6 patients achieved control of their ocular inflammation with methotrexate, azathioprine, or cyclosporine A.

AIN, acute interstitial nephritis; NSAIDs, nonsteroidal antiinflammatory drugs.

25 years ago. Several authors have expressed the need for better data on this subject for many years, but none are anticipated.

In treating a patient with AIN, it is obviously important to establish the diagnosis and then remove the suspected offending agent when possible. Continued exposure to a drug responsible for inducing AIN has been shown to result in significant irreversible damage, including the need for long-term dialysis. Although withdrawal of the offending agent often leads to improvement, it is not clear whether this improvement assures complete recovery. The duration of renal injury does have an impact on the eventual outcome: patients treated within the first 2 weeks of AIN returned to a serum creatinine level around 1 mg/dL, whereas those who were treated after 3 weeks had a final serum creatinine level around 3 mg/dL.[17] Given the knowledge that interstitial fibrosis represents irreversible injury and can occur as early as 7–14 days after the onset of AIN, it is understandable that therapeutic interventions must be instituted early.[10] This will potentially minimize irreversible injury and limit chronic renal dysfunction. To this end, the observation that corticosteroids may hasten recovery encourages their use.

Corticosteroids have been used as immunosuppressive agents for several decades. We now know that corticosteroids can effectively abrogate an ongoing immune response through their multiple actions, including stabilization of lysosomal membranes, reduction of nuclear factor (NF)-κB, and decreased transcription of several cytokines including interleukin 1 (IL-1), IL-2, IL-6, γ-interferon, and tumor necrosis factor-α.[41] There is, therefore, a rational scientific basis for using these drugs to treat AIN.

Perhaps the most quoted study, which demonstrated a beneficial effect of corticosteroids in AIN, involved 14 patients with methicillin-induced AIN.[28] In this retrospective analysis, in addition to withdrawal of methicillin, eight patients had received prednisone in an average dose of 60 mg/day for a mean duration of 9.6 days. Compared with the six patients who did not receive prednisone, the treated group showed a faster improvement in renal function. They reached their new baseline creatinine level in 9.3 days as opposed to 54 days in the untreated group. Even more important was the fact that six of eight treated patients returned to their previous normal creatinine level as opposed to only two of six in the untreated group.

There are numerous other reports in which recovery from AIN seemed to have been brought about by therapy with corticosteroids. To highlight a few, Linton et al[29] reported their experience with nine cases of drug-induced AIN. Seven patients failed to recover after the culprit drug was withdrawn, although these patients showed prompt diuresis and a return to baseline renal function within 10 days of receiving 60 mg/day of prednisone for 6–12 days. In another report of nine cases occurring over a period of 8 years, Pusey et al[30] describe remarkable diuresis and improvement in renal function within 12–72 h of receiving high-dose intravenous methylprednisolone in a regimen similar to that used for treatment of acute rejection in renal allografts (500–1000 mg/day); no major adverse effects were described. In a dramatic case report of a patient who developed acute renal failure due to AIN and was on hemodialysis for over 3 months, treatment with high-dose methylprednisolone led to a surprising improvement in renal function and discontinuation of dialysis.[42] Similar cases of improvement in renal function with corticosteroids in AIN due to carbamazepine, cimetidine, allopurinol, captopril, and co-trimoxazole have been reported (see Table 30.1).

Granulomatous inflammation may be seen in severe cases of drug-induced AIN and may carry a worse prognosis.[13] Granulomas are also seen with sarcoidosis, idiopathic AIN, and in AIN caused by infections like tuberculosis. Corticosteroids have been beneficial in the treatment of AIN due to sarcoid, TINU syndrome, and idiopathic AIN. In some cases of sarcoid, however, AIN may be steroid-dependent, and a relapsing course has been described.[10]

The literature is also replete with reports contesting the use of corticosteroids in AIN and demonstrating no benefit of therapy. This may be especially true of AIN due to NSAIDs.[34] Cases of rifampin-related AIN have been known to occur in patients on corticosteroids.[43] This may possibly be related to decreased effectiveness of steroids due to enhanced metabolism with concomitant rifampin use. It must be noted that the criticism applied to the reports professing benefit of corticosteroids in the therapy of AIN, namely the lack of prospective controlled data, is also applicable to the literature propounding their ineffectiveness. The decision to use corticosteroids must, therefore, be guided by clinical circumstances.

Corticosteroid therapy may be associated with adverse effects, including worsening hypertension, hyperglycemia, psychiatric disturbances, weight gain, and increased risk of infection. In the risk–benefit analysis of corticosteroid use, however, one has to weigh the problems associated with prolonged renal failure and the morbidity associated with dialysis when this is necessary.[10]

In a small pilot study from Europe, corticosteroids were reported as being effective in slowing the progression of renal failure in women with chronic interstitial nephritis with fibrosis, secondary to herbal-associated nephropathy.[44,45] This is an intriguing report that supports the need to further evaluate this strategy in patients with chronic interstitial nephritis.

As a second step, there is convincing experimental evidence that cyclophosphamide is effective in ameliorating renal dysfunction in animal models of interstitial nephritis.[46,47] It has been long suggested that cyclophosphamide be initiated in patients with AIN who do not respond to corticosteroid therapy,[10] as the risk of infertility and neoplasia is marginal with short-term use and may be worth taking given the morbidity and mortality associated with endstage renal disease and uremia. There is only anecdotal experience in the literature describing the use of cyclophosphamide in AIN and mainly with the variety associated with sarcoidosis.[10] We were unable to find any strong data describing the use of this drug in human interstitial nephritis. Nevertheless, based on experimental data, we believe cyclophosphamide may be considered in the appropriate setting and after involvement of the patient in the decision.

Finally, cyclosporine is also a potent immunosuppressive agent that is used extensively in the transplant population and also in other autoimmune disorders. There are experimental data that cyclosporine is effective in reversing AIN in animal models.[48-51] Limited clinical data on the use of cyclosporine (and perhaps methotrexate and azathioprine) for the treatment of TINU-associated interstitial nephritis suggest it may be efficacious.[40] However, high blood levels of cyclosporine and tacrolimus for prolonged periods may worsen the fibrogenesis one is trying to suppress.[52]

In AIN due to infectious agents, therapy for the infection is usually sufficient to treat the renal disease. It is unclear whether corticosteroids should be used in this situation.

Specific recommendations

1. It is key to establish the diagnosis of AIN early and with certainty. There are no diagnostic clinical features or laboratory tests with adequate sensitivity or specificity to effectively rule out the diagnosis of AIN. The bedside clinician must maintain a high index of suspicion in the appropriate clinical setting and in the absence of convincing evidence that supports an alternative diagnosis. An effort must be made to rule out other potential causes of renal dysfunction such as obstruction or acute tubular necrosis.

2. In the algorithm outlined in Fig. 30.1, we suggest that potential offending agents that may be responsible for causing AIN be discontinued as soon as the diagnosis is suspected. It is important to identify drugs that commonly cause this problem and to discontinue those in patients on multiple medications.

3. We strongly favor the use of an early renal biopsy to establish the diagnosis of AIN. Provided the patient's general medical condition does not preclude performance of the procedure safely or the use of immunosuppressive therapy based on the diagnosis, a renal biopsy is likely to provide useful diagnostic and prognostic information. The presence of diffuse infiltrates or granulomatous inflammation may encourage the use of immunosuppressive agents, whereas the presence of significant fibrosis may favor withholding potentially toxic therapy for marginal potential benefit.

4. In patients who do not demonstrate improvement within several days of stopping potential offending drugs, we recommend a course of corticosteroids. Prednisone 1 mg/kg/day orally (or equivalent dose intravenously) should be initiated. In patients who have improved renal function within 7–10 days, the drug should be continued for 4–6 weeks and then tapered over the next several weeks. It is important to monitor patients for volume overload, hyperglycemia, gastric irritation, hypertension, hypercatabolism, and infections. In patients who do not show improvement within 2–3 weeks,

therapy can either be discontinued or additional cytotoxic therapy can be considered.

5. In patients with severe AIN that does not respond to corticosteroid therapy of 2–3 weeks' duration, cyclophosphamide 2 mg/kg/day may be considered. Some physicians start both drugs orally at the same time and stop cyclophosphamide therapy if there is dramatic improvement in the first few days of treatment, recognizing that the full effect of cyclophosphamide is not realized for several weeks. Although there are few clinical data to support this use, given the poor outcome of patients likely to develop endstage renal disease, it may be worth trying this therapy after obtaining informed consent from the patient. We believe that a trial of cyclophosphamide for 5–6 weeks is warranted and is unlikely to significantly increase the risk of neoplasia. There is a small risk of infertility; however, given the effects of uremia on fertility and overall quality of life, the patient may wish to accept this trial. If no response is seen within 5–6 weeks, the therapy may be discontinued. In patients who do respond, the drug may be continued for 1 year. Corticosteroids may be tapered to very low doses or discontinued in patients on cyclophosphamide. It is important to closely monitor the patient for leukopenia, infections, and microscopic hematuria. We recommend that the white blood cell count be maintained about 3500/mm^3.

6. Plasmapheresis has been suggested as an adjunctive therapy in patients who do not respond to corticosteroids alone and are started on cyclophosphamide.[7] There are few clinical data to help assess the efficacy of this intervention. The suggestion is based on the success of plasmapheresis in the treatment of patients with antiglomerular basement membrane disease, and it is speculated that plasmapheresis may be beneficial in patients with evidence of antitubular basement membrane antibodies.

7. Supportive therapy for patients with acute renal failure includes management of azotemia and electrolyte and acid–base disorders, with dialysis as necessary. Volume overload and hypertension may also require therapy. Dietary modifications like moderate protein restriction or the use of angiotensin-converting enzyme inhibitors to retard progressive renal insufficiency may be indicated in patients who are left with residual renal dysfunction.

Future directions

There has been an explosion of new information in the field of immunology during the past several years. We have developed key insights into T cell-mediated immune responses in the areas of T-cell activation and effector mechanisms.[12] Several new immunosuppressive agents, including tacrolimus, rapamycin, and mycophenolate mofetil, have been approved for use in transplantation. Since the pathology of subacute transplant rejection is reminiscent of some aspects of interstitial nephritis, we

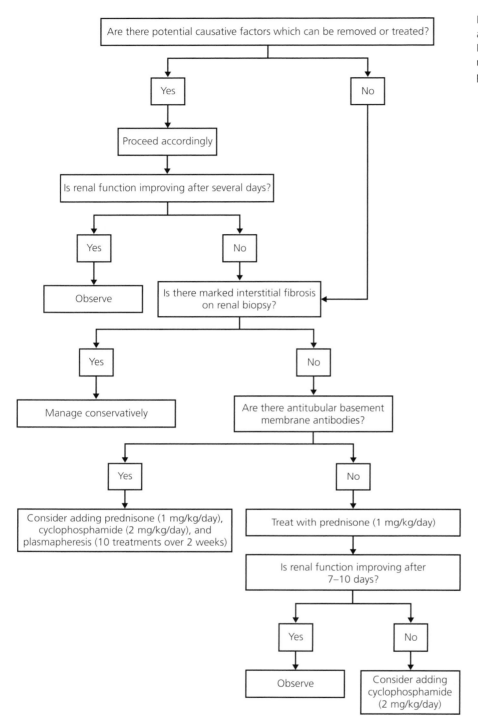

Figure 30.1 Algorithm for the treatment of acute interstitial nephritis. (From Neilson EG: Pathogenesis and therapy of interstitial nephritis. Kidney Int 1989;35:1257–1270, with permission.)

Are there potential causative factors which can be removed or treated?

Yes → Proceed accordingly → Is renal function improving after several days?

No

Yes → Observe

No → Is there marked interstitial fibrosis on renal biopsy?

Yes → Manage conservatively

No → Are there antitubular basement membrane antibodies?

Yes → Consider adding prednisone (1 mg/kg/day), cyclophosphamide (2 mg/kg/day), and plasmapheresis (10 treatments over 2 weeks)

No → Treat with prednisone (1 mg/kg/day) → Is renal function improving after 7–10 days?

Yes → Observe

No → Consider adding cyclophosphamide (2 mg/kg/day)

may eventually see the application of some of these new drugs to the therapy of primary interstitial nephritis.

It is hoped that any new approaches to the therapy of interstitial nephritis are tested in a randomized, controlled, prospective trial. This is understandably a tall order given the relative heterogeneity and scarcity of clinical material at any one center and the significant expense involved in the organization of a multicenter trial. It is not possible to be optimistic that such data will become available, given the fact that so many years have passed without the

appearance of a single reliable trial addressing corticosteroid use in AIN, despite convincing experimental and anecdotal clinical responses. In the meanwhile we may be forced to make do with acquiring further experimental data and applying lessons learned from other areas to the therapy of interstitial nephritis in the most pragmatic and practical manner in order to benefit our patients.

The forefront of research in immunology is rapidly advancing to involve the induction of regulatory T-cell responses, the creation of specific inhibitors of corecognition, and the tailoring of immunosuppressive therapy to target specific T-cell clones so as to reduce the need for global immunosuppression. New methods to attenuate fibrosis, such as pirfenidone[53] and ST1571,[54] may also be on the horizon. These approaches are far from clinical application but hold considerable promise for the future.

Acknowledgments

This work was supported in part by grants DK-46282 from the National Institutes of Health.

References

1. Kelly CJ, Neilson EG: Tubulointerstitial diseases in the kidney. *In* Brenner BM (ed): The Kidney. Philadelphia: WB Saunders, 2000, pp 1509–1536.
2. Strutz F, Okada H, Lo CW, et al: Identification and characterization of a fibroblast marker: FSP1. J Cell Biol 1995;130:393–405.
3. Okada H, Inoue T, Suzuki H, Strutz F, Neilson EG: Epithelial–mesenchymal transformation of renal tubular epithelial cells in vitro and in vivo. Nephrol Dial Transplant 2000;15(Suppl 6):44–46.
4. Rossert J: Drug-induced acute interstitial nephritis. Kidney Int 2001;60:804–817.
5. Murray KM, Keane WR: Review of drug-induced acute interstitial nephritis. Pharmacotherapy 1992;12:462–467.
6. Ditlove J, Werdmann P, Bernstein M, Massry SG: Methicillin nephritis. Medicine 1977;56:483–505.
7. Appel GB, Kunis CL: Acute tubulointerstitial nephritis. *In* Cotran RS, Brenner BM, Stein JH (eds): Contemporary Issues in Nephrology, Vol 10. New York: Churchill Livingstone, 1983, pp 151–185.
8. Corwin HL, Bray RA, Haber MH: The detection and interpretation of urinary eosinophils. Arch Pathol Lab Med 1989;113:1256–1258.
9. Bennett WM, Henrich WL, Stoff JS: The renal effects of nonsteroidal anti-inflammatory drugs: summary and recommendations. Am J Kidney Dis 1996;28:S56–S62.
10. Neilson EG: Pathogenesis and therapy of interstitial nephritis. Kidney Int 1989;35:1257–1270.
11. Kelly CJ: Cellular immunity and the tubulointerstitium. Semin Nephrol 1999;19:182–187.
12. Kelly CJ, Tomaszewski J, Neilson EG: Immunopathogenic mechanisms of tubulointerstitial injury. *In* Tisher CC, Brenner BM (eds): Renal Pathology. Philadelphia: WB Saunders, 1994, pp 699–723.
13. Viero RM, Cavallo T: Granulomatous interstitial nephritis. Human Pathology 1995;26:1347–1353.
14. Sessa A, Meroni M, Battini G, Vigano G, Brambilla PL, Paties CT: Acute renal failure due to idiopathic tubulo-intestinal nephritis and uveitis: "TINU syndrome". Case report and review of the literature. J Nephrol 2000;13:377–380.
15. Schwarz A, Krause PH, Kunzendorf U, Keller F, Distler A: The outcome of acute interstitial nephritis: risk factors for the transition from acute to chronic interstitial nephritis. Clin Nephrol 2000;54:179–190.
16. Haas M, Spargo BH, Wit EJ, Meehan SM: Etiologies and outcome of acute renal insufficiency in older adults: a renal biopsy study of 259 cases. Am J Kidney Dis 2000;35:433–447.
17. Laberke HG: Treatment of acute interstitial nephritis. Klin Wochenschr 1980;58:531–532.
18. Kelly CJ, Gold DP: Nitric oxide in interstitial nephritis and other autoimmune diseases. Semin Nephrol 1999;19:288–295.
19. Neilson EG, McCafferty E, Feldman A, Clayman MD, Zakheim B, Korngold R: Spontaneous interstitial nephritis in kdkd mice. I. An experimental model of autoimmune renal disease. J Immunol 1984;133:2560–2565.
20. Kelly CJ, Korngold R, Mann R, Clayman M, Haverty T, Neilson EG: Spontaneous interstitial nephritis in kdkd mice. II. Characterization of a tubular antigen-specific, H-2K-restricted Lyt-2+ effector T cell that mediates destructive tubulointerstitial injury. J Immunol 1986;136:526–531.
21. Joh K, Shibasaki T, Azuma T, et al: Experimental drug-induced allergic nephritis mediated by antihapten antibody. Int Arch Allergy Appl Immunol 1989;88:337–344.
22. Border WA, Lehman DH, Egan JD, Sass HJ, Glode JE, Wilson CB: Antitubular basement-membrane antibodies in methicillin-associated interstitial nephritis. N Engl J Med 1974;291:381–384.
23. Fasth A, Ahlstedt S, Hanson LA, Jann B, Jann K, Kauser B: Cross-reactions between the Tamm-Horsfall glycoprotein and *Escherichia coli*. Int Arch Allergy Appl Immunol 1980;63:303–311.
24. Neilson EG: Interstitial nephritis: another kissing disease? J Clin Invest 1999;104:1671–1672.
25. Remuzzi G, Bertani T: Pathophysiology of progressive nephropathies. N Engl J Med 1998;339:1448–1456.
26. Frishberg Y, Kelly CJ: TGF-beta and regulation of interstitial nephritis. Miner Electrolyte Metab 1998;24:181–189.
27. Chazan JA, Garella S, Esparza A: Acute interstitial nephritis. A distinct clinico-pathological entity? Nephron 1972;9:10–26.
28. Galpin JE, Shinaberger JH, Stanley TM: Acute interstitial nephritis due to methicillin. Am J Med 1978;65:756–765.
29. Linton AL, Clark WF, Driedger AA, Turnbull DI, Lindsay RM: Acute interstitial nephritis due to drugs: review of the literature with a report of nine cases. Ann Intern Med 1980;93:735–741.
30. Pusey CD, Saltissi D, Bloodworth L, Rainford DJ, Christie JL: Drug associated acute interstitial nephritis: clinical and pathological features and the response to high dose steroid therapy. Q J Med 1983;52:194–211.
31. Handa SP: Drug-induced acute interstitial nephritis: report of 10 cases. Can Med Assoc J 1986;135:1278–1281.
32. Buysen JG, Houthoff HJ, Krediet RT, Arisz L: Acute interstitial nephritis: a clinical and morphological study in 27 patients. Nephrol Dial Transplant 1990;5:94–99.
33. Joh K, Aizawa S, Yamaguchi Y: Drug-induced hypersensitivity nephritis: lymphocyte stimulation testing and renal biopsy in 10 cases. Am J Nephrol 1990;10:222–230.
34. Porile JL, Bakris GL, Garella S: Acute interstitial nephritis with glomerulopathy due to nonsteroidal anti-inflammatory agents: a review of its clinical spectrum and effects of steroid therapy. J Clin Pharmacol 1990;30:468–475.
35. Shibasaki T, Ishimoto F, Sakai O, Joh K, Aizawa S: Clinical characterization of drug-induced allergic nephritis. Am J Nephrol 1991;11:174–180.
36. Koselj M, Kveder R, Bren AF, Rott T: Acute renal failure in patients with drug-induced acute interstitial nephritis. Ren Fail 1993;15:69–72.
37. Bhaumik SK, Kher V, Arora P, et al: Evaluation of clinical and histological prognostic markers in drug-induced acute interstitial nephritis. Ren Fail 1996;18:97–104.
38. Vanherweghem JL, Abramowicz D, Tielemans C, Depierreux M: Effects of steroids on the progression of renal failure in chronic interstitial renal fibrosis: a pilot study in Chinese herbs nephropathy. Am J Kidney Dis 1996;27:209–215.
39. O'Riordan E, Willert RP, Reeve R, et al: Isolated sarcoid granulomatous interstitial nephritis: review of five cases at one center. Clin Nephrol 2001;55:297–302.
40. Gion N, Stavrou P, Foster CS: Immunomodulatory therapy for chronic tubulointerstitial nephritis-associated uveitis. Am J Ophthalmol 2000;129:764–768.
41. Boumpas DT, Chrousos GP, Wilder RL, Cupps TR, Balow JE: Glucocorticoid therapy for immune-mediated diseases: basic and clinical correlates. Ann Intern Med 1993;119:1198–1208.
42. Frommer P, Uldall R, Fay WP, Deveber GA: A case of acute interstitial nephritis successfully treated after delayed diagnosis. Can Med Assoc J 1979;121:585–586.
43. Qunibi WY, Godwin J, Eknoyan G: Toxic nephropathy during continuous rifampin therapy. South Med J 1980;73:791–792.
44. Yoshimura E, Fujii M, Koide S, et al: A case of Chinese herbs nephropathy in which the progression of renal dysfunction was slowed by steroid therapy. Nippon Jinzo Gakkai Shi 2000;42:66–72.
45. Vanherweghem JL, Abramowicz D, Tielemans C, Depierreux M: Rapidly progressive interstitial renal fibrosis in young women: association with slimming regimen including Chinese herbs. Lancet 1993;341:387–391.
46. Chen XM, Cheng QL: Treatment of rapid progressive glomerulonephritis (RPGN) with pulse methylprednisolone (MP) and urokinase (UK): a renal rebiopsy study. Zhonghua Nei Ke Za Zhi 1993;32:607–609.
47. Agus D, Mann R, Clayman M: The effects of daily cyclophosphamide

administration on the development and extent of primary experimental interstitial nephritis in rats. Kidney Int 1986;29:635–640.

48. Berden JH, Faaber P, Assmann KJ, Rijke TP: Effects of cyclosporin A on autoimmune disease in MRL/1 and BXSB mice. Scand J Immunol 1986;24:405–411.

49. Gimenez A, Leyva-Cobian F, Fierro C, Rio M, Bricio T, Mampaso F: Effect of cyclosporin A on autoimmune tubulointerstitial nephritis in the brown Norway rat. Clin Exp Immunol 1987;69:550–556.

50. Thoenes GH, Umscheid T, Sitter T, Langer KH: Cyclosporin A inhibits autoimmune experimental tubulointerstitial nephritis. Immunol Lett 1987;15:301–306.

51. Shih W, Hines WH, Neilson EG: Effects of cyclosporin A on the development of immune-mediated interstitial nephritis. Kidney Int 1988;33:1113–1118.

52. Morales JM, Andres A, Rengel M, Rodicio JL: Influence of cyclosporin, tacrolimus and rapamycin on renal function and arterial hypertension after renal transplantation. Nephrol Dial Transplant 2001;16(Suppl 1):121–124.

53. Shimizu T, Kuroda T, Hata S, Fukagawa M, Margolin SB, Kurokawa K: Pirfenidone improves renal function and fibrosis in the post-obstructed kidney. Kidney Int 1998;54:99–109.

54. Hasselbalch HC: A possible role for STI571 in the treatment of idiopathic myelofibrosis. Am J Hematol 2001;68:63–64.

New Horizons in the Treatment of Glomerulonephritis

Gunter Wolf

Development of innovative therapies requires a detailed pathophysiologic understanding of glomerulonephritis
Etiology of glomerular inflammation
Mediators of glomerular inflammation
Response phase of intrinsic glomerular cells
Resolution of glomerular injury
Conclusions

The currently applied immunodulatory therapeutic strategies for glomerulonephritis and vasculitis are unsatisfactory for several reasons. Although newer substances such as mycophenolate mofetil may exhibit a higher specificity for proliferating immune cells, all currently used drugs are more or less nonspecific. They generate a general immunosuppressive state and may even inhibit proliferation of nonimmune cells. An increased incidence of sometimes life-threatening infections is the logical consequence of such nonspecific immunosuppressive approaches. Moreover, alkylating agents such as cyclophosphamide that interfere with DNA structure have considerable gonadal toxicity and through cumulative adverse effects induce an increased risk of cancer. Other adverse effects of the currently used immunomodulatory substances are provided elsewhere in this book. Therefore, novel specific therapies are urgently needed that target only the pathophysiologic processes of glomerulonephritis and vasculitis, resulting hopefully in less general toxicity to the patient.

Development of innovative therapies requires a detailed pathophysiologic understanding of glomerulonephritis

Many innovative strategies have been tested in animal models of various types of glomerulonephritis.[1–3] Instead of providing a complete list of all these substances, I present a general conceptual framework of novel therapies. A better understanding of the mechanisms of glomerular immune injury is a necessary prerequisite for the development of more specific drugs. Indeed enormous progress has been made in this field during the last decade. Space does not allow description of these advances in detail and the reader is referred to several recent reviews.[1,3,4] However, a few key developments should be pointed out. Whatever the etiology, the pathophysiologic process of glomerulonephritis may be arbitrarily divided into four phases (a schematic overview of the mechanisms of glomerular injury is provided in Fig. 31.1). First, there is initiation of glomerular inflammation, for example through in situ formation or deposition of circulating immune complexes. Glomerular deposition of immunoglobulins is regulated by many factors, including the recently discovered protein uteroglobin that may reduce binding of IgA complexes to mesangial cells. Alternatively, circulating antibodies can bind directly to intrinsic glomerular antigens as found in Goodpasture disease. In other types of glomerulonephritis, such as minimal change disease, humoral factors, which are still incompletely characterized on a molecular level, induce injury of the glomerular ultrafiltration barrier resulting in proteinuria. Lastly, in the so-called "pauci" type of glomerulonephritis often associated with systemic vasculitis, no glomerular deposition of antibodies or immune complexes can be detected, although it is likely that various cytokines and growth factors contribute to the adhesion, infiltration of inflammatory cells, and proliferation of glomerular cells.[1] Although best established in immune complex nephritis, it is conceivable that humoral and cellular immune mechanisms are also important in this initial phase of glomerular nephritis via production of special cytokines, even in cases without glomerular deposition of antibodies. This initial phase of glomerular injury leads, via local activation of complement components, production of chemokines, and other inflammatory mediators such as leukotrienes, to the formation of a chemotactic gradient and local endothelial upregulation of adhesion molecules. The consequence is recruitment of inflammatory cells from the circulation into the glomerulus. Depending on the composition of these chemotactic factors, the inflammatory cells could be macrophages/monocytes, T cells, or granulocytes. The third phase of glomerular injury may be viewed as a response of intrinsic glomerular cells to the proinflammatory environment. The proinflammatory cells that have infiltrated the glomerulus further produce a host of harmful substances, including various cytokines, growth factors, enzymes, and reactive oxygen species among others. This phase includes injury and subsequent response such as activation and proliferation of local glomerular cells. The fourth phase may be either resolution of inflammation or development of glomerular sclerosis.

Many of the pathophysiologic processes that occur during the different phases of glomerular injury require that particular cells synthesize and release a distinct mediator, which then binds to a specific receptor on target cells, activating a signal transduction pathway that ultimately results in changes in gene transcription. These mediators could be cytokines, chemokines, growth factors, eicosanoids, nitric oxide, reactive oxygen species, or other humoral mediators; however, the general concept of specific ligand–receptor interaction also applies to antigen presentation to specific receptors on T or B cells as well as to coactivation of T cells, e.g. CD28–B7 interaction. Table 31.1

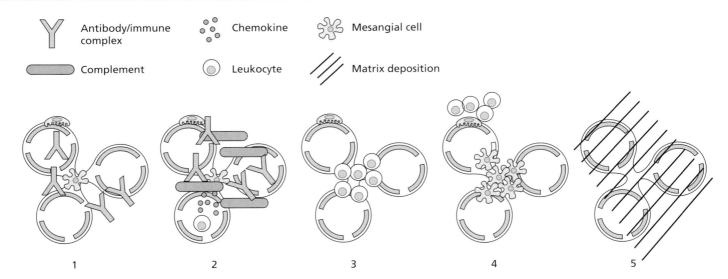

Figure 31.1 Schematic overview of the various stages of the development of glomerular inflammation and injury. 1, Deposition of antibodies against intrinsic glomerular antigens, immune complex deposition, or in situ formation of immune complexes start the injury process. 2, Activation of complement, via either the classical or alternative pathway, stimulates the release of chemotactic factors such as chemokines. 3, Recruitment of leukocytes and/or macrophages into the glomerulus occurs with release of many cytokines. 4, As a consequence of the local growth factor cytokine bath, intrinsic glomerular cells such as mesangial cells proliferate. In addition, macrophages together with epithelial cells may eventually form crescents. 5, Deposition of extracellular matrix proteins ultimately leads to glomerular sclerosis. Alternatively, glomerular inflammation may resolve, leaving only minor permanent damage.

summarizes the conceptual approaches for generally interfering with the activation of the receptor–ligand cascade at different levels using various therapeutic strategies or for promoting glomerular healing. These strategies have been successfully tested for several ligand–receptor pairs. However, it should be recognized that these approaches often stem from cell culture studies or rodent animal models. Indeed, very few of them have been tested in nonhuman primates, and the change from rodent models to primates remains a quantum leap in testing the efficiency of novel therapeutic approaches for glomerulonephritis. Gene therapy, a favorite of many investigators, may serve as a paradigm. Although elegant methods have been developed to interfere with gene expression in vitro, the delivery of DNA into kidneys is still unsatisfactory and the results are less than convincing (reviewed in reference 2). Thus, it remains highly questionable whether there will be efficient gene delivery to human kidneys in the near future, and the catastrophic results of recent human gene therapy studies in nonrenal monogenic diseases only underscore this problem. A fundamental reappraisal and development of new vector systems are necessary before gene therapy will be considered novel therapy for human glomerulonephritis.

Etiology of glomerular inflammation

The etiology of all forms of primary glomerulonephritis remains unclear, making therapy of the cause impossible. However, the identification of hepatitis C as a cause of cryoglobulinemia and membranoproliferative glomerulonephritis, which may be treated with appropriate antiviral therapy, serves as an example that future research may identify additional antigens in a minority of those cases currently considered as primary immune complex nephritis, with the potential for development of novel therapies. It is clear that close cooperation between T and B cells is necessary for the development of frank autoimmunity.[3–5] It has been known for many years that clonal deletion of all autoreactive cells is necessary for the normal development of the immune system. However, it now appears that a low level of autoreactivity is required for normal immune function.[4] Moreover, it has even been postulated that homeostasis of peripheral T cells depends on continuous self-recognition that requires a constant subthreshold signal provided by self-MHC–peptide ligands.[5] Such a provocative concept implies that in lymphopenic states, e.g. induced by the current armamentarium of nonspecific immunosuppressive drugs, self-MHC–peptide ligands provide a proliferative signal for self-reactive T cells that may actually foster autoimmunity after homeostatic reconstitution of the T-cell pool. A more antigen-specific immunomodulation can be achieved, at least experimentally, with altered peptide ligands.[6] The substitution of one amino acid can change certain antigens from T-cell agonists to antagonists that still bind specifically to the T-cell receptor but drive the cell into a suppressive state. The problem with this elegant therapy is that the majority of autoantigens in human glomerulonephritis are not well characterized and "antigen spreading" occurs during the development of disease, providing novel self-antigen–T-cell interactions.

Many genetic factors have been characterized that increase the susceptibility to autoimmune disease including glomerulonephritis. Some of these factors, e.g. defects in the apoptosis-mediating Fas pathway, lower the threshold for

Table 31.1 Potential approaches for treating glomerular inflammation

Inhibition of proinflammatory events

Ligand–mediator
Antisense gene therapy to inhibit expression
RNA interference to induce posttranscriptional gene silencing of the ligand
Aptamers
Neutralizing antibodies
Chimeric scavenger receptors

Receptor
Antisense gene therapy to interfere with receptor expression
RNA interference to induce posttranscriptional gene silencing of the receptor
Specific nonactivating receptor antagonists
Blocking antibodies directed against the ligand-binding site

Signal transduction pathways
Specific pharmacologic inhibitors of distinct signal transduction pathways (e.g. inhibition of tyrosine kinases)

Gene transcription
Gene therapy using decoy oligonucleotides that compete with binding of transcription factors for target genes
Antisense gene therapy to inhibit expression of target genes
RNA interference to induce posttranscriptional gene silencing of target genes

Harnessing the resolution phase of inflammation
Promoting the metabolism of proinflammatory mediators
Overexpression of certain proteases
Overexpression of clearance receptors for mediators

Mimicking the action of endogenous mediators that inhibit leukocyte recruitment
Overexpression of specific cytokines
Mimicking certain signal transduction pathways

Delineating and then mimicking the endogenous systems that restore normal glomerular structure
Overexpression of specific cytokines
Mimicking certain signal transduction pathways

the survival and activation of autoreactive B cells, resulting in systemic lupus erythematosus (SLE). In fact, reconstitution of the immune system with bone marrow ablation and replacement with stem cells has been successfully used in severe cases of SLE with renal involvement.

An attractive target for inhibiting T-cell activation is blockade of costimulatory pathways such as CD28, CTLA-4, and B7-1,2 molecules, ensuring more specific inhibition of only those T cells that have encountered an antigen. A soluble recombinant fusion protein (CTLA4-Ig) blocks the activation of T-cell costimulatory pathways and has been found to reduce autoantibody production and prevent renal injury in a model of nephrotoxic glomerulonephritis.[7] However, treatment with CTLA4-Ig exacerbated other autoimmune diseases such as diabetes in NOD mice and certain models of autoimmune encephalitis, probably by depleting immunoregulatory T cells.

Mediators of glomerular inflammation

Chemokines are key mediators in the recruitment of circulating proinflammatory cells into the glomerulus.[8,9]

These substances are synthesized by intrinsic glomerular cells, e.g. mesangial cells, after binding of antibodies to specific immunoglobulin receptors. Other cytokines, such as tumor necrosis factor (TNF)-α or reactive oxygen species, that could also be locally generated during the first wave of glomerular injury are additional strong inducers of glomerular chemokine expression. Even vasoactive peptides such as angiotensin II, endothelin 1, leukotrienes, and platelet-activating factor all stimulate renal production of these chemotactic factors. In addition, proinflammatory cytokines such as TNF-α also induce expression of specific chemokine receptors on intrinsic glomerular cells. The increase in local chemokine synthesis and additional chemokines produced by leukocytes recruited into the glomerulus could act as autocrine/paracrine factors that may stimulate proliferation of mesangial and local synthesis of profibrogenic factors, including transforming growth factor (TGF)-β. Thus, the various chemokines and their distinct receptor systems can be viewed as a link between early glomerular inflammation and subsequent responses of glomerular cells.

Studies in rodent models of various types of glomerulonephritis have provided evidence that neutralizing antibodies against certain chemokines or chemokine receptor antagonists (e.g. AOP-RANTES and Met-RANTES) reduce glomerular infiltration with macrophages/monocytes and partly prevent permanent glomerular injury.[9] In addition, viral proteins, glycosaminoglycans such as heparin, nonpeptide synthetic compounds (4-hydroxypiperidines), flavonoids, prostaglandin E, and small synthetic molecules such as bindarit have all been found to interfere with the chemokine network, although limited data are available to show whether these substances are effective in animal models of glomerulonephritis. An N-terminal deletion mutant of the chemokine monocyte chemoattractant protein (MCP)-1 that has been over-expressed in skeletal muscle binds to CCR2 receptors and attenuates the effect of endogenously produced MCP-1. Other therapeutic approaches have targeted nuclear factor (NF)-κB, a key transcription factor for various cytokines. NF-κB decoy oligonucleotides have been found, at least in vitro and in very limited in vivo approaches, to attenuate chemokine transcription in renal cells. However, proteasome inhibitors, thought to inhibit the NF-κB pathway by blocking degradation of IκB, unexpectedly stimulate transcription of chemokines under certain conditions.[10] Antioxidant therapy with radical scavengers, blockade of the renin–angiotensin system, pentoxifylline, and statins all partly prevent NF-κB-mediated chemokine expression. Blockade of the TNF-α cascade with either monoclonal antibodies or a soluble TNF-α receptor–IgG fusion protein that serves as a scavenger has been successfully used in other autoimmune disorders such as rheumatoid arthritis, but there are currently very few data for glomerulonephritis. However, clinical trials using etanercept, a TNF-α receptor–IgG fusion protein, are underway in antineutrophil cytoplasmic antibody-positive vasculitis.

There is increasing evidence that renal chemokine expression and excretion correlate with disease activity in various types of human glomerulonephritis, suggesting that these factors may also play a pivotal role in human renal disease. However, blockade of the complex chemokine network may not be straightforward. Recent studies in mice of disruption of the chemokine receptor CCR1, one of the various receptors for RANTES, macrophage inflammatory protein (MIP)-1α, MCP-3 and MCP-4, surprisingly revealed that nephrotoxic nephritis exhibited a more severe course in these mice compared with wild-type animals. These unexpected results have been interpreted as showing that the absence of CCR1 favors a Th1 immune response with stronger local inflammation, and provide a clear warning that further studies are necessary before the chemokine network should be manipulated in human glomerulonephritis.

Chemokines such as B-lymphocyte chemoattractant (BLC) and secondary lymphoid tissue chemokine (SLC), and their putative receptors (CXCR3, CXCR5, CCR7), control the migration of lymphocytes within primary lymphoid organs, from primary to secondary organs, and between secondary lymphoid organs.[11] Lymphotoxin α (also called TNF-β) is a key factor for homing of B and T cells via the induction of SLC and BLC and probably other chemokines. Recently it has been shown that BLC is highly expressed in the kidney of lupus mice, creating a lymphoid environment in a nonlymphoid organ that results in massive lymphocyte "homing" to the kidney. Two alternative therapeutic approaches might be developed from these observations. First, neutralization of BLC expression in target organs of autoimmunity may reduce local inflammation. Second, it is also imaginable that overexpression of homing chemokines in secondary lymphoid organs such as lymph nodes could provide an environment preventing lymphocytes from migrating to target organs, thus serving as a "sink" for immune cells.

Since the chemokine receptor CCR5 is preferentially expressed on immune cells of tissue inflammatory infiltrates and is not readily found on peripheral blood cells, specific deletion of those cells with bispecific antibodies and chemokine toxins appears to be an innovative strategy to deplete active immune cells more specifically.[12]

Finally, other strategies such as overexpression of complement inhibitors have been developed to prevent chronic inflammation of the kidney in experimentally induced glomerulonephritis (see reference 13 for an example).

Response phase of intrinsic glomerular cells

This phase of glomerular injury may be viewed as a response of intrinsic glomerular cells to the cytokine bath produced by infiltrating immune cells.[14,15] The final outcome may be either resolution of glomerular injury or the ultimate development of glomerular sclerosis. Cytokines such as platelet-derived growth factor (PDGF), released from thrombocytes during glomerular injury or directly produced by glomerular cells, are strong proliferative factors for mesangial cells that contribute to proliferative glomerulonephritis and crescent formation. Inhibition of the PDGF axis by different approaches, including the application of aptamer antagonists, ameliorates injury in various models of glomerulonephritis. Another way to antagonize the effects of these cytokines is interference with specific signal transduction pathways, such as pharmacologic inhibition of tyrosine kinases using quinoxalines for example. On the other hand, TGFβ is a potent profibrogenic cytokine that stimulates expression of extracellular matrix components, mediates fibroblast proliferation, and inhibits matrix turnover.[15] Glomerular TGFβ expression can be directly induced by chemokines, cytokines including PDGF, and angiotensin II. TGFβ activity has been neutralized in experimental models of glomerulonephritis with antibodies, chimeric scavenger receptors, overexpression of TGFβ binding proteins such as decorin, and antisense oligonucleotides. In general, these approaches have resulted in less severe glomerular sclerosis. Since angiotensin II is a major inducer of renal TGFβ synthesis, it is logical to inhibit the renin–angiotensin system in an attempt to interfere with renal profibrogenic processes. Vitamin D treatment also ameliorates injury in a rat model of mesangioproliferative glomerulonephritis by inhibition of TGFβ. However, TGFβ exhibits anti-inflammatory properties under certain conditions. Thus, neutralization of TGFβ may result in prolonged inflammation.

Injury to glomerular capillaries is an integral part of many types of glomerulonephritis. Infusion of vascular endothelial growth factor enhances glomerular capillary repair and accelerates resolution of anti-Thy1 nephritis in rats. These interesting studies suggest that application of distinct growth factors may stimulate remodeling of the already injured glomerulus and could enhance recovery of a normal renal architecture in glomerulonephritis.

Resolution of glomerular injury

In most patients with poststreptococcal glomerulonephritis the renal injury heals, although recent evidence suggests that long-term renal function is not optimal even years later. Yet as this disease indicates, the resolution phase of glomerular inflammation involves mechanisms for clearance of antigen, antibodies, and immune complexes, elimination of invading leukocytes, and even resolution of increased proliferation of local cells with crescent formation. It is currently unclear why such a distinct acute glomerular disease resolves whereas another type of glomerulonephritis progresses more chronically. It is reasonable to assume that certain cytokines exhibiting anti-inflammatory and antiproliferative effects, such as TGFβ, eicosanoids, IL-4 and IL-10, as well as others, contribute to this process. These factors also suppress helper T cells, although the anti-inflammatory effects may be partly traded off by the concurrent stimulation of renal fibrosis (e.g. via TGFβ). A better understanding of the mechanisms of resolution of glomerular injury may lead to the development of therapeutic strategies that facilitate healing of glomerular inflammation.

Conclusions

The nonspecific immunosuppression and adverse effects of the drugs currently used for treatment of glomerulonephritis demand the development of innovative, more specific therapies based on a comprehensive understanding of the pathophysiology of glomerulonephritis. While the etiology and pathogenesis of human glomerulonephritis remains poorly understood, many novel therapies have been studied in animal models. These therapeutic strategies aim to modulate the immune system directly, interfere with chemokines and their receptors in order to prevent recruitment of inflammatory cells into the glomerulus, or may interfere with cytokines involved in glomerular remodeling and scarring. Yet many of these promising studies have been performed only in rodent models of glomerulonephritis. However, lessons learned from transplantation immunology clearly indicate that there is a great difference in dealing with the immune systems of rodents and primates. Moreover, animal models of

glomerulonephritis are well characterized: the antigen for nephritis induction or the epitope for a nephrotoxic antibody is known; the experimental treatment interferes with glomerulonephritis during a small time-window shortly after or even before induction of nephritis. This is obviously not feasible in humans. The target antigens of glomerulonephritis are, with a few exceptions, not known and the duration of the subclinical course of the disease before diagnosis is often unclear. Thus it remains uncertain whether the strategies described may ever work in human glomerulonephritis. Finally, for practical applications such novel substances should be active after oral administration, a requirement not fulfilled by many currently used artificial fusion proteins and antibodies. An efficient and practical clinical approach could be the application of certain cytokines that might foster the resolution phase of an acute glomerular injury, although these mechanisms need to be more clearly defined.

The observation that angiotensin-converting enzyme inhibitors and statins may exhibit immunosuppressive properties provides a little help to the busy clinician who cannot wait for the more speculative treatments in animal models to make it to the bedside.

References

1. Schlöndorff D, Segerer S: Pathogenesis of glomerulonephritis, a perspective from the last 30 years. J Nephrol 1999;12(Suppl 2):S131–S141.
2. Kelley VR, Sukhatme VP: Gene transfer in the kidney. Am J Physiol 1999;276: F1–F9.
3. Davidson A, Diamond B: Autoimmune diseases. N Engl J Med 2001;345:340–350.
4. Parkin J, Cohen B: An overview of the immune system. Lancet 2001;357:1777–1789.
5. Theofilopoulos AN, Dummer W, Kono DH: T cell homeostasis and systemic autoimmunity. J Clin Invest 2001;108:335–340.
6. Bielekova B, Martin R: Antigen-specific immunomodulation via altered peptide ligands. J Mol Med 2001;79:552–565.
7. Salomon B, Bluestone JA: Complexities of CD28/B7: CTLA-4 costimulatory pathways in autoimmunity and transplantation. Annu Rev Immunol 2001;19:225–252.
8. Rossi D, Zlotnik A: The biology of chemokines and their receptors. Annu Rev Immunol 2000;18:217–242.
9. Rovin BH: Chemokine blockade as a therapy for renal disease. Curr Opin Nephrol Hypertens 2000;9:225–232.
10. Nakayama K, Furusu A, Xu Q, Konta T, Kitamura M: Unexpected transcriptional induction of monocyte chemoattractant protein 1 by proteasome inhibition: involvement of the c-jun N-terminal kinase-activator protein 1 pathway. J Immunol 2001;167:1145–1150.
11. Bachmann MF, Kopf M: On the role of the innate immunity in autoimmune disease. J Exp Med 2001;193:F47–F50.
12. Brühl H, Cihak J, Stangassinger M, Schlöndorff D, Mack M: Depletion of CCR5-expressing cells with bispecific antibodies and chemokine toxins: a new strategy in the treatment of chronic inflammatory diseases and HIV. J Immunol 2001;166:2420–2426.
13. Schiller B, Cunnighman PN, Alexander JJ, Bao L, Holers VM, Quigg RJ: Expression of a soluble complement inhibitor protects transgenic mice from antibody-induced acute renal failure. J Am Soc Nephrol 2001;12:71–79.
14. Cybulsky AV: Growth factor pathways in proliferative glomerulonephritis. Curr Opin Nephrol Hypertens 2000;9:217–223.
15. Floege J, von Ostendorf T, Wolf G: Growth factors and cytokines. In Couser W, Neilson EG (eds): Immunologic Renal Diseases, 2nd edn. Philadelphia: Lippincott-Raven, 2001, pp 415–463

PART III
Diabetic Nephropathy

CHRISTOPHER S. WILCOX

Prevention and Management of Diabetic Nephropathy

Carl Erik Mogensen

Prevention, early detection, and treatment of renal disease in diabetic patients are becoming major healthcare issues.[1] Therapeutic options such as optimized glycemic control and early antihypertensive treatment effectively prevent or slow the progression of renal disease in both types of diabetes. Management of elevated blood pressure must go hand in hand with the general management of diabetic patients (i.e. metabolic control with appropriate diet and treatment with insulin or oral agents), guided by blood glucose values, glycated hemoglobin, dietary discussions, and, importantly, systematic screening for microalbuminuria and early retinopathy. The desire for optimal management of hyperglycemia has been strongly reinforced by publication of the positive results from the American Diabetes Control and Complication Trial (DCCT) and the United Kingdom Prospective Diabetes Study (UKPDS), as well as studies in noninsulin-dependent diabetes mellitus (NIDDM) from Japan.[2–4] Although a sustained reduction of HbA_{1c} delays development of renal complications,[4] there are some reservations from the UKPDS trial.[5] Moreover, many patients in the intensified arm of the DCCT program

did not escape renal disease, very likely because glycemia was not adequately controlled. Familial factors, intrauterine malnutrition, and even genetic factors may be involved.[1,6,7]

Hemodynamic and metabolic risk factors are closely interrelated.[8] They should be managed by a specialized diabetes team, which encourages the patient to participate actively in the management. Increased blood pressure is likely to aggravate considerably all the vascular complications associated with diabetes, including stroke,[9] coronary and peripheral vascular disease, retinopathy, and nephropathy.[1,4]

Insulin- and noninsulin-dependent patients

Blood pressure increases early in diabetes, well before glomerular filtration rate (GFR) declines.[1] Patients with insulin-dependent diabetes mellitus (IDDM) typically develop hypertension after microalbuminuria, which is followed by a decline in GFR with clinical proteinuria. In contrast, hypertension, albeit often only moderate, is frequently present in NIDDM (or type 2 diabetes) at diagnosis.[10,11] Thus in these patients elevated blood pressure may be related not only to increasing age and obesity but also to hyperinsulinism as part of the so-called "metabolic syndrome," and this is perhaps linked by a common background in insulin resistance and dyslipidemia.[10] Contemporary studies show that nephropathy is an important feature in type 2 diabetics. It often leads to endstage renal disease (ESRD), the most common cause of which is type 2 diabetes.[11]

The management of hypertension is similar in patients with NIDDM and IDDM, although a somewhat higher blood pressure level may be acceptable in NIDDM patients than in young patients with IDDM. NIDDM shows a progressive reduction in insulin secretion.[4] Many patients start with dietary treatment but soon require oral agents and later insulin, as guided by HbA_{1c} levels. In many cases, treatment with insulin is postponed much too long. Similarly, hypertension also worsens without intervention and should be treated early.

Critical issues in management

The treatment of diabetic patients should be evaluated in relation to glycemia and blood pressure elevation as follows.

1. Classification of renal disease involvement.
2. Treatment of diabetes in general should be evaluated, with the emphasis on an early program for near-normal glycemia and detection of complications.

3. Analysis of blood pressure in relation to the stage of diabetic renal disease.
4. Evaluation of the requirement for a specific antihypertensive regimen, with consideration of likely adverse effects and concurrence with appropriate guidelines.

Classification of diabetic renal involvement or disease

A classification system for diabetic renal disease should comply with the following general criteria:

1. The system should imply predictive power with respect to progression of the disease.
2. It should relate to pathophysiologic changes.
3. Relationship to structural lesions is clearly important.
4. The system should also collate other abnormalities characteristic of, or related to, complications in general.
5. Clearly such a system should also be therapeutically orientated. That is, should insulin and the general diabetes treatment be optimized or is another diet relevant (e.g. low protein or low sodium)? Should blood pressure be monitored more closely? Should treatment be started, changed, or optimized?

The classification system for patients with IDDM shown in Table 32.1 does to a great extent meet the criteria indicated above, and there are presently no other alternatives in classifying patients. It generally also applies to patients with NIDDM, who may often die prematurely of cardiovascular disease rather than uremia (Fig. 32.1). Renal biopsy may help the clinician clarify the diagnosis in a few atypical diabetic patients but is very rarely indicated in the patient with NIDDM.[12] The clinical course of NIDDM itself usually reveals nondiabetic renal disease, and a biopsy is justified only if it has clear therapeutic consequences.[13] In the long term, patients with a normal urinary albumin excretion (UAE) rate are not protected against the development of diabetic nephropathy: approximately 2–4% of normoalbuminuric patients with IDDM develop microalbuminuria each year (and thus possibly later overt nephropathy). However, the prognosis of normoalbuminuric patients with regard to the development of overt nephropathy with clinical proteinuria and hypertension over the subsequent decade is much better than patients with microalbuminuria. With a normal UAE rate, the risk for development of overt proteinuric renal disease is small, whereas the risk in patients with microalbuminuria (and no intervention) may be approximately 8% per year, as recently confirmed in the DCCT. Indeed, new intervention modalities have appeared since these retrospective studies were published,[14,15] and the risk of subsequent nephropathy with appropriate optimized metabolic control and effective antihypertensive treatment is likely to be around 2% per year.[14]

As seen in Table 32.1, renal involvement can be traced throughout the course of diabetes and is related to long-term glycemic control. It is important to emphasize that the control and evaluation of diabetic nephropathy (including blood pressure and glycemic monitoring) must be implemented from the diagnosis of diabetes; these measures are also important in defining baseline values for the individual patient. If blood pressure, glycemic control, and evaluation of renal function are delayed until advanced nephropathy, the game is partly lost. In this situation the healthcare system must also favor preventive medicine, which is rarely the case, for example in the USA where, according to several surveys, screening for microalbuminuria is uncommon although recommended in guidelines.[15]

In the classification system described earlier, patients are categorized according to abnormal albuminuria. Because albuminuria is continuously (rather than categorically) variable, it could be considered advisable to use only numeric values for albuminuria. However, for practical communication reasons, the categories "normoalbuminuria," "microalbuminuria," and "macroalbuminuria" were introduced. Importantly, different measures of

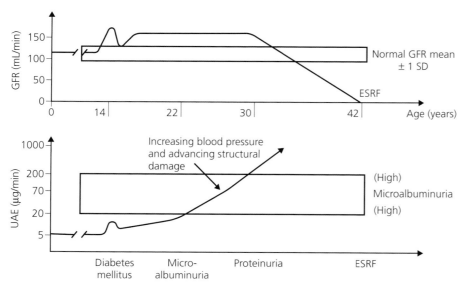

Figure 32.1 Typical natural history of diabetic nephropathy for a patient developing diabetes at age 14. For the first 8–10 years the patient remains normoalbuminuric, with a tendency for urinary albumin excretion (UAE) to increase. Glomerular filtration rate (GFR) remains significantly elevated in these years, as an expression of poor metabolic control. With progression to overt proteinuria, GFR starts to decline usually in a linear fashion and, without any intervention, the patient reaches endstage renal failure (ESRF) at age 42. Without development of diabetic nephropathy, patients usually have limited early hyperfiltration and remain normoalbuminuric or close to normoalbuminuric throughout their lives. With the development of microalbuminuria there is usually an increase in blood pressure, and advancing structural damage appears in the kidney and the vasculature elsewhere.

Table 32.1 Stages in the development of renal changes and lesions in type 1 diabetes (partly relevant also for type 2 diabetes)

Stage	Chronology	Main structural changes or lesions	GFR	Albumin excretion* (e.g. overnight UAE)	Blood pressure	Effects of strict insulin treatment	Role of antihypertensive treatment†
I Acute renal hypertrophy–hyperfunction	Present at diagnosis (reversible with good control)	Increased kidney and glomerular size	Increased by 20–50%	May be increased, reversible	Normal	Yes	No hypertension present
II Normoalbuminuria (< 20 µg/min)	Almost all patients normoalbuminuric in the first 5 years	On renal biopsy, increased BM thickness after 2 years	Increased by 20–40% related to HbA_{1c}	Normal by definition (15–20 µg/min may still be abnormal)	Normal (same as in background population). Increase by ~ 1 mmHg/year	Hyperfiltration reduced	Filtration fraction and UAE may be reduced by ACE inhibitors
III Incipient diabetic nephropathy (microalbuminuria)	Usually after 6–15 years (in 25–35% of patients)	Further BM thickness, mesangial expansion	Still supranormal, but declines with proteinuria	20–200 µg/min (increase ~ 20%/year) of glomerular origin	Incipient increase, usually ~ 3 mmHg/year (if untreated)	Microalbuminuria and GFR stabilized, if HbA_{1c} reduced	Microalbuminuria reduced; prevention of fall in GFR; DD genotype less responsive?
IV Proteinuria or overt diabetic nephropathy	After 15–25 years (in 25–35% of patients)	Clear and pronounced abnormalities	Decline ~ 12 mL/min/year with proteinuria‡	Progressive proteinuria of glomerular origin	High, increase by ~ 5 mmHg/year (if untreated)	Higher fall in GFR with poor HbA_{1c}	Progression reduced (aiming at 135/85 mmHg or less); DD genotype less responsive?
V Endstage renal failure	Final outcome after 25–30 years or more	Glomerular closure	< 10 mL/min	Often some decline due to nephron closure	High (if untreated)	No, but good glycemic control may relate to better outcome	Good blood pressure control relates to better late outcome

ACE, angiotensin-converting enzyme; BM, basement membrane; GFR, glomerular filtration rate; UAE, urinary albumin excretion.

*The best marker of early renal involvement.

†Mostly ACE inhibitors plus diuretics.

‡Without antihypertensive treatment. Smoking is a risk factor throughout the course, including in endstage renal failure.

albumin excretion can be used, and in clinical practice the ratio of albumin to creatinine must be preferred.[1]

Associated abnormalities of microalbuminuria in incipient renal and nonrenal diabetic nephropathy

Incipient diabetic nephropathy, as evidenced by microalbuminuria, is an important stage, the diagnosis of which is decisive because intensified treatment (especially antihypertensive treatment) is likely to be much more effective than when overt nephropathy is established.[15,16] Patients with microalbuminuria are in the process of developing multiple vascular lesions in addition, or related, to increased blood pressure. Because development of vascular changes may be related not only to glycemic control but also to blood pressure increase, and may interact with treatment, these changes are discussed briefly.

Blood pressure elevation

Many studies have shown that blood pressure elevation (usually about 10%) is present in patients with microalbuminuria, although there is considerable overlap between normoalbuminuric and microalbuminuric patients. This pattern has been confirmed in 24-h ambulatory blood pressure (AMBP) recording.[17] Studies using 24-h AMBP suggest that abnormal albuminuria frequently triggers blood pressure elevation, thus leading to a subsequent vicious circle.[17]

Renal structure and function

Many studies have clearly shown that patients with microalbuminuria exhibit early glomerulopathy.[18,19] Also, in the arterioles the extracellular matrix is increased relative to the total media in patients with microalbuminuria. This structural change may adversely influence the autoregulation of glomerular flow and subsequently the pressure, and may therefore be one of the key abnormalities in the pathogenesis of early glomerular albuminuria. Regarding type 2 diabetes, studies from Italy report that glomerular lesions and arteriolar hyalinosis are common in patients with microalbuminuria.[19] Hyperfiltration is often found at the stage of microalbuminuria, and GFR starts to decline late in the phase of incipient diabetic nephropathy or, more commonly, the stage of transition to overt nephropathy.

Retinopathy

Danish and recent Australian studies have documented that microalbuminuria strongly predicts proliferative diabetic retinopathy.[20] However, in these studies it is difficult to clearly separate the possible effect of increasing blood pressure, because patients who show progression in albuminuria rate and development of proliferative retinopathy clearly have increasing blood pressure.

Heart disease

Heart disease is very prevalent with hypertension and diabetic renal disease.[21] Echocardiographic studies showed increased left ventricular wall thickness in hypertensive diabetics, with a high prevalence of microvascular complications. Using multiple regression analysis it was found that blood pressure is the most important statistical determinant of left ventricular wall hypertrophy.[22] In overt nephropathy, cardiac hypertrophy is very prevalent.[23]

Choice of therapy related to mechanisms of blood pressure elevation

Based on some of the mechanisms that supposedly operate in the genesis of renal disease and hypertension in diabetes, interesting concepts regarding the selection of antihypertensive treatments are evolving. However, it must be emphasized that the pathophysiologic mechanisms underlying the association between diabetes and blood pressure elevation are still unclear and may involve many complex interactions.[24]

The early abnormalities in renal function in diabetes, where hyperperfusion, hyperfiltration, and increased glomerular pressures may be important phenomena, point to the use of angiotensin-converting enzyme (ACE) inhibitors or angiotensin receptor blockers (ARBs) because these agents tend to reduce efferent glomerular resistance. To some extent, this effect (i.e. reduction of glomerular pressure) may be partly independent of systemic hypertension or systemic blood pressure level, but not necessarily so. Sodium retention is observed not only in type 2 but also in type 1 diabetes and may suggest the use of diuretics or sodium restriction in antihypertensive programs for diabetes. This treatment may potentiate the effect of ACE inhibitors.[23] The early cardiac hyperfunction in microalbuminuric patients may point to the use of cardioselective β-blockers in order to reduce this hyperfunction[23] or benefit cardiac prognosis. Obviously, the generalized reduction in blood pressure seen with all these agents may be very important. The three mechanisms described could favor the use of triple therapy: ACE inhibitors, diuretics, and cardioselective β-blockers.[23] Calcium antagonists are used mainly in patients with NIDDM, although long-term trials suggest no beneficial effects as far as the kidney is concerned as shown in the irbesartan diabetic nephropathy trial (IDNT).[12]

Obviously, from a theoretical point of view, adverse effects should be balanced against potential additional beneficial effects (Table 32.2). For example, inhibitors of the renin–angiotensin system may, as suggested by animal studies, specifically reduce the local glomerular pressure increase thought to prevail in these patients. The common occurrence of edema favors the use of diuretics. It is suggested that arrhythmia may play a role in the early mortality in postmyocardial infarction trials, and β-blockers are notably effective in diabetic patients. This points to an additional beneficial effect of β-blockers in

Table 32.2 Adverse and favorable effects of antihypertensive treatment in diabetes (mainly type 1 diabetes mellitus)

	Diuretics (thiazide or loop)	Cardioselective β-blockers	ACE inhibitors	Triple therapy: diuretic, β$_1$-blocker, ACE inhibitor	Calcium channel blockers	Angiotensin receptor blockers*
Glucose intolerance	Yes, in NIDDM (related strongly to hypokalemia)	Limited problem	No adverse effects	Limited (with small dosages)	No	No
Hypoglycemic masking	No	May be a problem in IDDM	Not seen	Limited (with small dosages)	No	No
Unfavorable lipid effects	Yes (dose dependent)	Limited	No adverse effects	?	No	No
Other unfavorable effects	May cause sodium depletion	Less physical exercise capacity	Cough and drug-related adverse effects	Limited (with small dosages)	Foot edema seen in a few patients	Rare
Favorable effects (apart from blood pressure reduction)	Elimination of edema	Reduction of cardiovascular morbidity/ mortality?; normalization of cardiac arrhythmias	Elimination of sodium excess and possibly restoration of glomerular pressure gradients	Probably also combination of favorable effects (stable GFR)	?	Renoprotection
Effect on abnormal albuminuria	Now well documented for some agents	Yes, but relatively few studies; related to blood pressure reduction	Very consistent finding	Addition of ACE inhibitor reduces albuminuria	Not a consistent finding, but seen with some agents	Yes
Reducing rate of GFR decline in long-term studies	Not documented	Yes (often with diuretics)	Yes	GFR may be stable on this program	Not documented	Yes

ACE, angiotensin-converting enzyme; GFR, glomerular filtration rate; IDDM, insulin-dependent diabetes mellitus; NIDDM, noninsulin-dependent diabetes mellitus.
*Mainly type 2 diabetes mellitus.

Table 32.3 Combination of antihypertensive treatments in diabetes, with focus on type 2 diabetes mellitus

	Diuretics	β-Blockers	ACE inhibitors	Calcium channel blockers
β-Blockers	Yes (often required)	—	May be used	Yes
ACE inhibitors	Yes (often required)	Yes	—	Yes
Calcium channel blockers	Yes	Yes (rare)	Yes	—
Angiotensin receptor blockers	Yes (often used)	Yes	Yes, dual blockade	Yes, blood pressure reduction

α-Blockers may also be used in various combinations. Careful clinical metabolic and blood pressure monitoring is always required, including control of serum electrolytes and serum creatinine or the glomerular filtration rate index.
ACE, angiotensin-converting enzyme.

the management of hypertension and diabetes, as well as the use of ACE inhibitors after myocardial infarction[25] (Table 32.3).

Adverse effects are important and usually dose related (Table 32.4). For example, the well-known diabetogenic effect of diuretics may only be seen with high doses. Potassium loss is important and can clearly be restored by potassium supplementation or ACE inhibitors. However, with decreasing renal function potassium accumulation is a problem (often but not always counteracted by the use of diuretics). An adverse effect that has caused concern is unawareness of hypoglycemia. This is typically found with unselective β-blockers but to some extent is also observed with cardioselective β-blockers, and these drugs should

317

Table 32.4 Undesirable effects of antihypertensive treatment and management

Drug	Problems	Mechanism	Methods of amelioration	Significance
β-Blockers	Hypoglycemic awareness (but sweating is enhanced)	Autonomic neuropathy and long-term diabetes	Use of cardioselective blockers; reduction of dose; information to the patient	In some cases considerable
Diuretics (K⁺ loss)	Increase in blood glucose (in NIDDM) by hypokalemia	Urinary loss of potassium	K⁺ supplementation (or counteraction by ACE inhibitors)	May be considerable
Some diuretics and β-blockers	Dyslipoproteinemia	Unknown	Discontinuation or reduction of the dose of drug	Unknown, but theoretically important
ACE inhibitors	Increase in serum K⁺; with renal artery stenosis GFR may fall	Too low a blood pressure or too large a dose	Reduction of the dosage; high serum K⁺ ameliorated by diuretics	As in nondiabetics
Angiotensin receptor blockers	Adverse effects rare; hyperkalemia may occur	Unknown	Reduction of the dosage; high serum K⁺ ameliorated by diuretics	As in nondiabetics
Calcium antagonists	As in nondiabetics; some agents may increase albuminuria	Afferent vasodilatation	Reduction of the dosage or change of treatment	As in nondiabetics
Most antihypertensive drugs	Claudication, dizziness, and possibly reduced working capacity may occur, but rarely with new classes of drugs	General arteriosclerosis and high age	Discontinuation of treatment or reduction of the dosage	As in nondiabetics

ACE, angiotensin-converting enzyme; GFR, glomerular filtration rate; NIDDM, noninsulin-dependent diabetes mellitus.

be used in appropriate doses if necessary. They are quite useful in type 2 diabetes.[4]

ACE inhibitors do not seem to produce any significant diabetogenic effect or a clinically significant effect on insulin resistance. This neutral (or maybe even positive, according to the HOPE study[26,27]) glycemic pattern may therefore favor the use of ACE inhibitors in diabetic patients. Cough as an adverse effect is surprisingly rare in diabetic patients and is perhaps due to neuropathic changes; when explained to patients, this problem is easily accepted. Several antihypertensive agents may be combined,[26] as seen in Table 32.3. Indeed, many patients are on combination therapy, including dual blockade of the renin–angiotensin system[28] (Table 32.5).

What is good glycemic control and what is its importance for progression of renal disease in comparison with antihypertensive treatment?

There is limited evidence that glycemic indices need to be totally normalized in order to avoid late nephropathy. If reliable and specific methods are used (e.g. high-performance liquid chromatography), the normal reference mean of HbA_{1c} is 5.5%, with a standard deviation of 0.5 and a range of 4.5–6.5. These reference values are valid in most centers. Increasing evidence suggests that the risk of nephropathy or progression of nephropathy is low provided that glycemic control corresponds with an HbA_{1c} of less than 7.5–8% (i.e. 3–4 standard deviations above the mean reference for HbA_{1c}). Data from the DCCT suggest that there is no clear threshold for HbA_{1c} with respect to the development of nephropathy; however, progression is slow with HbA_{1c} lower than 7.5%. A less clear effect of glucose control compared with antihypertensive treatment was observed in the UKPDS.[4] Clearly, implementation of adequate control remains an enormous healthcare issue, and effective antihypertensive treatment may be easier to practice. Also, in overt diabetic nephropathy, progression is much less pronounced with good glycemic control.[29,30]

Clinical intervention trials with special reference to antihypertensive treatment

Several review articles on different intervention modalities have been published and all are discussed in a recent book.[1] Many trials using antihypertensive treatment, especially ACE inhibitors, have been completed in patients with microalbuminuria. When incipient diabetic nephropathy is developing (as evidenced by microalbuminuria),

Table 32.5   Results of dual renin–angiotensin system blockade on blood pressure[84]

Reference	No. of patients	Population	Study drug	Reduction in blood pressure (systolic/diastolic, mmHg)
Azizi et al[77]	177	Essential hypertension	Losartan 50 mg plus enalapril mg	3.4/3.6
Baruch et al[82]	55	Chronic heart failure	Valsartan 80–160 mg plus ACE inhibitor	11/*
McKelvie et al[80]	332	Chronic heart failure	Candesartan 4–8 mg plus enalapril	6.5/3.8
Mogensen et al[42]	199	Hypertensive, microalbuminuric diabetics	Lisinopril 20 mg plus candesartan 16 mg	10.0/6.0
Ruilope et al[81]	86	Chronic renal failure	Valsartan 160 mg plus benazepril 10 mg	21.5/13.0
Kincaid-Smith et al[78]	60	Normotensive nephropathy	Candesartan 8 mg plus ACE inhibitor	6.0/2.0
Rossing et al[79]	18	Diabetic nephropathy	Candesartan 8 mg plus ACE inhibitor	10/*
Weir et al[76]	473	Essential hypertension	Candesartan 16–32 mg plus ACE inhibitor	13.4/4.3

ACE, angiotensin-converting enzyme.
*Diastolic blood pressure not assessed.

elevation of blood pressure becomes increasingly important and studies suggest that the rate of progression of renal disease may be associated with blood pressure elevation as well as metabolic control. Therefore, antihypertensive and also glycemic treatments are a crucial area of intervention in these patients.

It is now possible to select normoalbuminuric patients at high risk for progression (high HbA_{1c}, UAE in the upper normal range, hyperfiltration, and increasing blood pressure) for such studies. In a European 2-year intervention study, normoalbuminuria was not significantly reduced and only patients with a UAE higher than 20 μg/min (definition for microalbuminuria) benefited from treatment, although there seemed to be an effect on retinopathy.[20,31] As far as progression in albumin excretion is concerned, a new study suggests effects even in normoalbuminuric patients.[32]

In many studies comprising patients with persistent microalbuminuria and normal or borderline elevation of blood pressure, ACE inhibition was shown to reduce or stabilize microalbuminuria; in contrast, microalbuminuria increased in the control groups.[33,34] GFR is generally stable during ACE intervention in these patients but tends to fall in control patients who develop proteinuria. In the first intervention study of microalbuminuric patients with IDDM, a combination of cardioselective β-blockers and diuretics was used also with positive effect.[35] Many subsequent studies have confirmed the reduction in microalbuminuria. Exercise-induced changes in blood pressure and microalbuminuria can also be relatively normalized.[36]

In patients with overt diabetic nephropathy, it has been shown that conventional treatment with cardioselective β-blockers and diuretics (in some cases combined with vasodilators) induces a dramatic reduction in the progression of nephropathy,[29,30] in accordance with the original observation made several years ago.[37] Indeed, the new long-term follow-up study by Parving et al[29,30,38] suggests that the progression of renal disease is very slow in diabetics on long-term antihypertensive treatment. It has been reported that ACE inhibitors are superior to other antihypertensive agents in slowing the progression of diabetic nephropathy.[29,30] Proteinuria can also be considerably reduced with this treatment modality. However, in other studies, ACE inhibitors and β-blockers had similar effects on the falling rate of GFR.[29] In the large study conducted by Lewis et al,[39] it was shown that ACE inhibitors were more efficacious in preventing doubling of serum creatinine. A significant effect was also obtained on mortality, combined with uremia.

It may be concluded that cardioselective β-blockers and ACE inhibitors can often be combined with diuretics and are useful in delaying the progression of renal disease in patients with type 1 diabetes and overt nephropathy. The rate of progression is reduced considerably when mean blood pressure during intervention is reduced to approximately 135/85 mmHg or lower ("the lower the better"). The Lewis study[39] indicates the superiority of ACE inhibitors. The adverse-effect profile of ACE inhibitors and β-blockers is different (see Table 32.2), and most clinicians now select ACE inhibition as the initial treatment.[15] One study combining ACE inhibitors with β-blockers and diuretics (combining beneficial effect?) has also shown positive preliminary results in early nephropathy with stable GFR over several years.[26]

Trials in patients with NIDDM

Several renal trials with early antihypertensive treatment in patients with NIDDM have recently been published.[34] A long-term study showed that over a 5-year period patients on the ACE inhibitor enalapril exhibited not only stabilization of albuminuria but also stable GFR (as indicated by reciprocal serum creatinine). This contrasted with the control group, who were treated with conventional antipressor agents and in whom a significant increase in albuminuria and a decline in GFR index were noticed. This study was subsequently analyzed after 7 years of follow-up, again with positive results that favored ACE inhibitors.[16]

New treatment strategies: microalbuminuria

The genesis of microalbuminuria is complex, being not only related to longstanding diabetes but also to blood pressure elevation, which is quite common in these patients. Loss of renal autoregulation may also be important due to lesions in the vasculature of the kidney; thus the systemic blood pressure may be transferred unhindered to the glomeruli.[40,41]

As with prevention, it is important to attain the best possible glycemic control in patients with microalbuminuria. However, antihypertensive therapy is a key feature of treatment in these patients, and blood pressure should probably be kept much lower in patients with microalbuminuria and overt renal disease, perhaps around 125/80 mmHg. Several studies show that ACE inhibitors or ARBs are effective in the treatment of these patients, although other agents may be used if antihypertensives do not achieve the desired goal.[42,43,51,84] Table 32.6 reviews results using ARBs in patients with microalbuminuric type

2 diabetes. An effect on insulin sensitivity as well as glomerular hemodynamics was recently observed with losartan.[52]

There are few reports of low-protein diets in diabetic patients. The studies so far performed are not positive in patients with type 2 diabetes.[53,54] While a low-protein diet may not be warranted, a low-sodium diet may be useful, especially if the patient does not respond to ordinary therapy. In some cases, restriction of sodium seems to be important in achieving the goal of antihypertensive treatment.[55]

There is little evidence that treatment of dyslipidemia protects renal function, and the few studies that do exist are somewhat conflicting. Obviously, treatment of hyperlipidemia is more important in the prevention of cardiac and vascular disease.

Cigarette smoking is also considered a risk factor and patients should be advised to stop smoking.[56]

Treatment in overt diabetic renal disease

The treatment strategy is essentially the same throughout the course of diabetic renal disease, from incipient to overt nephropathy. Two new important studies, the Renaal and Irbesartan trials, show that treatment with ARBs can postpone ESRD in proteinuric patients with type 2 diabetes.[57,58] Both studies showed that there is a considerable positive effect in these patients. However, prognosis unfortunately remains poor (Tables 32.7–32.9).

The Renaal study[57] showed a significant effect on all predefined endpoints considered together, namely ESRD, doubling of serum creatinine, and mortality. Mortality in itself was not significant, but mortality plus ESRD was positively affected by the treatment. This study may be a little more encouraging than the IDNT study,[58] although in principle the two studies, both of similar design, gave the same results. The IDNT study also included patients who were treated with a calcium channel blocker and

Table 32.6 Angiotensin receptor blockers: effects in patients with type 2 diabetes mellitus and microalbuminuria

Reference	No. of patients	Months	Drugs	Remarks
Muirhead et al[83]	122	12	Valsartan	Captopril also effective
Lacourcière et al[49]	92	12	Losartan	Enalapril also effective
Mogensen et al[42]	199	3	Candesartan	Lisinopril also effective. Dual blockade better
Esmatjes et al[47]	14	6	Losartan	TGFβ also reduced
Lozano et al[48]	422	6	Losartan	Open label
Parving et al[59]	590	104	Irbesartan	Dose–response
Viberti et al[60]	332	6	Valsartan	Amlodipine showed reduction in blood pressure but not microalbuminuria

TGF-β, transforming growth factor β.

Table 32.7 RENAAL and IDNT trials: comparison of cohort baseline characteristics

	RENAAL	IDNT
Age	60 ± 7.5 years	59 ± 8 years
Serum creatinine	1.9 ± 0.5 mg/dL	1.7 ± 0.6 mg/dL
Blood pressure	152/82 ± 19/10 mmHg	156/85 ± 18/11 mmHg
HbA$_{1c}$	8.5 ± 1.6% Urinary albumin/creatinine: 1867 ± 2701 mg/g (~ 3.9 g/24 h)	8.1 ± 1.7% Urinary protein excretion: 4.2 ± 4.1 g/24 h

Table 32.8 RENAAL and IDNT trials: comparison of racial characteristics

Race (%)	RENAAL* (n = 1513)	IDNT (n = 1715)
Caucasian	49	73
Hispanic	18	5
Asian	17	4
Black	15	14
Other	1	4

*More multiracial.

again the ARB was more successful in preventing or postponing the course of renal disease. The Renaal study also showed a beneficial effect of hospitalization for cardiac insufficiency, which is a noteworthy result.

Another study recently published, the IRMA-II trial,[59] showed that in patients with microalbuminuria irbesartan had a positive effect on reduction in albuminuria but did not prevent the fall in GFR since the study was too short for this purpose, as also seen in another trial.[60] From a theoretical point of view, it may be more advantageous to treat the patient with microalbuminuria early and perhaps even before the onset of microalbuminuria.[32,43,52] There is evidence to suggest that renal disease in diabetes is a self-perpetuating process, and with more advanced disease there may be less autoregulation and more transmission of systemic blood pressure to glomeruli.[40,41]

It is clear that antilipidemic treatment could also be important to these patients, although there is no clinical trial regarding renal endpoints. Obviously, any cardiovascular disease may well be positively affected by a lipid-lowering agent, especially statins. Further studies are needed in this area.

Evaluation before pharmacologic treatment

Before treatment, the following points need to be clarified.

1. What is the exact level of blood pressure at repeated measurement? Exact definition of blood pressure is important to avoid overtreatment. It is essential that a number of measurements of blood pressure over a period of time (e.g. 3–6 months) are done under relaxed circumstances, preferably by a nurse or technician. It is usually sufficient to measure multiple blood pressures in the sitting position. However, if autonomic neuropathy is suspected, blood pressure should also be measured in the supine as well as the standing position.

Table 32.9 RENAAL and IDNT trial results: comparison of primary endpoints and components

Components	Losartan vs. placebo (RR%)	Irbesartan vs. placebo (RR%)	Irbesartan vs. amlodipine (RR%)	Amlodipine vs. placebo (RR%)
Doubling of serum creatinine, ESRD, death	16 P = 0.024	20 P = 0.024	23 P = 0.006	−4 NS
Doubling of serum creatinine	25 P = 0.006	33 P = 0.003	37 P = 0.001	−6 NS
ESRD	28 P = 0.002	23 NS	23 NS	0 NS
Death	NS	NS	NS	NS
ESRD or death	20 P = 0.01	?	?	?

ESRD, endstage renal disease; NS, not significant; RR, risk reduction.[1]

2. What is the underlying cause of hypertension? Secondary causes should be excluded, preferably on the basis of a straightforward clinical and laboratory examination. From a clinical point of view, renal arterial stenosis is rare in patients under 70 years of age,[61] and monitoring of serum creatinine after intervention will reveal evidence of this abnormality. However, a slight increase in serum creatinine (about 10–15%) should be expected in patients without evidence of stenosis.

3. Are there contributory or modulating factors present, such as high salt intake, heavy smoking, alcohol intake, stressful situations, or an excessively sedentary lifestyle?

4. Is "white-coat hypertension" present? This can be excluded by 24-h AMBP on an outpatient basis. Usually blood pressure is not greatly elevated in diabetic patients, and therefore this procedure can be strongly recommended, especially when apparently high blood pressure is associated with normoalbuminuria.

5. What is the extent of damage to the eyes, heart, and peripheral vessels?

General measures should include encouraging weight loss, modifying smoking and dietary habits, reducing alcohol and salt intake, and altering a stressful lifestyle. Regular moderate exercise should be advised, and metabolism should be controlled in the best possible way. Long-term adherence to lifestyle modifications may be improved by contemporary patient diabetes education, which includes a special focus on hypertension.

Antihypertensive effect of diabetic diets

A modern diabetes diet, with low fat, high carbohydrate, moderately low protein, and reduced sodium content, has been shown to lower blood pressure in diabetic patients with moderate levels of hypertension.[62] A low-protein diet may be of some value in diabetic patients with incipient or overt nephropathy; this effect is related to the reduction in microalbuminuria and proteinuria but possibly not to the rate of decline in GFR.[63] Blood pressure is generally not changed by a low-protein diet but may fall, perhaps partly due to concomitant antihypertensive medication. Clarifying the specific effect of diet may therefore be difficult. The effect of diet in type 2 diabetes is limited or nonexistent. A low-salt diet seems to be beneficial.[55]

Pharmacologic treatment of hypertension in diabetes: advantages and disadvantages of the use of specific antihypertensive agents

Usually, it is possible to control hypertension in diabetic patients with relatively few agents; a simple conventional scheme of antihypertensive treatment with some modification should be used. Treatment is usually started with small or moderate doses of ACE inhibitors, but some may still prefer β-blockers or diuretics. Another alternative, especially for patients with NIDDM, may be calcium antagonists; certain calcium antagonists are highly preferable according to the experience of Bakris et al. Cardioselective β-blockers (compared with nonselective blockers) are strongly recommended if this class of drugs is preferred. Masking of hypoglycemia was found in propranolol-treated patients, and this drug should clearly be avoided. The relative safety of cardioselective β-blockers in diabetics, at least when used in moderate dosages, has been confirmed, although some patients on selective blockers still experience serious problems with unawareness of hypoglycemia. Therefore, it may be necessary to reduce the dosage or discontinue the drug. However, unawareness of hypoglycemia is not uncommon during the natural history of diabetes, even without β-blocker therapy. When diuretics are used in the treatment of diabetic patients, one should bear in mind the possible aggravation of metabolic control, particularly with NIDDM patients. This aggravation may relate to potassium loss (potentially counteracted by ACE inhibitors); therefore, serum potassium should be monitored frequently and regularly along with kidney function (serum creatinine). In overt diabetic nephropathy, loop diuretics (often in high dosages) are useful in eliminating edema as well as reducing blood pressure, even when GFR is almost normal. Diuretics are usually not administered as monotherapy but are quite often combined with other agents.

As discussed earlier, ACE inhibitors are likely to prove very useful in diabetics during long-term treatment. ACE inhibitors may be used as the main drug, often together with diuretics. The rationale for using ACE inhibitors are twofold: (1) they seem to be free of diabetes-related adverse effects; and (2) their administration is likely to reduce intraglomerular pressure, perhaps to a greater extent than the agents mentioned earlier. ACE inhibitors may be used in conjunction with cardioselective β-blockers and diuretics and also with certain calcium antagonists (see Table 32.3). A satisfactory reduction in blood pressure is usually possible with such a combination. ACE inhibitors are absolutely contraindicated in pregnancy and should be used with appropriate caution in women of childbearing age.

Table 32.4 provides an outline of the adverse effects that are specifically relevant for diabetic patients receiving antihypertensive treatment.

What is the optimal blood pressure during treatment in patients with IDDM?

The optimal blood pressure during antihypertensive treatment in patients with diabetic nephropathy is not clearly defined.[4,15,64] The smallest decline in renal function is found in the average patient aged about 40 years with blood pressure around 130/80 mmHg or less. This blood pressure is also easily obtainable during treatment in incipient diabetic nephropathy, before the decline in GFR has started. As a practical guideline it is therefore proposed that in relatively young patients (< 45 years of age), blood pressure during antihypertensive treatment should be reduced to 120–140/70–80 mmHg. The lower limit may depend on the dose or type of agent that the individual patient tolerates. No severe symptoms or complications due to low blood pressure are noted during clinical trials.

New approach using albuminuria to guide treatment

In most clinical trials on microalbuminuric patients, the inclusion criterion has been the finding of microalbuminuria in the absence of clear hypertension. This approach may also be used in the ordinary clinical situation, i.e. microalbuminuria or abnormal albuminuria is the main indication for antihypertensive treatment as indicated in recent algorithms[64] (Fig. 32.2). It is recommended that antihypertensive treatment be started when albuminuria is increasing. Several patients may stay microalbuminuric for a long time, when metabolic control is satisfactory and blood pressure is low. One advantage of using microalbuminuria as a guide for treatment is that this parameter is quite easy to record.

Final remarks

This chapter clearly documents that abnormal albuminuria, most often related to increased blood pressure, is associated with actual or subsequent organ damage, not only in the kidney but also other organs, especially the eyes and the heart. In the kidney, abnormal albuminuria,

initially in the microalbuminuric range, is a reflection of more advanced glomerular structural lesions, although the exact location of the permeability defect has not been defined at an ultrastructural level.[65] Blood pressure elevation may not initiate the glomerular permeability defect but high systemic blood pressure aggravates the course of established lesions. Transition from microalbuminuria to macroalbuminuria is associated with a reduction in GFR, the key parameter in evaluation of renal function.

Biochemical and hemodynamic hypotheses have been proposed and are supported by animal models. However, these ideas are difficult to substantiate in humans, where phenomena cannot be studied in isolation nor measured directly (e.g. glomerular wall charge and intraglomerular pressure). A unifying concept would be attractive,[1,8] linking biochemical aberrations (e.g. charge defects, changes in enzymatic activities and advanced glycation phenomena, growth factor and cytokine abnormalities, and activation of protein kinase C) to hemodynamic changes such as hyperfiltration with elevated glomerular pressure, aggravated by an early rise in systemic blood pressure. This may be seen together with vascular and endothelial changes, reflected by increases in von Willebrand factor, circulating prorenin, and increased transcapillary escape rate of albumin. A common pathway, based on the prolonged hyperglycemia and related molecular changes characteristic of the diabetic state, that explains all or most of these abnormalities should be investigated.[1,65–75]

References

1. Mogensen CE: Microalbuminuria, blood pressure and diabetic renal disease: origin and development of ideas. *In* Mogensen CE (ed): The Kidney and Hypertension in Diabetes Mellitus, 5th edn. Boston: Kluwer Academic Publishers, 2000, pp 655–706.

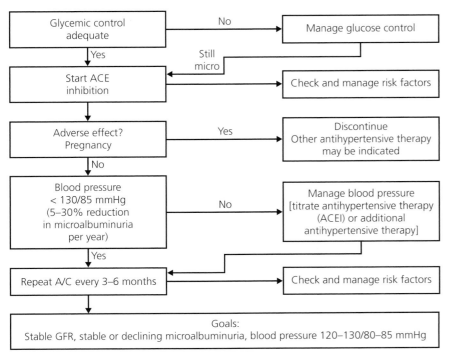

Figure 32.2 Algorithm for managing diabetes and microalbuminuria in diabetes (long-term poor control is the major risk factor for development of microalbuminuria). New studies suggest similar effects in the relatively young and lean NIDDM patients. A/C, albumin/creatinine ratio; ACE, angiotensin-converting enzyme; AHT, antihypertensive treatment; GFR, glomerular filtration rate.

2. Diabetes Control and Complication Trial Research Group: The effect of intensive treatment of diabetes on the development and progression of long-term complications in insulin-dependent diabetes mellitus. N Engl J Med 1993; 329:977–986.

3. Shichiri M, Ohkubo Y, Kishikawa H, et al: Long-term results of the Kumamoto study on optimal diabetes control in type 2 diabetic patients. Diabetes Care 2000;23(Suppl 2):B21–B29.

4. Mogensen CE: Combined high blood pressure and glucose in type 2 diabetes: double jeopardy. British trials shows clear effects of treatment, especially blood pressure reduction. Br Med J 1998;317:693–694.

5. Ewart RM: The case against aggressive treatment of type 2 diabetes: critique of the UK prospective diabetes study. Br Med J 2001;323:854–858.

6. Jones S, Nyengaard JR: Birth, Barker and Brenner: the concept of low birth weight and renal disease. In Mogensen CE (ed): The Kidney and Hypertension in Diabetes Mellitus, 5th edn. Boston: Kluwer Academic Publishers, 2000, pp 129–140.

7. Bain SC, Chowdhury TA: Genetics of diabetic nephropathy and microalbuminuria. J R Soc Med 2000;93:62–66.

8. Cooper ME: Pathogenesis, prevention and treatment of diabetic nephropathy. Lancet 1998;352:213–219.

9. Progress Collaborative Group: Randomised trial of perindopril-based blood-pressure-lowering regimen among 6105 individuals with previous stroke or transient ischaemic attack. Lancet 2001;358:1033–1041.

10. Reaven GM, Lithell H, Landsberg L: Hypertension and associated metabolic abnormalities: the role of insulin resistance and the sympathoadrenal system. N Engl J Med 1996;334:374–382.

11. Ritz E, Rychlik I: Diabetic nephropathy: the size of the problem. In Hasslacher C (ed): Diabetic Nephropathy. Chichester: John Wiley & Sons, 2001, pp 3–18.

12. Hostetter TH: Prevention of end-stage renal disease due to type 2 diabetes. N Engl J Med 2001;345:910–912.

13. Olsen S, Mogensen CE: How often is type II diabetes mellitus complicated with non-diabetic renal disease? A material of renal biopsies and an analysis of the literature. Diabetologia 1996;39:1638–1645.

14. The Diabetes Control and Complications Trial/Epidemiology of Diabetes Interventions and Complications Research Group: Retinopathy and nephropathy in patients with type 1 diabetes four years after a trial of intensive therapy. N Engl J Med 2000;342:381–389.

15. The ACE Inhibitors in Diabetic Nephropathy Trialist Group: Should all patients with type 1 diabetes mellitus and microalbuminuria receive angiotensin-converting enzyme inhibitors? A meta-analysis of individual patient data. Ann Intern Med 2001;134:370–379.

16. Ravid M, Lang R, Rachmani R, et al: Long-term renoprotective effect of angiotensin-converting enzyme inhibition in non-insulin-dependent diabetes mellitus: a 7-year follow-up study. Arch Intern Med 1996;156:286–289.

17. Hansen KW, Poulsen PL, Ebbehoj E: Blood pressure elevation in diabetes: the results from 24-h ambulatory blood pressure recordings. In Mogensen CE (ed): The Kidney and Hypertension in Diabetes Mellitus, 5th edn. Boston: Kluwer Academic Publishers, 2000, pp 339–362.

18. Osterby R: Lessons from kidney biopsies. Diabetes Metab Rev 1996;12:151–174.

19. Fioretto P, Mauer M, Brocco E, et al: Patterns of renal injury in type 2 (non insulin-dependent) diabetic patients with microalbuminuria. Diabetologia 1996;39:1569–1576.

20. Chaturvedi N, Fuller JH: Retinopathy in relation to albuminuria and blood pressure in IDDM. In Mogensen CE (ed): The Kidney and Hypertension in Diabetes Mellitus, 5th edn. Boston: Kluwer Academic Publishers, 2000, pp 29–38.

21. Grundy SM, Benjamin IJ, Burke GL, et al: Diabetes and cardiovascular disease. A statement for healthcare professionals from the American Heart Association. Circulation 1999;100:1134–1146.

22. Mogensen CE, Damsgaard EM, Froland A, et al: Reduced glomerular filtration rate and cardiovascular damage in diabetes: a key role for abnormal albuminuria. Acta Diabetol 1992;29:201–213.

23. Mogensen CE: The kidney in diabetes: how to control renal and related cardiovascular complications. Am J Kidney Dis 2001;37(Suppl 2):S2–S6.

24. Mogensen CE, Hansen KW, Nielsen S, et al: Monitoring diabetic nephropathy. Glomerular filtration rate and abnormal albuminuria in diabetic renal disease: reproducibility, progression, and efficacy of antihypertensive intervention. Am J Kidney Dis 1993;22:174–187.

25. Zuanetti G, Latini R, Maggioni A: The heart in diabetes: results of trial. In Mogensen CE (ed): The Kidney and Hypertension in Diabetes Mellitus, 5th edn. Boston: Kluwer Academic Publishers, 2000, pp 55–66.

26. Kennedy J, Mogensen CE, Ball SG, et al: What is the relevance of the HOPE study in general practice? Int J Clin Pract 2001;55:449–457.

27. Heart Outcomes Prevention Evaluation (HOPE) Study Investigators: Effects of ramipril on cardiovascular and microvascular outcomes in people with diabetes mellitus: results of the HOPE study and the MICROHOPE substudy. Lancet 2000;355:253–259.

28. Andersen NH, Mogensen CE: Inihibtion of the renin–angiotensin system with particular reference to dual blockade treatment. J Renin Angiotensin Aldosterone Syst 2001;2:146–152.

29. Parving H-H: Diabetic nephropathy: prevention and treatment. Kidney Int 2001;60:2041–2055.

30. Hovind P, Rossing P, Tarnow L, et al: Progression of diabetic nephropathy. Kidney Int 2001;59:702–709.

31. Euclid Study Group: Randomised placebo-controlled trial of lisinopril in normotensive patients with insulin-dependent diabetes and normoalbuminuria or microalbuminuria. Lancet 1997;349:1787–1792.

32. Kvetny J, Gregersen G, Pedersen RS: Randomized placebo-controlled trial of perindopril in normotensive, normoalbuminuric patients with type 1 diabetes mellitus. Q J Med 2001;94:89–94.

33. Marre M, Hadjadj S, Bouhanick B: The concept of incipient diabetic nephropathy and effect of early antihypertensive intervention. In Mogensen CE (ed): The Kidney and Hypertension in Diabetes Mellitus, 5th edn. Boston: Kluwer Academic Publishers, 2000, pp 423–434.

34. Cooper ME, McNally PG, Boner G: Antihypertensive treatment in NIDDM, with special reference to abnormal albuminuria. In Mogensen CE (ed): The Kidney and Hypertension in Diabetes Mellitus, 5th edn. Boston: Kluwer Academic Publishers, 2000, pp 441–460.

35. Christensen CK, Mogensen CE: Effect of antihypertensive treatment on progression of incipient diabetic nephropathy. Hypertension 1985;7(Suppl II):109–113.

36. Mogensen CE: Nephropathy: early. In Devlin JT, Schneider SH (eds): Handbook of Exercise in Diabetes. Alexandria, VA: American Diabetes Association, 2001, pp 433–449.

37. Mogensen CE: Long-term antihypertensive treatment inhibiting progression of diabetic nephropathy. Br Med J 1982;285:685–688.

38. Parving H-H, Andersen AR, Smidt UM, et al: Effect of antihypertensive treatment on kidney function in diabetic nephropathy. Br Med J 1987;294:1443–1447.

39. Lewis EJ, Hunsicker LG, Bain RP, et al: The effect of angiotensin converting enzyme inhibition on diabetic nephropathy. N Engl J Med 1993;329:1456–1462.

40. Christensen CK, Lund S, Parving H-H: Autoregulated glomerular filtration rate during candesartan treatment in hypertensive type 2 diabetic patients. Kidney Int 2001;60:1435–1442.

41. Christensen PK, Hansen HP, Parving H-H: Impaired autoregulation of GFR in hypertensive non-insulin dependent diabetic patients. Kidney Int 1997;52:1369–1374.

42. Mogensen CE, Neldam S, Tikkanen I, et al for the CALM study group: Randomised controlled trial of dual blockade of renin angiotensin system in patients with hypertension, microalbuminuria, and non-insulin-dependent diabetes: the candesartan and lisinopril microalbuminuria (CALM) study. Br Med J 2000;321:1440–1444.

43. Ravid M, Brosh D, Levi Z, et al: Use of enalapril to attenuate decline in renal function in normotensive, normoalbuminuric patients with type 2 diabetes mellitus. A randomized controlled trial. Ann Intern Med 1998;128:982–988.

44. Mogensen CE: Intervention strategies for microalbuminuria: the role of angiotensin II antagonists, including dual blockade with ACE-I and a receptor blocker. J Renin Angiotensin Aldosterone Syst 2000;1:63–67.

45. Parving H-H, Hovind P, Rossing K, et al: Evolving strategies for renoprotection: diabetic nephropathy. Curr Opin Nephrol Hypertens 2001;10:515–523.

46. De Pablos PL, Martin FJM: Effects of losartan and diltiazem on blood pressure, insulin sensitivity, lipid profile and microalbuminuria in hypertensive type 2 diabetic patients. Clin Drug Invest 1998;16:361–370.

47. Esmatjes E, Flores L, Inigo P et al: Effect of losartan on TGFβ1 and urinary albumin excretion in patients with type 2 diabetes mellitus and microalbuminuria. Nephrol Dial Transplant 2001;16(Suppl 1):90–93.

48. Lozano JV, Llisterri JL, Aznar J, et al: Losartan reduces microalbuminuria in hypertensive microalbuminuric type 2 diabetics. Nephrol Dial Transplant 2001;16(Suppl 1):85–89.

49. Lacourcière Y, Bélanger A, Godin C, et al: Long-term comparison of losartan and enalapril on kidney function in hypertensive type 2 diabetics with early nephropathy. Kidney Int 2000;58:762–769.

50. Chan JCN, Critchley JAJH, Tomlinson BM, et al: Antihypertensive and anti-albuminuric effects of losartan potassium and felodipine in Chinese elderly hypertensive patients with or without non-insulin-dependent diabetes mellitus. Am J Nephrol 1997;17:72–80.

51. Mann JFE. Gerstein HC, Pogue J, et al for the HOPE investigators: Renal insufficiency as a predictor of cardiovascular outcomes and the impact of ramipril: the HOPE Randomized Trial. Ann Intern Med 2001;134:629–636.

52. Nielsen S, Hove KY, Dollerup J, et al: Losartan modifies glomerular hyperfiltration and insulin sensitivity in type 1 diabetes. Diabetes Obesity Metab 2001;3:1–9.

53. Hermansen K: Diet, blood pressure and hypertension. Br J Nutr 2000;83(Suppl 1): S113–S119.

54. Pijls LTJ, de Vries H, Donker AJ, et al: The effect of protein restriction on albuminuria in patients with type 2 diabetes mellitus: a randomised trial. Nephrol Dial Transplant 1999;14:1445–1453.

55. Dodson PM, Beevers M, Hallworth R: Sodium restriction and blood pressure in hypertensive type 2 diabetics: randomised blind controlled and crossover studies of moderate sodium restriction and sodium supplementation. Br Med J 1989;298:227–230.

56. Orth SR, Ritz E, Schrier RW: The renal risks of smoking. Kidney Int 1997;51:1669–1677.

57. Brenner BM, Cooper ME, de Zeeuw D, et al for the Reduction of End-points in NIDDM with the Angiotensin II Antagonist Losartan (Renaal) Study Investigators: Effects of losartan on renal and cardiovascular outcomes in patients with type 2 diabetes and nephropathy. N Engl J Med 2001;345:861–870.

58. Lewis EJ, Hunsicker LG, Clarke WR, et al: Renoprotective effect of the angiotensin-receptor antagonist irbesartan in patients with nephropathy due to type 2 diabetes. N Engl J Med 2001;345:851–861.

59. Parving H-H, Lehnert H, Brochner-Mortensen J, et al: The effect of irbesartan on the development of diabetic nephropathy in patients with type 2 diabetes. N Engl J Med 2001;345:870–879.

60. Viberti G, Wheeldon NM, Microalbuminuria Reduction with VALsartan (MARVAL) Study Investigators: Microalbuminuria reduction with valsartan in patients with type 2 diabetes mellitus: a blood pressure-independent effect. Circulation 2002;106:672–678.

61. Williams B: Addendum regarding renovascular hypertension and renal artery stenosis (especially NIDDM). In Mogensen CE (ed): The Kidney and Hypertension in Diabetes Mellitus, 5th edn. Boston: Kluwer Academic Publishers, 2000, pp 458–459.

62. Dodson PM, Pacy PJ, Bal P, et al: A controlled trial of a high fibre, low fat and low sodium diet for mild hypertension in type 2 (non-insulin-dependent) diabetic patients. Diabetologia 1984;27:522–526.

63. Hansen HP, Tauber-Lassen E, Jensen BR, et al: Effect of protein restriction on prognosis in type 1 diabetic patients with diabetic nephropathy. Kidney Int 2002;62:220–228.

64. Mogensen CE, Keane WF, Bennet PH, et al: Prevention of diabetic renal disease with special reference to microalbuminuria. Lancet 1995;346:1080–1084.

65. Mogensen CE: The early detection of renal impairment in diabetes mellitus. The case for microalbuminuria and other biomarkers. In Trull AK, Price CP (eds): Biomarkers of Disease. Cambridge: Cambridge University Press, 2001, p 76.

66. McGowan T, McCue P, Sharma K: Diabetic nephropathy. Clin Lab Med 2001;21:111–146.

67. Tryggvason K, Wartiovaara J: Molecular basis of glomerular permselectivity. Curr Opin Nephrol Hypertens 2001;10:543–549.

68. Menè P, Festuccia F, Polci R, et al: Diabetic nephropathy and advanced glycation end products. Contrib Nephrol 2001;131:22–32.

69. Gambaro G, Van der Woude FJ: Glycosaminoglycans: use in treatment of diabetic nephropathy. J Am Soc Nephrol 2000;11:359–368.

70. Trevisan R, Viberti GC: Sodium-hydrogen antiporter: its possible role in the genesis of diabetic nephropathy. Nephrol Dial Transplant 1997;12:643–645.

71. Deinum J, Ronn B, Mathiesen E, et al: Increase in serum prorenin precedes onset of microalbuminuria in patients with insulin-dependent diabetes mellitus. Diabetologia 1999;42:1006–1010.

72. Greaves M, Malia RG, Goodfellow K, et al: Fibrinogen and von Willebrand factor in IDDM: relationships to lipid vascular risk factors, blood pressure, glycemic control and urinary albumin excretion rate. The EURODIAB IDDM Complications study. Diabetologia 1997;40:698–705.

73. Hofmann MA, Kohl B, Zumbach MS, et al: Hyperhomocyst(e)inemia and endothelial dysfunction in IDDM. Diabetes Care 1998;21:841–848.

74. Jager A, Kostense PJ, Nijpels G, et al: Microalbuminuria is strongly associated with NIDDM and hypertension but not with the insulin resistance syndrome: the Hoorn Study. Diabetologia 1998;41:694–700.

75. Flyvbjerg A: An update of the role of growth factors in the development of diabetic kidney disease. In Mogensen CE (ed): The Kidney and Hypertension in Diabetes Mellitus, 5th edn. Boston: Kluwer Academic Publishers, 2000, pp 295–312.

76. Weir MR, Weber MA, Neutel JM, et al: Efficacy of candesartan cilexetil as add-on therapy in hypertensive patients uncontrolled on background therapy: a clinical experience trial. ACTION Study Investigators. Am J Hypertens 2001;14:567–572.

77. Azizi M, Chatellier G, Guyene TT, et al: Additive effects of combined angiotensin-converting enzyme inhibition and angiotensin II antagonism on blood pressure and renin release in sodium-depleted normotensives. Circulation 1995;92:825–834.

78. Kincaid-Smith PS, Fairley KF, Packham DK: Effects on blood pressure, proteinuria and renal function of adding an angiotensin receptor antagonist (candesartab 8 mgs) to an ACE inhibitor in normotensive patients with renal disease. J Renin Angiotensin Aldosterone Syst 2001;2:50.

79. Rossing K, Christensen PK, Jensen BR, et al: Dual blockade of the renin-angiotensin system in diabetic nephropathy: a randomized double-blind crossover study. Diabetes Care 2002;25:95–100.

80. McKelvie RS, Yusuf S, Pericak D, et al: Comparison of Candesartan, Enalapril and their Combination in Congestive Heart Failure Randomized Evaluation of Strategies for Left Ventricular Dysfunction (RESOLVD) Pilot study. Circulation 1999;100:1056–1064.

81. Ruilope LM, Aldigier JC, Ponticelli C, et al: Safety of the combination of valsartan and benazepril in patients with chronic renal disease. European Group for the Investigation of Valsartan in Chronic Renal Disease. J Hypertens 2000;18:89–95.

82. Baruch L, Anand I, Cohen IS, et al for the Vasodilator Heart Failure Trial (V-HeFT) Study Group: Augmented short- and long-term hemodynamic and hormonal effects of an angiotensin receptor blocker added to angiotensin converting enzyme inhibitor therapy in patients with heart failure. Circulation 1999;99:2658–2664.

83. Muirhead N, Feagan BF, Mahon J, et al: The effects of valsartan and captopril on reducing microalbuminuria in patients with type 2 diabetes mellitus: a placebo-controlled trial. Curr Ther Res 1999;60:650–660.

84. Andersen NH, Mogensen CE: ACE inhibitors and angiotensin II receptor blockers: evidence for and against the combination in the treatment of hypertension and proteinuria. Curr Hypertens Rep 2002;4:394–402.

CHAPTER 33

Management of the Diabetic with Advanced and Endstage Renal Disease

David C. Wheeler

Despite the major advances in the prevention of diabetic nephropathy described in Chapter 32, diabetes mellitus has become the most important cause of endstage renal failure in industrialized countries, with approximately 90% of patients presenting with type 2 disease.[1] While the survival of diabetic patients with uremia has been greatly improved by the widespread availability of dialysis and renal transplantation, these individuals experience considerably higher morbidity and mortality than nondiabetics with endstage renal failure.[1] This is largely due to the high prevalence of extrarenal complications of diabetes (Table 33.1). As a consequence, many diabetics receiving renal replacement therapy are disabled as a result of visual impairment, limb amputation, angina, hemiparesis, and intractable gastrointestinal symptoms. Although the outlook for these patients is poor, much can be done from a therapeutic standpoint to improve outcomes. Therapy should be focused on slowing the progression of chronic renal failure (see Chapter 32), treating nonrenal complications of diabetes (Table 33.1) and of uremia, reducing the risk of cardiovascular disease, and preparing the patient for renal replacement therapy. Cooperation between primary care physicians, diabetologists, ophthalmologists, cardiologists, chiropodists, and nephrologists is in the interests of these patients and should help to optimize outcomes.

Management of progressive renal failure

The clinician should be sure of the nature of the kidney disease since a small proportion of diabetic patients will develop renal failure due to causes other than diabetes and may require specific therapy for these other conditions.[2] Assuming that the patient has diabetic nephropathy, if left untreated the rate of decline of renal function (measured as glomerular filtration rate, GFR) is likely to be 1 mL/min/month, making the interval between onset of nephropathy and endstage renal failure about 7 years.[3] The best practical approach for monitoring renal failure is to use a calculated GFR measurement, which can be derived from an equation such as the Cockcroft–Gault formula and which takes into account the patient's age, sex, and weight:[4]

creatinine clearance (mL/min) =

$$\frac{(140 - \text{age}) \times (\text{wt in kg})}{72 \times \text{serum creatinine (mg/dL)}} \times 0.85 \text{ if female}$$

or

$$= 1.2 \times \frac{(140 - \text{age}) \times (\text{wt in kg})}{\text{serum creatinine } (\mu\text{mol/L})} \times 0.85 \text{ if female}$$

Patients with diabetic nephropathy may develop acute and occasionally reversible declines in renal function. This may occur as a result of intercurrent urinary tract infection, which should be treated promptly with appropriate antibiotics, or contrast nephropathy, which can be largely prevented by prior intravenous hydration (see Chapter 5). Other causes for acute-on-chronic renal failure include prescription of angiotensin-converting enzyme (ACE) inhibitors or angiotensin II receptor antagonists to patients with renovascular disease or administration of nephrotoxic agents such as nonsteroidal anti-inflammatory drugs.

Table 33.1 Complications of diabetes associated with endstage renal failure

Retinopathy, cataracts, glaucoma
Sensory and motor neuropathy
Autonomic neuropathy
Myopathy
Atherosclerotic vascular disease
Cardiac failure
Depression

Glycemic control in advanced renal failure

Clear evidence from clinical studies demonstrates that strict control of glycemia slows the development of microvascular complications associated with diabetes (see Chapter 32). Since the kidneys, along with the liver and peripheral tissues, are responsible for the breakdown of insulin, renal failure leads to a reduced insulin requirement.[5] This is offset to a degree by the development of insulin resistance in association with uremia. Oral hypoglycemic agents should be used with extreme caution in patients with impaired renal function.[6] All sulfonylureas are partially excreted by the kidney and accumulate in renal failure, increasing the risk of hypoglycemia. Short-acting compounds (such as tolbutamide) and those predominantly excreted by the liver (gliquidone and gliclazide) should be used in the lowest recommended doses in patients with mild renal impairment and should be discontinued if possible once GFR falls below 10 mL/min. Similar problems occur with biguanides, which are contraindicated in patients with a GFR below 50 mL/min because of an increased risk of lactic acidosis. Early experience with the thiazolidinediones, which should be used in combination with other oral hypoglycemic agents, suggests that dose reductions may not be required in patients with impaired renal function, although the manufacturers recommend that rosiglitazone should be avoided in patients with severe renal impairment. Any diabetic with renal impairment undergoing an interventional procedure or developing a severe intercurrent illness will require temporary conversion to insulin.

Monitoring of glycemic control in patients with renal failure is complicated by carbamylation of hemoglobin, which leads to spurious elevation of hemoglobin A_{1c} concentrations.[7] Serum fructosamine concentrations can be used as an alternative, but are not a valid monitor of diabetic control if serum albumin levels fall below normal.[8]

Treatment of other diabetic complications

As nephropathy is a manifestation of diabetic microvascular disease, it is not surprising that other extrarenal complications are more common in diabetics with diabetic kidney disease than in those without (Table 33.1). As patients progress toward endstage renal failure and commence dialysis or receive organ transplants, the control of diabetes and management of these complications must remain a priority.

Retinopathy

The majority of diabetic patients commencing dialysis will have already needed laser treatment with or without vitrectomy and will require ongoing ophthalmologic review at least annually when on renal replacement therapy. Optimal management of diabetic eye disease includes tight control of blood pressure and glycemia along with early retinal photocoagulation to eradicate ischemic areas.[9] An active renin–angiotensin system has been demonstrated in the retina, suggesting a specific therapeutic role for ACE inhibitors or angiotensin II receptor antagonists.[10] These drugs should be started at the lowest recommended doses in patients with impaired renal function, and serum creatinine rechecked after 7–10 days in those who have not commenced dialysis. The use of aldose reductase inhibitors has not been supported by controlled clinical trials.[9] With improvements in the management of retinopathy, repeated heparinization during hemodialysis does not appear to have a major adverse impact on visual acuity.

Neuropathy

Neuropathy involves both sensorimotor and autonomic nerves and usually presents with loss of pain, temperature, vibration, and fine touch sensation in the feet in a "stocking" distribution.[11] Many patients develop rest pain, which may be helped by the prescription of carbamazepine. Although the manufacturers of this drug advise that it should be used with caution in patients with renal impairment, there is little evidence of increased toxicity. Autonomic neuropathy frequently leads to gastroparesis, which causes symptoms of nausea and vomiting; disturbances in bowel habit, with constipation or intermittent explosive nocturnal diarrhea; and cytopathy with impaired bladder emptying, which increases the risk of urinary tract infection. Treatment of these complications is generally unsatisfactory. Although nausea and vomiting may be improved by prescription of metoclopramide, this drug is not recommended for use in patients with renal failure unless there are compelling reasons.

The diabetic foot

Foot problems in diabetic patients result from neuropathy compounded by a poor blood supply due to peripheral vascular disease.[12] Diabetic patients should be trained to care for their feet, should wear appropriate footwear, should be instructed on how to manage minor foot lesions, and should receive regular chiropody. Ulcers are traditionally managed by immobilization but may heal if weight bearing is redistributed using a plaster cast. Infection should be treated with appropriate antibiotics (following bacterial culture) and radiographs taken if there is any suspicion of underlying osteomyelitis. Surgical debridement is often required, while vascular lesions may be amenable to angioplasty or bypass grafting. Extensive areas of necrosis must receive prompt surgical attention and frequently lead to amputation.

Treatment of uremic complications

Patients with advanced renal failure, including those with diabetic nephropathy, should be fully assessed for complications of uremia. These include dyslipidemia (Chapter 67), malnutrition (Chapter 70), anemia (Chapter 71), and abnormalities of calcium and phosphate metabolism (Chapter 73). Early management of such complications is likely to delay the onset of comorbid conditions such as bone disease and cardiovascular complications (see below). It should be stressed that metabolic and endocrine abnormalities associated with uremia develop when GFR falls below 60 mL/min, often long before patients are referred to a nephrologist.

Prevention of cardiovascular disease

Premature cardiovascular disease is a recognized complication of both chronic renal failure and diabetes, and patients with both diseases comprise a group at very high risk. Even before the development of advanced nephropathy, diabetic men have a three times and diabetic women a six times greater risk of cardiovascular mortality than nondiabetic individuals.[13] The risk of cardiovascular disease in the diabetic patient rises with the level of urinary albumin/protein excretion at all levels of proteinuria.[14] Thus efforts to prolong the lifespan of a diabetic patient should include the correction of reversible cardiovascular risk factors. Table 33.2 lists the randomized controlled trials designed to assess the impact of risk factor management on cardiovascular outcomes that have included diabetics or diabetic subgroups.

Hypertension

Hypertension is commonly associated with diabetes, particularly once patients develop nephropathy,[15] and there is now good evidence that control of blood pressure reduces the risk of complications. For example, in a subset of patients recruited to the UK Prospective Diabetes Study, those randomized to tight blood pressure control were less likely to suffer a stroke than those with less well controlled hypertension.[16] Similar results were obtained among diabetic patients recruited into the Hypertension Optimal Treatment study.[17] Most guidelines set targets of 140/80 mmHg, although there is still debate as to whether a lower threshold for benefit exists. Patients are likely to require more than one antihypertensive agent and any regimen should include an ACE inhibitor or angiotensin II receptor antagonist, particularly if patients have not yet reached endstage renal disease. Importantly, results obtained among diabetic patients recruited into the Heart Outcomes Prevention Evaluation (the MICRO-HOPE study) suggest that compared with placebo, treatment with the ACE inhibitor ramipril was associated with reductions in stroke, myocardial infarction, and all-cause mortality in diabetic patients despite similar levels of blood pressure control.[18]

Dyslipidemia

The pattern of dyslipidemia in diabetes and chronic renal failure is essentially similar and characterized by hypertriglyceridemia, reduced high-density lipoprotein

Table 33.2 Trials of cardiovascular risk factor management in diabetic patients

Intervention	Trial	Population	No. of patients	Conclusions	Reference
Glycemic control	UKPDS	Type 2 diabetic patients	3867	Intensive glycemic control reduced risk of microvascular but not macrovascular disease	25
Blood pressure control	UKPDS	Hypertensive type 2 diabetic patients	1148	Tight blood pressure control reduced risk of stroke	16
	HOT	Hypertensive diabetic patients	1501 (subgroup)	Tighter blood pressure control reduced risk of cardiovascular events	17
Statin therapy	4S	Diabetes, IHD, and high cholesterol	202 (subgroup)	Statin reduced risk of a recurrent IHD event	21
	CARE	Diabetes*, IHD, and average cholesterol	586 (subgroup)	Statin reduced risk of a recurrent IHD event	22
ACE inhibition	MICRO-HOPE	Type 2 diabetes with one additional cardiovascular risk factor	3654	Ramipril reduced risk of combined endpoint (myocardial infarction, stroke, cardiovascular death) vs. placebo	18
Aspirin	HOT	Hypertensive diabetic patients	1501 (subgroup)	Asprin reduced major cardiovascular events	17

ACE, angiotensin-converting enzyme; CARE, Cholesterol And Recurrent Events; HOPE, Heart Outcomes Prevention Evaluation; HOT, Hypertension Optimal Treatment; IHD, ischemic heart disease; 4S, Scandinavian Simvastatin Survival Study; UKPDS, United Kingdom Prospective Diabetes Study.
*Includes patients with glucose intolerance.

(HDL), and a shift of low-density lipoprotein (LDL) to the smaller denser subclasses thought to be more highly atherogenic.[19] Hypercholesterolemia is a less common feature, although at a given plasma cholesterol level a diabetic patient is at greater risk of a cardiovascular event than a nondiabetic.[20] Subgroup analysis of diabetic patients included in trials of statin therapy suggest that the benefits are comparable to those observed in nondiabetic individuals.[21,22] Since patients with renal failure have generally been excluded from these trials, safety data are lacking and these agents should be started at lowest recommended doses and used with caution. While fibrates may be a more logical choice for patients with hyper-triglyceridemia, the results of clinical trials, some of which have included diabetics, have been conflicting and risks of muscle injury are increased in renal impairment.[23] Studies specifically designed to assess the benefits of lipid-lowering therapy in diabetic patients with nephropathy are ongoing, but in the mean time statins are probably the safer class of drug to use. Although the National Cholesterol Education Program Adult Treatment Panel III guidelines recommend a target LDL cholesterol goal of 100 mg/dL (2.6 mmol/L) in patients with diabetes, whether this can be safely achieved in those with nephropathy is not yet clear.

Other cardioprotective therapies

While tight glycemic control has been shown to delay microvascular complications of diabetes and is therefore a desirable treatment goal, there has been no proven benefit in terms of macrovascular complications.[24,25] Available evidence, although limited, suggests that aspirin prevents cardiovascular events among diabetic individuals and that β-blockers should be used for secondary prevention, despite concerns about their ability to mask symptoms of hypoglycemia.[26,27] Antioxidant vitamins were not shown to prevent cardiovascular events in either diabetic or nondiabetic patients in the HOPE study.[18]

Options for renal replacement therapy

The options for patients with advanced diabetic nephropathy requiring renal replacement therapy are given in Table 33.3. No prospective trials have assessed outcomes in patients randomized to these treatment modalities and so all reported comparisons lack balanced treatment groups. In general, younger patients tend to be listed for renal transplantation, while older individuals with a greater burden of comorbid illness receive hemodialysis. To overcome such biases when assessing outcomes, investigators have attempted to match patients who have received kidney transplants with controls on dialysis. Such comparisons indicate that the mortality of diabetics on renal replacement therapy is at least twice that of the total dialysis population[28] and that patients who have had a transplant do better than those remaining on dialysis.[29] However, careful patient selection is likely to

Table 33.3 Options for renal replacement therapy in diabetic patients

Conservative therapy	Erythropoietin, palliative care
Peritoneal dialysis	Continuous ambulatory peritoneal dialysis
	Automated peritoneal dialysis
Hemodialysis	Facility-based hemodialysis
	Home hemodialysis
Organ transplantation	Renal transplantation
	Combined renal and pancreas transplantation (type 1)
	Islet-cell transplantation (type 1)

influence such results and to bias any nonrandomized studies.

Preparation for renal replacement therapy should begin early, ideally when calculated GFR drops below 30 mL/min. Factors that should be considered when planning the mode of dialysis treatment include age, severity of comorbidity, availability of resources, level of social support, and patient preference. In some cases, the clinician may recommend conservative therapy to the patient and their family.

Hemodialysis

Most diabetic patients treated in countries with well-developed healthcare systems will be offered hemodialysis (Chapter 81). Placement of temporary central venous lines for vascular access carries a risk of disseminated infection and an internal arteriovenous fistula should be created whenever possible and allowed to mature (for approximately 8 weeks) before use. This operation is generally thought to be more difficult in diabetics due to the presence of vascular disease, and higher rates of failure and digital ischemia have been reported.[30] Thus many diabetic patients will require prosthetic vascular grafts or will be managed in the longer term using central venous catheters, tunneled to minimize infection risk. Coexisting left ventricular disease and autonomic neuropathy contribute to intradialytic hypotension and arrythmias and increase the risk of cardiac death.[31]

Peritoneal dialysis

Motivated diabetic patients with good manual dexterity who wish to maintain some independence may initially choose continuous ambulatory peritoneal dialysis or automated peritoneal dialysis (Chapter 85). Peritoneal dialysis does not require vascular access, avoids the rapid fluid shifts associated with hemodialysis, and may be preferable in patients with severe cardiovascular instability and vascular disease. However, although blind patients can learn the technique, the majority of elderly type 2 diabetics will struggle to perform their exchanges and success rates are lower than among nondiabetics of similar

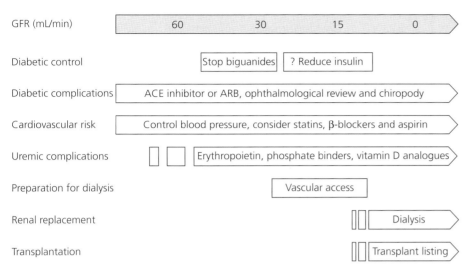

Figure 33.1 Management algorithm for the patient with advanced and endstage diabetic nephropathy. Treatment priorities at various levels of renal function are based on calculated glomerular filtration rate (GFR). Arrowheads depict the need for ongoing intervention once the patients are established on renal replacement therapy. ACE, angiotensin-converting enzyme; ARB, angiotensin II receptor antagonist.

age, usually due to recurrent peritonitis.[32] The intraperitoneal administration of insulin to diabetics on peritoneal dialysis has proved unpopular due to the risks of infection and hypoglycemia. Solutions based on amino acids, while having potential advantages, have not been widely adopted.

Kidney and pancreas transplantation

Because of improvements in quality of life and survival, renal transplantation is considered the optimal therapy for those patients with diabetic nephropathy who are fit enough to safely undergo surgery and to receive immunosuppressive therapy thereafter.[29] The use of live related or unrelated donors is becoming increasingly popular and is associated with better graft survival compared with cadaveric kidney donation.[33] Selection of patients for transplant waiting lists should take into account other comorbidities, particularly cardiovascular disease. Many centers now routinely perform coronary angiography on such patients before listing and can expect to find disease amenable to intervention in a high proportion.[34] Recommendations for screening methods have recently been published by the American Society of Transplantation and are discussed in Chapter 89.[35] Even with careful selection, diabetic patients are more prone to operative complications and at higher risk of mortality from cardiovascular disease in the post-transplant period.[36] All immunosuppressive drugs in routine clinical use are suitable for diabetics and there is no universally accepted regimen. Diabetic control needs to be closely monitored during the postoperative period and additional insulin may be required to cover treatment of acute rejection with high-dose steroids.

The place for whole-pancreas or islet-cell transplantation in type 1 diabetic patients receiving a kidney is still controversial and is not usually considered an option for those with type 2 disease. Combining whole-pancreas with kidney transplantation increases postoperative morbidity[37] but, if successful, can free the patient from dietary restrictions and insulin therapy, stabilize other diabetic complications such as neuropathy, and may prevent recurrence of diabetic nephropathy.[38] The problem of diverting exocrine secretions is now usually overcome by enteric drainage, although some surgeons favor bladder drainage thereby allowing assessment of pancreatic function by monitoring of urinary amylase concentrations.

Interest in islet-cell transplantation, first used in the 1970s, has recently been revived followed publication of promising results from a single center in Canada.[39] This group have refined their isolation techniques, use at least two donors per recipient, and have abandoned steroids and cyclosporine in their immunosuppressive regimen. A multicenter trial is underway to assess whether others can reproduce such results and, at present, islet-cell transplantation must still be regarded as an experimental therapy.

Conclusions

The management of the diabetic patient with advanced and endstage kidney failure provides a major challenge for healthcare professionals and demands a multidisciplinary approach. Efforts to improve the quality of life of these unfortunate individuals and to reduce mortality must include correction of cardiovascular risk factors, ongoing management of the extrarenal complications of diabetes and uremia, and early preparation for renal replacement therapy. Patients who are otherwise reasonably fit should be offered a kidney transplant. Future developments that may improve outcomes for suitable patients include advances in islet-cell transplantation and the increased availability of grafts through xenotransplantation.

References

1. Ritz E, Rychlik I, Locatelli F, Halimi S: End-stage renal failure in type 2 diabetes: a medical catastrophe of worldwide dimensions. Am J Kidney Dis 1999;34:795–808.
2. Olsen S: Identification of non-diabetic glomerular disease in renal biopsies from diabetics: a dilemma. Nephrol Dial Transplant 1999;14:1846–1849.

3. Biesenbach G, Janko O, Zazgornik J: Similar rate of progression in the predialysis phase in type I and type II diabetes mellitus. Nephrol Dial Transplant 1994;9:1097–1102.

4. Duncan L, Heathcote J, Djurdjev O, Levin A: Screening for renal disease using serum creatinine: who are we missing? Nephrol Dial Transplant 2001;16:1042–1046.

5. Alvestrand A: Carbohydrate and insulin metabolism in renal failure. Kidney Int 1997;62(Suppl):S48–S52.

6. Scheen AJ, Lefebvre PJ: Oral antidiabetic agents. A guide to selection. Drugs 1998;55:225–236.

7. Chachou A, Randoux C, Millart H, Chanard J, Gillery P: Influence of in vivo hemoglobin carbamylation on HbA1c measurements by various methods. Clin Chem Lab Med 2000;38:321–326.

8. Shoji T, Tabata T, Nishizawa Y, et al: Clinical availability of serum fructosamine measurement in diabetic patients with uremia. Use as a glycemic index in uremic diabetes. Nephron 1989;51:338–343.

9. Ferris FL, Davis MD, Aiello LM: Treatment of diabetic retinopathy. N Engl J Med 1999;341:667–678.

10. Chaturvedi N, Sjolie AK, Stephenson JM, et al: Effect of lisinopril on progression of retinopathy in normotensive people with type 1 diabetes. The EUCLID Study Group. EURODIAB Controlled Trial of Lisinopril in Insulin-Dependent Diabetes Mellitus. Lancet 1998;351:28–31.

11. Parry GJ: Management of diabetic neuropathy. Am J Med 1999;107(2B):27S–33S.

12. Schomig M, Ritz E, Standl E, Allenberg J: The diabetic foot in the dialyzed patient. J Am Soc Nephrol 2000;11:1153–1159.

13. Haffner SM, Lehto S, Ronnemaa T, Pyorala K, Laasko M: Mortality from coronary heart disease in subjects with type 2 diabetes and in nondiabetic subjects with and without prior myocardial infarction. N Engl J Med 1998;339:229–234.

14. Stephenson JM, Kenny S, Stevens LK, Fuller JH, Lee E: Proteinuria and mortality in diabetes: the WHO Multinational Study of Vascular Disease in Diabetes. Diabetic Med 1995;12:149–155.

15. Tarnow L, Rossing P, Gall MA, Nielsen FS, Parving HH: Prevalence of arterial hypertension in diabetic patients before and after the JNC-V. Diabetes Care 1994;17:1247–1251.

16. UK Prospective Diabetes Study Group: Tight blood pressure control and risk of macrovascular and microvascular complications in type 2 diabetes: UKPDS 38. Br Med J 1998;317:703–713.

17. Hansson L, Zanchetti A, Carruthers SG, et al: Effects of intensive blood-pressure lowering and low-dose aspirin in patients with hypertension: principal results of the Hypertension Optimal Treatment (HOT) randomised trial. The HOT Study Group. Lancet 1998;351:1755–1762.

18. Heart Outcomes Prevention Evaluation Study Investigators: Effects of ramipril on cardiovascular and microvascular outcomes in people with diabetes mellitus: results of the HOPE study and MICRO-HOPE substudy. Lancet 2000;355:253–259.

19. Shoji T, Emoto M, Kawagishi T, et al: Atherogenic lipoprotein changes in diabetic nephropathy. Atherosclerosis 2001;156:425–433.

20. Stamler J, Vaccaro O, Neaton JD, Wentworth D: Diabetes, other risk factors, and 12-year cardiovascular mortality for men screened in the Multiple Risk Factor Intervention Trial. Diabetes Care 1993;16:434–444.

21. Pyorala K, Pedersen TR, Kjekshus J, Faergeman O, Olsson AG, Thorgeirsson G: Cholesterol lowering with simvastatin improves prognosis of diabetic patients with coronary heart disease. A subgroup analysis of the Scandinavian Simvastatin Survival Study (4S). Diabetes Care 1997;20:614–620.

22. Goldberg RB, Mellies MJ, Sacks FM, et al: Cardiovascular events and their reduction with pravastatin in diabetic and glucose-intolerant myocardial infarction survivors with average cholesterol levels: subgroup analyses in the Cholesterol And Recurrent Events (CARE) trial. The CARE Investigators. Circulation 1998;98:2513–2519.

23. Feargeman O: Hypertriglyceridemia and the fibrate trials. Curr Opin Lipidol 2000;11:609–614.

24. The Diabetes Control and Complications Trial (DCCT) Research Group: Effect of intensive diabetes management on macrovascular events and risk factors in the Diabetes Control and Complications Trial. Am J Cardiol 1995;75:894–903.

25. UK Prospective Diabetes Study (UKPDS) Group: Intensive blood-glucose control with sulphonylureas or insulin compared with conventional treatment and risk of complications in patients with type 2 diabetes (UKPDS 33). Lancet 1998;352:837–853.

26. Antiplatelet Trialists' Collaboration: Collaborative overview of randomised trials of antiplatelet therapy I: prevention of death, myocardial infarction, and stroke by prolonged antiplatelet therapy in various categories of patients. Br Med J 1994;308:81–106.

27. Gottlieb SS, McCarter RJ, Vogel RA: Effect of beta-blockade on mortality among high-risk and low-risk patients after myocardial infarction. N Engl J Med 1998;339:489–497.

28. Rodriguez JA, Cleries M, Vela E and Renal Registry Committee: Diabetic patients on renal replacement therapy: analysis of Catalan Registry data. Nephrol Dial Transplant 1997;12:2501–2509.

29. Wolfe RA, Ashby VB, Milford EL, et al: Comparison of mortality in all patients on dialysis, patients on dialysis awaiting transplantation, and recipients of first cadaveric transplant. N Engl J Med 1999;341:1725–1730.

30. Prischl FC, Kirchgatterer A, Brandstatter E, et al: Parameters of prognostic relevance to the patency of vascular access in hemodialysis patients. J Am Soc Nephrol 1995;6:1613–1618.

31. Chen HS, Hwu CM, Kuo BI, et al: Abnormal cardiovascular reflex tests are predictors of mortality in type 2 diabetes mellitus. Diabetic Med 2001;18:268–273.

32. Passadakis P, Oreopoulos D: Peritoneal dialysis in diabetic patients. Adv Ren Replace Ther 2001;8:22–41.

33. Hariharan S, Johnson CP, Bresnahan BA, Taranto SE, McIntosh MJ, Stablein D: Improved graft survival after renal transplantation in the United States, 1988 to 1996. N Engl J Med 2000;342:605–612.

34. Manske CL, Thomas W, Wang Y, Wilson RF: Screening diabetic transplant candidates for coronary artery disease: identification of a low risk subgroup. Kidney Int 1993;44:617–621.

35. Kasiske BL, Vazquez MA, Harmon WE, et al: Recommendations for the outpatient surveillance of renal transplant recipients. American Society of Transplantation. J Am Soc Nephrol 2000;11(Suppl 15):S1–86.

36. Kasiske BL, Chakkera HA, Roel J: Explained and unexplained ischemic heart disease risk after renal transplantation. J Am Soc Nephrol 2000;11:1735–1743.

37. Friedman EA: Management choices in diabetic end-stage renal disease. Nephrol Dial Transplant 1995;10(Suppl 7):61–69.

38. Robertson RP, Davis C, Larsen J, Stratta R, Sutherland DE: Pancreas and islet transplantation for patients with diabetes. Diabetes Care 2000;23:112–116.

39. Shapiro AM, Lakey JR, Ryan EA, et al: Islet transplantation in seven patients with type I diabetes mellitus using a glucocorticoid-free immunosuppressive regimen. N Engl J Med 2000;343:230–238.

PART IV
Disorders of Fluid, Electrolyte, and Acid–Base Homeostasis

CHRISTOPHER S. WILCOX

Therapy of Dysnatremic Disorders

Joshua M. Thurman, Richard K. Halterman, and Tomas Berl

Abnormalities of the serum sodium concentration (S_{Na}) are the most common electrolyte disorders encountered in clinical medicine.[1] Collectively referred to as the dysnatremias, they represent disturbances in the control of the body's relative amount of water to sodium. In some settings, treatment must be prompt and judicious, because symptoms may be life-threatening and inappropriate therapy can be deleterious. Skilled management of these disorders requires an understanding of the normal control of the serum sodium, the pathologic settings in which dysnatremias occur, and the ability to quantify the disturbances in order to prescribe safe and effective treatment.

Plasma sodium concentration

The plasma sodium value only reflects the relative amount of sodium to water.[2] It cannot therefore be used to assess total body sodium (TB_{Na}). The S_{Na} is determined by TB_{Na}, total body potassium (TB_K) and total body water (TBW):

$$S_{Na} = \frac{(TB_{Na} + TB_K)}{TBW} \qquad (34.1)$$

Thus, hyponatremia can occur as a consequence of a decrease in the body's content of monovalent cations, an increase in TBW, or a combination of these. Overall, the dysnatremias should be viewed primarily as disturbances in water balance, with a variable component of negative solute balance.

The sodium concentration is a primary determinant of plasma osmolality (P_{osm}):

$$P_{osm} = 2[Na] + glucose/18 + BUN/2.8 \qquad (34.2)$$

where BUN represents blood urea nitrogen. Normally, the osmolality of body fluids can be estimated as twice the S_{Na} plus approximately 10 mosmol to account for other solutes. The addition of solutes to the extracellular fluid will increase its measured osmolality. However, the permeability of a solute across cell membranes determines whether it will cause water to be redistributed between the intracellular and extracellular compartments. Solutes that are permeable across cell membranes, such as urea, ethanol, methanol, or ethylene glycol, do not induce water movement and thus cause hyperosmolality without cellular dehydration. In contrast, the addition of impermeable solutes such as glucose (in an insulinopenic state) or mannitol establishes an effective gradient for water to leave the cell. This process lowers the S_{Na}, producing a "translocational" hyponatremia in the setting of either an isotonic or even hypertonic state, and leads to cellular dehydration. Conversely, when hyponatremia occurs as a consequence of an increase in TBW (hypotonic hyponatremia), water flows into cells causing increased cell volume and decreased intracellular osmolality.

Therapeutic approach to the hyponatremic patient

Although most hyponatremic patients are asymptomatic, severe hyponatremia is a medical emergency that may lead to cerebral edema, tentorial herniation, and death.[3] Surveys of severe symptomatic hyponatremia suggest high mortality rates in the absence of aggressive intervention.[4] In some patients, however, the treatment itself may result in central nervous system demyelination, producing permanent neurologic sequelae or even death. Safe treatment

Cerebral adaptation to hypotonicity

Due to the unyielding confines of the skull, the brain is the primary site of symptoms in acute hyponatremia. Decreases in extracellular osmolality cause water to flow into the intracellular space, and the resultant cellular edema within the fixed volume of the cranium produces an increase in intracranial pressure (ICP). Fortunately, the brain possesses adaptive mechanisms that defend against such increases in ICP, making overt neurologic manifestations infrequent.[5] The first protective mechanism, occurring early in hyponatremia (1–3 h), involves a decrease in cerebral extracellular fluid volume. As cellular volume expands, the resultant increase in interstitial pressure stimulates flow of extracellular fluid into the cerebrospinal fluid, which is shunted into the systemic circulation, effectively relieving some of the elevation of ICP. This mechanism protects against mild acute changes in hyponatremia. A second protective mechanism involves a reduction in intracellular solutes. This starts approximately 3 h after the onset of hypotonicity with the loss of cellular potassium. This is followed over the ensuing 72 h by the loss of organic solutes, including glutamate, taurine, myo-inositol, and glutamine.[6] Although some of the osmolyte losses occur within 24 h, the loss of such solutes becomes more marked in subsequent days and accounts for almost complete restoration of cerebral water.

The benefits afforded by cerebral adaptation are also the source of the problems encountered in the treatment of hyponatremia. The increase in plasma tonicity that accompanies correction of chronic hyponatremia requires a reversal of the adaptive process in order to prevent cellular dehydration. The rate at which the brain reverses this process and restores lost solutes is of great pathophysiologic importance. While brain sodium and chloride levels recover rapidly, the reaccumulation of osmolytes is considerably delayed. The process of increasing or restoring cellular electrolytes and accumulating organic osmolytes in the face of rising extracellular sodium concentration is less efficient in brains previously adapted to hypotonic conditions compared with those in normonatremic states. This is reflected by the greater cerebral water loss sustained by adapted brains.[7]

Correction of chronic hyponatremia with resultant cerebral dehydration correlates with the delayed appearance of severe neurologic deficits and the pathologic finding of foci of demyelination. While cerebral demyelination may be widespread, the historic observation of central basis pontis involvement has led to the syndrome being commonly referred to as central pontine myelinolysis (CPM). The typical clinical presentation is for patients to show an initial improvement in mental status after the start of correction, with subsequent deterioration and development of (1) motor abnormalities, sometimes progressing to flaccid quadriplegia and even respiratory paralysis; (2) pseudobulbar palsy; and (3) mental status or behavioral changes, including progressive loss of consciousness. The diagnosis of this "osmotic demyelination syndrome" is made through confirmation of foci of demyelination on head computed tomography or magnetic resonance imaging, although the radiologic findings may lag behind clinical findings by several weeks. Although survival without residual deficits is becoming more common, CPM frequently pursues a fatal course within 3–5 weeks, making this a dreaded complication of therapy.

Risk factors for neurologic complications of hyponatremia and its correction

Mortality estimates of inpatient hyponatremia range from 10 to 50%, although the contribution of the hypotonicity to poor outcome is difficult to separate from other underlying causes. The combination of hyponatremia and hypoxia may be particularly dangerous. In experimental animals, hypoxia abrogates the volume adaptive response to hyponatremia, therefore resulting in increased brain edema.[8] Oh et al[9] suggested that most patients dying of complications related to acute hyponatremia may already be brain dead at the time of diagnosis, further supporting need for careful monitoring and a high index of suspicion in making the diagnosis.

Symptoms of hyponatremia, such as gastrointestinal complaints, lethargy, apathy, agitation, and cramps, occur most commonly with rapid decreases in S_{Na} below 125 mequiv./L. Seizures and coma usually result from rapid decreases to levels below 110 mequiv./L. Conversely, hyponatremia usually needs to be present for at least 72 h in order to set the stage for complications related to treatment. Despite these generalizations, there is tremendous variation in the physiologic responses to water intoxication and the likelihood of suffering complications during correction. Clinical surveys and experimental data suggest that there are subgroups of patients at greatest risk for either acute cerebral edema or osmotic demyelination (Table 34.1).

Table 34.1 Patient groups at increased risk for neurologic complications of hyponatremia

Acute cerebral edema	Osmotic demyelination
Postoperative menstruating women	Alcoholics
Elderly women on thiazide diuretics	Malnourished patients
Polydipsic patients	Hypokalemic patients
Children	Burn patients
	Patients with previous hypoxic episodes
	Elderly women on thiazide diuretics

Risk factors for acute cerebral edema

Hospital-acquired hyponatremia in menstruating women

In the hospital setting, hyponatremic menstruating women are more symptomatic at higher sodium levels than other groups and appear to be at increased risk for neurologic complications related to acute hyponatremia. Although hyponatremia appears to develop with almost equal frequency in men and women, Ayus et al[10] reported that of 307 men with postoperative hyponatremia only one had an outcome of permanent cerebral dysfunction or death; in contrast, 33 of 367 women with hyponatremia had such outcomes. Experimental data support gender differences in arginine vasopressin (AVP) release and its cerebral action, including the process of cerebral adaptation. In female rats, AVP decreases high-energy phosphates and pH in the brain and increases mortality relative to male rats. Some of these effects may be related to female sex hormones, which can stimulate release of AVP, compared with male sex hormones, whose action may be inhibitory.[11] Studies in rabbits suggest that cellular adaptation may be less efficient in females than in males, perhaps due to decreased potassium extrusion. Synaptosomes obtained from females demonstrated lower levels of sodium transport and Na^+,K^+-ATPase activity than those obtained from males.

Patients on thiazide diuretics

Thiazide diuretics are a common cause of hyponatremia. These agents reduce electrolyte-free water clearance by inhibiting sodium reabsorption in the early distal tubule, and also induce sodium, potassium, and magnesium losses. They may also directly stimulate thirst. Occasionally, thiazides can cause severe hyponatremia, with levels below 115 mequiv./L. The majority of affected patients reach these levels within 2 weeks of starting the diuretic, although about one-third require less than 5 days.[12] These patients seem to have a predisposition towards thiazide-induced hyponatremia, as rechallenge with the drug can rapidly reinduce the hypotonic state. Sonnenblick et al[12] reported 12 deaths in a group of 129 patients with diuretic-induced severe hyponatremia. These deaths were directly related to the hyponatremia and were associated with a lower mean sodium level on presentation (103 mequiv./L) compared with those patients who recovered (108 mequiv./L). In most studies, the patients at greatest risk are elderly women with low body mass. This may be related to decreased body water at the start of therapy, but possibilities also include altered hypothalamic responses and intrarenal water excretion defects in this group. Of note, some elderly women may have a habitually increased water intake and low solute intake as described by the "tea and toast" diet. Low solute excretion impairs the ability to excrete the ingested water load, resulting in hyponatremia.

Polydipsia

Polydipsia, particularly in psychiatric patients, is a common cause of hyponatremia. Approximately 6–17% of all chronically ill psychiatric patients exhibit features of polydipsia, consuming 4–25 L of water per day. Most of these patients have schizophrenia, although associations with affective disorders, mental retardation, and alcoholism are also observed. Only a subgroup of polydipsic patients becomes hyponatremic; estimates range from 25 to 50%.[13] Hyponatremic patients who compulsively drink water frequently have increased circulating levels of AVP and defects in intrarenal water handling. These abnormalities may be related to antipsychotic medications, but some evidence suggests the presence of defects in water homeostasis even in the absence of pharmacotherapeutic agents.[14]

Children

Children are at risk of becoming hyponatremic because of either excessive dietary intake of hypotonic fluids (such as plain water or diluted formula) or the inappropriate use of hypotonic fluids during hospital admission.[15] Use of hypotonic fluids in children may overestimate their requirements, and also may not take into account nonosmotic release of vasopressin due to stimuli such as pain and nausea.[16] In the USA, hyponatremia is the primary cause of nonfebrile seizures and may also cause respiratory failure. Keating et al[17] reviewed 34 cases of water intoxication in infants and found that an inability to pay for formula was the most common reason given by caretakers for diluting the formula or substituting water.

Risk factors for osmotic demyelination

Several factors appear to increase the treated individual's susceptibility to osmotic demyelination (see Table 34.1). First, CPM is rarely observed in patients with S_{Na} > 120 mequiv./L and occurs only if hyponatremia has been present for at least 24 h and probably for 48 h. In addition, severely hyponatremic patients with alcoholism, malnutrition, or hypokalemia, as well as elderly women taking thiazide diuretics, appear to be at increased risk for osmotic demyelination.[18] Hypoxia or anoxia may also contribute[8].

Treatment strategies in hyponatremia

The optimal treatment of hyponatremia involves attention to four factors: (1) the presence of symptoms; (2) the duration of the hypoosmolality; (3) the volume status; and (4) the degree of hyponatremia.

Urine electrolytes and calculation of electrolyte-free water clearance can help predict how the kidney will handle the salt and water administered during therapy. If the urine sodium concentration (U_{Na}) is < 10 mequiv./L, the kidney is sodium avid and the patient will likely retain any sodium that is administered. Conversely, if U_{Na} is > 50 mequiv./L, the kidney will likely excrete any administered sodium, and the concentration at which it excretes this sodium will determine the change in the patient's S_{Na}.

For patients who are euvolemic and who will likely excrete the administered sodium, the electrolyte-free water clearance can be calculated in order to predict the resultant change in the relative amount of TBW to sodium. Urine flow (V) can be divided into two components. The first component is the urine volume needed to excrete electrolytes at the concentration of electrolytes in plasma (i.e. isotonic). The second component is any remaining urine volume, which represents electrolyte-free water (cH_2Oe). Because sodium and potassium contribute to the osmolality of urine and sodium is the primary determinant of osmolality in serum, the fraction of urine volume that is isotonic can be calculated as:

$$\frac{(U_{Na} + U_K)}{S_{Na}} \tag{34.3}$$

The electrolyte-free water can therefore be calculated as:

$$cH_2Oe = V\left[1 - \frac{(U_{Na} + U_K)}{S_{Na}}\right] \tag{34.4}$$

The cH_2Oe is negative when $U_{Na} + U_K > S_{Na}$, indicating that the kidney is producing urine with an electrolyte concentration greater than that of plasma and S_{Na} will decrease. Conversely, if $U_{Na} + U_K < S_{Na}$, cH_2Oe is positive and S_{Na} will rise.

Acute symptomatic hyponatremia

Prompt rapid correction is indicated for patients with acute (< 48 h) symptomatic hyponatremia, as the risks of cerebral edema exceed the risk of treatment complications (Fig. 34.1). Correction should aim for a rise in S_{Na} of ~ 2 mequiv./L/h. Although full correction is probably safe, it is by no means necessary (Table 34.2). A clinical case is described to illustrate the following principles.

1. In the setting of antidiuresis, $U_{Na} + U_K$ can exceed 150 mequiv./L, and the electrolyte-free water clearance is negative. Thus, if isotonic saline is infused, the body may excrete the infused sodium in a more concentrated form, possibly even worsening the hyponatremia.
2. The administration of hypertonic saline with furosemide ensures electrolyte-free water excretion while preventing volume expansion.

Case history

A 31-year-old, 60-kg woman with normal preoperative laboratory values underwent an elective hysterectomy with minimal intraoperative blood loss. During a 4-h

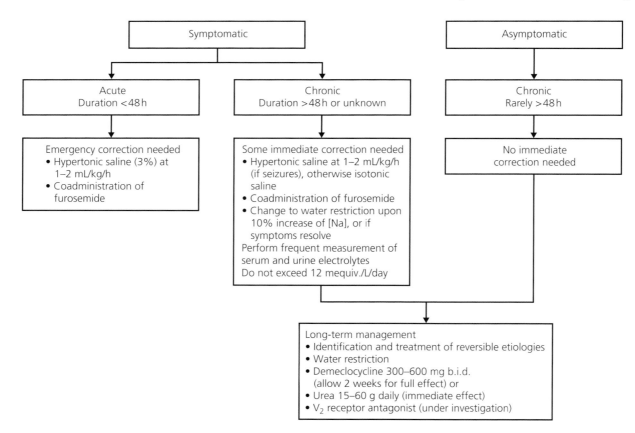

Figure 34.1 Treatment of severe (< 125 mequiv./L) euvolemic hyponatremia.

Table 34-2. General guidelines for the treatment of symptomatic hyponatremia

Acute hyponatremia (duration < 48 h)
Increase S_{Na} rapidly by ~ 2 mequiv./L/h until resolution of symptoms
Full correction probably safe but not necessary

Chronic hyponatremia (duration > 48 h)
Initial rapid increase in S_{Na} by 10% or 10 mequiv./L
Perform frequent neurologic evaluations; correction rate may be reduced with improvement in symptoms
At no time after initial increment should correction exceed rate of 1.5 mequiv./L/h or total increment of 12 mequiv./L/day
Hypotonic fluids, and even DDAVP, can be administered to prevent correction in excess of desired daily goal

The sum of urinary cations (UNa + UK) should be less than the concentration of infused sodium to ensure excretion of electrolyte-free water.
DDAVP, 1-deamino-8-d-arginine vasopressin.

period encompassing the surgery and recovery room care, she received 2 L of 0.9% normal saline. Thereafter, 125 mL/h of 0.45% normal saline was administered. Her total urine output for the 12 h after surgery was 1500 mL. The patient suffered progressively worsening abdominal pain and intermittent vomiting, for which she received meperidine (Demerol) and prochlorperazine (Compazine). At 30 h postoperatively, mental status changes developed and S_{Na} was 114 mequiv./L. Her intravenous orders were changed to 200 mL/h of 0.9% normal saline for 5 h, during which time the patient's urine output was 750 mL, U_{Na} 140 mequiv./L, and U_K 60 mequiv./L. The patient then had a seizure and respiratory arrest. The repeat S_{Na} was 112 mequiv./L.

Case analysis

Since preoperative S_{Na} was 140 mequiv./L and preoperative TBW was 30 L (50% of body weight), rearranging equation 35.1 gives:

$$\begin{aligned} TB_{Na} + TB_K &= S_{Na} \times TBW \\ &= 140 \times 30 \\ &= 4200 \text{ mequiv.} \end{aligned}$$

Postoperatively, when S_{Na} was 114 mequiv./L (assuming solute balance), the patient's new TBW would have been:

$$\begin{aligned} TBW &= \frac{(TB_{Na} + TB_K)}{S_{Na}} \\ &= \frac{4200 \text{ mequiv.}}{114 \text{ mequiv./L}} \\ &= 36.8 \text{ L} \end{aligned}$$

Therefore, a rough estimate of positive water balance would have been 36.8 − 30 = 6.8 L.

Even after the patient's hyponatremia was recognized and the hypotonic fluids were replaced by isotonic saline, the patient's S_{Na} continued to decrease. The following table is an analysis of water and solute balance during the 5 h of isotonic saline infusion.

	Water (L)	Solute (Na + K) (mequiv.)
Intake (0.9% saline at 200 mL/h)	1.00	150 Na
Output	0.75	105 Na + 45 K
Balance (intake − output)	+0.25	0

The resultant TBW is now 36.8 + 0.25 = 37.05 L. The S_{Na}, assuming essentially unchanged solute balance, would be:

$$\begin{aligned} S_{Na} &= \frac{(TB_{Na} + TB_K)}{TBW} \\ &= \frac{4200 \text{ mequiv.}}{37.05 \text{ L}} \\ &= 113 \text{ mequiv./L} \end{aligned}$$

This example illustrates that, in a patient with high AVP levels, the infusion of isotonic saline not only fails to correct hyponatremia but can further aggravate it. The correction of hyponatremia requires the excretion of electrolyte-free water, i.e., the sum of urinary sodium and potassium must be less than the sodium of the infusing fluid.

The administration of furosemide promotes such electrolyte-free water excretion. When combined with the infusion of hypertonic saline, S_{Na} can be promptly increased. The table below illustrates what would have happened if the patient had received 100 mL/h of 3% saline for 2 h and 40 mg of furosemide, with urine output of 1000 mL, U_{Na} 70 mequiv./L, and U_K 30 mequiv./L.

	Water (L)	Solute (Na + K) (mequiv.)
Intake (3% saline at 100 mL/h)	0.2	100 Na
Output	1.00	70 Na + 30 K
Balance (intake − output)	−0.8	0

Therefore TBW is 36.8 − 0.8 = 36 L. Since solute balance is unchanged:

$$\begin{aligned} S_{Na} &= \frac{(TB_{Na} + TB_K)}{TBW} \\ &= \frac{4200 \text{ mequiv.}}{36 \text{ L}} \\ &= 117 \text{ mequiv./L} \end{aligned}$$

Thus, rather than decreasing, the patient's S_{Na} has increased and has done so at an acceptable rate (~ 2 mequiv./L/h).

Chronic symptomatic hyponatremia

Symptomatic hyponatremia that has persisted for longer than 48 h or is of unknown duration must be treated with great caution. Neurologic symptoms, such as depressed sensorium or seizures, reflect cerebral dysfunction and the need for some correction, yet overly rapid correction puts the patient at risk for osmotic demyelination (see

Fig. 34.1). Various studies have attempted to resolve whether it is the rate or magnitude of correction that determines the risk for complications (Table 34.3). However, these two variables are not readily dissociated, because a rapid correction rate is usually accompanied by a greater absolute magnitude of correction over a given time period.

Several animal studies indicate that the daily absolute change may be the primary determinant of the risk for osmotic demyelination, and that correction by < 25 mequiv./L in the first 24 h correlates best with survival. Soupart et al[19] showed that in rats corrected over 48 h, 95% of the hyponatremic animals developed brain lesions when the daily absolute change in S_{Na} reached 20 mequiv./L/day. Below this limit, the incidence and severity of brain lesions were very low, even in the group corrected rapidly with bolus injections. In another study, hyponatremic rats treated with rapid correction (2.7 mequiv./L/h) but an absolute change in S_{Na} of < 25 mequiv./L/day had a lower mortality rate (95% survival) compared with rats treated with

rapid correction and an absolute change in S_{Na} of > 25 mequiv./L/day (15% survival).[20] Verbalis et al[21] have shown that in rats with hyponatremia of 19 days' duration, demyelination might be a function of both the rate and magnitude of correction. Demyelination was not observed in any rats in which the maximal correction rate was < 2.5 mequiv./L/h and the magnitude of increase in S_{Na} < 25 mequiv./L/day. If either of these limits was exceeded, the demyelination rate was 60%.

What is known about this subject in humans? Obviously, the potentially severe consequences make controlled clinical trials in humans impossible. Most retrospective studies indicate that demyelinating lesions are rare in patients who are corrected at a rate < 0.5 mequiv./L/h and a magnitude < 12 mequiv./L/day (see Table 34.3). Sterns et al[22] reported eight hyponatremic patients who developed the osmotic demyelination syndrome after being corrected by > 12 mequiv./L in 24 h. In a subsequent study,[18] Sterns reviewed 54 patients with

Table 34.3 Studies of patients with chronic hyponatremia

Reference	Type of study	No. of patients	Initial S_{Na} (mequiv./L)	Rate of correction (mmol/L/h)	Magnitude of correction (mmol/L/day)	No. of patients with neurologic complications
Sterns et al[22]	Retrospective	8 (duration of hyponatremia uncertain)	107		Average 21.5, all corrected > 12	8
	Literature review	51				22/38 of those corrected > 12 mmol/L/day; 0/13 corrected < 12 mmol/L/day
Sterns[18]	Retrospective	54 chronic cases	107	0.59	17 in those with neurologic complications	7 (two had demyelination)
		10 acute cases (defined as 2–4 days)	105	1.57		None
Ayus et al[26]	Prospective	33 (30 of whom had hyponatremia for > 24 h)	108 ± 1	1.3 ± 0.2 (in five patients, correction was 1.6–4.7)	20 ± 1 (two acute patients were corrected to 27 and 38 mmol/L, raising the average)	None
	Retrospective	12 (four with hepatic encephalopathy and only mild hyponatremia)	107 ± 4	1 ± 0.2	37 ± 3 (over 41 ± 3 h)	8
	Literature review	17	107 ± 2	0.7 ± 0.1	27 ± 2 (over 39 ± 4 h)	17 (11 with evidence of demyelination)
Sterns et al[23]	Retrospective	56	≤ 105	No complications if < 0.55	No complications if < 12 mmol/L/day	14
Ayus & Arieff[27]	Prospective	17	111	0.7	14	None
		22	103	0.8	22	14 died or had permanent neurologic sequelae
		14	109	0.1	3	11 died, three had permanent neurologic sequelae

chronic hyponatremia who underwent treatment. Seven of these patients developed neurologic complications after treatment. Those who developed neurologic complications had experienced a wide range of corrections (< 0.7 mequiv./L/h in three patients), but all had been corrected by > 12 mequiv./L in 24 h (mean correction 17 mequiv./L in 24 h). In another retrospective study of 56 patients, 14 developed neurologic complications, although there were no neurologic complications in patients corrected by < 0.55 mequiv./L/h and < 12 mequiv./L/day.[23] In a retrospective analysis of the literature, Ayus et al[24] initially found that patients treated "slowly" (< 0.7 mequiv./L/h) had a greater mortality than those corrected at a rate of 2 mequiv./L/h. However, this was based on case reports that may have included patients with acute hyponatremia, and the deaths were typically due to brain edema and herniation as one would expect with acute hyponatremia corrected too slowly.[25] In a combined prospective and retrospective analysis of patients with demyelinating lesions, Ayus et al[26] later showed that an increase in S_{Na} of > 25 mequiv./L in the initial 48 h was the primary risk factor for the development of cerebral lesions.

A more recent study by Ayus and Arieff[27] also highlights the risks of delaying therapy in symptomatic patients. The outcomes of 53 postmenopausal women with chronic symptomatic hyponatremia were compared based on whether they were treated promptly with saline, treated with saline only after the onset of respiratory insufficiency, or treated with fluid restriction only. The group treated promptly had no long-term neurologic sequelae, whereas those whose treatment was delayed until after the onset of respiratory insufficiency had significant morbidity and mortality, particularly in the group treated by fluid restriction alone.

The question of whether the process that leads to brain demyelination is reversible has significant clinical importance. This issue has been studied by Soupart et al.[28] Hyponatremic rats were submitted to an excessive correction (> 25 mequiv./L) with hypertonic saline during a single intraperitoneal infusion. This osmotic stress was maintained for 12 h. Next, hypotonic fluid was administered to maintain the total magnitude of correction below 20 mequiv./L/day. Mild brain lesions were noted in 20% of the treated group and in 100% of the control rats that did not receive hypotonic fluids. This experiment implies that, at least in animals, subsequent brain damage can be prevented in asymptomatic rats by early lowering of S_{Na}, provided that the final correction is maintained below 20 mequiv./L/day. Soupart et al[29] have also published a case report of a patient with chronic symptomatic hyponatremia who received hypotonic fluid and 1-desamino-8-D-arginine vasopressin (DDAVP) to lower the serum sodium after she had initially been overcorrected. The patient was reported to have had neurologic deterioration after the overcorrection, but after the sodium was relowered and allowed to correct slowly she recovered without neurologic deficits. This finding merits further investigation for its obvious clinical relevance.

The rate at which S_{Na} will increase depends on the rate of administration and electrolyte content of infused fluids as well as on the rate of production and electrolyte content of urine. The initial increment may be achieved with cautious infusion of hypertonic or normal saline and furosemide, with frequent determinations of S_{Na} and urinary electrolytes. If correction occurs at an inappropriately rapid rate, free water can be administered. After the desired increment is attained, therapy can continue in the form of water restriction.

These data lead us to propose the following guidelines for treating chronic hyponatremia (see Fig. 34.1 and Table 34.2).

1. Correction of S_{Na} should be undertaken without delay in symptomatic patients, particularly those experiencing seizures. Since cerebral water is only increased by about 10% in severe chronic hyponatremia, S_{Na} should be promptly increased by 10% or ~ 10 mequiv./L, followed by water restriction. Rapid correction of S_{Na} should only continue until symptoms resolve or until this 10% change is achieved.
2. After the initial correction, the rate should not exceed 1–1.5 mequiv./L/h and probably should be < 0.5 mequiv./L/h.
3. S_{Na} should not be increased by more than 12 mequiv./L/day.
4. If the patient has reached the desired rate or magnitude of correction yet is excreting hypotonic urine, hypotonic fluids and even DDAVP can be administered to prevent correction in excess of the desired daily goal. Calculation of the electrolyte-free water and attention to urine volume can be used to predict the patient's free water requirement.

Example

A 50-kg man with altered mental status is found to have an S_{Na} of 110 mequiv./L. The initial goal of therapy is to increase the patient's S_{Na} by 10% or to ~ 120 mequiv./L. If the patient is felt to be euvolemic, correction can be achieved via electrolyte-free water excretion without a significant change in total body osmoles.

For men, TBW $\cong 0.6 \times$ weight (kg). Rearranging equation 34.1 yields:

$$\frac{\text{Desired } S_{Na}}{S_{Na}} = \frac{\text{TBW}}{\text{Desired TBW}}$$

Since TBW $= 0.6 \times 50 = 30$ L,

$$\text{Desired TBW} = \frac{S_{Na} \times \text{TBW}}{\text{Desired } S_{Na}}$$
$$= \frac{110 \times 30}{120}$$
$$= 27.5 \text{ L}$$

Therefore, 2.5 L of electrolyte-free water must be excreted. If 500 mL/h of electrolyte-free water is lost, the load will be excreted in 5 h. This can be achieved by administering furosemide and replacing any sodium, potassium, and excess free water lost in the urine. The balance during the first hour is shown below.

	Water (L)	Solute (Na + K) (mequiv.)
Intake (500 mL normal saline + 100 mL D5W with 20 mequiv. KCl)	600	75/20
Output	1000	75/20
Balance	−400	0

D5W, 5% dextrose in water.

Continuing to replace urine electrolyte or excess electrolyte-free water losses, the balance during the second hour is shown below.

	Water (L)	Solute (Na + K) (mequiv.)
Intake (400 mL normal saline + 100 mL D5W with 20 mequiv. KCl)	500	60/20
Output	800	60/25
Balance	−300	−5

D5W, 5% dextrose in water.

The patient's TBW has decreased by about 700 mL, total body osmoles are essentially unchanged, and one can estimate S_{Na} as ~ 113 mequiv./L.

Asymptomatic euvolemic hyponatremia

(see Fig. 34.1)

Nonedematous asymptomatic hyponatremia should invoke a search for reversible etiologies. If indicated, thyroid or glucocorticoid replacement should be initiated. If the syndrome of inappropriate secretion of antidiuretic hormone (SIADH) is present, identification of reversible etiologies should be undertaken with subsequent removal of offending agents. If the aforementioned strategies are not attainable, then fluid restriction should be prescribed. An initial restriction of 1 L/day is often prescribed. In most patients, this will be adequate to allow net free water excretion. In some patients, however, such a volume exceeds insensible and urinary losses and does not result in improvement. Furst et al[30] described a patient whose S_{Na} fell from 121 to 117 mequiv./L over 24 h even though his fluid intake was limited to 1 L/day. This patient had a U_{Na} of 100 mequiv./L and a U_K of 66 mequiv./L, and produced 900 mL of urine over the 24 h. Using equation 34.4, net electrolyte-free water can be calculated as follows:

$$cH_2Oe = V \left[1 - \frac{U_{Na} + U_K}{S_{Na}} \right]$$
$$= 0.9 \left[1 - \frac{100 + 66}{121} \right]$$
$$= -0.33 \text{ L}$$

Unless his intake is less than insensible losses plus electrolyte-free water excretion (which is negative in this case), his S_{Na} will fall even further. The authors therefore proposed the following guide to therapy based on urine and serum electrolytes.

$(U_{Na} + U_K)/S_{Na}$	Water restriction
> 1	< 500 mL/day
~ 1	500–700 mL/day
< 1	Up to 1 L/day

Restricting fluid intake to 1 L/day or less is difficult to attain in the outpatient setting and pharmacologic therapy may be necessary. SIADH impairs the renal capacity for urine dilution, but pharmacologic agents that impair urinary concentration increase free water excretion. Lithium carbonate and demeclocycline hydrochloride have been used in the treatment of chronic hyponatremia. However, the nephrotoxicity and unwanted central nervous system effects of lithium have limited its usefulness.

Demeclocycline is currently the agent of choice,[31] although it has been noted to induce reversible diabetes insipidus in patients treated for bacterial infections. Administered in doses of 300–600 mg twice daily, demeclocycline interferes with the renal action of AVP and promotes maximal water diuresis after 1–2 weeks of therapy. To ensure adequate gastrointestinal absorption, the drug should be given at least 1–2 h after eating, and antacids that contain aluminum, calcium, or magnesium should be avoided. Once diuresis begins, dosage may be tapered to 150–300 mg twice daily to minimize toxicity. Additionally, water intake should be allowed to increase, thus preventing diabetes insipidus-induced dehydration. Nephrotoxicity may be observed in patients with liver disease. Azotemia independent of renal function may result from mild antianabolic effects. It may be associated with severe photosensitivity and should not be used in pregnant patients or children due to abnormalities in bone or enamel formation.

Urea has also been used in the treatment of SIADH.[32] Assume that a patient has an S_{Na} of 134 mequiv./L, a fixed urine concentration of 800 mosmol/day, an obligatory solute load of 500 mosmol/day, a dietary sodium intake of 100 mmol/day, and a potassium intake of 40 mmol/day. Calculation of the volume required to excrete the daily solute load at baseline reveals:

$$V = \frac{\text{solute excretion}}{U_{osm}}$$
$$= \frac{500 \text{ mosmol/day}}{800 \text{ mosmol/kg } H_2O}$$
$$= 0.625 \text{ L/day}$$

Urinary sodium and potassium concentrations can be determined as follows:

U_{Na} =100 mmol/0.625 L = 160 mmol/L
U_K = 40 mmol/0.625 L = 64 mmol/L

These values may then be inserted into equation 34.4 to compute the electrolyte-free water clearance:

$$cH_2Oe = V \left[1 - \frac{U_{Na} + U_K}{S_{Na}} \right]$$

$$= 0.625 \left[1 - \frac{160 + 64}{134} \right]$$

$$= -0.418 \text{ L/day}$$

The negative value for excretion of electrolyte-free water clearance implies net free water absorption, which could worsen hyponatremia.

Under the same conditions, administration of urea (30 g/day) adds approximately 500 mosmol/day to the obligatory solute load that must be excreted. This has a profound effect on electrolyte-free water clearance:

Volume required for excretion of solute load

$$= \frac{1000 \text{ mosmol/day}}{800 \text{ mosmol/kg } H_2O}$$

$$= 1.25 \text{ L/day}$$

As a result of the increased volume for solute clearance, urinary electrolyte concentrations decrease:

$$U_{Na} = \frac{100 \text{ mmol}}{1.25 \text{ L}} = 80 \text{ mmol/L}$$

$$U_K = \frac{40 \text{ mmol}}{1.25 \text{ L}} = 32 \text{ mmol/L}$$

Note the resultant changes in electrolyte-free water clearance:

$$cH_2Oe = V \left[1 - \frac{U_{Na} + U_K}{S_{Na}} \right]$$

$$= 1.25 \left[1 - \frac{80 + 32}{134} \right]$$

$$= 1.25 (1 - 0.83) = 0.21 \text{ L/day}$$

Thus, the administration of urea has altered this patient's water handling from net reabsorption to excretion of electrolyte-free water.[32] Without altering urinary concentration, the increase in urine flow allows for more liberal water intake without the danger of worsening hyponatremia. Urea administration at doses > 60 g is limited by gastrointestinal adverse effects such as gastric distress and diarrhea. A similar effect can be obtained by increasing salt intake (200 mequiv./day) in combination with furosemide. Because this combination is likely to result in high potassium losses, serum potassium needs to be monitored and potassium replacement should be provided.

A number of antagonists of the hydroosmotic effect of AVP (V_2 receptor antagonists) have been developed, four of which can be administered orally.[33] Although they differ in their relative V_1/V_2 selectivity, they all lower urinary osmolality and have no effect on sodium and potassium excretion. In animal studies these agents have been used to treat the hyponatremia of SIADH.[34,35] In humans they have also been shown to induce an effective water diuresis in healthy controls[36] and in patients with SIADH.[37,38] Saito et al[37] administered OPC-31260 intravenously to 11 patients with SIADH. The drug increased free water clearance and decreased urine osmolality. In the study by Decaux[38], six hyponatremic patients with SIADH and five hyponatremic patients with cirrhosis and ascites were treated with the V_2 receptor antagonist VPA-925. Both groups of patients had significant increases in S_{Na} compared with those who received placebo. In another study, Decaux[39] treated two patients with SIADH with the V_{1A}/V_2 receptor antagonist conivaptan for 3 months. In both patients treatment was well tolerated and as effective as treatment with urea and water restriction.

Whether the oral V_2 receptor antagonists can produce an effective and sustained increase in S_{Na} in patients with high circulating levels of AVP remains to be determined. More clinical experience will be necessary so that these drugs can be titrated to produce a reliable clinical response without correcting S_{Na} too quickly. V_2 receptor antagonists are an attractive alternative to water restriction.

Hypovolemic and hypervolemic hyponatremia (Table 34.4)

Hypovolemic hyponatremia results from the loss of both water and solute, with a greater relative loss of solute. The nonosmotic release of AVP in response to reduced effective circulating volume perpetuates the hyponatremia by producing antidiuresis. Patients with this type of hyponatremia are usually asymptomatic, probably because the losses of sodium and water limit the development of cerebral edema. The cornerstone of therapy is the administration of isotonic saline while also treating the underlying disturbance. Resolution of the volume disturbance removes the stimulus for AVP and restores normal S_{Na}.

Hypervolemic hyponatremia is observed when both water and solute are increased, but water is increased to a greater extent. This condition is very difficult to treat, because it often reflects severe irreversible dysfunction of the liver, heart, or kidney. In heart failure, cirrhosis, and nephrotic syndrome, reduced effective arterial volume results in the nonosmotic stimulation of AVP and an increase in thirst. Therefore compliance with water restriction is difficult. Diuretics are the primary therapeutic agents for edema, but caution must be used in selecting the appropriate regimen. While thiazide diuretics

Table 34.4 Treatment of noneuvolemic hyponatremia

Hypovolemic hyponatremia	Hypervolemic hyponatremia
Volume restoration with isotonic saline	Water restriction
Identify and correct etiology of water and sodium losses	Sodium restriction
	Substitute loop diuretics in place of thiazide diuretics
	Treatment of stimulus for sodium and water retention
	V_2 receptor antagonists (under investigation)

impair urinary dilution and may exacerbate hyponatremia, loop diuretics increase free water excretion and can improve S_{Na}. Correction of the underlying disturbances is usually not attainable. The oral V_2 antagonists effectively induce a water diuresis in hyponatremic subjects with congestive heart failure and cirrhosis.[40–42] In animal models of heart failure, V_2 antagonists improve survival and these agents may become a valuable form of therapy.[43] At present, therapy relies on fluid restriction, salt restriction, and loop diuretics.

The hypernatremic patient

Hypernatremia is defined as an $S_{Na} > 146$ mequiv./L. The presence of hypernatremia implies both extracellular hyperosmolality and, more importantly, hypertonicity, which produces central nervous system injury through cell shrinkage. The reported incidence of hypernatremia ranges from 0.65 to 2.23% of all hospitalized patients. Morbidity and mortality estimates in hypernatremic adults range from 42% to more than 70%, with approximately 10% mortality in chronic hypernatremia compared with 75% mortality in severe acute elevations of S_{Na} (> 160 mequiv./L). Unfortunately, even in survivors neurologic sequelae are common, especially in children in whom two-thirds may show long-term deficits. As with hyponatremia, correcting hypernatremia too rapidly may be as dangerous as allowing the condition to persist.

Treatment of the hypernatremic patient

Cerebral response to hypernatremia

Cellular dehydration is the primary basis of brain injury, as fluid shifts from the cellular compartment into the extracellular fluid. Neurologic symptoms ensue, with initial changes in sensorium potentially culminating in seizures, coma, or death. Although alterations of cellular fluid and solute balance likely contribute to these signs and symptoms, pathologic evidence demonstrates a variety of underlying anatomic derangements. Loss of brain cell volume places mechanical stress on cerebral vessels and supporting tissues, potentially leading to damage of vascular structures. This is supported by autopsy evidence of hypernatremia-related capillary and venous congestion, subcortical and subarachnoid bleeding, and venous sinus thrombosis.

Cellular adaptation to extracellular hypertonicity results in an increase in intracellular osmolality. This is achieved through events that mirror those described previously for adaptation to hyponatremia.[5] Within seconds the brain is protected from severe water loss by an increase in cellular sodium, potassium, and chloride content.[44] Thereafter, cerebral dehydration is further attenuated by the accumulation of osmolytes such as glutamine, glycerolphosphorylcholine, and myo-inositol.[45] As cellular adaptation requires a period of days to reach full effect, the rate and

severity of developing hypernatremia alter the degree of cell shrinkage and injury. Because it also takes several days for cells to reverse the accumulation of these organic osmolytes, treatment of chronic hypernatremia requires a gradual reduction of extracellular fluid tonicity in order to avoid treatment-induced cerebral edema.

Prevention

Hypernatremia occurs in predictable clinical settings (Table 34.5). Elderly persons, hospitalized patients receiving hypertonic infusions, those suffering increased insensible losses or undergoing osmotic losses, diabetics, and patients with previous symptoms of polydipsia and polyuria should invoke a high index of suspicion when displaying neurologic alterations, especially in periods of stress.

Geriatric patients have impaired thirst responses, decreased urinary concentrating ability, and lower baseline levels of TBW. As a result, elderly patients are the group most likely to develop severe hypernatremia in the outpatient setting, and hypernatremia in the elderly accounts for 1–2% of all hospital admissions.[46] The most common scenario is that of a debilitated patient with a febrile illness. Increased insensible losses are not compensated because of impaired access to free water. Recognition of mental status changes in settings of increased insensible losses should prompt close attention to S_{Na} and increased administration of free water.

Hospitalized patients are also susceptible to the development of hypernatremia. Individuals developing hypernatremia during hospital admission are more likely to be younger and to have an iatrogenic etiology.[47] Inpatients with high insensible losses (e.g. patients on mechanical ventilators) develop hypernatremia due to restricted access to water and inadequate fluid prescriptions. Hypertonic fluid administration (e.g. sodium bicarbonate) and osmotic diuretics including mannitol and urea may also result in hypertonicity. Hyperosmolar tube feedings may induce diarrhea and gastrointestinal water losses, and the large daily osmolar load may lead to increased electrolyte-free water losses. Palevsky et al[47] noted that despite frequent S_{Na} measurements, treatment of hypernatremia was often delayed. Of patients with S_{Na}

Table 34.5 Patient groups at increased risk for development of severe hypernatremia

Elderly patients
Hospitalized patients
Hypertonic infusions
Tube feedings
Osmotic diuretics
Lactulose
Mechanical ventilation
Patients with decreased baseline levels of consciousness
Patients with uncontrolled diabetes
Patients with underlying polyuric disorders

values > 150 mequiv./L, 50% did not receive hypotonic fluid within 24 h of becoming hypernatremic and only 36% were corrected within 72 h.

Patients with both type 1 and 2 diabetes frequently develop hypernatremia in the setting of diabetic keto-acidosis or hyperosmotic nonketotic coma. In both disorders, a relative deficiency in insulin with respect to increased basal requirements produces hyperglycemia and glucosuria. The ensuing osmotic diuresis and decreased fluid intake produce a state of hypovolemic hyper-natremia. The S_{Na} must be interpreted with caution since it may not reflect the actual degree of hyperosmolality. Hyperglycemia leads to the translocation of cellular water into the extracellular fluid and may cause a dilutional hyponatremia. New-onset hyperglycemia associated with decreases in mental status should invoke prompt eva-luation and therapy of both volume and free water deficits. However, the simultaneous administration of both insulin and free water can lead to a rapid fall in extracellular osmolality and can result in cerebral edema.[48] To prevent an excessively rapid fall in serum osmolality, isotonic fluids can be used until the serum glucose is only mildly elevated, at which point hypotonic saline can be administered to start correcting the free water deficit.[49]

Polyuric patients should undergo evaluation for defects in urinary concentration, because previous knowledge of such disorders can avert serious hypernatremia. In dia-betes insipidus, patients compensate for water losses by consuming large amounts of water, thus maintaining relatively normal osmolality. If an illness increases water losses or restricts access to water, hypernatremia will result. Patients at risk for diabetes insipidus include those with central nervous system disease or trauma and also those receiving lithium or amphotericin B.

Treatment strategies in hypernatremia (Fig. 34.2)

The keys to detection and treatment of hypernatremia are: (1) recognition of symptoms, when present; (2) correct identification of the underlying defects of water metabolism; (3) correction of volume disturbances; and (4) correction of hypertonicity. Treatment should be initiated promptly to avoid worsening of hypernatremia and increased risk of poor outcome. Once the condition has been stabilized, steps may be taken for long-term prevention.

Early signs and symptoms of hypernatremia are non-specific and primarily manifest as changes in mental status. These include restlessness, irritability, lethargy, confusion, and somnolence. Progression of neurologic injury may produce muscular twitching, hyperreflexia, seizures, coma, or even death. If corresponding mechan-isms are intact, patients may complain of intense thirst. As previously asserted, mental status changes related to hypernatremia may be difficult to differentiate from neurologic manifestations of other underlying illnesses. Therefore, a high index of suspicion is required for consistent diagnosis.

The rate of correction of hypernatremia depends on its rate of development and on the presence or absence of symptoms. As a general rule, the rate of correction should parallel the rate of development. Cerebral adaptation to chronic hypernatremia results in the generation of organic intracellular solutes.[45] If extracellular tonicity is rapidly reduced, water moves into brain cells producing cerebral edema. A slower rate of correction likely prevents these events by allowing time for dissipation of these solutes. Two studies in children suggest that correction of hyper-natremia should occur at ≤ 0.5 mequiv./L/h.[50,51] No seizures occurred in those corrected at this rate, whereas seizures occurred in nearly 20% of the patients in the group corrected more rapidly. If symptoms are present and the time-course of hypernatremia is acute, then rapid correction with resolution of hypernatremia over several hours is appropriate. It is generally recommended that half the deficit be replaced in 12–24 h as the neurologic status is carefully monitored (Table 34.6). Thereafter, the remaining deficit can be corrected during the ensuing 48 h. The maximum correction rate should not exceed 2 mequiv./L/h. Since ongoing fluid losses are difficult to estimate, frequent determinations of S_{Na} should be made during the course of treatment.

Therapy, like diagnosis, is categorized by extracellular volume status. The chief goals are initial correction of underlying volume disturbances and subsequent cor-rection of hypertonicity.

Euvolemic hypernatremia

The guiding principle in the treatment of euvolemic hypernatremia is the necessity of replacing the water deficit as well as ongoing losses with hypotonic fluids. However, the presence of such losses is not always obvious. The measurement of urinary osmolality can suggest the excretion of isotonic or even hypertonic urine despite continued electrolyte-free water losses.

For example, a patient has the following laboratory values: P_{Na} 146 mequiv./L, U_{osm} 320 mosmol/kg H_2O, P_{osm} 310 mosmol/kg, U_{Na} 40 mequiv./L, U_K 30 mequiv./L, and urine volume 2 L. $U_{osm} > P_{osm}$ might suggest that no free water is being excreted. However, using equation 34.4, calculation of electrolyte-free water clearance reveals the following:

Table 34.6 General guidelines for the treatment of symptomatic hypernatremia

Correct at rate of 2 mequiv./L/h
Replace half calculated water deficit over first 12–24 h
Replace remaining deficit over the next 24 h
Perform serial neurologic examinations; prescribed rate of correction can be decreased with improvement in symptoms
Perform measurements of serum and urine electrolytes every 1–2 h

$$cH_2Oe = V\left[1 - \frac{U_{Na} + U_K}{S_{Na}}\right]$$

$$cH_2Oe = V\left[1 - \frac{70}{146}\right]$$

$$= 2\,L \times 0.52 = 1.04\,L$$

Therefore, this individual is excreting over 1 L of free water over the time period of this urine collection. If this water is not replaced, S_{Na} will increase further. Replacement can be with oral cold water or infusion of 5% dextrose in water.

The water deficit can be calculated on the basis of the S_{Na} and the assumption that 60% of body weight is water.

$$\text{Water deficit} = 0.6 \times \text{body weight} \times \frac{S_{Na}}{140} - 1$$

For example, the water deficit of a 70-kg male with an S_{Na} of 156 mequiv./L would be:

$$0.6 \times 70\,\frac{156}{140} - 1 = 4.8\,L$$

This is the net positive water balance that needs to be achieved over about 48 h, not including ongoing losses that must also be replaced, as estimated by the electrolyte-free water clearance. The water deficit can be replaced orally or parenterally, using solutions such as 0.45% sodium chloride or 5% dextrose in water (see Table 34.6 and Fig. 34.2). Central diabetes insipidus may be treated by hormone replacement or pharmacologic agents (Table 34.7). In acute settings where renal water losses are extensive, aqueous vasopressin (Pitressin) is preferable. Its short duration of action allows for more careful monitoring and decreases the likelihood of complications such as water intoxication. An initial dose of 5 μg may be given subcutaneously, with quantification of its effect on S_{Na} and

urine output used to guide additional dosing. Pitressin activates vascular V_1 receptors and may produce coronary spasm, uterine contraction, gastrointestinal cramping, and pallor. Caution must therefore be used in patients with known coronary artery disease or peripheral vascular disease. In chronic settings, DDAVP is the agent of choice because of its long half-life and diminished V_1 receptor stimulation. It is conveniently administered intranasally in doses of 10–20 μg every 12–24 h, and a single dose may induce antidiuresis for 8–12 h. DDAVP may also be given intravenously or subcutaneously, especially during periods of upper respiratory disease or surgery. For patients who are converted from the intranasal to the injectable form, the dose should be reduced to 10% of the intranasal administration. Dosing regimens need to be tailored individually, with a bias toward undertreatment. The lowest dose that decreases polyuria to acceptable levels should be used, and the return of polyuria should be noted prior to repeat dosing in order to prevent hyponatremia. The drug appears to be safe for use in pregnancy and is resistant to degradation by increased circulating vasopressinases. DDAVP is usually tolerated extremely well but in very large doses may cause hypertension, headache, and abdominal cramping. Unfortunately, the agent is very expensive, and adjunctive measures may be used to reduce the required dose.

When the quantity of DDAVP available for treatment is limited, and in cases of partial central diabetes insipidus, circulating AVP may be increased by pharmacologic agents that potentiate its release. These drugs include chlorpropamide, clofibrate, and carbamazepine. When used alone these agents are not usually adequate to control polyuria, but when combined with hormonal therapy, decreased solute intake, or diuretic administration they prove very useful in the treatment of diabetes insipidus.

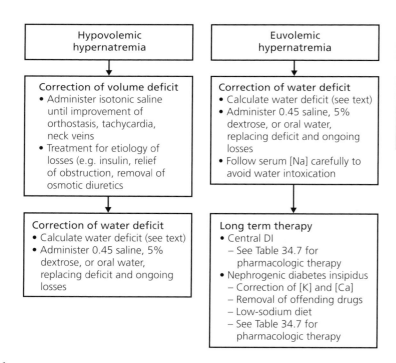

Figure 34.2 Therapeutic approach to hypernatremia.

Table 34.7   Therapeutic regimens for the treatment of diabetes insipidus*

	Drug	Dose
Complete central diabetes insipidus	DDAVP	10–20 μg intranasally every 12–24 h
		0.1–0.8 mg orally in divided doses. Start with
		0.05 mg orally every 12 h and adjust as needed
Partial central diabetes insipidus	Aqueous vasopressin	5–10 units s.c. every 4–6 h
	Chlorpropamide	250–500 mg/day
	Clofibrate	500 mg t.i.d. to q.i.d.
	Carbamazepine	400–600 mg/day
Nephrogenic diabetes insipidus	Thiazide diuretics	25–50 mg/day
	NSAIDs	Indomethacin 1–2 mg/kg/day
	Amiloride (for lithium-related disease)	5 mg daily
Gestational diabetes insipidus	DDAVP	As above

DDAVP, 1-deamino-8-D-arginine vasopressin; NSAIDs, nonsteroidal anti-inflammatory drugs.
*Adapted from Lanese D, Teitelbaum I: Hypernatremia. *In* Jacobson HR, Striker GE, Klahr S (eds): The Principles and Practice of Nephrology. Philadelphia: CV Mosby, 1998, pp 884–887.

It is interesting that chlorpropamide has been used to normalize S_{Na} by increasing water intake and has also been used to treat primary polydipsia. Although other agents such as thioridazine and benzodiazepines appear to increase water intake, they are not of practical use.

Nephrogenic diabetes insipidus does not respond to increased circulating levels of AVP. Initial therapeutic maneuvers should be focused on identifying reversible etiologies of impaired water conservation and, if possible, correcting them. This includes treatment of hypokalemia, hypercalcemia, or the withdrawal of drugs such as lithium, demeclocycline, glyburide, or colchicine. Because of its therapeutic benefits, lithium may be difficult to discontinue in some bipolar patients. In such cases, amiloride may attenuate water losses by blocking entry of lithium into the collecting tubule cell.[52] Thiazide diuretics may decrease polyuria related to nephrogenic diabetes insipidus by reducing the delivery of dilute urine to the distal collecting tubule. This seems to occur by inducing mild extracellular fluid volume contraction with a decreased glomerular filtration rate and increased proximal tubular reabsorption, and by diminishing sodium reabsorption in the diluting segment of the distal nephron. Another method of reducing renal water losses is by reducing oral solute intake in the form of a low-sodium diet. Finally, the polyuria of congenital nephrogenic diabetes insipidus may be attenuated by nonsteroidal anti-inflammatory drug-mediated inhibition of cyclooxygenase.

A rare form of diabetes insipidus may occur during pregnancy. This is related to the production of a vasopressinase by the placenta.[53] These patients respond to treatment with DDAVP, which is not subject to degradation by the enzyme.

Hypovolemic hypernatremia

When hypernatremia coexists with low TB_{Na} and physical evidence of hypovolemia, the primary goal is fluid resuscitation because the extracellular fluid volume contraction may be more life-threatening than the hypertonicity. Such patients should receive initial therapy with normal saline or other plasma expanders until signs of hypovolemia are no longer present. In states of hypernatremia, isotonic saline is actually hypotonic compared with the existing extracellular fluid and can lower plasma osmolality, although not significantly. Serial examinations of volume status should demonstrate the return of normal neck veins and improvement of orthostatic hypotension or tachycardia. Once intravascular volume depletion has been corrected, administration of 0.45% saline or 5% dextrose may be used for further correction of hypertonicity.

Hypervolemic hypernatremia

When the patient is hypervolemic and hypernatremic, the therapeutic goal is to remove the excess sodium. Natriuresis is likely to be present if renal function is normal but can be further enhanced by diuretics such as furosemide with 5% dextrose. Care must be taken not to reduce S_{Na} too rapidly with concomitant diuretic and hypotonic fluid administration. The rate of urine flow and calculation of electrolyte-free water clearance can help estimate free water requirements. If renal function is impaired, volume overload and hypertonicity may require treatment by dialysis.

References

1. Anderson RJ, Chung HM, Kluge R, et al: Hyponatremia: a prospective analysis of its epidemiology and the pathogenetic role of vasopressin. Ann Intern Med 1985;102:164–168.
2. Berl T, Robertson G: Pathophysiology of water metabolism. *In* Brenner BM (ed): The Kidney, 6th edn. Philadelphia: WB Saunders, 2000, pp 866–924.
3. Sterns RH: The management of symptomatic hyponatremia. Semin Nephrol 1990;10:503–514.
4. Ayus J, Krothapalli R, Arieff A: Treatment of hyponatremia: the case for rapid correction. *In* Narins R (ed): Controversies in Nephrology

and Hypertension. New York: Churchill Livingstone, 1984, pp 393–407.

5. Verbalis JG: Hyponatremia: epidemiology, pathophysiology, and therapy. Curr Opin Nephrol Hypertens 1993;2:636–652.

6. Sterns RH, Baer J, Ebersol S, et al: Organic osmolytes in acute hyponatremia. Am J Physiol 1993;264:F833–F836.

7. Berl T: Treating hyponatremia: damned if we do and damned if we don't. Kidney Int 1990;37:1006–1018.

8. Vexler ZS, Ayus JC, Roberts TP, et al: Hypoxic and ischemic hypoxia exacerbate brain injury associated with metabolic encephalopathy in laboratory animals. J Clin Invest 1994;93:256–264.

9. Oh MS, Kim HJ, Carroll HJ: Recommendations for treatment of symptomatic hyponatremia. Nephron 1995;70:143–150.

10. Ayus JC, Wheeler JM, Arieff AI: Postoperative hyponatremic encephalopathy in menstruant women. Ann Intern Med 1992;117:891–897.

11. Stone JD, Crofton JT, Share L: Sex differences in central adrenergic control of vasopressin release. Am J Physiol 1989;257:R1040–R1045.

12. Sonnenblick M, Friedlander Y, Rosin AJ: Diuretic-induced severe hyponatremia. Review and analysis of 129 reported patients. Chest 1993;103:601–606.

13. Illowsky BP, Kirch DG: Polydipsia and hyponatremia in psychiatric patients. Am J Psychiatry 1988;145:675–683.

14. Goldman MB, Luchins DJ, Robertson GL: Mechanisms of altered water metabolism in psychotic patients with polydipsia and hyponatremia. N Engl J Med 1988;318:397–403.

15. Bhalla P, Eaton FE, Coulter JB, et al: Lesson of the week: hyponatraemic seizures and excessive intake of hypotonic fluids in young children. Br Med J 1999;319:1554–1557.

16. Durward A, Tibby SM, Murdoch IA: Hyponatraemia can be caused by standard fluid regimens. Br Med J 2000;320:943.

17. Keating JP, Schears GJ, Dodge PR: Oral water intoxication in infants. An American epidemic. Am J Dis Child 1991;145:985–990.

18. Sterns RH: Severe symptomatic hyponatremia: treatment and outcome. A study of 64 cases. Ann Intern Med 1987;107:656–664.

19. Soupart A, Penninckx R, Stenuit A, et al: Treatment of chronic hyponatremia in rats by intravenous saline: comparison of rate versus magnitude of correction. Kidney Int 1992;41:1662–1667.

20. Ayus JC, Krothapalli RK, Armstrong DL: Rapid correction of severe hyponatremia in the rat: histopathological changes in the brain. Am J Physiol 1985;248:F711–F719.

21. Verbalis JG, Martinez AJ: Neurological and neuropathological sequelae of correction of chronic hyponatremia. Kidney Int 1991;39:1274–1282.

22. Sterns RH, Riggs JE, Schochet SS Jr: Osmotic demyelination syndrome following correction of hyponatremia. N Engl J Med 1986;314:1535–1542.

23. Sterns R, Cappuccio J, Silver S, et al: Neurologic sequelae after treatment of severe hyponatremia: a multicenter perspective. J Am Soc Nephrol 1994;4:1522–1530.

24. Ayus JC, Krothapalli RK, Arieff AI: Changing concepts in treatment of severe symptomatic hyponatremia. Rapid correction and possible relation to central pontine myelinolysis. Am J Med 1985;78:897–902.

25. Arieff AI: Hyponatremia, convulsions, respiratory arrest, and permanent brain damage after elective surgery in healthy women. N Engl J Med 1986;314:1529–1535.

26. Ayus JC, Krothapalli RK, Arieff AI: Treatment of symptomatic hyponatremia and its relation to brain damage. A prospective study. N Engl J Med 1987;317:1190–1195.

27. Ayus JC, Arieff AI: Chronic hyponatremic encephalopathy in postmenopausal women: association of therapies with morbidity and mortality. JAMA 1999;281:2299–2304.

28. Soupart A, Penninckx R, Crenier L, et al: Prevention of brain demyelination in rats after excessive correction of chronic hyponatremia by serum sodium lowering. Kidney Int 1994;45:193–200.

29. Soupart A, Ngassa M, Decaux G: Therapeutic relowering of the serum sodium in a patient after excessive correction of hyponatremia. Clin Nephrol 1999;51:383–386.

30. Furst H, Hallows KR, Post J, et al: The urine/plasma electrolyte ratio: a predictive guide to water restriction. Am J Med Sci 2000;319:240–244.

31. Forrest JN Jr, Cox M, Hong C, et al: Superiority of demeclocycline over lithium in the treatment of chronic syndrome of inappropriate secretion of antidiuretic hormone. N Engl J Med 1978;298:173–177.

32. Decaux G, Brimioulle S, Genette F, et al: Treatment of the syndrome of inappropriate secretion of antidiuretic hormone by urea. Am J Med 1980;69:99–106.

33. Gross P, Reimann D, Henschkowski J, et al: Treatment of severe hyponatremia: conventional and novel aspects. J Am Soc Nephrol 2001;12(Suppl 17):S10–S14.

34. Fujisawa G, Ishikawa S, Tsuboi Y, et al: Therapeutic efficacy of non-peptide ADH antagonist OPC-31260 in SIADH rats. Kidney Int 1993;44:19–23.

35. Fujita N, Ishikawa SE, Sasaki S, et al: Role of water channel AQP-CD in water retention in SIADH and cirrhotic rats. Am J Physiol 1995;269:F926–F931.

36. Ohnishi A, Orita Y, Okahara R, et al: Potent aquaretic agent. A novel nonpeptide selective vasopressin 2 antagonist (OPC-31260) in men. J Clin Invest 1993;92:2653–2659.

37. Saito T, Ishikawa S, Abe K, et al: Acute aquaresis by the nonpeptide arginine vasopressin (AVP) antagonist OPC-31260 improves hyponatremia in patients with syndrome of inappropriate secretion of antidiuretic hormone (SIADH). J Clin Endocrinol Metab 1997;82:1054–1057.

38. Decaux G: Difference in solute excretion during correction of hyponatremic patients with cirrhosis or syndrome of inappropriate secretion of antidiuretic hormone by oral vasopressin V2 receptor antagonist VPA-985. J Lab Clin Med 2001; 138:18–21.

39. Decaux G: Long-term treatment of patients with inappropriate secretion of antidiuretic hormone by the vasopressin receptor antagonist conivaptan, urea, or furosemide. Am J Med 2001;110:582–584.

40. Inoue T, Ohnishi A, Matsuo A, et al: Therapeutic and diagnostic potential of a vasopressin-2 antagonist for impaired water handling in cirrhosis. Clin Pharmacol Ther 1998;63:561–570.

41. Naitoh M, Suzuki H, Murakami M, et al: Effects of oral AVP receptor antagonists OPC-21268 and OPC-31260 on congestive heart failure in conscious dogs. Am J Physiol 1994;267:H2245–H2254.

42. Nishikimi T, Kawano Y, Saito Y, et al: Effect of long-term treatment with selective vasopressin V1 and V2 receptor antagonist on the development of heart failure in rats. J Cardiovasc Pharmacol 1996;27:275–282.

43. Schrier RW, Martin PY: Recent advances in the understanding of water metabolism in heart failure. Adv Exp Med Biol 1998;449:415–426.

44. McManus ML, Churchwell KB, Strange K: Regulation of cell volume in health and disease. N Engl J Med 1995;333:1260–1266.

45. Lien YH, Shapiro JI, Chan L: Effects of hypernatremia on organic brain osmoles. J Clin Invest 1990;85:1427–1435.

46. Snyder NA, Feigal DW, Arieff AI: Hypernatremia in elderly patients. A heterogeneous, morbid, and iatrogenic entity. Ann Intern Med 1987;107:309–319.

47. Palevsky PM, Bhagrath R, Greenberg A: Hypernatremia in hospitalized patients. Ann Intern Med 1996;124:197–203.

48. Silver SM, Clark EC, Schroeder BM, et al: Pathogenesis of cerebral edema after treatment of diabetic ketoacidosis. Kidney Int 1997;51:1237–1244.

49. Harris GD, Fiordalisi I, Harris WL, et al: Minimizing the risk of brain herniation during treatment of diabetic ketoacidemia: a retrospective and prospective study. J Pediatr 1990;117:22–31.

50. Blum D, Brasseur D, Kahn A, et al: Safe oral rehydration of hypertonic dehydration. J Pediatr Gastroenterol Nutr 1986;5:232–235.

51. Kahn A, Brachet E, Blum D: Controlled fall in natremia and risk of seizures in hypertonic dehydration. Intensive Care Med 1979;5:27–31.

52. Wells BG: Amiloride in lithium-induced polyuria. Ann Pharmacother 1994;28:888–889.

53. Durr J, Hoggard J, Hunt J, et al: Diabetes insipidus in pregnancy associated with abnormally high circulating vasopressinase activity. N Engl J Med 1987;316:1070–1074.

Treatment of Hypokalemia and Hyperkalemia

Kamel S. Kamel, Man S. Oh, and Mitchell L. Halperin

The dyskalemias are common and potentially life-threatening electrolyte disorders. Our objective is to apply principles of physiology to their therapy.[1] We highlight two categories of treatment: (1) emergency measures directed at averting the acute threat to the life of a patient; and (2) measures to return the body potassium (K^+) content to normal and reverse the abnormality in K^+ physiology. When considering specific disorders, emphasis is given to those that are common and/or those where new developments in the understanding of their pathophysiology have occurred. To facilitate the presentation, we begin with a brief review of two aspects of K^+ physiology: events at the interface between the extracellular fluid (ECF) and the intracellular fluid (ICF), and regulation of renal K^+ excretion.

Brief overview of K⁺ physiology

In a 70-kg adult, the ICF compartment contains close to 3500 mmol K^+ whereas the ECF compartment contains only 60 mmol K^+. Minor alterations in plasma K^+ concen-

tration (P_k) may be associated with major changes in the electrical gradient for K^+ across cell membranes.

Interface between ECF and ICF

A shift of K^+ between the ECF and ICF compartments is vital for survival on a moment-to-moment basis. K^+ remains largely in the ICF compartment because of the electrical force keeping it there (inside-negative orientation).

Resting membrane potential

The Na^+,K^+-ATPase causes three sodium ions (Na^+) to exit but only two K^+ to enter cells, so there is a net export of one-third of a positive charge per Na^+ transported (Fig. 35.1) (for review see reference 2). Two other points merit emphasis: (1) the majority of intracellular anions cannot cross cell membranes because they are large macromolecular organic phosphates; and (2) for every K^+ that exits cells via K^+ channels, there is a net export of one positive charge.

An abnormal shift of K^+ across cell membranes can be anticipated when the Na^+,K^+-ATPase does not function normally (e.g. hyperkalemia may occur if there is cell necrosis or hypoxia). K^+ may shift into cells when this pump is activated (mainly a β_2-adrenergic effect). Conversely, K^+ may shift out of cells when this ion pump is inhibited (e.g. α-adrenergic effect). Flux through the Na^+,K^+-ATPase will rise substantially when more Na^+ enter cells. The impact of this increase in pump activity on the net voltage depends on whether the Na^+ entry into cells is electroneutral or electrogenic.

Electroneutral Na⁺ entry into cells This may occur when Na^+ enters the cell via the Na^+/H^+ ion exchanger (NHE) (Fig. 35.2) (for review see reference 3). Because Na^+ exit the cell via the Na^+,K^+-ATPase, there is a net export of one-third of a positive charge per Na^+ pumped out of cells, rendering the cell interior more negative. This may explain why insulin induces a shift of K^+ into cells.[4]

It appears that NHE is normally *inactive* in cells because the concentrations of its substrates (Na^+ in the ECF compartment and H^+ in the ICF compartment) are considerably higher than that of its products (Na^+ in the ICF compartment and H^+ in the ECF compartment) at steady state (Fig. 35.2). Therefore activation of NHE is required to produce a gain of Na^+ (and loss of H^+) in the ICF compartment due to ion movement down their concentration gradients. There are two major activators of NHE: insulin[4] and a higher concentration of H^+ in the ICF compartment.[3]

Electrogenic Na⁺ entry into cells The Na^+ channel is normally gated by voltage; when open, one cationic charge

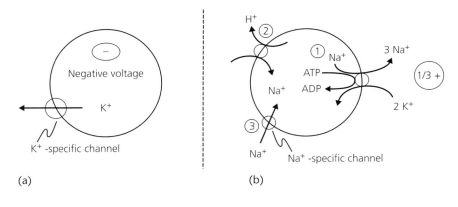

Figure 35.1 K^+ distribution at the interface between the extracellular fluid (ECF) and intracellular fluid (ICF). (a) The force retaining K^+ in the ICF is an electronegative ICF voltage. K^+ may leave the ICF via specific K^+ channels, carrying out positive charge. (b) One-third of a positive charge is exported per Na^+ pumped out of the cell. Two sources of Na^+ do result in positive charge exit: intracellular Na^+ (1) or Na^+ that entered the cell via the Na^+/H^+ ion exchanger (2). In contrast, there is net entry of two-thirds of a positive charge per Na^+ entry via the Na^+ channel (3) coupled with its exit via Na^+,K^+-ATPase. (From Halperin ML: The ACID Truth and Basic Facts: With a Sweet Touch, an enLYTEnment, 4th edn. Stirling, Ontario: Ross Mark Medical Publishers, 1997, with permission.)

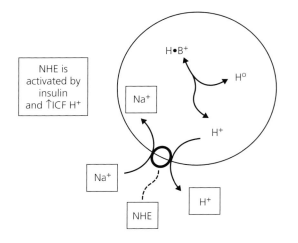

Figure 35.2 Role of the Na^+/H^+ ion exchanger (NHE) in the shift of K^+ into cells. NHE is normally inactive in cells. Activation of NHE is required to translocate Na^+ into the intracellular fluid (ICF) compartment. This higher concentration of Na^+ in the ICF compartment causes more Na^+ (and positive voltage) to be exported by Na^+,K^+-ATPase (see Fig. 35.1). There are two major activators of NHE, insulin and a higher concentration of H^+ in the ICF compartment. B, protein buffers.

enters the cell per Na^+. As only one-third of a charge exits per Na^+ ion pumped via Na^+,K^+-ATPase, this should diminish the degree of intracellular net negative valence and could lead to net K^+ exit and hyperkalemia. Examples of this depolarization include severe exercise,[5] and the hyperkalemia in patients with hyperkalemic periodic paralysis.[6]

Most K^+ is released locally into T-tubules during depolarization and taken back into cells during repolarization, preventing a large release of K^+ into the general circulation. Should this architecture be disturbed (e.g. in patients with cachexia), a greater degree of hyperkalemia might occur with exercise (e.g. fist-clenching during phlebotomy,[7] severe exhaustive exercise[5]). There are several families of K^+ channels; some are regulated by voltage, others by calcium ions (Ca^{2+}), and yet others by metabolites such as ATP.[8]

Renal regulation

Control of the rate of K^+ excretion occurs primarily in the late distal tubule and cortical collecting duct (CCD).[9] Secretion of K^+ requires the generation of a lumen-negative transepithelial voltage and the presence of K^+ channels in the apical membrane.[8] The excretion of a large quantity of K^+ requires a high flow rate through the terminal CCD.[10]

To generate the lumen-negative voltage in the CCD, the rate of reabsorption of Na^+ must occur at a faster rate than the accompanying anion, chloride (Cl^-).[11] The pathway for Na^+ reabsorption is via an epithelial Na^+ channel (ENaC) in the apical membrane of principal cells (for review see reference 12). The pathway for the absorption of Cl^- is likely paracellular.[13,14] Variations in the luminal Na^+ concentration do not play a major regulatory role in the net secretion of K^+.[15] On the other hand, the activity of ENaC is important in the control of K^+ secretion. When this channel is "open", the lumen could become more electronegative and the concentration of K^+ in luminal fluid may rise.[16] Examples of when ENaC is activated include high aldosterone levels, conditions where cortisol acts as a mineralocorticoid, and when there is an increased abundance of ENaC in the luminal membrane of principal cells (Liddle syndrome). On the other hand, other mutations in ENaC may lead to a channel with less opening probability (autosomal recessive form of type 1 pseudo-hypoaldosteronism). K^+-sparing diuretics and certain drugs such as trimethoprim and pentamidine decrease the opening probability of ENaC.

Aldosterone's stimulation of Na^+ reabsorption and K^+ secretion is mediated via binding of aldosterone to its cytoplasmic receptor in principal cells and entry of this hormone–receptor complex into the nucleus, which leads to the synthesis of new proteins.[17,18] Principal cells contain the enzyme 11β-hydroxysteroid dehydrogenase that converts cortisol to the inactive metabolite cortisone, a compound that does not bind the mineralocorticoid receptor.[19] Low activity of this enzyme (apparent mineralocorticoid excess syndrome) or its inhibition by glycyrrhizic acid (found in licorice[20]) or carbenoxolone allows cortisol to bind to the intracellular aldosterone receptor and exert a potent mineralocorticoid effect. 11β-Hydroxysteroid dehydrogenase activity may not be able to "detoxify" all endogenous cortisol in certain settings (adrenocorticotropic hormone-producing tumors, severe Cushing syndrome), and this could explain the excessive K⁺ excretion and hypokalemia observed in these settings.

Another factor that may modulate K⁺ secretion in the CCD is the delivery of Na^+ without Cl^-. Bicarbonaturia leads to an increase in the net secretion of K⁺, even when the concentration of Cl^- in the urine is greater than 15 mmol/L,[21,22] by an unknown mechanism.

Reabsorption of K⁺ from luminal fluid could be mediated by H^+,K^+-ATPase in intercalated cells.[23] For this transporter to operate, there must be luminal acceptors for H^+ ions. As there is little NH_3 and HPO_4^{2-} available in the lumen of the medullary collecting duct, this transport system may only reabsorb a small quantity of K⁺ and hence has a limited role in reducing K⁺ excretion unless there is a parallel increase in activity of the Cl^-/HCO_3^- anion exchanger in the CCD.

Approach to the patient with dyskalemia

Chronic dyskalemias almost always imply a defect in the renal regulation of K⁺ excretion. We use the following steps in the assessment of patients with disordered K⁺ homeostasis.

K⁺ excretion rate

There is no "normal" rate of K⁺ excretion; K⁺ excretion should simply reflect K⁺ intake. To assess the renal response to disordered K⁺ homeostasis, we use the "expected" rate of K⁺ excretion when hypokalemia or hyperkalemia is due to nonrenal causes (< 10–15 mmol/day during hypokalemia, > 200 mmol/day during hyperkalemia). If there is a disordered renal response to hypokalemia or hyperkalemia, the two components of K⁺

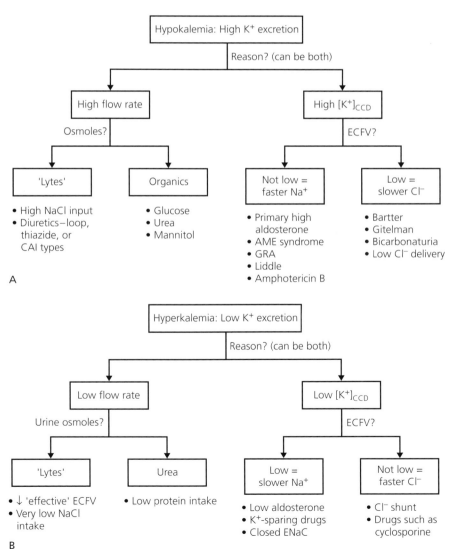

A

B

Figure 35.3 Approach to the patient with hypokalemia or hyperkalemia. (A) Causes of hypokalemia due to excessive excretion of K⁺. The causes of excessive K⁺ excretion (> 15–20 mmol/day) despite hypokalemia are an excessively high flow rate in the CCD (left side of diagram) and too high a $[K^+]_{CCD}$ (right side of diagram). Both flow rate and $[K^+]_{CCD}$ should be evaluated in each patient. Final considerations are shown by the bullet symbols. A slower Cl^- reabsorption in the CCD is suggested by high plasma renin activity and NaCl wasting despite low extracellular fluid volume (ECFV); the converse applies for faster Na^+ reabsorption. AME, apparent mineralocorticoid excess; CAI, carbonic anhydrase inhibitor; GRA, glucocorticoid-remediable aldosteronism. (B) Causes of hyperkalemia due to low excretion of K⁺. The causes of a low rate of K⁺ excretion (< 200 mmol/day) despite hyperkalemia are an exceedingly low flow rate in the CCD (left side of diagram) and too low a $[K^+]_{CCD}$ (right side of diagram). Both flow rate and $[K^+]_{CCD}$ should be evaluated in each patient. Final considerations are shown by the bullet symbols. A slower Na^+ reabsorption is suggested by high renin and NaCl wasting despite low ECFV; the converse applies for faster Cl^- reabsorption. In some cases of renal failure, the excessive flow rate per nephron limits electrogenic reabsorption of Na^+ and thus behaves as if there is relatively slower reabsorption of Na^+. ENaC, epithelial Na^+ channel. (A and B, From Halperin ML: The ACID Truth and Basic Facts: With a Sweet Touch, an enLYTEnment, 4th edn. Stirling, Ontario: Ross Mark Medical Publishers, 1997, with permission.)

excretion, the flow rate and the concentration of K^+ in the urine, are "translated" to reflect events in the lumen of the CCD.[11]

Flow rate in the CCD

A minimum estimate of the rate of flow in the terminal CCD is obtained by dividing the rate of excretion of osmoles by the osmolality of the fluid in the terminal CCD (equal to the osmolality of plasma (P_{osm}) when vasopressin acts):[1,24]

$$\text{Flow rate in CCD} = \text{urine osmole excretion rate}/P_{osm} \quad (35.1)$$

Assessment of concentration of K^+ in the CCD

The transtubular potassium gradient (TTKG) provides a semiquantitative way to assess the driving force for K^+ secretion in the terminal CCD (equation 35.2).[25] The expected value for TTKG in hypokalemia due to low K^+ intake is < 2, while that in hyperkalemia due to excessive K^+ intake is > 10.[25] The first step in the calculation of TTKG is to estimate the concentration of K^+ in the terminal CCD ($[K^+]_{CCD}$) (equation 35.2); the second step is to divide the $[K^+]_{CCD}$ by the P_K (equation 35.3).

$$[K^+]_{CCD} = [K^+]_{urine}/(U/P)_{osm} \quad (35.2)$$

$$TTKG = [K^+]_{CCD}/P_K \quad (35.3)$$

A $[K^+]_{CCD}$ that is inappropriate for the conditions produced by hypokalemia or hyperkalemia may be caused by an altered rate of electrogenic Na^+ reabsorption and/or an altered K^+ conductance (Fig. 35.4).

Hypokalemia

A higher than expected $[K^+]_{CCD}$ could be due to a relatively faster rate of Na^+ reabsorption or a relatively slower rate of Cl^- reabsorption. If the rate of Na^+ reabsorption is relatively faster, the ECF volume might be expanded. Measurement of plasma renin activity and plasma aldosterone levels provide clues to the cause of faster Na^+ reabsorption. In response to induced ECF volume contraction, Na^+- and Cl^--poor urine will be excreted.[1,24] Patients with slower Cl^- reabsorption in the CCD should have a low ECF volume and are usually unable to excrete Na^+- and Cl^--poor urine. Plasma renin activity is expected to be high.

Hyperkalemia

A lower than expected $[K^+]_{CCD}$ could be due to a relatively slower rate of Na^+ reabsorption or a relatively faster rate of Cl^- reabsorption (Fig. 35.4). Patients with a slower rate of Na^+ reabsorption should have renal salt wasting, ECF volume contraction, and a high plasma renin activity, as seen in patients with adrenal insufficiency for example but not in those with a primary defect in the production of renin. On the other hand, patients with a relatively faster rate of Cl^- reabsorption in the CCD would tend to have an

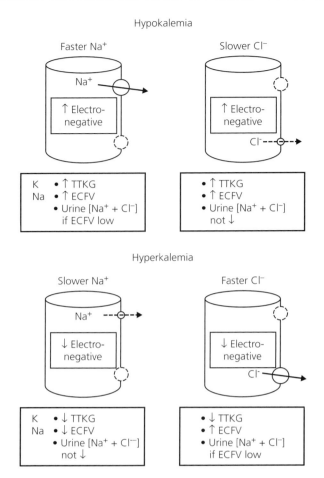

Figure 35.4 Components of K^+ excretion in the cortical collecting duct (CCD). The barrel-shaped structures represent the CCD. The normal pathway for Na^+ and Cl^- reabsorption are shown by the hatched circles in the luminal membrane. Slower pathways are indicated by smaller open circles with dashed lines and faster ones by larger open circles with bold arrows. ECFV, extracellular fluid volume; TTKG, transtubular potassium gradient. (From Halperin ML: The ACID Truth and Basic Facts: With a Sweet Touch, an enLYTEnment, 4th edn. Stirling, Ontario: Ross Mark Medical Publishers, 1997, with permission.)

expanded ECF volume and low plasma renin activity, and also be able to excrete Na^+- and Cl^--poor urine when their ECF volume is contracted.

Hypokalemia

General considerations for treatment of hypokalemia

Our approach is to first recognize those conditions in which hypokalemia may be life-threatening.

Medical emergencies

There are three potentially life-threatening circumstances that require aggressive therapy: cardiac arrhythmias;

extreme weakness involving the respiratory muscles, especially when respiratory acidosis or metabolic acidosis (e.g. hypokalemic distal renal tubular acidosis or severe diarrhea) is present; and hepatic encephalopathy.

Having decided that hypokalemia requires urgent therapy, enough K^+ must be given to raise the P_K quickly and sufficiently so that the dangers of hypokalemia, particularly an arrhythmia, are averted; the total body K^+ deficit should be replaced much more slowly. Because large doses and a high concentration of K^+ in the infusate might be needed, K^+ must be administered via a large central vein and the patient should be connected to a cardiac monitor. Unless otherwise indicated, the infusion should not contain glucose or HCO_3^- because they may aggravate an already severe degree of hypokalemia.

Illustrative example   We use this case[26] to illustrate how we would make a decision concerning the initial amount of KCl to administer when a profoundly low P_K is a medical emergency.[26] A patient fell five stories and sustained a serious head injury. While in intensive care, his P_K fell to 1.3 mmol/L over 30 min, and this led to ventricular tachycardia. This sudden and marked shift of K^+ into cells was likely due to the extreme adrenergic response from the head injury in conjunction with the adrenergic agents administered to maintain hemodynamics. Our aim in therapy would be to raise his P_K by 1 mmol/L in 1 min, recognizing the fact that this rise would be much smaller in the interstitial fluid bathing cardiac myocytes. Therefore we would infuse 3 mmol K^+ in 1 min (blood volume 5 L; cardiac output 5 L/min; 60% of blood volume is plasma, i.e. 3 L). However, the concentration of K^+ in the ECF compartment would rise by < 1 mmol/L because the infused K^+ mixes with the interstitial fluid. Following this initial K^+ bolus, we would reduce the rate of infusion of K^+ to 1 mmol/min and would repeat the measurement of P_K in 5 min (stopping the infusion for 60 s to avoid a spuriously high P_K). If the ECG changes did not improve and hypokalemia persisted, we would repeat the above procedure. It is interesting that the patient in this report was given 618 mmol K^+ intravenously but his P_K never rose above 2.4 mmol/L. This failure of therapy was explained because the predominant K^+ salt infused was a HCO_3^- derivative not KCl.[26]

No medical emergency

We consider the following issues in treatment.

Hypokalemic periodic paralysis   In the absence of a cardiac or respiratory emergency, the treatment of patients with hypokalemic periodic paralysis (HPP) is different because they do not have a large deficit of K^+. In the West, most cases of HPP have a positive family history, whereas others are sporadic in nature. In contrast, in Asian populations patients are most frequently young males who have hyperthyroidism.[27] A high-carbohydrate meal or an adrenergic surge precipitates attacks.[28] Typically, these patients have low rates of K^+ excretion and no plasma acid–base disorder. Plasma phosphate levels are usually low.

Small doses of KCl are usually needed for therapy. Recently Lin and Lin[29] used a nonselective β-blocker (propranolol 3 mg/kg) in the treatment of two patients with thyrotoxic HPP. It caused a prompt rise in P_K (within 2 h). Acetazolamide may be useful for prevention of HPP attacks, although its mechanism of action is not clear.

Magnitude of the K^+ deficit   A loss of 100–400 mmol K^+ lowers the P_K from 4.0 to 3.0 mmol/L, while a P_K of 2 mmol/L suggests a body deficit of K^+ as high as 800 mmol.[30] In an individual patient, there is no useful quantitative relationship between P_K and total body K^+ deficit. Hence careful monitoring of P_K during replacement of the K^+ deficit is mandatory.

Route of K^+ administration   The oral route is preferred. Certain factors may necessitate using the intravenous route, including the urgency of therapy, the level of consciousness, and the presence of gastrointestinal problems. As a rule, the concentration of K^+ should not be > 40 mmol/Lif infused peripherally because higher K^+ concentrations may irritate small veins; the rate of administration of K^+ should not exceed 60 mmol/h in most settings.

K^+ preparations   Most tablets are "slow release." Although usually well tolerated, they occasionally cause ulcerative or stenotic lesions in the gastrointestinal tract due to a high local K^+ concentration. Oral KCl can also be given in a crystalline form (e.g. salt substitutes like Co-salt, which provide 14 mmol K^+ per gram); this is generally well tolerated and is an inexpensive form of K^+ supplementation.

For electroneutrality, a deficit of K^+ must be accompanied by the loss of Cl^- or HCO_3^- or gain of Na^+. With a KCl deficit (e.g. due to chronic vomiting or diuretic use), KCl is needed; in contrast, with a $KHCO_3$ deficit (e.g. due to diarrhea), $KHCO_3$ is needed. A note of caution is necessary: the administration of HCO_3^- may cause a shift of K^+ into cells. Therefore in a patient who is markedly hypokalemic and acidemic, KCl should be given initially; alkali in the form of $NaHCO_3$ may then be administered after the P_K approaches a safe level (about 3 mmol/L). In conditions where K^+ loss is matched by Na^+ retention (e.g. in a patient with primary hyperaldosteronism), K^+ is usually given as KCl while measures are taken to ensure that NaCl will be excreted. The need for K^+ as its phosphate salt is most evident when there is rapid anabolism; examples include patients on nutritional support or those in the acute recovery phase of a catabolic disorder such as diabetic ketoacidosis. If given, phosphate should not be administered too rapidly (< 50 mmol in 8 h) because a large phosphate load has the danger of inducing metastatic calcification and hypocalcemia. We give K^+ as KCl in the treatment of diabetic ketoacidosis and rely on the patient's diet to supply the phosphate needed for ICF replacement, which occurs later.

While it sounds reasonable, increasing the intake of K^+-rich foods (e.g. bananas, fruit juice) is not an effective way to replace a K^+ deficit. A few centimetres of banana provides only about 1 mmol K^+, so it will take a true banana lover to consume enough bananas to provide 50 mmol K^+ each day. The calories in this quantity of bananas could add 22.5–45 kg to the patient's body weight in a year if the intake of "nonbanana food" is not diminished.

Adjuncts to therapy   Renal loss of K^+ can be reduced by using K^+-sparing diuretics. However, this is only useful on a chronic basis and not during the treatment of acute hypokalemia, when the rate of K^+ excretion is usually < 10 mmol/h. Amiloride and triamterene are better tolerated than spironolactone because they lack the gastrointestinal and hormonal (amenorrhea, gyneco-mastia, decreased libido) complications of spironolactone. When using the former two agents, the patient should be on a low NaCl intake because this leads to a lower delivery of osmoles to the CCD and thereby a lower flow rate. With a lower flow rate, the concentration of the drug near ENaC will be higher. A note of caution: hyperkalemia can develop when K^+ is given along with K^+-sparing diuretics, especially if other conditions that may compromise K^+ excretion are present; it is also to be noted that these drugs have a long half-life.

Risks of therapy   With prolonged hypokalemia, the CCD may become hyporesponsive to the kaliuretic effect of aldosterone (reviewed in reference 31). An increase in the "apparent" permeability for Cl^- or downregulation of K^+ channels may explain this phenomenon. This would allow aldosterone to continue to be a NaCl-retaining hormone while diminishing its kaliuretic effect.[16] Hence, it is important to monitor the P_K frequently during the treatment of hypokalemia.

Hyperkalemia has been observed in approximately 4% of patients taking K^+ supplements. The risk is highest in patients with renal failure and diabetes mellitus. The simultaneous use of angiotensin-converting enzyme inhibitors, β-blockers, or nonsteroidal anti-inflammatory drugs may also predispose to the development of hyperkalemia.

Specific causes of hypokalemia

A summary of the causes of hypokalemia is provided in Fig. 35.3. We only comment briefly on some of them because they are common or because new strides have been made in understanding their pathophysiology.

Diuretic-induced hypokalemia

The excessive excretion of K^+ with diuretics (and in diseases where the net effect is an endogenous diuretic action, such as Bartter and Gitelman syndromes) is due to increased delivery of Na^+ and Cl^- to the CCD. There is not only high flow in the CCD but also enhanced K^+ secretion because the ability to reabsorb Na^+ in the presence of aldo-sterone is stimulated and it exceeds that for Cl^- (see Fig. 35.4). Hypokalemia is usually modest. A fall in P_K to < 3 mmol/L occurs in less than 10% of patients and usually is present in the first 2 weeks of therapy.[32] Our view is that patients with hypokalemia in the setting of coronary heart disease, left ventricular hypertrophy, or digitalis therapy should be treated to minimize the risk of a ventricular arrhythmia.

There are several ways to minimize the degree of diuretic-induced hypokalemia. First, the lowest effective dose of diuretic should be used as the risk of hypokalemia is dose dependent. In most patients with essential hypertension, 12.5–25 mg of hydrochlorothiazide produces as great a fall in blood pressure as higher doses. Second, the intake of K^+ should not be low. Salt substitutes such as Co-salt (14 mmol K^+ per gram) are an inexpensive way to provide K^+ while limiting the intake of Na^+. Third, the degree of hypokalemia can be minimized by lowering K^+ excretion. This may be achieved in part by limiting the intake and thereby the excretion of NaCl to ~ 100 mmol/day. The renal loss of K^+ can be reduced with the use of K^+-sparing diuretics.

Primary hyperaldosteronism

This should be suspected when hypertension accompanies hypokalemia with renal K^+ wasting in patients who have low plasma renin activity. A poorly explained fact is that a significant number of patients with primary hyperaldos-teronism do not have hypokalemia.[33] Unilateral adrenal-ectomy is generally the preferred treatment in a patient with an adrenal adenoma. With bilateral adrenal hyperplasia, or when the patient has an adrenal adenoma but is not a candidate for surgery, medical therapy with a K^+-sparing diuretic (amiloride or spironolactone) is the preferred treatment.

Other disorders

The molecular basis for genetic causes of hypokalemia are summarized in Table 35.1.[34–40] An important step in this process is to rule out secondary causes (Fig. 35.5). A constellation of findings similar to those in Bartter syndrome result from inhibition of the luminal K^+ channel in the thick ascending limb of the loop of Henle. This may be acquired as a result of binding of cationic antibiotics (e.g. aminoglycosides[41–43]) to a basolateral Ca^{2+}-sensing receptor.[44] Nevertheless, when considering Bartter or Gitelman syndromes, the major differential diagnosis is occult vomiting, laxative abuse, and diuretic abuse. We use urine electrolytes to guide us here (Table 35.2). In the patient with occult vomiting, the key finding is a very low urine $[Cl^-]$; in the laxative abuser, helpful clues include a Cl^--rich, Na^+-poor urine, hyperchloremic metabolic acidosis, and possibly a high urine osmole gap and/or urine net charge. Diuretics should be suspected when most spot urines have abundant Na^+ and Cl^- but at least one spot urine has little Na^+ and Cl^-; this diagnosis is confirmed by a positive test for diuretics in a urine sample with abundant Na^+ and Cl^-.

Another cause of hypokalemia with renal K^+ wasting is hypomagnesemia. Aside from a very unusual diet, one should consider conditions where there is malabsorption of magnesium (Mg^{2+}) (e.g. alcohol abuse) and/or renal Mg^{2+} wasting (e.g. patients on cisplatin, gentamicin, or large doses of loop diuretics). In these settings, the hypo-magnesia is more likely an associated finding than a cause of hypokalemia. Treatment of the underlying lesion and correction of the Mg^{2+} deficit may reverse the hypo-kalemia.[45] We recently examined the role of hypomagne-semia as a factor that may aggravate the degree of renal K^+ wasting in patients with Gitelman syndrome.[45] The response to Mg^{2+} infusion was heterogeneous in that only four of six patients had a marked decline in TTKG when hypomagnesemia was corrected. Notwithstanding, one

Table 35.1 Hereditary diseases and hypokalemia*

	Gitelman syndrome	Bartter syndrome	Liddle syndrome	GRA[†]	AME syndrome
Site of lesion	DCT	mTAL in LOH	CCD	Adrenal gland	CCD
Molecular lesion	Low NCC Low ClCNB Low Na$^+$,K$^+$-ATPase	Low NKCC Low ROM-K Low ClCNB CaSR Barttin	High ENaC in the CCD	ACTH-driven mineralocorticoid synthesis	Low 11β-HSDH in principal cells
Presenting features	Tetany, unexpected laboratory finding	Failure to thrive, laboratory finding	High blood pressure Family history	High blood pressure Family history	High blood pressure Family history
Age of first symptoms	Teenage	Children	Young if severe	Young adult	Children
Mimicked by drugs	Thiazides	Loop diuretics	Amphotericin B	Mineralocorticoids	Licorice, carbenoxolone
Plasma Mg	Low	May be low	Normal	Normal	Normal
Extracellular fluid volume	Low	Low	High	High	High
Blood pressure	Normal	Normal	High	High	High
Key features	Hypocalciuria Normal maximum U_{osm}	Lower than expected maximum U_{osm}	High blood pressure Responds to amiloride but not spironolactone	Suppress with dexamethasone	Urine cortisone: cortisol ratio

ACTH, adrenocorticotropic hormone; AME, apparent mineralocorticoid excess; CCD, cortical collecting duct; ClCNB, basolateral Cl$^-$ channel; DCT, distal convoluted tubule; ENaC, epithelial Na$^+$ channel; GRA, glucocorticoid-remediable aldosteronism; 11β-HSDH, 11β-hydroxysteroid dehydrogenase, NCC, Na/Cl cotransporter; NKCC, Na$^+$/K$^+$/2Cl$^-$ cotransporter in thick ascending limb of loop of Henle; ROM-K, K$^+$ channel; CaSR, calcium-sensing receptor.
*All the disease categories present with hypokalemia and excessive excretion of K$^+$ associated with higher than expected urine [K$^+$].
[†]Some members of families with this disorder do not have hypokalemia.

usually cannot correct the hypomagnesemia with oral Mg^{2+} replacement therapy. We do not advise the use of nonsteroidal anti-inflammatory drugs in patients with Bartter or Gitelman syndromes because of their potential to cause chronic renal dysfunction. We are also cautious about using K$^+$-sparing diuretics (e.g. spironolactone, amiloride) as they might further aggravate an already contracted ECF volume.

Table 35.2 Urine electrolytes in the differential diagnosis of hypokalemia*

Condition	Urine electrolytes	
	Na$^+$	Cl$^-$
Vomiting		
Recent	High[†]	Low[‡]
Remote	Low	Low
Diuretics		
Recent	High	High
Remote	Low	Low
Diarrhea or laxative abuse	Low	High
Bartter or Gitelman syndrome	High	High

*Do not use the urine electrolytes in this fashion during polyuric states.
[†]High: urine concentration > 15 mmol/L.
[‡]Low: urine concentration < 15 mmol/L.

Hyperkalemia

General considerations for treatment of hyperkalemia

Medical emergencies

The major danger of hyperkalemia is cardiac arrhythmia. Because mild ECG changes may progress rapidly to a dangerous arrhythmia, any patient with an ECG abnormality related to hyperkalemia should be considered as a potential medical emergency. We would also treat patients with a severe degree of hyperkalemia (P_K > 7.0 mmol/L) aggressively, even in the absence of ECG changes (Fig. 35.6). A note of caution is needed: a severe degree of hyperkalemia is well tolerated in certain settings such as extremes of exercise (the super-marathon[5]) and in infants.

Antagonize the cardiac effects of hyperkalemia Ca^{2+} is the best agent and its effects should be evident within minutes. It is usually given as 20–30 mL of a 10% calcium gluconate solution (two to three ampoules) or 10 mL of 10% CaCl$_2$ (one ampoule). This dose can be repeated in 5 min if ECG changes persist. The effect may last 30–60 min. Extreme caution should be exerted using Ca^{2+} in patients on digitalis because hypercalcemia may precipitate digitalis toxicity.

Induce a shift of K$^+$ into the ICF

Insulin Insulin activates the NHE in cell membranes

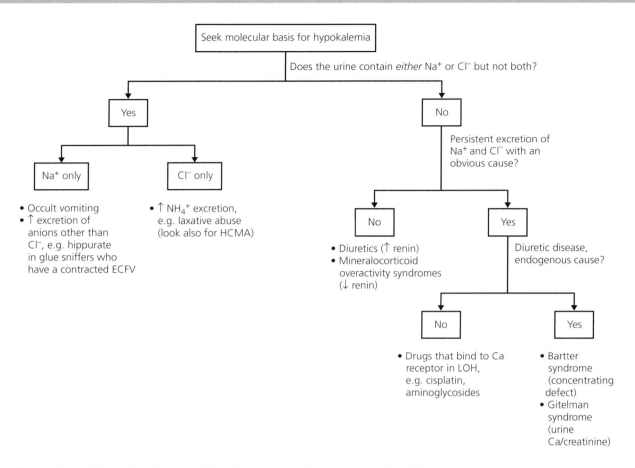

Figure 35.5 Differential diagnosis of hereditary causes of hypokalemia. The initial step is to rule out common causes of hypokalemia that may be denied by the patient. Here the urine electrolytes become very important (see Table 35.2). A finding of persistent excretion of Na⁺ and Cl⁻ despite a contracted extracellular fluid volume narrows the differential diagnosis. Failure to find an obvious cause for renal Na⁺ and Cl⁻ wasting suggests that Bartter or Gitelman syndrome may be present. HCMA, hyperchloremic metabolic acidosis; LOH, loop of Henle. (From Halperin ML: The ACID Truth and Basic Facts: With a Sweet Touch, an enLYTEnment, 4th edn. Stirling, Ontario: Ross Mark Medical Publishers, 1997, with permission.)

and increases the electroneutral entry of Na⁺ into the cell in exchange for H⁺ (see Fig. 35.2). The increase in intracellular Na⁺ stimulates Na⁺,K⁺-ATPase; the electrogenic export of Na⁺ out of the cell results in a more negative resting membrane potential.

Studies support the use of insulin in the treatment of acute hyperkalemia in patients with endstage renal disease (ESRD).[46–50] For example, Blumberg et al[46] studied 10 patients with ESRD on hemodialysis after an overnight fast prior to their regularly scheduled hemodialysis. The patients were treated on different occasions with ~ 20 units of intravenous regular insulin plus glucose, or NaHCO₃ at 4 mmol/min, or epinephrine 0.05 µg/kg/min, or hemodialysis. The P_K was followed for 60 min. Hemodialysis was the most effective modality in lowering P_K, reducing it from 5.6 to 4.3 mmol/L. Insulin with glucose also caused the P_K to fall rapidly from 5.6 to 4.7 mmol/L. Of note, epinephrine caused only a minor decline in the P_K, from 5.6 to 5.3 mmol/L, although 5 of 10 patients did not have a decline. Intravenous NaHCO₃ failed to lower the P_K. Similar beneficial effects of insulin have also been noted in a number of other recent studies.[47–50] Large doses of insulin are needed for maximal K⁺ shift into cells. In the study by Blumberg et al,[46] 20 units of regular insulin were given to raise the plasma insulin level to 300–400 milliunits/L. Hypoglycemia was a frequent complication.[46,47,48] One cannot overemphasize the need to give enough glucose to prevent hypoglycemia and to monitor blood glucose levels for a sufficient period of time.

We recommend insulin with glucose as initial therapy to induce a shift of K⁺ into cells in the emergency treatment of hyperkalemia. One could consider treating nondiabetic hyperkalemic patients with a bolus of glucose without exogenous insulin. We feel that this strategy is unwise because the high levels of insulin required to induce an adequate shift of K⁺ into cells might not be achieved without giving insulin. In addition, hypertonic glucose may cause K⁺ to shift out of cells in patients with inadequate insulin reserves, leading to a paradoxical rise in P_K.[51,52]

β₂-Adrenergic agonists β₂-Agonists stimulate Na⁺,K⁺-ATPase via a cyclic AMP-dependent pathway (see Fig. 35.2). This leads to the electrogenic export of Na⁺ and

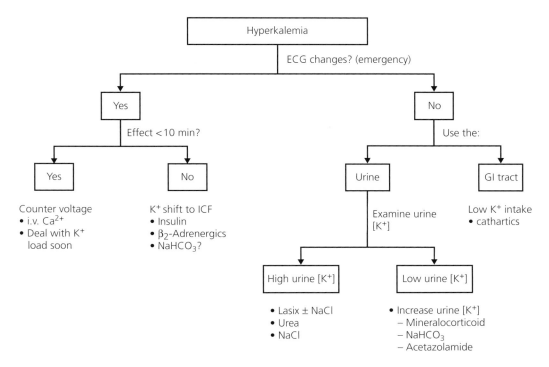

Figure 35.6 Treatment of the patient with hyperkalemia. If an emergency is present (usually cardiac), intravenous Ca^{2+} must be given. This treatment should act promptly. Efforts are now made to shift K^+ into cells with insulin and glucose. (See text for discussion). Longer-term strategies are to limit intake of K^+, prevent its absorption in the gastrointestinal (GI) tract, and promote its excretion. In this latter context, examine the urine $[K^+]$ and flow rate to decide leverage for therapy. ICF, intracellular fluid. (From Halperin ML: The ACID Truth and Basic Facts: With a Sweet Touch, an enLYTEnment, 4th edn. Stirling, Ontario: Ross Mark Medical Publishers, 1997, with permission.)

a more negative intracellular voltage. In normal subjects, infusion of physiologic doses of epinephrine lowers the P_K. However, patients with ESRD seem to be resistant to the hypokalemic effects of epinephrine. Epinephrine is a mixed α and β agonist: β_2-adrenergic stimulation increases cellular K^+ uptake, whereas α-adrenergic stimulation causes K^+ to shift from the ICF to the ECF.[53–56] A study by Allon and Shanklin[57] suggested that the impaired hypokalemic response to epinephrine in ESRD is caused by an enhanced hyperkalemic effect due to α-adrenergic stimulation.

The ability of β_2-adrenergic stimulation to lower the P_K in patients with renal failure has been demonstrated in a number of studies.[47,49,58–63] Montoliu et al[58] gave 20 patients on maintenance hemodialysis 0.5 mg of albuterol intravenously over 15 min. The mean P_K decreased from 5.6 to 4.5 mmol/L within 30 min. Eight patients developed tremors and six had minor ill-defined discomfort. In a second part of the study,[64] consecutive patients with acute or chronic renal failure were given intravenous albuterol 0.5 mg over 15 min. Their mean P_K decreased from 7.0 to 5.6 mmol/L within 30 min, and the effect was sustained for 3 h. Reversal of the ECG manifestations of hyperkalemia was documented in most patients and only minor adverse effects were noted. It was recognized, however, that there was considerable individual variation

in the response of the P_K to albuterol, although the data for individual patients were not shown. Similar results have been found in other studies where the selective β_2-agonist salbutamol was infused intravenously.[58–60]

A number of studies have examined nebulized β_2-agonists as therapy for hyperkalemia. In a study by Allon et al,[61] 10 ESRD patients on hemodialysis who had hyperkalemia were treated with 10 mg of nebulized albuterol, 20 mg of nebulized albuterol, or placebo on three separate occasions. After the administration of albuterol, the P_K decreased within 30 min and this fall in P_K was sustained for at least 2 h. The maximum decreases in P_K were 0.6 mmol/L with 10 mg nebulized albuterol and 1.0 mmol/L with the 20-mg dose. However, 2 of the 10 patients were resistant to the hypokalemic effects of albuterol. There was a minimal increase in heart rate and a notable absence of cardiovascular adverse effects. Similar observations were made by Liou et al[59] and Montoliu et al.[62] In a more recent study, Mandelberg et al[63] found that salbutamol 1200 mg via metered-dose inhaler given over 2 min also had similar hypokalemic and tachycardic effects as nebulized β_2-agonists. In a significant number of the patients the P_K rose by 0.1 mmol/L in the first 1–2 min of therapy.

While these studies suggest that nebulized β_2-agonists are effective in rapidly lowering the P_K, we do not recommend their use as preferred therapy in the emergency treatment of hyperkalemia for two main reasons. First, they are not effective in a significant proportion of patients; 20–40% of patients studied had a decline in P_K of < 0.5 mmol/L. It is unclear why certain patients do not exhibit a fall in P_K following the administration of β_2-agonists and it is not possible to predict which patients will respond. Second, we are concerned about the safety of these drugs in the doses used for the treatment of hyperkalemia, doses that are four to eight times those prescribed for the treatment of acute asthma. Although no severe adverse events were reported in the studies noted above, most were performed in stable patients with a mild degree of hyperkalemia prior to their regular hemodialysis session. A number of these studies excluded patients on β-blockers and selected those with no significant coronary heart disease or unstable heart rhythms. Therefore, the safety of these agents was determined in a group of patients that may not resemble the general ESRD population that has a high prevalence of cardiac disease.

Whether the effect of nebulized β_2-agonists in lowering P_K is additive to that of insulin has been examined by Allon and Copkney.[47] In a crossover design, 12 patients on maintenance hemodialysis who had predialysis P_K of > 5 mmol/L received 10 units of regular insulin plus glucose as an intravenous bolus or 20 mg nebulized albuterol over 10 min, or both. Insulin decreased P_K in 15 min and albuterol decreased P_K within 30 min. There was a similar decrease in P_K with insulin (0.65 mmol/L) or albuterol (0.66 mmol/L). However, 4 of 10 patients treated with albuterol had a mean decrease in P_K of < 0.5 mmol/L. There was a substantially greater fall in P_K with the combined regimen (1.2 mmol/L) compared with either agent alone. One should note, however, that only 10 units of intravenous regular insulin were given in this study, the plasma insulin level was only 40 milliunits/L at 60 min, and the magnitude of the decrease in P_K was lower than that observed in other studies when higher doses of insulin were used. Blumberg et al[46] administered 20 units of intravenous insulin and achieved a similar decrease in P_K (~ 1 mmol/L) as Allon and Copkney[47] with their combined therapy of 10 units of intravenous insulin and albuterol. Thus it remains uncertain whether β_2-agonists would have a P_K-lowering effect additive to that of insulin if insulin were given at the higher doses.

NaHCO$_3$ The utility of this therapy for acute hyperkalemia has been the subject of considerable controversy. The administration of $NaHCO_3$ decreases the concentration of H^+ in the ECF compartment. In theory, if the NHE were in an active mode and if the administration of $NaHCO_3$ were to favor the movement of H^+ out of cells via the NHE, more Na^+ would enter the cell in an electroneutral manner (see Fig. 35.2). The subsequent electrogenic exit of these Na^+ ions via Na^+,K^+-ATPase would render the resting membrane potential more negative and allow a shift of K^+ into the cell. Of note, the NHE antiporter catalyzes an electroneutral exchange and it is normally inactive, as evidenced by the higher concentration of Na^+ and lower concentration of H^+ in the ECF compared with the ICF compartments (see Fig. 35.2). One major activator of the NHE antiporter is intracellular

acidosis because H^+ are not only a substrate for the antiporter but they also bind to a modifier site that activates the NHE.

A number of recent studies have found $NaHCO_3$ therapy to be ineffective in the acute treatment of hyperkalemia.[46,64,65] Blumberg et al[44] studied 10 patients with ESRD on hemodialysis who had mild hyperkalemia (mean P_K close to 5.5 mmol/L). These patients were given 100–215 mmol of intravenous $NaHCO_3$ as either an isotonic or a hypertonic solution. Although the mean plasma HCO_3^- concentration (P_{HCO_3}) rose from 21 to 34 mmol/L, there was no change in P_K after 60 min, a time-frame during which an intervention used in a potentially life-threatening situation is expected to have a significant effect. In a subsequent study, Blumberg et al[65] infused 390 mmol of $NaHCO_3$ over 6 h in 12 patients with ESRD on hemodialysis. There was a moderate decline in P_K from 6.0 to 5.4 mmol/L, but only after 4 h of starting the $NaHCO_3$ infusion.

It is noteworthy that the studies that found a lack of effect of $NaHCO_3$ were performed in stable hemodialysis patients without significant acidosis. In other words, these studies examined the effect of $NaHCO_3$ when the NHE was presumably in an inactive mode. The question remains as to whether $NaHCO_3$ would be effective in patients with a more significant degree of acidosis, when the NHE is likely to become activated. There are limited data in the literature to answer this question. A report by Schwarz et al[66] described four uremic patients with P_K values ranging from 5.9 to 8.5 mmol/L associated with ECG changes attributable to hyperkalemia and a profound degree of acidosis (P_{HCO_3} 1.3–7.3 mmol/L). With infusion of 150–400 mmol $NaHCO_3$, all four patients showed a significant reduction in P_K and improvement of their ECG. Thus it is difficult to draw a definite conclusion from the available data in the literature. On the one hand, studies similar to those of Blumberg et al[46,63,65] examined patients with only a mild degree of hyperkalemia and no significant acidosis and concluded that there was no benefit. On the other hand, the report by Schwarz et al[66] demonstrated benefit using $NaHCO_3$, but this was evaluated in a small number of patients who had a severe degree of acidosis. We still use $NaHCO_3$ to treat acute hyperkalemia in patients with significant acidosis, but we would not use it as the only emergency therapy to shift K^+ into cells. Caution is warranted as excessive administration of $NaHCO_3$ should be avoided due to the risk of inducing hypernatremia, ECF volume expansion, carbon dioxide retention, and a fall in ionized serum calcium.

Studies that examined the combined use of $NaHCO_3$ with insulin have also produced conflicting results. Allon and Shanklin[48] found that the addition of $NaHCO_3$ did not enhance the P_K-lowering effects of insulin in their study of eight ESRD patients on hemodialysis. In this study, the mean P_K before therapy was 4.5 mmol/L and the mean P_{HCO_3} 22 mmol/L. In contrast, Kim[50] compared insulin, $NaHCO_3$, or both in eight patients with a predialysis P_K of > 6 mmol/L. There was no change in P_K with $NaHCO_3$ as sole therapy after 60 min. Insulin caused P_K to fall from 6.3 to 5.7 mmol/L. However, the combination of insulin and $NaHCO_3$ showed the greatest decline in P_K (from 6.2 to 5.2 mmol/L). It is unclear why Kim[50] found a synergistic effect of $NaHCO_3$ with insulin yet Allon and Shanklin[48] did not. It should be noted, however, that the patients studied by Allon and Shanklin were not hyperkalemic.

No medical emergency: removal of K^+ from the body

It is important to appreciate that to lower the P_K from 7.0 to 6.0 mmol/L requires very much less K^+ loss than that needed to lower the P_K from 6.0 to 5.0 mmol/L.[30] Hence creating a small K^+ loss can be very important when there is a severe degree of hyperkalemia.

Diuretics and/or mineralocorticoids There are two aspects to consider here. If K^+ excretion is low because of a low urine volume with a high concentration of K^+, a loop diuretic may induce a kaliuresis by increasing the flow rate in the CCD. One can avoid unwanted ECF volume contraction by replacing the NaCl lost in the urine. This NaCl should be given at the same tonicity as the urine in order to avoid dysnatremia. If the urine K^+ concentration is unduly low, giving a mineralocorticoid (100 μg fludrocortisone acetate) and inducing bicarbonaturia with the carbonic anhydrase inhibitor acetazolamide may cause substantial kaliuresis (HCO_3^- lost in the urine might need to be replaced).

Cation-exchange resins A cation-exchange resin is a cross-linked polymer with negatively charged structural units. The resin can exchange bound Na^+ (Kayexalate) or Ca^{2+} (calcium resonium) for cations including K^+. The purpose of using resins is to enhance the elimination of K^+ from the gastrointestinal tract. We first outline why resins cannot significantly enhance K^+ removal with regard to their relative affinities for Na^+ and K^+ and the concentrations of these cations throughout the gastrointestinal tract. This is followed by a critique of human studies that have examined the effects of resins and/or cathartics on fecal K^+ excretion.

The cation-exchange resin, Kayexalate, contains 4 mequiv. of Na^+ per gram. This Na^+ is theoretically exchangeable for 4 mequiv. of K^+. Thus, 30 g of Kayexalate could theoretically remove 120 mequiv. of K^+. However, this degree of exchange does not occur at the Na^+ and K^+ concentrations found in the gastrointestinal tract. Emmet et al[67] examined the in vitro binding characteristics of Kayexalate and found that the Na^+ and K^+ concentrations at which 50% of the initial Na^+ exchanged for K^+ were 65 and 40 mmol/L, respectively. With a higher concentration of Na^+ and/or a lower concentration of K^+, less exchange would be expected to take place. If one considers the concentrations of Na^+ and K^+ in the duodenum (110 and 15 mmol/L respectively), jejunum (140 and 5 mmol/L respectively), ileum (130 and 20 mmol/L respectively), and rectum (10 and 80 mmol/L respectively),[68,69] it seems that the only favorable location for the exchange of Na^+ for K^+ is in the lumen of the rectum. Because there is little absorption of K^+ in the rectum, there is no significant advantage to having the K^+ in its luminal fluid excreted in an ionic form or bound to a resin. Furthermore, normal fecal K^+ excretion is about 9 mequiv./day; uremic subjects

excrete only slightly more K^+ (an extra 2.3 mequiv./day) in their feces than normal subjects.[70]

In humans, active secretion of K^+ in the gastrointestinal tract occurs in the rectosigmoid portion of the colon. One possible theoretical benefit for the use of cation-exchange resins is if they were to lower the K^+ concentration in luminal water, thereby enhancing the net secretion of K^+ by the rectosigmoid colon. However, a number of factors limit the magnitude of this process. First, the volume of stool water is small. Second, in the colon, other cations are available to exchange for resin-bound Na^+ apart from K^+, including NH_4^+, Ca^{2+}, and Mg^{2+}. The concentration of NH_4^+ in stool water may be high in patients with ESRD as a result of their high blood urea levels and because of bacterial urease activity in the lumen of the gastrointestinal tract. Cations such as Ca^{2+} and Mg^{2+} have an even greater affinity for the resin than K^+ because of their divalent positive charge. In addition, resins are usually given with cathartics because of their notorious tendency to cause constipation. Cathartics can increase stool Na^+ concentration, leading to conditions even more unfavorable for K^+ binding to the resin. Third, the surface area of the rectum is small so the rate of rectal K^+ secretion would severely limit the ability of resins to remove K^+ from the gastrointestinal tract. In experiments where dialysis bags were placed into the rectum of subjects with chronic renal failure, the rate of net K^+ secretion was 1.5 μmol/h per cm^2 of rectal surface area.[70–72] Thus in a subject with an average rectal surface area of 100 cm^2, net K^+ secretion would be only 4 mmol daily.[70] Thus, from a theoretical point of view, resins would seem of little use in inducing a loss of K^+ from the gastrointestinal tract unless lowering of the stool K^+ concentration plays an important role in this process.

Two reports are commonly cited to support the use of resins for treatment of hyperkalemia. Flinn et al[73] examined 10 patients with oliguria and hyperkalemia. All were treated with a low K^+ diet consisting of 50% dextrose in water or Karo syrup and gingerale, up to 15 g of resin four times daily, and sorbitol to produce one to two diarrheal stools per day. P_K decreased in all patients over 5 days. Scherr et al[74] described 32 patients with acute or chronic renal failure and hyperkalemia. All were given K^+-restricted diets, 20–60 g/day of resin orally or 10–40 g of resin by enema, and cathartics for constipation. Three patients were also given insulin and glucose, and four patients were given $NaHCO_3$. Of the 32 patients, 23 showed a fall in their P_K of at least 0.4 mequiv./L within 24 h. Although the authors of both studies concluded that resins were useful for treating hyperkalemia, it is difficult to determine their exact role. It should be noted that several doses were given, sometimes for a number of days, and that the effect on P_K was noted after 1–5 days. Furthermore, it is not clear if the effect was due to the resin or merely to the induction of diarrhea with hypertonic glucose or other cathartics. Flinn et al[73] commented that sorbitol alone was as effective as the combination of resin and sorbitol in removing K^+, but that it was associated with a larger volume of "debilitating" diarrhea.

Two recent studies have reexamined the effect of cathartics and/or resins on fecal K^+ excretion.[67,75] Emmett et al[67] gave nine normal human subjects 60 or 120 g sorbitol, or 100 mmol sodium sulfate, or eight phenolphthalein/docusate tablets; each with and without 30 g of Kayexalate. Stool water, Na^+, and K^+ were followed over the ensuing 12 h. Phenolphthalein resulted in the highest stool K^+ excretion rate (37 mequiv. in 12 h) compared with the other laxatives. The addition of 30 g of Kayexalate to phenolphthalein increased stool K^+ excretion only modestly to 49 mequiv. in 12 h. The addition of the resin to sorbitol or sodium sulfate did not significantly increase stool K^+ excretion compared with either laxative alone. The results of this study suggest that the majority of K^+ excretion with cathartics and resins is due to the induction of diarrhea.

Gruy-Kapral et al[75] studied the effect of a single dose of cathartic and/or resin on fecal K^+ excretion and P_K in patients with renal failure. Six patients with ESRD on hemodialysis received placebo, 30 g of Kayexalate, eight tablets of phenolphthalein/docusate, eight tablets of phenolphthalein/docusate plus 30 g of Kayexalate, and 60 g of sorbitol plus 30 g of Kayexalate on different occasions. Four hours after the treatment, the patients also ingested a standard meal containing 21 mequiv. of K^+. Stools were collected and P_K levels followed for 12 h. The total stool K^+ excretion was 54 mequiv. with phenolphthalein alone, 49 mequiv. with phenolphthalein plus Kayexalate, and 31 mequiv. with sorbitol plus Kayexalate. The excreted resin bound K^+ at a ratio of 0.65 mequiv./g, which is far below its maximum of 4 mequiv./g. Although the patients were not initially hyperkalemic, none of the regimens reduced P_K compared with baseline levels. This study supports the argument that resins do not contribute to fecal K^+ excretion above the induction of diarrhea alone, and that single-dose resin/cathartic therapy is of no value in the management of acute hyperkalemia.

In summary, we do not recommend the use of resins for acute hyperkalemia. In the setting of chronic hyperkalemia, the addition of resins to cathartics adds little to the induction of diarrhea alone. One other point merits emphasis: there is evidence that the hypertonic sorbitol may cause colonic necrosis.[76,77]

Dialysis Hemodialysis is more effective than peritoneal dialysis for removing K^+. Removal rates of K^+ can approximate 35 mmol/h with a dialysate bath K^+ concentration of 1–2 mmol/L. A glucose-free dialysate is preferable in order to avoid the glucose-induced release of insulin and the subsequent shift of K^+ into cells, lessening the removal of K^+. For the same reason, one should consider discontinuing the insulin/glucose infusion once hemodialysis is initiated.

Specific causes of hyperkalemia

A clinical algorithm to the treatment of these patients is illustrated in Fig. 35.6.

Conditions that are heterogeneous in pathophysiology but are linked under a single inappropriate diagnostic category

Hyporeninemic hypoaldosteronism Although most commonly seen in patients with diabetic nephropathy, this syndrome has also been associated with many other renal diseases. On the one hand, a biosynthetic defect in the juxtaglomerular apparatus could cause renal salt wasting and ECF volume contraction; if present, the administration of aldosterone should lead to the expected rise in TTKG. Nevertheless, a large number of patients with this diagnosis probably have an expanded ECF volume and hence low plasma renin levels.[78,79] A rise in TTKG is not observed acutely after the administration of mineralocorticoids. A higher TTKG occurs with the induction of bicarbonaturia. These findings suggest a "Cl^- shunt" disorder as the underlying pathophysiology.[80] The increased electroneutral reabsorption of NaCl could lead to ECF volume expansion, suppression of renin–aldosterone, and hyperkalemia.

Characterization of the pathophysiology in each patient is important because it has implications with regard to therapy. Obviously the use of exogenous mineralocorticoids is of little acute benefit with respect to its kaliuretic effect in patients with a Cl^- shunt disorder. Because these agents may stimulate the reabsorption of NaCl, they may aggravate the patient's hypertension. In this group of patients, the administration of loop or thiazide diuretics should enhance kaliuresis and may also help with blood pressure control. Diuretic therapy would be a threat to the subgroup of patients with hyporeninemic hypoaldosteronism and a low ECF volume; these patients respond to fludrocortisone.[1,24] In practice, the level of blood pressure may be helpful in distinguishing these two groups: high in the Cl^- shunt group, and low in the group with a primary problem in renin–aldosterone release.

Hypertension with hyperkalemia The association of hypertension and hyperkalemia in patients with normal glomerular filtration rate is usually accompanied by a low plasma renin activity and plasma aldosterone levels that are not elevated considering the presence of hyperkalemia; this is the Cl^- shunt disorder.[81] Recent molecular studies have identified two potential WNK kinase candidates affecting Cl^- permeability via the paracellular route that may be involved in the underlying pathophysiology in patients with Gordon syndrome or type 2 pseudohypoaldosteronism.[13] Thiazide diuretics are helpful in these patients. In contrast, a patient with hypertension and hyperkalemia was described in whom the ECF volume was mildly contracted, and plasma renin and aldosterone levels were elevated.[82] Hyperkalemia in this patient was postulated to be due to "slow" Na^+ reabsorption in the CCD, perhaps an ENaC defect that led to a slower rate of electrogenic reabsorption of Na^+ (see Fig. 35.4). The renal salt wasting resulted in ECF volume contraction and the release of renin and aldosterone and possibly other vasoactive mediators that could have led to vasocontriction and hypertension in a patient who may have been unduly sensitive to vasoconstrictors. This hypothesis was supported by a fall in blood pressure when the patient's ECF volume was expanded, the opposite form of treatment for a patient with hypertension and hyperkalemia due to a Cl^- shunt disorder.

Cyclosporine-induced hyperkalemia

Hyperkalemia develops in some patients receiving cyclosporine following organ transplantation. Even though cyclosporine can lead to inhibition of Na⁺,K⁺-ATPase in vitro,[83,84] we favor the hypothesis that the pathophysiology of hyperkalemia in these patients resembles a Cl⁻ shunt disorder in the CCD.[85] Kaliuresis could be enhanced in these patients with the administration of a loop diuretic if it increased the flow rate in the CCD. Bicarbonaturia (presumably by decreasing the apparent permeability for Cl⁻ in the CCD) could also lead to a significant increase in TTKG; the use of acetazolamide may be considered if there is a reason not to give $NaHCO_3$.

Trimethoprim-induced hyperkalemia

Trimethoprim and pentamidine can cause hyperkalemia by blocking ENaC in the CCD.[86,87] Although frequently reported in patients with AIDS who received high doses of trimethoprim for the treatment of *Pneumocystis carinii* pneumonia, trimethoprim causes a rise in P_K even when used in conventional doses. Patients with AIDS might also have other causes that make them prone to the development of a more severe degree of hyperkalemia (shift of K⁺ from cells, decreased K⁺ excretion because of low flow in the CCD due to a low rate of osmole (urea) excretion[88]).

Use of a loop diuretic may help by increasing the volume delivered to the CCD, which will lower the concentration of trimethoprim in its lumen; enough NaCl administration will be required to defend ECF volume. Since trimethoprim only blocks ENaC when the drug is in its charged (protonated) form, increasing luminal fluid pH in the CCD should decrease the cationic form of trimethoprim and minimize the antikaliuretic effect of this drug.[89] Inducing bicarbonaturia with acetazolamide and the use of a loop diuretic are rational therapeutic options in a patient with hyperkalemia in whom continuation of trimethoprim is necessary. However, sufficient NaCl and $NaHCO_3$ would need to be given to avoid a contracted ECF volume and metabolic acidosis, respectively.

Addison disease

In a recent publication, Gagnon and Halperin[90] reported detailed data on a patient with Addison disease who did not have hyperkalemia on repeated examinations. Nevertheless, there was a relatively sudden rise in his P_K on one hospital visit. In fact, a lack of hyperkalemia is not uncommon because close to one-third of patients with Addison disease have P_K values in the normal range.[91]

When treatment is considered, both glucocorticoids as well as mineralocorticoids must be replaced. In addition, the deficit of NaCl must also be corrected; this permits the renal excretion of water and K⁺ that were retained in excess of body needs.

References

1. Kamel KS, Quaggin S, Scheich A, et al: Disorders of potassium homeostasis: an approach based on pathophysiology. Am J Kidney Dis 1994;24:597–613.
2. Clausen T: Regulation of active Na⁺-K⁺ transport in skeletal muscle. Physiol Rev 1986;66:542–580.
3. Soleimani M, Sing G: Physiologic and molecular aspects of the Na⁺/H⁺ exchangers in health and disease processes. J Invest Med 1995;43:419–430.
4. Moore RD: Stimulation of Na:H exchange by insulin. Biophys J 1981;33:203–210.
5. McKechnie JK, Leary WP, Joubert SM: Some electrocardiographic and biochemical changes recorded in marathon runners. S Afr Med J 1967;41:722–725.
6. Lehmann-Horn F, Iaizzo PA, Hatt H, et al: Altered gating and conductance of Na⁺ channels in hyperkalemic periodic paralysis. Pflugers Arch 1991;418:297–299.
7. Don BR, Sebastian A, Cheitlin M, et al: Pseudohyperkalemia caused by fist clenching during phlebotomy. N Engl J Med 1990;322:1290–1292.
8. Lang F, Rehwald W: Potassium channels in renal epithelial transport regulation. Physiol Rev 1992;72:1–32.
9. Giebisch G, Malnic G, Berliner R: Control of renal potassium excretion. In Brenner BM (ed): Brenner and Rector's The Kidney, 5th edn. Philadelphia: WB Saunders, 1996, pp 371–407.
10. Giebisch G: Renal potassium transport: mechanisms and regulation. Am J Physiol 1998;274:F817–F833.
11. Halperin ML, Kamel KS: Potassium. Lancet 1998;352:135–142.
12. Rossier BC, Canessa CM, Schild L, et al: Epithelial sodium channels. Curr Opin Nephrol Hypertens 1994;3:487–496.
13. Wilson FH, Disse-Nocodeme S, Choate KA, et al: Human hypertension caused by mutations in WNK kinases. Science 2001;293:1107–1112.
14. Stokes JB: Ion transport by the collecting duct. Semin Nephrol 1993;13:202–212.
15. Good DW, Velazquez H, Wright FS: Luminal influences on potassium secretion: low sodium concentration. Am J Physiol 1984;246:F609–F619.
16. Halperin ML, Kamel KS: Dynamic interactions between integrative physiology and molecular medicine: the key to understand the mechanism of action of aldosterone in the kidney. Can J Physiol Pharmacol 2000;78:587–594.
17. Rossier BC, Palmer LG: Mechanisms of aldosterone action on sodium and potassium transport. In Seldin DW, Giebisch G (eds): The Kidney: Physiology and Pathophysiology. New York: Raven Press, 1992, pp 1373–1409.
18. Garty H: Regulation of the epithelial Na⁺ channel by aldosterone: open questions and emerging answers. Kidney Int 2000;57:1270–1276.
19. Clore J, Schoolwerth A, Watlington CO: When is cortisol a mineralocorticoid? Kidney Int 1992;42:1297–1308.
20. Farese RV, Biglieri EG, Shackelton CHL: Licorice-induced hypermineralocorticoidism. N Engl J Med 1991;325:1223.
21. Velazquez H, Ellison DH, Wright FS: Chloride-dependent potassium secretion in early and late renal distal tubules. Am J Physiol 1987;253:F555–F562.
22. Carlisle EJF, Donnelly SM, Ethier J, et al: Modulation of the secretion of potassium by accompanying anions in humans. Kidney Int 1991;39:1206–1212.
23. Wingo CS, Armitage FE: Potassium transport in the kidney: regulation and physiologic relevance of H⁺, K⁺-ATPase. Semin Nephrol 1993;13:213–224.
24. Kamel KS, Halperin ML, Faber MD, et al: Disorders of potassium balance. In Brenner BM (ed): Brenner and Rector's The Kidney, 5th edn. Philadelphia: WB Saunders, 1996, pp 999–1037.
25. Ethier JH, Kamel KS, Magner PO, et al: The transtubular potassium concentration in patients with hypokalemia and hyperkalemia. Am J Kidney Dis 1990;15:309–315.
26. Schaefer M, Link J, Hannemann L, et al: Excessive hypokalemia and hyperkalemia following head injury. Intensive Care Med 1995;21:235–237.
27. Lin SH, Lin YF, Halperin ML: Hypokalemia and paralysis. Q J Med 2001;94:133–139.
28. Patcek LJ, Tawil R, Griggs RC, et al: Dihydropyridine receptor mutations cause hypokalemic periodic paralysis. Cell 1994;17:863–868.
29. Lin SH, Lin YF: Propranolol rapidly reverses paralysis, hypokalemia and hypophosphatemia in thyrotoxic periodic paralysis. Am J Kidney Dis 2001;37:620–624.
30. Sterns RH, Guzzo J, Feig PU, et al: Internal potassium balance and the control of the plasma potassium concentration. Medicine 1981;60:339–354.
31. Vasuvattakul S, Quaggin SE, Scheich AM, et al: Kaliuretic response to aldosterone: influence of potassium in the diet. Am J Kidney Dis 1993;21:152–160.

32. Tannen RL: Diuretic-induced hypokalemia. Kidney Int 1985;28:988–1000.

33. Gordon RD: Mineralocorticoid hypertension. Lancet 1994;344:240–243.

34. Lifton RP, Dluhy RG, Power M, et al: A chimaeric 11β-hydroxylase/aldosterone synthetase gene causes glucocorticoid-remediable aldosteronism and human hypertension. Nature 1992;355:262–265.

35. Simon DB, Nelson-Williams C, Bia MJ, et al: Gitelman's variant of Bartter's syndrome, inherited hypokalaemic alkalosis, is caused by mutations in the thiazide-sensitive Na-Cl contransporter. Nature Genetics 1996;12:24–30.

36. Simon DB, Karet FE, Hamdan JM, et al: Bartter's syndrome, hypokalaemic alkalosis with hypercalciuria, is caused by mutations in the Na-K-2Cl cotransporter NKCC2. Nature Genetics 1996;13:183–188.

37. Shimkets RA, Warnock DG, Bositis CM, et al: Liddle's syndrome: heritable human hypertension caused by mutations in the β subunit of the epithelial sodium channel. Cell 1994;79:407–414.

38. Funder JW: 11β-Hydroxysteroid dehydrogenase and the meaning of life. Mol Cell Endocrinol 1990;68:C3.

39. Vargas-Poussou R, Huang C, Hulin P, et al: Functional characterization of a calcium-sensing receptor mutation in severe autosomal dominant hypocalcemia with a Bartter-like syndrome. J Am Soc Nephrol 2002;13:2259–2266.

40. Watanabe S, Fukumoto S, Chang H, et al: Association between activating mutations of calcium-sensing receptor and Bartter's syndrome. Lancet 2002;360:692–694.

41. Shetty AK, Rogers NL, Hannick EE, et al: Syndromes of hypokalemic metabolic alkalosis and hypomagnesemia associated with gentamicin therapy: case reports. Clin Pediatr 2000;9:529–533.

42. Steiner RW, Omachi AS: A Bartter's-like syndrome from capneomycin, and a similar gentamicin to bulopathy. Am J Kidney Dis 1986;7:245–249.

43. Goodhart GL, Handelsman S: Gentamicin and hypokalemia. Ann Intern Med 1985;103:645–646.

44. Riccardi D, Park J, Lee W-S, et al: Cloning and functional expression of a rat kidney extracellular calcium/polyvalent cation-sensing receptor. Proc Natl Acad Sci USA 1995;92:131–135.

45. Kamel KS, Harvey E, Douek K, et al: Studies on the pathogenesis of hypokalemia in Gitelman's syndrome: role of bicarbonaturia and hypomagnesemia. Am J Nephrol 1998;18:42–49.

46. Blumberg A, Weidmann P, Shaw S, et al: Effect of various therapeutic approaches on plasma potassium and major regulating factors in terminal renal failure. Am J Med 1988;85:507–512.

47. Allon M, Copkney C: Albuterol and insulin for treatment of hyperkalemia in hemodialysis patients. Kidney Int 1990;38:869–872.

48. Allon M, Shanklin N: Effect of bicarbonate administration on plasma potassium in dialysis patients: interactions with insulin and albuterol. Am J Kidney Dis 1996;28:508–514.

49. Lens XM, Montoliu J, Cases A, et al: Treatment of hyperkalemia in renal failure: salbutamol v. insulin. Nephrol Dial Transplant 1989;4:228–232.

50. Kim HJ: Combined effect of bicarbonate and insulin with glucose in acute therapy of hyperkalemia in end-stage renal disease patients. Nephron 1996;72:476–482.

51. Nicolis GL, Kahn T, Sanchez A, et al: Glucose-induced hyperkalemia in diabetic subjects. Arch Intern Med 1982;141:49–53.

52. Conte G, Dal Canton A, Imperatore P, et al: Acute increase in plasma osmolality as a cause of hyperkalemia in patients with renal failure. Kidney Int 1990;38:301–307.

53. Rosa RM, Silva P, Young JB, et al: Adrenergic modulation of extrarenal potassium disposal. N Engl J Med 1980;302:431–434.

54. Brown MJ, Brown DC, Murphy MB: Hypokalemia from beta 2 receptor stimulation by circulating epinephrine. N Engl J Med 1983;309:1414–1419.

55. Williams ME, Rosa RM, Silva P: Impairment of extrarenal potassium disposal by alpha adrenergic stimulation. N Engl J Med 1984;311:145–149.

56. Williams ME, Gervino EV, Rosa RM, et al: Catecholamine modulation of rapid potassium shifts during exercise. N Engl J Med 1985;312:823–827.

57. Allon M, Shanklin N: Adrenergic modulation of extrarenal potassium disposal in men with end-stage renal disease. Kidney Int 1991;40:1103–1109.

58. Montoliu J, Lens XM, Revert L: Potassium-lowering effect of albuterol for hyperkalemia in renal failure. Arch Intern Med 1987;147:713–717.

59. Liou HH, Chiang SS, Wu SC, et al: Hypokalemic effects of intravenous infusion or nebulization of salbutamol in patients with chronic renal failure. Am J Kidney Dis 1994;23:266–270.

60. Kemper MJ, Harps E, Muller-Wiefel DE: Hyperkalemia: therapeutic options in acute and chronic renal failure. Clin Nephrol 1995;46:67–69.

61. Allon M, Dunlay R, Copkney C: Nebulized albuterol for acute hyperkalemia in patients on hemodialysis. Ann Intern Med 1989;110:426–429.

62. Montoliu J, Almirall J, Ponz E, et al: Treatment of hyperkalemia in renal failure with salbutamol inhalation. J Intern Med 1990;228:35–37.

63. Mandelberg A, Krupnik Z, Houri S: Salbutamol metered-dose inhaler with spacer for hyperkalemia: how fast? how safe? Chest 1999;115:617–622.

64. Guttierez R, Schlessinger F, Oster JR, et al: Effect of hypertonic versus isotonic sodium bicarbonate on plasma potassium concentration in patients with end-stage renal disease. Miner Electrolyte Metab 1991;17:297–302.

65. Blumberg A, Weidmann P, Ferrari P: Effect of prolonged bicarbonate administration on plasma potassium in terminal renal failure. Kidney Int 1992;41:369–374.

66. Schwarz KC, Cohen BD, Lubash GD, et al: Severe acidosis and hyperpotassemia treated with sodium bicarbonate infusion. Circulation 1959;19:215–220.

67. Emmett M, Hootkins RE, Fine KD: Effect of three laxatives and a cation exchange resin on fecal sodium and potassium excretion. Gastroenterology 1995;108:752–760.

68. Wingate DL, Krag E, Mekhjian HS, et al: Relationships between ion and water movement in the human jejunum, ileum and colon during perfusion with bile acids. Clin Sci Mol Med 1995;45:593–606.

69. Jeejeebhoy KN: Nutrient requirements and nutrient deficiencies in gastrointestinal disease. In Sleisenger MH, Fordtran JS (eds): Gastrointestinal Disease: Pathophysiology, Diagnosis, Management, 5th edn. Philadelphia: WB Saunders, 1993, pp 2017–2047.

70. Agarwal R, Afzalpurkar R, Fordtran J: Pathophysiology of potassium absorption and secretion by the human intestine. Gastroenterology 1994;107:548–571.

71. Salas-Coll CA, Kermode JC, Edmonds CJ: Potassium transport across the distal colon in man. Clin Sci Mol Med 1976;51:287–296.

72. Martin RS, Panese S, Virginillo M, et al: Increased secretion of potassium in the rectum of humans with chronic renal failure. Am J Kidney Dis 1988;8:105–110.

73. Flinn RB, Merrill JP, Welzant WR: Treatment of the oliguric patient with a new sodium-exchange resin and sorbitol. N Engl J Med 1961;264:111–115.

74. Scherr L, Ogden DA, Mead AW: Management of hyperkalemia with a cation-exchange resin. N Engl J Med 1961;264:115–119.

75. Gruy-Kapral C, Emmett M, Santa Ana CA: Effect of single dose resin–cathartic therapy on serum potassium concentration in patients with end-stage renal disease. J Am Soc Nephrol 1998;9:1924–1930.

76. Gerstman BB, Kirkman P, Platt R: Intestinal necrosis associated with postoperative orally administered soduim polystyrene sulfonate in sorbitol. Am J Kidney Dis 1992;20:159–161.

77. Shepard KU: Cleansing enemas after sodium polystyrene enemas (letter). Ann Intern Med 1990;112:711.

78. Phelps KR, Lieberman RL, Oh MS, et al: Pathophysiology of the syndrome of hyporeninemic hypoaldosteronism. Metabolism 1980;29:186–199.

79. Oh MS, Carroll HJ, Clemmens JE: A mechanism for hyporeninemic hypoaldosteronism in chronic renal disease. Metabolism 1974;23:1157–1166.

80. Kaiser UB, Ethier JH, Kamel KS, et al: Persistent hyperkalemia in a patient with diabetes mellitus: a reversible defect in kaliuresis during bicarbonaturia. Clin Invest Med 1992;15:187–193.

81. Schambelan M, Sebastian A, Rector FC Jr: Mineralocorticoid-resistant renal hyperkalemia without salt wasting (type II pseudohypoaldosteronism): role of increased renal chloride reabsorption. Kidney Int 1981;19:716–727.

82. Kamel KS, Halperin ML: Hyperkalemia with mild ECF volume contraction: studies to provide a possible physiologic interpretation. Clin Invest Med 1994;17:414–419.

83. Tumlin JA, Sands JM: Nephron segment-specific inhibition of Na^+/K^-

ATPase activity by cyclosporin A. Kidney Int 1993;43:246–251.

84. Deppe CE, Heering PJ, Tinel H, et al: Effect of cyclosporine A on Na$^+$/K$^+$-ATPase, Na$^+$/K$^+$/2 Cl$^-$ contransporter, and H$^+$/K$^+$-ATPase in MDCK cells and two subtypes, C7 and C11. Exp Nephrol 1997;5:471–480.

85. Kamel K, Ethier JH, Quaggin S, et al: Studies to determine the basis for hyperkalemia in recipients of a renal transplant who are treated with cyclosporin. J Am Soc Nephrol 1992;2:1279–1284.

86. Choi MJ, Fernandez PC, Patnaik A, et al: Trimethoprim induced hyperkalemia in a patient with AIDS. N Engl J Med 1993;328:703–706.

87. Kleyman TR, Roberts C, Ling BN: A mechanism for pentamidine-induced hyperkalemia: inhibition of distal nephron sodium transport. Ann Intern Med 1995;122:103–106.

88. Schreiber M, Halperin ML: Urea excretion rate as a contributor to trimethoprim-induced hyperkalemia. Ann Intern Med 1994;120:166–167.

89. Schreiber M, Schlanger LE, Chen CB, et al: Antikaliuretic action of trimethoprim is minimized by raising urine pH. Kidney Int 1996;49:82–87.

90. Gagnon RF, Halperin ML: Possible mechanisms to explain the absence of hyperkalemia in a patient with Addison's disease. Nephrol Dial Transplant 2001;16:1–5.

91. Orth DN, Kovacs WJ: The adrenal cortex. *In* Wilson JD, Foster DW, Kronenberg HM, Larsen PR (eds): Williams Textbook of Endocrinology, 9th edn. Philadelphia: WB Saunders, 1998, p 550, Table 12-8.

Metabolic and Respiratory Acidosis

Thomas D. DuBose Jr

Pathophysiology of acid–base disorders

Definition and fundamental concepts

Metabolic acidosis occurs when there is increased production of endogenous acid (e.g. lactic acid and ketoacids), loss of bicarbonate (HCO_3^-) in diarrhea, or a sustained inability to generate new bicarbonate by the kidney (renal failure and renal tubular acidosis). Metabolic acidosis is recognized by the co-occurrence of acidemia (pH < 7.35) and a low serum bicarbonate concentration (total CO_2 concentration). Metabolic acidosis may also be recognized by an elevated anion gap (AG), even in the face of normal values for pH and HCO_3^- in plasma. Two broad types of metabolic acidoses are recognized by consideration of the AG: (1) high AG acidoses; and (2) normal AG or hyperchloremic acidoses. The AG is defined as:

$$AG = Na^+ - (Cl^- + HCO_3^-) = 12 \text{ mequiv./L}$$

A flow diagram outlining the diagnostic approach to metabolic acidosis, in which the initial consideration is the AG, is displayed in Fig. 36.1.

When there is a primary decrease in plasma $[HCO_3^-]$, an increase in alveolar ventilation and thereby a decrease in $PaCO_2$ (respiratory compensation) is expected because the medullary chemoreceptors are stimulated by acidemia to invoke an increase in ventilation. The ratio of $[HCO_3^-]$ to

$PaCO_2$ and the subsequent pH will be returned toward, but not to, normal. This hypocapnic response to acidemia is predictable in simple acid–base disturbances, and blunts the magnitude of the decline in blood pH that would occur otherwise.

The degree of respiratory compensation expected in uncomplicated or "simple" metabolic acidosis was derived empirically and can be predicted from the relationship:

$$PaCO_2 = (1.5 \times HCO_3^-) + 8 \pm 2 \text{ mmHg}$$

Thus, in a patient with metabolic acidosis and a plasma $[HCO_3^-]$ of 12 mequiv./L, a $PaCO_2$ between 24 and 28 mmHg would be anticipated. Values for $PaCO_2 < 24$ or > 28 mmHg denote a mixed disturbance (metabolic acidosis and respiratory alkalosis, or metabolic acidosis and respiratory acidosis, respectively). While this relationship is reliable, the $PaCO_2$ can be estimated more conveniently by adding 15 to the patient's serum $[HCO_3^-]$.

Renal response to acidosis

The kidneys regulate plasma $[HCO_3^-]$ through three processes: (1) "reabsorption" of the filtered HCO_3^-; (2) excretion of titratable acidity; and (3) synthesis and excretion of NH_4^+. The sum of the last two processes represents net acid excretion. Approximately 80–90% of the filtered HCO_3^- is reabsorbed in the proximal tubule. Under normal conditions, the distal nephron reabsorbs the remainder of the filtered HCO_3^- (5–10%). The quantity of acids produced on a daily basis from metabolism and digestion of dietary protein is approximately 40–60 mequiv. Thus an equal amount of acid must be secreted by the collecting duct to prevent the development of chronic positive hydrogen ion balance and metabolic acidosis. NH_4^+ excretion, the major component of net acid excretion, is regulated by both NH_4^+ production and NH_4^+ transport by the kidney.

When renal function is normal, the kidney responds to chronic metabolic acidosis by increasing NH_4^+ production and excretion. NH_4^+ production and excretion is much less than normal in the face of chronic renal failure, hyperkalemia, and renal tubular acidosis (RTA). Therefore, a normal renal response to metabolic acidosis must be distinguished from a subnormal response in order to determine if the kidney is responding appropriately or is responsible for the acidosis. NH_4^+ excretion can be estimated from a spot urine sample by consideration of the urine anion gap (UAG) and/or the urinary osmolal gap. The UAG is defined as the difference between the concentrations of chloride (Cl^-) and the sum of the urinary cations Na^+ and K^+, i.e. $UAG = [Na^+ + K^+]_u - [Cl^-]_u$. In chronic metabolic acidosis of nonrenal origin (such as

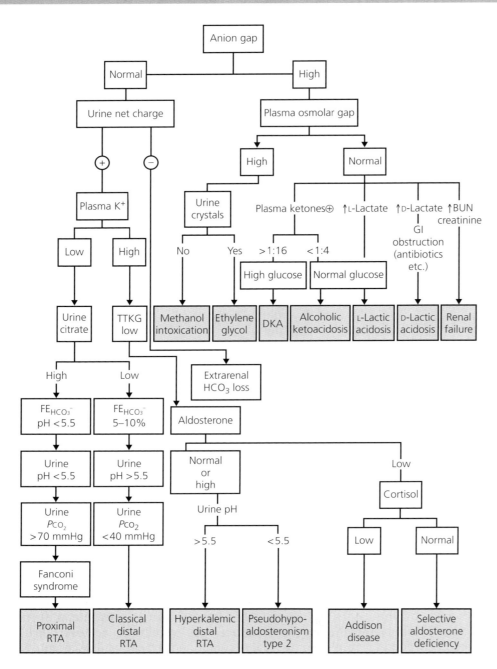

Figure 36.1 Flow diagram of approach to metabolic acidosis. The anion gap is the entry point and divides the types of metabolic acidoses into the high anion gap and normal anion gap categories. Final diagnoses are displayed in hatched boxes. BUN, blood urea nitrogen; DKA, diabetic ketoacidosis; $FE_{HCO_3^-}$, fractional excretion of bicarbonate; RTA, renal tubular acidosis; TTKG, transtubular potassium gradient.

diarrhea), the expected response by the kidney is to increase NH_4^+ production and excretion. The increase in $[NH_4^+]$ in the urine in this condition is manifest as an increase in the UAG (i.e. the urinary Cl^- would exceed the sum of $Na^+ + K^+$). In contrast, in hyperchloremic metabolic acidosis of renal origin (i.e. RTA) the UAG is expected to be zero or positive, denoting no increase in or minimal NH_4^+ in the urine, signifying an inappropriate renal response to the metabolic acidosis or a tubular defect in H^+ secretion. Caution is warranted with this test since ketonuria or the presence of drug anions or toxins (such as toluene metabolites) in the urine invalidates this method.

The urinary NH_4^+ ($U_{NH_4^+}$) may be estimated more precisely from the measured urine osmolality (U_{osm}), urine $[Na^+ + K^+]$, and urine urea and glucose:

$$U_{NH_4^+} = 0.5(U_{osm} - [2(Na^+ + K^+) + urea + glucose]$$ (all expressed in mmol/L)

Clinical settings for mixed acid–base disorders

Mixed acid–base disorders are commonly observed in patients in critical care units and may lead to dangerous extremes of pH or, conversely, a normal pH in the face of grossly abnormal values for $Paco_2$ and HCO_3^-. Mixed acid–base disorders can be distinguished from simple (single) disturbances by prediction of the respiratory compensatory response (as explained above), by comparison of the decrement in AG with the increment in serum bicarbonate, or by the use of clinical nomograms.

Clinical examples of metabolic acidosis

High anion gap acidosis (AG > 10 mequiv./L)

There are five major causes of a high AG acidosis: (1) ketoacidoses, (2) L-lactic acidosis, (3) acute and chronic renal failure, (4) ingested drugs and toxins, and rarely (5) gastrointestinal overproduction of organic acids (D-lactic acidosis) (Table 36.1 and Fig. 36.1). Identification of the underlying cause of a high AG acidosis is facilitated by consideration of the clinical setting and associated laboratory values. Initial screening to differentiate the high AG acidoses should include the following:

1. a careful history or other evidence for drug or toxin ingestion;
2. arterial blood gas measurement to detect coexistent respiratory alkalosis;
3. oxalate crystals in the urine plus an osmolal gap in the patient with a high AG acidosis suggest ethylene glycol ingestion;
4. historical evidence of diabetes mellitus (diabetic ketoacidosis);
5. evidence of alcoholism or increased levels of β-hydroxybutyrate (alcoholic ketoacidosis);
6. observation for clinical signs of uremia and determination of blood urea nitrogen (BUN) and creatinine (uremic acidosis);
7. recognition of the numerous settings in which L-lactate levels may be increased (hypotension, cardiac failure, drugs, leukemia, cancer);

Table 36.1 Causes of high anion gap acidosis

Ketoacidosis
Diabetic ketoacidosis
Alcoholic ketoacidosis
Starvation ketoacidosis

Lactic acidosis
L-Lactic acidosis
    Type A
    Type B
D-Lactic acidosis

Renal failure
Acute
Chronic

Toxins
Ethylene glycol
Methyl alcohol
Salicylates

8. appreciation of the possibility of accumulation of D-lactate in the presence of low gastrointestinal motility, gastrointestinal obstruction, gastrointestinal pouches, antibiotic therapy, and bacterial overgrowth;

The distinguishing features of high AG acidoses are outlined in Fig. 36.1.

Diabetic ketoacidosis

Pathophysiology Diabetic ketoacidosis is due to increased fatty acid metabolism and accumulation of acetoacetate and β-hydroxybutyrate, the consequences of insulin deficiency and relative excess of glucagon. An absence of insulin stimulates lipolysis and fatty acid release, while glucagon stimulates the hepatic metabolism of fatty acids to ketoacids.

Key diagnostic points Diabetic ketoacidosis (most often in insulin-dependent diabetes mellitus) is seen in association with an intercurrent illness, particularly infections, which increase insulin requirements temporarily and acutely. The diagnosis is confirmed by the concurrence of a metabolic acidosis, strongly positive plasma ketones in undiluted serum, hyperglycemia, extracellular fluid (ECF) volume depletion, and Kussmaul respiration. Although hyperchloremic acidosis may occur in patients who remain euvolemic, the majority of patients will have an AG acidosis, a consequence of buffering by bicarbonate of the H^+ from ketoacids released into the plasma.

Therapeutic options Therapy consists of insulin, to inhibit ketoacid production, and intravenous fluids for ECF volume restoration and correction of electrolyte deficits. Low-dose intravenous insulin therapy (0.1 units/kg/h) reduces plasma glucose, smoothly corrects the keto-nemia, lowers the elevated AG, and repairs the acidosis. While regular insulin may also be administered intramuscularly (0.2 mg/kg initially, then 6 units every hour), it should be noted that intramuscular insulin may not be effective in volume-depleted and/or hypotensive patients, as is often the case in ketoacidosis. Most, if not all, patients with diabetic ketoacidosis require correction of the ECF volume depletion that predictably accompanies the osmotic diuresis and ketoacidosis. Initiate therapy with isotonic saline at a rate of 1000 mL/h i.v. The usual ECF deficit in adults is in the range of 3 L of isotonic saline. When the pulse and blood pressure have stabilized and the corrected serum $[Na^+]$ is 130–135 mequiv./L, switch to 0.45% NaCl. Ringer's lactate should be avoided. If the blood sugar declines below 250–300 mg/dL, 0.45% NaCl with 5% dextrose should be administered.

Total body potassium depletion is usually present. Nevertheless, the serum potassium is usually elevated at admission, indicating that potassium replacement therapy must be individualized. A normal or reduced $[K^+]$ on admission, which is found in certain patients (e.g. where vomiting was a prominent prodromal symptom), indicates severe potassium depletion. Potassium depletion occurs as a result of osmotic diuresis, decreased dietary intake, and vomiting which accompanies diabetic ketoacidosis. Administration of saline, insulin, and alkali will cause the potassium level to decline further by enhancing renal K^+

excretion. Frequent monitoring (hourly) of the serum potassium is mandatory and a precise recipe is difficult to provide. Caution should be exercised in the presence of hyperkalemia, especially in the patient with renal insufficiency; withhold potassium as long as the serum level is > 5.0 mequiv./L. Nevertheless, when urine output has been established, 20 mequiv. KCl may be administered in each liter of intravenous fluid as long as the plasma [K$^+$] is < 3.8 mequiv./L. Monitor and record plasma concentrations of K$^+$, glucose, HCO$_3^-$, Na$^+$, and Cl$^-$ hourly.

Controversial points The routine administration of phosphate (usually as potassium phosphate) is not advised because of the potential for hyperphosphatemia and hypocalcemia. A significant number of patients with diabetic ketoacidosis will display hyperphosphatemia before initiation of therapy. In virtually all patients the elevated phosphate concentration on admission is followed by a fall in plasma phosphate levels within 2–6 h after initiation of therapy. In this circumstance phosphate should be replaced as neutral potassium phosphate (10–20 mmol per liter of intravenous fluids) unless hyperkalemia coexists, in which case neutral sodium phosphate should be used. Bicarbonate therapy is usually not necessary unless the acidosis is severe (pH < 7.1 and *Pa*CO$_2$ is low). In general, the increment in AG above normal represents "potential" bicarbonate, or that bicarbonate that will be realized when circulating ketones are metabolically converted to bicarbonate following primary therapy (insulin). Nevertheless, during therapy it is difficult to predict to what extent ketones will be converted back to bicarbonate before being lost in the urine when glomerular filtration rate (GFR) is normalized. If exogenous bicarbonate is administered, that amount of bicarbonate will be added to that produced endogenously so that an "overshoot alkalosis" may develop. Therefore, a prudent goal is to administer small amounts of bicarbonate (45–90 mequiv. i.v. slowly, or one to two ampoules) until the pH reaches ~ 7.2 or [HCO$_3^-$] is 10–12 mequiv./L. With exogenous bicarbonate therapy, additional potassium will be needed.

Alcoholic ketoacidosis

Pathophysiology and diagnostic points This relatively common but underappreciated disorder occurs in alcoholics, particularily binge drinkers. Ketoacidosis develops when alcohol consumption is abruptly curtailed, usually as a result of vomiting or abdominal pain. In association with starvation and metabolism of ethanol (which inhibits gluconeogenesis), the glucose concentration is frequently low or normal. When ECF volume depletion is pronounced, the acidosis may be severe. The AG value is elevated because of increased ketones, predominantly β-hydroxybutyrate. Mild lactic acidosis may coexist because of alteration in the redox state caused by ethanol or severe hypoxia. The nitroprusside ketone reaction (Acetest) can detect acetoacetic acid but not β-hydroxybutyrate, so the initial degree of ketosis and ketonuria may not be appreciated. Typically, insulin levels are low and levels of triglyceride, cortisol, glucagon, and growth hormone are increased, leading to ketoacidosis.

Therapeutic options The mainstay of therapy is intravenous normal saline to expand the ECF. Glucose is necessary if hypoglycemia is present. Insulin is obviously contraindicated, illustrating why the diagnosis of alcoholic ketoacidosis must not be mistaken for diabetic ketoacidosis. Intravenous replacement of potassium, phosphate, and magnesium deficits, as well as vitamin supplementation (thiamine 100 mg i.v.), are usually necessary and should be given as needed later in the course, particularly in the face of chronic alcoholism and malnutrition. Hypophosphatemia usually emerges several hours after admission, so the need for therapy can be overlooked, especially if the serum phosphate concentration on admission is normal. Profound hypophosphatemia may provoke aspiration, rhabdomyolysis, and coagulopathy. Phosphate should be replaced as either neutral sodium or potassium phosphate 10–20 mmol per liter of intravenous fluids, as dictated by plasma [K$^+$]. Upper gastrointestinal hemorrhage, pancreatitis, and pneumonia may accompany alcoholic ketoacidosis.

L-Lactic acidosis

Pathophysiology L-Lactic acidosis occurs in a diverse group of disorders that are recognized by an increase in plasma L-lactate concentration (normal venous levels < 1.8 mmol/L or 16 mg/dL). Brain, muscle, gastrointestinal tract, skin, and red cells produce lactate, while the liver is the major organ that participates in lactate disposal. Lactate synthesis is altered by changes in systemic pH, which control the rate of glycolysis by acting on the rate-limiting enzyme, phosphofructokinase. Acidosis decreases while alkalosis increases lactate production. The major determinants of plasma L-lactate levels include the concentration of pyruvate, the NADH:NAD$^+$ ratio, and the pH. Clinically significant L-lactic acidosis (plasma L-lactate > 4.0 mmol/L) is most often the result of tissue hypoxia; other causes include metabolic disorders, drugs, toxins, or hereditary defects. The accumulation of L-lactate may be secondary to an obvious cause of tissue hypoxia, e.g. cardiac arrest, cardiogenic shock hemorrhage, sepsis, carbon monoxide poisoning, severe asthma, and severe anemia; this is called type A L-lactic acidosis. Conversely, type B L-lactic acidosis may accompany disorders in which tissue hypoperfusion or hypoxia are absent, such as diabetes mellitus, ethanol poisoning, liver failure, mitochondrial diseases, thiamine deficiency, malignancies, and drug and toxin overdose (e.g. metformin, salicylates, cocaine, fructose, cyanide, nonnucleoside reverse transcriptase inhibitors, nitroprusside). Lactic acidosis in combination with respiratory alkalosis can be observed early in the development of septic shock and may be one of the few harbingers of this entity.

Treatment The basic principle of therapy is that the underlying condition initiating the disruption in normal L-lactate metabolism must first be corrected. Every attempt should be made to restore tissue perfusion. Vasoconstricting agents should be administered only when absolutely necessary and at the lowest feasible dose, since they potentiate the hypoperfused state. Alkali therapy is generally recommended for acute severe acidemia (pH < 7.2) to improve cardiac function and lactate utilization. However, the use of bicarbonate therapy is of only marginal value. Excess bicarbonate may depress cardiac performance and can even exacerbate the acidemia through increased phosphofructokinase activity. Thus attempts to normalize the pH or [HCO_3^-] by exogenous bicarbonate therapy is deleterious. One approach is to provide, by slow infusion over 30–40 min intervals, sufficient bicarbonate to raise the arterial pH to no more than 7.2, i.e. [HCO_3^-] is 10 mequiv./L. Despite initial enthusiasm for the use of dichloroacetate, a beneficial effect has not been substantiated. Similarly, no benefit is derived from administration of methylene blue. Thiamine should also be administered (50–100 mg) in patients with chronic malnutrition or alcoholism.

Fluid overload occurs with excessive bicarbonate therapy because the amount required is often massive when production of lactic acid is relentless. This complication may require slow continuous ultrafiltration, continuous venovenous hemodialysis, or acute intermittent hemodialysis. Lactate-containing dialysate should be avoided, which obviates the use of peritoneal dialysis. Unabated severe L-lactic acidosis in patients receiving large amounts of bicarbonate carries a very high mortality. If the underlying cause of the L-lactic acidosis can be corrected, the blood lactate will be reconverted to bicarbonate. Bicarbonate derived from lactate conversion in addition to any new bicarbonate generated by renal mechanisms during acidosis and from exogenous alkali therapy are additive and may result in an "overshoot" alkalosis.

D-Lactic acidosis

Pathophysiology   D-Lactate, which is not an endogenous metabolite in vertebrates, is produced by bacterial overgrowth in the gastrointestinal tract in association with jejunoileal bypass, intestinal obstruction, antibiotic therapy, or decreased gastrointestinal motility. The diagnosis of D-lactic acidosis requires measurement of D-lactate levels specifically, since it is not measured as L-lactate. The acid–base disturbance may consist of both an increased AG and hyperchloremia.

Treatment   Since the potential danger in D-lactic acidosis is from accumulation of toxic products and not the acidosis, initial therapy should include (1) cessation of feeding, (2) eradication of bacterial overgrowth by administration of appropriate oral antibiotics (metronidazole or neomycin) or intravenous vancomycin, and (3) enhanced gastrointestinal motility. Longer-term therapy may necessitate reversal of intestinal bypass if stasis and bacterial overgrowth persist or are recurrent.

Drug-induced acidosis

Salicylates   Aspirin overdose usually gives rise to a complex acid–base disturbance, in which respiratory alkalosis predominates (due to stimulation of respiration by salicylates) and a high AG may occur concomitantly. Only a portion of the increased AG can be attributed to the increased plasma salicylate concentration, e.g. a toxic salicylate level of 100 mg/dL can only account for an increase in AG of 7 mequiv./L. Lactic acid production is also often increased, partly as a direct effect of the drug and partly as a result of the decrease in P_{CO_2} induced by salicylate.

Treatment   The initial step in therapy should include vigorous gastric lavage followed by activated charcoal administration via a nasogastric tube. The mainstay of therapy is an alkaline diuresis to allow the relatively impermeant anionic form of salicylate to be trapped in tubular fluid and excreted in the urine. To facilitate removal of salicylate, intravenous sodium bicarbonate in amounts adequate to alkalinize the urine and maintain urine output is necessary (urine pH > 7.5). An alkaline diuresis may be induced by infusion of half-isotonic saline plus two ampoules of sodium bicarbonate (45 mequiv. each). While this form of therapy is straightforward in acidotic patients, alkalemia from respiratory alkalosis may make this approach hazardous. Arterial pH should be monitored and not allowed to increase above 7.55. Acetazolamide in small doses (250 mg) is recommended only when an alkaline diuresis cannot be achieved or when the pH exceeds 7.55, since larger doses may result in systemic metabolic acidosis if sodium bicarbonate is not given concomitantly. Moreover, acetazolamide and salicylates compete for binding sites on albumin. Coexisting metabolic acidosis greatly impedes salicylate clearance and enhances salicylate entry into the central nervous system (CNS), and must be avoided. Hypokalemia may occur as a result of alkaline diuresis from either sodium bicarbonate or acetazolamide and should be treated promptly. If renal failure prevents rapid clearance of salicylate or if salicylate levels remain in the toxic range (> 40–50 mg/dL), hemodialysis against a bicarbonate dialysate (35 mequiv./L) should be performed.

Toxin-induced acidosis: ethylene glycol and methyl alcohol and the osmolal gap

Pathophysiology   Plasma osmolality (mosmol/kg H_2O) is calculated according to the following expression:

$$P_{osm} = 2Na^+ + glucose/18 + BUN/2.8$$

where BUN and glucose are expressed in milligrams per deciliter. The calculated and determined osmolality should agree within 10–15 mosmol/kg. When the measured osmolality exceeds the calculated osmolality by more than 15–20 mosmol/kg, one of two circumstances prevails: (1) the serum sodium may be spuriously low, as occurs with hyperlipidemia or hyperproteinemia (pseudohyponatremia); or (2) osmolytes other than sodium salts, glucose, or urea have accumulated in plasma. Examples include the accumulation of solutes that can increase plasma osmolality, such as the alcohols ethylene glycol and methyl alcohol. Less commonly, mannitol or retained radiocontrast agents increase the osmolal gap. In these examples, the difference between the calculated osmolality and the measured osmolality is proportional to the concentration of the unmeasured solute (osmolal gap). With an appropriate clinical history and index of suspicion, the osmolal gap becomes a very helpful screening tool in poison-associated AG acidosis.

Ethylene glycol

Diagnostic points Ingestion of ethylene glycol (commonly used in antifreeze) leads to a metabolic acidosis and severe damage to the CNS, heart, lungs, and kidneys. Ethylene glycol (molecular mass 62 Da) increases the osmolal gap (> 10 mosmol/kg H_2O). The increased AG and osmolal gap are attributable to ethylene glycol and its metabolites oxalic acid, glycolic acid, and other organic acids. Lactic acid production increases secondary to inhibition of the tricarboxylic acid cycle and altered intracellular redox state. Diagnosis is facilitated by recognizing oxalate crystals in the urine, the presence of an osmolal gap in serum, and a high AG acidosis. Ethylene glycol ingested as antifreeze may be detected in the urine sample by use of Woods' light. Treatment should not be delayed while awaiting measurement of ethylene glycol levels in this setting.

Treatment The principles of treatment of ethylene glycol intoxication are to stop production of toxic metabolites by competitive inhibition of alcohol dehydrogenase using intravenous administration of ethanol, coupled with removal of the accumulated toxins. Immediate therapy is necessary to prevent irreversible CNS and renal toxicity. Ethanol (20% solution) 0.6 g/kg i.v. is given over 30–45 min followed by a maintenance infusion of 5% ethanol 110 mg/kg/h to produce a serum ethanol level of 100–150 mg/dL. A saline or osmotic diuresis should be initiated and the patient given thiamine and pyridoxine supplements, fomepizole or ethanol, and hemodialysis. During dialysis it is necessary to increase the rate of ethanol infusion. The intravenous administration of the new alcohol dehydrogenase inhibitor fomepizole (4-methylpyrazole) (7 mg/kg as a loading dose) or ethanol to produce a serum ethanol level of 100 mg/dL serves to lessen toxicity because they compete with ethylene glycol for metabolism by alcohol dehydrogenase. Fomepizole, although expensive, offers the advantage of a predictable decline in ethylene glycol levels without the adverse effects, such as excessive obtundation, associated with ethanol infusion.

Methyl alcohol

Ingestion of methyl alcohol, as wood alcohol or paint thinners, causes metabolic acidosis and severe optic nerve and CNS manifestations when methyl alcohol is metabolized to formaldehyde and then formic acid. Lactic acid, ketoacids, and other unidentified organic acids may contribute to the acidosis.

Diagnostic points This form of toxic acidosis should be considered when the "blind drunk" patient with a high AG metabolic acidosis is encountered. Nausea, vomiting, and abdominal pain are usually present. Lactic acids and ketoacids as well as other unidentified organic acids may contribute to the acidosis. Because of its high retention and low molecular mass (32 Da), an osmolal gap is usually present.

Treatment The treatment of methyl alcohol intoxication is generally similar to that for ethylene glycol intoxication, including ethanol or fomepizole administration, general supportive measures, volume expansion, and hemodia-lysis. Initiation of a saline diuresis is less of an issue with methyl alcohol than with ethylene glycol intoxication because renal toxicity is not a direct effect of methyl alcohol intoxication and crystals are not present in the urine.

Acute and chronic renal failure

Pathophysiology Progressive renal insufficiency will eventually convert the hyperchloremic acidosis of moderate renal insufficiency (discussed later) to the typical high AG acidosis of advanced renal failure. Low glomerular filtration, continued reabsorption of organic anions, and low NH_4^+ excretion all contribute to the pathogenesis of this metabolic disturbance. As functional renal mass is compromised in the relentless progression of renal disease, the number of functioning nephrons eventually becomes insufficient to maintain NH_4^+ excretion to the extent necessary to balance net acid production. Thus $[HCO_3^-]$ declines but rarely falls below 15 mequiv./L, and the AG rarely exceeds 20 mequiv./L. The acid retained in patients with chronic renal disease is buffered in part by alkaline salts derived from bone, resulting in loss of bone calcium carbonate that contributes to the skeletal demineralization seen with renal acidosis. In addition, chronic acidosis increases urinary calcium excretion to a level proportional to the degree of cumulative acid retention and is corrected with repair of the acidosis.

Treatment Both uremic acidosis and hyperchloremic acidosis of renal insufficiency require oral alkali replacement to maintain $[HCO_3^-]$ between 20 and 24 mequiv./L. This can usually be accomplished with relatively modest amounts of alkali (1–1.5 mequiv./kg/day). Sodium citrate (Shohl solution) has been shown to enhance the absorption of aluminum from the gastrointestinal tract and should never be administered to patients receiving aluminum-containing antacids because of the risk of aluminum intoxication. If hyperkalemia persists, furosemide (60–80 mg/day) should be added.

Hyperchloremic metabolic acidosis (normal anion gap acidosis)

Pathogenesis and differential diagnosis Alkali may be lost from the gastrointestinal tract (diarrhea) or from the kidneys (RTA). In these disorders (Table 36.2), reciprocal changes in chloride and bicarbonate result in a normal AG. In a pure form of simple hyperchloremic acidosis, therefore, the increase in chloride above the normal value equals the decrease in bicarbonate. The absence of such a relationship suggests a mixed disturbance. Diarrhea results in the loss of large quantities of HCO_3^- and further HCO_3^- depletion occurs by its reaction with organic acids. Instead of an acid urine pH, as often anticipated with diarrhea, a pH of 6.0 is usually observed because metabolic acidosis and hypokalemia increase renal NH_4^+ synthesis and excretion, thus providing more urinary buffer, which increases urine pH. Metabolic acidosis due to gastrointestinal losses with a high urine pH can be differentiated from RTA, since

Table 36.2 Causes of hyperchloremic metabolic acidosis*

Gastrointestinal bicarbonate loss
Diarrhea
External pancreatic or small bowel drainage
Ureterosigmoidostomy, jejunal loop
Drugs
    Calcium chloride (acidifying agent)
    Magnesium sulfate (diarrhea)
    Cholestyramine (bile acid diarrhea)

Renal tubular acidification defects
Hypokalemia
Proximal renal tubular acidosis (type 2 RTA)
Classical distal renal tubular acidosis (type 1 RTA)

Hyperkalemia
Generalized distal nephron dysfunction (type 4 RTA)
Mineralocorticoid deficiency
Mineralocorticoid resistance
Decreased delivery of Na^+ to the distal nephron
    Liver disease

Normokalemia or hyperkalemia
Early renal failure

Other
Acid loads (ammonium chloride, hyperalimentation with insufficient alkali infusion)
Loss of potential bicarbonate: ketosis with ketone excretion
Expansion acidosis (rapid saline administration)
Posthypocapnic state
Glue sniffing

*Must rule out hypoalbuminemia, pseudohyponatremia, pseudohyperchloremia, and paraproteinemia.

urinary NH_4^+ excretion is low in RTA and high in patients with diarrhea. Urinary NH_4^+ levels can be estimated by calculating the urine AG or the urine osmolal gap (see earlier). With extrarenal bicarbonate loss, $[Cl^-]$ in urine exceeds $[Na^+ + K^+]$ in urine. If urine $[Na^+ + K^+]$ exceeds $[Cl^-]$, urine $[NH_4^+]$ is low, a finding compatible with RTA. The distinguishing features of hyperchloremic acidoses are outlined in Table 36.3.

Hyperchloremic acidosis of chronic renal failure

Pathophysiology Loss of functioning renal parenchyma due to progressive renal failure is commonly associated with metabolic acidosis, which is typically hyperchloremic when GFR is 20–50 mL/min but may convert to the typical high AG acidosis of uremia with more advanced renal failure, i.e. when GFR is < 20 mL/min. The major defect in acidification with advanced renal failure is that ammoniagenesis is reduced in proportion to the loss of functional renal mass. In addition, medullary NH_4^+ accumulation and trapping in the medullary collecting duct is impaired. Because of adaptive increases in K^+ secretion by the collecting duct and colon, the acidosis of chronic renal insufficiency is typically normokalemic.

Renal tubular acidosis

Proximal renal tubular acidosis

Diagnostic points The majority of cases of proximal RTA fit into the category of generalized proximal tubular dysfunction with glycosuria, generalized aminoaciduria, hypercitraturia, and phosphaturia. The generalized failure of proximal tubular function is referred to as Fanconi syndrome. The diagnosis is confirmed by demonstrating an inappropriately high rate of bicarbonate excretion in the face of a low or normal plasma bicarbonate (> 10–15%). Causes of acquired proximal RTA include the dysproteinemias, heavy metal intoxication, vitamin D deficiency or resistance, cancer chemotherapeutic drugs (such as ifosfamide), and genetically transmitted systemic diseases (Wilson disease, hereditary fructose intolerance).

Treatment The treatment of proximal RTA is directed toward amelioration of, or improvement in, the fluid, electrolyte, and acid–base abnormalities. In patients with proximal RTA, massive amounts of exogenous bicarbonate

Table 36.3 Distinguishing features of hyperchloremic acidoses

	Proximal RTA (type 2 RTA)	Classical distal RTA (type 1 RTA)	Generalized distal defect (type 4 RTA)	Extrarenal bicarbonate loss
Anion gap	Normal	Normal	Normal	Normal
Plasma $[K^+]$	Low (with therapy)	Low	High	Low
Urine anion gap or urine osmolal gap	Low	Low	Very low	High
Urine pH	Low	High	Low or high	Low or high
Urine P_{CO_2} (mmHg)	> 70	< 40	< 40	> 70
$FE_{HCO_3^-}$	> 15% (with therapy)	5–10%	10–15%	< 5%
Urine citrate	High	Low	Low	Normal
TTKG	High	High	Low (not high)	Low

$FE_{HCO_3^-}$, fractional excretion of bicarbonate; RTA, renal tubular acidosis; TTKG, transtubular potassium gradient.

are required to correct the [HCO_3^-] to normal. Moreover, since bicarbonate absorption in the proximal tubule is abnormal, the increase in distal bicarbonate delivery results in enhanced renal potassium wasting and hypokalemia. Therefore, large alkali loads are not advised; rather, smaller amounts of alkali therapy may be provided as Shohl solution (one to two tablespoons t.i.d.) or sodium bicarbonate tablets (500 mg, one to two tablets t.i.d.). If there is a compelling necessity to correct the plasma bicarbonate (growing children with proximal RTA), hydrochlorothiazide may be added to enhance proximal bicarbonate absorption. Most children and some adults will require potassium supplementation (K-Shohl solution or Polycitra, or K-Lyte), particularly if larger doses of alkali are provided.

Classical distal renal tubular acidosis

Pathophysiology and diagnostic points   The typical findings in classical distal RTA include hypokalemia, hyperchloremic acidosis, an abnormally low excretion of urinary NH_4^+ (positive urine AG or low urinary osmolal gap), and, in contradistinction to proximal RTA, an inappropriately high urine pH in the face of systemic metabolic acidosis. Recently, the genetic bases of inherited forms of classical distal RTA have been elucidated. A number of patients in families with autosomal recessive distal RTA have been shown to have point mutations in the gene that encodes the basolateral HCO_3^-/Cl^- exchanger (or band 3 protein) in A-type intercalated cells of the collecting duct. Other families with inherited sensorineural deafness and classical distal RTA have been shown to have defects in the H^+-ATPase (Table 36.4). Finally, an inherited form not associated with hearing impairment has been associated with an abnormality of a unique subunit of the H^+-ATPase. Under a number of different circumstances, including acute acid infusion, patients with classical hypokalemic distal RTA are unable to acidify their urine below pH 5.5. Most patients with acquired distal RTA and many with inherited forms of distal RTA (except those with the HCO_3^-/Cl^- exchanger defect) uniformly display a lower urinary P_{CO_2} than normal subjects. These abnormalities suggest that one or both of the transporters in the collecting duct involved in bicarbonate absorption (H^+-ATPase or H^+,K^+-ATPase) are defective. In contrast, patients with the inherited HCO_3^-/Cl^- exchanger abnormality have been reported to have higher than normal urinary P_{CO_2}. This finding suggests that the HCO_3^-/Cl^- exchanger may be mistargeted to the apical membrane in these patients. With the exception of the gradient lesion (insertion of a leak pathway) that accompanies amphotericin B intoxication, most patients with distal RTA studied with dynamic tests of urinary acidification, such as urinary P_{CO_2}, have been shown to have a defect in H^+ secretion or a pump defect rather than the "gradient" or "leak" defect as proposed initially.

Hypokalemia and hypercalciuria often accompany this disorder but proximal tubule reabsorptive function is preserved. Thus, hypocitraturia is common, and the combination of hypercalciuria and hypocitraturia enhance urinary stone formation and nephrocalcinosis. Nephrocalcinosis is a marker of classical distal RTA since it does not occur with proximal RTA or the generalized dysfunction of the nephron associated with hyperkalemia. Nephrocalcinosis aggravates further the reduction in net acid excretion by impairing the transfer of NH_4^+ from loop of Henle to collecting duct.

The vast majority of patients with distal RTA have distal RTA in association with a systemic illness, which is referred to as "secondary" distal RTA. Conversely, distal RTA may occur as a part of an inherited defect in which there is no association with systemic disease.

Treatment   Correction of chronic metabolic acidosis can usually be achieved in patients with classical distal RTA by administration of alkali in an amount sufficient to neutralize the production of metabolic acids derived from the diet. In adult patients with distal RTA, this is usually equal to no more than 1 mequiv./kg/day as Shohl solution or sodium bicarbonate tablets. In patients with distal RTA, correction of acidosis with alkali therapy reduces urinary potassium excretion, and hypokalemia and sodium depletion may resolve without additional therapy. Frank wasting of potassium may occur in a minority of patients in association with secondary hyperaldosteronism despite correction of the acidosis by the alkali therapy. A major benefit of correction of the acidosis is that the renal failure should not progress, especially when nephrocalcinosis accompanies distal RTA. The frequency of nephrolithiasis, when present, is usually markedly reduced by alkali therapy.

Generalized distal nephron dysfunction (type 4 renal tubular acidosis)

Pathophysiology and diagnostic points   Although hyperchloremic metabolic acidosis and hyperkalemia occur with regularity in advanced renal insufficiency, patients with type 4 RTA have hyperkalemia that is disproportionate to the reduction in GFR. In such patients a generalized dysfunction of potassium and acid secretion by the collecting tubule is present. In this group of disorders, urinary NH_4^+ excretion is depressed and renal function often compromised at the time of diagnosis. Patients with renal insufficiency and hyperkalemia (> 5.0 mequiv./L) have hyperkalemia that is disproportionate to the reduction in GFR. The causes of type 4 RTA are listed in Table 36.4.

The transtubular potassium gradient (TTKG) = $(U_K/P_K)/(U/P)_{osm}$, where U represents urine values and P represents plasma values. TTKG is abnormally low in patients with this disorder, indicating that the collecting tubule is not responding appropriately to the prevailing hyperkalemia. Impaired NH_4^+ production and excretion, in part due to hyperkalemia, leads to impaired net acid excretion and systemic metabolic acidosis. This form of generalized distal tubule dysfunction with hyperkalemia is acquired with diabetic nephropathy, obstructive uropathy, sickle cell nephropathy, tubulointerstitial diseases, and transplant rejection (see Table 36.4).

A number of patients have been reported with hyperkalemia, hyperchloremic metabolic acidosis, hypertension, undetectable plasma renin activity, and low aldosterone levels (type 2 pseudohypoaldosteronism). These patients generally have not exhibited glomerular or tubulointerstitial disease. The acidosis in such patients is mild and

Table 36.4 Etiology of distal renal tubular acidosis

CLASSICAL DISTAL RENAL TUBULAR ACIDOSIS (TYPE 1 RTA)
Primary
Familial
Autosomal dominant
  AE1 gene defect
Autosomal recessive
  With deafness (ATP6V1B1 gene)
  Without deafness (rdRTA2 gene)

Endemic (northeastern Thailand, H$^+$,K$^+$-ATPase defect?)

Secondary to systemic disorders (acquired)
Autoimmune diseases
Hyperglobulinemic purpura
Cryoglobulinemia
Sjögren syndrome
Thyroiditis
HIV nephropathy
Fibrosing alveolitis
Chronic active hepatitis
Primary biliary cirrhosis
Polyarteritis nodosa

Hypercalciuria and nephrocalcinosis
Primary hyperparathyroidism
Hyperthyroidism
Medullary sponge kidney
Fabry disease
X-linked hypophosphatemia
Vitamin D intoxication
Idiopathic hypercalciuria
Wilson disease
Hereditary fructose intolerance
Hereditary sensorineural deafness

Drug and toxin induced
Amphotericin B
Cyclamate
Vanadate
Hepatic cirrhosis
Ifosfamide
Toluene
Mercury
Lithium
Classic analgesic nephropathy
Foscarnet

Tubulointerstitial diseases
Balkan nephropathy
Chronic pyelonephritis
Obstructive uropathy
Vesicoureteral reflux
Renal transplantation
Leprosy
Jejunoileal bypass with hyperoxaluria

Associated with genetically transmitted diseases
Ehlers–Danlos syndrome
Sickle cell anemia
Medullary cystic disease
Hereditary sensorineural deafness
Osteopetrosis with carbonic anhydrase II deficiency
Hereditary elliptocytosis
Marfan syndrome
Jejunal bypass with hyperoxaluria
Carnitine palmitoyltransferase I

GENERALIZED ABNORMALITY OF DISTAL NEPHRON WITH HYPERKALEMIA
Mineralocorticoid deficiency
Primary mineralocorticoid deficiency
Combined deficiency of aldosterone, desoxycorticosterone, and cortisol (Addison disease, bilateral adrenalectomy)
Isolated (selective) aldosterone deficiency
  Chronic idiopathic hypoaldosteronism
  Heparin or persistent hypotension and/or hypoxemia in critically ill patient
  Familial hypoaldosteronism
Angiotensin II-converting enzyme (ACE) inhibition
  ACE inhibitors and AT$_1$ receptor antagonists

Secondary mineralocorticoid deficiency
Hyporeninemic hypoaldosteronism
Diabetic nephropathy
Tubulointerstitial nephropathies
Nephrosclerosis
Nonsteroidal anti-inflammatory agents

Mineralocorticoid resistance
Type 1 pseudohypoaldosteronism: autosomal dominant

Renal tubular dysfunction (voltage defect)
Type 1 pseudohypoaldosteronism: autosomal recessive
Type 2 pseudohypoaldosteronism: autosomal recessive
Drugs that interfere with Na$^+$ channel function in cortical collecting duct
  Amiloride
  Pentamidine
  Trimethoprim
  Triamterene
Drugs that interfere with Na$^+$,K$^+$-ATPase in cortical collecting duct
  Cyclosporine
Drugs that inhibit aldosterone effect on cortical collecting duct
  Spironolactone
Disorders associated with tubulointerstitial nephritis and renal insufficiency
  Lupus nephritis
  Methicillin nephrotoxicity
  Obstructive nephropathy
  Kidney transplant rejection
  Sickle cell disease

can be accounted for by the magnitude of hyperkalemia. Renal potassium secretion is resistant to mineralocorticoid administration. Renin and aldosterone levels both increase if volume expansion is corrected by diuretics or salt restriction. This disorder appears to be the result of impaired function of the apical epithelial sodium channel in the cortical collecting duct. When the sodium channel is ineffective or inoperative, potassium cannot be secreted across the apical membrane and excreted ("voltage defect"). The hyperkalemia that follows depresses, in turn, NH_4^+ production and excretion and may result in hyperchloremic metabolic acidosis, especially in the face of even mild renal insufficiency. Impaired operation of the sodium channel can also occur as a result of drugs that physically occupy the sodium channel, such as amiloride, triamterene, pentamidine, or trimethoprim; as a result of conditions that alter sodium absorption indirectly, such as aldosterone resistance; or as a result of cyclosporine or tacrolimus administration. Nonsteroidal anti-inflammatory drugs and the angiotensin-converting enzyme inhibitors may also produce hyperkalemia and metabolic acidosis, particularly in patients with preexisting renal insufficiency, volume depletion, or in the elderly. Therefore, drugs should always be considered as a possible cause of hyperkalemia and metabolic acidosis in such patients.

Treatment A reduction in serum potassium enhances renal ammoniagenesis and NH_4^+ excretion, increasing net acid excretion and thus improving or correcting the metabolic acidosis. Treatment of patients with mild chronic hyperkalemia and metabolic acidosis with chronic renal insufficiency is not always necessary, and the decision to treat is often based on the severity of the hyperkalemia and acidosis, when present. Patients with combined glucocorticoid and mineralocorticoid deficiency should receive both adrenal steroids in replacement dosages. Patients with hyporeninemic hypoaldosteronism may respond to a cation-exchange resin (sodium polystyrene sulfonate 15 g orally b.i.d. or 50 g per rectum), alkali therapy (Shohl solution, one to two tablespoons b.i.d.), or a loop diuretic (furosemide 40–80 mg daily) to induce renal potassium and salt excretion. Mineralocorticoid replacement with 9α-fludrocortisone (0.1–0.3 mg/day) can theoretically improve net acid excretion. However, mineralocorticoid administration is contraindicated in the face of coexisting hypertension or congestive heart failure. Volume depletion should be avoided unless the patient is volume overexpanded or hypertensive. Higher doses of mineralocorticoids, if necessary, should be administered cautiously in combination with a loop diuretic in order to avoid volume overexpansion or aggravation of hypertension and to increase potassium excretion. Pseudohypoaldosteronism in children (type 1) should be treated with avid dietary sodium chloride intake, while pseudohypoaldosteronism in adults (type 2) responds to thiazide diuretics and dietary salt restriction. Since bicarbonate is not avidly absorbed in the distal nephron, administration of bicarbonate in sufficient quantity to induce a bicarbonaturia may reverse the "voltage defect" induced by amiloride, pentamidine, or trimethoprim by enhancing K^+ and H^+ secretion by the collecting duct.

Respiratory acidosis

Diagnostic points Respiratory acidosis can be due to severe pulmonary disease, respiratory muscle fatigue, or abnormalities in ventilatory control and is recognized by an increase in Pa_{CO_2} and a decrease in pH (Table 36.5). In acute respiratory acidosis, there is an immediate compensatory elevation (due to cellular buffering mechanisms) in $[HCO_3^-]$, which increases by 1 mmol/L for every 10-mmHg increase in Pa_{CO_2}. In chronic respiratory acidosis (> 24 h), renal adaptation increases the $[HCO_3^-]$ by 4 mmol/L for every 10-mmHg increase in Pa_{CO_2}. The serum $[HCO_3^-]$ usually does not increase above 38 mmol/L.

The clinical features vary according to the severity and duration of the respiratory acidosis, the underlying disease, and whether there is accompanying hypoxemia. A rapid increase in Pa_{CO_2} may cause anxiety, dyspnea, confusion, psychosis, and hallucinations and may progress to coma. Lesser degrees of dysfunction in chronic hypercapnia include sleep disturbances, loss of memory, daytime somnolence, personality changes, impairment of coordination, and motor disturbances such as tremor, myoclonic jerks, and asterixis. Headaches and other signs that mimic raised intracranial pressure, such as papilledema, abnormal reflexes, and focal muscle weakness, are due to vasoconstriction secondary to loss of the vasodilator effects of CO_2.

Depression of the respiratory center by a variety of drugs, injury, or disease can produce respiratory acidosis. This may occur acutely with general anesthetics, sedatives, and head trauma or chronically with sedatives, alcohol,

Table 36.5 Respiratory acidosis

Central
Drugs (anesthetics, morphine, sedatives)
Stroke
Infection

Airway
Obstruction
Asthma

Parenchyma
Emphysema
Pneumoconiosis
Bronchitis
Adult respiratory distress syndrome
Barotrauma

Neuromuscular
Poliomyelitis
Kyphoscoliosis
Myasthenia
Muscular dystrophies

Miscellaneous
Obesity
Hypoventilation
Permissive hypercapnia

intracranial tumors, and the syndromes of sleep-disordered breathing (e.g. primary alveolar and obesity hypoventilation syndromes). Abnormalities or disease in the motor neurons, neuromuscular junction, and skeletal muscle can cause hypoventilation via respiratory muscle fatigue. Mechanical ventilation, when not properly adjusted and supervised, may result in respiratory acidosis, particularly if CO_2 production suddenly rises (because of fever, agitation, sepsis, or overfeeding) or alveolar ventilation falls because of worsening pulmonary function. High levels of positive end-expiratory pressure in the presence of reduced cardiac output may cause hypercapnia as a result of large increases in alveolar dead space. Permissive hypercapnia is being used with increasing frequency because of studies suggesting lower mortality compared with conventional mechanical ventilation, especially with severe CNS or heart disease. Although the potential beneficial effects of permissive hypercapnia might be mitigated by correction of the acidemia, nevertheless it seems prudent to keep the pH in the range 7.2–7.3 by administration of sodium bicarbonate.

Acute hypercapnia follows sudden occlusion of the upper airway or generalized bronchospasm as in severe asthma, anaphylaxis, inhalational burn, or toxin injury. Chronic hypercapnia and respiratory acidosis occur in endstage obstructive lung disease. Restrictive disorders involving both the chest wall and the lungs can cause respiratory acidosis because the high metabolic cost of respiration causes ventilatory muscle fatigue. Advanced stages of intrapulmonary and extrapulmonary restrictive defects present as chronic respiratory acidosis.

The diagnosis of respiratory acidosis requires the measurement of Pa_{CO_2} and arterial pH. A detailed history and physical examination often indicate the cause.

Treatment The management of respiratory acidosis depends on its severity and rate of onset. Acute respiratory acidosis can be life-threatening, and measures to reverse the underlying cause should be undertaken simultaneously with restoration of adequate alveolar ventilation. This may necessitate tracheal intubation and assisted mechanical ventilation. Oxygen administration should be titrated carefully in patients with severe obstructive pulmonary disease and chronic CO_2 retention who are breathing spontaneously. When oxygen is used injudiciously, these patients may experience progression of the respiratory acidosis. Aggressive and rapid correction of hypercapnia should be avoided, because the falling Pa_{CO_2} may provoke the same complications noted with acute respiratory alkalosis (i.e. cardiac arrhythmias, reduced cerebral perfusion, and seizures). The Pa_{CO_2} should be lowered gradually in chronic respiratory acidosis, aiming to restore the Pa_{CO_2} to baseline levels and to provide sufficient Cl^- and K^+ to enhance the renal excretion of HCO_3^-.

Chronic respiratory acidosis is frequently difficult to correct, but measures aimed at improving lung function such as cessation of smoking, use of oxygen, bronchodilators, glucocorticoids, diuretics, and physiotherapy can help some patients and forestall further deterioration in most. The use of respiratory stimulants may be useful in selected patients, particularly if hypercapnia is out of proportion to the abnormality in lung function.

Further reading

DuBose TD Jr: Acid–base disorders. *In* Brenner BM (ed): Brenner and Rector's The Kidney, 6th edn. Philadelphia: WB Saunders, 2000, pp 925–997.

DuBose TD Jr, Alpern RJ: Renal tubular acidosis. *In* Scriver CR, Beaudet AL, Valle D, et al (eds): The Metabolic and Molecular Bases of Inherited Diseases, 8th edn. New York: McGraw-Hill, 2000, pp 4983–5021.

Hamm LL, Alpern RJ: Cellular mechanisms of renal tubular acidification. *In* Seldin DW, Giebisch G (eds): The Kidney: Physiology and Pathophysiology, 3rd edn. New York: Lippincott, Williams and Wilkins, 2000, pp 1935–1979.

Nagami GT: Renal ammonia production and excretion. *In* Seldin DW, Giebisch G (eds): The Kidney: Physiology and Pathophysiology, 3rd edn. New York: Lippincott, Williams and Wilkins, 2000, pp 1995–2013.

Laski ME, Wesson DW: Lactic acidosis. *In* DuBose TD, Hamm LL (eds): Acid–Base and Electrolyte Disorders. Philadelphia: Saunders, 2002, pp 83–108.

Halperin ML: The Acid Truth and Basic Facts: With a Sweet Touch, an Enlytenment. Montreal: LetroMac, 1991.

Bidani A, DuBose TD Jr: Cellular and whole-body acid–base regulation. *In* Arieff AI, DeFronzo RA (eds): Fluid, Electrolyte, and Acid–Base Disorders. New York: Churchill Livingstone, 1995, pp 69–104.

Narins RG, Kupin W, Faber MD, Goodkin DA, Dunfee TP: Pathophysiology, classification and therapy of acid–base disturbances. *In* Arieff AI, DeFronzo RA (eds): Fluid, Electrolyte, and Acid–Base Disorders. New York: Churchill Livingstone, 1995, pp 105–198.

Metabolic and Respiratory Alkalosis

John H. Galla

Metabolic alkalosis

Clinical features

Metabolic alkalosis is common and, when severe, is associated with high morbidity and mortality.[1] This acid–base disorder should be anticipated when conditions such as vomiting, diuretic use, or severe hypertension are present. Both deficits and surfeits of volume often accompany metabolic alkalosis depending on its etiology. Symptoms such as apathy, confusion, cardiac arrhythmias, and neuromuscular irritability are observed only when alkalosis is severe (arterial pH > 7.55).

Metabolic alkalosis is characterized by the primary tendency to retain bicarbonate in the extracellular compartment and is recognized by high bicarbonate and low chloride concentrations in the serum electrolyte profile. This anion pattern is usually accompanied by hypokalemia regardless of the etiology of the alkalosis. The anion gap may be increased by lactate and negatively charged albumin.

Proper examination of arterial blood gases is necessary to establish the diagnosis of metabolic alkalosis (Table 37.1). After the accuracy of the variables of the Henderson equation is confirmed, the pattern of elevated arterial pH, serum bicarbonate, and partial pressure of carbon dioxide (Pa_{CO_2}) establishes metabolic alkalosis as the predominant acid–base disturbance. If the observed magnitude of respiratory compensation is as predicted from published data,[2] one is dealing with a simple disorder irrespective of its etiology (Fig. 37.1). On the other hand, if the measured Pa_{CO_2} is more or less than ± 5 mmHg of the predicted value, at least one other primary respiratory acid–base disturbance is present.

Diagnostic considerations

Metabolic alkalosis, which can be divided into three phases[3] (generation, maintenance, and correction), is due largely to chloride depletion or potassium depletion usually coupled with mineralocorticoid excess. Disorders characterized by both chloride and potassium depletion can occur. For the major clinically relevant etiologic classification, the diagnostic approach begins with the determination of the urine chloride concentration to establish the presence or absence of chloride depletion (Table 37.2).

Chloride depletion is characterized by a urine chloride of < 10 mequiv./L except when a chloruretic diuretic is present in the urine or accompanying profound potassium depletion produces severe tubule dysfunction that induces a chloride leak.[4] It can be generated by losses usually from the gut or the kidney; exocrine glands can contribute to chloride losses in cystic fibrosis[5] in which renal chloride handling is normal.[6] A discussion of the mechanisms of alkalosis generated by gastric HCl losses, chloruretic diuretics, intestinal chloride losses, or renal losses in compensation for respiratory acidosis[7] is beyond the scope of this chapter, which focuses on correction.

From the standpoint of the maintenance and correction of chloride-depletion alkalosis (CDA), volume depletion is a commonly associated but not causative or essential factor that maintains the alkalosis.[8,9] Although the restoration of extracellular fluid (ECF) volume is of paramount importance in its own right, chloride administration with any of several cations, most often sodium or potassium, is necessary and sufficient for the correction of CDA, which probably occurs primarily in the collecting duct of the kidney.[10] Similarly, although concomitant potassium repletion is indicated to avoid other potentially harmful effects of hypokalemia, it is not essential for the correction of CDA when potassium depletion is modest (350–400 mequiv.).

When urine chloride is > 20 mequiv./L, potassium-depletion alkalosis (KDA) and other miscellaneous disorders are suggested. When potassium depletion is present, urine potassium excretion is normally < 20 mequiv./day. Thus, in the differential diagnosis of KDA, urine potassium excretion > 30 mequiv./day in the presence of hypokalemia establishes renal potassium wasting and indicates mineralocorticoid excess or an agent that promotes renal potassium wasting. Within this group, KDA can be further subdivided by the status of ECF volume and blood pressure. In those diseases characterized by persistent intravascular and ECF volume expansion and consequent hypertension, such as primary aldosteronism or syndromes of apparent mineralocorticoid excess,[11] escape from the sodium-retaining effect of mineralocorticoids occurs. However, escape does not occur from the potassium-wasting effects,[12] thereby promoting alkalosis. The transtubular potassium gradient (TTKG) is a fast and useful test for determining the presence of renal potassium wasting;

Table 37.1 Four steps to the diagnosis of alkalosis

1. Accuracy of data is confirmed

If the serum $[HCO_3^-]$ from arterial blood gas determinations or calculated from the Henderson equation

$[HCO_3^-]$ (mequiv./L) = 24 $[Paco_2]$ (mmHg)/$[H^+]$ (nmol/L)

approximates the measured value (± 3 mequiv./L) from the serum electrolyte profile, the data are accurate and internally consistent

2. Predominant disorder is classified

(a) If an elevated serum $[HCO_3^-]$, increased $Paco_2$, and increased arterial pH are present, a predominant metabolic alkalosis is established

(b) If a decreased serum $[HCO_3^-]$, decreased $Paco_2$, and increased arterial pH are present, a predominant respiratory alkalosis is established

3. Presence of a mixed disorder is tested by comparison of the predicted compensatory response with the observed response

(a) In a *simple* metabolic alkalosis, each 1-mequiv./L increment in serum $[HCO_3^-]$ above the normal value of 24 mequiv./L is accompanied by a 0.6–0.7 mmHg compensatory increment in $Paco_2$ above the normal value of 40 mmHg or as calculated in Fig. 37.1. If the observed $Paco_2$ does not approximate (± 5 mmHg) the predicted value for a simple disorder, one is dealing with a *mixed* disorder, an additional primary respiratory acidosis or alkalosis

(b) In a simple respiratory alkalosis, each 1-mmHg decrement in $Paco_2$ below the normal value of 40 mmHg is accompanied by a 0.2–0.25 mequiv./L decrement in serum $[HCO_3^-]$ below the normal value of 24 mequiv./L in the acute setting and by a 0.4–0.5 mequiv./L decrement in the chronic setting. If the observed serum $[HCO_3^-]$ does not approximate (± 5 mequiv./L) the predicted value, one is dealing with a mixed disorder, an additional primary metabolic acidosis or alkalosis

4. With the proper acid-base diagnosis in hand, the etiology is addressed

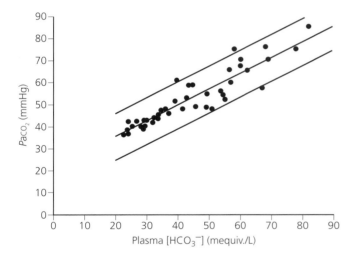

Figure 37.1 Respiratory compensation for simple metabolic alkalosis. The relationship between plasma $[HCO_3^-]$ and $Paco_2$ is depicted; the 95% confidence limits are indicated. If the measured $Paco_2$ does not conform to the value predicted from this regression (i.e. $Paco_2$ = 0.73 plasma $[HCO_3^-]$ + 20 ± 5), a mixed acid–base disorder is present with either a respiratory acidosis or alkalosis, at least, superimposed.

TTKG > 4 in the setting of hypokalemia is consistent with this abnormality.[13]

In contrast, in Bartter and Gitelman syndromes, sodium loss due to primary defects in the kidney is associated with normotension. Bartter syndrome is probably a group of disorders *in which both potassium and chloride losses occur.*[14] Heterogeneous mutations of the $Na^+/K^+/2Cl^-$ transporter in the thick ascending limb of the loop of Henle have now been shown to account for the renal sodium, potassium, and chloride wasting, macula-densa and volume depletion-stimulated activation of the renin–aldosterone system, and high renal prostaglandin production.[15] Gitelman syndrome is similar but less severe, usually presenting in adulthood and characterized by hypocalciuria not hypercalciuria as in Bartter syndrome. These features are consistent with several identified mutations of the thiazide-sensitive Na^+/Cl^- cotransporter in the distal nephron.[16] One should recognize that these uncommon syndromes could be confused with some of the commonly concealed causes of metabolic alkalosis, such as diuretic or laxative abuse, bulimia, or surreptitious vomiting.

When urine potassium excretion is < 20 mequiv./day, potassium depletion due solely to dietary or gut losses is established and is associated with metabolic alkalosis due to the intracellular shift of protons.[17] The alkalosis in these disorders is usually mild. More severe alkalosis should suggest additional causative factors, such as concomitant chloride depletion or base ingestion.

Causes of alkalosis other than CDA or KDA as listed in Table 37.2 are uncommon.

Treatment

In general terms, one should intervene as far as possible to prevent or blunt the continued generation of losses. Second, replacement of any continuing unpreventable losses as well as existing deficits are essential. Third, specific treatment, as discussed below, is generally indicated when arterial pH is > 7.55 or serum bicarbonate concentration > 33 mequiv./L.

Table 37.2 Causes of metabolic alkalosis

Chloride depletion (urinary [Cl⁻] < 10 mequiv./L)
Gastric acid losses: vomiting, mechanical drainage, bulimia, gastrocystoplasty
Chloruretic diuretics: bumetanide, chlorothiazide, metolazone, and their congeners
Diarrheal states: villous adenoma, congenital chloridorrhea
Posthypercapnic state
Dietary chloride deprivation with base loading: chloride-deficient infant formulas
Excessive sweating in cystic fibrosis

Potassium depletion/mineralocorticoid excess (urinary [Cl⁻] > 20 mequiv./L)
Urinary potassium excretion > 30 mequiv./day
With hypertension
    Primary aldosteronism: adenoma, hyperplasia, carcinoma, glucocorticoid-suppressible
    Primary deoxycorticosterone excess: 11β- and 17α-hydroxylase deficiencies
    Secondary aldosteronism
        Adrenal corticosteroid excess: primary, secondary, exogenous
        Severe hypertension: malignant, accelerated, renovascular
        Hemangiopericytoma, nephroblastoma, renal cell carcinoma
    Apparent mineralocorticoid excess: licorice, Liddle syndrome
With normotension
    Bartter syndrome, Gitelman syndrome
Urinary potassium excretion < 20 mequiv./day
Laxative abuse, clay ingestion, severe dietary potassium restriction

Miscellaneous
Hypercalcemia with suppressed parathyroid hormone
Acute or chronic milk alkali syndrome
Carbenicillin, ampicillin, penicillin
Administration of bicarbonate or its precursors usually with renal insufficiency
Recovery from starvation

Specific recommendations

Chloride depletion In CDA, the chloride deficit must be replaced, with selection of the accompanying cation (Na⁺, K⁺, or H⁺) based on (1) ECF volume status, (2) the degree of associated potassium depletion, and (3) the degree and reversibility of any depression of glomerular filtration rate (Fig. 37.2). Because the magnitude of the loss of each of these cations is difficult to assess, an empirical clinical approach is recommended in the order shown by the shaded boxes in Fig. 37.2. When chloride and severe potassium depletion coexist, both must be replenished to correct the alkalosis.[18] In patients with overt signs of ECF volume contraction, such as hypotension, tachycardia, and diminished skin turgor, administration of 3–5 L of 0.15 mol/L NaCl at a minimum is usually necessary to correct volume deficits and metabolic alkalosis. Once volume is replenished, further chloride replacement

should be accomplished with KCl unless contraindications are present.

Grave conditions such as hepatic encephalopathy, cardiac arrhythmia, digitalis cardiotoxicity, or altered mental status may be seen in the setting of severe alkalosis (arterial pH > 7.55). No clinical studies have specifically addressed the impact of the treatment of severe alkalosis on outcome in these states. However, the high reported mortality suggests that, to the extent that severe alkalosis may be a contributing factor, it should be corrected promptly. HCl (0.1 equiv./L) administration through a central venous catheter at rates up to 25 mequiv./h should be considered.[19] The amount of HCl needed to correct alkalosis is calculated using the formula: $0.5 \times$ body weight (kg) $\times$ desired decrement in plasma bicarbonate (mequiv./L), with additional amounts to replace any continuing losses of acid. With the goal being to rescue the patient from severe alkalosis, the plasma bicarbonate concentration should initially be restored halfway to normal. An alternative to HCl is ammonium chloride, which may be administered via a peripheral vein at a rate of not more than 300 mequiv. NH_4^+ daily but should be avoided in advanced renal or hepatic insufficiency. The HCl salts of lysine or arginine are available but have been associated with severe hyperkalemia; they are not recommended. Of the aforementioned agents, HCl is preferred and is to be used only as noted.

In the clinical setting of ECF volume overload, such as congestive cardiac failure in association with CDA, NaCl administration is contraindicated. KCl is the preferred alternative in this setting but it too may be contraindicated because of either concurrent hyperkalemia or renal insufficiency, which could precipitate hyperkalemia. If glomerular filtration rate is adequate in this setting (serum creatinine concentration < 4.0 mg/dL), acetazolamide 250 mg twice or thrice daily orally or 5–10 mg/kg intravenously[20] may be effective. Because the distal nephron can avidly reabsorb the excess sodium delivery promoted by acetazolamide, which inhibits sodium uptake in the proximal tubule, the carbonic anhydrase inhibitors are most effective when used in conjunction with diuretics that have more distal sites of action.[21,22] Acetazolamide could also be used intermittently to avoid or lessen CDA in edema-forming states such as congestive heart failure treated with loop diuretics. Plasma electrolyte composition should be followed serially during its administration as acetazolamide is usually associated with high urinary potassium losses. This approach could be used, for example, in a patient with chronic obstructive pulmonary disease and cor pulmonale who develops metabolic alkalosis after therapeutic correction of acute CO_2 retention and in the presence of hyperkalemia. Carbonic anhydrase in erythrocytes and along the pulmonary capillary endothelium participates in the dehydration of bicarbonate to CO_2 and its subsequent excretion by the lung. In vitro studies of inhibited erythrocytes[23] and lungs inhibited by acetazolamide[24] show significant decreases and delays in pulmonary CO_2 excretion. While these acute studies have been confirmed in normal human subjects,[25] studies in critically ill patients have shown only minor

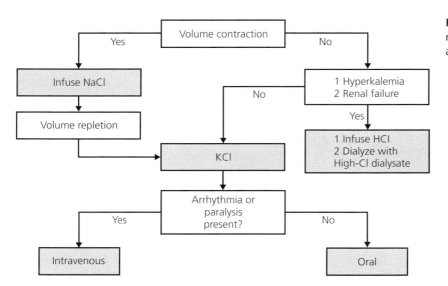

Figure 37.2 Algorithm for the general treatment of metabolic alkalosis. The shaded boxes indicate actions.

CO_2 retention.[26] Particularly in patients with impaired respiratory function, clinicians should be alert to the potential of CO_2 retention with carbonic anhydrase inhibitors. In such a case, the goal of treatment is the baseline plasma bicarbonate concentration for that patient and not a normal concentration.

Other primary or adjunctive therapies should be considered. Villous adenomas require surgical removal. Congenital chloridorrhea does not respond to antidiarrheal agents and dietary replenishment of fluid, chloride, and potassium losses is usually required.[27] However, as recently reported, omeprazole (an inhibitor of H^+/K^+ ATPase) 20 mg twice daily may substantially decrease diarrhea and obviate the need for dietary electrolyte supplementation; the reduction in the intestinal chloride load by inhibition of gastric chloride secretion is presumably the mechanism.[28] When continuing gastric acid losses cannot be prevented, e.g. Zollinger–Ellison syndrome, omeprazole or a histamine H_2-receptor blocker (e.g. cimetidine or ranitidine) will reduce output. These drugs have also been used to augment chloride replacement in patients with unremitting losses due to gastrocystoplasty;[29] on occasion, only surgical revision can correct the alkalosis in these patients.

If renal insufficiency compromises the effectiveness of the above therapies or in patients on maintenance dialysis, exchange of bicarbonate for high bath chloride concentration during hemodialysis or peritoneal dialysis is an effective mechanism for correcting metabolic alkalosis.[30]

Potassium depletion The magnitude of potassium depletion can be estimated from the serum potassium concentration (Table 37.3). The decrease in serum potassium concentration evoked by alkalosis per se (~ 0.5-mequiv. decrement for each 0.1 increment in arterial pH[31]) accounts for only a modest overestimation of the potassium deficit.

For KDA, oral replacement will often suffice unless ileus is present. Oral KCl in the liquid form diluted with fruit juice or the slow-release form can be given in doses of up to 40–60 mequiv. four or five times per day. Potassium

Table 37.3 Estimation of total body potassium deficit*

Serum potassium (mequiv./L)[†]	Potassium deficit (mequiv.)
3.5	100–250
3.0	150–350
2.5	300–600
2.0	500–750

*Adapted from Sterns RH, Cox M, Feig PU, et al: Internal potassium balance and the control of plasma potassium concentration. Medicine 1981;60:339–354.
[†]Serum and plasma concentrations differ by less than 10% unless hemolysis or marked thrombocytosis or leukocytosis is present.

salts such as citrate, gluconate, or bicarbonate are not appropriate.

However, if a serious cardiac arrhythmia or generalized paralysis is present, intravenous KCl in concentrations no greater than 60 mequiv./L at rates as high as 40 mequiv./h should be preferred. The downregulation of Na^+,K^+-ATPase in skeletal muscle with potassium-depletion states may slow the clearing of the potassium load.[32] Thus ECG monitoring and frequent determinations of serum potassium concentration are mandatory. Glucose should be omitted from infusions initially because stimulated insulin secretion may cause serum potassium to decrease even further. However, once replacement is begun, infused glucose facilitates cellular potassium replenishment. Because hypokalemic nephropathy may prevent concentration of the urine, plasma sodium concentration should also be monitored. If chloruretic diuretics or laxatives are contributing, they should be stopped.

Correction of the potassium deficit reverses the alkalinizing effects of potassium depletion, although blockade or removal of the source of mineralocorticoid excess is essential for definitive correction. If the source of aldosterone excess cannot be removed, potassium-sparing diuretics will effectively blunt its effects. Amiloride 5–10 mg daily, triamterene 100 mg twice daily, or spironolactone 25–50 mg in single or divided doses daily are all useful. Restriction of sodium and addition of potassium to the diet will also ameliorate the alkalosis[33] and associated hypertension.

In Bartter syndrome, the focus of therapy is to prevent urinary potassium loss. Converting enzyme inhibitors have been shown to be effective[34] and are a reasonable first approach. Because of concern for hypotension, low doses should be used initially. Other interventions may also partially correct the alkalosis. The potassium-sparing diuretics mentioned earlier are effective but dietary potassium supplementation is usually also needed. Spironolactone may produce unacceptable gynecomastia in men. Because renal production of prostaglandin E_2 is increased and may contribute to sodium, chloride, and potassium wasting, prostaglandin synthetase inhibitors, such as indomethacin or ibuprofen, may blunt but not completely correct the hypokalemic alkalosis. Since magnesium depletion may contribute to the increase in urinary potassium wasting, hypomagnesemia should be corrected and magnesium stores replenished, if clinically feasible. Oral magnesium oxide 250–500 mg four times daily (12.5–25 mequiv. Mg^{2+}) is recommended. However, the degree to which the correction of magnesium depletion blunts the alkalosis is uncertain and magnesium salts often produce an unacceptable degree of diarrhea that can worsen electrolyte imbalance.

Several of the primary disorders of mineralocorticoid excess are treated definitively by tumor ablation or by medication when that cannot be accomplished.

Miscellaneous In acute milk-alkali syndrome, cessation of alkali ingestion and the sources of calcium (milk, antacids, etc.) and replenishment of chloride and volume usually leads to the prompt resolution of these abnormalities.[35] For those alkaloses due to alkali loading, cessation of alkali administration and continuation of normal electrolyte intake usually suffices.

Respiratory alkalosis

Clinical features

Respiratory alkalosis is also common.[36] The defining feature of respiratory alkalosis is hyperventilation in which the pulmonary excretion of CO_2 exceeds the endogenous production rate. Symptoms are usually confined to the acute phase and include numbness and paresthesias, dizziness, and confusion. With increasing severity of the alkalosis, muscle cramps, hyperreflexia, or seizures may be seen.

Hyperventilation produces a decrease in Pa_{CO_2} that results in a rise in arterial blood pH, which is buffered within minutes by nonbicarbonate buffers in tissue such that the serum bicarbonate concentration falls by 2.0–2.5 mmol/L for each 10-mmHg decrement in Pa_{CO_2} below the nominal value of 40 mmHg (Table 37.1).[37,38] If hyperventilation is sustained, further renal compensation occurs with excretion of bicarbonate and reabsorption of

chloride. Full compensation occurs after 3–4 days, with a decrement of 4–5 mmol/L for a 10-mmHg decrement in Pa_{CO_2}.[39–41]

Diagnostic considerations

Hyperventilation is caused by central nervous system stimulation (pain, anxiety, fever, stroke, infection, tumor, trauma), hypoxemia or tissue hypoxia (pneumonia, pulmonary edema, anemia), pregnancy, salicylates, septicemia, hepatic failure, and mechanical and direct stimulation of chest receptors. Numerous drugs have been implicated in hyperventilation, particularly those used specifically to stimulate ventilation. The appropriate examination of body fluids and imaging of organs will reveal the cause of respiratory alkalosis in virtually all settings; the description of these examinations to determine the etiology is beyond the scope of this chapter.

Treatment

The treatment of respiratory alkalosis is directed at correction of the underlying cause. In the acute setting of anxiety-related hyperventilation, rebreathing into a closed system will help. If the hyperventilation persists and is severe, an increase in ventilatory dead space or paralysis with mechanical ventilation can be considered.

References

1. Anderson LE, Henrich WL: Alkalemia-associated morbidity and mortality in medical and surgical patients. South Med J 1987;80:729–733.
2. Javaheri S, Kazemi H: Metabolic alkalosis and hypoventilation in humans. Am Rev Respir Dis 1987;136:1101–1016.
3. Seldin DW, Rector FC Jr: The generation and maintenance of metabolic alkalosis. Kidney Int 1972;1:306–321.
4. Luke RG, Wright FS, Fowler N, et al: Effects of potassium depletion on tubular chloride transport in the rat. Kidney Int 1978;14:414–427.
5. Pedroli G, Leichti-Gallati S, Mauri S, et al: Chronic metabolic alkalosis: not uncommon in young children with severe cystic fibrosis. Am J Nephrol 1995;15:245–250.
6. Koch C, Høiby N: Pathogenesis of cystic fibrosis. Lancet 1993;339:1065–1069.
7. Schwartz WB, van Ypersele de Strihou C, Kassirer JP: Role of anions in metabolic alkalosis and potassium deficiency. N Engl J Med 1968;279:630–639.
8. Rosen RA, Julian BA, Dubovsky EV, et al: On the mechanism by which chloride corrects metabolic alkalosis in man. Am J Med 1988;84:449–458.
9. Kassirer JP, Schwartz WB: Correction of metabolic alkalosis in man without repair of potassium deficiency. Am J Med 1966;40:19–25.
10. Galla, JH, Gifford JD, Luke RG, et al: Adaptations to chloride-depletion alkalosis. Am J Physiol 1991;261:R771–R781.
11. Blumenfeld JD: Hypertension and adrenal disorders. Curr Opin Nephrol Hypertens 1993;2:274–282.
12. August JT, Nelson DH, Thorn GW: Response of normal subjects to large amounts of aldosterone. J Clin Invest 1958;37:1549–1555.
13. Ethier JH, Kamel KS, Magner PO, et al: The transtubular potassium gradient in patients with hypokalemia and hyperkalemia. Am J Kidney Dis 1990;15:309–315.
14. Kurtz I: Molecular pathogenesis of Bartter's and Gitelman's syndromes. Kidney Int 1998;34:1396.
15. Simon DB, Karet FE, Hamdan JM, et al: Bartter's syndrome, hypokalemic alkalosis with hypercalciuria, is caused by mutations in

the Na-K-2Cl cotransporter, NKCC2. Nature Genetics 1996;13:183–188.

16. Simon DB, Nelson-Williams C, Bia MJ, et al: Gitelman's variant of Bartter's syndrome, inherited hypokalemic alkalosis, is caused by mutations in the thiazide-sensitive Na-Cl cotransporter. Nature Genetics 1996;12:24–30.

17. Jones JW, Sebastian A, Hulter HN, et al: Systemic and renal acid–base effects of chronic dietary potassium depletion in humans. Kidney Int 1982;21:402–410.

18. Wall BM, Williams HH, Cooke CR: Chloride-resistant metabolic alkalosis in an adult with congenital chloride diarrhea. Am J Med 1988;85:570–572.

19. Kopel RF, Durbin CG Jr: Pulmonary artery catheter deterioration during hydrochloric acid infusion for the treatment of metabolic alkalosis. Crit Care Med 1989;17:688–689.

20. Marik PE, Kussman BD, Lipman J, et al: Acetazolamide in the treatment of metabolic alkalosis in critically ill patients. Heart Lung 1991;20:455–458.

21. Kahn MI: Treatment of refractory congestive heart failure and normokalemic hypochloremic alkalosis with acetazolamide and spironolactone. Can Med Assoc J 1980;123:883–887.

22. Knauf H, Mutschler E: Functional state of the nephron and diuretic dose–response: rationale for low-dose combination therapy. Cardiology 1994;84(Suppl 2):18–26.

23. Crandall ED, Mathew SJ, Fleischer RS, et al: Effects of inhibition of RBC HCO_3/Cl exchange on CO_2 excretion and downstream pH disequilibrium in isolated rat lungs. J Clin Invest 1981;68:853–862.

24. Schunemann HJ, Klocke RA: Influence of carbon dioxide kinetics on pulmonary carbon dioxide exchange. J Appl Physiol 1993;74:715–721.

25. Kowalchuk JM, Heigenhauser GJ, Sutton JR, et al: Effect of chronic acetazolamide administration on gas exchange and acid–base control after maximal exercise. J Appl Physiol 1994;76:1211–1219.

26. Berthelsen P, Gothgen I, Husum B, et al: Dissociation of renal and respiratory effects of acetazolamide in the critically ill. Br J Anaesth 1986;58:512–516.

27. Kagalwalla AF: Congential chloride diarrhea: a study in Arab children. J Clin Gastroenterol 1994;19:36–40.

28. Aichbichler BW, Zerr CH, Santa Ana CA, et al: Proton-pump inhibition of gastric chloride secretion in congenital chloridorrhea. N Engl J Med 1997;336:106–109.

29. Plawker MW, Rabinowitz SS, Etwaru DJ, et al: Hypergastrinemia, dysuria–hematuria and metabolic alkalosis: complications associated with gastrocystoplasty. J Urol 1995;154:546–549.

30. Ponce P, Santana A, Vinhas J: Treatment of severe metabolic alkalosis by "acid dialysis." Crit Care Med 1991;19:583–585.

31. Sterns RH, Cox M, Feig PU, et al: Internal potassium balance and the control of plasma potassium concentration. Medicine 1981;60:339–354.

32. Clausen T, Everts ME: Regulation of the Na,K-pump in skeletal muscle. Kidney Int 1989;35:1–13.

33. Krishna GG, Kapoor SC: Potassium supplementation ameliorates mineralocorticoid-induced sodium retention. Kidney Int 1993;43:1097–1103.

34. Hene RJ, Koomans HA, Dorhout Mees EJ, et al: Correction of hypokalemia in Bartter's syndrome by enalapril. Am J Kidney Dis 1987;9:200–205.

35. Abreo K, Adalkha A, Kilpatrick S, et al: The milk-alkali syndrome. A reversible form of acute renal failure. Arch Intern Med 1993;153:1003–1010.

36. Wilson RF, Gibson D, Percinal AK, et al: Severe alkalosis in critically ill surgical patients. Arch Surg 1972;105:197–203.

37. Adler S, Roy A, Relman A: Intracellular acid–base regulation. I. Response of muscle cells to changes in CO_2 tension or extracellular bicarbonate concentration. J Clin Invest 1965;44:8–20.

38. Arbus GS, Herbert LA, Levesque PR, et al: Characterization and clinical application of the "significance band" for acute respiratory alkalosis. N Engl J Med 1969;280:117–123.

39. Stanbury SW, Thomson AE: The renal response to respiratory alkalosis. Clin Sci 1952;11:357–374.

40. Gennari FJ, Goldstein MB, Schwartz WB: The nature of the renal adaptation to chronic hypocapnia. J Clin Invest 1972;51:1722–1730.

41. Krapf R, Beeler I, Hertner D, et al: Chronic respiratory alkalosis: the effect of sustained hyperventilation on renal regulation of acid–base equilibrium. N Engl J Med 1991;324:1394–1401.

38 Hypercalcemia, Hypocalcemia, and Other Divalent Cation Disorders

Shakil Aslam and Francisco Llach

changes in pH affect the ionized but not total S_{Ca}. Acidosis increases ionized calcium by decreasing its binding to albumin, whereas alkalosis has the opposite effect. A direct measurement of ionized S_{Ca} is preferred in patients who have combined changes in pH and serum albumin.

The S_{Ca} normally reflects a balance between the entry of calcium into the extracellular fluid (ECF) from the gastrointestinal tract, skeleton, and kidneys and its removal by renal excretion and deposition into the skeleton. The precise regulation of S_{Ca} is largely controlled by parathyroid hormone (PTH) and the highly active vitamin D_3 metabolite 1,25-dihydroxycholecalciferol ($1,25(OH)_2D_3$, also called calcitriol). Dietary calcium is absorbed in the proximal intestine via both active and passive processes. Absorption is enhanced by calcitriol, the principal hormonal regulator of intestinal absorption. In the kidneys, 99% of the filtered load of calcium is reabsorbed. Approximately 90% of reabsorption occurs passively in the proximal tubule and loop of Henle; the remaining 10% occurs in the distal tubule under the regulation of PTH. A fall in free S_{Ca} stimulates the release of PTH, which increases renal calcium reabsorption. PTH also mediates the hydroxylation of cholecalciferol (vitamin D_3) to calcitriol. The effects of S_{Ca} on PTH secretion are mediated via a calcium-sensing receptor. This cell-surface receptor is coupled with guanine-nucleotide regulatory G proteins and is expressed in parathyroid, kidney, brain, and other organs.[2]

Calcium disorders

Homeostasis

The adult human body contains approximately 1200 g of calcium, of which > 99% is within bone. The remaining 1% is distributed in three different plasma fractions: ~ 50% is bound to serum albumin; 10% is complexed to various serum anions (phosphate, bicarbonate, citrate, lactate); and 40% is free and ionized. Ionized calcium is the physiologically active form. Its concentration is tightly regulated by the endocrine system. Normal total serum calcium concentration (S_{Ca}) ranges from 8.5 to 10.5 mg/dL (2.1–2.5 mmol/L), whereas ionized S_{Ca} is approximately 5 mg/dL (1.2 mmol/L). A reduction in serum albumin lowers the total S_{Ca}, although the ionized fraction remains normal. A correction for hypoalbuminemia may be made by adding 0.8 mg/dL to the total S_{Ca} for every 1-g/dL drop in serum albumin concentration below 4 g/dL. Conversely, falsely elevated S_{Ca} may result from hemoconcentration and may be found in rare patients with multiple myeloma who produce calcium-binding paraproteins.[1] In contrast to changes in serum albumin, which affect only total S_{Ca},

Hypercalcemia
Pathophysiology, clinical features, and etiology

Hypercalcemia is almost always due to an increase in ionized S_{Ca}. Hypercalcemia develops when the rate of entry of calcium into the ECF exceeds its excretion into urine or deposition in bone. An increase in influx can result from increased absorption from either intestine or bone, or both. However, multiple sites can be involved. For example, hypervitaminosis D increases both intestinal calcium absorption and bone resorption. Primary hyperparathyroidism (PHP) increases reabsorption from bone and renal tubules and increases renal synthesis of calcitriol. The major causes of hypercalcemia are PHP and malignancy: PHP accounts for over 90% of cases in ambulatory patients, whereas in hospitalized patients cancer accounts for about 65% of cases.[3]

Clinical presentation of hypercalcemia depends on the magnitude and rapidity of the elevation in S_{Ca}. Mild hypercalcemia (10.6–12 mg/dL) accompanying PHP is generally asymptomatic.[4] More severe hypercalcemia is frequently associated with neurologic, gastrointestinal, and renal manifestations. Neurologic symptoms may range

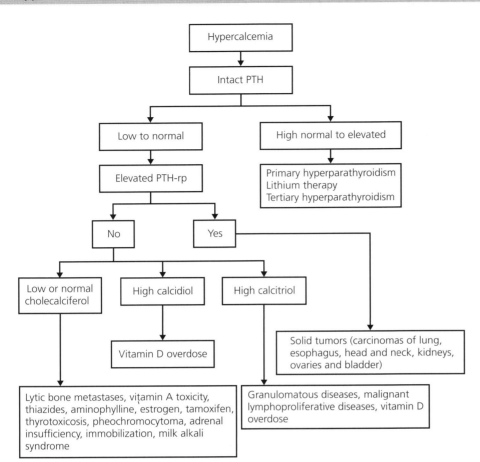

Figure 38.1 Diagnostic approach to hypercalcemia. PTH, parathyroid hormone; PTH-rp, PTH-related protein.

from subtle changes in concentration to depression, confusion, increased somnolence, and even coma. Gastro-intestinal symptoms are often prominent, with constipation, anorexia, nausea, and vomiting. The most important renal manifestations are nephrolithiasis, renal tubular dysfunction (particularly decreased concentrating ability[5]), and acute and chronic renal insufficiency. Nephrolithiasis has been reported in 20% of patients with PHP, while 4–5% of stone formers have PHP.[6] Increased calcitriol production may contribute to both hypercalciuria and stone formation.

Diagnosis

PHP and malignancy account for 80–90% of cases. Long-standing asymptomatic hypercalcemia suggests familial hypocalciuric hypercalcemia. An elevated serum intact PTH concentration (measured by immunoradiometric assay) indicates the presence of PHP or a patient taking lithium.[7] If the plasma PTH level is below normal, a neoplastic disorder should be strongly considered (Fig. 38.1). The diagnosis of humoral hypercalcemia of malignancy can be confirmed by demonstrating an elevated serum PTH-related protein. The serum levels of the vitamin D metabolites calcitriol and 25-hydroxycholecalciferol (calcidiol) should be measured if there is no obvious malignancy and neither PTH nor PTH-related protein levels are elevated. An elevated serum calcidiol is indicative of vitamin D intoxication due to the ingestion of either vitamin D or calcidiol itself. On the other hand, increased levels of calcitriol may be induced by direct intake of this metabolite, extrarenal production in granulomatous diseases or lymphoma, or increased renal production by PTH.

Treatment

Overview The definitive treatment of hypercalcemia depends on the treatment of the underlying disease, e.g. parathyroidectomy for PHP, and chemotherapy for a malignancy. The initial treatment can be instituted without a specific diagnosis. General measures include rapid mobilization and hydration. Volume depletion, by limiting renal calcium excretion, perpetuates a vicious circle and worsens acute hypercalcemia. Medications that worsen hypercalcemia, such as thiazide diuretics, should be discontinued. Volume expansion with isotonic saline usually reduces S_{Ca} by enhancing renal calcium excretion. Only after volume repletion should loop diuretics be used to enhance sodium and calcium excretion (Fig. 38.2). In patients with renal failure, dialysis effectively removes calcium from the ECF. Careful monitoring of cardiac function and serum electrolytes is necessary with both saline diuresis and dialysis treatment. Hypercalcemia can be divided into mild ($S_{Ca} < 12$ mg/dL), moderate (S_{Ca} 12–14 mg/dL), and severe ($S_{Ca} > 14$ mg/dL).[8]

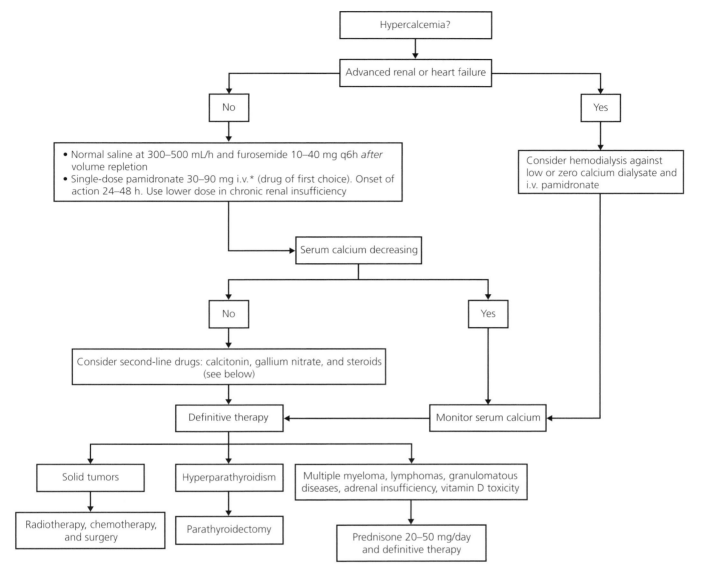

Figure 38.2 Treatment of hypercalcemia. S_{Ca}, serum calcium concentration.

Mild hypercalcemia Most cases of mild hypercalcemia are caused by PHP. All patients with PHP and symptomatic hypercalcemia who are surgical candidates should be referred to an experienced parathyroid surgeon for parathyroidectomy. Patients with familial hypocalciuric hypercalcemia require no therapy.

However, management of patients with asymptomatic PHP remains controversial.[9] Immediate intervention is not necessary. Surgery may be beneficial in patients with vertebral osteopenia, in whom parathyroidectomy may lead to a dramatic improvement (up to 20%) in bone density.[10] Consideration of parathyroidectomy should also be given to patients with PHP who are vitamin D deficient, because the loss of inhibition by calcitriol on the PTH gene worsens the PHP.[11] Replacement of vitamin D in face of hypercalcemia and/or hypercalciuria can be risky. Estrogen–progestin therapy is beneficial in postmeno-pausal women with PHP because it reduces bone resorp-tion and reduces S_{Ca} by 0.5–1.0 mg/dL and increases bone density modestly.[12] Estrogen–progestin therapy reduces urinary calcium and hydroxyproline excretion and serum alkaline phosphatase, indicating decreased bone resorption, without changes in PTH.[13]

Diuretics should not be used to treat patients with mild PHP. Loop diuretics increase calcium excretion in the urine but may induce volume depletion. Thiazide diuretics are contraindicated because they reduce urinary calcium excretion and increase S_{Ca}. Oral inorganic phosphates can effectively lower S_{Ca} but the resultant ectopic calcification is harmful to kidneys, blood vessels, and soft tissues. Thus inorganic phosphates are reserved for patients who are not candidates for or who have failed alternate therapies, and those who are moderately hypophosphatemic. The use of β-adrenergic blockers such as propranolol, H_2 receptor antagonists such as cimetidine, and progestin has been unsuccessful in lowering S_{Ca} in patients with PHP.

Bisphosphonates are potent inhibitors of bone but are rarely required for mild hypercalcemia. However, risedronate, a newer bisphosphonate that can be given orally, inhibits bone resorption and lowers fasting S_{Ca} in patients with PHP.[14] It may become the drug of choice for patients with PHP, particularly in those with osteoporosis. However, long-term benefit has not been documented (see section Severe hypercalcemia). Drugs under development include those that activate the calcium-sensing receptor in the parathyroid gland, thereby inhibiting PTH secretion;[15] calcitriol analogs that inhibit PTH secretion directly but do not stimulate gastrointestinal calcium or phosphate absorption;[16] and drugs that block the PTH receptor.[17]

Moderate hypercalcemia Moderate hypercalcemia (S_{Ca} 12–14 mg/dL) should be treated aggressively if there are signs or symptoms. The severity of the symptoms correlates with the rate of rise of S_{Ca}. In patients with few or mild symptoms, treatment of the underlying cause should be instituted while embarking on hydration and mobilization. When neurologic symptoms are the sole manifestation of hypercalcemia, other causes of an altered mental status must be excluded.[18]

The rationale for the use of normal saline for initial treatment is that volume depletion impairs glomerular filtration and increases sodium and calcium reabsorption in the proximal tubule. Normal saline should be administered to replenish volume and decrease proximal tubule calcium reabsorption. Occasional patients may become hypernatremic and require hypotonic fluids because of the relative resistance to antidiuretic hormone in hypercalcemia combined with impairment of thirst if they are confused. If congestive heart failure develops or more rapid lowering of S_{Ca} is desired, small doses of a loop diuretic may be added, e.g. furosemide 10–20 mg every 6 h. Diuretic-induced ECF depletion should be avoided, as this worsens hypercalcemia. Higher doses of loop diuretics may be required in patients with renal insufficiency. The combination of intravenous normal saline and loop diuretics should decrease S_{Ca} rapidly, by ~ 1–3 mg/dL, within 1–2 days. If the symptoms persist or hypercalcemia worsens, the treatment plan for severe hypercalcemia should be instituted.

Severe hypercalcemia When S_{Ca} exceeds 14 mg/dL, therapy should be initiated regardless of whether the patient has signs or symptoms of hypercalcemia, except in terminally ill patients. Therapy involves a combination of volume replenishment, enhanced renal calcium excretion, reduced bone resorption, and management of the underlying disease.

Patients with an elevated PTH should be referred for prompt parathyroidectomy after S_{Ca} has been lowered sufficiently for safe surgery. Excessive preoperative correction of hypercalcemia leads to postoperative hypocalcemia due to a fall in osteoclastic bone resorption and marked influx of calcium into unmineralized osteoid.

Malignancy is usually responsible for severe hypercalcemia. Specific treatment of tumors with radiation or chemotherapy should not be delayed. Mobilization and oral sodium chloride and water, while still helpful, are unlikely alone to correct hypercalcemia. The first step is replacement of ECF volume with 0.9% saline at 300–500 mL/h, reduced after volume deficit has been partially corrected. At least 3–4 L should be given in the first 24 h to achieve a positive fluid balance of at least 2 L. Caution is required in patients who are elderly and those with compromised cardiac or renal function. Saline infusion increases the delivery of sodium chloride, fluid, and calcium to the loop of Henle. Therefore a loop diuretic is used to block transport at this site. Furosemide (40–160 mg/day in divided doses) is given after the ECF volume has been replenished. Thiazide diuretics are contraindicated because they decrease renal calcium excretion. The patient's hemodynamic and electrolyte status (potassium, phosphate, and magnesium replenishment are usually required) must be monitored closely, often in an intensive care unit.

Concomitant measures to reduce osteoclastic bone resorption should be initiated because there is usually a marked enhancement of osteoclast-mediated bone resorption in patients with hypercalcemia. *Bisphosphonates* are analogs of pyrophosphate that are resistant to phosphatases. These bone-seeking compounds bind to hydroxyapatite and prevent its dissolution. They have a very long half-life. Since they are poorly absorbed (1–5% of an oral dose) they should be given with water on an empty stomach at least 30 min before food.[19] Approximately 80% of the absorbed bisphosphonate is cleared by the kidney. The remaining 20% is taken up by bone and this is enhanced by high bone turnover. Although the plasma half-life is only 1 h, bisphosphonates may persist in bone for the patient's lifetime.[19] Intravenous administration of bisphosphonate should be given in 500 mL over at least 4 h to dilute the precipitated calcium bisphosphonate that likely accounts for much of the nephrotoxicity.[20] In patients with renal insufficiency, therapy should be initiated with lower doses diluted in larger volumes of fluid with additional doses given if renal function remains stable.

Etidronate is given intravenously (7.5 mg/kg/day in saline over 4 h) for at least three consecutive days. Prolonging treatment to 5 days increases the response rate from 60 to 100% of patients. Therapy should be interrupted if S_{Ca} drops rapidly (2–3 mg/dL in the first 2–3 days) or normalizes in order to avoid hypocalcemia. Normocalcemia may persist for 1–7 weeks. Some patients can be maintained on oral etidronate (20 mg/kg/day). Prolonged administration has been associated with osteomalacia[21] and hyperphosphatemia due to increased tubular reabsorption of phosphate. The dosage of etidronate should be reduced by 50% in patients with renal insufficiency because some is excreted in the urine.

As p*amidronate* is more potent and long-lasting than etidronate, it is the bisphosphonate of choice.[21] A single injection of pamidronate is more effective in ameliorating hypercalcemia than a 3-day regimen of intravenous etidronate.[22] The intravenous dose of pamidronate depends on the degree of hypercalcemia: 30 mg if S_{Ca} < 12 mg/dL (3 mmol/L); 60 mg if S_{Ca} 12–13.5 mg/dL (3–3.4 mmol/L); and 90 mg if S_{Ca} is higher. It is usually given in isotonic saline as a single intravenous infusion over 4–24 h.[23] The dose should not be repeated in less than 7 days. Pamidronate is well tolerated, although a few patients develop fever. It is excreted by the kidney. Although not been approved for use in patients with renal failure, pamidronate seems to be safe and effective for the treatment of dialysis patients who have severe hypercalcemia induced by the combination of calcium carbonate and calcitriol,[24] providing that the dose does not exceed 30 mg. Pamidronate produces sustained normocalcemia for 15 days. In patients with cancer, the duration of hypocalcemic effect correlates inversely with serum PTH-related protein concentrations, with values > 12 pmol/L usually indicating a short-lived response.[25]

Clodronate (4–6 mg/kg/day infused over 2–4 h) is widely used in Europe but is not available in the USA. *Alendronate*, while very potent when administered intravenously, is approved only for oral therapy of osteoporosis. *Zolendronate* is pending approval by the Food and Drug Administration. A single 4–8 mg dose is more effective than 90 mg of pamidronate. The duration of normocalcemia is 32–43 days. *Risedronate*, a potent third-generation oral bisphosphonate, is being evaluated for treatment of hypercalcemia. It lowers S_{Ca} in mild PHP but its long-term utility remains to be determined.

Plicamycin (mithramycin) inhibits osteoclastic RNA synthesis and decreases osteoclastic bone resorption. It is given intravenously (15–25 µg/kg) over 3–6 h and repeated in 1–2 days if required. S_{Ca} begins to fall within 12 h, usually reaching a nadir by 48 h. The hypocalcemic effect lasts for several days. Repeated doses can be given at 3–7 day intervals. Use of mithramycin is limited by its toxicity, particularly in patients with liver, bone marrow, or kidney disease. It is rarely used.

Calcitonin inhibits osteoclastic bone resorption and enhances renal calcium excretion. The most potent form of the drug is salmon calcitonin, which is given intramuscularly or subcutaneously (4–8 units/kg every 6–12 h). It is safe, nontoxic, and acts rapidly within 4–6 h. Unfortunately, calcitonin is effective in only 60–70% of patients, most of whom then develop tachyphylaxis rapidly.[21] It is additive with bisphosphonates.

Gallium nitrate inhibits bone resorption by binding to bone, reducing hydroxyapatite crystal solubility and lowering S_{Ca}. Since it also inhibits PTH secretion, it may be particularly effective in the treatment of hyperparathyroidism. It is administered intravenously over 5 days at a dose of 200 mg/m²/day in 1 L of saline over 24 h. Like biphosphonates, there is a latent period of 6–8 days before a nadir in S_{Ca} is seen, with the effect lasting approximately 1 week. However, adverse effects are more frequent and more severe, with nephrotoxicity being common, as well as hypophosphatemia and anemia. The drug should be avoided in patients with renal insufficiency or those receiving concomitant nephrotoxic agents.

Glucocorticoids lower S_{Ca} by inhibiting cytokine release, by direct cytolytic effects on select tumor cells, by inhibiting intestinal calcium absorption, and by increasing renal calcium excretion. They are effective in hypercalcemia due to myeloma, other hematologic malignancies, sarcoidosis, and vitamin D intoxication. Other tumors rarely respond. The initial oral dose of prednisone is 20–50 mg b.i.d. The S_{Ca} may take 5–10 days to fall, after which the dose should be gradually reduced. Toxicity limits the usefulness of glucocorticoids for long-term therapy.

Hemodialysis, with little or no calcium in the dialysis fluid, and peritoneal dialysis, albeit slower, are both very effective modes of therapy for hypercalcemia. Dialysis is particularly useful in patients with renal insufficiency or congestive heart failure who cannot safely be given intravenous saline.

Inorganic phosphates, although effective, are not recommended for therapy of hypercalcemia because of the precipitation of calcium phosphate crystals in blood vessels and soft tissues.

Future therapies for cancer-induced hypercalcemia include noncalcemic analogs of calcitriol, e.g. 22-oxacalcitriol, that reduce the release of PTH-related protein. A calcimimetic agent, such as norcalcin, that binds to the calcium-sensing receptor and suppresses the release of PTH is being evaluated for PHP.

Hypocalcemia
Clinical features, pathophysiology, and etiology

The symptoms and signs of acute hypocalcemia include latent tetany, tetany, papilledema, and seizures. By comparison, ectodermal and dental changes, cataracts, basal ganglia calcification, and extrapyramidal disorders are features of chronic hypocalcemia.[27] Hypocalcemia can cause emotional instability, anxiety, depression, confusional states, hallucinations, and frank psychosis. Hypocalcemia characteristically causes prolongation of the QT interval on the ECG. Because the ST segment rather than the T wave is affected, the interval to the onset of the T wave (QoTc interval) may be a more sensitive indicator of hypocalcemia.[28] Hypocalcemia impairs the response to digitalis. Ventricular arrhythmias and congestive heart failure can occur. Chronic hypocalcemia, particularly when associated with hypophosphatemia and vitamin D deficiency, causes growth plate abnormalities in children (rickets) and defects in the mineralization of new bone. Severe symptomatic hypocalcemia requires immediate intervention.

Falsely low S_{Ca} due to hypoalbuminemia should first be excluded by measuring ionized S_{Ca}. The most common causes of hypocalcemia in hospital include magnesium deficiency, pancreatitis, sepsis, acute and chronic renal failure, hypoparathyroidism, vitamin D deficiency, and complexing of calcium with infused phosphate, citrate, or albumin[29] (Fig. 38.3).

Treatment

Rationale and overview Treatment of hypocalcemia varies with its severity, the rapidity with which it develops, and the underlying cause. At one end of the spectrum, an asymptomatic patient with mild hypocalcemia (7.5–8.5 mg/dL, 1.9–2.1 mmol/L) may warrant cautious observation and require only oral calcium supplements

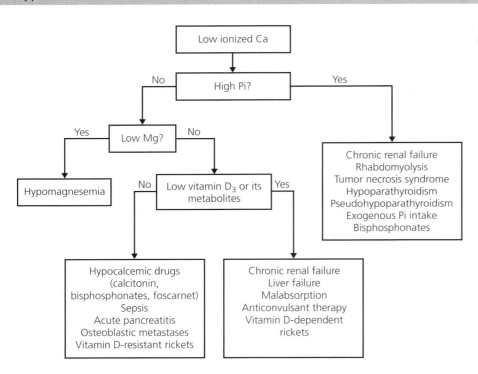

Figure 38.3 Diagnostic approach to hypocalcemia.

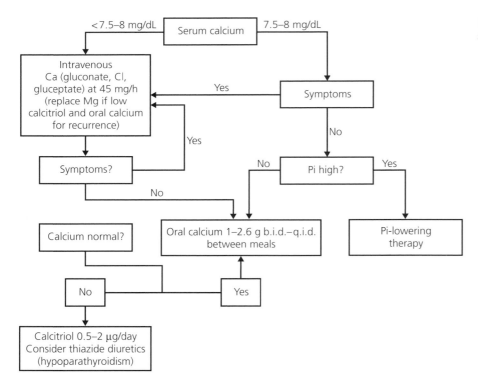

Figure 38.4 Treatment of hypocalcemia. S_{Ca}, serum calcium concentration.

(500–1000 mg elemental calcium every 6 h ingested between meals). In contrast, a patient with tetany, a sign of severe hypocalcemia, must be treated aggressively with intravenous calcium. Patients with $S_{Ca} < 7.5$ mg/dL, or any symptoms, require parenteral therapy (Fig. 38.4). Administration of calcium alone is only effective transiently. PTH is not available for clinical use; therefore patients with PTH deficiency are treated with calcium and vitamin D.

Investigation into the underlying cause for hypocalcemia should include the serum phosphate (high in renal failure and tumor lysis; low in hypomagnesemia, osteoblastic metastatic disease, and vitamin D-deficient states such as osteomalacia), creatinine, and alkaline phosphatase (high in renal osteodystrophy, osteoblastic metastatic disease, and osteomalacia).

Hypocalcemia is often associated with other electrolyte and acid–base disorders. Hypomagnesemia should be treated as needed (see section Hypomagnesemia). When metabolic acidosis is present, S_{Ca} must be corrected before acidosis because the treatment of acidosis reduces the ionized S_{Ca}, thereby precipitating problems such as tetany or cardiac arrest. Moreover, sodium bicarbonate and calcium salts must be administered in different intravenous lines to avoid precipitation of calcium carbonate. Since the administration of calcium potentiates digoxin toxicity, such patients should be monitored closely.

Hyperphosphatemia may accompany hypocalcemia in patients with hypoparathyroidism, renal disease, rhabdomyolysis, or tumor lysis. In order to avoid precipitation of calcium and phosphate, calcium supplementation must be given with phosphorus binders. By decreasing the fraction of calcium bound to phosphate, reduction of the serum phosphate improves ionized S_{Ca}. When hypocalcemia persists, it is best to delay calcium supplementation until the serum phosphate is below 6 mg/dL.

Acute hypocalcemia Patients with symptomatic hypocalcemia should be treated immediately. Many patients have symptoms when ionized S_{Ca} is < 2.8 mg/dL or total S_{Ca} is < 7 mg/dL. In general, the intravenous infusion of 15 mg/kg of elemental calcium over 4–6 h will raise total S_{Ca} by ~ 2–3 mg/dL.[30] Thus, a 70-kg patient with S_{Ca} of 6 mg/dL will require about 1 g of elemental calcium to raise S_{Ca} to 8 mg/dL. Several forms of calcium can be utilized for intravenous administration.

Calcium gluconate (10% in 10-mL ampoules containing 94 mg of elemental calcium) is given in emergency situations as one ampoule over 4 min followed by a calcium gluconate drip, if necessary. Solutions concentrated to greater than 200 mg (two ampoules) of calcium per 100 mL should be avoided because calcium is irritating to veins. Ten ampoules (100 mL) may be combined with 1000 mL of 5% dextrose and infused at 50 mL/h (45 mg of elemental calcium per hour), titrating the rate as needed. For a symptomatic 70-kg patient, calcium may be infused more rapidly until symptoms decline, when the infusion is decreased to 50 mL/h to achieve a low-normal calcium level within 8–18 h. If necessary, all 10 ampoules may be infused over 4–6 h.[30]

Calcium gluceptate (10%) is similar to calcium gluconate but provides 90 mg of elemental calcium in a 5-mL ampoule, which is useful in patients who cannot tolerate large volumes of fluid. Ten ampoules (50 mL) may be added to 450 mL of 5% dextrose as 1.8 mg/mL. A dose of 45 mg of calcium (half an ampoule) can be infused in 25 mL of fluid.

Calcium chloride (10%) provides more calcium per ampoule (272 mg per 10-mL ampoule) and is more bioavailable than either calcium gluconate or calcium gluceptate. Although this results in a more rapid elevation in S_{Ca}, which may be preferable in emergency situations, it is more irritant to veins thus rendering it less desirable for prolonged infusion.

Calcium glubionate (Neo-Calglucon) is an oral liquid that provides 23 mg of calcium per milliliter or 115 mg per teaspoon (5 mL). It is readily absorbed in the gastrointestinal tract and is well tolerated. It is an excellent supplement for hypocalcemic neonates and infants, and for adults who lack intravenous access.

Patients with hypocalcemia following elective parathyroidectomy for renal osteodystrophy may require emergency vitamin D therapy. When the excessive PTH stimulation is withdrawn suddenly, calcium and phosphate accumulate rapidly in healing bone lesions and osteoclastic bone resorption is decreased. These effects cause a dramatic reduction in S_{Ca} (hungry bone syndrome). The failed kidneys cannot increase calcitriol, so that intestinal calcium absorption remains low. Intravenous calcium is often required initially and is replaced with oral calcium supplements and calcitriol. Calcitriol is the vitamin D metabolite with the greatest potency and most rapid onset of action. It is available in oral (Rocaltrol) and intravenous (Calcijex) preparations. Initially, large intravenous doses are generally required (~ 1–2 µg/day), decreasing to maintenance oral daily doses or thrice weekly intravenous doses at dialysis of 0.2–1 µg.[29]

Chronic hypocalcemia This requires treatment with oral calcium supplementation and, if necessary, vitamin D to enhance intestinal calcium absorption. Calcium is available with carbonate, gluconate, lactate, acetate, citrate, glubionate, and phosphate, although absorption varies with the preparation and timing of ingestion. Treatment is usually started at a dose of 1000–2600 mg two to four times daily between meals, adjusted according to S_{Ca}. Calcium carbonate is available in tablets containing 500–750 mg of calcium. Calcium citrate is well absorbed but should not be used in patients taking aluminum-containing medications because it enhances aluminum absorption. Calcium glubionate is well absorbed but expensive. Calcium phosphate should be avoided because it exacerbates hyperphosphatemia and metastatic calcification.[31]

Patients with hypoparathyroidism may develop hypercalciuria with treatment since they lack the normal stimulatory effect of PTH on renal tubular calcium reabsorption and therefore excrete excessive calcium. This may cause nephrolithiasis, nephrocalcinosis, or chronic renal insufficiency. Therefore the dose of calcium should be adjusted to maintain S_{Ca} slightly below normal range and calcium excretion should be measured periodically. A few patients with hypoparathyroidism can be treated with a thiazide diuretic.

In disorders associated with insufficient vitamin D (e.g. hypoparathyroidism, osteomalacia, chronic renal failure), calcitriol acts rapidly because it requires no further metabolism to function. Administration of 0.5–1 µg/day is usually sufficient, although in extreme cases, such as immediately after parathyroidectomy, more may be required (2–3 µg). Calcitriol is more expensive than the parent vitamin D compounds vitamin D_2 (ergocalciferol) and vitamin D_3 (cholecalciferol), which are adequate for nutritional deficiency at doses of ~ 400 units/day or for malabsorption at higher doses (50 000–100 000 units/day). However, their action may be delayed for several weeks because they requires conversion to calcitriol. They are ineffective for diseases in which 25- or 1α-hydroxylation is impaired, such as liver and renal failure, hypoparathyroidism, and vitamin D-dependent rickets type 1. In contrast to the rapid elimination of calcitriol and calcidiol (within days), vitamins D_2 and D_3 may continue to function for several weeks after dosing, potentially resulting in hypervitaminosis D.[31]

Phosphate disorders

Homeostasis

Phosphate is the most abundant intracellular anion: ~ 80% is contained within bone mineral, 19% in cells, and about 1% in the ECF. Plasma phosphate concentrations are 2.5–4.5 mg/dL (0.81–1.45 mmol/L) in adults and 4.0–7.0 mg/dL (1.3–2.3 mmol/L) in children. Thus changes in serum phosphate concentration (S_{Pi}) may not reflect total body content. The majority (~ 70%) of S_{Pi} is organic and present mainly in phospholipids, while the remainder is inorganic. Approximately 15% of inorganic phosphate is bound to protein and is therefore not available for ultrafiltration by the kidneys. The remainder exists mainly in the monohydrogen (HPO_4^{2-}) and dihydrogen ($H_2PO_4^-$) forms in a ratio of 4:1 at a physiologic pH of 7.4. Small amounts are complexed to sodium, magnesium, and calcium.

S_{Pi} is not as tightly regulated as S_{Ca}. It varies with dietary intake, age (higher in infants and children, decreasing with adolescence), time of day (peak at 4 AM and nadir 6–7 h later), and hormonal status (higher in postmenopausal women). Phosphate is prevalent in meats, dairy products, and grains. Some 65% of ingested phosphate (800–1600 mg/day) is absorbed in the small intestine, both passively and by calcitriol-mediated active transport. Normally, phosphate transport occurs primarily through unregulated paracellular diffusive pathways. However, when luminal phosphate concentrations are low, absorption is by active sodium-dependent transport via a Na^+/P cotransporter that is secondarily active and utilizes the favorable sodium gradient from the basolateral Na^+,K^+-ATPase.[32] Phosphate egress is passive. Calcitriol enhances phosphate absorption, while PTH stimulates intestinal phosphate absorption indirectly by increasing the synthesis of calcitriol. Other factors that increase intestinal phosphate absorption include low phosphate intake, acidosis, bile salts, lactose, prolactin, thyroid hormone, and the acute effect of glucocorticoids. Calcium, magnesium, and aluminum decrease phosphate absorption by binding to phosphate. Hypophosphatemia stimulates production of calcitriol, which subsequently enhances phosphate and calcium absorption. Hyperphosphatemia increases PTH secretion and decreases calcitriol production.

Renal phosphate excretion generally equals phosphate absorption. Some 85% of phosphate reabsorption occurs in the proximal tubule, where the brush-border membrane phosphate transporter is secondarily active via the Na^+/P cotransporter.[33] Growth hormone, insulin-like growth factor 1 (IGF-1), insulin, epidermal growth factor, thyroid hormone, and calcitriol stimulate renal phosphate reabsorption. PTH, PTH-related protein, calcitonin, atrial natriuretic factor, transforming growth factors α and β, and glucocorticoids inhibit phosphate absorption.[20] Intravascular volume expansion and high-phosphate diets enhance phosphate excretion.

S_{Pi} can be decreased acutely by stimulating cellular uptake with intravenous glucose or insulin, ingestion of carbohydrate-rich meals, acute respiratory alkalosis, epinephrine, and rapid cell proliferation (e.g. neoplasia).[34] Conversely, S_{Pi} is increased by metabolic acidosis and intravenous infusion of calcium.

Hyperphosphatemia
Clinical features, pathophysiology, and etiology

Hyperphosphatemia (S_{Pi} > 4.5 mg/dL in adults, > 7 mg/dL in children) is most commonly caused by reduced renal phosphate excretion due to renal failure, i.e. glomerular filtration rate (GFR) below 20–25 mL/min. Hyperphosphatemia due to defective renal phosphate clearance also occurs with hypoparathyroidism, pseudohypoparathyroidism, increased growth hormone or IGF-1, bisphosphonate therapy, and a variety of rare inherited diseases.[19] Acidosis redistributes cellular phosphate to the plasma. Hyperphosphatemia can also occur during increased release of intracellular phosphate in acute tumor lysis or rhabdomyolysis coupled with acute renal failure[35] (Fig. 38.5).

In advanced renal failure, hyperphosphatemia is a universal finding. As GFR falls, fractional tubular phosphate excretion increases progressively, under the influence of PTH, to 60–90%. This maintains S_{Pi} until GFR falls to < 25 mL/min. The ensuing hyperphosphatemia and loss of functioning kidney mass suppress the production of calcitriol, thus decreasing intestinal absorption of calcium. The ensuing fall in S_{Ca} and rise in S_{Pi} decrease calcitriol and increase PTH secretion, which may aggravate hyperphosphatemia by release of calcium and phosphate from bone. The eventual parathyroid hyperplasia and excessive PTH action cause high-turnover bone disease.[35]

The rapid turnover of malignant tumors stimulated by chemotherapy releases intracellular potassium, uric acid, and phosphate. Uric acid precipitation in the renal tubules can cause acute renal failure, which may worsen the hyperphosphatemia and hyperkalemia. Raising the urine pH with intravenous alkaline sodium bicarbonate solubilizes the uric acid but may enhance calcium phosphate precipitation, which can cause nephrocalcinosis or nephrolithiasis.

Pseudohyperphosphatemia due to hyperglobulinemia, hyperlipidemia, hemolysis, and hyperbilirubinemia can be assessed by serum analysis after deproteinization.

The manifestations of acute severe hyperphosphatemia are related mainly to accompanying hypocalcemia and tetany caused by precipitation of calcium phosphate. In addition, hyperphosphatemia inhibits the activity of 1α-hydroxylase in the kidney. The resulting fall in calcitriol aggravates hypocalcemia further by impairing intestinal calcium absorption, inducing skeletal resistance to PTH. Profound hypocalcemia and tetany are occasionally

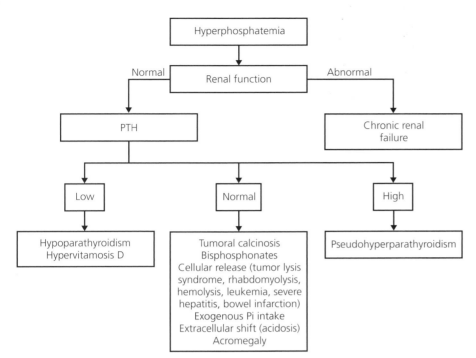

Figure 38.5 Diagnostic approach to hyperphosphatemia. PTH, parathyroid hormone.

observed during the early phase of the tumor lysis syndrome and rhabdomyolysis. When the (calcium × phosphate) product exceeds ~ 65, patients may develop metastatic calcification in the skin, cornea, blood vessels, myocardium, heart valves, and other organs.[35] Patients on maintenance dialysis may also develop premature coronary artery calcification.[36] An extreme case of metastatic calcification, acral calciphylaxis, is rapid occlusion of small-sized arteries with necrosis and gangrene of the digits. Parathyroidectomy is recommended if levels of PTH are extremely elevated.[35] Hyperphosphatemia is critical in the development of secondary hyperparathyroidism and renal osteodystrophy in chronic renal failure.

Treatment

Correction of the cause is the primary aim. Acute hyperphosphatemia in patients who do not have renal failure is treated by saline diuresis. Proximally acting diuretics, such as acetazolamide, are the most phosphaturic. Correction of acidosis or treatment of hyperglycemia with insulin promotes cellular phosphate uptake.

In patients with impaired renal function, S_{Pi} may be reduced by dietary phosphate restriction. Because phosphate is ubiquitous, severe dietary restriction is impractical. The average American diet contains 800–1600 mg of phosphate; restriction to 1000–1250 mg does not cause protein–calorie malnutrition.[35] In patients with endstage renal disease or severe acute renal failure, S_{Pi} may be reduced by dialysis. Although dialysis membranes are permeant to phosphate, there is only a slow phosphate efflux from the large intracellular phosphate stores. Hemodialysis removes only about 2–3 g of phosphate per week. Nocturnal hemodialysis improves control of S_{Pi}.[37] Peritoneal dialysis is more effective in eliminating phosphate but is still unable to match the dietary phosphate intake of most patients.

Phosphate binders form insoluble nonabsorbable compounds with phosphate in the intestines that are lost in stool. They must be ingested immediately before, during, or after the meal. Calcium, aluminum, and magnesium all bind phosphate, although magnesium is relatively weak and is avoided in renal insufficiency. Oral calcium carbonate and the more potent calcium acetate are preferred to calcium citrate because the latter enhances intestinal aluminum absorption. Calcium carbonate is available in 500 and 1000 mg tablets. The initial dose is 1 g with each meal three times daily. If S_{Pi} does not decrease, the dose is gradually increased up to 8–12 g/day. Persistent hyperphosphatemia may be due to incomplete dissolution of the tablets in the gastrointestinal tract, excessive phosphate intake, or noncompliance. Hypercalcemia is more likely if a vitamin D preparation is also given or if there is decreased bone turnover due to osteomalacia or adynamic bone disease.[38] Absorption of calcium promotes coronary arterial calcification, which is associated with coronary atherosclerosis.[37] If hypercalcemia develops or if the (calcium × phosphate) product exceeds 65, the therapy should be replaced by noncalcium-based phosphate binders (see below). Reducing the dialysate calcium to 2.5 mg/L or less is useful when large doses of calcium are required.[32,35] However, extended treatment with a low-calcium dialysate increases the risk of severe hyperparathyroidism. Aluminum hydroxide can cause aluminum intoxication, with vitamin D-resistant osteomalacia, a refractory microcytic anemia, bone and muscle pain, and dementia. It is no longer recommended.

Sevelamer (RenaGel) is a nonabsorbable agent that contains neither calcium nor aluminum. It is a cationic polymer that binds phosphate through ion exchange. It is as effective as calcium carbonate or calcium acetate but does not affect S_{Ca}.[39] It lowers total cholesterol concentration by 15%. Gastrointestinal adverse effects may limit its use in some patients. At present it is reserved for patients with hypercalcemia because of its considerable cost. The usual recommended dose is 800–1600 mg with meals three times a day.

Treatment of secondary hyperparathyroidism begins with reduction of S_{Pi} while maintaining the (calcium × phosphate) product below 65. Thereafter, pulse oral or intravenous calcitriol two to three times per week can reduce PTH secretion. To prevent adynamic bone disease, most investigators recommend that intact PTH should be maintained in a mildly elevated range (< 250 pg/mL).[40] Mild hyperparathyroidism (intact PTH 250–400 pg/mL) should be treated first with better control of S_{Pi}. If PTH continues to rise, calcitriol (intravenous Calcijex or oral Rocaltrol) is initiated at a dose of 1 μg three times weekly. For PTH above 600–700 pg/mL an increase in calcitriol dose to 2 μg or more three times weekly is required. Calcitriol may cause hypercalcemia and may exacerbate hyperphosphatemia. S_{Ca} may be reduced by lowering dialysate calcium concentrations. Patients with refractory secondary hyperparathyroidism or those who develop severe hypercalcemia require parathyroidectomy.[41]

Hypophosphatemia
Clinical features, pathophysiology, and etiology

Moderate hypophosphatemia (S_{Pi} 1–2.5 mg/dL, 0.32–0.81 mmol/L) is usually asymptomatic. Severe hypophosphatemia (S_{Pi} < 1 mg/dL or 0.32 mmol/L) indicates total body phosphate depletion and is potentially fatal. Numerous cellular mechanisms require phosphate, e.g. 2,3-diphosphoglycerate and adenosine triphosphate (ATP).[32,35] Clinical features include erythrocyte, leukocyte, and platelet dysfunction, myopathy, confusion, ataxia, seizures, and coma, respiratory insufficiency, osteomalacia, metabolic acidosis, cardiac arrhythmias, and cardiomyopathy. Hypophosphatemia may result from decreased intestinal phosphate absorption, increased renal phosphate losses, and a shift of phosphate to intracellular compartments (Fig. 38.6).

Alcoholism and alcohol withdrawal Up to 10% of chronic alcoholics are hypophosphatemic.[32,35] The causes include insufficient phosphate intake, use of phosphate-binding antacids for gastrointestinal disorders, emesis, hypomagnesemia, diarrhea, and excessive alcohol-induced renal phosphate excretion, as well as intracellular shifts due to hyperventilation or glucose infusion in patients with alcoholic cirrhosis or in acute abstinence.[32]

Nutritional repletion This may result in severe hypophosphatemia due to cellular phosphate uptake and utilization in anabolic tissue if sufficient amounts of phosphate are not provided. Phosphate requirements often exceed those provided in either enteral or parenteral feeds.[32,35]

Diabetes mellitus Patients with decompensated diabetes associated with ketoacidosis excrete excessive phosphate due to osmotic diuresis. The plasma level is usually maintained because of large shifts of phosphate from cells into plasma. Administration of insulin, fluids, and correction of ketoacidosis causes S_{Pi} to fall sharply. Patients with very low S_{Pi} usually require phosphate supplementation during correction of hyperglycemia and acidosis.[32]

Acute respiratory alkalosis Acute hyperventilation can reduce S_{Pi} to very low levels as phosphate enters muscle. Such a fall in S_{Pi} is not observed in acute metabolic alkalosis. Paradoxically, chronic hyperventilation causes hyperphosphatemia.[41]

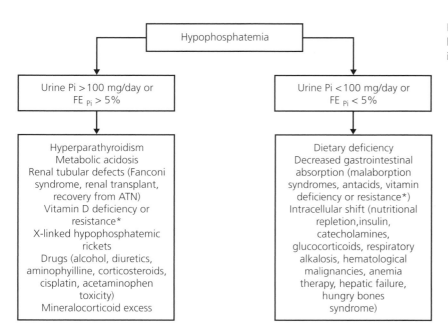

Figure 38.6 Diagnostic approach to hypophosphatemia. *More than one mechanism involved. FE_{Pi}, fractional excretion of phosphate.

Hypophosphatemia

Urine Pi >100 mg/day or FE_{Pi} > 5%

Urine Pi <100 mg/day or FE_{Pi} < 5%

Hyperparathyroidism
Metabolic acidosis
Renal tubular defects (Fanconi syndrome, renal transplant, recovery from ATN)
Vitamin D deficiency or resistance*
X-linked hypophosphatemic rickets
Drugs (alcohol, diuretics, aminophyilline, corticosteroids, cisplatin, acetaminophen toxicity)
Mineralocorticoid excess

Dietary deficiency
Decreased gastrointestinal absorption (malaborption syndromes, antacids, vitamin deficiency or resistance*)
Intracellular shift (nutritional repletion, insulin, catecholamines, glucocorticoids, respiratory alkalosis, hematological malignancies, anemia therapy, hepatic failure, hungry bones syndrome)

Table 38.1 Phosphate preparations*

	Phosphate	Sodium	Potassium
Oral preparations			
Skim milk	1 g/L	28 mequiv./L	38 mequiv./L
Neutra-Phos	250 mg/packet	7.1 mequiv./packet	7.1 mequiv./packet
Phospho-Soda	150 mg/mL	4.8 mequiv./mL	0
Neutra-Phos K	250 mg/capsule	0	14.25 mequiv./capsule
K-Phos Original	150 mg/capsule	0	3.65 mequiv./capsule
K-Phos Neutral	250 mg/tablet	13 mequiv./tablet	1.1 mequiv./tablet
Intravenous preparations			
Neutral sodium potassium phosphate	1.1 mmol/mL	0.2 mequiv./mL	0.02 mequiv./mL
Neutral sodium phosphate	0.09 mmol/mL	0.2 mequiv./mL	0
Sodium phosphate	3.0 mmol/mL	4.0 mequiv./mL	0
Potassium phosphate	3.0 mmol/mL	0	4.4 mequiv./mL

*From Subramanian R, Khardori R: Severe hypophosphatemia: pathophysiologic implications, clinical presentations, and treatment. Medicine 2000;79:1–8.

Treatment

Rationale and overview   The appropriate management of hypophosphatemia usually requires phosphate supplementation and diagnosis of the cause to prevent recurrence. Phosphate replacement can cause diarrhea (with oral supplements), hyperphosphatemia, and hypocalcemia.[32,35] Therefore replacement should be used cautiously. Diarrhea is uncommon in patients with severe phosphate deficiency, especially when daily doses of phosphate are less than 1 g and given four times a day. Hypophosphatemia should be seen as a marker of an underlying disorder for which evaluation and therapy may be necessary. Hypophosphatemia should be anticipated in patients receiving enteral or parenteral nutrition, malnourished patients receiving glucose-containing intravenous fluids, and alcoholics.

Oral replacement is preferred in asymptomatic patients, even those with very low phosphate levels (Table 38.1). Correction of any associated hypokalemia and hypomagnesemia reduces phosphaturia (Fig. 38.7). Milk provides 1 g/L (33 mmol/L) of inorganic phosphate. It is usually better tolerated than phosphate tablets.[32,35]

Mild hypophosphatemia   Mild hypophosphatemia (S_{Pi} > 2 mg/dL), especially when ascribed to intracellular shifts, usually resolves without pharmacologic intervention.

Moderate hypophosphatemia   Moderate hypophosphatemia (S_{Pi} > 1 mg/dL in adults, > 2 mg/dL in children) responds to oral supplementation. Patients receiving total parenteral nutrition should receive at least 1000 mg (32 mmol) of phosphate daily. Lactose and lipids are poorly tolerated in malnourished patients with lactose or fat intolerance. Therefore skim milk is preferable. With each 8-ounce serving (containing ~ 235 mg phosphate), most people can replenish their stores with four to eight glasses per day for 7–10 days.[32,35]

Severe hypophosphatemia   In general, S_{Pi} < 0.5 mg/dL reflects a phosphate deficit > 3 g; in the presence of symptoms, this deficit is > 10 g.[32] In asymptomatic

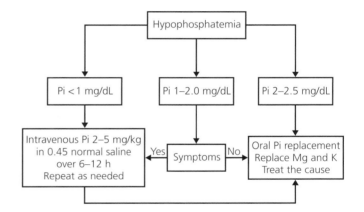

Figure 38.7   Treatment of hypophosphatemia. S_{Pi}, serum phosphate concentration.

patients, severe hypophosphatemia is treated with oral supplements of phosphate (6–10 g) over several days. Oral supplements are available as monobasic, dibasic, and acid sodium and potassium salts. Neutral potassium and sodium preparations (Neutraphos, K-Phos-Neutral) provide 250 mg of phosphate per tablet (Table 38.1) but also contain large amounts of sodium. Phosphate enemas are also available (Fleet Enema) for patients intolerant of oral supplements. Because of the high sodium content, laxative effect, and erratic absorption, enemas are not primary therapy. In symptomatic patients, intravenous supplementation is usually required in order to raise S_{Pi} to more than 1–1.5 mg/dL, at which point oral supplements may be given. The usual starting dose is 2 mg/kg i.v. infused in half-normal saline over 6 h, or 5 mg/kg over 12 h, checking S_{Pi} frequently and discontinuing the infusion when necessary. In symptomatic, severely hypophosphatemic patients, 1 g of phosphate in 1 L of fluid may be infused over 8–12 h.[32,35] Intravenous phosphate can precipitate with calcium and produce hypocalcemia, renal failure, and serious arrhythmias. Intravenous phosphate supplements are also available in combination with sodium or potassium.

Magnesium disorders

The normal body content of magnesium is ~ 1000 mmol or 22.66 g, of which 50–60% is contained in bone; extracellular magnesium accounts for only 1%. The normal serum magnesium concentration (S_{Mg}) is 1.7–2.2 mg/dL (0.75–0.95 mmol/L). Approximately 55% is ionized and 15% complexed to bicarbonate, citrate, and phosphate; the remaining 30% is protein-bound and thus is not available for ultrafiltration by the kidneys.

Magnesium is essential for the function of important enzymes, including those involved in the transfer of phosphate groups, all reactions that require ATP, and every step in the replication and transcription of DNA and translation of mRNA. Magnesium is also required for cellular energy metabolism and has an important role in membrane stabilization, nerve conduction, ion transport, and calcium channel activity.

Homoeostasis

Maintenance of normal magnesium levels depends on gastrointestinal absorption and renal excretion. Daily magnesium intake is 300–350 mg. Absorption is by saturable and passive systems. Absorption is reduced by phosphate in the diet and enhanced by calcitriol.

Daily renal excretion of magnesium averages 100 mg. The thick ascending limb of the loop of Henle reabsorbs 60–70%. Reabsorption in the thick ascending limb and distal tubule (~ 10%) is closely regulated by S_{Mg}. Reabsorption in the thick ascending limb is regulated by the calcium/magnesium-sensing receptor, located on the basolateral membrane of the thick ascending limb.[42]

Hypermagnesemia
Clinical features, pathophysiology, and etiology

Patients with renal insufficiency are susceptible to hypermagnesemia. Most cases are due to magnesium ingestion. Hypermagnesemia due to cellular release complicates tumor lysis syndrome, rhabdomyolysis, acidosis, and catecholamine excess. Mild hypermagnesemia complicates familial hypocalciuric hypercalcemia, Addison disease, hyperparathyroidism, and lithium therapy.[43] Hypomagnesemia causes mild hypotension, nausea, flushing, and loss of deep tendon reflexes, somnolence, weakness, lethargy, and ultimately apnea due to muscular paralysis. Cardiac manifestations include prolongation of PR, QRS, and QT intervals, bradycardia, complete heart block, and even cardiac arrest. Hypomagnesemia can lead to hypocalcemia. Symptoms may be treated by calcium administration.[44]

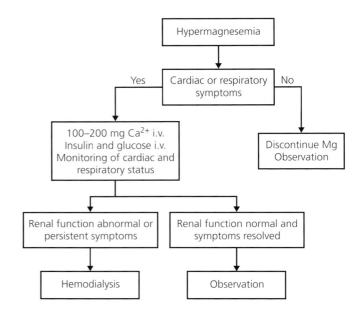

Figure 38.8   Treatment of hypermagnesemia.

Treatment

Patients with mild hypermagnesemia and normal renal function require only discontinuation of magnesium supplementation (Fig. 38.8). For those with severe symptoms of hypermagnesemia, intravenous calcium (100–200 mg) is the initial treatment. Glucose and insulin can shift magnesium intracellularly. Patients with S_{Mg} in excess of 8–9 mg/dL should have cardiac monitoring and consideration for ventilatory support. Hemodialysis against a low-magnesium dialysate is more effective than peritoneal dialysis in rapidly lowering S_{Mg} in patients with renal failure.[45]

Hypomagnesemia
Clinical features, pathophysiology, and etiology

Hypomagnesemia occurs in 12% of hospitalized patients.[45] Gastrointestinal depletion occurs during acute or chronic diarrhea or during malabsorption. Thiazide and loop diuretics inhibit tubular magnesium reabsorption, although hypomagnesemia is usually mild because of increased proximal tubular magnesium reabsorption induced by the volume depletion. Diabetes mellitus is the most common cause of hypomagnesemia, probably secondary to glycosuria and osmotic diuresis (Fig. 38.9).

The possibility of cellular magnesium depletion despite a maintained S_{Mg} should be considered as a possible cause of refractory hypokalemia or unexplained hypocalcemia. This is detected by demonstrating a low renal magnesium excretion (< 24 mg/day) or a low fractional excretion of magnesium (< 2%).

Magnesium deficiency causes neuromuscular irritability, with tremor, tetany, asterixis, myoclonus, seizures, muscular weakness, prolongation of PR and QT intervals, ventricular and supraventricular arrhythmias, and dimin-

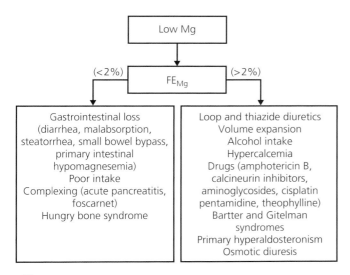

$$FE_{Mg}$$
(fractional excretion of Mg) $= \dfrac{\text{Urinary Mg} \times \text{plasma creatinine} \times 100}{(0.7 \times \text{plasma Mg}) \times \text{urinary creatinine}}$

Figure 38.9 Diagnostic approach to hypomagnesemia.

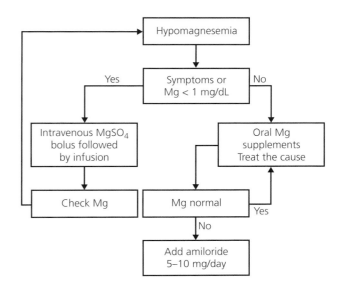

Figure 38.10 Treatment of hypomagnesemia. S_{Mg}, serum magnesium concentration.

ished response to digoxin. Accompanying hypokalemia or hypocalcemia can be refractory to therapy unless magnesium deficiency is corrected.

Treatment

Mild hypomagnesemia may be treated with oral replacement (Fig. 38.10) using a sustained-release preparation such as Slow Mag, containing magnesium chloride, or Mag-Tab SR, containing magnesium lactate (2.5–3.5 mmol or 60–84 mg of magnesium per tablet). Patients with severe magnesium deficiency require six to eight tablets daily, while those with mild asymptomatic disease require only two to four tablets daily. Patients with renal magnesium wasting due to loop diuretics benefit from a magnesium-sparing diuretic such as amiloride (5–10 mg/day). Amiloride is also used for the persistent renal magnesium wasting associated with Bartter or Gitelman syndromes or cisplatin nephrotoxicity. Adults with malabsorption may require daily magnesium supplementation of up to 50 mmol (~ 1 g); children with malabsorption may require up to 30 mmol (720 mg).

Patients with symptomatic or more severe hypomagnesemia require parenteral magnesium. Magnesium sulfate (2.1 mmol/mL) as a 50% solution is effective intramuscularly but should preferably be given intravenously. For life-threatening cardiac arrhythmias or seizures, 4–8 mmol (100–200 mg) of magnesium sulfate may be given intravenously over 5–10 min, followed by an intravenous infusion of 0.5 mmol/kg (12 mg/kg) daily or 4 mmol (~ 100 mg) intramuscularly every 3–4 h. About half of the administered magnesium will be excreted, and therapy may need to be continued for several days. The dose should be decreased in patients with renal insufficiency, who require close monitoring.[45]

References

1. Pearce CJ, Hine TJ, Peek K. Hypercalcemia due to Ca^{2+} binding by a polymeric IgA kappa paraprotein. Ann Clin Biochem 1991;28:229–234.
2. Brown EM, Pollak M, Seidman CE, et al: Calcium ion-sensing cell-surface receptors. N Engl J Med 1995;333:234–240.
3. Walls J, Ratcliffe WA, Howell A, et al: Parathyroid hormone and parathyroid hormone-related protein in the investigation of hypercalcemia in two hospital populations. Clin Endocrinol 1994;41:407–413.
4. Bilezikian JP. Management of hypercalcemia. J Clin Endocrinol Metab 1993;77:1445–1449.
5. Earm JH, Christensen BM, Frokiaer J, et al: Decreased aquaporin-2 expression and apical plasma membrane delivery in kidney collecting ducts of polyuric hypercalcemic rats. J Am Soc Nephrol 1998;9:2181–2193.
6. Parks J, Coe F, Favus M: Hyperparathyroidism in nephrolithiasis. Arch Intern Med 1980;140:1479–1481.
7. Haden ST, Stoll AL, McCormick S, Scott J, Fuleihan G el-H: Alterations in parathyroid dynamics in lithium-treated subjects. J Clin Endocrinol Metab 1997;82:2844–2848.
8. Favus MJ (ed): Primer on the Metabolic Bone Diseases and Disorders of Mineral Metabolism. Philadelphia: Lippincott-Raven, 1996, p 179.
9. NIH conference. Diagnosis and management of asymptomatic primary hyperparathyroidism: consensus development conference statement. Ann Intern Med 1991;114:593–597.
10. Silverberg SJ, Gartenberg F, Jacobs TP, et al: Increased bone mineral density after parathyroidectomy in primary hyperparathyroidism. J Clin Endocrinol Metab 1995;80:729–734.
11. Silverberg SJ, Shane E, Dempster DW, Bilezikian JP: The effects of vitamin D insufficiency in patients with primary hyperparathyroidism. Am J Med 1999;107:561–567.
12. Marcus R, Madvig P, Crim M, Pont A, Kosek J: Conjugated estrogens in the treatment of postmenopausal women with hyperparathyroidism. Ann Intern Med 1984;100:633–640.
13. Grey AB, Stapleton JP, Evans MC, Tatnell MA, Reid IR: Effect of hormone replacement therapy on bone mineral density in postmenopausal women with mild primary hyperparathyroidism. A randomized, controlled trial. Ann Intern Med 1996;125:360–368.
14. Reasner CA, Stone MD, Hosking DJ, Ballah A, Mundy GR: Acute changes in calcium homeostasis during treatment of primary hyperparathyroidism with risedronate. J Clin Endocrinol Metab 1993;77:1067–1071.
15. Silverberg SJ, Bone HG 3rd, Marriott TB, et al: Short-term inhibition of parathyroid hormone secretion by a Ca^{2+}-receptor agonist in patients with primary hyperparathyroidism. N Engl J Med 1997;337:1506–1510.

16. Finch JL, Brown AJ, Slatopolsky E: Differential effects of 1,25-dihydroxy-vitamin D3 and 19-nor-1,25-dihydroxy-vitamin D2 on calcium and Pi resorption in bone. J Am Soc Nephrol 1999;10:980–985.

17. Rosen HN, Lim M, Garber J, et al: The effect of PTH antagonist BIM-44002 on S_{Ca} and PTH levels in hypercalcemic hyperparathyroid patients. Calcif Tissue Int 1997;61:455–459.

18. Shane E: Hypercalcemia: pathogenesis, clinical manifestations, differential diagnosis and management. In: Favus MJ (ed): Primer on the Metabolic Bone Diseases and Disorders of Mineral Metabolism. Philadelphia: Lippincott-Raven, 1996, pp 171–181.

19. Agarwal R, Knochell JP: Hypophosphatemia and hyperphosphatemia. In Brenner BM (ed) Brenner and Rector's The Kidney, 6th edn. Philadelphia, WB Saunders, 2000, pp 1071–1114.

20. Tenenhouse H: Cellular and molecular mechanisms of renal phosphate transport. J Bone Miner Res 1997;12:159–164.

21. Bilezikian JP: Management of acute hypercalcemia. N Engl J Med 1992;326:1196–1203.

22. Gucalp R, Ritch P, Wiernik PH, et al: Comparative study of pamidronate disodium and etidronate disodium in the treatment of cancer-related hypercalcemia. J Clin Oncol 1992;10:134–142.

23. Gucalp R, Theriault R, Gill I, et al: Treatment of cancer-associated hypercalcemia. Double-blind comparison of rapid and slow intravenous infusion regimens of pamidronate disodium and saline alone. Arch Intern Med 1994;154:1935–1944.

24. Davenport A, Goel S, Mackenzie JC: Treatment of hypercalcaemia with pamidronate in patients with end stage renal failure. Scand J Urol Nephrol 1993;27:447–451.

25. Gurney H, Grill V, Martin TJ: Parathyroid hormone-related protein and response to pamidronate in tumour-induced hypercalcaemia. Lancet 1993;341:1611–1613.

26. Major P, Lortholary A, Hon J, et al: Zoledronic acid is superior to pamidronate in the treatment of hypercalcemia of malignancy: a pooled analysis of two randomized, controlled clinical trials. J Clin Oncol 2001;19:558–567.

27. Fonseca OA, Calverley JR: Neurological manifestations of hypoparathyroidism. Arch Intern Med 1967;120:202–206.

28. Colletti RB, Pan MW, Smith EW, Genel M: Detection of hypocalcemia in susceptible neonates: the QoTc interval. N Engl J Med 1974;290:931–935.

29. Shane E: Hypocalcemia: pathogenesis, clinical manifestations, differential diagnosis and management. In Favus MJ (ed): Primer on the Metabolic Bone Diseases and Disorders of Mineral Metabolism. Philadelphia: Lippincott-Raven, 1996, pp 217–219.

30. Pak CYC: Calcium disorders: hypercalcemia and hypocalcemia. In Kokko JP, Tannen RL (eds): Fluids and Electrolytes. Philadelphia: WB Saunders, 1990, pp 596–630.

31. Hruska KA, Connolly J: Hyperphosphatemia and hypophosphatemia. In Favus MJ (ed): Primer on the Metabolic Bone Diseases and Disorders of Mineral Metabolism. Philadelphia: Lippincott-Raven, 1996, pp 238–245.

32. Cross HS, Debiec H, Peterlik M: Mechanism and regulation of intestinal phosphate reabsorption. Miner Electrolyte Metab 1990;16:115–124.

33. Murer H, Biber J: Molecular mechanisms in renal phosphate reabsorption. Nephrol Dial Transplant 1995;10:1501–1504.

34. Mostellar ME, Tuttle EP: Effects of alkalosis on plasma concentration and urinary excretion of inorganic phosphate in man. J Clin Invest 1964;43:138–149.

35. Llach F, Felsenfeld AJ, Haussler MR: The pathophysiology of altered calcium metabolism in rhabdomyolysis-induced acute renal failure. Interactions of parathyroid hormone, 25-hydroxycholecalciferol, and 1,25-dihydroxycholecalciferol. N Engl J Med 1981;305:117–123.

36. Goodman WG, Goldin J, Kuizon BD, et al: Coronary-artery calcification in young adults with end-stage renal disease who are undergoing dialysis. N Engl J Med 2000;342:1478–1483.

37. Mucsi I, Hercz G, Uldall R, Ouwendyk M, Francouer R, Pierratos A: A control of serum phosphate without any phosphate binders in patients treated with nocturnal hemodialysis. Kidney Int 1998;53:1399–1404.

38. Kurz P, Monier-Faugere MC, Bognar B, et al: Evidence for abnormal calcium homeostasis in patients with adynamic bone disease. Kidney Int 1994;46:855–861.

39. Chertow GM, Burke SK, Lazarus JM, et al: Poly[allylamine hydrochloride] (RenaGel): a noncalcemic phosphate binder for the treatment of hyperphosphatemia in chronic renal failure. Am J Kidney Dis 1997;29:66–71.

40. Coburn JW, Frazao J: Calcitriol in the management of renal osteodystrophy. Semin Dial 1996;9:316–320.

41. Krapg R, Jaeger P, Hulter HN: Chronic respiratory alkalosis induced renal PTH-resistance, hyperphosphatemia and hypocalcemia in humans. Kidney Int 1992;42:727–734.

42. Quamme GA: Renal magnesium handling: new insights in understanding old problems. Kidney Int 1997;52:1180–1195.

43. Rude RK: Magnesium depletion and hypermagnesemia. In Favus MJ (ed): Primer on the Metabolic Bone Diseases and Disorders of Mineral Metabolism. Philadelphia: Lippincott-Raven, 1996, pp 234–238.

44. Subramanian R, Khardori R: Severe hypophosphatemia: pathophysiologic implications, clinical presentations, and treatment. Medicine 2000;79:1–8.

45. Wong ET, Rude RK, Singer FR, Shaw ST Jr: A high prevalence of hypomagnesemia and hypermagnesemia in hospitalized patients. Am J Clin Pathol 1983;79:348–352.

PART V
Nephrolithiasis

CHRISTOPHER S. WILCOX

Medical Management of Nephrolithiasis

Fredric L. Coe and Joan H. Parks

Background

Nephrolithiasis arises from increased urine supersaturations with respect to calcium oxalate, calcium phosphate, uric acid, cystine, and struvite. All known clinical causes of stones act through increased supersaturation, and all known treatments act by reducing supersaturation. A majority of stones are made primarily of calcium oxalate, often admixed with calcium phosphate salts. Uric acid admixtures occur in about 15% of calcium oxalate stones. Calcium phosphate and uric acid stones, without appreciable calcium oxalate, are less common, each occurring in about 10% of patients. Cystine stones arise entirely from hereditary cystinuria and account for less than 1% of all stone disease. Struvite stones, in humans at least, arise only from urinary infection with bacteria that produce urease and can therefore hydrolyze urea to ammonia, raising pH and causing precipitation of magnesium ammonium phosphate (struvite). In this chapter, trials and recommendations are grouped by type of stone and thence by cause, this being the best possible organization. All important references concerning these diseases can be found in the chapter on nephrolithiasis in *Brenner and Rector's The Kidney*[1] and in reviews and comprehensive books on stone disease.[2,3]

Clinical trials and specific recommendations

Calcium stones

Primary hyperparathyroidism

Parathyroid adenomas (85% of cases) and parathyroid hyperplasia (15% of cases) cause high parathyroid hormone (PTH) levels, elevating blood and urine calcium levels and urine pH. These two disorders raise urine supersaturation with respect to both calcium oxalate and calcium phosphate salts. Stones are therefore higher in phosphate content than in usual stone diseases. Diagnosis is from elevated blood and urine calcium levels without suppressed PTH levels.[4] Treatment is entirely surgical in that, given recurrent stones, no authority has heretofore supported any form of nonsurgical intervention. Success rates for solitary adenoma are nearly 100%; for multigland hyperplasia, cure rates for stones average 70%.[5] Given hypercalcemia without hypercalciuria, one must consider familial hypocalciuric hypercalcemia, a nonstone-forming condition caused by a disordered calcium receptor.[6] Alternatively, thiazide diuretics can cause this combination. Given suppressed PTH levels, sarcoidosis, malignant neoplasm, and vitamin D intoxication are clinical possibilities.

Idiopathic hypercalciuria

This hereditary disorder resembles hyperparathyroidism in having hypercalciuria but with normal blood calcium and PTH levels. Diagnosis is by hypercalciuria, i.e. > 250 or 300 mg/day in women and men respectively, or > 4 mg/kg/day or > 140 mg/g creatinine in either sex. Stones are typically calcium oxalate, because urine pH is neither high nor low compared with normal. Hypercalciuria arises from a complex mixture of excess intestinal calcium absorption and bone mineral lability.

Bone mineral lability leads to loss of bone mineral in urine given a low-calcium diet[7] and predicts that low bone mineral density should be a feature of idiopathic hypercalciuria. This finding has been documented in multiple trials (see Table 40.9 in reference 1). Low-calcium diet is not, therefore, a good choice for treatment except under special circumstances. Thiazide diuretics have been proved effective in three 3-year prospective trials,[8,9] with stone relapse rates falling from 50% to 20%. Short-term trials of 1 and 2 years fail to show effects of treatment, as do the first 2 years of the 3-year trials, because stones occur with a periodic interval of about 1–2 years. For this reason, treatment must aim at the long term.

Chlorthalidone 12.5–25 mg once daily or hydrochlorothiazide 25 mg twice daily is a reasonable starting dose. Follow-up is needed at 4–6 weeks to ensure a response of urine calcium, and dosage may be adjusted thereafter. Yearly follow-up is prudent to ensure that the drug is effective. Reduced sodium intake to 100 mequiv. daily will reduce potassium wasting and also sodium-driven calciuria; typical stone formers have urine sodium levels of 150–200 mequiv. daily. If potassium levels fall, urine citrate will also fall, offsetting the benefit of thiazide. Potassium repletion should be as the citrate (see later) or bicarbonate salt.

In some patients, incomplete renal tubular acidosis develops, presumably because of hypercalciuria and stones.[10] Stone composition will show a shift to higher (50% or more) calcium phosphate, urine citrate will fall, and urine pH will increase above 6.2 in the 24-h urine sample. Such patients are treated the same as those without renal tubular acidosis, but our experience suggests that stone recurrence is more likely and that stones will be larger than usual. For this reason, we are particularly diligent to control urine calcium as best we can.

Hypocitraturia

Compared with same-sex normal subjects, all stone-forming groups show a tendency toward low urine citrate.[11,12] Broadly speaking, the causes are acid retention, either renal or extrarenal in origin, so low citrate tends to occur with either low or high urine pH compared with normal. Low pH with low citrate occurs in extrarenal alkali-losing states such as ileostomy, short-bowel syndromes, malabsorption states, and inflammatory bowel disease. It also occurs in chronic renal diseases of all kinds, and especially in so-called type 4 renal tubular acidosis in association with reduced renal potassium excretion.[10] High pH with low citrate is from renal tubular acidosis, as noted before. Forms of renal tubular acidosis that we have encountered as a consequence of idiopathic hypercalciuria include Sjögren syndrome and cystic renal disease. In the low pH states, stones are often admixed with uric acid; when pH is unduly high, admixture is with calcium phosphate.[11] In general, the most common form of hypocitraturia is with a slightly low urine pH in patients with common calcium oxalate stones and no evidence of renal tubular acidosis. We presume that acid-ash diet or some hitherto undefined abnormality is responsible.

The diagnosis is by urine citrate < 450 or 500 mg daily in men and women, respectively. Whatever the cause, treatment is with a potassium citrate salt, 25–30 mequiv. twice daily; the dose may be increased if follow-up shows an incomplete response. Given type 4 renal tubular acidosis, the sodium salt is needed in the same dosage ranges. Given that citrate is an important calcium-binding ligand in urine and reduces supersaturation,[13] low urine citrate is functionally similar to hypercalciuria and presumably promotes stones in that manner.

Thus far, two 3-year trials have shown efficacy of citrate in hypocitraturic calcium oxalate stone-forming patients.[1,14] Given the excellent physicochemical rationale for the use of citrate and two positive prospective, doubleblind, 3-year trials, we have few reservations about its use. However a third trial of sodium potassium citrate did not show reduction in stone rates.[1] This failure is not explained, except perhaps by the use of a sodium salt.

Hyperuricosuria

Uric acid > 750 or 800 mg/day in men and women seems to promote calcium oxalate stones.[15] How it does so is a prolonged research issue, with at least two major theories extant. One holds that uric acid, or one of its salts, acts as a heterogeneous nucleus to promote crystallization of calcium oxalate, whereas the other holds that high levels of uric acid in urine salt out calcium oxalate salts by a direct salt–salt interaction.[16] The cause of high urine uric acid is mainly a high dietary intake of purine in the form of meat, fish, and poultry, and mere change of diet is in theory a reasonable treatment. We recommend this approach, with the reservation that no trial has ever documented an effect of such a diet change. Allopurinol 200 mg daily has been tried in a 3-year, prospective, double-blind trial involving calcium oxalate stone-forming patients with no other metabolic disorder.[17] The drug reduced relapse from 36.6% among placebo recipients to 18.8% among treated patients at the end of 3 years.

We use allopurinol only when stones are recurrent despite advice to change diet and when follow-up shows persistent hyperuricosuria despite such advice as well. Under these circumstances, we assume that the stones are of clinical importance and that either diet was not changed or the patient is a primary overproducer of uric acid. We use 100–200 mg daily as a starting dose and guide treatment by follow-up after 6 weeks.

Hyperoxaluria

Normal urine oxalate for both sexes is 20–40 mg daily. Values above this are common in practice and almost always due to diet. Common foods that raise oxalate excretion include nuts, chocolate, pepper, and dark green vegetables, but we give patients a comprehensive list of foods so that they can analyze their diets individually and make needed corrections. No trials have documented effects of diet, and no drugs exist as alternatives.

All disorders of small bowel absorption that involve fats, including short bowel, inflammatory bowel disease, bypass, and pancreatic insufficiency, can cause enteric hyperoxaluria in which the colon absorbs an excess of dietary oxalate and causes severe oxaluria. The diagnosis is made clinically and by documenting high urine oxalate. Fat absorption itself is not measured as a rule, because the presence of high urine oxalate and enteric disease are a presumed set of linked circumstances. Treatments are aimed at reducing oxalate absorption and include a low-fat, low-oxalate diet and oral calcium carbonate with each meal. Typically, 1 g of calcium as the carbonate with each meal will crystallize oxalate in the bowel lumen and hinder absorption. Cholestyramine, 2–4 g with each meal, is also effective. This resin binds oxalate and also binds fatty acids and bile acids that may injure the colon and lead to high oxalate absorption. Because nutrition is compromised in these patients, treatment is complex and usually requires a competent gastroenterologist as well as a physician treating the stone condition. No trials have documented the effects of treatment of these patients.

Primary hyperoxaluria arises from disorders of critical enzymes detailed elsewhere.[18] In the so-called type 1 disorder, some patients show an incomplete response to pyridoxine 10–200 mg daily, whereas others do not. No trials document the effectiveness of pyridoxine. Because the disease tends to cause renal failure and is rare, it is not treated except in centers with some experience. Segmental liver transplantation is the ideal treatment and has been shown to be clearly effective.[18] The other two types of primary hyperoxaluria are rare indeed and need not be discussed here.

Uric acid stones

Under this heading we include pure uric acid stones, and calcium oxalate stones with some uric acid solid phase in them. These phases are of at least three types. Undissociated uric acid is the most common and implies that a low urine pH has been present on a chronic basis.[11] Ammonium hydrogen urate is uncommon and is most often encountered among patients who overuse laxatives. Sodium acid urate is uncommon and implies a normal urine pH but high urine uric acid and sodium levels.

Undissociated uric acid, the usual phase encountered, is soluble to only 96 mg/L at 37°C (98.6°F).[19] The relevant pK_a is about 5.3; at this pH, 50% of uric acid is undissociated. Given a normal urine uric acid excretion of 700 mg daily in 1 L of urine, supersaturation would be extreme. On the other hand, at pH 6, the fraction of uric acid undissociated is small, and even marked hyperuricosuria is unlikely to produce supersaturation.[16] Accordingly, undissociated uric acid phases in calcium oxalate stones or pure uric acid stones almost always mean a chronically low urine pH, on a 24-h basis, which should be sought for and confirmed in such patients. Treatment is exactly as mentioned before for hypocitraturia with low urine pH, and the range of causes is similar. We prefer potassium citrate, 25–30 mequiv. twice daily, and recheck urine at 4 weeks to prove efficacy. Dosage is adjusted depending on follow-up results.

Cystine stones

Cystine stones always arise from cystinuria, a hereditary loss of function of the dibasic amino acid transporters in renal tubules.[20] Normal urine contains clinically trivial amounts of cystine, whereas levels range from 2 to > 8 mmol daily in cystinuria. The solubility of cystine in urine is about 1 mmol/L; using this value, plus urine volume and daily urine cystine excretion, one can plan therapy rationally. If the daily volume adequate to dissolve the cystine excretion is lower than 5 L, one may use water alone as a reasonable starting treatment, aiming at nocturnal as well as daytime polyuria. Raising urine pH above 7 increases cystine solubility, but this must be done only when stones are known to contain only cystine, not calcium salts, and when studies show normal urine calcium levels.

If cystine excretion is too great for water alone, or if stones develop or enlarge despite high water intake or when water intake cannot be maintained at high levels because of interference with quality of life, D-penicillamine or tiopronin (Thiola) can be used. These sulfhydryl-containing drugs form mixed disulfides with cysteine, preventing cysteine from combining with itself to form cystine. Penicillamine is available in 125- and 250-mg capsules, providing 0.83 and 1.68 mmol of drug respectively. Because the drug combines on a molar basis with cysteine and because excretion rates of cystine are in the range 2–8 mmol/day, one can estimate the reduction of cystine needed to bring the remaining amount into the range for dissolving in the clinically achievable urine volume. For example, given 8 mmol of excretion, 125 or 250 mg four times daily will in theory bind 3.3 or 6.6 mmol respectively at most, leaving 4.7 or 1.4 mmol for dissolving in 2 L of urine. For tiopronin, the 100-mg tablet provides 0.61 mmol of drug, and one tablet four times daily will complex, at most, 2.4 mmol of cystine.

Because stones will grow given any supersaturation at all, the combination of drug and water must be sufficient to reduce supersaturation below 1.0, i.e. to produce an undersaturated urine. In practice, this usually means a steady 4 L of urine for most patients, with drug for those with excretion rates > 4 mmol/day. Adverse effects of these drugs include serum sickness-like reactions, including nephrotic syndrome, and loss of taste and smell from zinc deficiency, which can be corrected with supplemental zinc.

Struvite stones

Proteus, *Klebsiella*, *Enterobacter*, and *Pseudomonas* species often express the gene for urease and hydrolyze urea to ammonia. The ammonia takes up protons to become the ammonium ion, thereby raising the pH of the urine. As pH rises, protons leave urine phosphate molecules, converting them into the trivalent anion form, and carbonate ions form because of the hydrolysis of urea followed by rising pH. As a result, magnesium crystallizes spontaneously with trivalent phosphate and ammonium ion to form struvite. Calcium crystallizes with the carbonate species to form calcium carbonate and with phosphate to form apatite. The resulting stones are large and often staghorn in shape, filling in or making an internal cast of the renal collecting system. The stones grow rapidly and injure kidneys from obstruction and local infection, as well as by extension into renal parenchyma.

Treatment is both surgical and medical. Stone fragments must be removed as completely as possible, and after treatment the initiating infection must be treated efficiently with the use of antibiotics appropriate for the specific organisms found in the urine. About half of patients form stones that contain calcium oxalate, not expected from the pathogenesis of struvite/carbonate apatite stones. On investigation these patients will have the same range of metabolic stone-forming conditions observed among routine calcium oxalate stone formers.[21] Presumably, they are routine stone formers who have become superinfected. They should be treated for their metabolic disorders to prevent more stones. The other half have stones without calcium oxalate. Such patients do not usually have metabolic disorders that lead to calcium oxalate stones.

Fine points of practice

Rather than future directions, we wish to comment on what clinicians can do to improve their chances of success in stone prevention. Most important is stone analysis, which is the backbone of this chapter. Stone type reflects average supersaturations[11] and is the perfect clue to where the pathogenesis must lie. All stones should be analyzed to get an average and to find changes, especially during treatment, that could reflect a changing cause for new stones.

Radiographs show the stone burden at the time of treatment. Whatever stones are present will not usually go away, but pass or grow. They must not be confused with new stone production, otherwise treatment that is successful will seem a failure and be changed or stopped for no reason. Radiologists will not always note exact stone numbers or location, so we ourselves draw stone radiographs for our own record.

Treatments are meant to be long term. We tell patients that all but the rare stone-forming conditions can be treated but not cured. To treat long term without some routine ascertainment of continued efficacy seems unreasonable to us, and we recheck relevant urine chemistries yearly when treatment is in progress. All patients are studied at 4–8 weeks of treatment to be sure that initial drug dosages or changes in diet have been effective. In trying to diagnose the metabolic causes of stone formation, we believe that at least two 24-h urine specimens should be obtained before treatment, given the importance of urine findings in directing long-term therapy.

Finally, we mention urine volume and work life. Supersaturations with calcium oxalate are dependent on urine volume, and we therefore seek to achieve 2 L of urine flow daily. For uric acid and calcium phosphate phases, volume dependence is less prominent.[11] Many kinds of work environment prevent adequate fluid intake to match losses, and the same is true for sports and some forms of travel. This is a problem usually solved only by clinical interview and persistence. A remarkable benefit of multiple 24-h urine measurements before treatment, and at initial and yearly follow-up, is detection of fall in urine volume, as the patient's interest in fluid intake wanes with the waning of stone recurrences.

Subsequent imaging of the kidneys is needed to ascertain silent recurrence, but the timing of these images as well as their type is an unsettled issue. We favor abdominal radiographs over ultrasound examination because the latter is operator dependent. Radiographs suffer from the well-known problems of patient preparation and poor visualization conditions from overlying bowel, but they still seem superior for practical purposes. Renal computed tomographic scanning without contrast enhancement is the ideal method for visualizing stones and will show uric acid stones (usually radiolucent) perfectly well. Cost makes this option impractical most of the time. We prefer yearly radiographs but usually settle for sporadic radiographs because of a mixture of fear of radiation, cost, and complacency in the presence of an apparent prevention of stones. Urinalysis yearly will disclose infection or bleeding as evidence of stones but is not helpful about recurrence if stones are present at the time of treatment.

Patients tire of medications and diet changes and in time gradually leave treatment. We find that 5 years is about the median for spontaneous decline, given an absence of stone activity. As therapists, we rail against such dismissal of our hard-won treatment effects but in another sense recognize that boredom and the subtle unpleasantness of medications cannot be denied forever. When stones return, as they often do, we have another opportunity.

References

1. Asplin JR, Favus MJ, Coe FL: Nephrolithiasis. In Brenner BM (ed): Brenner and Rector's The Kidney, 6th edn. Philadelphia: WB Saunders, 2000, pp 1774–1819.
2. Coe FL, Favus MJ, Pak CYC, et al (eds): Kidney Stones: Medical and Surgical Management. Philadelphia: Lippincott-Raven, 1996.
3. Coe FL, Favus MJ (eds): Disorders of Bone and Mineral Metabolism. New York: Raven Press, 1992.
4. Bilezikian JP: Nephrolithiasis in primary hyperparathyroidism. In Coe FL, Favus MJ, Pak CYC, et al (eds): Kidney Stones: Medical and Surgical Management. Philadelphia: Lippincott-Raven, 1996, pp 787–802.
5. Kaplan EL, Tanaka R, Younes N: Primary hyperparathyroidism. In Coe FL, Favus MJ, Pak CYC, et al (eds): Kidney Stones: Medical and Surgical Management. Philadelphia: Lippincott-Raven, 1996, pp 803–820.
6. Sutton RAL, Dirks JH: Disturbances of calcium and magnesium metabolism. In Brenner BM (ed): Brenner and Rector's The Kidney, 5th edn. Philadelphia: WB Saunders, 1996, pp 1038–1085.
7. Coe FL, Favus MJ, Crockett T, et al: Effects of low-calcium diet on urine calcium excretion, parathyroid function and serum $1,25(OH)_2D_3$ levels in patients with idiopathic hypercalciuria and in normal subjects. Am J Med 1982;72:25–32.
8. Coe FL, Parks JH, Asplin JR: The pathogenesis and treatment of kidney stones: medical progress. N Engl J Med 1992;327:1141–1152.
9. Borgji L, Meschi T, Guerra A, Novarini A: Randomized prospective study of a nonthiazide diuretic, indapamide, in preventing calcium stone recurrences. J Cardiovasc Pharmacol 1993;22(Suppl 6):S78–S86.
10. Buckalew VM Jr: Calcium nephrolithiasis and renal tubular acidosis. In Coe FL, Favus MJ (eds): Disorders of Bone and Mineral Metabolism. New York: Raven Press, 1992, pp 729–756.
11. Parks JH, Coward M, Coe FL: Correspondence between stone composition and urine supersaturation in nephrolithiasis. Kidney Int 1997;51:894–900.
12. Coe FL, Parks JH: New insights into the pathophysiology and treatment of nephrolithiasis: new research venues. J Bone Miner Res 1997;12:522–533.
13. Tiselius H: Solution chemistry of supersaturation. In Coe FL, Favus MJ, Pak CYC, et al (eds): Kidney Stones: Medical and Surgical Management. Philadelphia: Lippincott-Raven, 1996, pp 33–64.
14. Barcelo P, Wuhl O, Servitge E, et al: Randomized double-blind study of potassium citrate in idiopathic hypocitraturic calcium nephrolithiasis. J Urol 1993;150:1761–1764.
15. Coe FL: Hyperuricosuric calcium oxalate nephrolithiasis. Adv Exp Med Biol 1980;128:439–450.
16. Ettinger B: Hyperuricosuric calcium stone disease and mixed stones. In Coe FL, Favus MJ, Pak CYC, et al (eds): Kidney Stones: Medical and Surgical Management. Philadelphia: Lippincott-Raven, 1996, pp 851–858.
17. Ettinger B, Tang A, Citron JT, et al: Randomized trial of allopurinol in the prevention of calcium oxalate calculi. N Engl J Med 1986;315:1386–1389.
18. Danpure CJ, Smith LH: The primary hyperoxalurias. In Coe FL, Favus MJ, Pak CYC, et al (eds): Kidney Stones: Medical and Surgical Management. Philadelphia: Lippincott-Raven, 1996, pp 859–882.
19. Rodman JS, Sosa RE, Lopez MA: Diagnosis and treatment of uric acid calculi. In Coe FL, Favus MJ, Pak CYC, et al (eds): Kidney Stones: Medical and Surgical Management. Philadelphia: Lippincott-Raven, 1996, pp 973–990.

20. Sakhaee K, Sutton RAL: Pathogenesis and medical management of cystinuria. *In* Coe FL, Favus MJ, Pak CYC, et al (eds): Kidney Stones: Medical and Surgical Management. Philadelphia: Lippincott-Raven, 1996, pp 1007–1018.

21. Kristensen C, Parks JH, Lindheimer M, Coe FL: Reduced glomerular filtration rate and hypercalciuria in primary struvite nephrolithiasis. Kidney Int 1987;32:749–753.

Nephrolithiasis: Lithotripsy and Surgery

Gary C. Curhan and John M. Fitzpatrick

During the past 15 years, the management of urinary calculi has undergone revolutionary changes as a result of the increasing number and availability of nonsurgical therapeutic approaches. Pyelolithotomy, ureterolithotomy, and retrograde blind endoscopic procedures were previously the only treatment options for removal of symptomatic stones. Fortunately, the development of extracorporeal shock wave lithotripsy (SWL), percutaneous nephrolithotomy (PCNL), and ureteroscopic lithotripsy has provided urologists with less invasive and safer treatment possibilities. The use of SWL and PCNL has led to a dramatic reduction in morbidity and mortality and has hastened recovery and return to usual activities. Remarkable technologic advances in the methods of SWL and endourology have continued with the introduction of smaller and less expensive devices. Although new technology has rendered stone management safer and less invasive, the appropriate role of each modality remains unsettled and merits careful individualized consideration.

This chapter discusses the role of lithotripsy and surgery in the management of nephrolithiasis. All the procedures described require the skill of an experienced urologist. For a more detailed discussion of these techniques, there are several excellent reviews.[1,2]

Types of lithotripsy

There are two main categories of lithotripsy: extracorporeal and intracorporeal.

Extracorporeal shock wave lithotripsy

Extracorporeal SWL, the most common technique, is performed by the generation of shock waves external to the body that are transmitted through the skin and soft tissues and focused on the stone. The energy delivered causes fragmentation of the stone into smaller pieces, which can then be passed spontaneously or removed endoscopically by the urologist. The original lithotriptors required the patient to be immersed in water to transmit the shock wave through the body to the stone; however, newer generation machines require only a small water cushion. Although SWL is often referred to as noninvasive lithotripsy, cystoscopic placement of ureteral stents before treatment may be needed to relieve obstruction or allow passage of a large (> 1.5 cm) stone burden.

Intracorporeal lithotripsy

Intracorporeal lithotripsy is performed through a nephroscope or cystoscope and is therefore more invasive than extracorporeal SWL. The four types of device currently available for intracorporeal lithotripsy (electrohydraulic, ultrasonic, laser, and pneumatic) differ according to the manner in which the energy for fragmentation is generated and delivered to the stone.

Electrohydraulic lithotripsy

Electrohydraulic lithotripsy (EHL), the first method of intracorporeal lithotripsy to be introduced, fragments stones by the transfer of energy from the generated shock wave to the stone at the fluid–stone interface. An electrical spark vaporizes water and creates a shock wave. Ureteral damage may occur from exposure to the spark produced during shock wave generation.

Ultrasonic lithotripsy

Ultrasonic lithotripsy (USL) makes use of mechanical vibration to break stones into smaller fragments that may be aspirated with specialized probes. This method requires direct contact between the probe and the stone and has several drawbacks. For example, it is often necessary to ensnare the stone in a basket before treatment because pressure exerted on the stone during the procedure may cause upward migration of stone fragments. In addition, heat produced within the ureter by the probe may lead to the formation of ureteral strictures. Furthermore, the rigidity and large size of the probes prevent the use of small ureteroscopes.

Laser lithotripsy

The flexibility and fine caliber of the fibers used to deliver the laser energy have allowed remarkable miniaturization of ureteroscopes. Moreover, laser fragmentation of stones can be performed with greater precision and control than by other methods and without propulsion of fragments or damage to surrounding tissue.

A number of laser types are available for stone fragmentation. The susceptibility to fragmentation by laser energy is dependent on stone composition and physical factors specific to each type of laser, such as pulse duration and wavelength. For example, the energy delivered by the pulsed dye laser has proved to be useful in the disruption of most stones and has the advantage of sparing the ureter from damage. Although this laser type does not fragment cystine stones well, its effectiveness can be enhanced by staining the cystine stone with an absorbing dye. In contrast, the holmium laser effectively disintegrates the surface of any stone with minimal propulsion, gradually cracking or boring a hole through the stone. However, ureteral tissue may absorb the wavelength from the holmium laser and is thus vulnerable to injury.

Pneumatic lithotripsy

The Swiss Lithoclast, the least expensive intracorporeal device, has been used effectively for stone fragmentation at all levels of the urinary tract. Under direct visualization, a solid rigid probe is applied directly to the stone to cause mechanical disruption by repeated percussion of the probe tip, similar to the mechanical action of a pneumatic jackhammer. Grasping instruments may then be used to remove the stone fragments. However, retrograde displacement of a ureteral stone is a potential drawback of this procedure, and the precise positioning required to prevent tissue damage and the requirement for a rigid or semirigid endoscope limit its usefulness as well.

Efficacy of lithotripsy

Although there is general agreement that both extracorporeal and intracorporeal lithotripsy are effective, there are no large randomized controlled trials comparing these two methods. A recent small randomized trial of 64 patients found comparable success rates for SWL compared with ureteroscopy for the treatment of distal ureteral calculi of 1.5 cm or less.[3] Results from studies of the individual methods must be compared with caution because the success or effectiveness of treatment is not uniformly defined. Although "stone free" is the gold standard for a successful procedure, there is great variability in the ascertainment of this outcome with

respect to both the time of assessment (e.g. immediately after the procedure, after 7 days, after 3 months) and the imaging modalities employed (e.g. x-ray of the kidneys, ureter, and bladder (KUB), intravenous pyelography, ultrasonography, computed tomography). When SWL was first introduced, a treatment session that produced "clinically insignificant fragments" was deemed a success. However, this definition has fallen out of favor owing to its ambiguity and the reality that the retention of small fragments results in regrowth and recurrence of symptomatic stone disease. The definition of a treatment failure may vary as well, yet is most commonly defined as the need for a repeated treatment or another type of procedure.

Extracorporeal shock wave lithotripsy

The success of SWL depends on the location, size, and composition of the stone. Thus a comparison of success rates between different studies must consider all three of these factors. Stones in the kidney are treated with slightly greater success than are ureteral stones, and success rates are higher for proximal ureteral stones than for distal stones. Smaller stones, usually < 2 cm, are more easily treated with SWL than are larger stones. Softer stones (calcium oxalate dihydrate, uric acid, apatite, and struvite) are more easily fragmented with SWL than are harder stones (calcium oxalate monohydrate, brushite, and cystine).

SWL is the treatment of choice for most renal stones, and success rates as high as 90% have been reported.[4] However, further procedures may be necessary in up to 20% of patients with stones of 1–2 cm. In general, SWL is more effective in the treatment of stones in the renal pelvis than in the calyces and, depending on size, composition, calyceal configuration, and infundibular pelvic angle, is least effective in treating lower pole stones.

There is an inverse relationship between stone size and stone-free rates. Stones > 2 cm in diameter are rarely successfully treated with SWL alone and may best be removed by PCNL in the upper urinary tract and ureteroscopically in the lower tract.

Stone-free rates of more than 80% for calcium oxalate and uric acid stones (softer stones) have been reported, although no distinction was made on the basis of stone size.[5] A study of retreatment rates in patients with stones of known composition, 1–3 cm in diameter, and treated with SWL found that calcium oxalate monohydrate calculi (hard stones) required the greatest number of retreatment procedures (10%), followed by struvite (6%), and calcium oxalate dihydrate (3%).[6]

First-generation lithotriptors caused enough pain to require anesthesia, either general or epidural. Most patients treated with newer generation devices require only moderate intravenous analgesia while undergoing SWL.

The early complications of SWL have been well described and are generally minor, with pain and hematuria most commonly reported. Direct injury to the kidney and surrounding tissues as well as complications due to the passage of stone fragments may also occur. Much less information is available on the long-term effects of SWL because most follow-up efforts have focused only on the short-term results and complications.

The morphologic changes that may occur after SWL and their mechanisms have been studied by a variety of imaging techniques. Imaging by computed tomography or magnetic resonance reveals that more than 75% of treated patients have changes in renal tissue and demonstrate edema in and around the kidney, as well as intraparenchymal, subcapsular, or perirenal hemorrhage. Although damage to nonrenal tissues has been reported rarely, pancreatitis, gastric erosions, ecchymoses of the colonic mucosa, splenic rupture, pulmonary contusions, and cardiac arrhythmias may occur. Although there have been no reported adverse effects of SWL on fertility or the risk of birth defects, the impact of SWL on the reproductive tract, if any, has yet to be established. SWL should not be used on pregnant women.

Functionally, biochemical evidence of kidney damage directly after SWL has been documented. Although the results of these laboratory studies generally return to near-normal levels within days, it is unclear whether these changes represent only transient dysfunction or more consequential chronic damage. A small prospective randomized study suggested that pretreatment with nifedipine or allopurinol may protect the kidney from shock wave-induced renal damage.[7] Nevertheless, there is no clear evidence to indicate that SWL is associated with any long-term effect on renal function in humans.[8]

Ureteral stone fragments may cause obstruction after incomplete stone fragmentation or fragmentation of a large stone burden resulting in steinstrasse, literally "stone street." Typically, partially obstructing steinstrasse will clear spontaneously within 2–4 weeks in asymptomatic patients. Otherwise, percutaneous nephrostomy tube decompression, ureteroscopic manipulation, PCNL, repeated SWL, or even open ureterolithotomy may be necessary to clear the stone fragments. Repeated SWL is often attempted in patients with minimal symptoms and no evidence of infection. In contrast, emergency decompression of the collecting system with a percutaneous nephrostomy tube is necessary for symptomatic patients or asymptomatic patients with significant obstruction. Steinstrasse that persists for longer than 1 or 2 weeks after placement of the percutaneous nephrostomy tube may be relieved with repeated SWL, ureteroscopy, or intracorporeal lithotripsy.

Although it has been suggested that SWL is associated with new-onset hypertension, this connection is not supported by all studies. The most persuasive study demonstrated that the incidence of hypertension is not higher in patients treated with SWL compared with other methods of stone removal. Nevertheless, there was a statistically significant rise in diastolic blood pressure of just under 1 mmHg in SWL-treated patients.[9] This rise may be more pronounced in older patients.

To date, the safe upper limit of shock wave energy that can be delivered to one kidney during one session, the total amount of energy that can be delivered cumulatively, and the minimum safe interval between treatment sessions have yet to be defined. The variables to be considered include the number of shock waves and the power at which they are delivered. These vary for each type of machine and have not been standardized. However, despite these variations, there are few reports of renal injury to the hundreds of thousands of patients treated with SWL. Available data suggest that if chronic kidney damage does occur, it is most likely to be suffered by patients with some degree of preexisting renal dysfunction.[10]

Surgical modalities

Stone surgery has changed so considerably over the last decade that the term has almost dropped out of use. The percutaneous approach was then introduced, which involved new technology both to approach the kidney and to enter it without damaging vital structures and then to remove the stone if small, or to fragment and aspirate it if larger.

Percutaneous nephrolithotomy

The fact that stone removal from the kidney required an extensive flank incision long frustrated urologists. Eventually, the task was performed using a combination of radiographic and minimally invasive surgical techniques.[11]

The procedure is usually carried out in a single session with general anesthesia. A fine needle is inserted into the renal pelvis under ultrasound or x-ray guidance: the track is not made directly into the pelvis but through the parenchyma of the lower pole of the kidney, so that the track into the lower pole calyx is supported by the renal tissue itself. A nephroscope is passed, and if the stone is visualized it can be broken up by intracorporeal lithotripsy. The fragments are then evacuated, and a nonself-retaining nephrostomy tube is inserted and sutured to the skin.[12]

Failure to remove the stone fragments completely is uncommon, particularly with increasing experience. The overall success rate of 95% throughout the world shows that this technique is an excellent way of clearing by a single method all but the most refractory of stones.[13–15]

The complication rate is low: hemorrhage requiring blood transfusion or surgical intervention is seen in 1–3% of patients, and residual stones are left behind in 2–8%.[15] Sepsis can develop, especially if the preoperative urine culture is positive. In this case antibiotic prophylaxis is needed.[16]

Open surgery

The newer techniques for removing and fragmenting stones, alone or in combination, have eliminated the requirement for open surgery except in a small number of cases. The actual percentage of cases that today require open surgery is not known but is unlikely to be greater than 12%. Stones of large bulk and complexity should be managed in stone centers by urologists who have the experience required for this type of surgery.

One of two methods is used to incise the renal cortical tissue and to approach the peripheral stone fragments in the calyces: radical paravascular nephrotomy[17] and anatrophic nephrolithotomy.[18] In the former approach, incisions are made between the branches of the renal artery. The calyx is approached and the fragments are removed. Several of these nephrotomies may have to be made, placed laterally in the kidney on either the anterior or posterior surface. After complete removal of the stone, the nephrotomies are closed with a fine suture, aiming to close only the renal capsule.

In anatrophic nephrolithotomy, the incision follows the avascular line between the segments of the kidney that are supplied by the anterior and posterior segmented branches of the renal artery. After complete removal of the stone, the kidney incision is sutured and closed completely.

Effect of surgical approaches on renal function

The overall effect on renal function of PCNL is usually minimal. Although there is a potential risk that increases with the size of the access track, no studies have reported any serious postoperative loss of function.

Two aspects of open surgery may interfere with postoperative renal function: renal ischemia and parenchymal incisions. To prevent excessive hemorrhage when the renal parenchyma is incised, the renal artery is traditionally clamped, exposing the kidney to ischemia. If the ischemic period is longer than 20 min, irreversible renal damage may occur. A number of methods have been described to preserve renal function during ischemia of more than 20-min duration, including renal cooling and vasoactive agents. In a canine model, the function of kidneys subjected to radial paravascular nephrotomy was unchanged compared with that of controls.[19] There was a statistically significant difference in postoperative function when the anatrophic nephrotomy was compared with control kidneys.

Recommendations

Contemporary indications for intervention

The generally accepted indications for intervention for the treatment of urinary calculi are summarized in Table 40.1. Absolute indications include persistent or progressive high-grade obstruction by the stone, urinary tract infection, and intractable pain. Infection in the face of obstruction is a medical emergency that requires immediate intervention to relieve the obstruction before

Table 40.1 Indications for urologic intervention in nephrolithiasis

Absolute indications
Persistent obstruction
Urinary tract infection
Intractable pain

Relative indications
Failure of ureteral stone to progress
Significant hematuria
Stone growth despite optimal medical treatment
Social, economic, or occupational factors
Stone too large to pass spontaneously

SWL. Relative indications for intervention include occupational factors, significant hematuria requiring transfusion, substantial stone growth despite appropriate medical management, stone size judged too large to pass spontaneously, or failure of a ureteral stone to move during a 6-week period.

A finding of hydronephrosis, a sign of ureteral obstruction, at initial presentation is not necessarily an indication for intervention. However, if follow-up studies reveal a lack of improvement during a 1–2 week period, intervention is usually required whether or not symptoms are present.

The location, size, and composition of the stone are the most important factors guiding the decision to treat and with which method (Table 40.2). Realistically, the cost of purchasing and maintaining the different types of lithotripsy equipment is substantial, and most hospitals, even large academic centers, have only one extracorporeal and one or two intracorporeal lithotripsy devices available. Thus, treatment with extracorporeal or intracorporeal lithotripsy is the first decision to be made, based on the availability of devices. Second, the skill and familiarity of the treating urologist with the different methods are important. Third, the choice of approach depends on both economic factors and individual preferences (e.g. travel, time lost from work, retreatment rates). Fourth, other medical conditions, such as morbid obesity and severe scoliosis or kyphosis, and conditions associated with an

Table 40.2 Factors influencing choice of intervention

Stone characteristics
  Size
  Location
  Composition

Urinary tract anatomy
  Duplicated collecting system
  Horseshoe kidney
  Medullary sponge kidney
  Solitary kidney
  Transplanted kidney
  Pediatric patient

Availability of technology

Experience of urologist

increased risk of general anesthesia must be taken into consideration.

Renal calculi

The majority of patients with renal stones < 2 cm may be successfully managed with outpatient SWL and return to routine activities within 48 h. In contrast, SWL treatment of stones 2 cm or larger presents a substantial risk of ureteral obstruction from stone fragments; therefore, PCNL is extremely effective and is the procedure of choice. Depending on stone composition and other clinical circumstances, stones 2–3 cm in size may occasionally be treated with SWL. A treatment algorithm for the management of renal calculi is presented in Fig. 40.1.

Bilateral stones

In the setting of bilateral stone disease, each kidney is commonly treated individually in separate sessions. However, patients with symptomatic bilateral stones may require bilateral intervention and can be treated with SWL during a single session if the stone burden is not too large and renal function is normal.[10] Patients with abnormal renal function before bilateral SWL treatment may be more likely to develop acute renal failure.[10] Potentially, patients with normal renal function and asymptomatic large bilateral stones may undergo bilateral SWL by an experienced endourologist in a single session for economic, social, or medical reasons (e.g. risk of anesthesia).

Calyceal diverticula

Stones in calyceal diverticula are generally asymptomatic. Nevertheless, intervention is necessary in the setting of local symptoms such as pain, associated infection, hematuria, or progressive stone growth. Rarely, if there is adequate drainage from the calyceal diverticulum, SWL is the treatment of choice for stones < 1.5 cm. PCNL is recommended for stones 1.5 cm or larger.

The management of asymptomatic calyceal calculi is more of a problem. One study suggested that 30% of patients with asymptomatic calyceal stones will present with a symptomatic episode within 3 years and 50% within 5 years of the initial evaluation.[20] Most urologists recommend a conservative approach and observe patients with asymptomatic calyceal diverticuli with calculi.

Horseshoe kidney

About 20% of individuals with a horseshoe kidney form a stone at some time. These stones may be composed of struvite, the result of infection due to abnormal urinary drainage, or calcium oxalate. SWL can be attempted if it is anatomically feasible. PCNL may be used as a primary or adjunctive procedure, particularly for larger stones. In general, stones 2 cm or less may be treated with either a first-generation lithotriptor or PCNL, whereas PCNL is the treatment of choice for stones > 2 cm.[21]

Medullary sponge kidney

SWL may be attempted for the treatment of renal calculi in patients with medullary sponge kidney, although the data on its effectiveness are limited.[22] It is noteworthy that residual calcifications will likely be evident on a KUB film owing to the presence of parenchymal calcifications. Thus radiologic assessment of the success of the procedure and preventive medical therapies is difficult.

Staghorn calculi

Struvite staghorn calculi are particularly concerning because they arise from infected urine and the stones harbor infection. Struvite staghorn calculi that fill the major part of the collecting system should be treated with a combination of percutaneous stone removal and SWL. The assessment of overall and split renal function is important when choosing what treatment to offer. The American Urological Association's treatment guidelines state that for struvite staghorn calculi PCNL should be performed to debulk the stone mass occupying the renal pelvis, followed by SWL or flexible nephroscopy at a later date to remove fragments remaining in the calyces.[23] In experienced hands, the stone-free rates with the combined approach should exceed 80%.[21]

Solitary kidney

A solitary kidney, whether congenital or acquired, presents a unique set of difficulties. Obstruction of a solitary kidney can lead to acute renal failure. SWL with or without cystoscopic assistance is the best approach in this setting because it is preferable to avoid the use of a percutaneous nephrostomy owing to potential damage to the renal parenchymal tissue. Otherwise, the same criteria for treatment selection apply to a solitary kidney.

Transplanted kidney

Fortunately, renal calculi form in less than 2% of transplanted kidneys. Hyperparathyroidism and nonabsorbable sutures are the most important risk factors. As for the native solitary kidney, it is preferable to avoid a percutaneous approach in a transplanted kidney. The transplanted kidney is typically located in the right or left

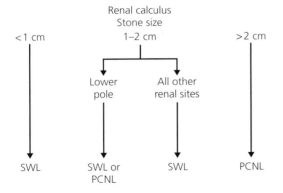

Figure 40.1 Treatment algorithm for the initial management of renal calculi. PCNL, percutaneous nephrolithotomy; SWL, shock wave lithotripsy.

lower quadrant of the abdomen and therefore is accessible to SWL. Alternatively, cystoscopic treatment with one of the intracorporeal methods may be attempted by an experienced endourologist.[24]

Ureteral calculi

Renal colic from a ureteral stone is the most frequent reason for a patient to present to a physician for acute treatment of nephrolithiasis. At the time of presentation, a radiographic study will usually be obtained that may consist of an intravenous pyelogram (also known as intravenous urogram) or an ultrasound examination; many centers have replaced these with the preferred spiral computed tomography, which is more rapid and provides greater resolution. For patients with a known history of stones whose renal and ureteral anatomy is known, a KUB film may be sufficient to identify a new stone.

The size of the ureteral calculus is an important factor in the determination of the need for intervention. Historically, ureteral stones 4 mm or less were observed, in anticipation of their spontaneous passage. However, recent data suggest that both size and location influence the likelihood of spontaneous passage.[25] In a retrospective study of 378 patients with ureteral stones, overall 60% of the stones passed without requiring intervention. Notably, the more proximal the stone, the lower the passage rate. For example, a 4-mm stone passed spontaneously only 20% of the time if it was located in the proximal ureter, whereas the same size stone in the distal ureter passed spontaneously in 55% of cases.[25] Currently, even with the new technology available, patients with stones 4 mm or less rarely undergo intervention because of the excellent chance of spontaneous passage. However, improvements in technology have altered the indications for intervention for those patients with slightly larger stones who in the past would have been observed expectantly.

When intervention is deemed necessary, the location of the stone within the ureter is an important consideration that influences the selection of the method to be used (Fig. 40.2). Approximately 70–80% of proximal ureteral stones (above the iliac vessels) can be successfully treated with extracorporeal SWL. Although there are no large prospective randomized trials that compare SWL with other methods of removal, SWL is a reasonable choice for the initial management of proximal ureteral stones because of safety, noninvasiveness, and observed high success rates. Complications from SWL for proximal ureteral stones often result from stone manipulation before treatment, and ureteral stent placement does not increase the efficacy of treatment. However, in the setting of ureteral calculi > 1.5 cm, urosepsis, or complete ureteral obstruction, the placement of a ureteral stent or nephrostomy tube is often necessary. If SWL alone is unsuccessful, retrograde approaches are indicated. If the stone still cannot be removed, an antegrade (percutaneous) approach may be attempted. PCNL is a highly effective yet much more invasive option for the removal of a proximal ureteral stone.

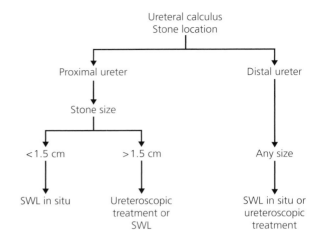

Figure 40.2 Treatment algorithm for the initial management of ureteral calculi. The proximal ureter is that portion above and the distal ureter that portion below the iliac vessels. SWL, shock wave lithotripsy.

The optimal treatment of distal ureteral stones is also controversial, primarily because of the lack of any prospective randomized controlled studies comparing SWL and ureteroscopy. SWL and endoscopic lithotripsy are both acceptable treatments of distal ureteral stones. SWL requires many more repeated treatments than endoscopic lithotripsy, but the latter is more invasive and occasionally may result in ureteral stricture formation.

SWL treatment of stones located in the distal ureter is technically more difficult than for stones in the renal pelvis or calyces. Thus some urologists still employ ureteroscopy to manipulate the stone retrogradely into the renal pelvis and then proceed with SWL (referred to as "push-bang"). However, data suggest that this more invasive technique does not yield substantially higher stone-free rates than does SWL alone.[26]

As with renal stones, the comparative efficacy of the different approaches to treatment of ureteral calculi is difficult to assess. Most likely, the choice of treatment will be based on availability and experience with the various methods. Similarly, the choice of ureteroscopic technique often depends on the availability of the equipment and the experience of the urologist. If it is available, the pulsed dye laser may be used for fragmentation of most ureteral calculi. However, USL may be more effective for the treatment of a calcium oxalate monohydrate stone > 1 cm. Small durile stones are best treated by grasping with forceps or a basket followed by extraction. Treatment of cystine stones is more easily performed by EHL or holmium laser than by coating with dye and fragmentation by the pulsed dye laser.[27]

The treatment of infants, pregnant women, or extremely obese individuals merits special consideration. Minimal invasiveness and radiation exposure are particularly important in pediatric and obstetric patients, and conservative management is prudent. SWL, preferably with ultrasound localization, may be used in infants. Ureteroscopic techniques are another treatment option.

Nevertheless, pregnant patients who present with symptomatic ureteral stones may require urgent treatment because of the increased risk to the fetus from systemic maternal infection or premature labor. The potential for serious complications and the technical difficulties involved in the treatment of infants and pregnant women demand care by only the most experienced endourologists. Although endoscopic treatment of distal calculi can be accomplished under local anesthesia in pregnant women, the most prudent approach is to insert an indwelling stent and allow the patient to complete the pregnancy. Extreme obesity, on the other hand, may impede SWL localization and the ability of the shock wave to reach the calculus; thus ureteroscopic methods are preferable in this setting.[28]

Antibiotics and shock wave lithotripsy

Historically, routine antimicrobial prophylaxis has been administered even in the absence of infection in the urinary tract. However, a prospective randomized trial involving 360 patients revealed that the incidence of urinary tract infection after SWL was low in patients with sterile urine before intervention and suggested that prophylactic antibiotics may be unnecessary.[29] If bacteriuria is associated with calculi, prophylactic antibiotics are required whatever the planned surgical procedure.

Acknowledgments

This work was supported in part by a grant to G.C.C. from the National Institutes of Health (R01-DK59583).

References

1. Lingeman JE, Preminger GM (eds): New Developments in the Management of Urolithiasis. New York: Igaku-Shoin Medical Publishers, 1996.
2. Coe F, Favus M, Pak C, et al (eds): Kidney Stones: Medical and Surgical Management. Philadelphia: Lippincott-Raven, 1996.
3. Pearle MS, Nadler R, Bercowsky E, et al: Prospective randomized trial comparing shock wave lithotripsy and ureteroscopy for management of distal ureteral calculi. J Urol 2001;166:1255–1260.
4. Dawson C, Whitfield HN: The long-term results of treatment of urinary stones. Br J Urol 1994;74:397–404.
5. Graf J, Deiderichs W, Schulze H: Long-term follow-up in 1003 extracorporeal shock wave lithotripsy patients. J Urol 1988;140:479–483.
6. Dretler SP: Stone fragility: a new therapeutic distinction. J Urol 1988;139:1124–1127.
7. Li B, Zhou W, Li P: Protective effects of nifedipine and allopurinol on high energy shock wave induced acute changes of renal function. J Urol 1995;153:596–598.
8. Liou LS, Streem SB: Long-term renal functional effects of shock wave lithotripsy, percutaneous nephrolithotomy and combination therapy: a comparative study of patients with solitary kidney. J Urol 2001;166:36, discussion 36–37.
9. Lingeman JE, Woods JR, Toth, PD: Blood pressure changes following extracorporeal shock wave lithotripsy and other forms of treatment for nephrolithiasis. JAMA 1990;263:1789–1794.
10. Lingeman JE, Newmark J: Adverse bioeffects of shock-wave lithotripsy. In Coe F, Favus M, Pak C, et al (eds): Kidney Stones: Medical and Surgical Management. Philadelphia: Lippincott-Raven, 1996, pp 605–614.
11. Fernstrom I, Johansson B: Percutaneous pyelolithotomy. A new extraction technique. Scand J Urol Nephrol 1976;10:257–259.
12. Marberger M: Percutaneous renal surgery: its role in stone management. In Krane RJ, Siroky MB, Fitzpatrick JM (eds): Clinical Urology. Philadelphia: JB Lippincott, 1994, pp 254–265.
13. Alken P: Teleskopbougierset zur perkutanen Nephrostomie. Akt Urol 1981;12:216.
14. Segura JW, Patterson DE, LeRoy AJ, et al: Percutaneous lithotripsy. J Urol 1983;130:1051–1054.
15. Marberger M, Stackl W, Hruby W, et al: Late sequelae of ultrasonic lithotripsy of renal calculi. J Urol 1985;133:170–173.
16. Marberger M: Disintegration of renal and ureteral calculi with ultrasound. Urol Clin North Am 1983;10:729–742.
17. Wickham JE, Coe N, Ward JP: One hundred cases of nephrolithotomy under hypothermia. J Urol 1974;112:702–705.
18. Boyce WH, Elkins IB: Reconstructive renal surgery following anatrophic nephrolithotomy: followup of 100 consecutive cases. J Urol 1974;111:307–312.
19. Fitzpatrick JM, Sleight MW, Braack A, et al: Intrarenal access: effects on renal function and morphology. Br J Urol 1980;52:409–414.
20. Glowacki LS, Beecroft ML, Cook R J, et al: The natural history of asymptomatic urolithiasis. J Urol 1992;147:319–321.
21. Pearle M, Clayman M: Outcomes and selection of surgical therapies of stones in the kidney and ureter. In Coe F, Favus M, Pak C, et al (eds): Kidney Stones: Medical and Surgical Management. Philadelphia: Lippincott-Raven, 1996, pp 705–755.
22. Fuchs G, Patel A, Tognoni P: Management of stones associated with anatomic abnormalities of the urinary tract. In Coe F, Favus M, Pak C, et al (eds): Kidney Stones: Medical and Surgical Management. Philadelphia: Lippincott-Raven, 1996, pp 1037–1057.
23. Segura JW, Preminger GM, Assimos DG, et al: Nephrolithiasis Clinical Guidelines Panel summary report on the management of staghorn calculi. The American Urological Association Nephrolithiasis Clinical Guidelines Panel. J Urol 1994;151:1648–1651.
24. Benoit G, Blanchet P, Eschwege P, et al: Occurrence and treatment of kidney graft lithiasis in a series of 1500 patients. Clin Transplant 1996;10:176–180.
25. Morse RM, Resnick MI: Ureteral calculi: natural history and treatment in an era of advanced technology. J Urol 1991;145:263–265.
26. Cass AS: Do upper ureteral stones need to be manipulated (push back) into the kidneys before extracorporeal shock wave lithotripsy? J Urol 1992;147:349–351.
27. Dretler SP: Modes of intracorporeal lithotripsy. In Coe F, Favus M, Pak C, et al (eds): Kidney Stones: Medical and Surgical Management. Philadelphia: Lippincott-Raven, 1996, pp 651–663.
28. Aso Y, Minowada S: Management of ureteral calculi. In Coe F, Favus M, Pak C, et al (eds): Kidney Stones: Medical and Surgical Management. Philadelphia: Lippincott-Raven, 1996, pp 665–679.
29. Ilker Y, Turkeri LN, Korten V, et al: Antimicrobial prophylaxis in management of urinary tract stones by extracorporeal shock-wave lithotripsy: is it necessary? Urology 1995;46:165–167.

PART VI
Genitourinary Infections, Malignancy, and Obstruction

HUGH R. BRADY

Therapy of Urinary Tract Infection

Nina E. Tolkoff-Rubin and Robert H. Rubin

The term "urinary tract infection" (UTI) encompasses a group of clinical disorders that are quite diverse and that, together, constitute the most common form of bacterial infection affecting humans throughout their life span. UTI is primarily an infection of females (both adult and pediatric), with males having a significant incidence of UTI only at the two extremes of life because of the higher incidence of urogenital anomalies among male babies and the effects of prostatic disease in the geriatric population.[1,2] More than 7 million women seek medical attention each year for acute, uncomplicated UTI (cystitis), with more than 100 000 hospital admissions each year for the care of pyelonephritis and a total cost of more than $1 billion dollars per year. The incidence of cystitis in sexually active young women is 0.5–0.7% per year. Approximately 50% of women will have at least one UTI in a lifetime.[3,4] Urinary tract infection may involve deep tissue infection of the kidney and/or the prostate gland, or superficial mucosal infection of the bladder; an estimated 90% of infections in males involve tissue invasion, whereas ≥ 70% of UTIs in females represent superficial mucosal infection. Clinically, UTIs may be symptomatic or asymptomatic, may or may not cause blood stream invasion, and may occur in anatomically normal or abnormal urinary tract anatomy or in persons with or without underlying renal disease.[1]

Over the years, it has been postulated that UTI, even if asymptomatic, had important effects beyond the inflammatory consequences of microbial invasion: hypertension, progressive renal disease, and an increased mortality being the most notable. There is now overwhelming evidence that UTI does not by itself cause these effects. However, when UTI is combined with other conditions such as vesicoureteral reflux, obstruction, and other significant conditions, it will accelerate the damage to the kidneys, particularly in children. As far as increased mortality is concerned, which has been studied most in the elderly, it appears that UTI is a marker of ill health and other significant disease, but by itself it does not cause increased mortality. In particular, antimicrobial therapy of asymptomatic bacteriuria is not associated with a decrease in mortality.[1,5–12]

Not surprisingly, then, different clinical syndromes of UTI require different patient management strategies. The purpose of this chapter is to outline the current concepts of pathogenesis, diagnosis, prevention, and treatment of this most common of human infections.

Pathogenesis of urinary tract infections

Although bacteremia with such virulent organisms as *Staphylococcus aureus*, *Pseudomonas aeruginosa*, and *Salmonella typhi* can infect the kidneys through the hematogenous route, more than 95% of UTIs occur because of ascension of organisms from the distal urethra to the bladder, the ureters, and, finally, the kidneys. Both bacterial virulence factors and certain host factors determine whether sustained infection is to occur. Gender is a major determinant of the incidence of UTI. In males with normal urinary tract anatomy and function, the incidence of UTI is quite low, at least in part due to the physical separation of the distal urethra from the fecal reservoir of bacteria and, perhaps, to the presence of antibacterial substances in the secretions of the normal prostate. In men, lack of circumcision, homosexual activity that involves anal intercourse, and, uncommonly, heterosexual vaginal intercourse with a women colonized with a uropathogen have been associated with an increased risk of UTI. However, because sustained colonization of the distal urethra in males is difficult to accomplish, bacteriuria is unusual in the absence of prostatic dysfunction or other urogenital abnormalities.[1]

Virtually all the studies of the pathogenesis of UTI have been carried out in women with *Escherichia coli* infection. However, the data that are clinically available now suggest that similar mechanisms are operative in males with UTI and also in other not uncommon bacterial causes of UTI such as *Proteus* and *Klebsiella*. Therefore, it is not unreasonable to base our discussion of the pathogenesis of UTI primarily on the data generated in females with *E. coli* infection. A few clones of *E. coli*, termed uropathogenic or nephritogenic *E. coli*, possess a variety of virulence properties that appear to be important in mediating the key steps in the pathogenesis of UTI in the normal urinary tract: sustained intestinal carriage, persistence in the vagina, and ascension and invasion of the urinary tract despite a normal urine output.[1,3,13]

These virulence properties are closely linked on the bacterial chromosome and are found in only a restricted number of E. coli serotypes (O1, O2, O4, O6, O7, O75, and O150 cause the majority of UTIs). The virulence properties of E. coli include the following: an intact O (somatic) antigen, a K (capsular) antigen, the production of hemolysin, the presence of the iron-binding protein aerobactin, the ability to resist the bactericidal effect of normal human serum, the production of colicin V, increased adherence to vaginal and uroepithelial cells, the production of both cytotoxic necrotizing factor type 1 and hemolysin, and the ability to induce an inflammatory response. Genes mediating these urovirulence factors are usually linked to large multigene chromosomal segments called pathogenicity islands and are absent in E. coli found in normal fecal flora.[14–20] The most important of these bacterial virulence factors are adhesions present on the surfaces of the uropathogenic strains that mediate attachment and adherence via specific receptors on the uroepithelium. Although a variety of bacterial adhesin–host receptor systems have been defined, the best studied (and probably most important) surface adhesins are the p-fimbriae (also known as p-pili, or type II pili), which bind to the globoseries of glycolipid receptors that have a common disaccharide $\alpha Gal(1-4)\beta Gal$. These receptors are identical to the glycosphingolipids of the P blood group system and are found on the epithelial cells of the vagina, urinary tract, kidneys, and large intestine, but not on phagocytic cells.[21–27]

Uropathogenic strains are able to attach to the host mucosal cells (thus effecting sustained carriage in the large intestine and adherence to the vaginal and uroepithelium) while avoiding binding to host polymorphonuclear cells.[21,28–30] Type I fimbriae bind to mannose epitopes, for example those found on such glycoproteins as secretory immunoglobulin A (IgA) and Tamm–Horsfall protein, and are thought to play a role in urovirulence in the presence of other virulence factors. In addition, there are uropathogenic strains that adhere in the absence of fimbriae.[31–34]

Recently, a single clone of uropathogenic E. coli has been identified as the cause of a large number of UTIs in individual communities. Isolates of these bacteria were identified initially by being trimethoprim–sulfamethoxazole resistant (generally associated with multidrug resistance). Epidemiologic studies have suggested that the source of this clonal outbreak is contaminated food or water. Prolonged colonization of the intestine is the first step in the pathogenesis of these infections, and it is possible that long-term intestinal carriage provides the opportunity for acquiring plasmids that mediate drug resistance. That this is an important phenomenon is shown by the fact that this single clone accounted for 10% of all UTIs in California, Minnesota, and Michigan and for 38–51% of trimethoprim–sulfamethoxazole-resistant strains. Similar clusters of cases have occurred in south London, UK, and St Louis, MO, and this clone has also been shown to be endemic in Barcelona. This clone (termed clone A) has played a significant role in the spread of antimicrobial resistance. A hitherto unusual stereotype to be isolated from the urinary tract, O15:K52:H1, is characteristic of this phenomenon. The epidemiologic pattern of this particular clone is very reminiscent of that seen when hemorrhagic enterocolitis due to E. coli O157:H7 was identified as a community-wide outbreak owing to the ingestion of contaminated food, and it is postulated that a similar epidemiologic pattern is operational here.[35,36]

Host factors are at least as important as bacterial virulence factors in the pathogenesis of UTI. These include the following:

1. Normal vaginal flora, particularly the presence of lactobacilli, plays an important role in preventing the colonization of the vaginal vestibule with uropathogenic strains. Such colonization is a necessary, although not sufficient, first step in the pathogenesis of UTI. It is estimated that ~ 8% of patients with uropathogen colonization of the vagina develop UTI, and when it occurs it is the same organism that is colonizing. Thus, spermicides, used with condoms or diaphragms for contraception, inhibit the normal flora, and the metabolic changes induced by menopause have a similar effect – the end result being an increased propensity to recurrent UTI. Sexual intercourse will regularly introduce distal urethral and vaginal flora into the bladder. If the organisms are so introduced, they will be quickly eliminated by local host defenses, including voiding. If uropathogens are present, they will adhere, and sexual activity will have played an important role in the development of sustained UTI.

2. The normally functioning bladder has a significant capacity for eliminating bacteria that have been introduced. Three factors appear to contribute significantly to this ability: the elimination of bacteria by voiding, the presence of bacteriostatic substances in the urine, and the intrinsic mucosal defense mechanisms (including the ability to mount an inflammatory response starting when the bacteria adhere to the mucosal lining). It is worth emphasizing that these defenses are greatly attenuated when there is a significant postvoiding residual.[37–41]

3. The ability to secrete blood group antigens into body fluids, including the urine and vaginal secretions, is an important host defense against UTI. These blood group antigens appear to block the adherence of bacterial adhesions to uroepithelial receptors and thus protect against the initiation of infection. Women who are nonsecretors have an increased incidence of recurrent UATi, and uropathogens have been shown to adhere to periurethral and vaginal mucosal cells from these women in much greater numbers than do those in women who are secretors.[42–45]

4. A competent ureterovesical junction provides significant protection against the reflux of both sterile and infected urine into the kidney.[1]

Thus, there are a number of conditions that predispose to urinary tract infection, and do so by overcoming the host defenses delineated above. These conditions either promote the occurrence of UTI or amplify its clinical impact. A corollary of these observations is that different antimicrobial programs are necessary for the prevention and treatment of UTI in patients with one or more of the following conditions:

1. Impedance of urine flow due to anatomic obstruction (e.g. a stone or an enlarged prostate gland) or a functional inability to empty the bladder (e.g. a neurogenic bladder due to spinal cord injury or neuropathy due to diabetes or multiple sclerosis) greatly increases the susceptibility to and the impact of UTI.[1]
2. Vesicoureteral reflux predisposes to the spread of infection to the kidney, and the combination of reflux and infection appears to be synergistic in terms of producing chronic renal injury, especially in children, and most particularly in children under the age of 5.[1]
3. The presence of such foreign bodies as an indwelling bladder catheter markedly increases the incidence of UTI. Even with modern closed drainage systems, once such a catheter is in place, after the first 3 days of its presence, there is an incidence of bacteriuria at a rate of 1–3% per day, with most patients becoming vacteriuric by the end of 1 month.[1]

Notable by their absence from this analysis are immunosuppressed states. Defects in T-cell, B-cell, and polymorphonuclear leukocyte function do not appear to be associated with an increased incidence of UTI, although the impact of any infections that do occur may be increased in the face of such conditions. Similarly, there is little evidence that conditions such as diabetes mellitus are associated with an increased incidence of UTI until diabetic neuropathy affecting bladder function develops.[1]

Diagnosis of urinary tract infection

The range of possible symptom complexes caused by UTI is very broad, ranging from asymptomatic bacteriuria to symptomatic abacteriuria (the acute urethral syndrome), from symptoms related to the lower urinary tract (dysuria and frequency) to symptoms suggesting kidney invasion and pyelonephritis (e.g. loin pain and costovertebral angle tenderness), to full-blown septic shock. The relationship of symptoms to the presence of bacteriuria and the anatomic site of infection is incomplete. Thus, 30% of women with symptoms of dysuria and frequency will have covert kidney involvement, while a similar or higher percentage of men with bacterial prostatitis will also have covert kidney involvement. Because the relationship between symptoms and either the presence of true infection or the anatomic site of infection is incomplete, the laboratory plays an important role in the diagnosis and management of UTI. This is particularly true given the difficulty of acquiring a voided urine specimen that is not contaminated by distal urethral or vaginal flora. The following observations can be utilized in deciding whether true UTI is present, and that treatment is indicated.[1,2]

In patients without bladder or ureteral catheters, more than 95% of infections are caused by a single species at any one time, with the Enterobacteriaceae, *Pseudomonas*

aeruginosa, enterococci, and *Staphylococcus saprophyticus* (this last being a particularly important uropathogen in sexually active young women) causing virtually all these infections. In contrast, the organisms that commonly colonize the distal urethra and skin of both men and women and the vagina of women (*Staphylococcus epidermidis*, diphtheroids, lactobacilli, *Gardnerella vaginalis,* and a variety of anaerobes) rarely cause UTI. The rare exception to this rule are patients with such complicating factors as an infarcted kidney or a necrotic tumor mass that has been invaded by these commensal organisms, particularly the anaerobes. Otherwise, the presence of one or more of these organisms in the urine suggests primarily a contaminated culture.[1,15]

In the adult patient who has urinary symptoms, the presence of pyuria correlates closely with UTI. The measurement of leukocyte esterase activity in the urine may be used as a screening technique, but the preferred method is to examine the unspun urine in a counting chamber, with more than 10 leukocytes/mm^3 being highly associated with true infection. The traditional method of testing for pyuria – by microscopic examination of spun urine – is fraught with error, carrying a high rate of both false positives and false negatives. A similarly useful, "low-technology" approach to the diagnosis of UTI is to examine under a light microscope a Gram stain of unspun urine. The presence of one or more organisms per oil immersion field correlates with the presence of $\geq 10^5$ bacteria/mL or urine (otherwise known as *significant bacteriuria*).[1,2,47,48]

The cornerstone of the diagnostic approach to UTI is the quantitative urine culture. More than four decades ago, Kass[48,49] defined the concept of significant bacteriuria ($> 10^5$ colony-forming units (CFU)/mL of a single uropathogenic species) as an epidemiologic tool for diagnosing "true" infection. However, it is now clear that, in as many as 20–30% of true bacterial UTIs in women with symptoms of infection, lesser numbers of organisms are present in the urine. These women respond appropriately to antibiotic therapy for the particular bacteria identified, just as those with significant bacteriuria do. The quantitative urine culture remains a useful diagnostic tool, however, but the guidelines have been revised, based on careful studies of patients who are symptomatic and respond to antimicrobial intervention:[2,50,51]

1. *Acute, uncomplicated UTI in women.* A diagnostic criterion of $> 10^5$ CFU/mL has a specificity of 99%, but a sensitivity of 51%. Particularly in the symptomatic patient, a more appropriate criterion appears to be $\geq 10^3$ CFU/mL, which has a sensitivity of ~80% and a specificity of ~90%.
2. *Acute urethral syndrome in women* (also called *symptomatic abacteriuria*). This entity is probably a variant of acute, uncomplicated UTI in that symptoms of dysuria and frequency predominate, with two major causes being noted – bacterial infection with the usual uropathogens but with smaller numbers (10^2–10^4 CFU/mL) being present or *Chlamydia trachomatis* infection. Patients from both these groups have pyuria on urinalysis and respond to appropriate antimicrobial therapy. It has

been suggested that those patients with low-count bacteriuria have early UTI, with increasing counts as time passes without therapy. Occasionally, patients with *Neisseria gonorrhoeae* infection or vaginitis will present with symptoms of dysuria and frequency, but cultures and vaginal examinations should permit these individuals to be distinguished from the others. In addition, there is a group of women with similar symptoms but who lack pyuria on urinalysis. These appear not to have a microbial basis to their symptoms, do not respond to antimicrobial therapy, and should be managed symptomatically.

3. *Acute, uncomplicated pyelonephritis in women.* Approximately 80% of patients will have $> 10^5$ CFU/mL in their urine; 10–15% will have 10^4–10^5 CFU/mL in their urine; and the remainder will have $< 10^4$ CFU/mL in their urine. Thus, $\geq 10^4$ CFU/mL of a single uropathogen is the usual requirement for the laboratory diagnosis of acute, uncomplicated pyelonephritis.

4. *Urinary tract infection in men.* A diagnostic threshold of $\geq 10^4$ CFU/mL offers a sensitivity and specificity of $> 90\%$.

5. *Particular infections.* Infections due to *S. saprophyticus* and *Candida* species (as well as other fungal pathogens, presumably) usually have organism counts in the 10^2–10^4 CFU/mL range.

Clinical management of urinary tract infection

Acute, uncomplicated urinary tract infection in women

Patients with this form of UTI are defined by their presenting symptom complex: symptoms of lower urinary tract inflammation (i.e. dysuria, frequency, urgency, or suprapubic discomfort) in the absence of signs and symptoms of vaginitis (vaginal discharge or odor, pruritus, dyspareunia, external dysuria without frequency, and vulvovaginitis on examination). Therapy for this form of UTI has three objectives: eradication of the lower UTI that is producing symptoms, identification of the minority of patients (~ 30%) who have silent renal infection and require more intensive therapy, and eradication of uropathogenic clones from the vaginal and gastrointestinal reservoirs that could produce rapid reinfection of the urinary tract.[52,53]

The cornerstone of therapy for this clinical syndrome in otherwise healthy women is a short course of therapy (3 days) with trimethoprim–sulfamethoxazole, trimethoprim, or a fluoroquinolone (e.g. ofloxacin, ciprofloxacin, and undoubtedly other fluoroquinolones that have not as yet been subjected to rigorous study). β-Lactams appear to be far less effective, both in terms of eliminating the bacteriuria and in clearing the uropathogens of interest from the vaginal and colonic reservoirs, thus predisposing to recurrence. The macrocrystals of nitrofurantoin have

not been studied as rigorously as the other compounds, but currently available information suggests that 3 days of therapy with this compound is not as effective as the recommended compounds, but that 7 days of therapy may yield results similar to those obtained with 3 days of trimethoprim–sulfamethoxazole. Another option would appear to be single-dose fosfomycin therapy. Although, at present, the standard of care is 3 days of trimethoprim–sulfamethoxazole therapy, the specter of resistance looms. If the incidence of resistance in a particular community is > 20%, then a fluoroquinolone would become the empiric (before sensitivity data are known) treatment of choice. Because of the importance of the fluoroquinolones in the treatment of prostatitis and other forms of complicated infection, the recently published guidelines for the management of acute, uncomplicated UTI in women has recommended the use of other drugs in order to delay the emergence of resistance to the fluoroquinolones.[52,53]

Because acute, uncomplicated UTI in healthy women is so common, and the efficacy, cost, and side-effects of short-course therapy so favorable, an efficient approach to such infections that minimizes laboratory studies and visits to the physician can be defined. The first step is to initiate short-course therapy in response to the complaint of dysuria and frequency without symptoms of vaginitis. If a urine specimen is readily available, a leukocyte esterase dipstick test can be carried out (which has a reported sensitivity of 75–96% in this clinical setting); urine culture and microscopic examination of the urine are reserved for the patient with an atypical presentation. Alternatively, a reliable patient who reports a typical clinical presentation by telephone should have short-course therapy prescribed without initial examination of the urine.[1,52,53]

The important patient–physician interaction comes after completion of the therapy: if the patient is asymptomatic, nothing further needs to be done. If the patient is still symptomatic, both urinalysis and urine culture are necessary. If both of these results are negative and no clear microbial cause of symptoms is present, symptomatic relief is prescribed and attention is directed toward sexual practices, gynecologic conditions, personal hygiene, allergy to clothing dyes, and the like. If the patient is pyuric but not bacteriuric, then the differential diagnosis includes *Chlamydia trachomatis* (common in sexually active, reproductively aged individuals), tuberculosis, systemic fungal infection, and intraabdominal inflammatory processes such as a diverticular abscess abutting the urinary tract. The presence of bacteriuria and pyuria should trigger a 10- to 14-day course of therapy, provided that the isolate was sensitive to the drug previously prescribed. If it has been resistant, then another trial of short-course therapy with an appropriate drug would be appropriate.[1,52–58]

Short-course therapy is prescribed for the eradication of superficial mucosal infection of the bladder and is contraindicated in patients with a high probability of tissue-invading infection. The following groups of patients, therefore, should never be considered as candidates for short-course therapy: any man with a UTI (tissue invasion of the prostate, kidney, or both should be assumed, and, as predicted, short-course therapy fails in men more than 80% of the time, even when both groups have identical presenting symptoms); patients with overt pyelonephritis; patients with symptoms of longer than 7 days' duration; patients with underlying structural or functional defects of the urinary tract; immunosuppressed individuals; and patients with indwelling catheters.[1]

Acute, uncomplicated pyelonephritis in women

The clinical syndrome in these patients includes recurrent rigors and fever; back and loin pain (with tenderness on percussion of the costovertebral angle), often with associated colicky abdominal pain; nausea and vomiting; dysuria; and frequency. These individuals, by definition, have invasive tissue infection, have or are at risk for bacteremia, and merit intensive antimicrobial therapy. The three goals of therapy in this group of individuals are control of possible urosepsis (bacteremia and its consequences), eradication of the invading organism, and prevention of recurrences. The therapeutic approach to acute, uncomplicated pyelonephritis can be divided into two parts: immediate control and final eradication of the process.[1,2]

The initial antimicrobial program prescribed should have a > 99% probability of being effective against the infecting organism. A urine Gram stain should be part of the initial evaluation. If a Gram-positive organism is responsible, then ampicillin or amoxicillin/clavulanic acid therapy would be reasonable. More likely would be a Gram-negative bacillus, with a variety of regimens then being useful: a fluoroquinolone, a β-lactam/aminoglycoside combination, or an advanced spectrum β-lactam alone (e.g. imipenem, ceftazidime, or piperacillin/tazobactam) can be prescribed to achieve this goal. Although parenteral therapy is usually prescribed to ensure the prompt achievement of therapeutic blood levels, it should be recognized that, in patients with milder disease who are free of nausea and vomiting, advantage can be taken of the excellent antimicrobial spectrum and oral bioavailability with oral administration (provided that the gastrointestinal tract is functioning adequately) of drugs such as fluoroquinolones and trimethoprim–sulfamethoxazole to employ oral therapy throughout the course of the treatment. At the present time, provided adequate blood levels are achieved, there is no evidence that any one of the regimens listed is better than any other in terms of accomplishing the first task – initial control of systemic sepsis.[1,2,52,53]

Following the establishment of control over sepsis, usually signaled by the temperature curve returning to a near normal level, oral therapy can be instituted. Failure of this to occur within 72 h of initiating therapy should trigger a search for some complicating problem – a stone, obstruction from any cause, poor bladder function, etc. Once evidence of improvement has occurred, prescription of trimethoprim–sulfamethoxazole or a fluoroquinolone to complete a 14-day course of therapy appears to be the most effective means of eradicating both tissue infection and residual clones of uropathogen present in the gastrointestinal tract, which could cause early recurrence if left in place.[1,2,52,53]

Urinary tract infection in pregnancy

Pregnant women constitute the one group in whom screening for asymptomatic bacteriuria – and subsequent treatment, if found – is justified to prevent adverse consequences for both mother and fetus: a risk of symptomatic pyelonephritis later in pregnancy that can induce premature onset of labor and delivery; some experts have attributed increased fetal loss and prematurity to UTI in the mother as well. Treatment of either asymptomatic infection or infection associated with symptoms of bladder inflammation is similar to that for nonpregnant women with acute, uncomplicated UTI, i.e. short-course therapy. However, there are two major differences in the overall management when compared with the management of nonpregnant women with UTIs: (1) the drugs that can be used safely are somewhat limited because of toxicity issues; and (2) continuing follow-up throughout pregnancy with treatment and prophylaxis instituted for positive cultures is indicated.[59]

There is extensive experience with sulfonamides, nitrofurantoin, ampicillin, and cephalexin in the treatment of UTI during pregnancy, with sulfonamides being avoided near term because of their possible contribution to the development of kernicterus in the newborn. Fluoroquinolones are avoided because of possible adverse effects on fetal cartilage developments. In pregnant women with overt pyelonephritis, hospital admission and parenteral therapy with β-lactam drugs and aminoglycosides should be considered the standard of care.[1]

Recurrent urinary tract infection in women

The great majority of recurrent UTIs in women of all ages are due to reinfection. The first steps in preventing such infections do not involve the use of antimicrobial agents. They do include voiding immediately after sexual intercourse and changing contraceptive practice to one in which a spermicide (which eliminates the normal protective flora in the vagina, increasing the potential for colonization with a uropathogen) is not required (e.g. from a diaphragm to oral contraceptives).[1,37–40] In postmenopausal women, two further measures have been shown to be of value: (1) local or systemic estrogen replacement, which will change the pH of the vagina, promotes the reappearance of the normal flora (particularly the lactobacilli) and protects against colonization with uropathogens;[60] and (2) ingestion of moderate amounts of cranberry or blueberry juice, which has been shown to have a marked protective effect against UTI owing to the secretion in the urine and the vagina of organic molecules that block the critical interaction of uropathogen surface adhesions to epithelial receptors – the first step in the invasion of the anatomically normal urinary tract.[61–63] Although the data supporting the use of cranberry juice have come primarily from studies of postmenopausal women, our anecdotal experience with reproductively aged women suggests efficacy in this population as well.

Despite the institution of the previously listed maneuvers, there remains a group of otherwise healthy women who are subject to recurrent symptomatic infection. A small minority of these will have recurrent infection owing to a sequestered focus within the kidney that causes relapsing infection after courses of therapy of ≤ 14 days. Such relapsing infections deserve at least one attempt at cure with an extended course (4–6 weeks) of therapy, preferably with trimethoprim–sulfamethoxazole or a fluoroquinolone to which the infecting organism is susceptible. If some predisposing factor such as a renal calculus is present, the intensive antimicrobial therapy should be carried out in conjunction with correction of the underlying abnormality. Patients with relapsing symptomatic infection that only derives temporary benefit from extended treatment courses usually can be kept symptom free with long-term suppressive therapy.[1]

The great majority of women (at least 85%) with recurrent UTI have repeated reinfection. There are basically three antimicrobial strategies that are effective in this situation:

1. Low-dose, long-term prophylaxis with either trimethoprim–sulfamethoxazole (one or two tablets) or a fluoroquinolone (e.g. ciprofloxacin 250 mg or ofloxacin 200 mg) at bed time. The efficacy of these prophylactic regimens is further delineated by their effectiveness in preventing UTI in the more challenging population of kidney transplant recipients.
2. A variant of continuous prophylaxis is for the woman to take a single dose of a fluoroquinolone or trimethoprim–sulfamethoxazole as postcoital prophylaxis.
3. Finally, many of these women prefer not to take antimicrobial drugs so continuously. These women may be given a supply of drug (again, either a fluoroquinolone or trimethoprim–sulfamethoxazole is preferable over other classes of drug in terms of efficacy) for single-dose therapy with the onset of symptoms of UTI.[1,54,64–67]

Urinary tract infection in men

UTI in men should always be assumed to mean tissue invasion of the prostate, kidney, or both. Thus, the standard of care is 10–14 days of fluoroquinolone or trimethoprim–sulfamethoxazole unless antimicrobial intolerance or an unusual pathogen requires an alternative approach. In men younger than 50 years, the following conditions are associated with an increased risk of UTI: anal intercourse, intercourse with women colonized with uropathogens, and AIDS with a CD4 lymphocyte count of < 200/mm^3. Men without one of these risk factors, particularly those with recurrent infection after an appropriate treatment course, merit a urologic evaluation as well as a more intensive treatment course: 4–6 weeks at a minimum.

Recurrent infection in men usually connotes a sustained focus within the prostate that is difficult to eradicate for one or more of the following reasons: many antimicrobial agents do not diffuse well across the prostatic epithelium into the prostatic fluid, where the infection lies; the prostate may harbor calculi, which can block drainage of portions of the prostate gland or act as foreign bodies around which persistent infection can be hidden; and an enlarged (and inflamed) prostate gland can cause bladder outlet obstruction, resulting in incomplete emptying and difficulty in eradicating infection.[1,2,13,68,69]

Complicated urinary tract infection

The term complicated UTI is used to describe a heterogeneous group of patients who have a wide variety of underlying structural and functional defects of the urinary tract. As a consequence, the range of organisms causing UTI is much greater than that for the general population, and antimicrobial resistance is common. As a result, the therapeutic principles employed in this patient population are somewhat different from those for other patient groups. In general, asymptomatic bacteriuria should not be treated, the major exception being when the bacteriuric patient is scheduled to undergo urinary tract manipulation – in this circumstance, sterilization of the urine before manipulation and continuation of antimicrobial therapy for 3–7 days after manipulation can prevent urosepsis.[1,2]

Acutely septic patients with complicated UTI merit initial broad-spectrum therapy (e.g. ampicillin plus gentamicin, imipenem/cilastin, piperacillin/tazobactam) until bacteriologic data are available and permit a more precise choice of therapy. For more subacutely ill individuals, a fluoroquinolone appears to be optimal initial therapy. In conjunction with antimicrobial therapy, thought should be given to correcting the abnormalities that led to the infection, whenever possible. If this can be accomplished, a prolonged 4- to 6-week "curative" course of therapy in conjunction with the surgical manipulation is appropriate. If such correction is not possible, shorter courses of therapy (7–14 days), aimed at controlling the symptoms, appear to be more reasonable. Spinal cord injury patients represent a particular challenge. In these patients, intermittent self-catheterization with clean catheters and methenamine prophylaxis has been shown to decrease the morbidity associated with UTI in this population.[1,2,13,70]

Candidal infection of the urinary tract

Candidal UTI has become increasingly common in recent years, particularly in individuals who are diabetic, have bladder catheters in place, and are receiving corticosteroids. Well-validated guidelines for managing candidal UTI are not available, particularly criteria for distinguishing trivial colonization from clinically significant infection. The following represents the approach we take at present, pending the availability of more data:[1,2,71,72]

1. The first step is the correction of the underlying conditions that led to the infection in the first place: removal of the catheter, correction of the hyperglycemia, cessation of broad-spectrum antibacterial therapy, and marked reduction in corticosteroid dose, if possible. Once these are accomplished, if candiduria is persistent, then further therapy can be considered.

2. If an indwelling bladder catheter is still required, it is reasonable to insert a three-way catheter and administer an amphotericin or a nystatin rinse to the bladder – this has an efficacy rate of ~ 50–60%. However, if a catheter is not required, it is far better to treat with systemic antifungal therapy to avoid the risk of other organisms being introduced because of the catheter.

3. Fluconazole, at a dose of 200–400 mg/day, is an effective therapy for candidal UTI caused by *Candida albicans, C. tropicalis,* and most of the other candidal species because of the extremely high concentrations that are delivered into the urine. The two organisms associated with fluconazole failure are *Candida krusei* and *Candida glabrata.*

4. In individuals who do not respond to fluconazole, the combination of low-dose systemic amphotericin (e.g. 10 mg/day) plus flucytosine at full doses (100 mg/kg/day in three or four divided doses) is quite effective when prescribed for a 10- to 14-day course. Flucytosine administered alone results in the rapid emergence of resistance, so the role of the low-dose amphotericin (which poorly penetrates the urine) is primarily to "protect" the flucytosine, which reaches quite high concentrations in the urine.

Summary

Improved understanding of the pathogenesis and impact of UTI has led to improved therapy. Perhaps the most important lessons of the past few decades are the following:

1. The normal vaginal flora in women is an important host defense against the occurrence of UTI, and strategies to reconstitute it (e.g. elimination of spermicides in premenopausal women and estrogen replacement in postmenopausal women) can be quite effective in preventing recurrent UTI.

2. The critical first step in the pathogenesis of UTI is adherence to the uroepithelium through the specific interaction of bacterial surface adhesions to specific receptors on the epithelial cell, and such strategies as the ingestion of cranberry juice (which delivers organic substances to the site that blocks such adhesions) can help prevent UTI.

3. Different clinical syndromes associated with UTI require different modes of antimicrobial prescription, although the optimal drugs for the treatment and prevention of UTI are trimethoprim–sulfamethoxazole and the fluoroquinolones.

4. In this regard, tissue-invasive infection (as all UTI in men should be assumed to be) needs more extended therapy than acute, uncomplicated UTI in women, for which the cornerstone of treatment is short-course therapy (3 days).

References

1. Rubin RH, Cotran RS, Tolkoff-Rubin NE: Urinary tract infection, pyelonephritis, and reflux nephropathy. *In* Brenner BM (ed): Brenner & Rector's The Kidney, 5th edn. Philadelphia: WB Saunders, 1996, pp 1597–1654.
2. Rubin RH, Shapiro ED, Andriole VT, et al: Evaluation of new anti-infective drugs for the treatment of urinary tract infection. Clin Infect Dis 1992;15(Suppl 1):S216–S227.
3. Hooton TM, Stamm WE: Management of acute uncomplicated urinary tract infection in adults. Med Clin North Am 1991;75:339.
4. Hooton TM, Scholes D, Hughes JP, et al: A prospective study of risk factors for symptomatic urinary tract infection in young women. N Engl J Med 1996;335:468–474.
5. Hansson S, Martinell J, Stokland E, Jodal U: The natural history of bacteriuria in childhood. Infect Dis Clin North Am 1997;11:499–512.
6. Gillenwater JY, Harrison RB, Kunin CM: Natural history of bacteriuria in school girls. A long-term case–control study. N Engl J Med 1979;301:396–399.
7. Bullen M, Kincaid-Smith P: Asymptomatic pregnancy bacteriuria: a follow-up study 4–7 years after delivery. *In* Kinkaid-Smith PK, Failey KF (eds): Renal Infection and Renal Scarring, 2nd edn. Melbourne: Mercedes, 1970, p 33.
8. Gower PE, Haswell B, Sidaway ME, et al: Follow-up of 164 patients with bacteriuria of pregnancy. Lancet 1968;1:990–994.
9. Asscher AW, Chick S, Radford N, et al: Natural history of asymptomatic bacteriuria in non-pregnant women. *In* Brumfitt W, Asscher AW (eds): Urinary Tract Infection. London: Oxford University Press, 1973, pp 51–61.
10. Dontas AS, Kasviki-Charvati P, Panayiotis CL, et al: Bacteriuria and survival in old age. N Engl J Med 1981;304:939–943.
11. Boscia JA, Abrutyn E, Kaya D: Asymptomatic bacteriuria in elderly persons. Treat or do not treat? Ann Intern Med 1987;106:764–766.
12. Boscia JA, Kay D: Asymptomatic bacteriuria in the elderly. Infect Dis Clin North Am 1987;3:1893–1905.
13. Lipsky BA: Urinary tract infections in men: epidemiology, pathophysiology, diagnosis, and treatment. Ann Intern Med 1989;100:138–150.
14. Roberts AP, Phillips R: Bacteria causing symptomatic urinary tract infection or bacteriuria. J Clin Pathol 1979;32:492–496.
15. Svanborg-Eden C, Hagberg L, Hanson LA, et al: Adhesion of *Escherichia coli* in urinary tract infection. Ciba Found Symp 1981;80:161–187.
16. Johnson JR, Orskov I, Orskov F, et al: O, K, and H antigens predict virulence factors, carboxylesterase B pattern, antimicrobial resistance and host compromise among *Escherichia coli* strains causing urosepsis. J Infect Dis 1994;169:119–126.
17. Dennenberg MS, Welsh RA: Virulence determinants of uropathogenic *Escherichia coli*. *In* Urinary Tract Infections: Molecular Pathogenesis and Clinical Management, Vol 4. Washington DC: American Society for Microbiology, 1996, pp 80–128.
18. Bjorksten B, Kaijser B: Interaction of human serum and neutrophils with *Escherichia coli* strains: differences between strains isolated from urine of patients with pyelonephritis or asymptomatic bacteriuria. Infect Immun 1978;22:308–311.
19. Johnson JR, Moseley SL, Roberts PL, et al: Aerobactin and other virulence factor genes among strains of *E. coli*. Infect Immun 1983;40:265–272.
20. Hull R, Hull SI: Nutritional requirements for growth of uropathogenic *Escherichia coli* in human urine. Infect Immun 1997;65:1960–1961.
21. Plos K, Connell H, Jodal U, et al: Intestinal carriage of P-fimbriated *Escherichia coli* and susceptibility to urinary tract infections in young children. J Infect Dis 1995;171:625–631.
22. Svanborg-Eden C, Gotschlich EC, Korhonen TK, et al: Aspects of structure and function of pili of uropathogenic *E. coli*. Prog Allergy 1983;33:189–202.
23. Iwahi T, Abe Y, Nakao M, et al: Role of type 1 fimbriae in the pathogenesis of ascending urinary tract infection induced by *Escherichia coli* in mice. Infect Immun 1983;40:265–315.
24. Hagberg L, Hull S, Hull R, et al: Contribution of adhesin to bacterial persistence in the mouse urinary tract. Infect Immun 1983;40:265–272.
25. Svanborg-Eden C, Eriksson B, Hanson LA: Adhesion of *Escherichia coli* to human uroepithelial cells in vitro. Infect Immun 1977;18:767–774.
26. Kallenius G, Molby R, Svensson SB, et al: Occurrence of P-fimbriated *Escherichia coli* in urinary tract infections. Lancet 1981;2:1369–1372.

27. Leffler H, Svanborg-Eden C: Glycolipid receptors for uropathogenic *Escherichia coli* binding to human erythrocytes and uroepithelial cells. Infect Immun 1981;34:920–929.
28. Johnson JR: Virulence factors in *Escherichia coli* urinary tract infection. Clin Microbiol Rev 1991;4:80–128.
29. Agace W, Hedges S, Andersson U, et al: Selective cytokine production by epithelial cells following exposure to *Escherichia coli*. Infect Immun 1993;61:602–609.
30. Hedges S, Agace W, Svanborg C: Epithelial cytokine responses and mucosal cytokine networks. Trends Microbiol 1995;3:266–270.
31. Pere A, Nowicki B, Saxen H, et al: Expression of P_1 type-1 and type 1_c fimbriae of *Escherichia coli* in the urine of patients with acute urinary tract infection. J Infect Dis 1987;156:567–574.
32. Nowicki B, Labigne A, Moseley S, et al: The Dr hemagglutinin, afimbrial adhesins AFA-1 and AFA-III, and F1845 fimbriae of uropathogenic and diarrhea-associated *Escherichia coli* belong to a family of hemagglutinins with Dr receptor recognition. Infect Immun 1990;58:279–281.
33. Goluszka P, Popov V, Selvarangan R: Dr Fimbriae operon of uropathogenic *Escherichia coli* mediate microtubule dependent invasion to the HeLa epithelial cell line. J Infect Dis 1997;176:158–167.
34. Zafriri D, Gron Y, Eisenstein BI, et al: Growth advantages and enhanced toxicity of *Escherichia coli* adherent to tissue culture cells due to restricted diffusion of products secreted by the cells. J Clin Invest 1987;79:1210–1216.
35. Manges AR, Johnson JR, Foxman B, et al: Widespread distribution of urinary tract infection caused by a multidrug-resistant *Escherichia coli* clonal group. N Engl J Med 2001;345:1007–1013.
36. Stamm WE: An epidemic of urinary tract infections? N Engl J Med 2001;345:1055–1057.
37. Hooton TM, Hillier S, Johnson C, et al: *Escherichia coli* bacteriuria and contraceptive method. JAMA 1991;265:64–69.
38. Strom BL, Collins M, West SL, et al: Sexual activity, contraceptive use, and other risk factors for systematic and asymptomatic bacteriuria: a case–control study. Ann Intern Med 1987;107:816–823.
39. Fihn SD, Latham RH, Roberts P, et al: Association between diaphragm use and urinary tract infection. JAMA 1985;254:240–245.
40. Stamm WE, Hooton TM: Management of urinary tract infections in adults. N Engl J Med 1993;329:1328–1334.
41. Raz R, Stamm WE: A controlled trial of intravaginal estriol in postmenopausal women with recurrent urinary tract infections. N Engl J Med 1993;329:753–756.
42. Sheinfeld J, Schaeffer AJ, Cordon-Cardo C, et al: Association of the Lewis blood group phenotype with recurrent urinary tract infections in women. N Engl J Med 1989;320:773–777.
43. Jantousch BA, Criss VR, O'Donnell, et al: Association of Lewis blood group phenotypes with urinary tract infection in children. J Pediatr 1994;124:863–868.
44. Navas EL, Venegas MF, Duncan JL, et al: Blood group antigen expression on vaginal cells and mucus in women with and without a history of urinary tract infections. J Urol 1994;152:345–349.
45. Hooton TM, Scholes D, Hughes JP, et al: A prospective of risk factors for symptomatic urinary tract infections in young women. N Engl J Med 1996;335:468–474.
46. Pollack HM: Laboratory techniques for detection of urinary tract infection and assessment of value. Am J Med 1983;75(18):79–84.
47. Stamm WE: Measurement of pyuria and its relation to bacteriuria. Am J Med 1983;75:53–58.
48. Kass EH: Bacteriuria and the diagnosis of infections of the urinary tract: with observations on the use of methionine as a urinary antiseptic. Arch Intern Med 1957;100:709–714.
49. Savage WE, Hajj SN, Kass EH: Demographic and prognostic characteristics of bacteriuria in pregnancy. Medicine (Baltimore) 1967;46:385–407.
50. Stamm WE, Wagner KF, Amsel R, et al: Causes of the acute urethral syndrome in women. N Engl J Med 1980;303:409–415.
51. Stamm WE, Counts GW, Running KR, et al: Diagnosis of coliform infection in acutely dysuric women. N Engl J Med 1982;307:463–468.
52. Warren JW, Abrutyn E, Hebel JR, et al: Guidelines for antimicrobial treatment of uncomplicated acute bacterial cystitis and acute pyelonephritis in women. Clin Infect Dis 1999;29:745–758.
53. Saint S, Scholes D, Fihn SD, et al: The effectiveness of a clinical practice guideline for the management of pressured uncomplicated urinary tract infection in women. Am J Med 1999;106:636–641.
54. Stamm WE, Hooton TM: Management of urinary tract infections in adults. N Engl J Med 1993;329:1328–1334.
55. Johnson JR, Stamm WE: Urinary tract infections in women: diagnosis and treatment. Ann Intern Med 1989;111:906–917.
56. Inter-Nordic Urinary Tract Infection Study Group: Double-blind comparison of 3-day versus 7-day treatment with norfloxacin in symptomatic urinary tract infections. Scand J Infect Dis 1988;20:619.
57. Hooton TM, Johnson C, Winter C, et al: Single dose and three day regimens of ofloxacin versus trimethoprim–sulfamethoxazole for acute cystitis in women. Antimicrob Agents Chemother 1991;35:1479–1483.
58. Norrby SR: Short term treatment of uncomplicated lower urinary tract infection in women. Rev Infect Dis 1990;12:458–467.
59. Zinner SH: Management of urinary tract infections in pregnancy: a review with comments on single dose therapy. Infection 1992;20 (Suppl 4):S280–S285.
60. Raz R, Stamm WE: A controlled trial of intravaginal estriol in postmenopausal women with recurrent urinary tract infections. N Engl J Med 1993;329:753–756.
61. Avorn J, Monane M, Gurwitz JH, et al: Reduction of bacteriuria and pyuria after ingestion of cranberry juice. JAMA 1994;271:751–754.
62. Zafriri D, Ofek I, Adar R, et al: Inhibitory activity of cranberry juice on adherence of type 1 and P fimbriated *Escherichia coli* to eukaryotic cells. Antimicrob Agents Chemother 1989;33:92–98.
63. Ofek I, Goldhar J, Zafriri D, et al: Anti-*Escherichia* adhesin activity of cranberry and blueberry juices. N Engl J Med 1991;324:1599.
64. Ronald AR, Harding GKM: Urinary infection prophylaxis in women. Ann Intern Med 1981;9:268–270.
65. Harding GKM, Buckwald FJ, Marrie TJ, et al: Prophylaxis of recurrent urinary tract infection in female patients: efficacy of low dose, thrice weekly therapy with trimethoprim–sulfamethoxazole. JAMA 1979;242:1975–1977.
66. Stapleton A, Latham RH, Johnson C, Stamm WE: Postcoital antimicrobial prophylaxis for recurrent urinary tract infection: a randomized, double-blind, placebo-controlled trial. JAMA 1990;264:703–706.
67. Wong ES, McKevitt M, Running K, et al: Management of recurrent urinary tract infections with patient-administered single dose therapy. Ann Intern Med 1985;102:302–307.
68. Wong ES, Stamm WE: Sexual acquisition of urinary tract infection in a man. JAMA 1983;250:3087–3088.
69. Hoepelman AI, van Buren M, van den Broek J, Borleffs JC: Bacteriuria in men infected with HIV-1 is related to their immune status (CD4+ cell count). AIDS 1992;6:179–184.
70. Abrutyn E, Mossey J, Berlin JA, et al: Does asymptomatic bacteriuria predict mortality and does antimicrobial treatment reduce mortality in elderly ambulatory women? Ann Intern Med 1994;120:827–833.
71. Jacobs LG, Skidmore EA, Cardoso LA, Ziv F: Bladder irrigation with amphotericin B for treatment of fungal urinary tract infections. Clin Infect Dis 1994;18:313–318.
72. Hibberd PH, Rubin RH: Clinical aspects of fungal infection in organ transplant recipients. Clin Infect Dis 1994;19 (Suppl 1):S33–S40.

Primary Neoplasms of the Kidney

Marc B. Garnick

Carcinoma of the kidney is perhaps one of the most enigmatic of cancers. The myriad presenting features, which include paraneoplastic phenomena, can challenge the most astute diagnostician.[1–3] The disease is typically diagnosed during the sixth and seventh decade with a male–female ratio of 2:1. Each year, it is estimated that there will be 30 000 newly diagnosed cases with an estimated 12 000 deaths.[4,5] Today, many renal cancers can be diagnosed at early, and potentially curable, stages owing to the more widespread use of ultrasound and computed tomography (CT) of the abdomen, which may pick up early, asymptomatic lesions of the kidney. Most malignant cancers of the kidney are adenocarcinomas; other pathologic varieties include transitional carcinomas of the renal pelvis and Wilms tumor in children.[6]

Risk factors

Risk factors for the development of renal cancer include cigarette smoking, occupational exposure to cadmium, obesity, excessive exposure to analgesics, acquired cystic disease in dialysis patients, adult polycystic kidney disease, and other industrial exposures, such as asbestos, leather tanning, and certain petroleum products. Genetic and familial forms of the disease occur, most notably with von Hippel–Lindau disease, an autosomal dominant disease characterized by the development of multiple tumors of the central nervous system, pheochromocytomas, and bilateral renal carcinomas.[7] Several families have also been reported with a high incidence of renal cancer. Genetic analyses of these patients demonstrate a balanced translocation between the short arm of chromosome 3 and either chromosome 6 or chromosome 8. Tuberous sclerosis may also be associated with a risk of developing renal cell cancer, but this is considerably less than that of von Hippel–Lindau disease. Other abnormalities have been reported.[8]

More recent genetic advances have identified the *RASSF1* gene, a Ras association family 1 gene, which may possess tumor-suppressor activity. In one study, abnormalities of this gene were identified in a high percentage of patients with primary clear-cell cancers.[9]

Presentation

Patients with renal cell cancer present with symptoms produced by the local neoplasm, with signs and symptoms of paraneoplastic phenomena, or by other aspects of systemic disease. Likewise, the patient may be totally asymptomatic and may be diagnosed by a radiologic abnormality detected on ultrasound or abdominal CT scanning. Fewer than 10% of patients present with the classic triad of hematuria, abdominal mass, and flank pain. The most common features include hematuria (70%), flank pain (50%), palpable mass (20%), fever (15%), and erythrocytosis (infrequent). Other features may include acute onset of lower extremity edema, or, in males, the presence of a left-sided varicocele, indicating an obstruction of the left gonadal vein at its point of entry into the left renal vein by a tumor thrombus. Other paraneoplastic/systemic manifestations include liver function abnormalities, high-output congestive failure, cachexia, fever, amyloidosis, anemia erythrocytosis, thrombocytosis, hypercalcemia, and manifestations of the secretion of substances such as prostaglandins, renin, glucocorticoids, and cytokines such as interleukin 6.

At presentation, a very small percentage of tumors are bilateral, whereas almost one-third of patients have demonstrable metastatic disease in almost any organ of the body. Most common sites of metastases include lung, bone, liver, and brain, but other sites such as the thyroid may be affected.

Pathology

In the past, renal carcinomas were divided pathologically into a classification that evaluated cell type and growth pattern. The former included clear-cell, spindle, and oncocytic types, whereas the latter included acinar, papillary, or sarcomatoid varieties. This classification has undergone a transformation to more accurately reflect the morphology and the histochemical and molecular bases of different types of adenocarcinomas.[10,11] Based on these studies, five distinct carcinoma types have been identified, including clear-cell (75–85% of tumors), chromophilic (15%), chromophobic (5%), oncocytic (uncommon), and collecting (Bellini's) duct (very rare) varieties. Each of these carcinoma types has a unique growth pattern, cell of origin, and cytogenetic characteristics. Table 42.1 summarizes this information and more accurately reflects

Table 42.1 Pathologic classification of renal cell carcinoma*

Carcinoma type	Growth pattern	Cell of origin	Cytogenetic characteristics Major	Minor	Incidence (%)
Clear cell	Acinar or sarcomatoid	Proximal tubule	3p–	+5, +7, +12, –6q,–8p, –9, –14q, –Y	75–85
Chromophilic[†]	Papillary or sarcomatoid	Proximal tubule	+7, +17, –Y	+12, +16, +20, –14	12–14
Chromophobic	Solid, tubular, or sarcomatoid	Intercalated cell of cortical collecting duct[‡]	Hypodiploid	–	4–6
Oncocytic	Typified by tumor nests	Intercalated cell of cortical collecting duct	Undetermined	–	2–4
Collecting duct	Papillary or sarcomatoid	Medullary collecting duct	Undetermined	–	1

*From Motzer RJ, Bander NH, Nanus DM: Renal-cell carcinoma. N Engl J Med 1996;335:865–875. Copyright 1996 Massachusetts Medical Society. All rights reserved.
[†]These tumors were previously classified as papillary tumors.
[‡]This classification is based on the work of Storkel and associates.[10]

the increased knowledge on molecular and genetic abnormalities of these lesions.

Diagnostic evaluation and staging

Evidence from the history or physical examination that suggests a renal abnormality should be followed by either an intravenous pyelogram or abdominal ultrasound. Often, however, evidence of a space-occupying lesion in the kidney is found incidentally during radiographic testing for other, unrelated conditions for which an ultrasound or abdominal CT scan is performed. Indeed, renal cancer, once dubbed the "internist's tumor" because of its multiple manifestations at presentation, can now be called the "radiologist's tumor" because many lesions are detected during radiographic evaluations. Renal ultrasound may help to distinguish simple cysts from more complex abnormalities. A simple cyst is defined sonographically by a lack of internal echoes, the presence of smooth borders, and the transmission of the ultrasound wave. If these three features exist, a benign cyst is most likely to be present. At one time, cyst puncture was utilized but seems to be unnecessary today in the asymptomatic patient without hematuria. Periodic repeat ultrasounds are suggested for follow-up. If a change occurs in the lesion, cyst puncture, needle aspiration, or CT scanning should be considered to further evaluate the lesion.

If the criteria for a simple sonographic cyst are not met, or the intravenous pyelogram suggests a solid or complex mass, a CT scan should be performed. If a renal neoplasm is demonstrated by CT scanning, renal vein or caval involvement should be assessed by CT scan or by magnetic resonance imaging. Although used frequently in the past, selective renal arteriography has assumed a more limited use, mainly in further evaluating the renal vasculature in patients who are to undergo partial nephrectomy ("nephron-sparing" surgery). CT scanning is also very helpful in determining the presence of lymphadenopathy.

Figure 42.1 illustrates a modern-day algorithm for the diagnostic evaluation of a renal mass.

The differential diagnosis of a renal mass detected on a CT scan includes primary renal cancers, metastatic lesions to the kidney, and benign lesions. The latter include angiomyolipomas (renal hamartomas), oncocytomas, and other rare unusual growths. If a renal cancer is considered based on the radiographic studies of the kidney, the patient should undergo a preoperative staging evaluation to assess the presence of metastases in the lung, bone, or brain. The operative and diagnostic approach may be dictated dependent on the preoperative stage of the patient. For example, the patient who presents with stage IV disease by virtue of a positive bone scan may need only a needle biopsy of either the kidney lesion or the bone lesion to establish the tissue diagnosis and thus avoid more extensive surgery on the kidney. In contrast, a patient with an isolated pulmonary lesion may be considered for both a nephrectomy and a pulmonary nodulectomy at one operative intervention.

Renal cell cancer can be staged using one of two systems that are in common use.[6] The tumor–node–metastasis (TNM) system has the advantage of being more specific but has the disadvantage of being cumbersome; a modification of the Robson staging system is more practical and more widely used in the USA. In this latter system, stage I represents cancer that is confined to the kidney capsule; stage II indicates invasion through the renal capsule, but not beyond Gerota's fascia; stage III reflects involvement of regional lymph nodes and the ipsilateral renal vein or the vena cava; and stage IV indicates the presence of distant metastases. Table 42.2 illustrates both systems. Other, newer staging systems utilized by the Eastern Cooperative Oncology Group have integrated the TNM classification with other variables such as performance status and histologic grade of the tumor. These systems provide prognostic categories and more accurately predict 2- and 5-year survival rates.[12,13]

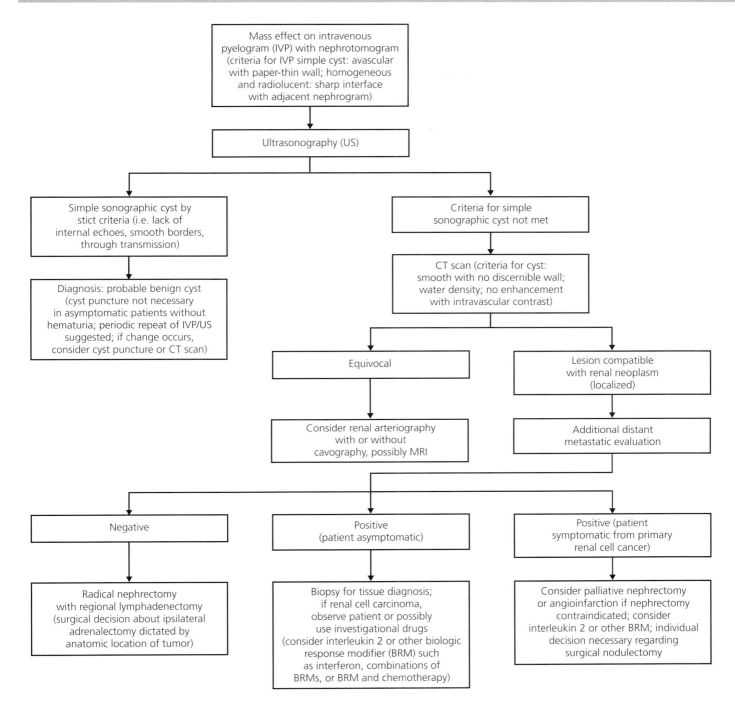

Figure 42.1 Algorithm for the diagnostic evaluation of a renal mass. (Modified from Garnick MB, Brenner BM: Tumors of the Urinary Tract. *In* Isselbacher KJ, Braumwald E, Wilson JD, et al (eds): Harrison's Principles of Internal Medicine, 13th edn. New York: McGraw Hill, 1994, p 1337.)

Clinical trials and specific recommendations

The standard therapy for localized renal cell carcinoma is radical nephrectomy, which includes removal of the kidney, Gerota's fascia, the ipsilateral adrenal gland, and regional hilar lymph nodes. The value of an extended hilar lymphadenectomy seems to be related to its ability to provide prognostic information because there is rarely a therapeutic reason for performing this portion of the operation. In the past, the removal of the ipsilateral adrenal gland was performed routinely; however, most data suggest that it is involved in fewer than 5% of cases and occurs most frequently with large upper pole lesions.[14] Therefore, ipsilateral adrenalectomy is reserved for patients with glands that appear to be abnormal or enlarged on CT scan or for those patients with large upper pole renal lesions, in whom the probability of

425

Table 42.2 Comparison of modified Robson and TNM staging systems for renal adenocarcinoma*

Modified Robson stage		T	N	M
I	Confined by renal capsule	T1 (small)	N0	M0
		T2 (large)		
II	Through renal capsule confined by Gerota's fascia	T3a	N0	M0
IIIa	Renal vein involvement	T3b	N0	M0
IIIb	Lymphatic involvement	T1–3b	N1–4	M0
IV	Contiguous organ involvement	T1–3b	N0–4	M0
	or			
	Metastatic spread	T1–3b	N0–4	M1

*From McDougal WS, Garnick MB: Clinical signs and symptoms of kidney cancer. *In* Vogelzang NJ, Scardino PT, Shipley WU, et al (eds): Comprehensive Textbook of Genitourinary Oncology. Baltimore: Williams & Wilkins, 1996, p 546.
TNM, tumor–node–metastasis.

direct extension of the tumor to the adrenal gland is more likely.

The surgical technique of performing a partial nephrectomy (nephron-sparing surgery) has become more popular, especially for patients with small tumors, for those at risk of developing bilateral tumors, or for patients in whom the contralateral kidney is at risk for other systemic diseases such as diabetes or hypertension.[15,16] The main concern associated with partial nephrectomy is the likelihood of tumor recurrence in the operated kidney because many renal cancers may be multicentric. Local recurrence rates of 4–10% have been reported, and even lower rates have been reported when a partial nephrectomy was performed for smaller lesions (< 3 cm with a normal contralateral kidney). Lesions that are centrally located, however, still require a radical nephrectomy. Frequent follow-up, usually with a CT scan or ultrasound, is necessary for patients who undergo a partial nephrectomy.

Renal cancer involving the inferior vena cava occurs more frequently with right-sided tumors and is associated with metastases in almost 50% of patients. Obstruction of the vena cava may lead to the diagnosis; symptoms include abdominal distention with ascites, hepatic dysfunction, nephrotic syndrome, abdominal wall venous collaterals, varicocele, malabsorption, or pulmonary embolus. The anatomic location of the caval thrombus is important prognostically: supradiaphragmatic lesions, which may involve the heart, can be resected, but the prognosis is poor; patients with subdiaphragmatic lesions enjoy a better 5-year survival, but this usually occurs in fewer than 50% of cases.[3] When approaching the surgical management of these patients, a team of specialists is required, especially if a cardiac tumor thrombectomy is contemplated.

The role of surgery in the management of metastatic disease, either at the initial presentation or later, remains controversial. Although most data that support nephrectomy plus metastatectomy are anecdotal, many patients with synchronous renal cell cancer and an isolated pulmonary nodule may be considered for surgical resection of both lesions. Likewise, patients who develop an isolated lesion in the liver or lung some time after the removal of the kidney may also be considered for surgical removal of the metastasis. Nevertheless, even when such vigorous surgery is carried out, most patients do poorly. Additional controversy surrounds the practice of performing a nephrectomy on patients with widespread metastatic disease as a means of potentially improving their response to systemic therapy. Many investigative programs require such resection; at this point, the practice should be considered investigational. However, a patient who does experience an excellent response to systemic therapy should be considered for a nephrectomy following the response. Finally, because many renal tumors can become quite large, consideration should be given to palliative nephrectomy (in the setting of metastatic disease), especially if the patient experiences uncontrollable hematuria or pain or is catabolic secondary to the sheer mass of the tumor.

Systemic management of advanced stages of renal cell cancer

The management of patients either with locally advanced renal cancer or with metastatic disease provides a great challenge to physicians and clinical investigators. Although chemotherapy and hormonal treatments have been studied extensively in patients with metastatic renal cancer, no single treatment protocol or program has been uniformly effective. Therefore, most physicians treating the disease usually rely on novel modalities of treatment, including biologic response modifiers, investigational anticancer agents, differentiation agents (e.g. retinoic acid), vaccines, or gene therapy.

It has been known for a long time that renal cancer may occasionally incite an immune response in the host, leading to spontaneous remissions of cancer. Although rare, this observation has led many to study agents that can augment the body's immune system. The agents that have been studied most extensively include the interferons, interleukins, cytokines, cellular-based therapies, and combinations of the aforementioned.

Interferon therapy with α-, β-, or γ-interferon moieties has led to responses in approximately 12–20% of treated patients.[17,18] Although their effects are numerous, interferons demonstrate antiproliferative activity against renal cell cancers in vitro, are stimulatory to immune cell function, and can modulate the expression of major histocompatibility complex molecules. Although patients' responses have been seen in many anatomic areas, patients who have had a prior nephrectomy with isolated pulmonary metastases and who are otherwise well may enjoy a higher response rate. The duration of the response is usually less than 2 years, although longer lasting remissions have been noted in a few selected patients. Interferons have been combined with other immune modifiers, as well as with chemotherapy agents, with no real improvement in patient outcome in larger scale trials. However, several smaller trials have combined interferon with interleukin 2 (IL-2) chemotherapy agents (e.g. 5-fluorouracil), and the preliminary results have been encouraging in some cases.

In a recent review of the utility of α-interferon, more than 450 patients with advanced renal cancer were studied. Again, there was a relatively short median duration of survival (13 months) and time to progression was less than 5 months. Further stratification of prognostic variables included Karnofsky performance status, lactate dehydrogenase (LDH) values, calcium values, hemoglobin levels, and time from diagnosis to initiation of interferon therapy. Risk assessment provides greater precision in predicting outcomes to treatment.[19]

IL-2 has received a great deal of attention as a potential advance in the treatment of renal cell cancer.[20] This agent enhances both the proliferation and the functioning of lymphocytes involved in antigen recognition and tumor elimination. Initial studies utilized very high doses of IL-2 in association with ex vivo populations of lymphoid cells that grew and matured under the influence of IL-2. These programs, despite early and encouraging therapeutic results, resulted in substantial toxicity, including patient deaths. Unfortunately, the initial encouraging results were not consistently observed in larger scale trials. Efforts have now been directed at selectively manipulating the immune-enhancing features of the treatment, with modification of the toxic effects. In several studies, lower doses of IL-2 *without* the cellular components have resulted in similar results with less toxicity.

The toxicity of IL-2 is related to alterations in vascular permeability, leading to a capillary leak-type syndrome. Although the drug is approved for the management of patients with metastatic renal cell cancer by the Food and Drug Administration, its use should be restricted to patients who can tolerate the side-effect profile and to patients with acceptable cardiac, renal, pulmonary, and hepatic function.

Investigational therapies continue to be studied for renal cell cancer.[21] Many such approaches are under investigation and include novel cytokines such as IL-12, combinations of biologic agents with or without chemo-therapeutic agents, circadian timing of chemotherapy administration, vaccine therapy, various forms of cellular therapy, and gene therapy. Although all of these approaches have a solid scientific preclinical rationale, none, unfortunately, can be considered as standard treatment. The sobering fact remains that almost 50% of patients diagnosed with renal cell cancer die of their disease within 5 years of diagnosis, and a substantial proportion initially present with advanced stages of cancer spread.

Wilms tumor (nephroblastoma) and neuroblastoma

Wilms tumor and neuroblastoma are the two most common pediatric kidney tumors.[2] Wilms tumor is usually found in children younger than 5 years of age and usually presents with abdominal mass, pain, hematuria, elevations in blood pressure, and systemic manifestations (e.g. fever). Genetic alterations of chromosome 11 have been associated with the disease. The diagnosis is usually established by a CT scan or by magnetic resonance imaging, identifying bilaterality in about 5% of patients. Fewer than 20% of patients have metastases at initial presentation; if they are found, metastases are usually in the lung and liver.

Neuroblastoma has many characteristics in common with Wilms tumor, but is characterized by an elevation of catecholamines, vanillylmandelic acid, and homovanillic acid in most patients. Both diseases are highly curable with a multimodal approach utilizing aggressive surgery, multiagent chemotherapy (with or without bone marrow transplantation), and selective use of radiation therapy.

Future directions

Clearly, the most important prognostic feature for a cure in managing renal cell cancers is the stage at which the cancer is diagnosed. Identification of high-risk patient populations, such as those with a strong family history or genetic predisposition, should be attempted in order to allow an earlier diagnosis and a potential cure. However, for most patients, additional research is needed to develop strategies for eradication of metastatic deposits. Further testing of biologic modifiers, gene therapy, and chemo-therapies directed at eliminating neoplastic cells are the ultimate goal, and patients should be encouraged to enter these types of clinical investigations.

References

1. Garnick MB: Bladder, renal and testicular cancer. Sci Am Med 1995;12(ixB):1–5.
2. Shapiro CL, Garnick MB, Kantoff PW: Tumors of the kidney, ureter, and bladder. *In* Bennett JC (ed): Cecil Textbook of Medicine, 20th edn. Philadelphia: WB Saunders, 1996, p 867.
3. McDougal WS, Garnick MB: Clinical signs and symptoms of kidney cancer. *In* Vogelzang NJ, Scardino PT, Shipley WU, et al (eds): Comprehensive Textbook of Genitourinary Oncology. Baltimore: Williams & Wilkins, 1996, p 546.
4. Motzer RJ, Bander NH, Nanus DM: Renal-cell carcinoma. N Engl J Med 1996;335:865–875.

5. Sokoloff MH, deKernion JB, Figlin RA, Belldegrun A: Current management of renal cell carcinoma. CA Cancer J Clin 1996;46:284–302.
6. Beahrs OH, Henson DE, Hutter RVP, et al: Handbook for the Staging of Cancer, 4th edn. Philadelphia: JB Lippincott, 1993.
7. Latif F, Tory K, Gnarra J, et al: Identification of the von Hippel–Lindau tumor suppressor gene. Science 1993; 260:1317–1320.
8. Olsson CA, Sawczuk IS (eds): Urologic cancer. Urol Clin North Am 1993;20(2).
9. Dreijerink K, Braga E, Kuzmin I, et al: The candidate tumor suppressor gene RASSF1A, from human chromosome 3p21.3 is involved in kidney tumorigenesis. Proc Natl Acad Sci USA 2001;98:7504.
10. Storkel S, Stearata PV, Drenckhaln D, Thoenes W: The human chromophobe cell renal carcinoma: its probable relation to intercalated cells of the collecting duct. Virchows Arch B Cell Pathol Incl Mol Pathol 1989;56:237–245.
11. Storkel S, van den Berg E: Morphologic classification of renal cancer. World J Urol 1995;13:153–158.
12. Zisman A, Pantuck A, Dorey F, et al: Improved prognostication of renal cell carcinoma using an integrated staging system. J Clin Oncol 2001;19:1649.
13. Motzer RJ, Mazumdar M, Bacik J, et al: Survival and prognostic stratification of 670 patients with advanced renal cell carcinoma. J Clin Oncol 1999;17:2530.
14. Shalev M, Cipolla B, Guille F, et al: Is ipsilateral adrenalectomy a necessary component of radical nephrectomy? J Urol 1995;153:1415–1417.
15. Licht MR, Novick AC, Goormastic M: Nephron sparing surgery in incidental versus suspected renal cell carcinoma. J Urol 1994;152:39–42.
16. Thrasher JB, Paulson DF: Prognostic factors in renal cancer. Urol Clin North Am 1993;20:247–262.
17. Nanus DM, Pfeffer LM, Bander NH, et al: Antiproliferative and antitumor effects of alpha-interferon in renal cell carcinomas: correlation with the expression of a kidney-associated differentiation glycoprotein. Cancer Res 1990;50:4190–4194.
18. Minasian LM, Motzer RJ, Gluck L, et al: Interferon alpha-2a in advanced renal cell carcinoma: treatment results and survival in 159 patients with long-term follow-up. J Clin Oncol 1993;11:1368–1375.
19. Motzer RJ, Bacik J, Murphy M, et al: Interferon-alfa as a comparative treatment for clinical trials of new therapies against advanced renal cell carcinoma. J Clin Oncol 2002;20:289.
20. Law TM, Motzer RJ, Mazumdar M, et al: Phase III randomised trial of interleukin-2 with or without lymphokine activated killer cells in the treatment of patients with advanced renal cell carcinoma. Cancer 1995;76:824–832.
21. Wigginton JM, Komschlies KL, Back TC, et al: Administration of interleukin 12 with pulse interleukin 2 and the rapid and complete eradication of murine renal carcinoma. J Natl Cancer Inst 1996;88:38–43.

43 Myeloma and Secondary Involvement of the Kidney in Dysproteinemias

Paul W. Sanders

This chapter reviews the current potential approaches to management of the renal lesions associated with multiple myeloma and Waldenström macroglobulinemia. A brief discussion of the broad spectrum of renal diseases associated with these plasma cell dyscrasias is offered, but the primary focus of discussion is the pathophysiology and treatment of cast nephropathy. Detailed discussions of cryoglobulinemia, amyloidosis, and light-chain deposition disease are included in other chapters.

Overview of light-chain metabolism by the kidney

Renal failure is a common occurrence in multiple myeloma; in one large series, 31% of the 1353 patients with newly diagnosed myeloma had associated renal failure. Deposition of immunoglobulin light chains in the kidney can cause several morphologic lesions with a wide range of clinical presentations.[1,2] In the necropsy study of kidneys of 57 patients by Iványi,[1] the most common renal lesion was cast nephropathy or "myeloma kidney" (65%), while 21% had AL-type amyloidosis and 11% had monoclonal light-chain deposition disease. In some patients, renal failure may be the only manifestation of disease or the presenting manifestation of occult malignancy. In particular, those patients with glomerular involvement can have strikingly few extrarenal manifestations of co-existent myeloma or other lymphoproliferative disorders. While most, if not all, patients with documented cast nephropathy have multiple myeloma, only about 20% of patients with primary (AL-type) amyloidosis have multiple myeloma.[3] In another series, 26% of patients with light-chain deposition disease manifested either myeloma or another lymphoproliferative disease over time.[4] Furthermore, patients with biopsy-proven light chain-related renal injury may even present with no evidence of light-chain proteinemia or proteinuria,[4–9] but all patients examined were found to produce abnormal monoclonal light chains when bone marrow cultures were performed.[7–10] These findings emphasize the central role of light chains in the pathogenesis of these diseases. Despite the absence of extrarenal manifestations, a therapeutic approach that decreases light-chain production appears to be warranted in all patients.

An understanding of the pathophysiology of immunoglobulin light chains is important in the specific diagnosis and intervention of this spectrum of conditions. The variable effects on the glomeruli, tubulointerstitium, and vasculature are responsible for this inconstant set of presenting problems. AL-type amyloidosis occurs when the immunoglobulin light chain, often the λ isotype, polymerizes to form amyloid. The λ6 subtype of light chains is particularly prone to form amyloid.[11] Only very rarely do heavy chains alone form amyloid.[12] Early studies suggested that intracellular proteases participated in the processing of the precursor proteins into amyloid.[13] Amyloidogenic light chains can aggregate intracellularly by a process that is modified by interaction of the light chain with cytoplasmic (Hsp70) and endoplasmic reticulum (BiP) heat-shock proteins.[14,15] Amyloid protein develops in the glomerulus following uptake and intracellular processing of the light chain by mesangial cells.[16] Amyloid expands the glomerular mesangium, compressing the capillary loops and subsequently producing the clinical manifestations of proteinuria and renal failure. Light-chain deposition disease, the second most common glomerular lesion associated with monoclonal gammopathies, is characterized by deposition of monoclonal light chain, typically κ isotype, in the mesangium. Occasionally, heavy chains may also be present, prompting some authors to describe this lesion as light- and heavy-chain deposition disease. Light chains from patients with light-chain deposition disease stimulate mesangial cells to produce transforming growth factor β, which then serves as an autacoid to stimulate mesangial cell production of extracellular matrix proteins.[17] Continued expansion of the mesangium compresses the capillary loops, which diminishes glomerular filtration and ultimately produces glomerulosclerosis.

With a molecular mass of 22 kDa (approximately one-third that of albumin), free light chains are filtered at the glomerulus. Filtered light chains enter the proximal tubule where low-molecular-mass proteins are endocytosed and hydrolyzed, and the constituent amino acids are returned to the circulation. Some pathologic light chains undergo a similar reabsorption process but are hydrolyzed poorly and accumulate in lysosomes. Clinical manifestations of this altered process can include renal failure from proximal tubular cell necrosis or, in less severe cases, acquired Fanconi syndrome.

As previously mentioned, cast nephropathy is the most common renal disease associated with monoclonal light chains. This disorder occurs in about one-third of patients with myeloma. Light chains secreted by these patients are unique in that they demonstrate specific binding to Tamm–Horsfall glycoprotein in vitro. The CDR3 domain in the variable region of the light chain determines binding to Tamm–Horsfall glycoprotein.[18] Nephrotoxic light chains that escape proximal tubular reabsorption enter the thick ascending limb of the loop of Henle, bind to Tamm–Horsfall glycoprotein, and produce casts that obstruct flow of tubule fluid. This results in proximal tubule atrophy and incipient renal failure.[19–21] Subsequent breaks in the epithelium produce the classic histiocytic giant cell formation.[22]

There are several clinically important factors that influence this interaction between monoclonal light chains and Tamm–Horsfall glycoprotein. Decreasing renal perfusion pressure influences the relative intratubular concentration of these constituents, increasing the likelihood of cast formation. Therefore, prerenal azotemia of any etiology is an important risk factor for the development of cast nephropathy. Infusion of radiocontrast agents and use of nonsteroidal anti-inflammatory agents are well-described risk factors for the precipitation of acute renal failure from cast nephropathy via this mechanism. Volume depletion is frequently complicated in myeloma by the presence of hypercalcemia, which may independently potentiate the interaction of light chains with Tamm–Horsfall glycoprotein. Further, increasing the ambient sodium concentration also facilitates binding in vitro. Furosemide facilitates this interaction by increasing intra-luminal sodium concentration and by binding directly to Tamm–Horsfall glycoprotein, and may precipitate acute renal failure in patients whose intravascular volume is diminished. Finally, the interaction between some light chains and Tamm–Horsfall glycoprotein diminishes as pH increases.[20]

Multiple myeloma

Approach to treatment

Therapeutic intervention for the monoclonal light chain-related renal diseases requires a multifaceted approach. Although renal failure in multiple myeloma generally responds to chemotherapy, identification of the nature of the renal injury allows tailoring of subsequent treatment (Table 43.1). The cornerstone of acute management of cast nephropathy is prevention of aggregation of light chains with Tamm–Horsfall glycoprotein. Volume repletion, normalization of electrolytes, and avoidance of complicating factors such as furosemide, radiocontrast material, and nonsteroidal anti-inflammatory agents are mainstays of therapy in cast nephropathy. Tubule fluid flow rates should be kept high to avoid obstruction from light chains.[21,23] Daily fluid intake up to 3 L in the form of free water should be encouraged as long as defects in osmoregulation do not manifest. Alkalinization of the urine prevents renal failure due to light chains in rats.[24] In one inadequately controlled trial in humans, however, alkalinization of the urine has not been shown to be readily beneficial,[25] perhaps because changing pH does not alter some of the interactions between light chain and Tamm–Horsfall glycoprotein. Until better studies

Table 43.1 Potential therapies for light chain-related renal diseases*

Renal lesion	Treatment
Cast nephropathy	Chemotherapy with or without autologous blood stem-cell transplant Plasmapheresis Maintain serum [Ca²⁺] within physiologic range Hydration Sodium bicarbonate (citrate) administration Avoid exposure to radiocontrast material, nonsteroidal anti-inflammatory agents, and loop diuretics Dialysis
Primary (AL-type) amyloidosis	Chemotherapy ± autologous blood stem-cell transplant Colchicine Dialysis Renal transplantation
Light-chain deposition disease	Chemotherapy Dialysis Renal transplantation
Waldenström macroglobulinemia	Chemotherapy Plasmapheresis

*See text for details.

are available, administration of sodium bicarbonate (or citrate) to keep urine pH > 7 could be considered an adjunct to the treatment of cast nephropathy.

Hypercalcemia develops in 20–30% of patients with multiple myeloma. Hypercalcemia is both directly nephrotoxic and enhances the nephrotoxicity of light chains.[20,21] For these reasons, aggressive intervention to achieve normalization of the serum ionized calcium concentration is necessary. Initial management includes volume expansion with 0.9% NaCl intravenously, provided renal function is not irreversibly impaired. Loop diuretics facilitate renal calcium excretion, but may facilitate nephrotoxicity from light chains.[21] Consequently, loop diuretics should be administered judiciously and only after the patient is clinically euvolemic. Glucocorticoids (prednisone, up to 60 mg/day) are frequently helpful for the management of hypercalcemia, although the response may not be dramatic. The bisphosphonates, particularly pamidronate, are used to treat moderate hypercalcemia (serum calcium > 3.25 mmol/L or 13 mg/dL) unresponsive to other measures. While hypercalcemia of myeloma responds to bisphosphonates, these agents are nephrotoxic and should be administered only to euvolemic patients. Pamidronate 60–90 mg may be infused intravenously over a minimum of 4 h; dosing may be repeated 7 days later if the patient remains hypercalcemic. This regimen also accommodates the management of mild hypercalcemia as an outpatient. Because bisphosphonates chelate calcium and may cause symptomatic acute hypocalcemia, intravenous infusion rates should be slow. The effect of these agents is transient, but often allows time for chemotherapy and hydration to prevent recurrence of hypercalcemia. Bisphosphonates have also been used to treat myeloma. In one prospective study, patients who received monthly intravenous infusions of pamidronate 90 mg had fewer skeletal events (pathologic fractures, cord compression, bone radiotherapy) and less bone pain with improved quality of life compared with the group that received placebo.[26] Many authorities recommend the use of monthly pamidronate therapy, particularly in those patients with advanced myeloma.

Specific therapies for cast nephropathy are those that decrease the serum concentration of monoclonal light chains (Table 43.1). This is accomplished through two general modalities: antitumor therapy and plasmapheresis. Standard treatment of myeloma employs alkylating agents and steroids. Melphalan 0.15–0.25 mg/kg/day plus prednisone 1.5 mg/kg/day for 4 days every 6 weeks decreases circulating levels of light chains and stabilizes or improves renal function in two-thirds of patients who present with renal failure.[27] Fanconi syndrome may also resolve with this therapy.[28] However, because the primary route of elimination of melphalan is through the kidneys, dosing is complicated by renal failure. Frequent monitoring of hemoglobin, platelet, and leukocyte counts is necessary, adjusting the dose to achieve mild leukopenia and prevent thrombocytopenia at mid-cycle. The difficulty in correctly dosing melphalan in renal failure, as well as unpredictable gastrointestinal absorption, prompted Aitchison et al[29] to suggest that melphalan can be avoided by use of vincris-

tine, adriamycin, and either methylprednisolone (VAMP) or dexamethasone (VAD). VAMP therapy (vincristine 0.4 mg and adriamycin 9 mg/m² in 1 L 5% dextrose over 24 h administered through a central venous catheter, and methylprednisolone 1 g/m² intravenously daily for 4 days and repeated every 3–4 weeks) produced a significant reduction in serum paraprotein concentration and improvement in renal function in the majority of the eight patients in this study. Three of the four patients who were dialysis-dependent at the start of study recovered sufficient renal function to discontinue dialysis. Because of the high incidence of relapse, maintenance chemotherapy is necessary.[29] VAD can induce a remission more rapidly than melphalan and prednisone, allowing faster reduction in the amount of circulating light chains. Often only two courses of treatment are necessary to determine whether a patient will respond to this chemotherapy.[30] VAD may be particularly beneficial in the setting of renal failure related to deposition of light chains, and the physician can rapidly determine the efficacy of such an approach in the patient.

The role of high-dose melphalan with autologous blood stem-cell transplantation has received increased attention, although randomized studies reporting the use of this modality in the setting of severe renal failure have not been reported. A randomized trial recently showed that patients who received high-dose therapy and autologous bone marrow transplantation had improved event-free survival and overall survival rates than did patients who received conventional chemotherapy. The mean serum creatinine of the patients at the time of entry into this study was 1.3 mg/dL (113 μmol/L).[31] Another randomized trial involving 185 patients with symptomatic myeloma demonstrated that high-dose chemotherapy plus autologous blood stem-cell transplantation produced results that were equivalent to initial treatment with standard chemotherapy followed by high-dose therapy/stem-cell support. In this study, patients were excluded if serum creatinine was more than 3.4 mg/dL (300 μmol/L).[32] High-dose chemotherapy early in the course may decrease the overall amount of chemotherapy that the patient will receive. While not considered a curative procedure, most authors have recommended this approach for the patient who is under 70 years of age and is considered a suitable candidate for transplantation. Myeloablative therapy with allogeneic stem-cell transplantation may also prove effective in controlling renal failure in myeloma, but has a significant mortality and is currently limited to a small population who are deemed suitable for such treatment and have an HLA-compatible relative.

Plasmapheresis appears to be particularly useful in the setting of acute renal failure related to nephrotoxicity of light chains.[33] Generally, acute renal failure in this setting represents cast nephropathy, although obstruction (nephrolithiasis, papillary necrosis, and amyloid deposition in the ureters), hypercalcemia, and hyperviscosity syndrome may also occur. The standard protocol consists of five daily plasma exchange sessions, with an additional exchange on days 7 and 10 if necessary. Zucchelli et al[33] randomized 29 patients with myeloma, light-chain proteinuria, and acute renal failure to receive either plasma exchanges with chemotherapy or chemotherapy alone. Plasmapheresis dramatically decreased light-chain proteinuria and increased urine output; 13 of 15 patients recovered renal function. Of the 14 patients who did not receive plasma exchange therapy, only two individuals recovered function. As a result, plasma exchange therapy significantly improved survival at 1 year post treatment. An uncontrolled nonrandomized study has also suggested that patients with advanced multiple myeloma (stage IIIB) and coexistent renal failure may benefit from plasma exchange therapy performed every 5 weeks on three consecutive days just prior to combination chemotherapy; survival in the plasmapheresis group improved compared with a group that received melphalan and prednisone alone (median survival 17 vs. 2 months).[34] At this time, however, there are insufficient data to recommend plasmapheresis for any situation other than acute renal failure and hyperviscosity syndrome.

Renal replacement therapy

Renal replacement therapy in the form of hemodialysis or peritoneal dialysis is generally recommended in patients with renal failure from monoclonal light chain-related renal diseases. Recovery of renal function sufficient to survive without dialysis occurs in as many as 5% of patients with multiple myeloma, although in some patients this requires months to achieve. Despite the susceptibility to infection in multiple myeloma, the peritonitis rate for continuous ambulatory peritoneal dialysis (one episode every 14.4 months) was not unacceptably high.[35] Neither peritoneal dialysis nor hemodialysis appears to provide a survival advantage in patients with myeloma.

Renal transplantation has also been successfully performed in highly selected patients with multiple myeloma. Extrarenal manifestations of the disease should be absent for more than 1 year before considering renal transplantation. Similarly, extrarenal manifestations should be absent in patients who have AL-type amyloidosis or light-chain deposition disease. Renal transplantation in these individuals may be particularly beneficial if the disease has remained limited to the kidney. In one study of 62 patients, eight of whom had AL-type amyloidosis, 65% were alive 5 years after renal allograft implantation. While amyloid was found to involve the graft in 10%, only 3% lost the graft as a result of this involvement.[36] Renal transplant experience in patients with light-chain deposition disease is even more limited, but the disease may also recur in the allograft and cause renal failure.[37] Recurrence of myeloma may also occur despite rigorous pretransplant surveillance. These complications notwithstanding, renal transplantation remains a valuable therapeutic option in selected patients.

Prognosis

Multisystem involvement and advanced age at the time of diagnosis of myeloma shorten lifespan, with death

occurring early in the course of treatment. Renal failure also decreases survival. In one series, median survival for patients with renal failure was 20 months compared with a median survival of 20–40 months for the general population of patients with myeloma. Major predictors of survival in this group with renal failure included the stage of the disease, decline in serum creatinine concentration at 1 month into treatment to < 300 μmol/L (3.4 mg/dL), and response to chemotherapy. Response to chemotherapy was important: median survival time was 36 months for responders but only 10 months for nonresponders.[27]

Monoclonal light chain-related renal diseases without multiple myeloma

A challenging situation for nephrologists is renal failure due to deposition of immunoglobulin light chains, frequently diagnosed by percutaneous renal biopsy, yet further evaluation demonstrates no other clinical or histologic evidence of multiple myeloma. Because the kidney filters and excretes light chains, it is perhaps not surprising that overproduction of monoclonal light chains that possess a tropism for a particular compartment of the kidney can produce clinical manifestations of renal injury long before the other features of a monoclonal gammopathy become manifest. Typically, these patients have AL-type amyloidosis or light-chain deposition disease. Again, the literature supports an approach that combats light chains.

Primary (AL-type) amyloidosis

For AL-type amyloidosis, a recent randomized trial compared colchicine therapy alone (0.6 mg twice daily) to colchicine plus melphalan and prednisone in doses used for multiple myeloma. Because melphalan has been associated with development of myelodysplastic syndromes and leukemia, the total dose was limited to 600 mg. Treatment continued for 1 year. Addition of melphalan and prednisone increased survival from 6.7 to 12.2 months, thus supporting the use of chemotherapy in AL-type amyloidosis not associated with multiple myeloma. Patients with AL-type amyloidosis should probably remain on colchicine indefinitely.[38] In the following year, Kyle et al[39] reported qualitatively similar effects of the same chemotherapeutic regimen. In an attempt to identify factors associated with response to chemotherapy, Gertz et al[40] examined the Mayo Clinic experience with AL-type amyloidosis. Interestingly, those patients with nephrotic syndrome, a normal serum creatinine concentration, and no echocardiographic evidence of cardiac amyloidosis had the best response rate (39%). Response in this subset required 11.7 months of treatment, but the median survival was 89.4 months with 78% surviving 5 years. Of 17 patients who responded to treatment, 11 had complete resolution of the nephrotic syndrome and six others had a 50% reduction in urinary protein excretion; only 3 of 17 had persistent nephrotic-range proteinuria. The major toxicity of treatment in this series was acute leukemia or myelodysplasia, which developed in seven of the responders.[40] At present, there are no controlled trials showing that patients who do not respond to melphalan and prednisone will respond to more aggressive chemotherapeutic regimens, but a negative study has been reported.[41]

The disappointing outcome and limitations of chemotherapy have prompted some authors to consider high-dose mephalan with blood stem-cell tranplantation in suitable patients. Comenzo et al[42] enrolled 25 patients with biopsy-proven AL-type amyloidosis; 40% had three or more organs involved. The patients received intravenous melphalan 200 mg/m^2 followed by blood stem-cell autograft. With a median follow-up of 24 months, 68% were alive. Evidence of improvement in organ function, including the kidney, was observed in two-thirds of the surviving patients, while in four patients the disease stabilized. Three patients experienced relapse of the plasma cell dyscrasia. This encouraging study was further supported by a recent report of the Mayo Clinic experience.[43] At present, it seems reasonable to consider this approach in those patients who are younger (< 70 years of age), have a cardiac septal wall thickness of ≤ 15 mm, an estimated left ventricular ejection fraction of > 55%, and a serum creatinine < 2 mg/dL.[43] Patients with clinical manifestations demonstrating involvement of fewer than two organs appeared to have a better prognosis with this approach than did patients with advanced amyloidosis.[44] The diagnosis of AL-type amyloidosis must be certain, since other types of amyloidosis will not respond to high-dose chemotherapy. Patients should be referred to those centers with significant experience with this approach, because treatment mortality will be minimized.

There are other therapeutic approaches that have not yet been shown to improve survival in patients with AL-type amyloidosis. Gianni et al[45] described use of 4'-iodo-4'-deoxydoxorubicin (I-DOX) in eight patients who had a plasma cell dyscrasia and progressive amyloidosis refractory to standard chemotherapy. The authors observed clinical improvement in five patients. Three individuals showed evidence of resorption of the amyloid deposits associated with binding of I-DOX to the amyloid protein; binding in some as yet poorly defined way facilitated degradation of the amyloid. A follow-up report, however, suggested that the I-DOX chemotherapy produced only transient improvement that was insufficient to alter the course of the disease.[46] Certainly, more studies are necessary before recommending this agent routinely for patients with amyloidosis.

Light-chain deposition disease

Light-chain deposition disease also occurs without overt myeloma at presentation, although some patients will develop extrarenal manifestations of multiple myeloma over time. Randomized controlled trials for treatment of this light chain-related renal disease are unavailable, but these patients appear to benefit from the same chemo-

therapy as that given for multiple myeloma, particularly if the renal failure is mild at presentation.[4,9,47] The 5-year survival is ~ 70%,[4] but is reduced by coexistent myeloma. The serum creatinine concentration at presentation is an important predictor of subsequent renal function: 5 of 8 patients with serum creatinine concentrations < 354 μmol/L (4.0 mg/dL) did not progress with chemotherapy, while 9 of 11 patients with creatinine concentrations > 354 μmol/L at presentation progressed to endstage renal failure despite therapy.

Waldenström macroglobulinemia

This disorder constitutes about 5% of monoclonal gammopathies and is characterized by the presence of a monoclonal population of lymphocytoid plasma cells. This condition clinically behaves more like lymphoma, although the malignant cell also secretes IgM (macroglobulin), which is usually responsible for the symptoms at presentation. This large molecule is not excreted and accumulates in plasma to produce hyperviscosity syndrome and cryoglobulinemia. Neurologic symptoms (headaches, dizziness, deafness, stupor), visual impairment (from hemorrhages and exudates and sluggish flow through the venous system), bleeding diathesis (complexed clotting factors with IgM and platelet dysfunction), renal failure, and symptoms of hypervolemia are classic manifestations of this disease. Osteolytic lesions of the bone are uncommon. Renal failure is usually mild but occurs in about 30% of patients. Although nephromegaly from lymphocytoid cell infiltration can produce renal failure, hyperviscosity syndrome and precipitation of IgM in the glomerular capillaries are the most common causes of renal failure. About 10–15% of patients also develop AL-type amyloidosis, but cast nephropathy is rare in these patients.

Therapy and prognosis

Because of the typically advanced age at presentation (sixth to seventh decade) and slowly progressive course, the major therapeutic goal is relief of symptoms. Treatment is generally plasmapheresis for hyperviscosity syndrome, followed by alkylating agents alone. All patients with monoclonal IgM levels > 3 g/dL should have a serum viscosity checked. A relative serum viscosity of > 0.004 Pa × s (normal < 0.0018 Pa × s) usually correlates with symptoms of hyperviscosity, although significant individual variation exists. Occasionally, clinically apparent hyperviscosity syndrome is associated with only mild increases in serum viscosity, particularly if the IgM forms cryoprecipitate and the serum viscosity is determined at room temperature. Alternatively, some patients with marked increases in serum viscosity manifest no symptoms. Plasmapheresis is indicated in symptomatic patients only and should be continued until symptoms resolve and serum viscosity normalizes. Blood transfusions, which can further increase viscosity, should be avoided in patients with hyperviscosity syndrome. Initial chemotherapy is usually chlorambucil 4 mg/day orally, with titration to control serum IgM concentration and organomegaly without inducing cytopenias. More aggressive chemotherapy (cyclophosphamide, vincristine, prednisone), given monthly, has also been used in patients who do not respond to chlorambucil. Severe renal failure requiring renal replacement therapy is uncommon in this disorder. Median survival is about 3 years and is related to the advanced age at onset of this disorder.

Summary

Advances in understanding the pathophysiology of the light chain-related renal diseases have produced improvements in management and prolongation of survival in this population. Approaches designed to lower circulating light chains and attack the basic mechanisms of renal damage, along with judicious use of renal replacement therapies, provide the best results. Even with these advances, however, overall prognosis remains suboptimal, so the clinician should remain receptive to new therapies for these renal lesions.

References

1. Iványi B: Frequency of light chain deposition nephropathy relative to renal amyloidosis and Bence Jones cast nephropathy in a necropsy study of patients with myeloma. Arch Pathol Lab Med 1990;114:986–987.
2. Knudsen LM, Hippe E, Hjorth M, et al: Renal function in newly diagnosed multiple myeloma: a demographic study of 1353 patients. Eur J Haematol 1994;53:207–212.
3. Kyle RA, Greipp PR: Amyloidosis (AL): clinical and laboratory features in 229 cases. Mayo Clin Proc 1983;58:665–683.
4. Heilman RL, Velosa JA, Holley KE, et al: Long-term follow-up and response to chemotherapy in patients with light-chain deposition disease. Am J Kidney Dis 1992;20:34–41.
5. Sanders PW, Herrera GA, Kirk KA, et al: Spectrum of glomerular and tubulointerstitial renal lesions associated with monotypical immunoglobulin light deposition. Lab Invest 1991;64:527–537.
6. van Ingen G, van Bronswijk H, Meijer CJLM, et al: Light chain deposition disease without detectable light chains in serum or urine. Report of a case and review of the literature. Neth J Med 1991;39:142–147.
7. Preud'homme J-L, Aucouturier P, Touchard G, et al: Monoclonal immunoglobulin deposition disease (Randall type). Relationship with structural abnormalities of immunoglobulin chains. Kidney Int 1994;46:965–972.
8. Matsuzaki H, Yoshida M, Akahoshi Y, et al: Pseudo-nonsecretory multiple myeloma with light chain deposition disease. Acta Haematol 1991;85:164–168.
9. Buxbaum JN, Chuba JV, Hellman GC, et al: Monoclonal immunoglobulin deposition disease: light chain and light and heavy chain deposition diseases and their relation to light chain amyloidosis. Ann Intern Med 1990;112:455–464.
10. Buxbaum J: Mechanisms of disease: monoclonal immunoglobulin deposition. Hematol Oncol Clin North Am 1992;6:323–346.
11. Solomon A, Frangione B, Franklin EC: Bence Jones proteins and light chains of immunoglobulins: preferential association of the $V_{\lambda VI}$ subgroup of human light chains with amyloidosis AL(λ). J Clin Invest 1982;70:453–460.
12. Eulitz M, Weiss DT, Solomon A: Immunoglobulin heavy-chain-associated amyloidosis. Proc Natl Acad Sci USA 1990;87:6542–6546.
13. Shirahama T, Cohen AS: An analysis of the close relationship of lysosomes to early deposits of amyloid. Am J Pathol 1973;73:97–114.
14. Davis DP, Khurana R, Meredith S, et al: Mapping the major interaction between binding protein and Ig light chains to sites within the variable domain. J Immunol 1999;163:3842–3850.
15. Dul JL, Davis DP, Williamson EK, et al: Hsp70 and antifrillogenic peptides promote degradation and inhibit intracellular aggregation of amyloidogenic light chains. J Cell Biol 2001;152:705–715.
16. Tagouri YM, Sanders PW, Picken MM, et al: In vitro AL-amyloid formation by rat and human mesangial cells. Lab Invest 1996;74:290–302.
17. Zhu L, Herrera GA, Murphy-Ullrich JE, et al: Pathogenesis of glomerulosclerosis in light chain deposition disease: role for transforming growth factor-β. Am J Pathol 1995;147:375–385.
18. Ying W-Z, Sanders PW: Mapping the binding domain of immunoglobulin light chains for Tamm–Horsfall protein. Am J Pathol 2001;158:1859–1866.
19. Huang Z-Q, Kirk KA, Connelly KG, et al: Bence Jones proteins bind to a common peptide segment of Tamm–Horsfall glycoprotein to promote heterotypic aggregation. J Clin Invest 1993;92:2975–2983.
20. Huang Z-Q, Sanders PW: Biochemical interaction of Tamm–Horsfall glycoprotein with Ig light chains. Lab Invest 1995;73:810–817.
21. Sanders PW, Booker BB, Bishop JB, et al: Mechanisms of intranephronal proteinaceous cast formation by low molecular weight proteins. J Clin Invest 1990;85:570–576.
22. Start DA, Silva FG, Davis LD, et al: Myeloma cast nephropathy: immunohistochemical and lectin studies. Modern Pathol 1988;1:336–347.
23. Sanders PW, Booker BB: Pathobiology of cast nephropathy from human Bence Jones proteins. J Clin Invest 1992;89:630–639.
24. Holland MD, Galla JH, Sanders PW, et al: Effect of urinary pH and diatrizoate on Bence Jones protein nephrotoxicity in the rat. Kidney Int 1985;27:46–50.
25. MRC Working Party on Leukemia in Adults: Analysis and management of renal failure in fourth MRC myelomatosis trial. Br Med J 1984;288:1411–1416.
26. Berenson JR, Lichtenstein A, Porter L, et al: Efficacy of pamidronate in reducing skeletal events in patients with advanced multiple myeloma. N Engl J Med 1996;334:488–493.
27. Ganeval D, Rabian C, Guérin V, et al: Treatment of multiple myeloma with renal involvement. Adv Nephrol 1992;21:347–370.
28. Uchida S, Matsuda O, Yokota T, et al: Adult Fanconi syndrome secondary to κ-light chain myeloma: improvement of tubular functions after treatment for myeloma. Nephron 1990;55:332–335.
29. Aitchison RG, Reilly IAG, Morgan AG, et al: Vincristine, adriamycin and high dose steroids in myeloma complicated by renal failure. Br J Cancer 1990;61:765–766.
30. Alexanian R, Dimopoulos M: The treatment of multiple myeloma. N Engl J Med 1994;330:484–489.
31. Attal M, Harousseau J-L, Stoppa A-M, et al: A prospective, randomized trial of autologous bone marrow transplantation and chemotherapy in multiple myeloma. N Engl J Med 1996; 335:91–97.
32. Fermand J-P, Ravaud P, Chevret S, et al: High-dose therapy and autologous peripheral blood stem cell transplantation in multiple myeloma: up-front or rescue treatment? Results of a multicenter sequential randomized clinical trial. Blood 1998;92:3131–3136.
33. Zucchelli P, Pasquali S, Cagnoli L, et al: Controlled plasma exchange trial in acute renal failure due to multiple myeloma. Kidney Int 1988;33:1175–1180.
34. Wahlin A, Löfvenberg E, Holm J: Improved survival in multiple myeloma with renal failure. Acta Med Scand 1987;221:205–209.
35. Shetty A, Oreopoulos DG: Continuous ambulatory peritoneal dialysis in end-stage renal disease due to multiple myeloma. Perit Dial Int 1995;15:236–240.
36. Hartmann A, Holdaas H, Fauchald P, et al: Fifteen years' experience with renal transplantation in systemic amyloidosis. Transpl Int 1992;5:15–18.
37. Howard AD, Moore J, Tomaszewski M-M: Occurrence of multiple myeloma three years after successful renal transplantation. Am J Kidney Dis 1987;10:147–150.
38. Skinner M, Anderson JJ, Simms R, et al: Treatment of 100 patients with primary amyloidosis: a randomized trial of melphalan, prednisone, and colchicine versus colchicine only. Am J Med 1996;100:290–298.
39. Kyle RA, Gertz MA, Greipp PR, et al: A trial of three regimens for primary amyloidosis: colchicine alone, melphalan and prednisone, and melphalan, prednisone, and colchicine. N Engl J Med 1997;336:1202–1207.
40. Gertz MA, Kyle RA, Greipp PR: Response rates and survival in primary systemic amyloidosis. Blood 1991;77:257–262.

41. Gertz MA, Lacy MQ, Lust JA, et al: Prospective randomized trial of melphalan and prednisone versus vincristine, carmustine, melphalan, cyclophosphamide, and prednisone in the treatment of primary systemic amyloidosis. J Clin Oncol 1999;17:262–267.

42. Comenzo RL, Vosburgh E, Falk RH, et al: Dose-intensive melphalan with blood stem-cell support for the treatment of AL (amyloid light-chain) amyloidosis: survival and responses in 25 patients. Blood 1998;91:3662–3670.

43. Gertz MA, Lacy MQ, Dispenzieri A: Immunoglobulin light chain amyloidosis and the kidney. Kidney Int 2002;61:1–9.

44. Moreau P, Leblond V, Bourquelot P, et al: Prognostic factors for survival and response after high-dose therapy and autologous stem cell transplantation in systemic AL amyloidosis: a report on 21 patients. Br J Haematol 1998;101:766–769.

45. Gianni L, Bellotti V, Gianni AM, et al: New drug therapy of amyloidoses: resorption of AL-type deposits with 4'-iodo-4'-deoxydoxorubicin. Blood 1995;86:855–861.

46. Merlini G, Anesi E, Garini P, et al: Treatment of AL amyloidosis with 4'-iodo-4'-deoxydoxorubicin: an update. Blood 1999;93:1112–1113.

47. Ganeval D, Noël L-H, Preud'homme J-L, et al: Light-chain deposition disease: its relation with AL-type amyloidosis. Kidney Int 1984;26:1–9.

Obstructive Uropathy

Saulo Klahr

General therapeutic considerations
Therapy
- Calculi
- Intramural causes of obstructive uropathy
- Extrinsic causes of obstructive uropathy
- Nephrostomy in the therapy of upper ureteral obstruction
- Lower urinary tract obstruction
  - Bladder neck and urethra
  - Bladder dysfunction
  - Postobstructive diuresis
  - Fetal uropathies

Since obstructive uropathy is generally a remediable cause of kidney failure, early and accurate diagnosis and prompt treatment are vital to the preservation or restoration of renal function. The clinical manifestations of obstructive uropathy are variable. Complete bilateral obstruction of urine flow is manifested as anuria. Partial obstruction can cause fluctuating urine output, alternating from oliguria to polyuria; urinary tract infections that are usually refractory to treatment; abdominal or flank pain; or unexplained acute or chronic renal failure. Obstruction must always be included in the differential diagnosis of acute renal failure, especially when urine output fluctuates or anuria occurs suddenly. The causes of upper and lower urinary tract obstruction are depicted in Tables 44.1 and 44.2.

General therapeutic considerations

After the diagnosis of obstructive uropathy is established, the next decision is whether or not surgical or instrumental procedures should be performed. High-grade or complete bilateral obstruction presenting as acute renal failure requires intervention as soon as possible. In these patients the site of obstruction frequently determines the approach. If the obstructive lesion is distal to the bladder, passage of a urethral catheter may suffice, although this may require the aid of a urologist. In some cases, suprapubic cystostomy may be necessary. On the other hand, if the lesion lies proximal to the bladder (upper tract lesion, e.g. malignant infiltration of the trigone by cervical or prostatic adenocarcinoma), placement of nephrostomy tubes at the time of ultrasonography or passage of a retrograde ureteral catheter should be undertaken. Tubes should be placed in both obstructed renal calyces because the potential for recovery of function by either kidney is not easily predicted at the time of the procedure. Such an

approach may circumvent the need for dialysis and allows the physician time to determine the specific site and nature of the obstructing lesion. Further, the nephrostomy tube may be used for local infusion of pharmacologic agents to treat infection, malignancy, or calculi. In patients with obstruction complicated by urinary tract infection and generalized sepsis, appropriate antibiotics and other supportive measures are indicated.

Table 44.1 Causes of upper urinary tract obstruction
Urolithiasis
Transitional cell cancer of the pelvis/ureter
Blood clot
Renal papillae
Fungus ball
Ureteral ligation
Primary obstruction of the ureteropelvic junction intrinsic (congenital) vs. acquired (vessel crossing postsurgical)
Ureteral valve
Ureteral polyp
Vascular lesions
Abdominal aortic aneurysm
Iliac artery aneurysm
Retrocaval ureter
Puerperal ovarian vein thrombophlebitis
Fibrosis following vascular reconstructive surgery
Diseases of the female reproductive tract
Pregnancy
Mass lesions of the uterus and ovary
Ovarian remnants
Gartner duct cyst
Tubo-ovarian abscess
Endometriosis
Uterine prolapse
Diseases of the gastrointestinal tract
Crohn disease
Diverticulitis
Appendiceal abscess
Pancreatic lesions
Diseases of the retroperitoneum
Retroperitoneal fibrosis
Tuberculosis
Sarcoidosis
Radiation fibrosis
Retroperitoneal hemorrhage
Primary retroperitoneal tumors (lymphomas, sarcomas, etc.)
Secondary retroperitoneal tumors (cervix, bladder, colon, prostate, etc.)
Lymphocele
Pelvic lipomatosis

Table 44.2 Causes of lower urinary tract obstruction

Phimosis
Meatal stenosis
Paraphimosis
Urethral stricture
Urethral stone
Urethral diverticulum
Periurethral abscess
Posterior urethral valves
Anterior urethral valves
Urethral surgery
Prostatic abscess
Prostatic calculi
Neurogenic bladder
Benign prostatic hyperplasia
Psychogenic urinary retention
Bladder calculus
Bladder cancer
Ureterocele
Trauma
   Straddle injury
   Pelvic fracture

In patients with low-grade acute obstruction or partial chronic obstruction, surgical intervention may be delayed for a few weeks or even months. However, prompt relief of partial obstruction is indicated when (1) there are multiple repeated episodes of urinary tract infection; (2) the patient has significant symptoms (flank pain, dysuria, voiding dysfunction); (3) there is urinary retention; and (4) there is evidence of recurrent or progressive renal damage. The presence of postvoid residual urine, urinary extravasation, ureterovesical reflux, or dilatation of the collecting system despite sterile urine is not an indication for surgical intervention.

Therapy

Calculi

Stones are the most common cause of ureteral obstruction (see also Chapters 39 and 40). Such calculi are frequently of the struvite type (magnesium, ammonium phosphate, calcium carbonate) resulting from the association of urinary infection with urea-hydrolyzing bacteria. The immediate treatment for ureteral stones consists of pain relief, elimination of obstruction, and control of infection. Relief of pain in this setting is best accomplished by intramuscular injection of adequate doses of a narcotic analgesic. If the diameter of the stone is under 4 mm, urologic instrumentation or surgical intervention is not required, since 80–90% of these stones pass spontaneously. However, if the diameter of the stone is 5–7 mm only 40–50% pass, while stones > 7 mm rarely pass spontaneously. High fluid intake designed to achieve urine volumes of at least 1.5–2.5 L daily helps pass the stone. The urine must be strained through a gauze sponge to

recover the calculi, which should be sent for analysis. If a stone completely blocks a ureter and does not move, surgical treatment should commence within a few days. However, if the obstruction is partial, the urine sterile, and the pain manageable, the patient may be observed for weeks before surgical therapy is undertaken. Stone removal is indicated when there is complete obstruction, unremitting colic, urinary tract infection, urosepsis, or a calculus that is too large to pass (> 7 mm) or that has failed to move despite a trial of time (usually months) and increased fluid intake.

The treatment of urolithiasis has changed dramatically during the past 20 years. A number of therapeutic modalities are now available to patients requiring stone removal, including extracorporeal shock wave lithotripsy (ESWL), percutaneous nephrolithotomy, or a combination of these two therapies; ureteroscopic removal; open surgery; laparoscopic surgery; and chemolysis. Treatment selection is based on size, position, and composition of the stone, anatomy of the collecting system, and the patient's health status and preferences.

The preferred therapeutic modality for patients with stones proximal to, or at the level of, the iliac vessels is ESWL. This treatment is effective and has a low complication rate. Individuals with stones distal to the iliac vessels that do not pass spontaneously are candidates for ESWL or ureteroscopic removal. The advantages of ureteroscopic removal are the high success rate (approaching 100%) of this procedure and its lower cost. New technologies, including smaller rigid and flexible ureteroscopes, electrohydraulic probes, the pulsed dye laser, and new basket extraction devices, have greatly improved ureteroscopic stone removal and decreased substantially the incidence of associated complications.

Patients with renal stones < 2 cm in size are usually treated with ESWL. Percutaneous nephrolithotomy is preferred for larger stones because the procedure provides a higher rate of stone-free results and fewer interventions are required. The composition of the stone should also be considered when selecting a given therapeutic modality. Brushite and cystine stones appear to be more resistant to shock-wave energy and hence to ESWL. Open surgery is employed in patients with large staghorn calculi who have extremely dilated renal collecting systems with or without infundibular stenosis, factors known to impair the likelihood of obtaining a stone-free status. The general use of open surgery for stone removal is relatively infrequent now. This is primarily due to the advent of ESWL and ureteroscopic and percutaneous stone removal. The use of open surgery after the establishment of ESWL has varied from 0.3% to 4.1% of patients requiring stone removal.

Broad-spectrum antibiotics are useful when infections complicate the presence of renal calculi. The choice of drugs should be based on sensitivity studies of the organism isolated from the urine. However, antimicrobial therapy without relief of obstruction is not effective in controlling the infection. Therefore when primary or secondary obstruction accompanies renal calculi, temporary relief of obstruction should be instituted promptly by insertion of a retrograde ureteral catheter. If the attempted retrograde catheter diversion is unsuccessful, a percutaneous nephrostomy tube can be placed. Whenever possible, relief of obstruction and infection should be achieved before stone manipulation and open surgery.

In summary, a stone < 4 mm in diameter is likely to be passed without surgical intervention. Even when stone removal appears necessary, in 95% of patients this can be achieved with ESWL or via a percutaneous nephrostomy alone, regardless of the size or location of the calculus. Surgical therapy is largely reserved for the few patients in whom these measures fail. Earlier intervention is certainly indicated for the patient whose history, laboratory data, and radiologic studies suggest complete obstruction, for the patient with infected urine, or for the patient with partial obstruction whose stone remains in the same position in the ureter for more than a few months.

Obstruction of the ureter by blood clots, a fungus ball, or papillary tissue can be managed by techniques similar to those employed in the treatment of stones. Significant obstruction attributable to neoplastic, inflammatory, and neurologic diseases must be treated aggressively since it is unlikely to remit spontaneously. The decision whether or not to divert the urine in patients who have metastatic malignant disease must be made on an individual basis.

Patients with sterile hydronephrosis secondary to advanced pelvic malignancy and a short life expectancy are usually not considered for percutaneous nephrostomy, while those with a reasonable prospect for tumor response to chemotherapy and radiotherapy are strong candidates for the procedure.

Intramural causes of obstructive uropathy

Intramural causes of upper urinary tract obstruction are managed by several diverse techniques. Infundibular stenosis is most commonly found following chronic infection of the renal parenchyma. This disorder can be managed either percutaneously by insertion of a nephrostomy tube (described later) into the affected infundibulum and subsequent infundibular dilatation or incision, or through open exposure of the infundibulum and spatulation. Intramural obstruction due to congenital causes, such as ureteropelvic or ureterovesical junction obstruction or upper ureteral valves, requires open surgery. Ureteropelvic junction obstruction is managed by pyeloplasty. This technique can create a widely patent ureteropelvic junction. Ureterovesical junction obstruction can be corrected by resection of the distal end of the ureter and reimplantation of the remaining ureter into the bladder. Congenital ureteral valves often require surgical excision and ureteroureterostomy. Intrinsic masses in the ureter or renal pelvis should be approached carefully, as if they were carcinomas, so as to avoid seeding and dissemination of the tumor. Treatment for high-grade transitional carcinoma requires nephroureterectomy with an en bloc resection of a 1-cm cuff of bladder around the ureteral orifice. Benign tumors (papillomas, polyps of the ureter) and certain low-grade transitional cell carcinomas may be treated using laser ablation.

Extrinsic causes of obstructive uropathy

Extrinsic obstruction of the ureter usually requires correction of the causative disease process. Ureteral obstruction as a result of an aneurysm of the abdominal aorta is treated by repair of the vascular lesion. Idiopathic retroperitoneal fibrosis is treated by open surgical ureteral lysis and intraperitoneal placement of the ureters. Distal ureteral obstruction from pelvic lipomatosis requires either ureteroneocystostomy into the anterior portion of the bladder or supravesical urinary diversion.

Nephrostomy in the therapy of upper ureteral obstruction

Nephrostomy is the insertion of a tube through the kidney into the renal pelvis to provide immediate urinary drainage. Until the 1950s all nephrostomy tubes were placed via an open surgical approach. This resulted in significant morbidity and mortality rates because patients requiring emergency nephrostomy tube placement were often quite debilitated. In 1955, Goodwin reported the first case of a needle-derived nephrostomy tube placed under fluoroscopic guidance. The technique did not gain popularity until the 1970s, when the advent of ultrasonography and improved methods of fluoroscopy made the percutaneous approach more feasible. Currently almost all nephrostomy tubes are placed percutaneously by an interventional radiologist or urologist. This is usually done with local anesthesia and takes less than 40 min.

The most common indications for placement of a nephrostomy tube are the need to provide a conduit to the kidney for percutaneous stone removal and the need to relieve ureteral obstruction secondary to neoplasia, inflammatory disease, or lower tract extrinsic or intrinsic obstruction in which the patient's condition does not permit a more definitive surgical procedure. Unmanageable infection in an obstructed system is another common indication. It is not unusual to note dramatic clinical improvement within hours of percutaneous drainage in the patient with urosepsis.

Potential early complications of nephrostomy are perirenal hemorrhage and acute obstruction from clot formation. One of the more serious delayed complications is dislodgement of the nephrostomy tube. This is considered an emergency; the tube should be replaced immediately or the tract will seal off, usually within 24 h. Another problem occurring after nephrostomy tube removal is an exsanguinating hemorrhage from a renal pseudoaneurysm. This occurs in 0.5–1% of patients and is best managed by immediate selective embolization of the affected vessel. Long-term complications, such as infection, calculus formation, and pyelonephritis, are significant and may lead to renal failure.

Except in unusual circumstances, long-term urinary diversion by the nephrostomy tube is not recommended. In many patients, however, several years may pass without the development of serious complications from their nephrostomy tubes. Also, in patients with extrinsic obstruction secondary to metastatic carcinoma, the nephrostomy tract can be used to manipulate a catheter into the bladder. A small tube can be placed through the affected flank and kidney with its pigtail end left in the bladder. The external portion of the stent can be clamped, thereby providing unobstructed flow from the affected kidney to the patient's bladder. This eliminates the need for external drainage bags and also facilitates changing the tube. In essence, all nephrostomy tubes or indwelling stents are changed every 3 months to decrease the build-up of concretions and to preclude breakage of ureteral stents within the collecting system.

For chronically obstructed kidneys a period of percutaneous drainage may permit significant restoration of renal function. With this knowledge and with periodic determination of split-renal function studies, treatment can be planned effectively. A lack of significant improvement in function would suggest that nephrectomy rather than reparative surgery should be undertaken.

Lower urinary tract obstruction
Bladder neck and urethra

Bladder neck and urethral obstruction can be surgically repaired in ambulatory patients who have recurrent infections, especially when associated with reflux, evidence of renal parenchymal damage, total urinary retention, repeated bleeding, or other severe symptoms. Difficulties with voiding due to benign prostatic hyperplasia do not always follow a progressive course. Therefore a man with minimal symptoms, no infection, and a normal upper urinary tract may be observed safely until he and his physician agree that surgery is desirable. Urethral stricture in men that is secondary to infection or trauma is frequently treated by simple dilation or direct-vision internal urethrotomy. In these patients, radiographic and endoscopic follow-up care is essential to rule out recurrence. The incidence of bladder neck and urethral obstruction in women is low and has been overestimated in the past; hence urethral dilation, internal urethrotomy, meatotomy, and revision of the bladder neck are seldom indicated. In some patients, suprapubic cystostomy may be necessary for bladder drainage. This is indicated in patients unable to void after sustaining injury to the urethra or who have an impassable urethral stricture.

Advances in urologic instrumentation have further decreased the indications for open surgery. Almost all suprapubic cystostomies are performed using a percutaneous approach under fluoroscopic guidance. Open cystostomy is rarely performed. In addition, a closed transurethral approach is used to treat the majority of patients with prostatic hyperplasia (60 g of tissue), urethral strictures, bladder neck contractures, bladder calculi, and superficial bladder tumors.

Bladder dysfunction

When obstructive uropathy is a consequence of neuropathic bladder function, urodynamic studies are essential to establish a treatment regimen. In all cases the main therapeutic goals are to establish the bladder as a site of urine storage without causing renal parenchymal injury and to provide a mechanism for bladder emptying acceptable to the patient. In general these patients fall into one of two groups: those with bladder atony secondary to lower motor neuron injury and those with unstable bladder function attributable to upper motor neuron disease. In both cases ureteral reflux and renal parenchymal injury may occur, although it is more common with the hyperactive upper motor neuron bladder. This problem may be potentiated by sphincter detrusor dyssynergia or by using external compression (Credé maneuver) or increasing abdominal pressure (Valsalva maneuver) to aid voiding.

Neurogenic bladder function caused by diabetes mellitus is a classic example of lower motor neuron disease. Voiding at regular intervals is one method to aid satisfactory bladder emptying in patients with the condition. Occasionally these individuals respond to cholinergic medications.

Overdistension of the bladder impairs emptying because detrusor contraction is essential to sphincter relaxation. Thus, bladder outlet obstruction may be a major problem. α-Adrenergic blockers such as phenoxybenzamine hydrochloride relax urethral sphincter tone but have only limited success because of adverse effects. Table 44.3 summarizes the drugs used in the treatment of lower urinary tract dysfunction and their proposed mechanism of action.

Table 44.3 Drugs used in the treatment of lower urinary tract dysfunction*

Drugs that facilitate urine storage
By increasing urethral tone
  β-Adrenergic antagonists (propranolol hydrochloride)
  α-Adrenergic agonists (imipramine hydrochloride, phenylpropanolamine hydrochloride)
By inhibiting bladder (detrusor) contractility
  Anticholinergic agents (propantheline hydrochloride)
  Smooth muscle depressants (imipramine hydrochloride, dicyclomine hydrochloride, oxybutynin chloride)
  α-Adrenergic antagonists (prazosin hydrochloride, phenoxybenzamine hydrochloride)

Drugs that facilitate voiding
By increasing bladder (detrusor) contractility
  Cholinergic agents (bethanechol chloride)
By decreasing sphincter tone
  α-Adrenergic antagonists (prazosin hydrochloride, phenoxybenzamine hydrochloride, clonidine hydrochloride)
  Skeletal muscle relaxants (diazepam, dantrolene sodium)

*Adapted from Klahr S: Obstructive uropathy. In Kassierer JP, Green HL (eds): Current Therapy in Adult Medicine, 4th edn. St. Louis: Mosby-Year Book, 1997, p 1135.

Another alternative for men with a flaccid bladder is external sphincterotomy. This transurethral procedure may be successful in relieving outlet obstruction and promoting bladder emptying, but it has the disadvantage of causing urinary incontinence and requires that the patient wear an external collection device. In men this problem can be obviated by the use of a penile clamp; however, the clamps often result in significant morbidity owing to urethral erosion and penile edema. In women the incontinence associated with external sphincterotomy precludes its use. In addition, the implantation of artificial urinary sphincters has been partially successful. Although these devices are useful, problems with their longevity have hindered their widespread acceptance.

The best treatment for patients with significant residual urine and recurrent bouts of urosepsis is clean intermittent catheterization (CIC) performed at regular intervals. Catheterization should be performed four to five times per day, so that the amount of urine drained from the bladder does not exceed 300–400 mL. This technique has met with considerable success in almost all age groups but requires patient acceptance and careful training.

In patients with unstable urine bladder function attributable to upper motor neuron lesions, the major goal is to improve the storage function of the bladder. Pharmacologic maneuvers include the use of anticholinergic agents such as oxybutynin chloride (Ditropan) (5 mg every 4–6 h). Adjunctive therapy such as CIC is frequently necessary to ensure complete bladder emptying and prevent incontinence.

In all patients with neurogenic bladders, chronic indwelling catheters are to be avoided if possible. In addition to problems of external drainage, bladder stones, urosepsis, and urethral erosion, chronic indwelling catheters are associated with the occurrence of squamous cell carcinoma of the bladder. Patients managed in this fashion for more than 5 years should get yearly cystoscopic examinations.

Surgical diversions are indicated for (1) deterioration of renal function despite conservative measures, (2) intractable incontinence, (3) a small contracted bladder, and (4) multiple bladder fistulas. The ileal conduit is the operation of choice for permanent diversion. Although many individuals do well after this procedure, operative mortality, postoperative intestinal obstruction, and stomal obstruction are complications that make the operation far from ideal. Further, recent studies have indicated that in as many as 80% of patients there is a progressive decline in renal function. A continent form of ileal diversion has become available: the Kock pouch. Using this procedure an ileal reservoir with a capacity of 300–500 mL is made. A continent stoma is placed in the right lower quadrant of the abdomen, which the patient must empty by catheterization four times per day. This method of diversion alleviates the need for any external collection devices.

In patients requiring short-term indwelling urethral catheters, good care is necessary to prevent urinary tract infection. Men are instructed to cleanse the glans twice daily with an antimicrobial soap and then to apply an antibiotic ointment. Given specific indications for catheter drainage, proper patient selection, aseptic technique, closed urinary drainage, the judicious use of systemic antimicrobials, and proper catheter care, the indwelling urethral catheter is a satisfactory means of short-term and, in rare instances, of long-term urinary diversion. The principles of closed drainage are that the system never be open, that the urine in the drainage tube never come in contact with the urine in the collecting bag, and that the bag be in a dependent position at all times. Cultures can be obtained by clamping the catheter for a few minutes and then using a small needle and syringe to aspirate urine from the lumen of the catheter. It is preferable not to break the drainage system for catheter irrigation or for the use of antibiotic irrigating solutions to reduce infection, as has been advocated by some. In patients requiring long-term catheter drainage, intermittent irrigation with an acid citrate solution reduces encrustation.

Postobstructive diuresis

Postobstructive diuresis refers to the marked polyuria that occurs after relief of urinary tract obstruction. This polyuria is usually associated with the excretion of large amounts of sodium, potassium, magnesium, and other solutes. Although self-limited (it may last several days), the losses of salt and water may be of such magnitude as to cause hypokalemia, hyponatremia or hypernatremia, hypomagnesemia and/or marked contraction of the extracellular fluid (ECF) volume, and peripheral vascular collapse. In many patients, however, a brisk diuresis after relief of urinary tract obstruction may be physiologically appropriate rather than the result of an inability of the postobstructed kidney to maintain volume and solute homeostasis. A postobstructive diuresis is appropriate and does not compromise the volume status of the patient when it is caused by excretion of excess salt, water, and urea retained during the period of obstruction. This diuresis is transient and usually subsides within the first day or two after relief of obstruction without causing depletion of the ECF volume. However, it is often impossible to distinguish patients experiencing benign postobstructive diuresis from those who have a true defect in tubular reabsorption of salt and water on the basis of urine volume and composition alone. Thus replacement therapy should be guided by clinical and laboratory evidence of the adequacy of the ECF volume and not by the volume of the urine only.

Postobstructive diuresis may be artificially prolonged by overzealous administration of salt and water after relief of obstruction. Replacement of excreted salt and water maintains a state of expansion of the ECF and hence results in continuous excretion of the excess salt and water administered. Thus, fluid replacement may be justified only after excessive losses of sodium and water that are inappropriate for the volume status of the patient and which are presumably caused by an intrinsic tubular defect in the reabsorption of sodium and water.

For patients with postobstructive diuresis, the appropriate fluid replacement depends largely on what is excreted. Although intravenous fluid administration may be necessary, urinary losses should be replaced only to the extent necessary to prevent hypovolemia, hypotension, hypokalemia, and hypomagnesemia. Excessive fluid administration only prolongs the duration of the postobstructive diuresis. Orthostatic hypotension and tachycardia are perhaps the best indicators of when intravenous fluid administration is needed. To distinguish between inappropriate diuresis and the excretion of fluid retained or excess fluid administration, it may be necessary to decrease the rate of intravenous fluid administration to levels below those of urinary output and observe the patient carefully for signs of volume depletion (hypotension, tachycardia, and stabilization or elevation of blood urea nitrogen, which was previously decreasing). In the case of inappropriate diuresis, appropriate fluid replacement consists of the prompt quantitative replenishment of urinary losses of water, sodium, potassium, and magnesium. This is best accomplished by frequent measurements of urine volume and serum and urine electrolytes. With massive diuresis, such measurements may be required every 6 h. The patient's body weight should be measured daily and occasionally even more often. Fluids administered should be tailored to match the urinary excretion of water and electrolytes.

Fetal uropathies

Modern real-time ultrasonography equipment and interpretation have presented physicians with a new type of patient: the fetus. One condition, obstructive uropathy, appears to be amenable in some cases to treatment in utero. The most common sites of obstruction found during development include the ureteropelvic junction, the ureterovesical junction, and the posterior urethral valves. Antenatal intervention is probably indicated whenever the function of both kidneys is threatened. The amount of amniotic fluid may represent an indirect guide to renal function in the fetus. The risk of invasive procedures for the mother and the fetus must be weighed against the potential benefits. Additional information is needed in this area of prenatal intervention before firm guidelines can be suggested.

Further reading

Chevalier RL, Klahr S: Therapeutic approaches in obstructive uropathy. Semin Nephrol 1998;18:652–658.

Klahr S: Nephrology forum: obstructive nephropathy. Kidney Int 1998;54:286–300.

Klahr S: Obstructive uropathy. *In* Giebisch GH, Seldin DW (eds): The Kidney: Physiology and Pathophysiology, 3rd edn. Philadelphia: Lippincott-Raven, 2000, pp 2473–2512.

Wasserstein AG: Nephrolithiasis. *In* Greenberg A (ed): Primer of Nephrology. New York: Academic Press, 2001, pp 348–354.

PART VII
Renal Disease and Pregnancy

CHRISTOPHER S. WILCOX

Hypertension in Pregnancy

Jason G. Umans

Hypertension is the most common medical complication of pregnancy. Importantly, its diagnosis, risks, goals of therapy, and approaches to treatment all differ considerably compared with hypertension in nonpregnant patients. This chapter focuses, in turn, on classification of hypertension in pregnancy (key to understanding limitations of many treatment trials), risks of hypertension, difficulties in diagnosis, approaches to secondary hypertension, monitoring and management of chronic mild-to-moderate hypertension remote from delivery, management of more severe hypertension, and efforts to prevent preeclampsia.

Classification and risks of hypertension in pregnancy

Until recently, most investigators failed to distinguish among the pathophysiologically distinct hypertensive disorders of pregnancy and used a variety of ill-defined terms that have made it difficult to interpret inclusion criteria and outcomes of many treatment trials. Published in 2000, the updated report of the National High Blood Pressure Education Program (NHBPEP) Working Group on High Blood Pressure in Pregnancy[1] recognizes four classes of hypertensive disorders in pregnancy: (1) chronic hypertension (essential and secondary), (2) preeclampsia–eclampsia, (3) preeclampsia superimposed on chronic hypertension, and (4) gestational hypertension. This schema is largely in accord with those of several national societies and that endorsed by the International Society for the Study of Hypertension in Pregnancy.[2] Absent are terms such as "gestosis," "toxemia," and "pregnancy-induced hypertension."

Chronic essential hypertension

Chronic hypertension is often difficult to diagnose in pregnancy. Many young women only seek medical care when pregnant, not having had baseline blood pressure measurement or clinical evaluation beforehand. The striking early (first-trimester) cardiovascular adaptations to normal pregnancy[3] include systemic vasodilation so profound that blood pressure falls despite 30–50% increments of cardiac output. Thus, while hypertension prior to conception, or documented early in pregnancy, establishes the diagnosis, blood pressures can appear deceptively normal, leading to the later misdiagnosis of preeclampsia or gestational hypertension when arterial pressure rises nearer to term.

Superimposed preeclampsia accounts for most of the morbidity associated with chronic hypertension as it complicates at least 15–20% of pregnancies in women with chronic hypertension and systolic blood pressure ≥ 140 mmHg or diastolic blood pressure ≥ 90 mmHg; this risk rises progressively at higher values.[4–6] Other risks that could conceivably justify treatment include: (1) placental abruption, whose risk is doubled in chronic hypertension and increases threefold further if preeclampsia supervenes;[5] (2) accelerated hypertension leading to hospitalization, target organ damage, or cerebral catastrophe; (3) fetal or perinatal mortality, which is increased threefold;[7] and (4) impaired fetal growth or early delivery based on concerns for maternal safety.

Secondary hypertension

Secondary hypertension, while rare, does occur in pregnancy and requires a high degree of suspicion to make a correct and potentially life-saving diagnosis.[8] Patients with hypertension in the setting of scleroderma, polyarteritis nodosa, or Cushing syndrome do poorly and should not contemplate pregnancy.

Pheochromocytoma may present during pregnancy; review of nearly 100 reported cases suggests high mortality near to term or during labor. Management includes α-adrenergic blockade, followed by β-blockade and resection of the tumor (if it can be localized by magnetic resonance imaging) during the first or second trimester, or resection coupled with operative delivery when the fetus is viable and the tumor discovered during the third trimester.[8]

Renovascular hypertension, usually due to fibromuscular dysplasia, seems to result uniformly in superimposed preeclampsia and such poor outcome as to merit diagnosis and correction by angioplasty during pregnancy, since treatment with angiotensin-converting enzyme (ACE) inhibitors is contraindicated. Diagnosis is sometimes problematic because plasma renin is elevated in normal pregnancy, Doppler ultrasound examinations are often so technically difficult as to miss small lesions, and it is usually difficult to convince radiology colleagues to perform the (single-dose) captopril renography, gadolinium-enhanced magnetic resonance angiography, or renal arteriography necessary for diagnosis. High clinical suspicion should lead first to measurement of plasma renin and to Doppler ultrasound examination, though negative results should not deter further investigation. Magnetic resonance angiography may define a likely lesion sufficient to limit intravenous contrast and x-ray exposure in a subsequent angioplasty.[9]

The clinical course of primary hyperaldosteronism is extraordinarily variable. Its diagnosis is often problematic in pregnancy. Aldosterone is quite elevated in normal pregnancy. There are only rare case reports of simultaneous renin and aldosterone measurements in pregnant women with proven aldosteronoma.[10] Further, pregnancy is often accompanied by mild hypokalemia, often worse in women with emesis. Finally, hypertension and hypokalemia may both be masked by an aldosterone-antagonistic effect of progesterone.[11] A rare mineralocorticoid receptor mutation may lead to first- or second-trimester hypertension when progesterone acts, paradoxically, as an agonist, leading to severe hypertension, salt retention, and hypokalemia with unmeasurable aldosterone levels.[12] Localization of aldosteronoma is often suboptimal during pregnancy as it is usually limited to magnetic resonance imaging. Adrenal vein sampling is avoided due to the large fetal x-ray exposure. Spironolactone is not used during pregnancy because animal studies show fetal virilization. There are physiologic concerns that weigh against use of amiloride. Blood pressure has most commonly been controlled with calcium entry blockers. Adenomas have been successfully resected during the second trimester when antihypertensive therapy has failed.

Preeclampsia–eclampsia

Preeclampsia, which occurs most commonly in the latter half of first pregnancies, is unique to human pregnancy. It is the disorder most apt to endanger the life of the mother and her fetus. Its cardinal features are de novo hypertension and proteinuria, often associated with hyperuricemia and sometimes with thrombocytopenia or abnormalities of liver function or coagulation tests. One should diagnose preeclampsia even in the absence of proteinuria when hypertension is accompanied by abdominal pain, headache, neurologic symptoms including headache or blurred vision, or any evidence of thrombocytopenia or liver function or coagulation abnormalities.[1] Preeclampsia can progress rapidly to a convulsive phase, termed "eclampsia." An especially threatening variant is the HELLP (*h*emolysis, *e*levated *l*iver enzymes, *l*ow *p*latelets) syndrome, which can present with minimal blood pressure elevations, mild proteinuria, and modest elevations of transaminases, but evolve over hours to microangiopathic hemolysis, plunging platelet counts, and marked hepatic damage.

Superimposed preeclampsia

While "pure" preeclampsia occurs in ~ 6% of (usually primigravid) pregnancies, it can be superimposed on up to 20–40% of underlying cases of chronic hypertension, or other predisposing medical diseases including renal disease (see Chapter 46), collagen vascular disease, inherited or acquired thrombophilia, or diabetes mellitus. This can be an especially difficult diagnosis, especially if some hypertension, proteinuria, or laboratory abnormalities were present at baseline. This difficulty is the basis for close monitoring in patients with these underlying conditions, repeatedly reestablishing baseline data in order to detect interval changes in blood pressure, proteinuria, symptoms, or blood test results that might suggest superimposed preeclampsia.

Throughout pregnancy, blood pressure should be measured at rest in the sitting position, using Korotkoff 5 as diastolic pressure. Automated oscillometric devices are notoriously inaccurate during pregnancy. The use of home blood pressure monitors is based more on their ability to detect significant changes in systolic pressure than on accuracy of the data.

Gestational (transient) hypertension

These women develop mild to moderate hypertension in the second half of pregnancy, usually close to term, without proteinuria or other manifestations of preeclampsia. The hypertension resolves post partum, often recurs in subsequent pregnancies, and predicts essential hypertension later in life.

Goals of antihypertensive therapy

Several recent and ongoing structured reviews prove sobering in suggesting that treatment of underlying hypertension fails to prevent superimposed preeclampsia, placental abruption, or reliably decrease perinatal mortality; these conclusions, however, are based on the results of several small trials whose results vary considerably.[7,13–16] The major apparent benefit is the prevention of later severe hypertension.[13–16] Severe hypertension is the major indication for hospital admission and a prime cause of early delivery. Most studies fail to address this important endpoint. It is well established that blood pressure elevations to 170/110 mmHg can lead to cerebrovascular hemorrhage during pregnancy, making treatment of such pressures a medical emergency. "Hard" clinical endpoints are few in mild hypertension and scarcer still over the short duration of a pregnancy. None of the available trials are adequately powered to guide therapy. Thus one must depend on consensus statements,[1,17,18] meta-analyses,[7,13,15,16,19] and clinical experience.[14]

There are no prospective studies to guide the goal for blood pressure. The Australasian Society for the Study of Hypertension in Pregnancy suggests maintaining blood pressures below 140/90 mmHg.[17] The Canadian Hypertension Society suggests similarly tight control only for some groups of women.[18] By contrast, the NHBPEP

Working Group on Hypertension in Pregnancy suggests (re)instituting drug therapy at pressures of 150–160/100–110 mmHg, targeting lower pressures in selected patients with end-organ damage or underlying renal disease.[1] None of the targets is as low as those recently advocated in nonpregnant patients with diabetic nephropathy or proteinuric renal disease. There is controversy as to whether placental blood flow is autoregulated. A recent regression metaanalysis of 14 trials concluded that fetal growth restriction worsened with tighter control of maternal hypertension, irrespective of the specific agents used.[20] Our lack of enthusiasm for tight control, in accord with that of the NHBPEP Working Group, is further tempered by the still limited information regarding fetal and remote childhood risks of exposure to most antihypertensive drugs in utero. Even the acknowledged long-term safety of methyldopa is based on a single study with 7.5-year follow-up of only a small number of children.[21]

No antihypertensive drugs have been conclusively proven safe in early pregnancy. Normal gestational vasodilation lowers mean arterial pressure by ~ 10 mmHg in normotensive women and by 15–20 mmHg in women with essential hypertension. Such decrements are usually adequate to allow discontinuation of some or all antihypertensives in most women with either stage 1 or 2 hypertension. Therapy can then be reinstituted when pressure rises later, usually during the second trimester. Women who fail to exhibit the early gestational vasodilation and fall in blood pressure or who require multidrug therapy during the first trimester seem especially likely to have a stormy pregnancy with guarded outcome.

Selection of antihypertensive agents

Oral agents for initial blood pressure control

Details of individual agents and their use in hypertension are given in Chapters 54, 56, 57, and 58. Each of the three recent consensus statements[1,17,18] recognize methyldopa as the preferred agent with the greatest experience in pregnancy. Methyldopa has been studied in both placebo-controlled and comparative trials,[1,7,13–15,17] appears well tolerated, is without adverse effects on uteroplacental or fetal hemodynamics,[22] and is the best-studied drug for subsequent childhood development.[21] Its use is further bolstered by elegant studies demonstrating increased autonomic outflow in preeclamptic hypertension.[23] While clonidine appears similarly effective as methyldopa, it may be embryopathic in early pregnancy and a small study detected subsequent sleep disturbances in clonidine-exposed infants.[24] However, a recent metaanalysis found no overall effect of antihypertensive therapy on perinatal mortality but suggested that other drugs might be superior to methyldopa in preventing this outcome.[15] Marked heterogeneity in the included trials should temper our willingness to favor this metaanalysis over the consensus statements and long clinical experience.

The β-blockers approach methyldopa in their use in pregnancy. They are advocated by many as preferred therapy. They have been assessed in several randomized trials and in an ongoing Cochrane metaanalysis.[16] Early preclinical and clinical observations raised concerns of impaired uteroplacental perfusion, fetal growth restriction, and harmful cardiovascular effects on the fetus. However, most prospective studies, focusing on β-blocker use in the third trimester, have shown effective blood pressure control, prevention of more severe hypertension, and no significant adverse effects on the fetus.[1,7,13–15,17,18] By contrast, earlier use of atenolol in one controversial trial[25] led to striking fetal growth restriction. Moreover, this conclusion is supported by several more recent reviews and meta-analyses.[15,16,26] More recently, a large non-randomized single-center series noted improved perinatal outcome with β-blockers (primarily atenolol) compared with other agents (primarily nifedipine or methyldopa).[27] Finally, there was a suggestion in one recent metaanalysis of several small trials that β-blockers might decrease, and calcium channel blockers increase, the incidence of proteinuria or superimposed preeclampsia.[15] This preliminary observation should provoke further study rather than a change in practice. While atenolol may be the β-blocker most commonly used in pregnancy, the NHBPEP Working Group advocated labetalol (a combined α- and β-blocker) as an alternative to methlydopa, and the Australasian group advocated use of β-blockers with intrinsic sympathomimetic activity, such as oxprenolol (not available in the USA) or pindolol.[17,28]

Calcium channel blockers are widely used, effective in pregnancy, and appear not to be teratogenic.[1] Most studies have focused on nifedipine, though there are reports of other dihydropyridine and nondihydropyridine agents, including a reassuring but small study with 18 months of infant follow-up.[29] Even though these are tocolytic agents, there are no data to suggest that use of calcium channel blockers for blood pressure control interferes with labor or delivery. While data remain sorely lacking, nifedipine is now widely recognized as an alternative agent to methyldopa or β-blockers for chronic use during pregnancy.

Hydralazine is the most commonly used second-line agent (following combinations of those discussed above). It is used only in combination with a sympatholytic to limit reflex tachycardia. There seems little basis for use of α-adrenergic blockers other than in the setting of suspected pheochromocytoma. Diuretics may be continued, if used before pregnancy, and may be combined with other agents, especially when volume overload is apparent. They appear safe in pregnancy[30] but seem ill-advised in preeclampsia, where hemodynamics are characterized by volume depletion, decreased cardiac output, and primary systemic vasoconstriction. Finally, while there have been several case reports and small series of ACE inhibitor use as "salvage therapy" during pregnancy,[31,32] there seems to be no justification for use of these agents or of angiotensin

Table 45.1 Drugs for chronic hypertension in pregnancy

Drug	FDA risk*†	Dose	Concerns or comments
Most commonly used preferred agents			
Methyldopa	C	0.5–3.0 g/day in two divided doses	Preferred agent of the NHBPEP Working Group; safety after first trimester well documented, including long-term follow-up of offspring
Labetalol (or other β-receptor blockers)	C	200–1200 mg/day in two to three divided doses. For other β-blockers, depends on specific agent	Labetalol is preferred by NHBPEP Working Group as alternative to methyldopa. β-Blockers may cause fetal bradycardia and decrease uteroplacental blood flow; this effect may be less for agents with partial agonist activity. They may all impair fetal growth, especially when started in first or second trimester
Nifedipine	C	30–120 mg/day of a slow-release preparation	May inhibit labor and potentiate effects of magnesium sulfate. Less experience with other calcium entry blockers
Adjunctive agents			
Hydralazine	C	50–300 mg/day in two to four divided doses	Few controlled trials; long experience with few adverse events documented; useful only in combination with sympatholytic agent. May cause neonatal thrombocytopenia
Thiazide diuretics	C	Depends on specific agent	Most studies in normotensive gravidas; can cause volume depletion and electrolyte disorders. May be useful in combination with methyldopa and vasodilator to mitigate compensatory fluid retention
Contraindicated			
ACE inhibitors and AT1 receptor antagonists	D‡		Leads to fetal loss in animals; human use associated with fetopathy, oligohydramnios, growth retardation, and neonatal anuric renal failure, which may be fatal

ACE, angiotensin-converting enzyme; FDA, Food and Drug Administration; NHBPEP, National High Blood Pressure Education Program.

*No antihypertensive has been proven safe for use during the first trimester, i.e. FDA category A.

†FDA classifies risk for most agents as C: "Either studies in animals have revealed adverse effects on the fetus (teratogenic or embryocidal effects or other) and there are no controlled studies in women, or studies in women and animals are not available. Drugs should only be given if the potential benefit justifies the potential risk to the fetus." This nearly useless classification unfortunately still applies to most drugs used during pregnancy.

‡FDA risk category D notes that "there is positive evidence of human fetal risk, but the benefits of use in pregnant women may be acceptable despite the risk (e.g. if the drug is needed in a life-threatening situation or for a serious disease for which safer drugs cannot be used or are ineffective)" and requires a "warning" in the labeling.

receptor blockers as antihypertensives during the second or third trimester. Table 45.1 summarizes those agents most commonly used for chronic blood pressure control in pregnancy.

Oral and parenteral agents for urgent control of more severe hypertension

Parenteral hydralazine, intravenous labetalol, and oral (immediate release) nifedipine are the agents most commonly used for urgent control of severe hypertension late in pregnancy (Table 45.2).[1,14,19] Hydralazine, which must be used in small (5–10 mg) repeated doses or as a continuous infusion, is preferred by many obstetricians and by the NHBPEP Working Group, based more on clinical experience than on compelling data. Indeed, several small studies have highlighted concerns regarding precipitous decreases in cardiac output, blood pressure, and renal function along with an excess of fetal distress. Parenteral labetalol, by continuous intravenous infusion

or in repeated boluses, has replaced hydralazine at many centers and appears to have similar safety and efficacy, though comparative studies are few. Despite never having been approved by the Food and Drug Administration for the treatment of hypertension, the NHBPEP Working Group, along with other workers,[1,33] have advocated oral (or sublingual) nifedipine as an acceptable alternative to hydralazine or labetalol in these patients. Its efficacy and safety appear similar to the other agents. There are conflicting data regarding its effects on uteroplacental perfusion.[34,35] Some animal data raise cautions regarding possible fetal toxicity.[36] Nevertheless, ongoing metaanalysis does not favor one of the agents over the others.[19] Choice is based on the experience of the physician.[1]

Diazoxide has inferior outcomes in several small trials, difficult dose titration, and concerns of possible fetal toxicity. Several reports have suggested ketanserin (not available in the USA) as an alternative, although it seems less effective than hydralazine.[19] Isolated reports of intravenous nicardipine[37] and sublingual nitrates[38] are too scanty to guide therapy. There are no reports of

Table 45.2 Preferred drugs for urgent control of severe hypertension in pregnancy

Drug	FDA risk*	Dose and route	Concerns or comments[†]
Hydralazine	C	5 mg i.v. or i.m., then 5–10 mg every 20–40 min; or constant infusion of 0.5–10 mg/h	Preferred by NHBPEP Working Group; long experience of safety and efficacy. Higher doses or more frequent administration often precipitates fetal distress
Labetalol	C	20 mg i.v., then 20–80 mg every 20–30 min, up to maximum of 300 mg; or constant infusion of 1–2 mg/min	Probably less risk of tachycardia and arrhythmia than with other vasodilators
Nifedipine	C	5–10 mg p.o., repeat in 30 min if needed, then 10–20 mg every 2–6 h	Possible interference with labor; may interact synergistically with magnesium sulfate

FDA, Food and Drug Administration; NHBPEP, National High Blood Pressure Education Program.
*FDA risk category C: see footnote to Table 45.1.
†Adverse effects for all agents, except as noted, may include headache, flushing, nausea, and tachycardia (primarily due to precipitous hypotension and reflex sympathetic activation).

fenoldopam in this clinical setting and nitroprusside remains a relatively contraindicated agent of last resort.[39]

Expectant management and definitive therapy in preeclampsia

Due to its unpredictable and sometimes rapidly progressive course, women should be hospitalized for evaluation at the suspicion of preeclampsia. With fetal maturity near to term, delivery is the treatment of choice for preeclampsia. Remote from term, one is often tempted to control blood pressure, monitor laboratory and clinical status closely, and attempt to prolong pregnancy to gain several weeks of additional fetal maturation. The literature on such temporizing strategies is confusing. Such approaches are

Table 45.3 Threatening maternal signs and symptoms that should suggest proceeding to delivery in women with preeclampsia

Rising blood pressure (systolic ≥ 160 mmHg or diastolic ≥ 105 mmHg) despite oral antihypertensives
Rapid increase in (nephrotic-range) proteinuria coupled with decreasing serum albumin
Increasing serum creatinine or any evidence of acute renal failure
Falling platelet counts, thrombocytopenia < 10⁵/mm³
Any evidence of microangiopathic hemolysis (schistocytes, elevated LDH, elevated direct bilirubin), or coagulopathy
Upper abdominal (epigastric or right upper quadrant) pain
Headache, visual disturbance, or any CNS signs
Retinal hemorrhage or papilledema
Pulmonary edema or acute heart failure

CNS, central nervous system; LDH, lactate dehydrogenase.

best reserved for tertiary centers. Regardless of gestational age, any of a variety of unfavorable signs or symptoms (Table 45.3) should lead to immediate delivery. Accelerated hypertension should be treated at systolic levels of 160 mmHg or diastolic levels of 105 mmHg in order to avoid the cerebral catastrophes reported at pressures of 170/110 mmHg. Central nervous system signs or symptoms should provoke treatment at lower pressures.

Finally, several large, well-designed, and unequivocal trials have demonstrated that parenteral magnesium sulfate is superior to phenytoin or diazepam for prevention or treatment of eclamptic convulsions.[40,41] It is not known whether such prophylactic therapy should be offered to all preeclamptic women prior to delivery. This has been the subject of a large ongoing trial sponsored by the World Health Organization and the British Medical Research Council. The Magpie trial randomized over 10,000 women with preeclampsia to 24 hours of treatment with parenteral magnesium sulfate, which halved the risk of convulsions (eclampsia) and probably reduced the risk of maternal death with no apparent substantive short-term harmful effects to mother or baby.[42] Treatment usually consists of a loading dose of 4–6 g magnesium sulfate (infused over 10 min, never as a bolus), followed by continuous infusion of 1–2 g/h to achieve plasma levels (which should be monitored) of 5–9 mg/dL. Lower doses of magnesium sulfate are required and should be used with great caution in women with any degree of renal insufficiency. A vial of calcium gluconate should be kept at the patient's bedside to treat magnesium toxicity.

Table 45.4 presents an approach to evaluation, management, and treatment of pregnant women with underlying essential hypertension. It expands upon recommendations made by the NHBPEP Working Group.[1] The key principles focus on control of blood pressure adequate to assure maternal safety, serial monitoring to favor early recognition

Table 45.4 An approach to monitoring and therapy (in addition to usual high-risk obstetric care) in pregnant women with chronic essential hypertension

- Stop ACE inhibitors and angiotensin receptor blockers at diagnosis of pregnancy
- Monitor blood pressure closely with aim of rapidly decreasing or stopping all antihypertensive drugs early in first trimester (if blood pressure can be maintained < 150/100 mmHg). Note that failure to exhibit improved blood pressure and increased GFR early in pregnancy may predict especially high risk of difficulties later in pregnancy
- Baseline measurement of creatinine clearance, 24-h protein excretion, electrolytes, BUN and creatinine, uric acid, ALT, AST, LDH, albumin, CBC with platelets. These baseline values and repeated "baselines" (usually only including blood tests and spot-urine protein/creatinine ratios) obtained at 2–4 week intervals later in pregnancy may be important in early recognition of superimposed preeclampsia
- Consider screening for thrombophilia, especially if previous early superimposed preeclampsia or mid-trimester pregnancy loss
- Encourage and instruct in home blood pressure monitoring; otherwise check blood pressure in office (by auscultation) at least every 2 weeks
- If hypertension persists or when it recurs (to levels ≥ 150 mmHg systolic or ≥ 100 mmHg diastolic) restart therapy, favoring methyldopa or labetalol as initial agents, titrating them to maximal doses or dose-limiting adverse effects, then adding a second agent as needed. Preferred second-line agents could be nifedipine or modest doses of the preferred agent not chosen initially (heart rate permitting). Aim is to achieve blood pressure reliably < 160/105 mmHg at all times, considering lower levels (140/90 mmHg) in the setting of significant baseline renal insufficiency or target organ damage
- During the third trimester, increase frequency of visit to every 1–2 weeks
- Admit to hospital for evaluation and add a third agent (hydralazine ± a diuretic) if blood pressure is inadequately controlled. Such severe hypertension occurring remote from term suggests a pregnancy that may not safely succeed in a live birth
- Admit to hospital for evaluation of any clinical or laboratory evidence suggestive of accelerated hypertension, new target organ damage, or superimposed preeclampsia
- Diagnosis of superimposed preeclampsia near to term should lead to expeditious delivery
- Accelerated hypertension, or hypertension not controlled on a reasonable two or three drug oral regimen, should lead to admission, blood pressure control using agents chosen from Table 45.2, and expeditious delivery
- One can delay delivery in cases of "mild" preeclampsia remote from term only if patient can be monitored closely in a tertiary care setting, blood pressure well controlled, and delivery effected for any fetal or maternal deterioration or for threatening findings as listed in Table 45.3
- Consider seizure prophylaxis, with close monitoring, using parenteral magnesium sulfate in all but mild preeclampsia

ACE, angiotensin-converting enzyme; ALT, alanine aminotransferase; AST, aspartate aminotransferase; BUN, blood urea nitrogen; CBC, complete blood cell count; GFR, glomerular filtration rate; LDH, lactate dehydrogenase.

of superimposed preeclampsia, and expeditious delivery (with or without magnesium prophylaxis) in the face of preeclampsia or accelerated hypertension with threat to maternal well-being.

Efforts to prevent preeclampsia

There have been several strategies to prevent preeclampsia or to abort it before it becomes clinically evident. A 1985 metaanalysis of trials including ~ 7000 women claimed that sodium restriction or prophylactic diuretics prevented preeclampsia.[30] Unfortunately, this conclusion was based on flawed definitions as there was no effect on proteinuric hypertension, only less edema and modest reductions in blood pressure.

Low-dose aspirin (60–100 mg/day), started at week 12 of gestation, has been studied extensively, based upon early observations suggesting an imbalance favoring thromboxane over prostacyclin production in preeclampsia. Several early small studies were remarkably encouraging. A 1991 metaanalysis concluded that there was a 76% reduction in proteinuric hypertension. Unfortunately, two large and well-designed trials, including over 12 000 gravidas, showed only trivial effects on maternal or fetal outcome or on the occurrence of preeclampsia.[43,44] Subsequent studies

have focused on aspirin prophylaxis in "high-risk" groups such as women with preeclampsia in a prior pregnancy, chronic essential hypertension, multifetal gestation, or type 1 diabetes mellitus. Again, there was no significant effect on proteinuric hypertension. Current metaanalyses[45] include over 30 000 women. Some have disclosed trivial favorable effects but have failed to identify any group of patients that would benefit from this therapy. Trials in which aspirin dose is altered, sustained-release preparations utilized, or dose schedule altered to take advantage of apparent circadian effects[46] are planned.

Observations that preeclamptic women are hypocalciuric and that preeclampsia is increased in populations with low dietary calcium intake provoked trials of calcium supplementation during pregnancy. Two large and well-designed trials, including over 5500 women, failed to detect any decrease in proteinuric hypertension.[47,48] Subsequent analyses suggested that there might be some effect in women with extremely low calcium intake, prompting a new World Health Organization trial focused on women in developing countries.

More recently, observations of increased oxidant stress in preeclampsia led to a small study of vitamins C and E in women at high risk.[49] This study, in which preeclampsia was but a secondary endpoint, suggested an effect on proteinuria but apparently not on hypertension and, of great concern, seemed to result in an excess of low birth-weight in the treatment group. Two large trials are underway.

Finally, the high incidence of recurrent early-onset preeclampsia in women with inherited or acquired thrombophilias[50] has led many obstetricians to screen for and treat these disorders. Most strategies use low molecular weight heparin or aspirin, while patients with hyperhomocysteinemia receive high-dose folic acid. These strategies may have some benefit in preventing recurrent mid-trimester pregnancy loss, but effects on preeclampsia are yet to be demonstrated.

References

1. Report of the National High Blood Pressure Education Project Working Group on High Blood Pressure in Pregnancy. NIH Publication No. 00-3029, July 2000 (available at www.nhlbi.nih.gov/health/prof/heart/hbp_preg.htm).
2. Brown MA, Lindheimer MD, DeSwiet M, Van Assche A, Moutquin J-M: The classification and diagnosis of the hypertensive disorders of pregnancy: statement from the International Society for the Study of Hypertension in Pregnancy. Hypertens Pregnancy 2001;20:ix–xiv.
3. McLaughlin MK, Roberts JM: Hemodynamic changes. In Lindheimer MD, Roberts JM, Cunningham FG (eds): Chesley's Hypertensive Disorders in Pregnancy, 2nd edn. Stamford: Appleton & Lange, 1999, pp 69–102.
4. Sibai BM, Abdella TN, Anderson GD: Pregnancy outcome in 211 patients with mild chronic hypertension. Obstet Gynecol 1983;61:571–576.
5. Sibai BM, Lindheimer M, Hauth J, et al: Risk factors for preeclampsia, abruptio placentae, and adverse neonatal outcomes among women with chronic hypertension. N Engl J Med 1998;339:667–671.
6. Rey E, Couturier A: The prognosis of pregnancy in women with chronic hypertension. Am J Obstet Gynecol 1994;171:410–416.
7. Ferrer RL, Sibai BM, Mulrow CD, et al: Management of mild chronic hypertension during pregnancy: a review. Obstet Gynecol 2000;96:849–860 (full report available at www.ahcpr.gov/clinic/evrptfiles.htm).
8. August P, Lindheimer MD: Chronic hypertension. In Lindheimer MD, Roberts JM, Cunningham FG (eds): Chesley's Hypertensive Disorders in Pregnancy, 2nd edn. Stamford: Appleton & Lange, 1999, pp 605–633.
9. Le TT, Haskal ZJ, Holland GA, Townsend R: Endovascular stent placement and magnetic resonance angiography for management of hypertension and renal artery occlusion during pregnancy. Obstet Gynecol 1995;85:822–825.
10. August PA, Seeley JE: The renin angiotensin system in normal and hypertensive pregnancy and in ovarian function. In Laragh JH, Brenner BM (eds): Hypertension: Pathophysiology, Diagnosis, and Management, 2nd edn. New York: Raven Press, 1995, pp 2225–2244.
11. Lindheimer MD, Richardson DA, Ehrlich EM, Katz AI: Potassium homeostasis in pregnancy. J Reprod Med 1987;32:517–532.
12. Geller DS, Farhi A, Pinkerton N, et al: Activating mineralocorticoid receptor mutation in hypertension exacerbated by pregnancy. Science 2000;289:119–123.
13. Magee LA, Ornstein MP, von Dadelszen P: Management of hypertension in pregnancy. Br Med J 1999;318:1332–1336.
14. Sibai BM: Treatment of hypertension in pregnant women. N Engl J Med 1996;335:257–265.
15. Abalos E, Duley L, Steyn DW, Henderson-Smart DJ: Antihypertensive drug therapy for mild to moderate hypertension during pregnancy. Cochrane Database Syst Rev 2001;2:CD002252.
16. Magee LA, Duley L: Oral beta blockers for mild to moderate hypertension during pregnancy. Cochrane Database Syst Rev 2000;4:CD002863.
17. Brown MA, Hague WM, Higgins J, et al: The detection, investigation and management of hypertension in pregnancy: full consensus statement. Aust N Z J Obstet Gynecol 2000;40:139–155.
18. Rey E, LeLorier J, Burgess E, et al: Report of the Canadian Hypertension Society consensus conference. 3. Pharmacologic treatment of hypertensive disorders in pregnancy. Can Med Assoc J 1997;157:1245–1254.
19. Duley L, Henderson-Smart DJ: Drugs for rapid treatment of very high blood pressure during pregnancy. Cochrane Database Syst Rev 2000;2:CD001449.
20. von Dadelszen P, Ornstein MP, Bull SB, et al: Fall in mean arterial pressure and fetal growth restriction in pregnancy hypertension: a meta-analysis. Lancet 2000;355:87–92.
21. Cockburn J, Moar VA, Ounsted M, Redman CW: Final report of study on hypertension during pregnancy: the effects of specific treatment on the growth and development of the children. Lancet 1982;i:647–649. (Earlier follow-up papers from this trial appeared in Early Hum Dev 1977;1:47–57, 59–67.)
22. Montan S, Anandakumar C, Arulkumaran S, et al: Effects of methyldopa on uteroplacental and fetal hemodynamics in pregnancy-induced hypertension. Am J Obstet Gynecol 1993;168:152–156.
23. Schobel HP, Fischer T, Heuszer K, Geiger H, Schmieder RE: Preeclampsia: a state of sympathetic overactivity. N Engl J Med 1996;335:1480–1485.
24. Huisjes HJ, Hadders-Algra M, Touwen BC: Is clonidine a behavioural teratogen in the human? Early Hum Dev 1986;14:43–48.
25. Butters L, Kennedy S, Rubin PC: Atenolol in essential hypertension during pregnancy. Br Med J 1990;301:587–589.
26. Lip GY, Beevers M, Churchill D, Shaffer LM, Beevers DG: Effect of atenolol on birthweight. Am J Cardiol 1997;79:1436–1438.
27. Ray JG, Vermeulen MJ, Burrows EA, Burrows RF: Use of antihypertensive medications in pregnancy and the risk of adverse perinatal outcomes: McMaster Outcome Study of Hypertension In Pregnancy 2 (MOS HIP 2). BMC Pregnancy Childbirth 2001;1:6.
28. Gallery EDM, Ross MR, Gyory AZ: Antihypertensive treatment in pregnancy: analysis of different responses to oxprenolol and methyldopa. Br Med J 1985;291:563–566.
29. Bortolus R, Ricci E, Chatenoud L, Parazzini F: Nifedipine administered in pregnancy: effect on the development of children at 18 months. Br J Obstet Gynaecol 2000;107:792–794.
30. Collins R, Yusuf S, Peto R: Overview of randomised trials of diuretics in pregnancy. Br Med J 1985;290:17–23.
31. Tomlinson AJ, Campbell J, Walker JJ, Morgan C: Malignant primary hypertension in pregnancy treated with lisinopril. Ann Pharmacother 2000;34:180–182.
32. Easterling TR, Carr DB, Davis C, Diederichs C, Brateng DA, Schmucker B: Low-dose, short-acting, angiotensin-converting enzyme inhibitors as rescue therapy in pregnancy. Obstet Gynecol 2000;96:956–961.
33. Gallery ED, Gyory AZ: Sublingual nifedipine in human pregnancy. Aust N Z J Med 1997;27:538–542.
34. Visser W, Wallenburg HC: A comparison between the hemodynamic effects of oral nifedipine and intravenous dihydralazine in patients with severe preeclampsia. J Hypertens 1995;13:791–795.
35. Fenakel K, Fenakel G, Appelman Z, Lurie S, Katz Z, Shoham Z: Nifedipine in the treatment of severe preeclampsia. Obstet Gynecol 1991;77:331–337.
36. Blea CW, Barnard JM, Magness RR, Phernetton TM, Hendricks SK: Effect of nifedipine on fetal and maternal hemodynamics and blood gases in the pregnant ewe. Am J Obstet Gynecol 1997;176:922–930.
37. Aya AG, Mangin R, Hoffet M, Eledjam JJ: Intravenous nicardipine for severe hypertension in preeclampsia: effects of treatment on mother and foetus. Intensive Care Med 1999;25:1277–1281.
38. Martinez-Abundis E, Gonzalez-Ortiz M, Hernandez-Salazar F, Huerta-J-Lucas MT: Sublingual isosorbide dinitrate in the acute control of hypertension in severe preeclampsia. Gynecol Obstet Invest 2000;50:39–42.
39. Shoemaker CT, Meyers M: Sodium nitroprusside for control of severe hypertensive disease of pregnancy: a case report and discussion of potential toxicity. Am J Obstet Gynecol 1984;149:171–173.
40. The Eclampsia Collaborative Group: Which anticonvulsant for women with eclampsia? Evidence from the collaborative eclampsia trial. Lancet 1995;345:1455–1463.
41. Lucas MJ, Leveno KJ, Cunningham FG: A comparison of magnesium sulfate with phenytoin for the prevention of eclampsia. N Engl J Med 1995;333:201–205.
42. The Magpie Trial Collaborative Group: Do women with preeclampsia, and their babies, benefit from magnesium sulphate? The Magpie Trial: a randomised placebo-controlled trial. Lancet 2002;359:1877–1890.
43. Sibai BM, Caritis SN, Thom E, et al: Prevention of preeclampsia with low-dose aspirin in healthy, nulliparous pregnant women. N Engl J Med 1993;329:1213–1218.
44. CLASP (Collaborative Low-dose Aspirin Study in Pregnancy)

Collaborative Group: CLASP: a randomised trial of low-dose aspirin for the prevention and treatment of among 9364 pregnant women. Lancet 1994;343:619–629.

45. Duley L, Henderson-Smart D, Knight M, King J: Antiplatelet drugs for prevention of pre-eclampsia and its consequences: systematic review. Br Med J 2001;322:329–333.

46. Hermida RC, Ayala DE, Fernandez JR, et al: Administration time-dependent effects of aspirin in women at differing risk for preeclampsia. Hypertension 1999;34:1016–1023.

47. Belizan JM, Villar J, Gonzalez L, Campodonico L, Bergel E: Calcium supplementation to prevent hypertensive disorders of pregnancy. N Engl J Med 1991;325:1399–1405.

48. Levine RJ, Hauth JC, Curet LB, et al: Trial of calcium to prevent preeclampsia. N Engl J Med 1997;337:69–76.

49. Chappell LC, Seed PT, Briley AL, et al: Effect of antioxidants on the occurrence of pre-eclampsia in women at increased risk: a randomised trial. Lancet 1999;354:810–816.

50. Dekker GA, de Vries JI, Doelitzsch PM, et al: Underlying disorders associated with severe early-onset preeclampsia. Am J Obstet Gynecol 1995;173:1042–1048.

46 Renal Disease in Pregnancy

Jason G. Umans

Urinary tract infection
Nephrolithiasis
Acute renal failure
Woman with underlying kidney disease or renal
insufficiency
Pregnancy in woman with end-stage renal disease
Pregnancy in woman with a renal allograft

This chapter reviews the evaluation and management of pregnant women with renal abnormalities. Pregnancy leads to major changes in renal physiology.[1] Severe hypertension or preeclampsia are the most common complications in the high-risk pregnancies of women with underlying renal disease (see Chapter 45). This chapter begins with a discussion of urinary infection and nephrolithiasis, both of which are importantly influenced by gestational changes in renal structure. The remainder of the chapter focuses on pregnancy in women with underlying renal disease.

Urinary tract infection

Urinary infection is among the most common medical complications of pregnancy. Asymptomatic bacteriuria progresses to overt infection in up to 40% of untreated gravidas, with pyelonephritis complicating 1–2% of all pregnancies. Normal pregnancy is accompanied by striking dilation of the intrarenal collecting system and ureters during the first trimester which persists for 3 months post partum. Urinary stasis favors the high incidence of pyelonephritis, with bacterial growth enhanced further by gestational glucosuria and aminoaciduria. Not only is bacteriuria often asymptomatic, but normal (uninfected) gravidas manifest symptoms of frequency and nocturia that might suggest cystitis. Standard obstetric practice thus includes urine screening by week 16 of gestation.

Asymptomatic or overt cystitis is treated for 7–10 days using an antibiotic based on sensitivity testing. The most commonly used first-line agents are nitrofurantoin, trimethoprim–sulfamethoxazole, or a first-generation cephalosporin. An ongoing metaanalysis discloses no preferred agent in pregnancy.[2] Such short-course therapy will eradicate most infections. By contrast, single-dose or 3-day regimens are usually inadequate in pregnancy. Several antibiotics present specific risks to the fetus: sulfonamides should be avoided for several weeks before delivery, fluoroquinolones can result in an arthropathy, tetracyclines cause dental problems, and aminoglycosides entail a 2–3% risk of ototoxicity.

Treatment of bacteriuria or cystitis appears to decrease the incidence of preterm birth,[3] fetal death,[4] and perhaps mental retardation and developmental delay in infancy. Animal studies suggest that preterm delivery may be due to clinically silent seeding of the genital tract and placenta.[5] Relapse of infection with the same organism requires an additional 2–3 weeks of antibiotic therapy, followed by suppressive therapy until delivery. By contrast, pyelonephritis occurring in pregnancy requires hospitalization and initial treatment with a combination of intravenous antibiotics to provide broad-spectrum coverage and narrowing antibiotic coverage when specific sensitivities become available. In the absence of complications, a recent randomized trial suggested that treatment could be completed with 2–3 weeks of oral antibiotics on an outpatient basis.[6] Treatment is then followed by either suppressive therapy or frequent-surveillance urine cultures to term.

Nephrolithiasis

Pregnancy is characterized by an absorptive hypercalciuria, in part associated with increased intake of calcium and vitamin D as well as by placental vitamin D hydroxylation. Normal urinary calcium excretion is doubled in pregnancy to ~ 250 mg/day. There is supersaturation of calcium oxalate and brushite.[7,8] This predisposition to nephrolithiasis does not lead to widespread stone disease, perhaps due to augmented excretion of urinary inhibitors of crystallization, adhesion, or aggregation. Few of the episodes of symptomatic stone during pregnancy occur in women with previously diagnosed stone disease. In many cases, stone disease remains undiagnosed, noted only as recurrent urinary infection.

Suppressive therapy with thiazide diuretics or allopurinol in known stone formers should be discontinued during pregnancy and replaced with a high fluid intake to maintain urine volumes in excess of 2.5 L/day. Oral alkali is used judiciously in women with uric acid nephrolithiasis. Several large series report an incidence of 1 in 1500–3500 deliveries, with most admissions for nephrolithiasis occurring in mid-gestation. Initial ultrasound evaluation successfully visualizes 60% of stones. The remainder can be detected by single-shot intravenous pyelography.[9] While 75% of symptomatic women respond to conservative management with intravenous fluids and analgesics, the remainder require urologic intervention, including stenting or percutaneous drainage. Finally, while none would advocate extracorporeal shock-wave lithotripsy during pregnancy, there are several case reports of such procedures being performed inadvertently during the first month of gestation without apparent harm.[10]

Acute renal failure

Acute renal failure (ARF) was a common and often fatal accompaniment of illlegal septic abortion. Dialysis is now required in only about 1 in 20 000 pregnancies. While most severe ARF is due to acute tubular necrosis (ATN), up to 1 in 4 of these dialysis-requiring cases are associated with usually irreversible cortical necrosis, most often in women with placental abruption occurring after 32 weeks of gestation. This should be suspected in the setting of anuria, hematuria, or persisting oliguria. Definitive diagnosis is most commonly made by renal angiography.

While most ARF is to due to familiar causes such as hemorrhage, infection, volume depletion, nephrotoxins, or obstruction, etiologies peculiar to pregnancy include acute fatty liver of pregnancy (which requires prompt evacuation of the uterus) and the HELLP (hemolysis, elevated liver function tests, low platelets) variant of preeclampsia. ATN only occurs in 1–2% of women with preeclampsia, but in one large series complicated > 7% of women with HELLP syndrome.[11] Finally, "idiopathic postpartum renal failure" is a rare disorder that can occur following delivery or present up to 6 weeks post partum as a thrombotic microangiopathy, clinically indistinguishable from hemolytic–uremic syndrome. Standard therapy now requires plasma infusion or plasmapheresis.

Recognition of the normal gestational dilation of the collecting system and ureters is key to avoiding misdiagnosis of obstructive uropathy in the absence of clinical correlation. Rarely, however, women will present with a "distension syndrome" characterized by abdominal pain, marked hydronephrosis, small decrements in glomerular filtration rate (GFR), and mild hypertension that resolve with stenting or delivery.

Women with underlying kidney disease or renal insufficiency

Subtle renal insufficiency often goes unrecognized in pregnancy. This is due to normal first-trimester renal vasodilation, with both GFR and effective renal plasma flow rising 30–50% even in most women with chronic renal insufficiency. A serum creatinine of 0.5 mg/dL is normal in pregnancy. Thus a serum creatinine > 0.8 mg/dL or blood urea nitrogen > 13 mg/dL should be viewed with suspicion. Failure of women with known renal insufficiency to augment their renal hemodynamics early in pregnancy predicts risk later in pregnancy.

An old literature fostered the notions that pregnancy had an adverse effect on the progression of chronic renal insufficiency, rarely succeeded in a live birth, and entailed intolerable risks to the gravida. Several large retrospective studies and careful case series have changed these impressions entirely. The degree of prior renal insufficiency and hypertension largely predict outcome.[12] Over 95% of pregnancies will succeed in a live birth without adverse impact on renal disease progression in those women whose renal function is stable and well preserved (serum creatinine ≤ 1.4 mg/dL) and in whom hypertension is absent or well controlled. These remain high-risk pregnancies, as up to 30% will suffer superimposed preeclampsia. Most women with glomerular disease have increases in proteinuria, often to nephrotic range, that sometimes complicate management, certainly make diagnosis of preeclampsia difficult, but rarely herald progressive loss of renal function. By contrast, while urinary protein excretion doubles in normal gravidas, increments in albuminuria rarely reach clinical significance.[1]

Women with lower GFR prior to conception (serum creatinine 1.4–2.8 mg/dL) still have a 90% likelihood of a live birth, although the incidence of prematurity and fetal growth restriction are increased dramatically.[12–15] Of great concern, 40% of these women will suffer precipitous and often irreversible loss of GFR due to the pregnancy. Many will progress to endstage renal disease within 1 year post partum. Over 30% of these pregnancies will be complicated by severe or difficult-to-control hypertension. Finally, in this group preexisting hypertension seems to predict poor outcome even more strongly than the severity of renal insufficiency.

Women with severe renal insufficiency (serum creatinine > 2.8 mg/dL) should avoid pregnancy as fewer than half will have live births, nearly all will suffer complications including severe hypertension, and a majority will have accelerated loss of renal function.

Some specific renal diseases may deviate from these rules. Women with polyarteritis nodosa or scleroderma are sufficiently likely to suffer functional loss or life-threatening hypertensive crises to merit counseling against pregnancy. There is disagreement as to whether the renal prognosis is worse in women with reflux nephropathy, focal segmental glomerulosclerosis, IgA nephropathy, or membranoproliferative glomerulonephritis, although the data seem more consistent in the case of membranoproliferative glomerulonephritis.[14–16] Patients with reflux require either frequent-surveillance urine cultures or suppressive antibiotic therapy for the duration of pregnancy. While outcome appears predicted by renal function and blood pressure control in women with autosomal dominant polycystic kidney disease, those with hepatic cysts often find that the cysts grow significantly during pregnancy.

Lupus nephropathy may fare worse than other glomerular diseases, although several recent small case series have been more encouraging.[17,18] Prognosis is most favorable when patients are in remission at least 6 months prior to conception. Disease flares may be difficult to differentiate from superimposed preeclampsia. Antiphospholipid antibodies lead to recurrent, usually midtrimester, pregnancy loss; standard therapy now includes low molecular weight heparin and aspirin.

While pregnancy outcome in diabetic nephropathy is excellent in normotensive women with baseline creatinine < 1.4 mg/dL, these remain high-risk pregnancies as roughly three-fourths will be complicated by nephrotic syndrome, a majority by hypertension, and one-third by reversible decrements in renal function.[19,20] Angiotensin-converting enzyme (ACE) inhibition or angiotensin II receptor blockade is contraindicated during pregnancy because of a specific fetopathy and the risk of neonatal acute renal failure. While these drugs are usually discontinued when pregnancy is planned, they are not teratogenic and can be stopped during the first trimester if pregnancy is detected early.

Nephrotic syndrome predicts poor fetal outcome. A recent small series suggests that proteinuria > 2 g/day might predict renal functional loss better than the classic criteria of residual function and blood pressure.[21] Even though serum albumin will usually fall and edema worsen during pregnancy, diuretic therapy should be avoided if possible. In normal pregnancy, total body water increases 6–9 L (4–7 L of which is extracellular), accompanied by cumulative retention of ~ 900 mequiv. of sodium, a 50% increase in plasma volume, and the occurrence of some clinically evident dependent edema, even in the absence of any disease. Diuretic-induced intravascular volume depletion may impair uteroplacental perfusion and fetal growth.

Nephrotic syndrome and pregnancy are each hypercoagulable states, together presenting increased risk of venous thrombosis or pregnancy loss due to placental infarction. While warfarin is contraindicated during pregnancy and heparin may lead to osteoporosis, many now advocate low molecular weight heparin in such hypercoagulable gravidas. The hyperlipidemia that accompanies nephrosis is rarely treated during pregnancy because hydroxymethylglutaryl CoA reductase inhibitors are contraindicated. Animal models show adverse effects of a low-protein diet on fetal development, arguing strongly against such diets in pregnant women. Finally, due to increased risk of infection, women with nephrotic proteinuria should have repeated screening for asymptomatic bacteriuria.

When renal disease presents during pregnancy, treatment depends on a specific pathologic diagnosis. The most common indications for biopsy include unexplained and progressive renal insufficiency or symptomatic nephrotic syndrome.[22]

Pregnancy in women with endstage renal disease

Fewer than half of desired pregnancies in dialysis patients lead to live births, with most infants being born early, small, and at increased risk for developmental problems, although not for congenital abnormalities. Pregnancies are characterized by a high incidence of hectic hypertension and by a real risk of maternal death. These pregnancies are rarely planned, usually not recognized early, and most commonly end in spontaneous abortion or termination.

Knowledge regarding dialysis in pregnancy has been enhanced by an American Registry,[23] to which all patients should be reported. It appears that women fare equally well with peritoneal dialysis or hemodialysis, although this may be confounded by greater residual renal function in women on peritoneal dialysis that favors successful pregnancy. It is common practice to increase dialysis delivery during pregnancy. Registry data support this, with

a significantly decreased prematurity and a trend toward increased infant survival in women receiving > 20 h of hemodialysis per week. Increased clearances in peritoneal dialysis will usually require use of a cycler, aiming for six to eight exchanges per day. Hemodialysis will usually include at least five and preferably six treatments per week. Such a strategy minimizes transient hypotension due to fluid removal, which has been associated with fetal distress. Suggested modifications of the dialysis prescription are listed in Table 46.1.

Pregnancy in women with a renal allograft

Renal transplantation reverses the impaired fertility of chronic renal failure. Approximately 12% of women of childbearing age with renal allografts will become pregnant. Over 14 000 pregnancies are reported to registries in the USA, Europe, and the UK. Pregnancy per se does not adversely affect long-term graft survival, nor does it increase rejection episodes or short-term loss of well-functioning allografts.[24,25] These pregnancies nevertheless have a high rate of complications, and require close monitoring and careful attention to the diagnosis and treatment of decreased clearance or hypertension.

Of the two-thirds of pregnancies that progress beyond the first trimester, 95% will lead to a live birth. Living donor kidneys, lower steroid dosage, and better allograft function all predict better outcome. These remain high-risk pregnancies, with a 30% incidence of new or worsened hypertension or of superimposed preeclampsia, and approximately half of the infants suffering preterm birth and fetal growth restriction.[24] A recent single-center experience further suggested that both proteinuria and chronic rejection are associated with poor outcome. Graft loss was accelerated in all women with baseline serum creatinine > 2.2 mg/dL.[25]

In anticipation of pregnancy, it is reasonable to ensure stable graft function, without recent (preceding 6 months) acute rejection; defer conception until 2 years after a cadaveric and 1.5 years after a living donor transplant; minimize immunosuppressive drug dosages (prednisone < 15 mg/day, cyclosporine < 4 mg/kg/day), establish tight glucose control in diabetic patients; and control blood pressure to < 140/90 mmHg without use of ACE inhibitors or angiotensin receptor blockers.

While much of the published experience includes women receiving prednisone and azathioprine in the "pre-cyclosporine" era, both registry and single-center data suggest similar outcomes in women on cyclosporine-based regimens, save for a tendency toward somewhat earlier delivery of slightly smaller infants.[24] Remote follow-up of infants exposed to cyclosporine in utero identified a possible excess of developmental delay.[26] There are now additional registry data to suggest similar outcomes in women receiving tacrolimus as in those receiving cyclosporine-based regimens.[24,27] Data with mycophenolate mofetil and sirolimus are so limited as to favor change to a regimen based on "older" agents prior to pregnancy.

Table 46.1 Modifications of hemodialysis prescription during pregnancy

Modification	Rationale
Intensified or daily dialysis to keep BUN < 50 mg/dL or achieve Kt/V > 1.7 in each of six dialyses per week. Avoid large fluid shifts and intradialytic hypotension	Increased dialysis delivery with ≥ 20 h/week of efficient hemodialysis appears to improve infant outcome in registry data
Increase estimated dry weight by 0.5–1.0 kg/month during the first 6 months and by 0.25–0.5 kg/week during the last trimester, with close monitoring of blood pressure	To mimic the usual physiologic volume expansion of normal pregnancy
Decrease dialysate Na^+ to 134 mequiv./L	To mimic the hypotonic hyponatremia due to the "reset osmostat" which characterizes normal pregnancy
Increase dialysate K^+ to 3.0–3.5 mequiv./L, based on serum chemistries	To avoid hypokalemia with increased dialysis
Decrease dialysate Ca^{2+} to 2.5 mequiv./L, decrease or discontinue calcitriol, and monitor serum Ca^{2+} weekly	Increased Ca^{2+} absorption due to vitamin D hydroxylation along with increased dialysis can lead to hypercalcemia
Decrease dialysate HCO_3^- to 25 mequiv./L; if not feasible, increase ultrafiltration and replace with saline	To avoid severe alkalosis, given the primary respiratory alkalosis that characterizes normal pregnancy
Double erythropoietin at conception and increase as needed to keep hematocrit > 30%	Anemia per se leads to poor pregnancy outcome and circulating volume is increased
Intravenous iron (only in 100–200 mg doses) to keep transferrin saturation > 15%	Normal pregnancy requires ~ 1 g of iron. Small doses to limit placental transfer
Monitor serum phosphorus weekly and decrease oral binders or supplement phosphorus during dialysis if low	Daily dialysis and phosphorus utilization can lead to unexpected hypophosphatemia
Double folate supplementation	To prevent neural tube defects

BUN, blood urea nitrogen.

Table 46.2 Evaluation and management of decreased renal function in pregnant transplant patients

Working diagnosis and suggestive findings	Initial interventions
Presumed toxicity High cyclosporine or tacrolimus level, variable hypertension, bland urine sediment, no recent increase in proteinuria or hepatic transaminases, and normal platelets and peripheral smear	Empiric decrease in cyclosporine or tacrolimus dose. Biopsy if not improved
Presumed rejection Variable hypertension, no recent increase in proteinuria or hepatic transaminases, and normal platelets and peripheral smear	Biopsy and treat empirically with high-dose steroids. If diagnosis confirmed, continue then taper steroids. May use OKT3 in refractory cases
Presumed preeclampsia New or worsened hypertension, new or worsened proteinuria, usually > 20 weeks' gestation, variable evidence of hemoconcentration or of HELLP syndrome (hemolysis by smear or LDH, elevated transaminases, thrombocytopenia)	Delivery is definitive treatment for preeclampsia. Treat severe hypertension prior to delivery and consider magnesium (dosed cautiously) for seizure prophylaxis. Biopsy if not improved; HELLP syndrome, hemolytic–uremic syndrome, and vascular rejection may be difficult to distinguish even with biopsy

HELLP, hemolysis, elevated liver function tests, low platelets; LDH, lactate dehydrogenase.

Routine maternal screening is required for infections transmissible to the fetus. These women are best followed with daily home blood pressure monitoring, frequent (2–4 weeks) monitoring of trough cyclosporine or tacrolimus levels, and frequent assessment of renal function, proteinuria, complete blood count, and serum chemistries that might aid in the diagnosis of superimposed preeclampsia (e.g., uric acid, lactate dehydrogenase, aspartate aminotransferase, alanine aminotransferase). They should have monthly fetal ultrasound examinations, once or twice weekly assessments of fetal well-being (nonstress test or biophysical profile) after week 26, and repeated screening (each trimester) for cytomegalovirus, toxoplasmosis and herpes simplex IgM (in seronegative patients).

It is often difficult to distinguish preeclampsia from acute rejection or calcineurin inhibitor toxicity. Registry data suggest that immunosuppressive dose adjustments are required in a majority of pregnant women receiving Neoral brand of cyclosporine and in about half of women on tacrolimus[24] (Table 46.2). Evaluation should also include efforts to rule out new cytomegalovirus infection or reactivation. Half of these infections will spread to the fetus, many with tragic consequences. Ganciclovir does not benefit proven fetal infections, causes fetal ocular toxicity, and should be used for maternal indications.

In the absence of graft dysfunction, new or worsened hypertension along with any degree of proteinuria should be considered as superimposed preeclampsia. Patients should be hospitalized, observed closely, and blood pressure controlled to a safe level. Temporizing to avoid immediate delivery should only be contemplated in a tertiary setting where maternal safety can be assured (see Chapter 45). Finally, the allograft itself presents no obstacle to vaginal delivery.

One can now be optimistic regarding fetal and maternal outcome in many pregnancies complicated by renal disease. However, difficulties in diagnosing and managing superimposed preeclampsia along with complications specific to individual disorders still make these high-risk pregnancies, requiring the cooperation of nephrologists and maternal and fetal medicine specialists, often in tertiary centers.

References

1. Conrad KP, Lindheimer MD: Renal and cardiovascular alterations. *In* Lindheimer MD, Roberts JM, Cunningham FG (eds): Chesley's Hypertensive Disorders in Pregnancy, 2nd edn. Stamford: Appleton and Lange, 1999, pp 262–326.
2. Vazquez JC, Villar J: Treatments for symptomatic urinary tract infections during pregnancy. Cochrane Database Syst Rev 2000;3:CD002256.
3. Smaill F: Antibiotics for asymptomatic bacteriuria in pregnancy. Cochrane Database Syst Rev 2000;2:CD000490.
4. McDermott S, Daguise V, Mann H, Szwejbka L, Callaghan W: Perinatal risk for mortality and mental retardation associated with maternal urinary-tract infections. J Fam Pract 2001;50:433–437.
5. Ovalle A, Levancini M: Urinary tract infections in pregnancy. Curr Opin Urol 2001;11:55–59.
6. Wing DA, Hendershott CM, Debuque L, Millar LK: Outpatient treatment of acute pyelonephritis in pregnancy after 24 weeks. Obstet Gynecol 1999;94:683–688.
7. Maikranz P, Lindheimer M, Coe F: Nephrolithiasis in pregnancy. Baillieres Clin Obstet Gynaecol 1994;8:375–386.
8. Smith CL, Kristensen C, Davis M, Abraham PA: An evaluation of the physicochemical risk for renal stone disease during pregnancy. Clin Nephrol 2001;55:205–211.
9. Butler EL, Cox SM, Eberts EG, Cunningham FG: Symptomatic nephrolithiasis complicating pregnancy. Obstet Gynecol 2000;96:753–756.
10. Asgari MA, Safarinejad MR, Hosseini SY, Dadkhah F: Extracorporeal shock wave lithotripsy of renal calculi during early pregnancy. BJU Int 1999;84:615–617.
11. Sibai BM, Ramadan MK: Acute renal failure in pregnancies complicated by hemolysis, elevated liver enzymes, and low platelets. Am J Obstet Gynecol 1993;168:1682–1687.
12. Lindheimer MD, Grunfeld J-P, Davison JM: Renal disorders. *In* Baron WM, Lindheimer MD (eds): Medical Disorders During Pregnancy. Chicago: Mosby, 2000, pp 39–70.
13. Jones DC, Hayslett JP: Outcome of pregnancy in women with moderate or severe renal insufficiency. N Engl J Med 1996;335:226–232.
14. Jungers P, Houillier P, Forget D, Henry-Amar M: Specific controversies concerning the natural history of renal disease in pregnancy. Am J Kidney Dis 1991;17:116–122.
15. Abe S, Amgasaki Y, Konishi K, et al: The influence of antecedent renal disease on pregnancy. Am J Obstet Gynecol 1985;153:508–514.
16. Barcelo P, Lopez-Lillo J, Cabero L, Del Rio G: Successful pregnancy in primary glomerular disease. Kidney Int 1986;30:914–919.
17. Julkunen H: Pregnancy and lupus nephritis. Scand J Urol Nephrol 2001;35:319–327.
18. Huong DL, Wechsler B, Vauthier-Brouzes D, Beaufils H, Lefebvre G, Piette JC: Pregnancy in past or present lupus nephritis: a study of 32 pregnancies from a single centre. Ann Rheum Dis 2001;60:599–604.
19. Kitzmiller JL, Brown ER, Phillippe M, et al: Diabetic nephropathy and perinatal outcome. Am J Obstet Gynecol 1981;141:741–751.
20. Reece EA, Coustan DR, Hayslett JP, et al: Diabetic nephropathy: pregnancy performance and fetomaternal outcome. Am J Obstet Gynecol 1988;159:56–66.
21. Hemmelder MH, de Zeeuw D, Fidler V, de Jong PE: Proteinuria: a risk factor for pregnancy-related renal function decline in primary glomerular disease? Am J Kidney Dis 1995;26:187–192.
22. Chen HH, Lin HC, Yeh JC, Chen CP: Renal biopsy in pregnancies complicated by undetermined renal disease. Acta Obstet Gynecol Scand 2001;80:888–893.
23. Hou S: Pregnancy in chronic renal insufficiency and end-stage renal disease. Am J Kidney Dis 1999;33: 235–252.
24. Armenti VT, Moritz MJ, Radomski JS, Davison JM: Pregnancy and transplantation. Graft 2000;3:59–63.
25. Crowe AV, Rustom R, Gradden C, et al: Pregnancy does not adversely affect renal transplant function. Q J Med 1999;92:631–635.
26. Stanley CW, Gottlieb R, Zager J, et al: Developmental well-being in offspring of women receiving cyclosporin post-renal transplant. Transplant Proc 1999;31:241–242.
27. Kainz A, Harabacz I, Cowlrick IS, Gadgil SD, Hagiwara D: Review of the course and outcome of 100 pregnancies in 84 women treated with tacrolimus. Transplantation 2000;70:1718–1721.

PART VIII
Pediatric Nephrology

HUGH R. BRADY

Management of Pediatric Kidney Disease

Nancy M. Rodig and Michael J.G. Somers

Proteinuria
Nephrotic syndrome
- Minimal-change disease
- Focal segmental glomerulosclerosis
- Congenital nephrotic syndrome
Hematuria
- Etiology and evaluation
  – Laboratory and radiographic studies
- Benign familial hematuria and Alport syndrome
- Idiopathic hypercalciuria
- Glomerulonephritis
- Henoch–Schönlein purpura
- IgA nephropathy
- Postinfectious glomerulonephritis
- Membranoproliferative glomerulonephritis
Hemolytic–uremic syndrome
- Epidemiology
- Clinical manifestations
- Therapy
- Outcome
Hypertension
Urinary tract infection and vesicoureteral reflux

Although few children are afflicted by serious renal disease, a wide variety of nephrologic problems may present in childhood. Many of these same problems may also be found in adults, but in children there are often significant differences in the etiology, the approach to diagnostic evaluation, and therapy. Moreover, the low incidence of pediatric renal disease has often precluded the execution of large controlled studies to provide evidence-based assessments of specific treatments. As a result, many therapies in children are either empiric or based on experiences drawn from treating adults. An additional distinguishing and important feature of the approach to therapy in the child is the need to consider the effect of any intervention on the child's ongoing physical and cognitive development. In this chapter, many of the more common renal conditions in children are discussed, with particular attention to aspects of diagnosis or management most germane to the pediatric patient that may contrast with the approach to the adult patient with a similar problem.

Proteinuria

As a common and readily detected sign of renal disease, proteinuria often triggers a diagnostic evaluation for significant underlying renal pathology. As with adults, all children excrete a small amount of protein daily in their urine. Normal parameters are related to both size and age and, as

a general rule, children under 10 years of age rarely excrete more than 100 mg of urinary protein per day.[1] In older children and adolescents, urinary protein excretion can increase up to the 150–200 mg/day threshold considered normal in adults.[2]

In most children, proteinuria is asymptomatic and detected as part of a general examination during which a random sample of urine is assayed by a qualitative colorimetric test strip. In urine samples in which a more precise estimation of protein excretion is needed, a urinary protein to creatinine ratio can prove more useful and has been demonstrated to be an accurate method for assessing daily protein excretion in children.[3] A ratio ≤ 0.5 in a child less than 2 years old or ≤ 2 in an older child is considered normal. These ratios can be followed to assess changes in proteinuria over time and have, for the most part, replaced routine 24-h urine collections, which are often cumbersome to collect and inaccurate in pediatric patients.

Isolated proteinuria is a relatively common finding in children. As reported in several studies, mass screening of schoolchildren for proteinuria points toward a prevalence between 5 and 10%.[4,5] Proteinuria appears to be more common in adolescence than early childhood. Most proteinuria in childhood is transient and not indicative of renal disease. When nearly 9000 schoolchildren in Helsinki were followed for 1 year with intermittent urine samples, 10% were found to have proteinuria $\geq 1+$ on urinary dipstick on an initial screen.[6] Only 2.5% were found to have persistent proteinuria on one of an additional three follow-up collections. Similarly, in a large survey done in pediatric office practice, only 10% of children initially found to have proteinuria on dipstick still manifested proteinuria 1 year later.[4] Such studies have called into question the utility of regular urinary screenings to detect early kidney disease since, in the vast majority of asymptomatic children, any detected abnormality tends to clear spontaneously.

Transient proteinuria often accompanies stress, acute febrile illness, or exercise. Such isolated proteinuria is thought to be most likely mediated by intrarenal hemodynamic changes, reducing renal plasma flow out of proportion to glomerular filtration rate (GFR) and enhancing the concentration gradient of protein into Bowman's space.[7] There is no long-term residual renal damage with transient proteinuria and these children do not require a diagnostic evaluation.

With persistent proteinuria, fixed proteinuria should be distinguished from orthostatic proteinuria. With fixed proteinuria, every urine sample has significant proteinuria; with orthostatic proteinuria, protein excretion is linked to body position. Thus, with orthostatic proteinuria, abnormally high rates of protein excretion occur while the child is upright or ambulatory and normal protein excretion ensues when the child is recumbent. The mechanism of orthostatic proteinuria is thought to arise from an enhanced renal sensitivity to the normal hemodynamic and hormonal alterations that occur with changes in position, resulting in enhanced glomerular protein permeability.[8]

Orthostatic proteinuria is quite common and accounts for up to two-thirds of pediatric proteinuria, especially in adolescents. Generally, in orthostatic proteinuria, excretion of urinary protein is below 1 g/day.[5,6] Many children go on to clear their postural proteinuria with time, but some may always demonstrate orthostatic proteinuria. Most follow-up studies of individuals found to have postural proteinuria point to no increased incidence of long-term renal disease as long as the proteinuria is an isolated finding and not accompanied by hematuria, an active urinary sediment, or hypertension.[9] However, some patients with orthostatic proteinuria followed for over 35 years did demonstrate late-onset renal insufficiency.[10]

With persistent nonorthostatic proteinuria, a diagnostic evaluation usually ensues to rule out any underlying glomerular or renal parenchymal disease. With increasing daily excretion of urinary protein > 1 g in the adolescent or > 600 mg/m^2 in the younger child, there must be an increased index of clinical suspicion that there may be more serious ongoing renal disease and these children often proceed to renal biopsy.[11]

In children with lower-grade fixed isolated proteinuria, the majority exhibit no evidence of progressive renal disease. Most of these children demonstrate normal or nonspecific changes on renal biopsy. However, some children will have evidence of focal segmental glomerulosclerosis on renal biopsy.[12,13] These children often have higher levels of proteinuria that may exceed nephrotic range over time and nearly 50% progress to end-stage renal disease (ESRD). Thus, in children with any element of fixed proteinuria, there should be long-term follow-up to monitor the degree of proteinuria and to assess for the development of hematuria, hypertension, or renal insufficiency.

The diagnostic evaluation of the child with proteinuria is best done in phases (Table 47.1). The evaluation is focused on confirming and quantifying proteinuria, distinguishing fixed proteinuria from orthostatic proteinuria, and identifying whether the proteinuria is isolated or if there are accompanying clinical signs or symptoms suggestive of increased likelihood of renal disease. The child who has proteinuria as part of the nephrotic syndrome should be considered separately since the evaluation as well as the management and prognosis varies.

Nephrotic syndrome

Because of the overwhelming preponderance of minimal-change disease as the etiology of nephrosis in the prepubertal child (Table 47.2), the initial evaluation and management of nephrotic syndrome in children differs from the approach seen in adults.[14] It is much less likely for children to undergo an extensive initial laboratory evaluation or a renal biopsy and much more likely for them to be placed on empiric steroid therapy. Moreover, the vast majority of children with nephrotic syndrome eventually outgrow this problem, with no long-term compromise of renal function.[15]

Nephrotic syndrome in children is characterized by massive proteinuria exceeding 50 mg/kg/day or 40 mg/m^2/h. Serum albumin levels will be less than 2.5 g/dL and may often be profoundly depressed (< 0.5 g/dL). Edema may be quite problematic especially at presentation or during protracted relapses. Hyperlipidemia may also be quite pronounced, especially in light of normal pediatric cholesterol levels rarely exceeding 180 mg/dL.

Table 47.1 Diagnostic evaluation of asymptomatic proteinuria in the child

Phase 1
Reconfirm proteinuria in random urine sample
Microscopic urinalysis to assess for red or white cells, casts, or crystals
Focused history and physical examination: urinary tract infection, family history of renal disease, growth parameters, blood pressure, presence of edema or rash

Phase 2
Serum creatinine
Assess for postural proteinuria by comparing proteinuria in first morning urine sample to random void later in day
If postural proteinuria confirmed with normal renal function, no further evaluation. Child needs annual follow-up

Phase 3
Quantitate proteinuria with urinary protein:creatinine ratio or timed collection
Other blood work as clinically indicated: albumin, cholesterol, antinuclear antibody, serologies
Renal ultrasound
Consider voiding cystourethrogram if ultrasound suggests reflux or scarring

Phase 4
Consider renal biopsy if active urinary sediment, significant microhematuria or macrohematuria, fixed proteinuria that is exacerbating or > 600 mg/m^2/day, hypertension, renal insufficiency, or family history of end-stage renal disease

Table 47.2 Etiology of nephrotic syndrome in children biopsied at presentation*

Histologic category	Frequency (%)
Minimal change	77
Focal and segmental glomerulosclerosis	9
Membranoproliferative glomerulonephritis	7
Other or unclassified	5
Mesangioproliferative glomerulonephritis	2

*Based on data from International Study of Kidney Disease in Children: Nephrotic syndrome in children: prediction of histopathology from clinical and laboratory characteristics at time of diagnosis. Kidney Int 1981;13:159–165.

Table 47.3 Frequency of clinical characteristics in pediatric nephrosis at presentation*

Clinical characteristic	Minimal change sclerosis (%)	Focal (%)
Age ≤ 6 years	80	50
Male gender	60	70
Hypertension	20	50
Microhematuria	25	50
Elevated serum creatinine	30	40

*Based on data from International Study of Kidney Disease in Children: Nephrotic syndrome in children: prediction of histopathology from clinical and laboratory characteristics at time of diagnosis. Kidney Int 1981;13:159–165.

In children under 16 years of age, the annual incidence of nephrotic syndrome is 2 per 100 000, with a cumulative prevalence of just under 20 per 100 000.[16] Presentation in the first year of life is uncommon and should raise the suspicion of congenital nephrotic syndrome, a condition quite unlike minimal-change nephrosis both in its etiology and long-term prognosis.[14] Typically, most children with nephrosis present between 2 and 6 years of age, and in younger children there is up to a 2:1 ratio of affected boys to girls.[17] In older children or adolescents who present with nephrotic syndrome, this ratio is closer to 1:1.[18] There appear to be racial differences in the virulence of nephrotic syndrome in children. For instance, in North America, data suggest that African-American and Hispanic children are more likely to have steroid-resistant disease that progresses to end stage renal failure.[19]

Minimal-change disease

The typical child with minimal-change disease presents following a nonspecific viral illness. Many children are first brought to medical attention because of periorbital edema and it is quite common to elicit a history that the child has been given diphenhydramine for "allergies" but the edema has not abated. Clinically, minimal-change disease can be distinguished from nephritis or other chronic glomerulopathies by the absence of signs or symptoms consistent with glomerular inflammation. Thus it is quite uncommon to see a child with minimal-change disease present with macroscopic hematuria, severe hypertension, or azotemia.[14] Pertinent clinical characteristics and their frequency in minimal-change disease are outlined in Table 47.3.

In a prepubertal child with nephrosis, normal blood pressure, nonnephrotic urinary sediment, and normal renal function, the presumed diagnosis is minimal-change disease and empiric steroid therapy is indicated. Most pediatric centers initiate such children on 60 mg/m^2/day of prednisone or its equivalent up to a maximum dose of 80 mg/day. The steroid dose may be given in one total daily dose or divided according to local practice or parental preference. Most children with minimal-change disease respond to steroid therapy within 2 weeks, and more than 90% of children who are steroid responsive respond by 4 weeks of daily steroid therapy.[20] Lack of response to oral steroids after 6–8 weeks of daily therapy should prompt reassessment of the treatment regimen and may call for renal biopsy.

Various treatment lengths are utilized for the child who presents with presumed minimal-change disease but there is evidence to suggest that an initial 3-month steroid regimen combining daily and then alternate-day therapy may result in fewer relapses.[21] In relapses, daily steroid therapy is often used until remission is induced and then a tapering steroid course initiated over weeks to months depending on the patient's individual history. With frequent relapses, long-term use of low-dose alternate-day therapy may actually reduce overall steroid burden by sustaining remission and minimizing exposure to daily high-dose steroid therapy.

Minimal-change disease in children is a relapsing condition. Fewer than 10% of affected children have only one episode of nephrosis while nearly 50% frequently relapse, with three or more relapses within 6 months of presentation.[22] Between 30% and 40% of children become steroid dependent, i.e. they relapse while still being treated with steroids or within 2 weeks of concluding steroid therapy. Sequelae of steroid therapy are common and include hypertension, loss of bone density, cataracts, gastritis, emotional lability, and increased susceptibility to infection. An adverse effect of chronic steroid use of particular concern in children is growth impairment. A child's somatic growth must be monitored quite closely and standardized growth charts utilized to assess growth velocity.

The development of significant steroid sequelae is the most common impetus for consideration of alternative drug therapy in minimal-change disease. Most commonly, alkylating agents such as cyclophosphamide or chlorambucil are used. A daily dose of 2–3 mg/kg of cyclophosphamide for 8–12 weeks up to a cumulative dose of 168 mg/kg has proved quite effective.[23,24] Nearly 70% of steroid-sensitive children remit for at least 1 year and 40% stay in a sustained remission for at least 5 years.[23] Alkylating agents seem most efficacious in steroid-sensitive children who are frequent relapsers but are somewhat less effective in inducing long-term remission in children with steroid-dependent disease.[25] Cyclophosphamide has also been shown to be effective in converting approximately one-third of children with steroid-resistant disease to steroid responsiveness.[26,27] In steroid-sensitive children, these agents seem to work best if given while the child is in remission and on concomitant steroid therapy.

There are multiple toxicities associated with the use of alkylating agents. Acutely, bone marrow suppression is common and patients must be monitored for leukopenia. Other acute toxicities include alopecia, gastrointestinal discomfort, and hemorrhagic cystitis. With chlorambucil, there is also a small risk of idiosyncratic seizures. Longer-term complications include dose-related gonadal toxicity and potential increased risk of future malignancies.

In children with particularly recalcitrant minimal-change disease, calcineurin inhibitors such as cyclosporine may induce remission.[28–30] An initial dose of 6 mg/kg/day divided into two doses often induces and sustains a remission and, in most children with minimal-change disease, steroid therapy can be weaned and steroid sequelae will improve. After a period of remission, cyclosporine may be weaned or discontinued. If relapses occur, the child may be placed back on steroids to see if the nephrotic syndrome now follows a less relapsing and more steroid-sensitive course or, if necessary, returned to cyclosporine therapy. Cyclosporine levels need to be monitored closely and changes in renal function carefully assessed. Some children on long-term cyclosporine with increasing serum creatinine values may require interval renal biopsies to assess for histologic changes compatible with cyclosporine-induced nephrotoxicity. Interestingly, cyclosporine-associated arteriopathy seems to recede after cessation of cyclosporine in children with nephrotic syndrome, whereas tubulointerstitial changes and focal glomerular lesions do not regress.[31]

In an attempt to prolong remission and to spare overall steroid burden, multiple medications have been used as adjunctive therapy in minimal-change disease. Levamisole, an anthelminthic immunostimulant, appears to be beneficial in maintaining remissions.[32,33] Levamisole is generally given orally concurrently with weaning doses of steroids over the course of many months to several years. Unlike the alkylating agents, levamisole does not seem to have a dramatic effect on the natural history of minimal-change disease and children who are frequent relapsers tend to begin to relapse more frequently after levamisole therapy is discontinued. Although widely used in parts of Europe and Asia, the drug has been employed less commonly in North America due to problems with its availability and clinician inexperience with its prescription. Adverse effects are rare with levamisole therapy but include agranulocytosis, liver function abnormalities, and an antineutrophil cytoplasmic antibody (ANCA)-positive vasculitis syndrome following protracted therapy.[34]

Azathioprine and, more recently, mycophenolate mofetil have also been used as steroid-sparing agents. Although there is no indication that azathioprine is advantageous as monotherapy, its concurrent use with steroids may allow tapering of steroids to low enough doses to ameliorate or preclude steroid sequelae.[35] With mycophenolate mofetil, there has yet to be a controlled study of its efficacy in minimal-change nephrotic syndrome compared with other more conventional agents.

Most children with minimal-change disease eventually outgrow their disease and by early adulthood are in long-term remission and considered cured. These children do not appear to be at increased risk of other renal disease or the development of functional renal impairment. Nearly 15% of affected children may continue to have relapses as an adult.[15] Most often, the relapses are infrequent and continue to follow a steroid-sensitive pattern.

Focal segmental glomerulosclerosis

Approximately 10–15% of prepubertal children with nephrotic syndrome have focal segmental glomerulosclerosis (FSGS). This incidence increases to over one-third of affected adolescents.[36] The median age at onset of FSGS is 6 years and, similar to minimal-change disease, there seems to be a male gender predisposition in young children. Most affected children present acutely with nephrotic syndrome but nearly one-quarter of children can present initially with asymptomatic proteinuria. Children with FSGS are more likely to manifest microhematuria, hypertension, and renal insufficiency at presentation than children with minimal-change disease[14] (see Table 47.3).

Almost all children with FSGS are likely to have the idiopathic or primary form. On renal biopsy there is focal involvement, with some areas of the kidney appearing absolutely normal and other areas showing segmental capillary collapse, mesangial matrix proliferation, and frank sclerosis.[37] The same histology may be seen in secondary FSGS, in which focal glomerular disease arises as a result of a concomitant renal insult, nephrotoxin, or systemic disease such as reflux nephropathy, heroin-induced nephropathy, or HIV.[38]

The clinical course of idiopathic FSGS in children is often characterized by steroid-resistant disease. Although up to one-third of children with FSGS respond to an 8-week trial of oral steroids, many initial responders later go on to become steroid unresponsive.[39] With steroid-unresponsive disease, there are few data to suggest that an oral alkylating agent by itself is likely to have a beneficial effect; in fact, one study comparing alternate-day steroid therapy with alternate-day steroids and cyclophosphamide found equivalent remission rates.[40] Children who do show sensitivity to initial oral therapy with steroids or alkylating agents are more likely to have less aggressive disease and may follow a course with few relapses or with sustained remissions.[41,42]

In children with FSGS who do not respond to initial therapy, more aggressive immunosuppressive regimens have met with some success in inducing partial or complete remission. Unfortunately, evaluation of treatment efficacy and comparison of treatment approach has been complicated by the lack of randomized or well-controlled studies in children with this disease. Many clinicians now utilize a 10-week induction course of frequent pulse intravenous methylprednisolone and concomitant oral prednisone to achieve a remission and then attempt to maintain a remission with continued oral steroids and less frequent intravenous pulses.[43] Initial treatment failure or any improvement with relapse leads to reinduction and the addition of a 3-month course of oral cyclophosphamide. In some reports, nearly three-fourths of children achieve a long-term partial or complete remission of their FSGS following this sort of protocol.[44] Other reports have demonstrated considerably less long-term efficacy and have also raised the issues that black children may not respond as well to such treatment and that there may be serious clinical complications that arise related to the high-dose steroids and potential for repeated course of alkylating agents.[45,46]

Cyclosporine has also been shown capable of inducing a partial or complete remission in many children with FSGS.[47–49] Doses of 5–6 mg/kg in one single daily dose or divided into two equal daily doses have been used. Although this approach avoids many of the sequelae of therapy with high-dose steroids or alkylating agents, children with FSGS who respond to cyclosporine almost always relapse if cyclosporine therapy is withdrawn and thus remain cyclosporine dependent. As a result, some children treated with cyclosporine are at risk of developing long-term nephropathy due to chronic exposure to calcineurin inhibitors.[50] As a result, attention to cyclosporine levels and serum creatinine must be part of the regular follow-up, and some patients may require intermittent renal biopsy to assess possible drug nephrotoxicity.

Many clinicians have begun to utilize angiotensin-converting enzyme (ACE) inhibitors or angiotensin receptor blockers (ARBs) as adjunctive therapy in children with FSGS.[51,52] These agents reduce glomerular filtration through their interaction with the homeostatic mechanisms involved with maintaining glomerular perfusion. As a result of the decrease in GFR, there is concomitantly less proteinuria. Although serum albumin levels may increase with the decreased proteinuria, they do not generally become normal in children with FSGS. However, the decreased proteinuria and the alteration in glomerular hemodynamics are thought to be beneficial in reducing the rate of glomerulosclerosis.

Similar to the experience with minimal-change disease, there are limited data as to the utility of therapy with mycophenolate mofetil in FSGS.[53,54] Some reports point toward its efficacy in children with FSGS who have been unresponsive to oral steroids or a combination of oral steroids and alkylating agents. It is often used in combination with ACE inhibitors or ARBs to see if there is a synergistic effect on reducing proteinuria.

Unlike the uniformly excellent long-term prognosis seen in minimal-change disease, a substantial number of children with FSGS manifest eventual renal insufficiency. Approximately one-quarter of affected children reach ESRD as soon as 5 years after disease onset.[55] Pediatric registry data confirm that FSGS is the most common glomerular disease leading to renal replacement therapy in children.[56]

In children undergoing renal transplantation for FSGS, recurrent disease may commonly be seen, often in the immediate postoperative period. Although recurrent disease can be treated successfully, generally utilizing a combined approach of plasmapheresis and intensification of immunosuppression, there is accelerated graft loss in recurrent FSGS and the usual graft survival advantage seen with kidneys donated from living donors is lost in children with FSGS who undergo transplantation.[56]

The etiology of idiopathic FSGS in children is unknown. However, in many children with FSGS a circulating lymphokine has been isolated that increases the albumin permeability of perfused rat glomeruli in vitro.[57] Some children with recurrent FSGS after renal transplantation appear to manifest more permeability in this assay, leading to speculation that they may have a more virulent circulating factor. The ability to induce a remission with the use of therapies aimed at immunomodulation and lymphokine removal, such as pheresis, also seems to support the role of some systemic factor in this disease.[58]

Recent genetic studies in children with FSGS point toward both an autosomal dominant and autosomal recessive mode of inheritance in some children with steroid-resistant disease.[59–62] These studies arose initially from the observation that although nephrotic syndrome is rare in the sibling of an affected child, in those cases of apparent familial nephrosis steroid-unresponsive FSGS was the common lesion. Unlike idiopathic FSGS, this form of the disease is unlikely to recur in a renal allograft. As the molecular genetics of this condition continue to be discerned, it may lead to an ability to screen children with nephrotic syndrome and avoid exposure to unnecessary and potentially toxic drug therapies in children with certain genotypes.

Congenital nephrotic syndrome

Congenital nephrotic syndrome is a rare condition generally diagnosed in the initial months of life. Although prenatal diagnosis has been reported as a result of alterations in amniotic fluid volume and protein content, infants may also present with edema and the associated proteinuria and hypoalbuminemia is then discerned. Etiology of congenital nephrotic syndrome generally follows one of three subtypes: (1) related to intrauterine or congenital infection, (2) related to diffuse mesangial sclerosis (DMS) as part of Denys–Drash syndrome, or as an isolated mutation in the WT1 gene, or (3) related to a defect in the podocyte protein nephrin as part of a mutation in the NPHS1 gene commonly referred to as Finnish-type congenital nephrotic syndrome (CNF).

History and physical examination often help guide the initial diagnostic evaluation and renal biopsy can provide a definitive histologic diagnosis. Congenital infections such as syphilis can be excluded with negative TORCH titers and the absence of early rash, jaundice, or hepatosplenomegaly in the baby. In the extremely rare instance of congenital infection, treatment of the underlying infection should lead to resolution of nephrosis. With other forms of congenital nephrotic syndrome, the long-term renal prognosis is guarded and most of these children inevitably progress to ESRD.

DMS may be isolated or related to Denys–Drash syndrome with associated pseudohermaphroditism and Wilms tumor. Mutations in the WT1 gene, a transcription factor that plays a key role in normal development and function of the urogenital tract, are associated with Denys–Drash syndrome.[63] Abnormalities in WT1 are well described in Wilms tumor and other urogenitary anomalies, but its exact role as a mediator of glomerular pathology in DMS is unclear.

Detection and appropriate resection and follow-up of Wilms tumor or other urogenitary malignancy are critical components of the care of an infant with DMS due to Denys–Drash syndrome. Other therapy is aimed at management of the sequelae of nephrotic-range proteinuria and may involve frequent infusion of 25% albumin, intensive nutritional therapy, and other supportive care. Children with DMS may have slower progression of their renal insufficiency than children with CNF and may have less profound protein losses, making their management somewhat less complex and more open to options such as unilateral nephrectomy or the use of high-dose ACE inhibitors or prostaglandin inhibitors to reduce glomerular filtration and reduce overall protein losses in the urine to more acceptable levels.[64]

Renal transplantation is the ultimate treatment for children with DMS. Most children do well post transplant without disease recurrence.[65] Because of concerns regarding an incomplete Denys–Drash syndrome, even in children with apparently isolated DMS, bilateral nephrectomy at the time of transplantation or onset of ESRD is recommended.[66]

CNF is an autosomal recessive disorder most common in, but not exclusive to, people of Finnish heritage. It results from genetic mutations in the NPHS1 gene that encodes for nephrin, an adhesion protein exclusively expressed in the podocyte and a main component of the slit diaphragm.[67] The exact mechanism of nephrosis due to nephrin anomalies remains unclear. If there is no family history of CNF, it may be suspected in a baby with congenital nephrotic syndrome and none of the manifestations of Denys–Drash syndrome. Babies with CNF are often born prematurely and have a large placenta, weighing more than 25% of the infant's birthweight.[66] There is often elevated maternal serum or amniotic fluid α-fetoprotein in the absence of neural tube defects or other structural abnormalities.[68]

Babies with CNF are at significant risk of morbidity and mortality if not treated aggressively for the sequelae of their nephrosis (Table 47.4).[69] They must receive intravenous albumin and diuretics to manage edema and are at profound risk of sepsis and thrombosis due to loss of immunoglobulin and coagulation factors in the urine. Significant improvement in long-term outcome has been accomplished by intensive medical support through early infancy until the child reaches 6–9 months of age, at which point bilateral nephrectomy can be performed and chronic peritoneal dialysis initiated for several months until the child reaches an appropriate size for renal transplantation. Some babies may need to be nephrectomized earlier in infancy if they have life-threatening infections, severe thrombotic events, or failure to thrive despite intensive therapy aimed at minimizing these complications.[70]

Long-term neurodevelopmental and renal allograft outcome is quite good in children with CNF managed in this fashion.[71] In a subset of children, there can be recurrent proteinuria within a year after renal transplantation that may progress and cause renal allograft loss.[72] This posttransplant proteinuria appears to be related to the extent of the initial nephrin mutation and whether the child has immunologically encountered nephrin prior to renal transplant. In the absence of native nephrin, as seen with some CNF mutations, there may be production of antinephrin antibodies and ensuing damage to the slit diaphragms and podocytes of the transplanted kidney.[73] Some children with recurrent proteinuria have been successfully treated with plasmapheresis or the addition of cyclophosphamide to their immunosuppressive regimen.[71]

Table 47.4 Management of congenital nephrotic syndrome in early infancy*

Infusion of 25% albumin at dose up to 2 g/kg/day. Loop diuretic midway and at end of infusion. Supplemental oral loop or thiazide diuretics may be considered

Minimal caloric intake of 120 kcal/kg/day with 3–4 g/kg/day protein. Increase caloric density for fluid restriction

Aggressive treatment of any fever. Initiate broad-spectrum antibiotics awaiting cultures. Infusion of intravenous immunoglobulin 200–400 mg/kg/day during antibiotic therapy

Thyroid function tests monthly and initiation of thyroxine for thyroid-stimulating hormone elevation

Chronic anticoagulation with coumadin or salicylate if any thrombotic complications

Early initiation of erythropoietin with doses two to three times normal

Consider therapeutic trial with captopril, gradually increasing dose up to 5 mg/kg/day with or without concomitant indomethacin up to 4 mg/kg/day. Response to therapy monitored with urinary protein/creatinine ratios

Consider early supplementation with activated vitamin D

Nephrectomies and initiation of peritoneal dialysis at 6–9 months of age. Consider earlier if any life-threatening complications of nephrosis such as sepsis, thrombosis, or severe failure to thrive

*Based in part on recommendations and data outlined by Holmberg C, Antikainen M, Ronnholm K, et al: Management of congenital nephrotic syndrome of the Finnish type. Pediatr Nephrol 1995;9:87–93.

Hematuria

Despite its rare association with malignancy or a renal condition that is progressive or requires treatment, the presence of blood in a child's urine sample often provokes significant anxiety and requires a thoughtful, cost-effective evaluation. The increased availability and use of very sensitive urinary dipsticks for screening has facilitated the identification of children with microhematuria.

In general pediatric practice, isolated microscopic hematuria is now a relatively frequent finding, with an overall prevalence rate of 1.5% of asymptomatic children screened. In a 5-year prospective study of hematuria in 12 000 schoolchildren between the ages of 6 and 12 years, the prevalence was up to 3.3% when hematuria was defined as five or more erythrocytes per high-power microscopy field occurring in at least two of three consecutive urine samples.[74] Hematuria frequency increased steadily with advancing age and was found more often in girls. In a Finnish study of nearly 9000 healthy children, 4.2% had more than six erythrocytes per high-power microscopy field.[75] However, this number decreased to 1.1% when hematuria was defined as occurring in two or more specimens. Of note, the number of children with isolated microscopic hematuria in these studies is disproportionately large compared with the number of children who have serious functional kidney disease or threatening anatomic anomaly, suggesting that the majority of children with microhematuria have benign or self-limited conditions.

Gross hematuria occurs far less frequently in children than microhematuria. The frequency of gross hematuria in a pediatric emergency department over a period of 24 months was 0.13% of all patient encounters.[76] Urinary tract infection (UTI) was documented or suspected in 49% of these cases. The combined diagnoses of perineal irritation, meatal stenosis, and trauma accounted for an additional 25% of cases. Apparent glomerular disease accounted for only 9% of cases of gross hematuria. At the time of this study, it was not routine to screen for hypercalciuria in children. In a later study, 43% of children presenting with gross hematuria were found to be hypercalciuric.[77] Thus it is likely that a significant number of these children may also have had excessive urinary calcium excretion.

Etiology and evaluation

The differential diagnosis of pediatric hematuria is large (Table 47.5). The ability to localize the source of hematuria greatly facilitates further evaluation. Urine that is tea- or cola-colored with concomitant proteinuria suggests glomerular pathology. Urine that is red or pink and is associated with clots or dysuria is most consistent with lower urinary tract bleeding. Phase-contrast microscopy allows assessment of urinary erythrocyte morphology and the presence of red cell casts is pathognomonic of glomerular hematuria. Hematuria in urine samples from a parent or sibling points to an inherited etiology. Crystalluria may connote abnormal solute excretion predisposing to nephrolithiasis.

Table 47.5 Etiology of childhood hematuria

Renal parenchymal disease
Glomerular
Inherited
  Benign familial hematuria
  Alport syndrome
Primary
  IgA nephropathy
  Focal segmental glomerulosclerosis
  Membranoproliferative glomerulonephritis
  Membranous glomerulonephritis
Systemic
  Hemolytic–uremic syndrome
  Henoch–Schönlein purpura
  Systemic lupus erythematosus
  Wegener granulomatosis
  Microscopic polyarteritis
  Goodpasture syndrome
Infectious
  Poststreptococcal glomerulonephritis
  Hepatitis B-associated glomerulonephritis
  Shunt nephritis
  Subacute bacterial endocarditis

Tubulointerstitial
Inherited
  Polycystic kidney disease
  Juvenile nephronophthisis
  Cystinosis
  Oxalosis
  Tuberous sclerosis
Acquired
  Hypercalciuria
  Nephrotoxic drugs
  Interstitial nephritis
  Renal transplant rejection

Vascular
Renal vein thrombosis
Renal artery thrombosis
Sickle cell disease

Urinary tract disorders
Nephrolithiasis
Urinary tract infection
Urethritis
Trauma

Coagulation disorders
Anticoagulant use
Hemophilia
Thrombocytopenic purpura

The evaluation of hematuria begins with a careful history and physical examination. In infants, the history should include questions regarding birth asphyxia, umbilical vessel catheterization, and abnormalities detected on prenatal ultrasound. In older children, the history should include questions regarding pain and accompanying voiding symptoms. If macroscopic hematuria exists, determining the timing of the visible hematuria during voiding is important. Gross hematuria at initiation of urination that subsequently clears suggests urethral irritation. Terminal gross hematuria suggests trigonitis. Urine that is persistently tea-colored or brown is likely due to glomerulonephritis. In many children who are already independently toilet trained, there may be a significant delay between the onset of symptoms and evaluation because of the failure of the child to recognize the ramifications of hematuria.

As some causes of hematuria may be inherited, a thorough family history is invaluable. A family history of isolated microhematuria without progression to renal insufficiency would suggest benign familial hematuria (BFH). However, a family history of hematuria, proteinuria, and progressive renal failure with associated high-frequency sensorineural hearing loss or visual impairment would raise concern for a familial nephritis such as Alport syndrome (AS). A family history of cystic kidney disease, IgA nephropathy, nephrolithiasis, coagulopathies, and sickle cell disease would also be significant.

Associated signs and symptoms often provide further etiologic clues. Dysuria, frequency, flank pain, and fever point toward UTI. Radiating pain in the loin or groin is consistent with renal colic from nephrolithiasis. The presence of acute edema formation and hypertension would suggest glomerulonephritis. As glomerular disease can be part of a systemic illness, the presence of rash, abdominal pain, and joint inflammation may suggest Henoch–Schönlein purpura, systemic lupus erythematosus, or a vasculitis.

Laboratory and radiographic studies

If the child has at least five urinary erythrocytes per high-power microscopy field on at least two samples over a 2–3 week period, further investigation should proceed. Urine studies include culture and quantification of urinary calcium and creatinine. If there is a history of nephrolithiasis, quantification of urinary citrate, oxalate, and uric acid should also be considered. If the protein is greater than trace on dipstick, especially in a dilute sample, then urinary protein and creatinine should also be quantified. Recommended serum studies include creatinine and C3 complement level to screen for renal insufficiency and chronic hypocomplementemic glomerulonephritis. When clinically appropriate, screening for systemic lupus, hepatitis, or coagulopathies should be considered. Renal ultrasound should be checked in all children less than 7 years of age to rule out Wilms tumor and in older children if there are concerns regarding structural anomalies or stones. Urine samples from parents and siblings should also be assessed for the presence of a familial hematuria.

In the absence of a history suggestive of lower urinary tract bleeding, cystoscopy is seldom indicated in the child with isolated microhematuria. Unlike adults, bladder malignancies are quite uncommon and sonography usually suffices as a screen to detect rare structural anomalies.

Benign familial hematuria and Alport syndrome

In children, the differential diagnosis of isolated microscopic hematuria often includes BFH and AS. The ability to distinguish between these two conditions is critical because it allows accurate prognosis, although this may be difficult as the microscopic examination of the urine and early glomerular basement membrane (GBM) changes may be identical.

The renal biopsy in patients with BFH is normal by light microscopy and immunofluorescence. The abnormality in BFH is apparent by electron microscopy, which demonstrates thinning of the lamina densa of the GBM. Thinning of the GBM may also be the only abnormality seen in patients with early AS or in female carriers of X-linked AS. However, the GBM abnormalities in AS continue to evolve, resulting in areas of irregular thinning, thickening, splitting, and multilamination, clearly distinguishing AS from BFH.[78,79]

Whereas BFH is inherited in an autosomal dominant manner, AS is most often inherited in an X-linked pattern. An autosomal recessive form of AS accounts for 15% of cases, while the autosomal dominant form is quite rare.[78] Type IV collagen is the major structural component of the GBM and mutations of this gene are the molecular basis for AS. X-linked AS has been attributed to mutations of the COL4A5 gene, while the recessive and dominant forms are linked to mutations of the COL4A3–COL4A4 locus.[78] Two families with BFH have had their disease linked to the COL4A4 gene.[80,81] These reports suggest that these BFH patients may be "carriers" of autosomal recessive AS. Those patients who are heterozygous for certain COL4A4–COL4A3 locus mutations have BFH, whereas patients who have homozygous or compound heterozygous mutations in the same locus develop autosomal recessive AS.

Clinical features and family history are critical in distinguishing between BFH and AS.[79,82] Unlike patients with AS, who typically develop proteinuria and progressive renal failure, patients with BFH do not develop significant proteinuria and preserve renal function over time. In addition, patients with AS may have a family history of high-frequency sensorineural hearing loss and lenticonus. Although BFH can be distinguished from AS with some certainty based on clinical features and family history, without a confirmatory renal biopsy it is a diagnosis of exclusion. Thus, in children with BFH as a putative diagnosis, regular follow-up must make sure that no concerning clinical or laboratory features, such as the development of proteinuria or declining renal function, evolve. In this event, a diagnostic renal biopsy should be performed.

Idiopathic hypercalciuria

Hypercalciuria is present in approximately 5% of healthy Caucasian children and is diagnosed in up to 35% of children evaluated for hematuria.[77,83] Hypercalciuria may be secondary to hyperparathyroidism, metabolic acidosis, distal renal tubular acidosis, vitamin D intoxication, immobilization, and therapy with loop diuretics. Most children, however, have normocalcemic idiopathic hypercalciuria. The pathogenesis of idiopathic hypercalciuria is unknown and could be secondary to increased intestinal absorption, reduced renal tubular reabsorption, increased osseous resorption, or a combination of these factors.[84]

Hypercalciuria exists when urinary calcium excretion exceeds 4 mg/kg/day. In young children, a 24-h collection may be impractical and calcium excretion can be estimated by a spot-urine calcium:creatinine ratio. Younger children normally excrete higher levels of calcium, with urinary calcium–creatinine ratios up to 0.5–0.8; after 2 years of age, however, the expected spot-urine calcium–creatinine ratio is ≤ 0.2.[85]

Presenting clinical features of hypercalciuria include microscopic hematuria, gross hematuria, frequency dysuria, abdominal or flank pain, and urolithiasis.[85] Although there is considerable clinical overlap, macroscopic hematuria and a family history of urolithiasis have been found to be more common in hypercalciuric patients. The reported incidence of documented urolithiasis at presentation varies depending on the population studied. In a report of the Southwest Pediatric Nephrology Study Group, all children with painless isolated hematuria and hypercalciuria underwent excretory urography or renal ultrasound at presentation and no child had urolithiasis at diagnosis.[77] In comparison, another study focused on children with hypercalciuria who presented with painless microhematuria, dysuria, recurrent abdominal or flank pain, and a family history of nephrolithiasis.[86] All children had renal ultrasound at entry; 57% had microcalculi and 5% had urolithiasis.

The natural history of idiopathic hypercalciuria is persistent hematuria and possible urolithiasis. In a longitudinal study of 58 untreated children with hematuria and hypercalciuria, 40% continued to have hematuria and 70% had hypercalciuria at 1 year.[87] At 2 and 3 years, 21 children were available for study; 40% still had hematuria and 50% had hypercalciuria. During the follow-up period, 16% of children developed urolithiasis. Children who developed stones were older when initially evaluated, were more likely to present with macroscopic hematuria, and all had a family history of urolithiasis. In the Southwest Pediatric Nephrology Study Group study, 13% of hypercalciuric patients developed urolithiasis or "stone-like episode" over a follow-up period up to 4 years.[77]

Hypercalciuria and hematuria clearly identify a group of children at high risk for subsequent urolithiasis. Conservative measures should be taken, including high fluid intake and a diet low in sodium. A restricted calcium diet is not recommended and may even predispose to increased stone formation.[88] If citrate excretion is found to be low, citrate supplementation should be provided, preferably as the potassium salt.[89] If such measures are unsuccessful, thiazide diuretics can be considered. However, thiazides can predispose to electrolyte abnormalities and elevation of the total cholesterol and low-density lipoprotein. Decisions regarding the use of thiazides for idiopathic hypercalciuria should take into consideration the clinical circumstances of the individual case, such as personal or family history of urolithiasis.

Glomerulonephritis

Glomerulonephritis is the leading cause of acquired chronic renal failure during childhood.[90] As with adults, glomerulonephritis may be a manifestation of systemic disease, such as vasculitis or lupus, or may be due to a primary renal process. Similarly, the clinical course may be acute with subsequent full recovery or may progress to renal insufficiency. Certain forms of glomerulonephritis, such as Henoch–Schönlein purpura nephritis, are seen more commonly in children. In other chronic forms of glomerulonephritis, such as membranoproliferative glomerulonephritis (MPGN) and IgA nephropathy, therapeutic approaches in children have often differed from those used in adults.

Henoch–Schönlein purpura

Henoch–Schönlein purpura (HSP) is a multisystem IgA-mediated vasculitis predominantly affecting the skin, joints, gastrointestinal tract, and kidneys. HSP and IgA nephropathy share many immunologic and pathologic features, although HSP is a systemic disease and IgA nephropathy is clinically confined to the kidneys. Despite great research efforts, the exact pathogenesis of HSP and IgA nephropathy remains unclear. Both enhanced IgA synthesis and decreased IgA clearance have been implicated.[91] Total serum IgA levels are increased in 40–50% of these patients. In a recent study, patients who develop HSP nephropathy were found to have abnormal glycosylation of serum IgA, and it has been proposed that the abnormal glycosylation may contribute to the immune complex deposition.[92]

Histologically, both IgA nephropathy and HSP nephritis are characterized by mesangial proliferation and matrix expansion with varying degrees of epithelial cell crescent formation. Unlike IgA nephropathy, HSP nephritis may be associated with polymorphonuclear leukocyte infiltration of the glomerular tufts. Tubulointerstitial changes may be apparent but generally reflect the severity of the glomerular lesions. Immunofluorescence staining invariably reveals IgA in the mesangium, often with weaker staining for C3 and IgG. Deposits may also be seen segmentally in the capillary wall.

Though HSP can occur at any age, most cases affect children between the ages of 2 and 10 years.[93–95] Unlike HSP in adults, which affects men and women equally, boys are up to two times more likely to develop HSP than girls. The disease is somewhat more prevalent during the winter months and early spring. The onset is usually sudden, frequently preceded by an acute illness that often involves a mucosal upper respiratory tract infection.

The clinical manifestations of HSP are due to the small-vessel vasculitis of affected organs. Hallmark signs and symptoms are a nonthrombocytopenic purpuric rash, arthralgias or a nonerosive arthritis, abdominal pain, and nephritis. The rash is often the most distinctive feature of the disease and characteristically involves the buttocks and extensor surfaces of the lower extremities in a symmetric pattern. When skin biopsies are performed, the pathology reveals leukocytoclastic vasculitis. The rash can persist for weeks, with some patients having recurrent episodes of new lesions. Angioedema may be present and involves the eyelids, lips, and dorsa of the hands and feet. Approximately two-thirds of patients have arthralgias or arthritis. Ankles and knees are the most commonly affected joints. The arthritis is nonerosive and not deforming. Gastrointestinal symptoms occur in approximately two-thirds of patients and one study found the abdominal symptoms preceded the rash in as many as 14% of patients. The most frequent abdominal symptoms are periumbilical pain, vomiting, diarrhea, and hematochezia. Surgical emergencies develop in about 5% of patients, with ileoileal intussusception being the most common.[96] The acute morbidity of HSP is usually related to severe gastrointestinal complications.

The exact prevalence of nephritis in children is unknown, although rates up to 54% have been reported.[97,98] The long-term outlook for children with HSP depends on the extent of renal involvement but the overall prognosis of HSP is good. In a long-term study of 270 patients with HSP, 1.1% developed chronic renal insufficiency.[97] Poor prognosis has been associated with the development of nephritic or nephrotic syndrome, initial renal insufficiency, and > 50% crescent formation on biopsy.[99–102] The majority of children manifest their nephritis as microscopic hematuria with or without proteinuria, and these patients have a good long-term prognosis.[101] In one series, 33% of patients with HSP nephritis had nephritic features or a combined nephritic–nephrotic syndrome.[97] Long-term follow-up of a similar cohort of more severely affected patients found that 44% developed chronic hypertension or renal insufficiency.[101]

The majority of children manifest a mild nephritis, recover fully, and require no specific therapy. Once HSP has developed, there are conflicting reports about the efficacy of early prednisone therapy to prevent significant nephritis.[102,103] There is controversy, however, regarding treatment of children with more extensive renal disease. Numerous uncontrolled studies have shown benefit when patients are treated with steroids with or without other agents such as azathioprine, cyclophosphamide, or anticoagulants.[104–108] ACE inhibitors have also been used for patients with persistent proteinuria and glomerular scarring. Plasmapheresis has also been reported to improve prognosis in a small number of children with rapidly progressive HSP nephritis.[109,110] However, well-designed, randomized, controlled studies are needed to look at outcomes of patients treated with various regimens.

IgA nephropathy

IgA nephropathy is the most common form of pediatric primary glomerulopathy. Initially considered a benign disease, long-term follow-up studies suggest that a signifi-

cant proportion of adult patients progress to ESRD. Similarly, study of the natural history of IgA nephropathy diagnosed in childhood demonstrates progression in many patients. In a study of 103 American children diagnosed with IgA nephropathy before 18 years of age, ESRD developed in 6% of children by 5 years, 13% by 10 years, 18% by 15 years, and 30% by 20 years.[111] Similarly, a report from Japan found that 5% of children with IgA nephropathy developed chronic renal failure by 5 years after diagnosis and 11% by 15 years from onset.[112]

The clinical presentation of IgA nephropathy varies from asymptomatic hematuria to a mixed nephritic–nephrotic syndrome.[113] The presence of heavy proteinuria and more active urinary sediment indicates more severe glomerular changes. The incidence of macroscopic hematuria is higher in children than adults and often occurs in association with a mucosal infection of the upper respiratory tract. The interval between the precipitating illness and episode of macroscopic hematuria is generally 1–2 days. Acute renal failure is sometimes seen in flares of IgA nephropathy, although it is usually reversible. However, a small subset of patients with significant crescentic changes have a rapidly progressive course to renal failure. Other histologic correlates with poor clinical outcome include diffuse mesangial proliferation, a high proportion of glomeruli with sclerosis or capsular adhesions, and moderate to severe tubulointerstitial disease.[114] Persistent hypertension and heavy proteinuria also predict a more progressive course.[115]

As the outcome of IgA nephropathy may be so variable, therapy remains challenging. Well-controlled studies are lacking, especially those focusing on children. Selecting the patients most likely to benefit from therapy is critical. Patients with more severe histologic changes, heavy proteinuria, persistent hypertension, and reduced GFR at presentation should be considered for specific therapy. Studies assessing the benefit of tonsillectomy alone or in combination with other therapies have arrived at conflicting conclusions.[116–118] A regimen of alternate-day prednisone and daily azathioprine has been successful in children with severe IgA nephropathy.[119] Therapy resulted in significant reductions in proteinuria and improvement in biopsy results, most notably decreased cellular crescents. Benefits from corticosteroids, including decreased proteinuria and lower incidence of chronic renal failure, were also seen in another small cohort of children with risk factors for progressive IgA nephropathy.[120] More recently, the Japanese Pediatric IgA Nephropathy Treatment Study Group treated 78 children with IgA nephropathy with either a combination of prednisolone, azathioprine, heparin–warfarin, and dipyridamole (group 1) or heparin–warfarin and dipyridamole (group 2) for 2 years.[121] Children in group 1 showed reduced proteinuria and a tendency toward decreased progression of glomerulosclerosis compared with group 2. Although use of fish oil and concomitant ACE inhibition has been studied in adults with IgA nephropathy and appear to reduce the loss of renal function, similar studies have not yet been performed in children.[122–125] Nonetheless, these agents are often used in children with IgA nephropathy as primary or adjunctive therapy, and studies of ACE polymorphisms have demonstrated that genotypes leading to higher levels of ACE are associated with more progressive disease.[126,127]

Postinfectious glomerulonephritis

Postinfectious glomerulonephritis is the leading cause of acute glomerulonephritis in children and has been associated with a host of bacteria, viruses, and parasites. In children, group A β-hemolytic streptococci are the most frequently implicated organisms and pyoderma and pharyngitis are the classic preceding illnesses. Streptococcal pharyngitis occurs most frequently in school-age children during the cooler months. The latent period from onset of pharyngitis to acute poststreptococcal glomerulonephritis (APSGN) is typically a few weeks. Streptococcal impetigo occurs more frequently in younger children during the warmer months, and APSGN after impetigo has a longer latent period of 2–6 weeks. Over the last two decades, the prevalence of APSGN has been declining in children in the USA.[128]

In children who become symptomatic with APSGN, the clinical onset is typically abrupt. Approximately 85% of patients develop edema, up to 80% have varying degrees of hypertension, up to one-third have gross hematuria, and oliguria is common.[129] Hypertension may be severe during the first week of clinical nephritis, with accompanying headaches, somnolence, or seizures, and should be aggressively treated. Generally, the clinical symptoms of APSGN begin to resolve within 1–2 weeks as evidenced by diuresis and normalization of blood pressure. The gross hematuria fades rapidly but microscopic hematuria may persist for years. Proteinuria typically improves rapidly and resolves within 6 months. Recurrences are rare but have been reported.[130–132] More commonly, recurrence of gross hematuria should raise the suspicion for an underlying chronic glomerulonephritis such as IgA nephropathy, MPGN, or membranous glomerulonephritis.

Laboratory studies during a typical episode of APSGN reflect a nephritic process with activation of the alternative complement pathway. The urine sediment shows erythrocytes, leukocytes, and may contain red cell casts. Proteinuria is found frequently but is rarely in the nephrotic range. GFR is often reduced, although severe azotemia is rare and should raise the concern for a rapidly progressive process. If azotemia is significant, electrolyte abnormalities including hyponatremia, hyperkalemia, and acidemia may be present. Serologic tests to document recent streptococcal infection are helpful but do not prove causation. When interpreting serologies, it is important to realize that antibiotic use may blunt the rise in titer and that a significant number of children are asymptomatic carriers of streptococci.[133–135] Serologic tests available include antibodies against streptolysin-O (ASO) and the streptozyme test. The streptozyme test assesses several antibodies including ASO, anti-deoxyribonuclease B (anti-DNase B), and anti-hyaluronidase. Streptolysin O binds to lipids in the skin and results in blunting of the immune response in cases of streptococcal impetigo. The anti-

DNase B titer is therefore more sensitive in detecting evidence of recent streptococcal skin infection. The majority of patients have a low total hemolytic complement and a low C3 complement with a normal C4. The C3 level typically recovers in 6–8 weeks, although prolonged hypocomplementemia has been reported in as many as one-quarter of patients.[136] If the C3 remains depressed after 3 months or the C4 is low, diagnostic considerations include chronic forms of nephritis such as MPGN and lupus nephritis. The possibility of a chronic form of glomerulonephritis warrants close surveillance and a renal biopsy should be considered. Renal biopsy is generally not indicated in typical APSGN, but may be necessary if the diagnosis is in question or if the course is consistent with rapidly progressive glomerulonephritis (RPGN). The biopsy shows diffuse endocapillary proliferation, predominant IgG and C3 deposition in the capillary loop on immunofluorescence, and subepithelial dense humps on electron microscopy.

The mainstay of therapy for APSGN is supportive care. Hospitalization is recommended if the child is hypertensive or has a reduced creatinine clearance. Blood pressure should be checked regularly early in the illness and, if hypertension is present, diuretic therapy with concomitant salt and fluid restriction is considered. If needed, short-acting calcium channel blockers or hydralazine can also be used. In most cases, significant improvement in hypertension, edema, and azotemia is seen within 2 weeks. In children whose course is consistent with RPGN, an immediate renal biopsy and more aggressive therapy are warranted. Although well-designed randomized control studies are lacking, several reports have shown benefits using high-dose intravenous methylprednisolone, with or without other agents such as cyclophosphamide, in the therapy of RPGN of various etiologies in children.[137,138]

In the absence of rapidly progressive disease, the prognosis for complete recovery is considered to be good. Several groups have studied long-term prognosis of patients who initially recovered and found that 3.4–20% of patients developed mild residual symptoms, including proteinuria, hematuria, and hypertension.[139–141] Azotemia develops in less than 3% of patients.[142] Though outcomes are good overall, these results indicate the need for regular monitoring to detect late sequelae.

Membranoproliferative glomerulonephritis

MPGN is a chronic glomerulonephritis characterized histologically by diffuse thickening of the GBM and endocapillary proliferation and subcategorized by the location of deposits on electron microscopy. Most MPGN in children is idiopathic, although occasional secondary cases of MPGN related to hepatitis virus or other infectious etiologies occur.

Either the classical or alternative complement pathways may be involved, resulting in a low serum C3 and, less commonly, a normal or low serum C4. Hypocomplementemia has been reported in up to 95% of children at presentation.[143-146] MPGN is primarily a disease of older children, adolescents, and young adults and is rarely reported in children less than 6 years of age. MPGN was diagnosed in 7.5% of children referred to tertiary centers for renal biopsy for evaluation of nephrotic syndrome.[14] At presentation, one-third of children had macroscopic hematuria or hypertension, up to two-thirds had nephrosis, and one-third had renal insufficiency.[143-146] The long-term renal prognosis in children with MPGN is guarded and natural history studies suggest that as many as 50% progress to ESRD within 10 years of onset.[143]

The small number of affected children has hampered evaluation of putative therapies. Treatment regimens have included corticosteroids, alkylating agents, and anticoagulants. Corticosteroids have not proven beneficial in adults, although various combinations of aspirin, dipyridamole, and warfarin have resulted in diminished proteinuria and an inconsistent impact on maintaining GFR.[147-150] In the pediatric population, corticosteroids have shown greater benefit.[151,152] In 71 children followed at a single center for an average of 7.7 years and mainly treated with alternate-day oral steroids, the cumulative renal survival was 82% at 10 years and 56% at 20 years after onset.[151]

The International Study of Kidney Disease in Children conducted a randomized, double-blind, placebo-controlled clinical trial in children with primary MPGN.[153] Criteria for enrollment included nephrotic-range proteinuria and normal renal function. Children received alternate-day oral prednisone or a lactulose placebo for a mean duration of 41 months. At 130 months, 61% of patients receiving prednisone showed stable renal function compared with only 12% of patients receiving placebo. Intravenous pulses of methylprednisolone followed by alternate-day oral prednisone have also been used in children, with improvement of hematuria, proteinuria, serum albumin, and creatinine clearance.[152]

Though these studies support the use of alternate-day corticosteroids in children with MPGN with nephrotic-range proteinuria, benefit of the same therapy in MPGN with nonnephrotic-range proteinuria is less clear. In a retrospective study of 39 children with MPGN, the outcome of the 11 nonnephrotic patients was excellent, with 100% renal survival at 10 years;[145] of these nonnephrotic patients, seven were untreated. In this report, absence of nephrosis was predictive of good long-term outcome, regardless of therapy, and suggests that a more tailored treatment approach in nonnephrotic children with MPGN may be useful.

Hemolytic–uremic syndrome

Hemolytic–uremic syndrome (HUS) consists of the classic clinical triad of microangiopathic hemolytic anemia, thrombocytopenia, and acute renal failure. HUS is the cause of ESRD in 2–4% of children on chronic dialysis and is the most frequent cause of acute renal failure in children.[154] HUS can be broadly divided into "typical" forms associated with prodromal diarrhea (D+ HUS) and "atypical" cases without diarrhea (D- HUS). Atypical HUS generally has a poorer prognosis and may be familial or can result from numerous triggers, including drugs, malignancies, nonenteric infections such as streptococcal pneumonia, and following bone marrow transplantation. However, the overwhelming majority of childhood cases of HUS include a diarrheal prodrome and are frequently due to infection with enterohemorrhagic Escherichia coli (EHEC).[155]

Epidemiology

Although outbreaks of diarrhea-associated HUS are dramatic and draw considerable public attention, only about 10% of cases in children arise from epidemics.[156,157] A variety of organisms have been implicated in the pathogenesis of HUS, including Shigella dysenteriae type 1, Salmonella, and Yersinia. The majority of cases, however, have been linked with EHEC, which produce a potent cytotoxin known as shiga-like toxin or verotoxin. E. coli 0157:H7 is the serotype isolated in more than 90% of EHEC infections in the USA.[155] EHEC may be carried in the intestines of asymptomatic cattle and higher carriage rates are noted in the summer months and early fall, mimicking the seasonal variation of human disease that peaks from June through September.[158]

Ground beef, vegetables, unpasteurized milk or juice, and water all serve as possible vectors of disease via contamination with bovine feces. Rarely, child-to-child transmission also occurs via oral–fecal contamination.[159] Although children of all ages can be infected, the highest attack rate for E. coli 0157:H7 infection occurs among children younger than 5 years of age.[160] Infected children may excrete the organism in stool for as long as 3 weeks. Approximately 10–15% of children who develop culture-confirmed E. coli 0157:H7 gastroenteritis progress to HUS.[156]

Central to the pathogenesis of HUS is microvascular endothelial cell injury. Only a small inoculum of 50–100 EHEC organisms is required to colonize the intestine.[160] Once established, EHEC elaborates verotoxin leading to intestinal hemorrhagic and ulcerative lesions. With the integrity of the intestinal mucosa compromised, verotoxin gains access to the circulation and extraintestinal sites. Verotoxin is composed of one A subunit and five B subunits. The B subunits are required for binding of the toxin to the high-affinity glycolipid receptor glycosphingolipid globotriosyl ceramide (Gb3), a protein especially expressed on renal microvascular endothelium. After binding, the A subunit is internalized and undergoes partial proteolysis to become an active enzyme capable of inactivating the 60S ribosome, thereby suppressing protein synthesis.[161]

During the acute phase of HUS, numerous proinflammatory cytokines (e.g. tumor necrosis factor α) are elaborated. Along with released bacterial products, these cytokines activate and promote adhesion of leukocytes and platelets to vascular endothelium. The pathogenic cascade results in swollen and detached endothelial cells, exposing the thrombogenic basement membrane and promoting microvascular thrombosis.

Host factors have been studied to determine their influence on the development and outcome of D+ HUS in children. The P1 blood group antigen has been proposed as a protective factor against the development of HUS. The terminal disaccharide structure of the P1 antigen is similar to the disaccharide structure of the Gb3 receptor. Verotoxins are known to bind to the P1 antigen on erythrocytes, which competes with the Gb3 receptor for verotoxin binding. This competitive binding potentially reduces the exposure of endothelia to verotoxin in P1-positive patients, and in fact the P1 group has been found to be protective against development of HUS after hemorrhagic colitis in some studies.[162] However, these findings were not supported in subsequent studies and no relationship has been found between severity of outcome and the P1 phenotype.[163–167]

The B blood group antigen has also been found to bind to verotoxin and has been proposed as a protective host factor. Although the expression of the B antigen appears to have a protective effect against the development of HUS, this expression does not affect the severity of the disease in individuals who go on to develop HUS.[168]

Clinical manifestations

In most children, a few days prior to the development of the classic triad of HUS, colitis manifests as watery diarrhea that then becomes bloody.[155,169] The child may have vomiting and complain of colicky or severe abdominal pain. The diarrhea often resolves at the time HUS becomes clinically apparent. Gastrointestinal complications include bowel wall necrosis, toxic megacolon, intussusception, and rectal prolapse.[169–171]

The severity of the acute nephritis varies widely. The clinical course ranges from microscopic hematuria and mild proteinuria without renal insufficiency to fulminant renal failure. In a retrospective review of D+ HUS in Utah over a 20-year period, 60% of children experienced anuria or oliguria lasting a median of 6 days (range 1–32 days).[172] Dialysis was performed in 43% of cases. Hypertension was present in two-thirds of children but was usually mild and resolved by the time of discharge. Severe disease, including oliguria for more than 14 days, anuria for more than a week, or extrarenal structural damage such as central nervous system (CNS) infarct, occurred in one-quarter of children and was found to be associated with age < 2 years, anuria during the diarrheal prodrome, and an elevated white blood count at presentation. With oliguria, metabolic derangements including metabolic acidosis, hyperkalemia, and dilutional hyponatremia can be seen.

The hematologic abnormalities reflect the microangiopathic process with microthrombi formation. Laboratory studies show a falling hemoglobin, elevated reticulocyte, and elevated lactate dehydrogenase coupled with a blood smear demonstrating fragmented erythrocytes and schistoctyes. Coagulation studies are generally normal, distinguishing HUS from sepsis and disseminated intravascular coagulation. The indirect and direct Coombs test should be negative. Thrombocytopenia may be severe, although a small minority of patients have a normal platelet count. The degree of hemolysis and thrombocytopenia does not correlate with the degree of renal involvement. An increase in the platelet count is one of the first signs of recovery, denoting decreased microangiopathy.

Special mention of CNS involvement in HUS is warranted because this results in significant morbidity and is the most common cause of death in children. As in other organs, the major insult to the CNS is thrombotic microangiopathy. The majority of children demonstrate some degree of encephalopathy as irritability and somnolence. Seizures and cerebral infarct occur in 10% and 4% of children respectively.[172]

Essentially any organ can be affected by the microangiopathy of HUS to varying degrees. Pancreatitis occurs and can be associated with transient or permanent diabetes mellitus. Liver involvement results in hepatomegaly and elevated transaminases. Clinical involvement of the heart or lung is not usually apparent, although rare cases of severe myocardial suppression have been reported.

Therapy

Although plasmapheresis has shown benefit in the course of D− HUS, the mainstay of therapy in D+ HUS is meticulous supportive care. Strict attention should be given to the patient's fluid status, with daily assessment of weight and accurate accounting of fluid input and urine output. As children often present after several days of gastrointestinal losses and poor oral intake, judicious fluid resuscitation with isotonic saline may be warranted to ameliorate prerenal physiology.

In the oligoanuric child, both intravenous and oral intake should match any measurable output and insensible water losses, estimated at $300 \text{ mL/m}^2/\text{day}$. The choice of replacement fluid can be guided by serum and urine electrolytes, with avoidance of potassium and phosphorus supplementation. If oligoanuria develops despite expansion of the intravascular volume, one or two doses of furosemide (1–3 mg/kg) are justified. A renal and bladder ultrasound should be obtained in patients with progressive renal failure to rule out rare instances of urinary tract obstruction.

A large percentage of children with acute HUS will need renal replacement therapy. Indications for dialysis include clinically significant volume overload such as evolving pulmonary edema or congestive heart failure, progressive azotemia, hyperkalemia unresponsive to conservative therapy, and the need for blood product transfusions or nutritional support in the oligoanuric patient. Adequate nutritional support is imperative to reverse the catabolic state associated with the acute disease. Many patients are unable to tolerate enteral nutrition, necessitating the use of total parenteral nutrition.

Packed red blood cell transfusions should be provided for symptomatic anemia or vigorous hemolysis with a hematocrit falling below 20%. Directed transfusions from blood relatives should be avoided as this may sensitize the patient against a potential kidney donor should ESRD develop. In the setting of thrombotic microangiopathy, transfused platelets will be consumed quickly and not result in a sustained increase in the platelet count. Platelets should therefore be transfused only if the patient is actively bleeding with significant clinical sequelae.

Hypertension is common in acute HUS. If there are prolonged episodes of blood pressure > 95th percentile for a child's height and age, medical therapy should be considered. Vasodilatory agents such as hydralazine or calcium channel blockers are effective and are preferred over ACE inhibitors in the setting of fluctuating glomerular perfusion.

D+ HUS is a potentially preventable disease. Ground beef should be cooked thoroughly and unpasteurized food products should be avoided. Children who are infected should be excluded from daycare, and enteric precautions should be taken until stool cultures are negative. Antibiotic treatment of E. coli 0157:H7 infection is not recommended as this has been shown to increase the risk of developing HUS.[173]

A potential therapeutic intervention involves an innovative and specific therapy for verotoxin-associated HUS. Synsorb Pk is a synthetic molecule composed of silicon dioxide particles covalently linked to verotoxin receptors. Phase I study showed that oral ingestion of Synsorb Pk was safe and well tolerated.[174] The phase II randomized controlled trial by the Canadian Pediatric Kidney Disease Research Center found no difference in the development of HUS between the treatment groups of children with documented E. coli 0157 infection, although the subset of children who entered the study early (< 4 days of diarrhea) showed a relative risk reduction of 54%.[175] More recently, a large multicenter clinical trial assessed the efficacy of Synsorb Pk in reducing the frequency of death, serious extrarenal events, or need for dialysis in children with D+ HUS, but the trial was terminated prior to full enrollment secondary to lack of efficacy.

Outcome

Although the majority of children with D+ HUS recover fully from the acute illness, the long-term renal prognosis is guarded. Acute mortality rates up to 5% have been reported and a small percentage of children remain dialysis dependent from the onset of disease.[172,176] In a study of 140 cases of pediatric D+ HUS over a 20-year period, after the acute HUS episode half of the children went on to develop one or more abnormalities including hypertension, proteinuria, and chronic renal insufficiency. ESRD had already developed in another 4% of patients.[172]

A study of 29 French children with a distant history of D+ HUS also suggested significant long-term sequelae.[177] After 15–25 years of follow-up, only 35% had no renal abnormalities, whereas 41% had hypertension, significant proteinuria, or mildly reduced GFR, 10% had chronic renal insufficiency, and 14% had already progressed to ESRD. The best indicator of prognosis was the extent of patchy cortical necrosis on renal biopsy performed at the time of recovery from the acute HUS episode. These studies underscore the importance of long-term and regular follow-up of children following D+ HUS.

In children with ESRD secondary to D+ HUS, renal transplantation is generally quite successful. The North American Pediatric Renal Transplant Cooperative Study reviewed the data from 61 patients with 68 renal transplants.[178] HUS recurred in six (8.8%) allografts in five patients. Four of these patients had D− HUS. In all but one graft, the HUS recurred within 33 days. The time elapsed before transplantation and the use of cyclosporine did not seem to affect the risk of HUS recurrence. In support of this relatively low rate of recurrent disease in children transplanted after D+ HUS, another review of 18 children in Argentina found no recurrences.[179]

Hypertension

In marked contrast to the adult population, the prevalence of hypertension in children is quite low (1–3%) and its etiology is much less likely to be essential and quite likely to be due to an underlying renal anomaly.[180] Unlike adults, in whom normal blood pressure values have been established based on epidemiologic assessment of end-organ damage, blood pressure parameters in children are based on screening data aimed at identifying the normal distribution of blood pressures in the pediatric population. In 1996, the National High Blood Pressure Education Program Working Group on Hypertension Control in Children and Adolescents updated blood pressure tables for children based on the screening of over 61 000 children.[181] These data demonstrated that there are several clinical factors that affect blood pressure in children, particularly age, gender, and height. Blood pressure increases with age during childhood and reaches "adult" levels as the child becomes an adolescent. For any given age, boys tend to have somewhat higher normal blood pressures than girls. Heavier and taller children also have higher blood pressures than their more average-sized peers.

These tables statistically defined hypertension as blood pressure > 95th percentile for readings obtained in children of the same age, gender, and height. Normal blood pressure is a reading < 90th percentile and high-normal is between the 90th and 95th percentiles. Children are considered hypertensive if blood pressure readings are > 95th percentile on three occasions. These tables serve as a resource for the clinician in determining if a child should be considered hypertensive in comparison to his or her peers of a similar size. Blood pressure tends to fall with repeated measurements due to accommodation; thus although 5% of pediatric blood pressure readings are statistically in the hypertensive range by definition, a significantly smaller number of children will be persistently hypertensive.

Most children should have their blood pressure checked annually as part of their visit to the pediatrician. In addition, blood pressure should be assessed in any child hospitalized or in an emergency facility, not only because hypertension may complicate an acute illness but also because the detection of transient hypertension in children during stressful occasions may serve as a marker for the development of future hypertension. Abnormal blood pressure readings require follow-up. High-normal or marginally elevated readings should prompt a repeat blood pressure in 3–6 months. Asymptomatic blood pressure readings up to 10 mmHg above normal require follow-up within 2–4 weeks. Higher blood pressure elevations demand speedier follow-up or, in the case of a child with potential symptomatic hypertension or complicating comorbid medical conditions, immediate attention.

Measuring blood pressure in children can be problematic. The cuff must be appropriately sized, with the width of the cuff's bladder equaling 40% of the mid-upper arm circumference or the cuff bladder encircling three-fourths of the upper arm length as measured from the olecranon to the acromion.[181] Some surveys have estimated that up to 50% of patients have their blood pressure measured with an incorrectly sized cuff.[182] Prior to blood pressure measurement, children should be inactive and acclimated to the examination room for at least 5 min. With auscultation, systolic blood pressure is the first Korotkoff sound (K1) and diastolic pressure in all children and adolescents is the fifth Korotkoff sound (K5) when all sounds disappear. In some small children, the diastolic pressure may be auscultated down to 0 mmHg. Although this is not the true diastolic pressure, it does eliminate any concern of diastolic hypertension.

Small uncooperative children or older children suspected of anxiety-induced hypertension may be relaxed by allowing a parent or nurse to measure their blood pressure in a familiar setting, so that the reading is more representative of the child's usual blood pressure. Some facilities have access to ambulatory blood pressure monitors, small devices worn by the patient that measure and record blood pressure frequently. Advantages of ambulatory monitoring include the ability to record blood pressure during a child's usual daily routine and during sleep so as to determine if hypertension exists, how often it exists and how extensive it may be, and if the measured blood pressure manifests a normal circadian variation.[183]

Since an organic etiology to hypertension is more common in a child, the diagnostic evaluation is slanted very much toward excluding renal parenchymal or vascular diseases. In fact, more than three-fourths of hypertensive children can be found to have a renal etiology to their hypertension (Table 47.6).[184] The child's history is elicited with emphasis on potential renal insults or other medical conditions suggesting a secondary cause of hypertension (Table 47.7). The physical examination includes careful general assessment for a unifying condition such as Williams or Turner syndrome or a disorder such as tuberous sclerosis or neurofibromatosis that may have been overlooked and which commonly includes renally mediated hypertension. Four extremity blood pressures should be measured and a focused examination conducted for pertinent findings such as adenoma sebaceum, café-au-lait marks, abdominal bruits, retinal vessel abnormalities, peripheral pulse variations, and aberrant sexual characteristics.

A phased laboratory evaluation consists of some general studies in almost every hypertensive child and tailored follow-up studies that depend on these results and the child's history, physical findings, and overall level of clinical suspicion. Baseline screening test should include a microscopic urinalysis of a freshly voided urine, serum electrolytes to rule out acidosis or hypokalemia, as seen in some of the mineralocorticoid-excess states, serum creatinine to assess renal function, and renal ultrasound to assess renal anatomy.

In some children, screening tests will be normal and a diagnosis of essential hypertension strongly suspected. Although essential hypertension in children is often consi-

Table 47.7 Pertinent medical history in pediatric hypertension

Birth history: prematurity, prolonged ventilation, umbilical catheter
Past medical history: urinary tract infection, unexplained fevers, recent systemic infections, changes in appearance of urine
Family history: hypertension in first- and second-degree relatives, history of stroke or myocardial infarction, history of endocrine or neurocutaneous disease, history of renal disease
Medication history: decongestants, oral contraceptives, street drugs, chewing tobacco, cigarettes, ethanol
Review of systems: headache, palpitations, sweating, flushing, visual changes

Table 47.6 Causes of hypertension in children

Etiology	Specific diagnoses	Frequency (%)
Renal parenchymal disease	Acute or chronic glomerulonephritis, reflux nephropathy, cystic disease, hemolytic–uremic syndrome	70
Renal vascular disease	Renal artery stenosis, vascular thrombosis	10
Essential hypertension		10
Cardiovascular disease	Aortic coarctation	5
Endocrine disease	Pheochromocytoma, hyperthyroidism, hyperaldosteronism, Cushing syndrome	3
Central nervous system anomaly	Increased intracranial pressure	0.5
Medication effect	Sympathomimetics	0.01

dered a diagnosis of exclusion, many children with essential hypertension follow a typical clinical profile: older child or adolescent, low-grade hypertension, cardiovascular reactivity with stress, high resting pulse rates, obesity, and a family history of essential hypertension.[185] In these children, no further diagnostic work-up is needed immediately; after a review of cardiac risk factors, the child's hypertension should be treated if necessary and followed with regular blood pressure checks and emphasis on adjunctive therapies for hypertension, such as weight reduction, exercise, and dietary counseling.

In children who do not meet the clinical profile for essential hypertension and who have otherwise unremarkable screening test results, further renal imaging with renal scintigraphy can be useful to determine if there is any renal scarring. If this is negative and the patient is significantly hypertensive, renal arteriography should be performed to diagnose any renal vascular abnormalities. Ideally, arteriography should be carried out by a physician experienced with transluminal angioplasty so that this technique may be performed at the same time if an appropriate lesion is identified.

Other laboratory evaluation is of low yield unless there are appropriate concerns from the child's history or physical evaluation. For instance, random serum renin and aldosterone levels are rarely useful. In some families with a pedigree suggestive of glucocorticoid-remediable aldosteronism (difficult to treat, early-onset hypertension in many family members), a random low plasma renin level may prompt more specific genetic testing. Similarly, in rare patients there may be consideration of urinary catecholamine measurement or abdominal magnetic resonance imaging for a catecholamine-secreting tumor.

Therapy for hypertension is tailored toward two basic populations of children. If there is relatively mild hypertension, a cardiac echocardiogram should be considered to rule out left ventricular hypertrophy or other evidence of end-organ effect of sustained high blood pressure. In the absence of end-organ damage, nonpharmacologic therapy could be instituted involving weight reduction, exercise, and dietary counseling. If the blood pressure remains elevated despite these interventions or if there is significantly elevated blood pressure, then pharmacologic therapy should be instituted along with counseling about weight, diet, and exercise.

As with adults, drug therapy in pediatric hypertension involves selecting an initial therapeutic agent and then stepping up therapy if it proves inadequate. In general, an agent based on the underlying presumed physiology is chosen. A submaximal dose of the drug is begun and then titrated up to a maximal dose as needed, aiming to reduce the blood pressure to at least the 90th percentile for age, gender, and height. If there is an inadequate response to the maximal dose of the first medication, a second medication is usually begun, also in a gradual fashion.

Most antihypertensive drugs have not been studied in children. Thus the doses that are used have arisen more from clinical experience than from any scientifically based trials. As with most medications in children, dosing is based on body weight rather than standard dosing amounts. Moreover, with the pediatric population, there can be limitations in the ability of the patient to take a medication: the drug may not be available in a liquid or crushable form if pills cannot be swallowed, and issues of palatability are often troublesome. Table 47.8 lists some of the more commonly utilized antihypertensive medications and their effective doses in children.

Rarely, children present with a hypertensive urgency or a hypertensive crisis. Often, these children have concomitant significant renal pathology, such as an acute nephritis or renal insufficiency. The initial aim of therapy is to reduce the blood pressure by about 30% over the first few hours of care to prevent or minimize end-organ or CNS damage. Table 47.9 lists medications and dosing guidelines that are often effective in treating hypertensive emergencies in children. After the child's blood pressure has been stabilized, it can then be returned more deliberately to an acceptable range by use of more routine antihypertensive medications.

Urinary tract infection and vesicoureteral reflux

Unlike adults, in whom UTI and especially cystitis is more commonly encountered, UTI in children is infrequent, affecting 3–8% of girls and 1–2% of boys. Of more concern, however, is that up to half of girls and two-thirds of boys with UTIs have accompanying high fever, suggestive of an upper tract UTI or pyelonephritis rather than simple cystitis.[186] The propensity for upper tract infection in children stems in part from the association between UTI and vesicoureteral reflux (VUR). In some series, up to half of children with UTI have VUR, whereas in children with no history of UTI only 2% have VUR.[187]

The signs and symptoms of UTI and pyelonephritis may be far less specific in children than in adults. Infants and young children generally have fever but their symptoms are otherwise often vague and include anorexia, lethargy, and irritability. In older children and adolescents, there is an increased likelihood of localizing symptoms such as dysuria, frequency, and flank pain. Since significant delay in the diagnosis and treatment of pyelonephritis in children has been associated with an increased likelihood of significant long-term renal damage, appropriate diagnostic and therapeutic interventions become all the more crucial.

The clinical diagnosis of pyelonephritis in children is usually based on finding bacteria and white cells in the urine of a febrile child. Subsequent urine culture confirms the diagnosis and helps tailor therapy. Obtaining the best possible urine specimen for culture poses more problems in the pediatric patient than with adults. In toilet-trained children, meticulous attention in collecting a midstream urine sample is usually successful. In younger children and infants, a catheterized specimen or a suprapubic aspirate may be required. Urine collected from a bag taped to the child's perineum is easily contaminated and is only useful if there is ultimately no bacterial growth.

Table 47.8 Blood pressure medication in children

	Initial dose (mg/kg/day)	Maximal dose (mg/kg/day)	Dosing frequency
ACE inhibitors			
Captopril (neonate)	0.03–0.15	2	b.i.d./t.i.d.
Captopril (child)	1.5	6	b.i.d./t.i.d.
Enalapril	0.15	Up to 40 mg/day total	q.d./b.i.d.
Calcium channel blockers			
Nifedipine	0.25	3	XL or SR forms b.i.d.
Amlodipine	0.1	0.4	q.d./b.i.d.
Diuretics			
Hydrochlorothiazide	1	2–3	q.d./b.i.d.
Furosemide	0.5–1.0	10	q.d./b.i.d.
Spironolactone	1	3	b.i.d./t.i.d.
Adrenergic agents			
Atenolol (β-blocker)	0.5	2–3	q.d./b.i.d.
Propranolol (β-blocker)	1	6–8	b.i.d.
Labetalol (αβ-blocker)	1	3	b.i.d.
Prazosin (α-blocker)	0.05–0.1	0.5	b.i.d./t.i.d.
Vasodilators			
Hydralazine	0.5	10	t.i.d./q.i.d.
Minoxidil	0.1–0.2	1	q.d./b.i.d.
α-Agonist			
Clonidine	0.05–0.1 mg/day total	0.6 mg/day total	b.i.d./t.i.d., patch every week

ACE, angiotensin-converting enzyme.

Table 47.9 Medications for hypertensive emergencies in children

	Mechanism	Dose	Onset	Duration
Hydralazine	Arteriolar dilator	0.15–0.25 mg/kg i.v. to maximum dose of 20 mg	5–15 min	3–8 h
Labetalol	αβ-Blocker	Initial i.v. bolus 0.25 mg/kg; repeat every 15 min at increasing doses up to 1.0 mg/kg until effective or total dose of 4 mg/kg Maintenance i.v. infusion: 1–3 mg/kg/h	5 min	2–6 h
Nifedipine	Calcium channel blocker	0.25–0.5 mg/kg oral or sublingual	10–20 min	3–6 h
Diazoxide	Arteriolar dilator	Rapid i.v. bolus 1 mg/kg; repeat after 10–15 min if insufficient response; maximum dose 5 mg/kg	3–10 min	4–10 h
Nitroprusside	Venous and arteriolar dilator	Start at 0.5 μg/kg/min i.v.	1–2 min	3–5 min

Most UTIs in children are caused by Gram-negative bacteria of the family Enterobacteriaceae, such as *Escherichia*, *Klebsiella*, *Enterobacter*, and *Citrobacter*.[188] Less commonly, Gram-positive bacteria may be pathogens, especially in patients with urinary tract malformations, voiding dysfunction, or instrumentation.

In the child with a febrile UTI, antibiotic therapy should be started quickly. In neonates and older infants and children with more complicated illness, hospitalization for parenteral therapy is warranted. Empiric therapy is most often a third-generation cephalosporin, an aminoglycoside, or ampicillin, pending urine culture results. In older children who do not appear toxic, therapy can commence on an ambulatory basis with an injection of a third-generation cephalosporin such as ceftriaxone and then transition to appropriate oral therapy to complete a

10–14 day course of therapy. In children with suspected cystitis, oral therapy may commence with a medication such as trimethoprim–sulfamethoxazole, nitrofurantoin, or cefixime that has antimicrobial coverage for the usual Gram-negative organsims associated with UTI. Ultimate oral therapy can be chosen after appropriate sensitivities are obtained from urine culture. In all children treated for UTI, a repeat urine culture should be obtained sometime after appropriate therapy has been initiated in order to document sterilization of the urinary tract.

In any child with a first episode of febrile UTI, renal ultrasonography should be performed to assess urinary tract anatomy. In children older than age 7 years, a normal renal ultrasound may preclude further urinary tract imaging. In the younger child or the older child with sonographic abnormalities such as hydronephrosis or renal scarring, a voiding cystourethrogram (VCUG) should be performed to exclude VUR. A VCUG may be performed at any time after the child is no longer symptomatic and the urine is sterile. If the child has completed the therapeutic course of antibiotics prior to VCUG, prophylactic antibiotic therapy with once-daily trimethoprim–sulfamethoxazole or nitrofurantoin should be initiated until VCUG is perfomed.

If the diagnosis of pyelonephritis is in question, renal scintigraphy with technetium-labeled dimercaptosuccinic acid is a sensitive and specific test. Renal scintigraphy has been shown to be superior to intravenous pyelography, computed tomography, or ultrasound in documenting renal cortical injury.[189] Its use is most helpful in children with chronic or recurrent infections to determine if parenchymal scarring is occurring.

In children with VUR, higher grades of reflux and especially intrarenal reflux predispose to renal scarring. Less than 5% of children with grade I VUR manifest renal scars compared with 50% of children with grade V VUR.[190] In a series of 200 children followed for up to 20 years after an episode of pyelonephritis, renal scarring was almost always associated with moderate to severe VUR.[191] Infants and young children appear more prone to developing renal scars with pyelonephritis. As children reach elementary school age, it becomes increasingly less common to see renal scarring, even in the presence of continued VUR.[192]

Most children with low-grade VUR (grades I–III) can be managed with nightly oral antibiotic prophylaxis and monitored with an annual VCUG or radionuclide cystogram to determine if VUR has spontaneously resolved. In children with higher-grade reflux, VUR is less likely to spontaneously resolve. All children less than 1 year of age are usually managed initially with oral antibiotic prophylaxis. In children with persistent grade V VUR, ureteral reimplantation is generally recommended given its infrequent spontaneous resolution. In children with grade IV VUR, there seems to be no advantage to reimplantation over medical therapy in terms of preventing further episodes of UTI or renal scarring.[193] Over time, there is a decreasing incidence of VUR even in children with higher grades of reflux at presentation, leading many to favor medical therapy unless repeated breakthrough infection, poor compliance, or parental request favor surgical correction.[194,195]

Children who develop extensive renal scarring have an increased incidence of proteinuria, hypertension, and renal insufficiency. The risk of developing these sequelae seems to be most closely linked to the severity of the scarring and the length of follow-up.[196] In children with significantly reduced renal reserve due to parenchymal scarring, there is the risk of hyperfiltration injury in remnant glomeruli and the development of secondary focal glomerulosclerosis and renal insufficiency. Such a consequence of chronic pyelonephritis or reflux nephropathy accounts for 10% of the cases of pediatric ESRD.[197]

References

1. Miltenyi M: Urinary protein excretion in healthy children. Clin Nephrol 1979;12:216–221.
2. Peterson PA, Evrin P, Berggard I: Differentiation of glomerular, tubular and normal proteinuria: determination of urinary excretions of beta-2 microglobulin, albumin and total protein. J Clin Invest 1968;48:1189–1198.
3. Houser M: Assessment of proteinuria using random urine samples. J Pediatr 1984;104:845–848.
4. Randolph MF, Greenfield M: Proteinuria: a six year study of normal infants, preschool and school-aged populations previously screened for urinary tract disease. Am J Dis Child 1967;114:631–638.
5. Wagner MA, Smith FG Jr, Tinglof BO, et al: Epidemiology of proteinuria. J Pediatr 1968;73:825–832.
6. Vehaskari VM, Rapola J: Isolated proteinuria: analysis of a school-age population. J Pediatr 1982;104:661–668.
7. Brenner BM, Baylis C, Deen WM: Transport of molecules across renal glomerular capillaries. Physiol Rev 1976;56:502–534.
8. Kim M: Proteinuria. Clin Lab Med 1988;8:527–539.
9. Rytand DA, Spvieter S: Prognosis in postural (orthostatic) proteinuria. N Engl J Med 1981;305:618–621.
10. Martin-Arevalo DL, Yee J, Pugh J, et al: Fixed and reproducible orthostatic proteinuria: a 35 year follow-up study (abstract). J Am Soc Nephrol 1996;7:1323.
11. Vehaskari VM, Robson AM: Proteinuria. In Edelmann CM (ed): Pediatric Kidney Disease. Boston: Little, Brown, 1992, pp 531–551.
12. Yoshikawa N, Kitagawa K, Ohta K, et al: Asymptomatic constant isolated proteinuria in children. J Pediatr 1991;119:375–379.
13. Habib R: Proteinuria. In Royer P (ed): Pediatric Nephrology. Philadelphia: WB Saunders, 1974, pp 247–252.
14. International Study of Kidney Disease in Children: The nephrotic syndrome in children. Prediction of histopathology from clinical and laboratory characteristics at the time of diagnosis. Kidney Int 1978;13:159–165.
15. Trompeter RS, Hicks J, Lloyd BW, et al: Long term outcome for children with minimal change nephrotic syndrome. Lancet 1985;i:368–370.
16. Sclesinger ER, Sulz HA, Mosher WE, et al: The nephrotic syndrome. Its incidence and implications for the community. Am J Dis Child 1968;116:623–632.
17. White RHR, Glasgow EF, Mills RJ: Clinicopathological study of nephrotic syndrome in childhood. Lancet 1970;i:1353–1359.
18. Clark AG, Barratt TM: Steroid-responsive nephrotic syndrome. In Barratt TM, Avner ED, Harmon WE (eds): Pediatric Nephrology, 4th edn. Baltimore: Lippincott, Williams and Wilkins, 1999, pp 731–747.
19. Ingulli E, Tejani A: Racial differences in the incidence and renal outcome of idiopathic focal segmental glomerulosclerosis in children. Pediatr Nephrol 1991;5:393–397.
20. Arbeitsgemeinschaft fur Padiatrische Nephrologie: Short versus standard prednisone therapy for initial treatment of idiopathic nephrotic syndrome in children. Lancet 1988;i:380–383.
21. Ehrich JH, Brodehl J: Long versus standard prednisone therapy for initial treatment of idiopathic nephrotic syndrome in children. Arbeitsgemeinschaft fur Padiatrische Nephrologie. Eur J Pediatr 1993;152:357–361.

22. Koskimies O, Vilska J, Rapola J, et al: Longterm outlook of primary nephrotic syndrome. Arch Dis Child 1982;57:544–548.

23. Barratt TM, Bercowsky A, Osofsky SG, et al: Cyclophosphamide treatment in steroid sensitive relapsing nephrotic syndrome of childhood. Lancet 1975;i:55–58.

24. Arbeitsgemeinschaft fur Padiatrische Nephrologie: Cyclophosphamide treatment of steroid dependent nephrotic syndrome: comparison of eight week with 12 week course. Arch Dis Child 1987;62:1102–1106.

25. Garin EH, Pryor ND, Fennell RS, et al: Pattern of response to prednisone in idiopathic minimal lesion nephrotic syndrome as a criterion in selecting patients for cyclophosphamide therapy. J Pediatr 1978;92:304–308.

26. Siegel NJ, Gur A, Krassner LS: Minimal lesion nephrotic syndrome with early resistance to steroid therapy. J Pediatr 1975;87:377–380.

27. Bergstrand A, Bollgren I, Samuelson A: Idiopathic nephrotic syndrome of childhood. Cyclophosphamide induced conversion from steroid refractory to highly steroid sensitive disease. Clin Nephrol 1973;1:302–306.

28. Niaudet P, French Society of Pediatric Nephrology: Comparison of cyclosporin and chlorambucil in the treatment of steroid-dependent idiopathic nephrotic syndrome: a multicentre controlled trial. Pediatr Nephrol 1992;6:1–3.

29. Smoyer WE, Gregory MJ, Bajwa RS, et al: Quantitative morphometry of renal biopsies prior to cyclosporine in nephrotic syndrome. Pediatr Nephrol 1998;12:737–743.

30. Neuhaus TJ, Burger HR, Klingler M, et al: Long-term low-dose cyclosporin A in steroid dependent nephrotic syndrome of childhood. Eur J Pediatr 1992;151:775–778.

31. Hamahira K, Iijima K, Tanaka R, et al: Recovery from cyclosporine-associated arteriopathy in childhood nephrotic syndrome. Pediatr Nephrol 2001;16:723–727.

32. Bragga A, Sharma A, Srivastava RN: Levamisole therapy in corticosteroid-dependent nephrotic syndrome. Pediatr Nephrol 1997;11:415–417.

33. Tenbrock K, Muller-Berghaus J, Fuchshuber A, et al: Levamisole treatment in steroid-sensitive and steroid-resistant nephrotic syndrome. Pediatr Nephrol 1998;12:459–462.

34. Bragga A, Hari P: Levamisole-induced vasculitis. Pediatr Nephrol 2000;14:1057–1058.

35. Hiraoka M, Tsukahara H, Hori C, et al: Efficacy of long-term azathioprine for relapsing nephrotic syndrome. Pediatr Nephrol 2000;14:776–778.

36. Gulati S, Sural S, Sharma RK, et al: Spectrum of adolescent-onset nephrotic syndrome in Indian children. Pediatr Nephrol 2001;16:1045–1048.

37. Chesney RW, Novello AC: Forms of nephrotic syndrome more likely to progress to renal impairment. Pediatr Clin North Am 1987;34:609–627.

38. Niaudet P: Steroid resistant idiopathic nephrotic syndrome. In Barratt TM, Avner ED, Harmon WE (eds): Pediatric Nephrology, 4th edn. Baltimore: Lippincott, Williams and Wilkins, 1999, pp 749–763.

39. Tune BM, Lieberman E, Mendoza SA: Steroid-resistant nephrotic focal segmental glomerulosclerosis: a treatable disease. Pediatr Nephrol 1996;10:772–778.

40. Tarshish P, Tobin JN, Bernstein J, et al: Cyclophosphamide does not benefit patients with focal segmental glomerulosclerosis. A report of the International Study of Kidney Disease in Children. Pediatr Nephrol 1996;10:590–593.

41. Arbus GS, Poucell S, Bacheyie GS, et al: Focal segmental glomerulosclerosis with idiopathic nephrotic syndrome: three types of clinical response. J Pediatr 1982;101:40–45.

42. Mongeau J-G, Corneille L, Rabitaille P, et al: Primary nephrosis in childhood associated with focal glomerular sclerosis: is long-term prognosis that severe? Kidney Int 1981;20:743–746.

43. Mendoza SA, Reznik VM, Griswold W, et al: Treatment of steroid resistant focal segmental glomerulosclerosis with pulse methylprednisolone and oral alkylating agents. Pediatr Nephrol 1990;4:303–307.

44. Tune BM, Kirpekar R, Sibley RK, et al: Intravenous methylprednisolone and oral alkylating agent therapy of prednisone-resistant pediatric focal segmental glomerulosclerosis: a long-term follow-up. Clin Nephrol 1995;43:84–88.

45. Guillot AP, Kim MS: Pulse steroid therapy does not alter the course of focal glomerulosclerosis (abstract). J Am Soc Nephrol 1993;4:276.

46. Waldo FB, Benfield MR, Kohaut EC: Methylprednisolone treatment of patients with steroid-resistant nephrotic syndrome. Pediatr Nephrol 1992;6:503–505.

47. Chishti AS, Sorof JM, Brewer ED, et al: Long-term treatment of focal segmental glomerulosclerosis in children with cyclosporine given as a single daily dose. Am J Kidney Dis 2001;38:754–760.

48. Singh A, Tejani C, Tejani A: One-center experience with cyclosporine in refractory nephrotic syndrome in children. Pediatr Nephrol 1992;13:26–32.

49. Lieberman KV, Tejani A: A randomized double-blind placebo-controlled trial of cyclosporine in steroid-resistant idiopathic focal segmental glomerulosclerosis in children. J Am Soc Nephrol 1996;7:56–63.

50. Gregory MJ, Smoyer WE, Sedman A, et al: Long-term cyclosporine therapy for pediatric nephrotic syndrome: a clinical and histologic analysis. J Am Soc Nephrol 1991;5:587–590.

51. Milliner DS, Morgenstern BZ: Angiotensin converting enzyme inhibitors for reduction of proteinuria in children with steroid resistant nephrotic syndrome. Pediatr Nephrol 1991;5:587–590.

52. Fitzwater DS, Brouhard BH, Cunningham RJ 3rd: Use of angiotensin converting inhibitors for the treatment of focal segmental glomerulosclerosis. Am J Dis Child 1990;144:522.

53. Briggs WA, Choi MJ, Scheel PJ Jr: Succesful mycophenolate mofetil treatment of glomerular disease. Am J Kidney Dis 1998;31:364–365.

54. Chandra M, Susin M, Abitbil C: Remission of relapsing childhood nephrotic syndrome with mycophenolate mofetil. Pediatr Nephrol 2000;14:224–226.

55. Broyer M, Meyrier A, Niaudet P, et al: Minimal changes and focal segmental glomerulosclerosis. In Cameron S, Davison AM, Grunfield JP, Kerr D, Ritz E (eds): Oxford Textbook of Clinical Nephrology. Oxford: Blackwell Scientific Publications, 1992, pp 298–339.

56. Baum MA, Stablein DM, Panzarino VM, et al: Loss of living donor renal allograft survival advantage in children with focal segmental glomerulosclerosis. Kidney Int 2001;59:328–333.

57. Savin VJ, Sharma R, Sharma M, et al: Circulating factor associated with increased glomerular permeability to albumin in recurrent focal segmental glomerulosclerosis. N Engl J Med 1996;334:878–883.

58. Artero M, Sharma R, Savin V, et al: Plasmapheresis reduces proteinuria and serum capacity to injure glomeruli in patients with recurrent focal segmental glomerulosclerosis. Am J Kidney Dis 1994;23:574–581.

59. Mathis B, Kim S, Calabrese K, et al: A locus for inherited focal segmental glomerulosclerosis maps to chromosome 19q13. Kidney Int 1998;53:282–286.

60. Kaplan J, Kim S, North K, et al: Mutations in ACTN4, encoding alpha-actinin-4, cause familial focal segmental glomerulosclerosis. Nature Genetics 2000;24:251–256.

61. Tsukaguchi H, Yager H, Dawborn J, et al: A locus for adolescent and adult onset familial focal segmental glomerulosclerosis on chromosome 1q25–31. J Am Soc Nephrol 2000;11:1674–1680.

62. Caridi G, Bartelli R, DiDuca M, et al: Prevalence, genetics, and clinical features of patients carrying podocin mutations in steroid-resistant nonfamilial focal segmental glomerulosclerosis. J Am Soc Nephrol 2001;12:2742–2746.

63. Little M, Wells CA: Clinical overview of WT1 gene mutations. Hum Mutat 1997;9:209–225.

64. Heaton PA, Smales O, Wong W: Congenital nephrotic syndrome responsive to captopril and indomethacin. Arch Dis Child 1999;81:174–175.

65. Habib R. Nephrotic syndrome in the 1st year of life. Pediatr Nephrol 1993;7: 347–353.

66. Holmberg C, Jalanko H, Tryyvason K, et al: Congenital nephrotic syndrome. In Barratt TM, Avner ED, Harmon WE (eds): Pediatric Nephrology, 4th edn. Baltimore: Lippincott, Williams and Wilkins, 1999, pp 765–777.

67. Kestila M, Lenkkeri U, Lamerdin J, et al: Positionally cloned gene for a novel glomerular protein – nephrin – is mutated in congenital nephrotic syndrome. Mol Cell 1998;1:575–582.

68. Seppala M, Aula P, Rapola J, et al: Congenital nephrotic syndrome: pre-natal diagnosis and genetic counseling by estimation of amniotic fluid and maternal serum alpha-fetoprotein. Lancet 1976;ii:123–124.

69. Holmberg C, Antikainen M, Ronnholm K, et al: Management of congenital nephrotic syndrome of the Finnish type. Pediatr Nephrol 1995;9:87–93.

70. Kim MS, Primack W, Harmon WE: Congenital nephrotic syndrome: preemptive bilateral nephrectomy and dialysis before renal transplantation. J Am Soc Nephrol 1992;3:260–263.

71. Holmberg C, Patrakka J, Laine J, et al: Post-transplant proteinuria in Finnish type nephrotic syndrome. In Cochat P (ed): Recurrence of the Disease in the Renal Graft. Paris: John Libby Eurotext, 2001, pp 35–38.

72. Lane J, Jalanko H, Holthofer H, et al: Post-transplantation nephrosis in congenital nephrotic syndrome of the Finnish type. Kidney Int 1993;44:867–874.

73. Patrakka J, Ruotsalainen V, Reponen P, et al: Recurrence of nephrotic syndrome in kidney grafts of patients with congenital nephrotic syndrome of the Finnish type: role of nephrin. Transplantation 2002;73:394–403.

74. Dodge W, West E, Smith E, et al: Proteinuria and hematuria in schoolchildren: epidemiology and early natural history. J Pediatr 1976;88:327–347.

75. Vehaskari V, Rapola J, Koskimies O, et al: Microscopic hematuria in schoolchildren: epidemiology and clinicopathologic evaluation. J Pediatr 1979;95:676–684.

76. Ingelfinger J, Davis A, Grupe W: Frequency and etiology of gross hematuria in a general pediatric setting. Pediatrics 1977;59:557–561.

77. Stapleton F: Idiopathic hypercalciuria: association with isolated hematuria and risk for urolithiasis in children. Kidney Int 1990;37:807–811.

78. Smeets H, Knoers V, van de Heuvel L, et al: Heredity disorders of the glomerular basement membrane. Pediatr Nephrol 1996;10:779–788.

79. Gubler M, Knebelmann B, Antignac C: Inherited glomerular disease. In Barrat T, Avner E, Harmon W (eds): Pediatric Nephrology, 4th edn. Baltimore: Lippincott, Williams and Wilkins, 1999, pp 475–484.

80. Ozen S, Ertoy D, Heidt L, et al: Benign familial hematuria associated with a novel COL4A4 mutation. Pediatr Nephrol 2001;16:874–877.

81. Lemmink H, Nillesen W, Mochizuki T, et al: Benign familial hematuria due to mutation of the type IV collagen alpha 4 gene. J Clin Invest 1996;98:1114–1118.

82. Pajari H, Kaariainen H, Muhohnen T, et al: Alport's syndrome in 78 patients: epidemiological and clinical study. Acta Paediatr 1996;85:1300–1306.

83. Stapleton F, Roy S, Noe N, et al: Hypercalciuria in children with hematuria. N Engl J Med 1984;310:1345–1348.

84. Ordonez F, Fernandez P, Rodriquez J, et al: Rat models of normocalcemic hypercalciuria of different pathogenic mechanisms. Pediatr Nephrol 1998;12:201–205.

85. Stapleton F: Hematuria associated with hypercalciuria and hyperuricosuria: a practical approach. Pediatr Nephrol 1994;8:756–761.

86. Polito C, La Manna A, Cioce F, et al: Clinical presentation and natural course of idiopathic hypercalciuria in children. Pediatr Nephrol 2000;15:211–214.

87. Garcia C, Miller L, Stapleton F: Natural history of hematuria associated with hypercalciuria in children. Am J Dis Child 1991;145:1204–1207.

88. Borghi L, Schianchi T, Meschi T, et al: Comparison of two diets for the prevention of recurrent stones in idiopathic hypercalciuria. N Engl J Med 2002;346:77–84.

89. Lemann J, Pleuss J, Gray R, et al: Potassium administration increases and potassium deprivation reduces urinary calcium excretion in healthy adults. Kidney Int 1991;39:973–983.

90. United States Renal Data Service: Pediatric end stage renal disease. Am J Kidney Dis 1994;24(Suppl 2):S112–S127.

91. Rai A, Nast C, Alder S: Henoch–Schonlein purpura nephritis. J Am Soc Nephrol 1999;10:2637–2644.

92. Allen A, Willis F, Beattie T, et al: Abnormal IgA glycosylation in Henoch–Schonlein purpura restricted to patents with clinical nephritis. Nephrol Dial Transplant 1998;13:930–934.

93. Meadow S, Glasgow E, White R, et al: Schönlein–Henoch nephritis. Q J Med 1972;41:241–258.

94. Cream J, Gumpel J, Peachey R: Schonlein–Henoch purpura in the adult. A study of 77 adults with anaphylactoid Schonlein–Henoch purpura. Q J Med 1970;39:461–484.

95. Balmelli C, Laux-End R, Di Rocco D, et al: Anaphylactoid purpura nephritis in childhood: natural history and immunopathology. Adv Nephrol Necker Hosp 1976;6:183–228.

96. Choong C, Beasley S: Intra-abdominal manifestations of Henoch–Schonlein purpura. J Paediatr Child Health 1998;34:405–409.

97. Stewart M, Savage J, Bell B, et al: Long term renal prognosis of Henoch–Schonlein purpura in an unselected childhood population. Eur J Pediatr 1988;147:113–115.

98. Calvino M, Llorca J, Garcia-Porrua C, et al: Henoch–Schonlein purpura in children from northwestern Spain. Medicine 2001;80:279–290.

99. Farine M, Poucell S, Geary D, et al: Prognostic significance of urinary findings and renal biopsies in children with Henoch–Schonlein nephritis. Clin Pediatr 1986;25:257–259.

100. Austin, H, Balow J: Henoch–Schonlein nephritis: prognostic features and the challenge of therapy. Am J Kidney Dis 1983;2:512–520.

101. Goldstein A, White R, Akuse R, et al: Long-term follow-up of childhood Henoch–Schonlein nephritis. Lancet 1992;339:280–282.

102. Mollica F, LiVolti S, Garozzo R, et al: Effectiveness of early prednisone treatment in preventing the development of nephropathy in anaphylactoid purpura. Eur J Pediatr 1992;151:140–144.

103. Saulsbury F: Corticosteroid therapy does not prevent nephritis in Henoch–Schonlein purpura. Pediatr Nephrol 1993;7:69–71.

104. Flynn J, Smoyer W, Bunchman T, et al: Treatment of Henoch Schonlein purpura glomerulonephritis in children with high-dose corticosteroids plus oral cyclophosphamide. Am J Nephrol 2001;21:128–133.

105. Foster B, Bernard C, Drummond K, et al: Effective therapy for severe Henoch Schonlein purpura nephritis with prednisone and azathioprine: a clinical and histopathologic study. J Pediatr 2000;136:370–375.

106. Oner A, Tinaztepe K, Erdogan O: The effect of triple therapy on rapidly progressive type of Henoch–Schonlein nephritis. Pediatr Nephrol 1995;9:6–10.

107. Niaudet P, Habib R: Methylprednisolone pulse therapy in the treatment of severe forms of Schonlein–Henoch purpura nephritis. Pediatr Nephrol 1998;12:238–243.

108. Iijima K, Ito-Kariya S, Nakamura H, et al: Multiple combined therapy for severe Henoch–Schonlein nephritis in children. Pediatr Nephrol 1998;12:244–248.

109. Hattori M, Ito K, Konomoto T, et al: Plasmapheresis as the sole therapy for rapidly progressive Henoch Schonlein purpura nephritis in children. Am J Kidney Dis 1999;33:427–433.

110. Schrarer K, Krmar R, Querfeld U, et al: Clinical outcome of Schonlein–Henoch purpura nephritis in children. Pediatr Nephrol 1999;13:816–823.

111. Wyatt R, Krichevsky S, Woodford S, et al: IgA nephropathy: long-term prognosis for pediatric patients. J Pediatr 1995;127:913–919.

112. Yoshikawa N, Ito H, Yoshira S, et al: IgA nephropathy in children from Japan. Child Nephrol Urol 1989;9:191–199.

113. Yoshikawa N, Tanaka R, Iijima K: Pathophysiology and treatment of IgA nephropathy in children. Pediatr Nephrol 2001;16:446–457.

114. Yoshikawa N, Ito H, Nakamura H: Prognostic indicators in childhood IgA nephropathy. Nephron 1992;60:60–67.

115. Hogg R, Silva F, Wyatt R, et al: Prognostic indicators in children with IgA nephropathy: report of the Southwest Pediatric Nephrology Study Group. Pediatr Nephrol 1994;8:15–20.

116. Hotta O, Furuta T, Chiba S, et al: Regression of IgA nephropathy: a repeat biopsy study. Am J Kidney Dis 2002;39:493–502.

117. Hotta O, Miyazaki M, Furuta T, et al: Tonsillectomy and steroid pulse therapy significantly impact on clinical remission in patients with IgA nephropathy. Am J Kidney Dis 2001;38:736–743.

118. Rasche F, Schwarz A, Keller F: Tonsillectomy does not prevent a progressive course in IgA nephropathy. Clin Nephrol 1999;51:147–152.

119. Andreoli S, Bergstein J: Treatment of severe IgA nephropathy in children. Pediatr Nephrol 1989;3:248–253.

120. Waldo F, Wyatt R, Kelly D: Treatment of IgA nephropathy in children: efficacy of alternate-day oral prednisone. Pediatr Nephrol 1993;7:529–532.

121. Yoshikawa N, Ito H, Sakai T: A controlled trial of combined therapy for newly diagnosed severe childhood IgA nephropathy. The Japanese Pediatric IgA Nephropathy Treatment Study Group. J Am Soc Nephrol 1999;10:101–109.

122. Donadio J, Bergstralh E, Offord K, et al: A controlled trial of fish oil in IgA nephropathy. N Engl J Med 1994;331:1194–1199.

123. Donadio J, Grande J, Bergstralh E, et al: The long-term outcome of patients with IgA nephropathy treated with fish oil in a controlled trial. J Am Soc Nephrol 1999;10:1772–1777.

124. Donadio J, Larson T, Bergstralh E, et al: A randomized trial of high-dose compared with low-dose omega-3 fatty acids in severe IgA nephropathy. J Am Soc Nephrol 2001;12:791–799.

125. Wolf G, Neilson E: Angiotensin II as a renal growth factor. J Am Soc Nephrol 1993;3:1531–1540.

126. Hunley T, Julian B, Phillips J, et al: Angiotensin converting enzyme gene polymorphism: potential silencer motif and impact on progression in IgA nephropathy. Kidney Int 1996;49:571–577.

127. Stratta P, Canavese C, Ciconne G, et al: Angiotensin I-converting enzyme genotype significantly affects progression of IgA glomerulonephritis in an Italian population. Am J Kidney Dis 1999;33:1071–1079.

128. Cole B, Salinas-Madrigal L: Acute proliferative glomerulonephritis and crescentic glomerulonephritis. In Barrat T, Avner E, Harmon W (eds): Pediatric Nephrology, 4th edn. Baltimore: Lippincott, Williams and Wilkins, 1999, pp 669–678.

129. Nissensona, Baraff L, Fine R, et al: Poststreptococcal acute glomerulonephritis: fact and controversy. Ann Intern Med 1979;91:76–86.

130. Watanabe T, Yoshizawa N: Recurrence of acute poststreptococcal glomerulonephritis. Pediatr Nephrol 2001;16:598–600.

131. Velhote V, Saldanha L, Malheiro P, et al: Acute glomerulonephritis: three episodes demonstrated by light and electron microscopy, and immunofluorescence studies. A case report. Clin Nephrol 1986;26:307–310.

132. Rosenberg H, Donoso P, Vial S, et al: Clinical and morphological recovery between two episodes of acute glomerulonephritis: a light and electron microscopy study with immunofluorescence. Clin Nephrol 1984;21:350–354.

133. Navaneeth B, Ray N, Chawda S, et al: Prevalence of beta hemolytic streptococci carrier rate among schoolchildren in Salem. Indian J Pediatr 2001;68:985–986.

134. Pichichero M, Marsocci S, Murphy M, et al: Incidence of streptococcal carriers in private pediatric practice. Arch Pediatr Adolesc Med 1999;153:624–628.

135. Begovac J, Bobinac E, Benic B, et al: Asymptomatic pharyngeal carriage of beta-hemolytic streptococci and streptococcal pharyngitis among patients at an urban hospital in Croatia. Eur J Epidemiol 1993;9:405–410.

136. Dedeoglu I, Springate J, Waz W, et al: Prolonged hypocomplementemia in poststreptococcal acute glomerulonephritis. Clin Nephrol 1996;46:302–305.

137. Bolton W, Sturgill B: Methylprednisolone therapy for acute crescentic rapidly progressive glomerulonephitis. Am J Nephrol 1989;9:368–375.

138. Kunis C, Kiss B, Williams G, et al: Intravenous "pulse" cyclophosphamide therapy of crescentic glomerulonephritis. Clin Nephrol 1992;37:1–7.

139. Kasahaa T, Hayakawa H, Okubo S, et al: Prognosis of acute poststreptococcal glomerulonephritis (APSGN) is excellent in children, when adequately diagnosed. Pediatr Int 2001;43:364–367.

140. Popovic-Rolovic M, Kosic M, Antic-Peco A, et al: Medium- and long-term prognosis of patients with acute poststretococcal glomerulonephritis. Nephron 1991;58:393–399.

141. Clark G, White R, Glasgow E, et al: Poststreptococcal glomerulonephritis in children: clinicopathological correlations and long-term prognosis. Pediatr Nephrol 1988;2:381–388.

142. Baldwin D, Gluck M, Schacht R, et al: The long-term course of post-streptococcal glomerulonephritis. Ann Intern Med 1974;80:342–358.

143. Cameron S, Turner R, Heaton J, et al: Idiopathic mesangiocapillary glomerulonephritis. Am J Med 1983;74:175–192.

144. Habib R, Kleinknecht C, Gubler M, et al: Idiopathic membranoproliferative glomerulonephritis in children. Report of 105 cases. Clin Nephrol 1973;1:194–214.

145. Somers M, Kertesz S, Rosen S, et al: Non-nephrotic children with membranoproliferative glomerulonephritis: are steroids indicated? Pediatr Nephrol 1995;9:140–144.

146. Iitaka K, Ishidate T, Hojo M, et al: Idiopathic membranoproliferative glomerulonephritis in Japanese children. Pediatr Nephrol 1995;9:272–277.

147. Donadio J, Anderson C, Mitchell J, et al: Membranoproliferative glomerulonephritis: a prospective clinical trial of platelet-inhibitor therapy. N Engl J Med 1984;310:1421–1426.

148. Zimmerman S, Moorthy A, Dreher W, et al: Prospective trial of warfarin and dipyridamole in patients with membranoproliferative glomerulonephritis. Am J Med 1983;75:920–927.

149. Catran D, Cardella C, Roscoe J, et al: Results of a controlled drug trial in membranoproliferative glomerulonephritis. Kidney Int 1985;27:436–441.

150. Zauner I, Bohler J, Braun N, et al: Effect of asprin and dipyridamole on proteinuria in idiopathic membranoproliferative glomerulonephritis: a multicentre prospective clinical trial. Nephrol Dial Transplant 1994;9:619–622.

151. McEnery P: Membranoproliferative glomerulonephritis: the Cincinnati experience. Cumulative renal survival from 1957 to 1989. J Pediatr 1990;116:S109–S114.

152. Bergstein J, Andreoli S: Response of type I membranoproliferative glomerulonephritis to pulse methlprednisone and alternate-day prednisone therapy. Pediatr Nephrol 1995;9:268–271.

153. Tarshish P, Bernstein J, Tobin J, et al: Treatment of mesangiocapillary glomerulonephritis with alternate-day prednisone: a report of the International Study of Kidney Disease in Children. Pediatr Nephrol 1992;6:123–130.

154. Quan A, Sullivan E, Alexander S: Recurrence of hemolytic uremic syndrome after renal transplantation in children (a report of the North American pediatric renal transplant cooperative study). Transplantation 2001;72:742–745.

155. Seigler R: The hemolytic uremic syndrome. Pediatr Clin North Am 1995;42:1505–1529.

156. Brandt J, Fouser L, Watkins S, et al: Escherichia coli 0157:H7-associated hemolytic–uremic syndrome after ingestion of contaminated hamburgers. J Pediatr 1994;125:519–526.

157. Seigler R: Hemolytic uremic syndrome in children. Curr Opin Pediatr 1995;7:159–163.

158. Hancock D, BesserT, Kinsel M, et al: The prevalence of Escherichia coli 0157:H7 in dairy and beef cattle in Washington state. Epidemiol Infect 1994;113:199–207.

159. Belongia E, Osterholm M, Soler J, et al: Transmission of Escherichia coli 0157:H7 infection in Minnesota child day-care facilities. JAMA 1993;269:883–888.

160. Kaplan B, Meyers K, Schulman S: The pathogenesis and treatment of hemolytic uremic syndrome. J Am Soc Nephrol 1998;9:1126–1133.

161. Moake J: Haemolytic–uraemic syndrome: basic science. Lancet 1994;343:393–397.

162. Taylor M, Milford D, Rose P, et al: The expression of blood group P1 in post-enteropathic haemolytic uraemic syndrome. Pediatr Nephrol 1990;4:59–61.

163. Jelacic S, Wobbe C, Boster D, et al: ABO and P1 blood group antigen expression and stx genotype and outcome of childhood Escherichia coli 0157:H7 infections. J Infect Dis 2002;185:214–219.

164. Ashida A, Matsui K, Chizaki T, et al: Erythrocyte P1 group antigen expression in VTEC-associated hemolytic uremic syndrome. Clin Nephrol 1999;51:73–76.

165. Orr H, Dong V, Schroeder M, et al: P1 blood group antigen expression and epidemic hemolytic uremic syndrome. Pediatr Nephrol 1995;9:612–613.

166. Robson W, Leung A, Bowen T, et al: The P1 blood group and the severity of diarrhea-associated hemolytic uremic syndrome. Clin Nephrol 1994;42:288–290.

167. Green D, Murphy W, Uttley W: Haemolytic uraemic synrome: prognostic factors. Clin Lab Haematol 2000;22:11–14.

168. Shimazu T, Shimaoka M, Sugimoto H, et al: Does blood type B protect against haemolytic uraemic syndrome? An analysis of the 1996 Sakai outbreak of Escherichia coli 0157:H7 (VTEC 0157) infection. The Osaka HUS Critical Care Study Group. J Infect 2000;41:45–49.

169. Grodinsky S, Telmesani A, Robson W, et al: Gastrointestinal manifestations of hemolytic uremic syndrome: recognition of pancreatitis. J Pediatr Gastrenterol Nutr 1990;11:518–524.

170. Brandt M, O'Regan S, Rousseau E, et al: Surgical complications of the hemolytic–uremic syndrome. J Pediatr Surg 1990;25:1109–1112.

171. Tochen M, Campbell J: Colitis in children with the hemolytic–uremic syndrome. J Pediatr Surg 1977;12:213–219.

172. Siegler R, Pavia A, Christofferson R, et al: A 20-year population-based study of postdiarrheal hemolytic uremic syndrome in Utah. Pediatrics 1994;94:35–40.

173. Wong C, Jelacic S, Habeeb R, et al: The risk of the hemolytic–uremic syndrome after antibiotic treatment of Escherichia coli 0157:H7 infections. N Engl J Med 2000;32:1930–1936.

174. Armstrong G, Rowe P, Goodyer P, et al: A phase I study of chemically synthesized verotoxin (Shiga-like toxin) Pk-trisaccharide

receptors attached to chromosorb for preventing hemolytic–uremic syndrome. J Infect Dis 1995;171:1042–1045.

175. Rowe P, Milner R, Orrbine E, et al: A phase II randomized controlled trial of Synsorb Pk for the prevention of hemolytic uremic syndrome in children with verotoxin-producing E. coli (VTEC) gastroenteritis. Pediatr Res 1997;41:283A.

176. Spizzirri F, Rahman R, Biblioni N, et al: Childhood hemolytic uremic syndrome in Argentina: long-term follow-up and prognostic features. Pediatr Nephrol 1997;11:156–160.

177. Gagnadoux M, Habib R, Gubler M, et al: Long-term (15–25 years) outcome of childhood hemolytic–uremic syndrome. Clin Nephrol 1996;46:39–41.

178. Quan A, Sullivan E, Alexander S: Recurrence of hemolytic uremic syndrome after renal transplantation in children. A report of the North American Pediatric Renal Transplant Cooperative Study. Transplantation 2001;72:742–745.

179. Bassani C, Ferraris J, Gianantonio C, et al: Renal transplantation in patients with classical haemolytic–uraemic syndrome. Pediatr Nephrol 1991;5:607–611.

180. Sinaiko AR, Gomez-Marin O, Prineas RJ: Prevalence of significant hypertension in junior high school-aged children. The children and adolescent blood pressure program. J Pediatr 1989;114:664–669.

181. National High Blood Pressure Education Program Working Group on Hypertension Control in Children and Adolescents: Update on the 1987 task force report on high blood pressure in children and adolescents: a working group report from the national high blood pressure education program. Pediatrics 1996;98:649–658.

182. Matoo TK: Arm cuff in the measurement of blood pressure. Am J Hypertens 2002;15:67S–68S.

183. Lurbe E, Redon J: Reproducibility and validity of ambulatory blood pressure monitoring in children. Am J Hypertens 2002;15:69S–73S.

184. Swinford RD, Ingelfinger JR: Evaluation of hypertension in childhood diseases. In Barratt TM, Avner ED, Harmon WE (eds): Pediatric Nephrology, 4th edn. Baltimore: Lippincott, Williams and Wilkins, 1999, pp 1007–1030.

185. Sadowski RH, Falkner B: Hypertension in pediatric patients. Am J Kidney Dis 1996;27:305–315.

186. Hellstrom AL, Hanson E, Hansson S, et al: Association between urinary symptoms at 7 years old and previous urinary tract infection Arch Dis Child 1991;66:232–234.

187. Bailey RR: Vesicoureteral reflux in healthy infants and children. In Hodson J, Kincaid-Smith P (eds): Reflux Nephropathy. New York: Masson, 1979, pp 59–61.

188. Rushton HG: Urinary tract infections in children: epidemiology, evaluation, and management. Pediatr Clin North Am 1997;44:1133–1169.

189. Lavocat MP, Granjon D, Allard D, et al: Imaging of pyelonephritis. Pediatr Radiol 1997;27:159–165.

190. Skoog SJ, Belman AB, Majd M: A nonsurgical approach to the managemnt of primary vesicoureteral reflux. J Urol 1987;138:941–946.

191. Smellie JM, Normand JC, Katz G: Children with urinary infections: a comparison of those with and those without vesicoureteric reflux. Kidney Int 1981;20:717–722.

192. Olbing H, Claesson I, Ebel KD, et al: Renal scars and parenchymal thinning in children with vesicoureteral reflux: a 5-year report of the International Reflux Study in Children (European branch). J Urol 1992;148:1653–1656.

193. Tamminen-Mobius T, Bruner E, Ebel KD, et al: Cessation of vesicoureteral reflux for 5 years in infants and children allocated to medical treatment. J Urol 1992;148:1662–1666.

194. Smellie JM, Jodal U, Lax H, et al: Outcome at 10 years of severe vesicoureteric reflux managed medically: report of the International Reflux Study in Children. J Pediatr 2001;199:656–663.

195. Wennerstrom M, Hansson S, Jodal U, et al: Disappearance of vesicoureteric reflux in children. Arch Pediatr Adolesc Med 1998; 152:879–883.

196. Rushton HG: Vesicoureteral reflux and scarring. In Barratt TM, Avner ED, Harmon WE (eds): Pediatric Nephrology, 4th edn. Baltimore: Lippincott, Williams and Wilkins, 1999, pp 851–871.

197. Benfield MR, McDonald R, Sullivan EK, et al: The 1997 annual renal transplantation in children: Report of the North American Pediatric Renal Transplant Cooperative Study (NAPRTCS). Pediatr Transplant 1999;3:152–167.

CHAPTER 48

Management of Endstage Renal Disease in Childhood and Adolescence

Joana E. Kist-van Holthe and David M. Briscoe

Special clinical issues in children with ESRD
- Nutrition
- Growth and other endocrine disorders
- Renal osteodystrophy
- Anemia
- Hypertension and cardiovascular disease
- Neurodevelopment outcome and psychosocial adjustment
- Mortality of children on renal replacement therapy

Dialysis therapy
- Peritoneal dialysis
  - Dialysis prescription
  - Dialysis adequacy
  - Complications
- Hemodialysis
  - Dialysis prescription
  - Dialysis adequacy
  - Complications

Renal transplantation
- Causes of graft failure in pediatric recipients
  - Acute rejection
  - Chronic rejection
- Preparation for pediatric renal transplantation
  - Donor
  - Recipient
- Immunosuppressive therapy

Summary

The management of children and adolescents with endstage renal disease (ESRD) differs from that for adults. Children have unique problems that are not only associated with renal failure itself but can also be related to current therapies. The optimal treatment of ESRD in a child is one that not only reverses biochemical and hematologic abnormalities related to the disease but also achieves normal physiologic patterns of growth and neurodevelopment. Such a treatment facilitates maximal educational opportunity and optimizes the quality of life of the child.

ESRD occurs in 1–3 per million total population of children per year.[1,2] The most common diagnoses of ESRD in small children are noted in Table 48.1.[3] Chronic renal insufficiency in children is associated with many biochemical and hematologic abnormalities as well as hypertension, hyperparathyroidism, anemia, and growth retardation, all of which require specific therapeutic interventions. Indications for renal replacement therapy include hypervolemia, hyperkalemia, symptoms of uremia not responsive to conservative therapy, failure to thrive

due to limitations in total caloric intake, severe refractory hypertension, growth retardation not responsive to growth hormone therapy, and delayed psychomotor development.[4] In contrast to adults, initiating renal replacement therapy in children does not depend on a specific cutoff point for glomerular filtration rate (GFR) or serum urea nitrogen but is more associated with other abnormalities in physiology. All children can undergo dialysis therapy, although the mortality associated with dialysis can be especially high in very young children under the age of 2 years. In older children, the mortality of dialysis is similar to that seen in adults.

Renal transplantation is a feasible treatment for ESRD and is widely recognized as the treatment of choice for all children.[5] In contrast to children on dialysis, children with a functioning renal transplant can have adequate growth, psychomotor development, and school achievements.[6–12] Absolute contraindications for renal transplantation are few but include active malignancy, active infection with hepatitis B or HIV, severe multiorgan failure, and a positive direct cross-match within the previous 3–12 months.[4]

Table 48.1 Primary diagnoses (%) of children with endstage renal disease who received a renal allograft*

Congenital abnormalities of the urinary tract	40.4
Obstructive uropathy	16.3
Aplastic/hypoplastic/dysplastic kidneys	15.7
Reflux nephropathy	5.6
Prune belly syndrome	2.8
Glomerulonephritis	17.7
Focal segmental sclerosis	11.7
Membranoproliferative glomerulonephritis	2.1
Idiopathic crescentic glomerulonephritis	2.0
Membranous nephropathy	0.5
Systemic lupus erythematosus	1.4
Chronic glomerulonephritis	4.0
Medullary cystic/juvenile nephronophthisis	2.8
Hemolytic–uremic syndrome	2.7
Congenital nephrotic syndrome	2.7
Polycystic kidney disease	2.7
Miscellaneous	27.0

*Adapted from Seikaly M, Ho PL, Emmett L, Tejani A: The 12th Annual Report of the North American Pediatric Renal Transplant Cooperative Study: renal transplantation from 1987 through 1998. Pediatr Transplant 2001;5:215–231.

Special clinical issues in children with ESRD

Nutrition

Inadequate nutrition in children with ESRD inevitably results in growth failure when caloric intake is < 70% of the recommended daily allowance.[13,14] Current recommendations are that children on dialysis should receive an energy intake that is at least 100% of the recommended daily allowance (Table 48.2).[15,16] For infants on peritoneal dialysis a slightly higher caloric intake (130–140% recommended daily allowance) and a high protein intake of 2.5–3 g/kg/day is needed for adequate growth.[16–19] Likewise for prepubertal and pubertal children receiving peritoneal dialysis, high protein intakes (1.5–2 g/kg/day) are advised to maintain physiologic growth patterns and to obviate protein malnutrition. The higher protein intake may result in a slightly higher blood urea nitrogen level, which needs to be treated with adequate and efficient dialysis. Urea kinetic modeling is thus an important tool for monitoring optimal protein intake and delivery of dialysis.[20]

The management of fluid intake can be difficult in children, especially those with minimal urine output. In these children, as discussed above, high-calorie nutrition must be administered. To achieve nutritional goals without problems of fluid overload, small volumes of high-calorie supplements containing additional glucose polymers and/or medium-chain triglycerides are required. Many infants and small children are treated through either nasogastric or gastrostomy tubes to ensure adequate intake, as they may be unwilling to consume the required amount of nutrition orally.[19,21,22] It is important to note that gastrostomy feeding is not contraindicated for children receiving peritoneal dialysis.[23] Several studies have documented that this nutritional strategy is effective, and long-term enteral nutrition may prevent or reverse

weight loss and growth retardation in infants and young children. Furthermore, if growth failure has already occurred, adequate nutrition can result in catch-up growth if started before the age of 2 years.[19,24] In addition, aggressive nutritional therapy can contribute to favorable psychomotor development in infants who develop ESRD in early infancy.[12] Together these data suggest that provision of adequate nutrition is critical for effective treatment of ESRD in children.

Growth and other endocrine disorders

Growth retardation is common in children with ESRD and occurs even with mild renal insufficiency. The correction of growth is of paramount importance in the treatment of ESRD in children. Growth is calculated as centimeters of growth per year and is measured frequently and plotted on a standard growth curve chart, as is typical for any normal child. As GFR decreases, the rate of growth decreases; it is at this time that treatment must begin to correct any rate of decline in linear growth. If untreated, growth failure will be progressive and catch-up is difficult to acheieve. Treatment involves ensuring that (1) recommended caloric and protein intakes are achieved, (2) metabolic disturbances (e.g. acidosis, hyponatremia) are normalized, and (3) parathyroid hormone (PTH), calcium intake, and phosphorus load are normalized to correct any problems related to renal osteodystrophy. These factors may all contribute to decreased linear growth. For children on dialysis, more efficient clearance can also improve growth.[25] If growth retardation occurs despite these treatment measures, growth hormone therapy is indicated. Growth hormone therapy significantly accelerates short- and long-term growth.[26,27] Over the last 10 years it has also been demonstrated that the majority of patients now achieve normal adult height with the use of growth hormone therapy.[28,29] Thus the clinician must not wait until growth retardation has occurred but must maintain normal growth patterns with the use of growth hormone. Growth hormone therapy consists of 1 unit (0.33 mg)/kg weekly (± 0.05 mg/kg/day) or 4 units/m² injected subcutaneously as a daily dose (usually in the evening).[28,29] The dose of growth hormone is adjusted to achieve normal growth patterns; some children require decreased dosing whereas others require increased dosing. Children receiving growth hormone should be monitored regularly for response, including assessment of growth velocity and bone age.[30]

As discussed above, achievement of normal growth rates is a mainstay of therapy for children with chronic renal insufficiency either before or during dialysis as well as after transplantation. Renal transplantation alone was once thought to be a good treatment for growth retardation as catch-up growth could occur, whereas this was not possible on dialysis. However, recent reports of renal transplantation with regard to growth have been disappointing. Results of multicenter studies have demonstrated that catch-up growth after renal transplantation occurs in only 25% of children, predominantly young children. Indeed,

Table 48.2 Recommended dietary allowances of energy and protein for children with renal disease*

Age (years)	Energy (kcal/kg)	Protein (g/kg)	Protein intake for peritoneal dialysis (g/kg)
0–0.5	108	2.2	3.0
0.5–1	98	1.6	2.4
1–3	102	1.2	2.0
4–6	90	1.2	2.0
7–10	70	1.1	1.8
11–14 (M)	55	1.0	1.8
11–14 (F)	47	1.0	1.8
15–18 (M)	45	0.9	1.5
15–18 (F)	38	0.8	1.5

M, male; F, female.
* From Clinical practice guidelines for nutrition in chronic renal failure: pediatric guidelines. Am J Kidney Dis 2000;35:S105–S136.

even in this group, catch-up growth is seen in only 47% of children aged 0–5 years.[3,31] This implies that the treatment of growth retardation must begin prior to the initiation of renal replacement therapy, whether this therapy is dialysis or renal transplantation. Following renal transplantation, ongoing clinical studies suggest that growth hormone can be given to children and can improve final adult height, without adversely affecting renal function.[32–34] Also following renal transplantation, the use of alternate-day steroid dosing vs. daily dosing can result in improved growth patterns without increased rejection or allograft loss.[35] To optimize growth, several centers in the USA are currently participating in a randomized, placebo-controlled, steroid-withdrawal trial to assess its potential for optimizing growth patterns without altering long-term graft function.

In addition to its effects on growth, ESRD is also associated with other endocrine disorders. These are thought to be related to inappropriate circulating hormone concentrations or changed hormonal action at the target site. Children with ESRD have an average delay of puberty of 2.5 years and two-thirds of adolescents with ESRD enter puberty beyond the normal range.[36] Furthermore, in children with ESRD there is a marked decrease in tissue sensitivity to insulin, in glucose uptake, and in metabolic clearance of insulin that can lead to glucose intolerance. There have also been reported thyroid abnormalities associated with ESRD. All these endocrine disorders should be managed according to standard therapeutic regimens to achieve normal patterns of hormonal homeostasis.

Renal osteodystrophy

Renal osteodystrophy is an important problem in children with chronic renal failure. Its incidence increases as GFR approaches 50% of normal. Once established, osteodystrophy leads to deceleration of linear growth, muscle weakness, and bone pain; when severe it results in skeletal deformities such as bowing of lower extremities, fractures, and epiphyseal slipping. Renal osteodystrophy occurs in children due to a lack of 1,25-dihydroxyvitamin D_3, hypocalcemia, and hyperphosphatemia. All children with renal insufficiency (GFR < 70 mL/min per 1.73 m^2) should be monitored by assessment of serum calcium, phosphorus, alkaline phosphatase, and PTH, and by occasional radiographs of the hand to assess bone age.

Renal osteodystrophy represents a spectrum of activity, from "high-turnover" to "low-turnover" bone disease. A detailed review of these lesions can be found in Chapter 73. The most common type of renal osteodystrophy seen in children is high-turnover bone disease, which is associated with high PTH levels and/or secondary hyperparathyroidism. In recent years, aggressive management of calcium and phosphorus has led to a decreasing incidence of both secondary hyperparathyroidism and low-turnover bone disease, including adynamic bone disease, osteitis fibrosa, and osteomalacia.[37]

Prevention of renal osteodystrophy consists of avoidance of hyperphosphatemia using phosphate restriction and/or phosphate binders such as calcium acetate and calcium carbonate taken with all meals. Plasma phosphate levels should be maintained at normal levels.[38] Aluminum-containing phosphate binders should be avoided because the aluminum accumulates in bone and can lead to low-turnover aluminum bone disease. Excess aluminum can also lead to central nervous system dysfunction.[39] Optimal management also involves following PTH levels carefully, administration of active 1,25-dihydroxyvitamin D_3, and assessment of biochemical response. Various active forms of vitamin D are also used to maintain calcium absorption and serum calcium levels. Preparations include dihydrotachysterol, 25-hydroxyvitamin D_3 (calcidiol), 1α-hydroxyvitamin D_3 (alfacalcidol), and 1,25-dihydroxyvitamin D_3 (calcitriol).[40] Although changes in serum PTH and calcium vary with different preparations, oral, intravenous, or intraperitoneal administration of calcitriol (the most potent vitamin D metabolite) is effective.[41] To avoid adynamic bone disease, serum PTH should be maintained at a level three to four times above the upper limit of normal, and plasma calcium at the upper end of the normal range.[16,38,42] Hypercalcemia as a result of excessive vitamin D supplementation must be avoided because calcium deposits can form in various tissues.

Bone disease also occurs in children following renal transplantation. Steroid therapy has been shown to exacerbate preexisting bone disease; 70% of young children who received a renal transplant in childhood already have osteopenia. In a multiple regression analysis it was found that the cumulative dose of steroids was inversely related to bone mineral density score.[43] Steroids are associated with osteoporosis and avascular bone necrosis after transplantation.[43]

Anemia

The management of anemia in the pediatric population is similar to that in adults (discussed in Chapter 71). Most pediatric patients with ESRD (GFR < 30 mL/min) require erythropoietin therapy to maintain normal hematocrit. The use of erythropoietin has dramatically improved the outcome of dialysis in children and has abolished the typical iron-overload syndromes that were associated with frequent transfusions as a result of dialysis anemia.[44,45]

In children, erythropoietin 50–150 units/kg is administered subcutaneously one to three times weekly.[16] For children on hemodialysis, intravenous administration is preferred because it is less painful.[45] Although infrequently performed, patients on peritoneal dialysis can have erythropoietin administered in the peritoneal dialysis fluid; however, the amount required to correct anemia is much higher.[46] Subsequently the dose is titrated to achieve a hemoglobin concentration of 10–11 g/dL (6–7 mmol/L) and hematocrit of ~ 36%. The median maintenance dose is age dependent and is higher for younger children.[47] Dosing recommendations for erythropoietin are 50 units/kg once to three times weekly, starting at 120 units/kg/week for children weighing more than 30 kg, 225 units/kg/week for children weighing 20–30 kg, and 300 units/

kg/week for children weighing less than 20 kg.[48,49] Iron deficiency is common in children receiving erythropoietin therapy and supplementation with oral or intravenous iron is often necessary.[45,49-52] Serum iron levels should be maintained in the normal range, transferrin saturation > 20%, and serum ferritin levels > 150 ng/mL. When starting therapy with erythropoietin, blood pressure and hematocrit should be measured regularly.[16,53]

Hypertension and cardiovascular disease

Although isolated blood pressure measurements are typically used in children with ESRD, it is recommended that 24-h ambulatory blood pressure is monitored at intervals.[54,55] When evaluated by ambulatory blood pressure monitoring, 70% of peritoneal dialysis and 33% of hemodialysis patients were found to be hypertensive. In contrast, isolated blood pressure measurements demonstrated hypertension in only 47% of peritoneal dialysis and 44% of hemodialysis patients.[54] Nevertheless, the primary goal of antihypertensive therapy is to reduce blood pressure below the 95th percentile for age and gender (Table 48.3).[56] Choice of medication depends on the likely cause of the hypertension. For instance, an angiotension-converting inhibitor is a good choice for treatment of hypertension associated with renal insufficiency. In contrast, a vasodilator and/or β-blocker is the most usual choice for therapy in a dialysis patient where hypertension may be associated with fluid overload. Blood pressure elevations can be marked and very difficult to control. It is thus most important to be aggressive and to lower blood pressure into the normal range in all children. One-third of all deaths in children with ESRD are related to cardiovascular causes.

In children with hypertension, one should consider evaluation of cardiac function and structure with echocardiography at initial presentation and yearly thereafter.[57,58] Severe left ventricular hypertrophy is seen in almost half of all young dialysis patients. Better control of blood pressure, anemia, and hypervolemia may be important in preventing left ventricular hypertrophy and improving long-term cardiac outcome.[59] ESRD patients less than 20 years of age rarely have evidence of coronary artery calcification, whereas patients aged 20–30 years are more likely to show disease.[60]

Neurodevelopmental outcome and psychosocial adjustment

It is well established in the literature that neurodevelopmental delay, cognitive and motor abnormalities, cerebral cortical atrophy, and progressive encephalopathy are associated with chronic renal insufficiency in children, especially within the first year of life.[7] However, improvements in nutrition, elimination of aluminum binders from treatment regimens, psychomotor therapy, and access to play specialists have all been shown to improve cognitive function and long-term outcome.[12] Furthermore, early renal transplantation is known to be beneficial for normalization of neurodevelopmental outcome.[10,61]

Current data indicate that 77% of children on peritoneal dialysis and 46% on hemodialysis attend school full-time.[62] Furthermore, dialysis patients function below age and grade levels in all areas. In contrast, transplant recipients achieve at or above the levels achieved by dialysis patients.[9] Data suggest that ESRD not dialysis/transplant status is still a risk factor for lower IQ and academic achievement. Cognitive development or low IQ is most notable in younger children and in children whose mothers/caregivers have lower educational levels.[63]

Lastly, it is important to note that children with chronic renal disease are at risk for psychosocial adjustment disturbances, as occurs with many chronic diseases. In addition, low self-esteem, anxiety, and depressed mood are more severe in children on dialysis than children not on dialysis.[64] Thus most pediatrics centers involve psychologists and social workers in the treatment of children with ESRD.

Mortality of children on renal replacement therapy

There is a high mortality associated with dialysis therapy in children, especially young children. Indeed, mortality in children has been shown to be related to age at initiation of dialysis. Furthermore, it is clear that time on dialysis is associated with mortality. Recent data suggest that after 1 year of dialysis children < 2 years of age have the highest mortality (39%), the rate decreasing with age: 22% at 2–5 years, 8.5% at 6–12 years, 11% at 13–17 years, and 3.5% at > 17 years.[44] The overall mortality for all children on dialysis at 24 months is 15.4%. The most common causes of death in children are infection, cardiopulmonary disease, and malignancy. In children < 2 years of age, it has been shown that ESRD associated with oliguria or anuria, multiorgan failure, and presence of nonrenal disease especially pulmonary disease and/or pulmonary hypoplasia are all risk factors for mortality.[65]

Table 48.3 Blood pressure in children (mean ± SD)*

Age	Male Systolic (mmHg)	Male Diastolic (mmHg)	Female Systolic (mmHg)	Female Diastolic (mmHg)
Newborn	72.7 ± 9.6	51.1 ± 8.9	71.8 ± 9.3	50.5 ± 8.4
1 year	93.6 ± 12.2	53.0 ± 9.0	93.0 ± 12.8	52.4 ± 9.2
3 years	93.5 ± 12.7	54.3 ± 9.4	92.6 ± 12.7	55.1 ± 9.8
5 years	94.3 ± 10.9	57.4 ± 9.7	94.1 ± 10.6	57.3 ± 9.9
10 years	101.9 ± 10.5	63.6 ± 9.5	101.8 ± 10.9	63.1 ± 9.9
12 years	105.8 ± 10.8	65.6 ± 9.8	107.5 ± 11.5	67.1 ± 9.7

*Adapted from National High Blood Pressure Education Program Working Group on Hypertension Control in Children and Adolescents: Update on the 1987 Task Force Report on High Blood Pressure in Children and Adolescents: a working group report from the National High Blood Pressure Education Program. Pediatrics 1996;98:649–658.

In contrast, patient survival following transplantation is excellent. Overall patient survival at 1, 2, and 5 years after transplantation is 97, 96, and 93.5% respectively.[3] When patient survival is analyzed by age, it appears that younger children are more at risk for death following transplantation. Infants who receive cadaver donor transplants have a higher mortality than those who receive living donor renal transplants. However, for all children there are no significant differences in patient survival when analyzed by donor source.[3] Patient survival after transplantation is illustrated in Fig. 48.1,[3] which shows that even in the youngest age groups the mortality

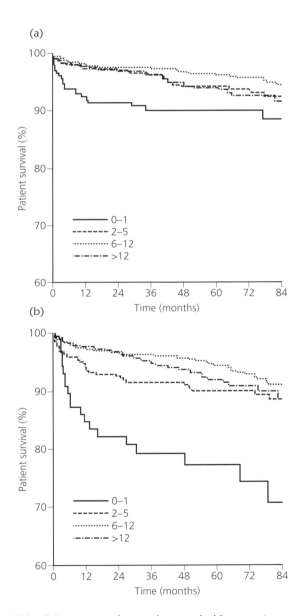

Figure 48.1 Primary transplant patient survival by age at transplantation and donor source: (a) living donor; (b) cadaver donor. (From Seikaly M, Ho PL, Emmett L, Tejani A: The 12th Annual Report of the North American Pediatric Renal Transplant Cooperative Study: renal transplantation from 1987 through 1998. Pediatr Transplant 2001;5:215–231.)

following renal transplantation is less than that seen with dialysis alone.

Dialysis therapy

All children are candidates for peritoneal dialysis or hemodialysis. In general, the decision to perform either form of dialysis involves patient preference, distance from a pediatric hemodialysis center, and center bias. In young children, there is a bias toward peritoneal dialysis because hemodialysis is associated with access problems in infants and young children and also involves significant expertise on the part of personnel. Thus, peritoneal dialysis has become the more common treatment in many centers. Some reports suggest that younger children fare better with peritoneal dialysis, although data indicate that so long as efficiency is maintained there are no significant therapeutic differences between peritoneal dialysis and hemodialysis.

Peritoneal dialysis

Peritoneal dialysis is discussed in great detail in Chapters 85–87. Here, we focus on specific issues pertaining to peritoneal dialysis in childhood. Approximately two-thirds of the pediatric dialysis population are currently maintained on peritoneal dialysis. Peritoneal dialysis is preferred for infants as it obviates the need for vascular access, which can be especially difficult in this group of children.[44] Another advantage of peritoneal dialysis over hemodialysis is that it requires less fluid restriction. As discussed earlier, this may be important for adequate administration of nutrition. Automated continuous cycler-assisted peritoneal dialysis at night is used most frequently in younger children.[44]

In older children and especially adolescents, compliance with dialysis prescription can be a problem and can thus affect dialysis efficiency. The requirement for a permanent intraabdominal catheter can distort body image and its presence become unwanted. This can lead to treatment issues and puts parents in a compromising situation if they wish to be caregivers. Therefore peritoneal dialysis in an adolescent needs careful monitoring. Hemodialysis has become the more common form of renal replacement therapy in this group because it provides adequate treatment and also enables assessment of compliance and adequacy.

Initiation of peritoneal dialysis in all children involves the use of a standard straight or curled catheter. In younger children with lax abdominal musculature, the catheter preferably has two cuffs to avoid leakage and infections. The catheter and cuff are typically allowed to heal for a minimum of 2 weeks before the initiation of dialysis in order to prevent leakage. Omentectomy during the insertion of the catheter is especially important in young children because it decreases the incidence of obstruction to 2% compared with the risk of obstruction in the absence of omentectomy (15–32%).[68]

Dialysis prescription

When prescribing peritoneal dialysis, volume input according to nutritional needs, residual urine output, and renal function must all be taken into account. In children a peritoneal dialysis exchange volume of 1100–1500 mL/ m^2 (35–45 mL/kg) is used.[69] Typically in young children, eight to ten exchanges are performed over 12–16 h at night by an automated peritoneal dialysis cycler. In older children, continuous ambulatory peritoneal dialysis is the usual mode of therapy, performed in a similar manner to adults. In addition to normalizing biochemical abnormalities, it must also be administered in a manner to facilitate growth. With all forms of peritoneal dialysis, ultrafiltration is adjusted in order to facilitate adequate volume intake according to nutritional needs. Typically, the ultrafiltration goal depends on analysis of the nutritional needs and the requirement for administration of volume.

Dialysis adequacy

A peritoneal equilibration test (PET) can be used to study the transport capacity of the peritoneal membrane. PET values for children have been calculated.[70,71] Warady found that the peritoneal membrane was stable in children over a mean interval of 20 months.[72,73] However, peritonitis is a risk factor for peritoneal dialysis failure. Follow-up of peritoneal solute kinetics is recommended in patients with a history of peritonitis in order to permit early identification of patients at risk for dialysis failure.[72,73] Dialysis adequacy can be expressed as urea Kt/V, calculated as the ratio of 24-h dialysate (+ urinary) urea clearance divided by total body water, where K is urea clearance (L/h), t is time on dialysis (h), and V is urea distribution volume and equals total body water volume (L). The target dialysis adequacy in children is a total weekly urea Kt/V 2.0 and a creatinine clearance 60 L per 1.73 m^2. Higher values for weekly urea Kt/V up to 2.75–3.1 can be achieved and have been correlated with improved clinical outcome.[16,74–76] However, a report from the Endstage Renal Disease Network of New England indicates that a urea $Kt/V > 2.75$ may result in albumin loss and may thus hinder nutrition.[77]

Complications

Complications of peritoneal dialysis in children include exit-site/tunnel infections, peritonitis, catheter-related problems (leakage and blockage), and the development of hernias due to increased intraabdominal pressure and relatively weak musculature. In one report, 11% of pediatric patients on peritoneal dialysis had an exit-site/ tunnel infection at 1 month, 26% between 1 and 6 months, and 30% between 6 months and 1 year of follow-up.[78] Patients with tunnel infections have twice the risk of developing peritonitis and the need for access revision.

Peritonitis is the major complication of peritoneal dialysis in children. The mean occurrence of peritonitis has been reported to be once every 13.2 patient-months.[44,78] Peritonitis rates decrease with age and are significantly less frequent when catheters with two cuffs and downward-pointed exit sites are used.[44,62,79] There is no difference in peritonitis in children treated with curled or straight catheters. Overall, 25% of patients on peritoneal dialysis switch to hemodialysis and in most patients the switch is due to repeated infections.[44]

Hemodialysis

Improvements in technology have enabled pediatric centers to perform hemodialysis in infants and young children effectively and efficiently. Furthermore, the ability to perform hemodialysis has decreased mortality and improved success in the long term. Important advances relate to dialysis access catheters and lines, complex machines that allow control of low blood volume, the ability to metrically control ultrafiltration, and compatible dialysis membranes and the composition of dialysates.[80,81]

Hemodialysis is the preferred dialysis modality for children older than 12 years of age, who comprise 64% of all children requiring dialysis.[44] In contrast, only 12% of children under 5 years of age receive hemodialysis. Overall, one-third of children who receive dialysis utilize hemodialysis.

Hemodialysis is mostly accomplished via an external percutaneous catheter placed in the subclavian or jugular veins. Other vascular access routes include internal arteriovenous fistula and grafts, used in approximately 12% of patients.[44] In Europe, arteriovenous fistula is still the preferred vascular access.[82] In younger children, a variety of shunts have been used in the past, e.g. the Thomas femoral shunt was placed into large groin vessels and was quite successful. However, more recently the use of percutaneous catheters has obviated the need for shunt placement.

Dialysis prescription

For all patients, the dialysis prescription is calculated by dialyzer type, blood flow, and dialysate flow. The duration of each treatment can be easily calculated to optimize urea clearance. In infants and small children, blood flow rates as low as 50 mL/min can be used such that the dialysis prescription can be calculated according to the ability of the patient to tolerate a given flow rate. In older children and adults, blood flow rates of 200–300 mL/min are frequently used. Knowledge of the clearance curve of the dialyzer is essential in estimating the total urea clearance at a given blood flow rate. Good clearances can be achieved in young children < 2 years of age with hemodialysis for 1–2 h. Older or larger children require more time with adequate blood flow rates. Extracorporeal blood volume (dialyzer priming volume plus blood tubing volume) should be kept under 8 mL/kg (< 10% of total blood volume) to avoid hemodynamic instability and hypoxemia. Adequate anticoagulation can be achieved with standard heparin dosing. To attain adequate clearance three hemodialysis treatments are usually given each week.

Dialysis adequacy

Adequate dialysis combined with adequate nutrition reduces mortality and promotes growth in children.[25,83] Urea kinetic modeling is used to assess dialysis adequacy and nutritional status.[20] Hemodialysis efficiency is expressed as Kt/V, where K is urea clearance (L/h), t is session length (h), and V is urea distribution volume and equals total body water volume (L). Goldstein et al[84] found no difference between the results of a formal urea kinetic modeling technique for obtaining Kt/V and results obtained by using Daugirdas' formula for the single-pool natural logarithm approximation equation for Kt/V.[85] Thus the ease with which Kt/V can be calculated using the natural logarithm supports its regular use in the monitoring of children on hemodialysis.[16,86] An appropriate goal is to achieve a single-pool Kt/V of 1.3, at least equal to that recommended for adults.[16,74] Higher Kt/V values may be necessary for growing children.[16,25]

Complications

The most common complications of hemodialysis are clotting and infection of the hemodialysis catheter, arteriovenous fistula, or graft. Infection of the hemodialysis access site can easily lead to septicemia, which is the most frequent cause of death in children on hemodialysis.[44] Other complications, such as disequilibrium syndrome, hypotension, anaphylactic reactions, hemolysis, and hypoxemia, are discussed in detail in Chapter 84.

Renal transplantation

Renal transplantation is the optimal treatment for ESRD in children because it offers the best hope for normalization of physiologic processes. Most important is the ability of renal transplantation to normalize growth and cognitive function and to enable a child to enjoy a relatively normal quality of life. Because of the mortality associated with dialysis therapy in young children and the risk/benefit ratio, the National Organ Allocation System in the USA has given preference to children on waiting lists to receive cadaver transplants.

In the USA an approximately equal number of renal transplants are performed with living and cadaver donors.[3] As a therapy, renal transplantation is very successful and, with current immunosuppressive regimens, 1- and 5-year graft survival rates are excellent: 5-year graft survival is currently 80% for living related donor grafts and 65% for cadaver donors[3] (Fig. 48.2). The projected half-life of renal transplants in pediatric recipients is equal or even better than adult recipients.[87,88] However, as discussed below, rejection remains a major cause of graft loss in the first post-transplant year.[3,89,90] Newer immunosuppressive agents have decreased the incidence of acute rejection and have improved 1-year graft survival rates, especially for recipients of cadaver donor transplants. The current 1-year graft survival rates for cadaver donor and living related donor transplants are approximately equal at 93 and 94%.[3] Unfortunately, graft survival rate beyond 1 year has remained stable for the past 10 years.[91] Interestingly, while the youngest recipients (< 2 years) have higher risks for early graft loss, their risk for later graft attrition is the lowest.[89]

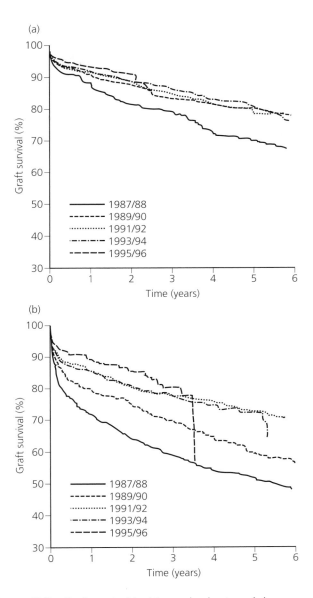

Figure 48.2 Graft survival by biannual cohorts and donor source: (a) living related donor; (b) cadaver donor. (From Seikaly M, Ho PL, Emmett L, Tejani A: The 12th Annual Report of the North American Pediatric Renal Transplant Cooperative Study: renal transplantation from 1987 through 1998. Pediatr Transplant 2001;5:215–231.)

Causes of graft failure in pediatric recipients

The North American Pediatric Renal Transplant Cooperative Study (NAPRTCS), which includes data on over 6500 transplants, analyzes risk factors for graft loss following pediatric renal transplantation (Fig. 48.3).[3,92–94] The most common cause of graft failure is chronic rejection.[3] Vascular thrombosis is also a major cause of graft failure, especially in young children, and accounts for ~ 12% of all pediatric renal allograft failures. Risk factors for vascular thrombosis include recipient age and cadaver donor age, especially donors under 6 years of

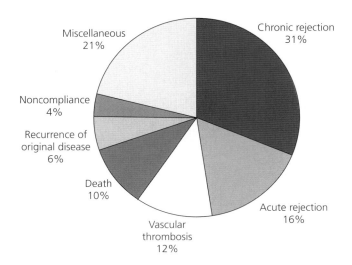

Figure 48.3 Causes of graft loss after pediatric renal transplantation. (Adapted from Seikaly M, Ho PL, Emmett L, Tejani A: The 12th Annual Report of the North American Pediatric Renal Transplant Cooperative Study: renal transplantation from 1987 through 1998. Pediatr Transplant 2001;5:215–231.)

age.[3,95] Although 1-year graft survival rates for teenage recipients are comparable to those for adults, adolescents have a significantly higher incidence of late acute rejection episodes than any other age group. Noncompliance among teenagers is well recognized.[89,96,97]

Acute rejection

Acute rejection episodes occur frequently following pediatric transplantation. Indeed, even in the current era of new immunosuppressive agents where acute rejection rates are 20–30% in adults, as many as 40–60% of pediatric recipients develop an acute rejection episode over the first post-transplant year. Moreover, many rejection episodes, especially those in young children, are only partially reversible with effective therapy. Furthermore, there is a higher instance of irreversible rejection episodes in pediatric recipients compared with adult recipients of renal transplants. Many factors have been postulated to account for the increased incidence of acute rejection in pediatric patients. These include the possibility of a heightened immune response,[98,99] altered absorption and metabolism of immunosuppressive agents, and/or a later diagnosis of rejection.[92] It has become evident that more aggressive therapy, including the use of induction therapy regimens, and surveillance biopsies to establish a diagnosis of "silent" rejection are associated with improved short-term outcome.[100,101] The high incidence of acute rejection in pediatric recipients is of special concern because of its relationship to the development of chronic rejection.[3] Even one episode of acute rejection increases the risk for the development of chronic rejection very significantly. Thus, strategies that decrease acute rejection rates and improve short-term graft survival rates can translate into improved long-term survival.[102] This possibility is currently being tested in large multicenter studies.

Chronic rejection

Chronic rejection is characterized histologically by progressive fibrosis and mononuclear cell infiltration with interstitial cell atrophy. Chronic rejection can be diagnosed as early as 3 months post transplant, and its presence in biopsy specimens 6 months post transplant is prognostic for the development of chronic rejection and long-term outcome.[103] Thus, early biopsy at 3–6 months post transplant can be used as a surrogate marker for the ultimate development of chronic rejection.[103] Once established, chronic rejection is progressive and ultimately leads to graft failure. For pediatric patients receiving a renal allograft, chronic rejection is responsible for ~ 31% of graft losses (Fig. 48.3).

Understanding risk factors for chronic rejection in pediatric patients has been a major undertaking of NAPRTCS. Preventing or minimizing risk factors has been proposed to impact long-term graft survival. Risk factors for chronic rejection have been defined and are multifactorial. They include HLA mismatch, ischemia reperfusion injury, repeat transplants, acute rejection, and other factors such as hypertension and hyperlipidemia. However, an extensive study established that acute rejection is the most important risk factor for the development of chronic rejection. Even a single acute rejection episode increases the risk for chronic rejection threefold, and two or more episodes of acute rejection increase the risk for chronic rejection by fivefold or more.[102] These data are similar to studies performed in adults that also identified acute rejection as a harbinger of chronic rejection.[87] Late acute rejection is also a major risk factor for the development of chronic rejection and graft failure.[102] It is proposed that acute rejection establishes an immune reaction within the graft that facilitates positive feedback loops and the production of fibrogenic cytokines (e.g. transforming growth factor β).[104] Another possible etiology contributing to the development of chronic rejection is decreased renal mass leading to hyperfiltration, which has a damaging effect on the renal parenchyma and produces the characteristic histology of chronic rejection.[104]

Currently there is no specific therapy for chronic rejection, so efforts must be directed toward preventing major risk factors. Current ideas include limiting calcineurin inhibitor-based immunosuppressive therapy, which is associated with progressive renal injury as a result of profound nephrotoxicity.[104] Other studies are using rapamycin or aggressive induction therapy to prevent acute rejection that may ultimately translate into better long-term survival.[105]

Preparation for pediatric renal transplantation

Every transplant center has its own practices regarding the preparation of a child for renal transplantation. However, there are certain issues that have been recommended as key factors for consideration. These have been reviewed and detailed elsewhere.[4] Of paramount importance is the evaluation of living donors, who must be carefully

Table 48.4   Risk factors for graft failure by donor source*

	Living donor RR increase	P	Cadaver donor RR increase	P
Recipient age (< 2 years)			1.95	< 0.001
Donor age (< 6 years)			1.22	0.025
Prior transplant			1.32	0.003
No ATG/ALG induction			1.26	0.001
More than five lifetime transfusions	1.6	< 0.001	1.29	0.001
No HLA-B matches	1.6	< 0.002	1.21	0.009
No HLA-DR matches			1.25	0.002
African-American race	2.0	< 0.001	1.41	< 0.001
Prior dialysis			1.37	0.012
Cold ischemia > 24 h			1.18	0.023

ATG/ALG, antithymocyte/antilymphocyte globulin; HLA, human leukocyte antigen; RR, relative risk.
*From Seikaly M, Ho PL, Emmett L, Tejani A: The 12th Annual Report of the North American Pediatric Renal Transplant Cooperative Study: renal transplantation from 1987 through 1998. Pediatr Transplant 2001;5:215–231.

examined by an independent advocate such that they are not put at risk for the sake of transplantation. Living donor advocacy is such an important issue that it was recently reviewed and a national consensus has been published.[107] Living donor advocacy is uniquely important in pediatrics because donors tend to be parents; they are highly motivated and are very disappointed if not eligible. Siblings can also feel pressure to donate. Thus the concept of donor advocacy (that of being a separate individual from those in the transplant program) ensures that donors are treated in a fair manner.

Donor

If available, a living donor has clear advantages over a cadaver donor. Living donation ensures adequate transplant preparation and optimizes elective transplantation particularly for pediatric patients. Preemptive transplantation is much easier to accomplish and improves graft survival.[108] Furthermore, the survival of living donor renal allografts is superior to cadaver donor allografts. For details of selection and preparation of a living donor see Chapter 89. Contrary to early reports, it has become clear that allografts from young cadaver donors (< 6 years of age) do not fare well in young recipients and that the best donor for a young child is an adult donor. A cadaver donor for children should ideally be 20–40 years of age and not younger than 6 years of age because the youngest donors are associated with an increased risk of graft failure.[3] Thus the best donor is an adult, whether living or dead (Table 48.4).

Recipient

An important aspect of renal transplantation is that success can also be determined by careful management of the recipient prior to the transplant procedure. Most pediatric centers utilize a multispecialty team to ensure that hematologic, biochemical, neurologic, and urologic parameters and potentially serious infections are corrected prior to transplantation. Many centers have adopted specific screening mechanisms and some of the major

considerations are reviewed in Table 48.5. Assessment of bladder function and correction of bladder dysfunction prior to transplantation is essential for patients in whom bladder disease or obstructive uropathy was the original etiology of ESRD. Some patients may require bladder augmentation and/or medication to improve bladder function prior to transplantation. Transplantation into a dysfunctional bladder or the use of ileal loops or other forms of urinary drainage are not optimal for long-term success. Thus it is important to have a pediatric urology

Table 48.5   Preparation of pediatric renal transplant recipient

Nutrition	Adjustment of caloric, protein, sodium, and potassium balance
Growth	Supply adequate nutrition, correct metabolic disturbances (e.g. acidosis, hyponatremia), renal osteodystrophy; consider growth hormone therapy
Renal osteodystrophy	Phosphate binders, calcium supplement, active 1,25-dihydroxyvitamin D_3
Anemia	Correct iron deficiency, consider erythropoietin
Infection prevention	Check titers of DTP, MMR, Hib, VZV, HBV, HCV, CMV, EBV, and HIV. Vaccinate if necessary (e.g. VZV, pneumococcus, HBV, influenza). Check tuberculosis status
Bladder work up	VCUG and bladder work
Psychosocial status	Social work assessment

CMV, cytomegalovirus; DTP, diphtheria/tetanus/polio; EBV, Epstein–Barr virus; HBV, hepatitis B virus; HCV, hepatitis C virus; Hib, *Haemophilus influenzae* B; MMR, measles/mumps/rubella; VCUG, voiding cystourethrogram; VZV, varicella zoster virus.

team assess a child prior to transplantation and be involved with the entire transplantation process.

Prevention of infections, especially viral infections, involves analysis of patient status and the use of chemoprophylaxis. This is a high priority with all pediatric patients as they typically acquire these infections during childhood and are not immune to many viruses prior to transplantation.[109] Knowledge of titers of varicella zoster virus, cytomegalovirus (CMV), Epstein–Barr virus (EBV), diphtheria, tetanus, poliovirus, measles, mumps, rubella, *Haemophilus influenzae* B, hepatitis B, hepatitis C, and HIV before transplantation is of paramount importance. Vaccination can prevent morbidity and mortality post transplantation.[110,111] CMV and EBV prophylaxis must be considered for patients at high risk, i.e. seronegative recipients receiving seropositive organs and patients who have received antilymphocyte antibodies.[109] Pneumococcal vaccination can be administered before transplantation in high-risk children (e.g. post splenectomy). Trimethoprim prophylaxis has reduced the incidence of *Pneumocystis carinii* pneumonia post transplantation from 3.7% to 0%.[112]

Bilateral native kidney nephrectomy prior to transplantation is currently performed in 24% of patients in the USA in order to avoid urinary tract infection in patients with reflux nephropathy, native kidney-related hypertension, and a steal syndrome resulting in diminished blood flow through the allograft.[3] Most renal allografts are transplanted extraperitoneally into the retroperitoneal cavity, even when a large adult kidney is used for a small child recipient. This technique does not seem to affect surgical complication rates and has the advantage of less gastrointestinal complications.[114–117] However, occasionally adult-sized kidneys are transplanted intraperitoneally in small children. There are other issues that require consideration but these are beyond the scope of this chapter and have been discussed in detail elsewhere.[4]

Immunosuppressive therapy

There are currently many immunosuppressive agents available to the transplant physician. This has resulted in multiple protocols each with a center bias, such that therapy can be center dependent. In addition, the advent of new immunosuppressive agents has enabled therapy to be administered on an individual basis and on the basis of risk. The newer more potent immunosuppressive agents and protocols that have been shown to limit acute rejection have provided tremendous advantages for the transplant recipient but also come at a price. This is the risk of posttransplant infections and posttransplant lymphoproliferative disease (PTLD). Efficacy of antilymphocyte antibody induction therapy is currently under study. Triple therapy, consisting of a calcineurin inhibitor, an antiproliferative agent, and steroids, is used in most patients in the USA.[94] The calcineurin inhibitor cyclosporine is the primary immunosuppressant, with 82% of pediatric renal transplant recipients receiving the drug during the first month; 11% of recipients receive tacrolimus although the number is increasing. Recently

azathioprine has been replaced by mycophenolate mofetil, which is currently given to 70% of transplant recipients in the USA. Approximately one-third of patients who receive maintenance steroid therapy in the long term receive alternate-day therapy in order to achieve better catch-up growth.[3,93,94]

Other new immunosuppressive drugs have been introduced into practice based on their ability to further decrease acute rejection. It is also hoped that they will improve long-term graft survival. The most exciting agents include rapamycin, which is thought to provide immunosuppression in the absence of associated nephrotoxicity.[118,119] Interleukin 2 (IL-2) receptor blockers have been introduced to limit acute rejection in the early posttransplant period. Protocols under investigation include donor-specific transfusion, IL-2 receptor blockers, rapamycin, and protocols to eliminate calcineurin inhibitors. Since these new protocols are currently in clinical trials, the "optimal" immunosuppressive strategy will be forthcoming.[119]

Complications of immunosuppressive therapy include infection, cancer, and in the case of chronic steroid use growth failure. Other adverse effects include hypertension, hyperlipidemia, diabetes mellitus, and osteoporosis.[120] Tacrolimus, cadaver donor source, and white race are risk factors for PTLD.[121–124] Treatment consists of reduction of immunosuppression, long courses of ganciclovir, and occasionally interferon-α or chemotherapy.[109] Experimental data suggest that rapamycin may inhibit growth of EBV-infected B cells and may be helpful in PTLD.[125]

Summary

In this chapter, we discuss unique problems associated with the management of ESRD in children. We discuss strategies to understand and prevent malnutrition and growth retardation in children with ESRD. In addition, we review important issues for the optimization of neuro-development and cognitive function. Lastly, we review current available treatment options including peritoneal dialysis and hemodialysis, and we discuss renal transplantation as a successful therapeutic option. All of these treatments are options for children with ESRD.

References

1. United States Renal Data System (USRDS): 1996 Annual Data Report. Bethesda, MD: USRDS, 1996.
2. Broyer M, Chantler C, Donckerwolcke R, et al: The paediatric registry of the European Dialysis and Transplant Association: 20 years' experience. Pediatr Nephrol 1993;7:758–768.
3. Seikaly M, Ho PL, Emmett L, Tejani A: The 12th Annual Report of the North American Pediatric Renal Transplant Cooperative Study: renal transplantation from 1987 through 1998. Pediatr Transplant 2001;5:215–231.
4. Davis ID, Bunchman TE, Grimm PC, et al: Pediatric renal transplantation: indications and special considerations. A position paper from the Pediatric Committee of the American Society of Transplant Physicians. Pediatr Transplant 1998;2:117–129.
5. Fine RN: Renal transplantation for children: the only realistic choice. Kidney Int 1985;Suppl 17:S15–S17.
6. Mendley SR, Zelko FA: Improvement in specific aspects of

neurocognitive performance in children after renal transplantation. Kidney Int 1999;56:318–323.

7. Rotundo A, Nevins TE, Lipton M, et al: Progressive encephalopathy in children with chronic renal insufficiency in infancy. Kidney Int 1982;21:486–491.

8. McGraw ME, Haka-Ikse K: Neurologic–developmental sequelae of chronic renal failure in infancy. J Pediatr 1985;106:579–583.

9. Lawry KW, Brouhard BH, Cunningham RJ: Cognitive functioning and school performance in children with renal failure. Pediatr Nephrol 1994;8:326–329.

10. Davis ID, Chang PN, Nevins TE: Successful renal transplantation accelerates development in young uremic children. Pediatrics 1990;86:594–600.

11. Kramer L, Madl C, Stockenhuber F, et al: Beneficial effect of renal transplantation on cognitive brain function. Kidney Int 1996;49:833–838.

12. Warady BA, Belden B, Kohaut E: Neurodevelopmental outcome of children initiating peritoneal dialysis in early infancy. Pediatr Nephrol 1999;13:759–765.

13. Simmons JM, Wilson CJ, Potter DE, Holliday MA: Relation of calorie deficiency to growth failure in children on hemodialysis and the growth response to calorie supplementation. N Engl J Med 1971;285:653–656.

14. Betts PR, Magrath G: Growth pattern and dietary intake of children with chronic renal insufficiency. Br Med J 1974;2:189–193.

15. Clinical practice guidelines for nutrition in chronic renal failure: pediatric guidelines. Am J Kidney Dis 2000;35:S105–S136.

16. Warady BA, Alexander SR, Watkins S, et al: Optimal care of the pediatric end-stage renal disease patient on dialysis. Am J Kidney Dis 1999;33:567–583.

17. Geary DF, Ikse KH, Coulter P, Secker D: The role of nutrition in neurologic health and development of infants with chronic renal failure. Adv Perit Dial 1990;6:252–254.

18. Edefonti A, Picca M, Damiani B, et al: Dietary prescription based on estimated nitrogen balance during peritoneal dialysis. Pediatr Nephrol 1999;13:253–258.

19. Ledermann SE, Scanes ME, Fernando ON, et al: Long-term outcome of peritoneal dialysis in infants. J Pediatr 2000;136:24–29.

20. Harmon WE: Urea kinetic modeling to prescribe hemodialysis in children. In Nissenson AR, Fine RN (eds): Dialysis Therapy. Philadelphia: Hanley and Belfus, 2002, pp 462–466.

21. Ellis EN, Yiu V, Harley F, et al: The impact of supplemental feeding in young children on dialysis: a report of the North American Pediatric Renal Transplant Cooperative Study. Pediatr Nephrol 2001;16:404–408.

22. Warady BA: Gastrostomy feedings in patients receiving peritoneal dialysis. Perit Dial Int 1999;19:204–206.

23. Ramage IJ, Harvey E, Geary DF, et al: Complications of gastrostomy feeding in children receiving peritoneal dialysis. Pediatr Nephrol 1999;13:249–252.

24. Kari JA, Gonzalez C, Ledermann SE, et al: Outcome and growth of infants with severe chronic renal failure. Kidney Int 2000;57:1681–1687.

25. Tom A, McCauley L, Bell L, et al: Growth during maintenance hemodialysis: impact of enhanced nutrition and clearance. J Pediatr 1999;134:464–471.

26. Tonshoff B, Mehis O, Heinrich U, et al: Growth-stimulating effects of recombinant human growth hormone in children with end-stage renal disease. J Pediatr 1990;116:561–566.

27. Hokken-Koelega AC, Stijnen T, de Muinck Keizer-Schrama SM, et al: Placebo-controlled, double-blind, cross-over trial of growth hormone treatment in prepubertal children with chronic renal failure. Lancet 1991;338:585–590.

28. Haffner D, Schaefer F, Nissel R, et al: Effect of growth hormone treatment on the adult height of children with chronic renal failure. German Study Group for Growth Hormone Treatment in Chronic Renal Failure. N Engl J Med 2000;343:923–930.

29. Hokken-Koelega A, Mulder P, De Jong R, et al: Long-term effects of growth hormone treatment on growth and puberty in patients with chronic renal insufficiency. Pediatr Nephrol 2000;14:701–706.

30. Gipson DS, Kausz AT, Striegel JE, et al: Intraperitoneal administration of recombinant human growth hormone in children with end-stage renal disease. Pediatr Nephrol 2001;16:29–34.

31. Fine RN: Growth post renal-transplantation in children: lessons from the North American Pediatric Renal Transplant Cooperative Study (NAPRTCS). Pediatr Transplant 1997;1:85–89.

32. Hokken-Koelega AC, Stijnen T, de Jong RC, et al: A placebo-controlled, double-blind trial of growth hormone treatment in prepubertal children after renal transplant. Kidney Int 1996;Suppl 53:S128–S134.

33. Hokken-Koelega AC, Stijnen T, de Ridder MA, et al: Growth hormone treatment in growth-retarded adolescents after renal transplant. Lancet 1994;343:1313–1317.

34. Mentser M, Breen TJ, Sullivan EK, Fine RN: Growth-hormone treatment of renal transplant recipients: the National Cooperative Growth Study experience. A report of the National Cooperative Growth Study and the North American Pediatric Renal Transplant Cooperative Study. J Pediatr 1997;131:S20–S24.

35. Jabs K, Sullivan EK, Avner ED, Harmon WE: Alternate-day steroid dosing improves growth without adversely affecting graft survival or long-term graft function. A report of the North American Pediatric Renal Transplant Cooperative Study. Transplantation 1996;61:31–36.

36. Scharer K: Growth and development of children with chronic renal failure. Study Group on Pubertal Development in Chronic Renal Failure. Acta Paediatr Scand 1990;Suppl 366:90–92.

37. Salusky IB, Ramirez JA, Oppenheim W, et al: Biochemical markers of renal osteodystrophy in pediatric patients undergoing CAPD. Kidney Int 1994;45:253–258.

38. Rigden SP: The treatment of renal osteodystrophy. Pediatr Nephrol 1996;10:653–655.

39. Sedman A: Aluminum toxicity in childhood. Pediatr Nephrol 1992;6:383–393.

40. Hamdy NA, Kanis JA, Beneton MN, et al: Effect of alfacalcidol on natural course of renal bone disease in mild to moderate renal failure. Br Med J 1995;310:358–363.

41. Sanchez CP: Prevention and treatment of renal osteodystrophy in children with chronic renal insufficiency and end-stage renal disease. Semin Nephrol 2001;21:441–450.

42. Salusky IB, Goodman WG: The management of renal osteodystrophy. Pediatr Nephrol 1996;10:651–653.

43. Boot AM, Nauta J, Hokken-Koelega AC, et al: Renal transplantation and osteoporosis. Arch Dis Child 1995;72:502–506.

44. Lerner GR, Warady BA, Sullivan EK, Alexander SR: Chronic dialysis in children and adolescents. The 1996 annual report of the North American Pediatric Renal Transplant Cooperative Study. Pediatr Nephrol 1999;13:404–417.

45. Van Damme-Lombaerts R, Herman J: Erythropoietin treatment in children with renal failure. Pediatr Nephrol 1999;13:148–152.

46. Jacobs C: Starting r-HuEPO in chronic renal failure: when, why, and how? Nephrol Dial Transplant 1995;10:43–47.

47. Scigalla P, Bonzel KE, Bulla M, et al: Therapy of renal anemia with recombinant human erythropoietin in children with end-stage renal disease. Contrib Nephrol 1989;76:227–240.

48. Gagnadoux MF, Loirat C, Bertheleme JP, et al: Treatment of anemia in hemodialyzed children using recombinant human erythropoietin (Eprex). Results of a French multicenter clinical trial (in French). Nephrologie 1994;15:207–211.

49. Van Damme-Lombaerts R, Broyer M, Businger J, et al: A study of recombinant human erythropoietin in the treatment of anaemia of chronic renal failure in children on haemodialysis. Pediatr Nephrol 1994;8:338–342.

50. Greenbaum LA, Pan CG, Caley C, et al: Intravenous iron dextran and erythropoietin use in pediatric hemodialysis patients. Pediatr Nephrol 2000;14:908–911.

51. Tenbrock K, Muller-Berghaus J, Michalk D, Querfeld U: Intravenous iron treatment of renal anemia in children on hemodialysis. Pediatr Nephrol 1999;13:580–582.

52. National Kidney Foundation-Dialysis Outcomes Quality Initiative: Clinical practice guidelines for the treatment of anemia of chronic renal failure. Am J Kidney Dis 1997;30:S192–S240.

53. Fishbane S, Maesaka JK: Iron management in end-stage renal disease. Am J Kidney Dis 1997;29:319–333.

54. Lingens N, Soergeld M, Loirat C, et al: Ambulatory blood pressure monitoring in pediatric patients treated by regular haemodialysis and peritoneal dialysis. Pediatr Nephrol 1995;9:167–172.

55. Soergel M, Kirschstein M, Busch C, et al: Oscillometric twenty-four-hour ambulatory blood pressure values in healthy children and adolescents: a multicenter trial including 1141 subjects. J Pediatr 1997;130:178–184.

56. National High Blood Pressure Education Program Working Group on Hypertension Control in Children and Adolescents: Update on

the 1987 Task Force Report on High Blood Pressure in Children and Adolescents: a working group report from the National High Blood Pressure Education Program. Pediatrics 1996;98:649–658.

57. United States Renal Data System (USRDS): The USRDS 1998 Annual Report: pediatric ESRD. Am J Kidney Dis 1998;32:S98–S108.

58. United States Renal Data System (USRDS): The USRDS 1998 Annual Report: pediatric ESRD. Am J Kidney Dis 1998;32:S81–S88.

59. Mitsnefes MM, Daniels SR, Schwartz SM, et al: Severe left ventricular hypertrophy in pediatric dialysis: prevalence and predictors. Pediatr Nephrol 2000;14:898–902.

60. Goodman WG, Goldin J, Kuizon BD, et al: Coronary-artery calcification in young adults with end-stage renal disease who are undergoing dialysis. N Engl J Med 2000;342:1478–1483.

61. Hulstijn-Dirkmaat GM, Damhuis IH, Jetten ML, et al: The cognitive development of pre-school children treated for chronic renal failure. Pediatr Nephrol 1995;9:464–469.

62. Warady BA, Hebert D, Sullivan EK, et al: Renal transplantation, chronic dialysis, and chronic renal insufficiency in children and adolescents. The 1995 Annual Report of the North American Pediatric Renal Transplant Cooperative Study. Pediatr Nephrol 1997;11:49–64.

63. Brouhard BH, Donaldson LA, Lawry KW, et al: Cognitive functioning in children on dialysis and post-transplantation. Pediatr Transplant 2000;4:261–267.

64. Garralda ME, Jameson RA, Reynolds JM, Postlethwaite RJ: Psychiatric adjustment in children with chronic renal failure. J Child Psychol Psychiatry 1988;29:79–90.

65. Wood EG, Hand M, Briscoe DM, et al: Risk factors for mortality in infants and young children on dialysis. Am J Kidney Dis 2001;37:573–579.

66. Reissman P, Lyass S, Shiloni E, et al: Placement of a peritoneal dialysis catheter with routine omentectomy: does it prevent obstruction of the catheter? Eur J Surg 1998;164:703–707.

67. Chadha V, Warady BA: What are the clinical correlates of adequate peritoneal dialysis? Semin Nephrol 2001;21:480–489.

68. Twardowski ZJNK, Khanna R, Prowant BF, Ryan LP, Moore HL, Nielson MP: Peritoneal equilibration test. Perit Dial Int 1987;7:378–383.

69. Warady BA, Alexander SR, Hossli S, et al: Peritoneal membrane transport function in children receiving long-term dialysis. J Am Soc Nephrol 1996;7:2385–2391.

70. Andreoli SP, Leiser J, Warady BA, et al: Adverse effect of peritonitis on peritoneal membrane function in children on dialysis. Pediatr Nephrol 1999;13:1–6.

71. Warady BA, Fivush B, Andreoli SP, et al: Longitudinal evaluation of transport kinetics in children receiving peritoneal dialysis. Pediatr Nephrol 1999;13:571–576.

72. NFK-DQOI: Clinical guidelines for hemodialysis adequacy. Am J Kidney Dis 1997;30:S15–S57.

73. Schaefer F, Klaus G, Mehls O: Peritoneal transport properties and dialysis dose affect growth and nutritional status in children on chronic peritoneal dialysis. Mid-European Pediatric Peritoneal dialysis Study Group. J Am Soc Nephrol 1999;10:1786–1792.

74. Holtta T, Ronnholm K, Jalanko H, Holmberg C: Clinical outcome of pediatric patients on peritoneal dialysis under adequacy control. Pediatr Nephrol 2000;14:889–897.

75. Brem AS, Lambert C, Hill C, et al: Outcome data on pediatric dialysis patients from the end-stage renal disease clinical indicators project. Am J Kidney Dis 2000;36:310–317.

76. Furth SL, Donaldson LA, Sullivan EK, Watkins SL: Peritoneal dialysis catheter infections and peritonitis in children: a report of the North American Pediatric Renal Transplant Cooperative Study. Pediatr Nephrol 2000;15:179–182.

77. Warady BA, Sullivan EK, Alexander SR: Lessons from the peritoneal dialysis patient database: a report of the North American Pediatric Renal Transplant Cooperative Study. Kidney Int 1996;Suppl 53:S68–S71.

78. Fischbach M, Terzic J, Menouer S, et al: Hemodialysis in children: principles and practice. Semin Nephrol 2001;21:470–479.

79. Bunchman TE: Pediatric hemodialysis: lessons from the past, ideas for the future. Kidney Int 1996;Suppl 53:S64–S67.

80. Bourquelot P, Cussenot O, Corbi P, et al: Microsurgical creation and follow-up of arteriovenous fistulae for chronic haemodialysis in children. Pediatr Nephrol 1990;4:156–159.

81. Innes A, Charra B, Burden RP, et al: The effect of long, slow haemodialysis on patient survival. Nephrol Dial Transplant 1999;14:919–922.

82. Goldstein SL, Sorof JM, Brewer ED: Natural logarithmic estimates of Kt/V in the pediatric hemodialysis population. Am J Kidney Dis 1999;33:518–522.

83. Daugirdas JT: Second generation logarithmic estimates of single-pool variable volume Kt/V: an analysis of error. J Am Soc Nephrol 1993;4:1205–1213.

84. Hingorani S, Watkins SL: Dialysis for end-stage renal disease. Curr Opin Pediatr 2000;12:140–145.

85. Hariharan S, Johnson CP, Bresnahan BA, et al: Improved graft survival after renal transplantation in the United States, 1988 to 1996. N Engl J Med 2000;342:605–612.

86. Cecka JM: The UNOS Scientific Renal Transplant Registry. Clin Transpl 1999:1–21.

87. Cecka JM, Gjertson DW, Terasaki PI: Pediatric renal transplantation: a review of the UNOS data. Pediatr Transplant 1997;1:55–64.

88. Mehls O, Rigden S, Ehrich JH, et al: Report on management of renal failure in Europe, XXV, 1994. The child–adult interface. The EDTA-ERA Registry. European Dialysis and Transplant Association/European Renal Association. Nephrol Dial Transplant 1996;11:22–36.

89. Dharnidharka VR, Turman MA, Briscoe DM: Unique aspects of chronic rejection in pediatric renal transplant recipients. Graft 1998;2:82–88.

90. Benfield MR, McDonald R, Sullivan EK, et al: The 1997 Annual Renal Transplantation in Children Report of the North American Pediatric Renal Transplant Cooperative Study (NAPRTCS). Pediatr Transplant 1999;3:152–167.

91. McDonald R, Donaldson L, Emmett L, Tejani A: A decade of living donor transplantation in North American children: the 1998 annual report of the North American Pediatric Renal Transplant Cooperative Study (NAPRTCS). Pediatr Transplant 2000;4:221–234.

92. Elshihabi I, Chavers B, Donaldson L, et al: Continuing improvement in cadaver donor graft survival in North American children: the 1998 annual report of the North American Pediatric Renal Transplant Cooperative Study (NAPRTCS). Pediatr Transplant 2000;4:235–246.

93. Murphy BG, Hill CM, Middleton D, et al: Increased renal allograft thrombosis in CAPD patients. Nephrol Dial Transplant 1994;9:1166–1169.

94. Meyers KE, Thomson PD, Weiland H: Noncompliance in children and adolescents after renal transplantation. Transplantation 1996;62:186–189.

95. Morgenstern BZ, Murphy M, Dayton J, et al: Noncompliance in a pediatric renal transplant population. Transplant Proc 1994;26:129.

96. Ettenger RB: Age and the immune response in pediatric renal transplantation. Eur J Pediatr 1992;151:S7–S8.

97. Strehlau J SV, Pavlakis M: Do children have a heightened immune response to acute allograft rejection? A preliminary comparative study of intragraft gene transcription of immune activation markers in adult and pediatric graft rejection. Am Soc Transplant Physicians 1997:85A.

98. Tejani AH, Stablein DM, Sullivan EK, et al: The impact of donor source, recipient age, pre-operative immunotherapy and induction therapy on early and late acute rejections in children: a report of the North American Pediatric Renal Transplant Cooperative Study (NAPRTCS). Pediatr Transplant 1998;2:318–324.

99. Melter M, Briscoe DM: Challenges after pediatric transplantation. Semin Nephrol 2000;20:199–208.

100. Tejani A, Sullivan EK: The impact of acute rejection on chronic rejection: a report of the North American Pediatric Renal Transplant Cooperative Study. Pediatr Transplant 2000;4:107–111.

101. Nickerson P, Jeffery J, Gough J, et al: Identification of clinical and histopathologic risk factors for diminished renal function 2 years posttransplant. J Am Soc Nephrol 1998;9:482–487.

102. Tejani A, Emmett L: Acute and chronic rejection. Semin Nephrol 2001;21:498–507.

103. Tejani A: Chronic rejection in pediatric renal transplantation: where are we? Pediatr Transplant 2000;4:83–85.

104. Abecassis M, Adams M, Adams P, et al: Consensus statement on the live organ donor. JAMA 2000;284:2919–2926.

105. Vats AN, Donaldson L, Fine RN, Chavers BM: Pretransplant dialysis status and outcome of renal transplantation in North American children: a NAPRTCS Study. North American Pediatric Renal Transplant Cooperative Study. Transplantation 2000;69:1414–1419.

106. Dharnidharka VR, Harmon WE: Management of pediatric postrenal transplantation infections. Semin Nephrol 2001;21:521–531.

107. Webb NJ, Fitzpatrick MM, Hughes DA, et al: Immunisation against varicella in end stage and pre-end stage renal failure. Trans-Pennine Paediatric Nephrology Study Group. Arch Dis Child 2000;82:141–143.

108. Furth SL, Neu AM, Sullivan EK, et al: Immunization practices in children with renal disease: a report of the North American Pediatric Renal Transplant Cooperative Study. Pediatr Nephrol 1997;11:443–446.

109. Elinder CG, Andersson J, Bolinder G, Tyden G: Effectiveness of low-dose cotrimoxazole prophylaxis against *Pneumocystis carinii* pneumonia after renal and/or pancreas transplantation. Transpl Int 1992;5:81–84.

110. Healey PJ, McDonald R, Waldhausen JH, et al: Transplantation of adult living donor kidneys into infants and small children. Arch Surg 2000;135:1035–1041.

111. Nahas WC, Mazzucchi E, Scafuri AG, et al: Extraperitoneal access for kidney transplantation in children weighing 20 kg or less. J Urol 2000;164:475–478.

112. Tanabe K, Takahashi K, Kawaguchi H, et al: Surgical complications of pediatric kidney transplantation: a single center experience with the extraperitoneal technique. J Urol 1998;160:1212–1215.

113. Valdes R, Munoz R, Bracho E, et al: Surgical complications of renal transplantation in malnourished children. Transplant Proc 1994;26:50–51.

114. Kahan BD, Podbielski J, Napoli KL, et al: Immunosuppressive effects and safety of a sirolimus/cyclosporine combination regimen for renal transplantation. Transplantation 1998;66:1040–1046.

115. Sho M, Samsonov DV, Briscoe DM: Immunologic targets for currently available immunosuppressive agents: what is the optimal approach for children? Semin Nephrol 2001;21:508–520.

116. Tejani A, Harmon WE: Clinical transplantation. *In* Barratt TM, Avner ED, Harmon WE (eds): Pediatric Nephrology. Baltimore: Lippincott, Williams & Wilkins, 1999, pp 1309–1337.

117. Dharnidharka VR, Sullivan EK, Stablein DM, et al: Risk factors for posttransplant lymphoproliferative disorder (PTLD) in pediatric kidney transplantation: a report of the North American Pediatric Renal Transplant Cooperative Study (NAPRTCS). Transplantation 2001;71:1065–1068.

118. Leblond V, Sutton L, Dorent R, et al: Lymphoproliferative disorders after organ transplantation: a report of 24 cases observed in a single center. J Clin Oncol 1995;13:961–968.

119. Newell KA, Alonso EM, Whitington PF, et al: Posttransplant lymphoproliferative disease in pediatric liver transplantation. Interplay between primary Epstein–Barr virus infection and immunosuppression. Transplantation 1996;62:370–375.

120. Alfrey EJ, Friedman AL, Grossman RA, et al: A recent decrease in the time to development of monomorphous and polymorphous posttransplant lymphoproliferative disorder. Transplantation 1992;54:250–253.

121. Majewski M, Korecka M, Kossev P, et al: The immunosuppressive macrolide RAD inhibits growth of human Epstein–Barr virus-transformed B lymphocytes in vitro and in vivo: a potential approach to prevention and treatment of posttransplant lymphoproliferative disorders. Proc Natl Acad Sci USA 2000;97:4285–4290.

PART IX
Inherited Renal Disease

CHRISTOPHER S. WILCOX

Renal Cystic Disorders

CHAPTER **49**

Arlene Chapman

Extrarenal manifestations
- Polycystic liver disease
- Intracranial aneurysms

Renal manifestations
- Infections
- Hypertension

Autosomal dominant polycystic kidney disease (ADPKD) is a systemic disorder affecting 1 in 700–1000 individuals.[1] It is the most common inherited renal disorder and the third most common cause of endstage renal disease (ESRD) in the USA after hypertension and diabetes. Half of ADPKD individuals reach ESRD by the fifth decade of life, at an annual cost of $1 billion for renal replacement therapy alone.[2] ADPKD is a systemic disorder (Table 49.1) characterized by the presence of hepatic cystic disease, intracranial aneurysms, inguinal and ventral hernias, and cardiac valvular abnormalities (mitral valve prolapse, aortic insufficiency).[3] Renal manifestations of ADPKD are multiple and include pain, gross hematuria, cyst hemorrhage, nephrolithiasis, infections, and a common and early presence of hypertension.

Table 49.1 Manifestations of autosomal dominant polycystic kidney disease

Extrarenal manifestations
Hepatic cystic disease
    Cholangiocarcinoma
    Congenital hepatic fibrosis
    Caroli disease
    Budd–Chiari syndrome
    Hepatocellular carcinoma
Intracranial aneurysms
    Dolichoectasis
    Fusiform dilations
    Pineal cysts
Cardiac valve abnormalities
    Aortic insufficiency
    Mitral valve prolapse
Hernias (inguinal and ventral)

Renal manifestations
Infection
Hypertension
Hematuria
Pain
Nephrolithiasis

ADPKD is a polygenic disorder, with the PKD1 gene located on chromosome 16 and the PKD2 gene located on chromosome 4.[4] PKD1 occurs in 85% and PKD2 in approximately 14%. The PKD2 form is milder, with a later age of diagnosis and age of onset of ESRD.[4,5]

Extrarenal manifestations

Polycystic liver disease

Polycystic liver disease (PLD) is a common manifestation of ADPKD, presenting approximately 10 years later than renal cystic disease.[7,8] PLD (defined as the presence of two or more hepatic cysts in an individual with ADPKD) occurs in both men and women and is present in the majority (~ 65%) of patients by the age of 50 years.[3,7–10] Autosomal dominant PLD without renal manifestations has been reported and its gene located on chromosome 19.[11] PLD occurs more frequently and earlier in women. It is not surprising therefore that estrogen exposure, including duration of oral contraceptive use, and pregnancy number are associated with more frequent and severe occurrence of PLD.[7,9] In a small series of 11 patients, 1 year of postmenopausal estrogen therapy was associated with greater liver cyst growth and number compared with placebo-treated controls (*n* = 8).[12] Of note, no effect on renal cyst growth or number was found.

Liver cyst growth can be massive (Fig. 49.1) and associated with significant morbidity, including pain, shortness of breath, early satiety, weakness, and fatigue. Although PLD can result in massive involvement of the liver, noncystic hepatic parenchymal volume remains normal and liver function remains intact, with minimal loss of drug clearance or metabolism.[13] Rarely, massive

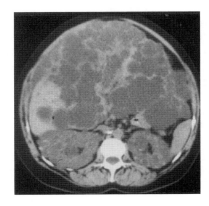

Figure 49.1 Axial computed tomography of the abdomen in an autosomal dominant polycystic kidney disease patient demonstrating massive hepatic cystic involvement.

PLD can be fatal secondary to inferior vena caval obstruction, infection, or Budd–Chiari syndrome or due to the development of endstage liver disease with portal hypertension.[14]

Current approaches to the treatment of PLD have been partially preventative but more often interventional. Attempts to avoid extensive estrogen exposure include minimizing use of the oral contraceptive pill have been implemented. Postmenopausal estrogen replacement therapy (lower in estrogen content than oral contraceptives) should be administered as topical or transdermal estrogen patches in order to avoid the higher estradiol concentrations in the biliary circulation that follow oral ingestion.

In those with massive PLD and associated morbidity, surgical fenestration resection or partial hepatic resection results in overall improvement.[15] Laparoscopic liver cyst decortication is also available; its advantages include shorter recovery and smaller surgical incisions.[16] Both surgical procedures have met with marginal success for diffuse PLD where multiple small cysts predominate.[17] Complications include the development of pleural effusions, ascites, lower extremity edema, hypertension, and infection. Finally, individuals have undergone either liver or combined liver–renal transplantation for massive polycystic liver disease.[18]

Intracranial aneurysms

Intracranial aneurysm (ICA) occurs more frequently in ADPKD (5–8%) than in the general population (1–2%).[19,20] ICA is not the most common cause of cerebrovascular death: hypertensive strokes and subarachnoid hemorrhage are responsible for the majority (75%) of deaths.[21] Dolichoectasia is found in increased frequency (~ 3%)[22] and subarachnoid or pineal cysts are not uncommon in ADPKD.

Accurate diagnosis of the cause of a cerebrovascular event is often impossible, making it difficult to identify individuals from a family with ICA. However, when in doubt, a positive or suspicious family history should be assigned to that individual. Saccular as opposed to fusiform dilation is the most frequent ICA in ADPKD. ICAs are distributed in the anterior portion of the circle of Willis in approximately 75% of cases. Multiple ICAs are not uncommon in ADPKD patients, unlike the general population where isolated ICAs are the rule.

Of these risk factors, only a family history of ICA is associated with the presence of ICA.[19] Although ICAs occur in less than 5% of ADPKD families, specific mutations on the PKD1 or PKD2 gene are not related to the presence of ICA. These data suggest that other genetic modifiers may be responsible for ICA in ADPKD.

Four-vessel cerebral angiography remains the gold standard for finding and identifying the location of ICA in ADPKD individuals. However, this procedure requires access to the arterial system and, specific to ADPKD individuals, is associated with significant vasospasm.[19] Currently, magnetic resonance imaging (MRI), also called magnetic resonance angiography (MRA), can identify ICAs as small as 3 mm. Dynamic computed tomography (CT) has also been used successfully. MRI/MRA is the preferred method of screening for the presence of ICA in an asymptomatic ADPKD individual. Given the low frequency of occurrence of ICA in ADPKD individuals, it is cost-effective to screen only those at risk for ICA (a positive family history) or whose current occupation (e.g., airline pilot) or lifestyle (e.g., scuba diving) would significantly increase the likelihood or consequences of rupture. In addition, for those individuals where knowledge of a positive or negative result would improve their quality of life, a screening test for the presence of ICA is warranted.

The value of an initial negative screening has been tested in ADPKD. Of 130 asymptomatic ADPKD individuals with an initial negative imaging study, imaging studies performed 3–15 years later (mean 9.7 years) were also negative. These findings suggest that repeat screening in ADPKD subjects can wait at least 5 years if the patient is symptom-free. The characteristics of surviving ADPKD individuals suffering from ICA rupture have also been evaluated.[20] Women are more commonly affected than men, with a mean age of 34 years, and there is a family history of ICA increasing in frequency to 20%. When radiographic imaging is repeated in patients who have suffered a ruptured ICA, the finding of new ICA is not uncommon (~ 12%).

Given that mortality and morbidity associated with ruptured ICA remain in excess of 50% in ADPKD, intervention is important. In the general population, 50% of ICAs remain intact during the individual's lifetime. The risk for rupture of ICA in ADPKD is related to the size of the aneurysm and is similar to the general population. The risk of rupture for ICAs > 10 mm increases exponentially, with an estimated rupture rate of 1 in 5 patient-years. Longitudinal information is also available for asymptomatic ADPKD individuals where intact ICAs have been found. In small identified ICAs (< 5 mm), little or no change in size of the ICA occurs. However, isolated reports of rupture of small ICAs in ADPKD exist. When small ICAs (< 5 mm) are followed over time, little if any change in size is apparent. ICAs > 5 and < 10 mm also appear not to change; however the number of individuals studied is small. Outcome of surgical interventions in individuals with intact ICAs is extremely good in comparison to those presenting with rupture. Surgical complications are typically reported as death or cerebrovascular accident with permanent neurologic sequelae. However, recovery from elective neurosurgery for ICAs may involve significant neurocognitive functional abnormalities as well as mood and sleep disorders lasting up to 6–12 months. Therefore, the decision to undergo elective surgical clipping, coiling, or injection of intact small ICAs should be done only after thorough discussion with the neurosurgeon, neurologist, and nephrologist and after taking into account the patient's overall health and comorbidities.

Renal manifestations

Infections

Lower and upper urinary tract infections are common and may be associated with a faster rate of functional loss in

ADPKD. Differentiating upper from lower tract infections is important. Upper urinary tract infections may be due to pyelonephritis, nephrolithiasis, obstruction, or cyst infection. Differentiating among these conditions relies on laboratory and radiographic studies.[21] Pyelonephritis and renal stone-related infections often have urinary abnormalities (leukocyturia and bacteriuria) and positive urine cultures compared with renal cyst infections.[21] In individuals with renal cyst infections, blood cultures are more likely to be positive than urine cultures, with the offending bacterium identified in ~ 50% of cases. The triad of localized pain, fever, and the presence of a complex cyst on ultrasound, MRI, or CT helps to diagnose renal cyst infection and rules out the presence of hepatic cyst infection, which occurs rarely. Nephrolithiasis can be identified using CT with care to rule out cyst rim calcifications.[22] Complex cysts (either consolidated hemorrhage or infection) can be identified by ultrasound but more often by CT. If symptoms are present in the area of the complex cyst, empiric antibiotic coverage is warranted for the treatment of a presumed cyst infection.

The majority of cysts are no longer attached to their parent nephron and therefore antibiotics typically used to treat organisms causing pyelonephritis (*Escherichia coli*, *Klebsiella*, *Proteus*, *Pseudomonas*, etc.), such as aminoglycosides, penicillins, or cephalosporins, do not provide adequate intracystic drug levels.[23] Aminoglycosides are easily filtered by the glomerulus but are distributed widely throughout the kidney, resulting in insufficient concentrations to adequately treat cyst infection. In noninflammatory studies (during elective surgical cyst reduction procedures), antibiotic levels adequate to treat cyst infections have been demonstrated with trimethoprim–sulfamethoxazole, ciprofloxacin, other fluoroquinolones, chloramphenicol, and vancomycin.

Cyst infections are equivalent to abscesses and therefore prolonged antibiotic therapy (4–6 weeks) is necessary to ensure successful treatment. In individuals where large cysts (> 5 cm) become infected, antibiotic therapy alone is often unsuccessful and percutaneous or surgical cyst decompression with parenteral antibiotic treatment may be necessary. Early identification of cyst infection and prolonged treatment with antibiotics is the key to successful eradication of cyst infections in ADPKD. Failure to use this approach can result in pyonephritis and loss of the kidney.

Hypertension

Hypertension is common and occurs early in individuals with ADPKD.[1,24] Approximately 60% of adults with normal renal function and 10–15% of children have hypertension.[25] The frequency of hypertension in ADPKD children increases to approximately 33% when 24-h ambulatory blood pressure monitoring is used. Hypertension is associated with a faster rate of progression to renal failure and is the most treatable risk factor associated with disease progression. Cardiovascular disease is the most common cause of death in ADPKD individuals,

indicating that hypertension is a comorbid condition in ADPKD. Importantly, when other factors related to progression are taken into account, age, renal volume, and blood pressure appear to be important risk factors for progression to ESRD. Although hypertension is common and a risk factor for progression to ESRD, it is not severe and blood pressure is usually adequately controlled (mean arterial pressure, MAP, 93 mmHg) using a mean of 1.2 antihypertensive medications.

Mechanisms responsible for the development of hypertension in ADPKD have been sought.[26] The most consistent information points to activation of the renin–angiotensin–aldosterone system.[27] ADPKD individuals with hypertension and normal renal function demonstrate larger renal volumes than their age- and gender-matched ADPKD normotensive counterparts. These findings led to the hypothesis that cyst growth and expansion leads to compression and stretch of renal arterioles, resulting in activation of the intrarenal renin– angiotensin–aldosterone system similar to bilateral renal artery stenosis. In support of this, barium-injected ADPKD kidneys and angiograms performed at the time of nephrectomy demonstrate increased tortuosity and compression of intrarenal vessels and a paucity of cortical vascularization. Tissue renin levels and renin-secreting granules are increased in ADPKD kidneys. When individuals with essential hypertension and hypertensive ADPKD individuals with normal renal function and similar sodium intake are compared, increased supine and upright plasma renin activity and aldosterone concentrations are found in ADPKD individuals.[27] After stimulation with captopril, renin activities are significantly increased in ADPKD compared with essential hypertensives. Improvement in effective renal plasma flow and a decline in filtration fraction are found in hypertensive ADPKD subjects undergoing single-dose or short-term therapy with angiotensin-converting enzyme (ACE) inhibitors compared with matched essential hypertensives.

End-organ damage related to the presence of hypertension occurs early in ADPKD. Left ventricular hypertrophy (LVH) is present in ~ 50% of hypertensive ADPKD individuals.[28] Increased left ventricular mass index (LVMI) is also present in normotensive ADPKD individuals compared with age-matched control subjects as well as in ADPKD children compared with age-matched controls. LVMI correlates with systolic and ambulatory blood pressure in ADPKD children and in ADPKD adults with normal renal function.

Proteinuria, an uncommon feature of ADPKD (~ 17%), is present more often in hypertensive than in normotensive ADPKD individuals and is related to the level of blood pressure control.[29] Proteinuria > 1 g/day is unusual in ADPKD and the presence of other renal diseases should be sought. Surprisingly, proteinuria is more common in ADPKD children (~ 27%) and is also related to blood pressure.[30] Microalbuminuria is present in approximately 27% of ADPKD adults and 34% of ADPKD children and is related to the hypertensive state. Importantly, hypertension and proteinuria are risk factors for progression to renal failure in ADPKD.

Treatment of hypertension in ADPKD has demonstrated salutory effects on LVMI and frequency of LVH as well as the presence of albuminuria. Long-term (5-year) therapy with ACE inhibitors in hypertensive ADPKD individuals with creatinine clearances > 30 mL/min per 1.73 m^2 results in a significant reduction in albuminuria, greater than that found with dihydropyridine therapy.[31] The greatest reduction in albuminuria was found in those whose treatment lowered blood pressure to < 120/75 mmHg. Long-term ACE inhibitor therapy (7 years) is effective in reducing LVMI and correcting LVH in the same individuals. The improvement in LVMI and frequency of LVH following treatment may not be specific to ACE inhibitors, because rigorous (MAP < 93 mmHg) compared with moderate (MAP 100–107 mmHg) blood pressure control demonstrates beneficial effects on LVMI independent of the type of antihypertensive agent used. Importantly, although treating ADPKD individuals with ACE inhibitors has renoprotective effects with regard to proteinuria, no clear benefit in slowing the rate of progression to renal failure has been demonstrated.

Three prospective longitudinal studies of ACE inhibitors, one with randomization, have failed to demonstrate an improvement in the rate of loss of renal function in ADPKD. However, these studies followed subjects for only a short period of time and multiple interventions were employed simultaneously (such as protein restriction and different blood pressure levels). Finally, the ADPKD individuals studied have been very advanced with regard to their renal disease, where benefit of any intervention may be lost. Importantly, in observational studies the use of diuretics as opposed to ACE inhibitors was associated with faster progression to ESRD, whereas β-blockers as opposed to ACE inhibitors (both of which inhibit the renin–angiotensin–aldosterone system) demonstrate similar effects on rate of progression. These studies indicate that more work needs to be done to determine if blockade of the renin–angiotensin–aldosterone system in ADPKD will result in slowing progression to ESRD. At present, it appears that ACE inhibitors have protective effects on cardiac structure and level of proteinuria and should be included in the treatment of hypertension in ADPKD patients.

References

1. Gabow PA: Autosomal dominant polycystic kidney disease. N Engl J Med 1993;329: 332–342.
2. Agodoa LYC, Held PJ, Port FK: United States Renal Data System 1998 Annual Data Report. Bethesda, MD: National Institutes of Health, National Institute of Diabetes and Digestive and Kidney Diseases, 1998.
3. Gabow PA: Autosomal dominant polycystic kidney disease: more than a renal disease. Am J Kidney Dis 1990;16:403–413.
4. Kimberling W, Fain PR, Kenyon JB, et al: Linkage heterogeneity of autosomal dominant polycystic kidney disease. N Engl J Med 1988;319:913–918.
5. Parfrey PS, Bear JC, Morgan J, et al: The diagnosis and prognosis of autosomal dominant polycystic kidney disease. N Engl J Med 1990;323:1085–1090.
6. Hanaoka K, Qian F, Boletta A, et al: Co-assembly of polycystin-1 and -2 produces unique cation-permeable currents. Nature 2000;408:990–994.
7. Gabow PA, Johnson AM, Kaehny WD, et al: Risk factors for the development of hepatic cysts in autosomal dominant polycystic kidney disease. Hepatology 1990;11:1033–1037.
8. Gabow PA, Ikle DW, Holmes JH: Polycystic kidney disease: prospective analysis of nonazotemic patients and family members. Ann Intern Med 1984;101:238–247 .
9. Ramos A, Torres V, Holley K, et al: The liver in autosomal dominant polycystic kidney disease. Arch Pathol Lab Med 1990;114:180–184.
10. Grunfeld JP, Bennett WM: Clinical aspects of autosomal dominant polycystic kidney disease. Curr Opin Nephrol Hypertens 1995;4:114–120.
11. Iglesias DM, Palmitano JA, Arrizurieta E, et al: Isolated polycystic liver disease not linked to polycystic kidney disease 1 and 2. Dig Dis Sci 1999;44:385–388.
12. Sherstha R, McKinley C, Russ P, et al: Postmenopausal estrogen therapy selectively stimulates hepatic enlargement in women with autosomal dominant polycystic kidney disease. Hepatology 1997;26:1282–1286.
13. Everson GT, Scherzinger A, Berger-Leff N, et al: Polycystic liver disease: quantification of parenchymal and cyst volumes from computed tomography images and clinical correlates of hepatic cysts. Hepatology 1988;8:1627–1634.
14. Nakanuma Y, Hoso M, Hayashi M, Hirai N: Adult polycystic liver presenting with progressive hepatic failure. J Clin Gastoenterol 1989;11:592–594.
15. Que F, Nagorney DM, Gross JB Jr, et al: Liver resection and cyst fenestration in the treatment of severe polycystic liver disease. Gastroenterology 1995;108:487–494.
16. Katkhouda N, Hurwitz M, Gugenheim J, et al: Laparoscopic management of benign solid and cystic lesions of the liver. Ann Surg 1999;229:460–466.
17. Turnage RH, Eckhauser FE, Knol JA, et al: Therapeutic dilemmas in patients with symptomatic polycystic liver disease. Am Surg 1988;54:365–372.
18. Jeyarajah DR, Gonwa TA, Testa G, et al: Liver and kidney transplantation for polycystic disease. Transplantation 1998;66:529–532.
19. Chapman AB, Rubenstein D, Hughes R, et al: Intracranial aneurysms in autosomal dominant polycystic kidney disease: a prospective study. N Engl J Med 1992;327:916–920.
20. Investigators of the International Study of Unruptured Intracranial Aneurysms: Unruptured intracranial aneurysms, risk of rupture and risks of surgical intervention. N Engl J Med 1988;339:1725–1733.
21. Fick GM, Johnson AM, Hammond WS, et al: Causes of death in autosomal dominant polycystic kidney disease. J Am Soc Nephrol 1995;5:2048–2056.
22. Schievink WI, Torres VE, Wiebers DO, et al: Intracranial arterial dolichoectasia in autosomal dominant polycystic kidney disease. J Am Soc Nephrol 1997;8:1298–1303.
23. Chapman AB, Thickman D, Gabow PA: Percutaneous cyst puncture in the treatment of cyst infection in autosomal dominant polycystic kidney disease. Am J Kidney Dis 1990;16:252–255.
24. Gabow PA, Johnson AM, Strain J: Children with autosomal dominant polycystic kidney disease. J Am Soc Nephrol 1995;6:720.
25. Chapman AB, Johnson AM, Duley I, et al: Hypertension occurs frequently in children with autosomal dominant polycystic kidney disease. J Am Soc Nephrol 1991;2:251.
26. Wang D, Strandgaard S: The pathogenesis of hypertension in autosomal dominant polycystic kidney disease. J Hypertens 1997;15:925–933.
27. Chapman AB, Johnson AM, Gabow PA, et al: The renin–angiotensin–aldosterone system and autosomal dominant polycystic kidney disease. N Engl J Med 1990;323:1091–1096.
28. Chapman AB, Johnson AM, Rainguet S, et al: Left ventricular hypertrophy in autosomal dominant polycystic kidney disease. J Am Soc Nephrol 1997;8:1292–1297.
29. Chapman AB, Johnson AM, Gabow PA, et al: Overt proteinuria and microalbuminuria in autosomal dominant polycystic kidney disease. J Am Soc Nephrol 1994;5:1349–1354.
30. Sharp C, Johnson A, Gabow P: Factors relating to urinary protein excretion in children with autosomal dominant polycystic kidney disease. J Am Soc Nephrol 1998;9:1908–1914.
31. Ecder T, Chapman AB, Brosnahan GM, et al: Effect of antihypertensive therapy on renal function and urinary albumin excretion in hypertensive patients with autosomal dominant polycystic kidney disease. Am J Kidney Dis 2000;35:427–432.

Noncystic Hereditary Diseases of the Kidney

Russell W. Chesney

Aminoacidurias
Glycosurias
Classical pseudohypoaldosteronism
Hereditary phosphaturias
• Primary or X-linked hypophosphatemic rickets
• Hypophosphatemic nonrachitic bone disease
• Hereditary hypophosphatemic rickets with hypercalcemia
• Oncogenous rickets with phosphaturia
• Adult sporadic osteomalacia
Magnesurias
Fanconi syndrome
Bartter syndrome
Liddle syndrome
Chloride shunt syndrome

The techniques of gene cloning, chromosomal localization, and gene "chips" have permitted a much more definitive understanding of many of the inherited renal disorders. This chapter reviews a number of clinical disorders that have as their basis a defect in some transport function of the renal tubular epithelium. Using the model of inherited disorders of renal tubular transport, one is able to define conditions in which single or multiple substances are lost, in which inorganic ions or organic solutes are excessively excreted, and in which the whole body pool of these substances is diminished due to excessive urinary losses (Table 50.1). The basic genetic and pathophysiologic mechanisms underlying these transport defects are detailed elsewhere.[1–4] The intent of this chapter is to describe current therapeutic approaches.

It is important to define certain principles of therapy because they are relevant for every disorder and because they must be borne in mind when approaching the patient with renal tubular disorders with a view toward therapy.

Principle 1. These disorders are frequently inherited and are found in families. The inheritance pattern may be autosomal recessive, autosomal dominant, X-linked recessive, X-linked dominant, or complex, such as multigenic or maternal (chromosomal DNA).
Principle 2. Because these disorders are genetic they may be evident at birth or during childhood, although sometimes they may not present clinically for many years.
Principle 3. The substances lost are usually natural body constituents, ions found in the extracellular or intracellular fluid, common organic solutes, and metabolites of carbohydrates, lipids and proteins.
Principle 4. Because the excessive loss of ions obligates water excretion, many of these patients may be polyuric and excrete a dilute urine.
Principle 5. Because of the excessive loss of ions and solutes, many of the conditions presenting in childhood result in growth failure.
Principle 6. Diagnosis can usually be made by measuring renal clearance of the substance lost *or* the fractional excretion of that substance.[2,4]
Principle 7. Some of these disorders are clinically inconsequential and thus require no therapy, e.g. familial glucosuria.
Principle 8. Therapy often consists of provision of the lost metabolite in quantities sufficient to increase body pool size and/or plasma concentration.
Principle 9. On occasions, the metabolite lost in the urine (e.g. cystine) may lead to renal damage due to its physicochemical properties.

Table 50.1 Inherited noncystic tubular disorders
Aminoacidurias
Iminoglycinuria
Hartnup disease
Cystinuria
Glycosurias
Pseudohypoaldosteronism
Phosphaturias
X-linked hypophosphatemic rickets
Hypophosphatemic bone disease (autosomal dominant)
Hypophosphatemia with hypercalciuria
Oncogenous rickets
Adult sporadic hypophosphatemic rickets
Magnesurias
Renal magnesium wasting: infantile and childhood
Gitelman syndrome: magnesium wasting and hypokalemia
Fanconi syndrome: many forms (see Table 50.4)
Bartter syndrome: infantile
Classical Bartter syndrome
Childhood Bartter syndrome
Gitelman syndrome
Liddle syndrome
Chloride shunt syndrome

Aminoacidurias

The aminoacidurias may be specific to a single amino acid or to a group of amino acids whose structure and charge are similar.[2,4] In recent years virtually all amino acid transporters have been cloned and localized to a specific human chromosome.[3] The technique of amino acid analysis of urine or plasma permits diagnosis of these disorders, particularly the measurement of urinary clearance or fractional excretion. Several of the aminoacidurias, such as iminoglycinuria in which excessive amounts of L-proline, hydroxy-L-proline, and glycine are found in the urine, are benign traits requiring no treatment.[1] In dicarboxylic aminoaciduria, there are no apparent clinical features and hence no recommended therapy.[1]

Hartnup disease is an autosomal recessive disorder characterized by massive urinary losses and intestinal malabsorption of the neutral monoamino–monocarboxylic amino acids. Affected patients develop features of pellagra[4] because of inability to synthesize minimal concentrations of nicotinamide as a result of bowel and urinary L-tryptophan losses. Thus, insufficient absorption and reabsorption of L-tryptophan results in vitamin deficiency. Treatment consists of providing nicotinamide (40–150 mg daily) or an American diet containing leafy green vegetables. With the provision of nicotinamide, the red scaly rash heals and neurologic problems improve.

Renal and urinary tract stones develop in cystinuria, an autosomal recessive disorder in which the poorly soluble disulfide amino acid is excreted into the urine in increased amounts.[5] The genes for the cystine transporter have recently been cloned.[3] Cystinuria is a relatively frequent cause of nephrolithiasis, found in 1 in 12 000 persons worldwide. The treatment of this condition has been modified by several advances.[5] The initial goal of therapy is to reduce the urinary concentration of cystine below its solubility limit and is generally accomplished by a forced high fluid intake. Unfortunately, this form of therapy requires strenuous compliance, with frequent ingestion of fluids and noctural rising to empty the bladder and imbibe additional fluids. Patients should also receive oral alkali therapy, since the solubility of cystine is pH dependent (urinary solubility of cystine rises steeply at pH values > 7.5). A suggested dose is 650 mg sodium bicarbonate every 6–8 h.

Should these more conservative measures fail, the next line of therapy is the thiol-containing agents. The most tested is oral D-penicillamine (dimethylcystine), a mercaptan that undergoes an in vivo disulfide exchange reaction with cystine, causing urinary excretion of a more readily soluble penicillamine–cystine mixed disulfide. In parallel, the concentration of cystine in the urine of a cystinuric subject actually falls.[4] Treatment with oral D-penicillamine at 1–2 g/day in the adult and 30 mg/kg in the child is highly effective in reducing urinary cystine excretion below 200–300 mg daily, but patient tolerance is poor and adverse effects are frequent.[5] Serious adverse effects that result in discontinuance of the drug occur in 30–50% of patients and include skin rash, membranous or linear IgG antiglomerular basement membrane antibody-induced nephropathy, nausea, vomiting, impairment or loss of taste or smell, and pemphigus.[4]

Because of these serious adverse effects, other disulfide compounds have been used. Most experience has been gained with 2-mercapto-propionylglycine (α-MPG), which is 1.5 times as effective as D-penicillamine in reducing free cystine and in increasing the quantity of mixed disulfide appearing in the urine.[5] α-MPG also results in adverse effects, including nausea, vomiting, and rash, but far less frequently than D-penicillamine. Development of the nephritic syndrome is rare. The final dose of α-MPG needed to reduce urinary cystine varies from 100 to 200 mg daily. While patients may experience adverse effects, it is seldom necessary to discontinue therapy, and only 6% of patients receiving α-MPG because of D-penicillamine toxicity are required to stop taking it.[4,5] Another compound containing a sulfhydryl group similar to D-penicillamine is the angiotensin-converting enzyme inhibitor captopril. Its clinical effectiveness remains controversial.[5]

The report that glutamine can induce a marked reduction in urinary cystine excretion has been difficult to confirm.[4] Reinvestigation of the anticystinuric influence of glutamine in cystinuric patients demonstrates that glutamine reduces urinary cystine excretion only in association with high dietary sodium intake.[2] With dietary sodium restriction of less than 150 mmol/day, no anticystinuric action of glutamine exists, suggesting that this therapy would not benefit patients on a normal diet and indicating that sodium restriction per se may also lower urinary cystine excretion.

Surgery for staghorn calculi or obstructing stones can potentially be avoided by the use of percutaneous ultrasonic or extracorporeal shock-wave lithotripsy (ESWL).[6] In ultrasonic lithotripsy, an ultrasound probe is passed up the ureter during cystoscopy; it is 97% effective in removing an obstructing calculus. ESWL employs a totally external technique, with patients placed in a special bath, anesthetized, and then undergoing thousands of precisely directed shock waves. The main drawbacks are hematuria, failure of stone passage, and mild-to-moderate obstruction and infection, although most patients pass the stone fragments with lesser symptoms of colic. Cystine stones are less effectively fragmented than are calcium oxalate stones.[6]

Hypercystinuria probably requires no treatment, since patients do not excrete the same quantities of cystine as patients with classical cystinuria.[6] Conditions such as histidinuria, oasthouse syndrome (urinary and intestinal methionine malabsorption), isolated glycinuria, and dicarboxylic aminoaciduria (lysine, arginine, ornithine) do not require therapy.[4]

Glycosurias

The renal glycosurias are a group of conditions where excessive urinary excretion of glucose occurs in the absence of hyperglycemia. The glycosurias occur because of abnormal renal tubular reabsorption of glucose due to mutations in the two renal isoforms of the sodium-dependent glucose transporter. The clinical course of the primary renal glycosurias is benign, as there is neither progressive renal deterioration nor serious metabolic derangement, and there is no specific therapy. It is important to distinguish the primary renal glycosurias from diabetes mellitus, which has serious consequences and which obviously requires insulin or other hypoglycemic therapy.

Classical pseudohypoaldosteronism

Classical pseudohypoaldosteronism is a condition described 30 years ago in which both renal tubular salt wasting and hyperkalemia are observed, despite normal renal and adrenal function.[4] The defect relates to abnormalities of the renal aldosterone or mineralocorticoid receptor, with an ultimate defect in the epithelial sodium channel (ENaC).[7] Salt wasting does not respond to exogenous mineralocorticoids alone, so sodium chloride supplements must be provided. This hyperkalemic state occurs in infancy and 24-h Na^+ and Cl^- losses are as high as 10–15 mequiv./kg, despite hypovolemia and hyponatremia. The administration of glucocorticoids, deoxycorticosterone acetate, or fluorinated glucocorticoids (which have extensive mineralocorticoid activity) even in large doses do little to reverse hyponatremia and hyperkalemia because of defective ENaC. The most effective therapy is supplemental sodium chloride based on the magnitude of measured urinary losses (mequiv./kg per 24 h).[4] Salt supplements normalize growth and correct serum Na^+ and Cl^- concentrations, despite the finding of persistently elevated plasma renin and aldosterone concentrations. A potassium-binding resin may be required to correct the concomitant hyperkalemia and oral bicarbonate or citrate therapy is necessary to correct the acidosis. Patients can frequently have their salt supplements reduced or discontinued after infancy without effect, and they continue to grow at a normal rate.[2]

Hereditary phosphaturias

Phosphorus is the most prevalent mineral anion found in bone (75–85% of total body phosphate pool) and is also essential for numerous life processes, including DNA metabolism, energy storage (ATP, GTP, etc.), maintenance of cell membrane stability, second messenger activity (cyclic AMP and inositol phosphates), and cellular intermediary metabolites (glycolysis, gluconeogenesis).[1] Since phosphate is the key anion for these important systems, biologic processes designed to maintain phosphate homeostasis are important. The renal proximal tubule is the major site in the nephron that regulates phosphate homeostasis.[2] A number of clinically distinguishable phosphaturic syndromes have been defined,[4] all of which result in excess renal phosphate wasting and in hypophosphatemic osteomalacia (Table 50.2). If these conditions present during childhood, the result is incomplete mineralization and the radiologic appearance of rickets.

Since the fundamental pathogenic mechanisms of the major phosphaturic syndromes differ, their treatment is also different (Table 50.2).

Primary or X-linked hypophosphatemic rickets

This X-linked dominant disorder is the most common of the phosphaturic syndromes and involves a double renal tubular defect: (1) failure of Na^+/PO_4^{3-} cotransport across the brush border membrane of the proximal tubule and (2) reduction in the conversion of 25-hydroxyvitamin D_3 to 1,25-dihydroxyvitamin D_3 by proximal tubule cell mitochondria.[2,4] A defective phosphate regulatory protein (PHEX) is the cause of this condition.

The current recommendation regarding the most appropriate form of treatment is a combination of oral 1,25-dihydroxyvitamin D_3 in as low a dose as possible (5–50 ng/kg/day) plus oral phosphate supplements (70 mg/kg/day).[4,8,9] Although this therapy has been shown to improve calcium and phosphate retention, phosphate must be administered every 4–5 h because the renal phosphate leak persists (Table 50.3). Therapy is probably needed throughout the life of the patient. Not only will the rachitic growth plate lesion be improved but endosteal bone trabecular lesions will also improve, a change not apparent when using vitamin D_2 or D_3 alone. Oral phosphate can be administered as Joulie solution[8] or as neutral phosphate.[9] The latter is far easier to use. This form of therapy should be given during childhood. Medical noncompliance is a major problem, as are excessively loose stools due to oral sodium phosphate. Hydrochlorothiazide and amiloride may be used in some cases where there appears to be resistance to the combination of vitamin D and phosphate supplementation.[9]

No long-term studies have been reported that confirm the role of lifetime phosphorus in adults with this disorder. However, studies indicate that calcification of ligaments and joints (enthesopathy) can occur in untreated adult patients,[10] suggesting the need for therapy during adult life. Severely affected adults who continue to have osteodystrophy, stress fractures, and dental caries require prolonged treatment, yet those who are asymptomatic may not always need to continue with treatment into adulthood. Normal pregnancies have been reported both in mothers treated with vitamin D/phosphate supplementation and in those not treated. The concomitant use of recombinant human growth hormone may be useful as an adjunct to standard therapy to improve growth.

Hypophosphatemic nonrachitic bone disease

Hypophosphatemic nonrachitic bone disease is an autosomal dominant or possibly sporadic disorder in which hypophosphatemia is milder than in X-linked hypophosphatemia and rickets is absent.[2,4] Both the $T_m PO_4/GFR$

Table 50.2 Features of different forms of primary hypophosphatemic rickets

Condition	Pattern of inheritance	Gene defect	Associated findings	Salient clinical features	Age detected	Therapy
X-linked hypophosphatemic rickets (vitamin D-dependent or familial)	X-linked dominant (rarely dominant or AR)	Presumed defect in PHEX, a regulator of protein coded Xp22.1–22.2	Occasional parathyroid adenoma/hyperplasia	Bowing lower segment, short stature, no myopathy; more severe in males (Lyon effect)	9–13 months	Oral phosphate 70–100 mg/kg/day (four to five times daily) Oral 1,25-(OH)$_2$D$_3$ 5–50 ng/kg/day
Hypophosphatemic nonrachitic bone disease	AD or sporadic	Unknown	Glycinuria	No radiologic evidence of rickets; mild short stature may develop late	3 years to adult	Oral phosphate and vitamin D; 1,25-(OH)$_2$D$_3$ may heal osteomalacia
Hereditary hypophosphatemic rickets and hypercalciuria	AR; consanguinity frequent	Unknown	High plasma 1,25-(OH)$_2$D$_3$; increased intestinal calcium absorption, hypercalciuria, low urine cAMP	Rickets, short stature, osteomalacia, equal sex distribution	Early childhood	Oral phosphate
Oncogenous rickets with phosphaturia	Sporadic or AD/AR	Presumed defect in phosphatonin activity	Neurofibromatosis, polyostotic fibrous dysplasia, epidermal nevus syndrome	Rickets healed by removal of tumor; where measured, serum 1,25-(OH)$_2$D$_3$ values are usually low	Birth onwards	Oral phosphate and 1,25-(OH)$_2$D$_3$ reverse hypophosphatemia; surgery may be curative
Adult sporadic hypophosphatemic osteomalacia	Sporadic	Not relevant	Glycinuria	Severe bone pain, vertebral flattening, Looser zones, severe myopathy/weakness	Adult	Oral phosphate and vitamin D (any form)

AD, autosomal dominant; AR, autosomal recessive; cAMP, cyclic adenosine monophosphate; 1,25-(OH)$_2$D$_3$, 1,25-dihydroxyvitamin D$_3$; PHEX, phosphate regulating gene on the X chromosome with homologies to endopeptidases.

Table 50.3 Phosphate preparations for therapy of phosphaturic syndromes and Fanconi syndrome

	Constituents	Phosphate content
K-Phos M.F.	Potassium acid phosphate Sodium acid phosphate	125.6 mg per tablet
K-Phos No. 2	Potassium acid phosphate Sodium acid phosphate	250 mg per tablet
K-Phos Neutral	Potassium acid phosphate, monobasic Sodium acid phosphate, monobasic/dibasic	250 mg per tablet
Neutra Phos	Potassium acid phosphate, monobasic Sodium acid phosphate, monobasic/dibasic	1 g per 300 mL
Neutra Phos (capsules)	Potassium acid phosphate, monobasic Sodium acid phosphate, monobasic/dibasic	250 mg per capsule (dissolve in water)
Joulie solution*	Sodium phosphate Phosphoric acid	30.4 mg/mL

*Must be prepared by a pharmacist.

(glomerular filtration rate) in hypophosphatemic patients and serum $1,25\text{-}(OH)_2$ D_3 concentrations are normal. Therapy with vitamin D_2 and oral phosphate salts appear to mineralize bone; however, oral 1,25-dihydroxyvitamin D_3 can be used in place of vitamin D_2 or D_3.

Hereditary hypophosphatemic rickets with hypercalcemia

This is a familial disorder that manifests as rickets, short stature, phosphaturia, hypercalciuria (8 mg/kg per 24 h), and augmented intestinal calcium and phosphate absorption.[12] Circulating 1,25-dihydroxyvitamin D_3 concentrations are two to five times normal, as compared with reduced concentrations in X-linked hypophosphatemic rickets and normal concentrations in hypophosphatemic bone disease. It has been speculated that this disorder represents a renal phosphate leak that results in hypophosphatemia, stimulating 1,25-dihydroxyvitamin D_3 synthesis. Higher vitamin D metabolite concentrations lead to increased active intestinal calcium absorption, suppression of parathyroid hormone (PTH) secretion, and hypercalciuria. As 1,25-dihydroxyvitamin D_3 concentrations in plasma are elevated, vitamin D therapy is not indicated. Long-term oral phosphate alone reverses the biochemical features of this rare disorder.[12]

Oncogenous rickets with phosphaturia

This is a sometimes hereditary but otherwise sporadic disorder in which tumors of mesenchymal origin or associated with neurocutaneous syndrome (neurofibromatosis) appear to elaborate a substance that promotes phosphaturia and hypophosphatemic osteomalacia.[13] These mesenchymal tumors may be found in soft tissue or bone. The levels of 1,25-dihydroxyvitamin D_3 in plasma are extremely low, usually below 5 pg/mL, and rise to normal values within a few hours of tumor removal.[4] Therapy with 1,25-dihydroxyvitamin D_3 2.5–3.0 µg daily and oral phosphate 1–4 g daily improve calcium and phosphate balance and sometimes result in bone healing.[2,4] This therapy should be used only in cases where the tumor is inoperable or when surgery must be postponed. The most appropriate form of therapy is resection of the tumor.

Adult sporadic osteomalacia

Hypophosphaturic osteomalacia arising de novo in adults is termed adult sporadic osteomalacia.[4] The diagnosis is based on a history of muscle, bone, and joint pains (the "princess-and-the-pea" syndrome), and common signs include a myopathy, Looser–Milkman zones, and collapsed "codfish" vertebrae. Pathogenesis is uncertain but does not involve hyperparathyroidism or hypercalcitoninemia, nor changes in vitamin D metabolism.[2] Although 1,25-dihydroxyvitamin D_3 therapy improves intestinal calcium absorption, this agent alone will not heal osteomalacia and completely reverse hypophosphatemia. Treatment with vitamin D and oral phosphate supplements improve all signs and symptoms. Vitamin D dosage regimens are 1–2 mg/day of 1,25-dihydroxyvitamin D_3, 50–100 mg/day of 25-hydroxyvitamin D_3, and 100 000–300 000 units/day i.v. of vitamin D_2, in addition to several grams of oral phosphate. With rare exceptions,[4] therapy must be for life. Because of the similar signs between this syndrome and oncogenous rickets, an exhaustive search for a tumor is necessary.

Magnesurias

Magnesium depletion is an uncommon mineral disorder and is frequently overlooked because it usually arises within a complex clinical setting. Renal magnesium wasting may be part of a primary inherited disorder (Gitelman syndrome),[14,15] a single defect in magnesium reabsorption,[16] or may be associated with several other clinical disorders.[2,4] Excessive urinary losses of magnesium can also be associated with diabetic ketoacidosis, hyperaldosteronism, hypercalciuria (with concomitant use of loop diuretics), Gitelman syndrome, and the use of several therapeutic agents such as cisplatin, aminoglycoside antibiotics, diuretics, and cyclosporine.[17] Hereditary isolated renal magnesium wasting is due to defects in two genes: a Na^+,K^+-ATPase subunit (a routing defect); and paracellin,[1] a protein located on the tight junction.[16] Gitelman syndrome is discussed later.

A predominant feature of magnesium deficiency is hypocalcemia related to altered parathyroid gland function. Hypomagnesemia alters end-organ (bone) responsiveness to PTH[17] and hence contributes to hypocalcemia. Further, the provision of intravenous magnesium supplements to magnesium-deficient hypocalcemic patients has been shown to augment serum values of PTH.[17] Magnesium may also be an important factor in the action and/or metabolism of vitamin D, in that some hypomagnesemic patients respond to 1α-vitamin D metabolites only after correction of serum magnesium values.[4,17] Serum concentrations of 1,25-dihydroxyvitamin D_3 are reduced in many magnesium-depleted patients.[17] Thus the mineral abnormalities can include reduced serum concentrations of magnesium, calcium, 1,25-dihydroxyvitamin D_3, and PTH, all of which may be restored to normal by infusion or oral ingestion of magnesium. Therapy with magnesium oxide 1–5 g (50–250 mequiv.) in three divided doses daily causes the following changes: increased serum and urine magnesium and calcium, reduced serum phosphate, increased urine phosphate, and increased serum 1,25-dihydroxyvitamin D_3 and PTH.[18] Although the doses of oral magnesium required vary from one patient to the next, improved magnesium homeostasis can usually be achieved. Magnesium should be taken three to four times a day as magnesium oxide or magnesium pyrrolidine carboxylate because urinary magnesium losses occur continuously, and patients who have magnesium wasting continue to excrete large amounts until they are magnesium depleted.

Infants who have hypomagnesemic tetany should receive 0.4–0.8 mg/kg of a 50% solution of magnesium sulfate either intramuscularly or intravenously. Intravenous magnesium should be infused slowly with monitoring, and calcium gluconate should be on hand to reverse dysrhythmias. Finally, renal magnesium wasting can occur in conjunction with varying degrees of renal insufficiency,[18] and these patients may also require oral vitamin D analogs and calcium salts. A daily dose of 0.25–1.0 μg of 1,25-dihydroxyvitamin D_3 may be needed as well as calcium lactate, carbonate, or acetate.

Fanconi syndrome

Fanconi syndrome is a generalized disorder of proximal tubule function that can occur as either a primary disorder

Table 50.4 Hereditary disorders associated with Fanconi syndrome

Primary or idiopathic (no identifiable associated disorder)
Familial
Sporadic

Hereditary
Cystinosis (Lignac–Fanconi disease) or infantile nephropathic cystinosis
Lowe syndrome
Hereditary fructose intolerance
Tyrosinemia: type 1 (tryosinosis)
Galactosemia
Glycogen storage disease (untyped): defect in GLUT-4
Wilson disease
Subacute necrotizing encephalomyelopathy (Leigh syndrome)
Hereditary mitochondrial myopathy with lactic acidemia
Other conditions
    Familial nephrotic syndrome (focal sclerosing glomerulonephritis): defective NHP2
    Metachromatic leukodystrophy
    Hereditary nephritis (Alport syndrome)
    Medullary cystic disease

or secondary to a number of inherited conditions[2,4] (Table 50.4). Patients always show hyperexcretion of substances that are reabsorbed and diminished excretion of substances that are secreted.[1-4] The manifestations of Fanconi syndrome often vary depending on the underlying disorder leading to tubular disease. Tubular dysfunction typically involves glycosuria, phosphaturia, generalized aminoaciduria, proteinuria, polyuria, and proximal renal tubular acidosis (RTA). Other substances frequently excreted in increased quantities include uric acid, sodium, potassium, magnesium, citrate, and proteins of molecular mass < 45 000 kDa.[16] Because of phosphaturia, hypophosphatemia, and sometimes renal insufficiency, various bone disorders may be found, including rickets, osteomalacia, osteoporosis, and osteitis fibrosa.[19] Adult patients may have severe osteomalacia and may present with intense bone pain and muscle weakness.[1-4] Symptomatic hypokalemia is manifested by muscle weakness, growth failure, dehydration, unexplained fevers due to volume depletion, and profound metabolic acidosis.[19]

Therapy of Fanconi syndrome depends on the underlying etiology. Symptomatic therapy includes large doses of oral alkali (sodium bicarbonate, often as much as 10–15 mequiv./kg/day), phosphate supplements given four to five times daily, a vitamin D analog, adequate water, and adequate sodium and potassium replacement to correct volume depletion and signs of hypokalemia. Indomethacin may reduce urine volume.[20]

Patients with infantile nephropathic cystinosis have specific therapeutic needs. Cystine deposition within the cornea leads to photophobia, which may be improved with dark glasses, wetting solutions, and the possible use of cyteamine eye drops that can dissolve cystine deposits.[19] The defect in this disorder involves reduction in the rate of efflux of cystine, but not cysteine, from within a lysosomal compartment; the oxidized (–S–S–) form of this sulfur amino acid remains trapped, thus forming intralysosomal cystine crystals. The defective gene encodes the lysosomal cystine transporter.[16] At least two cystine-depleting agents, cysteamine and pantethine (its precursor), can be used to deplete the lysosomes, creating mixed disulfides with cystine that are freely permeable across the lysosomal membrane. The reduced SH form is then free to exit the lysosome as well and thus intracellular cystine falls.[19,20] The results of the Collaborative Cysteamine Study indicated that 98 patients receiving cysteamine showed a real slowing of the progression toward renal failure and improved linear growth compared with more than 100 historic control cystinotic subjects.[19] A recent analysis of 88 patients followed for more than 10 years identified not only uremia but also hepatomegaly, splenomegaly, neurologic disease, progressive ocular disease, and continuing poor growth despite a functioning renal allograft.[19] These results suggest the need for continuing cysteamine therapy, but this is only now being addressed by clinical trials. The drug Cystagon (cysteamine bitartrate) in capsule form has been approved by the Food and Drug Administration for use in patients with cystinosis at a daily dose of 1.3 g/m^2. Patient compliance should be assured by measuring leukocyte cystine content.[19]

Because of glandular cystine crystal deposition, hypothyroidism is universal in cystinosis and therefore low-dose thyroxine is needed to prevent the clinical features of this endocrinopathy.[4] The dose of L-thyroxine is chosen by determining the amount needed to suppress thyroid-stimulating hormone levels into the normal range. Cystinotic patients have also been shown to lose massive amounts of carnitine and therefore have a deficiency of this acyl-transporting compound. Oral carnitine therapy may reverse muscle carnitine depletion and the histologic features of the deficiency.[4] Finally, recall that cystinosis is a lifelong disorder with continuing cystine deposition. The long-term involvement of organs other than the kidney is only now being appreciated since long-term survivors of renal transplantation became available for study.[19,20]

Lowe syndrome is an X-linked disorder that presents with cataracts, glaucoma, growth impairment, hypotonia, severe mental retardation, and features of Fanconi syndrome. It is caused by defective inositol polyphosphate 5′-phosphatase activity, presumably involving the phosphatidylinositol signaling pathway.[1] Treatment is directed at correcting the metabolic derangements of Fanconi syndrome. Renal dysfunction begins with tubular dysfunction but can progress to chronic renal failure. Tubular dysfunction eventually diminishes because of the decline in GFR. Patients with this syndrome usually die of infection or renal insufficiency but have a lifelong need for ophthalmologic evaluations. Most patients are boys, although girls with Lowe syndrome have been described due to chromosomal translocations.[1,4]

Patients with galactosemia, an autosomal recessive deficiency of galactose 1-phosphate uridyltransferase, develop a Fanconi syndrome that is totally reversible when patients are maintained on a galactose- and lactose-free diet.[4] This diet is a lifelong necessity.

Tyrosinosis is due to an autosomal recessive defect in fumarylacetoacetate fumaryl hydrolase, with the accumulation of succinylacetone and succinylacetoacetate, which in turn leads to hepatomegaly, cirrhosis, and full-blown Fanconi syndrome.[1,2] The disorder has a poor prognosis and usually results in death in children due to cirrhosis and/or hepatoblastomas. A low-tyrosine, low-phenylalanine diet can treat the Fanconi syndrome and prevent rickets but does not prevent cirrhosis. The definitive form of therapy is liver transplant or liver–kidney transplant.[21]

Hereditary fructose intolerance is an autosomal recessive disorder caused by mutations in the aldolase B gene, resulting in diminished aldolase B activity in the liver, renal cortex, and small intestine and leading to accumulation of fructose 1-phosphate.[1,4] Diagnostic clues to this condition include an aversion to sweets, a lack of dental caries, and hepatomegaly. Development of Fanconi syndrome is temporally related to exposure to fructose, and treatment is directed at assiduously avoiding this sugar in the diet. As in galactosemia, development of Fanconi syndrome may occur within a few minutes to hours after ingestion of fructose and patients may become gravely ill with profound acidosis. Patients generally quickly recognize the advantage of avoiding fructose-containing foods.

Fanconi syndrome can be seen in certain children with an as yet untyped glycogen storage disease that is associated with hepatomegaly, massive glycosuria, glucose and galactose intolerance, and a mutation in the glucose transporter GLUT-4.[16,22] These patients are also profoundly growth retarded. Treatment consists of controlling the symptoms of Fanconi syndrome with sodium bicarbonate, phosphate, potassium chloride, and vitamin D, and patients tend to improve with age.

Wilson disease is an autosomal recessive hepatocellular disorder of copper metabolism that presents with hepatomegaly and Fanconi syndrome. Copper deposits are noted in the brain, liver, and kidney.[1] Patients with Wilson disease also have, in addition to proximal RTA, findings that can only be explained as distal RTA, and urinary calculi are common. Hypoparathyroidism has also been described in a single patient with Wilson disease, possibly related to copper deposits in the parathyroid gland.[4] Therapy of Wilson disease consists of D-penicillamine, which can be troublesome in some patients, as noted in the section on cystinuria. Whenever D-penicillamine cannot be used, triethylene tetramine dihydrochloride can be used without fear of the same allergic manifestations.[4]

When Fanconi syndrome appears in conjunction with the nephrotic syndrome, it is usually found in association with a familial pattern and with focal segmental glomerulosclerosis. Tubular atrophy and interstitial fibrosis are prominent.[4] Treatment of this glomerulopathy is unsatisfactory and features of Fanconi syndrome continue until renal failure ensues.

Finally, Fanconi syndrome is associated with mutations of the mitochondrial genome,[23] particularly if the respiratory chain is affected. Treatment is symptomatic as described above.

Bartter syndrome

Bartter syndrome is characterized by hyperplasia of the juxtaglomerular apparatus, increased circulating angiotensin II concentrations, normal blood pressure with diminished pressor response to infused angiotensin II, hyperaldosteronism, hypokalemic alkalosis, and vasopressin-resistant polyuria.[2,4] This condition is very heterogeneous and most patients present in childhood or adolescence, although a presentation over the age of 40 has occurred.[4] The inheritance pattern is sporadic or autosomal recessive.

Recent progress in molecular biology has clarified certain aspects of this syndrome.[16,24–26] The genetic mutations that underlie Bartter syndrome involve defects in (1) the luminal $Na^+/K^+/2Cl^-$ cotransporter (NKCC2), (2) the outwardly directed K^+ channel (ROMK), or (3) the Cl^- channel (ClCNKB). These transport proteins are all located in the thick ascending limb of the loop of Henle: NKCC2 and ROMK are in the luminal membrane and ClCNKB in the peritubular membrane.[25] Gitelman syndrome is caused by a mutation in the thiazide-sensitive Na^+/Cl^- cotransporter in the lumen of the distal convoluted tubule. Differences in the function of these four ion-transport systems help explain the clinical heterogeneity in Bartter and Gitelman syndromes.

Children may present with growth failure as well as weakness, muscle cramps, polyuria, and abdominal pain; delayed or slowed mentation is seen in all children with Bartter syndrome. The laboratory features are also heterogeneous in that patients show variable degrees of increased urinary losses of potassium, sodium, chloride, magnesium, calcium, and kallikrein, and increased production and excretion of prostaglandin $(PG)E_2$.[15] The differential diagnosis includes Fanconi syndrome, incomplete distal RTA, use of diuretics, abuse of laxatives, cyclical vomiting, chloride-deficient diets, and cystic fibrosis. Alkalosis is associated with administration of impermeable anions, mineralocorticoid excess, and primary renal magnesium wasting (Gitelman syndrome).[25] Because of abnormalities in the concentration of prostaglandins in plasma and urine, it was once felt that the primary defect was one of prostaglandin metabolism;[4] this was before the genetic basis was understood.[15,25] Elevated prostaglandin levels could potentially explain vasodilation, the lack of responsiveness to pressors, the inhibition of chloride transport in the loop of Henle, and potassium hyperexcretion and metabolic alkalosis. However, prostaglandin inhibition does not always correct the defect in these patients, and continued use of prostaglandin inhibitors may not result in continued therapeutic benefit.[15] Moreover, in disorders that mimic familial Bartter syndrome, such as bulimia, chronic diuretic abuse, and chloride-deficient formula-induced disease, the same plasma and urine profile is found.[4]

Recent studies suggest that at least five different pathogenetic mechanisms produce this syndrome.[24]

1. Patients with isolated potassium transport defects with normal sodium and chloride reabsorption.

2. Sodium and chloride transport defects may occur at multiple sites along with nephron. Urinary potassium loss would be the result of enhanced Na^+/K^+ exchange in the distal tubule and increased urine flow within the tubule lumen.

3. Perhaps the most common variant is a defect in chloride transport and hence in sodium transport by the thick ascending limb of the loop of Henle. Potassium loss would take place by the same mechanism as in (2) above.

4. As mentioned previously, magnesium-wasting syndromes can lead to virtually all the features of Bartter syndrome, with prominent renal potassium wasting.[20]

5. Patients with increased production of PGE_2 and $PGF_{2\alpha}$ can have abnormalities of chloride reabsorption and hypokalemia as a result of renal hyperprostaglandinism.[24] These patients do not have hyperplasia of the juxtaglomerular apparatus but show hypertrophy of prostaglandin-producing cells[24] or dense cytoplasm, compact mitochondria, pyknotic nuclei, and hypertrophy of the basement membrane. This latter group does not appear to have abnormal chloride reabsorption and has a defective ROMK.

Therapy of Bartter syndrome is problematic.[19,20,24] Potassium supplementation is necessary and large doses of potassium chloride may be required. Prostaglandin inhibitors have short-lived effects when used alone, unless the patients have one of the hyperprostaglandinuric syndromes;[24] indomethacin has been used most often. The prostaglandin inhibitors appear to work best in most patients if they are considered an adjunct therapy that limits the need for potassium chloride supplements.[19,20,24]

Patients with Gitelman syndrome have renal magnesium wasting, hypokalemia, metabolic alkalosis, and hypocalciuria.[7,16,26] Some patients may have a tendency toward hypocalcemia.[26] If magnesium wasting is present, magnesium supplementation is clearly indicated, as noted previously. Supplementation with magnesium oxide or magnesium pyrrolidine carboxylate 30 mmol/L daily improves hypomagnesemia, sometimes corrects hypokalemia, and raises hypocalcemia.[26]

Patients with either Bartter or Gitelman syndrome are difficult to treat, require frequent serum chemistry tests, and compliance is essential. In a subset of patients the use of supplemental potassium chloride and treatment with a prostaglandin synthetase inhibitor may not fully correct hypokalemia, which should be the primary aim of therapy. In these cases, a potassium-sparing diuretic such as amiloride or triamterene in the usual doses can be useful.[4,7] If constantly applied, these therapeutic approaches usually result in improved growth and development in children and improved symptoms in adult patients with Bartter syndrome.

Liddle syndrome

Liddle syndrome is a rare familial cause of hypokalemia associated with failure to thrive, sodium retention, hypertension, and suppressed plasma levels of renin and aldosterone.[27] Patients with this syndrome have an enhanced influx of sodium into red blood cells, although there does not appear to be a generalized increase in sodium permeability across cell membranes, as the ratio of sodium to potassium in saliva and sweat is normal and fecal potassium wasting is not apparent.[4] A report of amelioration of the syndrome after renal transplantation suggests that the disorder is not related to an unidentified mineralocorticoid but is rather a transport defect. The specific transport defect is located in the cytoplasmic region of the β or γ subunit of the sodium channel or the amiloride-sensitive channel in the distal nephron segments.[27,28] Sodium reabsorption is excessive even with dietary salt excess. Therapy is aimed at reducing dietary salt intake and the use of amiloride.[27]

Chloride shunt syndrome

The chloride shunt syndrome (type 2 pseudohypoaldosteronism) is almost a mirror image of Bartter syndrome. The principal metabolic derangement is a hyperkalemic, hyperchloremic metabolic acidosis.[29] The primary etiology is unknown. Clinical variants include Gordon syndrome and Spitzer–Weinstein syndrome.[4] Constant features of Gordon syndrome include hyperkalemia, hyperchloremia, normal GFR, and, in adults, hypertension. The hypertension is associated with low plasma aldosterone and plasma renin activity; blood pressure is often normal in children. Muscular weakness may be a presenting symptom of this disorder and hypercalciuria is sometimes present. Hypotheses proposed to explain Gordon syndrome include hypoprostaglandinism and an insensitivity of the proximal tubule to atrial natriuretic peptide. However, none has been proven.[30,31]

A similar syndrome of metabolic acidosis with hyperkalemia was described by Spitzer et al in 1973 and Weinstein et al in 1974.[32,33] This entity is also associated with short stature and has been called Spitzer–Weinstein syndrome. The proposed defect is one of decreased distal tubular potassium secretion with a secondary metabolic acidosis. Thiazide diuretics have been used in the management of both Gordon syndrome and Spitzer–Weinstein syndrome, with variable results.

References

1. Section on membrane transport systems. *In* Scriver CR, Beaudet AL, Valle D, et al (eds): The Metabolic Basis of Inherited Disease, 8th edn. New York: McGraw Hill, 2001, Vol IV, pp 4891–5240.
2. Chesney RW, Novello AC: Defects of renal tubular transport. *In* Massry SG, Glassock R (eds): Textbook of Nephrology, 4th edn. Baltimore: Lippincott, Williams and Wilkins, 2001, pp 462–476.
3. Malandro MS, Kilberg MS: Molecular biology of mammalian amino acid transporters. Annu Rev Biochem 1996;65:305–336.
4. Chesney RW: Inherited renal tubular disorders. *In* Bennett C, Plum F (eds): Cecil Textbook of Medicine, 21st edn. Philadelphia: WB Saunders, 1999, pp 594–599.
5. Chow GK, Streem SB: Medical treatment of cystinuria: results of contemporary clinical practice. J Urol 1996;156:1576–1578.
6. Chesney RW: Cystinuria. *In* Glassock R (ed): Current Therapy in Nephrology and Hypertension, 5th edn. St Louis: BC Decker, 2000, pp 96–98.
7. Stokes JB: Disorders of the epithelial sodium channel: insights into the regulation of volume and blood pressure. Kidney Int 1999;56:2318–2333.
8. Glorieux FM, Scriver CR, Reade TM, Goldman H, Roseborough A: Use of phosphate and vitamin D to prevent dwarfism and rickets in X-linked hypophosphatemic rickets. N Engl J Med 1972;287:481–485.
9. Latta K, Hisano S, Chan JCM: Therapeutics of X-linked hypophosphatemic rickets. Pediatr Nephrol 1993;7:744–748.
10. Polisson RB, Martinez SJ, Khoury M, et al: Calcification of enthesis associated with X-linked hypophosphatemic osteomalacia. N Engl J Med 1985;313:1–6.
11. Wilson DM, Lee PDK, Morris AH, et al: Growth hormone therapy in hypophosphatemic rickets. Am J Dis Child 1991;145:1165–1170.
12. Teder M, Modai D, Samuel R, et al: Hereditary hypophosphatemic rickets with hypercalciuria. N Engl J Med 1985;312:611–616.
13. Kumar R: Inhibition of renal phosphate transport by a tumor product in a patient with oncogenic osteomalacia. N Engl J Med 1994;330:1645–1649.
14. Gitelman HJ, Graham JB, Welt LG: A new familial disorder characterized by hypokalemia and hypomagnesemia. Trans Assoc Am Physicians 1966;79:221–228.
15. Lemmink HH, van den Heuvel LPW, van Dijk HA, et al: Linkage of Gitelman syndrome to the thiazide-sensitive sodium-chloride cotransporter gene with identification of mutations in Dutch families. Pediatr Nephrol 1996;10:403–407.
16. Zelikovic I: Molecular pathophysiology of tubular transport disorders. Pediatr Nephrol 2001;16:919–935.
17. Carpenter TO, Key LL Jr: Disorders of the metabolism of calcium, phosphorus, and other divalent ions. *In* Ichikawa I (ed): Pediatric Textbook of Fluids and Electrolytes. Baltimore: Williams and Wilkins, 1990, pp 237–268.
18. Zelikovic I, Dabbagh S, Friedman AL, Goelzer ML, Chesney RW: Severe renal osteodystrophy without elevated serum immunoreactive parathyroid hormone concentrations in hypomagnesemia due to renal magnesium wasting. Pediatrics 1987;79:403–409.
19. Schneider JA, Clark KF, Green AA, et al: Recent advances in the treatment of cystinosis. J Inherit Metab Dis 1995;18:387–397.
20. Clark KF: A comparative study of indomethacin for treatment of the Fanconi syndrome in cystinosis. J Rare Dis 1996;2:5–12.
21. Cochat P, Guinbaud P, Baverel G: Renal involvement in type I tyrosinemia. Arch Pediatr 1994;1:417–418.
22. Chesney RW, Kaplan BS, Teitel D, et al: Metabolic abnormalities in the idiopathic Fanconi syndrome: studies of carbohydrate metabolism in two patients. Pediatrics 1981;67:113–118.
23. Singh PJ, Santella RS, Zawada ET: Mitochondrial genome mutations and kidney disease. Am J Kidney Dis 1996;28:140–146.
24. Karolyi L, Ziegler A, Pollak M, et al: Gitelman's syndrome is genetically distinct from other forms of Bartter's syndrome. Pediatr Nephrol 1996;10:551–554.
25. Calo L, Punzi L, Semplicini A: Hypomagnesemia and chondrocalcinosis in Bartter's and Gitelman's syndrome: review of pathogenetic mechanisms. Am J Nephrol 2000;20:347–350.
26. Bettinelli A, Basilico E, Metta MG, Borella P, Jaeger P, Bianchetti MG: Magnesium supplementation in Gitelman syndrome. Pediatr Nephrol 1999;13:311–314.
27. Warnock DG: Polymorphism with beta subunit and Na⁺ transport. J Am Soc Nephrol 1996;7:2490–2494.
28. Kamynina E, Debonneville C, Hirt RP, Staub O: Liddle's syndrome: a novel mouse Nedd4 isoform regulates the activity of the epithelial Na⁺ channel. Kidney Int 2001;60:466–471.
29. Rodriquez-Soriano J, Valle A, Dominguez MJ: "Chloride-shunt" syndrome: an overlooked cause of renal hypercalciuria. Pediatr Nephrol 1989;3:113–121.
30. Klemm SA, Hornych A, Tunny TJ, Gordon RD: The syndrome of hypertension and hyperkalemia with normal glomerular filtration rate: is there a deficiency in vasodilator prostaglandins? Clin Exp Pharmacol Physiol 1991;18:309–313.
31. Klemm SA, Gordon RD, Tunny TJ, et al. Levels of atrial natriuretic peptide are not always consistent with atrial pressure: is there alternative regulation as evidenced in Gordon's and Bartter's syndromes? Clin Exp Pharmacol Physiol 1989;16:269–274.
32. Spitzer A, Edelmann CM Jr, Goldberg LD, Henneman PH: Short stature, hyperkalemia and acidosis: A defect in renal transport of potassium. Kidney Int 1973;3:251–257.
33. Weinstein SF, Allan DM, Mendoza S: Hyperkalemia, acidosis, and short stature associated with a defect in renal potassium excretion. J Pediatr 1974;85:355–358.

Prospects for Gene Therapy

Vikas P. Sukhatme and Enyu Imai

The primary goal of this chapter is to discuss prospects for gene therapy in the kidney.[1–4] We start with a brief review of general concepts and vectors, and then cite specific considerations unique to the kidney that affect gene therapeutic approaches to renal diseases. A review of current data on gene delivery to the kidney follows. We conclude with a discussion of potential applications.

General concepts

In-vivo vs. ex-vivo therapy

The complexities, both medical and ethical, of germline or in-utero gene therapy make it likely that these modalities will be preceded by clinical experience in somatic cell therapy administered postnatally to nongermline cells. Such therapy can be in vivo or ex vivo. In-vivo gene therapy utilizes either viral or nonviral vectors for gene delivery: the therapy is treated as a drug to be administered systemically or perhaps regionally. Even localized delivery can have systemic effects, e.g. skeletal muscle has been used as a tissue for gene transfer.[5] Ex-vivo gene therapy refers to the genetic modification of cells or possibly organs by gene transfer outside the body and the subsequent placement of genetically engineered tissue into a patient. The source of cells may be from the patient or be generic, i.e. a human or animal cell appropriately altered genetically. The major advantages of in-vivo therapy are simplicity and cost. However, if "universal" donor cells could be developed and/or the problems of (xeno)transplantation surmounted, the cost of ex-vivo therapy would decline.

General considerations

Three critical general considerations underlie any gene therapy protocol whether in vivo or ex vivo: delivery, expression, and safety.[6] Delivery refers to the ability to introduce the gene of interest where it is needed to affect the disease process. How many cells need to be transduced and in what tissues? How promiscuous is the delivery system? What unintended targets are being transduced? Expression entails an assessment of the level of therapeutic protein made. Is it enough to achieve the desired biologic effect? How tightly need levels be regulated? How long does expression last and what limits duration? Safety issues can arise in the patient as well as in the population at large. "Toxic" effects such as inflammation, injury, and other mechanisms leading to functional damage to the transduced organ are particularly important issues for the therapy of chronic disorders. All these considerations have to be examined in the context of the disease in question: its severity and time-course (chronic vs. acute), alternative treatments available, organs affected, genetics, pathophysiology, etc. Moreover, careful consideration needs to be given to selecting patients at certain stages of disease or perhaps those with the worst prognosis when gene transfer protocols are initially devised, so as to carefully weigh risks and benefits.

Vectors

Since excellent detailed articles exist on this subject, only a brief summary is provided. Clearly, vector development (viral and nonviral) that achieves suitable delivery, expression, and safety profiles will be critical if gene therapy is to proceed to the clinic. The advantages and disadvantages of various systems have been discussed extensively[1–4] and are subjects of intense ongoing investigations. Briefly, retroviruses are well suited for ex-vivo applications because of their broad host range and their ability to give long-term expression through proviral integration into the host genome. However, in-vivo fragility and low titers (typically 10^5–10^6 transducing units/mL but up to 10^9/mL in a stock of concentrated pseudotyped vector) limit in-vivo applications, as does the requirement for cell division for DNA integration. Interestingly, HIV, a member of the lentivirus subclass of retroviruses, can infect nondividing cells, and lentiviral-based vectors have successfully transduced nondividing cells.[7]

Adenoviruses are DNA viruses that have a wide host range and survive robustly in the circulation.[8] High titers (~ 10^{13}/mL) of replication-deficient adenovirus can easily be generated and the virus can infect nondividing cells. Duration of expression in vivo is largely limited by a T-cell response to low levels of adenoviral proteins and transgene (if nonself) produced in the transduced cell. Newer versions of the virus with E3 deleted (along with E1) allow inserts up to 8 kb in size. The E2 mutant version is less immunogenic. Recent E4 deletion variants accept an additional 3 kb of insert DNA and may turn out to be even less immunogenic. The ideal vector would contain only the cis elements required for packaging, namely the so-called inverted terminal repeats and the packaging signal, and progress toward the construction of such a vector has been reported.[9] However, these advances do not circumvent the antibody response to adenoviral proteins, which precludes secondary infection with the same serotype but not with a different serotype.[10] The nonspecific inflammatory response (that can be produced even by empty virus) may also limit the amount of adenovirus that can be delivered.

Recombinant adeno-associated virus (AAV) has emerged as an attractive alternative to retroviral vectors. AAV, a parvovirus, is a single-stranded DNA virus. It has the ability to integrate specifically into chromosome 19 in humans.[11] However, this property is lost in a recombinant viral vector devoid of certain AAV genes.[12] AAV can infect both nondividing and dividing cells. Infection has not been associated with toxicity. Replication of wild-type AAV requires a helper virus such as adenovirus. Therefore, the possibility of contamination needs to be addressed carefully. One major drawback is that the generation of recombinant AAV is generally intricate and results in low viral titers.

Naked plasmids, liposomes, modified liposomes with peptides, and hemagglutinating virus of Japan (HVJ)-liposomes have been used as "nonviral" vectors. Such vectors are relatively nontoxic and nonimmunogenic, but generally transduction efficiency in vivo is far less than with adenoviruses. Moreover, duration is usually transient (days), although use of replication origins and nuclear retention signals have extended this period to 8 weeks.[13] The HVJ-liposome method was used for gene transfer to various tissues and organs and showed significant transfection efficiency.[14] However, the procedure is still hampered by the fact that the viral genome has to be efficiently destroyed by ultraviolet irradiation.

Recently, high-efficiency transfection by electroporation-mediated gene transfer has been developed. Gene therapy targeting skeletal muscle has been extensively studied in various experimental models. Several electric pulses at 70–100 V of short duration (50 ms) are usually used for gene transfer to skeletal muscle.[5,15] Plasma concentration of the transgene product is sufficiently high to achieve a biologic action (200 ng/mL) using this method.[16]

In summary, there is an emerging realization that significant improvements in vector design are needed in order to ensure the success of many contemplated gene therapy protocols.

Considerations that apply to renal disease

The kidney is a complex organ whose function depends on its architecture. As a consequence, it is not possible to introduce genes into all its various cell types by a single method. In principle, there are four routes to effect gene transfer into the kidney whether by ex-vivo or in-vivo methods: via the renal artery, subcapsularly, retrograde from the ureter, or by parenchymal injection. Combinations of these routes can also be considered. It is conceivable that introduction of cells or vectors into the peripheral circulation could be targeted to the kidney. Recently, Pasqualini and Ruoslahti[17] have used a phase display library to identify sequences that selectively bind to renal vasculature in vivo.

Clearly, an initial database, describing which cells are transduced by various gene therapy vectors, is needed urgently. In building this database, it should be borne in mind that delivery in a disease context may differ from that in a normal kidney. The reasons for this can be many: different populations of dividing cells, the presence of an inflammatory response, alterations in vascular permeability, etc. Thus, it will be important to generate data in an appropriate preclinical disease model.

Given that overexpression of a therapeutic protein may cause harmful effects in experimental and clinical settings, control of transgene expression is an important issue to be considered. Kitamura[18] introduced a tetracycline-dependent, reversible on–off system into mesangial cells. He inserted the tetracycline-controlled transactivator (tTA) gene in a regulator plasmid and cotransfected it with a reporter plasmid encoding the LacZ gene driven by a promoter containing a tTA binding element. Furthermore, Kitamura and Kawachi[19] created a gene expression system responsive to "inflammation" in mesangial cells using so-called CArG box elements. They placed three CArG box copies in the promoter region of the LacZ reporter gene and transfected this construct into mesangial cells. β-Galactosidase activity was increased in about 40% of the glomeruli where the mesangial cells lodged for up to 3 days after induction of Thy-1 glomerulonephritis.

Data on gene transfer into the kidney

Tomita[20] has utilized a Sendai virus, HVJ, for in-vivo gene therapy. Plasmid DNA and a nucleoprotein coencapsulated in liposomes was fused to the inactivated Sendai virus. Gene transfer was accomplished by inserting a catheter proximal to the right renal artery with the abdominal aorta clipped distally beneath the left renal artery. Four days after injection of the liposome suspension containing the SV40 T antigen reporter gene, SV40 T antigen was detected immunohistochemically in 15% of glomerular cells, although it was difficult to ascertain whether expression was in endothelial, epithelial, or mesangial cells. Interestingly, no expression of the foreign gene was detected outside the glomerulus. Expression of the T antigen declined rapidly over the ensuing 2–3 days. The success of this method for gene transfer was predicated on the ability of the HMG1 nucleoprotein, a high-mobility group 1 nonhistone nuclear protein, to enhance plasmid DNA passage into nuclei.[21] The HVJ virus contains a fusogenic protein on its surface and is responsible for neutral pH-mediated cell fusion. This approach was used to "investigate" glomerular pathophysiology by Isaka et al.[22] The transfer of cDNAs for transforming growth factor β1 (TGF-β1) and platelet-derived growth factor (PDGF) into the rat renal artery resulted in the expected phenotypic changes in mesangial cells.[22]

Tsujie et al[23] used electroporation to target gene transfer to the kidney. A LacZ gene-containing plasmid was injected into the renal artery followed by electroporation; 75% of glomeruli expressed β-galactosidase. LacZ gene was mainly expressed in mesangial cells. No tissue damage was observed in the kidney after the procedure.

Another approach to in-vivo gene therapy involves the use of retroviruses. Fine and colleagues[24] obtained no gene transfer into a normal kidney, which generally has a very low mitotic index. However, in a kidney subjected to toxic doses of folic acid, thereby leading to a significant amount of tubular damage and subsequent proliferation, β-galactosidase staining was seen in some proximal cells when a retrovirus containing the β-galactosidase gene was utilized.

Moullier[25] was the first to report adenoviral-mediated gene transfer into the rat kidney using two methods. The first involved selective perfusion into the renal artery of a replication-deficient adenovirus carrying the β-galactosidase gene, which resulted in an occasional blue proximal tubular cell. No expression was observed in vasculature. In contrast to our method (see below),[26] no venous clamping was utilized. More dramatic was the data using retrograde injection into the renal pelvis: many collecting tubular cells showed significant gene transfer. Expression lasted typically for 1–2 weeks.

Thompson and colleagues[27] have utilized adenovirus as an adjunct for gene transfer. Their scheme is the first genetic transfection of isolated human kidneys under conditions of organ preservation. By utilizing an adenovirus polylysine DNA complex, they were able to insert a cDNA expression vector encoding β-galactosidase into the intact human kidney. In their protocol, a pump was used to maintain pulsatile perfusion. A solution of adenoviral particles admixed with polylysine and the expression cassette was perfused over a period of approximately 2 days. Immunohistochemical and in-situ enzymatic analyses showed that gene delivery and expression were localized to a significant fraction of proximal tubular epithelial cells. Though expression appeared to be patchy, it was largely relegated to the cortex in proximal tubular epithelial cells. The investigators also conducted in-situ hybridization analysis using a β-galactosidase antisense probe, although no sense probe controls were shown. Of some concern is the fact that the pattern noted by in-situ hybridization appeared to be either interstitial or vascular

and not tubular as suggested by the enzymatic analysis. Moreover, the controls used were pretransfection kidneys. No controls were done in the absence of either adenovirus or polylysine. Finally, the investigators used reverse transcriptase polymerase chain reaction (RT-PCR) to demonstrate β-galactosidase mRNA expressed in the biopsied kidney at various time points following gene transfer into the isolated perfused kidney. These findings and the antegrade data of Moullier raise the intriguing question of how adenovirus infects tubular cells when injected into the renal artery. Is virus able to traverse the glomerular basement membrane (GBM) or does it pass through the postglomerular capillary network or vasa recta and escape from the vascular bed?

Tryggvason and colleagues[28] have also reported the use of a perfusion system for adenoviral gene transfer into the kidney. Several models were used. They showed that isolated glomeruli can be very efficiently transduced by adenovirus in culture. Secondly, they isolated a pig kidney in vivo and perfused it for 2–12 h with a replication-deficient adenovirus. They then reconnected the kidney and examined expression 3 days later. Marked expression noted by histochemistry was largely located in the glomeruli, although the cell type could not be determined. They also showed that the kidney could be maintained ex vivo with continuous perfusion over this period of time and that examination on the day following perfusion demonstrated glomerular gene transfer. These data are the first to report glomerular gene transfer using recombinant adenovirus. Although no in-situ hybridizations were performed in these studies, it is unlikely that their data represent endogenous β-galactosidase activity because that activity is not known to be localized in the glomerulus.

Zhu et al[26] have demonstrated adenovirus-mediated gene transfer into the normal rat kidney. Their technique utilized two manipulations: (1) the use of cold incubation (following antegrade injection and cross-clamping) to prolong contact time of the adenovirus while limiting ischemic injury; and (2) the use of vasodilators. These two methods resulted in different localization patterns of transferred gene expression. They were able to transfer successfully a β-galactosidase reporter gene into the vasculature without ischemic injury to the kidney. Transfer occurred largely in the cortex (periglomerular capillaries) when cold was used alone, whereas with the use of cold and vasodilators transfer was accomplished efficiently into the outer medulla in both the inner and outer stripe.

It is unclear why various studies have produced such remarkably different results. Details of the protocol may well be responsible for the differences noted, e.g. injection vs. injection with clamping[26] vs. perfusion.[28] It will be particularly important to dissect these issues in the future.

Lipkowitz et al[29] reported that AAV delivered in vivo by intraparenchymal injection resulted in at least 3 months of reporter gene expression in tubular epithelial cells but not in glomeruli or vascular cells. The expression was limited to the vicinity of the injection.

Considering ex-vivo kidney transfer, as noted earlier Kitamura[30] reported on mesangial cells that had been transduced with a β-galactosidase-expressing plasmid. These cells were then injected into the left renal artery and the effects examined. Expression was noted throughout the kidney in about 50% of glomeruli and was detectable over a 4–8 week period. The mesangial cells lodged in the glomerular capillary. Interestingly, they expressed β-galactosidase at high levels when amplified "in situ" by introduction of an anti-Thy-1 antibody. Kitamura and Suto[31] demonstrated that genetically modified macrophages accumulated in inflamed glomeruli in experimental glomerulonephritis. Yokoo et al[32] used CD11/CD18-positive monocyte lineage cells of bone-marrow origin as a vector for delivery to inflamed glomeruli. After intraperitoneal injection, genetically modified monocytes accumulated in glomeruli of mice treated with lipopolysaccharide. This method may target inflamed glomeruli selectively.

Kelley et al[33] have reported on tubular cells injected subcapsularly in the mouse kidney. Various cytokine genes were expressed for weeks or months. The expected phenotypic effects of these proteins were noted. Rabbit fibroblasts transferred with a human growth hormone construct and injected subcapsularly into a nude mouse continue to express human growth hormone for over a year.[34] The implant site was particularly well vascularized.

Ex-vivo systems suffer from the obvious need to procure cells from the patient or a suitable "universal donor." If heterotransplants are utilized, attendant problems of rejection will need to be addressed.

Applications in the kidney

Kidney transplantation

Genes could be transferred into the kidney (or other organs) ex vivo or in vivo just prior to harvest from a brain-dead patient. If adenovirus was used, as in the protocol above,[26] it could be flushed out prior to organ removal from the body or prior to transplantation, so that inadvertent delivery to other sites would be of no consequence. Moreover, the fact that gene delivery occurs into the vasculature would be of clear benefit in the transplant situation. Three types of gene products could be delivered: those designed to decrease organ antigenicity and/or to induce tolerance, those designed to blockade the effector arm of the immune system, or those designed to improve organ preservation. Candidate genes (given individually or in combination) (see review in reference 35) might include donor MHC class I or II molecules,[36,37] CTLA4-Ig,[38,39] interleukin 4 (IL-4), (viral) IL-10,[40] Fas ligand, galactin,[41] adenoviral E3 gene,[42] soluble tumor necrosis factor (TNF) receptor, IL-1 receptor antagonist, soluble cell adhesion molecules (vascular cell adhesion molecule or intercellular cell adhesion molecule), TGF-β,[43] hepatocyte growth factor (HGF),[44] and catalase.[45] The Fas ligand has shown dramatic results in a model of islet cell allogeneic transplant.[46] It is also conceivable that molecules such as Fas ligand, aimed at eliminating effector T cells, may find use in the treatment of autoimmune diseases affecting the kidney. Tomasoni et al[47] reported the

use of CTLA4-Ig for gene therapy in a rat model of acute rejection. They introduced an adenoviral vector encoding CTLA4-Ig into a Norway rat kidney ex vivo and transplanted the kidney into a Lewis rat. Kidney survival was significantly prolonged to 20–40 days in rats receiving the CTLA4-Ig gene therapy, whereas control rats died in a week. Azuma et al[44] demonstrated that 4 weeks of intravenous treatment with recombinant HGF completely protected the transplant kidney in a rat chronic rejection model. Short-term expression over weeks to one or more of these gene products may be adequate to produce tolerance. Since kidney subcapsular cell implants "take" well and are nicely vascularized, the use of this site for ex-vivo application (e.g. islet cell transplants) is also worthy of consideration.[34] Additional problems related to xenotransplantation will need to be addressed, namely preformed antibody to targets (such as the gal α-1,3 epitope) and complement-mediated hyperacute rejection.[48] Here, too, ex-vivo gene transfer of human genes encoding the H-transferase (to address the first issue)[48] and CD59 or decay-accelerating factor (to address the latter) is worthy of consideration.[49]

Polycystic kidney disease

The recent identification of the cDNAS for PKD1[50,51] and PKD2[52] suggests that transduction of this cDNA might provide a future approach to the therapy of autosomal dominant polycystic kidney disease (ADPKD) caused by mutation in the PKD1 and PKD2 genes. However, this approach is fraught with problems. These include the genetics of ADPKD, which is haplotype insufficiency rather than a dominant-negative mechanism; the requirement for highly efficient tubular cyst transduction; and problems of vector capacity and stability, since the open reading frame for the PKD1 cDNA is 13 kb. On the other hand, a more realistic notion may be to antagonize downstream events, for example the inflammatory process, epithelial cell proliferation, or the fibrotic process. Gene transfer into a small number of cells (vascular and/or epithelial) of agents working in a paracrine manner might achieve a therapeutic effect. However, safety concerns will be paramount since ADPKD is a chronic nonlethal disorder. Though similar considerations apply to the autosomal recessive form of PKD, the disease phenotype, genetics, and population affected are clearly different and even limited gene transfer to kidney (and liver) could be beneficial once the appropriate disease gene(s) is identified.

Our data in the Han:SPRD rat model[26] is a first step in gene therapy in cystic disease. The Han:SPRD rat is an excellent model of ADPKD, with genetic and histologic features resembling those of the human disease.[53–55] A replication-deficient adenovirus carrying a β-galactosidase reporter was introduced into the renal artery. Of note, some of the cysts stained blue. Those that did were often entirely blue, suggesting that adenovirus had reached the cyst lumen. Moreover, some interstitial cells were also positive in addition to the vascular staining noted in normal animals. One explanation for these findings is that vascular permeability/integrity in cystic kidneys is compromised. In very recent studies, we have shown that pelvic (retrograde) injection into cystic kidneys leads to substantial interstitial expression, with the highest density of β-galactosidase cells in areas of greatest disease activity.[8] These studies underscore the importance of assessing gene delivery in the context of pathology.

Renal cancer

The most challenging problem in renal cancer is that of metastatic disease. Nevertheless, it is worth reviewing all the gene therapy modalities that might impact on the treatment of cancer. Several options exist.

1. A gene correction strategy such as the replacement of an intracellularly acting tumor suppressor gene. However, this would likely require transduction of 100% of tumor cells unless there were a bystander effect, as recently suggested for p53.
2. Introduction of an agent that causes cell differentiation, acting intracellularly or extracellularly.
3. Cytotoxic therapy, for example with herpes simplex virus – thymidine kinase (HSV-TK), which has a bystander effect, or with a paracrine factor such as TNF.

All these options are useful for the treatment of local disease. For localized renal cell carcinoma, nephrectomy is a reasonable choice. Therefore, these gene therapies would have to be better than this approach. This is not an easily attainable goal. For the treatment of metastatic disease by gene therapy, "immunotherapy" is the main rational approach. This could be delivered either ex vivo or in vivo. Given the sensitivity of renal cancer to systemic IL-2, a gene therapy approach aimed at introduction of IL-2 certainly merits further study. Other treatment modalities could include antiangiogenic therapy or cytoprotective gene therapy. For example, the introduction of the gene for multidrug resistance into bone marrow or gut epithelial cells might allow more vigorous chemotherapy or might reduce the toxicity of current regimens.

Acute glomerular disease

The notion of utilizing gene therapy, perhaps delivered as antisense oligonucleotides, to counter the action of various inflammatory, proliferative, or profibrotic cytokines in acute glomerulonephritides is reasonable. The rapidly progressive glomerulonephritides may provide a suitable first setting because disease progression is rapid, thereby making the efficacy of therapy easy to judge. It is possible that retroviral vectors may be particularly advantageous in this context, since they transduce dividing cells selectively. Moreover, gene therapy to muscle or liver, with the aim of creating a transient source of circulating protein, could also be useful in glomerular disease. Isaka et al[56] have utilized the HVJ system in skeletal muscle to deliver a cDNA for decorin, a proteoglycan known to bind to TGF-β1, -β2, and -β3. Decorin gene

therapy ameliorated disease in the anti-Thy-1 glomerulonephritis model. Isaka et al[57] also demonstrated that therapy with the gene for a soluble receptor, composed of the extracellular domain of the type 2 TGF-β receptor and IgG-Fc, inhibited TGF-β activity in glomeruli in the anti-Thy-1 glomerulonephritis model. This leads to a reduction in extracellular matrix expansion. They showed further that therapy using a similar gene for a chimeric soluble receptor for PDGF-BB reduced glomerular lesions in anti-Thy-1 glomerulonephritis.[16]

Yokoo et al[58] introduced the IL-1ra gene into bone-marrow cells to generate genetically modified monocytes for delivering this IL-1 antagonist to sites of inflammation. Prophylactic injection of monocytes secreting IL-1ra suppressed glomerular injury in a mouse model of anti-GBM glomerulonephritis. Kluth et al[59] reported that gene therapy with IL-4-producing macrophages in the anti-GBM model of glomerulonephritis diminished necrosis and mesangial cell proliferation, and reduced proteinuria.

Chronic interstitial disease

The degree of interstitial fibrosis is the best correlate of long-term renal prognosis, irrespective of initiating insult. Approaches to reduce the fibrotic response have been reviewed recently.[60] Long-term therapy will be needed. However, there are some 500 000 patients in the USA. Therapy could be delivered to one kidney and renal function assessed over 2–3 years. Urgently needed are pre-clinical studies on (1) vectors for sustained delivery, (2) delivery modalities, (3) cell types transduced, and (4) reagents for antagonizing the action of target molecules such as TGF-β1, basic fibroblast growth factor, and PDGF. Since fibrosis is a key component of chronic rejection, the transplanted kidney would also be a suitable target for such interventions. The studies of retrograde application with adenovirus injected into the pelvis of a cystic (and fibrotic) kidney highlights the relative ease of transducing interstitial cells in the kidney.[8] This might be used advantageously in this setting.

Miscellaneous

Applications outside the kidney but of interest to nephrologists would include vascular access and the problem of graft stenosis,[61] and genes such as erythropoietin expressed from liver utilizing adenovirus and muscle as a "depot" source.[62,63] Even without the ability to regulate gene expression quantitatively, gene therapy for the anemia of chronic disease could be used to raise the baseline hematocrit in a patient with end-stage renal disease, with fine tuning accomplished by erythropoietin injections. Primary hyperoxaluria is another disease that affects the kidney but where definitive therapy would be directed to the liver. Cloning of the relevant genes would clearly be a first step. Long-term transduction of a significant number of liver cells would likely be needed. Finally, in the study of renal development, gene transfer techniques will help define cis regulatory elements. For studying the pathophysiology of renal disease in animal models, gene transfer technologies will help ascertain the importance of a given gene product in the disease model, thereby providing key guideposts for future clinical studies.[64]

In summary, gene transfer technology for the treatment of certain kidney diseases will be feasible but a large database on vectors and transfer methods in the normal kidney and in disease models is an essential first step.

Acknowledgment

The authors thank their colleagues for lively discussions.

References

1. Crystal R: Transfer of genes to humans: early lessons and obstacles to success. Science 1995;270:404–410.
2. Mulligan R: The basic science of gene therapy. Science 1993;260:926–932.
3. Culver K: Gene Therapy. A Handbook for Physicians. New York: Mary Ann Liebert, 1994.
4. Vos J-M: Viruses in Human Gene Therapy. Durham, NC: Carolina Academic Press, 1995.
5. Imai E, Isaka Y: New paradigm of gene therapy: skeletal muscle targeting gene therapy for kidney disease. Nephron 1999;83:296–300.
6. Sukhatme V: Prospects for gene therapy in the kidney. In Bonventre DSJ (ed): Molecular Nephrology: Kidney Function in Health and Disease. New York: Marcel Dekker, 1995.
7. Naldini L, Blomer U, Gallay P, et al: In vivo gene delivery and stable transduction of nondividing cells by a lentiviral vector. Science 1996;272:263–267.
8. Sukhatme VP, Cowley BD, Zhu G: Gene transfer into kidney tubules and vasculature by adenoviral vectors. Exp Nephrol 1997;5:137–143.
9. Kochanek S, Clemens P, Mitani K, Chen H-H, Chan S, Caskey C: A new adenoviral vector: replacement of all viral coding sequences with 28 kb of DNA independently expressing both full-length dystrophin and β-galactosidase. Proc Natl Acad Sci USA 1996;93:5731–5736.
10. Mastrangeli A, Harvey B-G, Yao J, et al: "Sero-switch" adenovirus-mediated in vivo gene transfer: circumvention of anti-adenovirus vector administration by changing the adenovirus serotype. Hum Gene Ther 1996;7:79–87.
11. Surosky R, Urabe M, Godwin S, et al: Adeno-associate virus rep proteins target DNA sequences to a unique locus in the human genome. J Viol 1997;71:7951–7959.
12. Rivadeneira E, Popescu N, Zimonjic D, et al: Recombinant adeno-associated virus integrates at diverse sites in the human genome. Int J Oncol 1999;12:805–810.
13. Tsujie M, Isaka Y, Nakamura H, Kaneda Y, Imai E, Hori M: Prolonged transgene expression in glomeruli using an Epstein–Barr virus replicon vector system combined with AVE type liposomes. Kidney Int 2001;59:1390–1396.
14. Isaka Y, Akagi Y, Kaneda Y, Imai E: The HVJ liposome method. Exp Nephrol 1998;6:144–147.
15. Aihara H, Miyazaki J: Gene transfer into muscle by electroporation in vivo. Nature Biotechnol 1998;16:867–870.
16. Nakamura H, Isaka Y, Tsujie M, et al: Electroporation-mediated PDGF receptor-IgG chimera gene transfer ameliorates experimental glomerulonephritis. Kidney Int 2001;59:2134–2145.
17. Pasqualini R, Ruoslahti E: Organ targeting in vivo using phage display peptide libraries. Nature 1996;380:364–366.
18. Kitamura M: Creation of a reversible on/off system for site-specific in vivo control of exogenous activity in the renal glomerulus. J Clin Invest 1996;93:7387–7391.
19. Kitamura M, Kawachi H: Creation of an in vivo cytosenser using engineered mesangial cells. J Clin Invest 1997;100:1394–1399.
20. Tomita N: Directed in vivo gene introduction into rat kidney. Biochem Biophys Res Commun 1992;186:129–134.
21. Kaneda Y, Iwai K, Uchida T: Increased expression of DNA cointroduced with nuclear protein in adult rat liver. Science 1989;243:375–378.
22. Isaka Y, Fujiwara Y, Ueda N, Kaneda Y, Kamada T, Imai E: Glomerulosclerosis induced by in vivo transfection of transforming growth factor-β or platelet-derived growth factor gene into the rat kidney. J Clin Invest 1993;92:2597–2601.
23. Tsujie M, Isaka Y, Nakamura H, Imai E, Hori M: Electroporation mediated gene transfer targeting glomeruli. J Am Soc Nephrol 2001;12:949–954.
24. Bosch R, Woolf A, Fine L: Gene transfer into the mammalian kidney: direct retrovirus transduction of regenerating tubular epithelial cells. Exp Nephrol 1993;1:49–54.
25. Moullier P: Adenoviral-mediated gene transfer to renal tubular cells in vivo. Kidney Int 1994;45:1220–1225.
26. Zhu G, Nicolson AG, Cowley B, Rosen S, Sukhatme VP: In vivo adenovirus-mediated gene transfer into normal and cystic rat kidneys. Gene Ther 1996;3:298–304.
27. Zeigler S, Kerby J, Curiel D, Diethelm A, Thompson J: Molecular conjugate-mediated gene transfer into isolated human kidneys. Transplantation 1996;61:812–817.
28. Heikkila P, Parpala T, Lukkarinen O, Weber M, Tryggvason K: Adenovirus-mediated gene transfer into kidney glomeruli using an ex vivo and in vivo kidney perfusion system: first step towards gene therapy of Alport syndrome. Gene Ther 1996;3:21–27.
29. Lipkowitz M, Hanss B, Tulchin N, et al: Transduction of renal cells in vitro and in vivo by adeno-associated virus gene therapy vectors. J Am Soc Nephrol 1999;10:1908–1915.
30. Kitamura M: Gene transfer into the rat renal glomerulus via a mesangial cell vector: site-specific delivery, in situ amplification, and sustained expression of an exogenous gene in vivo. J Clin Invest 1994;94:497–505.
31. Kitamura M, Suto T: Transfer of genetically engineered macrophages into the glomerulus. Kidney Int 1997;51:1274–1279.
32. Yokoo T, Utsunomiya Y, Ohashi T, et al: Inflamed site-specific gene delivery using bone marrow-derived CD11b+CD18+ vehicle cells in mice. Hum Gene Ther 1998;9:1731–1738.
33. Naito T, Yokoyama H, Moore KJ, Dranoff G, Mulligan RC, Kelley VR: A gene transfer system establishing interleukin-6 neither promotes nor suppresses renal injury. Am J Physiol 1996;271:F603–F609.
34. Heartlein M, Roman V, Jiang J, et al: Long-term production and delivery of human growth hormone in vivo. Proc Natl Acad Sci USA 1994;91:10967–10971.
35. Anegon I, David A, Charreau B, Soulillou J-P: Somatic gene transfer in transplantation. In Tilney NL, Strom TB, Paul LC (eds): Transplantation Biology: Cellular and Molecular Aspects. Philadelphia and New York: Lippincott, Raven, 1996, pp 689–699.
36. Sykes M, Sachs D, Nienhuis A, Pearson D, Moulton A, Bodine D: Specific prolongation of skin graft survival following retroviral transduction of bone marrow with an allogeneic major histocompatibility complex gene. Transplantation 1993;55:197–202.
37. Madsen J, Superina R, Wood K, Morris P: Immunological unresponsiveness induced by recipient cells transfected with donor MHC genes. Nature 1988;332:161–164.
38. Baliga P, Chavin Y, Qin L, et al: CTLA4Ig prolongs allograft survival while suppressing cell-mediated immunity. Transplantation 1994;58:1082–1090.
39. Lenschow D, Zeng Y, Thistlethwaite J, et al: Long-term surivival of xenogenetic pancreatic islet grafts induced by CTLA4Ig. Science 1992;257:789–792.
40. Abramowicz D, Durez P, Gerard C, et al: Neonatal induction of transplantation tolerance in mice is associated with in vivo expression of IL-4 and -10 mRNAs. Transplant Proc 1993;25:312–313.
41. Perillo N, Pace K, Sellhamer J, Baum L: Apoptosis of T cells mediated by galectin-1. Nature 1995;378:736–738.
42. Efrat S, Fejer G, Brownlee M, Horwitz M: Prolonged survival of pancreatic islet allograft mediated by adenovirus immunoregulatory transgenes. Proc Natl Acad Sci USA 1995;92:6947–6951.
43. Qin L, Chavin K, Ding Y, et al: Gene transfer for transplantation. Prolongation of allograft survival with transforming growth factor-β1. Ann Surg 1994;220:508–518.
44. Azuma H, Takahara S, Matsumoto K, et al: Hepatocyte growth factor prevents the development of chronic allograft nephropathy in rats. J Am Soc Nephrol 2001;12:1280–1292.
45. Erzurum S, Lemarchand P, Rosenfeld M, Yoo J-H, Crystal R: Protection of human endothelial cells from oxidant by adenovirus-mediated transfer of the human catalase cDNA. Nucleic Acids Res 1993;21:1607–1612.

46. Lau HT, Yu M, Fontana A, Stoeckert CJ Jr: Prevention of islet allograft rejection with engineered myoblasts expressing fasl in mice. Science 1996;273:109–112.

47. Tomasoni S, Azzollini N, Casiraghi F, Capogrossi M, Remuzzi G, Benigni A: CTLA4Ig gene transfer prolongs survival and induces donor-specific tolerance in a rat renal allograft. J Am Soc Nephrol 2000;11:747–752.

48. Sandrin M, Fodor W, Mouhtouris E, et al: Enzymatic remodelling of the carbohydrate surface of a xenogenic cell substantially reduces human antibody binding and complement-mediated cytolysis. Nature Med 1995;1:1261–1267.

49. McCurry KR, Kooyman DL, Alvarado CG, et al: Human complement regulatory proteins protect swine-to-primate cardiac xenografts from humoral injury. Nature Med 1995;1:423–427.

50. The European Polycystic Kidney Disease Consortium: The polycystic kidney disease 1 gene encodes a 14 kb transcript and lies within a duplicated region on chromosome 16. Cell 1994;77:881–894.

51. The International Polycystic Kidney Disease Consortium: Polycystic kidney disease: the complete structure of the PKD1 gene and its protein. Cell 1995;81:289–298.

52. Mochizuki T, Wu G, Hayashi T, et al: PKD2, a gene for polycystic kidney disease that encodes an integral membrane protein. Science 1996;272:1339–1342.

53. Kaspareit-Rittinghausen J, Rapp K, Deerberg F, Wcislo A, Messow C: Hereditary polycystic kidney disease associated with osteorenal syndrome in rats. Vet Pathol 1989;26:195–201.

54. Kaspareit-Rittinghausen J, Deerberg F, Wcislo A: Adult polycystic kidney disease associated with renal hypertension, renal osteodystrophy, and uremic enteritis in SPRD rats. Am J Pathol 1991;139:693–696.

55. Cowley B Jr: Autosomal dominant polycystic kidney disease in the rat. Kidney Int 1993;43:522–534.

56. Isaka Y, Brees D, Ikegaya K, Imai E, Noble N, Border W: Gene therapy by skeletal muscle expression of decorin prevents fibrotic disease in rat kidney. Nature Med 1996;2:418–423.

57. Isaka Y, Akagi Y, Ando Y, et al: Gene therapy by transforming growth factor-β receptor-IgG Fc chimera suppressed extracellular matrix accumulation in experimental glomerulonephritis. Kidney Int 1999;55:465–475.

58. Yokoo T, Ohashi T, Utsunomiya Y, et al: Prophylaxis of antibody-induced acute glomerulonephritis with genetically modified bone marrow-derived vehicle cells. Hum Gene Ther 1999;10:2673–2678.

59. Kluth D, Ainslie C, Pearce W, et al: Macrophages transfected with adenovirus to express IL-4 reduce inflammation in experimental glomerulonephritis. J Immunol 2001;166:4728–4736.

60. Sukhatme VP: Fibrosis. In Tilney N, Strom T, Paul LC (eds): Transplantation Biology: Cellular and Molecular Aspects. Philadelphia and New York: Lippincott, Raven, 1996, pp 249–255.

61. Sukhatme VP: Stenosis of vascular access revisited: pathobiology and prospects for prevention and therapy. Kidney Int 1996;49:1161–1174.

62. Tripathy S, Black H, Goldwasser E, Leiden J: Immune responses to transgene-encoded proteins limit the stability of gene expression after injection of replication-defective adenovirus vectors. Nature Med 1996;2:545–550.

63. Tripathy SK, Svensson EC, Black HB, et al: Long-term expression of erythropoietin in the systemic circulation of mice after intramuscular injection of a plasmid DNA vector. Proc Natl Acad Sci USA 1996;93:10876–10880.

64. Fine L: Gene transfer into the kidney: promise for unravelling disease mechanisms, limitations for human gene therapy. Kidney Int 1996;49:612–619.

PART X
Management of Essential Hypertension

CHRISTOPHER S. WILCOX

Treatment Decisions for Hypertension

Lawrence R. Krakoff

Who is and who is not really hypertensive?
Which blood pressures are most important: the systolic, diastolic, or pulse pressure?
The absolute risk concept: blood pressure, nonhypertensive risk factors, and target-organ damage
- Low-risk profiles: the role of nondrug strategies (lifestyle change)
- High-risk patients who need drug treatment
  - Very high blood pressure
  - Minimal hypertension, very high risk
  - Special importance of diabetes
Conclusions

- Which blood pressures are the most important for diagnosis and treatment? What is the role of supplemental pressures? Are systolic pressure, diastolic pressure, and pulse pressure equally important?
- Apart from pressure, what determines future cardiovascular risk and the benefit of antihypertensive treatment?
- Can nondrug therapies (lifestyle change) play a greater role as initial and even continuing treatment?
- Is the benefit of antihypertensive treatment related only to reduced blood pressure or do different approaches, especially drug classes, have greater or lesser value, independent of their effect on pressure?
- Are different goals for treating with antihypertensive drugs appropriate to certain high-risk subgroups?

These questions imply that the strategies and decisions related to initiating, maintaining, and changing antihypertensive therapy are, in many instances, highly complex (Fig. 52.1).

Treatment of systemic arterial hypertension is one of the most frequently performed actions by which primary-care practitioners and the medical subspecialties of cardiology, nephrology, or endocrinology benefit their adult patients. In offices and clinics it is a cornerstone for prevention of both cardiovascular and end-stage renal disease (ESRD) wherever modern medicine is available. Increased application of treatment to lower blood pressure has followed the succession of randomized clinical trials of antihypertensive therapy in mild to moderate hypertension. These trials, taken individually or in aggregate via metaanalysis, demonstrate that compared with lack of treatment antihypertensive drug therapy for both middle-aged and elderly hypertensives is predictably effective with regard to prevention of fatal and nonfatal cerebrovascular disease (stroke) and cardiac disease (myocardial infarction and heart failure).[1-3] With regard to the prevention of ESRD, recent clinical trials have shown progress with antihypertensive treatment using either angiotensin-converting enzyme (ACE) inhibitors or angiotensin receptor blockers, particularly in diabetic nephropathy.[4-6] For nondiabetic renal disease, especially with proteinuria, there is suggestive (but not decisive) evidence that antihypertensive therapy with ACE inhibitors also delays progression.[8,9] Thus there is no longer doubt that antihypertensive therapy is beneficial.

The success of antihypertensive treatment might seem to make any discussion of decisions regarding treatment limited to the somewhat simple imperative: "If hypertensive, then treat." However, several important issues have emerged to modify prior concepts about which patients should receive which type of antihypertensive therapy and how the lessons of recent trials and research can be focused to increase prevention of disease events, and minimize or even eliminate any risk of treatment. These issues are as follows.

Who is and who is not really hypertensive?

Are the few measurements of blood pressures made in the highly contrived atmosphere of a busy medical practice sufficient for a diagnosis of hypertension? The best answer is no. Greater certainty is needed,[10] given the long-term implications of the diagnosis with regard to cardiovascular risk, consequences of treatment, and psychologic effects. Furthermore, it is the average pressure that is best related to risk. Thus the value of supplemental measurement using ambulatory blood pressure monitoring or home blood pressure recording has become evident. Several studies have established the superiority of ambulatory blood pressure recording for predicting future cardiovascular morbidity based on average pressures.[11-13]

The distribution of blood pressures in a population is nearly normal. The various cut-points for blood pressure that have been used to divide high-normal from hypertensive are all on the upper part of the downslope of these distributions. In other words, a large fraction of those with high-normal pressures may be falsely labeled as hypertensive, given a small error (5–10 mmHg) in measurement. It is less likely that a patient with hypertension will be falsely classified as normal or high-normal, but this remains a worrisome possibility. For those with initial or first screen pressures just above the limit of the normal range (i.e. 140–150 mmHg systolic, 90–100 mmHg diastolic), the likelihood of a false-positive diagnosis of hypertension is a distinct possibility unless additional measurements are made that then achieve regression to the mean and

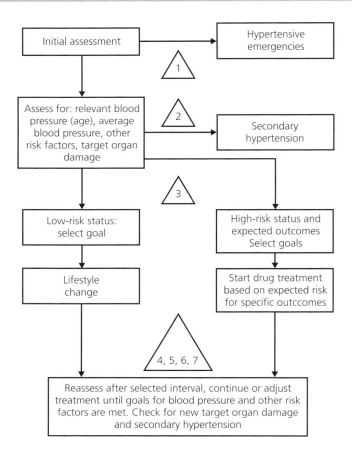

Figure 52.1 Flow diagram for hypertensive patients. The diagnostic and management process is a continuum from the initial evaluation to short- and long-term surveillance, reassessment, and change in strategy as needed for the benefit of each patient. The triangles indicate where major decisions are made for diagnosis and treatment. (1) During initial assessment, is an emergency present? (2) Should secondary hypertension be considered? (3) After the initial risk profiling, is the patient's present risk status low enough for *only* lifestyle change or is it high enough for drug treatment? During follow-up: (4) Have treatment goals been met so that there is no need for change in treatment or, if goals not met, what changes in treatment are required? (5) Has risk status changed (e.g. new diabetes)? (6) Are there changes of new target-organ damage (e.g. coronary heart disease)? (7) Are there signs of secondary hypertension (e.g. renal artery stenosis)?

downward classification of the pressure to the high-normal or normal range. Conversely, some with normal or high-normal pressure in the clinic will have much higher pressures during usual activities including work (so-called "reverse white coat syndrome"). The clinic pressures for these latter individuals may be viewed as a false-negative result, in that upward reclassification to a higher-risk status can be revealed by ambulatory pressures and is correlated with more target organ damage.[14]

As ambulatory blood pressure monitoring is not yet easily available, there is increasing interest in the use of selfmeasured home blood pressures. The potential utility of this strategy requires that patients be trained properly and that the devices have memory to preserve and replay all measurements (recorded home blood pressures), rather than relying on patients to select measurements on their own.[15-17] A new development in this area is the availability of home blood pressure devices that store measurements and transmit them via a modem to a central computer, which can issue periodic reports to treating physicans and patients for feedback.[19,20] Use of this technique may be helpful for both determination of pretreatment average pressures outside the clinic and for initiation and adjustment of antihypertensive therapy with far greater efficiency and accuracy than has been possible in the past.

Many past studies have shown that those with higher clinic pressures and normal ambulatory pressures (white coat hypertensives) tend to be younger, more often women, and have far less target-organ pathology. By contrast, those with higher usual pressures, either similar to or even higher than clinic pressures (lacking the white coat element and considered reverse white coat types), may be older and have more target-organ pathology. Whether the variation between clinic and usual or average pressure has any clinical significance is still uncertain.[13] There remains some disagreement as to the location of an exact cut-point between "normal" and "high" blood pressure that determines when supplemental pressures are required; several values have been suggested in the range 130–137 mmHg for systolic pressure and 85–90 mmHg for diastolic pressure. Perhaps a definition of hypertension using specific cut-points for systolic and diastolic pressure is less important than determining the average pressure with greater precision and relating it to other factors that determine future risk of cardiovascular disease.

Which blood pressures are most important: the systolic, diastolic, or pulse pressure?

Clinical trials of therapy that focus on isolated or predominant systolic hypertension in the elderly support the epidemiologic evidence for the importance of systolic pressure.[21-23] However, retrospective analysis of some databases has suggested that the pulse pressure may be a superior predictor of later cardiovascular disease and that a higher diastolic pressure confers less risk than a lower one, at least for older patients.[24,25] Further reanalysis of age-related trends in the Framingham study indicates that in those under 50 years of age, diastolic pressure remains the better predictor of risk; between 50 and 59 years both systolic and diastolic pressure are directly related to risk, while above 59 years systolic and pulse pressures are the best predictors.[26]

To summarize: (1) the age of the patient must be considered in determining which measurement of pressure has the greatest clinical relevance; and (2) those with clinic pressures in the range 130–160/80–100 mmHg should have their usual daily pressure assessed using ambulatory blood pressure monitoring (the gold standard), home blood pressure recording, or repeated clinic measurement using standardized conditions.[27] Perhaps 20–30% of those with "hypertensive" clinic pressures will be found to have normal averages according to supplemental measurements. Some 10–15% of those with normal or high-normal clinic pressures will have "hypertensive" average pressures revealed by ambulatory recording or home blood pressure measurement. It is the usual or average pressures that should be used as the basis for assigning risk related to pressure.

The absolute risk concept: blood pressure, nonhypertensive risk factors, and target-organ damage

The likelihood of future cardiovascular disease depends on a composite assessment of treatable factors including (1) those related to blood pressure, (2) those related to other reversible risk factors, and (3) those indicative of existing target organ damage (Table 52.1). Each separate risk factor enhances the burden of others in a multiplicative way. Thus, for the same average pressure, the likelihood of a fatal cardiovascular event over the subsequent 10 years may be as high as 20% for 55-year-old men who smoke and have a low-density lipoprotein (LDL) cholesterol > 160 mg/dL (4 mmol/L) but is < 2% for 45-year-old nonsmoking women with LDL cholesterol < 130 mg/dL (3.25 mmol/L). The *relative risk* (expressed as a risk ratio or percentage) may differ substantially from the *absolute risk* (defined as fraction of a population or subpopulation). A 20% decrease in relative risk achieved by treatment for a disease that affects 1% of a population would lead to one protected patient for 500 treated; the same decrease in relative risk for a condition that affected 20% of a population would benefit 1 in 25.

The "absolute risk concept" is useful for classification of hypertensive patients by taking age, serum cholesterol, smoking history, and diabetes into account.[28-30] This approach has been adopted for several widely distributed guidelines.[31,32]

Low-risk profiles: the role of nondrug strategies (lifestyle change)

For those under 50 years of age with blood pressures in the range 130–150/80–95 mmHg, who are not diabetic, and have no other cardiovascular risk factors or target-organ damage, the risk of future cardiovascular or renal disease is very low. If overweight, this is a reversible risk factor, since weight loss lowers blood pressure and improves lipid status and diabetic control even in older groups.[33] Recent studies indicate that blood pressure can be significantly reduced, without weight reduction, by diets rich in fruit and vegetables but with limited dairy products. This is more effective when salt intake is restricted.[34] There is optimism that many with minimal elevations of pressure and low-risk profiles might benefit from such approaches.[35,36]

High-risk patients who need drug treatment
Very high blood pressure

By 1980 it was certain that in middle-aged subjects the current antihypertensive medications were effective in preventing death and cardiovascular disease, primarily stroke, in those with pretreatment pressures above 160 mmHg systolic and 90–95 mmHg diastolic.[1] More recently, the benefit of antihypertensive drug treatment has been extended to older patients (60–80 years) with isolated or predominant systolic hypertension (> 160 mmHg at entry).[2] Antihypertensive drug treatment may also be effective for prevention of nonfatal stroke in older groups (> 80 years at entry).[37] In all these studies and others,[38] the major source of risk for cardiovascular disease was the very high pretreatment blood pressure itself.

Table 52.1 Factors to be assessed in establishing cardiovascular and renal risk status

Related to blood pressure	Nonpressure risk factors	Target organ pathology
Supplemental pressures For all ages, estimate of usual/average pressures. Consideration of abnormal diurnal pattern in selected patients	*Best established* Presence of type 1 or 2 diabetes History of smoking Lipid status: elevated LDL, low HDL cholesterol	*Cardiac* Left ventricular enlargement, ischemia, prior myocardial infarction or angina, abnormal stress test, impaired systolic function, arrhythmia
Age < 50 Diastolic pressure most important	*Less well established but may be useful* Plasma renin profile, triglyceride level	*Renal* Microalbuminuria or proteinuria, reduced GFR, elevated creatinine
Age 50–60 Both systolic and diastolic pressure equally important	*Suggested by recent research* C-reactive protein, fibrinogen, lipoprotein(a), homocysteine	*Peripheral vascular* Ankle–arm index, claudication, arterial bruits, aortic aneurysm
Age > 60 Systolic pressure and pulse pressure more important		*Cerebrovascular* History of TIA or stroke, carotid bruit

GFR, glomerular filtration rate; HDL, high-density lipoprotein; LDL, low-density lipoprotein; TIA, transient ischemic attack.

For those with very high pressures (> 160 mmHg systolic or > 100 mmHg diastolic) does it matter which antihypertensive drugs are used?[38,40–42] The overall results for primary endpoints suggest that there are very few differences between treatment strategies and that reduction of pressure per se is the important factor for prevention of stroke and cardiovascular mortality. Subgroup analysis reveals some interesting trends. For example, in the CAPP trial, initial treatment with captopril prevented the appearance of new diabetes. However, there were slightly more strokes in the captopril-treated group, which might have been due to higher pretreatment pressures.[41] One conclusion is that when blood pressure is very high, stroke is the more likely outcome and the benefit of antihypertensive drug treatment is a consequence of lowering pressure rather than the pharmacologic properties of any one drug class.[43] If the likelihood of stroke is far higher than that of cardiac disease, as in Asian populations, perhaps calcium channel blockers are superior as antihypertensives.[44] However, when events related to coronary heart disease become more likely, metaanalyses suggest that primary therapy with calcium channel blockers is less effective than alternate drug classes.[43,45] Thus even among those with very high pressure, attention to the most likely outcomes may be a guide to appropriate treatment.

Minimal hypertension, very high risk

When blood pressure is in the range 135–155 mmHg systolic and 80–100 mmHg diastolic, future risk of cardiovascular and renal disease is highly dependent on age and the presence of other risk factors, particularly type 2 diabetes and target-organ damage including evidence of ischemic cardiac disease and peripheral vascular disease. Thus high-risk patients can be identified who might benefit from antihypertensive drugs, despite blood pressures that are minimally elevated or even normal. These patients have a lesser risk of stroke (compared to those with higher pressure) but a higher risk of myocardial infarction, ischemic heart disease, and congestive heart failure. Several studies have explored the differences among the major classes of antihypertensive drugs, from which some conclusions can be drawn[46–48] (Table 52.2).

1. In the HOPE study, ACE inhibition was remarkably effective in preventing cardiovascular disease in high-risk patients despite little or no reduction in pressure.
2. In the ALLHAT study, initial treatment with the α_1-receptor blocker doxazosin was associated with a significantly worse outcome compared with the effect of a low-dose diuretic, particularly with regard to the appearance of congestive heart failure.
3. In the PROGRESS study, combined use of an ACE inhibitor and a diuretic was more effective than the alternate strategy for those with either normal or high entry pressures and high-risk status due to prior stroke or transient ischemic attacks.

Thus in those older patients (> 50 years) with high-risk status primarily due to presence of other risk factors plus target-organ damage due to coronary artery disease, peripheral vascular disease, or stroke, diuretics and ACE inhibitors are highly beneficial out of proportion to their effect on arterial pressure. In addition, one should not overlook the well-established value of β-receptor blockers for those with evidence of coronary heart disease.[49]

Special importance of diabetes

No discussion about decisions for treatment of hypertension would be complete without emphasis on the importance of diabetes, the presence of which (usually as type 2 diabetes) invariably increases risk of cardiovascular disease and renal failure. Antecedent hypertension doubles the likelihood of type 2 diabetes. Therefore, all hypertensives should be followed up for diabetes.[50] The presence of type 2 diabetes actually enhances the effect of antihypertensive therapy (in terms of absolute risk) in middle-aged and elderly hypertensive patients as shown in the UKPS,[51] Syst-Eur,[52] and SHEP[53] trials. The value of lower on-treatment blood pressure goals in diabetics was suggested by subgroup analyses in the HOT trial,[39] where optimal results were associated with on-treatment diastolic pressures < 80 mmHg. However, the MICRO-HOPE study reported that an ACE inhibitor was highly effective for prevention of cardiovascular disease in type 2 diabetes, with no clinically significant reduction of pressure from slightly elevated pretreatment levels (142/80 mmHg).[54] Some urge very low treatment goals for diabetic hypertensives (< 130/80 mmHg) based on extrapolation from the available trials.

For type 2 diabetics with diabetic nephropathy, angiotensin receptor blockers delay progression of renal disease and seem to reduce cardiovascular disease when compared with a dihydropyridine calcium channel blocker at equal on-treatment pressures.[4,6,55] Taking all available studies together, it is likely that optimal prevention of cardiovascular disease and delay of diabetic nephropathy require therapy with drugs that block the renin–angiotensin system (ACE inhibitors or angiotensin II type 1 receptor blockers) and whatever other antihypertensive drugs are needed to achieve the lowest acceptable on-treatment pressures.

Conclusions

Physicians evaluate patients one by one. The lessons learned from epidemiology and clinical trials need translation to management decisions. Treatment decisions became more precise by taking age into account when establishing which pressure is most relevant, by determining a patient's usual blood pressure, and by characterizing other risk factors and target-organ damage. Effective strategies include lifestyle interventions and many classes of drug. Careful clinical assessment leading to appropriate selection of therapy now has extraordinary power for prevention of cardiovascular and renal mortality and morbidity in those with elevated blood pressure.

Table 52.2 Clinical trials of high-risk patients due to combination of risk factors and/or target-organ damage

Reference	Entry criteria	Treatment strategies	Entry blood pressures (mmHg)	Outcomes assessed	Results
Heart Outcomes Prevention Evaluation (HOPE)[48]	Age ≥ 55 years. Past diabetes, coronary disease, stroke, or peripheral vascular disease, and one other risk factor: hypertension, high cholesterol, smoking, or albuminuria	Low-dose ramipril run in, then randomize to placebo vs. ramipril 10 mg. All other medications permitted on open basis	Ramipril group: 139/79 Placebo group: 139/79	*Primary endpoint* Composite of MI, stroke, or cardiovascular death	*Primary endpoint* Ramipril group: 14.0% Placebo group: 17.8% ARR: 3.8% RRR: 22% NNT: 26 *Conclusion* Benefit for ramipril vs. placebo as initial treatment
Antihypertensive and Lipid-Lowering Treatment to Prevent Heart Attack Trial (ALLHAT)[47]	Age ≥ 55 years. Blood pressure ≥ 140/90 mmHg or treated. One additional risk factor for coronary artery disease: prior MI, stroke, LVH, type 2 diabetes, smoking, low HDL cholesterol	Withdrawal from current treatment. Randomize to initial treatment: chlorthalidone, lisinopril, doxazosin, or amlodipine. Titrate, then add other drugs per protocol, atenolol or reserpine, then others	Chlorthalidone group: 140/83 Doxazosin group: 140/84	*Primary endpoint* Fatal coronary heart disease or nonfatal MI *Secondary* Combined CHD, stroke, combined CVD (includes heart failure)	*Primary endpoint* Equal for doxazosin and chlorthalidone *Secondary; combined CVD* Doxasosin: 25.5% Chlorthalidone: 21.8% ARR: 3.7% RRR: 14% NNT: 27 *Conclusion* Benefit of chlorthalidone vs. doxazosin as initial treatment
PROGRESS[46]	Any patient with history of cerebrovascular accident (stroke) or TIA, without heart failure or uncontrolled hypertension	Low-dose perindopril run in. Randomize to active: perindopril 4 mg, flexible addition of indapamide 2.5 mg or placebo for both. Treating physicians given options for other treatment as needed	Active: 147/86 Placebo: 147/86 Prespecified combination: 149/87 Prespecified single drug, perindopril: 144/84	*Primary endpoint* Fatal or nonfatal stroke *Secondary* Total major vascular events (nonfatal MI, stroke, or vascular death)	*Primary endpoint* Placebo: 14% Active: 10% ARR: 4% RRR: 28% NNT: 25 *Total vascular events* Placebo: 19.8% Active: 15.0% ARR: 4.8% RRR: 26% NNT: 21 *Conclusion* Benefit of perindopril and indapamide strategy vs. placebo

ARR, absolute risk reduction; CHD, coronary heart disease; CVD, cardiovascular disease; HDL, high-density lipoprotein; LVH, left ventricular hypertrophy; MI, myocardial infarction; NNT, number needed to treat for benefit of one patient; RRR, relative risk reduction; TIA, transient ischemic attack.

References

1. Collins R, Peto R, MacMahon S, et al: Blood pressure, stroke, and coronary heart disease. Part 2, short-term reductions in blood pressure: overview of randomized drug trials in their epidemiological context. Lancet 1990;335:827–838.
2. Staessen J, Gasowski J, Wang JG, et al: Risks of untreated and treated isolated systolic hypertension in the elderly: meta-analysis of outcome trials. Lancet 2000;355:865–872.
3. Mulrow CD, Lau J, Cornell J, et al: Pharmacotherapy for hypertension in the elderly (Cochrane Review). The Cochrane Library 2001.
4. Brenner BM, Cooper ME, de Zeeuw D, et al: Effects of losartan on renal and cardiovascular outcomes in patients with type-2 diabetes and nephropathy. N Engl J Med 2001;345:861–869.
5. Lewis EJ, Hunsicker LG, Bain RP, et al: The effect of angiotensin-converting-enzyme inhibition on diabetic nephropathy. N Engl J Med 1993;329:1456–1462.
6. Lewis EJ, Hunsicker LG, Clarke WR, et al: Renoprotective effect of the angiotensin-receptor antagonist irbesartan in patients with nephropathy due to type-2 diabetes. N Engl J Med 2001;345:851–860.
7. Ruggenenti P, Pema A, Gherardi G, et al: Renoprotective properties of ACE-inhibition in non-diabetic nephropathies with non-nephrotic proteinuria. Lancet 1999;354:359–364.
8. Jafar TH, Schmid CH, Landa M, et al: Angiotensin-converting enzyme inhibitors and progression of nondiabetic renal disease. A meta-analysis of patient-level data. Ann Intern Med 2001;135:73–87.
9. Schrier RW, Estacio RO: The effect of angiotensin-converting enzyme inhibitors on the progression of nondiabetic renal disease: a pooled analysis of individual data from 11 randomized controlled trials. Ann Intern Med 2001;135:138–139.
10. Perry HM Jr, Miller JP: Difficulties in diagnosing hypertension: implications and alternatives. J Hypertens 1992;10:887–896.
11. Perloff D, Sokolow M, Cowan R: The prognostic value of ambulatory blood pressures. JAMA 1983;249:2792–2798.
12. Verdecchia P, Schillaci G, Boldrini F, Zampi I, Porcellati C: Variability between current definitions of "normal" ambulatory blood pressure. Hypertension 1992;20:555–562.
13. Verdecchia P, Borgioni C, Ciucci A, et al: Prognostic significance of blood pressure variability in essential hypertension. Blood Pressure Monit 1996;1:3–11.
14. Liu JE, Roman MJ, Pini R, Schwartz JE, Pickering TG, Devereux RB: Cardiac and arterial target organ damage in adults with elevated ambulatory and normal office blood pressure. Ann Intern Med 1999;131:564–572.
15. Campbell NRC, Milkovich L, Burgess E, McKay DW: Self-measurement of blood pressure: accuracy, patient preparation for readings, technique and equipment. Blood Pressure Monit 2001;6:133–138.
16. Mengden T, Hernandez RM, Beltran B, Alvarez E, Kraft K, Vetter H: Reliability of reporting self-measured blood pressure values by hypertensive patients. Am J Hypertens 1998;11:1413–1417.
17. Myers MG: Self-measurement of blood pressure at home: the potential for reporting bias. Blood Pressure Monit 1998;3(Suppl 1):S19–S22.
18. Rogers MAM, Small D, Buchan DA, et al: Home monitoring service improves mean arterial pressure in patients with essential hypertension. Ann Intern Med 2001;134:1024–1032.
19. Broege PA, James GD, Pickering TG: Management of hypertension in the elderly using home blood pressures. Blood Pressure Monit 2001;6:139–144.
20. Artinian NT, Washington OG, Templin TN: Effects of home telemonitoring and community-based monitoring on blood pressure control in urban African Americans: a pilot study. Heart Lung 2001;30:191–199.
21. Izzo JL Jr, Levy D, Black HR: Importance of systolic blood pressure in older Americans. Hypertension 2000;35:1021–1024.
22. Sagie A, Larson MG, Levy D: The natural history of borderline isolated systolic hypertension. N Engl J Med 1993;329:1912–1917.
23. Mulrow CD, Cornell JA, Herrera CR, Kadri K, Farnett L, Aguilar C: Hypertension in the elderly. Implications and generalizability of randomized trials. JAMA 1994;272:1932–1938.
24. Alderman MH, Cohen H, Madhavan S: Distribution and determinants of cardiovascular events during 20 years of successful antihypertensive treatment. J Hypertens 1998;16:761–769.
25. Franklin SS, Khan SA, Wong ND, Larson MG, Levy D: Is pulse pressure useful in predicting risk for coronary heart disease? The Framingham Heart Study. Circulation 1999;100:354–360.
26. Franklin SS, Larson MG, Kahn, SA, et al: Does the relation of blood pressure to coronary heart disease risk change with aging? The Framingham Heart Study. Circulation 2001;103:1245–1249.
27. Jula A, Puukka P, Karanko H: Multiple clinic and home blood pressure measurements versus ambulatory blood pressure monitoring. Hypertension 1999;34:261–266.
28. Baker S, Priest P, Jackson R: Using thresholds based on risk of cardiovascular disease to target treatment for hypertension: modelling events averted and number treated. Br Med J 2000;320:680–685.
29. Levy D: Have expert panel guidelines kept pace with new concepts in hypertension? Lancet 1995;346:1112–1113.
30. Ogden LG, He J, Lydick E, Whelton PK: Long-term absolute benefit of lowering blood pressure in hypertensive patients according to the JNC VI risk stratification. Hypertension 2000;35:539–543.
31. The Sixth Report of the Joint National Committee on Prevention, Detection, Evaluation, and Treatment of High Blood Pressure. Arch Intern Med 1997;157:2413–2445.
32. Guidelines Subcommittee: 1999 World Health Organization/International Society of Hypertension Guidelines for the Management of Hypertension. J Hypertens 1999;17:151–183.
33. Whelton PK, Appel LJ, Espeland MA, et al: Sodium reduction and weight loss in the treatment of hypertension in older persons: a randomized controlled trial of nonpharmacologic interventions in the elderly (TONE). TONE Collaborative Research Group. JAMA 1998;279:839–846.
34. Sacks FM, Svetkey LP, Vollmer WM, et al: Effects on blood pressure of reduced dietary sodium and the dietary approaches to stop hypertension (DASH) study. N Engl J Med 2001;344:3–10.
35. Greenland P: Beating high blood pressure with low-sodium DASH. N Engl J Med 2001;344:53–54.
36. Chobanian AV: Control of hypertension: an important national priority. N Engl J Med 2001;345:534–535.
37. Gueyffier F, Bulpitt C, Boissel JP, et al: Antihypertensive drugs in very old people: a subgroup meta-analysis of randomized controlled trials. Lancet 1999;353:793–796.
38. Hansson L, Lindholm LH, Ekbom T, et al: Randomised trial of old and new antihypertensive drugs in elderly patients: cardiovascular mortality and morbidity. The Swedish Trial in Old Patients with Hypertension, STOP 2. Lancet 1999;354:1751–1756.
39. Hansson L, Zanchetti A, Carruthers G, et al: Effects of intensive blood-pressure lowering and low-dose aspirin in patients with hypertension: principal results of the Hypertension Optimal Treatment (HOT) randomized trial. Lancet 1998;351:1755–1762.
40. Brown MJ, Palmer CR, Castaigne A, et al: Morbidity and mortality in patients randomised to double-blind treatment with a long-acting calcium-channel blocker or diuretic in the International Nifedipine GITS study: Intervention as a Goal in Hypertension Treatment (INSIGHT). Lancet 2000;356:366–372.
41. Hansson L, Lindholm LH, Niskanen L, et al: Effect of angiotensin-converting-enzyme inhibition compared with conventional therapy on cardiovascular morbidity and mortality in hypertension: the Captopril Prevention Project (CAPP) randomised trial. Lancet 1999;353:611–616.
42. Hansson L, Hedner T, Lund-Johansen P, et al: Randomized trial of effects of calcium antagonists compared with diuretics and beta-blockers on cardiovascular morbidity and mortality in hypertension: the Nordic Diltiazem (NORDIL) Study. Lancet 2000;356:359–365.
43. Blood Pressure Lowering Treatment Trialists Collaboration: Effects of ACE inhibitors, calcium antagonists, and other blood-pressure-lowering drugs: results of prospectively designed overviews of randomized trials. Lancet 2000;356:1955–1964.
44. He J, Whelton PK: Selection of initial antihypertensive drug therapy. Lancet 2000;356:1942–1943.
45. Pahor M, Psaty BM, Alderman MH, et al: Therapeutic effects of calcium antagonists and other antihypertensive drugs. Lancet 2000;356:1949–1954.
46. PROGRESS Collaborative Group: Randomised trial of a perindopril-based blood-pressure lowering regimen among 6105 individuals with previous stroke or transient ischemic attack. Lancet 2001;358:1033–1041.
47. The ALLHAT Officers and Coordinators for the ALLHAT Collaborative Research Group: Major cardiovascular events in

hypertensive patients randomized to doxazosin vs chlorthalidone: the Antihypertensive and Lipid-Lowering Treatment to Prevent Heart Attack Trial (ALLHAT). JAMA 2000;283:1967–1975.

48. The Heart Outcomes Prevention Evaluation Study Investigators: Effects of an angiotensin-converting-enzyme inhibitor, ramipril, on death from cardiovascular causes, myocardial infarction, and stroke in high-risk patients. N Engl J Med 2000;342:145–153.

49. Gottlieb SS, McCarter RJ, Vogel RA: Effect of beta-blockade on mortality among high-risk and low-risk patients after myocardial infarction. N Engl J Med 1998;339:489–497.

50. Gress TW, Nieto J, Shahar E, et al: Hypertension and antihypertensive therapy as risk factors for type 2 diabetes. N Engl J Med 2000;342:905–912.

51. UK Prospective Diabetes Study (UKPDS) Group: Tight blood pressure control and risk of macrovascular and microvascular complications in type 2 diabetes (UKPDS 38). Br Med J 1998;317:703–713.

52. Tuomilehto J, Rastenyte D, Birkenhager WH, et al: Effects of calcium-channel blockade in older patients with diabetes and systolic hypertension. N Engl J Med 1999;340:677–684.

53. Curb JD, Pressel SL, Cutler JA, et al: Effect of diuretic-based antihypertensive treatment on cardiovascular disease risk in older diabetic patients with isolated systolic hypertension. Systolic Hypertension in the Elderly Program Cooperative Research Group. JAMA 1996;276:1886–1892.

54. Heart Outcomes Prevention Evaluation (HOPE) Study Investigators: Effects of ramipril on cardiovascular and microvascular outcomes in people with diabetes mellitus: results of the MICRO-HOPE substudy. Lancet 2000;355:253–259.

55. Parving HH, Lehnert H, Brochner-Mortensen J, et al: The effect of irbesartan on the development of diabetic nephropathy in patients with type 2 diabetes. N Engl J Med 2001;345:870–878.

Nonpharmacologic Treatment

CHAPTER
53

Paul R. Conlin

There is a continuum of risk between increases in blood pressure and cardiovascular events. While 27% of the US adult population have hypertension and often receive some form of therapy,[1] these numbers do not include the substantial group of individuals with high-normal blood pressure whose likelihood of developing hypertension is great. Nonpharmacologic interventions, such as weight reduction, sodium restriction, and changes in dietary patterns, have the ability to reduce the incidence and prevalence of hypertension. Clinicians often do not emphasize these maneuvers, as acceptance and adherence by patients is often low.

Lifestyle and environmental factors affect the risk of death due to coronary heart disease (CHD). CHD mortality as a function of blood pressure has been determined in men from six international sites.[2] Over a 25-year period, the relative risk of death from CHD was quite similar but the absolute risk of CHD death was different, ranging from 20 deaths per 10 000 person-years in Japan and Mediterranean southern Europe to 70 deaths per 10 000 person-years in the USA and northern Europe. Thus, while high blood pressure is an extremely important predictor of CHD mortality, other factors such as dietary and environmental influences also play a significant role.

The treatment of hypertension has evolved considerably over the last 30 years, generating changes in strategies, approaches, and pharmacologic options. One aspect that has remained constant is the recognition that lifestyle modifications are a cornerstone of treatment. While clinical trials of nonpharmacologic treatment in hypertension have not had sufficient power to detect differences in cardiovascular events, epidemiologic studies have strongly supported the effects of these lifestyle modifications based on the observed cardiovascular risk reduction. Several recent studies have evaluated the effects of dietary patterns, sodium restriction, and weight loss on blood pressure in normal and hypertensive individuals.

Effects of dietary patterns

Dietary Approaches to Stop Hypertension study

The rationale for studying dietary patterns and blood pressure stems from observational studies and clinical trials showing that a vegetarian diet or one that replaces animal products with vegetable products lowers blood pressure. However, a practical reality is that vegetarian diets are not widely accepted. Features have been identified in the vegetarian diet (such as higher fiber, potassium, and magnesium content and lower fat content) that may affect blood pressure. All these individual nutrients are associated with lower blood pressure, but trials that have tested the blood pressure-lowering effects of individual nutrients have observed that the change in blood pressure is typically small. This may be due to the fact that each nutrient by itself has a small effect and only when all are consumed together is a clinically significant effect observed.

The Dietary Approaches to Stop Hypertension (DASH) study[3] was designed to identify a diet that lowers blood pressure and is also palatable and acceptable to the general population. In this study, 459 individuals with diastolic blood pressure (DBP) 80–95 mmHg and systolic blood pressure (SBP) < 159 mmHg were randomized to receive one of three intervention diets. Participants were provided with all their meals for an 11-week period. After a 3-week run-in period in which participants were fed a typical American control diet, they were then randomized to continue with the control diet or receive (1) a diet enriched in fruits and vegetables (FV diet) but otherwise similar to the control diet in fat and carbohydrate content or (2) a diet that combined the increased fruits and vegetables of the FV diet with increased low-fat dairy products and overall reduced total and saturated fat and cholesterol (DASH diet). All diets had similar sodium content (~ 3 g/day). The diets and feeding protocols were designed to prevent significant weight change, which might confound the interpretation of changes in blood pressure.

Participants randomized to the DASH diet had a significant fall in both SBP and DBP and the FV diet produced an intermediate effect.[3] The DASH diet lowered blood pressure by –5.5/–3.0 mmHg. The response was greater in African-Americans (–6.9/–3.7 mmHg) than in whites (–3.3/–0.4 mmHg) and those with hypertension benefited the most (–11.6/–5.3 mmHg).[4] Of hypertensives eating the DASH diet 70% had normal blood pressure (SBP

< 140 mmHg and DBP < 90 mmHg) at the end of the study compared with only 23% of those eating the control diet.[5] Ambulatory blood pressure measured in a subset of patients ($n = 354$) both at baseline and after the intervention period showed similar results.[6] The DASH diet was well accepted and compliance during the feeding phase was in excess of 90%.

These favorable effects of the DASH diet on blood pressure have been followed by studies showing that it has added benefits. It is associated with increased serum antioxidant capacity, which may protect against lipid peroxidation,[7] and lower plasma homocysteine levels, possibly related to an increase in serum folate associated with the DASH diet.[8]

While the DASH study was a short-term trial that assessed effects on blood pressure, other studies have recently confirmed the favorable long-term effects of similar lifestyle modifications on cardiovascular disease outcomes. The favorable effects of modifying dietary fat intake on secondary prevention of CHD was confirmed in the Lyon Diet Heart Study, which showed that a Mediterranean-type diet, reduced in saturated fat but enriched in α-linolenic acid, lowered CHD mortality by 70%.[9] A recent clinical trial showed that part of the mechanism of action of a Mediterranean-type diet is through improvement in endothelial function.[10]

Data from two large ongoing cohort studies, the Nurses Health Study (> 75 000 women) and the Health Professionals' Follow-up Study (> 38 000 men), indicated that risk of ischemic stroke was reduced by 31%[11] and risk of CHD was reduced by 20%[12] among individuals consuming the highest quintile for daily intake of fruits and vegetables (approximately five to six servings per day) compared with those in the lowest quintile. In other analyses from the Nurses Health Study, a dietary pattern similar to the DASH diet was associated with a 24% lower risk of CHD over a 12-year period.[13] In the same study cohort, higher fiber intake was associated with a 47% risk reduction for CHD events[14] and higher whole-grain intake with a 43% reduction in ischemic stroke.[15]

Thus the DASH diet lowers blood pressure without weight loss or sodium restriction. Components of the DASH diet are associated with a reduced incidence of cardiovascular events. These findings provide ample evidence that the DASH diet is an effective, well-tolerated, nonpharmacologic treatment for individuals with high-normal blood pressure and stage 1 hypertension.

Effects of sodium restriction

Sodium restriction has been well documented to lower blood pressure in hypertensive individuals. "Sodium sensitivity" is frequently used to describe the blood-pressure response to alteration in dietary sodium in hypertensive individuals, yet this term is variably defined and no specific clinical tool can be applied to predict a given patient's blood pressure response to sodium. Guidelines for the prevention and treatment of hypertension have advocated restriction of dietary sodium intake in the general population.[16] This has generated substantial debate on both sides of the issue.[17–19]

Most would agree that although there is significant interindividual variability, reduced sodium intake is associated with lower blood pressure among older, hypertensive, or African-American individuals. Whether young and normotensive individuals have a response to sodium restriction has been debated. Contributing to this discussion is the association between higher dietary sodium intake and risk of cardiovascular disease, confirmed in data obtained from a follow-up of overweight persons in the National Health and Nutrition Examination Survey (NHANES I).[20] There is concern that the accompaniments of sodium restriction, such as increased plasma renin activity, sympathetic nervous system activity, and insulin resistance, may impose adverse effects that counterbalance or exceed any net benefit.

DASH-Sodium study

The DASH-Sodium study added significant new information on the role of sodium restriction in lowering blood pressure while also confirming the results of the DASH study.[21] The DASH-Sodium study was a feeding trial that compared the effects on SBP of three levels of sodium intake in two dietary patterns, a control diet and the DASH diet. The three sodium levels were defined as "higher" (target 150 mmol/day, typical of US consumption), "intermediate" (target 100 mmol/day, the upper limit of current US recommendations), and "lower" (target 50 mmol/day, a possible optimal level). Using similar eligibility criteria as the DASH study, participants entered a 2-week run-in period eating the control diet with higher sodium and were then randomized to one of the two dietary patterns with higher, intermediate, and lower sodium levels for 30 days each, with the sequence determined randomly.

When compared with the control diet, the DASH diet significantly lowered SBP at each sodium level: –5.9 mmHg with higher, –5.0 mmHg with intermediate, and –2.1 mmHg with lower sodium intake. The effects were significant in nonhypertensives, hypertensives, African-Americans, all other races, men, and women.[22] When compared with the control diet with higher sodium, the DASH diet with lower sodium lowered blood pressure in hypertensives (–11.5/–5.7 mmHg) and nonhypertensives (–7.1/–3.7 mmHg).

Thus the DASH-sodium study showed that sodium reduction to levels below the current recommendation of 100 mmol/day, either alone or in conjunction with the DASH diet, substantially lowers blood pressure. The effect is greater with the two interventions in combination, the DASH diet and sodium restriction, than with either alone. However, the long-term health benefits that might accrue with chronic adherence to the DASH-sodium diet at the lowest level of sodium intake are unproven.

Effects of weight loss

Weight loss as a lifestyle modification has long been advocated to lower blood pressure and also reduce other cardiovascular risk factors. This has been explored in relationship to blood pressure in recent trials.[23–28] In each of these trials, weight loss (particularly among obese participants) lowered blood pressure, prevented the development of hypertension, or potentiated the effect of antihypertensive medications. Results from a few of these trials are highlighted.

The Trials of Hypertension Prevention (TOHP) Phase 1 was an 18-month lifestyle modification trial in which individuals with high-normal blood pressure were randomized to weight loss, sodium restriction, or a control group.[25] Follow-up examinations (7 years after randomization) were conducted in 181 of the 208 participants studied at Johns Hopkins University in Baltimore.[26] During the original 18-month study, significant weight loss was achieved in the group randomized to the weight-loss intervention and this was associated with a significant reduction in blood pressure. However, after 7 years of follow-up, the weight-loss group did not differ in body weight or urinary sodium excretion from the other intervention groups. Despite this apparent loss of effect, the weight-loss group had an incidence of hypertension that was reduced by 77%.

The TOHP Phase 2 study had a similar design but enrolled more patients and had 3–4 years of follow-up.[27] The group randomized to weight loss (595 individuals with high-normal blood pressure who were 110–165% of ideal body weight) had a 2-kg weight difference at 3 years of follow-up compared with the control group. This modest weight loss was associated with a risk ratio of 0.81 (19% risk reduction) for the development of hypertension; those with a sustained 4.5-kg weight loss had a risk ratio of 0.35 (65% risk reduction).

In a substudy of the Hypertension Optimal Treatment (HOT) study, obese hypertensive patients were randomly assigned to receive a weight-loss intervention, including individual and group counseling, and compared with those receiving no intervention.[28] Those in the weight-loss group lost significantly more weight than the control group during the initial 6 months following randomization but at 30 months of follow-up there was no significant difference between the groups. Despite this, patients in the weight-loss group used fewer medications to achieve the same level of blood pressure.

These results show that dietary modifications implemented as part of a weight-loss intervention, even without producing sustained weight loss, may facilitate control of blood pressure and prevent the progression to hypertension or control blood pressure with fewer antihypertensive medications.

Effects of exercise

Exercise is frequently promoted as a tool to facilitate weight loss and with independent favorable effects on blood pressure. Indeed, exercise and weight loss together result in lower blood pressure than either alone.[29] The mechanisms that mediate lowering of blood pressure with exercise are not fully understood but the effects appear to be independent of changes in weight or body composition. Several studies have evaluated the effects of moderate-intensity aerobic exercise or resistance training on blood pressure.

Among individuals with high-normal or stage 1 hypertension, aerobic exercise significantly lowers blood pressure, although the effects tend to be smaller than those seen with moderate sodium restriction.[30] Among postmenopausal women[31] or elderly individuals,[32] low- to moderate-intensity aerobic exercise (e.g., walking) significantly lowers blood pressure. Among postmenopausal women, increased frequency of moderate physical activity was associated with a 30% lower risk of mortality during a 7-year follow-up period.[33]

Three metaanalyses have analyzed results from clinical trials that assessed the effects of walking, aerobic exercise, and resistance exercise on blood pressure. From these studies one may conclude that regular aerobic exercise produces the greatest reduction in blood pressure (–7/–6 mmHg)[34] compared with walking (–3/–2 mmHg)[35] or resistance exercise (–3/–3 mmHg).[36]

Thus the optimum exercise program for blood-pressure reduction should include moderate-intensity aerobic exercise three to five times per week for 30–60 min per session. Resistance exercise has limited effects on blood pressure and should not be recommended as the sole form of exercise. There is no apparent age- or sex-related difference in the response to exercise. Weight loss is facilitated by exercise programs that expend 1255–2090 kJ/day. Exercise intensity and duration should be appropriate to the individual's abilities and concomitant medical conditions. In some cases an assessment of cardiovascular risk, by completing a supervised exercise test, may be appropriate before participation in a regular exercise program. The most benefits on blood pressure occur in individuals with high-normal or stages 1–2 hypertension.

Conclusion and recommendations

Several studies have conclusively demonstrated the favorable effects on blood pressure of sodium restriction and consumption of low-fat diets enriched in fruits and vegetables, the sustained effects of weight-loss interventions, and the benefits of aerobic exercise. The results of the DASH and DASH-Sodium studies have broad applicability to the US population. If a population-wide reduction in blood pressure were achieved to the extent observed with the DASH diet, this would reduce the incidence of CHD by 15% and stroke by 27%.[16] The long-term effects on blood pressure of weight-loss interventions, with or without aerobic exercise, provide a strong case to continue advocating that obese individuals receive weight management counseling. A secondary benefit of these lifestyle changes (2–3 kg weight loss) includes a reduced incidence of type 2 diabetes mellitus, particularly in those with impaired glucose tolerance.[37]

The foods prepared and fed to participants during the DASH and DASH-Sodium studies are generally available, although low-sodium foods are more difficult to identify (Table 53.1). Importantly, the cost of eating a DASH diet is not expensive. It has been estimated that the cost for a family of four to eat the DASH diet, using items purchased at a typical grocery store, would be between "low cost"

Table 53.1 Sodium content of common foods before and after processing*

Food groups	Sodium (mg)
Grains and grain products	
Cooked cereal, rice, pasta, unsalted, ½ cup	0–5
Ready-to-eat-cereal, 1 cup	100–360
Bread, 1 slice	110-175
Vegetables	
Fresh or frozen, cooked without salt, ½ cup	1–70
Canned or frozen with sauce, ½ cup	140–460
Tomato juice, canned ½ cup	820
Fruit	
Fresh, frozen, canned, ½ cup	0–5
Low-fat or fat-free dairy foods	
Milk, 1 cup	120
Yogurt, 8 oz	160
Natural cheeses, 1½ oz	110–450
Processed cheeses, 1½ oz	600
Nuts, seeds, and dry beans	
Peanuts, salted, ⅓ cup	120
Peanuts, unsalted, ⅓ cup	0–5
Beans, cooked from dried or frozen, without salt, ½ cup	0–5
Beans, canned, ½ cup	400
Meats, fish, and poultry	
Fresh meat, fish, poultry, 3 oz	30–90
Tuna canned, water pack, no salt added, 3 oz	35–45
Tuna canned, water pack, 3 oz	250–350
Ham, lean, roasted, 3 oz	1020

*From National Institutes of Health: Facts about the DASH Diet. Bethesda, MD: National Institutes of Health, NIH Publication No. 01-4082, 2001.

and "moderate cost" based on the typical food costs for a family of four as estimated by the United States Department of Agriculture.[38] Eating the DASH diet requires attention to food groups, caloric requirements, and the calorie and sodium content of foods (Table 53.2). The servings of fruits and vegetables (8–10 daily) are approximately twice the typical daily consumption of four servings by US adults. Likewise, the three servings of dairy products are twice the typical daily US consumption.[39] More detailed summaries of the findings of the DASH and DASH-Sodium studies and some menus that employ the DASH diet have been developed for a lay audience.[40,41]

While the results of the DASH and DASH-Sodium studies are relevant to the care of patients with high-normal and established hypertension, it is important to keep in mind a few points that were not addressed.

1. Each study involved only 8–11 weeks of intervention feeding. It is not known whether the blood-pressure changes observed are sustained over longer periods of time, particularly when adherence to the diet may decline. It is also not known whether full compliance with the dietary pattern is necessary to produce the full effect.
2. The DASH study tested the effects of eating a dietary pattern rather than individual nutrients. One cannot conclude that specific food items and/or nutrients produced the effects of the diet.
3. These studies were conducted in individuals with high-normal or stage 1 hypertension. It is not known if similar or greater effects would be seen in patients with higher levels of blood pressure.
4. The DASH diet is enriched in potassium, magnesium, and protein, which should be limited in patients with kidney disease. Therefore, the DASH diet should be implemented with caution in these patients.

Table 53.2 Following the DASH diet*

Food group	Daily servings (except as noted)	Serving sizes	Examples and notes	Significance of each food group to the DASH eating plan
Grain and grain products	7–8	1 slice bread 1 oz dry cereal† ½ cup cooked rice, pasta, or cereal	Whole wheat bread, English muffin, pitta bread, bagel, cereals, grits, oatmeal, crackers, unsalted pretzels, popcorn	Major sources of energy and fiber
Vegetables	4–5	1 cup raw leafy vegetable ½ cup cooked vegetable 6 oz vegetable juice	Tomatoes, potatoes, carrots, green peas, squash, broccoli, turnip greens, collards, kale, spinach, artichokes, green beans, lima beans, sweet potatoes	Rich sources of potassium, magnesium, and fiber
Fruits	4–5	6 oz fruit juice 1 medium fruit ½ cup dried fruit ½ cup fresh, frozen, or canned fruit	Apricots, bananas, dates, grapes, oranges, orange juice, grapefruit, grapefruit juice, mangoes, melons, peaches, pineapples, prunes, raisins, strawberries, tangerines	Important sources of potassium, magnesium, and fiber

Table 53.2 (*cont'd*)

Food group	Daily servings (except as noted)	Serving sizes	Examples and notes	Significance of each food group to the DASH eating plan
Low-fat or fat-free dairy foods	2–3	8 oz skim milk 1 cup yogurt $1\frac{1}{2}$ oz cheese	Fat-free (skim) or low-fat (1%) milk, fat-free or low-fat buttermilk, fat-free or low-fat regular or frozen yogurt, low-fat and fat-free cheese	Major sources of calcium and protein
Meats, poultry, and fish	2 or less	3 oz cooked meats, poultry, or fish	Select only lean; trim away visible fats; broil, roast, or boil instead of frying; remove skin from poultry	Rich sources of protein and magnesium
Nuts, seeds, and dry beans	4–5 per week	$\frac{1}{3}$ cup or $1\frac{1}{2}$ oz nuts 2 tbsp or $\frac{1}{2}$ oz seeds $\frac{1}{2}$ cup cooked dry beans	Almonds, filberts, mixed nuts, peanuts, walnuts, sunflower seeds, kidney beans, lentils, peas	Rich sources of energy, magnesium, potassium, protein, and fiber
Fats and oils‡	2–3	1 tsp soft margarine 1 tbsp low-fat mayonnaise 2 tbsp light salad dressing 1 tsp vegetable oil	Soft margarine, low-fat mayonnaise, light salad dressing, vegetable oil (such as olive, corn, canola, or safflower)	DASH has 27% of calories as fat, including that in or added to foods
Sweets	5 per week	1 tbsp sugar 1 tbsp jelly or jam $\frac{1}{2}$ oz jelly beans 8 oz lemonade	Maple syrup, sugar, jelly, jam, fruit-flavored gelatin, jelly beans, hard candy, fruit punch, sorbet, ices	Sweets should be low in fat

*The DASH eating plan is based on an intake of 2000 kcal/day. The number of daily servings in a food group may vary based on the caloric needs of the individual. From National Institutes of Health: Facts about the DASH Diet. Bethesda, MD: National Institutes of Health, NIH Publication No. 01-4082, 2001.

†Equals $\frac{1}{2}$ to $1\frac{1}{4}$ cup, depending on cereal type. Check the product's nutrition label.

‡Fat content changes serving counts for fats and oils, e.g., 1 tbsp of regular salad dressing equals one serving; 1 tbsp of a low-fat dressing equals $\frac{1}{2}$ serving; 1 tbsp of a fat-free dressing equals zero servings. tbsp, tablespoon; tsp, teaspoon.

5. The blood pressure-lowering effects of sodium restriction and the DASH diet were greater than either alone. It is not known if the addition of other nonpharmacologic treatments such as weight loss and exercise lowers blood pressure further.

Nonpharmacologic treatment can be implemented by patients on their own, involves minimal risk (and may have a positive impact on quality of life), and also may be less expensive than medications. The long-term beneficial effects of dietary patterns like the DASH diet on the incidence of cardiovascular events has been demonstrated. While debate continues about whether sodium restriction should be recommended to all in the general population, the DASH-Sodium study showed that individuals with high-normal blood pressure have favorable effects. Weight loss and regular aerobic exercise lead to lower blood pressure even in the absence of sustained weight loss. Clearly, the role of lifestyle modifications as both preventive and adjunctive means to lower blood pressure has been reaffirmed.

References

1. Hyman DJ, Pavlik VN: Characteristics of patients with uncontrolled hypertension in the United States. N Engl J Med 2001;345:479–486.
2. van den Hoogen PCW, Feskens EJM, Nagelkerke NJD, et al: The relation between blood pressure and mortality due to coronary heart disease among men in different parts of the world. N Engl J Med 2000;342:1–8.
3. Appel LJ, Moore TJ, Obarzanek E, et al: A clinical trial of the effects of dietary patterns on blood pressure. N Engl J Med 1997;336:1117–1124.
4. Svetkey LP, Simons-Morton D, Vollmer WM, et al: Effects of dietary patterns on blood pressure: subgroup analysis of the Dietary Approaches to Stop Hypertension (DASH) randomized clinical trial. Arch Intern Med 1999;159:285–293.
5. Conlin PR, Chow D, Miller ER, et al: The effect of dietary patterns on blood pressure control in hypertensive patients: results from the Dietary Approaches to Stop Hypertension (DASH) Trial. Am J Hypertens 2000;13:949–955.
6. Moore TJ, Vollmer WM, Appel LJ, et al: Effect of dietary patterns on ambulatory blood pressure: results from the DASH study. Hypertension 1999;34:472–477.
7. Miller ER III, Appel LJ, Risby TH: Effect of dietary patterns on measures of lipid peroxidation: results from a randomized clinical trial. Circulation 1998;98:2390–2395.

8. Appel LJ, Miller III ER, Jee SH, et al: Effect of dietary patterns on serum homocysteine: results of a randomized, controlled feeding study. Circulation 2000;102:852–857.

9. de Lorgeril M, Salen P, Martin J-L, et al: Mediterranean diet, traditional risk factors, and the rate of cardiovascular complications after myocardial infarction: final report of the Lyon Diet Heart Study. Circulation 1999;99:779–785.

10. Fuentes F, Lopez-Miranda J, Sanchez E, et al: Mediterranean and low-fat diets improve endothelial function in hypercholesterolemic men. Ann Intern Med 2001;134:1115–1119.

11. Joshipura KJ, Ascherio A, Manson JE, et al: Fruit and vegetable intake in relation to risk of ischemic stroke. JAMA 1999;282:1233–1239.

12. Joshipura KJ, Hu FB, Manson JE, et al: The effect of fruit and vegetable intake on risk for coronary heart disease. Ann Intern Med 2001;134:1106–1114.

13. Fung TT, Willet WC, Stampfer MJ, et al: Dietary patterns and the risk of coronary heart disease in women. Arch Intern Med 2001;161:1857–1862.

14. Wolk A, Manson JE, Stampfer MJ, et al: Long-term intake of dietary fiber and decreased risk of coronary heart disease among women. JAMA 1999;281:1998–2004.

15. Liu S, Manson JE, Stampfer MJ, et al: Whole grain consumption and risk of ischemic stroke in women: a prospective study. JAMA 2000;284:1534–1540.

16. The Sixth Report of the Joint National Committee on Prevention, Detection, Evaluation, and Treatment of high blood pressure. Arch Intern Med 1997;157:2413–2445.

17. Swales J: Population advice on salt restriction: the social issues. Am J Hypertens 2000;13:2–7.

18. MacGregor GA, de Wardener HE: "Salt": a commentary. Am J Hypertens 2000;13:313–316.

19. Alderman MH: Salt, blood pressure and human health. Hypertension 2000;36:890–893.

20. He J, Ogden LG, Vupputuri S, et al: Dietary sodium intake and subsequent risk of cardiovascular disease in overweight adults. JAMA 1999;282:2027–2034.

21. Sacks FM, Svetkey LP, Vollmer WM, et al: A clinical trial of the effects on blood pressure of reduced dietary sodium and the DASH dietary pattern (The DASH-Sodium Trial). N Engl J Med 2001;344:3–10.

22. Vollmer WM, Sacks FM, Ard J, et al: Effects of dietary patterns and sodium intake on blood pressure: subgroup analysis of the DASH-Sodium trial. Ann Intern Med 2001;135:1019–1028.

23. Whelton PK, Appel LJ, Espeland MA, et al: Sodium reduction and weight loss in the treatment of hypertension in older persons: a randomized controlled trial of nonpharmacologic interventions in the elderly (TONE). JAMA 1998;279:839–846.

24. The Trials of Hypertension Prevention Collaborative Research Group: Effects of weight loss and sodium reduction intervention on blood pressure and hypertension incidence in overweight people with high-normal blood pressure: the Trials of Hypertension Prevention, Phase II. Arch Intern Med 1997;157:657–667.

25. Trials of Hypertension Prevention Collaborative Research Group: The effects of non-pharmacologic interventions on blood pressure of persons with high normal levels: results of the Trials of Hypertension Prevention, Phase 1. JAMA 1992;267:1213–1220.

26. He J, Whelton PK, Appel LJ, et al: Long-term effects of weight loss and dietary sodium reduction on incidence of hypertension. Hypertension 2000;35:544–549.

27. Stevens, VJ, Obarzanek E, Cook NR, et al: Long-term weight loss and changes in blood pressure: results of the Trials of Hypertension Prevention, phase II. Ann Intern Med 2001;134:72–74.

28. Jones DW, Miller ME, Wofford MR, et al: The effect of weight loss intervention on antihypertensive medication requirements in the Hypertension Optimal Treatment (HOT) Study. Am J Hypertens 1999;12:1175–1180.

29. Steffen PR, Sherwood A, Gullette EC, Georgiades A, Hinderliter A, Blumenthal JA: Effects of exercise and weight loss on blood pressure during daily life. Med Sci Sports Exerc 2001;33:1635–1640.

30. Seals DR, Tanaka H, Clevenger CM, et al: Blood pressure reductions with exercise and sodium restriction in post-menopausal women with elevated systolic pressure: role of arterial stiffness. J Am Coll Cardiol 2001;38:506–513.

31. Seals DR, Silverman HG, Reiling MJ, Davy KP: Effect of regular aerobic exercise on elevated blood pressure in postmenopausal women. Am J Cardiol 1997;80:49–55.

32. Ehsani AA: Exercise in patients with hypertension. Am J Geriatr Cardiol 2001;10:253–259.

33. Kushi LH, Fee RM, Folsom AR, Mink PJ, Anderson KE, Sellers TA: Physical activity and mortality in postmenopausal women. JAMA 1997;277:1287–1292.

34. Kelley G, McClellan P: Antihypertensive effects of aerobic exercise: a brief meta-analytic review of randomized controlled trials. Am J Hypertens 1994;7:115–119.

35. Kelley GA, Kelley KS, Tran ZV: Walking and resting blood pressure in adults: a meta-analysis. Prev Med 2001;33:120–127.

36. Kelley GA, Kelley KS: Progressive resistance exercise and resting blood pressure: a meta-analysis of randomized controlled trials. Hypertension 2000;35:838–843.

37. Tuomilehto J, Lindstrom J, Eriksson J, et al: Prevention of type 2 diabetes mellitus by changes in lifestyle among subjects with impaired glucose tolerance. N Engl J Med 2001;344:1343–1350.

38. Center for Nutrition Policy and Promotion, Washington, DC www.usda.gov/fcs/cnpp.htm

39. Cleveland LE, Goldman JD, Borrud LG: Data Tables: Results from the USDA's 1994 Continuing Survey of Food Intakes by Individuals and the 1994 Diet and Health Knowledge Survey. Riverdale, MD: Food Surveys Research Group, 1996.

40. National Institutes of Health: Facts about the DASH Diet. Bethesda, MD: National Institutes of Health, NIH Publication No. 01-4082, 2001.

41. Moore TM, Pao-Hwa L, Karanja N, Svetkey L, Jenkins M: The DASH Diet for Hypertension. New York: Free Press, 2001.

536

CHAPTER 54

Diuretics and β-Blockers

Hamish Dobbie, Giovambattista Capasso, and Robert Unwin

The original large clinical trials that demonstrated unequivocally the benefit of drug treatment for hypertension were carried out using diuretics and β-blockers. In recent years a succession of newer antihypertensive drugs have become available and the role of these older drugs has been called into question. Much research has been carried out into the mechanisms of action of these drugs; the mode of action of diuretics is discussed in Chapter 95. The β-blockers act by reducing both heart rate and cardiac output and the production of renin by the kidneys. In this chapter we summarize the data currently available on diuretics and β-blockers and show that they still have a central role to play in the treatment of most hypertensive patients in the twenty-first century.

Randomized trials of diuretic or β-blocker treatment against placebo

The results of randomized trials comparing diuretics or β-blockers with placebo are discussed extensively in the recent metaanalysis and review by Psaty et al.[1] The 18 trials identified included 48 220 patients, followed up for an average of 5 years. The earlier trials were mainly carried out on middle-aged adults and involved the use of higher doses of diuretics or β-blockers; trials from the late 1980s

and the 1990s were largely in older adults and involved the use of lower doses of diuretics. High-dose diuretics, low-dose diuretics, and β-blockers all reduced the risk of stroke, with relative risks (RR) in the metaanalysis of 0.49, 0.66, and 0.71 respectively. The risk of coronary heart disease was reduced in the low-dose diuretic trials (RR 0.72) but not in the high-dose diuretic trials or the β-blocker trials. These results are somewhat surprising in view of the proven benefits of β-blockers in secondary prevention of coronary heart disease. It is not clear if this difference in rate of coronary events is due to the difference in patient groups included in these trials or a real biologic difference between these therapies. Cardiovascular mortality was significantly reduced by high-dose and low-dose diuretic therapy, although the reduction was not significant for β-blockers. There was a trend toward reduced overall mortality for all therapies but in no case did this reach statistical significance.

In a 22-year follow-up of hypertensive men identified and treated in the 1970s a significant excess of deaths due to cardiovascular disease and stroke has been shown, despite good control of blood pressure on treatment.[2] This suggests that even patients well treated with current therapies do not return to the cardiovascular risk of the general population. An overview and metaanalysis of drug treatment of hypertension, comparing treated groups with placebo controls, concluded that even over the short term (a few years) effective treatment of hypertension reduces the risk of stroke in treated patients by almost exactly the amount expected on the basis of epidemiologic studies.[3] However, the reduction in risk of coronary heart disease, although clinically and statistically significant, is less than might have been expected for the observed fall in blood pressure. This failure of (predominantly diuretic-based) treatment to reverse the increased mortality associated with hypertension may be due to their adverse metabolic effects.[4] Other explanations for this finding include the fact that hypertensive patients also often have multiple additional risk factors for cardiovascular disease and the fact that arteriosclerosis develops over decades so it may not be realistic to expect a few years of treatment to reverse it.

Randomized trials of diuretics or β-blockers against other antihypertensive treatments

There is now general agreement about the benefits to be expected from the treatment of hypertension in the middle-aged and elderly. Further placebo-controlled trials are probably no longer ethically justifiable. Recent trials have concentrated on comparing therapeutic strategies with one another. A number of trials have compared diuretic-based regimens with newer therapies. In no large trial has there been any significant advantage in clinical endpoints when treatment with a newer agent is compared with β-blockers or diuretics. In two large trials, one arm was halted when a newer agent, doxazosin[5] or amlodipine,[6] was found to be inferior. In the metaanalysis of trials comparing angiotensin-converting enzyme (ACE) inhibitors with diuretics or β-blockers conducted by the Blood Pressure Lowering Treatment Trialists Collaboration, diuretics or β-blockers were found to be associated with no significant difference in the risk of stroke, coronary heart disease, heart failure, cardiovascular death, or all-cause mortality compared with ACE inhibitors.[7] Comparing dihydropyridine calcium channel antagonists with diuretic or β-blocker therapy shows a slightly reduced risk of heart failure (RR 0.89) and coronary heart disease (RR 0.89) with diuretics or β-blockers, but these differences did not reach statistical significance.[7] The risk of stroke was slightly raised on diuretics or β-blockers compared with calcium channel blockers (RR 1.12); this difference just reached significance. However, there was no difference in cardiovascular or all-cause mortality. In summary, with the exception of certain well-defined subgroups discussed later, there is no evidence that any other treatment for hypertension is superior to diuretics or β-blockers in terms of any important clinical outcome.

Adverse effects of diuretics and β-blockers

One reason for the fall in popularity of diuretics and β-blockers is the belief that these drugs have detrimental adverse effects. In fact many of these adverse effects are much less of a problem at the lower doses now recommended.

Hypokalemia

Thiazide diuretics deplete potassium in a dose-dependent fashion. In the Multiple Risk Factor Intervention Trial, in a subgroup of patients with abnormal ECGs at baseline, there was an increase in the risk of death due to coronary heart disease in patients randomized to more intensive management including high-dose thiazide diuretics.[8] However, in patients with normal ECGs there was a lower mortality in the intensively treated group. The incidence of diuretic treatment in the control group is not known but was probably considerable. In the Systolic Hypertension in the Elderly Program (SHEP) trial, patients randomized to diuretics had significantly lower potassium levels than those on placebo (average reduction 0.36 mmol/L) and significantly more of them were frankly hypokalemic (7.2% vs. 1%).[9] Hypokalemic patients had higher event rates that were similar to patients on placebo. A case–control study found that patients on high-dose diuretics were at an increased risk of cardiac arrest compared with patients on lower doses.[10] The lowest risk of all was found in patients taking thiazides in combination with a potassium-sparing diuretic. It is clearly important to measure serum potassium,

and if necessary correct hypokalemia, in patients taking thiazide diuretics.

Dyslipidemia

It has long been recognized that diuretics are associated with modest changes in serum lipids in short-term studies. In a metaanalysis there was a significant increase in total and low-density lipoprotein cholesterol but no change in high-density lipoprotein cholesterol in patients treated with diuretics.[11] These changes were much more marked in patients on high diuretic doses. Moreover, in longer-term studies, the effects do not seem to persist beyond 1 year.[12,13] In the Treatment Of Mild Hypertension Study (TOMHS), the placebo and diuretic groups showed no difference in their lipids after the first year.[13] In the Multicentre Isradipine Diuretic Atherosclerosis Study (MIDAS), the differences in lipids noted in the first year between patients treated with thiazides and those treated with calcium channel blockers had disappeared by the third year. Overall, it is reasonable to conclude that the effects of both thiazides and β-blockers on serum lipids are small and of little clinical significance.[14]

Insulin resistance/diabetes

There is evidence that both diuretics and β-blockers can worsen glucose tolerance. However, in a prospective study of nondiabetic adults followed for 6 years, there was no increased risk of diabetes in those who received a thiazide.[15] In this study, taking β-blockers was associated with a 28% increase in the risk of developing diabetes, although as the study was not randomized differences in patient selection for these drug classes cannot be ruled out. Patients who were hypertensive at baseline were almost 2.5 times more likely to develop diabetes over the next 6 years. In the SHEP trial, there was no difference in mean fasting glucose levels between patients treated for 3 years with low-dose thiazides and those given placebo.[16] In a subgroup analysis, diabetic patients had exactly the same relative reduction in cardiovascular events on treatment as nondiabetic patients.[17] Since they were at a greater risk of cardiovascular events, diabetic patients had twice the absolute benefit from treatment. In the United Kingdom Prospective Diabetes Study (UKPDS) 38, diabetic patients randomized to a β-blocker-based regimen did as well as those treated with ACE inhibitors.[18]

Hyperuricemia

Diuretics raise serum urate by decreasing renal excretion and increasing reabsorption. Gout is one of the few contraindications to thiazide therapy for hypertension. Hyperuricemia per se is a recognized risk factor for cardiovascular disease,[19] although in the Framingham cohort it was no longer significant once allowance had been made for other risk factors.[20] Some have suggested that urate itself is toxic, perhaps through generation of free radicals,[21] while others maintain that the association is noncausal.[20] The influence of serum uric acid on cardiovascular events has been examined in the patients randomized in the SHEP trial.[22] In this group, the baseline serum urate level did predict subsequent events, although the relative risk of the highest versus the lowest quintile of serum urate was only 1.32. Baseline urate levels did not affect the demonstrable benefits of active treatment in this trial. Treatment with a thiazide increased serum urate by a median 0.06 mmol/L. When patients were divided into two groups according to the increase in serum urate level, those with a small change in serum urate (< 0.06 mmol/L) had a highly significant reduction in event rates on treatment, whereas those with a larger increase in urate had no decrease in event rates on active treatment. These data suggest that patients can be stratified in terms of their cardiovascular risk according to the response of their serum urate to thiazides. However, there is no direct evidence that the increases in urate seen in patients taking thiazides are in themselves harmful. Moreover, thiazides have the same effects on risk of cardiac death as β-blockers and ACE inhibitors, which do not affect serum urate.

Sexual dysfunction

Impotence was reported with considerable frequency in the Medical Research Council trial of mild hypertension, leading to the withdrawal of 12.6% of male patients from the diuretic arm compared with 6.3% in the β-blocker arm and 1.3% in the placebo arm.[23] The incidence of this adverse effect seems to be less in more recent trials, although whether this relates to the lower doses of diuretics used or the older patient populations studied in more recent trials is not clear. There is evidence that the incidence of sexual dysfunction is increased in men with hypertension, whether they are on treatment or not: the incidence of complete erectile dysfunction is 15% in those with treated hypertension and 14% in those with untreated hypertension in a population sample of American men in whom the overall incidence of impotence was 9.6%.[24] A post-hoc subanalysis of patients in trials of sildenafil who were taking antihypertensives concluded that sildenafil was as effective in these patients as in those not taking antihypertensives and no more likely to cause adverse effects.[25] Whether antihypertensive treatment causes sexual dysfunction in women is less clear, although most investigators have reported no significant problems. Prisant et al[26] review this area and conclude that only high-dose diuretics consistently cause sexual dysfunction.

Increased risk of cancer

An association between diuretic use and renal or colonic cancer has been suggested.[27] Case–control studies have suggested an increased risk of renal cell carcinoma. The largest of the case–control studies found that the excess risk associated with being hypertensive was larger than that associated with any drug exposure, and that the risk associated with diuretic use disappeared once adjustment

had been made for the risk associated with hypertension.[28] Three large cohort studies have also suggested some risk, although the most recent and largest such study suggested the increased risk applied to women only and was not seen in patients on monotherapy. No clinical trial of these agents has demonstrated an increased risk of cancer in treated patients, although as most trials are followed up for less than 5 years and many patients take antihypertensives for decades this issue is still open. In a cohort of hypertensive men treated for more than two decades with therapy based on diuretics and β-blockers, there was no increase in cancer mortality.[2] At present the proven benefits of blood pressure reduction outweigh the unproven and rather poorly defined risks of cancer.

Effects on bone

Thiazide diuretics reduce urinary calcium excretion and are thought to reduce postmenopausal bone loss. Numerous case–control studies have demonstrated a reduction in risk of fractures in patients taking thiazides.[29] It has been suggested that hypertension itself is a risk factor for bone mineral loss.[30] A recent randomized controlled trial demonstrated that thiazides slow cortical bone loss in postmenopausal women, although the effect was small.[31]

Diuretic and β-blocker use in specific groups of patients

The elderly

The evidence for the benefits of drug treatment of isolated systolic hypertension in the elderly is now overwhelming.[9,32,33] The most dramatic reductions are in risk of stroke, both ischemic and hemorrhagic,[34] but there are also reductions in the risk of coronary heart disease and heart failure. Elderly patients also benefit from the treatment of diastolic hypertension.[35] There is some residual uncertainty about the treatment of patients over the age of 80, although a subgroup metaanalysis of patients over this age included in the trials of the last 20 years concluded that they too benefit from treatment.[36] Thiazide diuretics are well tolerated by the elderly and are of proven effectiveness.[35] A systematic review of the risk of falls in elderly patients on antihypertensive drugs found a modestly increased risk with diuretics (odds ratio 1.08) and nonsignificant differences for β-blockers and other classes of antihypertensives.[37] None of the studies was randomized and overall the effects found were small. Because of their high absolute risk of stroke and cardiovascular events, elderly patients have much to gain from effective treatment. In most older patients a low-dose thiazide is the preferred treatment; β-blockers are less well tolerated by older persons and should probably be avoided unless there is a specific indication, for example after myocardial infarction.[38] An appropriate second or additional treatment would be a calcium channel blocker.

Black patients

There is considerable evidence that black people have higher rates of hypertension than the population as a whole.[39] They also have higher risks of stroke and renal failure, although (at least in the UK) not of coronary artery disease.[40] Black patients are more likely to have salt-sensitive hypertension and are less likely to have high renin levels.[41] Hypertensive black men have a larger blood pressure response to hydrochlorothiazide than to propranolol, whereas this difference is not significant in white men.[42] Studies have usually found that black patients respond well to diuretics[12] but require higher doses of ACE inhibitors to obtain a given level of blood pressure control. A recently published trial from South Africa[43] concluded that in black patients calcium channel blockers were more effective as monotherapy than either diuretics or ACE inhibitors, although these patients were rather younger than those in most other published studies. However, current UK and US guidelines recommend using thiazides as preferred treatment in black patients.

Patients with cardiovascular disease

In patients who have suffered a heart attack, subsequent prescription of a β-blocker reduces mortality by about 20%.[44] This also applies to diabetic patients.[45] ACE inhibitors also benefit this group of patients. Many patients should be taking both drugs as well as aspirin.[46] The Heart Outcomes Prevention Evaluation (HOPE) study showed that the ACE inhibitor ramipril reduced the risk of death, myocardial infarction, and stroke each by about 20% in patients at high vascular risk.[47] Although 80% of patients in this trial had previously suffered a myocardial infarction, only 40% were on a β-blocker. Patients in the HOPE study had acceptable control of blood pressure at study entry and the investigators concluded that the effects of ACE inhibition were not due to blood pressure reduction. The recent trial of secondary prevention of stroke using a perindopril-based regimen recorded a lower risk of subsequent stroke among actively treated patients, although subgroup analysis found that only those treated with both ACE inhibitors and diuretics had significant benefit.[48] The American Heart Association now recommends β-blockers for all patients recovering after myocardial infarction and acute coronary syndromes, and ACE inhibitors for all patients recovering after myocardial infarction and to be considered in all patients with coronary or peripheral vascular disease.[49] On balance it is clear that all patients with hypertension and established coronary disease should receive treatment with β-blockers and probably ACE inhibitors also.

Patients with heart failure

The β-blockers are negatively inotropic and can worsen or precipitate heart failure, especially at high doses. For this reason heart failure was long regarded as a contraindication to β-blocker therapy. Recent trials have shown that closely supervised β-blocker treatment is associated with reduced mortality in patients with moderate[50,51] and severe heart failure. This is partly due to a reduction in the incidence of sudden death. Trials have used the cardioselective β-blockers bisoprolol and metoprolol and the nonselective αβ-blocker carvedilol. It remains unclear whether these have the same benefit: a head-to-head comparison showed a greater improvement in left ventricular ejection fraction with carvedilol but a greater increase in exercise capacity with metoprolol.[50] The most appropriate strategy based on currently published data is to treat with both ACE inhibitors and β-blockers if tolerated, and to aim for a blood pressure target of 130/70 mmHg or below. Diuretics can be added to control fluid overload, although there is no evidence that they alter outcomes.

Patients with left ventricular hypertrophy

Left ventricular hypertrophy (LVH) is an independent risk factor for cardiovascular events and sudden cardiac death.[52] Patients with hypertension often have LVH. In the Framingham Heart Study of persons over 40 less than 1% had an ECG suggesting LVH, but 15.5% of men and 21% of women had LVH on echocardiography.[52] Some of the newer antihypertensives may be better at inducing regression of LVH than diuretics or β-blockers. A metaanalysis of randomized studies concluded that ACE inhibitors are more effective at reducing LVH than β-blockers, calcium channel antagonists, or diuretics.[53] Direct head-to-head trial evidence suggests that diuretics are as effective as other drugs in inducing regression of LVH, but β-blockers seem less effective. In the Veterans Study, hydrochlorothiazide was at least as effective as any other drug in reversing LVH; in the TOMHS trial, diuretic treatment was superior to any other.[54]

Hypertension in pregnancy

The treatment of hypertension in pregnancy is an especially difficult area and there is still disagreement about the most suitable treatment strategy (see Chapter 45). The β-blockers have been widely used in treating hypertension in pregnancy, particularly in the USA. Atenolol is effective and well tolerated by the mother, although metaanalysis of the published trials indicates a negative effect on fetal growth.[55] A recent paper reported that therapy based on atenolol, with the dose adjusted and additional therapy added according to cardiac output, is a safe and effective strategy.[56] Diuretics have not been widely used in pregnancy-associated hypertension because of concern about contraction of circulating volume; however, they can be safely continued during pregnancy in those taking them for hypertension prior to conception.

Patients with chronic renal disease

There is incontrovertible evidence that control of blood pressure is of major importance in preserving renal function in patients with chronic renal disease and following renal transplantation. In patients with significant protein-uria, ACE inhibitors are the agents of choice.[57] Diabetic patients with renal disease should always be given ACE inhibitors.[58] However, UKPDS 38 noted no differences between patients randomized to captopril or atenolol as their first antihypertensive agent; this trial emphasized the key importance of good blood pressure control, however achieved, in diabetic patients.[18] In patients with less pro-teinuria, the evidence is not so clear-cut. Stratum II of the Ramipiril Efficacy In Nephropathy (REIN) study demon-strated most advantage for ramipril over placebo in patients with proteinuria > 1.5 g/day.[59] The ongoing African American Study of Kidney Disease trial of black Americans with hypertensive renal disease originally compared amlo-dipine, metoprolol, and ramipril. The amlodipine arm was stopped after an interim analysis revealed an advantage for ACE inhibitors, especially in proteinuric patients.[6] A recent metaanalysis found that regimens containing ACE inhibitors were more effective in slowing the progression of renal disease than those not containing these drugs, but for the subset of patients with proteinuria < 0.5 g/day no definite advantage of ACE inhibitors was evident.[60] This is probably at least partly because the rate of decline of renal function in patients with minimal proteinuria is very low. In practice, patients with renal disease often require multiple drugs to obtain control of blood pressure (77% of patients required additional hypertensives, as well as ramipril, to keep their diastolic blood pressure below 90 mmHg in the REIN follow-up study[61]). Many patients are currently undertreated.[62] Treatment based on a combi-nation of ACE in-hibitors and loop diuretics, β-blockers, or calcium channel blockers is required for most renal patients to achieve the lower blood pressure targets.

Patients outside the developed world

The vast majority of patients in trials of hypertension have come from western Europe, North America, Australia, and New Zealand. One major exception is the Sys-China trial, which demonstrated significant benefits for stroke risk and reduced mortality when older Chinese patients with isolated systolic hypertension were treated.[63] The Global Burden of Disease Study attempted to look at premature mortality and at disability worldwide. This study found that in 1990 ischemic heart disease was the fifth leading cause of disability-adjusted life years lost and that cerebrovascular disease was the sixth leading cause.[64] Projections for 2020 are that cardiovascular disease will be the leading cause of disability-adjusted life years lost and cerebrovascular disease will be the fourth leading cause.[65] The overall burden of cerebrovascular and cardiovascular disease worldwide is projected to almost double between 1990 and 2020, with the major increase occurring in the developing world. There is evidence from Africa that urbanization leads to a considerable increase in the incidence of hypertension.[66] Very high age-adjusted rates of stroke are seen in sub-Saharan Africa,[67] and because other cardiovascular risk factors are largely absent these have been attributed to untreated hypertension. The countries of eastern Europe are currently suffering an epidemic of cardiovascular disease.[68,69] There is clearly a great need for effective and inexpensive treatment of hypertension in these popula-tions. In view of their low cost and documented effec-tiveness, thiazides and β-blockers are the drugs of choice, although outcome trials in these populations are urgently needed.

Conclusions and treatment algorithm

A number of epidemiologic studies in Europe and the USA have shown that many patients known to be hypertensive have poorly controlled blood pressure, either because they are not on treatment or because their treatment is inade-quate.[70] These findings have been confirmed in a study of 24-h blood pressure control.[71] It is becoming increasingly clear that a very significant proportion of all patients requiring treatment for hypertension need a combination of drugs to bring their blood pressure down to a desirable level.[38] The sixth report of the Joint National Committee on Prevention, Detection, Evaluation, and Treatment of High Blood Pressure comes down strongly in favor of diuretics or β-blockers as the best treatment of hyper-tension unless there are specific indications for another drug.[72] The guidelines of the British Hypertension Society also favor β-blockers or diuretics unless there are contra-indications or a specific indication for an alternative drug.[73] The 1999 World Health Organization/International Society of Hypertension Guidelines are less specific and do not recommend any drug or class of drugs as the first choice, preferring to recommend that "the physician tailors the choice of drug to the individual patient."[74]

For most patients with hypertension over the age of 70, a thiazide diuretic is the drug of first choice. For patients under 70, treatment should begin with either a β-blocker or a thiazide. A low dose of a thiazide (e.g. hydrochlorothi-azide 12.5 mg or bendrofluazide 1.25 mg) or a β-blocker (e.g. atenolol 25 mg) is appropriate. If after 4 weeks the blood pressure is not well controlled, these doses should be doubled. There is little further gain, in terms of blood pressure control, in increasing the doses beyond this and good evidence that more adverse effects will be encoun-tered.[75] Patients on diuretics should have their urate and potassium checked within the first month of treatment and at least annually thereafter. Significant hypokalemia is not very common on low-dose thiazide diuretics and its occurrence should raise the possibility of underlying endocrine abnormalities. Patients who become hypokalemic should have this corrected; there is no clear evidence as to whether oral potassium supplementation or the addition of a potassium-sparing diuretic is the better way of doing this, although both have been shown to be effective.[76] Our practice is to add amiloride.

Patients in whom blood pressure control is still poor after 3 months of treatment require a change of therapy. There is controversy as to whether the best choice at this point is to add a further agent[77] (with good trial evidence of the

Table 54.1 Diuretics for the treatment of hypertension

	Initial dose	Maximum dose
Hydrochlorothiazide	12.5 mg once daily	50 mg once daily (perhaps only 25 mg)
Bendrofluazide	1.25 mg once daily	5 mg once daily
Chlorthalidone	12.5 mg once daily	25 mg once daily
Trichloromethiazide	2 mg once daily	4 mg once daily
Amiloride	5 mg once daily	10 mg once daily

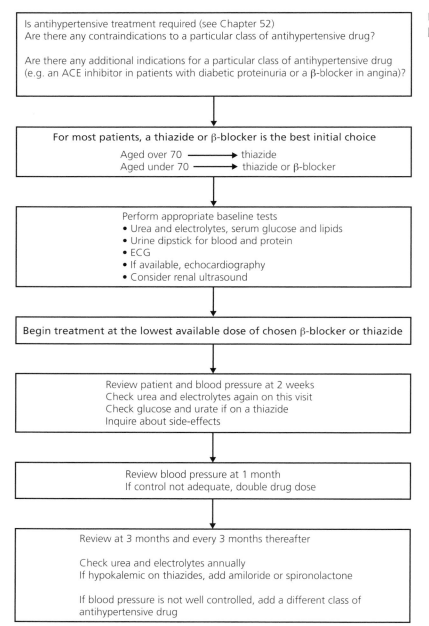

Is antihypertensive treatment required (see Chapter 52)
Are there any contraindications to a particular class of antihypertensive drug?

Are there any additional indications for a particular class of antihypertensive drug
(e.g. an ACE inhibitor in patients with diabetic proteinuria or a β-blocker in angina)?

For most patients, a thiazide or β-blocker is the best initial choice
Aged over 70 ⟶ thiazide
Aged under 70 ⟶ thiazide or β-blocker

Perform appropriate baseline tests
• Urea and electrolytes, serum glucose and lipids
• Urine dipstick for blood and protein
• ECG
• If available, echocardiography
• Consider renal ultrasound

Begin treatment at the lowest available dose of chosen β-blocker or thiazide

Review patient and blood pressure at 2 weeks
Check urea and electrolytes again on this visit
Check glucose and urate if on a thiazide
Inquire about side-effects

Review blood pressure at 1 month
If control not adequate, double drug dose

Review at 3 months and every 3 months thereafter

Check urea and electrolytes annually
If hypokalemic on thiazides, add amiloride or spironolactone

If blood pressure is not well controlled, add a different class of
antihypertensive drug

Figure 54.1 Algorithm for the use of thiazides or β-blockers in the treatment of hypertension.

Table 54.2 β-Blockers for the treatment of hypertension*

	Initial dose	Maximum dose
Atenolol	25 mg once daily	100 mg once daily
Metoprolol	50 mg once daily	100 mg once daily
Propranolol	40 mg twice daily	80 mg three times daily
Bisoprolol	2.5 mg once daily	10 mg once daily
Carvedilol	12.5 mg once daily	25 mg twice daily

*Low doses of β-blockers are appropriate for the treatment of hypertension, as discussed in the text. Higher doses (if tolerated) are of proven benefit in the treatment of heart failure and should be employed in this situation.

effectiveness and safety of combinations of thiazides and β-blockers,[78] thiazides and ACE inhibitors,[79] and thiazides and calcium channel antagonists[33]) or simply to switch to monotherapy with a drug from a different class.[80] In practice, many, perhaps most, patients need a combination of antihypertensive drugs to obtain their target blood pressure.[38] We therefore recommend adding another agent sooner rather than later and before the maximum dose of the initial agent has been reached.

The available diuretics and β-blockers for use in hypertension are detailed in Tables 54.1 and 54.2. An algorithm for the use of diuretics or β-blockers in the treatment of hypertension is shown in Fig. 54.1.

References

1. Psaty BM, Smith NL, Siscovick DS, et al: Health outcomes associated with antihypertensive therapies used as first-line agents. A systematic review and meta-analysis. JAMA 1997;277:739–745.
2. Andersson OK, Almgren T, Persson B, et al: Survival in treated hypertension: follow up study after two decades. Br Med J 1998;317:167–171.
3. Collins R, Peto R, MacMahon S, et al: Blood pressure, stroke, and coronary heart disease. Part 2, Short-term reductions in blood pressure: overview of randomised drug trials in their epidemiological context. Lancet 1990;335:827–838.
4. Kaplan NM: How bad are diuretic-induced hypokalemia and hypercholesterolemia? Arch Intern Med 1989;149:2649.
5. ALLHAT Collaborative Research Group: Major cardiovascular events in hypertensive patients randomized to doxazosin vs chlorthalidone: the antihypertensive and lipid-lowering treatment to prevent heart attack trial (ALLHAT). JAMA 2000;283:1967–1975.
6. Agodoa LY, Appel L, Bakris GL, et al: Effect of ramipril vs amlodipine on renal outcomes in hypertensive nephrosclerosis: a randomized controlled trial. JAMA 2001;285:2719–2728.
7. Neal B, MacMahon S, Chapman N: Effects of ACE inhibitors, calcium antagonists, and other blood-pressure-lowering drugs: results of prospectively designed overviews of randomised trials. Blood Pressure Lowering Treatment Trialists' Collaboration. Lancet 2000;356:1955–1964.
8. Trial Research Group: Multiple Risk Factor Intervention Trial. Risk factor changes and mortality results. JAMA 1982;248:1465–1477.
9. Anonymous: Prevention of stroke by antihypertensive drug treatment in older persons with isolated systolic hypertension. Final results of the Systolic Hypertension in the Elderly Program (SHEP). SHEP Cooperative Research Group. JAMA 1991;265:3255–3264.
10. Siscovick DS, Raghunathan TE, Psaty BM, et al: Diuretic therapy for hypertension and the risk of primary cardiac arrest. N Engl J Med 1994;330:1852–1857.
11. Kasiske BL, Ma JZ, Kalil RS, et al: Effects of antihypertensive therapy on serum lipids. Ann Intern Med 1995;122:133–141.
12. Materson BJ, Reda DJ, Cushman WC, et al: Single-drug therapy for hypertension in men. A comparison of six antihypertensive agents with placebo. The Department of Veterans Affairs Cooperative Study Group on Antihypertensive Agents. N Engl J Med 1993;328:914–921.
13. Grimm RHJ, Flack JM, Grandits GA, et al: Long-term effects on plasma lipids of diet and drugs to treat hypertension. Treatment of Mild Hypertension Study (TOMHS) Research Group. JAMA 1996;275:1549–1556.
14. Weir MR, Moser M: Diuretics and beta-blockers: is there a risk for dyslipidemia? Am Heart J 2000;139:174–183.
15. Gress TW, Nieto FJ, Shahar E, Wofford MR, Brancati FL: Hypertension and antihypertensive therapy as risk factors for type 2 diabetes mellitus. Atherosclerosis Risk in Communities Study. N Engl J Med 2000;342:905–912.
16. Savage PJ, Pressel SL, Curb JD, et al: Influence of long-term, low-dose, diuretic-based, antihypertensive therapy on glucose, lipid, uric acid, and potassium levels in older men and women with isolated systolic hypertension: The Systolic Hypertension in the Elderly Program. SHEP Cooperative Research Group. Arch Intern Med 1998;158:741–751.
17. Curb JD, Pressel SL, Cutler JA, et al: Effect of diuretic-based antihypertensive treatment on cardiovascular disease risk in older diabetic patients with isolated systolic hypertension. Systolic Hypertension in the Elderly Program Cooperative Research Group. JAMA 1996;276:1886–1892.
18. UK Prospective Diabetes Study Group: Tight blood pressure control and risk of macrovascular and microvascular complications in type 2 diabetes: UKPDS 38. Br Med J 1998;317:703–713.
19. Alderman MH, Cohen H, Madhavan S, et al: Serum uric acid and cardiovascular events in successfully treated hypertensive patients. Hypertension 1999;34:144–150.
20. Culleton BF, Larson MG, Kannel WB, et al: Serum uric acid and risk for cardiovascular disease and death: the Framingham Heart Study. Ann Intern Med 1999;131:7–13.
21. McCord JM: Oxygen-derived free radicals in postischemic tissue injury. N Engl J Med 1985;312:159–163.
22. Franse LV, Pahor M, Di Bari M, et al: Serum uric acid, diuretic treatment and risk of cardiovascular events in the Systolic Hypertension in the Elderly Program (SHEP). J Hypertens 2000;18:1149–1154.
23. Medical Research Council Working Party: MRC trial of treatment of mild hypertension: principal results. Br Med J 1985;291:97–104.
24. Feldman HA, Goldstein I, Hatzichristou DG, et al: Impotence and its medical and psychosocial correlates: results of the Massachusetts Male Aging Study. J Urol 1994;151:54–61.
25. Kloner RA, Brown M, Prisant LM, et al: Effect of sildenafil in patients with erectile dysfunction taking antihypertensive therapy. Sildenafil Study Group. Am J Hypertens 2001;14:70–73.
26. Prisant LM, Carr AA, Bottini PB, et al: Sexual dysfunction with antihypertensive drugs. Arch Intern Med 1994;154:730–736.
27. Grossman E, Messerli FH, Goldbourt U: Does diuretic therapy increase the risk of renal cell carcinoma? Am J Cardiol 1999;83:1090–1093.
28. McLaughlin JK, Chow WH, Mandel JS, et al: International renal-cell cancer study. VIII. Role of diuretics, other anti-hypertensive medications and hypertension. Int J Cancer 1995;63:216–221.

29. Ray WA, Griffin MR, Downey W, et al: Long-term use of thiazide diuretics and risk of hip fracture. Lancet 1989;i:687–690.
30. Cappuccio FP, Meilahn E, Zmuda JM, et al: High blood pressure and bone-mineral loss in elderly white women: a prospective study. Study of Osteoporotic Fractures Research Group. Lancet 1999;354:971–975.
31. Reid IR, Ames RW, Orr-Walker BJ, et al: Hydrochlorothiazide reduces loss of cortical bone in normal postmenopausal women: a randomized controlled trial. Am J Med 2000;109:362–370.
32. Staessen JA, Gasowski J, Wang JG, et al: Risks of untreated and treated isolated systolic hypertension in the elderly: meta-analysis of outcome trials. Lancet 2000;355:865–872.
33. Staessen JA, Fagard R, Thijs L, et al: Randomised double-blind comparison of placebo and active treatment for older patients with isolated systolic hypertension. The Systolic Hypertension in Europe (Syst-Eur) Trial Investigators. Lancet 1997;350:757–764.
34. Perry HMJ, Davis BR, Price TR, et al: Effect of treating isolated systolic hypertension on the risk of developing various types and subtypes of stroke: the Systolic Hypertension in the Elderly Program (SHEP). JAMA 2000;284:465–471.
35. MRC Working Party: Medical Research Council trial of treatment of hypertension in older adults: principal results. Br Med J 1992;304:405–412.
36. Pahor M, Psaty BM, Alderman MH, et al: Health outcomes associated with calcium antagonists compared with other first-line antihypertensive therapies: a meta-analysis of randomised controlled trials. Lancet 2000;356:1949–1954.
37. Leipzig RM, Cumming RG, Tinetti ME: Drugs and falls in older people: a systematic review and meta-analysis: II. Cardiac and analgesic drugs. J Am Geriatr Soc 1999;47:40–50.
38. Morgan TO, Anderson AI, MacInnis RJ: ACE inhibitors, beta-blockers, calcium blockers, and diuretics for the control of systolic hypertension. Am J Hypertens 2001;14:241–247.
39. Cooper RS, Liao Y, Rotimi C: Is hypertension more severe among U.S. blacks, or is severe hypertension more common? Ann Epidemiol 1996;6:173–180.
40. Wild S, McKeigue P: Cross sectional analysis of mortality by country of birth in England and Wales, 1970–92. Br Med J 1997;314:705–710.
41. Preston RA, Materson BJ, Reda DJ, et al: Age–race subgroup compared with renin profile as predictors of blood pressure response to antihypertensive therapy. Department of Veterans Affairs Cooperative Study Group on Antihypertensive Agents. JAMA 1998;280:1168–1172.
42. Veterans Administration Cooperative Study Group on Antihypertensive Agents: Comparison of propranolol and hydrochlorothiazide for the initial treatment of hypertension. I. Results of short-term titration with emphasis on racial differences in response. JAMA 1982;248:1996–2003.
43. Sareli P, Radevski IV, Valtchanova ZP, et al: Efficacy of different drug classes used to initiate antihypertensive treatment in black subjects: results of a randomized trial in Johannesburg, South Africa. Arch Intern Med 2001;161:965–971.
44. Yusuf S, Wittes J, Friedman L: Overview of results of randomized clinical trials in heart disease. I. Treatments following myocardial infarction. JAMA 1988;260:2088–2093.
45. Chen J, Marciniak TA, Radford MJ, et al: Beta-blocker therapy for secondary prevention of myocardial infarction in elderly diabetic patients. Results from the National Cooperative Cardiovascular Project. J Am Coll Cardiol 1999;34:1388–1394.
46. Mehta RH, Eagle KA: Secondary prevention in acute myocardial infarction. Br Med J 1998;316:838–842.
47. Yusuf S, Sleight P, Pogue J, et al: Effects of an angiotensin-converting-enzyme inhibitor, ramipril, on cardiovascular events in high-risk patients. The Heart Outcomes Prevention Evaluation Study Investigators. N Engl J Med 2000;342:145–153.
48. PROGRESS Collaborative Group: Randomised trial of a perindopril-based blood-pressure-lowering regimen among 6105 individuals with a previous stoke or transient ischaemic attack. Lancet 2001;358:1033–1041.
49. Smith SCJ, Blair SN, Bonow RO, et al: AHA/ACC Scientific Statement: AHA/ACC guidelines for preventing heart attack and death in patients with atherosclerotic cardiovascular disease: 2001 update. A statement for healthcare professionals from the American Heart Association and the American College of Cardiology. Circulation 2001;104:1577–1579.
50. Metra M, Giubbini R, Nodari S, et al: Differential effects of beta-blockers in patients with heart failure: a prospective, randomized, double-blind comparison of the long-term effects of metoprolol versus carvedilol. Circulation 2000;102:546–551.
51. Effect of metoprolol CR/XL in chronic heart failure: Metoprolol CR/XL Randomised Intervention Trial in Congestive Heart Failure (MERIT-HF). Lancet 1999;353:2001–2007.
52. Levy D, Garrison RJ, Savage DD, et al: Prognostic implications of echocardiographically determined left ventricular mass in the Framingham Heart Study. N Engl J Med 1990;322:1561–1566.
53. Schmieder RE, Martus P, Klingbeil A: Reversal of left ventricular hypertrophy in essential hypertension. A meta-analysis of randomized double-blind studies. JAMA 1996;275:1507–1513.
54. Liebson PR, Grandits GA, Dianzumba S, et al: Comparison of five antihypertensive monotherapies and placebo for change in left ventricular mass in patients receiving nutritional–hygienic therapy in the Treatment of Mild Hypertension Study (TOMHS). Circulation 1995;91:698–706.
55. Magee LA, Elran E, Bull SB, et al: Risks and benefits of beta-receptor blockers for pregnancy hypertension: overview of the randomized trials. Eur J Obstet Gynecol Reprod Biol 2000;88:15–26.
56. Easterling TR, Carr DB, Brateng D, et al: Treatment of hypertension in pregnancy: effect of atenolol on maternal disease, preterm delivery, and fetal growth. Obstet Gynecol 2001;98:427–433.
57. The GISEN Group (Gruppo Italiano di Studi Epidemiologici in Nefrologia): Randomised placebo-controlled trial of effect of ramipril on decline in glomerular filtration rate and risk of terminal renal failure in proteinuric, non-diabetic nephropathy. Lancet 1997;349:1857–1863.
58. The EUCLID Study Group: Randomised placebo-controlled trial of lisinopril in normotensive patients with insulin-dependent diabetes and normoalbuminuria or microalbuminuria. Lancet 1997;349:1787–1792.
59. Ruggenenti P, Perna A, Gherardi G, et al: Renoprotective properties of ACE-inhibition in non-diabetic nephropathies with non-nephrotic proteinuria. Lancet 1999;354:359–364.
60. Jafar TH, Schmid CH, Landa M, et al: Angiotensin-converting enzyme inhibitors and progression of nondiabetic renal disease. A meta-analysis of patient-level data. Ann Intern Med 2001;135:73–87.
61. Ruggenenti P, Perna A, Gherardi G, et al: Renal function and requirement for dialysis in chronic nephropathy patients on long-term ramipril: REIN follow-up trial. Gruppo Italiano di Studi Epidemiologici in Nefrologia (GISEN). Ramipril Efficacy in Nephropathy. Lancet 1998;352:1252–1256.
62. Messerli FH, Frohlich ED, Dreslinski GR, et al: Serum uric acid in essential hypertension: an indicator of renal vascular involvement. Ann Intern Med 1980;93:817–821.
63. Liu L, Wang JG, Gong L, et al: Comparison of active treatment and placebo in older Chinese patients with isolated systolic hypertension. Systolic Hypertension in China (Syst-China) Collaborative Group. J Hypertens 1998;16:1823–1829.
64. Murray CJ, Lopez AD: Global mortality, disability, and the contribution of risk factors: Global Burden of Disease Study. Lancet 1997;349:1436–1442.
65. Murray CJ, Lopez AD: Alternative projections of mortality and disability by cause 1990–2020: Global Burden of Disease Study. Lancet 1997;349:1498–1504.
66. Poulter NR, Khaw KT, Hopwood BE, et al: The Kenyan Luo migration study: observations on the initiation of a rise in blood pressure. Br Med J 1990;300:967–972.
67. Walker RW, McLarty DG, Kitange HM, et al: Stroke mortality in urban and rural Tanzania. Adult Morbidity and Mortality Project. Lancet 2000;355:1684–1687.
68. Sarti C, Rastenyte D, Cepaitis Z, et al: International–trends in mortality from stroke, 1968 to 1994. Stroke 2000;31:1588–1601.
69. Notzon FC, Komarov YM, Ermakov SP, et al: Causes of declining life expectancy in Russia. JAMA 1998;279:793–800.
70. Hyman DJ, Pavlik VN: Characteristics of patients with uncontrolled hypertension in the United States. N Engl J Med 2001;345:479–486.
71. Mancia G, Sega R, Milesi C, et al: Blood-pressure control in the hypertensive population. Lancet 1997;349:454–457.
72. The sixth report of the Joint National Committee on Prevention, Detection, Evaluation, and Treatment of High Blood Pressure. Arch Intern Med 1997;157:2413–2446.
73. Ramsay LE, Williams B, Johnston GD, et al: British Hypertension Society guidelines for hypertension management 1999: summary. Br Med J 1999;319:630–635.

74. Guidelines Subcommittee: 1999 World Health Organization/ International Society of Hypertension Guidelines for the Management of Hypertension. J Hypertens 1999;17:151–183.

75. Carlsen JE, Kober L, Torp-Pedersen C, et al: Relation between dose of bendrofluazide, antihypertensive effect, and adverse biochemical effects. Br Med J 1990;300:975–978.

76. Schnaper HW, Freis ED, Friedman RG, et al: Potassium restoration in hypertensive patients made hypokalemic by hydrochlorothiazide. Arch Intern Med 1989;149:2677–2681.

77. Ruilope LM, de la Sierra A, Moreno E, et al: Prospective comparison of therapeutical attitudes in hypertensive type 2 diabetic patients uncontrolled on monotherapy. A randomized trial: the EDICTA study. J Hypertens 1999;17:1917–1923.

78. Hansson L, Hedner T, Lund-Johansen P, et al: Randomised trial of effects of calcium antagonists compared with diuretics and beta-blockers on cardiovascular morbidity and mortality in hypertension: the Nordic Diltiazem (NORDIL) study. Lancet 2000;356:359–365.

79. Chrysant SG: Antihypertensive effectiveness of low-dose lisinopril–hydrochlorothiazide combination. A large multicenter study. Lisinopril–Hydrochlorothiazide Group. Arch Intern Med 1994;154:737–743.

80. Dickerson JE, Hingorani AD, Ashby MJ, et al: Optimisation of antihypertensive treatment by crossover rotation of four major classes. Lancet 1999;353:2008–2013.

The Kidney and Angiotensin-converting Enzyme Inhibitors, Angiotensin Receptor Blockers, and Aldosterone Antagonists

Norman K. Hollenberg

Pharmacology of the ACE inhibitors
Pharmacology of the angiotensin receptor blockers
Renal actions of renin–angiotensin system blockers
Renin–angiotensin system blockade and the natural
history of renal injury
Use of these agents in patients with renal failure
Aldosterone antagonists
Mechanisms and pharmacology

When pharmacological interruption of the renin–angiotensin system first became possible through the development of angiotensin-converting enzyme (ACE) inhibitors, even the wildest enthusiast could not have predicted the evolution of this field.[1,2] Agents that block the renin system were thought by many at that time to hold promise only in a small patient population – those with hypertension associated with an elevated plasma renin activity (PRA). This group of patients is important as it includes those with accelerated hypertension and those in whom hypertension tends to be difficult to treat, but these processes are relatively uncommon. This class of drug, therefore, was perceived to occupy an important but rather small niche.

That niche has grown, and indeed continues to grow. The introduction of ACE inhibitors involved their early successful use in patients with extremely high blood pressure resistant to the effect of triple-drug regimens. A series of studies over the past two decades has identified a much broader range of efficacy, indicating that these drugs were also remarkably helpful in patients with advanced heart failure, those with a large anterior myocardial infarction, and those at risk of diabetic nephropathy, other forms of nephropathy, and, with the Heart Outcome Prevention Evaluation (HOPE) study, the consequences of atherosclerosis.[2] ACE inhibitors have gradually emerged, therefore, as the leading class for the treatment not only of complicated patients described above but also of patients with mild-to-moderate essential hypertension who are free of any identifiable target organ damage and who are at rather low risk. Although this chapter appears in the part of this book entitled *Management of Essential Hypertension*, and there are separate and relevant chapters on drug dosing and renal failure, prevention of progressive renal failure, cardiovascular complications, control of cardiovascular risk factors in hypertension, individualization of pharmacological therapy, management of diabetic nephropathy, immunoglobulin A (IgA) nephropathy, and other forms of glomerulonephritis, and clinical trials in nephrology and hypertension – with inevitable overlap as each author develops their chapter – it will be necessary to touch on many of these subjects as this chapter evolves. As the drugs are not the subject of any other individual chapter, greater emphasis will be given to their pharmacology and to their handling in patients who have lost kidney function.

Despite this remarkable record of success, it is important to recognize that ACE inhibition was not the product of a planned pharmacological approach, but rather was an accidental byproduct of snake venom toxicology. A pharmacologist examining the renin cascade would first have chosen two alternative points as candidates for blockade.[3] In principle, blockade of a system is most effective at the rate-limiting step. In the renin cascade, the rate-limiting step is the interaction between renin and its substrate, angiotensinogen. Renin inhibitors were developed and were efficacious, but poor bioavailability and cost of synthesis brought development programs to a halt. Blockade at the level of the angiotensin II (AII) receptor is also attractive, especially if non-ACE-dependent pathways for AII generation exist. Evidence for such pathways in the intact human is growing, especially in the kidney,[3] which makes blockade of the renin system at the level of the angiotensin II receptor an important therapeutic step.

There is another factor that is likely to shape future use of these agents. The angiotensin II antagonists are products of imidazole chemistry, and imidazole derivatives have a wide range of pharmacological activity.[4] Thus, no one could have anticipated how remarkably well tolerated this class of agents is. In study after study, AT_1 (one of the subtypes of the angiotensin II receptor) receptor blockers compare favorably with placebo in frequency of adverse reactions,[1,5] a statement that could never have been made about antihypertensive agents in the past. At a recent symposium, over 90% of 800 physicians queried indicated that they would choose an angiotensin receptor blocker first if their own blood pressure needed lowering.

Pharmacology of the ACE inhibitors

Angiotensin-converting enzyme is a widely distributed zinc metallopeptidase that represents the final enzymatic step in the lysis of angiotensin I (AI) to produce angiotensin II. There are three main ACE isoforms: somatic ACE, plasma ACE, and testicular ACE. Somatic ACE is attached to the cell membrane and has an extracellular region that consists of two homologous domains,[6,7] each of which contains an active catalytic site. The testicular ACE, conversely, has only one catalytically active site. Plasma ACE is thought to be derived from the somatic ACE, but lacks the transmembrane domain and intracellular portion. Like somatic ACE, plasma ACE contains two active sites. The fact that there are two catalytic sites in somatic ACE – each capable of converting angiotensin I to angiotensin II, but displaying different kinetics – has raised the interesting possibility that ACE inhibitors could differ in their affinity for the two sites. The C-terminal site accounts for about 75% of total ACE,[7] and is largely responsible for the conversion of angiotensin I to angiotensin II. It has been suggested that the N-terminal site has greater responsibility for the metabolism of other peptide substrates.[8]

ACE inhibitors interact differently with ACE-active sites, depending on their structure.[9,10] Lisinopril, for example, shows affinity for only one binding site on both somatic and testicular ACE, suggesting that it binds only the C-terminal active site of ACE. Conversely, cilazapril has affinity for the two binding sites on somatic ACE. These findings suggest that the two active sites of somatic ACE have different structural requirements. Although of interest, at the moment, there are no compelling data to indicate a functional or therapeutic implication of these findings.

ACE generally functions as a carboxyl-dipeptide hydrolase, having as its substrates not only AI and bradykinin but also a wide range of peptides, including enkephalins, substance P, and the β-chain of insulin.[11] It is widely believed that there are consequences to the broad range of peptide substrates degraded by ACE for the specificity of ACE inhibitor function. A number of studies in animal models, not yet supported by information from studies in humans, have suggested that bradykinin might play a role in the tissue-sparing effects of ACE inhibitors. Conversely, it is thought that the same mechanism might underlie the cough so often induced by ACE inhibitors, which represents their main drawback.[11]

The first effective ACE inhibitor, captopril, is a sulfhydryl-containing compound that is relatively rapid in onset and short acting.[11] Thereafter, all of the ACE inhibitors developed are longer acting and, with the exception of lisinopril and captopril, undergo metabolic conversion into an active diacid form. There is no evidence that this conversion is ever rate limiting. The ACE inhibitors are structurally heterogeneous both in their primary binding sites to the ACE receptor and in the side chains capable of binding ACE. The sulfhydryl group in captopril was replaced by a carboxyl group in most of the remainder, with the exception of a phosphinyl group in fosinopril. Although there are a number of claims that these substitutions have functional significance, for example the reduced frequency of cough claimed for fosinopril and free radical scavenging for the sulfhydryl group on captopril, in fact clinically meaningful difference remains to be proved. Indeed, beyond the frequency of dosing and handling of these agents in the patient with renal failure, there are few persuasive differences.

For all of the ACE inhibitors with the exception of fosinopril and trandolapril, the diazaform is excreted primarily via renal clearance, involving both filtration and tubular secretion.[11,12] In the case of fosinopril and trandolapril, excretion is more balanced, and hepatic excretion rises with a reduction in renal function (Table 55.1).

Although there are many claims that ACE inhibitors differ in functionally important ways, such as tissue penetration and action on endothelial function, in fact the available evidence for such differences is not persuasive, and there is no clear evidence that these differences have therapeutic implications. Most of the impetus for such claims has come from industry. There are quantitatively important differences in the duration of action and metabolism of these drugs that have implications for their use in the patient with renal failure (see below for reviews of the features of the individual agents).

Pharmacology of the angiotensin receptor blockers

The first antagonists to angiotensin II and its receptor were peptide analogs of angiotensin II that had been developed as byproducts of analyses of the structural requirements for binding of angiotensin II to its receptor and as a result of the synthesis of many structural analogs of angiotensin II.[1,5] The most widely studied, saralasin, is an octapeptide that differs in structure from angiotensin II at the eighth amino acid, where alanine is the residue, and at the first amino acid, where sarcosine – an amino acid that does not

Table 55.1 Clinical pharmacology of ACE inhibitors

Drug	Elimination route	Serum half-life (h)	Effect of food	Protein binding (%)
Benazepril	Renal, some biliary	10–11	None	> 95
Captopril	Renal, as disulfides	< 2	Reduced	25–30
Enalapril	Renal	11	None	50
Fosinopril	Renal = hepatic	11	None	95
Lisinopril	Renal	13	None	10
Moexipril	Renal, some biliary	2–9	Reduced	50
Perindopril	Renal	7	None	60%
Quinapril	Renal > hepatic	2	Reduced	97
Ramipril	Renal	13–17	Reduced	73
Trandolapril	Renal > hepatic	16–24	None	80–94

occur in mammals – was employed to slow the degradation of the molecule. Because saralasin could only be given intravenously, was a partial agonist, and was very expensive to manufacture, it never had a major role in therapy or diagnostics.

In 1982, an unanticipated advance was made through the application of high-throughput screening at the Takeda laboratory in Japan.[13] A series of imidazole derivatives were identified that bound specifically to the angiotensin II receptor. Structure–action work at the Dupont laboratories led to the development of losartan, the first of a new class of nonpeptide, clinically effective, angiotensin receptor blockers.[14] Most of the antihypertensive action of losartan in vivo involves conversion of the parent compound to EXP-3174, the carboxylic acid metabolite of losartan.[15] Further structural modifications led to the identification of valsartan, irbesartan, candesartan, and telmisartan,[5] all of which are biphenyl tetrazoles. Investigators at Smith Kline Beecham pursued an alternative pathway from the original Takeda compound to produce eprosartan, which is a nonbiphenyl nontetrazole.[16]

One clear difference among the available agents involves structure. All of the currently marketed AT_1 receptor antagonists, with the exception of eprosartan, are biphenyl tetrazoles.[4,5] Eprosartan also differs from all of the other marketed drugs in its interaction with the AT_1 receptor. Eprosartan is a pure competitive antagonist, the action of which is surmountable by a sufficiently high angiotensin II concentration.[17] Valsartan, irbesartan, candesartan, telmesartan, and the active metabolite of losartan, EXP-3174, all show noncompetitive kinetics, which suggests a nonequilibrium relation to the receptor.[18] When the binding is sufficiently tight, the equilibrium conditions required to show competitive antagonism are not in place and the kinetics become insurmountable. In the case of losartan, the parent molecule is a weak competitive antagonist, and virtually all of the blockade after the first several hours depends on the 15% that is converted to a much more potent nonequilibrium antagonist – EXP-3174. One clinically relevant effect of the tight binding is the very long duration of action of the nonequilibrium angiotensin receptor blockers. The half-life in plasma predicts poorly the duration of the blockade because of the long sojourn of the blocker on the receptor. In studies that we have performed in healthy human volunteers and in patients with type 2 diabetes mellitus, for example, the duration of action of irbesartan and candesartan was 48 h after a single dose. Thus, with daily dosing of these agents, the patient can enjoy prolonged blockade even with the occasional missed dose.

The available angiotensin II receptor antagonists differ from one another in their oral bioavailability, metabolism, and elimination.[1,5] Candesartan cilexetil is a true prodrug, the active agent being candesartan, which is freed from the complex during passage through the gut wall. Losartan is an active agent – a very weak competitive antagonist with an active metabolite (EXP-3174) that is substantially more potent and long acting. Bioavailability ranges from about 25% for valsartan to 80% for irbesartan (Table 55.2). The absorption of candesartan or irbesartan is not influenced by food, whereas valsartan and losartan do show interference of absorption by food. With the exception of candesartan, which has a 60% renal route of elimination, for most of the agents the primary route of excretion is biliary (Table 55.2). Only one of the agents, losartan, has a tubular action that leads to increased uric acid excretion.

The angiotensin II receptors are divided into AT_1 and AT_2 subtypes, which have been characterized both pharmacologically and by cloning. All of the clinically important, well-defined actions of angiotensin on the kidney are mediated via the AT_1 receptor. Studies in animal models where AT_2 receptor competitive antagonists are available have suggested that the renal actions supported by the AT_2 receptor are opposite to those of the AT_1 receptor, including vasodilatation, natriuresis, and growth inhibition.[19] The AT_2 receptor is prominent during embryogenesis in the kidney and elsewhere, but becomes rapidly and progressively more sparse after birth. Any discussion of the role played by the AT_2 receptor in humans is speculative, as there are no direct data available from studies in humans. Species differences in the contribution of the renin–angiotensin system to renal control mechanisms are discussed below, and may well be relevant. For example, there is a single AT_1 receptor and responsible gene in humans, and two AT_1 receptor isoforms in the rat.[20]

Table 55.2 Clinical pharmacology of angiotensin receptor blockers

Drug	Elimination route	Effect of food	Protein binding (%)	Uricosuric
Candesartan	Renal (60%)	No	99	No
Eprosartan	Biliary (70%)	No	90	No
Irbesartan	Biliary (99%)	No	90	No
Losartan	Biliary (90%)	Yes	98	Yes
EXP-3174	Renal (50%)	–	99	Yes
Telmesartan	Biliary (99%)	No	99	No
Valsartan	Biliary (70%)	Yes	95	No

Renal actions of renin–angiotensin system blockers

The renal response to blocking the renin–angiotensin system with any of the three classes of blocker that have been studied depends on three factors. The first factor is the action of angiotensin II on the kidney in the setting of the study. Thus, for example, salt intake is a major determinant of the response to blocking the renin system, as salt intake influences the production and action of angiotensin II on the kidney. Second, the completeness of the blockade induced by the agent is a crucial factor. In many studies, a somewhat arbitrary dose of a blocker has been employed, often much less than the optimal dose for blockade. The third major force involves additional actions of the pharmacological agent employed. Achieving an overall synthesis of the data is complicated further by the fact that there are important species differences both in the renin–angiotensin system pathways and in the additional effects of the agents used to block the system.[20] Moreover, in protocols performed in animals, anesthesia is often used, which further modifies both the state of the renin–angiotensin system and the condition of the kidney.[21]

Shortly after the first ACE inhibitor – the peptide teprotide – became available, studies in dogs and rabbits made it clear that, when the renin system was activated by a low-salt diet, the administration of the ACE inhibitor would lead to striking and consistent renal vasodilation and natriuresis, with little or no change in the glomerular filtration rate.[3] In studies performed in trained animals that could be studied without anesthesia, it became apparent that the responses were much smaller when the animals studied were on a high-salt diet to suppress the renin–angiotensin system. The angiotensin II antagonist available at that time, saralasin, was a partial agonist with substantial angiotensin-like activity – especially when the dose was pushed. When used properly, saralasin revealed a qualitatively similar, albeit smaller, renal vasodilator response to the ACE inhibitor. Essentially, identical findings were found with teprotide, captopril, and saralasin in humans.[22]

The striking influence of salt intake on the renal vasodilator response to ACE inhibition, recognized early, supported a dominant role for the angiotensin II mechanism.[20] If the renal vasodilator response induced by ACE inhibitors in humans included a substantial component due to bradykinin, prostaglandins, nitric oxide, or some other vasodilator pathway, several conclusions follow. First, if alternative vasodilator pathways were engaged, the vasodilatation should have been associated with blunting of the renal vascular response to angiotensin II. Conversely, if the vasodilator response reflected a reduction in angiotensin II formation, the expectation would be enhancement of the renal vascular response to angiotensin II. As enhancement of the renal vascular response to angiotensin II was found, it seemed likely that the other vasodilator pathways were less important.

A second consequence would have been that the renal vasodilator response to renin inhibition would have been substantially less than the response to ACE inhibition. In fact, in humans the renal vasodilator response to two renin inhibitors exceeded expectations from earlier experience with ACE inhibition.[3] Because of the notorious risk of employing historic controls, a study was performed in which volunteers received an ACE inhibitor or a renin inhibitor or placebo during the same week. The study was coded and double blinded. The response was unambiguous: renin inhibition induced a substantially larger renal vasodilator response than did ACE inhibition. As a result, there was no opportunity for ACE inhibition-induced activation of renal vasodilator pathways, but this did not explain why the response to renin inhibition was substantially larger. In this case, the angiotensin II receptor antagonist provided a "tie breaker." If the renin inhibitor did, indeed, operate via the renin–angiotensin system cascade, one would anticipate a similar or larger renal vasodilator response to the angiotensin II antagonist in studies performed with an identical protocol. This is precisely what was found in studies performed with an identical model, protocol, and technique. Three angiotensin II receptor antagonists – eprosartan, irbesartan, and candesartan – induced a renal vasodilator response that matched or slightly exceeded the response to renin inhibition in healthy humans in balance on a low-salt diet.[20] All of the studies were performed at the top of the relationship between drug dose and renal vascular response.

From this observation, a series of conclusions are reasonable. The renal hemodynamic response to ACE inhibition has underestimated systematically the contribution of angiotensin II to renal vascular tone in humans. The effectiveness of renin inhibition suggests that this response represents interruption of primarily renin-dependent but non-ACE-dependent pathways, probably involving chymase. From quantitative considerations – a response to ACE inhibition was 90–100 mL/min per 1.73 m^2 in this model compared with 140–150 mL/min per 1.73m^2 induced by renin inhibition or angiotensin II receptor blockers – it follows that 30–40% of angiotensin-dependent renal vascular tone reflects angiotensin generated via a non-ACE pathway.[3] That percentage is higher when the renin system is suppressed by a high-salt diet in healthy humans.[23]

Species variation was mentioned earlier, and several important species differences merit discussion at this point.[20] The first involves pathways for non-ACE generation. In humans and other primates, the enzyme chymase has a single substrate, angiotensin I, and a single product, angiotensin II. Indeed, it should have been called "angiotensin-converting enzyme," but that name was used for another enzyme in the 1950s. The primate separated from other mammals in phylogeny millions of years ago. Since then, there has been ample opportunity for shifts in the metabolic pathways. In the rat and rabbit, chymase has angiotensin II, rather than angiotensin I, as its substrate and the degradation products of angiotensin II as its products. Thus, the actions of chymase in humans and in small animals are opposite to each other. One would anticipate that ACE inhibitors and angiotensin II receptor blockers would have similar actions. In these small creatures, they do.

A second major species-dependent difference involves the mechanism by which ACE inhibition influences the renal blood supply. In rats and dogs, there is considerable evidence to indicate that bradykinin and other vasodilator pathways make a substantial contribution to the renal vasodilator response to ACE inhibition. Conversely, in the rabbit and humans, available evidence suggests that the dominant action, by far, involves a reduction in angiotensin II production with little evidence of activation of these alternative pathways.[24] The biochemical explanation underlying these differences is not yet available.

Renin–angiotensin system blockade and the natural history of renal injury

Opinion will vary on the first observation that pointed to a specific renal action of ACE inhibitors, especially their potential for preserving renal function. One can argue that this was first recognized in 1979 in a description of the maintenance of renal function with blood pressure control during captopril treatment of two patients with unequivocal scleroderma renal crisis.[25] As this process is characterized by a rapidly progressive downhill course, with no exceptions in the literature, it was clear that something special had happened. The outcome did raise the debate on whether it was the result of blood pressure control, which was improved with ACE inhibition that led to improvement of the renal course, or whether ACE inhibition offered other renal protective qualities.

In 1985, studies in animal models and in patients with proteinuria led to the first discussion of the possibility that ACE inhibition might be renal protective and to discussions of a possible ambitious therapeutic trial in patients with type 1 diabetes mellitus. It is important that the decision to focus on patients with type 1 diabetes did not depend on the special role that ACE inhibitor therapy had in that process, but rather that these patients represent a very attractive target for establishing a principle. The disease course is relatively predictable based on renal function and level of proteinuria, and the patient population is relatively homogeneous and young; therefore, the natural history of nephropathy is less likely to be complicated by cardiovascular events. Thus, one could isolate a specific renal influence and thereby establish a principle. In part because the study was planned as a collaboration between a corporate sponsor and the National Institutes of Health (NIH), several years were required before the study was launched, and the data did not become available until late 1993.[26] During that time, a large literature had accrued both in animal models and in humans, reported as a meta-analysis of 100 clinical studies performed over the interval. With the 1993 publication policy changed, for the first time a regulatory agency approved a drug for a specific renal-protective indication. Since that time, studies on ACE inhibition have been extended to studies in patients with noninsulin diabetes mellitus and nondiabetic renal disease.[27]

What of the angiotensin receptor blockers? Until recently, their potential utility in preventing the progression of renal disease was a construct. The predicted outcome depended on whether non-ACE angiotensin II generation (in which case, the angiotensin receptor blockers would be better) or the nonangiotensin-dependent actions of ACE inhibition (in which case, the ACE inhibitors would be better) was considered to be the most quantitatively important. In May 2001, three presentations were made at the American Society of Hypertension, all of which appeared in a single issue of the *New England Journal of Medicine*.[22,27–31] In patients with type 2 diabetes and nephropathy, both irbesartan and losartan reduced the frequency of progression to a renal endpoint – doubling serum creatinine, need for dialysis, or death – by about 20%. In the study in which irbesartan was employed, there were three limbs, including irbesartan in one limb, placebo add on in the second limb, and amlodipine add on in the third limb. Amlodipine proved to be essentially identical to placebo. Perhaps the most exciting finding was in the third study, in which two doses of irbesartan were employed in patients with type 2 diabetes mellitus and microalbuminuria to assess the frequency with which the patients would progress to frank proteinuria.[30] The results were extraordinarily striking. The 150-mg irbesartan dose reduced the frequency of progression from about 15% to about 10%. An increase in the irbesartan dose to 300 mg reduced the frequency of progression further – to about 5%. Overall, at the highest dose, the protective effect was a 70% reduction, much the largest reduction in risk induced by blockade of the renin–angiotensin system in any clinical condition. The important message seems to be that it is better, indeed far better, to treat early.

Use of these agents in patients with renal failure

There are two reasons why ACE inhibitors are used in patients who have lost renal excretory function: to control hypertension and to retard the progression of renal injury. There is much less clinical experience with the angiotensin receptor blockers but the goal of their use is the same, and preliminary data indicate that their efficacy is probably similar. ACE inhibitors are effective antihypertensive agents in most patients with renal insufficiency, but their use is complicated by their tendency to increase azotemia in certain patients. This is especially likely to occur in patients who have been treated aggressively with restriction of salt intake or diuretic therapy, and it may be difficult to manage in patients who are already very azotemic. Too often, physicians are tempted to discontinue ACE inhibitor therapy because of an abrupt rise in serum creatinine during the initiation of treatment.[11] Whenever possible, and generally when the patient is free of symptoms of azotemia, it is worthwhile maintaining ACE inhibitor therapy. In the Collaborative Study Group Trial of captopril in patients with type 1 diabetes mellitus, it was the patients who were already azotemic at baseline who showed the greatest benefit from captopril treatment,[26] and who showed the highest increase in azotemia during initial therapy.

In such patients, it is important to be aware of the possibility of drug accumulation during treatment because of renal excretion.[12] Although it is not entirely predictable, in general dosage modification is not required for fosinopril, trandolapril, or quinipril. When using perindopril, benazepril, enalapril, lisinopril, and ramipril, a 50–75% reduction in dose is recommended. For captopril, the dose should be reduced by 50–75% and administered only once daily.

In general, the principles for the use of angiotensin receptor blockers are the same, although only candesartan is excreted by the kidney by more than 50%, and there is little information to suggest that dose adjustment is crucial in the patient with renal failure for any of these agents.[5]

Another consideration in the use of drugs that block the renin–angiotensin system in patients with renal failure involves the potential development of hyperkalemia.[11,12] Patients at greatest risk have diabetes mellitus, mild to moderate azotemia, and evidence of hyporeninemic hypoaldosteronism, often evident in a high-baseline serum potassium concentration. In addition, there is often evidence of metabolic acidosis that is more severe than expected for the degree of renal failure. Such patients should be treated cautiously and reviewed within 48 h of beginning ACE inhibitor therapy for repeat serum potassium and creatinine measurement as these patients can develop a life-threatening rise in serum potassium. The use of cyclooxygenase inhibitors in such patients can precipitate hyporeninemic hypoaldosteronism, and so patients should be cautioned about their use.

For reasons that are not entirely clear, the angiotensin receptor blockers appear to cause less hyperkalemia than ACE inhibitors.[1,5,32] Because a close correlation was found between the uricosuric effect and kaliuretic effect when losartan was used, it was believed, initially, that the potassium effect of losartan reflected a tubular action rather than angiotensin receptor blockade. This explanation has been called into question by the recent observation that valsartan, which has no tubular action, also appears to spare potassium.[32] In patients for whom hyperkalemia is an important threat, the uses of one of these two angiotensin receptor blockers in place of an ACE inhibitor should be considered.

The ideal blood pressure for such patients is the subject of substantial debate, remains controversial, and is addressed in greater detail elsewhere. Most advisory groups now recommend a blood pressure of less than 130/80 mmHg in patients at risk of progression of endstage renal disease, and it will not be surprising to find groups recommending systolic blood pressures of 120 mmHg or lower – if only we can find a way to achieve these levels.

Aldosterone antagonists

The first aldosterone antagonist, spironolactone, was introduced in 1959, well before ACE inhibitors were developed. The agent, a 17-spirolactone steroid, was an unanticipated byproduct of progesterone chemistry and pharmacology.

It was quickly shown to be a specific competitive antagonist of aldosterone at the receptor level, and was developed as a potassium-sparing diuretic. Because of frequent side-effects, it was of limited therapeutic interest until approximately 10 years ago. Interest in specifically interrupting aldosterone production or action has risen during the past 10 years for three major reasons. The first involves a series of studies in the heart and kidney which indicated that aldosterone leads to substantial fibrosis and tissue injury via a mechanism that could be interrupted by an aldosterone antagonist.[34–36] Indeed, in some studies, a substantial portion of the tissue sparing provided by ACE inhibition involved the reduction in plasma aldosterone concentration.

The second investigation that led to renewed interest in blocking the effects of aldosterone was the RALES Trial in patients with advanced heart failure. In this study, the addition of spironolactone in very low doses – averaging 25 mg/day – reduced the incidence of cardiovascular events by a striking 30%.[37] Because the doses were very low, the agent was well tolerated; however, the doses are probably too low to have a major influence on blood pressure or electrolyte homeostasis. Thus, another mechanism must be sought.

The third reason for renewed interest in aldosterone antagonists as a therapeutic area involved the development of a new aldosterone antagonist, eplerenone, which is much better tolerated than spironolactone. Eplerenone doses that substantially influence blood pressure and electrolyte homeostasis – similar to the peak of the spironolactone dose–response, which is believed to be about 150 mg/day – have little or no effect on libido, gynecomastia, or breast pain and tenderness. Currently, a series of clinical studies comparing the efficacy and adverse effect profiles of antihypertensive agents is under way: eplerenone is being compared with spironolactone in patients with primary aldosteronism, with other antihypertensive agents in patients with essential hypertension, and for its influence on natural history in patients with heart failure.

Mechanisms and pharmacology

Until recently, attention has mostly focused on the distal tubules in the nephron, however aldosterone receptors are found in many tissues. Spironolactone acts as a competitive inhibitor of aldosterone binding to its receptor. Spironolactone is extensively metabolized in humans. Some of its metabolites – especially canrenone – have antialdosterone effects, but the dominant effect appears to be due to the parent compound.

Partly because it was developed in the 1950s, the pharmacokinetics of spironolactone are not well known. Concomitant food intake enhances bioavailability by increasing the absorption of spironolactone and decreasing the first-pass effect.[38] There is a gradual onset of diuretic action, requiring 3 days to reach its maximum, and the diuretic response persists for 2–3 days.[39] It is unlikely that the tissue-sparing effect involves sodium or potassium handling, and little is known about the kinetics of that action.

The most troubling adverse effect of spironolactone has been gynecomastia. This adverse effect is dose sensitive. In a systematic comparison of spironolactone doses of 100, 200, and 400 mg/day, the 200 and 400 mg/day doses were associated with a striking increase of gynecomastia, and no greater antihypertensive effect than that associated with 100 mg/day.[40] In general, spironolactone has much more often been used in combination with a thiazide diuretic, as much for the potassium-sparing effect as for the primary diuretic action.

The adverse effect of greatest concern is hyperkalemia. The risk of hyperkalemia was found to be greatly increased in patients with renal insufficiency, and those in whom there was simultaneous exposure to potassium supplements.[41] In one large survey, 8.6% of patients taking spironolactone developed hyperkalemia. The frequency was only 2.8% in those with normal blood urea nitrogen (BUN) levels in that study and rose to 42.1% in those in whom BUN exceeded 50 mg/dL.[41]

At least in part because of the interaction between azotemia and hypokalemia, there have been few studies in patients with renal failure. The glomerular filtration rate has been shown to be stable during 3 months of spironolactone therapy.[42]

Substantially fewer data have been published on eplerenone, which is not yet marketed. Presumably, many of the issues addressed in this chapter will be discussed in the medical literature before it is approved for human use.

Acknowledgment

I am grateful to Ms Diana Capone for her assistance in the preparation and submission of this chapter.

References

1. Burnier M, Brunner HR: Angiotensin II receptor antagonists. Lancet 2000;355:637–645.
2. The Heart Outcome Prevention Evaluation (HOPE) Study Investigators: Effects of an angiotensin-converting enzyme inhibitor, ramipril, on death from cardiovascular causes, myocardial infarction and stroke in high risk patients. New Engl J Med 2000;342:145–153.
3. Hollenberg NK, Fisher NDL, Price DA: Pathways for angiotensin II generation in intact human tissue. Evidence from comparative pharmacological interruption of the renin system. Hypertension 1998;32:387–392.
4. Nickerson M, Hollenberg NK: Blockade of alpha-adrenergic receptors. In Root W (ed): Physiological Pharmacology. New York: Academic Press, 1967, pp 243–305.
5. Ruddy MC, Kostis JB: Angiotensin II receptor antagonist. In Oparil S, Weber MA (eds): Hypertension: a Companion to Brenner and Rector's The Kidney. 1999, pp 621–637.
6. Perich RB, Jackson B, Rogerson FM, Mendelsohn FA, Paxton D, Johnston CI: Two binding sites on angiotensin converting enzyme: evidence from radioligand binding studies. Mol Pharmacol 1992;42:286–293.
7. Wei L, Alhenc-Gelas F, Corvol P, Clauser E: The two homologous domains of human angiotensin I-converting enzyme are both catalytically active. J Biol Chem 991;266:9002–9008.
8. Ehlers MRW, Riordan JF: Angiotensin-converting-enzyme: zinc and inhibitor binding stoichiometries of the somatic and testis isozymes. Biochemistry 1991;30:7118–7126.
9. Wei L, Clauser E, Alhenc-Gelas F, Corvol P: The two homologous domains of human angiotensin I-converting enzyme interact differently with competitive inhibitors. J Biol Chem 1992;267:1398–13405.
10. Perich RB, Jackson B, Attwood MR, et al: Angiotensin-converting enzyme inhibitors act at two different binding sites on angiotensin-converting enzyme. Pharm Pharmacol Lett 1991;1:41–43.
11. Sica DA, Todd W, Gehr B: Angiotensin-converting enzyme inhibitors. In Oparil S, Weber M (eds): Hypertension. A Companion to Brenner and Rector's The Kidney. Philadelphia: W.B. Saunders, 1996, pp 599–609.
12. Wilcox CS: Management of hypertension in patients with renal disease. In Smith TW (ed): Cardiovascular Therapeutics. A Companion to Braunwald's Heart Disease. Philadelphia: W.B. Saunders, 1996, pp 538–545.
13. Furakawa Y, Kishimoto S, Nishikawa K: Hypotensive imidazole derivatives and hypotensive imidazole 5-acetic acid derivatives. Takeda Chemical Industries Ltd. US Patent nos 4,340,598 and 4,355,040, Osaka, Japan, 1982.
14. Wexler RR, Greenlee WJ, Irvin JD, et al: Nonpeptide angiotensin II receptor antagonists: the next generation in antihypertensive therapy. J Med Chem 1996;39:626–656.
15. Wong PC, Price WA, Chiu AT, Ardecky RJ, Smith RD, Timmermans PB: Nonpeptide angiotensin antagonists. IX. Pharmacology of EXP3174: an active metabolite of DuP 753, an orally active antihypertensive agent. J Pharmacol Exp Ther 1990;255:211–217.
16. Keenan RM, Weinstock J, Finkelstein JA, et al: Potent nonpeptide angiotensin II receptor antagonists: 1-(carboxybenzyl)imidazole-5-acrylic acids. J Med Chem 1993;36:1880–1892.
17. Edwards RM, Aiyer N, Chilstein EH, et al: Pharmacological characterization of the nonpeptide angiotensin II receptor antagonist SK&F 108566. J Pharmacol Exp Ther 1992;260:175–181.
18. Vauquelin G, Fierens F, Vanderheyden P: Distinction between surmountable and insurmountable angiotensin II AT_1 receptor antagonists. In Epstein M, Brunner HR (eds): Angiotensin II Receptor Antagonists. Philadelphia: Hanley & Belfus, 2001, pp 105–118.
19. Navar LG, Harrison-Bernard LM, Imig JD, Mitchell KD: Renal actions of angiotensin II and AT_1 receptor blockers. In Epstein M, Brunner HR (eds): Angiotensin II Receptor Antagonists. Philadelphia: Hanley & Belfus, 2001, pp 189–214.
20. Hollenberg NK, Arthur C: Corcoran Lecture. Implications of species difference for clinical investigation. Studies on the renin–angiotensin system. Hypertension 2000;35:150–154.
21. Burger BM, Hollenberg NK: Barbiturate anesthesia reduces renal blood flow and its response to angiotensin II via RAS activation. Int Nephrol Soc 1975;6:522.
22. Weinberg MS, Weinberg AJ, Zappe DH: Effectively targeting the renin–angiotensin–aldosterone system in cardiovascular and renal disease: rationale for using angiotensin II receptor blockers in combination with angiotensin-converting enzyme inhibitors. JRAAS 2000;1:217–233.
23. Hollenberg NK, Osei SY, Lansang MC, Price DA, Fisher ND: Salt intake and non-ACE pathways for intrarenal angiotensin II generation in man. JRAAS 2001;2:14–18.
24. Lansang MC, Hollenberg NK: ACE inhibition and the kidney: species variation in the mechanisms responsible for the renal hemodynamic response. JRAAS 2000;1:119–124.
25. Hollenberg NK, Raij L: Angiotensin-converting enzyme inhibition and renal protection. An assessment of implications for therapy. Arch Intern Med 1993;153:2426–2435.
26. Lewis EJ, Hunsicker LG, Bain RP, Rohde RD: The effect of angiotensin-converting-enzyme inhibition on diabetic nephropathy. The Collaborative Study Group. N Engl J Med 1993;329:1456–1462.
27. Giatras I, Lau J, Levey AS: Effect of angiotensin-converting enzyme inhibitors on the progression of nondiabetic renal disease: a meta analysis of randomized trials. Angiotensin-converting-enzyme inhibition and progressive renal disease study group. Ann Intern Med 1997;127:337–345.
28. Lewis EJ, Hunsicker LG, Clarke WR, et al for the Collaborative Study Group: Renoprotective effect of the angiotensin-receptor antagonist irbesartan in patients with nephropathy due to type 2 diabetes. N Engl J Med 2001;345:851–860.
29. Parving H-H, Lehnert H, Brochner-Mortensen J, Gomis R, Andersen S, Arner P for the Irbesartan in Patients with Type 2 Diabetes and Microalbuminuria Study Group: The effect of irbesartan on the development of diabetic nephropathy in patients with type 2 diabetes. N Engl J Med 2001;345:870–878.
30. Brenner BM, Cooper ME, DeZeeuw D, et al for the RENAAL Study Investigators: Effects of losartan on renal and cardiovascular outcomes in patients with type 2 diabetes and nephropathy. N Engl J Med 2001;345:861–869.

31. Hostetter TH: Prevention of end-stage renal disease due to type 2 diabetes. N Engl J Med 2001;345:910–912.

32. Bakris GL, Siomos M, Richardson D, et al: ACE inhibition or angiotensin receptor blockade: impact on potassium in renal failure. Kidney Int 2000;58:2084–2092.

33. Karim A: Spironolactone: deposition, metabolism, pharmacodynamics, and bioavailability. Drug Metab Rev 1978;8:151–158.

34. Brilla CG, Weber KT: Mineralocorticoid excess, dietary sodium and myocardial fibrosis. J Lab Clin Med 1992;120:893–901.

35. Greene EL, Kren S, Hostetter TH: Role of aldosterone in the remnant kidney model in the rat. J Clin Invest 1996;98:1063–1068.

36. Rocha R, Stier CT, Kifor I, et al: Aldosterone: a mediator of myocardial necrosis and renal arteriopathy. Endocrinology 2000;141:3871–3878.

37. Pitt B, Zannad F, Remme WJ, et al: The effect of spironolactone on morbidity and mortality in patients with severe heart failure. Randomized aldactone evaluation study investigators. N Engl J Med 1999;341:709–717.

38. Overdiek HW, Merkus FW: Influence of food on the bioavailability of spironolactone. Clin Pharmacol Ther 1986;40:531–536.

39. Shackelton CR, Wong NLM, Sutton RAL: Distal (potassium-sparing) diuretics. In Dirks JH, Sutton RAL (eds): Diuretics, Physiology, Pharmacology and Clinical Use. Philadelphia: W.B. Saunders, 1986, pp 117–134.

40. Schrijver G, Weinberger MH: Hydrochlorothiazide and spironolactone in hypertension. Clin Pharmacol Ther 1979;25:33–42.

41. Greenblatt DJ, Koch-Weser J: Adverse reactions to spironolactone. A report from the Boston Collaborative Drug Surveillance Program. JAMA 1973;225:40–43.

42. Roos JC, Doarhout Mees EJ, Koomans HA, Boer P: Intrarenal sodium handling during chronic spironolactone treatment. Nephron 1984;38:226.

Calcium Channel Blockers

Lance D. Dworkin and Douglas G. Shemin

Calcium channel blockers were developed in the 1960s, introduced in the 1980s, and are widely used for the treatment of hypertension, angina, and cardiac arrhythmias. Calcium channel blockers are structurally heterogeneous but share the universal property of blocking the transmembrane flow of calcium ions through voltage-gated channels (L-type channels) in vascular and nonvascular smooth muscle.[1] Blockade of these channels may result in smooth muscle relaxation, decreased peripheral vascular resistance, dilation of coronary arteries, and a decrease in myocardial contractility.

Clinical pharmacology

Calcium channel blockers can be divided into two classes by structure and function: dihydropyridines and nondihydropyridines. Verapamil, a phenylalkylamine, and diltiazem, a benzothiazepine, are the currently available nondihydropyridine agents. Mibefradil, another nondihydropyridine agent, was removed from the market by its manufacturer in 1998 due to adverse cytochrome P450-associated drug interactions[2] (Table 56.1). Dihydropyridine calcium channel antagonists block L-type channels selectively in peripheral vascular tissue and therefore act primarily by dilating resistance vessels. Nondihydropyridine calcium channel antagonists block L-type channels in both vascular and cardiac tissue and therefore affect the atrioventricular node in addition to causing vasodilation. They decrease heart rate and prevent reflex tachycardia. Nondihydropyridine agents may also decrease glomerular protein and albumin sieving and therefore urinary protein excretion rate.[1]

The newer agents and formulations of most calcium channel blockers have a relatively long half-life and time to peak effect. There are also immediate-release, relatively short-acting preparations of diltiazem, verapamil, nifedipine, and nicardipine. Because of the potential risks of short-acting agents (see later), only the long-acting preparations are recommended for use in hypertension. Calcium channel blockers are primarily metabolized by the liver and have similar half-lives in individuals with normal renal function or with renal insufficiency. In general, dose adjustment is not required in renal failure; however, there are reports of toxicity with long-acting verapamil in patients with endstage renal disease (ESRD).[3]

Clinical studies of calcium channel blockers in hypertensive patients have examined three issues: their efficacy in controlling hypertension, their use in reducing cardiovascular morbidity and mortality, and their effect on progression of renal disease. These data are summarized below and in Table 56.2.

Efficacy in the treatment of essential hypertension

In short-term studies in which blood pressure was the primary outcome, calcium channel blockers, as single agents, were as effective or more effective in lowering blood pressure than other antihypertensive agents. In the VA Cooperative Study, hypertensive patients were randomized to placebo or one of six agents as monotherapy. Those randomized to diltiazem had the highest rate of success compared with those given hydrochlorothiazide, atenolol, captopril, clonidine, or prazosin.[4] In a similar study, amlodipine was as effective as chlorthalidone, acebutolol, doxazosin, or enalapril in hypertensive men and women.[5] In the German HANE study, hydrochlorothiazide, atenolol, nitrendipine, or enalapril all provided similar degrees of blood pressure reduction.[6]

Prevention of cardiovascular morbidity and mortality

In most of the studies summarized in Table 56.2, calcium channel blockers appear to be as effective as, or somewhat inferior to, other agents in preventing most cardiovascular events, particularly when prescribed as sole agents. The Verapamil in Hypertension and Atherosclerosis study randomized patients to verapamil or a diuretic and found no difference in morbid and mortal outcomes.[7] In the Fosinopril versus Amlodipine Cardiovascular Events Randomized Trial, hypertensive type 2 diabetics were randomized to fosinopril or amlodipine; the rate of cardiovascular morbid and mortal events was greater in the

Table 56.1 Calcium channel blockers: recommended doses for hypertension

	Trade name	Half-life (hours) (normal/ESRD)	Dosage	Comment*
Amlodipine	Norvasc	35–50/50	Initial: 2.5 mg daily Maintenance: 2.5–10 mg daily	Dihydropyridine. Combination form with benazapril available. Dosage adjustment for impaired liver function
Diltiazem	Dilacor Cardizem Cartia Tiazac (q.i.d.)	2–8/3.5	Initial: 120–180 mg SR daily Maintenance: 120–480 mg SR daily Initial: 30 mg q.i.d. Maintenance 120–360 mg daily	Benzothiazepine. Greater potential than dihydropyridines for inducing conduction defects or interfering with left ventricular function. Dosage adjustment for impaired liver function
Felodipine	Plendil	10–14/21	5–10 mg daily	Dihydropyridine. Combination form with enalapril available. Dosage adjustment for liver disease and in geriatric patients
Isradipine	Dynacirc	1.9–4.8/10–11	Initial: 2.5 mg b.i.d. Maintenance: 2.5–10 mg b.i.d. Initial: 5 mg (CR) daily Maintenance: 5–20 mg (CR) daily	Dihydropyridine
Nicardipine	Cardene	5/5–7	20–40 mg p.o. t.i.d. 30–60 mg SR b.i.d. 1–15 mg/h i.v. infusion	Dihydropyridine. Can be given as a constant infusion in malignant/accelerated hypertension
Nifedipine	Adalat Procardia	4–5.5/5–7	Initial: 30–60 mg SR daily Maintenance: 30–90 mm SR daily	Dihydropyridine. Short-acting preparation hypertension
Nimodipine	Nimotop	1–2.8/22	60 mg q4h × 21 days	Dihydropyridine. Not approved for hypertension. Used to treat neurologic deficits due to cerebral artery spasm in patients with subarachnoid hemorrhage
Nisoldipine	Sular	6.6–7.9/6.8–9.7	Initial: 20 mg daily Maintenance: 20–40 mg daily	Dihydropyridine. Dose adjustments in liver disease and in geriatric patients
Nitrendipine		4.6/3.3–5.8	Initial: 10 mg daily Maintenance: 10–40 mg daily	Dihydropyridine. Investigational drug in the USA. Dose adjustments in liver disease and in geriatric patients
Verapamil	Calan Covera Isoptin Verelan	3–7/2.4–4	180–480 mg SR daily (divide q.d. to b.i.d.)	Phenylalkylamine. Dose adjustments in liver disease and in geriatric patients; 74% excreted in urine mostly as metabolites. Use with caution in patients with impaired renal function

*No dose adjustments are necessary for any of the calcium channel blockers in patients with renal insufficiency or for dialysis.

group assigned to amlodipine.[8] In the STOP-2 trial, 6614 elderly patients with hypertension were randomized to a calcium antagonist (isradipine or felodipine), an angiotensin-converting enzyme (ACE) inhibitor, or conventional therapy with diuretics and β-blockers. Calcium channel blockers were found to be equivalent to ACE inhibitors and conventional therapies in preventing most cardiovascular endpoints, but they were inferior to ACE inhibitors in preventing congestive heart failure or myocardial infarction.[9] In the Intervention as a Goal in Hypertension Treatment (INSIGHT) study, patients were randomized to long-acting nifedipine or a thiazide diuretic; the risk of stroke was lower in the nifedipine group but the risk of myocardial infarction or any cardiovascular mortality was increased.[10] In the Appropriate Blood Pressure Control in Diabetes (ABCD) Trial, 470 subjects with type 2 diabetes, hypertension, and nephropathy were randomized to the calcium channel blocker nisoldipine or enalapril.[11] The study was stopped prematurely because of a significant increase in the risk of nonfatal myocardial infarction in the nisoldipine group. There was no significant difference in overall mortality and the original assessment of relative risk was subsequently lowered significantly when additional patient follow-up data became available.[12] In the Multicenter Isradipine Diuretic Atherosclerosis (MIDAS) study, 883 hypertensive patients

Table 56.2 Studies of calcium channel blockers in prevention of cardiovascular (CV) disease in hypertensive patients

Study and reference	No. of patients	Drugs studied	Relative risk for calcium antagonist for:		
			CV morbidity	CV mortality	Stroke
VHAS[7]	1414	Verapamil vs. diuretic			
FACET[8]	380	Amlodipine vs. ACE inhibitor		2.04 (1.05–3.84)	2.56 (0.81–8.33)
STOP-2[9]	6614	Isradipine/felodipine vs. diuretic/β-blocker vs. ACE inhibitor	0.99 (0.87–1.12)	0.97 (0.80–1.17)	0.88 (0.73–1.06)
INSIGHT[10]	6321	Nifedipine vs. diuretic	1.11 (0.90–1.36)	1.16 (0.80–1.69)	0.87 (0.61–1.26)
ABCD[11,12]	470	Nisoldipine vs. ACE inhibitor	3.3 (1.5–7.1)	NS	
MIDAS[13]	883	Isradipine vs. diuretic	1.78 (0.94–3.38)		2.00 (0.50–7.93)
SYST-EUR[14]	4695	Nitrendipine vs. placebo	0.69 (0.55–0.86)	0.73 (0.52–1.02)	0.58 (0.40–0.83)
NORDIL[15]	10 881	Diltiazem vs. diuretic/β-blocker	1.04 (0.91–1.18)	1.11 (0.87–1.43)	0.80 (0.65–0.99)

ACE, angiotensin-converting enzyme.

were randomized to the calcium channel blocker isradipine or hydrochlorothiazide. Carotid artery thickness progressed similarly in both groups of patients, but adverse cardiovascular events occurred more often in the isradipine group.[13]

On the other hand, some studies have shown improved results with calcium channel blockers, particularly in prevention of cerebrovascular disease. In the SYST-EUR study, 4695 elderly patients with systolic hypertension were randomized to the calcium channel blocker nitrendipine or placebo; ACE inhibitors and diuretics were added as needed in both groups to lower the systolic blood pressure to below 150 mmHg. The risk of cardiovascular events and strokes was reduced by nitrendipine.[14] In the Nordic Diltiazem study, patients were randomized to diltiazem or conventional therapy with a β-blocker and diuretic. Major cardiovascular events occurred at equal rates in the two groups, but there was a lower risk of stroke in the diltiazem group. Other cardiovascular events and deaths from cardiovascular disease occurred more often in the diltiazem group, although this was not statistically significant.[15] In the Hypertension Optimal Treatment (HOT) trial, almost 19 000 adults with hypertension were assigned to three different diastolic blood pressure goals, from less than 80 mmHg to less than 90 mmHg. The long-acting dihydropyridine felodipine was given to every patient; other agents were added as needed to reach the blood pressure goal. Patients whose diastolic blood pressure fell below 85 mmHg benefited from therapy including a calcium channel blocker. In diabetic subjects, cardiovascular risk was significantly reduced in those patients assigned to the lowest diastolic blood pressure target. Of note, the rate of cardiovascular events in HOT was lower than reported previously in other studies, suggesting that calcium channel blockers, in conjunction with other agents, specifically improve outcomes when blood pressure is aggressively lowered.[16]

Safety

Beginning in the 1980s, short-acting calcium channel blockers were linked, in a series of cases, to a number of serious acute cardiovascular morbid events. This was especially true for sublingually administered nifedipine in severe hypertension, perhaps because of reflex activation of the adrenergic system induced by sudden changes in blood pressure. Therefore, the use of short-acting calcium channel blockers for the treatment of hypertension is not recommended and has been largely abandoned.[17] In parallel with these reports, a series of observational studies described an increased risk of cardiovascular morbidity associated with the use of calcium channel blockers, raising concern about the safety of these agents. One example was the Nurses Health Study of over 14 000 women, in which subjects taking a calcium antagonist had a higher risk of death and myocardial infarction than those taking other antihypertensive agents.[18] Another retrospective analysis suggested a link between calcium channel blockers and myocardial infarction in hypertensives with cardiovascular disease.[19] Furberg et al[20] performed a metaanalysis of 16 studies involving the dihydropyridine nifedipine and found an increased dose-dependent relationship between nifedipine and cardiovascular mortality. In most of these studies, a large group of heterogeneous patients was examined and the choice of antihypertensive agent was not controlled. Therefore it is likely that differences in patient characteristics may have explained the different outcomes. For example, in the Nurses Health Study calcium channel blockers were more likely to be given to women with underlying heart disease.[18] Similarly, a number of these studies did not differentiate between the use of long-acting vs. short-acting calcium channel blockers.

In the mid 1990s, a higher risk of cancer of all types and a higher risk of gastrointestinal bleeding was observed in two population-based studies of hypertensive patients taking calcium channel blockers as compared to β-blockers or ACE inhibitors. Increased risk was primarily observed in elderly individuals.[21,22] Conversely, three large studies from Europe and the USA found no relationship between calcium channel blockers and the development of cancer.[23–25] Because of the controversy in the literature regarding the safety of calcium channel blockers, particularly with regard to the risk of cancer, gastrointestinal bleeding, and acute coronary syndromes, a subcommittee of the World Health Organization and the International Society of Hypertension formed an ad hoc committee to review the topic. After review of the literature, the committee concluded that the available evidence did not establish any relationship between the use of calcium channel blockers and the development of cancer, bleeding, or acute myocardial infarction.[26]

Progression of chronic renal disease

Calcium channel blockers modulate the progression of chronic renal disease by diverse mechanisms, including alterations in renal hemodynamics and renal growth and by direct effects on the production and/or responses to various cytokines, growth factors, and vasoconstrictor substances by glomerular and tubular cells. The effect of calcium channel blockers on progression of experimental chronic renal disease has been the subject of numerous studies. Although a protective effect was often found, the results of these studies are somewhat inconsistent. The explanations for these divergent findings are not always apparent but have been attributed to differences in the model studied, the particular drug or dose administered, concomitant variability in systemic and/or intraglomerular pressure, and/or other relevant parameters. A detailed discussion of these data, as well as the potential mechanisms by which calcium channel blockers reduce renal injury, is beyond the scope of this chapter and the reader is referred to several recent reviews.[27–30] The effects of calcium channel blockers on progression of renal disease in humans have now been examined in several randomized, controlled, clinical trials. These studies in patients with diabetic or nondiabetic renal disease have provided sufficient data to make rational recommendations regarding the use of calcium channel blockers to preserve kidney function.

Studies in which calcium channel blockers were compared with drugs that block the renin–angiotensin–aldosterone system (Table 56.3)

Most studies have compared the effects of calcium channel blockers with ACE inhibitors. Zucchelli et al[31] conducted a prospective randomized clinical trial in 121 patients with hypertension and chronic renal disease. Most patients had glomerulonephritis; patients with diabetes, proteinuria > 5 g, or systemic diseases were excluded. Patients were observed for 1 year on standard therapy and then randomized to receive either captopril or slow-release nifedipine for an additional 3 years of follow-up. Blood pressure and creatinine clearance were monitored. Mean blood pressure was approximately 165/100 mmHg prior to randomization and declined significantly by about 20 mmHg with addition of captopril or nifedipine. There was no significant sustained decline in protein excretion rate from the baseline value of 1.5 g/day with either drug. Creatinine clearance declined similarly in both groups but by a relatively small amount (only 5–6 mL/min) over the entire 3-year period of observation. Following randomization and with improved blood pressure control, the mean rate of decline in creatinine clearance was cut by half; captopril and nifedipine had similar effects. Most likely, the slowing in the rate of progression resulted more from the marked decline in blood pressure achieved after randomization than from the use of either agent specifically. More patients in the nifedipine group reached dialysis, but the study was insufficiently powered to examine this endpoint and the difference was not statistically significant. Therefore, the data demonstrate that both ACE inhibitors and calcium channel blockers have a renal protective effect when hypertension is aggressively treated.

Velussi et al[32] studied 44 patients with hypertension and noninsulin-dependent diabetes mellitus (NIDDM). Of these patients, 26 had normal amounts of albumin in their urine and 18 had microalbuminuria. Patients were randomly assigned to receive the calcium channel blocker amlodipine or the ACE inhibitor cilazapril and treated to a target blood pressure of < 140/85 mmHg. Diuretics were added as needed. Albumin excretion rate and EDTA clearance (a measure of glomerular filtration rate, GFR) were measured at 6–12 month intervals for a period of 3 years. Blood pressure was aggressively lowered, declining from about 170–185/90–95 mmHg at baseline without therapy to about 130–135/75 mmHg with either agent. Associated with this marked reduction in blood pressure, there was a significant reduction in GFR over the first 6–12 months of follow-up. Thereafter, GFR stabilized and was not different in patients taking the calcium channel blocker or the ACE inhibitor. In patients with microalbuminuria, albumin excretion rate declined modestly in both groups. None of the patients studied had overt nephropathy and the data may not be relevant to renal disease progression in that setting. However, it has been suggested that dihydropyridine calcium channel blockers

Table 56.3 Summary of long-term randomized clinical trials examining the effects of calcium channel blockers on progression of chronic renal disease

Reference	Renal disease	No. of patients	Duration	Drugs	Effect on proteinuria	Effect on GFR decline
Zucchelli et al[31]	Nondiabetic	121	3 years	Nifedipine vs. captopril	Declined if MAP < 100 mmHg	50% reduction in rate of decline compared with baseline
Velussi et al[32]	Early NIDDM	44	3 years	Amlodipine vs. cilazapril	Declined	Annual rate of decline ~ 2 mL/min on therapy
Bakris et al[33]	Hypertensive NIDDM	52	63 months	Diltiazem or verapamil vs. lisinopril vs. atenolol	Decreased	Annual rate of decline 1.44 mL/min on calcium channel blockers
Estacio et al[34]	Hypertensive NIDDM	470	5 years	Nisoldipine vs. enalapril	No change	Stable in patients with microalbuminuria. Annual rate of decline 5–6 mL/min in patients with overt albuminuria
Agodoa et al[36]	African-Americans with hypertensive nephrosclerosis	653	3 years	Amlodipine vs. ramipril	Increased	Annual rate of decline 3.22 mL/min for all patients. Faster for those with proteinuria > 300 mg/day or GFR < 40 mL/min
Lewis et al[37]	NIDDM with nephropathy	1715	2.6 years	Amlodipine vs. irbesartan vs. placebo	Declined by 6%, similar to placebo, inferior to irbesartan	Serum creatinine slope with amlodipine similar to placebo, inferior to irbesartan
Bakris et al[40]	NIDDM with nephropathy	37	1 year	Verapamil plus trandolapril	Declined by 27% on verapamil alone, 62% on combination therapy	GFR unchanged
Ruggenenti et al[42]	Nondiabetic nephropathies	117	18 months	Various dihydropyridines ± ramipril	Increased by ~ 20% but not in patients also on ACE inhibitor or with good blood pressure control	30% faster than noncalcium channel blockers but not in patients also on ACE inhibitor or with good blood pressure control
Brenner et al[38]	NIDDM with nephropathy	1513	3.4 years	Various ± losartan	No adverse impact on beneficial response to ARB	No adverse impact on beneficial response to ARB

ACE, angiotensin-converting enzyme; ARB, angiotensin receptor blocker; GFR, glomerular filtration rate; MAP, mean arterial pressure; NIDDM, noninsulin-dependent diabetes mellitus.

may increase renal plasma flow and augment proteinuria. Therefore, it is notable in this study that when blood pressure was truly normalized, both GFR and protein excretion rate were reduced by amlodipine in a manner exactly comparable to the ACE inhibitor.

In another relatively small study, Bakris et al[33] compared treatment with diltiazem or verapamil to the ACE inhibitor lisinopril or the β-blocker atenolol in 52 patients with NIDDM and associated nephropathy. Median blood pressure declined from about 155/97 mmHg at baseline to 132–138/82–86 mmHg during therapy; there were no

significant differences in blood pressure between the groups. Over 63 months of follow-up, the rate of decline in creatinine clearance was modest and similar in patients receiving either lisinopril or one of the calcium channel blockers. Proteinuria was also similarly reduced by the ACE inhibitor and the calcium channel blockers. Once again, the data suggest that both calcium channel blockers and ACE inhibitors protect renal function in diabetic patients.

The Appropriate Blood Pressure Control in Diabetes (ABCD) trial was a prospective, randomized, blinded clinical trial comparing the effects of the dihydropyridine calcium channel blocker nisoldipine with enalapril on the rate of change in creatinine clearance in 470 hypertensive type 2 diabetic subjects.[34] Additional antihypertensive agents were added as needed to achieve the target blood pressure. The study was stopped 67 months after the first patient was enrolled because of a significant difference in incidence of nonfatal myocardial infarction between the groups[11,12] (see earlier). The renal endpoint data were subsequently presented separately.[34] Blood pressure at entry, off medication, averaged approximately 160/77 mmHg. Most patients were without diabetic nephropathy at entry; creatinine clearance averaged about 85 mL/min per 1.73 m^2 and less than 20% of patients had overt albuminuria. A decline in creatinine clearance was observed but occurred primarily during the first year, and may have represented an acute hemodynamic response to blood pressure reduction rather than a specific effect on progression of nephropathy per se. There was no significant difference in renal outcomes between patients randomized to nisoldipine vs. enalapril. Of note, enalapril did produce an initial decline in urinary albumin excretion of relatively modest degree. However, by the end of the study, there was no significant difference in protein excretion rate between the groups. Importantly, there was no significant difference in the number of patients with normoalbuminuria progressing to microalbuminuria or in those with microalbuminuria progressing to overt proteinuria. Thus the study demonstrates similar renal outcomes with the use of an ACE inhibitor or a dihydropyridine calcium channel blocker.

The Modification of Diet in Renal Disease (MDRD) study examined the effects of a low blood pressure target on progression of nondiabetic types of chronic renal disease.[35] Post-hoc subset analysis suggested that African-Americans with hypertension and nephropathy specifically benefited from the low blood pressure target, although the number of subjects was too small to permit a firm conclusion. To further address this question, the African American Study of Kidney Disease and Hypertension (AASK) was launched.[36] Participants were 1094 African-Americans with hypertension and presumed nephrosclerosis, with a GFR between 20 and 63 mL/min per 1.73 m^2. The subjects were randomized to a usual (102–107 mmHg) vs. a low (92 mmHg) blood pressure goal and to one of three antihypertensive agents as preferred therapy: a sustained-release form of the β-blocker metoprolol, the ACE inhibitor ramipril, or the dihydropyridine calcium channel blocker amlodipine. Additional antihypertensive agents were added as needed to achieve the target pressure. The primary endpoint of this study was the rate of change in GFR (slope) as determined by iothalamate clearance. The amlodipine intervention was discontinued prematurely because of an apparent increase in the rate of decline in GFR in proteinuric patients randomized to this group. The mean duration of follow-up for the GFR data was about 3 years at the time the study was discontinued. To date, only the comparison between ramipril and amlodipine has been reported[36] and the study is ongoing.

In total, 436 patients were randomized to ramipril and 217 to amlodipine. Outcomes were analyzed separately for the patients with a baseline urine protein/creatinine ratio > 0.22. There were 144 such patients in the ramipril group and 69 in the amlodipine arm. Baseline blood pressure off therapy was similar in all the groups and averaged approximately 151/96 mmHg. Baseline GFR was about 45 mL/min in all the groups and slightly lower (38–40 mL/min) in the proteinuric patients. Of interest, 46% of the patients were receiving a calcium channel blocker at entry. Blood pressure was significantly and similarly reduced by either therapy, on average to 134/82 mmHg with ramipril vs. 132/81 mmHg with amlodipine. Of note, additional agents were necessary to reduce blood pressure to these levels in both groups; the average patient took four blood pressure medications. Over the entire study, there were no significant differences in the GFR slope from baseline to the stopping point between patients receiving amlodipine vs. ramipril; however, subset analysis suggested that ramipril was superior to enalapril. In nonproteinuric patients, GFR actually increased by about 10% following initiation of amlodipine and then declined at a slightly faster rate. This acute vasodilator effect of amlodipine may not be associated with long-term preservation of GFR, but was responsible for the fact that both groups finished the study with similar GFR. Patients with proteinuria greater than about 300 mg/day and patients with initial GFR less than 40 mL/min did not experience this initial rise in GFR and had an even faster rate of decline on amlodipine than nonproteinuric patients, consistent with the notion that amlodipine was inferior to ramipril in this setting. In addition to a more rapid chronic rate of decline in GFR, subjects on amlodipine experienced an increase in protein excretion rate. Even more striking, significantly more patients on amlodipine reached the clinical endpoints of death or ESRD than in the ramipril group.

Thus in several categories, ramipril appeared to be superior to amlodipine in African-Americans with hypertensive nephrosclerosis. It should be noted, however, that this study does not demonstrate any adverse effect of amlodipine, except perhaps a mild increase in proteinuria. For the amlodipine group as a whole, GFR declined at an annual rate of only 3.2 mL/min per 1.73 m^2, which is relatively slow. Due to the initial increase in GFR, patients with proteinuria < 300 mg per 24 h on amlodipine actually concluded the study with a higher GFR on average than patients on ramipril. Amlodipine was probably inferior to ramipril in proteinuric patients and those with moderate to severe renal functional impairment at baseline; however, it still may have been significantly superior to placebo or therapy with a combination of drugs that did not include amlodipine. Therefore, these data should not be interpreted as implying that calcium channel blockers are unsafe in this patient population.

Lewis et al[37] examined the relative blood pressure-independent capacity of the angiotensin II receptor antagonist irbesartan and amlodipine to slow progression of renal disease in patients with type 2 diabetes, hypertension, and nephropathy. To enter, the 1727 subjects had to have a creatinine between 1.0 and 3.0 mg/dL and greater than 900 mg of urinary protein. Patients were randomly assigned to irbesartan, amlodipine, or placebo. At baseline, blood pressure was approximately 160/87 mmHg. Thus patients in the "placebo" group received on average 3.3 antihypertensive agents, including diuretics, β-blockers, and peripheral and/or central α-blockers. Subjects were followed for an average of 2.6 years. The primary endpoint was doubling of serum creatinine, development of ESRD, or death. With treatment, blood pressure was similarly reduced in all three groups to an average value of 140–144/77 mmHg. The risk of reaching the primary endpoint was significantly reduced by 23% in the irbesartan group compared with placebo or amlodipine. In contrast, outcomes in the amlodipine group were not significantly different from placebo. The risk of experiencing a doubling of serum creatinine was 37% lower in the irbesartan compared with the amlodipine group. Protein excretion rate also declined more markedly with irbesartan compared with amlodipine. However, patients taking amlodipine also experienced a modest decline in proteinuria. There were no significant differences in deaths between the three groups. However, the study was not sufficiently powered to examine cardiovascular events.

Taken together, these data support the conclusion that irbesartan is superior to amlodipine in slowing progression of diabetic renal disease. Of note, two other recent studies support a beneficial effect of angiotensin receptor blockers in this setting.[38,39] Once again, it is important to note that administration of amlodipine was equivalent to therapy with diuretics and α- and β-blockers and probably beneficial in this population, albeit slightly less so than irbesartan. There was no increase in proteinuria in the amlodipine group, and GFR declined at an annual rate of only about 1 mL/min per 1.73 m^2 faster than that seen in the irbesartan group.

In some respects, the discussion surrounding the use of calcium channel blockers in patients with renal disease may have been incorrectly framed and somewhat misguided. Most investigators and reviewers have focused on the effects of calcium channel blockers as preferred agents for preservation of kidney function compared with drugs that block the renin–angiotensin–aldosterone system (RAAS). As discussed above, it seems clear that at present the data favor using ACE inhibitors or angiotensin receptor blockers as preferred agents, particularly in proteinuric patients. However, it is important to note that blood pressure is almost never controlled with a single agent in patients with hypertension and renal disease. In the studies discussed above, most patients were taking combinations of three to four blood pressure medications in order to reach target blood pressure. Beyond the scope of this chapter, a variety of data suggest that a relatively low blood pressure target of < 130/80 mmHg is associated with superior outcomes in diabetic patients or those with nondiabetic renal disease and proteinuria > 500 mg/day. Practically speaking, these low targets are almost never reached without combination therapy. Therefore, similar to combination chemotherapy for the treatment of malignancy, the key question is what combination of antihypertensive agents is associated with the best cardiovascular and renal outcomes for patients. This combination should include a drug that blocks the RAAS, but the best second, third, and fourth drugs to use are not clear. The effect of combination therapy with a drug that blocks the RAAS and a calcium channel blocker has been examined in a few studies.

Studies in which calcium channel blockers were combined with drugs that block the renin–angiotensin–aldosterone system (Table 56.3)

Bakris et al[40] randomly assigned 37 patients with hypertension and diabetic nephropathy to receive the ACE inhibitor trandolapril, the calcium channel blocker verapamil, or both drugs in combination for 1 year. Blood pressure was similarly reduced in all three groups, from a baseline off therapy of approximately 170/105 mmHg to less than 140/90 mmHg. Almost all patients required the addition of a diuretic to achieve this goal. Protein excretion rate fell significantly in subjects on the ACE inhibitor (–33%) or verapamil (–7%) alone, but the greatest reduction was seen in the 14 patients on combination therapy (–62%). GFR was stable in all groups during the 1-year period of follow-up. This study was not powered to examine progression of chronic renal failure and relied on a surrogate endpoint, proteinuria, to assess efficacy. Nevertheless, the data are consistent with the hypothesis that combination therapy with an ACE inhibitor and a calcium channel blocker is safe and well tolerated and may have additive if not synergistic antiproteinuric effect.

The Ramipril Efficacy in Nephropathy (REIN) study examined the hypothesis that proteinuria and its modification by an ACE inhibitor influences the progression of renal disease.[41] REIN investigators stratified patients with nondiabetic chronic glomerular disease (GFR 20–70 mL/min, proteinuria > 1 g) according to protein excretion rate and then randomly assigned them to receive an ACE inhibitor or placebo. Antihypertensive drugs other than ACE inhibitors included the dihydropyridine calcium channel blockers and these were administered as needed to reach the target diastolic blood pressure of < 90 mmHg. The primary endpoints were the change in GFR and risk of endstage renal failure. The basic finding was that proteinuria was reduced and progression slowed by administration of the ACE inhibitor, with the greatest benefit accruing to those patients with the heaviest proteinuria.[41] In a subsequent report, Ruggenenti et al[42] described the changes in protein excretion rate and GFR decline in 117 patients in this study that were given a calcium channel blocker. Subjects in the placebo group (not receiving an ACE inhibitor) who were given a calcium channel blocker experienced about a 20% increase in protein excretion rate as well as a more rapid rate of decline in GFR. However, if blood pressure was well controlled (MAP < 100 mmHg) or if patients received an ACE inhibitor, there was no adverse effect of being treated with a dihydropyridine calcium channel blocker. These data suggest that calcium channel blockers can be safely administered to patients with hypertension, proteinuria, and chronic renal disease if combined with an ACE inhibitor or even in the absence of ACE inhibition as long as blood pressure is tightly controlled.

A similar outcome was observed in patients with type 2 diabetes in the recently reported Reduction of Endpoints in NIDDM with the Angiotensin II Antagonist Losartan (RENAAL) trial.[38] The study enrolled 1500 patients with type 2 diabetes and nephropathy and randomly assigned them to receive the angiotensin receptor blocker losartan or placebo; they were followed for a mean duration of 3.4 years. Subjects were treated to a target blood pressure of < 140/90 mmHg and additional non-RAAS blocking agents were given as needed to reach this goal. The primary outcome was a composite endpoint of doubling of serum creatinine, ESRD, or death. The study was positive, demonstrating that losartan reduced the numbers of patients experiencing a doubling of serum creatinine or ESRD. There were no significant differences in overall mortality between the groups. Almost all patients required additional antihypertensive medications to control blood pressure; calcium channel blockers were the most common additional agents and were given to about 80% of patients. Most often these were dihydropyridine calcium channel blockers (about 60% of all patients). In this study, simultaneous therapy with calcium channel blockers did not detract from the beneficial effects of losartan.

Conclusions

Calcium channel blockers are effective, generally well tolerated antihypertensive agents; their long duration of action and favorable adverse-effect profile are benefits. Earlier concerns that they increase the risk of acute myocardial infarction or other cardiovascular mortality seem not to be valid, especially with the use of long-acting agents, and they do not appear to be associated with an increased risk of cancer or bleeding. They are as efficacious as diuretics, β-blockers, or ACE inhibitors in lowering blood pressure. Although some studies are encouraging, the bulk of evidence suggests that they are inferior to ACE inhibitors or diuretics in preventing cardiac disease in hypertensive subjects, including myocardial infarction and congestive heart failure. However, calcium channel blockers may be associated with a lower risk of stroke, particularly in elderly patients with systolic hypertension.

The results of studies of progression of chronic renal disease are also largely consistent in both diabetic and nondiabetic patients. Calcium channel blockers are safe and well tolerated in patients with hypertension and renal disease. Progression of renal disease is probably slowed when blood pressure is well controlled with a combination of agents including a calcium channel blocker. This effect may not be as great as that seen when the combination of drugs administered includes an agent that specifically blocks the RAAS, i.e., an ACE inhibitor or angiotensin receptor blocker; however, this has not been consistent in all studies. The magnitude of the additional benefit associated with RAAS blocking drugs is likely to be small, perhaps

an additional decrease in the annual rate of decline in GFR of about 1–2 mL/min. However, this difference may become quite significant with time. Clinically important increases in protein excretion rate are not typically observed with dihydropyridine calcium channel blockers. Furthermore, the evidence that nondihydropyridine calcium channel blockers have superior renal protective effects is not sufficiently compelling to recommend preferential use of these agents in a subset of kidney patients.

An increasing number of clinical trials and the most recent JNC-VI guidelines support aggressive lowering of the blood pressure to 130/80 mmHg or below in individuals at high risk for cardiovascular events, with dibetes, or with proteinuria. It is difficult to reach these blood pressure targets with ACE inhibitors, angiotensin receptor antagonists, diuretics, or β-blockers as single agents. Calcium channel blockers are excellent second- or third-line agents, in combination with ACE inhibitors and/or diuretics, for the treatment of hypertension in individuals with cardiovascular and/or renal disease.

Acknowledgment

L.D.D. was partially supported by an NIH RO1 grant DK52314 during the preparation of this manuscript.

References

1. Abernathy DR, Schwartz JB: Calcium antagonist drugs. N Engl J Med 1999;341:1447–1457.
2. Mullins ME, Horowitz BZ, Linden D et al: Life threatening interaction of mibefradil and beta blockers with dihydropyridine calcium channel blockers. JAMA 1998;280:157–158.
3. Pritza DR, Bierman MH, Hammeke MD: Acute toxic effects of sustained release verapamil in chronic renal failure. Arch Intern Med 1991;151:2081–2084.
4. Materson BJ, Reda DJ, Cushman WC, et al: Single drug therapy for hypertension in men. N Engl J Med 1993;328:914–921.
5. Neaton JD, Grimm RH, Prineas RJ, et al: Treatment of mild hypertension study: final results. JAMA 1993;270:713–724.
6. Philipp T, Anlauf M, Distler A, et al: Randomized, double blind, multicenter controlled comparison of hydrochlorthiazide, atenolol, nitrendipine, and enalapril in antihypertensive treatment: the results of the HANE Study: Hane Trial Research Group. Br Med J 1997;315:154–159.
7. Zanchetti A, Rosei EA, Dal Palu C, et al: The Verapamil in Hypertension and Atherosclerosis Study (VHAS): results of long term randomized treatment with either verapamil or chlorthalidone on carotid intima-media thickness. J Hypertens 1998;16:1667–1676.
8. Tatti P, Pahor M, Byington RP: Outcome results of the fosinopril versus amlodipine cardiovascular events randomized trial (FACET) in patients with hypertension and NIDDM. Diabetes Care 1998;21:597–603.
9. Hansson L, Lindholm LH, Ekbom T, et al: Randomized trial of old and new antihypertensive drugs in elderly patients: cardiovascular mortality and morbidity. The Swedish Trial in Old patients with Hypertension 2 study. Lancet 1999;354:1751–1756.
10. Brown MJ, Palmer CR, Castaigne A, et al: Morbidity and mortality in patients randomised to double blind treatment with a long acting calcium channel blocker or diuretic in the International Nifedipine GITS Study: Intervention as a Goal in Hypertension Treatment (INSIGHT). Lancet 2000;356:366–372.
11. Estacio RO, Jeffers BW, Hiatt WR, et al: The effect of nisoldipine as compared with enalapril on cardiovascular outcomes in patients with non-insulin-dependent diabetes and hypertension. N Engl J Med 1998;338:645–652.

12. Schrier RW, Estacio RO: Additional follow-up from the ABCD trial in patients with type 2 diabetes and hypertension. N Engl J Med 2000;343:1969.
13. Borhani NO, Mercuri M, Borhani PA, et al: Final outcome results of the Multicenter Isradipine Diuretic Atherosclerosis Study (MIDAS): a randomized placebo controlled trial. JAMA 1996;276:785–791.
14. Staessen JA, Fagard R, Thijs L, et al: Randomized double blind comparison of placebo and active treatment for elderly patients with isolated systolic hypertension. Lancet 1997;350:757–764.
15. Hansson L, Hedner T, Lund-Johansen P, et al: Randomised trial of the effects of calcium antagonists compared with diuretics and beta blockers on cardiovascular morbidity and mortality in hypertension: the Nordic Diltiazem (NORDIL) study. Lancet 2000;356:359–365.
16. Hansson L, Zanchetti A, Carruthers SG: Effects of intensive blood pressure lowering and low dose aspirin in patients with hypertension: principal results of the Hypertension Optimal Treatment (HOT) randomized trial. Lancet 1998;351:1755–1762.
17. Grossman E, Messerli FH, Grodzicki T, et al: Should a moratorium be placed on sublingual nifedipine capsules given for hypertensive emergencies and pseudoemergencies? JAMA 1996;276:1328–1331.
18. Michels K, Rosner B, Manson J: Prospective study of calcium channel blocker use, cardiovascular disease, and total mortality among hypertensive women. Circulation 1998;97:1540–1548.
19. Psaty BM, Heckbert SR, Koepsel TD: The risk of myocardial infarction associated with antihypertensive drug therapies. JAMA 1995;274:620–625.
20. Furberg C, Psaty B, Meyer J: Nifedipine: dose related increase in mortality in patients with coronary heart disease. Circulation 1995;92:1326–1331.
21. Pahor M, Guralnik JM, Corti M, et al: Calcium channel blockade and incidence of cancer in aged populations. Lancet 1996;348:493–497.
22. Pahor M, Guralnik JM, Furberg C, et al: Risk of gastrointestinal hemorrhage with calcium antagonists in hypertensive patients over 67 years old. Lancet 1996;347:1061–1065.
23. Olson JH, Sorenson HT, Fiis S: Cancer risk in users of calcium channel blockers. Hypertension 1997;29:1091–1094.
24. Hole DJ, Gillis CR, McCallum JR: Cancer risk of hypertensive patients taking calcium antagonists. J Hypertens 1998;16:119–124.
25. Rosenberg L, Rao S, Palmer JR, et al: Calcium channel blockers and the risk of cancer. JAMA 1998;279:1000–1004.
26. Ad hoc subcommittee of the World Health Organization/International Society of Hypertension Liaison Committee: Effects of calcium antagonists on the risks of coronary heart disease, cancer, and bleeding. J Hypertens 1997;15:105–115.
27. Epstein M: Calcium antagonists and renal disease. Kidney Int 1998;54:1771–1784.
28. Kloke HJ, Branten AJ, Hyysmanns FT, et al: Antihypertensive treatment of patients with proteinuric renal diseases: risks or benefits of calcium channel blockers? Kidney Int 1998;53:1559–1573.
29. Wier MR, Dworkin LD: Antihypertensive drugs, dietary salt and renal protection: how low should you go and with which therapy? Am J Kidney Dis 1998;32:1–22.
30. Griffin KA, Bidani AK: Calcium-channel blockers and the progression of renal disease. Curr Hypertens Rep 1999;1:436–445.
31. Zucchelli P, Zuccala A, Borghi M, et al: Long-term comparison between captopril and nifedipine in the progression of renal insufficiency. Kidney Int 1992;42:452–458.
32. Velussi M, Brocco E, Frigato F, et al: Effects of cilazapril and amlodipine on kidney function in hypertensive NIDDM patients. Diabetes 1996;45:216–222.
33. Bakris GL, Copley JB, Vicknair N, et al: Calcium channel blockers versus other antihypertensive therapies on progression of NIDDM associated nephropathy. Kidney Int 1996;50:1641–1650.
34. Estacio RO, Jeffers BW, Gifford N, et al: Effect of blood pressure control on diabetic microvascular complications in patients with hypertension and type 2 diabetes. Diabetes Care 2000;23:B54–B64.
35. Klahr S, Breyer JA, Beck GJ, et al: Dietary protein restriction, blood pressure control, and the progression of polycystic kidney disease. Modification of Diet in Renal Disease Study Group. J Am Soc Nephrol 1995;5:2037–2047.
36. Agodoa LY, Appel L, Bakris GL, et al: Effect of ramipril vs amlodipine on renal outcomes in hypertensive nephrosclerosis: a randomized controlled trial. JAMA 2001;285:2719–2728.
37. Lewis EJ, Hunsicker LG, Clarke WR, et al: Renoprotective effect of the angiotensin-receptor antagonist irbesartan in patients with nephropathy due to type 2 diabetes. N Engl J Med 2001;345:851–860.
38. Brenner BM, Cooper ME, de Zeeuw D, et al: Effects of losartan on renal and cardiovascular outcomes in patients with type 2 diabetes and nephropathy. N Engl J Med 2001;345:861–869.
39. Parving HH, Lehnert H, Brochner-Mortensen J, et al: The effect of irbesartan on the development of diabetic nephropathy in patients with type 2 diabetes. N Engl J Med 2001;345:870–878.
40. Bakris G, Weir MR, DeQuattro V, et al: Effects of an ACE inhibitor/calcium antagonist combination on proteinuria in diabetic nephropathy. Kidney Int 1998;54:1283–1289.
41. The Gisen Group: Randomized placebo-controlled trial of effect of ramipril on decline in glomerular filtration rate and risk of terminal renal failure in proteinuric, nondiabetic nephropathy. Lancet 1997;349:1857–1863.
42. Ruggenenti P, Perna A, Benini R, et al: Effects of dihydropyridine calcium channel blockers, angiotensin-converting enzyme inhibition, and blood pressure control on chronic, nondiabetic nephropathies. J Am Soc Nephrol 1998;9:2096–2101.

Individualization of Pharmacologic Therapy

Norman M. Kaplan

Individualized therapy
The elderly
The diabetic hypertensive
Other common compelling indications
Conclusion

All drugs approved for use in the treatment of hypertension will, in moderate doses, lower elevated blood pressure by ~ 10% in about two-thirds of patients.[1] This uniformity of response is inherent in the approval process: each drug must have been shown to lower blood pressure significantly compared with placebo and to have an efficacy equal to other antihypertensive drugs. Doses are chosen to provide sufficient but not excessive drug concentrations so that patients will tolerate them and achieve a demonstrable effect.

Comparisons between various antihypertensive drugs almost always demonstrate similar efficacy. The best comparison was performed in the Treatment of Mild Hypertension Study (TOMHS).[2] TOMHS involved random allocation of five drugs: the diuretic chlorthalidone, the β-blocker acebutolol, the α-blocker doxazosin, the calcium channel blocker amlodipine, and the angiotensin-converting enzyme (ACE) inhibitor enalapril. Each drug was given to almost 200 mild hypertensives, while another group took a placebo and all patients remained on a nutritional-hygienic program. The overall antihypertensive efficacy of the five drugs over 4 years was virtually equal.

Under this overall umbrella, each drug provides equal protection from the major cardiovascular diseases induced by hypertension.[3] However, individual patients show considerable differences in their response to one drug or another. Some of this variability can be accounted for by patient characteristics, including age and race, which in turn could be mediated by differences in activity of the renin–angiotensin system. In a Veterans Administration (VA) cooperative 1-year trial, 1292 men were randomly given one of six drugs from each major class. Overall and in the black patients the calcium channel blocker was most effective, while the ACE inhibitor was best in younger whites and the β-blocker best in older whites.[4] Similarly, in a randomized crossover trial of elderly patients with isolated systolic hypertension given a representative of four major classes (ACE inhibitor, β-blocker, calcium channel blocker, and diuretic) each for 1 month, diuretic and calcium channel blocker were more effective than β-blocker or ACE inhibitor.[5] In a similarly designed trial of younger patients with combined systolic and diastolic hypertension, the ACE inhibitor and β-blocker were more effective than the calcium channel blocker or diuretic.[6]

A general pattern emerges from these various comparative trials. Younger and white patients, who have higher renin levels, respond better to β-blockers and ACE inhibitors, drugs that work in large part by blocking the renin–angiotensin system. Conversely, older and black patients, who tend to have lower renin levels, respond better to diuretics and calcium channel blockers, which work in ways independent of initial renin levels. Some would argue that the hypertension in younger and white patients is more related to vasoconstriction whereas the hypertension in older and black patients is more related to volume excess.[7]

In clinical practice, these nuances often do not hold up[8] and are largely irrelevant because, as I argue later, a diuretic should be the foundation of all therapy, thereby raising the responsiveness of older and black patients to renin-inhibiting agents. Therefore, age and race are not sufficient criteria for choosing specific drugs for therapy.

Individualized therapy

Increasingly, the choice of initial therapy is being based on the presence of "compelling" indications that are, in turn, based on extensive clinical trial data.[9,10] The 1997 Joint National Committee (JNC) report[9] provided four such compelling indications and contraindications, whereas the 1999 World Health Organization/International Society of Hypertension report broadened this number[10] (Table 57.1). As seen in Table 57.1, each class of drug has one or more compelling indications and less certain indications for its use, as well as contraindications that are absolute (compelling) or relative (possible).

The list in Table 57.1 needs a few revisions based on clinical trial data published in the last 3 years. Specifically, β-blockers should be switched from "possible" indication to "compelling" indication for heart failure,[11] and angiotensin II antagonists can now be considered to have a compelling indication alongside ACE inhibitors for diabetic nephropathy.[12] Some would argue that ACE inhibitors should, on the basis of the HOPE trial,[13] be considered to have a compelling indication for all patients at high risk for atherothrombotic cardiovascular events.[14]

Obviously, more sharply defined indications for individual drugs will evolve from the multiple comparative trials now in progress, including ALLHAT. However, the data now available are sufficient to cover the majority of hypertensive patients, namely the elderly and the diabetic.

The elderly

More than half of people over age 60 have hypertension and, in almost two-thirds of the elderly, the nature of the

Table 57.1   Guidelines for selecting drug treatment of hypertension*

Class of drug	Compelling indications	Possible indications	Compelling contraindications	Possible contraindications
Diuretics	Heart failure Elderly patients Systolic hypertension	Diabetes	Gout	Dyslipidemia Sexually active males
β-Blockers	Angina After myocardial infarction Tachyarrhythmias	Heart failure Pregnancy Diabetes	Asthma and COPD Heart block†	Dyslipidemia Athletes and physically active patients Peripheral vascular disease
ACE inhibitors	Heart failure Left ventricular dysfunction After myocardial infarction Diabetic nephropathy		Pregnancy Hyperkalemia Bilateral renal artery stenosis	
Calcium antagonists	Angina Elderly patients Systolic hypertension	Peripheral vascular disease	Heart block‡	Congestive heart failure§
α-Blockers	Prostatic hypertrophy	Glucose intolerance Dyslipidemia		Orthostatic hypotension
Angiotensin II antagonists	ACE inhibitor cough	Heart failure	Pregnancy Bilateral renal artery stenosis Hyperkalemia	

ACE, angiotensin-converting enzyme; COPD, chronic obstructive pulmonary disease.
*Guidelines Subcommittee: 1999 World Health Organization/International Society of Hypertension guidelines for the management of hypertension. J Hypertens 1999;17:151–183.
†Grade 2 or 3 atrioventricular block.
‡Grade 2 or 3 atrioventricular block with verapamil or diltiazem.
§Verapamil or diltiazem.

disease is isolated systolic hypertension (ISH) from large-artery atherosclerosis.[15] As people live longer and follow lifestyles that engender atherosclerosis, ISH will become even more common.

As shown in Table 57.1, low-dose diuretics and dihydropyridine calcium channel blockers are recommended for the elderly with ISH because they have been shown to protect them from cardiovascular morbidity and mortality.[16] JNC-VI recommends a low-dose diuretic first and a dihydropyridine calcium channel blocker as an alternative.

An elderly man with prostatism would logically be given an α-blocker along with the low-dose diuretic. The use of an α-blocker alone in high-risk patients already prone to heart failure may push the patient into overt failure,[17] so a diuretic is a logical accompaniment.

A β-blocker alone provides less cardioprotection to the elderly than other drugs,[18] although in those who have overt coronary disease they are clearly indicated for their proven secondary cardioprotective effect.[19]

The diabetic hypertensive

As described in Chapter 32, the most common cause of end-stage renal disease is diabetic nephropathy. The hypertension that almost invariably accompanies the progressive renal insufficiency adds a major additional accelerator for further renal damage, setting up a vicious cycle. As described, the progression can be averted by multiple therapies but most effectively by inhibitors of the renin–angiotensin system that preferentially dilate the efferent arterioles, lowering intraglomerular pressure and slowing glomerular sclerosis.

Table 57.1 indicates the compelling indication for ACE inhibitors in diabetic nephropathy. As noted, recent trials with angiotensin receptor blockers likely place them in a similar status to ACE inhibitors, at least for this indication.

ACE inhibitor or angiotensin receptor blocker, separately or together, will rarely be enough to bring blood pressure down to the currently accepted goal of therapy for such high-risk patients (< 130/80 mmHg). A diuretic

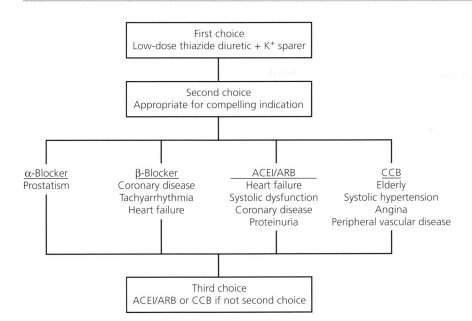

Figure 57.1 An algorithm for initial and subsequent choices of antihypertensive therapy. Those patients with renal insufficiency likely require a more potent diuretic, e.g. metolazone. ACE, angiotensin-converting enzyme; ACEI, angiotensis-converting enzyme inhibitor; ARB, angiotensin receptor blocker.

adequate to work in the face of renal insufficiency is almost always needed. As a third drug, calcium channel blockers have proven their ability to serve as an effective additive to ACE inhibitors/angiotensin receptor blockers.[20]

Other common compelling indications

Most of these relate to coronary disease, manifested by angina and myocardial infarction, which are in turn the most common path to congestive heart failure. As seen in Table 57.1, angina usually calls for β-blockers and calcium channel blockers; postmyocardial infarction almost always demands a β-blocker and an ACE inhibitor, congestive heart failure a diuretic (logically combined with spironolactone), ACE inhibitor, and likely a β-blocker.

Often combinations are appropriate. As noted in JNC-VI:[9]

Combinations of low doses of two agents from different classes have been shown to provide additional antihypertensive efficacy, thereby minimizing the likelihood of dose-dependent side effects. Very low doses of a diuretic (e.g. 6.25 mg hydrochlorothiazide) can potentiate the effect of the other agent without producing adverse metabolic effects.[21] Low-dose combinations with an ACE inhibitor and a nondihydropyridine calcium antagonist may reduce proteinuria more than either drug alone.[22] Combinations of a dihydropyridine calcium antagonist and an ACE inhibitor induce less pedal edema than does the calcium antagonist alone.[23] In some instances, drugs with similar modes of action may provide additive effects, such as metolazone and a loop diuretic in renal failure.

Conclusion

A strong argument can be made for starting almost all hypertensives (without renal insufficiency) on a low-dose thiazide diuretic (Fig. 57.1). For the half whose blood

pressure is not controlled with diuretics alone and for the many who have a compelling indication for other drugs, the individualization of therapy should provide the most efficacy and protection against the cardiovascular consequences of hypertension.

References

1. Kaplan NM: Treatment of hypertension: drug therapy. *In* Kaplan NM (ed): Kaplan's Clinical Hypertension, 8th edn. Lippincott, Williams and Wilkins, 2002, pp 237–338.
2. Neaton J, Grimm RH Jr, Prineas RJ, et al: Treatment of mild hypertension study (TOMHS). JAMA 1993;270:713–724.
3. Blood Pressure Lowering Treatment Trialists' Collaboration: Effects of ACE inhibitors, calcium antagonists, and other blood-pressure-lowering drugs. Lancet 2000;355:1955–1960.
4. Materson BJ, Reda DJ, Cushman WC: Department of Veterans Affairs single-drug therapy of hypertension study. Am J Hypertens 1995;8:189–192.
5. Morgan TO, Anderson AIE, MacInnis RJ: ACE inhibitors, beta-blockers, calcium blockers, and diuretics for the control of systolic hypertension. Am J Hypertens 2001;14:241–247.
6. Dickerson JEC, Hingorani AD, Ashby MJ, et al: Optimization of antihypertensive treatment by crossover rotation of four major classes. Lancet 1999;353:2008–2013.
7. Laragh J: Laragh's lessons in pathophysiology and clinical pearls for treating hypertension. Lesson I. A brief history of hypertension research: renin is twice rejected. Am J Hypertens 2001;14:186–189.
8. Donnelly R, Elliott HL, Meredith PA: Antihypertensive drugs: individualized analysis and clinical relevance of kinetic–dynamic relationships. Pharmacol Ther 1992;53:67–79.
9. Joint National Committee: The sixth report of the Joint National Committee on detection, evaluation, and treatment of high blood pressure (JNC VI). Arch Intern Med 1997;157:2413–2446.
10. Guidelines Subcommittee: 1999 World Health Organization/International Society of Hypertension guidelines for the management of hypertension. J Hypertens 1999;17:151–183.
11. Gomberg-Maitland M, Baran DA, Fuster V: Treatment of congestive heart failure. Arch Intern Med 2001;161:342–352.
12. Parving H-H, Lehnert H, Bröchner-Mortensen J, et al: The effect of irbesartan on the development of diabetic nephropathy in patients with type 2 diabetes. N Engl J Med 2001;345:870–878.
13. Heart Outcomes Prevention Evaluation (HOPE) Study Investigators: Effects of an angiotensin-converting-enzyme inhibitor, ramipril,

on cardiovascular events in high-risk patients. N Engl J Med 2000;342:145–153.

14. Yasuf S: Clinical, public health, and research implications of the Heart Outcomes Prevention Evaluation (HOPE) study. Eur Heart J 2001;22:103–104.

15. Izzo JL Jr, Levy D, Black HR: Clinical Advisory Statement. Importance of systolic blood pressure in older Americans. Hypertension 2001;35:1021–1024.

16. Wang J-G, Staessen JA: The benefit of treating isolated systolic hypertension. Curr Hypertens Rep 2001;3:333–339.

17. ALLHAT Officers and Coordinators for the ALLHAT Collaborative Research Group: Major cardiovascular events in hypertensive patients randomized to doxazosin vs chlorthalidone. JAMA 2000;283:1967–1975.

18. Messerli FH, Grossman E, Goldbourt U: Are β-blockers efficacious as first-line therapy for hypertension in the elderly? JAMA 1998;279:1903–1907.

19. Rochon PA, Tu JV, Anderson GM, et al: Rate of heart failure and 1-year survival for older people receiving low-dose β-blocker therapy after myocardial infarction. Lancet 2000;356:639–644.

20. Ruggenenti P, Perna A, Benini R, et al: Effects of dihydropyridine calcium channel blockers, angiotensin-converting enzyme inhibition, and blood pressure control on chronic, nondiabetic nephropathies. J Am Soc Nephrol 1998;9:2096–2101.

21. Frishman WH, Bryzinski BS, Coulson LR, et al: A multifactorial trial design to assess combination therapy in hypertension. Arch Intern Med 1994;154:1461–1468.

22. Bakris GL, Williams M, Dworkin L, et al: Preserving renal function in adults with hypertension and diabetes: a consensus approach. Am J Kidney Dis 2000;36:646–661.

23. Gradman AH, Cutler NR, Davis PJ, et al: Combined enalapril and felodipine extended release (ER) for systemic hypertension. Am J Cardiol 1997;79:431–435.

Hypertensive emergencies

Samuel J. Mann

The term hypertensive emergency covers an array of clinical situations, with the degree of urgency determined by either: (1) the severity or acuteness of onset of blood pressure elevation; or (2) the presence of a critical underlying medical condition (e.g. acute aortic dissection), when even modest degrees of blood pressure elevation may require immediate treatment.

True hypertensive "emergencies" (Table 58.1) require lowering of blood pressure within minutes to 1 h. The drug employed should act immediately and be predictably effective. In contrast, more gradual lowering of blood pressure, from 30 min to hours, is appropriate in treating medical "urgencies" (Table 58.2); rapidly acting drugs requiring intraarterial monitoring are not necessary.

Rapid lowering of blood pressure greatly increases the risk of unwanted adverse effects. The risk can exceed the benefit, particularly in the elderly and in patients in whom urgent treatment confers no benefit. Despite common practice, patients with severe but asymptomatic elevation of blood pressure usually do not require urgent therapy to lower blood pressure.

Natural history of untreated severe hypertension

Accelerated or malignant hypertension

The classic hypertensive crisis of accelerated or malignant hypertension is characterized by severe elevation of arterial pressure (usually with diastolic pressure > 140 mmHg) and vascular damage manifest by retinal hemorrhages and exudates.[1] The term "accelerated" signifies the absence, and "malignant" the presence, of papilledema. The

Table 58.1 Hypertensive emergencies

Hypertension associated with acute myocardial ischemia or infarct
Hypertensive encephalopathy
Hypertension associated with intracranial hemorrhage
Hypertension associated with stroke
Hypertension associated with pulmonary edema
Adrenergic crisis
Dissecting aortic aneurysm
Eclampsia
Perioperative hypertension
Severe epistaxis

Table 58.2 Hypertensive urgencies

Hypertension associated with left ventricular failure
Accelerated or malignant hypertension
Hypertension associated with angina
Perioperative hypertension
Preeclampsia
Acute glomerulonephritis
Scleroderma renal crisis

pathogenesis, management, and prognosis of accelerated and malignant hypertension are similar.[2]

The syndrome usually occurs as an accelerated phase of preexisting hypertension.[3] Severe and inadequately treated essential hypertension, particularly in smokers,[2] is the most common antecedent. Among other causes, renovascular and renal parenchymal disorders are most common. In recent-onset hypertension, in the absence of protective vascular thickening, the risk for encephalopathy or hemorrhage may be present at relatively modest blood pressure elevation.

Why some individuals with hypertension proceed to this accelerated phase and others do not is not entirely clear. A vicious cycle is postulated whereby vascular damage from severe hypertension causes renal ischemia, which stimulates renin secretion and renin-mediated vasoconstriction, which in turn worsen renal ischemia and further stimulate renin secretion.[3] Intravascular volume contraction due to pressure natriuresis may further stimulate renin secretion. Consistent with this, elevations of plasma renin activity and of aldosterone secretion are commonly found, and angiotensin-converting enzyme (ACE) inhibitors usually lower blood pressure.[2]

Hypertensive encephalopathy

Hypertensive encephalopathy is characterized by a reversible alteration in neurologic function in the setting of severe or abrupt blood pressure elevation. Although frequently a complication of malignant hypertension, it can also occur as a result of acute elevation from other causes, such as acute glomerulonephritis, clonidine withdrawal, cocaine, monoamine oxidase (MAO) inhibitor/tyramine interaction, and others. Manifestations include headache, altered mental status, visual impairment, nausea, and seizures.[4] Focal neurologic signs can also occur.[4]

Encephalopathy is ascribed by some to cerebral ischemia as a result of luminal narrowing and spasm[2] and possibly occlusion,[4] and by others to breakdown (or failure) of autoregulation at high systemic pressures leading to localized hyperperfusion and eventually edema.[4,5] Cerebral edema is a constant finding.[2] Pathologic findings include cerebral microinfarctions and petechial hemorrhages.[2]

Treatment of hypertensive emergencies

General considerations

Two important considerations are how quickly and how much to lower blood pressure. Normalization of blood pressure has been associated with reversible and irreversible complications, particularly in patients with cerebrovascular or coronary artery disease. Unintended hypotension may further exaggerate this risk. Therefore, rapid normalization of blood pressure should generally not be the goal of acute management.

The choice of antihypertensive agents should take into consideration the following factors.

Age

Elderly patients are at greater risk for adverse effects of acute blood pressure lowering. Known or occult coronary and cerebrovascular disease, together with reduced autoregulatory capacity, contributes to hypoperfusion as blood pressure is lowered. In addition, increased sensitivity to the pharmacologic effect of drugs is often seen. The use of lower drug doses, selection of a higher target blood pressure, and more careful monitoring are indicated in elderly patients.

Volume status

Severe hypertension, particularly in the malignant phase, is often characterized by a reduced intravascular volume,[2,6] and this may be exaggerated by prior use of diuretics, nausea, vomiting, or reduced oral intake. Potent vasodilators can cause a precipitous fall in blood pressure in this setting, in which case aggressive crystalloid infusion, up to 1–2 L or more, may be required. Because of this, in the absence of evident volume overload, the early use of diuretics is usually not advisable.

In contrast, in the setting of volume overload, such as hypertension associated with left ventricular failure, renal parenchymal disease, acute glomerulonephritis, or iatrogenic volume overload, diuretics are required. They may also need to be added as a second or third drug, particularly after prolonged administration of vasodilators that induce sodium retention.

Concurrent antihypertensive treatment

Antihypertensive medications taken before presentation, although failing to lower blood pressure, may have blocked compensatory mechanisms. Addition of the acutely administered drug may then drastically lower blood pressure. Therefore, it may be preferable to use short-acting drugs administered by infusion.

Duration of hypertension

Autoregulation of cerebral blood flow is impaired in chronic hypertension,[7] and rapid normalization of blood pressure can produce cerebral ischemia. In malignant hypertension, localized areas of ischemia may occur as a result of luminal narrowing of small vessels. Thus, cerebral ischemia can occur at blood pressures that are at or above normal, even in the absence of large-vessel cerebrovascular disease.

Underlying medical conditions

In addition to specific contraindications to a particular agent, there are some additional caveats in hypertensive crises (see section Drugs for hypertensive emergencies). Drugs with significant depressant effects on the central nervous system, such as clonidine, methyldopa, and reserpine, are best avoided in patients requiring neurologic monitoring. Drugs that increase myocardial oxygen consumption or cardiac contractility can be harmful in myocardial ischemia or dissecting aortic aneurysm. Other specific examples are considered later.

Oral vs. parenteral agents

Despite widespread assumptions, oral agents are not always safer than those administered parenterally. Some oral agents (e.g. captopril or nifedipine) can lower blood pressure precipitously, whereas agents with short half-lives that are infused intravenously can be accurately titrated.

Certainty of response

In true emergencies, a universally effective agent should be employed. Intravenous nitroprusside and labetalol are more predictably effective than enalaprilat, which is effective in only about 60% of urgencies.[8,9] An ACE inhibitor seems better suited in urgencies in which it can provide both diagnostic information and therapeutic benefit (i.e. in assessing renin dependency as well as the likelihood of renovascular hypertension) or in urgencies in which it may have a unique therapeutic advantage (e.g. hypertension with heart failure).

Cost efficacy

Treatment with agents such as labetalol, captopril, or others that do not require intraarterial monitoring in an intensive care unit reduces costs. Agents such as nitroprusside should be reserved for true emergencies.

Drugs for hypertensive emergencies

Drugs for the treatment of hypertensive emergencies are outlined in Table 58.3.

Sodium nitroprusside

In hypertensive emergencies, sodium nitroprusside provides rapid onset and offset of action, ease of titration, and almost universal effectiveness. It is an arterial and venous dilator, reducing both cardiac preload and afterload as well as myocardial oxygen requirement, which makes the drug highly suitable for patients with coronary artery disease. Adverse effects are attributed to both the rapidity of blood pressure lowering and toxic effects. The risk of unintended hypotension mandates intraarterial monitoring in an intensive care unit. Computer-controlled infusion facilitates blood pressure control.[10]

Thiocyanate toxicity, which can be manifested by blurred vision, tinnitus, confusion, and seizures, occurs rarely at infusion rates below 3 µg/kg/min for up to 72 h, except in patients with renal insufficiency. Blood thiocyanate levels should be monitored during high-dose or prolonged treatment. Cyanide accumulation can occur when the infusion rate is above 2 µg/kg/min, and concern about undiagnosed and hazardous cyanide toxicity has been raised.[11] Thiosulfate infusion can prevent or treat cyanide toxicity.[12,13] However, because the frequency of cyanide toxicity is unclear and because thiosulfate infusion can cause thiocyanate accumulation, particularly in patients with reduced renal function, the use of prophylactic thiosulfate infusion remains controversial. Bolus infusion of 150–200 mg/kg over 15 min is recommended when cyanide toxicity is suspected.[12]

Labetalol

Intravenous labetalol, a combined α- and β-receptor blocker, is usually effective, has a rapid onset of action and a sustained effect, is of low toxicity, and does not require intraarterial monitoring. The use of large initial boluses (1–2 mg/kg) has been associated with precipitous falls in blood pressure.[2] An initial bolus of 10–20 mg or an infusion of 1–2 mg/min is used to lower blood pressure within 15 min.[2]

Labetalol reduces peripheral resistance without reflex stimulation of cardiac output. Because of its β-blocking effect, it can cause deterioration in patients with preexisting left ventricular dysfunction.[2] It is useful in the treatment of hyperadrenergic states, including hypertension after coronary artery bypass graft, pheochromocytoma, and clonidine withdrawal.[2] However, in patients with pheochromocytoma, it is generally preferable to first establish α-blockade and then add a β-blocker because of the risk of a paradoxical pressor response associated with β-blockade.

Diazoxide

The use of diazoxide, an arterial vasodilator, fell into disfavor because of reports of precipitous falls in blood pressure resulting in cerebral and coronary complications after administration of 300 mg as a rapid bolus.[2] However, the use of repeated smaller (e.g. 50 mg) boluses or a continuous infusion appears safer.[2]

Diazoxide is almost universally effective. Its sustained effect obviates the need for minute-to-minute monitoring once blood pressure reduction has been achieved. A precipitous fall in blood pressure is unlikely to occur beyond 5 min after administration, enabling repeated boluses to be given as frequently as every 5–10 min.[2] Obviously, the sustained action is undesirable in situations in which blood pressure lowering may cause clinical deterioration.

Because of reflex increases in cardiac rate, contractility, and output, diazoxide should not be used in the setting of coronary disease or dissecting aneurysm. Adjunctive treatment with a diuretic and sympatholytic agent is generally required. The drug may cause hyperglycemia by inhibiting insulin release. Monitoring of blood glucose is advisable.[2]

Nitroglycerin

Intravenous nitroglycerin reduces blood pressure, afterload, left ventricular filling pressures, and myocardial oxygen consumption. For an equivalent degree of blood pressure reduction, it reduces myocardial oxygen consumption more and preserves coronary perfusion better than nitroprusside, favoring its use in the setting of coronary insufficiency.[13] It is also suitable in treating perioperative hypertension, including that following coronary artery bypass graft.[13] In the setting of severe hypertension, however, nitroprusside is more effective.

Phentolamine

Phentolamine, a nonselective α-adrenergic blocker, is most effective in situations of catecholamine excess, such

Table 58.3 Drugs for the treatment of hypertensive emergencies or urgencies*

	Method of administration	Initial dose	Dosage range or interval	Onset	Duration	Precautions and adverse effects
Direct vasodilators						
Sodium nitroprusside†	i.v. infusion	0.3–0.5 μg/kg/min	0.5–10 μg/kg/min	Immediately	2–3 min	Shield infusate from light Thionate toxicity
Diazoxide	i.v. bolus	50–100 mg	50–100 mg at 5–10 min intervals to maximum 600 mg	1–2 min	3–15 h	Hypotension: hyperglycemia, fluid retention, reflex tachycardia
Hydralazine	i.v. infusion i.v. bolus	10 mg/min 10 mg	10–30 min 10–50 mg at 10–20 min intervals	5–10 min	2–6 h	Reflex tachycardia
	i.m.	10–25 mg	10–50 mg at 20–30 min intervals	10–20 min	2–6 h	
Nitroglycerin	i.v. infusion	5 μg/min	5–100 μg/min	Minutes	Minutes	Tachyphylaxis
ACE inhibitors						
Captopril	Oral	6.25–50 mg	12.5–50 mg at 30–45 min intervals	10–15 min	2–6 h	Hypotension; renal failure (if bilateral renal artery stenosis)
Enalaprilat	i.v. bolus	0.625 mg	0.625–2.5 mg	10–15 min	2–6 h	Hypotension; renal failure (if bilateral renal artery stenosis
Dopamine antagonists						
Fenoldopam	i.v. infusion	0.03–0.1 μg/kg/min	0.1–1.6 μg/kg/min	15 min	1–4 h	Increased intraocular pressure
α-Adrenergic blockers						
Phentolamine	i.v. infusion	0.5–1 mg bolus or 1 mg/min	1–5 mg/min	1–2 min	15–60 min	Hypotension; tachycardia
Labetalol	i.v. bolus	10–20 mg	20–80 mg at 5–10 min intervals	5 min	2–6 h	Hypotension
Prazosin	i.v. infusion Oral	0.5 mg/min 1 mg	0.5–2 mg/min 1–2 mg at 1-h intervals	5–30 min 15–60 min	2–6 h 2–6 h	Hypotension

Table 58.3 (cont'd)

	Method of administration	Initial dose	Dosage range or interval	Onset	Duration	Precautions and adverse effects
Calcium channel blockers						
Nicardipine	i.v. infusion	5 mg/h	5–15 mg/h	5–20 min	1–2 h	Tachycardia, headache
Nifedipine (not recommended)	Sublingual or oral	10 mg	10–20 mg at 30 min intervals	10–20 min	3–6 h	Hypotension, headache
Ganglionic blockers						
Trimetaphan	i.v. infusion	0.5 mg/min	0.5–5 mg/min	1–5 min	5–10 min	Urinary retention, ileus; respiratory arrest
Sympatholytic agents						
Clonidine	Oral	0.1–0.2 mg	0.05–0.1 mg	1–2 h	8–12 h	Drowsiness
Methyldopa	i.v.	250 mg	250–500 mg at 4–8 h intervals	1–2 h	8–12 h	Drowsiness

*Adapted from Mann SJ, Atlas SA: Hypertensive emergencies. In Laragh JH, Brenner BM (eds): Hypertension: Pathophysiology, Diagnosis and Management, 2nd edn. New York: Raven Press, 1995, pp 3009–3022.
†Preferred drug for true emergency.
‡Not approved for use in hypertensive emergencies.

as pheochromocytoma. Phentolamine can be useful in diagnosing a pheochromocytoma but can lower blood pressure precipitously. A test dose of 0.5–1 mg infused in 1 min is generally advised, followed by infusion at 1 mg/min or more. The absence of a dramatic response virtually rules out the diagnosis.

Trimetaphan camsylate

Although rapidly acting and titratable, trimetaphan, a ganglionic blocking agent, is rarely used because of adverse effects resulting from autonomic blockade and rare unpredictable reactions including respiratory arrest. Because it impairs pupillary reflexes, it is contraindicated in patients requiring neurologic monitoring. Its use requires intraarterial monitoring of blood pressure in an intensive care unit. Finally, it is more difficult to achieve stable blood pressure with trimetaphan than with nitroprusside.

Its use has been generally limited to the following special situations: (1) hypertension associated with dissecting aortic aneurysm, for which the lack of a sympathetically mediated increase in ejection velocity is advantageous; (2) cases in which nitroprusside has been ineffective or is suspected of causing toxicity; and (3) cases in which alternative therapy is not effective or available.

New agents

Fenoldopam The vasodilator fenoldopam, a DA_1 dopamine agonist, lowers blood pressure, with an increase in cardiac output, heart rate, and urinary sodium excretion, and preservation of glomerular filtration rate.[14] The antihypertensive effect of fenoldopam is comparable to that of nitroprusside, with a slower onset of action but a similar time to achievement of target blood pressure.[14] In contrast, fenoldopam offers the advantages of lack of toxicity, a lower likelihood of hypotension, and lack of need for intraarterial monitoring of blood pressure.[15]

Fenoldopam is an alternative for nitroprusside in most hypertensive urgencies. The most common adverse effects are headache and increase in heart rate.[15] Fenoldpam increases intraocular pressure and its use may be contraindicated in patients with glaucoma.

Urapidil Urapidil is a combined α_1-adrenergic blocker and central serotonin antagonist ($5HT_{1A}$ receptors), which prevents reflex tachycardia.[16] Urapidil has been shown to lower blood pressure in hypertensive urgencies, although the onset of effect and time to achievement of target blood pressure is slower than that of nitroprusside.[17] Its potential place among other drugs used in treating hypertensive emergencies requires further study.

Drugs for hypertensive urgencies

ACE inhibitors Captopril is most effective in patients with an activated renin–angiotensin system resulting from conditions such as accelerated or malignant hypertension, scleroderma, and other forms of renal vasculitis.[2] The hypotensive response is dependent on volume status.[2] In the face of volume depletion, hypotension requiring

aggressive intravenous fluid replacement can occur. Conversely, in volume-expanded patients, characterized by suppressed plasma renin activity, the blood pressure response is smaller or absent.

The blood pressure response is evident quickly and is usually predictive of the chronic response; nonresponders can be switched to a different class of drug (Fig. 58.1). Measurement of plasma renin activity can guide therapy: responsiveness to an ACE inhibitor or angiotensin receptor blocker (ARB) is more likely in high-renin patients.

Enalaprilat, the bioactive form of the prodrug enalapril, acts within 5 min when given intravenously.[18] Doses higher than 0.625 mg increase the duration but not the magnitude of the initial response.[9,18] However, because enalaprilat is not universally effective,[9] it is generally not a preferred drug in the treatment of true emergencies.

Direct vasodilators

Intravenous hydralazine has been used for rapid reduction of blood pressure in urgent situations, particularly preeclampsia. However, in a true emergency, more universally effective agents are preferable. Minoxidil may be effective within 4 h of oral administration at doses of 5–20 mg. Marked sodium retention and tachycardia require addition of a diuretic and adrenergic blocker, and discourage its more widespread use. Sympathetically mediated increases in cardiac contractility and heart rate associated with both of these drugs contraindicate their use in patients with coronary insufficiency or dissecting aortic aneurysm.

Calcium channel blockers

Nifedipine The dihydropyridine nifedipine, given orally or sublingually, has been widely used in hypertensive urgencies.[19] However, the rapid fall in blood pressure has been associated with symptomatic coronary and cerebrovascular insufficiency, even at a "normal" blood pressure.[19] Consequently, the use of short-acting nifedipine in hypertensive urgencies is not recommended, particularly in elderly patients and patients with suspected coronary or cerebrovascular disease. Reflex sympathetic discharge and tachycardia are also contraindications to its use in patients with coronary insufficiency or dissecting aneurysm. Nondihydropyridine calcium channel blockers are less well studied.

Nicardipine Nicardipine, also a dihydropyridine calcium channel blocker, is available in parenteral form. Compared with nitroprusside, continuous infusion of nicardipine requires fewer dose adjustments, is associated with fewer adverse effects, and appears equally effective.[20,21] The infusion rate can be increased at intervals as short as 5–15 min. The mean time to response is 11.5 min.[22] It has high selectivity for vascular tissue, with little negative inotropic effect, and increases cardiac output.[22] It causes less headache and tachycardia than nitroprusside.[22]

Adrenergic blocking agents

Labetalol Intravenously administered labetalol can be used in urgencies. Orally administered labetalol, at doses of 100–400 mg, can lower blood pressure within 1–3 h.[2] A second dose can be administered after 3–4 h.

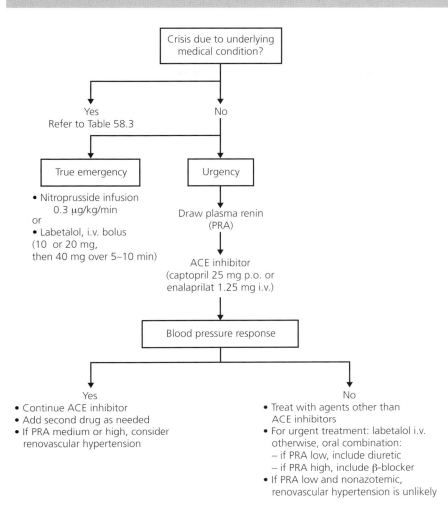

Other β-receptor blockers   Intravenous propranolol, metoprolol, and esmolol have little acute blood pressure-lowering effect but minimize reflex cardiac stimulation. These agents are useful in combination with vasodilators such as nitroprusside, in patients with acute aortic dissection or coronary insufficiency and, when indicated, in combination with phentolamine in patients with pheochromocytoma.

Sympatholytic agents

Clonidine lowers blood pressure with a maximal response within 2–4 h and little risk of a precipitous fall. However, the acute response and dosage used do not necessarily predict the long-term response. In addition, the high frequency of bothersome adverse effects (drowsiness, dry mouth, impotence) may contribute to noncompliance, with possible rebound hypertension if the drug is stopped abruptly.

Management of specific
conditions (see Table 58.4 for recommended agents)
Accelerated or malignant hypertension

In the absence of complications such as encephalopathy, symptomatic coronary insufficiency, or severe congestive heart failure, malignant hypertension constitutes a medical urgency, and instantaneously acting intravenous drugs requiring intraarterial monitoring, such as nitroprusside, are not indicated. A target diastolic blood pressure of 100–110 mmHg or higher, to be achieved during the first 24–48 h of treatment, has been recommended. When time allows, observation of the response to agents that attack a specific pathophysiologic mechanism, such as an ACE inhibitor, can provide useful diagnostic information. A different agent can then be given if there is no response within 30 min.

Hypertensive encephalopathy

The risk of imminent brain damage necessitates rapid lowering of blood pressure. Treatment can rapidly ameliorate the signs and symptoms of encephalopathy,[4] but if blood pressure falls below the autoregulatory limit cerebral ischemia can worsen.[23] Therefore, use of drugs such as nitroprusside is recommended. If neurologic status deteriorates, the blood pressure should be allowed to rise. Such deterioration should also prompt consideration of other diagnoses, such as cerebrovascular accident, head injury, or other cerebral pathologic processes accompanied rather than caused by severe blood pressure elevation.

It is generally recommended that mean blood pressure

Table 58.4 Drugs of choice*

	Drugs	Relative contraindications
Hypertensive encephalopathy	Nitroprusside, labetalol i.v.	Centrally acting sympatholytic agents
Malignant hypertension	ACE inhibitor, labetalol i.v., clonidine, ? fenoldopam	
Hypertension associated with	Nitroprusside, labetalol i.v.	Diazoxide, nifedipine
Intracranial hemorrhage	Nitroprusside, labetalol i.v.	Diazoxide, nifedipine
Stroke		
Left ventricular failure		
Pulmonary edema	ACE inhibitor + loop diuretic ± nitroprusside or nitroglycerin	β-Blocker, verapamil
Congestive heart failure	ACE inhibitor + loop diuretic	β-Blocker, verapamil
Coronary insufficiency		
Acute myocardial infarction	Nitroglycerin ± β-blocker Nitroprusside ± β-blocker	Diazoxide, hydralazine
Unstable angina	Nitrates (sublingual, oral, or transdermal) ± β-blocker, or as for myocardial infarction	Diazoxide, hydralazine
Adrenergic crisis	Nitroprusside, phentolamine ± β-blocker, ? i.v. labetalol	β-Blocker monotherapy
Dissecting aortic aneurysm	Nitroprusside + β-blocker; labetalol	Diazoxide, hydralazine, nifedipine
Perioperative hypertension	Nitroprusside, nitroglycerin, labetalol; ? fenoldopam, ? nicardipine	

*Adapted from Mann SJ, Atlas SA: Hypertensive emergencies. In Laragh JH, Brenner BM (eds): Hypertension: Pathophysiology, Diagnosis and Management, 2nd edn. New York: Raven Press, 1995, pp 3009–3022.

be reduced initially (during the course of 1 h) by a maximum of 20%, or to a diastolic blood pressure of 100–110 mmHg, although even higher target blood pressures may be advisable in selected patients. In previously normotensive patients, rapid normalization of blood pressure is generally not hazardous.

Cerebrovascular accident

Blood pressure elevation commonly accompanies thrombotic stroke.[24] Increased sympathetic tone and intracranial pressure may contribute. Whether blood pressure elevation has the beneficial effect of increasing flow through stenotic or collateral vessels or a harmful one by aggravating local edema formation is unclear.

Acute lowering of blood pressure might reduce cerebral blood flow and exacerbate the neurologic deficit, particularly in the setting of stroke and in the elderly, when cerebral autoregulation is impaired. Therefore, the wisdom of treating the blood pressure is unclear.

There is general agreement that mild blood pressure elevation should not be treated. The treatment of acute and severe blood pressure elevation is more controversial. Gradual blood pressure reduction is recommended if the diastolic pressure is above 130 mmHg, with a target diastolic pressure of no lower than 100 mmHg. Many prefer to use rapidly acting drugs whose effects can be easily titrated should neurologic signs worsen as pressure is lowered.

There is insufficient evidence to support the use of nimodipine.

Antihypertensive treatment in patients with hemorrhagic infarction after thrombotic stroke should follow the preceding guidelines. Stroke due to hypertensive hemorrhage may be treated more aggressively, although careful differentiation between hemorrhagic stroke and hemorrhagic infarction after thrombotic stroke should precede such measures.

Subarachnoid hemorrhage

Acute management of blood pressure elevation remains controversial. Acute lowering might prevent rebleeding and reduce edema formation but could reduce cerebral perfusion, particularly in patients with chronic hypertension or increased intracranial pressure. Mortality and rebleeding are reportedly higher in patients presenting with a systolic pressure exceeding 160 mmHg.[25] However, the effect of blood pressure lowering on mortality is uncertain.

It seems reasonable to treat acutely and severely elevated blood pressure with rapidly acting and easily titratable drugs. However, in patients with mildly elevated blood pressure, particularly in chronic hypertensives, benefits of blood pressure reduction are unproven. Nimodipine has recently been shown to improve neurologic outcome, presumably mediated by its counteractive effects on cerebral vasospasm rather than by blood pressure reduction.[26] Nicardipine, although reducing vasospasm, did not affect the long-term outcome.[27] Propranolol may improve outcome.[28]

Hypertension associated with left ventricular failure

Left ventricular failure is associated with physiologic increases in vasoconstrictor hormones, including catecholamines and angiotensin II, which combined with elevation of peripheral vascular resistance can severely impair left ventricular performance. Vasodilators, including nitrates and ACE inhibitors, can dramatically improve cardiac output.

Acute pulmonary edema generally requires parenteral therapy. Either nitroglycerin or nitroprusside can be used initially, although nitroprusside is more effective. Administration of an ACE inhibitor (oral captopril or intravenous enalaprilat), with or without a loop diuretic (e.g. furosemide), assists weaning from parenteral therapy.

In less urgent situations, ACE inhibitors combined with diuretics can rapidly improve heart failure. Nifedipine can also be effective[2] but can aggravate underlying coronary insufficiency.

Hypertension associated with myocardial infarction or coronary ischemia

The goal of acute antihypertensive therapy is to reduce myocardial oxygen demand and increase myocardial blood supply. Intravenous nitroglycerin, which induces a greater reduction of myocardial oxygen consumption than does nitroprusside and which appears to better sustain regional blood flow distal to a stenosis, is the preferred drug. The β-blockers generally have little acute antihypertensive effect but can reduce heart rate and oxygen consumption. The combined effects of β-blockers and nitrates are advantageous. The use of nifedipine, which can aggravate ischemia, is contraindicated.

Dissecting aortic aneurysm

Acute blood pressure reduction reduces shear forces on the damaged aorta. Arterial vasodilators, such as hydralazine, diazoxide, and nifedipine, which cause a reflex increase in the rate and velocity of left ventricular ejection, are contraindicated. Nitroprusside, combined with a β-blocker, has replaced trimetaphan as the treatment of choice.

Adrenergic crises

Increased catecholamine levels and sympathetic tone mediate acute hypertension associated with clonidine (and possibly methyldopa) withdrawal, pheochromocytoma, cocaine abuse, MAO inhibitor/tyramine interaction, and sympathomimetics such as phenylpropanolamine.

Acute blood pressure elevation is largely due to α-mediated vasoconstriction, with β-adrenergic cardiac stimulation playing a secondary role.

Although the use of phentolamine is logical, nitroprusside is equally effective and preferred by many because of greater familiarity with its use. However, if adjunctive therapy with β-blockers is indicated (e.g. because of severe tachycardia or ventricular ectopy), establishment of α-blockade (with phentolamine or perhaps prazosin) should be accomplished first to avoid a pressor response due to unopposed α tone and loss of β-mediated vasodilation. Intravenous labetalol appears effective, although further experience with its use in pheochromocytoma is needed. If time allows, oral clonidine is an effective alternative for hypertension caused by clonidine withdrawal.

Postoperative hypertension

Postoperative hypertension is characterized by increased sympathetic tone and vascular resistance. Pain and overhydration can also contribute to blood pressure elevation.

Nonspecific vasodilators are generally effective. Intravenous nitroglycerin and nitroprusside are of nearly equal efficacy.[29] After coronary artery bypass surgery, nitroglycerin might be preferable. Isradipine,[30] nicardipine,[31] fenoldopam,[14,15] and, in patients with preserved left ventricular function, labetalol[32] provide alternatives.

In some cases, postoperative hypertension appears to be a consequence of overzealous hydration. When there is evidence of a markedly positive fluid balance, diuresis with an intravenous loop diuretic merits consideration.

Renal failure

Many factors contribute to the hypertension associated with renal insufficiency, and treatment directed at them can help normalize blood pressure. First and foremost is the need to address reduced sodium excretion. Loop diuretics are often effective in patients who are unresponsive to thiazides; doses as high as 80–240 mg of furosemide are sometimes necessary. Adding a thiazide diuretic such as metolazone to a loop diuretic can further promote sodium excretion and lower blood pressure. Aggressive volume control may of necessity be accompanied by an increase in serum creatinine.

The renin–angiotensin system also frequently contributes to hypertension in patients with renal failure. In such patients, ACE inhibitors and/or ARBs are usually needed to lower blood pressure and also provide some degree of renoprotection. An elevated plasma renin activity increases the likelihood that an ACE inhibitor or ARB will be effective. In contrast to diuretics, high doses of ACE inhibitors are not indicated because their excretion is reduced in renal failure, although dosage of ACE inhibitors such as fosinopril, or ARBs such as candesartan, is unaffected by renal failure. ACE inhibitors can be combined with ARBs, although combining either agent with a drug from a different class is likely to be more effective. Other agents, including calcium channel blockers, β-blockers, and α-blockers, are also effective; studies unfortunately provide little guidance as to which agent to choose. In many cases, combination therapy with two or more agents is needed.

Erythropoietin is also associated with blood pressure elevation, sometimes severe. The mechanism and treatment are unclear, although, again, volume control may be crucial.[33,34]

Of patients who require hemodialysis, 72% have hypertension.[35] All classes of antihypertensive agents lower blood pressure to some extent.[35] Nevertheless, hypertension remains uncontrolled in 62% of dialysis patients.[36] Prominent reasons include failure to achieve dry weight, interdialytic weight gain (although study results vary), inadequate medication, and withholding of medication prior to dialysis.[36] If hypotension during dialysis prevents attainment of dry weight, discontinuation or withholding of antihypertensive agents such as ACE inhibitors may be helpful.

The blood levels of renally excreted agents such as atenolol persist longer in patients with renal failure, and lower dosage is usually sufficient.[37] Atenolol is dialyzable, and it makes sense to dose the atenolol after dialyses.[37]

"Severe" hypertension

Severe hypertension, as usually encountered in a physician's office, usually does not constitute an emergency or urgency. If a patient presents with a blood pressure of 180–220/110–130 mmHg but is asymptomatic, with neither retinal hemorrhages or exudates nor renal insufficiency, prescription of oral agents with close follow-up is appropriate.

In such patients, the low likelihood of achieving control with a single agent argues for initiating treatment with at least two agents. Although no specific regimen is universally recommended, an ACE inhibitor or ARB makes sense, given the renal arteriolar changes that accompany longstanding or severe hypertension. ACE inhibitor/diuretic and ARB/diuretic combinations are widely employed. Many other combinations provide attractive alternatives. In most cases, an ACE inhibitor (or ARB) and/or a diuretic, at adequate dose, is likely to be a necessary component of any multidrug regimen. Normalization of blood pressure may require a three- or four-drug regimen.

Failure to control hypertension may be related to inadequate dosage, whether of a diuretic, ACE inhibitor, or β-blocker. Addition of a potassium-sparing diuretic such as spironolactone or amiloride, or in patients with renal insufficiency substitution of a loop diuretic, can greatly enhance control of blood pressure and volume.

Conclusions

Hypertensive "crises" can be viewed as a spectrum, from nonurgent, to urgent, to true emergency. Most instances of severe but asymptomatic hypertension need not be treated urgently unless required by underlying conditions. Hypertensive urgencies can be treated with oral or intravenous agents, whereas in true emergencies short-acting intravenous agents such as sodium nitroprusside remain the drugs of choice. In the treatment of accelerated or malignant hypertension, there is usually sufficient time to use agents that can help identify pathogenetic mechanisms and guide subsequent treatment (see Fig. 58.1). The need for therapeutic restraint is emphasized in order to avoid complications from unnecessary and overzealous lowering of blood pressure.

References

1. Kincaid-Smith P: Malignant hypertension: mechanisms and management. Pharmacol Ther 1980;9:245–269.
2. Mann SJ, Atlas SA: Hypertensive emergencies. In Laragh JH, Brenner BM (eds): Hypertension: Pathophysiology, Diagnosis and Management, 2nd edn. New York: Raven Press, 1995, pp 3009–3022.
3. Kincaid-Smith P: Understanding malignant hypertension. Aust N Z J Med 1981;11(Suppl 1):64–68.
4. Chester EM, Agamanolis DP, Banker BQ: Hypertensive encephalopathy: a clinicopathologic study of 20 cases. Neurology 1978;28:928–939.
5. Johansson B, Strandgaard S, Lassen NA: On the pathogenesis of hypertensive encephalopathy. The hypertensive "breakthrough" of autoregulation of cerebral blood flow with forced vasodilatation, flow increase, and blood-brain-barrier damage. Circ Res 1974;34/35(Suppl 1):I-167–I-171.
6. Kincaid-Smith P, McMichael J, Murphy EA: The clinical course and pathology of hypertension with papilledema. Q J Med 1958;27:117–154.
7. Strandgaard S, Olesen J, Skinhoj E, et al: Autoregulation of brain circulation in severe arterial hypertension. Br Med J 1973;1:507–510.
8. Huey J, Thomas P, Hendricks DR, et al: Clinical evaluation of intravenous labetalol in the treatment of hypertensive urgency. Am J Hypertens 1988;1:284S–289S.
9. Hirschl MM, Binder M, Bur A, et al: Clinical evaluation of different doses of intravenous enalaprilat in patients with hypertensive crisis. Arch Intern Med 1995;155:2217–2223.
10. Chitwood WR Jr, Cosgrove DH III, Lust RM: Multicenter trial of automated nitroprusside infusion for postoperative hypertension. Titrator Multicenter Study Group. Ann Thorac Surg 1992;54:517–522.
11. Robin ED, McCauley R: Nitroprusside-related cyanide poisoning: time (long past due) for urgent, effective interventions. Chest 1992;102:1842–1845.
12. Friederich JA, Butterworth JF: Sodium nitroprusside: twenty years and counting. Anesth Analg 1995;81:152–162.
13. Fremes SE, Weisel RD, Mickle DAG: A comparison of nitroglycerin and nitroprusside: I. Treatment of post-operative hypertension. Ann Thorac Surg 1985;39:53–60.
14. Oparil S, Aronson S, Deeb GM, Taylor A: Fenoldopam: a new parenteral antihypertensive: consensus roundtable on the management of perioperative hypertension and hypertensive crises. Am J Hypertens 1999;12:653–664.
15. Frishman WH: Fenoldopam: a new dopamine agonist for the treatment of hypertensive urgencies and emergencies. J Clin Pharmacol 1998;38:2–13.
16. Hirschl MM: Guidelines for the drug treatment of hypertensive crises. Drugs 1995;50:991–1000.
17. Hirschl MM, Binder M, Bur A, et al: Safety and efficacy of urapidil and sodium nitroprusside in the treatment of hypertensive emergencies. Intensive Care Med 1997;23:885–888.
18. Dipette DJ, Ferraro JC, Evans RR, et al: Enalaprilat, an intravenous angiotensin-converting enzyme inhibitor in hypertensive crises. Clin Pharmacol Ther 1985;38:199–204.
19. Grossman E, Messerli FH, Grodzicki T, Kowey P: Should a moratorium be placed on sublingual nifedipine capsules given for hypertensive emergencies and pseudoemergencies? JAMA 1996;276:1328–1331.
20. Neutel JM, Smith DHG, Wallin D, et al: A comparison of intravenous nicardipine and sodium nitroprusside in the immediate treatment of severe hypertension. Am J Hypertens 1994;7:623–628.

21. Habib GB, Dunbar LM, Rodrigues R, et al: Evaluation of the efficacy and safety of oral nicardipine in treatment of urgent hypertension: a multicenter, randomized, double-blind, parallel, placebo-controlled clinical trial. Am Heart J 1995;129:917–923.
22. Erstad BL, Barletta JF: Treatment of hypertension in the perioperative patient. Ann Pharmacother 2000;34:66–79.
23. Strandgaard S, Paulson OB: Cerebral autoregulation. Stroke 1984;15:413–415.
24. Wallace JD, Levy LL: Blood pressure after stroke. JAMA 1981;246:2177–2180.
25. Nibbelink DW: Antihypertensive and antifibrinolytic therapy following subarachnoid hemorrhage from ruptured intracranial aneurysm. *In* Sahs AL, Nibbelink DW, Torner JC (eds): Aneurysmal Subarachnoid Hemorrhage: Report of the Cooperative Study. Baltimore: Urban and Schwartzenberg, 1981, pp 287–296.
26. Wong MCW, Haley EC Jr: Calcium antagonists: stroke therapy coming of age. Stroke 1990;21:494–501.
27. Haley EC Jr, Kassell NF, Torner JC, et al: A randomized controlled trial of high dose intravenous nicardipine in aneurysmal subarachnoid hemorrhage. A report of the Cooperative Aneurysm Study. J Neurosurg 1993;78:537–547.
28. Neil-Dwyer G, Walter P, Cruikshank JM: β-Blockade benefits patients following a subarachnoid hemorrhage. Eur J Clin Pharmacol 1985;28(Suppl):25–29.
29. Hackman BB, Griffin B, Mills M, et al: Comparative effects of fenoldopam mesylate and nitroprusside on left ventricular performance in severe systemic hypertension. Am J Cardiol 1992;69:918–922.
30. Ruegg PC, David D, Loria Y: Isradipine for the treatment of hypertension following coronary artery bypass graft surgery: a randomized trial versus sodium nitroprusside. Eur J Anaesthesiol 1992;9:293–305.
31. Halpern NA, Goldberg M, Neely C, et al: Postoperative hypertension: a multicenter, prospective, randomized comparison between intravenous nicardipine and sodium nitroprusside. Crit Care Med 1992;20:1637–1643.
32. Cruise CJ, Skrobik Y, Webster RE, et al: Intravenous labetalol versus sodium nitroprusside for treatment of hypertension post coronary bypass surgery. Anesthesiology 1989;71:835–839.
33. Luft FC: Erythropoietin and arterial hypertension. Clin Nephrol 2000;53(Suppl):S61–S64.
34. Dorhout Mees EJ, Ok E: Erythropoietin hypertension: fact or fiction? Int J Artif Organs 1997;20:415–417.
35. Salem MM: Hypertension in the hemodialysis population: a survey of 649 patients. Am J Kidney Dis 1995;26:461–468.
36. Rahman M, Dixit A, Donley V, et al: Factors associated with inadequate blood pressure control in hypertensive hemodialysis patients. Am J Kidney Dis 1999;33:498–506.
37. Agarwal R: Strategies and feasibility of hypertension control in a prevalent hemodialysis cohort. Clin Nephrol 2000;53:344–353.

Cardiovascular Risk factors in Patients with Essential Hypertension

Vasilios Papademetriou

Influence of dyslipidemias
Role of low HDL-cholesterol
Cholesterol and blood pressure regulation
Smoking and hypertension
Diabetes in patients with hypertension
Diet, weight loss, and exercise in patients with hypertension
Emerging cardiovascular risk factors
• Lipoprotein (a)
• Homocysteine

Hypertension is a major contributor to cardiovascular disease (CVD). While some CVD endpoints such as encepholopathy, hemorrhagic strokes, and acute renal failure may be directly attributable to elevated blood pressure, the most common consequence of chronic hypertension is progressive atherosclerosis. Hypertension plays a significant and independent role in atherogenesis but its impact is greatly exaggerated by the presence of other risk factors. The independent role of hypertension is supported by many lines of evidence: the risk of developing initial clinical manifestations of vascular events is related to the previous level of blood pressure and the complications of CVD are clearly higher in patients with hypertension. Furthermore, it seems that there is a threshold of blood pressure required for the development of atherosclerosis. Lesions do not appear in normally low-pressure vascular beds, such as the pulmonary vasculature, but do appear in patients with pulmonary hypertension. Veins do not develop atherosclerosis until they are utilized as grafts in the systemic circulation. Animal experiments strongly suggest that the process of atherosclerosis can be altered by manipulation of blood pressure.[1,2]

The presence of other CVD risk factors can greatly influence the risk of complications in patients with hypertension.[3] For example in the Framingham heart study, the risk of coronary heart disease over a 10-year period was greatly influenced by other risk factors as shown in Fig. 59.1.[4] The presence of other CVD risk factors is important for other reasons: (1) they may influence the decision to treat, how aggressively, and with what agents; (2) they may affect the response of hypertension to therapy; and (3) they may influence the expected benefit on CVD endpoints (Table 59.1).

Influence of dyslipidemias

Lipids and lipoproteins greatly affect the impact of hypertension on atherogenesis. A synergistic effect on the risk for CVD events has been found between systolic blood pressure and low-density lipoprotein (LDL) cholesterol. High-density lipoprotein (HDL) cholesterol greatly influences the rate of removal of oxidized LDL from the tissues and an inverse relationship between HDL-C and systolic blood pressure has been demonstrated.[5,6] The interaction of LDL, HDL cholesterol, and blood pressure is shown in Fig. 59.2. Several large randomized trials have demonstrated conclusively that effective lowering of LDL cholesterol can substantially reduce the risk of myocardial infarction (MI) and coronary events,[6–10] in patients with and without pre-existing CVD. Post-hoc analysis of most of these trials has also demonstrated a substantial risk reduction for stroke with lowering of LDL, although epidemiologic observations have not detected a relationship between the two.[11] In these studies, women, minorities, diabetics, and the elderly have been underrepresented. Among the primary prevention

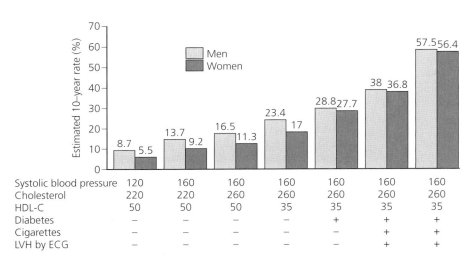

Systolic blood pressure	120	160	160	160	160	160	160
Cholesterol	220	220	260	260	260	260	260
HDL-C	50	50	50	35	35	35	35
Diabetes	–	–	–	–	+	+	+
Cigarettes	–	–	–	–	–	+	+
LVH by ECG	–	–	–	–	–	+	+

Figure 59.1 Estimated risk of coronary heart disease over 10 years according to various combinations of risk factors for men and women. HDL, high-density lipoprotein; LVH, left ventricular hypertrophy. (From Anderson KM, Wilson PWF, Odell PM, et al: An updated coronary risk profile. Statement for health professionals. Circulation 1991;83:357–363.)

Table 59.1 Cardiovascular risk factors that may interact with hypertension

Major risk factors	Emerging risk factors
High LDL cholesterol (> 130 mg/dL)	High lipoprotein (a)
Low HDL cholesterol (< 40 mg/dL)	Homocysteine
Cigarette smoking	Prothrombotic factors
Diabetes mellitus	Proinflammatory factors
Physical activity	Impaired fasting glucose
Obesity	Subclinical atherosclerosis
	High uric acid
	Vascular calcification

HDL, high-density lipoprotein; LDL, low-density lipoprotein.

trials, three are most commonly quoted: the Helsinki Heart Study,[12] the West of Scotland Coronary Prevention Study (WOSCOPS),[9] and the Air Force/Texas Coronary Atherosclerosis Prevention Study (AFCAPS/TexCAPS) trial.[13]

In the Helsinki Heart Study,[13] the upper age limit was 55 years and the baseline LDL cholesterol 270 mg/dL. Using the fibric acid derivative gemfibrozil, this study demonstrated a 34% reduction in combined CVD events. WOSCOPS was also limited to middle-aged men, with an upper age limit of 64 years and mean baseline LDL cholesterol of 272 mg/dL. Using pravastatin as the lipid-lowering intervention, this study also demonstrated a reduction of combined coronary events, CVD death, non-fatal MI, and all cardiovascular deaths by nearly one-third. The AFCAPS/TexCAPS included a lower risk but more

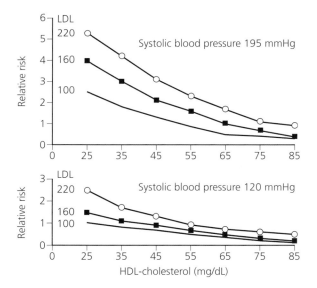

Figure 59.2 Relative risk of coronary heart disease according to high-density lipoprotein cholesterol (HDL), low-density lipoprotein cholesterol (LDL), and systolic blood pressure in the Framingham Study. All subjects were men aged 50–70 years. (From Gordon T, Kannel WB, Castelli WP, et al: Lipoproteins, cardiovascular disease, and death: the Framingham Study. Arch Intern Med 1981;252:1123–1131.)

representative population: the average age was 58.2 years but 21% were over 65, 15% were women, 3% blacks, and 7% Hispanics. The average LDL cholesterol at baseline was 150 mg/dL. Treatment with lovastatin reduced the risk of coronary events, MIs, and revascularization across the board, but the number of participants in the subgroups was too small to allow definite conclusions.

Three major secondary prevention trials established the benefit of lipid-lowering therapy in patients with known CVD. Although these studies also focused primarily on middle-aged men, they included women and patients aged over 65 years; they also included patients with LDL cholesterol from the high-normal range (110 mg/dL) and the very high range (232 mg/dL). The Scandinavian Simvastatin Survival Study (4S) included patients with established CVD and LDL cholesterol 174–232 mg/dL (average 188 mg/dL), of whom 19% were women and 23% aged over 65 years.[7] Simvastatin resulted in a significant reduction in total mortality, coronary events, CVD deaths, revascularization procedures, and strokes. The Cholesterol and Recurrent Events (CARE) trial included patients post MI with LDL cholesterol 116–174 mg/dL (mean 139 mg/dL), of whom 14% were women and 31% aged over 65 years. In this study, treatment with pravastatin resulted in a 24% risk reduction of fatal coronary events and nonfatal MI and a 25% reduction in the need for revascularization.[10,14] The Long-term Intervention with Pravastatin in Ischemic Heart Disease (LIPID) study included patients with a broad range of serum cholesterol (155–271 mg/dL).[15] Average LDL at baseline was 150 mg/dL. Of the patients in this study, 17% were women and 39% aged over 65 years. As with the previous trials this study also demonstrated that treatment with pravastatin reduced the risk of major cardiovascular events including stroke by about 25%.

In a recent metaanalysis, LaRosa et al[16] examined the data from the five large trials that used statins as the lipid-lowering intervention (4S, WOSCOPS, CARE, AFCAPS/TexCAPS, LIPID), with primary focus on risk reduction in women and elderly patients. Collectively, these trials included 30 817 patients, of whom 13% were women and 29% aged over 65 years. The overall proportional risk reduction for major cardiovascular events was equally reduced in men and women, in younger and older patients, and in patients with or without hypertension. However, the effect on coronary deaths remained unclear. Overall, only two of the studies (4S and LIPID) showed significant reduction in coronary deaths, whereas the subgroups of women and the elderly were too small for definite conclusions.

The lipid-lowering trial of ALLHAT is powered to address primarily the effect of lipid lowering on total mortality in elderly patients. In addition it will provide a unique opportunity to assess risk reduction in several subgroups that have been intentionally overrepresented in ALLHAT, such as women, blacks, Hispanics, and diabetics.

Role of low HDL-cholesterol

Considerable epidemiologic data demonstrate that low HDL-cholesterol is a major risk factor for CVD and stroke.[17–20] Low HDL-cholesterol is the most common lipid abnormality in men with CVD in the USA. Furthermore, low HDL-cholesterol better distinguishes populations with coronary artery disease from those without. Recently the Veterans Administration High-density Lipoprotein Intervention Trial (VA-HIT) established substantial benefits of interventions to raise low HDL-cholesterol. The VA-HIT included 2531 men with known coronary artery disease, low HDL-cholesterol, and fairly normal LDL-cholesterol. Approximately 45% were also hypertensives. Patients were randomized to receive gemfibrozil 600 mg twice daily or placebo. At baseline, the average total cholesterol was 175 mg/dL, triglycerides 162 mg/dL, LDL-cholesterol 111 mg/dL, and HDL-cholesterol 32 mg/dL. After 1 year of treatment and throughout the study, therapy with gemfibrozil reduced triglycerides by 31% and increased HDL-cholesterol by 6%. No change in LDL-cholesterol or total cholesterol was noted. During a median follow-up of 5.1 years gemfibrozil therapy resulted in a significant 22% reduction in the primary endpoint of nonfatal MI and CVD death and a 31% reduction in atherothrombotic strokes.[21] Further extensive analysis of the data demonstrated that the reduction in the primary endpoint was significantly related with on-therapy changes in HDL-cholesterol but not LDL-cholesterol or triglycerides.[22] The benefits observed were similar among all subgroups analyzed including hypertensives and diabetics. Thus this study established for the first time that raising HDL-cholesterol in patients with CVD and no major other lipid abnormality is beneficial. This was true even though the change in HDL-cholesterol was only 6%.

Greater increases in HDL-cholesterol can be achieved with niacin. Improvements of up to 30% have been noted with daily doses of 3 g. However, several problems have limited the widespread use of niacin. Short-acting preparations need be administered three times a day with food and/or acetylsalicylic acid to avoid flashing and gastrointestinal symptoms. Slow-release preparations are well tolerated but are associated with substantial hepatotoxicity.[23] A recently developed intermediate-release niacin (NIASPAN) given at night with a snack is well tolerated and is devoid of liver toxicity. Changes in lipid profile noted with this intermediate-release preparation are similar to the short-acting niacin and include up to 30% increase in HDL-cholesterol, 15% reduction in triglycerides, 20% reduction in LDL-cholesterol, and 28% reduction in lipoprotein (Lp)(a). These lipid improvements may confer substantial improvements in CVD outcomes, particularly when combined with a statin.[24]

Cholesterol and blood pressure regulation

Therapy with a statin attenuates the onset and progression of hypertension and renal disease in Dahl salt-sensitive rats.[25,26] More recent data demonstrated a similar effect of long-term treatment with lovastatin in spontaneously hypertensive rats.[27] The mechanism by which statin therapy attenuates the development of hypertension may not be directly related to lipid lowering. Treatment shifts the relation between renal perfusion pressure and sodium excretion toward lower blood pressure. This effect has been attributed to the ability of statins to prevent vascular hypertrophy, thus improving pressure natriuresis. The effect of statins is largely related to their ability to inhibit synthesis of mevalonate, a precursor of isoprenoids,[27] and not to reduction of LDL-cholesterol. A review of the literature suggested that a reduction of plasma cholesterol in humans was associated with a significant 3–5 mmHg reduction in diastolic blood pressure.[28] Statin therapy resulted in the greatest reduction of blood pressure and patients with the highest cholesterol benefited the most. In the Brisighella Heart Study, over 1500 hyperlipidemic patients were randomly treated with either a statin or other lipid-lowering therapy (fibrates or cholestyramine) for 5 years.[29] Changes in lipid profile and blood pressure were assessed every 6 months. Lipid lowering was associated with a significant reduction of both systolic and diastolic blood pressure (10–15 mmHg) only among hypertensive patients in the higher two quartiles. There was only a weak correlation between changes in total cholesterol and blood pressure ($r = 0.16$, $P < 0.044$).

Glorioso et al[30] conducted a double-blind crossover study of patients with untreated hypertension and hypercholesterolemia. Participants were randomly assigned to either pravastatin or placebo. Pravastatin resulted in a significant reduction of systolic, diastolic, and pulse pressure and blunted the pressor response to the cold pressor test. This study too found that the effect of statin therapy on blood pressure was largely independent of the effect on LDL and total cholesterol.

These data strongly suggest that treatment of hyperlipidemic hypertensive patients with a statin may result in better regulation of blood pressure. The most plausible mechanism is a vasodilatory effect of statins due to improvement in endothelial dysfunction. Increased cholesterol contributes to reduced arterial compliance[31] and increased blood pressure. Reduction in cholesterol with statins can therefore contribute to improved arterial compliance and blood pressure regulation and also may contribute to upregulation of nitric oxide.[32]

Smoking and hypertension

Epidemiologic data indicate that smoking and hypertension are additive major CVD risk factors. Approximately 30% of the US population and 35% of hypertensives smoke.[33] The relative risk for death attributable to hypertension in MRC participants was 1.9 for men and 1.7 for women smokers as opposed to 1.3 and 1.2 in nonsmokers. The acute short-term effects of smoking on blood pressure are related to nicotine, carbon monoxide, and other constituents of tobacco smoke. Heart rate and blood pressure increase within 1 min of smoking and rise about 30% during the first 10 min. The effects of nicotine are maintained for several minutes after smoking has ceased. The half-life of nicotine is over 2 h. Thus heavy smokers may maintain elevated heart rates and blood pressures for most of their waking hours.[34] Several studies have suggested that infrequent and moderate smokers may have lower blood pressure than nonsmokers.[35] However in most of these studies patients abstained from smoking prior to blood pressure determination. The lower blood pressure found in smokers persists after adjustments are made for body weight.[36] A recent study examined the effect of smoking cessation on blood pressure and the incidence of hypertension in 8170 healthy male employees of a steel manufacturing company.[37] Mildly hypertensive patients were excluded from this analysis. Adjustments were made for baseline age, body mass index, cigarette smoking, alcohol consumption, exercise, family history of hypertension, systolic blood pressure, and change in body mass index over the follow-up period of 4 years. The adjusted relative risks of hypertension in those who had quit smoking for < 1, 1–3, and > 3 years were 0.6, 1.5, and 3.5 respectively compared with nonsmokers. The trends were similar among those who lost or gained weight during the follow-up period. The mechanism by which long-term smoking lowers blood pressure or prevents hypertension and by which smoking cessation increases the frequency of hypertension is not clear but it should not distract from the well-known harmful effects of cigarette smoking. Cigarette smokers may not derive the expected benefits from hypertension control. In the MRC trial β-blocker therapy was less effective in preventing strokes than thiazide diuretics.[38] In the Heart Attack Primary Prevention in Hypertension (HAPPHY) trial, β-blockers failed to improve coronary morbidity in smokers.[39] It is important therefore to inform patients of the importance of smoking cessation, and encourage them to do so at every visit. Smoking cessation is an important intervention in reducing CVD risk in patients with hypertension. Use of various smoking deterrents may be helpful.

Diabetes in patients with hypertension

Diabetes and hypertension commonly coexist. In the USA, more than 60% of diabetics have hypertension and approximately 20% of hypertensives have diabetes.[40] Diabetics are two to three times more likely to have hypertension than nondiabetics. The incidence is even higher among African-Americans. Diabetes is the most common cause of endstage renal disease and a major contributor to CVD.[41] Even mild elevations of blood pressure in diabetics increases the risk of CVD and renal disease dramatically. It is therefore of utmost importance to control both blood pressure and glycemia tightly in diabetics with hypertension.

Aggressive treatment of blood pressure in diabetics has been largely ignored, although it may confer greater reduction of CVD events than glycemic control. The goal of blood pressure reduction has been set at lower levels in diabetics, mostly because studies have shown continued benefit with lower blood pressure. The Appropriate Blood Pressure Control in Diabetics[42] and the Hypertension Optimal Treatment[43] trials indicated that aggressive reduction of diastolic blood pressure to below 80 mmHg provides greater reduction in CVD events. Similarly the UK Prospective Diabetes Study (UKPDS) demonstrated that tight control of blood pressure had greater impact on CVD events than tight glycemic control.[44] The impact on CVD events included a 44% reduction in strokes and a 24% reduction in diabetes-associated endpoints, and a 32% reduction in deaths. For every 10-mmHg reduction in systolic blood pressure there was an associated risk reduction of 12% for any complication related to diabetes.[45] For these reasons the recommended target blood pressure in patients with diabetes is < 130/80 mmHg. Angiotensin-converting enzyme (ACE) inhibitors and more recently angiotensin receptor blockers (ARBs) provide better vascular and renal protection, although most patients require combinations of three to four drugs to achieve target blood pressure control.

The UKPDS study compared the effects of intensive blood glucose control with conventional treatment on microvascular and macrovascular complications of diabetes over 10 years in over 4000 patients.[46,47] Average HbA$_{1c}$ was reduced to 7% in the intensive-treated group and to 7.9% in the conventional group. This difference resulted in a 12% reduction in diabetes-related endpoints, a 10% reduction in deaths, and a 25% reduction in microvascular complications. There was minimal reduction in macrovascular disease. For every 1% reduction in HbA$_{1c}$ there was a 21% reduction in any endpoint related to diabetes, a 21% reduction in deaths, a 14% reduction in MIs, and a 37% reduction in microvascular complications. There was no threshold for any of the endpoints.

These observations suggest that aggressive glycemic and blood pressure control is warranted in patients with diabetes and hypertension.

Diet, weight loss, and exercise in patients with hypertension

Epidemiologic studies have consistently shown substantial correlation between hypertension, excess body weight, and physical inactivity. Although all three variables are independently associated with increased CVD risk,[48,49,50] their coexistence increases the risk for complications cumulatively. Guidelines for the management of hypertension recommend lifestyle changes for nonpharmacologic treatment of hypertension.[48,51] Dietary changes are effective even without weight loss. The DASH (SR) study showed that a combination diet of fruits and vegetables low in saturated fats reduced blood pressure in patients in the high-normal range. This diet was more effective in African-Americans and patients with established hypertension.[52] It has been shown that there is roughly 1-mmHg reduction in diastolic blood pressure for every kilogram of weight loss in obese subjects. The World Health Organization/International Society of Hypertension guidelines recommend at least 5 kg of weight loss in order to induce blood pressure reduction.[51]

Numerous observational studies have shown an inverse relation between physical activity and blood pressure.[53,54] In a recent review of the literature we identified 12 prospective randomized trials completed in the last 10 years.[55] Significant reduction in resting blood pressure was reported with aerobic exercise in 10 of these studies. The average blood pressure reduction was 8.7/7.0 mmHg in the exercise group compared with 3.8/1.3 mmHg in the controls despite body weight remaining unchanged. An important observation is that low- to moderate-intensity exercise may be more effective in lowering blood pressure than high-intensity exercise. Exercise appears safe and effective in improving hypertension in treated patients with severe hypertension and left ventricular hypertrophy. In a study of 46 African-Americans with severe hypertension, we found that regular aerobic exercise for 30–60 min, at least three times per week, resulted in significant reduction of blood pressure despite a decrease of antihypertensive medication by 30–40%. The body weight in the exercise and control groups and the blood pressure in the controls remained unchanged at 32 weeks.[55] Blumenthal et al[56] studied 134 patients with stage 1 hypertension. They compared the effect of aerobic exercise alone with weight management including exercise. Aerobic exercise was more effective and reduced blood pressure by 7/5 mmHg.

These data indicate that diet, weight reduction, and exercise can reduce blood pressure independently. However, reductions are modest. A combination can be more effective. However, their feasibility and application in clinical practice remains to be demonstrated.

Emerging cardiovascular risk factors

Emerging CVD risk factors have appeared in the literature in recent years. These risk factors have been associated with high risk for coronary atherosclerosis, CVD complications, and cardiac death. These new risk factors include Lp(a), homocysteine, inflammatory markers, high triglycerides, coronary calcifications, high uric acid, and others. Extensive coverage of these risk factors is beyond the scope of this chapter. In general, clinical associations have been well established with all these factors but interventional data conclusively demonstrating benefit is lacking in most instances.

Lipoprotein (a)

Lp(a) resembles LDL but additionally contains a highly glycosylated protein, apoA. Elevated Lp(a) has been associated with coronary artery disease in most but not all studies. Some studies suggested gender differences in the prognostic significance of Lp(a). In a large cohort study, 4967 men and 4968 women free of atherosclerosis were followed for up to 14 years. There was a significant increase in the adjusted hazards ratio for coronary artery disease with increased Lp(a) (1.9 for women, 1.6 for men), but the association with cerebrovascular disease was less certain.[57] Lp(a) can be reduced significantly with niacin (up to 30% reduction) but the clinical importance of such an intervention has not been demonstrated.

Homocysteine

Homocysteinemia is an independent predictor of coronary artery disease, MI, and peripheral vascular disease. One recent study examined the association of homocysteine levels with recurrent events in 110 young patients (< 56 years old) who had suffered a prior MI. Over a 7-year follow-up, patients with normal homocysteine levels had significantly fewer combined events (26% vs. 72%), lower mortality (1.6% vs. 6%), lower morbidity (14% vs. 36%), and less need for revascularization (18% vs. 48%).[58] Definite interventional data with treatment to reduce homocysteine (vitamin B_6, vitamin B_{12} or folic acid) is lacking. Similar deficiencies exist for all other emerging CVD risk factors.

References

1. Dustan HP: Role of hypertension and its control: experimental aspects. Prog Biochem Pharmacol 1983;19:177–191.
2. Tobian LJ: Interrelationships of sodium volume, CNS and hypertension. Prog Biochem Pharmacol 1983;19:208–229.
3. Kannel WB, Sorlie P: Hypertension in Framingham. In Paul O (ed): Epidemiology and Control of Hypertension. Symposia Specialists, 1993.
4. Anderson KM, Wilson PWF, Odell PM, et al: An updated coronary risk profile. Statement for health professionals. Circulation 1991;83:357–363.
5. Kannel WB, Castelli WP, Gordon T: Cholesterol in the prediction of atherosclerotic disease. New perspectives based on the Framingham Study. Ann Intern Med 1979;90:85–91.
6. Gordon T, Kannel WB, Castelli WP, et al: Lipoproteins, cardiovascular disease, and death: the Framingham Study. Arch Intern Med 1981;252:1123–1131.
7. Scandinavian Simvastatin Survival Study Group. Randomized trial of cholesterol lowering in 4444 patients with coronary heart disease. Lancet 1994;344:1383–1389.
8. Miettinen TA, Pyorala K, Olsson AG, et al: Cholesterol-lowering therapy in women and elderly patients with myocardial infarction or angina pectoris. Circulation 1997;96:4211–4218.
9. Shepherd J, Cobbe SM, Ford I, et al: Prevention of coronary heart disease with pravastatin in men with hypercholesterolemia. N Engl J Med 1995;333:1301–1307.
10. Sacks FM, Pfeffer MA, Moye LA, et al: The effect of pravastatin on coronary events after myocardial infarction in patients with average cholesterol levels. N Engl J Med 1996;335:1001–1009.
11. Prospective Studies Collaboration: Cholesterol, diastolic blood pressure and stroke. Lancet 1995;346:1647–1653.
12. Cholesterol Treatment Trialists' Collaboration: Protocol for a prospective collaborative overview of all current and planned randomized trials of cholesterol treatment regimens. Am J Cardiol 1995;75:1130–1134.
13. Downs JR, Clearfield M, Weis S, et al: Primary prevention of acute coronary events with lovastatin in men and women with average cholesterol levels: results of AFCAPS/TexCAPS. JAMA 1998;279:1615–1622.
14. Lewis SJ, Sacks FM, Mitchell JS, et al: Effect of pravastatin on cardiovascular events in women after myocardial infarction. J Am Coll Cardiol 1998;32:140–146.
15. Long-term Intervention With Pravastatin in Ischaemic Disease (LIPID) Study Group: Prevention of cardiovascular events and death with pravastatin in patients with coronary heart disease and a broad range of initial cholesterol levels. N Engl J Med 1998;339:1349–1357.
16. LaRosa JC, He J, Vupputuris S: Effect of statins on risk of coronary disease. JAMA 1999;282:2340–2346.
17. Gordon DJ, Probstfield JL, Garrison RJ, et al: High-density lipoprotein cholesterol and cardiovascular disease: four prospective American Studies. Circulation 1989;79:8–15.
18. Tanne D, Yaari S, Goldbourt U: High-density lipoprotein cholesterol and risk of ischemic stroke mortality: a 21-year follow-up of 8586 men from the Israeli Ischemic Heart Disease Study. Stroke 1997;28:83–87.

19. Wannamethee S, Shaper AG, Ebrahim S: HDL-cholesterol, total cholesterol, and the risk of stroke in middle-aged British men. Stroke 2000;31:1882–1888.
20. Rubins HB, Robins SJ, Collins D, et al: Gemfibrozil for the secondary prevention of coronary heart disease in men with low levels of high-density lipoprotein cholesterol. N Engl J Med 1999;341:410–418.
21. Rubins HB, Davenport J, Babikian V, et al: Reduction in stroke with gemfibrozil in men with coronary heart disease and low HDL cholesterol. Veterans Affairs HDL Intervention Trial (VA-HIT). 2000.
22. Robins SJ, Collins D, Wittes JT, et al: Relation of gemfibrozil treatment and lipid levels with major coronary events. VA-HIT: a randomized controlled trial. 2001
23. Golberg A, Alagona P, Capuzzi DM, et al: Multiple-dose efficacy and safety of an extended-release form of niacin in the management of hyprlipidemia. Am J Cardiol 2000;85:1100–1105.
24. Brown G, Zhao XO, Chait A, et al: Simvastatin and niacin, antioxidant vitamins, or the combination for the prevention of coronary disease. N Engl J Med 2001;345:1583–1592.
25. O'Donnell MP, Kasiske BL, Katz SA, et al: Lovastatin but not enalapril reduces glomerular injury in Dahl salt-sensitive rats. Hypertension 1992;20:651–658.
26. Wilson TW, Alonso-Galicia M, Roman RJ: Effects of lipid-lowering agents in the Dahl salt-sensitive rat. Hypertension 1998;31:225–231.
27. Jiang J, Roman RJ: Lovastatin prevents development of hypertension in spontaneously hypertensive rats. Hypertension 1997;30:968–974.
28. Goode GK, Miller JP, Heagerty AM: Hyperlipidemia, hypertension, and coronary heart disease. Lancet 1995;345:362–364.
29. Borghi C, Gaddi A, Ambrosini E, et al: Improved blood pressure control in hypertensive patients treated with statins. J Am Coll Cardiol 2001;37(Suppl A):233A–234A.
30. Glorioso N, Troffa C, Filigheddu F, et al: Effect of the HMG-CoA reductase inhibitors on blood pressure in patients with essential hypertension and primary hypercholesterolemia. Hypertension 1999;34:1281–1286.
31. Lewis TV, Cooper BA, Dart AM, et al: Responses to endothelium-dependent agonists in subcutaneous arteries excised from hypercholesterolaemic men. Br J Pharmacol 1998;124:222–228.
32. Kaesemeyer WH, Caldwell RB, Huang J, et al: Pravastatin sodium activates endothelial nitric oxide synthase independent of its cholesterol-lowering actions. J Am Coll Cardiol 1999;33:234–241.
33. De Cesaris R, Ranieri G, Filitti V, et al: Cardiovascular effects of cigarette smoking. Cardiology 1992;81:233–237.
34. Groppelli A, Giorgi DM, Omboni S, et al: Persistent blood pressure increase induced by heavy smoking. J Hypertens 1992;10:495–499.
35. Green MS, Jucha E, Lz Y: Blood pressure in smokers and non-smokers: epidemiologic findings. Am Heart J 1986;111:932–940.
36. Savdie E, Grosslight GM, Adena MA: Relation of alcohol and cigarette consumption to blood pressure and serum creatinine levels. J Chron Dis 1984;37:617–623.
37. Duk-Hee L, Myung-Hwa H, Jang-Rak K, et al: Effects of smoking cessation on changes in blood pressure and incidence of hypertension. Hypertension 2001;37:194–198.
38. Dollery C, Brennan PJ: The Medical Research Council Hypertension Trial: the smoking patient. Am Heart J 1988;115:276–281.
39. Wilhelmsen L, Berglund G, Elmfeldt D, et al: Beta-blockers versus diuretics in hypertensive men: results from the HAPPHY atrial. J Hypertens 1987;5:561–570.
40. Bloomgarden ZT: Perspective on the news: cardiovascular disease in type 2 diabetes. Diabetes Care 1999;22:1739–1744.
41. American Diabetes Association: National Diabetes Fact Sheet, December 1997.
42. Estacio RO, Jeffers BW, Hiatt WR, et al: The effect of nosoldipine as compared with enalapril on cardiovascular outcomes in patients with non-insulin-dependent diabetes and hypertension. N Engl J Med 1998;338:645–652.
43. Hansson L, Zanchetti A, Carruthers G, et al: Effects of intensive blood-pressure lowering and low-dose aspirin in patients with hypertension: principal results of the Hypertension Optimal Treatment (HOT) randomized trial. Lancet 1998;351:1755–1762.
44. UK Prospective Diabetes Study Group: Tight blood pressure control and risk of macrovascular and microvascular complications in type 2 diabetes (UKPDS 38). Br Med J 1998;317:703–713.
45. Adler AI, Stratton IM, Neil HA, et al: Association of systolic blood pressure with macrovascular and microvascular complications of type 2 diabetes (UKPDS 36): prospective observational study. Br Med J 2000;321:412–419.
46. UK Prospective Diabetes Study (UKPDS) Group: Intensive blood-glucose control with sulphonylureas or insulin compared with conventional treatment and risk of complications in patients with type 2 diabetes (UKPDS 33). Lancet 1998;352:837–853.
47. Straton IM, Adler AI, Neil AW, et al: Association of glycaemia with macrovascular and microvascular complications of type 2 diabetes (UKPDS 35): prospective observational study. Br Med J 2000;321:405–412.
48. The Sixth Report of the Joint National Committee on Prevention, Detection, Evaluation, and Treatment of High Blood Pressure. Arch Intern Med 1997;157:2413–2446.
49. Eckel RH: Obesity and heart disease: a statement for healthcare professionals from the Nutrition Committee, American Heart Association. Circulation 1997;96:3248–3250.
50. Appel LJ, Moore TJ, Obarzanek E, et al: A clinical trial of dietary patterns on blood pressure. N Engl J Med 1997;336:1117–1124.
51. Guidelines Subcommittee: 1999 World Health Organization/ International Society of Hypertension Guidelines for the Management of Hypertension. J Hypertens 1999;17:151–183.
52. Svetky LP, Simons-Morton D, Vollmer WM, et al: Effects of dietary patterns on blood pressure: subgroup analysis of the Dietary Approaches to Stop Hypertension (DASH) randomized clinical trial. Arch Intern Med 1999;159:285–293.
53. Hickey N, Mulcahy R, Bourke GJ, et al: Study of coronary risk factors related to physical activity in 15,171 men. Br Med J 1975;3:507–509.
54. Miall WE, Oldham PD: Factors influencing arterial blood pressure in the general population. Clin Sci 1958;17:409–444.
55. Papademetriou V, Kokkinos P: The role of exercise in the control of hypertension and cardiovascular risk. Curr Opin Nephrol Hypertens 1996;5:459–462.
56. Blumenthal JA, Sherwood A, Gullette ECD, et al: Exercise and weight loss reduce blood pressure in men and women with mild hypertension: effects on cardiovascular, metabolic, and hemodynamic functioning. Arch Intern Med 2000;160:1947–1958.
57. Nguyen TT, Ellefson RD, Hodge DO, et al: Predictive value of electrophoretically detected lipoprotein (a) for coronary heart disease and cerebrovascular disease in a community-based cohort of 9936 men and women. Circulation 1997;96:1390–1397.
58. Reis RP, Azinheira J, Reis HP, et al: Prognosis significance of blood homocysteine after myocardial infarction. Rev Port Cardiol 2000;19:581–585.

PART XI
Management of Secondary Hypertension

CHRISTOPHER S. WILCOX

Medical Management of Renovascular Hypertension and Ischemic Nephropathy

Christopher S. Wilcox

Introduction

The effects of medical treatment on the control of blood pressure and on stabilization or improvement of renal function in trials of patients with renovascular disease have been reviewed comprehensively.[1–3]

Renal artery stenosis (RAS) is defined as a narrowing of one or both renal arteries or their branches (usually by more than 70–80% to be functionally significant).[4] Renovascular hypertension is defined as hypertension that is caused by RAS; in practice, it is defined as hypertension that is improved or cured after correction of RAS. The term ischemic nephropathy defines progressive renal failure due to RAS. There is little evidence that ischemia is critical for progressive loss of renal function. Therefore, this condition is better referred to as azotemic renovascular disease. Most cases of renovascular hypertension, and almost all cases of azotemic renovascular disease, are due to atherosclerosis. In order to plan for rational therapy, it is essential to understand the anticipated natural history of untreated subjects, and the underlying pathophysiology.

Natural history of untreated patients

Fibromuscular dysplasia has numerous subtypes. The most common is medial fibroplasia, which is not normally progressive. Thus, the aim of therapy is to improve or cure hypertension rather than to prevent azotemic renovascular disease. Approximately half of carefully selected patients may be cured of hypertension by percutaneous transluminal renal angioplasty (PTRA) or reconstructive surgery.[5] In contrast, cure of hypertension after correction of RAS due to atherosclerosis occurs in less than 20% of patients.[6] Studies with duplex ultrasound measurements over 5 years reported progression of atherosclerotic RAS in more than one-third of patients, and complete occlusion in 15%.[7] Contemporary studies indicate that less than 10–15% of patients with RAS treated medically develop intractable hypertension, progressive renal insufficiency, or total arterial occlusion.[7–9] Following intervention with PTRA and stenting (PTRAS) or reconstructive surgery numerous observational studies[1,2] show that ~ 30% have a worthwhile improvement in glomerular filtration rate (GFR) matched by a reduction in serum creatinine concentration (S_{Cr}) and blood urea nitrogen (BUN), ~ 50% have a stable GFR, and ~ 20% have a deterioration in GFR. The outcome in most studies is no overall benefit from the intervention. However, this conclusion conceals the fact that some patients derive substantial benefit while others deteriorate, either because of – or despite – the intervention.

These considerations give rise to the following conclusions regarding the choice of medical therapy or intervention:

1. Medical therapy is appropriate for patients with fibromuscular disease as it is not progressive and does not lead to significant loss of renal function; on the other hand, rates of cure of hypertension following intervention are high, and complications of PTRAS (such as atheroembolism) are quite uncommon. Therefore, most patients with troublesome hypertension are offered an intervention, but this can be preceded by a prolonged trial of medical therapy.

2. Among patients with atherosclerotic RAS, only some will benefit from intervention (see Chapters 61 and 62). Medical therapy in atherosclerotic RAS is used either as a primary treatment for those who are stable during close observation, or as an adjunct for those who have had an intervention, or as sole therapy for those who are deemed unsuitable for intervention.

3. A "wait-and-see" policy carries a small but significant risk of progression to total renal arterial occlusion after which definitive intervention may not be possible.

4. Certain categories of patient have an absolute indication for intervention. These include patients with high grade bilateral renal artery stenosis or stenosis of a single or dominant kidney, whose course is complicated by recurrent fluid retention and "flash" pulmonary edema.[1,2]

Pathophysiologic basis for therapy

Animal models provide a rational basis for medical therapy. The two-kidney, one-clip (2K, 1C) Goldblatt model of unilateral RAS is characterized by an early rise in blood pressure and plasma renin activity. Hypertension initially is entirely dependent on angiotensin II (Ang II). It can be rapidly restored to normal by an angiotensin converting enzyme inhibitor (ACEI) or an angiotensin receptor blocker (ARB). After 2–12 months, the blood pressure increases further and some experimental animals perish from malignant hypertension. The remainder develop normal renin hypertension complicated by vascular and renal damage. At this stage, acute administration of an ACEI or ARB does little to the blood pressure. However, prolonged administration over 3 days can restore blood pressure to a nearly normal level.[10]

The one-kidney, one-clip (1K, 1C) Goldblatt model of bilateral RAS or stenosis of a single or dominant kidney is characterized by an early rise in blood pressure. The level of PRA depends on salt intake. The hypertension depends on the combined effects of salt intake and Ang II.[11]

Human renovascular disease usually has components of both models. Therefore, therapy directed at an overactive renin–angiotensin system on the one hand, and inappropriate renal salt and water retention on the other, is usually required for full control of hypertension, but carries risks of adverse changes in renal function, as described in Specific agents: Angiotensin converting enzyme inhibitors and angiotensin receptor blockers.

The role of Ang II in maintaining blood pressure and renal hemodynamics in Goldblatt hypertension has been studied with the use of ARBs and ACEIs.[11–13] As shown in Fig. 60.1 compared with spontaneously hypertensive rats (SHR) an ACEI causes a larger fall in mean arterial pressure (MAP) in 2K, 1C rats.[12,13] The GFR and the excretion of fluid and sodium ions (Na^+) increase with the ACEI in the contralateral kidney (CK), but decrease in the postclipped kidney. There is an increase in renal blood flow (RBF) at both kidneys. Therefore the filtration fraction (FF) falls quite sharply at the postclip kidney.

The renal microvessels downstream from a functionally significant RAS are under two dominant influences (Fig. 60.2). One is renal autoregulation, which is a vasodilation, especially of the afferent but also of the efferent arterioles, that maintains the RBF. The second is the release of renin from the juxtaglomerular cells in the afferent arteriole in response to decreased stretch and decreased sodium chloride (NaCl) delivery to the macula densa.[14] (Fig. 60.2) The ensuing increase in the generation of angiotensin I (Ang I) from angiotensinogen (A_0), and the action of angiotensin-converting enzyme (ACE), increase the interstitial generation of Ang II in the kidney. Ang II acts on angiotensin type 1 (AT_1) receptors to constrict preferentially the efferent arterioles, thereby maintaining a reasonable pressure for ultrafiltration (P_{Uf}) at the glomerular capillaries despite a fall in MAP. Therefore, an ACEI or an ARB may prevent an increase in efferent arteriolar

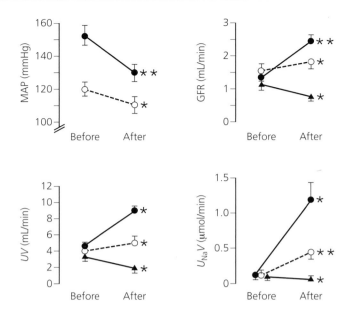

Figure 60.1 Mean ± SEM values for mean arterial pressure, renal excretion of fluid and sodium, and glomerular filtration rate in anesthetized rats. Data are shown for spontaneously hypertensive rats (open symbols and broken lines) and for rats with Goldblatt two-kidney, one-clip hypertension (solid symbols and lines) for the contralateral kidney (solid circles); and post-clip kidney (solid triangles). Each panel shows values before and after administration of an angiotensin converting enzyme inhibitor, compared to before *$P < 0.05$; **$P < 0.01$. (Drawn from data from Huang et al[12] with permission.)

resistance, leading to a fall in P_{Uf} with a consequent fall in the GFR. However, the RBF will be maintained or improved because of the reduction in overall renal vascular resistance. These effects have been confirmed in studies of split renal function in patients with unilateral RAS.[15,16]

A recent study compared responses to an ACEI and an ARB in 1K, 1C hypertensive rats.[17] Both lowered the blood pressure similarly, but the fall in GFR was greater with the ACEI. This was attributed to accumulation of bradykinin and its effects on the bradykinin type 2 (B_2) receptor, since the greater fall in GFR after ACEI was prevented by a B_2-receptor antagonist. These results have yet to be confirmed clinically, but suggest the possibility of some advantage of ARBs over ACEIs in patients with renovascular disease who experience a reduction in GFR during treatment.

Calcium antagonists (CAs) administered to animals with angiotensin-induced hypertension substantially reduce blood pressure and renal vascular resistance. However, in contrast to ACEIs and ARBs, CAs increase the GFR.[18] This is attributed to a preferential effect of CAs on vasodilation of afferent – rather than efferent – arterioles because of selective distribution of voltage-gated calcium channels to the afferent arteriole (Fig. 60.2).[19] These effects of CAs have been confirmed in studies of split renal function in patients with renovascular hypertension.[15]

ACEIs and CAs should have contrasting effects on glomerular hemodynamics in the clipped kidney. Two studies compared therapy with ACEIs and CAs in Goldblatt

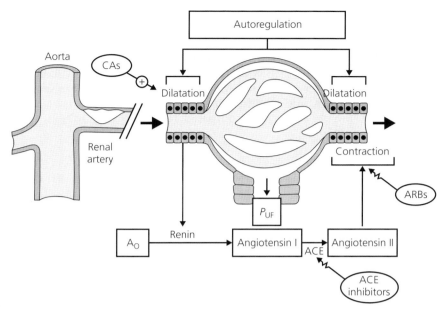

Figure 60.2 Diagrammatic representation of factors affecting the pressure for ultrafiltration (P_{Uf}) in the glomerulus downstream from a functional renal artery stenosis. Autoregulation leads to vasodilation of the afferent and efferent arterioles. Afferent arteriolar vasodilation is further enhanced by a calcium antagonist (CA). Renin release from the afferent arteriole acts on angiotensinogen (A_O) to form angiotensin I (Ang I) which, after action by angiotensin converting enzyme (ACE), forms angiotensin II (Ang II). Ang II constricts preferentially the efferent arteriole. ACEIs or ARBs prevent these effects of Ang II on type I receptors and reduce the P_{Uf}.

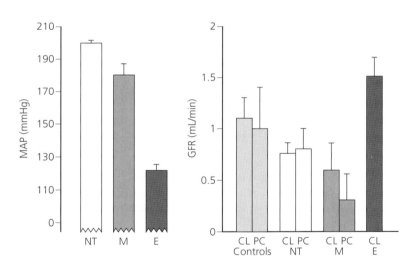

Figure 60.3 Mean ± SEM values for mean arterial pressure, glomerular filtration rate in the contralateral (CL) and postclipped (PC) kidneys, the weight of the PC kidney, and number of animals surviving for control (Cont), and two-kidney, one-clip Goldblatt hypertensive rats given for 1 year either no treatment (NT), a vasodilator (minoxidil, M), or an angiotensin-converting enzyme inhibitor (enalapril, E). (Drawn from data by Jackson et al[22] with permission.)

hypertensive rats over 5–6 weeks.[20,21] ACEI therapy prevented glomerular hypertrophy and glomerular sclerosis in the contralateral kidney, whereas CA therapy worsened these changes.[20] Only the ACEI reduced proteinuria from the clipped kidney.[21] Interestingly, the CA worsened the lesions in the clipped kidney to the same extent as the ACEI.[21] These data suggest the possibility of a trade-off: ACEI therapy may reduce the GFR, and perhaps enhance irreversible atrophy in the poststenotic kidney, but may improve function in the contralateral kidney through better antihypertensive action, better control of glomerular capillary hypertension, and prevention of the fibrotic and sclerotic effects of Ang II. The role of CAs in therapy is not yet clear.

Further insight into potential therapeutic differences between ACEIs and ARBs on the one hand, and vasodilators or CAs on the other, comes from longer-term studies. In the 2K, 1C model, both minoxidil (M), a vasodilator, and an ACEI, enalapril (E), compared with no treatment (NT) reduced the BP, although the ACEI was more effective (Fig. 60.3).

After 1 year, the postclipped kidney of the ACEI-treated rats was atrophic and had no residual function, but that of the minoxidil-treated rats retained some residual GFR. This led to the concept of "pharmacologic nephrectomy" with ACEIs.[22] This adverse effect of ACEIs was, however, offset by two benefits. First, there was a significant increase in the GFR of the contralateral kidney (CL) with the ACEI, but not with the vasodilator. This resulted in an overall GFR of animals treated with an ACEI that was better preserved than those treated with minoxidil. Second, the 1-year survival was 15% in untreated rats, 48% in minoxidil-treated rats, and 84% in ACEI-treated rats. This study poses very elegantly the clinical dilemma: can a loss of GFR, with potential structural atrophy of the postclipped kidney during ACEI therapy be considered a reasonable trade-off for improved function of the contralateral kidney, overall better blood pressure control, and better cardiovascular survival? These issues will be discussed in the context of data from human subjects with renovascular disease (see Specific agents).

Clinical studies have shown that there is a critical level of vascular occlusion beyond which the RBF and GFR fall with any further reduction in blood pressure because the renal perfusion pressure is below the autoregulatory limits.[23,24] Revascularization can restore the ability of such kidneys to tolerate a reduction of blood pressure to normal levels. The Sixth Report of the Joint National Commission (JNC VI)[25] explicitly recognizes the potential for blood pressure reduction to slow renal disease progression. It sets reduced goals (< 130/75 mmHg) for blood pressure reduction in azotemic patients with proteinuria. However, a reduction of systemic pressures in patients with a critical renal artery stenosis can cause a sharp fall in GFR, regardless of the type of antihypertensive agent used. Hence, chronic azotemic renovascular disease must be considered and excluded when necessary, before vigorous blood pressure reduction is undertaken in patients with renal disease.

Aims of treatment

Treatment has the following aims:

1. to reverse hypertension and associated cardiovascular morbidity and mortality;
2. to improve or preserve kidney function;
3. to prevent the irreversible loss of kidney function that follows renal artery occlusion;
4. to prevent or treat dangerous complications such as recurrent pulmonary edema.

Outcomes of medical therapy

To date, no placebo-controlled trials have evaluated specific medical therapies for renovascular disease. However, three controlled trials and many observational trials have compared the outcomes of patients treated medically with those treated by intervention.

Hypertension

Three groups measured the blood pressure of patients with renovascular hypertension during steady-state treatment with an ACEI and compared it with blood pressure recorded after intervention by PTRA or reconstructive surgery.[26] There was a close correlation between the systolic and diastolic blood pressure achieved by these two forms of treatment. This implies that therapy with an ACEI is generally as effective in controlling hypertension as an intervention.

Three groups performed controlled trials in which patients were randomized to receive medical therapy or intervention with PTRA.[8,27] Blood pressure was measured with automated devices. Each group concluded that patients randomized to intervention had a similar reduction in blood pressure as those randomized to medical therapy, although those receiving the intervention required fewer antihypertensive drugs.[8,27] Apparently, modern antihypertensive drug therapy given under protocol conditions is effective in controlling hypertension in the majority of patients with renovascular disease. These relatively short-term trials (6–12 months) were not convincing about the need for intervention to control BP. However, they leave several unresolved issues: whether the conclusions will hold over a longer time period, and whether the choice of antihypertensive agent (an ACEI or ARB compared to a CA) will influence the outcome.

Renal function

Most trials that have compared an intervention by PTRA alone or combined with stenting (PTRAS) with medical therapy have failed to show statistically significant differences in renal function at followup.[1,2] To date, only one controlled trial has compared renal function of patients randomized to medical therapy on PTRA. Van Jaarsveld et al[8] randomized ~ 100 patients over 1 year. Overall, at completion there were no differences in creatinine clearance between the two groups, leading to the conclusion that there was no clear benefit of PTRA over medical therapy. However, closer inspection highlights the difficulty of pursuing a nonintervention policy in patients with known renovascular disease; 44% of the patients randomized to medical therapy required a PTRA during the one year of study, thereby confounding very seriously the interpretation of the results. Moreover, 12% of patients in the medical treatment group suffered complete occlusion of a renal artery, and twice as many suffered significant decline in renal function, as indicated by a doubling of S_{Cr} or a need for hemodialysis. This trial included patients with refractory hypertension and an RAS of > 50%. Recent studies show clearly that a narrowing of 75–80% is required to produce renovascular disease.[4] Thus, many patients in this study may not have had functional renovascular disease and therefore could not have benefited from therapy. However, similar outcomes for renal function after treatment with medical therapy or interventions, lead to the conclusion that medical therapy is an acceptable choice, at least in the short term. Medical therapy is less expensive and less likely to produce serious adverse affects.[27] This has kindled increased interest in medical therapy for renovascular disease.

Despite many inconclusive studies,[1,2] Watson et al[29] identified a group of patients with global renal ischemia and progressive renal impairment. After treatment with PTRAS, the decline in renal function was arrested and reversed. Thus patients with documented progression of renal insufficiency during medical therapy should be considered for intervention.

There are no trials comparing survival among patients receiving other forms of treatment for renovascular disease.

Specific agents

There is a lack of controlled trials in patients with renovascular disease that compare classes of agents.

Diuretics

Renovascular disease is a high-renin state. It has been considered resistant to diuretic therapy. However, there are good reasons for selecting a diuretic with dietary salt restriction as first-line therapy for many patients. The poststenotic kidney has sharply reduced perfusion pressure, which is a powerful stimulus for salt and water retention. The contralateral kidney, although perfused at high pressure, is under the influence of unusually high levels of circulating Ang II and aldosterone. Its pressure natriuresis mechanism is also reset to favor salt retention. Moreover, the contralateral kidney may be damaged by nephrosclerosis or may develop a stenosis of its artery, which will leave no normal kidney to regulate salt balance. Severe and unpredictable episodes of primary renal salt and fluid retention can occur, leading to overflow flash pulmonary edema.[30] Diuretics and salt restriction enhance the antihypertensive response to all other medical therapies, except perhaps CAs. For these reasons, dietary salt should be restricted and a diuretic agent used at an early stage in most treatment regimens. Since diuretics cause a further stimulation of plasma renin activity, with enhancement of Ang II and aldosterone, additional measures to combat renin secretion or inhibit its effects are usually necessary. Renin secretion can be inhibited by a beta-blocker, and the effects of Ang II and aldosterone blunted by an ACEI, ARB, or spironolactone.

Dietary salt restriction and diuretics have little effect on the GFR of normal subjects.[31] However, in patients with renal disease and hypertension such treatment reduces the GFR – at least initially.[32] Therefore, some increase in S_{Cr} and BUN after initiating diuretic therapy should be anticipated. Diuretic therapy for hypertension in discussed in Chapter 54.

Beta-blockers

Beta-blockers are most effective in patients with high-renin hypertension, making them a rational treatment for renovascular hypertension. Moreover, beta-blockers powerfully inhibit renin secretion[33] so it is rational to combine beta-blockers with diuretics to prevent the further rise in plasma renin activity that would otherwise occur. Beta-blockers are strongly indicated in patients with angina or with prior myocardial infarction. Beta-blocker therapy for hypertension is discussed in Chapter 54.

Central agents and beta-blockers

Central agents such as clonidine, or peripheral beta-blockers such as labetalol or carvetolol, are effective in hypertension that is associated with increased sympathetic drive. During renovascular or renal parenchymal hypertension, there is increased neural input from the affected kidney, which engages a central sympathetic drive that maintains the hypertension.[34] Therefore, the use of these agents is rational, and usually effective as adjunctive treatment for more severe forms of renovascular disease. Comparison of the short-term response to clonidine and an ACEI in patients with renovascular disease showed that both agents reduced the BP, although the ACEI was more effective.[35] However, the ACEI reduced the GFR in the poststenotic kidney, whereas this remained stable with clonidine.

Calcium antagonists

CAs reverse the hypertension and renal vasoconstriction associated with prolonged Ang II infusion, and selectively vasodilate the afferent arteriole.[18] They should, therefore, be ideal for patients with renovascular disease by controlling hypertension without compromising GFR in the poststenotic kidney. Moreover, they have mild natriuretic actions, and can blunt the aldosterone response to Ang II.[36] The role of CAs in treatment is not yet clear. The effects of CAs seen in animal models are confirmed in acute studies of patients with renovascular disease. In studies of patients with RAS[37] or post–renal-transplant stenosis[38] the GFR in the poststenotic kidney is reduced by ACEIs but unchanged by CAs. During longer-term studies in patients with unilateral RAS, both ACEIs and CAs reduce the blood pressure and increase the RBF in the contralateral kidney.[15] The total GFR is not affected significantly by either treatment, but the GFR of the poststenotic kidney is reduced by 54% during the ACEI therapy compared to only 21% during the CA therapy. Hence, there can be a relative sparing of the GFR of the poststenotic kidney with a CA. Therefore, CAs are indicated in patients with renovascular hypertension where renal function is already compromised, or has been unacceptably reduced by an ACEI or ARB. Moreover, CAs can be used in azotemia without modification of the dosage. Further study is needed on the role of CAs in long-term management of patients with renovascular disease. CA therapy for hypertension is discussed in Chapter 56.

Angiotensin-converting enzyme inhibitors and angiotensin receptor blockers

When these agents are given to patients with essential hypertension, they normally increase the GFR. They block the sodium and fluid retention that normally accompanies a fall in BP. On the other hand, they can cause a sharp fall in GFR in some patients with chronic renal failure due to polycystic kidney disease[39] or nephrosclerosis[40] when given with salt-depleting therapy. When given to patients with renovascular hypertension they can reduce the GFR in the poststenotic kidney.[15,35,37,38,41] There may be unacceptable worsening of azotemia if these drugs are given to patients with bilateral RAS or stenosis of a single or dominant kidney. Where the stenosis is critical, a sharp fall in blood pressure produced by any antihypertensive drug reduces the GFR.[23,42] Even the effects of Ang II on enhancing efferent arteriolar resistance cannot maintain the P_{Uf} of the glomerular capillaries in the presence of a tight stenosis and a sharp fall in arterial pressure.

Van de Ven et al[43] studied 108 patients at high risk for renovascular disease. All patients received a 2-week course of ACEI therapy. This increased the S_{Cr} by more than 20% in all 52 patients with severe bilateral RAS, providing volume retention was prevented by diuretic therapy. These authors proposed that a reversible increase in S_{Cr} could be used as a safe clinical test for bilateral renovascular disease. However, these interesting results also show that caution is needed when using ACEIs in patients with bilateral RAS and azotemia, especially during diuretic therapy.

Long-term studies over 6–24 months in a small number of patients with renovascular disease have shown that ACEI therapy is effective in reducing or normalizing BP, and does not lead (in the group as a whole) to progressive deterioration in renal function, or to a decrease in size of the poststenotic kidney.[44,45] In a worldwide study of 269 patients treated with captopril, 40% were azotemic before therapy and a similar fraction had either a solitary kidney or advanced bilateral renovascular disease.[46] Even within this latter group, clinically significant renal failure developed in only 12% during captopril therapy. Overall, there was good control of BP.

In another study, 75 patients with renovascular hypertension were randomized to triple therapy (hydrochlorothiazide, beta-blocker, and hydralazine), or to an ACEI and a diuretic. Antihypertensive control was clearly better in the group given an ACEI plus diuretic; some 80% of this group maintained their GFR over a mean follow-up period of 7.5 months. However, 10 patients – mostly with very high-grade RAS – had deterioration of renal function.[47]

In a 4-year study of patients with renovascular hypertension, Losito et al[48] found a cumulative survival of only 60%. Cerebrovascular and cardiovascular disease caused 92% of the deaths. A multivariate analysis identified treatment with ACEIs as the only factor associated with significantly better survival. Their observational data highlights once more the dilemma facing physicians using medical therapy for renovascular disease. Do the benefits from better control of hypertension and prevention of associated cardiovascular disease with ACEIs or ARBs outweigh the likely reduction in the GFR of the poststenotic kidney?

An important issue is whether reductions in the GFR of poststenotic kidneys in long-term ACEI-treated RAS patients leads to irreversible renal atrophy, as in the animal model.[22] In a study of split renal function in six patients with RAS, Miyamori et al[49] reported the individual kidney responses to 1 week and 1 year of captopril therapy (Fig. 60.4). After 1 week, the GFR of the poststenotic kidney was reduced, but renal plasma flow to the two kidneys was maintained or increased. These changes remained stable over 1 year. This study is reassuring because it shows that progressive loss of GFR leading to renal atrophy is quite

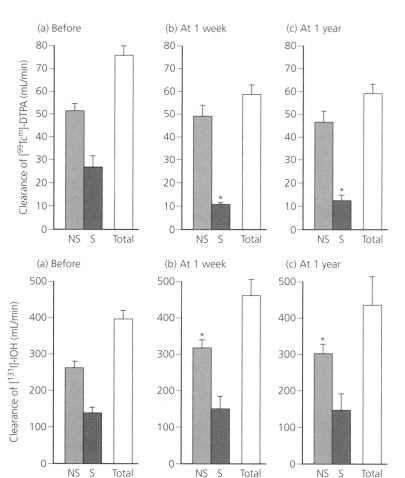

Figure 60.4 Mean ± SEM values from four patients with unilateral renal artery stenosis studied (a) before, (b) 1 week after, and (c) 1 year after starting therapy with captopril. Using split renal function for glomerular filtration rate and effective renal plasma flow, data were obtained for the overall function (Total) and individual functions in the nonstenotic (NS) and stenotic (S) kidneys. Compared with before *$P < 0.05$. (After Miyamori et al[49] with permission.)

unlikely in RAS patients treated with ACEIs. However, this conclusion may not hold for patients with high-grade RAS. The use of ACEIs and ARBs in hypertension is discussed in Chapter 55.

Conclusions and recommendations

The two controlled clinical trials in patients with renovascular disease have not shown any particular benefit of intervention over medical management for short term changes in blood pressure or renal function over 6–12 months.[8,27] This indicates that a short-term trial of medical management is a reasonable choice to initiate treatment of patients with newly diagnosed renovascular disease. There are no long-term comparisons between specific drugs in patients with renovascular disease; therefore, strong recommendations cannot be made. Nevertheless, as in other forms of hypertension, many patients benefit from a reduction in dietary salt intake and a low dose of diuretic. A reasonable goal for daily dietary salt intake is 100 mmol. It can be monitored by measuring 24-hour excretion of Na^+, even in patients who are on steady-state diuretic therapy, as renal excretion reflects current dietary intake. The trade-off hypothesis for beneficial and adverse effects of therapy with ACEIs or ARBs in patients with renovascular hypertension is summarized in Fig. 60.5.

The first step in planning prolonged treatment for patients with hypertension and atherosclerotic renovascular disease is initiation of a life-long regimen to improve blood-vessel structure and function, preventing cardiovascular disease. The appropriate choice of remedy depends on the clinical circumstances, concurrent disease, and identified cardiovascular risk factors (see Chapter 59). Consideration should be given to all patients for life-long therapy with low-dose aspirin (e.g. 80 mg once daily), three to four periods of exercise of 20–30 min each week, and a diet to limit intake of saturated fats and salt and, if necessary, lower body weight. If the patient is a current smoker, a therapeutic anti-smoking program must be a high priority. All patients require a lipid profile with correction of any identified increases in low-density lipoprotein (LDL) cholesterol and lipoprotein(a) with appropriate use of statins, slow-release nicotinic acid, or other treatments (see Chapter 67).

Nontraditional cardiovascular risk factors have been identified in patients with renal insufficiency.[50] These include hyperhomocystinemia, oxidative stress, and nitric oxide deficiency related to accumulation of asymmetric dimethyl arginine[51,52] (see Chapters 59, 68, and 69).

The next step is to initiate effective antihypertensive therapy for those in whom salt restriction and a low dose of diuretic are not sufficient. For patients with mild hypertension, administration of a beta-blocker, a calcium antagonist or central agent, or an alpha/beta-blocker, is often effective. In any subject who sustains a rapid reduction in BP, there may be a temporary decline in GFR with a rise of S_{Cr} and BUN. This usually peaks in 3–7 days and returns to baseline over the few weeks that follow. This is not normally an indication to withdraw or change treatment.

Once a steady-state antihypertensive regimen has been established, quantitative assessment should be made of blood pressure and renal structure and function. An automated BP-recorder should be prescribed, and the patient educated to record their blood pressure daily at home. Where this is impractical, or if there are persistent doubts about the validity of measurements, an ambulatory 24-hour blood pressure profile should be made. Renal function should be assessed by 24-hour measurement of urinary creatinine clearance and microalbumin excretion. Plasma renin activity should be measured. Kidney length should be quantified using renal ultrasound. Peak renal arterial blood flow velocity should be recorded by duplex Doppler velocimetry. These quantitative measures are used

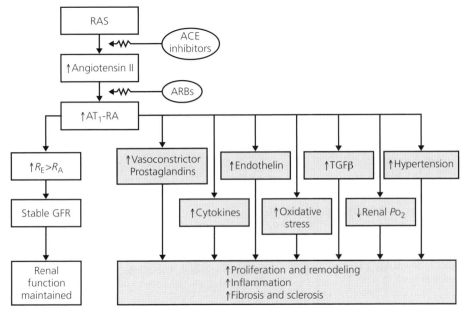

Figure 60.5 A diagrammatic representation of the contrasting effects of angiotensin converting enzyme inhibition (ACEI) or angiotensin receptor blocker (ARB) therapy in patients with renovascular disease. Such therapy reduces the glomerular filtration rate (GFR) due to the effect of angiotensin II (Ang II) increasing resistance of the efferent arteriole (R_E) compared to the afferent arteriole (R_A) of the poststenotic kidney. However, it counteracts many of the adverse mediators generated in response to Ang II action on type I receptors (AT_1-R) in blood vessels and kidneys. These include endothelin (ET), vasoconstrictor prostaglandins, transforming growth factor beta (TGF-β) and numerous cytokines, as well as physiologic changes related to hypertension, hypoxia and oxidative stress.

to establish whether the clinical course is stable or progressive. They should be repeated initially at 4 months, and later at every 6 months, or at any point at which there is evidence of deterioration in clinical state (e.g. deterioration in blood pressure control or development of azotemia). If these measurements remain stable, the physician can elect for a trial of therapy with an ACEI or ARB. It is ideal to quantify split renal function by nuclear renogram, prior to a trial of ACEI, to monitor the effects of therapy on the function of the individual kidneys. Patients developing a sharp rise in BUN and serum creatinine (> 25%) should be followed very carefully. Withdrawal of ACEI or ARB therapy is required if the rise does not abate in 5 or 10 days.

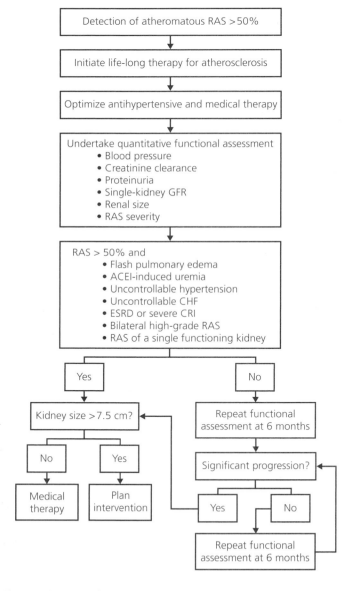

Patients who are established on medical therapy who do not have evidence of functional deterioration can often be managed by continued therapy under close medical supervision with regular quantitative assessments as indicated in Fig. 60.6. Those who require intervention with PTRA(S) or reconstructive surgery also require close follow-up using similar quantitative measures, since there is a high rate of restenosis, even in those treated by stenting, and a significant probability of developing a stenosis in the contralateral kidney.

There is a group of patients who either cannot be controlled adequately by medical therapy or who experience dangerous complications, such as recurrent flash pulmonary edema. There are others who have less to lose from a failed intervention, namely those who are already receiving dialysis therapy, or are very close to endstage renal disease. These are patients who may benefit from an intervention with PTRA(S) or reconstructive surgery. (This is discussed further in Chapters 61 and 62.)

The individual steps in the algorithm shown in Fig. 60.6 have not been subjected to properly controlled clinical trials. Therefore, they represent only an attempt at providing rational advice.

References

1. Textor SC, Wilcox CS: Ischemic nephropathy or azotemic renovascular disease. Semin Nephrol 2000;20:489–502.
2. Textor SC, Wilcox CS: Renal artery stenosis: A common, treatable cause of renal failure? Annu Rev Med 2001;52:421–442.
3. Textor SC: Renovascular disease: epidemiology and clinical presentation. Semin Nephrol 2000;20:426–431.
4. Simon G: What is critical renal artery stenosis? Am J Hypertens 2000;13:1189–1193.
5. Davidson RA, Barri Y, Wilcox CS: Predictors of cure of hypertension in fibromuscular renovascular disease. Am J Kidney Dis 1996;28:334–338.
6. Barri YM, Davidson RA, Senler S, et al: Prediction of cure of hypertension in atherosclerotic renal artery stenosis. South Med J 1996;89:679–683.
7. Caps MT, Zierler RE, Polissar NL, et al: Risk of atrophy in kidneys with artherosclerotic renal artery stenosis. Kidney Int 1998;53:735–742.
8. van Jaarsveld, B, Krijnen P, Pieterman H, et al: The effect of balloon angioplasty on hypertension in atherosclerotic renal artery stenosis. N Eng J Med 2000;342:1007–1014.
9. Chabova V, Schirger A, Stanson AW, et al: Outcomes of atherosclerotic renal artery stenosis managed without revascularization. Mayo Clin Proc 2000;75:437–444.
10. Wilcox CS, Cardozo J, Welch WJ: AT_1 and TxA_2 /PGH_2 receptors maintain hypertension throughout 2K,1C Goldblatt hypertension in the rat. Am J Physiol 1996;271:R891–R896.
11. Ploth DW: Angiotensin-dependent renal mechanisms in two-kidney, one-clip renal vascular hypertension. Am J Physiol 1983;14:F131–F141.
12. Huang WC, Ploth DW, Bell PD, et al: Bilateral renal function responses to converting enzyme inhibitor (SQ 20,881) in two-kidney, one clip Goldblatt hypertensive rats. Hypertension 1981;3:285–293.
13. Huang WC, Ploth DW, Navar LG: Angiotensin-mediated alterations in nephron function in Goldblatt hypertensive rats. Am J Physiol 1982;243:F553–F560.
14. Welch WJ: The pathophysiology of renin release in renovascular hypertension. Semin Nephrol 2000;20:394–401.
15. Miyamori I, Yasuhara S, Matsubara T, et al: Comparative effects of captopril and nifedipine on split renal function in renovascular hypertension. Am J Hypertens 1988;1:359–363.
16. Mimran A, Ribstein J, DuCailar G: Converting enzyme inhibitors and renal function in essential and renovascular hypertension. Am J Hypertens 1991;4:7S–14S.

Figure 60.6 An algorithm for the approach to medical management of patients with renovascular disease (ACEI, angiotensin-converting enzyme inhibitor; BP, blood pressure; CHF, congestive heart failure; CRF, chronic renal failure; ESRD, end-stage renal disease; GFR, glomerular filtration rate; RAS, renal artery stenosis).

17. Demeilliers B, Jover B, Mimran A: Contrasting renal effects of chronic administrations of enalapril and losartan on one-kidney, one-clip hypertensive rats. J Hypertens 1999;16:1023–1029.

18. Huelsemann JL, Sterzel RB, McKenzie DE, et al: Effects of a calcium entry blocker on blood pressure and renal function during angiotensin-induced hypertension. Hypertension 1985;7:374–379.

19. Carmines PK, Navar LG: Disparate effects of Ca channel blockade on afferent and efferent arteriolar responses to ANG II. Am J Physiol 1989;256:1015–1020.

20. Wenzel UO, Troschau G, Schoeppe W, et al: Adverse effect of the calcium channel blocker nitrendipine on nephrosclerosis in rats with renovascular hypertension. Hypertension 1992;20:233–241.

21. Veniant M, Heudes D, Clozel JP, et al: Calcium blockade versus ACE inhibition in clipped and unclipped kidneys of 2K,1C rats. Kidney Int 1994;46:421–429.

22. Jackson B, Franze L, Sumithran E, et al: Pharmacologic nephrectomy with chronic angiotensin converting enzyme inhibitor treatment in renovascular hypertension in the rat. J Lab Clin Med 1990;115:21–27.

23. Textor SC, Novick AC, Tarazi RC, et al: Critical perfusion pressure for renal function in patients with bilateral atherosclerotic renal vascular disease. Ann Int Med 1985;102:309–314.

24. Textor SC, Smith-Powell L: Post-stenotic arterial pressure, renal haemodynamics and sodium excretion during graded pressure reduction in conscious rats with one- and two-kidney coarctation hypertension. J Hypertens 1998;6:311–319.

25. JNC Committee: Sixth Report of the Joint National Committee on Prevention, Detection, Evaluation and Treatment of High Blood Pressure. Bethesda, MD: National Institutes of Health, 1997.

26. Wilcox CS: Use of angiotensin-converting-enzyme inhibitors for diagnosing renovascular hypertension. Kidney Int 1993;44:1379–1390.

27. Plouin PF, Chatellier G, Darne B, et al: blood pressure outcome of angioplasty in atherosclerotic renal artery stenosis: a randomized trial. Essai Multicentrique Medicaments vs Angioplastie (EMMA) Study Group. Hypertension 1998;1:823–829.

28. Xue F, Bettman MA, Langdon DR, et al: Outcome and cost comparison of percutaneous transluminal renal angioplasty, renal arterial stent placement, and renal arterial bypass grafting. Radiology 1999;212:378–384.

29. Watson PS, Hadjipetrou P, Cox SV, et al: Effect of renal artery stenting on renal function and size in patients with atherosclerotic renovascular disease. Circulation 2000;102:1671–1677.

30. Pickering TG, Herman L, Devereux RB, et al: Recurrent pulmonary oedema in hypertension due to bilateral renal artery stenosis: treatment by angioplasty or surgical revascularisation. Lancet 1988;2:551–552.

31. Wilcox CS, Mitch WE, Kelly RA, et al: The response of the kidney to furosemide. I. Effects of salt intake and renal compensation. J Lab Clin Med 1983;102:450–458.

32. Cianciaruso B., Bellizzi V, Minutolo R, et al: Renal adaptation to dietary sodium restriction in moderate renal failure resulting from chronic glomerular disease. J Am Soc Nephrol 1996;7:306–313.

33. Wilcox CS, Lewis PS, Peart WS, et al: Renal function, body fluid volumes, renin, aldosterone, and noradrenaline during treatment of hypertension with pindolol. J Cardiovasc Pharmacol 1981;3:598–611.

34. Converse RL Jr, Jacobsen TN, Toto RD, et al: Sympathetic overactivity in patients with chronic renal failure. N Engl J Med 1992;27:1912–1918.

35. Wilcox CS, Smith TB, Frederickson ED, et al: The captopril GFR renogram in renovascular hypertension. Clin Nucl Med 1988;14:1–7.

36. Wilcox CS, Loon NR, Ameer B, et al: Renal and hemodynamic responses to bumetanide in hypertension: effects of nitrendipine. Kidney Int 1989;36:719–725.

37. Ribstein J, Mourad G, Mimran A: Contrasting acute effects of captopril and nifedipine on renal function in renovascular hypertension. Am J Hypertens 1988;1:239–244.

38. Mourad G, Ribstein J, Argiles A, et al: Contrasting effects of acute angiotensin converting enzyme inhibitors and calcium antagonists in transplant renal artery stenosis. Nephrol Dial Transplant 1989;4:66–70.

39. Chapman AB, Gabow PA, Schrier RW: Reversible renal failure associated with angiotensin-converting enzyme inhibitors in polycystic kidney disease. Ann Intern Med 1991;15:769–773.

40. Toto RD, Mitchell HC, Lee HC, et al: Reversible renal insufficiency due to angiotensin converting enzyme inhibitors in hypertensive nephrosclerosis. Ann Intern Med 1991;115:513–519.

41. Textor SC, Tarazi RC, Novick AC, et al: Regulation of renal hemodynamics and glomerular filtration in patients with renovascular hypertension during convering enzyme inhibition with captopril. Am J Med 1984;76:29–37.

42. Textor SC, Novick AC, Steinmuller DR, et al: Renal failure limiting antihypertensive therapy as an indication for renal revascularization. Arch Intern Med 1983;143:2208–2211.

43. Van de Ven, PJG, Beutler JJ, Kaatee R, et al: Angiotensin converting enzyme inhibitor-induced renal dysfunction in atherosclerotic renovascular disease. Kidney Int 1998;3:986–993.

44. Arzilli F, Giovannetti R, Meola M, et al: ACE-inhibition vs surgical treatment in the outcome of ischmeic kidney of renovascular patients: a one year follow-up. High blood pressure 1992;1:47–50.

45. Fyhrquist F, Gronhagen-Riska C, Tikkanen I, et al: Long-term monotherapy with lisinopril in renovascular hypertension. J Cardiovasc Pharmacol 1987;9:S61–S65.

46. Hollenberg NK: Medical therapy of renovascular hypertension: efficacy and safety of captopril in 269 patients. Cardiovasc Res 1983;4:852–879.

47. Franklin SS, Smith RD: Comparison of effects of enalapril plus hydrochlorothiazide versus standard triple therapy on renal function in renovascular hypertension. Am J Med 1985;79:14–23.

48. Losito A, Gaburri M, Errico R, et al: Survival of patients with renovascular disease and ACE inhibition. Clin Nephrol 2000;52:339–343.

49. Miyamori I, Yasuhara S, Takeda Y, et al: Effects of converting enzyme inhibition on split renal function in renovascular hypertension. Hypertension 1986;8:415–421.

50. Kitiyakara C, Gonin J, Massy Z, et al: Non-traditional cardiovascular disease risk factors in end-stage renal disease: oxidative stress and hyperhomocysteinemia. Curr Opin Nephrol 2001;9:477–487.

51. Kielstein JT, Boger RH, Bode-Boger SM, et al: Asymmetric dimethylarginine plasma concentrations differ in patients with end-stage renal disease: relationship to treatment method and atherosclerotic disease. J Am Soc Nephrol 1999;10:594–600.

52. Miyazaki H, Matsuoka H, Cooke JP, et al: Endogenous nitric oxide synthase inhibitor: a novel marker of atherosclerosis. Circulation 1999;99:1141–1146.

Renovascular Hypertension and Ischemic Nephropathy: Angioplasty and Stenting

Stephen C. Textor and Michael McKusick

Introduction

Few problems pose more opportunities and challenges than decisions about whether to undertake revascularization for renal artery stenosis (RAS). Although minor degrees of stenosis may be detected "incidentally", high-grade RAS can lead to renovascular hypertension, which remains one of the most common secondary causes of hypertension, and to critical loss of renal perfusion in the form of "ischemic nephropathy," a potentially treatable form of progressive renal failure. Recent advances in detection and imaging of RAS, in medical therapy of hypertension, and in endovascular methods, including vascular stents, make this a rapidly changing field. The introduction of endovascular stents makes restoring renal circulation a realistic possibility in patients with ostial lesions who were previously considered at unacceptable risk for major surgical procedures.

The purpose of angioplasty with or without stenting is to restore blood flow and perfusion pressure to the kidney beyond a stenotic lesion. Fundamentally, this is intended to allow improved blood pressure control – in principle, to allow "cure" of renovascular hypertension – and to salvage kidney function beyond a "critical" RAS. While these goals seem simple enough, it is still difficult to identify individual patients with the greatest likelihood of obtaining benefit. Nephrologists in practice recognize that invasive renal vascular procedures present hazards even in the best of circumstances. Complications from atheroemboli,

contrast, and other adverse events sometimes worsen renal function and aggravate hypertension, such that renovascular procedures cannot be undertaken casually. Hence, the risks and benefits of each patient's situation require careful consideration.

Demographics of renovascular disease

Patients with fibromuscular diseases of the renal arteries are more commonly young and female, in contrast to those with atherosclerosis. The former constitute 16–20% of renovascular lesions referred for vascular procedures, at least for refractory hypertension. It should be emphasized that patients with fibromuscular disease usually have normal renal function and appear to be at low risk for progressive occlusive disease and renal functional loss.[1,2]

By contrast, the prevalence of RAS from atherosclerosis seems to be increasing with the advancing age of the US population.[3] Whether the true prevalence is increasing or whether older subjects are living longer and developing clinical manifestations of progressive renovascular occlusion is not known. What is certain, however, is that the mean ages of reported series of renal revascularization dating from the 1970s have increased to older ages by more than 15 years[4-13] (Fig. 61.1).

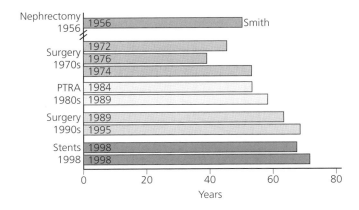

Figure 61.1 Mean ages of selected series of surgical (Nx, nephrectomy) or endovascular intervention for renal artery stenosis. Early data using unilateral nephrectomy are included as a reference point. The techniques available have changed, with a marked increase in the use of angioplasty and stenting in recent years. The ages and associated comorbid disease risks have increased considerably during this period. Reasons for the change in demographics include changes in survival from coronary disease and stroke, changes in medical therapy and the ability to intervene safely in patients considered at unacceptable risk in the past (see text).

As a result, patients with atherosclerosis have a longer background history of hypertension, and greater risk of comorbid disease (including diabetes, peripheral vascular, coronary, and carotid diseases) than ever before. It is recognized that atherosclerosis is a systemic disease and the likelihood of some degree of atherosclerosis affecting the kidney when it is detected elsewhere (e.g. during coronary or lower extremity angiography) is 30–50%.[14] The benefits and goals of renal revascularization, then, must be weighed up in the context of "competing" risk from other cardiovascular diseases. These competing risks sometimes offset the benefits of restoring the renal circulation in marginal cases.

Risks of disease progression

One of the compelling reasons to restore renal artery patency is the potential for untreated lesions to progress further, potentially to total occlusion and functional loss of the entire kidney. Such arguments have led to speculation that unsuspected renal artery occlusive disease may account for up to 14–20% of patients reaching endstage renal disease (ESRD), particularly Caucasians.[15,16] Recent Doppler studies conducted between 1990 and 1997 confirm that stenotic lesions can progress, as evidenced by increases in blood flow velocities over time (Fig. 61.2).[17] The likelihood of progression is directly related to the severity of the initial stenosis. Remarkably, total occlusion was observed in only 9/295 vessels (3%), fewer than had been reported in earlier angiographic series.[18] Whether progressive vascular stenosis by Doppler translates into clinical progression is less clear. Reports of incidentally detected, high-grade renal artery disease from The

Netherlands suggest that none later resulted in renal failure.[19] Follow-up studies of patients with incidental high-grade RAS (> 70% lumen affected), who were managed without revascularization during 1989–93 in the US, indicate that only 10–15% come to revascularization based upon progressive renal dysfunction or uncontrollable hypertension.[20] It must be emphasized that the hazards associated with RAS differ between unilateral disease (one kidney affected by stenosis, the other without stenosis) and bilateral disease (usually identified as high-grade stenosis to both kidneys, or stenosis to a solitary functioning kidney).[21] In the former, vascular progression, even to loss of one kidney, is buffered by a "spare" contralateral kidney. The change in renal function associated with unilateral disease therefore may be minor. In the instance of renal artery stenosis to the entire renal mass, however, progressive loss of blood supply threatens renal function overall, making renal failure, and circulatory congestion, or "flash" pulmonary edema genuine concerns.[22]

Understanding the true magnitude of progression risk is crucial to identifying the risk–benefit ratio regarding angioplasty and stenting. It is likely that current levels of disease progression will continue to fall. This may reflect more intense efforts at blood pressure control, smoking cessation, and intensive efforts to lower lipids with HMGCo-A reductase inhibitors.

Diagnostic considerations in renal artery disease

Most physicians in the US follow recommendations of the Joint National Commission (JNC) to minimize testing and focus on reduction of blood pressure after obtaining basic information.[23] With the widespread application of effective antihypertensive medications, including agents that interrupt the renin–angiotensin system, such as angiotensin-converting enzyme inhibitors (ACEIs) and angiotensin receptor blockers (ARBs), many individuals with RAS are treated effectively and are never detected. One result of this process is that most patients being considered for renal revascularization have been treated for hypertension for a long time and may be developing recognizable syndromes of progressive renovascular disease, as summarized in Table 61.1. Most of these include a combination of

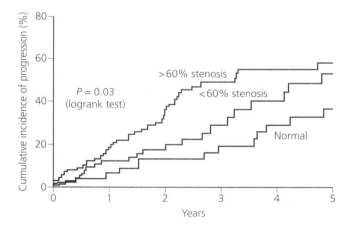

Figure 61.2 Rates of progressive vascular disease as evidenced by increased flow velocities in 295 arteries measured prospectively at 6-month intervals between 1990 and 1997. The probability of disease progression was related to the initial severity of stenosis, but remarkably few proceeded to total occlusion (9/295 vessels, or 3%). Estimates of change in vessel characteristics are higher than the number demonstrating clinical progression either in the form of intractable hypertension or by renal dysfunction (see text). (With permission from Caps et al[17])

Table 61.1 Clinical syndromes of renal artery stenosis

Asymptomatic
Incidental renal artery stenosis
Easily treated hypertension
Symptomatic
Treatment-resistant hypertension
Bilateral disease/solitary function kidney
Progressive renal failure in treated hypertension
Renal failure limiting antihypertensive therapy
Pulmonary vascular congestion – "flash" pulmonary edema
Endstage renal disease

resistance to antihypertensive therapy and/or deterioration of renal function. Often, these signal more severe stenoses or the development of bilateral disease in previously stable situations.

Diagnostic studies now focus primarily upon establishing whether (1) high-grade RAS is present, (2) it affects both kidneys or the entire functioning renal mass, and (3) it is amenable to endovascular repair and/or is associated with more widespread aortic disease, such as an abdominal aortic aneurysm. Biochemical studies to determine renin release and/or lateralization are less commonly performed than before. In many centers, angiography is reserved until these issues are resolved, with the intention of undertaking endovascular repair at the same sitting if needed. As a result, most individuals undergo some form of vascular staging, which may consist of Doppler ultrasound, captopril renography, and more recently, magnetic resonance angiography (MRA). The last is suitable for individuals with impaired renal function, using contrast without nephrotoxicity (gadolinium). Each of these methods has advantages and disadvantages,[24,25] some of which are specific to the institution in which they are performed (Fig. 61.3).

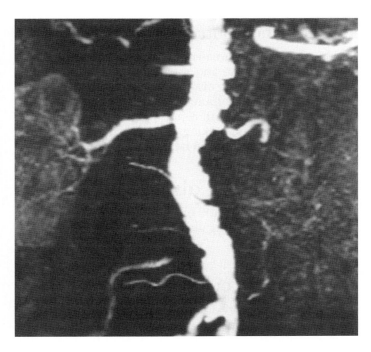

Figure 61.3 Magnetic resonance angiogram (MRA) in an 81-year-old woman with deteriorating renal function and accelerated hypertension. This study illustrates extensive aortic disease associated with high-grade stenoses of both renal arteries, and a delayed nephrogram in the left kidney. These images could be obtained without toxicity despite a serum creatinine level of 3.1 mg/dL because of the relative safety of gadolinium-based contrast.

Renal angioplasty and stenting

Goals of renal angioplasty and stenting

The goals of correcting RAS include (1) improving blood pressure levels, and (2) preservation of renal function. Note that these goals are distinct from whether or not "technical success" regarding restoring vessel patency is achieved.

Angioplasty alone has been advocated for fibromuscular disease affecting the renal arteries.[26] This disease often affects the mid-portion segments of the renal artery and may comprise "webs" with partial obstructive effects in series. Such individuals often have normal kidney function and may have clinical benefit more commonly than patients with parenchymal renal disease. It should be noted that occasionally fibromuscular disease and atherosclerosis may coexist and must be addressed separately.

Atherosclerosis commonly affects the proximal portion of the renal artery, particularly at the ostium. It may represent extension of an aortic plaque into the renal artery. Such lesions typically do not respond well to balloon angioplasty alone, and tend to recoil immediately after dilation. For that reason, stents have been employed to maintain vessel patency for ostial lesions. Randomized, prospective studies indicate that stents do, in fact, allow much improved primary patency of ostial renal artery stenoses.[27] Although in the US no stents are yet approved by the Food and Drug Administration (FDA) for use in the renal arteries, interventional radiologists and cardiologists commonly employ them for such lesions.

Techniques of renal angioplasty and stenting

Renal arteriography with angioplasty and stent placement should be performed in a peripheral vascular suite with digital-subtraction capability by an individual who is properly trained and skilled in percutaneous vascular intervention. In general, these procedures are done under i.v. conscious sedation from a transfemoral approach. Diagnostic arterial imaging is often performed at the same sitting as the therapeutic maneuvers. It is important to establish the baseline level of serum creatinine (S_{Cr}). For patients with chronic renal insufficiency, especially those who are diabetic, an alternative to iodinated contrast material for arteriography should be considered. Although regarded less good than traditional agents with respect to image quality, carbon dioxide (CO_2) and gadolinium provide sufficient enhancement for diagnostic imaging and intervention and lack the nephrotoxicity of iodine.[28]

Unless a preoperative MRA or computed tomography (CT) angiogram of good quality is available, it is best to proceed with a flush abdominal aortogram prior to selective renal arteriography. This overall view gives a global impression of the status of the patient's vascular system and an assessment of the relative risk of intervention. The presence of an aortic aneurysm, extent of atheromatous disease, kidney size, number of renal arteries, and the location and condition of the renal artery ostia are all well evaluated by the aortogram.

Selective renal images should include the origin of the renal artery as well as all peripheral branches. Lesions resulting in stenosis greater than 60% or 70% are generally considered hemodynamically significant and suitable for treatment. As a practical matter, if the appropriate patient has been chosen for arteriography, the offending lesion is usually obvious and little time need be spent on measuring gradients, or otherwise "quantifying" the percentage of stenosis.

Patients with fibromuscular dysplasia are treated with balloon angioplasty alone. Those with nonostial atheromatous disease are often ballooned first to see the response of simple PTRA, and stented only if needed. Reasons for stent placement include: residual stenosis visually greater than 20%, or pressure gradient of 5–10 mmHg measured with a side-hole catheter, or a flow-limiting dissection after PTRA. Stent placement is required in renal artery ostial disease because simple PTRA has been shown ineffective due to lesion recoil.[27] Stents should also be placed in the setting of restenosis following simple balloon angioplasty.

Following stent placement, a final selective renal artery image is helpful to document not only the stent position and improved lumen patency, but also preservation of distal branch filling and exclusion of peripheral embolization. The frequency of cholesterol and atheromatous debris embolization is unknown but may at least partially account for the worsened renal function found in up to 30% of azotemic patients after stent placement.[27,29]

Most patients should be placed on an antiplatelet agent for a month after renal artery stenting. Clopidogrel 75 mg/day is a potent regimen that has proven beneficial in preventing early restenosis in the coronary bed.[30] However, one aspirin daily (325 mg) is also effective and useful in the rare patient sensitive to clopidogrel, or in those patients for whom an open surgical procedure is required within a month.

Outcomes of renal artery angioplasty and stenting

Endovascular procedures are evaluated by considering the benefits regarding blood pressure control, renal function, and complications of the procedure.

Fibromuscular disease

As noted above, fibromuscular disease is much more common in women. "Technical success" is the rule and is reported to exceed 90% (Fig. 61.4) in patients attempted, although these lesions can be made more complicated if they extend beyond the renal artery bifurcations into segmental branches. Occasionally fibromuscular disease is associated with aneurysmal dilation, which does not benefit from angioplasty. Dilation of dysplastic webs occasionally leads to arterial dissection and/or occlusion of the small segmental vessels.

Blood pressure outcomes

Clinical effectiveness has been rated as high, with some patients needing no further antihypertensive medications (Table 61.2),[31,32] and many others needing less medication than before are considered "improved". As a result, many authors consider balloon angioplasty as standard therapy for fibromuscular disease when feasible. As noted by Aurell and Jensen,[31] Ramsay and Waller[33] and others, reported response rates to PTRA differ widely between studies and between different time periods. This may be the case for several reasons that are worth emphasizing:

1. Target blood pressure levels are changing, generally to lower levels. Earlier studies used criteria of achieved blood pressures < 160/95 mmHg, or simply diastolic pressure < 90 mmHg, whereas more recent targets seek to achieve blood pressure levels < 140/90 mmHg. Consequently, fewer patients are allowed to remain medication-free during long-term follow-up and therefore are not considered "cured".
2. Standards for measuring blood pressure and administering antihypertensive therapy are highly variable between studies. Therefore, interpretation of "benefit" is inconsistent.
3. Patient selection varies between studies, including such factors as duration of hypertension and urgency of intervention.

Renal function outcomes

Most patients with isolated fibromuscular disease have normal renal function and total arterial occlusion rarely develops. The lesions of medial fibroplasia, the most common variant of fibromuscular disease, rarely progress to produce renal insufficiency. Hence, there is little justification for undertaking balloon dilation of these lesions for preservation of renal function alone.

Atherosclerotic disease

The results of PTRA with or without stents for atherosclerosis are more ambiguous and merit close consideration.

Blood pressure outcomes

Much of the literature in this field is based upon retrospective, observational consideration of blood pressure levels recorded before and at intervals after the procedure, without standardization of conditions or antihypertensive therapy. Several summaries have been published comprising more than 1000 people subjected to PTRA, and more recently stenting. Some of these are summarized in Table 61.2. Lack of standard medical therapy, however, has led to reports of reduced "number of medications" with little regard for differences between medication regimens. This point deserves emphasis because three recent prospective,

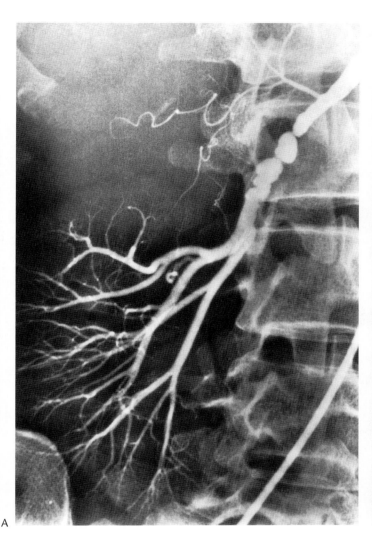
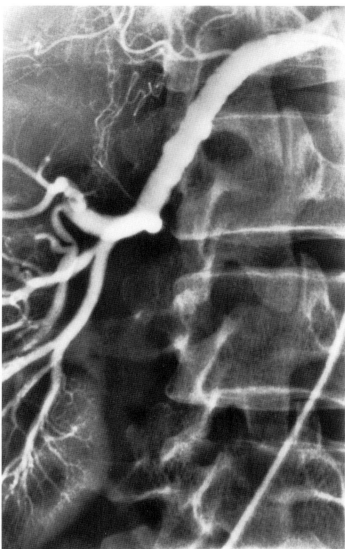

A   B

Figure 61.4 (A) and (B) show focal fibromuscular disease in the mid-portion of the left renal artery in a 42-year-old woman. Note that distal vessels are well preserved with normal renal function, but severe hypertension. This lesion was dilated successfully using percutaneous transluminal renal angioplasty with an excellent technical result (B) and clinical outcome.

randomized controlled trials (RCTs) comparing medical therapy of atherosclerotic renal artery disease with PTRA, in which therapy and blood pressure measurement were standardized, found only minor blood pressure benefits from PTRA. The major features of these prospective RCTs are summarized in Table 61.3.[34–36] These studies were small, and limited by patient selection, but they underscore the effectiveness of current drug regimens and the relative infrequency of "cure" in patients with atherosclerosis. All of these were limited in size and excluded many patients with (1) progressive renal dysfunction, (2) accelerated hypertensive disease, or (3) recent cardiovascular events.

The largest of these studies was published in 2000 as the DRASTIC study (Dutch RAS Intervention Cooperative Study Group). It included 106 patients with relatively resistant hypertension, randomized to either medical

therapy or PTRA. The lack of difference in blood pressure after 1 year between patients treated with PTRA and those treated medically led the authors to conclude that "angioplasty has little advantage over antihypertensive drug therapy".[36] This study was analyzed under "intention to treat" statistical rules, in which 22/50 patients assigned to medical therapy (44%) crossed over to the PTRA arm due to uncontrolled blood pressure levels at 3 months. Despite the inclusion of this group in the medical arm, many authorities reviewing the data might argue that they offer compelling evidence of medical treatment failure in some instances, and the benefit of the renal revascularization for such individuals.

However, the ambiguity of these recent studies highlights differences between medical practice now as compared with 20 years ago. In the era before the arrival of potent

Table 61.2 Outcomes of percutaneous transluminal renal angioplasty and stenting (PTRAS)*

Fibromuscular disease

Blood pressure	"Cured"	Improved	Failed
Aurell (n = 245)	42.4%	36.2%	21.4%
Bonelli (n = 105)	22%	41%	37%

Atherosclerotic disease

Blood pressure	"Cured"	Improved	Failed
Stent (n = 678)	20%	49%	31%
PTRA (n = 644)	10%	53%	37%

Renal function	"Improved"	Stable	Worse
Stent (n = 678)	30%	38%	32%
PTRA (n = 674)	38%	49%	21%
Surgery (n = 733)	25–30%	45–50%	20–25%

*Summary of recent published outcomes of PTRAS for fibromuscular and atherosclerotic renal artery stenosis. Interpretation of these reports must be considered in the context of highly variable definitions of "cure" and "improved" blood pressure responses, which lead to high variability between reports (see text).[31–33] Results in patients with atherosclerosis are generally worse than those with fibromuscular disease. The results with PTRAS are adapted from a recent metaanalysis of published series.[49]

Table 61.3 Summarized comparison of medical therapy and percutaneous transluminal renal angioplasty in atherosclerotic renal artery stenosis*

References	Number of subjects	Features	Outcome
Webster et al[34]	55 (Unilateral = 27)	Run-medical treatment	No differences in BP, renal function, or survival ?Crossover?
Plouin et al[35]	49 (All unilateral)	Multicenter Ambulatory BP at 6 months No ACE inhibitors	No difference in BP Slightly fewer medicines used in PTRA group More complications Crossover in medical therapy 7/26 (27%)
van Jaarsveld et al[36]	106	Multicenter Office and automated BP Lateralization studies (scan, renal vein renin)	No difference in BP at 12 months Crossover in medical therapy 22/50 (44%)

*Summary of three recent prospective, randomized controlled trials. These series were limited to selected groups of patients, but had the benefit of careful prospective use of antihypertensive medications, standardized blood pressure measurement and definitions of outcomes. The results of these trials were less dramatic than those of observational reports.

antihypertensives, capable of blocking the renin–angiotensin system and/or calcium channel blocking drugs, renovascular hypertension commonly presented as refractory to treatment, with accelerated or malignant-phase manifestations. Reports from emergency departments suggested that nearly 30% of hypertensive emergencies in white people were derived from individuals with renovascular hypertension. Some of these were refractory to therapy with the agents then available and suffered recurrent episodes of malignant hypertension, leading to occasional bilateral nephrectomy as a life-saving measure.[37] With the introduction of more effective and tolerable antihypertensive regimens, particularly those capable of blocking activation of the renin–angiotensin system, inability to control blood pressure is far less often the motivation for renal revascularization.[38] What must be considered in each case, of course, is whether the limits of antihypertensive therapy have been reached and whether progressive occlusive disease poses a hazard for the individual in question.

Renal function outcomes

Some authors argue that the primary motivation for renal revascularization is now "preservation of renal function".[39] This premise is based upon (1) the potential for progressive loss of renal function beyond critical levels of RAS and (2) the possibility of restoring blood flow with effective procedures, including the use of stents. Dramatic proof of this concept is available from case studies of individual patients with advanced renal insufficiency regaining viable kidney function after successful PTRA or surgery.[40,41] In some instances, this has meant removal from dialysis dependence to adequate endogenous renal function. Few experiences are more rewarding to nephrologists than the restorating independent renal function to someone previously requiring dialytic support. Even when advanced renal dysfunction is not present, it is sometimes prudent to revascularize the kidney to protect it from future progressive vascular occlusion. An example of this is illustrated in Fig. 61.5 and Fig. 61.6.

This argument is tempered by review of the available data, however. Review of renal functional outcomes in several recent series is summarized in Table 61.2. Remarkably, group mean measures of renal function, as reflected by S_{Cr}, are rarely changed by renal revascularization, with either surgery or PTRA. Mean values obscure several distinctly different outcomes, however, as we have recently reviewed.[29] Some patients experience major improvements in renal function (20–25%). Most have no detectable change in function (50%). Unfortunately, the first group is offset by a substantial fraction (15–22%) who rapidly lose

renal function after revascularization procedures.

Results in the latter group remain the "Achilles heel" of general application of renal revascularization. One must reckon with the possibility that nearly one in five subjects will lose renal function, sometimes drastically, as a result of the procedure. The precise reasons for this are not well understood, although it is agreed that atheroemboli commonly develop within the renal parenchyma, sometimes producing irreversible renal injury.[42,43] Importantly, adverse renal outcomes may not be apparent immediately after a seemingly successful revascularization procedure; in fact they may only unfold over the following days or weeks. Patients who follow this course have a far worse prognosis, in terms of both renal and patient survival, than those who do not.[44,45] Hence, the clinician must weigh the potential hazards of an adverse outcome of renal revascularization against the true potential for disease progression, and/or adverse events from uncontrolled hypertension.

Until now it has been difficult to predict who will gain from renal revascularization procedures. It is accepted that greatly advanced renal dysfunction (S_{Cr} above 3.0 mg/dL) is an adverse sign, as are small kidneys (less than 7 cm in length). Recent studies using Doppler "resistive index"

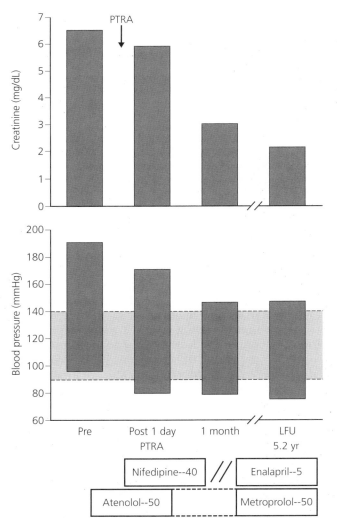

Figure 61.5 Blood pressure (BP) and serum creatinine (S_{Cr}) levels in a patient with bilateral renal artery stenosis treated with percutaneous transluminal renal angioplasty. BP control improved during more than 5 years of follow-up (LFU), although medication was still required, including an ACE inhibitor. Most importantly, far advanced renal dysfunction ($S_{Cr} > 6$ mg/dL) improved, avoiding need for renal replacement therapy. Although not uniformly observed, such cases establish the concept that angioplasty and stenting can provide major clinical benefits in selected cases. (Adapted from Textor and Wilcox[53] with permission.)

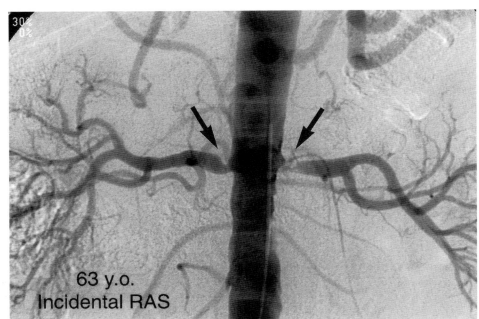

A

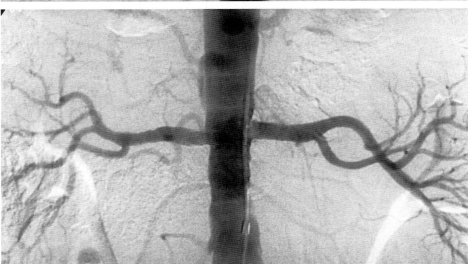

B

Figure 61.6 (A) Bilateral ostial atherosclerotic disease in a 63-year-old man, first detected incidentally, then later associated with accelerated hypertension. (B) Post-stent films indicate excellent vessel patency despite their proximal location, which would previously have made them unlikely to remain patent after percutaneous transluminal renal angioplasty alone.

suggest that high vascular resistance within the post-stenotic kidney is an adverse sign also.[46] The duration and rapidity of onset of renal dysfunction appear to be relevant factors, although these are difficult to quantify. Some individuals appear to have preserved renal parenchyma via capsular arteries and have been successfully restored to viable renal function after years on dialysis, although this is rare.

Complications of angioplasty and stenting

Procedure-related complications from PTRA intervention without or with stenting (PTRAS) are common, usually clinically insignificant, and directly proportional to the experience and skill of the operator.[47] During these procedures, a variety of untoward events can occur, related to catheter insertion and aortoiliac manipulation, guidewire and catheter negotiation of the renal artery and branches, balloon angioplasty and stent placement itself, and adverse affects of contrast material on renal function. Some of these are summarized in Table 61.4.

Groin hematoma following renal PTA and stent placement probably occurs in at least 20% of patients but is most often only a nuisance. False aneurysms of the common femoral artery occur far less frequently and are now readily treated with ultrasound compression or thrombin injection. More serious is cholesterol or atheromatous embolization of either the lower extremities or kidneys, which can occur in as many as 10% of patients.[48] This can lead to a permanent reduction in renal function, or even death.

Review of data from the Mayo Clinic in Rochester, MN during a 3-year period (1997–2000) indicates an overall major complication rate of 7.5% per attempted procedure in 140 consecutive patients. No deaths were directly

Table 61.4 Complications of percutaneous transluminal renal angioplasty and stenting

Most common
Groin hematoma
Contrast toxicity
Renal artery dissection
Segmental infarction/thrombosis

Most severe
Cholesterol embolism
Cerebral hemorrhage
Bowel infarction

Vascular events
Iliac artery dissection
Aortic dissection
Peripheral atheroemboli

Miscellaneous
Sepsis
Stent migration
Perinephric hematoma

attributable to renal PTRAS. Complications included renal artery rupture in 2%, partial kidney infarction in 2.7%, transient or permanent elevation of serum creatinine of 20% or more in 9.5%, procedure-induced requirement of hemodialysis in 2.7%, and blood transfusion in 2.7%.

As serious as these complications were, it is noteworthy that none of these patients required open surgical rescue. In fact, stents allowed treatment of balloon-induced renal artery rupture, or wire perforation, and renal artery dissection, without surgical intervention. From this standpoint renal artery stent placement is probably safer than balloon angioplasty alone. These data are supported by observations from a metaanalysis comparing 678 patients after renal artery stent placement and 644 patients treated with PTRA alone. The authors concluded that technical success, vessel patency rates, and restenosis were improved by the use of stents. Remarkably, the clinical outcomes in the short term (6–15 months) were no different between stent-treated and PTRA-alone groups.[49]

Restenosis

Although implantable metallic stents have expanded the population of patients eligible for PTRA(S) intervention, restenosis rates remain substantial. A recent metaanalysis of 14 published series reporting on a total of 678 patients revealed an angiographically proved mean restenosis rate of 17% (range 0% to 39%) during a follow-up period that ranged from 6 to 29 months.[49] As might be expected, restenosis is at least partially related to renal artery size. Henry et al[50] reported restenosis in 17.6% of stents less than or equal to 5 mm in diameter, while those 6 mm or larger had a 10.2% rate. This limits the use of these devices in patients with multiple smaller renal arteries or severely atrophic kidneys (Fig. 61.7). These rates also temper the enthusiasm for stent placement in "incidental" lesions of

marginal clinical significance. In such cases, the probability of requiring reintervention for restenosis may exceed the actual probability of progressive disease needing intervention at all.[20]

Restenosis can usually be detected clinically, although periodic Doppler ultrasound can be useful to evaluate persistent vessel patency and detect in-stent stenosis.[51] The decision to redilate should be based upon the clinical response to the initial intervention. Secondary patency rates are well over 85% and usually do not require additional stent placement. The overall costs of additional intervention are not trivial, however, and need to be factored into the treatment equation.

Selection of patients for percutaneous transluminal renal angioplasty and stenting

As should be apparent from the previous section, selection for endovascular renal revascularization involves a considered judgement of risks and benefits for each patient. There is sufficient ambiguity that randomized, prospective trials are being planned to better define these issues. Until

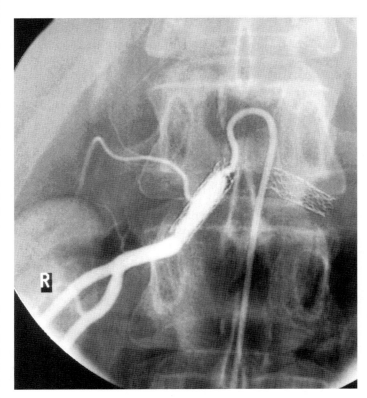

Figure 61.7 Angiogram demonstrating development of restenosis within an endovascular stent, and development of a stenotic lesion at the distal portion of the stent. The latter may relate to movement of the kidney relative to a fixed stent. Such lesions may account for worsening hypertension and declining renal function, and may require repeat intervention. Rates of restenosis currently appear to be 14–20% within the first year.

results from such trials are available, clinicians will continue to apply their best judgement to individual cases.

Several points merit re-emphasis in this regard: patients with unilateral renovascular disease with reasonable blood pressure control and stable kidney function may gain little from vascular procedures; most will continue to need anti-hypertensive therapy. Every effort should be directed to medical management of their condition, including limiting atherosclerosis by using statin-class drugs, and meticulous control of blood pressure and risk factors, such as cessation of smoking.

There is a particular risk for patients with bilateral disease (or stenosis to a solitary functioning kidney) of both deterioration of renal function, and unsatisfactory blood pressure control, with medical management alone.[20] It should be emphasized that a recent study indicating benefits to renal function after endovascular stenting was limited to patients with stenosis affecting the entire functioning renal mass.[52] While many individuals with bilateral disease can be managed without clinical evidence of progression, they may have more to gain from successful renal revascularization than other groups, although this has not been proven.

Many patients fall between these limits, with relatively stable blood pressure and kidney function, but who are at risk for progressive disease and have extensive comorbid risk factors. Such individuals merit close follow-up and reconsideration based upon demonstrated vascular progression. In this respect, RAS is analogous to other vascular lesions, such as an abdominal aneurysm or carotid stenoses, both of which may exist for many years without posing a true hazard. Evidence of progression may be the critical determinant of who will gain the most from angioplasty or stenting in the kidney also.

Summary

The endovascular techniques of angioplasty and stenting offer effective alternatives for restoring renal blood flow to a wider group of patients than ever before. Interventional procedures should be considered for patients with progressive hypertension and/or loss of renal parenchymal function due to renal artery lesions. There is a potential for recurrence (restenosis) and for serious adverse effects, although these are not common. Most importantly, for best results, clinicians need to balance the potential for true benefit against the potential for adverse effects.

References

1. Textor SC: Renal artery disease: epidemiology and clinical presentation. Semin Nephrol 2000;20:426–431.
2. Bloch MJ, Pickering T: Renal vascular disease: medical management, angioplasty and stenting. Semin Nephrol 2000;20:474–488.
3. Schneider E, Guralnik J: The aging of America: impact on health care costs. JAMA 1990;263:2335–2340.
4. Smith HW: Unilateral nephrectomy in hypertensive diseases. J Urol 1956;76:685–701.
5. Lazarus JM, Hampers CL, Bennett AH, et al: Urgent bilateral nephrectomy for severe hypertension. Ann Intern Med 1972;76:733–739.
6. Graham RM, Sebel EF, Stokes GS: Surgical intervention in severe and complicated renal hypertension: Report of the Sydney Renal Hypertension Group (1969–1975). Clin Sci Molec Med 1976;51:231S–233S.
7. Hunt JC, Sheps SG, Harrison EG, et al: Renal and renovascular hypertension: a reasoned approach to diagnosis and management. Arch Int Med 1974;133:988–999.
8. Tegtmeyer CJ, Kellum CD, Ayers C: Percutaneous transluminal angioplasty of the renal artery: results and long-term follow-up. Radiology 1984;153: 77–84.
9. Canzanello VJ, Millan VG, Spiegel JE, et al: Percutaneous transluminal renal angioplasty in management of atherosclerotic renovascular hypertension: results in 100 patients. Hypertension 1989;13:163–172.
10. Hallett JW, Fowl R, O'Brien PC, et al: Renovascular operations in patients with chronic renal insufficiency: do the benefits justify the risks? J Vasc Surg 1987;5:622–627.
11. Hallett JW, Textor SC, Kos PB, et al: Advanced renovascular hypertension and renal insufficiency: trends in medical comorbidity and surgical approach from 1970 to 1993. J Vasc Surg 1995;21:750–759.
12. Dorros G, Jaff M, Mathiak L, et al: Four-year follow-up of Palmaz-Schatz stent revascularization as treatment for atherosclerotic RAS. Circulation 1998;98:642–647.
13. Tuttle KF, Chouinard RF, Webber JT, et al: Treatment of atherosclerotic ostial RAS with the intravascular stent. Am J Kidney Dis 1998;32:611–622.
14. Jaff MR, Olin JW: Atherosclerotic stenosis of the renal arteries. Tex Heart Inst J 1998;25: 34–39.
15. Greco BA, Breyer JA: The natural history of RAS: who should be evaluated for suspected ischemic nephropathy? Semin Nephrol 1996;16:2–11.
16. Scoble JE: The epidemiology and clinical manifestations of atherosclerotic renal disease. In Novick AC, Scoble J, Hamilton G (eds): Renal Vascular Disease. London: WB Saunders Co Ltd, 1996, pp 303–314.
17. Caps MT, Perissinotto C, Zierler RE, et al: Prospective study of atherosclerotic disease progression in the renal artery. Circulation 1998;98:2866–2872.
18. Schreiber MJ, Pohl MA, Novick AC: The natural history of atherosclerotic and fibrous renal artery disease. Urolog Clin N Amer 1984;11:383–392.
19. Leertouwer TC, Pattynama PMT, van den Berg-Huysmans A: Incidental RAS in peripheral vascular disease: a case for treatment? Kidney Int 2001;59:1480–1483.
20. Chabova V, Schirger A, Stanson AW, et al: Outcomes of atherosclerotic RAS managed without revascularization. Mayo Clin Proc 2000;75:437–444.
21. Bloch MJ, Trost DW, Pickering TG, et al: Prevention of recurrent pulmonary edema in patients with bilateral renovascular disease through renal artery stent placement. Am J Hypertens 1999;12:1–7.
22. Hricik DE, Browning PJ, Kopelman R, et al: Captopril-induced functional renal insufficiency in patients with bilateral renal-artery stenosis or renal-artery stenosis in a solitary kidney. N Engl J Med 1983;308:377–381.
23. JNC Committee: Sixth Report of the Joint National Committee on Prevention, Detection, Evaluation and Treatment of High Blood Pressure. Bethesda, MD: National Institutes of Health, 1997.
24. King BF: Diagnostic imaging evaluation of renovascular hypertension. Abdom Imaging 1995;20:395–405.
25. Safian RD, Textor SC: Medical progress: RAS. N Engl J Med 2001;344:431–442.
26. Tegtmeyer CJ, Selby JB, Hartwell GD, et al: Results and complications of angioplasty in fibromuscular disease. Circulation 1991;83(suppl.):I155–I161.
27. van de Ven PJ, Kaatee R, Beutler JJ, et al: Arterial stenting and balloon angioplasty in ostial atherosclerotic renovascular disease: a randomised trial. Lancet 1999;353:282–286.
28. Spinosa DJ, Hagspiel KD, Angle JF, et al: Gadolinium-based contrast agents in angiography and interventional radiology: uses and techniques. J Vasc Inter Radiol 2000;11:985–990.
29. Textor SC, Wilcox CS: RAS: a common, treatable cause of renal failure? Ann Rev Med 2001;52:421–442.
30. Taniuchi M, Kurz HI, La Sala JM: Randomized comparison of ticlodipine and clopidogrel after intracoronary stent implantation in a broad patient population. Circulation 2001;104:539–543.

31. Aurell M, Jensen G: Treatment of renovascular hypertension. Nephron 1997;75:373–383.
32. Bonelli FS, McKusick MA, Textor SC, et al: Renal artery angioplasty: technical results and clinical outcome in 320 patients. Mayo Clinic Proc 1995;70:1041–1052.
33. Ramsay LE, Waller PC: Blood pressure response to percutaneous transluminal angioplasty for renovascular hypertension: an overview of published series. Br Med J 1990;300:569–572.
34. Webster J, Marshall F, Abdalla M, et al: Randomised comparsion of percutaneous angioplasty vs continued medical therapy for hypertensive patients with atheromatous RAS. J Hum Hypertens 1998;12:329–335.
35. Plouin PF, Chatellier G, Darne B, et al: Blood pressure outcome of angioplasty in atherosclerotic RAS: a randomized trial. Hypertension 1998;31:822–829.
36. Van Jaarsveld BC, Krijnen P, Pieterman H, et al: The effect of balloon angioplasty on hypertension in atherosclerotic renal artery stenosis. N Engl J Med 2000;342:1007–1014.
37. Bennett AH, Lazarus JM: Bilateral nephrectomy performed on an emergency basis for life-threatening malignant hypertension. Surg Gynecol Obstet 1973;137:451–452.
38. Pohl MA: Medical management of renovascular hypertension. *In* Novick A, Scoble J, Hamilton G (eds): Renal Vascular Disease. London: WB Saunders Co Ltd, 1996, pp 339–349.
39. Schreiber MJ, Pohl MA, Novick AC: Preserving renal function by revascularization. Ann Rev Med 1990;41:423–429.
40. Kaylor WM, Novick AC, Ziegelbaum M, et al: Reversal of endstage renal failure with surgical revascularization in patients with atherosclerotic renal artery occlusion. J Urol 1989;141:486–488.
41. Hansen KJ, Thomason RB, Craven TE, et al: Surgical management of dialysis-dependent ischemic nephropathy. J Vasc Surg 1995;21:197–209.
42. Meyrier A, Hill GW, Simon P: Ischemic renal diseases: new insights into old entities. Kidney Int 1998;54:2–13.
43. Thadhani RI, Camargo CA, Xavier RJ, et al: Atheroembolic renal failure after invasive procedures: Natural history based on 52 histologically proven cases. Medicine 1995;74:350–358.
44. Hansen KJ, Cherr GS, Craven TE, et al: Management of ischemic nephropathy: Dialysis-free survival after surgical repair. J Vasc Surg 2000;32:472–482.
45. Textor SC: Revascularization in atherosclerotic renal artery disease. Kidney Int 1998;53:799–811.
46. Radermacher J, Chavan A, Bleck J, et al: Use of Doppler ultrasonography to predict the outcome of therapy for renal-artery stenosis. N Engl J Med 2001;344:410–417.
47. Palmaz JC: The current status of vascular intervention in ischemic nephropathy. J Vasc Intervent Radiol 1998;9:539–543.
48. Beek FJ, Kaatee R, Beutler JJ, van der Ven PJ, Mali WP: Complications during renal artery stent placement for atherosclerotic ostial stenosis. Cardiovasc Intervent Radiol 1997;20:184–190.
49. Leertouwer TC, Gussenhoven EJ, Bosch JP, et al: Stent placement for renal arterial stenosis: where do we stand? A meta-analysis. Radiology 2000;216:78–85.
50. Henry M, Amor M, Henry I, et al: Stents in the treatment of RAS: long-term follow-up. J Endovasc Surg 1999;6:42–51.
51. Tullis MJ, Zierler RE, Glickerman DJ, et al: Results of percutaneous transluminal angioplasty for atherosclerotic RAS: a follow-up study with duplex ultrasonography. J Vasc Surg 1997;25:46–54.
52. Watson PS, Hadjipetrou P, Cox SV, et al: Effect of renal artery stenting on renal function and size in patients with atherosclerotic renovascular disease. Circulation 2001;102:1671–1677.
53. Textor SC, Wilcox CS: Ischemic nephropathy/azotemic renovascular disease. Semin Nephrol 2000;20:489–502.

Surgical Treatment of Renovascular Hypertension and Ischemic Nephropathy

David A. Goldfarb and Andrew C. Novick

Surgical renal revascularization is well established for treating patients with renovascular hypertension (RVH), ischemic nephropathy, or both. A variety of factors must be assessed to determine if surgical treatment is appropriate for a given patient. These include the causal relationship of renal vascular disease to hypertension, the adequacy of blood pressure control with medical therapy, the natural history of untreated renal vascular disease with attention to the risk of renal functional impairment, the medical condition of the patient, and the known results of surgical therapy and other interventions such as percutaneous transluminal renal angioplasty (PTRA) or renal artery stents.

Indications for surgical treatment

Renovascular hypertension

The coexistence of hypertension and renal artery disease does not always imply a causal relationship between the two. Renal artery disease is far more common than renovascular hypertension. Classically, renovascular hypertension is a retrospective diagnosis made when hypertension resolves after intervention to correct a renal artery lesion. It now commonly refers to renin-mediated hypertension as a result of renal artery disease. Clinical clues that suggest renovascular hypertension include age of < 30 or > 50 years, abrupt onset and short duration of hypertension, the presence of extrarenal vascular disease, end-organ damage, such as left ventricular hypertrophy or high-grade hypertensive retinopathy, a systolic–diastolic abdominal bruit, and deterioration of renal function in response to angiotensin-converting enzyme inhibitors (ACEIs).

In patients with a moderate clinical suspicion for RVH, a number of noninvasive tests have been developed that identify patients with RVH and help to predict the outcome of interventions. The response of peripheral plasma renin to administration of an ACEI is a simple test with acceptable accuracy for identifying patients with RVH.[1] Conditions for this test must be carefully controlled, and no information on individual kidney function is obtained. The most useful test to identify patients with RVH is ACEI renography.[2] After administration of an ACEI, changes in the renogram curve predict successfully the blood pressure response to intervention in nearly 90% of patients with a positive test. Differential renal vein renin studies which require cannulation of the vena cava have largely been replaced by less invasive procedures such as ACEI renography.

For patients with RVH due to fibrous dysplasia, candidacy for surgical intervention is guided by the specific pathology, as determined by angiographic findings and its associated natural history.[3] Medical management of medial fibroplasia is the initial approach because loss of renal function from progressive obstruction is uncommon, and intervention is reserved for patients with difficult-to-control hypertension. Renal artery disease due to intimal or perimedial fibroplasia is often associated with progressive obstruction that can result in ischemic renal atrophy. Therefore, early intervention is recommended to improve blood pressure control and to preserve renal function.

The known results of PTRA are important in assessing the need for surgery in patients with fibrous dysplasia. The technical and clinical success rates of PTRA for fibrous disease of the main renal artery are 90–95%[4] – no different from results obtainable with surgery.[5,6] Nonetheless, up to 30% of patients may present with branch disease, or an aneurysm that is not amenable for PTRA. Surgery is then reserved for patients with peripheral, complex branch disease, or for those who have failed PTRA.

Renal artery aneurysms may require repair if they result in significant hypertension, or to prevent rupture when they are > 2 cm and noncalcified.[5] This is a particular concern in women of reproductive age because aneurysms have a tendence to rupture during pregnancy.

For patients with atherosclerosis and RVH, the indications for intervention are more limited because of the frequent presence of concomitant extrarenal vascular disease. More vigorous attempts at medical management for this group is warranted. Surgical revascularization is reserved for those patients whose hypertension cannot be satisfactorily controlled with medication, or when renal function becomes threatened by advanced vascular disease. While PTRA is associated with a successful blood pressure result for nonostial atherosclerosis, the long-term success rate with ostial lesions is poor, because of a higher incidence of restenosis.[7] Surgical revascularization is useful for patients with RVH and ostial atherosclerosis.

Ischemic nephropathy

Recent epidemiological studies suggest that atherosclerotic renovascular disease is quite common in patients with generalized atherosclerosis obliterans, regardless of the presence of renovascular hypertension.[8] The development of chronic renal insufficiency from atherosclerotic renal artery disease, known as ischemic nephropathy, has become an important clinical issue, which is separate and distinct from the problem of RVH. Knowledge of the natural history of atherosclerotic renal artery disease permits identification of patients at risk for ischemic nephropathy.[3] Those at highest risk are patients with high-grade stenosis (> 75%) involving the entire renal mass (bilateral disease, or disease in a solitary kidney). Intervention in these patients is for the purpose of preservation of renal function. Many of these patients are older, with diffuse extrarenal vascular disease, and ostial renal artery disease. This is a group of patients where the results of PTRA have been disappointing and surgical revascularization can be performed safely and successfully.[9,10] The outcomes of renal function after surgery for ischemic nephropathy are depicted in Table 62.1.

Long-term survival of these patients has been recently assessed.[11] In 222 patients operated on from 1974 to 1987 the 5-year patient survival was 81% and was comparable to the age-matched general population. The 10-year survival was 53% and lower than the expected age-matched survival. Long-term stabilization or improvement in renal function was achieved in 71.3% of patients. The most important factors, corresponding to diminished survival, included age > 60 years, coronary artery disease, and previous vascular operations. These outcomes substantiate the effectiveness of the surgical approach.

Clinical clues suggesting ischemic nephropathy include azotemia (unexplained, or in association with ACEI treatment), diminished renal size, and the presence of vascular disease in other sites (cerebrovascular disease, coronary artery disease, or peripheral vascular disease). Azotemic patients with clinical suspicion for the disease are screened with duplex ultrasonography of the renal arteries.[12] This technique, used successfully by many centers, allows identification of patients with 0–59% stenosis, 60–99% stenosis, and total occlusion. Angiography can then be applied selectively to those patients with > 60% stenosis, avoiding a contrast study in patients with a low likelihood of disease.

When considering a patient for revascularization, the potential for renal salvability must be determined.[13] The testing for this aims to identify the presence of severe underlying renal parenchymal disease, in which case restoration of renal blood flow would not result in recovery of renal function. Successful revascularization usually results when the affected kidney size is > 9 cm, and demonstrates some evidence of function (usually assessed by isotopic renal scan). Total occlusion of the renal artery is not a contraindication for repair as the viability of the kidney can be maintained by a collateral circulation that can be seen by angiography. Patients with mild-to-moderate renal dysfunction are acceptable surgical candidates; however, surgical revascularization is generally not worthwhile for patients with advanced azotemia (S_{Cr} > 4.0 mg/dL) owing to the presence of significant underlying renal parenchymal disease. An exception to this rule is the small number of patients with significant renal functional impairment and bilateral total renal artery occlusion, where one or both kidneys remain viable on the basis of collateral circulation.[14] Such kidneys otherwise meet the criteria for revascularization (i.e. adequate size and minimal parenchymal disease). While such a presentation is uncommon, these patients can have favorable outcomes with surgical revascularization. Finally, in equivocal cases, a renal biopsy is performed at the time of revascularization.[13] Preservation of the majority of glomeruli is the most important element of a favorable biopsy. Excessive hyalinization of the glomeruli precludes surgical revascularization. The presence of tubular atrophy, interstitial fibrosis, and arteriolar sclerosis are less important and do not preclude consideration for revascularization.

Atheroembolic renal disease, as a feature of the renal biopsy, can be an important determinant of outcome.[15] In a recent study, histopathological evidence of atheroemboli were observed in 16 patients (group I) and absent in 28 patients (group II). The 5-year patient survival was significantly worse in group I (54% versus 85%) and the incidence of systemic atherosclerotic complications was

Table 62.1 Renal functional results of surgery for atherosclerotic renovascular disease

Reference	No. patients	Improved (%)	Stabilized (%)	Deteriorated (%)	Mortality (%)
Hallett et al[29]	98	29	48	16	7.1
Novick et al[19]	161	58	31	11	2.1
Bredenberg et al[30]	50	36	48	16	0
Hansen et al[31]	70	49	36	15	3.1
Liberteno et al[32]	97	49	35	16	6
Fergany et al[24]	158	35	47	18	2.9
Cambria et al[33]	139	76*	–	26	–
Steinbach et al[11]	195	71*	–	29	2.2
Hansen et al[34]	215	58	35	7	7.3

*Improved and stable combined.

also higher in group I (85% versus 58%). These results indicate a poorer long-term outcome and more aggressive atherosclerosis in those patients with atheroembolic disease.

Preoperative considerations

Patients with atherosclerotic renal artery disease who are considered for surgical revascularization should undergo screening and correction of significant associated extrarenal vascular disease, such as coronary and carotid disease. With aggressive treatment of coexisting extrarenal vascular disease prior to surgical renal revascularization, perioperative morbidity and mortality can be minimized.

All patients require arteriography prior to surgery. For most patients we use digital subtraction angiography with iodinated contrast material because accurate anatomic information can be obtained with limited contrast exposure. In addition to anteroposterior views of the renal artery and aorta, we routinely obtain a lateral aortogram, to assess the celiac artery, and a view of the lower thoracic aorta. These additional views are obtained in anticipation of the use of extraanatomic bypass procedures.

There have been successful reports of renal artery surgery on the basis of clinical profiling and magnetic resonance angiography (MRA) as the sole radiographic evaluation.[16] This approach avoids potential morbididty from iodinated contrast as well as the arterial puncture. In selected cases carbon dioxide angiography can be used, which eliminates the risk for contrast-related nephrotoxicity.

Many patients will have bilateral disease, especially those with ischemic nephropathy. Since the morbidity of bilateral procedures is greater and disease is frequently asymmetric, we usually perform unilateral renal revascularization. In cases of RVH, the more extensively diseased artery is repaired, and for ischemic nephropathy the larger kidney is repaired.

Surgical treatment

Nephrectomy

Nephrectomy or partial nephrectomy are rarely needed because of advancements in renal arterial surgical reconstruction. Still, an occasional patient may require such treatment as a result of renal infarction, severe arteriolar nephrosclerosis, ischemic renal atrophy, or an uncorrectable renovascular lesion. While an extraperitoneal flank approach has been routinely employed in these circumstances, there is increasing enthusiasm for the use of laparoscopic nephrectomy.[17] This minimally invasive technique is particularly useful because such kidneys are often small and severely ischemic. Laparoscopic nephrectomy is associated with a shorter postoperative hospital stay and convalescence.

Aortorenal bypass

In the absence of a significantly diseased aorta, aortorenal bypass is the preferred method of surgical revascularization.[18] The optimal graft material is autogenous artery, such as the hypogastric artery. However, this vessel is often short or severely atherosclerotic, rendering it unusable. The most common graft is autogenous saphenous vein (see Fig. 62.1) and excellent clinical results have been obtained.[19] In the absence of autogenous material, a synthetic graft may be used. Polytetrafluoroethylene (PTFE) has become the synthetic graft material of choice.[20]

Techniques for the surgically difficult aorta

Aortorenal bypass may be technically difficult or hazardous in patients with severe atherosclerosis, aneurysmal disease, or a prior aortic procedure.[21] Aortic replacement with concomitant renal artery reconstruction has been associated historically with a mortality rate of 10% or more,[22] although this has improved in recent years.[23] This procedure is now reserved for those candidates with a significant aortic aneurysm or symptomatic aortoiliac occlusive disease. Several extraanatomic bypass techniques have been developed that are successful in cases of a surgically difficult aorta.[24]

Splenorenal bypass is the preferred approach for left renal revascularization (see Fig. 62.2).[25] The preoperative

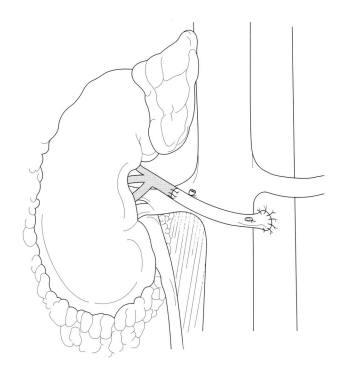

Figure 62.1 Aortorenal bypass using a saphenous vein graft. (With permission from Novick AC: Aortorenal bypass. *In* Novick AC, Streem SB, Pontes JE (eds): Stewart's Operative Urology: Vol 1, 2nd edn. Baltimore: Williams & Wilkins, 1989.)

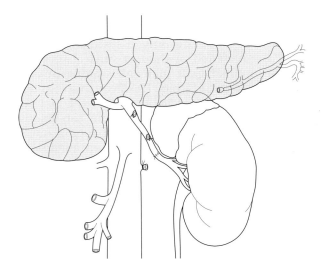

Figure 62.2 Splenorenal bypass for the left kidney. (With permission from Novick AC: Splenorenal bypass. *In* Novick AC, Streem SB, Pontes JE (eds): Stewart's Operative Urology: Vol 1, 2nd edn. Baltimore: Williams & Wilkins, 1989.)

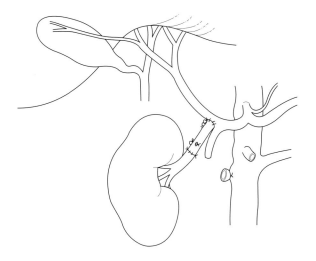

Figure 62.3 Hepatorenal bypass to the right kidney. (With permission from Novick AC: Alternative bypass techniques for renal revascularization. *In* Novick AC, Scoble J, Hamilton G (eds): Renal Vascular Disease. London: WB Saunders Co Ltd, 1996.)

angiogram must demonstrate patent celiac and splenic arteries, emphasizing again the need for a lateral aortogram. The splenic artery must be carefully inspected at surgery for atherosclerotic disease which can preclude its use for revascularization. The distal splenic artery can be ligated without the need for concomitant splenectomy. Ischemic time to the kidney is minimized because the operation involves a single anastamosis away from the aorta.

Hepatorenal bypass is the preferred approach for right renal revacularization.[26] Analogous to the splenorenal bypass, the preoperative lateral aortogram must demonstrate patent celiac and hepatic arteries. An additional prerequisite is the biochemical demonstration of normal liver function. The most common procedure uses a saphenous vein graft, anastamosed proximally end-to-side to the hepatic artery, just distal to the gastroduodenal artery, and distally an end-to-end anastamosis to the renal artery (see Fig. 62.3). This technique preserves the continuity of the hepatic circulation. When the hepatic artery is diminutive, or the right and left hepatic arteries have a separate origin, the end-to-side anastomosis as previously described may not be feasible. In such cases an end-to-end anastamosis to either the common, right or left hepatic artery can be performed.[27] This is usually a direct anatamosis, although a saphenous vein interposition graft may be needed. Ischemic damage to the liver is rare because the portal circulation is its major source of oxygenation; however, patients may show transient elevations of liver function tests in the postoperative period. When the right hepatic arterial circulation is interrupted, a cholecystectomy should be performed to prevent perioperative necrosis of the gallbladder. Finally, the gastroduodenal artery can occasionally be used as an inflow source, using an end-to-end technique, with or without a sphenous vein interposition graft.

In a review of 254 angiograms performed at our institution from 1989 to 1993, 54% demonstrated significant stenosis of the celiac artery.[24] This effectively limits the use of splenorenal or hepatorenal bypass in approximately one-half of patients who may benefit from surgical revascularization. We have observed that the lower thoracic aorta is much less involved with atherosclerosis than the abdominal aorta. In patients with significant celiac stenosis the preferred approach is a thoracic aortorenal bypass (see Fig. 62.4).[28] This is easily achieved on the left side using a thoracoabdominal incision; on the right a subcostal incision is used. Using partial aortic clamping, thus avoiding the need for systemic heparinization, a long saphenous vein graft is anastamosed to the lower thoracic aorta. This graft is passed through the aortic hiatus into the retroperitoneum and anastamosed end-to-end to the cut end of the renal artery. Excellent results have been obtained in 23 patients in whom this procedure has initially been performed. There was one operative death due to a myocardial infarction. Of the remaining 22 patients, 86% showed cure or improvement in blood pressure, and 95% had stable or improved renal function.

Iliorenal bypass is another alternative when the celiac artery has significant stenosis.[21] This is performed using a saphenous vein graft as a conduit from the ipsilateral iliac artery to the affected kidney (see Fig. 62.5). A prerequisite for this approach is adequate blood flow through the abdominal aorta and minimal atherosclerosis of the iliac artery. Currently this procedure is considered when splenorenal, hepatorenal, or thoracic aortorenal bypass are not feasible. This preference arises because atherosclerosis will continue to progress, most likely to involve the infrarenal abdominal aorta, which might compromise blood flow to a kidney with its primary blood supply from the iliac arteries.

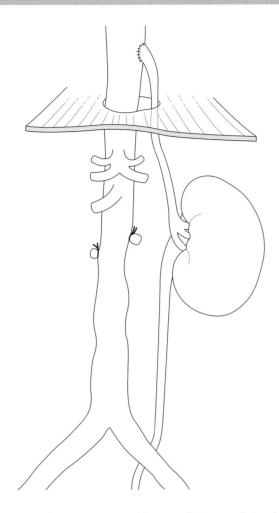

Figure 62.4 Thoracic aortorenal bypass. (With permission from Novick et al.[28])

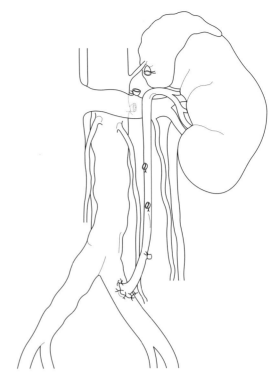

Figure 6.5 Iliorenal bypass. (With permission from Novick AC: Iliorenal and mesenterorenal bypass. *In* Novick AC, Streem SB, Pontes JE (eds): Stewart's Operative Urology: Vol 1, 2nd edn. Baltimore: Williams & Wilkins, 1989.)

We reviewed our results with extraanatomic bypass procedures between 1980 and 1992.[24] There were 175 procedures in 171 patients including hepatorenal bypass ($n = 59$), splenorenal bypass ($n = 54$), iliorenal bypass ($n = 37$), thoracic aortorenal bypass ($n = 23$), renal autotransplantation ($n = 1$), and superior mesenterorenal bypass ($n = 1$). Most patients were operated for preservation of renal function ($n = 158$) while a smaller group underwent revascularization for hypertension ($n = 13$). The perioperative mortality rate was 2.9% and graft thrombosis occurred in 4% of cases. All patients with poorly controlled hypertension were cured or improved postoperatively. For the patients with ischemic nephropathy, postoperative renal function improved in 35%, stabilized in 47%, and deteriorated in 18%. The best results were obtained in those patients with S_{Cr} < 2.0 mg/dL, where 90% of patients had improvement or stablization of renal function. These results confirm the efficacy of alternate bypass procedures in appropriately selected patients.

Extracorporeal microvascular reconstruction

Improvements in renal preservation and microvascular techniques, as an extension of the field of renal allotransplantation, have facilitated development of extracorporeal renal surgery for renal artery disease. The advantages of extracorporeal surgery include optimal exposure in a bloodless surgical field, improved protection from renal ischemia, easier use of microvascular techniques, and optimal magnification. Extracorporeal microvascular repair should only be applied to cases with intrarenal branch disease for whom an in situ repair is not feasible.[5] This includes patients with branch fibrous dysplasia, renal artery aneurysm, renal arteriovenous fistula, or renal artery dissection. This technique is rarely applicable to atherosclerotic lesions. Preoperative evaluation should accurately demonstrate the anatomy of the renal arterial, confirm the absence of disease in the iliac vessels, and assess the

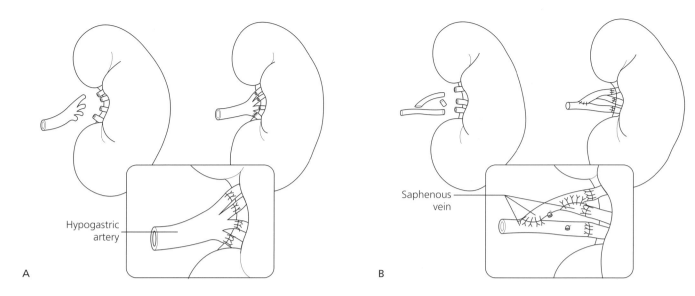

Figure 62.6 (A) Extracorporeal renal arterial repair using autogenous hypogastric artery. (B) Extracorporeal renal arterial repair with branched saphenous vein graft. (With permission from Novick AC: Extracorporeal microvascular branch renal artery reconstruction. In Novick AC, Streem SB, Pontes JE (eds): Stewart's Operative Urology: Vol 1, 2nd edn. Baltimore: Williams & Wilkins, 1989.)

hypogastric artery and branches as a possible interposition graft. At surgery the kidney is flushed with an intracellular preservation solution and maintained using surface hypothermia in an iced basin. Arterial disease is resected and repaired with autogenous graft material. Hypogastric artery is preferred, but must be of the appropriate length, with appropriate branch anatomy, and be free of arterial disease (see Fig. 62.6A); in cases where suitable artery is not available the saphenous vein may be fashioned into a branched graft (see Fig. 62.6B). The repaired kidney is then autotransplanted to the iliac fossa in a manner analogous to renal allotransplantation.

We reviewed our experience with extracorporeal microvascular reconstruction and autotransplantation in 66 patients between 1976 and 1991.[5] Renal artery pathology included fibrous dysplasia ($n = 42$), aneurysm ($n = 13$), atherosclerosis ($n = 7$), primary dissection ($n = 2$), arteriovenous fistula ($n = 1$), and arteritis ($n = 1$). The indications for reconstruction were renovascular hypertension ($n = 58$), prevention of aneurysm rupture ($n = 7$), and asymptomatic arteriovenous fistula ($n = 1$). A total of 187 diseased branches were repaired (mean = 2.8 branches per patient). The cold renal ischemic period ranged from 1 to 3.5 h. All but two patients had a technically successful repair, and those two had a normal contralateral kidney. At current follow-up all 66 patients are normotensive, but 11 patients require low doses of antihypertensive medication. Renal function was stabilized or improved in all patients. These results confirm the efficacy of extracorporeal microvascular revascularization for patients with complex branch renal artery disease.

References

1. Nally JV: Provocative captopril testing in the diagnosis of renovascular hypertension. Urol Clin North Am 1994;21:227–234.
2. Taylor A, Nally J, Aurell M, et al: Consensus report on ACE inhibitor renography for detecting renovascular hypertension. J Nucl Med 1996;37:1876–1882.
3. Schreiber MJ, Pohl MA, Novick AC. The natural history of atherosclerotic and fibrous renal artery disease. Urol Clin N Am 1984;11:383–392.
4. Tegtmeyer CJ, Matsumoto AH, Angle JF: Percutaneous transluminal angioplasty in fibrous dysplasia and children. In Novick AC, Scoble J, Hamilton G, (eds): Renal Vascular Disease. London: WB Saunders Co Ltd, 1996, pp 363–384.
5. Novick AC. Extracorporeal microvascular reconstruction and autotransplantation for branch renal artery disease. In Novick A, Scoble J, Hamilton G (eds): Renal Vascular Disease: WB Saunders Co Ltd, 1996, pp 497–509.
6. Ramsay LE, Waller PC: Blood pressure response to percutaneous transluminal angioplasty for renovascular hypertension: an overview of published series. BMJ 1990;300:569–572.
7. Hayes J, Risius B, Novick A, et al: Experience with percutaneous transluminal angioplasty for renal artery stenosis at the Cleveland Clinic. J Urol 1988;139:488–492.
8. Olin J, Melia M, Young J, et al: Prevalence of atherosclerotic renal artery stenosis in patients with atherosclerosis elsewhere. Am J Med 1990;188:46–51.
9. Novick A, Pohl M, Schreiber M, et al: Revascularization for the preservation of renal function in patients with atherosclerotic renovascular disease. J Urol 1983;129:907–912.
10. Ziegelbaum M, Novick A, Hayes J, et al: Management of renal arterial disease in the elderly. Surg Gynecol Obstet 1987;165:130–134.
11. Steinbach F, Novick AC, Campbell S, et al: Long-term survival after surgical revascularization for atherosclerotic renal artery disease. J Urol 1997;158:38–41.
12. Olin J: Role of duplex ultrasonography in screening for significant renal artery disease. Urol Clin N Am 1994;21:215–226.
13. Novick A. Patient selection for intervention to preserve renal function in ischemic renal disease. In Novick A, Scoble J, Hamilton G (eds): Renal Vascular Disease. London: WB Saunders Co Ltd, 1996, pp 323–335.
14. Kaylor W, Novick A, Ziegelbaum M, et al: Reversal of end-stage renal failure with surgical revascularization in patients with atherosclerotic renal artery occlusion. J Urol 1989;141:486–488.
15. Krishnamurthi V, Novick AC, Myles JL: Atheroembolic renal disease: effect on morbidity and survival after revascularization for atherosclerotic renal artery stenosis. J Urol 1999;161:1093–1096.
16. Cambria RP, Kaufman JL, Brewster DC, et al: Surgical renal artery reconstruction without contrast arteriography: the role of clinical profiling and magnetic resonance angiography. J Vasc Surg 1999;29:1012–1021.

17. Gill IS, Schweizer D, Hobart MG, et al: Retroperitoneal laparoscopic radical nephrectomy: the Cleveland Clinic experience. J Urol 2000;163:1665–1670.

18. Novick A, Khauli R, Vidt D. Diminished operative risk and improved results following revascularization for atherosclerotic renovascular disease. Urol Clin North Am 1984;11:435–449.

19. Novick A, Ziegelbaum M, Vidt D, et al: Trends in surgical revascularization for renal artery disease: ten years experience. J Am Med Assoc 1987;257:498–501.

20. Khauli R, Novick A, Coseriu G: Renal revascularization with polytetrafluoroethylene grafts. Cleve Clin Q 1984;51:365–369.

21. Novick A. Alternative bypass techniques for renal revascularization. In Novick A, Scoble J, Hamilton G (eds): Renal Vascular Disease. London: WB Saunders Co Ltd, 1996, pp 465–480.

22. Tarazi R, Hertzer N, Beven E, et al: Simultaneous aortic reconstruction and renal revascularization: risk factors and late results in eighty-nine patients. J Vasc Surg 1987;5:707–714.

23. Cambria R, Brewster D, L'Italien G, et al: Simultaneous aortic and renal artery reconstruction: evolution of an eighteen-year experience. J Vasc Surg 1995;21:916–925.

24. Fergany A, Kolettis P, Novick A. The contemporary role of extra-anatomical surgical revascularization in patients with atherosclerotic renal artery disease. J Urol 1995;153:1798–1802.

25. Khauli R, Novick A, Ziegelbaum M: Splenorenal bypass in the treatment of renal artery stenosis: experience with sixty-nine cases. J Vasc Surg 1985;2:547–551.

26. Chibaro E, Libertino J, Novick A. Use of hepatic circulation for renal revascularization. Ann Surg 1984;199:406–411.

27. Novick A, McElroy J: Renal revascularization by end-to-end anastamosis of the hepatic and renal arteries. J Urol 1985;134:1089–1093.

28. Novick A, Stewart R, Hodge E, et al: Use of the thoracic aorta for renal arterial revascularization. J Vasc Surg 1994;19:605–609.

29. Hallett JW, Jr, Fowl R, O'Brien PC, et al: Renovascular operations in patients with chronic renal insufficiency: do the benefits justify the risks? J Vasc Surg 1987;5:622–627.

30. Bredenberg CE, Sampson LN, Ray FS, et al: Changing patterns in surgery for chronic renal artery occlusive diseases. J Vasc Surg 1992;15:1018–1023.

31. Hansen KJ, Starr SM, Sands RE, et al: Contemporary surgical management of renovascular disease. J Vasc Surg 1992;16:319–330.

32. Libertino JA, Bosco PJ, Ying CY, et al: Renal revascularization to preserve and restore renal function. J Urol 1992;147:1485–1487.

33. Cambria RP, Brewster DC, L'Italien GJ, et al: Renal artery reconstruction for the preservation of renal function. J Vasc Surg 1996;24:380–382.

34. Hansen KJ, Cherr GS, Craven TE, et al: Management of ischemic nephropathy: dialysis-free survival after surgical repair. J Vasc Surg 2000;32:481–482.

CHAPTER

63 Hypertension in Renal Transplant Recipients

Robert S. Gaston and John J. Curtis

Clinical features
Approach to the patient with hypertension after renal transplantation
Management
- Calcium antagonists
- Angiotensin-converting enzyme inhibitors and angiotensin receptor blockers
- Diuretics
- Other agents
- Refractory post-transplant hypertension

Management of hypertension is a common challenge for physicians involved in the care of renal allograft recipients. Hypertension may appear at any time following engraftment, and ultimately afflicts 75–80% of patients in the current era of immunosuppressive therapy.[1] In recent years, advances in therapeutics for transplantation patients mean that graft loss due to rejection is significantly less common.[2] Now recipients are older and have more comorbid disease, the most common cause of transplant failure is death with a functioning allograft, and the most common cause of death is cardiovascular disease. Like anyone with chronic renal disease, risk of cardiovascular mortality in transplant recipients greatly exceeds that of the general population.[1] Clearly hypertension is a significant risk factor for accelerated atherosclerosis and premature coronary disease, and the impact of hypertension and other variables on cardiovascular risk is exaggerated in transplant recipients.[3,4] In addition, hypertension increases the risk of allograft failure and may accelerate deterioration of graft function over time.[5,6] Thus the primary objectives for management of post-transplant hypertension include reducing cardiovascular morbidity and mortality, and preserving allograft function.

Clinical features

Unlike elevated blood pressure in the general population (which in > 90% of cases is *essential* hypertension), identifiable causes of post-transplant hypertension are evident in most recipients. Factors such as age, sex, and race are usually thought to predispose patients to essential hypertension, but they do not significantly influence development of post-transplant hypertension. Similarly, the nature of a recipient's original renal disease is of little importance. Although post-transplant hypertension may manifest as a hypertensive crisis, it is usually mild to moderate in severity.[7]

In the past, hypertension was noted most frequently in renal transplant recipients with retained native kidneys, or with a cadaveric organ, or both. However, under current immunosuppressive protocols the impact of calcineurin-inhibitor therapy with cyclosporine or tacrolimus may override the influence of other factors.[8] Definable causes of post-transplant hypertension may be grouped conveniently as either intrinsic or extrinsic to the allograft (Table 63.1). Several pathogenic factors often coexist in an individual patient. Some causes are amenable to specific diagnosis and correction, and others are relatively fixed, needing long-term antihypertensive therapy. Virtually all causes of post-transplant hypertension share the common mechanism of impaired renal allograft function.

Approach to the patient with hypertension after renal transplantation

The initial challenge in hypertensive renal transplant recipients is to identify any potentially correctable cause. Immediately after transplantation, delayed graft function (with sodium and volume excess) may be the main cause of elevated blood pressure. Inadequately controlled post-operative pain may also contribute. Thereafter new or worsening hypertension may represent the onset of acute rejection. Alternatively, since cyclosporine and tacrolimus levels are usually kept highest during the early post-transplant period, a dose-dependent elevation in systemic pressure often results. Beyond 6 months post transplant, acute rejection becomes less likely and, in the recipient

Table 63.1   Causes of post-transplant hypertension

Intrinsic
Delayed graft function
Acute rejection
Chronic rejection
Cyclosporin nephropathy – chronic
Recurrent primary renal disease

Extrinsic
Native kidneys
Immunosuppression
   Cyclosporine
   Tacrolimus
   Corticosteroids
Transplant renal artery stenosis
Hypercalcemia

619

with de novo or worsening hypertension, other causes should be considered; these include toxicity from calcineurin inhibitors, recurrent disease, chronic rejection, or transplant renal artery stenosis (TRAS). Finally, retained native kidneys may contribute to hypertension at any time.[7]

With this timeframe in mind, initial studies aim to document the adequacy of allograft function (Fig. 63.1). Measurement should be made not only of serum creatinine (S_{Cr}) levels, but also 24-h urinary protein excretion, with some reliable estimates of glomerular filtration rate (GFR) and/or renal plasma flow (RPF). Control of extracellular volume should be optimized. If allograft dysfunction is present, renal biopsy may be required to distinguish specific causes.

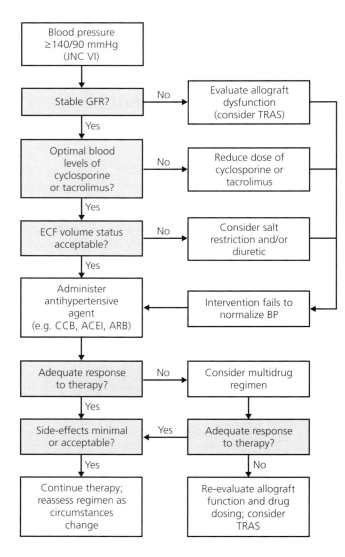

Figure 63.1 Diagnosis and management of hypertension in the renal allograft recipient. ACEI, angiotensin-converting enzyme inhibitor; ARB, angiotensin receptor blocker; CCB, calcium channel blocker; ECF, extracellular fluid; GFR, glomerular filtration rate; JNC VI, Joint National Committee VI;[12] TRAS, transplant renal artery stenosis.

Immunosuppressants play a major role in the pathogenesis of post-transplant hypertension, so the patient's antirejection therapy might need reassessment. Calcineurin phosphatase inhibitors (either cyclosporine or tacrolimus) remain the cornerstone of current immunosuppressive regimens. Although recent data indicate that hypertension is slightly less common with tacrolimus, both agents are nephrotoxic and – particularly at high blood levels – elevate systemic blood pressure.[9] The dose of cyclosporine or tacrolimus should be optimized in post-transplant hypertension, and it should be noted that excessive reduction of the dose to reduce elevated systemic blood pressure may increase the risk of acute rejection. When given in combination with cyclosporine, the immunosuppressant sirolimus may potentiate hypertension, but independently it does not appear to cause high blood pressure in transplant recipients.[10] Although corticosteroids clearly contribute to hypertension, the pathogenetic influence of prednisone at a maintenance dose of 5–10 mg/day seems minimal, and withdrawal of steroids remains controversial.[11] Other immunosuppressants, such as azathioprine and mycophenolate mofetil, seemingly have no adverse effect on systemic blood pressure.

Late onset of hypertension, particularly in a previously stable recipient, is suggestive of TRAS. Administration of an angiotensin-converting enzyme inhibitor (ACEI) or an angiotensin receptor blocker (ARB) may be helpful in screening for hemodynamically significant stenosis: when patients with TRAS are given a low dose of ACEI, there is often an immediate and marked decline in GFR. Patients who respond in this fashion to an ACEI often demonstrate TRAS at angiography. Although radionuclide scanning and Doppler imaging may be useful adjuncts, availability of magnetic resonance angiography has greatly simplified evaluation for TRAS. Conventional angiography and its risks can now be limited to patients with a high chance of benefiting from angioplasty and/or surgery.

Management

In the hypertensive transplant recipient with stable allograft function, and in cases of chronic rejection, normalization of blood pressure (< 140/90 mmHg) has always been the goal. However, given recent recommendations from the Joint National Committee (JNC) VI[12] and the World Health Organization/International Society of Hypertension,[13] a more aggressive target may be in order. Commensurate with these recommendations, and acknowledging the increased risk of end-organ damage in renal transplant recipients, a recent Task Force endorsed target blood pressures of < 130/85 mmHg for patients without proteinuria, and 125/75 mmHg for those excreting more than 1 g of urinary protein per day.[1]

Because of varying doses of steroids and calcineurin inhibitors, as well as changes in GFR, blood pressure may fluctuate considerably in the transplant recipient, requiring vigilance by the physician, and continuous reevaluation of treatment. While JNC VI emphasizes the role of "lifestyle modifications" in treating hypertension (including smoking cessation, weight loss, limited sodium intake, and exercise), renal transplant recipients will generally require pharmacologic therapy to achieve adequate blood pressure control.[1,12]

Calcium antagonists

Calcium antagonists, or calcium channel blockers (CCBs), effectively reduce blood pressure in most patients and have been shown to attenuate both cyclosporine- and endothelin-induced vasoconstriction.[14] In practice, these agents reduce renal vascular resistance, preventing the acute deterioration in RPF and GFR that may accompany elevated cyclosporine blood levels. Theoretically, their other benefits include enhancement of immunosuppression, preventing delayed graft function, and improving GFR in cyclosporine-treated allograft recipients.[15]

Currently available CCBs have significantly different effects on the metabolism of cyclosporine and tacrolimus, and on blood levels of the immunosuppressant sirolimus.[10] Verapamil and diltiazem, along with the dihydropyridine nicardipine, interfere with the hepatic metabolism of cyclosporine, increasing its blood level by 40–50%. While some investigators have found this interaction beneficial, it clearly complicates immunosuppressive management: dosages of the CCB and the immunosuppressant must be altered concurrently. For this reason, others prefer to use nifedipine or isradipine, which have little effect on blood levels of cyclosporine or tacrolimus. Amlodipine has an intermediate effect on cyclosporine metabolism and the dose does not usually need adjustment.[16]

Although CCBs are generally well tolerated in this population, peripheral edema can be a complication, and they may exacerbate cyclosporine-induced gingival hyperplasia. As previously noted for the general population, a recent retrospective study found increased risk of cardiac mortality in renal transplant recipients on dihydropyridine CCBs.[3] The implications of this observation remain unclear.

Angiotensin-converting enzyme inhibitors and angiotensin receptor blockers

Use of ACEIs and ARBs to treat hypertension in transplant recipients is becoming increasingly common.[17,18] While these agents effectively reduce blood pressure and exert a salutary impact on renal hemodynamics, their use in cyclosporine-treated patients has been associated with acute renal failure, hyperkalemia, and anemia. Another theoretical basis for avoiding ACEIs and ARBs in such patients involves the physiologic similarity of TRAS and cyclosporine-induced afferent arteriolar vasoconstriction. Angiotensin is critical for maintaining glomerular perfusion in both situations, so in theory inhibition of its effect in the postglomerular circulation would adversely affect GFR. Indeed, in a recent crossover study comparing amlodipine with losartan, there was a similar efficacy in blood pressure reduction, but an increase in GFR with amlodipine versus a slight (though not statistically signif-

icant) decline with the ARBs.[17] However, only losartan significantly reduced proteinuria and plasma levels of transforming growth factor β_1 (TGF-β_1) – effects that may prove beneficial in preserving renal function and reducing risk of cardiovascular disease.

While therapy with these agents must be introduced cautiously, paying close attention to renal function, potassium levels, and blood counts, the vast majority of transplant recipients tolerate ACEIs and ARBs quite well. In some of the 10–15% of patients who develop anemia while receiving these drugs, we have at times prescribed recombinant erythropoietin (rHuEpo) in order to continue what appears to be beneficial therapy. Post-transplant erythrocytosis, a late complication seen most often in stable recipients with well-functioning grafts, resolves with ACEI or ARB therapy in most patients.[19]

Diuretics

In light of the volume expansion and salt sensitivity that often accompany post-transplant hypertension, diuretics are an important therapeutic option. Although salt restriction may pose less of a medical risk, it is rarely adequate to achieve or enhance blood pressure control in this population. Diuretics are a useful adjunct for those who respond to a CCB or another vasodilator with only suboptimal blood pressure control, or worsening edema. In this setting, a loop diuretic (furosemide or bumetanide) may be required to achieve adequate natriuresis. Thiazides increase the risk of hyperuricemia and/or hypercalcemia, but may also be effective. Given the predisposition of transplant recipients to hyperkalemia, there is little role for potassium-sparing agents.

Other agents

There appear to be no distinct advantages or disadvantages associated with use of other antihypertensive agents; these are described extensively in Part XI: Management of Secondary Hypertension.

Refractory post-transplant hypertension

Transplant recipients with refractory hypertension, or those who require more than three drugs to normalize blood pressure, should undergo evaluation for TRAS. When TRAS is demonstrated, it appears that surgical repair offers the best hope for both immediate and long-term cures (92% and 82% respectively). However, angioplasty may be successful in as many as three-quarters of patients, with long-lasting remissions in 40–50%. Most transplant physicians would thus offer angioplasty as a first intervention, particularly for those patients with lesions removed from the vascular anastomosis. Proximal lesions or stenoses at the vascular anastomosis may more frequently require surgical intervention.

When TRAS is excluded in the patient with well-preserved allograft function and no evidence of rejection, bilateral native kidney nephrectomy is an option for intractable hypertension. In experienced hands this substantial operation can be performed safely and – for most patients – will improve control of post-transplant hypertension. Unfortunately, there is no diagnostic study that accurately predicts who will, or will not, benefit from surgery. With the currently available medical therapies, native kidney nephrectomy is rarely indicated.

References

1. Levey AS, Beto JA, Coronado BE, et al: Controlling the epidemic of cardiovascular disease in chronic renal disease: What do we know? What do we need to learn? Where do we go from here? Am J Kidney Dis 1998;32:853–906.
2. USRD 2000: Excerpts from the United States Renal Data System Annual Data Report: 2000. Am J Kidney Dis 2000;36(Suppl 2):S15–S181.
3. Kasiske BL, Chakkera HA, Roel J: Explained and unexplained ischemic heart disease risk after renal transplantation. J Am Soc Nephrol 2000;11:1735–1743.
4. Massry ZA, Kasiske BL: Post-transplant hyperlipidemia: mechanisms and management. J Am Soc Nephrol 1996;7:971–977.
5. Brazy PC, Pirsch JD, Belzer FO: Factors affecting renal allograft function in long-term recipients. Am J Kidney Dis 1992;19:558–566.
6. Sanders CE, Curtis JJ: Role of hypertension in chronic allograft dysfunction. Kidney Int 1995;48(Suppl 52):S43–S47.
7. Gaston RS, Curtis JJ: Hypertension following renal transplantation. In Massry SG, Glassock RJ (eds): Textbook of Nephrology. Philadelphia: Lippincott Williams & Wilkins, 2001, pp 1677–1681.
8. Curtis JJ, Luke RG, Jones P: Hypertension in cyclosporin-treated renal transplant recipients is sodium-dependent. Am J Med 1988, 85:134–138.
9. Ligtenberg G, Hene RJ, Blankestijn PJ, et al: Cardiovascular risk factors in renal transplant patients: cyclosporin versus tacrolimus. J Am Soc Nephrol 2001;12:368–373.
10. Saunders RN, Metcalfe MS, Nicholson ML: Rapamycin in transplantation: a review of the evidence. Kidney Int 2001;59:3–16.
11. Steroid Withdrawal Study Group: Prednisone withdrawal in kidney transplant recipients on cyclosporin and mycophenolate mofetil – a prospective randomized study. Transplantation 1999;68:1865–1874.
12. JNC VI: Report of the Joint National Committee on prevention, detection, evaluation, and treatment of high pressure. Arch Intern Med 1997;157:2413–2446.
13. WHO–ISH Committee. World Health Organization–International Society of Hypertension 1999: Guidelines for the Management of Hypertension. J Hypertens 1999;17:151–183.
14. Ruggenenti P, Perico N, Mosconi L, et al: Calcium channel blockers protect transplant patients from cyclosporin-induced daily renal hypoperfusion. Kidney Int 1993;43:706–711.
15. Weir MR: Therapeutic benefits of calcium channel blockers in cyclosporin-treated organ transplant recipients: blood pressure control and immunosuppression. Am J Med 1991;90(Suppl 5A):32S–36S.
16. Pesavento TE, Jones PA, Julian BA, et al: Amlodipine increases cyclosporin levels in hypertensive renal transplants: results of a prospective study. J Am Soc Nephrol 1996;7:831–835.
17. Inigo P, Campistol JM, Lario S, et al: Effects of losartan and amlodipine on intrarenal hemodynamics and TGF-beta1 plasma levels in a crossover trial in renal transplant recipients. J Am Soc Nephrol 2001;12:822–827.
18. Mourad G, Ribstein J, Mimran A: Converting-enzyme inhibition versus calcium antagonist in cyclosporin-treated renal transplants. Kidney Int 1993;43:419–425.
19. Gaston RS, Julian BA, Curtis JJ: Posttransplant erythrocytosis: an enigma revisited. Am J Kidney Dis 1994;24:1–11.

CHAPTER 64

Management of Hypertension in Patients Receiving Dialysis Therapy

Christopher S. Wilcox

Pathophysiology
- Salt and fluid retention
- Structural changes and endothelial dysfunction
- Endogenous sodium/potassium-adenosine triphosphatase inhibitor
- Renin–angiotensin–aldosterone system
- Sympathetic nervous system

Blood pressure goals

Nonpharmacologic treatment

Pharmacologic management
- Diuretics
- Calcium channel blockers
- β-Adrenergic blocking agents
- Angiotensin-converting enzyme inhibitors
- Angiotensin II receptor blockers
- Centrally acting drugs
- Adrenergic blocking agents
- Nonspecific vasodilators

Overview of hypertension management in ESRD

Hypertension is an increasingly common cause of end-stage renal disease (ESRD).[1] The prevalence of hypertension increases with declining renal function. When renal disease reaches endstage, approximately 80–90% of patients suffer from significant hypertension. Diseases that affect the renal interstitium predominantly may produce a salt-losing state, with normotension or even episodes of hypotension and hypovolemia, whereas the more common arterial and glomerular diseases almost invariably cause hypertension.

Blood pressure control usually improves after initiation of dialysis therapy. However, in practice, more than 75% of people receiving outpatient hemodialysis are receiving antihypertensive drug therapy. Cheigh et al[2] used ambulatory blood pressure monitoring and reported adequate control in only 15% of their patients monitored over 48 hours despite widespread use of antihypertensive agents. The US Renal Data System (USRDS) analyzed predialysis blood pressure data on 5369 patients: even with antihypertensive therapy 63% of patients were hypertensive: mild in 27%, moderate in 25%, and severe in 11%.[3] Multivariate analysis showed that higher blood pressure was associated with greater intradialytic weight gain, with noncompliance with the dialysis regimen, and younger age. This last surprising finding perhaps reflects the observation that patients with congestive heart failure (CHF) or coronary artery disease (CAD) are generally older and have low blood pressure. Therefore, younger age groups, containing fewer people with these diseases, have higher blood pressures.

Dialysis patients tend to be more prone to accelerated atherosclerosis, independently of comorbid conditions or age.[4] Longitudinal observation studies suggest that atherosclerosis may be retarded by better control of blood pressure, which also appears to increase life expectancy. Indeed, cardiovascular and cerebrovascular disease are the major causes of mortality in the ESRD population. Among patients receiving hemodialysis (HD) or peritoneal dialysis (PD), left ventricular hypertrophy (LVH) is seen in 75%, CAD in 40% and cardiac chamber dilation and CHF in 40%. Rates of CVD mortality are 3–20 times higher than in age-matched subjects.[4] These changes have been related to many factors such as anemia with intravascular volume overload, which increases left ventricular wall stress, redistributes coronary flow, and eventually leads to systolic and diastolic dysfunction and CHF.

When analyzing factors associated with survival on dialysis, it becomes clear how difficult it is to assess the importance of hypertension. Some observational studies show that improved dialysis time and efficiency translate into improved survival. Remarkably, despite the very high prevalence of CVD and hypertension in the dialysis population, the largest studies have failed to show that blood pressure is a predictor of total cardiovascular death in these patients.[5–7] Closer examination of the data provides some insight into this paradox. First, the overall relationship between relative risk and blood pressure is U-shaped (Fig. 64.1).[5,6] The patients with a predialysis systolic blood pressure below 120 mmHg (> 10%) had a sharply increased risk. Likewise, the relatively few (> 5%) who had dialysis-resistant, severe hypertension with a postdialysis systolic blood pressure above 180 mmHg also had an increased risk. There is no trend for increased risk among the many patients with moderate hypertension, or even among the 10% with severe predialysis hypertension. The sharply increased risk among those with low blood pressure was explained by the high proportion of patients with CHF and CAD in this group. Whereas CHF may present with signs and symptoms of fluid overload in the general population, in the dialysis population this is managed by fluid removal at dialysis. Therefore, hypotension becomes a frequent clinical sign. As anticipated, cerebrovascular death is predicted by predialysis hypertension.[6] A Japanese study found that death from cerebral hemorrhage and the size of the intracerebral hematoma are predicted by blood pressure in dialysis patients.[8] This confirms the very close association between incident blood pressure and the occurrence and severity of cerebral hemorrhage in the general population. However, what is not confirmed is the well-known association in the general population between cardiac causes of death and hypertension.

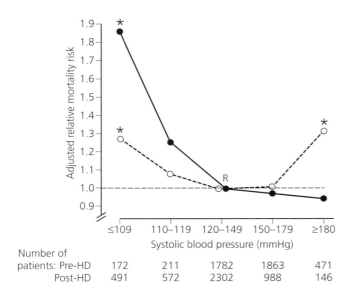

Number of patients:	≤109	110–119	120–149	150–179	≥180
Pre-HD	172	211	1782	1863	471
Post-HD	491	572	2302	988	146

Figure 64.1 The adjusted relative risk for mortality in endstage renal disease patients established on maintenance hemodialysis as a function of systolic blood pressure (SBP), measured predialysis (solid circles and continuous lines) or postdialysis (open circles and broken lines). Compared to reference values at SBP 120–149 mmHg; *P < 0.06. Data are from 4500 patients. (Drawn from Port et al[6] with permission.)

In another study, mortality was related to hypertension in established HD patients. However, during the first 2 years of HD, low systolic blood pressure was associated with a sharp increase in mortality.[5] During a more prolonged follow-up, increased mortality was apparent in those with a high systolic blood pressure. This suggests that those with low blood pressure are at risk for early death from CHF and CAD. If this group is excluded and later deaths are examined, at least a modest enhancing effect of hypertension on cardiovascular death becomes apparent. These results are probably influenced by the very high prevalence of prolonged hypertension and atherosclerosis in this population before they reach HD. This presumably contributes to the greatly increased risk of CVD in those receiving HD even at a normal level of blood pressure.

There are no controlled interventional trials that determine whether CVD is reduced by controlling hypertension in the HD population. Good control of blood pressure with antihypertensives can cause regression of LVH in patients with ESRD, as in those with essential hypertension. Indeed, a controlled trial of angiotensin-converting enzyme inhibitor (ACEI) therapy in normotensive HD patients over 2 years demonstrated regression of LVH in the treatment group, without a change in the control group.[9]

Sleep apnea is common in HD patients. Nocturnal oxygen desaturation is related to "nondipper" blood pressure status and predicts LVH in these patients.[10] Since nocturnal blood pressure is not routinely assessed, the high incidence of "nondipping" may confound the relationship between blood pressure measured during the day at dialysis sessions and CVD mortality. Indeed, in a small study of ambulatory 48-h blood pressure monitoring in HD patients, this meas-

ure of blood pressure was shown to be a much better predictor of LVH than predialysis blood pressure.[11] Finally, another study has shown a significant correlation between predialysis hypertension and cerebral atrophy in HD patients.[12]

These complex data suggest that low blood pressure is a very serious prognostic sign in HD patients. Such patients should be worked up urgently for occult CHF and CAD. Severe hypertension that is resistant to dialysis-induced fluid loss is also an established risk for CVD. Failure to detect a relationship between CVD death and more modest elevations of blood pressure may arise from a failure to detect nocturnal hypertension accompanying sleep apnea, the irreversible effect of pre-ESRD hypertension and atherosclerosis, and confounding effects due to early CV deaths from low blood pressure. At this time, it seems quite reasonable to treat hypertension aggressively in patients receiving HD. Many may benefit from ambulatory blood pressure recording, to assess their true blood pressure burden, and to diagnose and assess the effects of therapy on nocturnal hypertension or nondipper status.

Pathophysiology

The pathophysiology of hypertension in renal failure has been reviewed[13] and is summarized in Fig. 64.2. Blood pressure is a reflection of cardiac output (CO) and total peripheral resistance (TPR). A third factor that determines systolic blood pressure and pulse pressure, and which becomes important in patients with decreased arterial compliance, is the reflection of the systolic pressure wave retrograde from the resistance vessels.[14] In the elderly, in diabetics, and in people with advanced atherosclerosis and vascular calcification, this pressure wave travels sufficiently fast to reach the ascending aorta during systole, thereby accentuating the systolic blood pressure and widening the pulse pressure. Many different factors interact in patients with ESRD to produce hypertension.

Salt and fluid retention

A reduction in renal function, associated with a fall in the glomerular filtration rate (GFR), restricts the excretion of salt (NaCl) and fluid. Early in renal failure, there is generally an increase in cardiac output with a relatively low TPR that may partly be a response to the development of anemia. With further declines in the GFR, the TPR begins to increase, reflecting an autoregulatory response to a sustained increase in cardiac output. This phenomenon is known as total body autoregulation. However, activation of specific vasoconstrictor mechanisms and inhibition of vasodilator mechanisms also are important.

Most studies of body fluid volumes in patients with renal insufficiency have shown an expansion of plasma, extracellular and intracellular fluid volumes, and of total body sodium and water.[15] Prolonged expansion of extracellular fluid volume (ECV) may be the major factor underlying hypertension in ESRD. As the GFR declines, the fraction of patients with salt-sensitive hypertension

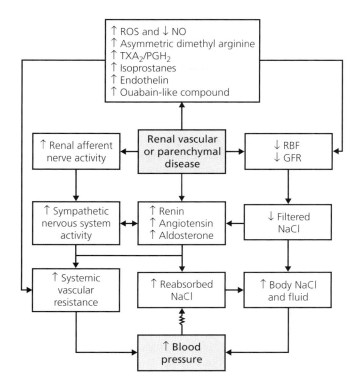

Figure 64.2 Some pathophysiologic mechanisms identified in patients, or animal models, that can increase blood pressure in chronic renal insufficiency. BP, blood pressure; GFR, glomerular filtration rate; NO, nitric oxide; PGH₂, prostaglandin H₂; RBF, renal blood flow; ROS, reactive oxygen species; TxA₂, thromboxane A₂; For full explanation, see text.

increases exponentially. Scrupulous control of ECV by dialysis can reverse hypertension in many patients. In a multivariate analysis of a large USRDS database, large intradialytic weight gain and noncompliance with the dialysis regimen were significant determinants of hypertension.[3] These effects were most pronounced in those free of CHF and with established hypertension. In an analysis over 1 year, patients were switched from conventional dialysis to HD six times a week; they showed a significant reduction in blood pressure, despite using fewer antihypertensive drugs.[16] There was an excellent survival rate in this selected group of compliant and motivated patients.

Another small study compared patients receiving conventional dialysis with those treated for a shorter time with high-flux dialysis; this showed similar levels of blood pressure.[17] These data suggest that the duration and efficiency of dialysis and the patient's ability to resist fluid intake between treatments are important to maintain a more normal level of ECV and moderating hypertension. Indeed, hypertension is remarkably rare in patients receiving daily overnight hemodialysis.[18] Another technique to reduce thirst and ECV is to reduce the dialysate sodium concentration ([Na]). However, this is associated with hypotension, dizziness, fatigue and cramp. In a crossover study, variable sodium dialysis (in which the dialysate [Na] was reduced exponentially from 155 to 135 mequiv./L over 3 h and maintained at 135 mequiv./L for the last hour) was tolerated well and resulted in reduced intradialytic weight gain, reduced need for antihypertensives and lower blood pressure.[19]

Structural changes and endothelial dysfunction

Hypertension in ESRD is associated with functional and morphologic changes in the resistance vessels. Vasodilation is limited by an increase of the media-to-lumen ratio in arterioles. There are increased levels of asymmetric dimethyl arginine (ADMA; an endogenous nitric oxide synthase inhibitor), and endothelin (ET), and diminished endothelium-dependent vasodilation in patients on dialysis. Thus, there is impaired endothelial control of vascular smooth muscle tone.

Endogenous sodium/potassium-adenosine triphosphatase inhibitor

An ouabain-like factor has been extracted from uremic serum that might be an endogenous natriuretic substance that can inhibit Na⁺/K⁺-adenosine triphosphatase (ATPase) in renal tubules, thus promoting salt excretion.[20] Elevated levels, as seen in uremia, could cause more generalized inhibition of Na⁺,K⁺-ATPase, leading to increased intracellular [Na⁺] in vascular smooth muscle cells (VSMCs), diminished Na⁺/Ca²⁺ exchange and increased intracellular calcium concentration [Ca²⁺], thereby increasing vascular tone. Inhibition of ion pump activity at synaptic neuronal clefts could reduce norepinephrine uptake, prolong activation of VSMC, and further enhance vasoconstriction.

Renin–angiotensin–aldosterone system

Renin, angiotensin, and aldosterone are important in the pathogenesis of hypertension in most patients with chronic renal failure. In selected patients with intractable hypertension blood pressure control improves after bilateral nephrectomy and correlates with the prenephrectomy levels of plasma renin activity (PRA). Although PRA is normal or mildly elevated in most dialysis-dependent patients, the PRA is inappropriately high for the expansion of ECV and the high blood pressure. Moreover, tissue angiotensin II (Ang II) may be important in patients in whom hypertension responds to ACEIs yet the PRA is normal. Ang II may potentiate vascular and cardiac hypertrophy both as a vasoconstrictor and by trophic actions.

Sympathetic nervous system

The sympathetic nervous system is implicated in the pathogenesis of hypertension in ESRD. Total autonomic blockade, or selective inhibition of norepinephrine with debrisoquine, reduces TPR and blood pressure. However, plasma norepinephrine levels are variously reported as low, normal, or high, perhaps reflecting the complex nature of catecholamine release, reuptake, metabolism, and excretion in chronic renal failure. Converse et al[21] made direct recordings of postganglionic sympathetic nerve activity in nerves distributed to skeletal muscle blood vessels using implanted microelectrodes. They reported that the frequency of sympathetic nerve discharge was nearly three times greater in patients receiving HD than in normal subjects. Interestingly, after bilateral nephrectomy, there was lower blood pressure and peripheral vascular resistance, and normal rates of sympathetic nerve discharge. These investigators concluded that chronic renal failure activates the sympathetic nervous system via afferent nerve signals arising in the failing kidney.

These studies demonstrate the complexity of the underlying pathophysiology of hypertension in ESRD. They provide a rational basis for using therapies aimed at reducing ECV, for using calcium channel blockers (CCBs), and therapies that interrupt the renin–angiotensin–aldosterone system or the sympathetic nervous system.

Blood pressure goals

Values for lying and standing blood pressure and heart rate should be obtained before and after dialysis treatment. Ideally, blood pressure should be monitored periodically between HD sessions by 48-hour ambulatory monitoring because casual measures of blood pressure do not reflect interdialytic blood pressure control and cannot assess nondipper status.

The ideal target level for reducing blood pressure is controversial. Studies are lacking on blood pressure goals that are safe and effective in minimizing cardiovascular events in ESRD. However, the Modification of Diet in Renal Disease (MDRD) study demonstrated that it was both feasible and safe, at least under protocol conditions, to have a reduced blood pressure goal of approximately 120/75 mmHg in patients with moderate or severe CHF.[22] However, this study used a selected group that was free of recent cardiovascular or cerebrovascular disease.

We recommend a target blood pressure of 135/85 mmHg in uncomplicated ESRD patients. This is based on experience gained by the MDRD, results from normal subjects in the epidemiological study by MacMahon and Rodgers[23] and hypertensive subjects in a trial by Hansson et al[24] in which morbidity and mortality increased with blood pressure levels above this target. It seems probable that many patients who have end-organ damage or LVH, and those with diabetes, would benefit from a lower blood pressure goal of 125/75 mmHg. However, some elderly patients will not tolerate this lower blood pressure; in such cases, a target of 140/90 mmHg should be selected. Moreover, lower blood pressures are dangerous for patients who have recently sustained a stroke, or an episode of coronary ischemia or myocardial infarction.

Nonpharmacologic treatment

The first step in nonpharmacologic treatment is to set and to achieve a true target dry weight. Dry weight is one at which intravascular volume is optimal. Weight above the target is accompanied by fluid overload, edema, and hypertension, whereas weight below target is accompanied by fatigue, orthostatic dizziness, hypotension during dialysis, excessive thirst, and cramps.[25]

The dry weight must be maintained by a combination of scrupulous attention to salt and water restriction between treatments and effective dialytic fluid removal. Some studies suggest that, when this goal is achieved, 85% of hemodialysis patients no longer need antihypertensive medication. In practice this ideal is rarely achieved. Generally, daily sodium salt restriction to 2 g and daily fluid restriction to 1.0–1.25 L produces a tolerable interdialytic weight gain of 2–3 kg.

During initiation of dialysis it is advisable to remove fluid gradually over 6–8 weeks to achieve the target weight and to prevent hypotension and severe cramps. Overuse of antihypertensives at this time can complicate the removal of fluid because of severe falls in blood pressure. Therefore, a stepwise withdrawal of antihypertensive agents is recommended as body weight is reduced toward the target dry weight. Some HD patients who do not tolerate removal of fluid by conventional ultrafiltration respond to sequential hemofiltration and hemodialysis, or to treatment with isolated ultrafiltration on consecutive days until the target dry weight is achieved. Others respond to a variable sodium bath regimen.[19]

Patients treated by continuous ambulatory peritoneal dialysis (CAPD) generally have better controlled blood pressure, probably because of the continuous and smooth ultrafiltration of fluid. Because daily NaCl and fluid losses are greater in CAPD, restriction of salt and water can be less stringent.

Other nonpharmacologic measures that help to control hypertension include reduction of body weight in overweight patients, regular exercise, avoidance of drugs causing hypertension (e.g. over-the-counter nasal decongestants and nonsteroidal antiinflammatory drugs), and stress reduction. It is critical to tackle other cardiovascular risk factors, including smoking, dyslipidemia, and coagulopathy states (see Chapter 59).

Pharmacologic management

Diuretics

Diuretics are reviewed in Chapters 54 and 95. Thiazide diuretics are generally ineffective when the GFR falls below 20–40 mL/min. Loop diuretics require increasing dosage with reduced GFR and become ineffective when the GFR falls below 5 mL/min. In some HD patients, an increase in urine output can be achieved by using high doses of loop diuretics that will reduce the interdialytic weight gain. However, because of the high doses needed in ESRD (e.g. 100–250 mg of furosemide), plasma levels will be elevated and the likelihood of ototoxicity increased. Moreover, in a study of CAPD patients with residual renal function, loop diuretics did not influence the rate of loss of residual renal function, or the outcome.[26] In general, diuretics should be withdrawn as dialysis is initiated.

Calcium channel blockers

These agents are reviewed in Chapter 56 (and see Table 64.1). They inhibit voltage-dependent Ca^{2+} channels in VSMCs and to some extent in cardiac cells. Three classes of chemical compounds and eight agents are currently approved for use in the USA.

These agents are readily absorbed after oral administration. No dose adjustments of CCBs are required in dialysis patients as they are metabolized extensively in the liver, are not renally excreted, and are not significantly removed by hemodialysis or CAPD.

CCBs are among the most frequently prescribed antihypertensive drugs in ESRD patients. Their antihypertensive efficacy, unlike all other classes of agents, is relatively well preserved in patients with volume expansion.

CCBs are generally well tolerated in dialysis patients. Minor side-effects relate to vasodilation and include dizziness, intradialytic hypotension (more markedly in patients with high interdialytic weight gain), headache, flushing, and edema. Less common effects are nausea, constipation, skin rash, somnolence, and transient abnormalities in liver function tests. Studies in hypertensive patients without ESRD have implicated short-acting CCBs in increased cardiovascular morbidity and mortality. Short-acting agents are not recommended even for hypertensive urgencies. Verapamil and diltiazem have negative inotropic and chronotropic actions. Therefore they should be used with

great caution in patients with poor cardiac function, or in those receiving β-blockers.

Because of their efficacy, their safety in renal failure, and generally low profile of adverse effects, long-acting CCBs are appropriate for hypertension in dialysis patients. They have added benefits in patients with ischemic heart disease, dilated cardiomyopathy, peripheral vascular disease, Raynaud syndrome, and vascular headaches. Further information is needed about their risk–benefit ratio for this group of patients.

β-Adrenergic blocking agents

β-Adrenergic blocking agents are reviewed in Chapter 54 (and see Table 64.2). They block renin release, reduce cardiac output with autoregulatory decreases in TPR, reduce central adrenergic drive, and limit norepinephrine release. Labetalol and carvetolol also block α-adrenergic receptors, and carvetolol is an anti-oxidant drug. These additional actions promote vasodilation and maintain cardiac output. Early in the course of β-blocker therapy in patients with essential hypertension, blood pressure reduction is achieved primarily by reducing cardiac output. However, prolonged administration leads to a fall in TPR. Whether this pattern is preserved in ESRD remains unclear.

β-Blocking agents are either predominantly lipid-soluble (lipophilic) or water-soluble (hydrophilic). Lipophilic β-blockers such as propranolol or metoprolol are metabolized extensively in the liver and have a short duration of action. However, the metabolites may be active and may be hydrophilic, as in the case of acebutolol. Hydrophilic β-blockers such as atenolol and nadolol are long-acting, are excreted by the kidneys, and are removed during hemodialysis or CAPD. They are likely to accumulate in

Table 64.1 Calcium channel blockers

Agent	Daily dose in ESRD (mg)	ESRD dose modification	Special adverse effects	Removal with dialysis	
				HD	PD
Phenylalkylamine					
Verapamil SR	120–240	None	Bradycardia	N	U
	max 480 q.d.		Constipation	N	U
Benzodiazepam					
Diltiazem CD	120–360 q.d.	None	Bradycardia	N	U
Dihydropyridines					
Amlodipine	5–10 q.d.	None		N	U
Bepridil	200–400 q.d.	None	Prolonged Q–T, torsades de pointes, agranulocytosis	U	U
Felodipine	5–20 q.d.	None	Tachyarrhythmia	N	U
Isradipine	2.5–10 b.i.d.	None		N	U
Nicardipine SR	30–60 b.i.d.	None		N	U
Nifedipine XL	30–120 q.d.	None	Tachycardia	N	N
Nisoldipine	20–50 q.d.	None		U	U

CD, controlled diffusion; ESRD, endstage renal disease; HD, hemodialysis; N, not dialyzed; PD, peritoneal dialysis; Q–T, interval on EEG; SR, slow release; XL, extended length; U, unknown.

Table 64.2 β-Blocking agents

Agent	ISA/CS/α+β	Daily dose in ESRD (mg)	ESRD dose modification	Special adverse effects	Removal with dialysis HD	Removal with dialysis PD
Acebutolol	+/+/0*	NR			Y	U
Atenolol	0/+/0	NR			Y	Y
Betaxolol	0/+/0	NR			N	N
Bisoprolol	0/+/0	NR			N	N
Carvedilol	0/0/+	6.25–12.5 b.i.d		Orthostasis	N	N
Labetalol	0/0/+	200–600 t.i.d.	None	Orthostasis	N	N
Metoprolol	0/+/0	50–100 b.i.d	Additional dose post HD		Y	U
Nadolol	0/0/0	NR			Y	U
Pindolol	+/0/0	NR			Y	N
Propanolol	0/0/0	80–160 b.i.d	Additional dose post HD		N	N
Sotalol	0/0/0	NR		Torsades de pointes	Y	N
Timolol	0/0/0	10 b.i.d		Hypotension	U	U

*+, present; 0, not present at therapeutic doses.
ESRD, endstage renal disease; HD, hemodialysis; ISA, intrinsic sympathomimetic activity; CS, cardioselectivity; α+β, alpha- and beta-blocking activity; N, not dialyzed; NR, not recommended for initial therapy in ESRD because the drug is cumulative and, if used, needs careful monitoring and dose reduction. PD, peritoneal dialysis; U, unknown.

patients with renal failure and to be removed by dialysis. Therefore, nadolol, atenolol, acebutolol, and sotalol must be used with extra caution in patients with ESRD. Some noncompliant or confused patients may not be able to manage a daily intake of antihypertensives. For them, a dose of long-acting atenolol after HD provides a measure of blood pressure control between dialysis.

β-Blockers produce a spectrum of dose-dependent adverse effects. They can increase insulin resistance and dyslipidemia – correlates of cardiovascular mortality. However, these effects are less obvious with cardioselective agents such as metoprolol, or those with intrinsic sympathomimetic activity such as pindolol. Other adverse effects include hyperkalemia, bradycardia, Raynaud's phenomenon, and central nervous system effects including nightmares, fatigue, and depression. β-Blockers may exaggerate cardiac failure in poorly compensated patients, or produce bronchospasm in patients with asthma, and may mask the symptoms of hypoglycemia in patients with diabetes. Some patients experience impotence.

β-Blockers are useful antihypertensive agents in patients with ESRD. Antihypertensive efficacy in essential hypertension is greater in white than in black patients, in young than in old, and in those with high plasma renin levels. Therefore, they are most effective in ESRD patients who are maintained at a low target weight. Their beneficial effect on cardiovascular morbidity and mortality, on symptomatic angina, and in preventing death in patients who have had a myocardial infarction have not been studied in ESRD. However, because of the experience of

these drugs in other areas, they are our preferred treatment for ESRD patients with these conditions, even in a patient without significant hypertension.

Angiotensin-converting enzyme inhibitors

ACEIs (Table 64.3) are reviewed in Chapter 55. They lower the blood pressure by reducing the peripheral vascular resistance. They not only inhibit conversion of angiotensin I to angiotensin II (Ang II) in the circulation and tissues, but also inhibit bradykinin degradation by blocking kinase II. The increased bradykinin levels stimulate nitric oxide and prostaglandin synthesis. ACEIs reset the baroreflex and dampen the sympathetic nervous system so that heart rate does not normally change.

ACEIs are divided into three broad groups: sulfhydryl-containing (captopril is the only one); dicarboxyl-containing (lisinopril, benazepril, quinapril, ramipril, spirapril, perindopril, enalapril, and cilazapril); and phosphorus-containing (fosinopril). Only captopril and lisinopril are active drugs; the others are prodrugs that are converted in vivo to the active compounds.

Absorption of captopril is markedly affected by food. It should be taken 1 h before meals. The active form of most ACEIs, and their metabolites, are largely excreted by the kidney. However, another important route of elimination for fosinopril, spirapril, and benazepril is by hepatic metabolism. In renal failure, this compensates for lack of renal excretion and prevents substantial accumulation of these agents. Quinapril is tightly bound to tissue angiotensin-

Table 64.3 Angiotensin-converting enzyme inhibitors

Agent	Daily dose in ESRD (mg)	Dose modification in ESRD	Removal with dialysis HD	PD
Benazepril*	2.5–20 q.d.	50–75% dose reduction	No	Unknown
Captopril	12.5–25 q.d.	50% dose reduction, and once daily dosing; additional dose post HD	Yes	No
Enalapril	2.5–10 b.i.d	50% dose reduction, and additional dose post HD	Yes	No
Fosinopril*	10–40 q.d.	Additional dose post HD	Yes	No
Lisinopril	2.5–20 q.d.	50–75% dose reduction, and additional dose post HD	Yes	No
Moexipril	7.5–15 q.d.		Unknown	Unknown
Quinapril*	10–40 q.d.	0–25% dose reduction, and additional dose post HD	Yes	No
Ramipril	2.5–10 q.d.	50–75% dose reduction, and additional dose post HD	Yes	No
Spirapril*	3–6 q.d.	None	Unknown	Unknown
Trandelapril	1–3 q.d.	50% dose reduction	Unknown	Unknown

*Preferred agents in endstage renal disease (ESRD) because major modifications of dose are not required. HD, hemodialysis; PD, peritoneal dialysis.

converting enzyme, which prevents major accumulation in ESRD. Therefore, only modest dose reduction is required.

ACEIs are generally well tolerated. Common side-effects include cough in 5–20%. Serious hyperkalemia can occur but is uncommon in HD patients. Other side-effects are quite rare but include skin rashes, angioedema, abnormal taste, neutropenia, and hepatotoxicity. Anaphylactoid reactions have been reported in patients on ACEIs treated with the high-flux membrane AN 69. Therefore, this membrane should be avoided in patients receiving ACEIs.

ACEIs (or β-blockers) are particularly effective in treating hypertension that is resistant to dialysis where high levels of plasma renin activity are encountered; in contrast, they have little antihypertensive action in patients who are overloaded with fluid and salt and in those who have very low levels of plasma renin activity. Other beneficial actions of ACEIs in treating essential hypertension include an increase in large artery compliance, reduction in LVH, and improvement in insulin resistance. These drugs can moderate the excessive thirst that plagues some people with ESRD.

Angiotensin II receptor blockers

These drugs (Table 64.4) are reviewed in Chapter 55. They act by blocking the binding of Ang II to its type 1 receptors (AT₁). The role of Ang II type 2 receptors (AT₂) is unclear. No therapeutic AT₂ receptor antagonists are available.

ARBs reduce blood pressure, inhibit the effects of Ang II on the kidney, sympathetic nervous system, and aldosterone secretion.

Losartan is absorbed readily. It has a bioavailability of 33%. It is metabolized in the liver to active metabolites. Losartan and its metabolite have plasma half-lives of 2 h and 6–9 h respectively. Only 4–7% is excreted through the kidney, thus accumulation in renal failure is not likely. The safety and efficacy of losartan in ESRD has been established in a controlled study.[27] Unlike an ACEI, losartan does not produce cough or angioedema, but it has other side-effects that are similar to those of ACEIs and may also cause headache, lightheadedness, and gastrointestinal problems. Other ARBs appear well tolerated and effective in patients with ESRD. As none is excreted significantly in an active form by the kidney, they do not accumulate in HD patients.

Centrally acting drugs

These agents (Table 64.5) reduce blood pressure by activating α₂-adrenergic receptors and imidazoline-preferring receptors in the brain. This reduces sympathetic outflow and thus reduces systemic vascular resistance.

Centrally acting drugs are well absorbed after oral administration. α-Methyldopa is metabolized to α-methylnorepinephrine, which is the active compound in the brain. The active metabolites of methyldopa and 50% of the dose of clonidine and guanfacine are excreted by the kidneys. Therefore, these drugs accumulate modestly in ESRD.

Sedation and dry mouth are dose-dependent side-effects that usually improve after several weeks of treatment. Sexual dysfunction with decreased libido is quite com-

Table 64.4 Angiotensin receptor blockers

Agent	Daily dose in ESRD (mg)	Removal with HD	Removal with PD
Candesartan	8–32	Not dialyzed	Not dialyzed
Eprosartan	400–800	Not dialyzed	Not dialyzed
Irbesartan	150–300	Not dialyzed	Not dialyzed
Losartan	25–100	Not dialyzed	Not dialyzed
Telmisartan	40–80	Not dialyzed	Not dialyzed
Valsartan	80–320	Not dialyzed	Not dialyzed

ESRD, endstage renal disease; HD, hemodialysis; PD, peritoneal dialysis. None of these agents requires major dose reductions in HD patients.

Table 64.5 Centrally acting agents

Agent	Daily dose in ESRD (mg)	ESRD dose modification	Special adverse effects	Removal with dialysis HD	PD
Methyldopa	250–500 q.d.	Increase dose interval to once daily dosing; additional dose of 250 mg post HD	Hepatotoxicity, HUS, Coombs-positive hemolytic anemia, LE-like syndrome retroperitoneal fibrosis, pancreatitis, bone marrow suppression	Yes	Yes
Clonidine	0.1–0.3 b.i.d	25–50% dose reduction, and b.i.d dosing	Contact dermatitis with patch	No	No
Guanfacine	0.5–1.5 q.d.	25–50% dose reduction		No	No

ESRD, endstage renal disease; HD, hemodialysis; HUS, hemolytic–uremic syndrome; LE, lupus erythematosus; PD, peritoneal dialysis.

mon. Bradycardia, especially in patients with sinoatrial nodal disease, may necessitate discontinuation of treatment.

Clonidine has been used extensively in ESRD. It is an effective antihypertensive. A clonidine transdermal patch is particularly beneficial when compliance is a problem. It provides useful background antihypertensive action in patients undergoing hemodialysis.

Adrenergic blocking agents

These agents (Table 64.6) antagonize the action of catecholamines at postjunctional α_1-receptors, thereby inhibiting vasocontriction. This results in dilation of arterial (resistance) and venous (capacitance) vessels that reduce peripheral vascular resistance and blood pressure. Cardiac output and heart rate are not usually affected.

These drugs are well absorbed, metabolized extensively in the liver, and excreted in the bile. Very small amounts are excreted unchanged in urine. They do not accumulate in ESRD.

Short-acting adrenergic blocking agents can cause a first-dose phenomenon, in which marked hypotension and syncope occur 30–90 min after taking the medica-

tion. Other side-effects such as headache, dizziness, drowsiness, and nausea are usually transient. However, their use in ESRD can exacerbate hypotension during dialysis-induced fluid removal. Therefore they require careful monitoring, and are not the drugs of first choice for these patients.

Nonspecific vasodilators

These drugs (Table 64.7) lower blood pressure by acting directly on vascular smooth muscle cells (VSMCs). Minoxidil produces vasodilation through its metabolite that activates adenosine triphosphate-dependent potassium channels in VSMCs, thereby increasing cellular potassium ion influx. This leads to cell membrane hyperpolarization, exit of calcium ions, and vasodilation. Minoxidil is readily absorbed and metabolized in the liver. Only 10–20% is excreted unchanged in urine.

Minoxidil remains an important agent for short-term treatment of severe and refractory hypertension in ESRD despite a side-effect profile that includes pericardial effusion, hypertrichosis, tachycardia, sympathetic excitation, and postural hypotension. It is contraindicated in patients with diastolic dysfunction and severe LVH where it can

Table 64.6 Adrenergic blocking agents

Agent	Daily dose in ESRD (mg)	Dose modification in ESRD	Removal with dialysis HD	PD
Doxazosin	1–16 q.d.	None	Not dialyzed	Not dialyzed
Prazosin	1–15 b.i.d	None	Not dialyzed	Not dialyzed
Terazosin	1–20 q.d.	None	Unknown	Unknown

ESRD, endstage renal disease; HD, hemodialysis; PD, peritoneal dialysis.

cause cardiac failure. It can induce nonspecific T-wave changes, rashes, Stevens–Johnson syndrome, glucose intolerance, formation of antinuclear antibodies, and thrombocytopenia.

Hydralazine is also a direct vasodilator, but its mechanism of action is not well understood. It causes quite marked tachycardia due to reflex sympathetic activation. It is well absorbed. It is inactivated by acetylation in the liver and bowel. The rate of acetylation is genetically determined. The drug is excreted hepatically, but its metabolite is excreted primarily by the kidneys. It has a longer duration of action in patients with ESRD. Side-effects include headache, flushing, hypotension, palpitations, tachycardia, dizziness, and angina pectoris. Other important but less common reactions include drug-induced lupus, hemolytic anemia, serum sickness, and vasculitis. The use of hydralazine in ESRD has diminished with the advent of more effective agents that have fewer side-effects.

Sodium nitroprusside is a nitrovasodilator with considerable value in hypertensive emergencies. It is converted in smooth muscle to nitric oxide, which activates guanyl cyclase, providing cyclic guanosine monophosphate, which leads to vasorelaxation. It is used parenterally in hypertensive emergencies (see Chapter 58). The thiocyanate produced during its metabolism is excreted solely through the kidneys. It accumulates in patients with ESRD and can cause lactic acidosis, central nervous system disturbance, seizures, and coma.

Overview of hypertension management in ESRD

Our approach is reviewed in Fig. 64.3. The first step toward controlling hypertension in ESRD is fluid management. Removal of salt and water with dialysis should be complemented by educating patients about restriction of their salt and water intake. If medications are required, they should be tailored according to the needs of each patient, and their own associated medical conditions (see Chapter 57). Blood pressure control is improved by judicious use of ambulatory monitoring to review control of arterial pressure and to make appropriate adjustment of

treatment. Long-term studies of blood pressure control in dialysis populations and the relative importance of different agents, in particular the role of ACEIs and ARBs, are urgently required.

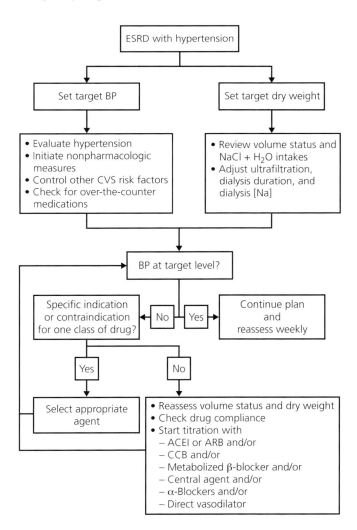

Figure 64.3 Algorithm for management of hypertension in hemodialysis patients. ACEI, angiotensin-converting enzyme inhibitor; BP, blood pressure; CCB, calcium channel blocker; CVS, cardiovascular system; ESRD, endstage renal disease.

Table 64.7 Vasodilators

Agent	Daily dose in ESRD (mg)	ESRD dose modification	Special adverse effects	Removal with dialysis	
				HD	PD
Hydralazine	25–50 b.i.d	b.i.d dosing	Lupus-like syndrome	No	No
Minoxidil	5–30 b.i.d	Additional dose post HD	Pericardial effusion	Yes	Yes
Nitroprusside	0.25–8 µg/kg/min	Not be used for more than 36–72 h	Thiocyanate toxicity	Yes	Yes

ESRD, endstage renal disease; HD, hemodialysis; PD, peritoneal dialysis.

References

1. Renal Data System: Annual Report of 1999. NIH National Institute of Diabetes and Digestive and Kidney Diseases. Bethesda, MD: National Institutes of Health, 1999.
2. Cheigh JS, Milite C, Sullivan JF, et al: Hypertension is not adequately controlled in hemodialysis patients. Am J Kidney Dis 1992;19:453–459.
3. Rahman M, Fu P, Sehgal AR, et al: Interdialytic weight gain, compliance with dialysis regimen, and age are independent predictors of blood pressure in hemodialysis patients. Am J Kidney Dis 2000;35:257–265.
4. Foley RN, Parfrey PS, Sarnak MJ: Clinical epidemiology of cardiovascular disease in chronic renal disease. Am J Kidney Dis 1998;32:S112–S119.
5. Mazzuchi N, Carbonell E, Fernández-Cean J: Importance of blood-pressure control in hemodialysis patient survival. Kidney Int 2000;58:2147–2154.
6. Port FK, Hulbert-Shearon TE, Wolfe RA, et al: Predialysis blood pressure and mortality risk in a national sample of maintenance hemodialysis patients. Am J Kidney Dis 1999;33:507–517.
7. Zager PG, Nikolic J, Brown RH, et al: "U" curve association of blood pressure and mortality in hemodialysis patients. Kidney Int 1998;54:561–569.
8. Kawamura M, Fijimoto S, Hisanaga S, et al: Incidence, outcome, and risk factors of cerebrovascular events in patients undergoing maintenance hemodialysis. Am J Kidney Dis 1998;31:991–996.
9. Cannella G, Paoletti E, Delfino R, et al: Prolonged therapy with ACE inhibitors induces the regression of left ventricular hypertrophy of dialysed uremic patients independently from hypotensive effects. Am J Kidney Dis 1997;5:659–664.
10. Zoccali C, Benedetto FA, Tripepi G, et al: Nocturnal hypoxemia, night–day arterial pressure changes and left ventricular geometry in dialysis patients. Kidney Int 1998;53:1078–1084.
11. Cannella G, Paoletti E, Ravera G, et al: Inadequate diagnosis and therapy of arterial hypertension as causes of left ventricular hypertrophy in uremic dialysis patients. Kidney Int 2000;58:260–268.
12. Savazzi GM, Cusmano F, Bergamaschi E, et al: Hypertension as an etiopathological factor in the development of cerebral atrophy in hemodialysed patients. Nephron 1998;81:17–24.
13. Wilcox CS: Management of hypertension in patients with renal disease. In: Smith TS (ed.): Cardiovascular Therapeutics. Cambridge, UK: WB Saunders Co Ltd, 1996, pp 538–545.
14. O'Rourke MF, Kelly RP: Wave reflection in the systemic circulation and its implications in ventricular function. J Hypertens 1993;11:327–337.
15. Mitch WE, Wilcox CS: Disorders of body fluids, sodium and potassium in chronic renal failure. Am J Med 1982;72:536–550.
16. Woods JD, Port FK, Orzol S, et al: Clinical and biochemical correlates of starting "daily" hemodialysis. Kidney Int 1999;55:2467–2476.
17. Velasquez MT, von Albertini B, Lew SQ, et al: Equal levels of blood-pressure control in ESRD patients receiving high-efficiency hemodialysis and conventional hemodialysis. Am J Kidney Dis 1998;31:618–623.
18. Charra B, Calemard E, Ruffet M, et al: Survival as an index of adequacy of dialysis. Kidney Int 1992;41:1286–1291.
19. Flanigan MJ, Khairullah QT, Lim VS: Dialysate sodium delivery can alter chronic blood pressure management. Am J Kidney Dis 1997;29:383–391.
20. Huang BS, Veerasingham SJ, Leenen FH: Brain "ouabain," Ang II, and sympathoexcitation by chronic central sodium loading in rats. Am J Physiol 1998;274:H1269–H1276.
21. Converse RL Jr, Jacobsen TN, Toto RD, et al: Sympathetic overactivity in patients with chronic renal failure. N Engl J Med 1992;327:1912–1918.
22. Klahr S, Levey AS, Beck GJ, et al: The effects of dietary protein restriction and blood-pressure control on the progression of chronic renal disease. N Engl J Med 1994;330:877–884.
23. MacMahon S, Rodgers A: The effects of blood pressure reduction in older patients: an overview of five randomized controlled trials in elderly hypertensives. Clin Exp Hypertens 1993;15:967–978.
24. Hansson L, Zanchetti A, Carruthers SG, et al: Effects of intensive blood-pressure lowering and low-dose aspirin in patients with hypertension: principal results of the Hypertension Optimal Treatment (HOT) randomised trial. Lancet 1998;351:1755–1762.
25. Mailloux LU, Fields S, Campese VM: Hypertension in chronic dialysis patients. In: Nissenson AR, Fine RN (eds): Dialysis Therapy. Philadelphia: Hanley & Belfus, Inc, 2000, pp 341–352.
26. Medcalf JF, Harris KP, Walls J: Role of diuretics in the preservation of residual renal function in patients on continuous ambulatory peritoneal dialysis. Kidney Int 2001;59:1128–1133.
27. Shahinfar S, Simpson RL, Carides AD, et al: Safety of losartan in hypertensive patients with thiazide-induced hyperuricemia. Kidney Int 1999;56:1879–1885.

Hypertensive Adrenal Disorders

Emmanuel L. Bravo

Adrenocortical disorders

The adrenal cortex can cause hypertension through overproduction of deoxycorticosterone (DOC), aldosterone, or cortisol. DOC and aldosterone are mineralocorticoids that produce hypertension primarily through salt and water retention. Cortisol is a glucocorticoid that can cause hypertension, in part, by exerting a mineralocorticoid effect because of incomplete metabolism at target sites.

Hypertensive syndromes due to excess production of deoxycorticosterone

Adrenocortical enzyme deficiency of either 11β-hydroxylase[1] or 17α-hydroxylase[2] results in reduced production of cortisol. This leads to uninhibited secretion of adrenocorticotropic hormone (ACTH), which drives the zona fasciculata to increase production of DOC. In deficiency disorders of both 11β- and 17α-hydroxylase, physiologic replacement doses of dexamethasone (0.5–0.75 mg/day) inhibit ACTH release and decrease DOC production, resulting in normalization of arterial blood pressure and serum potassium concentration.

In generalized glucocorticoid resistance, cortisol secretion remains ACTH-dependent but is reset to a higher than normal level.[3] There is an ACTH-dependent increase in mineralocorticoids (primarily DOC) and adrenal androgens. As there is no peripheral resistance to these hormones, they produce clinical effects. Therefore, hypertension and hypokalemia (together with signs of excess androgens) are prominent features of this disorder. There are two strategies for treating generalized glucocorticoid resistance. The first employs large doses of dexamethasone (i.e., supraphysiologic amounts) to suppress ACTH secretion. Alternatively, mineralocorticoid and/or androgen antagonists can be used.

Hypertensive syndromes due to excess production of aldosterone
Primary aldosteronism

Medical therapy is indicated in patients with adrenal hyperplasia, in those with adenoma who are poor surgical risks, and in those with bilateral adrenal adenomas that may require bilateral adrenalectomy. Total bilateral adrenalectomy has no place in the management of primary aldosteronism because adrenal insufficiency may be more difficult to treat than hypertension caused by aldosteronism. The hypertension associated with primary aldosteronism is salt- and water-dependent and is best treated by sustained salt and water depletion (Fig. 65.1).[4] The usual doses of diuretics are hydrochlorothiazide 25–50 mg/day or furosemide 80–160 mg/day in combination with either spironolactone 100–200 mg/day or amiloride 10–20 mg/day. These combinations usually result in prompt correction of hypokalemia and normalization of blood pressure within 2–4 weeks (Fig. 65.2).[5] In some cases, the addition of either a β-adrenergic blocker or a vasodilator may be needed to normalize arterial pressure.

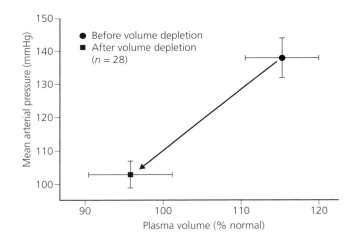

Figure 65.1 The effect of adequate volume depletion on the blood pressure of patients with primary aldosteronism and resistant hypertension. Spironolactone (200 mg/day) and hydrochlorothiazide (50–100 mg/day) were added to current therapy. Blood pressure and plasma volume values were those obtained before and after 8–12 weeks of continued therapy. Mean arterial pressure (MAP) was significantly reduced in all. For the group as a whole, it fell from 138 ± 2 to 103 ± 9 (SEM) mmHg ($P < 0.01$). Associated with the reduction in MAP were decreases in plasma volume from 114% ± 3% to 97% ± 2% (SEM) of normal ($P < 0.01$). (From Bravo EL: Primary aldosteronism. Endocrinol Metab Clin North Am 1994;23:271.)

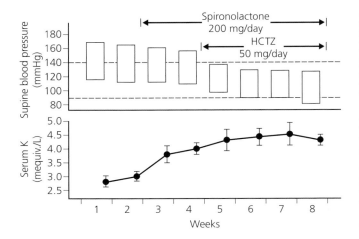

Figure 65.2 Diuretic therapy in primary aldosteronism. The effect of spironolactone combined with hydrochlorothiazide (HCTZ) on blood pressure and serum potassium concentrations in patients with aldosterone-producing tumors. (From Bravo EL, Dustan HP, Tarazi RC: Spironolactone as a nonspecific treatment for primary aldosteronism. Circulation 1973;48:491–498, with permission from the American Heart Association.)

Spironolactone and amiloride are both capable of controlling blood pressure and normalizing serum potassium concentration in patients with primary aldosteronism. However, spironolactone may be more efficacious.[6] In 11 of 25 patients who had taken both amiloride and spironolactone at different times in the course of long-term (≥ 5 years) medical therapy, the blood pressure was 123 ± 46 (standard error; SE) mmHg systolic and 82 ± 18 (SE) diastolic on spironolactone and 134 ± 3.9 (SE) systolic and 80 ± 2.5 (SE) diastolic on amiloride. The serum potassium concentration on spironolactone was 4.6 ± 0.2 (SE) mequiv./L and 4.1 ± 0.1 (SE) mequiv./L on amiloride. None of the differences was statistically significant, perhaps because of the small number of patients. However, spironolactone was associated with more adverse effects. In 17 patients started on spironolactone, the most common complaints included breast tenderness in 13, breast engorgement in 8, muscle cramps in 7, and sexual dysfunction in 5. These adverse events had no relationship to the dose. The only adverse effect noted with amiloride was muscle cramping, which was usually dose-related.

Agents that block transmembrane calcium influx and inhibit in vitro aldosterone production induced by angiotensin II (Ang II), ACTH, and potassium[7] are potent direct arteriolar vasodilators, and in some studies, are reported to have natriuretic properties.[8] For these reasons, calcium entry-blocking agents should be ideally suited for treating the hypertension associated with excessive aldosterone production. In a study by Bravo et al[9], nifedipine (30–80 mg/day) was given to eight hypertensive patients with solitary adenomas for at least 4 weeks, followed by the addition of spironolactone (100–200 mg/day) for 4 weeks, after which nifedipine was discontinued and patients remained on spironolactone alone. The following factors were assessed in the fourth week of each phase of the study: weekly averages of supine home blood pressures, plasma volume, plasma renin activity, plasma aldosterone concentration, and serum electrolyte levels. Nifedipine decreased blood pressure (157/97 ± 4/4 SE), but not to normal levels, and did not alter plasma volume, plasma renin activity, aldosterone, or serum potassium concentration. Spironolactone normalized blood pressure (122/80 ± 5/3) and serum potassium concentration, reduced plasma volume, and increased plasma renin activity and aldosterone concentration. Nifedipine plus spironolactone did not result in greater antihypertensive effect than spironolactone alone. These results suggest that nifedipine is not as efficacious as spironolactone in the treatment of primary aldosteronism.

In the majority of patients, surgical excision of an aldosterone-producing adenoma leads to normotension as well as reversal of the biochemical defects. At the very least, surgery renders arterial pressure easier to control with medications. Neither the duration and severity of hypertension, nor the degree of target-organ involvement has any relationship to the arterial pressure response after surgery.[10] One year postoperatively, about 70% of patients remained normotensive, but 5 years postoperatively only 53% remained normotensive. The restoration of normal potassium homeostasis is permanent.

Patients undergoing surgery should receive drug treatment for at least 8–10 weeks both to decrease blood pressure and to correct metabolic abnormalities. These patients have significant potassium deficiency that must be corrected preoperatively because hypokalemia increases the risk of cardiac arrhythmias during anesthesia. Prolonged control of blood pressure (at least 3 months before surgery) permits the use of intravenous fluids during surgery, without producing hypertension, and decreases morbidity. Administration of antihypertensive medications is usually continued until surgery, and glucocorticoid administration is not needed before surgery. After removal of an aldosterone-producing adenoma, selective hypoaldosteronism usually occurs, even in patients whose plasma renin activity has been stimulated with chronic diuretic therapy.[11] Potassium supplementation should, therefore, be given cautiously, and serum potassium values should be monitored closely. Residual mineralocorticoid activity is often sufficient to prevent excessive renal retention of potassium provided that sodium intake is adequate (at least 150 mequiv./day). If hyperkalemia does occur, furosemide in doses of 80–160 mg/day should be started. Treatment with fludrocortisone is not often necessary. If it is required, 0.1 mg/day may be used as the initial dose and adequate salt intake continued. Abnormalities in aldosterone production can persist for as long as 3 months after tumor removal.

Glucocorticoid-remediable aldosteronism

Glucocorticoid-remediable aldosteronism (GRA) is an inherited autosomal disorder that mimics primary aldosteronism.[12] The disorder is caused by a genetic mutation that results in a hybrid or chimeric gene product fusing nucleotide sequence of the 11β-hydroxylase and aldosterone synthase genes.[13] The structure of the duplicated gene contains 5' regulatory sequences conferring the ACTH responsiveness of 11β-hydroxylase fused to more distal coding sequences of the aldosterone synthase gene. This hybrid gene is expected to be regulated by ACTH and to have aldosterone synthase activity. It allows ectopic expression of aldosterone synthase activity in the ACTH-regulated zona fasciculata, which normally produces cortisol.[13]

No controlled studies on treatment of patients with GRA have been carried out. Theoretically, the suppression of ACTH with exogenous glucocorticoid should correct all GRA abnormalities. However, this therapy may be limited by complications of glucocorticoid administration. Another concern with glucocorticoid treatment is that patients may undergo a brief period of mineralocorticoid insufficiency when therapy is initiated before the renin-angiotensin axis recovers fully. Additional treatment modalities include mineralocorticoid receptor blockade with spironolactone, or inhibition of the mineralo-corticoid-sensitive sodium channel of the distal tubule with amiloride.

Activation of mineralocorticoid receptors by excessive circulating cortisol

Mineralocorticoid receptors in the distal nephron have equal affinity for their two ligands – aldosterone and cortisol – but are protected from cortisol by the presence of 11β-hydroxysteroid dehydrogenase (11β-OHSD) which inactivates cortisol by converting it to cortisone.[14] The 11,18-hemiacetal structure of aldosterone protects it from the action of 11β-OHSD so that aldosterone gains specific access to the receptors. Intrarenal levels of cortisol increase when this mechanism fails because of congenital 11β-OHSD deficiency, enzyme inhibition (by either licorice or carbenoxolone), or excessive circulating cortisol over-whelming the enzyme (e.g., ACTH excess syndrome), causing inappropriate activation of mineralocorticoid receptors.[15] The resulting antinatriuresis and kaliuresis lead to hypertension and hypokalemia. The signs and symptoms are reversed by spironolactone or dexamethasone and are exacerbated by administration of physiologic doses of cortisol.

Pheochromocytoma

The management of pheochromocytoma has been dominated by attempts to prevent hypertensive crises and associated complications mediated by catecholamine-induced stimulation of α-adrenergic receptors, and to diminish the magnitude of postoperative hypotension. For control of blood pressure, the use of α-blocking agents has been advocated. Phenoxybenzamine hydrochloride (10–20 mg, three or four times daily) is given in increasing doses until the blood pressure is controlled and symptomatic paroxysms are prevented. The theoretical advantages of phenoxybenzamine concern its ability to permit vascular volume repletion and to block α-receptors that noncompetitively make it difficult for released catechola-mines to overcome its blocking effect.[16] It produces significant orthostatic hypotension and reflex tachycardia, however. Moreover, it may prolong and contribute to the reduction in blood pressure that follows removal of the tumor. Despite adequate α-blockade, total elimination of cardiovascular disturbance is seldom achieved, and significant elevations of blood pressure are to be anticipated during manipulation of the tumor.[17]

Other α-adrenergic antagonists have been used to circumvent some disadvantages of phenoxybenzamine. Prazosin hydrochloride, a selective α₁-receptor antagonist, does not produce reflex tachycardia and has a shorter duration of action, thereby allowing more rapid adjustment of dosage and decreasing the duration of post-operative hypotension.[18] The initial dosage of prazosin is 1 mg, three or four times daily. This dose may be increased to a total daily dose of 20 mg. Labetalol, an α-adrenergic and β-adrenergic receptor blocker, has been reported to be effective at controlling blood pressure and clinical manifestations associated with pheochromocytoma.[19] The initial dosage is 100 mg four times daily, and is increased stepwise to a maximum of 800–1600 mg/day. Its safety has been questioned, however, because it has precipitated hypertensive crises in some people.

In 1990, Boutros et al[20] reported findings of a retro-spective study in 60 patients with proven pheochromo-cytoma who underwent 63 surgical procedures at the Cleveland Clinic from 1978 to 1988. Six patients received phenoxybenzamine preoperatively, 28 patients received prazosin, and 29 patients received neither. Intravenous sodium nitroprusside and nitroglycerin, alone or in combination, were used in all but 10 patients to control intraoperative hypertensive episodes. One patient died after surgery from a pre-existing intracranial malignant tumor. The other patients were discharged with no evidence of stroke or myocardial infarction. These findings indicated that pheochromocytoma patients can undergo successful surgery without profound and long-lasting preoperative α-adrenergic blockade.

Calcium channel blockers (CCBs) have also been successful in controlling blood pressure in patients with pheochromocytoma.[21] They have the advantage of not producing overshoot hypotension or orthostatic hypotension and therefore may be used safely in patients who are normotensive but who have occasional episodes of paroxysmal hypertension. They are useful for managing cardiovascular complications because they may also prevent catecholamine-induced coronary vasospasm and myocarditis.[22] In addition, they have none of the compli-cations associated with chronic use of α-adrenergic blockers. In doses of 40–60 mg/day, nifedipine normalizes basal blood pressure in hypertensive patients and prevents the hypertensive response to provocative challenge. Vera-pamil and diltiazem produce the same results (Fig. 65.3).[23] It is likely that they reduce arterial pressure by inhibiting norepinephrine-mediated transmembrane calcium influx in vascular smooth muscle – not by decreasing catecholamine synthesis in tumors.

Hypertensive crises may be managed with intravenous phentolamine mesylate or sodium nitroprusside. Nifedipine,

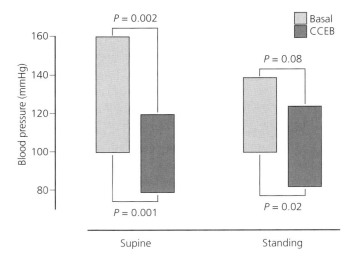

Figure 65.3 Blood pressure response to calcium antagonists in pheochromocytoma. Bars represent the mean systolic and diastolic blood pressures from 10 patients with surgically-diagnosed pheochromocytoma. Patients received either verapamil SR (120–240 mg daily; n = 5) or nifedipine XL (30–90 mg daily; n = 5) for 6–8 weeks. The blood pressure values reported here were obtained immediately before drug administration and before the surgical procedure. Calcium antagonists maintained blood pressure at normal levels, and patients were symptom-free throughout the study period. Before drug treatment, patients had reduction in systolic blood pressure with standing. This reduction was completely eliminated during treatment. CCEB, calcium channel entry blocker; Basal, baseline blood pressure. (With permission from Bravo EL: Secondary hypertension: adrenal and nervous systems. In Hollenberg NK, (ed). Atlas of Heart Diseases, 3rd edn. Philadelphia, Current Medicine, 2001, pp 118–143.)

10 mg (orally or sublingually) has also been successfully used.

Patients with pheochromocytoma have a high plasma volume requirement, both during and after surgery. Expansion of intravascular volume approximately 12 h before operation, with generous replacement of blood lost during the procedure, greatly reduces the frequency and severity of postoperative hypotension. Persistence of hypotension may be caused by hemorrhage, sudden increases in venous capacitance, inadequate volume repletion, or residual effects of preoperative α-adrenergic blockade. Fluids should be administered first, keeping in mind that these patients require large amounts of volume after tumor resection. Pressor agents are not usually effective in the presence of persistent hypovolemia. In addition, it is often difficult to withdraw vasopressors once they have been started.

Until recently, pheochromocytoma removal was only through an open approach. With technological advances and experience of minimally invasive techniques, the tumor can now be removed safely and successfully with laparoscopic surgery. Fourteen pheochromocytoma patients who underwent laparoscopic surgery were compared with 20 patients who underwent the traditional open approach.[24] (Table 65.1). The intraoperative hemodynamic values during laparoscopic surgery (adrenalectomy) were comparable to those of open surgery. However, in patients undergoing laparoscopy, intraoperative hypotension was less severe (mean lowest blood pressure 98/57 mmHg versus 80/50 mmHg, $P = 0.05$) and hypotensive episodes were less frequent (median 0 versus two episodes, $P = 0.005$). The median estimated blood loss was 100 mL (range 100–200 mL) in the laparoscopy group

Table 65.1 Perioperative hemodynamic variables

Patients	Open (n = 20)	Laparoscopic (n = 14)	P-value
Blood pressure (mmHg)			
Mean preoperative*	140 ± 18/78 ± 10	144 ± 13/74 ± 14	0.50
Highest*	191 ± 33/98 ± 25	194±19/106 ± 19	0.50
Hypertension†	0.5 (0–5)	1.0 (0–3)	0.41
Systolic ≥ 200†	0 (0–4)	0 (0–2)	0.70
Lowest*	88 ± 14/50 ± 13	98 ± 19/57 ± 8	0.05
Hypotension (episodes)	2.0 (0–6)	0 (0–2)	0.005
Heart rate (beats/min)			
Highest	104 ± 15	101 ± 24	0.78
≥ 110†	0 (0–3)	0 (0–3)	0.36
Lowest	61 ± 11	60 ± 9	0.81
≤ 50†	0 (0–1)	0 (0–5)	0.81
No. requiring treatment for hypertension‡	17	13	0.63
No. requiring treatment for hypotension§	9	1	0.02

*Systolic and diastolic blood pressure presented as the standard deviation; P-value based on the t-test test.
†Median number of episodes for one patient, with the range in parentheses; P-value based on the Mann–Whitney U-test.
‡Includes patients who intraoperatively received at least one of the following treatments; nitroglycerin, sodium nitroprusside, β-blocker, α/β-blocker, and/or calcium antagonist.
§Includes patients who intraoperatively received at least one of the following treatments: phenylephrine, dopamine, and/or epinephrine. (From Sprung et al.[24])

and 400 mL (range 150–1500 mL) in the open group ($P = 0.0001$). Surgery time was no different between the two groups (196 ± 69 min for open versus 177 ± 59 min for laparoscopy). Patients who underwent laparoscopy had a faster postoperative course. Time to ambulation was 1.5 days versus 4 days ($P = 0.002$); resumption of oral food intake was quicker (median 1 day versus 3.5 days, $P = 0.001$) and duration of hospitalization was much shorter (median 3 days versus 7.5 days, $P = 0.001$). This study indicates that laparoscopic removal of pheochromocytoma is not only safe but also has marked advantages over the open approach: patients recover more quickly, have a shorter hospital stay, and better cosmetic outcome.

References

1. White PC, Speiser PW: Steroid 11 beta-hydroxylase deficiency and related disorders. Endocrinol Metab Clin N Am 1994;23:325–339.
2. Biglieri EG, Herron MA, Brust N: 17-hydroxylation deficiency in man. J Clin Invest 1966;45:1946–1954.
3. Malchoff CD, Malchoff DM: Glucocorticoid resistance in humans. Trends Endo Metab 1995;6:89–95.
4. Bravo EL, Fouad-Tarazi FM, Tarazi RC, et al: Clinical implications of primary aldosteronism with resistant hypertension. Hypertension 1988;11:I207–I211.
5. Bravo EL, Dustan HP, Tarazi RC: Spironolactone as a nonspecific treatment for primary aldosteronism. Circulation 1973;48:491–498.
6. Ghose RP, Hall PM, Bravo EL: Medical management of aldosterone-producing adenomas. Ann Intern Med 1999;131:105–108.
7. Schiffrin EL, Lis M, Gutkowska J, et al: Role of Ca^{2+} in response of adrenal glomerulosa cells – angiotensin II, ACTH, K^+ and ouabain. Am J Physiol 1981;241:E42–E46.
8. Kiowski W, Bertel O, Erne P, et al: Hemodynamic and reflex responses to acute and chronic antihypertensive therapy with the calcium entry blocker nifedipine. Hypertension 1983;5:I70–I74.
9. Bravo EL, Fouad FM, Tarazi RC: Calcium channel blockade with nifedipine in primary aldosteronism. Hypertension 1986;8(Suppl 1):1–191.
10. Bravo EL: Pheochromocytoma and mineralocorticoid hypertension. *In* Glassock RJ (ed): Current Therapy in Nephrology and Hypertension, 4th edn. St Louis: Mosby Year Book Inc, 1998, pp 330–334.
11. Bravo EL, Dustan HP, Tarazi RC: Selective hypoaldosteronism despite prolonged pre- and postoperative hyperreninemia in primary aldosteronism. J Clin Endocrinol Metab 1975;41:611–617.
12. Lifton RP, Dluhy RG, Powers M, et al: A chimaeric 11 beta-hydroxylase/aldosterone synthase gene causes glucocorticoid-remediable aldosteronism and human hypertension. Nature 1992;355:262–265.
13. Lifton RP, Dluhy RG, Powers M, et al: Hereditary hypertension caused by chimaeric gene duplications and ectopic expression of aldosterone synthase. Nat Genet 1992;2:66–74.
14. Edwards CR, Stewart PM, Burt D, et al: Localisation of 11 beta-hydroxysteroid dehydrogenase tissue specific protector of the mineralocorticoid receptor. Lancet 1988;2(8618):986–989.
15. Funder JW, Pearce PT, Smith R, et al: Mineralocorticoid action: target tissue specificity is enzyme, not receptor, mediated. Science 1988;242:583–585.
16. Hoffman BB: Catecholamines, sympathomimetic drugs, and adrenergic receptor antagonists. *In* Hardman JG, Lombard LE (eds): The Pharmacological Basis of Therapeutics, 10th edn. Philadelphia: McGraw-Hill, 2001, pp 215–268
17. Stenstrom G, Haljamae H, Tisell LE: Influence of pre-operative treatment with phenoxybenzamine on the incidence of adverse cardiovascular reactions during anaesthesia and surgery for phaeochromocytoma. Acta Anaesthesiol Scand 1985;29:797–803.
18. Nicholson JP Jr, Vaughn ED Jr, Pickering, TG, et al: Pheochromocytoma and prazosin. Ann Intern Med 1983;99:477–479.
19. Oates JA, Brown NJ: Antihypertensive agents and the drug therapy of hypertension. *In* Hardman JG, Lombard LE (eds): Goodman & Gillman's The Pharmacological Basis of Therapeutics. Philadelphia: McGraw-Hill, 2001, pp 871–900.
20. Boutros AR, Bravo EL, Zanettin G, et al: Perioperative management of 63 patients with pheochromocytoma. Cleve Clin J Med 1990;57:613–617.
21. Serfas D, Shoback DM, Lorell BH: Phaeochromocytoma and hypertrophic cardiomyopathy: apparent suppression of symptoms and noradrenaline secretion by calcium-channel blockade. Lancet 1983;2:711–713.
22. van Vliet PD, Burchell HB, Titus JL: Focal myocarditis associated with pheochromocytoma. N Engl J Med 1966;274:1102–1108.
23. Bravo EL: Secondary hypertension: adrenal and nervous systems. *In* Hollenberg NK, (ed): Atlas of Heart Diseases, 3rd edn. Philadelphia: Current Medicine, 2001, pp 118–143.
24. Sprung J, O'Hara JF, Jr., Gill IS, et al: Anesthetic aspects of laparoscopic and open adrenalectomy for pheochromocytoma. Urology 2000;55:339–343.

PART XII
Chronic Renal Failure and its Systemic Manifestations

CHRISTOPHER S. WILCOX

Prevention of Progressive Renal Failure

Maarten W. Taal and Barry M. Brenner

Despite substantial advances in medical science over the past 50 years, there are few effective treatments for specific renal diseases. Consequently, many cases progress to chronic renal failure (CRF) and the population of patients requiring renal replacement therapy continues to grow rapidly worldwide. In the USA alone, about 300 000 people require chronic dialysis and 80 000 are renal transplant recipients.[1] Moreover the annual mortality rate on dialysis is 20–25% and there is a worldwide shortage of organs for transplantation. In an attempt to address this problem, attention has focused on the mechanisms whereby chronic renal disease (CRD) progresses to endstage renal failure. It has been appreciated for several decades that renal diseases of diverse etiology that result in substantial loss of functioning nephrons provoke a common syndrome characterized by systemic hypertension, proteinuria, and a progressive decline in glomerular filtration rate (GFR), the rate of which depends more upon the individual's characteristics than specific disease etiology.[2,3] These observations suggest that CRD progresses via a common pathway of mechanisms and that therapeutic interventions inhibiting this pathway may successfully slow down the rate of progression of CRD, irrespective of the initiating cause. In this chapter we review experimental and clinical evidence in support of this hypothesis and propose a comprehensive strategy for achieving maximal renoprotection with currently available interventions.

Mechanisms underlying progression of chronic renal disease

When rats are subjected to surgical ablation of five-sixths of their renal mass (5/6 nephrectomy model), they develop hypertension, proteinuria, and a progressive loss of GFR, features similar to those of human CRD. This model has therefore been used widely to study the mechanisms of progression of CRD.[4] Hostetter, Brenner and colleagues[5] used micropuncture techniques to measure glomerular capillary hydraulic pressure (P_{GC}) and GFR in single nephrons (single nephron GFR; SNGFR). They showed experimentally that when nephrons were lost, the remaining glomeruli underwent hemodynamic adaptations resulting in substantial increases in SNGFR (glomerular hyperfiltration) and P_{GC} (glomerular capillary hypertension). Furthermore, the observation of structural injury to glomerular cells as early as 1 week after 5/6 nephrectomy suggested that these hemodynamic changes, although initially adaptive, eventually cause glomerular damage that results in a further loss of nephrons, thereby establishing a vicious cycle of progressive renal injury.[6]

Support for this hypothesis came from experimental studies showing that interventions resulting in protection of remnant kidneys from progressive injury were associated with attenuation of the glomerular hemodynamic changes. Low-protein feeding was associated with normalization of SNGFR and P_{GC} and substantial protection from progressive glomerular injury.[5,7] Treatment with an angiotensin-converting enzyme inhibitor (ACEI) had little effect on SNGFR but did normalize P_{GC} and afforded effective renoprotection, suggesting that P_{GC} rather than SNGFR was the critical determinant of glomerular injury in the remnant kidney.[8] Moreover, combination treatment with hydralazine, hydrochlorothiazide, and reserpine was associated with a similar reduction of systemic blood pressure to ACEI, but not with a lower P_{GC} or renoprotection.[9]

The pathogenesis of diabetic nephropathy is multifactorial and is discussed in more detail in Chapter 31. Nevertheless, micropuncture studies in a rodent model of diabetic nephropathy showed that glomerular hypertension and hyperfiltration are also present in this form of CRD. The importance of these hemodynamic factors in the pathogenesis of diabetic nephropathy was confirmed by experimental studies showing that normalization of P_{GC} by low-protein diet or treatment with ACEI resulted in prevention of progressive renal injury despite persistent chronic hyperglycemia.[10,11]

Although angiotensin II (Ang II) is an important mediator of the glomerular hemodynamic changes associated with progressive renal injury, experimental studies have revealed several nonhemodynamic effects of Ang II that may also be important in CRD progression. These include proliferation of mesangial cells and induction of transforming growth factor beta (TGF-β) expression, stimulation of production of plasminogen activator inhibitor 1 by endothelial and vascular smooth muscle cells, macrophage activation and increased phagocytosis, as well as adrenal production of aldosterone, a recently recognized contributor to renal injury.[12] Ang II has thus emerged as a central factor in the pathogenesis of progressive renal injury and it is a logical target for interventions to slow progression of CRD (Fig. 66.1). Further mechanisms that may contribute to progressive renal injury are discussed below and are summarized in Fig. 66.1.

Interventions to slow the rate of progression of chronic renal disease

Antihypertensive therapy

The treatment of systemic hypertension was the first intervention shown to significantly slow the rate of CRD progression. It remains the fundamental tenet of renoprotective strategies. Initial studies showed that among insulin-dependent diabetic patients with diabetic nephropathy, the initiation of antihypertensive therapy results in a marked reduction in the rate of GFR decline,[13,14] implying that hypertension – an almost universal consequence of impaired renal function – also contributes to the progression of CRD. Similar observations were later reported among patients with nondiabetic forms of CRD.[15–17] Furthermore, data from the MRFIT[18] study, which identified elevated blood pressure as a strong, independent risk factor for ESRD in 332 544 prospectively evaluated men, confirmed that systemic hypertension is important in the pathogenesis of the progression of nondiabetic CRD. Uncertainty remained, however, as to what degree of blood pressure lowering was required to achieve optimal renoprotection.

The Modification of Diet in Renal Disease (MDRD)[19] study sought to resolve this issue. It directly evaluated whether lower than previously recommended blood pressure targets gave greater renoprotection than "usual" blood pressure control among patients with predominantly nondiabetic CRD. In addition to the dietary interventions described below, patients were randomized to a target mean arterial pressure (MAP) of 107 mmHg or 92 mmHg. The primary analysis did not show any overall difference in rate of GFR decline between these groups, but patients randomized to the low blood pressure group showed an early rapid decrease in GFR, likely due to associated renal hemodynamic effects. This result obscured a later significantly slower rate of GFR decline than that observed in the "usual" blood pressure target group. Furthermore, a higher level of baseline proteinuria was associated with a greater difference in GFR decline between the "usual" and low blood pressure groups.

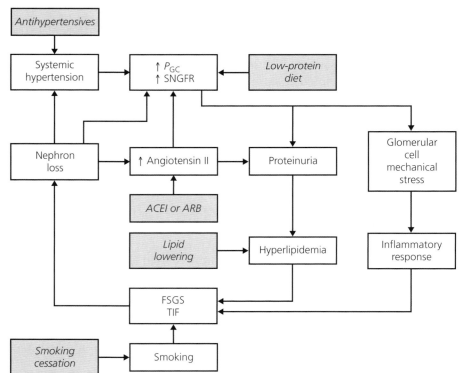

Figure 66.1 Scheme depicting the proposed mechanisms resulting in a common pathway of progressive nephron loss in chronic renal disease and illustrating the actions of different interventions (in italics) in interrupting this pathway. ACEI, angiotensin-converting enzyme inhibitor; Ang II, angiotensin II; ARB, angiotensin receptor blocker; FSGS, focal and segmental glomerulosclerosis; P_{GC}, glomerular capillary hydraulic pressure; SNGFR, single nephron glomerular filtration rate; TIF, tubulointerstitial fibrosis.

Secondary analysis revealed significant correlations between the rate of GFR decline and achieved blood pressure, an effect that was also more marked among those with greater baseline proteinuria. In study I of the MDRD[20] (patients with GFR of 25–55 mL/min/1.73 m^2), rates of decline in GFR increased above a MAP of 98 mmHg among patients with baseline proteinuria of 0.25–3.0 g/day, and above 92 mmHg in those with baseline proteinuria > 3.0 g/day. In MDRD study II[20] (patients with GFR of 13–24 mL/min/m^2), higher achieved blood pressure was associated with greater rates of GFR decline at all levels in those with baseline proteinuria > 1 g/day. The authors recommended a blood pressure goal of < 125/75 mmHg (MAP = 92 mmHg) for CRD patients with > 1 g/day of proteinuria, and a goal of < 130/80 mmHg (MAP = 98 mmHg) for those with proteinuria of 0.25–1.0 g/day.[20] Since not all the patients in the MDRD study received ACEI, it remains unclear how important the blood pressure level attained is in CRD patients receiving ACEI or angiotensin receptor blockers (ARBs). However, experimental studies have found systolic blood pressure to be a major determinant of glomerular injury in rats receiving either ACEIs or ARBs.[21,22] Moreover, in patients with type 1 diabetes and established nephropathy receiving ACEIs, randomization to a low (MAP = 92 mmHg) versus "usual" (MAP = 100–107 mmHg) target blood pressure was associated with significantly lower levels of proteinuria after 2 years, although there was no significant difference in GFR.[23] Based on this (admittedly incomplete) evidence, we would recommend that the blood pressure goals derived from the MDRD study should also be applied to patients receiving ACEIs or ARBs for renoprotection. Care should be taken, however, to avoid potentially dangerous hypotension in patients with autonomic neuropathy, labile blood pressure, or arteriosclerosis (resulting in decreased vascular compliance), which were excluded from the MDRD study.

There has been some controversy over the role of calcium channel blockers (CCBs) as antihypertensive agents in patients with CRD. There is concern that the dihydropyridine class of CCBs may in fact have adverse effects on the progression of CRD. In experimental studies, dihydropyridine CCBs allowed greater transmission of systemic blood pressure to the renal microcirculation, and were associated with more rapid progression of renal injury than ACEIs in the 5/6 nephrectomy model.[24] Whereas one relatively small study found no difference between the renoprotective effects of the dihydropyridine CCB, nifedipine, and the ACEI, captopril,[25] two larger studies reported adverse outcomes with the use of dihydropyridine CCB.[26] A secondary analysis of data from the Ramipril Efficacy in Nephropathy (REIN)[26] study found that treatment with a dihydropyridine CCB (nifedipine or amlodipine) was associated with greater proteinuria and more rapid GFR decline than with other antihypertensives, in those patients who failed to achieve a MAP of < 100 mmHg and who were not receiving an ACEI.

In the African American Study of Kidney Disease and Hypertension (AASK)[27] patients with CRD and hypertension were randomized to treatment with an ACEI or amlodipine or a β-blocker. The amlodipine therapy arm of the study was stopped prematurely because of more rapid decline in GFR among these patients compared with those receiving β-blocker or ACEI therapy, particularly among those with >1 g/day of proteinuria.

Based on the above evidence we recommend that dihydropyridine CCBs should not be used in patients with CRD unless they are required as combination therapy with other antihypertensive agents to achieve the targets for blood pressure control outlined above, and unless they are used in combination with an ACEI. The AASK study implies that this is particularly true for African American patients. On the other hand, available data suggest that nondihydropyridine CCBs may contribute to renoprotection. In one study involving patients with type 2 diabetes and overt nephropathy, treatment with nondihydropyridine CCBs reduced proteinuria and improved glomerular permselectivity whereas nifedipine did not.[28] In another similar study a nondihydropyridine CCB had an antiproteinuric effect, additive to that of ACEI treatment.[29]

Pharmacological inhibitors of the renin–angiotensin system

Over the past decade a large number of clinical studies have been published that together provide strong support for using pharmacological inhibitors of the renin–angiotensin (RA) system as an essential component of any strategy that aims for maximal renoprotection in patients with CRD (summarized in Table 66.1).

Angiotensin-converting enzyme inhibitors

Diabetic nephropathy

Following experimental evidence of the specific renoprotective effects of ACEIs, several reports (including one small prospective study) suggested that ACEIs afford renoprotection in type 1 diabetics with established nephropathy.[30] In 1993, the Captopril Collaborative Study Group published the first large prospective randomized controlled trial to clearly show specific renoprotection attributable to ACEI treatment in human CRD.[31] In this study, 409 patients with type 1 diabetes and established nephropathy (proteinuria > 0.5 g/day; serum creatinine < 2.5 mg/dL) were randomized to receive captopril or placebo. A blood pressure goal of < 140/90 mmHg was set for all patients. After a median follow-up of 3 years, captopril treatment was associated with a 50% reduction in the risk of the combined endpoint of death, dialysis, and renal transplantation, and a 48% reduction in the risk of doubling serum creatinine levels. Moreover, this additional renoprotection was not attributable simply to the antihypertensive effects of ACEI, as blood pressure control was not statistically different between the groups.

This landmark study prompted several further studies to investigate whether ACEI may also benefit type 1 diabetic patients with the increased risk of developing nephropathy

Table 66.1 Summary of studies showing the renoprotective effects of angiotensin-converting enzyme inhibitors and angiotensin receptor blockers in diabetic and nondiabetic chronic renal disease

CRD type	Trial outcome	Reference
Angiotensin-converting enzyme inhibitors		
Type 1 DM + CRD	50% ↓ risk of dialysis, transplant or death	31
Type 1 DM + MA	↓ risk of overt nephropathy (OR = 0.38)	32,33
Type 1 DM + NA	12.7% ↓ in albuminuria (NS)	34
Type 2 DM + CRD	Benefit in only one study	35–38
Type 2 DM + MA	24–67% ↓ risk of overt nephropathy	39–45
Type 2 DM + NA	12.5% ↓ risk of developing MA	46
Nondiabetic CRD	↓ creatinine doubling / ESRD (RR = 0.52)	49,50,52,53
Angiotensin receptor blockers		
Type 2 DM + MA	↓ risk of overt nephropathy (HR = 0.30)	63
Type 2 DM + CRD	25–37% ↓ risk of creatinine doubling	61,62
	23–28% ↓ risk of ESRD	

CRD, chronic renal disease; DM, diabetes mellitus; ESRD, endstage renal disease; HR, hazard ratio; OR, odds ratio; MA, microalbuminuria; NA, normoalbuminuria; NS, not significant; RR, risk ratio.

associated with microalbuminuria. A metaanalysis of 12 such studies included 689 patients with type 1 diabetes, followed for at least a year. The analysis found that ACEI treatment was associated with a significant reduction in the risk of progression to overt nephropathy (odds ratio (OR) 0.38) and with three times the incidence of complete normalization of microalbuminuria.[32] Furthermore, another study showed that the effect of ACEIs in preventing progression to overt nephropathy was sustained over 8 years and was associated with preservation of a normal GFR.[33] Finally, subgroup analysis of the EUCLID study[34] found that ACEI treatment reduced albuminuria by 12.7% among normotensive, normoalbuminuric type 1 diabetic people. However, this trend was not statistically significant and was associated with a statistically lower blood pressure in the ACEI-treated group.[34]

Data on the renoprotective effects of ACEI in patients with type 2 diabetes are, to some extent, conflicting. Studies comparing ACEI and other antihypertensives among patients with type 2 diabetes with overt nephropathy have included relatively small numbers of patients. Only one study[35] was able to show a greater reduction in GFR decline associated with ACEI versus other antihypertensives.[36–38] By contrast, several studies – including the diabetic subgroup analysis of the Heart Outcomes Prevention Evaluation (HOPE) study[39] – have reported beneficial effects of ACEIs on decreasing microalbuminuria,[40–42] or reducing the number of type 2 diabetes patients who progress from microalbuminuria to overt proteinuria (risk reduction 24–67%).[43–45] In addition, the HOPE study reported a 25% reduction in the combined primary endpoint of myocardial infarction, stroke, or cardiovascular death in ramipril-treated type 2 diabetic patients with risk factors for cardiovascular disease.[39] Finally, at least one study has reported a beneficial role for ACEI in the primary prevention of nephropathy among 156 normotensive, normoalbuminuric type 2 diabetics. Patients receiving enalapril over a 6–year period had an absolute risk reduction of 12.5% versus placebo for developing microalbuminuria.[46] On the other hand, one relatively large study found no renoprotective benefit of ACEI over β-blocker treatment in hypertensive type 2 diabetic people with normoalbuminuria or microalbuminuria.[47]

Based on the above data, we recommend ACEI treatment for all type 1 diabetic patients with microalbuminuria or overt nephropathy. At present, insufficient data exist to support the use of ACEIs in normoalbuminuric type 1 diabetics. Although there is no clear evidence of specific benefit associated with ACEIs in slowing the progression of established nephropathy in type 2 diabetes, this may be due to the lack of adequately powered studies. There is sufficient evidence, however, to recommend the use of ACEI for reducing progression to overt nephropathy in type 2 diabetic patients with microalbuminuria. On a final point, since cardiovascular disease is the most common cause of morbidity and mortality among type 2 diabetics, ACEI treatment should be considered for the reduction of cardiovascular risk.

Nondiabetic chronic renal disease

Following the publication of studies that show the renoprotective effects of ACEIs in diabetics, investigators sought to study the potential of ACEIs for renoprotection in nondiabetic forms of CRD. Maschio et al[48] randomized 583 patients with CRD of diverse etiology to treatment with benazepril or placebo. After 3 years of follow-up, the study found a 53% reduction in the risk of reaching the combined endpoint of doubling baseline serum creatinine or the need for dialysis associated with ACEI treatment. However, significantly lower blood pressure in those receiving ACEIs versus placebo made it impossible to separate the beneficial effects of lowered blood pressure from any unique effects of ACEI treatment.[48]

By contrast, in the REIN study,[49] 352 patients with nondiabetic CRD randomized to either ACEI or placebo achieved similar control of blood pressure. The study was stopped early in patients with ≥ 3 g/day of proteinuria at baseline, because of a significantly lower rate of decline in GFR in patients receiving the ACEI (0.53 versus 0.88 mL/min/month). Further analysis showed a significant reduction in the risk of the combined endpoint of doubling serum creatinine or ESRD in the ACEI group (risk ratio = 1.91 for the placebo group). In the next phase of this study,[50] patients who had received placebo were switched to ACEI and those already on ACEI continued treatment. Consistent with the findings of the first phase of the study, there was a significant reduction in the rate of decline in GFR of patients switched to ACEI. In addition, patients continuing on ACEI treatment showed a further reduction in the rate of GFR decline, to levels similar to those associated with normal aging. Patients who received ACEI from the start of the REIN study had a significantly lower risk of reaching endstage renal failure than those switched to ACEI after the initial phase of the study (relative risk for placebo group = 1.86). Indeed from 36 to 54 months of follow-up, no further patients in the former group reached endstage renal failure. Interestingly, a small number of patients who continued on ACEI actually showed an increase in GFR after prolonged treatment.[51] In stratum 2 of the REIN study[52], 186 patients with < 3 g/day of proteinuria were followed for a median of 31 months after randomization. Similar to the findings among those with more severe proteinuria, ACEI treatment significantly reduced the incidence of endstage renal failure (relative risk for placebo group = 2.72), particularly among those with a GFR of < 45 mL/min at baseline.[52]

The findings of these individual studies were recently confirmed by a metaanalysis of 11 studies that included 1860 patients with nondiabetic CRD.[53] Antihypertensive regimens that included ACEIs resulted in significantly greater reductions in blood pressure and proteinuria, but even after statistical adjustment for these factors ACEI treatment was associated with significantly lower risks of reaching ESRD (relative risk = 0.69; confidence interval (CI) 0.51–0.94) and the combined endpoint of doubling baseline serum creatinine or ESRD (relative risk = 0.70; CI = 0.55–0.88). These data indicate that the renoprotective effects of ACEI are mediated by factors in addition to their antihypertensive and antiproteinuric effects.

Moreover, on further analysis the benefits of ACEI treatments were shown to be greater in patients with higher levels of baseline proteinuria. We therefore agree with the authors of this study that ACEI treatment is indicated in most patients with CRD. In addition to the renoprotective benefits of ACEI treatment, the recent HOPE study[54] reported substantial reductions in overall mortality (relative risk = 0.84) and cardiovascular mortality (relative risk = 0.74), as well as myocardial infarction (relative risk = 0.80) and stroke (relative risk = 0.68). This study used an ACEI versus placebo in 9297 patients who were at increased risk of cardiovascular disease.[54] Although the HOPE study did not include large numbers of patients with nondiabetic CRD, cardiovascular disease remains the single largest cause of morbidity and mortality among these patients. These data therefore provide a further rationale for the use of ACEI therapy as

the single most important intervention in patients with CRD.

Practical considerations in prescribing ACE inhibitors in chronic renal disease

Despite the clear trial evidence of the renoprotective effects of ACEIs, many physicians remain reluctant to prescribe ACEIs in CRD patients due to concerns about a potential rise in serum creatinine or potassium. It should be noted, however, that the incidence of these complications in published trials is low. Discontinuation of therapy due to uncontrolled hyperkalemia has been reported in only 0–4% of patients and the overall incidence was no different in ACEI versus non-ACEI treated patients when data from six studies were combined.[55] The discontinuation of potassium supplements, avoidance of potassium-sparing diuretics, and dietary advice to avoid high-potassium foods may all help to reduce the incidence of hyperkalemia. Similarly, a progressive rise in serum creatinine is seldom seen in patients without bilateral renal artery stenosis (in whom ACEIs and ARBs are contraindicated). Moreover, it is important to appreciate that an initial increase in serum creatinine probably results from the renal hemodynamic effects of ACEIs and predicts greater renoprotective efficacy.[56] Thus, provided that the increase is less than 30% and is not progressive, an initial rise in serum creatinine should not be regarded as an indication for discontinuing ACEI therapy.

Patients in whom renal perfusion is compromised due to intravascular volume depletion or other factors are most likely to exhibit a serious decline in renal function following the introduction of ACEI therapy. It is therefore important to ensure adequate hydration, to omit diuretics for 48–72 hours, and to avoid nonsteroidal anti-inflammatory drugs prior to starting an ACEI in CRD patients. In addition, the ACEI should be started at a low dose and titrated upward with repeated monitoring. Figure 66.2 represents an algorithm that should facilitate safe use of ACEIs in the vast majority of CRD patients.

Angiotensin receptor blockers

Angiotensin receptor blockers (ARBs) inhibit the RA system by blocking angiotensin II subtype 1 (AT_1) receptors. Thus ACEIs and ARBs differ significantly in their effects on the RA system in ways that may be therapeutically relevant.

First, ACEIs are able to inhibit only angiotensin-converting enzyme (ACE)-dependent Ang II production, whereas an ARB blocks the effect of Ang II from any source at the receptor level. In the presence of ACE inhibition, studies have shown that Ang II is produced by other proteases, including chymase and other serine proteases.[57]

Second, there are at least two subtypes of the Ang II receptor. Thus, blockade of AT_1 receptors in the presence of elevated Ang II levels can be expected to result in stimulation of subtype 2 (AT_2) receptors. Whereas AT_1 receptors mediate most of the known effects of Ang II, including vasoconstriction, stimulation of aldosterone synthesis and release, and renal tubule sodium and water

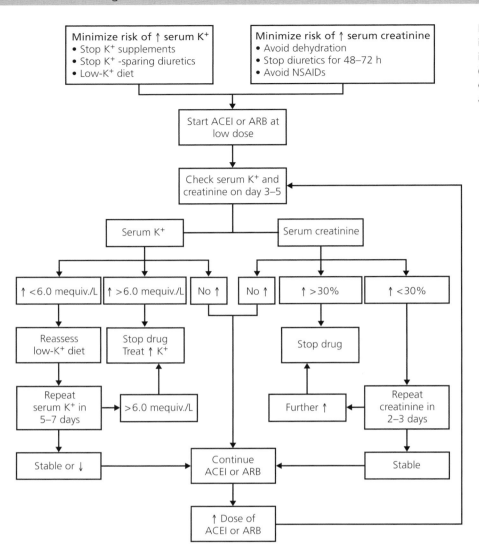

Figure 66.2 An algorithm for the safe introduction of angiotensin-converting enzyme inhibitor (ACEI) or angiotensin receptor blocker (ARB) treatment in patients with chronic renal disease. K+, potassium; NSAIDs, nonsteroidal anti-inflammatory drugs.

reabsorption, the role of AT_2 receptors is not clearly defined. Although they do not appear to be involved in any of the main effects of Ang II, AT_2 receptors are important in the fetal kidney, in modulation of pressure-natriuresis, mediation of Ang II-induced renal production of nitric oxide, and renal conversion of prostaglandin E_2 to prostaglandin F_2 (reviewed in detail in Taal and Brenner[12]).

Despite these theoretical differences, experimental studies have found that ACEIs and ARBs produce similar changes in glomerular hemodynamics and afford equivalent renoprotection in a variety of experimental CRD models.[12] In small preliminary clinical studies, ARBs and ACEIs produced similar antihypertensive and antiproteinuric effects among patients with essential hypertension,[58] nondiabetic CRD,[59] or type 2 diabetes and early nephropathy.[60]

Recently, the publication of three large randomized studies has clearly established a role for ARB therapy in achieving renoprotection for patients with type 2 diabetes. In the Reduction of Endpoints in NIDDM with Angiotensin II Antagonist Losartan (RENAAL) trial,[61] 1513 patients with established diabetic nephropathy were randomized

to losartan or placebo and followed for a mean of 3.4 years.[61] Losartan treatment was associated with significant reductions in the incidence of a doubling of baseline serum creatinine (risk reduction = 25%) and ESRD (risk reduction = 28%) as well as a 35% reduction in proteinuria. In the Irbesartan Diabetic Nephropathy Trial (IDNT),[62] 1715 patients with hypertension and established diabetic nephropathy were randomized to treatment with irbesartan, amlodipine or placebo. After a mean of 2.6 years, irbesartan was associated with a 33% lower risk of doubling of baseline serum creatinine versus placebo, and a 37% reduction versus amlodipine. Although not statistically significant, irbesartan was associated with a 23% reduction in the risk of ESRD versus placebo and amlodipine. Importantly, close matching of achieved blood pressure between groups in both these trials implies that, as with ACEI studies, the additional renoprotective effects of ARB treatment could not be attributed merely to their antihypertensive effects.

A third study examined the renoprotective effects of irbesartan in 590 type 2 diabetics with hypertension and microalbuminuria.[63] Patients were randomized to irbesartan at two different doses (300 or 150 mg/day) or placebo, and followed for 2 years. During this period significant differences emerged in the incidence of overt proteinuria (5.2% versus 9.7% versus 14.9%) and the higher dose of irbesartan was associated with a substantial reduction in the risk of developing overt nephropathy (hazard ratio = 0.30; CI 0.14–0.61 versus placebo). Although significantly lower blood pressures were achieved with irbesartan, the risk reduction was similar after adjustment for the baseline level of microalbuminuria and blood pressure.

Whereas clear evidence of the renoprotective effects of ACEIs in type 2 diabetics with overt nephropathy is lacking, there are now two large studies showing the benefits of ARBs in this population.[61,62] A single large study[63] supports the notion that ARB treatment is as effective as ACEI treatment in preventing progression from microalbuminuria to overt nephropathy. Although large randomized clinical trials of the renoprotective effects of ARBs in type 1 diabetics or nondiabetic CRD are not yet available, these data suggest that the ARBs will duplicate renoprotection achieved by ACEIs in these populations.

One important advantage of ARBs over ACEIs is their more favorable side-effect profile. In clinical trials ARBs have been reported to have side-effect profiles similar to placebo.[64,65] Importantly, ARBs are not associated with the cough that may occur in up to 20% of patients receiving ACEIs. Among patients converted from ACEI to ARB therapy, recurrence of cough was significantly lower than in patients rechallenged with an ACEI.[66,67] Thus, even in the absence of clinical trials in type 1 diabetes or nondiabetic CRD, the available evidence supports use of ARBs as an alternative in patients who are unable to tolerate ACEI due to side-effects. Furthermore, the favorable side-effect profile of ARBs suggests that it may be possible to administer higher doses. Preliminary data have shown that doubling the dose of an ARB may cause greater lowering of proteinuria without a further reduction in blood pressure.[59]

The differing effects of ACEIs and ARBs on the RA system imply that in combination they may have additive or even synergistic effects. Eight patients with immunoglobulin A (IgA) nephropathy were treated consecutively with an ACEI, an ARB, and combination therapy. The combination was associated with greater antiproteinuric effects than either treatment alone, without significant additional antihypertensive effects.[68] Addition of an ARB to prior ACEI therapy in 11 patients with CRD was associated with a 6 mmHg fall in MAP and a further 30% reduction in proteinuria.[69]

Finally, in the largest study to date among 199 type 2 diabetic patients with hypertension and microalbuminuria, combination therapy with an ACEI and ARB afforded greater reductions in blood pressure and albuminuria than either treatment alone.[70] Although more data are required before firm recommendations can be made, evidence is accumulating that combination ACEI and ARB therapy may offer additional renoprotection to that afforded by either agent alone.

Reduction of proteinuria

Proteinuria has traditionally been seen as a marker of integrity of the glomerular filtration barrier. The extent of proteinuria has therefore been used as an indicator of glomerular disease severity. Recently, however, it has been proposed that proteinuria per se also contributes to progressive renal injury.[71]

In the REIN study,[49] higher levels of baseline proteinuria were associated with more rapid rates of GFR decline. Among patients with initial proteinuria of > 3 g/day, ACEI treatment reduced proteinuria to an extent that correlated inversely with the subsequent rate of GFR decline.[49]

Furthermore, the MDRD study[20] showed that a reduction in proteinuria, independent of blood pressure, was associated with slower progression of CRD, and that the degree of benefit achieved through blood pressure lowering depended on the extent of baseline proteinuria.

Experimental observations suggest mechanisms whereby an excess of filtered proteins may contribute to renal damage. Culture of tubular epithelial cells in the presence of a variety of plasma proteins has been shown to induce production of proinflammatory cytokines and extracellular matrix proteins,[71] responses that may contribute to tubulointerstitial fibrosis. Proteinuria induced by protein overload in vivo was associated with renal expression of cell adhesion molecules and chemoattractants, resulting in interstitial inflammation and fibrosis.[72]

Together, these clinical and experimental data provide considerable support for the hypothesis that excessive filtration of serum proteins by injured glomeruli directly contributes to progressive renal damage. Whether or not proteinuria contributes directly to renal injury, the strong association between the achievement of proteinuria reduction and renoprotection in clinical studies implies that minimization of proteinuria should be regarded as an important independent therapeutic goal in renoprotective strategies.

Low-protein diet

Based on the notion that reducing the excretory burden on the kidneys would slow the rate of progressive injury, dietary protein restriction was one of the first interventions proposed to slow CRD progression. Experimental studies showed that a low-protein diet normalized glomerular hemodynamics in the remnant kidney model[5] and resulted in effective long-term renoprotection.[7] Unfortunately, clinical studies to date have failed to provide similar unambiguous evidence in support of protein restriction in human CRD.

Several smaller studies were published that generally suggested a beneficial effect from protein restriction, but they suffered from deficiencies in design or patient compliance. Subsequently, a large, multicenter, randomized study, the Modification of Diet in Renal disease (MDRD) study[19] was conducted to finally resolve the issue.

It included 585 patients with moderately severe chronic renal failure (GFR = 25–55 mL/min/1.73 m^2) who were randomized to "usual" (1.3 g/kg/day) or "low" (0.58 g/kg/day) protein diets (MDRD study I), and 255 patients with severe CRD (GFR = 13–24 mL/min/1.73 m²) who were randomized to "low" (0.58 g/kg/day) or "very low" (0.28 g/kg/day) protein diets (MDRD study II). The MDRD study included all causes of CRD, but excluded patients with diabetes mellitus requiring insulin therapy. Patients were also assigned to different levels of blood pressure control.

After a mean of 2.2 years follow-up, the primary analysis revealed no difference in the mean rate of GFR decline in MDRD study I, and showed only a trend towards a slower rate of decline in the "very low" protein group in MDRD study II.[19] Secondary analyses of the MDRD data, however, revealed that dietary protein restriction probably did achieve beneficial effects. In MDRD study I, the "low-protein" diet was associated with an initial reduction in GFR that likely resulted from the functional effects of decreased protein intake and not from loss of nephrons. This initial reduction in GFR obscured a later reduction in the rate of GFR decline that was evident after 4 months in the "low-protein" group, and that may have resulted in more robust evidence of renoprotection had follow-up been continued for a longer period.

Further analysis of data from MDRD study I also showed that dietary protein restriction achieved the greatest renoprotective effect in those with the highest initial rates of decline in GFR.[73] In MDRD study II, analysis of achieved protein intakes revealed that patients assigned to the "very low-protein" diet achieved an intake of only 0.66 g/kg/day versus 0.73 g/kg/day in the "low-protein" group. When data from both diet groups were combined and analyzed according to achieved dietary-protein intake, a reduction in protein intake of 0.2 g/kg/day correlated with a 1.15 mL/min/year reduction in the rate of GFR decline, equivalent to a 29% reduction in mean rate of GFR decline, and implying a 41% prolongation in renal survival.[74]

Several factors have been identified that may account for the inconclusive results of the study, including the generally slow rate of decline in GFR (4 mL/min/year, or less), relatively short follow-up, high proportion of patients with adult polycystic kidney disease, and unrestricted use of ACEIs.

Further evidence supporting a renoprotective effect of a low-protein diet was provided by two metaanalyses of randomized studies.[75] Among 1413 patients with nondiabetic CRD from five studies (including those from the MDRD study 1) a low-protein diet was associated with a relative risk of 0.67 for ESRD or death. Similarly, among 108 type 1 diabetics from five studies, a low-protein diet significantly slowed the increase in albuminuria or the decline in GFR/creatinine clearance.

In conclusion, although no single study has yet provided conclusive evidence of the renoprotective effect of dietary protein restriction in humans, we believe that sufficient evidence exists to recommend moderate protein restriction of 0.6 g/kg/day in patients with CRD and evidence of disease progression. The decision to institute dietary protein restriction should be tailored for the individual, and should be avoided in patients with low serum albumin due to severe nephrotic syndrome or malnutrition.

Treatment of hyperlipidemia

CRD is commonly associated with abnormalities of plasma lipids characterized by elevated levels of the triglyceride-rich very low-density lipoproteins (VLDL) and low-density lipoproteins (LDL), and reduced levels of high-density lipoproteins (HDL).[76] In addition to placing CRD patients at increased risk of cardiovascular disease, these lipid abnormalities may also accelerate the progression of CRD. In the MDRD study, low serum HDL-cholesterol was an independent predictor of more rapid decline in GFR.[77] In another study elevated levels of triglyceride-rich apolipoprotein-B-containing lipoproteins correlated significantly with the rate of deterioration of renal function.[78]

Hypercholesterolemia has been associated with more rapid progression of renal disease among patients with diabetic[79–81] and nondiabetic forms of CRD.[82] Recently, analysis of data from 12 728 patients without significant renal disease found that elevated baseline serum triglyceride levels and low HDL-cholesterol levels were independent predictors of a rise in serum creatinine over the following 2.9 years, suggesting that dyslipidemias may also be involved in the initiation of CRD.[83] The mechanisms whereby hyperlipidemia my contribute to renal injury are the subject of ongoing research, but studies to date have identified several different mechanisms, including stimulation of mesangial cell proliferation, cytokine expression, and extracellular matrix synthesis,[84,85] oxidation of LDL to form reactive oxygen species[86] and elevations in P_{GC}.[87] In experimental studies, treatment of hyperlipidemia has resulted in attenuation of renal injury in a variety of models of CRD.[88,89]

Although large randomized clinical trials of lipid-lowering therapy in CRD are awaited, a recent meta-analysis of 12 small studies that included both diabetic and nondiabetic renal disease found that lipid-lowering therapy significantly reduced the rate of decline in GFR (mean reduction 1.9 mL/min/year).[90]

These data, plus the fact that patients with CRD are at substantially increased risk for cardiovascular disease, support a policy of active dietary and drug intervention to correct hyperlipidemia in all patients with CRD. Future studies should focus on confirming this finding in larger numbers of patients, and on defining appropriate levels for intervention as well as therapeutic targets.

Smoking cessation

Smoking has been identified as a risk factor for the development of microalbuminuria, overt proteinuria, and renal disease progression in type 1 and 2 diabetics.[91–93] Similarly, smoking is a risk factor for progression of a variety of forms of nondiabetic CRD: among patients with adult polycystic kidney disease, or IgA nephropathy, smokers had a 10–fold increased risk of progression to ESRD compared with nonsmokers;[94] the median time to ESRD was almost halved in smokers versus nonsmokers in patients with lupus nephritis;[95] patients with primary glomerulonephritis and serum creatinine > 1.7 mg/dL were significantly more likely to be smokers than those with normal creatinine;[96] smoking was the most powerful predictor of a rise in serum creatinine among patients with severe essential hypertension.[97]

Moreover, smoking has been associated with increased albuminuria as well as both increased and decreased GFR in a large population-based study of nondiabetic people.[98] Proposed mechanisms whereby smoking may exacerbate renal injury include glomerular hyperfiltration, endothelial dysfunction, and increased albuminuria. Although there is a lack of prospective studies showing renal benefit from smoking cessation, this evidence suggests that the kidney is another organ adversely affected by smoking. The well-established benefits of smoking cessation for prevention of lung and cardiovascular disease, as well as malignancy, mandate that all patients with CRD should be counseled to stop smoking and should be assisted in achieving this goal.

Control of hyperglycemia

The role of glycemic control in diabetic renoprotection is discussed more fully in Chapter 31. Briefly, the Diabetes Control and Complications Trial (DCCT)[99] provided unequivocal evidence that tight glycemic control significantly reduced the development of microalbuminuria and overt nephropathy among type 1 diabetic patients. Similar results were obtained in a smaller study on type 2 diabetes.[100]

Unfortunately, the benefits of improved glycemic control are less well established for those who already have microalbuminuria. Only two of five small randomized studies[101–105] have shown a reduction in progression to overt nephropathy with tight versus "normal" glycemic control among type 1 diabetics with microalbuminuria.

On the other hand, evidence of histological reversal of diabetic glomerulopathy lesions in type 1 diabetics with normo- or microalbuminuria following pancreatic transplantation attests to the importance of tight glycemic control in achieving renoprotection in this group.[106] Furthermore, the UK Prospective Diabetes Study[107] showed a benefit of tight glycemic control in delaying the development of overt proteinuria and slowing the rate of rise in serum creatinine in type 2 diabetics with microalbuminuria.

No data are available to assess the renoprotective effect of tight glycemic control among diabetics with established nephropathy. Based on the above data we recommend tight glycemic control (target hemoglobin A_{1C} (HBA_{1C}) < 6.5%) in all diabetics for the prevention of microvascular complications including nephropathy. Despite the somewhat conflicting evidence, we also recommend continued tight glycemic control in diabetics who develop microalbuminuria or overt nephropathy.

Future therapies

Currently available renoprotective therapies have in general achieved a slowing in the rate of progression of CRD, but relatively few patients have achieved complete cessation of progression, and still fewer have evidenced a reversal of renal injury. There is therefore a need for more effective treatments and many novel renoprotective interventions are currently being investigated in experimental studies. Here we discuss some of the more promising potential additions to our renoprotective armamentarium.

Vasopeptidase inhibitors

Vasopeptidase inhibitors (VPIs) are a new class of drugs comprising single molecules that simultaneously inhibit both ACE and neutral endopeptidase (NEP). This latter ectoenzyme is localized principally in the brush border membrane of renal tubule cells and it catabolizes several vasodilator molecules including the natriuretic peptides, adrenomedullin, and bradykinin. Thus, VPI treatment is associated with reduced production of the vasoconstrictor, Ang II, and accumulation of the above-mentioned vasodilators.

In experimental[108,109] and clinical[110] studies, VPIs have been effective antihypertensive agents in both low- and high-renin states. Recently we reported that in rats subjected to 5/6 nephrectomy, the VPI omapatrilat produced greater lowering of P_{GC} than an ACEI. Furthermore, VPI treatment of rats with established renal injury after 5/6 nephrectomy almost doubled the delay in progression of CRD achieved with an ACEI, despite equivalent control of systemic blood pressure.[111] If clinical studies produce similar results, this new class of drugs may have a major impact in reducing the number of CRD patients progressing to endstage renal failure.

Antiinflammatory therapies

In recent years attention has focused on the role of cytokines and other inflammatory molecules in mediating the cellular events involved in progressive renal injury.[112] Glomerular and interstitial infiltration by macrophages is characteristically present in the 5/6 nephrectomy model and in human CRD. Furthermore, several studies have observed the apparently coordinated upregulation of a number of cytokines, cell adhesion molecules, and profibrotic growth factors in this model. If these inflammatory elements do in fact play a role in progressive renal injury in CRD, then anti-inflammatory therapies or interventions directed at inhibiting specific inflammatory or fibrotic molecules may result in additional renoprotection. Interestingly, several studies have now shown that treatment of 5/6 nephrectomized rats with the immunosuppressive agent, mycophenolate mofetil, was associated with substantial renoprotection.[113–115] Clearly, the potential benefits of this approach must be weighed against the obvious risks of immunosuppression. It is likely that a wide range of specific inhibitors of cytokines and profibrotic growth factors will soon be available, providing new tools for investigating this emerging field.

Table 66.2 A comprehensive strategy and therapeutic goals for achieving maximal renoprotection in patients with chronic renal disease

Intervention	Goal
1. ACEI or ARB treatment (consider combination therapy if goals not achieved with monotherapy)	Proteinuria < 0.5 g/day GFR decline < 1 mL/min/month
2. Additional antihypertensive therapy	BP < 125/75 if proteinuria >1 g/day BP < 130/80 if proteinuria < 1 g/day
3. Dietary protein restriction	0.6 g/kg/day
4. Tight glycemic control	HBA_{1C} < 6.5%
5. Smoking cessation	
6. Lipid-lowering therapy	

ACEI, angiotensin-converting enzyme inhibitor; ARB, angiotensin receptor blocker; BP, blood pressure; GFR, glomerular filtration rate; HBA_{1C}, hemoglobin A_{1C}.

A strategy for maximal renoprotection

In this chapter we have considered individually a variety of interventions shown to slow the rate of progression of CRD. At best, however, each intervention slows the rate of progression by about 50%. We therefore suggest that to achieve maximal long-term renoprotection a comprehensive strategy is required, using multiple elements directed at different aspects of the pathogenesis of progressive renal injury (Fig. 66.1).

Once treatments have been introduced, it is essential to frequently monitor blood pressure, proteinuria, and GFR, so that therapy can be escalated until therapeutic goals have been achieved (Table 66.2). In this regard, our approach is analogous to that applied in modern oncologic chemotherapy strategies, where multiple agents are used and treatment is directed towards correcting all signs of disease activity until the patient is said to be in "remission".

Moreover, data from a small number of patients suggest that if remission can be maintained in the long term, some recovery of renal function or "regression" of renal disease may be achieved.[51] Limited data already indicate that significant improvements in renoprotection can be achieved with this strategy. Among 160 type 2 diabetics with microalbuminuria,[116] a combined approach of intensive therapy resulted in a marked reduction in the risk of overt nephropathy (OR 0.27). Similarly, 9 of 13 patients with resistant nephrotic range proteinuria and CRD (referred to a "remission clinic") achieved reduction of proteinuria to < 1 g/day and stabilization of renal function after application of a similar intensive therapy protocol.[55]

It should be noted that the above recommendations are based on currently available interventions and the measurements required for monitoring are already widely used. Thus, a comprehensive approach to renoprotection is an achievable goal for all patients with CRD. Although it has been argued that there is a need for new renoprotective agents, it is also true that the available therapies have not yet been applied to all patients with CRD.[117] If widely implemented, a comprehensive renoprotective strategy may not only delay the need for dialysis in many patients, but may also substantially reduce the number of CRD patients progressing to ESRD.

References

1. USRDS 2001: Annual Data Report US Renal Data System: Atlas of End-stage Renal Disease in the United States. Bethesda, MD: National Institutes of Health, National Institute of Diabetes and Digestive and Kidney Diseases, 2001.
2. Mitch WE, Walser M, Buffington GA, et al: A simple method for estimating progression of chronic renal failure. Lancet 1976;2:1326–1328.
3. Rutherford WE, Blondin J, Miller JP, et al: Chronic progressive renal disease: rate of change of serum creatinine. Kidney Int 1977;11:62–70.
4. Shimamura T, Ashton B, Morrison MD: A progressive glomerulosclerosis occurring in partial five-sixths nephrectomized rats. Am J Pathol 1975;79:95–106.
5. Hostetter TH, Olson JL, Rennke HG, et al: Hyperfiltration in remnant nephrons: a potentially adverse response to renal ablation. Am J Physiol 1981;241: F85–F93.
6. Brenner BM, Meyer TW, Hostetter TH: Dietary protein intake and the progressive nature of kidney disease: the role of hemodynamically mediated glomerular injury in the pathogenesis of progressive glomerular sclerosis in aging, renal ablation, and intrinsic renal disease. N Engl J Med 1982;307:652–659.
7. Hostetter TH, Meyer TW, Rennke HG, et al: Chronic effects of dietary protein in the rat with intact and reduced renal mass. Kidney Int 1986;30:509–517.
8. Anderson S, Meyer TW, Rennke HG, et al: Control of glomerular hypertension limits glomerular injury in rats with reduced renal mass. J Clin Invest 1985;76:612–619.
9. Anderson S, Rennke HG, Brenner BM: Therapeutic advantage of converting enzyme inhibitors in arresting progressive renal disease associated with systemic hypertension in the rat. J Clin Invest 1986;77:1993–2000.
10. Zatz R, Meyer TW, Rennke HG, et al: Predominance of hemodynamic rather than metabolic factors in the pathogenesis of diabetic glomerulopathy. Proc Natl Acad Sci USA 1985;82:5963–5967.
11. Zatz R, Dunn BR, Meyer TW, et al: Prevention of diabetic glomerulopathy by pharmacological amelioration of glomerular capillary hypertension. J Clin Invest 1986;77:1925–1930.
12. Taal MW, Brenner BM: Renoprotective benefits of RAS inhibition: from ACEI to angiotensin II antagonists. Kidney Int 2000;57:1803–1817.
13. Mogensen CE: Progression of nephropathy in long-term diabetics with proteinuria and effect of initial anti-hypertensive treatment. Scand J Clin Lab Invest 1976;36:383–388.

14. Parving HH, Andersen AR, Smidt UM, et al: Early aggressive antihypertensive treatment reduces rate of decline in kidney function in diabetic nephropathy. Lancet 1983;1:1175–1179.

15. Bergstrom J, Alvestrand A, Bucht H, et al: Progression of chronic renal failure in man is retarded with more frequent clinical follow-ups and better blood pressure control. Clin Nephrol 1986;25:1–6.

16. Brazy PC, Fitzwilliam JF: Progressive renal disease: role of race and antihypertensive medications. Kidney Int 1990;37:1113–1119.

17. Kes P, Ratkovic-Gusic I: The role of arterial hypertension in progression of renal failure. Kidney Int Suppl 1996;55:S72–S74.

18. Klag MJ, Whelton PK, Randall BL, et al: Blood pressure and end-stage renal disease in men. N Engl J Med 1996;334:13–18.

19. Klahr S, Levey AS, Beck GJ, et al: The effects of dietary protein restriction and blood-pressure control on the progression of chronic renal disease. Modification of Diet in Renal Disease Study Group. N Engl J Med 1994;330:877–884.

20. Peterson JC, Adler S, Burkart JM, et al: Blood pressure control, proteinuria, and the progression of renal disease. The Modification of Diet in Renal Disease Study Group. Ann Intern Med 1995;123:754–762.

21. Bidani AK, Griffin KA, Bakris G, et al: Lack of evidence of blood pressure-independent protection by renin–angiotensin system blockade after renal ablation. Kidney Int 2000;57:1651–1661.

22. Taal MW, Chertow GM, Rennke HG, et al: Mechanisms underlying renoprotection during renin-angiotensin system blockade. Am J Physiol 2001;280:F343–F355.

23. Lewis JB, Berl T, Bain RP, et al: Effect of intensive blood pressure control on the course of type 1 diabetic nephropathy. Collaborative Study Group. Am J Kidney Dis 1999;34:809–817.

24. Griffin KA, Picken MM, Bidani AK: Deleterious effects of calcium channel blockade on pressure transmission and glomerular injury in rat remnant kidneys. J Clin Invest 1995;96:793–800.

25. Zucchelli P, Zuccala A, Borghi M, et al: Long-term comparison between captopril and nifedipine in the progression of renal insufficiency. Kidney Int 1992;42:452–458.

26. Ruggenenti P, Perna A, Benini R, et al: Effects of dihydropyridine calcium channel blockers, angiotensin-converting enzyme inhibition, and blood pressure control on chronic, nondiabetic nephropathies. Gruppo Italiano di Studi Epidemiologici in Nefrologia (GISEN). J Am Soc Nephrol 1998;9:2096–2101.

27. Agodoa LY, Appel L, Bakris GL, et al: Effect of ramipril vs amlodipine on renal outcomes in hypertensive nephrosclerosis: a randomized controlled trial. J Amer Med Assoc 2001;285:2719–2728.

28. Smith AC, Toto R, Bakris GL: Differential effects of calcium channel blockers on size selectivity of proteinuria in diabetic glomerulopathy. Kidney Int 1998;54:889–896.

29. Bakris GL, Weir MR, DeQuattro V, et al: Effects of an ACE inhibitor/calcium antagonist combination on proteinuria in diabetic nephropathy. Kidney Int 1998;54:1283–1289.

30. Bjorck S, Nyberg G, Mulec H, et al: Beneficial effects of angiotensin converting enzyme inhibition on renal function in patients with diabetic nephropathy. Br Med J (Clin Res Ed) 1986;293:471–474.

31. Lewis EJ, Hunsicker LG, Bain RP, et al: The effect of angiotensin-converting-enzyme inhibition on diabetic nephropathy. N Engl J Med 1993;329:1456–1462.

32. The ACE Inhibitors in Diabetic Nephropathy Trialist Group: Should all patients with type 1 diabetes mellitus and microalbuminuria receive angiotensin-converting enzyme inhibitors? A meta-analysis of individual patient data. Ann Intern Med 2001;134:370–379.

33. Mathiesen ER, Hommel E, Hansen HP, et al: Randomised controlled trial of long-term efficacy of captopril on preservation of kidney function in normotensive patients with insulin dependent diabetes and microalbuminuria. Br Med J 1999;319:24–25.

34. The EUCLID Study Group: Randomised placebo-controlled trial of lisinopril in normotensive patients with insulin-dependent diabetes and normoalbuminuria or microalbuminuria. Lancet 1997;349:1787–1792.

35. Bakris GL, Copley JB, Vicknair N, et al: Calcium channel blockers versus other antihypertensive therapies on progression of NIDDM-associated nephropathy.Kidney Int 1996;50:1641–1650.

36. Lebovitz HE, Wiegmann TB, Cnaan A, et al: Renal protective effects of enalapril in hypertensive NIDDM: role of baseline albuminuria. Kidney Int 1994;45:S150–S155.

37. Nielsen FS, Rossing P, Gall MA, et al: Long-term effect of lisinopril and atenolol on kidney function in hypertensive NIDDM subjects with diabetic nephropathy. Diabetes 1997;46:1182–1188.

38. Fogari R, Zoppi A, Corradi L, et al: Long-term effects of ramipril and nitrendipine on albuminuria in hypertensive patients with type II diabetes and impaired renal function. J Hum Hypertens 1999;13:47–53.

39. Heart Outcomes Prevention Evaluation (HOPE) Study investigators: Effects of ramipril on cardiovascular and microvascular outcomes in people with diabetes mellitus: results of the HOPE and MICRO-HOPE substudy. Lancet 2000; 355:253-259.

40. Sano T, Kawamura T, Matsumae H, et al: Effects of long-term enalapril treatment on persistent micro-albuminuria in well-controlled hypertensive and normotensive NIDDM patients. Diabetes Care 1994;17:420–424.

41. Trevisan R, Tiengo A: Effect of low-dose ramipril on microalbuminuria in normotensive or mild hypertensive noninsulin-dependent diabetic patients. North-East Italy Microalbuminuria Study Group. Am J Hypertens 1995;8:876–883.

42. Agardh CD, Garcia-Puig J, Charbonnel B, et al: Greater reduction of urinary albumin excretion in hypertensive type II diabetic patients with incipient nephropathy by lisinopril than by nifedipine. J Hum Hypertens 1996;10:185–192.

43. Ravid M, Lang R, Rachmani R, Lishner M: Long-term renoprotective effect of angiotensin-converting enzyme inhibition in noninsulin-dependent diabetes mellitus. A 7–year follow-up study. Arch Intern Med 1996;156:286–289.

44. Ahmad J, Siddiqui MA, Ahmad H: Effective postponement of diabetic nephropathy with enalapril in normotensive type 2 diabetic patients with microalbuminuria. Diabetes Care 1997;20:1576–1581.

45. Andersen S, Tarnow L, Rossing P, et al: Renoprotective effects of angiotensin II receptor blockade in type 1 diabetic patients with diabetic nephropathy. Kidney Int 2000;57:601–666.

46. Ravid M, Brosh D, Levi Z, et al: Use of enalapril to attenuate decline in renal function in normotensive, normoalbuminuric patients with type 2 diabetes mellitus. A randomized, controlled trial. Ann Intern Med 1998;128:982–988.

47. UK Prospective Diabetes Study Group: Efficacy of atenolol and captopril in reducing risk of macrovascular and microvascular complications in type 2 diabetes (UKPDS 39): Br Med J 1998;317:713–720.

48. Maschio G, Alberti D, Janin G, et al: Effect of angiotensin-converting-enzyme inhibitor benazepril on the progression of chronic renal insufficiency. The ACE Inhibition in Progressive Renal Insufficiency Study Group. N Eng J Med 1996;334:939–945.

49. Gruppo Italiano di Studi Epidemiologici in Nefrologia: Randomised placebo-controlled trial of effect of ramipril on decline in glomerular filtration rate and risk of terminal renal failure in proteinuric, nondiabetic nephropathy. Lancet 1997;349:1857–1863.

50. Ruggenenti P, Perna A, Gherardi G, et al: Renal function and requirement for dialysis in chronic nephropathy patients on long-term ramipril: REIN follow-up trial. Gruppo Italiano di Studi Epidemiologici in Nefrologia (GISEN). Lancet 1998;352:1252–1256.

51. Ruggenenti P, Perna A, Benini R, et al: In chronic nephropathies prolonged ACE inhibition can induce remission: dynamics of time-dependent changes in GFR. Gruppo Italiano Studi Epidemiologici in Nefrologia (GISEN). J Am Soc Nephrol 1999;10:997–1006.

52. Ruggenenti P, Perna A, Gherardi G, et al: Renoprotective properties of ACE-inhibition in nondiabetic nephropathies with nonnephrotic proteinuria. Lancet 1999;354:359–364.

53. Jafar TH, Schmid CH, Landa M, et al: Angiotensin-converting enzyme inhibitors and progression of nondiabetic renal disease. A meta-analysis of patient-level data. Ann Int Med 2001;135:73–87.

54. The Heart Outcomes Prevention Evaluation Study Investigators: Effects of an angiotensin-converting-enzyme inhibitor, ramipril on cardiovascular events in high-risk patients. N Engl J Med 2000;342:145–153.

55. Ruggenenti P, Schieppati A, Remuzzi G: Progression, remission, regression of chronic renal diseases. Lancet 2001;357:1601–1608.

56. Bakris GL, Weir MR: Angiotensin-converting enzyme inhibitor-associated elevations in serum creatinine: is this a cause for concern? Arch Int Med 2000;160:685–693.

57. Arakawa K: Serine protease angiotensin II systems. J Hypertens 1996;Suppl 5:S3–S7.

58. Nielsen S, Dollerup J, Nielsen B, et al: Losartan reduces albuminuria in patients with essential hypertension. An enalapril controlled 3 months study. Nephrol Dial Transplant 1997;2:19–23.

59. Gansevoort RT, de Zeeuw D, de Jong PE: Is the antiproteinuric effect of ACE inhibition mediated by interference in the renin-angiotensin system? Kidney Int 1994;45:861–867.

60. Lacourciere Y, Belanger A, Godin C, et al: Long-term comparison of losartan and enalapril on kidney function in hypertensive type 2 diabetics with early nephropathy. Kidney Int 2000;58:762–769.

61. Brenner BM, Cooper ME, de Zeeuw D, et al: Effects of losartan on renal and cardiovascular outcomes in patients with type 2 diabetes and nephropathy. New Engl J Med 2001;345:861–869.

62. Lewis EJ, Hunsicker LG, Clarke WR, et al: Renoprotective effect of the angiotensin-receptor antagonist irbesartan in patients with nephropathy due to type 2 diabetes. New Engl J Med 2001;345:851–860.

63. Parving HH, Lehnert H, Brochner-Mortensen J, et al: The effect of irbesartan on the development of diabetic nephropathy in patients with type 2 diabetes. New Engl J Med 2001;345:870–878.

64. Goldberg AI, Dunlay MC, Sweet CS: Safety and tolerability of losartan potassium, an angiotensin II receptor antagonist, compared with hydrochlorothiazide, atenolol, felodipine ER, and angiotensin-converting enzyme inhibitors for the treatment of systemic hypertension. Am J Cardiol 1995;75:793–795.

65. Weber M: Clinical safety and tolerability of losartan. Clin Ther 1997;19:604–616.

66. Lacourciere Y, Brunner H, Irwin R, et al: Effects of modulators of the renin-angiotensin-aldosterone system on cough. Losartan Cough Study Group. J Hypertens 1994;12:1387–1393.

67. Benz J, Oshrain C, Henry D, et al: Valsartan, a new angiotensin II receptor antagonist: a double-blind study comparing the incidence of cough with lisinopril and hydrochlorothiazide. J Clin Pharmacol 1997;37:101–117.

68. Russo D, Pisani A, Balletta MM, et al: Additive antiproteinuric effect of converting enzyme inhibitor and losartan in normotensive patients with IgA nephropathy. Am J Kidney Dis 1999;33:851–856.

69. Zoccali C, Valvo E, Russo D, et al: Antiproteinuric effect of losartan in patients with chronic renal diseases. (Letter.) Nephrol Dial Transplant 1997;12:234–235.

70. Mogensen CE, Noltham S, Tikkanen I, et al: Randomised controlled trial of dual blockade of renin-angiotensin system in patients with hypertension, microalbuminuria, and noninsulin dependent diabetes: the candesartan and lisinopril microalbuminuria (CALM) study. Br Med J 2000;321:1440–1444.

71. Remuzzi G, Bertani T: Pathophysiology of progressive nephropathies. N Engl J Med 1998;339:1448–1456.

72. Eddy AA, Giachelli CM: Renal expression of genes that promote interstitial inflammation and fibrosis in rats with protein-overload proteinuria. Kidney Int 1995;47:1546–1557.

73. Levey AS, Adler S, Greene T, et al: Effects of dietary protein restriction on the progression of moderate renal disease in the Modification of Diet in Renal Disease Study. J Am Soc Nephrol 1996;7:2616–2626.

74. Levey AS, Adler S, Caggiula AW, et al: Effects of dietary protein restriction on the progression of advanced renal disease in the Modification of Diet in Renal Disease Study. Am J Kidney Dis 1996;27:652–663.

75. Pedrini MT, Levey AS, Lau J, et al: The effect of dietary protein restriction on the progression of diabetic and nondiabetic renal diseases: a meta-analysis. Ann Intern Med 1996;124:627–632.

76. Monzani G, Bergesio F, Ciuti R, et al: Lipoprotein abnormalities in chronic renal failure and dialysis patients. Blood Purif 1996;14:262–272.

77. Hunsicker LG, Adler S, Caggiula A, et al: Predictors of progression of renal disease in the Modification of Diet in Renal Disease Study. Kidney Int 1997;51:1908–1919.

78. Samuelsson O, Attman PO, Knight-Gibson C, et al: Complex apolipoprotein B-containing lipoprotein particles are associated with a higher rate of progression of human chronic renal insufficiency. J Am Soc Nephrol 1998;9:1482–1488.

79. Krolewski AS, Warram JH, Christlieb AR: Hypercholesterolemia – a determinant of renal function loss and deaths in IDDM patients with nephropathy. Kidney Int 1994;Suppl 45:S125–S131.

80. Ravid M, Brosh D, Ravid-Safran D, et al: Main risk factors for nephropathy in type 2 diabetes mellitus are plasma cholesterol levels, mean blood pressure, and hyperglycemia. Arch Intern Med 1998;158:998–1004.

81. Mulec H, Johnson S-A, Bjorck S: Relation between serum cholesterol and diabetic nephropathy. Lancet 1990;335:1537–1538.

82. Maschio G, Oldrizzi L, Rugiu C, et al: Serum lipids in patients with chronic renal failure on long-term, protein-restricted diets. Am J Med 1989;87:51N–54N.

83. Muntner P, Coresh J, Smith JC, et al: Plasma lipids and risk of developing renal dysfunction: the atherosclerosis risk in communities study. Kidney Int 2000;58:293–301.

84. Grone EF, Abboud HE, Hohne M, et al: Actions of lipoproteins in cultured human mesangial cells: modulation by mitogenic vasoconstrictors. Am J Physiol 1992;263:F686–F696.

85. Rovin BH, Tan LC: LDL stimulates mesangial fibronectin production and chemoattractant expression. Kidney Int 1993;43:218–225.

86. Wheeler DC, Chana RS, Topley N, et al: Oxidation of low density lipoprotein by mesangial cells may promote glomerular injury. Kidney Int 1994;45:1628–1636.

87. Kasiske B, O'Donnell MP, Schmitz PG, et al: Renal injury of diet-induced hypercholesterolemia in rats. Kidney Int 1990;37:880–891.

88. Kasiske BL, O'Donnel MP, Garvis WJ, et al: Pharmacologic treatment of hyperlipidemia reduces injury in rat 5/6 nephrectomy model of chronic renal failure. Circ Res 1988;62:367–374.

89. O'Donell MP, Kasiske BL, Kim Y, et al: Lovastatin retards the progression of established glomerular disease in obese Zucker rats. Am J Kidney Dis 1993;22:83–89.

90. Fried LF, Orchard TJ, Kasiske BL: Effect of lipid reduction on the progression of renal disease: a meta-analysis. Kidney Int 2001;59:260–269.

91. Chase HP, Garg SK, Marshall G, et al: Cigarette smoking increases the risk of albuminuria among subjects with type I diabetes. J Amer Med Assoc 1991;265:614–617.

92. McKenna K, Thompson C: Microalbuminuria: a marker to increased renal and cardiovascular risk in diabetes mellitus. Scott Med J 1997;42:99–104.

93. Muhlhauser I, Overmann H, Bender R, et al: Predictors of mortality and end-stage diabetic complications in patients with type 1 diabetes mellitus on intensified insulin therapy. Diabetic Medicine 2000;17:727–734.

94. Orth SR, Stockmann A, Conradt C, et al: Smoking as a risk factor for end-stage renal failure in men with primary renal disease. Kidney Int 1998;54:926–931.

95. Ward MM, Studenski S: Clinical prognostic factors in lupus nephritis. The importance of hypertension and smoking. Arch Intern Med 1992;152:2082–2088.

96. Stengel B, Couchoud C, Cenee S, Hemon D: Age, blood pressure and smoking effects on chronic renal failure in primary glomerular nephropathies. Kidney Int 2000;57:2519–2526.

97. Regalado M, Yang S, Wesson DE: Cigarette smoking is associated with augmented progression of renal insufficiency in severe essential hypertension. Am J Kidney Dis 2000;35:687–694.

98. Pinto-Sietsma SJ, Mulder J, Janssen WM, et al: Smoking is related to albuminuria and abnormal renal function in nondiabetic persons. Ann Int Med 2000;133:585–591.

99. The Diabetes Control and Complications (DCCT) Research Group: The effect of intensive treatment of diabetes on the development and progression of long-term complications in insulin-dependent diabetes mellitus. N Engl J Med 1993;329:977–986.

100. Ohkubo Y, Kishikawa H, Araki E, et al: Intensive insulin therapy prevents the progression of diabetic microvascular complications in Japanese patients with noninsulin-dependent diabetes mellitus: a randomized prospective 6–year study. Diabetes Res Clin Prac 1995;28:103–117.

101. Feldt-Rasmussen B, Mathiesen ER, Deckert T: Effect of two years of strict metabolic control on progression of incipient nephropathy in insulin-dependent diabetes. Lancet 1986;2:1300–1304.

102. Reichard P, Nilsson BY, Rosenqvist U: The effect of long-term intensified insulin treatment on the development of microvascular complications of diabetes mellitus. New Engl J Med 1993;329:304–309.

103. Bangstad HJ, Osterby R, Dahl-Jorgensen K, et al: Improvement of blood glucose control in IDDM patients retards the progression of morphological changes in early diabetic nephropathy. Diabetologia 1994;37:483–490.

104. Microalbuminuria Collaborative Study Group, UK: Intensive therapy and progression to clinical albuminuria in patients with insulin dependent diabetes mellitus and microalbuminuria.. Br Med J 1995;311:973–977.

105. The Diabetes Control and Complications (DCCT) Research Group: Effect of intensive therapy on the development and progression of diabetic nephropathy in the Diabetes Control and Complications Trial. Kidney Int 1995;47:1703–1720.

106. Fioretto P, Steffes MW, Sutherland DE, et al: Reversal of lesions of diabetic nephropathy after pancreas transplantation. New Engl J Med 1998;339:69–75.

107. UK Prospective Diabetes Study (UKPDS) Group: Intensive blood-glucose control with sulphonylureas or insulin compared with conventional treatment and risk of complications in patients with type 2 diabetes (UKPDS 33). Lancet 1998;352:837–653.

108. Trippodo NC, Robl JA, Asaad MM, et al: Effects of omapatrilat in low, normal, and high renin experimental hypertension. Am J Hypertens 1998;11:363–372.

109. Intengan HD, Schiffrin EL: Vasopeptidase inhibition has potent effects on blood pressure and resistance arteries in stroke-prone spontaneously hypertensive rats. Hypertension 2000;35:1221–1225.

110. Weber M: Emerging treatments for hypertension: potential role for vasopeptidase inhibition. Am J Hypertens 1999;12:139S–147S.

111. Taal MW, Nenov VD, Wong W, et al: Vasopeptidase inhibition affords greater renoprotection than angiotensin-converting enzyme inhibition alone. J Am Soc Nephrol 2001;12:2051–2059.

112. Taal MW, Omer SA, Nadim MK, Mackenzie HS: Cellular and molecular mediators in common pathway mechanisms of chronic renal disease progression. Curr Opin Nephrol Hypertens 2000;9:323–331.

113. Fujihara CK, Malheiros DM, Zatz R, et al: Mycophenolate mofetil attenuates renal injury in the rat remnant kidney. Kidney Int 1998;54:1510–1519.

114. Romero F, Rodriguez-Iturbe B, Parra G, et al: Mycophenolate mofetil prevents the progressive renal failure induced by 5/6 renal ablation in rats. Kidney Int 1999;55:945–955.

115. Remuzzi G, Zoja C, Gagliardini E, et al: Combining an antiproteinuric approach with mycophenolate mofetil fully suppresses progressive nephropathy of experimental animals. J Am Soc Nephrol 1999;10:1542–1549.

116. Gaede P, Vedel P, Parving HH, et al: Intensified multifactorial intervention in patients with type 2 diabetes mellitus and microalbuminuria: the Steno type 2 randomised study. Lancet 1999;353:617–622.

117. McClellan WM, Knight DF, Karp H, et al: Early detection and treatment of renal disease in hospitalized diabetic and hypertensive patients: important differences between practice and published guidelines. Am J Kidney Dis 1997;29:368–375.

CHAPTER
67 Cholesterol Management in Patients with Chronic Kidney Disease

Robert Toto, Gloria Lena Vega, and Scott M. Grundy

Summary of ATP III guidelines as related to chronic kidney disease
- Low-density lipoprotein cholesterol: the primary target of therapy
- Risk assessment: first step in risk management
- High-risk conditions: established coronary heart disease and risk equivalents
- Low-density lipoprotein-lowering therapies
- Atherogenic dyslipidemia and the metabolic syndrome
  - Primary nephrotic syndrome
  - Diabetic nephropathy
  - Chronic renal failure (before dialysis)
  - Chronic renal failure (on dialysis)
  - Chronic renal failure (postrenal transplant)

In the past few decades several important clinical trials have documented that lowering of serum cholesterol levels reduces the risk for development of myocardial infarction and other complications of coronary heart disease (CHD). These trials have added strength to national recommendations for detection and treatment of high serum cholesterol levels. In the USA, the National Cholesterol Education Program (NCEP) has published guidelines on the clinical management of elevated serum cholesterol. The most recent, called Adult Treatment Panel III (ATP III),[1] was published in 2001. ATP III did not provide specific advice on treating lipid disorders in patients with renal disease. However, the general framework of the guidelines may apply to many patients with renal disease, who are almost certainly at increased risk for CHD. In this chapter, the general features of ATP III will first be reviewed for background information. It must be pointed out, however, that therapies for patients with complex medical conditions such as renal disease require clinical judgement when using ATP III guidelines. Therefore, this chapter will not attempt to provide "hard-and-fast" rules for management of lipid disorders in patients with renal disease. It will however review available information about the nature of lipid disorders in different types of renal disease, and it will outline areas for potential intervention.

Many patients with chronic kidney disease are at increased risk for major coronary events, either because they already have established atherosclerotic disease, or because they have concomitant risk factors for CHD. In addition, chronic kidney disease itself may impart a higher risk independently of the usual CHD risk factors. The extent of incremental risk likely depends on the type of chronic kidney disease. Regardless, patients with most forms of chronic kidney disease commonly have multiple cardiovascular risk factors. Among these are a variety of abnormalities in plasma lipoproteins. For these reasons, physicians who care for patients with renal disease often are faced with the need to make decisions whether to intervene on a given patient's lipid disorder, and if so how.

Summary of ATP III guidelines as related to chronic kidney disease

Low-density lipoprotein cholesterol: the primary target of therapy

There are several classes of lipoproteins, such as low-density lipoproteins (LDL), very-low-density lipoproteins (VLDL), high-density lipoproteins (HDL), and lipoprotein(a) (Lp(a)). Of these, elevated serum LDL has the most robust relationship to CHD.[1] LDL is usually identified in clinical practice as LDL-cholesterol, which is recognized by ATP III as the primary target of lipid-lowering therapy. ATP III provides a detailed listing of the evidence to support the concept that LDL-cholesterol should be the primary target of therapy. Highest on this list is evidence from recent clinical trials. Among them are five major clinical trials[2–6] which have documented that LDL-lowering therapy will reduce risk for developing CHD by about one-third. Nevertheless, other lipoproteins are potential secondary targets of therapy. For example, many patients with chronic kidney disease have a lipoprotein abnormality called *atherogenic dyslipidemia*.[1] This disorder is characterized by raised serum triglyceride, small LDL, and low HDL-cholesterol. It seems likely that LDL-cholesterol should be the primary target of therapy in patients with renal disease, but the question of whether to intervene on atherogenic dyslipidemia becomes an important issue for many patients with renal disease. Table 67.1 summarizes the ATP III classification of lipids, lipoproteins, and atherogenic dyslipidemia.

Risk assessment: first step in risk management

ATP III recognizes that the intensity of risk-reduction therapy should be adjusted to the patient's absolute risk. Assessment of risk depends on identification of medical conditions that impart higher risk and risk factors for CHD. Several renal diseases may well increase the risk for CHD independently of the major risk factors; nonetheless, patients with renal disease often have multiple, major risk factors (Table 67.2). Further, they may have one or more of the emerging risk factors that also are common in patients with CHD (Table 67.3). Some patients with renal disease will have a constellation of risk factors, called the *metabolic syndrome* (Table 67.4). This condition includes several borderline risk factors that when combined confer higher risk. In patients without CHD, ATP III recommends that risk assessment be carried out using the Framingham risk

Table 67.3 Emerging risk factors

Lipid risk factors
    Lipoprotein(a) (Lp(a))
    Apolipoproteins (CIII, B, AI)
    Small lipoprotein particles (small LDL, small HDL)

Inflammatory markers
    High-sensitivity C-reactive protein (hs-CRP)
    Cytokines
    Fibrinogen

Prothrombotic markers
    Plasminogen activator inhibitor-1 (PAI-1)
    Fibrinogen
Homocysteine

Table 67.1 Adult Treatment Panel (ATP) III classification of total, LDL-, and HDL-cholesterol, triglycerides (mg/dL), and atherogenic dyslipidemia

LDL-cholesterol	
Optimal	<100
Above optimal/near optimal	100–129
Borderline high	130–159
High	160–189
Very high	≥190
Total cholesterol	
Desirable	<200
Borderline-high	200–239
High	≥240
HDL-cholesterol	
Low	<40
High	>60
Triglycerides	
Normal	< 150
Borderline high	150–199
High	200–499
Very high	≥ 500
Atherogenic dyslipidemia	
Raised triglycerides	≥ 150
Small LDL	
Reduced HDL-cholesterol	< 40 (men)
	< 50 (women)

Table 67.4 Risk factors of the metabolic syndrome

Atherogenic dyslipidemia
    Elevated triglycerides (≥ 50 mg/dL)
    Small LDL particles
    Elevated nonHDL-cholesterol (1≥ 30 mg/dL)
    Low HDL-cholesterol (< 40 mg/dL in men; < 50 mg/dL in women)

High-normal blood pressure (130–139/15–89 mmHg)

Insulin resistance

± Impaired fasting glucose (110–126 mg/dL)

Proinflammatory*
Prothrombotic state†

*Indicated by one or more of elevated high sensitivity C-reactive protein (hs-CRP) (> 3.0 mg/L), homocysteine (≥ 15 mmol/L) or lipoprotein(a) (Lp(a)) (≥ 30 mg/dL), and fibrogen. Elevated hs-CRP appears to be the most reliable indicator of proinflammatory state. Lp(a) can be elevated on a genetic basis.
†Indicated by elevated plasminogen activator inhibitor-1 (PAI-1), fibrogen, or clotting factor VIIc.

Table 67.2 Categorical classification of major risk factors

Cigarette smoking (any smoking in past year)

Hypertension (blood pressure ≥ 140/90 mmHg or on antihypertensive medication)

High LDL-cholesterol (≥ 160 mg/dL)*

Low HDL-cholesterol (< 40 mg/dL)†

High plasma glucose (≥ 126 mg/dL)‡

Family history of premature coronary heart disease (CHD) (in male first-degree relative < 55 years; in female first-degree relative < 65 years)

Age (men ≥ 50 years; women ≥ 55 years)

*High LDL-cholesterol is not included in the "risk factor" count in ATP III because it is the target of therapy based on other risk factors.
†HDL-cholesterol > 60 mg/dL counts as a "negative" risk factor; its presence removes one risk factor from the total count.
‡High plasma glucose is not included in the "risk factor" count in ATP III because its presence identifies a patient as having diabetes, which is counted as a CHD risk equivalent.

algorithm.[7] In patients with renal disease, however, Framingham scores may not accurately predict future CHD events. If anything, the presence of multiple risk factors likely raises the risk for major coronary events in patients with renal disease even more than suggested by Framingham scoring.

High-risk conditions: established coronary heart disease and risk equivalents

Conditions at highest risk deserve the most intensive lipid-lowering therapy. ATP III recognizes two categories of high-risk patients: those with established CHD and those with CHD risk equivalents. According to ATP III, LDL-cholesterol should be lowered to the optimal range in high-risk patients, to an LDL-cholesterol < 100 mg/dL (Table 67.1). Many patients with chronic kidney disease will fall into one of these categories. The conditions that constitute established CHD are: (1) history of acute coronary syndromes (unstable angina or myocardial infarction); (2) history of angina pectoris; and (3) history of coronary artery procedures (coronary angioplasty or coronary artery by-pass grafting).

Any patient with chronic kidney disease who has one of these forms of established CHD can be considered at high risk for future events. Such a patient thus would be a candidate for intensive lowering of LDL, with an LDL-cholesterol goal of < 100 mg/dL.

LDL-lowering therapy is only one of several possible modes of intervention in patients with established CHD. The American Heart Association has published general guidelines for risk reduction in patients with CHD or other atherosclerotic diseases.[8] These guidelines are summarized in Table 67.5. They include smoking cessation, blood pressure regulation, physical activity as part of a program of cardiac rehabilitation, weight loss in overweight patients, appropriate antiplatelet therapy, and cardio-protective drugs [β-blockers and angiotensin-converting enzyme inhibitors (ACEIs)]. A large body of data supports benefit from each of these regimens.[8] Particular attention should be given to using a full range of risk-reduction modalities in patients with chronic kidney disease who also have established CHD.

Patients with CHD risk equivalents are those with one of the following: (1) noncoronary forms of atherosclerotic disease (peripheral arterial disease, carotid artery disease (carotid transient ischemic attacks), carotid stroke, > 50% obstruction of carotid artery), and abdominal aortic aneurysm; (2) diabetes mellitus; and (3) multiple risk factors with 10-year risk for CHD > 10% (by Framingham risk scoring).

Some investigators have speculated that various forms of chronic kidney disease constitute a CHD risk equivalent

Table 67.5 Risk reduction strategy in patients with coronary and other vascular disease (modified from American Heart Association recommendations)

Smoking
    Goal to stop tobacco use altogether
    Encourage patient and family to stop smoking
    Provide counseling and use cessation programs as appropriate

Hypertension
    Blood pressure goal < 130/85 mmHg
    Modify life habits to lower blood pressure (weight control, exercise, alcohol moderation, moderate sodium restriction)
    Add blood pressure medication if needed to achieve blood pressure goal (consider ACEIs and β-blockers for concomitant benefits – see below)

Physical activity
    Minimum goal of 30 min three or four times per week
    Assess overall risk to guide prescription
    Encourage use of cardiac rehabilitation programs for patients with CHD (when available)
    Encourage moderate intensity exercise

Weight management
    Goal to achieve desirable body weight
    Provide counseling and use of professional dietitian as appropriate

Antiplatelet agents/anticoagulants
    Start aspirin 80–325 mg/day if not contraindicated

Beta-blockers
    Start and continue for 6 months minimum in high-risk patients (arrhythmia, LV dysfunction, include ischemia)

ACE inhibitors
    Start early in stable high-risk patients (anterior MI, previous MI, Killip class II: S3 gallop, radiographic CHF)

ACEIs, angiotensin-converting enzyme inhibitors; CHD, coronary heart disease; LV, left ventricular; MI, myocardial infarction.

similar to the case for diabetes. Certainly a sizable fraction of patients with chronic kidney disease will have diabetes, which warrants their inclusion in the category of CHD risk equivalent. Whether renal-disease per se without diabetes or noncoronary forms of atherosclerosis confers a high-risk status probably depends on the type of renal disease. Two questions must be considered, namely (1) what is the absolute risk for patients with various forms of chronic kidney disease? and (2) how effective is LDL-lowering for reducing major coronary events in such patients? For both questions, the literature is limited, and generalizations are difficult; therefore, clinical judgement is required as to whether it is appropriate to classify particular patients as CHD risk equivalents. Framingham risk scoring probably underestimates the 10-year risk for CHD patients with renal disease and therefore is of limited value in assessing absolute 10-year risk. Nevertheless, it is reasonable to assume that most patients with chronic kidney disease, who have several major risk factors, belong in the category of CHD risk equivalents. If a patient is judged to be so, it is reasonable to lower LDL-cholesterol into the optimal range (< 100 mg/dL).

For patients with established CHD and CHD risk equivalents, ATP III recommends starting LDL-lowering drug therapy simultaneously with dietary therapy when LDL-cholesterol levels > 130 mg/dL. If baseline (or on-treatment) LDL-cholesterol levels are in the range of 100–129 mg/dL, dietary therapy can be intensified first before starting (or intensifying) LDL-lowering drugs; in some cases, the LDL goal may be achieved without the need for starting (or changing) drug therapy.

When patients with chronic kidney disease do not have established CHD or have uncertain CHD risk equivalent, the physician has the option of reducing LDL to near optimal levels (100–129 mg/dL) rather than to the optimal range (< 100 mg/dL). This lesser reduction in LDL-cholesterol is justified because of a lack of clinical trials showing the efficacy of achieving optimal LDL levels renal disease. Decisions about the intensity of drug therapy should take into consideration safety issues and the potential dangers of high doses of LDL-lowering drugs, or the use of drugs in combination.

Low-density lipoprotein-lowering therapies

Two modalities of LDL-lowering therapy are recognized by ATP III: *therapeutic lifestyle changes (TLC)* and *drug therapy*. Therapeutic lifestyle changes go beyond LDL-lowering by dietary therapy to achieve maximal risk reduction; these changes include: (1) maximal reduction of saturated fats and cholesterol; (2) adding LDL-lowering adjuncts (plant stanol or sterols and/or increased viscous fiber); (3) weight reduction (in overweight or obese patients); (4) increased physical activity.

When therapeutic lifestyle changes are recommended, dietary saturated fatty acids should be reduced to < 7% of total energy intake, and dietary cholesterol to < 200 mg/day. Physicians are advised to seek consultation from a registered dietitian or other qualified nutritional professional to provide patients with appropriate *medical nutrition therapy*. A cholesterol-lowering diet is only one component of medical nutrition therapy for patients with chronic kidney disease. Adding LDL-lowering adjuncts can provide another 10–15% reduction in LDL-cholesterol levels; these include plant stanols or sterols (2 g/day) and increased viscous fiber (10–25 g/day). Medical nutrition therapy should include caloric restriction in overweight patients. To match the patient's clinical needs the physician can prescribe regular physical activity. Four drugs are available for LDL lowering (Table 67.6). Two drug classes (statins and bile acid sequestrants) mainly lower LDL. Fibrates and nicotinic acid can moderately reduce LDL levels, but they are used primarily for treatment of atherogenic dyslipidemia. The use of these drugs will be considered for each category of chronic kidney disease discussed below.

Atherogenic dyslipidemia and the metabolic syndrome

Atherogenic dyslipidemia, which is common in patients with chronic kidney disease, is a potential secondary target of lipid-lowering therapy. It consists of raised tri-glycerides, small LDL particles, and low HDL-cholesterol levels. In some patients, weight reduction and increased physical activity may help to normalize levels of triglyceride and HDL. However, in some forms of renal disease, atherogenic dyslipidemia results mainly from metabolic defects secondary to renal disease.[9–11] The standard drugs for treatment of atherogenic dyslipidemia are fibrates and nicotinic acid. Unfortunately, both fibrates and nicotinic acid can cause side-effects that may be accentuated in patients with chronic kidney disease. For example, when fibrates are combined with statins, there is increased risk for severe myopathy. This side-effect is particularly dangerous in patients with renal disease because it may result in myoglobinuria and acute tubular necrosis.

In patients with atherogenic dyslipidemia the primary target of therapy is still LDL. Nonetheless, the ATP III guidelines note that elevated VLDL-cholesterol also may contribute substantially to the risk for CHD when triglycerides are raised. For this reason, the ATP III identified LDL + VLDL-cholesterol (also called nonHDL-cholesterol) as a secondary target of therapy in patients with raised triglyceride. The goal for reduction of nonHDL-cholesterol is a level 30 mg/dL higher than for LDL-cholesterol. For example, with an LDL-cholesterol goal of < 100 mg/dL, the nonHDL-cholesterol goal would be < 130 mg/dL.

Some patients with chronic kidney disease have the metabolic syndrome (Table 67.4). The ATP III proposed criteria for clinical diagnosis of the metabolic syndrome (see Table 67.7); when a patient has three of the five abnormalities shown in this table, a diagnosis of the metabolic syndrome can be made. If a patient with chronic kidney disease has the metabolic syndrome, more intensive intervention on serum lipids seems warranted.

Table 67.6 Drugs for lipid management

Drug class	Drugs and daily doses	Lipid/lipoprotein effects	Side-effects	Contraindications	Clinical trial results
Bile acid sequestrants	Cholestyramine 4–16 g Colestipol 5–20 g Colesevelam 2.6–3.8 g	LDL-C ↓15–30% HDL-C ↑3–5% TG No change or increase	Gastrointestinal distress, constipation, decreased absorption of other drugs	Absolute: dysbetalipoproteinemia TG > 400 mg/dL Relative: TG > 200 mg/dL	Reduced major coronary events and CHD deaths
HMG-CoA reductase inhibitors (statins)*	Lovastatin 20–80 mg Pravastatin 20–40 mg Simvastatin 20–80 mg Fluvastatin 20–80 mg Atorvastatin 10–80 mg	LDL-C ↓18–55% HDL-C ↑5–15% TG ↓7–30%	Myopathy, increased liver enzymes	Absolute: active or chronic liver disease Relative: concomitant use of certain drugs†	Reduced major coronary events, CHD deaths, need for coronary procedures, stroke, and total mortality
Nicotinic acid	Immediate release crystalline 1.5–3 g Extended release niaspan 1–2 g Sustained release 1–2 g	LDL-C ↓5–25% HDL-C ↑15–35% TG ↓20–50%	Flushing, hyperglycemia, hyperuricemia (gout), upper gastrointestinal distress, hepatotoxicity	Absolute: chronic liver disease, severe gout Relative: diabetes, hyperuricemia, peptic ulcer disease	Reduced major coronary events, and (possibly) total mortality
Fibric acids	Gemfibrozil 600 mg b.i.d. Fenofibrate 200 mg Clofibrate 1000 mg b.i.d.	LDL-C ↓5–20% (may be increased in patients with high TG) HDL-C ↑10–20% TG ↓10–50%	Dyspepsia, gallstones, myopathy	Absolute: severe renal disease, severe hepatic disease Relative: severe renal disease	Reduced major coronary events, increased nonCHD mortality (in 2/5 clinical trials)

*Standard starting doses of statins are lovastatin (40 mg), pravastatin (40 mg), simvastatin (20 mg), fluvastatin (40 mg), and atorvastatin (10 mg).
†Cyclosporine, gemfibrozil (or niacin), macrolide antibiotics, various antifungal agents and cytochrome P450 inhibitors.
CHD, coronary heart disease; HDL, high-density lipoproteins; HMG-CoA, a-hydroxy-g-methylglutaryl coenzyme A; LDL, low-density lipoproteins; TG, triglycerides.

Table 67.7 Clinical diagnosis of the metabolic syndrome based on any three of the following

Risk factor	Defining level
Abdominal obesity (waist circumference)*†	
Men	> 102 cm (> 40 inches)
Women	> 88 cm (> 35 inches)
Triglycerides	≥ 150 mg/dL
HDL-cholesterol	
Men	< 40 mg/dL
Women	< 50 mg/dL
Blood pressure	≥ 130/≥ 85 mmHg
Fasting glucose	≥ 110 mg/dL

*Overweight and obesity are associated with insulin resistance and the metabolic syndrome. However, the presence of abdominal obesity is more highly correlated than elevated body mass index (BMI) with metabolic risk factors. Therefore, the simple measure of waist circumference is recommended to identify the body weight component of the metabolic syndrome.
†Some male patients can develop multiple metabolic risk factors when the waist circumference is only marginally increased (e.g. 94–102 cm; 37–39 inches). Such patients may have a strong genetic contribution to insulin resistance. They should benefit from changes in life habits, similarly to men with categorical increases in waist circumference.

Primary nephrotic syndrome

Hyperlipidemia is a typical feature of the nephrotic syndrome. In most patients, serum LDL-cholesterol levels are raised;[12–14] in some cases, VLDL-cholesterol and VLDL-triglycerides are increased as well.[10,15] The mechanisms of nephrotic hyperlipidemia are not fully understood and appear to be multiple. Hepatic overproduction of lipoproteins is a response to depletion of serum albumin. In vivo and in vitro studies support this mechanism.[16,17] Moreover, research in humans,[10,15] as well as in experimental animals,[18,19] indicates that catabolism of VLDL can be impaired, accentuating triglyceride elevation. Removal of LDL via LDL receptors also may be delayed;[10] this change will further raise LDL-cholesterol levels. Nephrotic patients apparently have increased serum levels of cholesterol ester transport protein (CETP).[20] This abnormality could account for the high content of cholesterol in LDL particles.[10] Thus, a single mechanism probably cannot explain nephrotic hyperlipidemia.

Prolonged severe hyperlipidemia in patients with irreversible nephrotic syndrome almost certainly promotes coronary atherosclerosis and predisposes to premature CHD.[21–24] For such patients, application of the NCEP guidelines (National Cholesterol Education Program)[1] for primary prevention seems appropriate. If LDL-cholesterol levels exceed 190 mg/dL (or nonHDL-cholesterol > 220 mg/dL), cholesterol-lowering drugs can be employed in most patients. If the LDL-cholesterol level ranges from 160 to 189 mg/dL (nonHDL-cholesterol 190–219 mg/dL), drug therapy can be considered if other risk factors are present. The goal of therapy for primary prevention is to reduce LDL-cholesterol levels to < 130 mg/dL (nonHDL-cholesterol to < 160 mg/dL).

Several studies[15,25–27] have demonstrated that the hyperlipidemia of nephrotic syndrome is responsive to statin drugs. Statins lower both LDL-cholesterol and VLDL-cholesterol levels. Bile acid sequestrants also reduce LDL levels, and enhance LDL lowering when given in combination with statins.[28] Even if triglycerides are concomitantly elevated in nephrotic patients, statins still are the preferred therapy because of their ability to lower levels of VLDL remnants as well as LDL.[15,29] Nicotinic acid also reduces triglyceride levels,[30] and may have additive effects with statins. The combination of statins plus fibrates has received little attention for patients with the nephrotic syndrome. Finally, it has been reported that LDL-pheresis can be used successfully to lower LDL in nephrotic patients with severe hypercholesterolemia.[31,32]

Recommendations In patients with nephrotic syndrome, LDL is the primary target of therapy. Statins are first-line therapy and can be used safely in most patients at moderate doses. There is little experience with high-dose statins. In nephrotic patients with severe hypercholesterolemia, it may not be possible to reduce LDL-cholesterol to the near-optimal or optimal levels as shown in Table 67.1. The LDL lowering that can be achieved with statin therapy nonetheless can be enhanced by adding a bile acid sequestrant. Statins also lower VLDL remnants and thus remain the preferred therapy in patients with combined elevations of LDL-cholesterol and triglycerides. Addition of nicotinic acid to statin therapy can be considered for patients with combined hyperlipidemia. The combination of statin plus fibrate, however, should be used with caution, or probably best not at all, because of the increased risk for severe myopathy, rhabdomyolysis, and acute renal failure.

Diabetic nephropathy

One cause of the nephrotic syndrome is diabetic nephropathy. This syndrome can develop in patients with either type 1 or type 2 diabetes, but lipid disorders are more common in type 2 diabetes than in type 1 diabetes. Diabetic dyslipidemia is essentially identical to atherogenic dyslipidemia (Table 67.1).[1] When the nephrotic syndrome comes into play in patients with diabetes, LDL-cholesterol levels are raised, and VLDL elevations are accentuated;[33] combined hyperlipidemia therefore is common. In patients with type 1 diabetes, the development of the nephrotic syndrome apparently produces a lipoprotein pattern resembling that of the primary nephrotic syndrome, i.e. predominant hypercholesterolemia.[34]

Patients with diabetes are at high risk for CHD even before development of nephropathy.[1] This high-risk status is due to at least two factors: (1) metabolic risk factors that are especially common in type 2 diabetes,[35] and (2) hyperglycemia, which appears to accelerate atherogenesis. Because of the high risk for major coronary events, the ATP III designated diabetes as a CHD risk equivalent. This designation was partly due to a high risk for future CHD events, but there were other reasons too. In particular, once patients with diabetes develop CHD, they have a poor prognosis for survival compared to non-diabetics with CHD.[36] Identifying a CHD risk equivalent for a patient with diabetes evokes an LDL-cholesterol goal of < 100 mg/dL. Since many patients with diabetes also have elevated triglycerides, a nonHDL-cholesterol goal of < 130 mg/dL further is indicated.[37] These goals are independent of whether established CHD is present. The use of cholesterol-lowering drugs to achieve LDL-cholesterol goals in patients with diabetes is supported by the favorable outcomes of statin therapy in diabetic patients in secondary prevention trials.[38,39]

Available evidence indicates that the onset of nephropathy in patients with diabetes enhances CHD risk even more.[36] This observation certainly justifies cholesterol-lowering therapy. Although combining fibric acid with a statin seems attractive, increased risk for myopathy must be kept in mind. Therefore, prudence favors the use of a statin alone for most patients with diabetic nephropathy.

Recommendations When a patient with diabetes also has chronic kidney disease, this patient should be designated as having a CHD risk equivalent, even if established CHD is not present. Regardless of whether CHD is present, the LDL-cholesterol goal is < 100 mg/dL, and the nonHDL-cholesterol goal is < 130 mg/dL. To achieve these goals, LDL-lowering drugs usually are required. The usual drug is a statin (Table 67.6). Although combining a statin with a fibrate is attractive, this combination carries a moderately high risk for severe myopathy. In most cases of diabetic nephropathy this combination should probably be avoided. An alternative drug is nicotinic acid. A recent multicenter trial demonstrated that relatively low doses of extended-release nicotinic acid are well tolerated in patients with diabetes.[40] Note that if nicotinic acid is used in patients receiving statins, lower doses of nicotinic acid are required to prevent a worsening of diabetes.

Chronic renal failure (before dialysis)

It is uncertain whether chronic renal failure before institution of dialysis independently raises CHD risk beyond that associated with major risk factors. At the very least, nevertheless, full attention should be given to modifying existing cardiovascular risk factors. Among these are cigarette smoking, hypertension, and low HDL-cholesterol levels (Table 67.2). Many patients with chronic renal failure exhibit hypertriglyceridemia;[9] here the underlying metabolic abnormality is a defective catabolism of VLDL triglycerides.[41] This defect leads to an accumulation of VLDL remnants.[9] Some investigators speculate that remnant lipoproteins are particularly atherogenic[42] and should be treated independently of LDL-cholesterol levels. This is an attractive hypothesis, although evidence that therapeutic reduction of VLDL levels will reduce CHD risk is lacking from clinical trials.

Recommendations If a patient with chronic renal failure prior to dialysis has multiple CHD risk factors but no clinically manifested atherosclerotic disease, the LDL-cholesterol target goal is < 130 mg/dL (nonHDL-cholesterol < 160 mg/dL).[1] Long-term data are not available on absolute risk for CHD in patients with chronic

renal failure before dialysis, so it is not possible to justify setting an LDL-cholesterol goal of < 100 mg/dL (nonHDL-cholesterol < 130 mg/dL). For untreated patients with LDL-cholesterol (or nonHDL-cholesterol) levels above target for high-risk primary prevention, the preferred drug is a statin. On the other hand, if nonHDL-cholesterol levels are below target without statin therapy, but hyper-triglyceridemia is present, use of a fibric acid can be considered.[43–45] The dose of fibric acid should be adjusted down as recommended in the package insert to reduce the risk for myopathy. In general, it is not appropriate to use a statin in combination with fibric acid in patients with chronic renal failure because of the increased danger of rhabdomyolysis and acute renal failure.

Chronic renal failure (on dialysis)

Risk for acute coronary events and CHD death goes up dramatically in patients with chronic renal failure who have begun on hemodialysis or peritoneal dialysis.[46] The mechanisms underlying this increase in risk are poorly understood. Two pathological factors acting at the level of coronary arteries likely play a role. First, coronary plaques may become more fragile and hence prone to erosion or rupture; and second, a hypercoagulable state may exist, which will increase the size of any newly formed thrombus. These two abnormalities should increase both the frequency and size of myocardial infarction. It is almost certain that patients on hemodialysis have an absolute risk for major coronary events high enough to justify classification as a CHD risk equivalent. To date, however, no clinical trials have documented how much risk reduction occurs from LDL-lowering therapy in patients or renal disease. Nonetheless, reduction of LDL-cholesterol (and nonHDL-cholesterol) levels may help to stabilize coronary plaques and to reduce the high frequency of acute coronary syndromes in this population.

The major lipoprotein abnormality in dialysis patients with chronic renal failure is a high VLDL level, reflected by increased VLDL-cholesterol and triglycerides.[41,47,48] This abnormality results mainly from defective catabolism of VLDL particles.[41] In patients on peritoneal dialysis, high VLDL-triglyceride levels are particularly common; these higher levels result from both hepatic overproduction of VLDL-triglycerides due to a high carbohydrate content in dialysis fluid, and from defective clearance of VLDL due to renal disease. VLDL remnants in patients on dialysis may be unusually atherogenic; if so, efforts to reduce VLDL levels would be warranted. However, no clinical trials have investigated whether lowering of serum VLDL levels in dialysis patients will reduce risk for major coronary events. Nonetheless, considering the high absolute risk for CHD in these patients, it is reasonable to institute therapy to decrease VLDL levels as part of an overall regimen to control CHD risk factors.

Recommendations Since patients on dialysis are at higher risk for CHD, reduction of LDL-cholesterol into the optimal range seems warranted. However, considering the complexity of the clinical problem, a blanket recommendation for an LDL goal cannot be made. In fact, many patients on dialysis already have optimal or near-optimal levels of LDL-cholesterol. A few reports indicate that statin therapy can be employed in patients on dialysis without an unusually high incidence of myopathy.[49–51] In addition, a recent study[52] suggested that statin therapy reduces total mortality in patients with endstage renal disease (ESRD). Even so, patients on dialysis are probably at higher risk for myopathy with statin therapy because of renal dysfunction combined with multiple medications. For these reasons, statins should be employed with reasonable caution, and higher doses probably avoided.

Many patients on dialysis have elevated triglycerides, and statin therapy can reduce levels of VLDL as well as LDL. Hence, statins can be used as single-drug therapy. An alternate approach is to reduce VLDL levels with a fibric acid instead of with a statin.[11,53,54] Fibrates may in fact be more widely used in clinical practice than statins, because of the high frequency of elevated triglycerides. Even so, it is uncertain whether reduction of VLDL levels by fibric acids gives as great a decrease in CHD risk as statins. A recent report[52] found no benefit from fibrate therapy in patients with ESRD, whereas statin therapy was apparently associated with a reduction in total mortality.

Chronic renal failure (postrenal transplant)

Cardiovascular disease appears to be a major cause of death in postrenal transplant patients.[46] A different set of factors may be responsible for this increased CHD risk compared with dialysis patients. For one thing, post-transplant patients are more likely than dialysis patients to have high cholesterol levels.[55,56] Higher cholesterol levels seemingly relate to the use of immunosuppressive agents.

Recommendations The aim of therapy in postrenal transplant patients is to reduce LDL-cholesterol levels to target goals, i.e. to < 100 mg/dL in patients with established CHD and CHD risk equivalents, and to < 130 mg/dL in those who do not otherwise appear at high risk. Parallel reductions of nonHDL-cholesterol levels are recommended for patients with hypertriglyceridemia. If drug therapy to lower serum cholesterol levels is required for posttransplant patients, statins appear to be the preferred agents.[55,56] Certainly they are more effective than fibric acids for lowering LDL and VLDL-cholesterol levels. Nevertheless it must be kept in mind that the combination of a statin with cyclosporine is accompanied by increased risk for severe myopathy.

References

1. Expert Panel on Detection Evaluation,and Treatment of High Blood Cholesterol in Adults: Executive summary of the third report of the National Cholesterol Education Program (NCEP) expert panel on detection, evaluation, and treatment of high blood cholesterol in adults (Adult Treatment Panel III). J Amer Med Assoc 2001;285:2508–2509.
2. Scandinavian Simvastatin Survival Study Group: Randomised trial of cholesterol lowering in 4444 patients with coronary heart disease: the Scandinavian Simvastatin Survival Study (4S). Lancet 1994;344:1383–1389.
3. Sacks FM, Pfeffer MA, Moye LA, et al: The effect of pravastatin on coronary events after myocardial infarction in patients with average cholesterol levels. N Engl J Med 1996;335:1001–1009.
4. The Long-Term Intervention with Pravastatin in Ischaemic Disease (LIPID) Study Group: Prevention of cardiovascular events and death with pravastatin in patients with coronary heart disease and a broad range of initial cholesterol levels. N Engl J Med 1998;339:1349–1357.
5. Shepherd J, Cobbe SM, Ford I, et al: Prevention of coronary heart disease with pravastatin in men with hypercholesterolemia. West of Scotland Coronary Prevention Study Group. N Engl J Med 1995;333:1301–1307.
6. Downs JR, Clearfield M, Whitney E, Shapiro D, Beere PA, Gotto AM: Primary prevention of acute coronary events with lovastatin in men and women with average cholesterol levels. Results of AFCAPS/TexCAPS. J Amer Med Assoc 1998;279:1615–1622.
7. Grundy SM, D'Agostino RB, Mosca L, et al: Cardiovascular risk assessment based on US cohort studies: findings from a National Heart Lung and Blood Institute Workshop. Circulation 2001;104:491–496.
8. Smith SCJr, Blair SN, Bonow RO, et al: AHA/ACC guidelines for preventing heart attack and death in patients with atherosclerotic cardiovascular disease: 2001 update. A statement for healthcare professionals from the American Heart Association and the American College of Cardiology. J Am Coll Cardiol 2001;38:1581–1583.
9. Nestel PJ, Fidge NH, Tan MH: Increased lipoprotein-remnant formation in chronic renal failure. N Engl J Med 1982;307:329–333.
10. Vega GL, Toto RD, Grundy SM: Metabolism of low-density lipoproteins in nephrotic dyslipidemia: comparison hypercholesterolemia alone and combined hyperlipidemia. Kidney Int 1995;47:579–586.
11. Elisaf MS, Dardamanis MA, Papagalanis ND, Siamopoulos KC: Lipid abnormalities in chronic uremic patients. Response to treatment with gemfibrozil. Scand J Urol Nephrol 1993;27:101–108.
12. Baxter JH: Hyperlipoproteinemia in nephrosis. Arch Intern Med 1962;109:742–757.
13. Warwick GL, Caslake MJ, Boulton-Jones JM, Dagen M, Packard CJ, Shepherd J: Low- density lipoprotein metabolism in the nephrotic syndrome. Metabolism 1990;39:187–192.
14. Joven J, Villabona C, Vilella E, Masana L, Albert R, Valles M: Abnormalities of lipoprotein metabolism in patients with the nephrotic syndrome. N Engl J Med 1990;323:579–584.
15. Vega GL, Grundy SM: Lovastatin therapy in nephrotic hyperlipidemia: effects on lipoprotein metabolism. Kidney Int 1988;33:1160–1168.
16. Marsh JB, Drabkin DL: Experimental reconstruction of metabolic pattern of lipid nephrosis: key role of hepatic protein synthesis in hyperlipidemia. Metabolism 1960;9:946–955.
17. Davis RA, Englhorn SC, Weinstein DB, Steinberg D: Very-low-density lipoprotein secretion by cultured rat hepatocytes: Inhibition by albumin and other macromolecules. J Biol Chem 1980;255:2039–2045.
18. Furukawa S, Hirano T, Mamo JCL, Nagano S, Takahashi T: Catabolic defect of triglyceride is associated with abnormal very-low-density lipoprotein in experimental nephrosis. Metabolism 1990;39:101–107.
19. Garber DW, Gottlieb BA, Marsh JB, Sparks CE: Catabolism of very-low-density lipoproteins in experimental nephrosis. J Clin Invest 1984;74:1375–1383.
20. Moulin P, Appel GB, Ginsberg HN, Tall AR: Increased concentration of plasma cholesteryl ester transfer protein in nephrotic syndrome: role in dyslipidemia. J Lipid Res 1992;33:1817–1822.
21. Berlyne GM, Mallick NP: Ischaemic heart-disease as a complication of nephrotic syndrome. Lancet 1969;2:399–400.
22. Alexander JH, Schapel GJ, Edwards KDG: Increased incidence of coronary heart disease associated with combined elevation of serum triglyceride and cholesterol concentrations in the nephrotic syndrome in man. Med J Aust 1974;2:119–122.
23. Mallick NP, Short CD: The nephrotic syndrome and ischemic heart disease. Nephron 1981;27:54–57.
24. Ordonez JD, Hiatt RA, Killebrew EJ, Fireman BH: The increased risk for coronary heart disease associated with nephrotic syndrome. Kidney Int 1993;44:638–642.
25. Toto RD, Grundy SM, Vega GL: Pravastatin treatment of very low density, intermediate density and low-density lipoproteins in hypercholesterolemia and combined hyperlipidemia secondary to the nephrotic syndrome. Am J Nephrol 2000;20:12–17.
26. Kasiske BL, Velosa JA, Halstenson CE, La Belle P, Langendorfer A, Keane WF: The effects of lovastatin in hyperlipidemic patients with the nephrotic syndrome. Am J Kidney Dis 1990;15:8–15.
27. Biesenbach G, Zazgornik J: Lovastatin in the treatment of hypercholesterolemia in nephrotic syndrome due to diabetic nephropathy stage IV–V. Clin Nephrol 1992;37:274–279.

28. Rabelink AJ, Erkelens DW, Hene RJ, Joles JA, Koomans HA: Effects of simvastatin and cholestyramine on lipoprotein profile in hyperlipidemia of nephrotic syndrome. Lancet 1988;II:1335–1338.

29. Massy ZA, Ma JZ, Louis TA, Kasiske BL: Lipid-lowering therapy in patients with renal disease. Kidney Int 1995;48:188–198.

30. Martin-Jadraque R, Tato F, Mostaza JM, Vega GL, Grundy SM: Effectiveness of low-dose crystalline nicotinic acid in men with low high-density lipoprotein cholesterol levels. Arch Intern Med 1996;156:1081–1088.

31. Muso E, Mune M, Fujii Y, et al: Low-density lipoprotein apheresis therapy for steroid- resistant nephrotic syndrome. Kansai-FGS-Apheresis Treatment (K-FLAT) Study Group. Kidney Int Suppl 1999;71:S122–S125.

32. Stenvinkel P, Alvestrand A, Angelin B, Eriksson M: LDL-apheresis in patients with nephrotic syndrome: effects on serum albumin and urinary albumin excretion. Eur J Clin Invest 2000;30:866–870.

33. Ravid M, Neumann L, Lishner M: Plasma lipids and the progression of nephropathy in diabetes mellitus type II: Effect of ACE inhibitors. Kidney Int 1995;47:907–910.

34. Borch-Johnsen K, Kreiner S: Proteinuria: value as predictor of cardiovascular mortality in insulin dependent diabetes mellitus. Br Med J 1987;294:1651–1654.

35. Bierman EL: Atherogenesis in diabetes: George Lyman Duff memorial lecture. Arterioscler Thromb 1992;12:647–656.

36. Wingard DL, Barrett-Connor E: Heart disease and diabetes. In Diabetes in America. Bethesda, MD: National Institutes of Health/ NIDDKD, 1995, pp 429–448.

37. Garg A, Grundy SM: Management of dyslipidemia in NIDDM. Diabetes Care 1990;13:153–169.

38. Pyorala K, Pederson TR, Kjekshus J, et al: Cholesterol lowering with simvastatin improves prognosis of diabetic patients with coronary heart disease: a subgroup analysis of the Scandinavian Simvastatin Survival Study (4S). Diabetes Care 1997;20:614–620.

39. Goldberg RB, Mellies MJ, Sacks FM, et al: Cardiovascular events and their reduction with pravastatin in diabetic and glucose-intolerant myocardial infarction survivors with average cholesterol levels. Subgroup analyses in the Cholesterol and Recurrent Events (CARE) Trial. Circulation 1998;98:2513–2519.

40. Grundy SM, Vega GL, McGovern M, et al: Efficacy, safety, and tolerability of extended-release niacin (Niaspan) for the treatment of dyslipidemia associated type 2 diabetes. Arch Intern Med 2002 (in press).

41. Sanfelippo M, Grundy SM, Henderson L: Transport of very-low-density lipoprotein triglyceride (VLDL-TG) metabolism. Circulation 1979;60:11a–74a.

42. Havel RJ: Triglyceride-rich lipoproteins and atherosclerosis – new perspectives. Am J Clin Nutr 1994;59:795–799.

43. Pasternack A, Vanttinen T, Solakivi T, Kuusi T, Korte T: Normalization of lipoprotein lipase and hepatic lipase by gemfibrozil results in correction of lipoprotein abnormalities in chronic renal failure. Clin Nephrol 1987;27:163–168.

44. Williams AJ, Baker F, Walls J: The short-term effects of bezafibrate on the hypertriglyceridaemia of moderate to severe uraemia. Br J Clin Pharmacol 1984;18:361–367.

45. Norbeck HE, Anderson P: Treatment of uremic hypertriglyceridaemia with bezafibrate. Atherosclerosis 1982;44:125–136.

46. US Renal Data System (USRDS) 2001 Annual Data Report: Atlas of End-Stage Renal Disease in the United States. Bethesda, MD: National Institutes of Health, National Institute of Diabetes and Digestive and Kidney Diseases, 2001.

47. Sanfelippo ML, Swenson RS, Reaven GM: Response of plasma triglycerides to dietary change in patients on hemodialysis. Kidney Int 1978;14:180–186.

48. Cattran DC, Steiner G, Fenton SSA, Ampil M: Dialysis hyperlipemia: response to dietary manipulations. Clin Nephrol 1980;13:177–182.

49. Nishizawa Y, Shoji t, Tabata T, Inoue T, Morii H: Effects of lipid-lowering drugs on intermediate-density lipoprotein in uremic patients. Kidney Int Suppl 1999;71:S134–S136.

50. Malyszko J, Malyszko JS, Hyrszko T, Mysliwiee M: Effects of long-term treatment with simvastatin on some hemostatic parameters in continuous ambulatory peritoneal dialysis patients. Am J Nephrol 2001;21:373–377.

51. Wanner C, Krane V, Metzger T, Quaschning T: Lipid changes and statins in chronic renal insufficiency and dialysis. J Nephrol 2001;14(Suppl 4):S76–S80.

52. Seliger SL, Weiss NS, Gillen DL, et al: HMG-CoA reductase inhibitors are associated with reduced mortality in ESRD patients. Kidney Int 2002;61:297–304.

53. Sherrard DJ, Goldberg AB, Haas LB, Brunzell JD: Chronic clofibrate therapy in maintenance hemodialysis patients. Nephron 1980;25:219–221.

54. De Giulio S, Boulu R, Drueke T, Nicolai A, Zingraff J, Crosnier J: Clofibrate treatment of hyperlipidemia in chronic renal failure. Clin Nephrol 1977;8:504–509.

55. Yoshimura N, Ohmori Y, Tsuji T, Oka T: Effect of pravastatin on renal transplant recipients treated with cyclosporine – 4-year follow-up. Transplant Proc 1994;26:2632–2633.

56. Cheung AK, Devault GA Jr, Gregory MC: A prospective study on treatment of hypercholesterolemia with lovastatin in renal transplant patients receiving cyclosporine. J Am Soc Nephrol 1993;3:1884–1891.

Hyperhomocysteinemia
Christopher S. Wilcox

Metabolism
Pharmacologic therapy

Homocysteine is a sulfa-containing amino acid that circulates in oxidized, reduced and complex forms. About 75% is bound to albumin. Routine assays measure total homocysteine (tHcy).[1,2] Homocysteine is manufactured in cells including erythrocytes. Consequently, it is exported into plasma after blood sampling. Blood samples must, therefore, be cooled to 4 °C, then centrifuged, and the plasma separated rapidly to avoid artificially high values. Reported normal values vary widely between laboratories but are on average 6–10 µmol/L. Hyperhomocysteinemia implies a value more than two standard deviations above normal; this is typically 12–16 µmol/L.

More than 90% of patients with endstage renal disease (ESRD) receiving hemodialysis (HD) or continuous ambulatory peritoneal dialysis (CAPD) have hyperhomocysteinemia. Very severe hyperhomocysteinemia (> 100 µmol/L) occurs as a genetic metabolic defect. It is associated with early and severe atherosclerosis. Mild hyperhomocysteinemia (12–20 µmol/L) occurs in otherwise normal people, often as a manifestation of vitamin B deficiency. Patients with ESRD usually have moderate hyperhomocysteinemia (20–100 µmol/L). Homocysteine may contribute to the markedly elevated risk of cardiovascular disease in ESRD. Indeed, conclusions from five retrospective[3,4–6] and two prospective studies[7,8] concur that tHcy is an independent risk factor for the development of cardiovascular disease in patients with ESRD. Plasma levels of tHcy appear similarly elevated in patients with CAPD and HD.[9–11] Following renal transplantation, tHcy levels fall, but less than anticipated from the improvement in renal function.[12]

In patients with chronic renal failure, the major determinant of tHcy is an increase in the serum creatinine concentration or a reduction in the glomerular filtration rate (GFR).[13] Among patients with ESRD, malnutrition and low serum albumin concentration predict lower levels of tHcy.[14] Levels of tHcy also are lower in patients receiving high-flux hemodialysis.[15] The polymorphism status for 5,10-methylene tetrahydrofolate reductase (MTHFR) has a relatively minor effect on tHcy levels in ESRD.[16]

The mechanism of hyperhomocysteinemia in ESRD remains obscure.[2] Therefore, therapy is empiric, and remains highly unsatisfactory. Since no effective treatment has been devised that normalizes tHcy in this patient population, it has not been possible to establish whether reversal of hyperhomocysteinemia reverses the associated risk of cardiovascular disease.

Metabolism

Homocysteine is metabolized to methionine via the "remethylation pathway;" alternatively, it may be metabolized by transsulfuration (Fig. 68.1).[1] Kinetic studies have defined a defect in remethylation in patients with ESRD, but there is also a failure to upregulate the transsulfuration pathway in response to hyperhomocysteinemia.[17] Remethylation via methionine synthase depends on the active form of folate, 5-methyltetrahydrofolate (5-Me-THF), and the active form of vitamin B_{12}. The transsulfuration pathway is initiated by cystathionine β-synthase, which catalyzes the conjugation of homocysteine and serine to form cystathionine. This is a vitamin B_6-dependent pathway. Therefore, folate, vitamins B_{12} and B_6, or their active metabolites, are essential for homocysteine metabolism. Indeed, defects in these three vitamins account for most cases of mild hyperhomocysteinemia in the general population.[18]

B vitamins are water-soluble and are removed significantly during dialysis. Dialysis patients normally receive a vitamin mix. Among the many choices, one widely used capsule, Nephrocap, contains folic acid 1 mg, vitamin B_6 10 mg, and vitamin B_{12} 6 µg. Such a prescription should maintain plasma vitamin levels in the normal range for most dialysis patients.[19] There is a strong inverse relationship between the log of plasma folate concentration and the log of plasma tHcy concentration, in both healthy people and those with ESRD. However, the relationship is shifted to higher plasma levels of homocysteine in patients with ESRD.[4] This has prompted a hypothesis that ESRD is a state of folate- and B vitamin-resistance, and should be reversed by supranormal doses of these vitamins.

Pharmacologic therapy

Prospective trials in patients with ESRD have evaluated the effects on hyperhomocysteinemia of folic acid (or its derivatives), vitamins B_6 and B_{12}, serine, and betaine.

The efficacy of supplementation of B vitamins in patients with ESRD has been the subject of 16 prospective clinical trials.[10,11,16,20–32] Despite this wealth of information, it is regrettable that no firm statements can be made about the role of vitamin supplementation in doses above those routinely recommended (folic acid 1 mg, B_6 10–50 mg, and B_{12} 5–50 µg daily). Although no consistent conclusions can be drawn from these trials, some trends are apparent.

1. All trials except two[30,31] report a statistically significant reduction in total homocysteine during folate supplementation. However, those two negative trials are

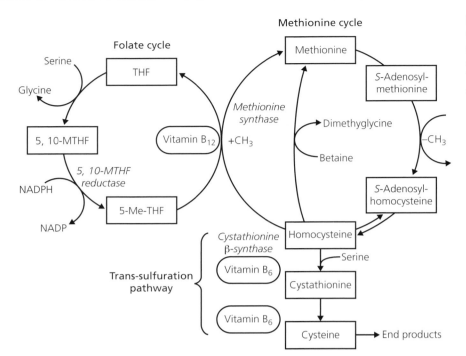

Figure 68.1 A diagrammatic representation of the pathways for methionine and homocysteine metabolism. 5,10-MTHF, 5,10-methyltetrahydrofolate; 5-Me-THF, 5-methyltetrahydrofolate; THF, tetrahydrofolate (Reproduced from Kitiyakara et al.[1])

among the only three that are placebo-controlled,[20,30,31] and both used very high doses of folic acid (30 or 60 mg daily)[31] or folate metabolite (intravenous leucovorin 100 mg, three times per week).[30]

2. Larger falls in total homocysteine usually occur during active treatment when routine vitamin supplementation is withdrawn before the trial starts. However, participants in the two negative trials,[30,31] as well as those from some positive trials,[10,20,23,25,28] were studied while maintaining the standard-of-care prescription with folate. In some studies, the routine supplement was withdrawn before the trial.[11,21,22,25,26] On the whole, participants in these trials had the highest pretreatment values for total homocysteine, probably reflecting some B-vitamin deficiency caused by dialytic losses. Consequently, they generally had the most robust responses to folate therapy (Fig. 68.2A).

3. There is no clear benefit from further supplements of vitamins B_6 and B_{12} that exceeds the effects of folic acid alone. This issue was studied specifically in one controlled trial in which groups of hemodialysis patients received either placebo, folic acid 30 mg or 60 mg, vitamins B_6 and B_{12}, or all three treatments together. There was no significant difference in any group relative to the placebo control.[31]

4. Although there are substantial and largely unexplained variations in the values for total homocysteine before supplementation, all trials report values during supplementation of 12–27 μmol/L (Fig. 68.2A).

5. The trials that used folate metabolites (5 Me-THF)[21,25,27] or folinic acid (leucovorin)[23,26,28,30,32] produced similar results to folic acid. Indeed, within-trial comparisons of folic acid and its metabolic derivatives have shown no significant differences.[23,25,27,28]

6. In only one trial were the values for total homocysteine normalized in the majority of patients. Touam et al[26] supplemented patients with a single post-dialysis injection of folinic acid (50 mg) given once weekly and 250 mg of vitamin B_6 after each dialysis session; they reported normalization of total homocysteine levels. However, a subsequent study found no benefit of equimolar folinic acid over folic acid.[28]

7. Supplementation with serine alone or in addition to folate metabolites produced no further fall in total homocysteine levels.[30]

8. No relationship is apparent between the fractional change in plasma total homocysteine concentration during therapy, and the daily dose of folate (or metabolite) that is given as a supplement (Fig. 68.2B). For example, one trial compared no vitamin supplementation to supplementation with folic acid 1 mg daily, and found that it reduced levels of total homocysteine by 32%, but 10 mg daily produced no further change.[22] The highest doses tested of folic acid (60 mg daily) or folinic acid (100 mg/day intravenously three times per week) are reported variously to reduce plasma total homocysteine by 38%[16] or to have no significant effect whatsoever.[30,31]

These considerations lead to the following conclusions:

1. Presently there is no rational justification for recommending more than routine vitamin supplementation with a daily dose of folic acid (1 mg), B_6 (10–50 mg) and B_{12} (5–50 g) in ESRD patients.

2. There is no benefit from active folate metabolites or folate analogs over folic acid itself.

3. There must be powerful, uncontrolled and presently unrecognized factors in the studies to date that account for the high degree of variability reported in responses to vitamin supplementation.

Figure 68.2A demonstrates that ESRD patients should normally be able to achieve a predialysis total homocysteine

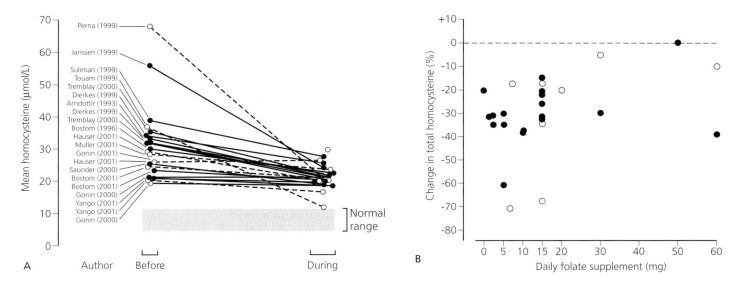

Figure 68.2 Mean data from prospective trials of supplementation with folic acid (solid symbols), or folate metabolites or analogs (open symbols) given with or without other treatments such as vitamins B_6 and B_{12}. (A) Mean total homocysteine (tHcy) for trial subjects before and during folate supplementation; the shaded area represents the normal range. (B) Relationship between the mean fractional change of plasma tHcy concentration during therapy and the daily dose of folate or folate metabolite or analog used.

concentration of below 30 μmol/L. Patients with higher values require assessment to ensure that they have been prescribed, and are indeed receiving, the routine vitamin supplement. If this does not explain the above average plasma level of total homocysteine, the plasma levels of folate, B_{12} and B_6 should be assessed to ensure that they are within the normal range. Occasionally patients present with very high values for total homocysteine due to unrecognized concurrent disease, such as pernicious anemia, or hypothyroidism, or because of concurrent therapy with antifolate drugs such as methotrexate. An algorithm for evaluation and treatment of hyperhomocysteinemia in renal disease is presented in Fig. 68.3.

Clearly, the present state of knowledge concerning hyperhomocysteinemia in patients with ESRD is highly unsatisfactory. On the one hand, hyperhomocysteinemia is almost universal in these patients, and is a powerful predictor of associated or future cardiovascular disease. On the other, treatment is generally ineffective in normalizing hyperhomocysteinemia and available clinical trials are so discordant that strong conclusions concerning the need for more than routine supplementation with folate and B vitamins are not warranted. Therapeutic advances may have to await the outcome of scientific studies that disclose the mechanism of hyperhomocysteinemia in ESRD.

References

1. Kitiyakara C, Gonin J, Massy Z, et al: Non-traditional cardiovascular disease risk factors in end-stage renal disease: oxidative stress and hyperhomocysteinemia. Curr Opin Nephrol 2001;9:477–487.
2. Friedman AN, Bostom AG, Selhub J, et al: The kidney and homocysteine metabolism. J Am Soc Nephrol 2001;12:2181–2189.

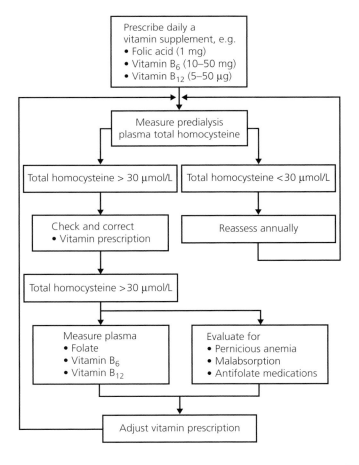

Figure 68.3 Algorithm for routine evaluation and management of hyperhomocysteinemia in patients with endstage renal disease. tHcy, total homocysteine.

3. Robinson K, Gupta A, Dennis V, et al: Hyperhomocysteinemia confers an independent increased risk of atherosclerosis in end-stage renal disease and is closely linked to plasma folate and pyridoxine concentrations. Circulation 1996;94:2743–2748.

4. Dennis VW, Robinson K: Homocysteinemia and vascular disease in end-stage renal disease. Kidney Int 1996;50:S11–S17.

5. Manns BJ, Burgess ED, Hyndman ME, et al: Hyperhomocyst(e)inemia and the prevalence of atherosclerotic vascular disease in patients with end-stage renal disease. Am J Kid Diseases 1999;34:669–677.

6. Bachmann J, Tepel M, Zidek W, et al: Hyperhomocysteinemia and the risk for vascular disease in hemodialysis patients. J Am Soc Nephrol 1995;6:121–125.

7. Ducloux D, Motte G, Challier B, et al: Serum homocysteine and cardiovascular disease occurrence in chronic, stable renal transplant recipients: a prospective study. J Am Soc Nephrol 2000;11:134–137.

8. Moustapha A, Naso A, Nahlawi M, et al: Prospective study of hyperhomocysteinemia as an adverse cardiovascular risk factor in end-stage renal disease. Circulation 1998;97:138–141.

9. Vychytil A, Fodinger M, Wolfl G, et al: Major determinants of hyperhomocysteinemia in peritoneal dialysis patients. Kidney Int 1998;53:1775–1782.

10. Arnadottir M, Brattstrom L, Simonsen O, et al: The effect of high-dose pyridoxine and folic acid supplementation on serum lipid and plasma homocysteine concentrations in dialysis patients. Clin Nephrol 1993;40:236–240.

11. Janssen MJ, van Guldener C, de Jong GM, et al: Folic acid treatment of hyperhomocysteinemia in dialysis patients. Miner Electrolyte Metab 1996;22:110–114.

12. Arnadottir M, Hultberg B, Wahlberg J, et al: Serum homocysteine concentration before and after renal transplantation. Kidney Int 1998;54:1380–1384.

13. Wollesen F, Brattstrom L, Refsum H, et al: Plasma homocysteine and cysteine in relation to glomerular filtration rate in diabetes mellitus. Kidney Int 1999;55:1028–1035.

14. Suliman ME, Qureshi AR, Barany P, et al: Hyperhomocysteinemia, nutritional status, and cardiovascular disease in hemodialysis patients. Kidney Int 2000;57:1727–1735.

15. van Tellingen A, Grooteman MP, Bartels PC, et al: Long-term reduction of plasma homocysteine levels by super-flux dialyzers in hemodialysis patients. Kidney Int 2001;59:342–347.

16. Sunder Plassmann G, Födinger M, Buchmayer H, et al: Effect of high-dose folic acid therapy on hyperhomocysteinemia in hemodialysis patients: results of the Vienna Multicenter study. J Am Soc Nephrol 2000;11:1106–1116.

17. Guttormsen AB, Ueland PM, Svarstad E, et al: Kinetic basis of hyperhomocysteinemia in patients with chronic renal failure. Kidney Int 1997;52:495–502.

18. Hoogeveen EK, Kostense PJ, Jager A, et al: Serum homocysteine level and protein intake are related to risk of microalbuminuria: The Hoorn Study. Kidney Int 1998;54:203–209.

19. Descombes E, Hanck AB, Fellay G: Water soluble vitamins in chronic hemodialysis patients and need for supplementation. Kidney Int 1993;43:1319–1328.

20. Bostom AG, Shemin D, Lapane KL, et al: High dose B-vitamin treatment of hyperhomocysteinemia in dialysis patients. Kidney Int 1996;49:147–152.

21. Perna AF, Ingrosso D, De Santo NG, et al: Metabolic consequences of folate-induced reduction of hyperhomocysteinemia in uremia. J Am Soc Nephrol 1997;8:1899–1905.

22. Tremblay R, Bonnardeaux A, Geadah D, et al: Hyperhomocysteinemia in hemodialysis patients: Effects of 12-month supplementation with hydrosoluble vitamins. Kidney Int 2000;58:851–858.

23. Hauser AC, Hagen W, Rehak PH, et al: Efficacy of folinic versus folic acid for the corrections of hyperhomocysteinemia in hemodialysis patients. Am J Kidney Dis 2001;37:758–765.

24. Dierkes J, Domrose U, Ambrosch A, et al: Response of hyperhomocysteinemia to folic acid supplementation in patients with end-stage renal disease. Clin Nephrol 1999;51:108–115.

25. Bostom AG, Shemin D, Gohh RY, et al: Treatment of hyperhomocysteinemia in hemodialysis patients and renal transplant recipients. Kidney Int 2001;59:S246–S252.

26. Touam M, Zingraff J, Jungers P, et al: Effective correction of hyperhomocysteinemia in hemodialysis patients by intravenous folinic acid and pyridoxine therapy. Kidney Int 1999;56:2292–2296.

27. Bostom A, Shemin D, Bagley P, et al: Controlled comaprison of L-5-methyltetrathydrofolate versus folic acid for the treatment of hyperhomocysteinemia in hemodialysis patients. Circulation 2000;101:2829–2832.

28. Yango A, Shemin D, Hsu N, et al: L-folinic acid versus folic acid for the treatment of hyperhomocysteinemia in hemodialysis patients. (Rapid communication.) Kidney Int 2001;59:324–327.

29. Suliman ME, Filho JCD, Barany P, et al: Effects of high-dose folic acid and pyridoxine on plasma and erythrocyte sulfur amino acids in hemodialysis patients. J Am Soc Nephrol 1999;10:1287–1296.

30. Gonin JM, Nguyen HT, Michels AM, et al: Evaluation of folinic acid and serine in hyperhomocysteinemia in ESRD: A Prospective placebo-controlled randomized study. J Am Soc Nephrol 2001;12:356A.

31. Gonin, JM, Sarna A, Loya A, et al: A double-blind, controlled study of folate and vitamin therapy for hyperhomocysteinemia in hemodialysis (abstract). J Am Soc Nephrol 2000;11:269A.

32. Mueller TF, Mueller N, Moser R, et al: Effect of oral substitution of reduced folates on homocysteine, neopterin, and lipid levels in patients treated with hemodialysis (abstract). J Am Soc Nephrol 2001;12:360A–361A.

CHAPTER 69

Oxidative Stress

Ziad A. Massy and Tilman B. Drüeke

Management of oxidative stress

Several lines of evidence indicate that chronic renal failure (CRF) is a pro-oxidant state. There is evidence (1) that lipid, protein, and DNA oxidation markers are increased in the plasma of CRF patients (Table 69.1);[1-5] and (2) there are oxidative markers in the atherosclerotic lesions of CRF patients, such as hypochlorous acid-modified lipoproteins[6] and advanced glycation endproducts (AGEs).[7] However, the prevalence of oxidative stress among CRF patients remains undetermined, since population-based studies are lacking. The pathogenesis of oxidative stress in CRF patients is multifactorial and includes several possible causes (Fig. 69.1). Uremia-related factors (e.g. hyperhomocysteinemia, or AGEs), and dialysis-related factors (e.g. bioincompatible membranes or endotoxin-contaminated dialysate) may contribute to the genesis of oxidative stress in these patients.[8-10] However, the close relationship between plasma levels of highly sensitive C-reactive protein and lipid oxidation markers in CRF patients suggests a possible role of inflammation in the genesis of oxidative stress.[1,2] The underlying mechanisms responsible for oxidative stress in CRF patients include increased production and decreased clearance of reactive oxygen species, as well as a dysfunctional antioxidant defense system.[1,11-13] In this chapter, we will focus on the management of oxidative stress in CRF patients.

Management of oxidative stress

Several antioxidant maneuvers aimed to modify the oxidative status in CRF patients are available (Table 69.2).

Short-term as well as long-term administration of vitamin E has been reported to reduce levels of circulating oxidative markers in CRF patients.[14-17] It should be noted that the ideal dosage and the long-term efficacy and safety of antioxidant molecules remain to be determined. The induction of oxidative stress by high doses of antioxidant agents remains possible, since several of them were shown to exert antioxidant or prooxidant effects, depending on their concentrations in vitro, or on various environmental conditions. Vitamin E-coated membranes and synthetic biocompatible membranes exhibited antioxidant effects as evaluated by the decrease of 8-hydroxy-2'-deoxyguanosine (8-OHdG) levels and the preservation of plasma vitamin E levels in hemodialysis patients.[18] Vitamin E-coated membrane and high-flux polysulfone have also been shown to decrease serum AGEs levels in hemodialysis patients.[5,19] Hemolipodialysis is a technique that uses dialysate con-

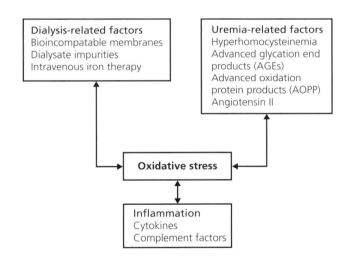

Figure 69.1 Potential factors responsible for oxidative stress in chronic renal failure patients.

Table 69.1 Examples of circulating markers of oxidative stress in chronic renal failure patients

Lipid oxidation markers
Malondialdehyde (MDA)[1]
Oxidized low-density lipoproteins, and reactive antibodies directed against them[3]
F_2-isoprostanes[2]

Protein oxidation markers
Advanced oxidation protein products (AOPP)[4]
Advanced glycation endproducts (AGEs)[8]
Carbonyls[1]

DNA oxidation markers
8-Hydroxy-2'-deoxyguanosine (8-OHdG)[5]

Table 69.2 Antioxidant maneuvers in chronic renal failure patients

Antioxidant molecules
High flux-biocompatible membrane
Vitamin E-coated dialyzer
Hemolipodialysis
Angiotensin II-converting enzyme inhibitors
Statins
Folate supplementation

Table 69.3 Clinical trial of antioxidant maneuvers (AOM) in the prevention of cardiovascular disease (CVD) in chronic renal failure patients

Trial	Antioxidant maneuvers	Number of subjects	Follow-up	Prevention	Oxidative status effects	Cardiovascular disease effects
Miyazaki et al[27]	Vitamin E-coated membrane	12	Single dialysis session	Primary	Prevention of dialysis-induced increased plasma levels of oxidized LDL	Prevention of dialysis-induced impaired flow-mediated vasodilation
Mune et al[15]	Vitamin E-coated membrane	50	2 years	Not defined	Reduction of plasma levels of LDL-MDA and oxidized LDL	Reduction of percentage increase in the aortic calcification index
Boaz et al[28]	Vitamin E 800 IU/day	196	1.4 years	Secondary	ND	Reduction of composite cardiovascular disease and myocardial infarction

LDL, low-density lipoprotein; MDA, malondialdehyde.

taining ascorbic acid and polyunsaturated, unilamellar liposomes filled with vitamin E; in a short-term preliminary study using this technique there was a significant decrease in levels of advanced oxidation protein products (AOPP) in eight patients.[20] In a few uncontrolled studies, the use of angiotensin II-converting enzyme inhibitors or statins was associated with modification of oxidative stress markers.[21,22] However, the results obtained with antioxidant maneuvers in CRF patients suffer from various methodological problems, which preclude firm clinical recommendations, regarding their efficacy and safety, at this point.

The issue of using antioxidant agents, aimed at reducing the dramatic, early incidence of cardiovascular disease in CRF patients, is still unresolved. The claimed causal relationship between oxidative stress and cardiovascular disease has not yet been firmly established for these patients. There have only been a few inconclusive epidemiological studies to evaluate the potential association between oxidative markers and cardiovascular disease. The presence of AGEs has been shown recently in aortic atherosclerotic lesions of CRF patients.[7] Increased oxidative stress, as evaluated by the presence of high serum antibody titer against oxidized low-density lipoproteins, or by low vitamin E levels, was found to be associated with the degree of presence of carotid plaques and the thickness of the intima media, respectively, in predialysis CRF patients.[23] In a cross-sectional study, serum malondialdehyde (MDA) was positively associated with prevalent cardiovascular disease in hemodialysis patients.[24] However, in a very recent study there was no significant correlation between lipid oxidation and endothelial dysfunction in CRF patients before or after the initiation of dialysis treatment.[25] Moreover, no prospective epidemiological study is available to evaluate the association between oxidative stress markers and cardiovascular disease in CRF patients, in contrast to a wide range of epidemiological studies in the general population which have linked the intake of dietary antioxidants to cardiovascular risk.[26]

Similarly, limited data are available regarding the success of interventional trials with antioxidant maneuvers, which aim to reduce cardiovascular disease in CRF patients (Table 69.3).[15,27,28] Miyazaki et al claim that the impairment of endothelial function induced by the hemodialysis procedure could be prevented by coating the dialysis membrane with vitamin E.[27] However, they compared vitamin E-coated cellulosic membrane with uncoated cellulosic, bioincompatible membrane, instead of using a biocompatible membrane as control. Only one study, that is the Secondary Prevention with Antioxidants of Cardiovascular Disease in Endstage Renal Disease (SPACE) trial, has demonstrated a reduction of cardiovascular events as an endpoint.[28] This trial was small and of limited duration. Moreover, the effects of vitamin E supplementation on oxidative status were not determined. In the general population, the cardiovascular benefit of antioxidant administration remains a debated issue as well, since positive and negative results with respect to cardiovascular protection have been reported.[26] Taken together, at this stage, the limited data available provide no clearcut evidence in favor of the clinical benefit of antioxidant maneuvers aimed to reduce cardiovascular disease in CRF patients.

References

1. Nguyen-Khoa T, Massy ZA, et al: Oxidative stress and haemodialysis: role of inflammation and duration of dialysis treatment. Nephrol Dial Transplant 2001;16:335–340.
2. Handelman GJ, Walter MF, Adhikarla R, et al: Elevated plasma F2–isoprostanes in patients on long-term hemodialysis. Kidney Int 2001;59:1960–1966.
3. Holvoet P, Donck J, Landeloos M, et al: Correlation between oxidized low density lipoproteins and von Willebrand factor in chronic renal failure. Thromb Haemost 1996;76:663–669.
4. Witko-Sarsat V, Friedlander M, Capeillere-Blandin C, et al: Advanced oxidation protein products as a novel marker of oxidative stress in uremia. Kidney Int 1996;49:1304–1313.
5. Satoh M, Yamasaki Y, Nagake Y, et al: Oxidative stress is reduced by the long-term use of vitamin E-coated dialysis filters. Kidney Int 2001;59:1943–1950.

6. Malle E, Woenckhaus C, Waeg G, et al: Immunological evidence for hypochlorite-modified proteins in human kidney. Am J Pathol 1997;150:603–615.

7. Sakata N, Imanaga Y, Meng J, et al: Increased advanced glycation endproducts in atherosclerotic lesions of patients with end-stage renal disease. Atherosclerosis 1999;142:67–77.

8. Miyata T, Sugiyama S, Saito A, et al: Reactive carbonyl compounds related uremic toxicity ("carbonyl stress"). Kidney Int Suppl 2001;78:S25–S31.

9. Massy ZA, Ceballos I, Chadefaux-Vekemens B, et al: Homocyst(e)ine, oxidative stress, and endothelium function in uremic patients. Kidney Int Suppl 2001;78:S243–S245.

10. Nguyen AT, Lethias C, Zingraff J, et al: Hemodialysis membrane-induced activation of phagocyte oxidative metabolism detected in vivo and in vitro within microamounts of whole blood. Kidney Int 1985;28:158–167.

11. Roselaar SE, Nazhat NB, Winyard PG, et al: Detection of oxidants in uremic plasma by electron spin resonance spectroscopy. Kidney Int 1995;48:199–206.

12. Nagase S, Aoyagi K, Hirayama A, et al: Favorable effect of hemodialysis on decreased serum antioxidant activity in hemodialysis patients demonstrated by electron spin resonance. J Am Soc Nephrol 1997;8:1157–1163.

13. Dantoine TF, Debord J, Charmes JP, et al: Decrease in paraoxonase activity in chronic renal failure. J Am Soc Nephrol 1998;9:2082–2088.

14. Cristol JP, Bosc JY, Badiou S, et al: Erythropoietin and oxidative stress in haemodialysis: beneficial effects of vitamin E supplementation. Nephrol Dial Transplant 1997;12:2312–2317.

15. Mune M, Yukawa S, Kishino M, et al: Effect of vitamin E on lipid metabolism and atherosclerosis in ESRD patients. Kidney Int Suppl 1999;71:S126–S129.

16. Maccarrone M, Meloni C, Manca-Di-Villahermosa S, et al: Vitamin E suppresses 5–lipoxygenase-mediated oxidative stress in peripheral blood mononuclear cells of hemodialysis patients regardless of administration route. Am J Kidney Dis 2001;37:964–969.

17. Islam KN, O'Byrne D, Devaraj S, et al: Alpha-tocopherol supplementation decreases the oxidative susceptibility of LDL in renal failure patients on dialysis therapy. Atherosclerosis 2000;150:217–224.

18. Tarng DC, Huang TP, Liu TY, et al: Effect of vitamin E-bonded membrane on the 8-hydroxy 2'-deoxyguanosine level in leukocyte DNA of hemodialysis patients. Kidney Int 2000;58:790–799.

19. Jadoul M, Ueda Y, Yasuda Y, et al: Influence of hemodialysis membrane type on pentosidine plasma level, a marker of "carbonyl stress". Kidney Int 1999;55:2487–2492.

20. Wratten ML, Navino C, Tetta C, et al: Haemolipodialysis. Blood Purif 1999;17:127–133.

21. de Cavanagh EM, Ferder L, Carrasquedo F, et al: Higher levels of antioxidant defenses in enalapril-treated versus non-enalapril-treated hemodialysis patients. Am J Kidney Dis 1999;34:445–455.

22. Nishikawa O, Mune M, Miyano M, et al: Effect of simvastatin on the lipid profile of hemodialysis patients. Kidney Int Suppl 1999;71:S219–S221.

23. Stenvinkel P, Heimburger O, Paultre F, et al: Strong association between malnutrition, inflammation, and atherosclerosis in chronic renal failure. Kidney Int 1999;55:1899–1911.

24. Boaz M, Matas Z, Biro A, et al: Serum malondialdehyde and prevalent cardiovascular disease in hemodialysis. Kidney Int 1999;56:1078–1083.

25. Bolton CH, Downs LG, Victory JG, et al: Endothelial dysfunction in chronic renal failure: roles of lipoprotein oxidation and pro-inflammatory cytokines. Nephrol Dial Transplant 2001;16:1189–1197.

26. Faggiotto A, Poli A, Catapano AL: Antioxidants and coronary artery disease. Curr Opin Lipidol 1998;9:541–549.

27. Miyazaki H, Matsuoka H, Itabe H, et al: Hemodialysis impairs endothelial function via oxidative stress: effects of vitamin E-coated dialyzer. Circulation 2000;101:1002–1006.

28. Boaz M, Smetana S, Weinstein T, et al: Secondary Prevention with Antioxidants of Cardiovascular disease in End-stage renal disease (SPACE): randomised placebo-controlled trial. Lancet 2000;356:1213–1218.

Nutritional Therapy of Patients with Chronic Renal Failure and its Impact on Progressive Renal Insufficiency

Tahsin Masud and William E. Mitch

Dietary protein requirements
- Metabolic acidosis
- Dietary phosphates
- Dietary calcium
- Energy requirements
- Potassium
- Sodium
- Trace elements and vitamin requirements
- Compliance

Low-protein diets and progression of chronic renal failure

Evidence of malnutrition and a low serum albumin concentration is common in dialysis patients with chronic renal failure (CRF). Numerous studies of several illnesses have found that a low serum albumin level is associated with increased morbidity and mortality. The same is true for dialysis, which is associated with even higher mortality than certain types of cancer.

The problems of uremia involve the accumulation of unexcreted waste products of protein metabolism. This is important for two reasons.

First, the net amount of protein catabolized each day (the protein catabolic rate or PCR) can be readily estimated because it is directly related to the rate of urea production. Thus, the PCR is simply the daily amount of urea nitrogen produced plus a constant representing the nonurea nitrogen excreted.[1] The total amount of waste nitrogen produced is then converted to protein equivalents by dividing by 0.16, as protein is 16% nitrogen (see Compliance).

Second, restriction of dietary protein reduces production of waste nitrogen and hence ameliorates uremia. As might be expected, some patients with advancing renal insufficiency spontaneously reduce their protein intake. The link between uremic symptoms and waste-product accumulation from excess dietary protein has led some clinicians to make the astonishing suggestion that patients who spontaneously reduce their dietary protein should begin dialysis therapy.[2] Presumably, this conclusion arose from an unsubstantiated fear that dietary restriction will cause malnutrition. On the contrary, there is abundant evidence that *proper use of dietary protein restriction* for predialysis patients will reduce complications of uremia without perturbing nitrogen balance, and indices of nutritional status are stabilized or improved.[3–5] For some patients, dietary manipulation can slow the rate of loss of renal function. The physician must design an appropriate diet and monitor protein intake and nutritional status to achieve compliance and prevent malnutrition.[6]

Dietary protein requirements

Dietary protein restriction has been a mainstay of therapy for CRF since at least 1869.[5] The goals of dietary therapy are to diminish the accumulation of nitrogenous waste, to limit the metabolic disturbances characteristic of uremia, to prevent malnutrition, and to slow the progression of renal failure.

In healthy adults performing moderate physical activity, the average minimum daily protein requirement is ~ 0.6 g/kg body weight, if they eat sufficient calories. The "safe level of protein intake," defined as the average minimum requirement plus two standard deviations is ~ 0.75 g/kg/day protein. This meets the protein requirements of 97.5% of normal adults.[7] Although most adults in the western world consume greater amounts of protein, the excess does not increase stores of body protein. Instead, the excess is catabolized to nitrogen-containing products that must be excreted, otherwise they will accumulate as uremic toxins.

The term PCR is confusing because it does not measure the daily amount of protein that is degraded – it estimates the amount of protein that is ingested. Adults synthesize and degrade about 4 g/kg/day protein, which is substantially more than is in the diet.[8] Rather than total protein catabolism, PCR measures the net protein catabolism (the difference between synthesized and degraded protein plus the amount eaten). If nitrogen balance is neutral, protein synthesis equals protein degradation and the net nitrogen excreted equals dietary protein intake.

Nonacidotic patients with CRF are remarkably efficient in adapting to dietary restriction. Goodship et al[9] showed that such patients reduce rates of amino acid oxidation and protein degradation in the same fashion as normal adults when their protein diet is restricted from 1.0 to 0.6 g/kg/day. The same adaptive metabolic responses are activated when the diet is restricted to only 0.3 g/kg/day, and a supplement of essential amino acids or their nitrogen-free analogues (ketoacids) is given. Such a dietary regimen maintains both neutral nitrogen balance and indices of adequate nutrition over 1 year of observation.[10] The supplement is required when the diet is so restricted in order to meet the requirements for essential amino acids.

Despite these encouraging findings, there has been concern about the nutritional safety of low-protein diets prescribed for CRF patients. More than 20 years ago, Kopple and Coburn[11] demonstrated that the nitrogen balance of patients with advanced CRF was neutral or positive when they consumed a daily diet containing about 0.6 g protein and 35 kcal/kg of body weight. Diets containing less protein but a supplement of either essential amino acids or ketoacids, and sufficient calories, can maintain neutral nitrogen balance.[12] Normal values of serum proteins, anthropometrics, and neutral nitrogen balance are maintained during long-term therapy.[3,4,10] In the Modification of Diet in Renal Disease (MDRD) study[12] in patients prescribed different low-protein diets, there were a few small – but statistically significant – changes in some nutritional parameters, including an increase in serum albumin but a decrease in transferrin and anthropometric measurements. Most importantly, only two patients had to discontinue the MDRD study because of nutritional abnormalities. There was no association between low-protein diets and higher rates of death, hospitalization, accelerated loss of kidney function, serum albumin below 3.0 g/dL, or weight loss below 75% standard body weight.[12]

Aparicio et al[4] followed 165 patients treated with a very low-protein diet supplemented with essential amino acids or ketoacids for an average of 29 months. In this group, body weight, body mass index, and serum albumin concentration were unchanged. They continued to observe the patients after they began hemodialysis and found that 54 months later the mortality was low and independent of nutritional parameters measured at the initiation of dialysis. A low-protein diet also ameliorates metabolic acidosis and renal osteodystrophy, and limits proteinuria.[5] Maroni et al[13] reported that dietary protein restriction is safe even in patients with the nephrotic syndrome. They treated patients with a daily diet of 0.8 g protein/kg of ideal body weight plus 1 g dietary protein for each gram of proteinuria. Nitrogen balance was neutral and hypoalbuminemia was diminished. Others have confirmed that hypoalbuminemia is prevented by proper restriction of dietary protein.[3–5] Properly implemented low-protein diets can also improve survival of patients with CRF after beginning dialysis.[3,4]

We recommend that CRF patients with symptoms attributable to uremia or with uncontrolled progressive renal insufficiency be treated with a well-planned low-protein diet providing 0.6 g protein/kg/day. The protein intake should not exceed 0.75 g/kg/day because excess protein will be converted to waste products. At least 50% of the protein intake for all these patients should be of high biological value.[7] The diet should be designed by an experienced CRF nutritionist to allow for the patient's food preferences, and to ensure an adequate intake of calories and vitamins. Malnourished patients with CRF may require more protein intake while they are being monitored by a skilled nutritionist (see Compliance).

Protein intake for nephrotic patients of 0.8 g/kg/day (plus 1 g protein for each gram of proteinuria) promotes neutral nitrogen balance and reduces proteinuria while ameliorating hypoalbuminemia and hypercholesterolemia.[5,13,17] The recommendation that nephrotic patients should have a high-protein diet, to compensate for urinary albumin losses and to promote anabolism, should be discarded. The ensuing increase in proteinuria is a risk factor for progressive renal insufficiency.

The requirement for dietary protein is strikingly higher for dialysis patients (Table 70.1); this is for several reasons: there is a loss of nutrients into the dialysate, and there is increased protein catabolism due to chronic inflammation, metabolic acidosis, and dialysis itself.[14–16] Measurements of nitrogen balance indicate that hemodialysis patients require a protein intake of 1 g/kg/day, and that peritoneal dialysis patients require 1.2 g/kg/day.[18] Unfortunately, a high-protein diet invariably increases the intake of sodium, potassium and phosphate.

Table 70.1 Recommended nutrient intake in patients with chronic renal failure and those on dialysis

Nutrient	Chronic renal failure	Peritoneal and hemodialysis
Protein* (g/kg of ideal body weight)	GFR (mL/min/1.73 m^2) > 25–50, no restriction recommended 0.6–0.75 < 25, 0.6	Hemodialysis, 1.2 CAPD, 1.2–1.3 Revise goals to 1.0–1.1 if serum phosphorus difficult to control
Energy (kcal/kg of ideal body weight)	For nephrotic patient† < 60 years old, 35 > 60 years old, 30 to 35	< 60 years old, 35 > 60 years old, 30 to 35
Carbohydrates	35% of nonprotein calories	35% of nonprotein calories
Fats	Polyunsaturated to saturated ratio of 2:1	Polyunsaturated to saturated ratio of 2:1
Phosphorus (mg)	800–1200	800–1200
Potassium	Individualized	Individualized
Sodium and water	As tolerated, to maintain body weight and blood pressure	As tolerated, to maintain body weight and blood pressure

*At least 50% of proteins should be of high biological value.
†For nephrotic patients, 0.8 g of protein/kg and add 1 g of protein/g of proteinuria.
CAPD, continuous ambulatory peritoneal dialysis; GFR, glomerular filtration rate.

Patients with CRF often suffer from anorexia.[19] Some unidentified circulating factor can suppress the appetite and thereby decrease the protein intake with advancing renal insufficiency.[2] Diabetic patients may have impaired gastrointestinal function, causing anorexia. Hemodialysis patients often experience hemodynamic instability and fatigue after dialysis, causing anorexia. Patients treated by peritoneal dialysis absorb glucose from the dialysate that provides 15–30% of the total energy intake;[18] this can suppress appetite. New dialysate formulations that substitute amino acids for glucose show promise in limiting the negative nitrogen balance that has been the bane of peritoneal dialysis therapy.

Anorexia with an inadequate intake of protein and calories may affect the patient in more subtle ways. For example, serum creatinine level does not rise above the normal range until the glomerular filtration rate (GFR) has declined by as much as 60%;[6] because creatinine is largely produced from muscle creatine, the clinician must interpret laboratory data in the context of body weight and anthropometric measurements of muscle mass. A parallel situation can occur in dialysis patients. If the dialysis prescription is too low, a patient may develop anorexia and decrease the intake of dietary protein. This will reduce the net rate of urea production and lower the serum urea nitrogen (SUN) level, leading to the false conclusion that the dialysis prescription is satisfactory. Because of a reduced accumulation of waste products, initially the patient may feel better and request even less dialysis, thereby aggravating the problem. If the SUN is < 60 mg/dL and the serum albumin is subnormal, the nephrologist must determine if there is concurrent illness, an inadequate dialysis prescription, or delivery of dialysis or some other factor, that is perturbing nutritional status. What other factors affect protein metabolism?

Metabolic acidosis

Acidosis has many deleterious consequences. Therefore a concerted effort should be undertaken to correct it. Acidosis increases the catabolism of essential amino acids and protein, resulting in a negative nitrogen balance and a loss of muscle protein.[15] Metabolic acidosis stimulates parathyroid hormone secretion and suppresses the production of 1,25-dihydroxyvitamin D_3 leading to osteopenia. It can depress cardiac function and perturb insulin, growth hormone, and glucocorticoids.[15]

The principal source of acid is catabolism of dietary proteins. When excessive acid is generated, it is buffered in bone, leading to dissolution of the bone matrix. Restricting dietary protein in predialysis patients will often ameliorate this response, sodium bicarbonate should be given if required as even modest acidemia can be detrimental. In dialysis patients, correction of metabolic acidosis also reduces the accelerated protein degradation. Optimizing the dialysis regimen, and prescription of sodium bicarbonate are the mainstays of therapy. Care is essential when prescribing sodium citrate because it increases aluminum absorption. It must never be used in patients treated with aluminum hydroxide. Calcium carbonate has been used for sodium-intolerant patients but it is less effective.

Dietary phosphates

A protein-restricted diet also reduces the intake of phosphates, calcium, calories, potassium, and vitamins. Secondary hyperparathyroidism can cause inanition in patients with CRF. It develops early in the disease as an adaptive response to maintain a normal serum phosphorus level, since parathyroid hormone increases the fractional excretion of phosphates (see Chapter 73). A prolonged elevation of serum phosphorus, a high calcium–phosphorus product, and secondary hyperparathyroidism result in vascular and visceral calcification, which contributes to the risk of cardiovascular death in the endstage renal disease population.[25] Restriction of dietary phosphorus to 800 mg is recommended for CRF patients.[19] Since even a slightly high serum phosphorus level stimulates parathyroid hormone production, dietary phosphorus should be restricted early in renal failure and if necessary a phosphate-binder should be added (Chapter 73). For patients with a high serum calcium–phosphorus product, a noncalcium-containing phosphorus binder should be selected. Aluminum hydroxide should be used only briefly (especially in dialysis patients) to limit the risk of aluminum toxicity. When serum calcium is low, calcium salts (e.g. calcium carbonate or calcium acetate) are ideal. The binder should be taken with food.

Dietary calcium

Patients with CRF often have an inadequate intake of calcium, aggravated by reduced intestinal calcium absorption because of vitamin D deficiency. CRF patients require a daily calcium intake of 1.5 g.[20] Dairy products and high-protein foods are an excellent source of calcium. However, they must be restricted to reduce dietary phosphates. Calcium intake can be increased by calcium-containing phosphate binders. Calcium carbonate requires an acidic gastric milieu to be effective. Calcium acetate is effective even with gastric atrophy. If serum phosphorus is controlled and calcium intake is adequate, supplemental vitamin D may not be necessary. However, supplements of vitamin D are beneficial for growing children and young adults; in those with established hyperparathyroidism, serum phosphorus and calcium levels must be maintained within the normal range to prevent hypercalcemia, calciphylaxis, and even cardiovascular complications of CRF.[25] Dietary indiscretion can raise the calcium–phosphorus product to a level sufficient to increase the spontaneous precipitation of calcium and phosphorus throughout the body.

Energy requirements

There have been few systematic investigations of the caloric requirements of CRF patients. In predialysis patients fed a low-protein diet containing approximately 0.6 g/kg/day, nitrogen balance improves when calories are raised. The optimal level is 30–35 kcal/kg/day.[7] The same calorie intake is recommended for hemodialysis patients. There are several caveats: first, only a few patients have been studied; second, the impact of exercise has not been defined; third, a diet containing too few calories will compromise the ability of a patient to achieve nitrogen balance and lead to loss of muscle mass. Unfortunately, it is difficult to obtain reliable estimates of calorie intake. The nephrologist must rely on repeated measurements of weight and muscle mass.

Potassium

Even in patients at an advanced stage of CRF receiving angiotensin-converting enzyme inhibitors or angiotensin receptor blockers, serious hyperkalemia generally does not occur unless there is an abrupt increase in potassium intake.[22,23] Dietary restriction is normally unnecessary until the renal insufficiency is advanced.[23] A large portion of the daily potassium intake is excreted in the gut of patients with CRF. Thus, constipation can aggravate hyperkalemia.

Dietary potassium restriction to 2 g/day is almost always required for dialysis patients. This means avoiding brightly colored fruits and vegetables, chocolates, nuts, and potatoes. No doubt the increase in sudden deaths of dialysis patients that occur in the summer months is related to dietary potassium lapses occasioned by sampling the season's fruits and vegetables!

Sodium

A salt-restricted diet potentiates the efficacy of antihypertensive medicines.[23,20] A high-protein diet invariably contains an excess of sodium. Therefore, it is easier to achieve the standard daily Na^+ restriction to 2 g when dietary protein is restricted. For patients with edema, it is difficult, if not impossible, to achieve a net loss of sodium (and, hence, extracellular volume) with diuretics unless dietary sodium is restricted. For dialysis patients, dietary sodium restriction is mandatory to minimize the interdialytic weight gain, to control blood pressure, and to reduce fluid losses at each dialysis. Patients should be urged to monitor their weight as a sign of fluid retention from dietary indiscretion.

Trace elements and vitamin requirements

Uremia alters the blood and tissue concentrations of trace elements and vitamins.[24] These derangements are due to a decrease in glomerular filtration, and impaired tubular function and protein binding of micronutrients. In addition, an inadequate diet or altered gastrointestinal absorption may limit absorption. Dialysis can remove micronutrients, depending on their water solubility, the membrane's permeability, and the gradient between the free fraction of an element in the serum and its concentration in the dialysate. Water-soluble vitamins can be lost during dialysis, but the limited number of studies examining this indicate that the need of dialysis patients for water-soluble vitamins are no different from healthy

adults. Pharmacological doses of folic acid are recommended by some for lowering plasma homocysteine levels but whether this decreases cardiovascular risk is not yet established.[24] A vitamin C intake above 100 mg/day can lead to tissue deposition of oxalate crystals that may hasten renal insufficiency, increase the risk of myocardial infarction, or contribute to the failure of dialysis access shunts, and muscle weakness. Plasma levels of vitamin A and retinol-binding protein are increased in renal patients. Therefore, vitamin A-containing multivitamin preparations should be avoided in patients with kidney disease. The use of vitamin E to reduce the risk of cardiovascular events[25] is discussed in Chapter 69. Patients with kidney disease who have an inadequate diet should take a multivitamin preparation that is formulated specifically for renal patients. For dialysis patients, deficiencies of water-soluble vitamins are common due to vitamin losses in the dialysate, poor oral intake, and/or altered metabolism. In summary, daily requirements for most trace elements and vitamins in renal patients differ little from the healthy population (Table 70.2).[24]

Compliance

A skilled dietitian is essential for treating the CRF patient. The nutritionist should be familiar with problems specific to kidney patients and knowledgable about the use of seasonings that can make meals appetizing, thus facilitating compliance.

To assess compliance with salt and protein intake, a 24-h urine is collected from patients with stable renal function for sodium, potassium, and urea nitrogen excretion.[1] The calculation of protein intake is detailed in Table 70.3. There are limitations to these calculations: first, they assume that the patient is in the steady state with no change in body weight or SUN; and, second, they assume minimal day-to-day variation in the diet. A change in the diet requires 5–7 days to establish a new steady-state.[1] This method provides a more accurate estimate of dietary protein than dietary questionnaires. However, there is no reliable means to estimate the intake of calories or other nutrients. This is another reason to enlist the assistance of a skilled nutritionist.

Low-protein diets and progression of chronic renal failure

Many of the reports examining the influence of dietary protein restriction on the progression of renal disease suffer from problems in design, from differences in measurement of efficacy, limited sample size, the type of diet, and degrees of compliance with the diet.[6] Randomized trials of nondiabetic and noninsulin dependant diabetic patients with CRF have not demonstrated consistently that dietary protein restriction slows progression (Table 70.4). Most randomized controlled trials have shown improved preservation of kidney function in insulin-dependent diabetic patients assigned to a low-protein diet.[26-30] Metaanalyses published by Fouque et al[31,33] and Pedrini et al[32] indicate a significant benefit from low-protein diets in preserving the renal function of diabetic patients.

The largest trial in nondiabetic patients was the Modification of Diet in Renal Disease (the MDRD study).[34] This was designed to test the effects of dietary protein restriction and different levels of blood pressure control on the progression of renal insufficiency in 840 patients. In study A, patients with GFRs of 25–55 mL/min/1.73 m^2 were randomly assigned to a normal protein diet (1.3 g/kg/day) or a low-protein diet (0.58 g/kg/day). In study B, patients with GFRs of 13–24 mL/min/1.73 m^2 were randomly assigned to the same low-protein diet or to a very low-protein diet (0.28 g/kg/day) plus a mixture of ketoacids (to supply essential amino acids). There was no control group eating an unrestricted diet in the group of patients with more advanced renal insufficiency. GFR was assessed every 4 months by measuring the renal clearance of [^{125}I]iothalamate. The patients were followed for an average of 2.2 years and the results extrapolated to 3 years. There was no significant difference in the loss of GFR between the two diet groups in either study A or study B, but there was a trend towards a slower decline in GFR in patients assigned to the lower-protein diets.

Table 70.2 Comparison of the recommended daily allowances (RDA) for micronutrients in healthy subjects and the measured intake by hemodialysis patients, with recommended intake as the percent of RDA for endstage renal disease patients

Micronutrient	RDA in healthy population	Observed intake in hemodialysis patients[*]	Recommended supplement as % of RDA
Zinc	Women 8 mg/men 11 mg	NA	None
Selenium	55 mg	NA	None
Copper	900 mg	NA	None
Thiamin	Women 1.1 mg/men 1.2 mg	0.78–2.36 mg	100 mg
Riboflavin	Women 1.1 mg/men 1.3 mg	0.69–2.29 mg	100 mg
Folic acid[†]	400 mg	71–378 mg	200–1000 mg
Vitamin B$_6$	1.3 mg	0.64–2.14 mg	100 mg
Vitamin B$_{12}$	2.4 mg	1.2–7.5 mg	100 mg
Vitamin C	Women 75 mg/men 90 mg	14–125 mg	120 mg
Vitamin A	Women 700 mg/men 900 mg	285–1385 mg	None
Vitamin E[‡]	15 mg	NA	None

[*]Intake values from Rocco MV and Makoff R. Appropiate vitamin therapy for dialysis patients. Semin Dial 1997;10:272–277.
[†]Expressed as dietary folate equivalent.
[‡]Represents α-tocopherol form only.

Table 70.3 Estimation of protein intake for a patient prescribed a diet containing 1 g protein/kg/day

A patient weighs 70 kg and the 24-h urinary collection contains:
    Volume 2400 mL
    Creatinine 1100 mg
    Protein 7 g
    Urea nitrogen 7.9 g

Nitrogen balance (B$_N$) = nitrogen intake (IN) – urea nitrogen appearance (U) – nonurea nitrogen excretion (NUN)*
    = IN – U – NUN

(Nitrogen in feces, urine creatinine, uric acid, other unmeasured nitrogen-containing compounds and urinary protein > 5 g)*

If the patient is in steady state, and is compliant, nitrogen input equals output, therefore:
    IN = U + NUN
    = 7.9 g N/day + (70 kg × 0.031 g N/kg/day + 7 g urinary protein × 0.16)
    = 7.9 g N/day + (2.17 g N/kg/day + 1.12 g N/kg/day)
    = 11.19 g N/day

Assuming that protein is 16% nitrogen (i.e. conversion factor is 1/0.16 = 6/25), the patient is eating:
    11.19 x 6.25 = 70 g protein/day

*Nitrogen in feces, urine creatinine, uric acid, other unmeasured nitrogen-containing compounds, and urinary protein > 5 g.

Table 70.4 Randomized controlled trials of effect of protein restricted diets on the progression of renal failure.

Reference	No. of patients	Mean follow-up (months)	Prescribed protein for randomized groups (g/kg/day)	Actual protein intake (g/kg/day)	Outcome of trial
Junger et al[40]	14	9	0.6 vs 0.4 plus KA	0.7 vs 0.4 plus KA	Time to dialysis longer and mean slope of $1/S_{Cr}$ lower in KA group
Bergstörm et al[41]	16	12–24	Unrestricted vs 0.4 plus EAA	0.86 vs 0.65	Slope of $1/S_{Cr}$ and drop in CrCl were similar
Ihle et al[42]	64	18	Unrestricted vs 0.4	> 0.75 vs 0.4	Significantly less decrease in GFR and progression to end-stage in low-protein group
Rosman et al[43]	239	48	Unrestricted vs 0.4–0.6	No data available	Renal survival better in low-protein group after 2 years but no difference after 4 years
Locatelli et al[44]	456	24	1.0 vs 0.6	0.9 vs 0.78	No difference in renal survival
Williams et al[45]	95	19	> 0.8 vs 0.6	1.0–1.14 vs 0.69	Rate of fall of CrCl and $1/S_{Cr}$ similar
Klahr et al,[34] study A	585	26	1.3 vs 0.58	1.1 vs 0.77	The intention-to-treat analysis revealed no difference in GFR decline. When analyzed by degree of compliance low-protein group has significant slowing in GFR
Klahr et al,[34] study B	255	26	0.58 vs 0.28 plus KA	0.73 vs 0.48	No difference in slowing of GFR, on secondary analysis lower protein intake caused slower mean decline in GFR but no independent effect of KA
D'Amico et al[46]	128	27	1.0 vs 0.6	1.1 vs 0.8	Low-protein group had significant lower risk of progression

CrCl, creatinine clearance; EAA, essential amino acids; GFR, glomerular filtration rate; KA, ketoacids; S_{Cr}, serum creatinine.

Do the MDRD study results provide the last word on the influence of low-protein diets in preserving kidney function? Because of the shortcomings of the MDRD study, we do not believe these results prove that there is no benefit from low-protein diets.

First, the hypothesis tested by the study was that eating a protein-restricted diet will slow the loss of residual renal function. However, the conclusions were based on the diet assignment, rather than achieved intake (Table 70.4). Indeed, when the MDRD results were analyzed according to compliance with the low-protein diets, there was a significant slowing of the loss of GFR and a delay until patients needed dialysis.[35]

Second, the criteria for entering the MDRD study did not include the requirement that patients were losing renal function. Approximately 15% of the control group in study A had no evidence of progressive loss of GFR. This increases the number of patients required to demonstrate a benefit from the dietary manipulations. Moreover, the rate of loss of renal function was slower than predicted. Meta-analyses of results from several studies[31–33] concluded that dietary protein restriction preserves residual renal function.

Third, about 20% of patients had polycystic kidney disease; they derived no benefit from the dietary restriction or from treatment of hypertension.

Fourth, patients in the MDRD study were randomly given angiotensin-converting enzyme inhibitors. The beneficial effects of these drugs[36] may obscure a benefit from the low-protein diet.

Finally, the MDRD study lasted only 2.2 years. Patients in study A had an initial rapid loss of GFR after institution of the low-protein diet followed by a slower loss of GFR. If this slowing had persisted, statistically significant slowing of progression may have been detected over time. In a trial that examined the influence of strict control of hyperglycemia, (the DCCT trial)[36] no benefit was apparent until after 4 years of therapy. Likewise, slowing of the loss of renal function in patients with IgA-nephropathy during treatment with a fish-oil supplement was not apparent until 3 years.[38]

Fouque et al[31] analyzed results from 890 randomly assigned patients participating in six different studies. The outcome event was initiation of dialysis, or death (i.e. "renal death"). The low-protein diet reduced the number of "renal deaths" (61 for low-protein diet groups versus 95 for control groups), yielding a calculated odds ratio of 0.54 ($P < 0.002$) for the likelihood of progressing to endstage renal disease. Pedrini et al[32] performed a metaanalysis of the course of renal failure in 1413 nondiabetic patients in five studies and 108 insulin-dependent diabetic patients participating in five studies.[34] For nondiabetic patients, assignment to a low-protein diet reduced the risk for renal failure or death by one-third ($P < 0.007$). For diabetic patients, the risk of a decrease in GFR or an increase in proteinuria was reduced by almost a half ($P < 0.001$). Notably, angiotensin-converting enzyme inhibitors were used in only 9 of 108 diabetic patients. Any benefits were independent of this drug.

Others have argued that although dietary protein restriction ameliorates uremic signs and symptoms, and therefore delays the need to initiate dialysis, it does slow the rate of decline in renal function. Kasiske et al[39] conducted a metaanalysis of 13 randomized control trials involving 1919 patients. Dietary protein restriction slowed the rate of decline in estimated GFR by only 0.53 mL/min/year. However, if the loss of GFR in the control group is about 4 mL/min/year and a low-protein diet was initiated at a GFR of 50 mL/min, the time to reach a GFR of 10 mL/mim GFR would be prolonged by 1.5 years in those given a low-protein diet. This metaanalysis also indicated a greater benefit of the low-protein diet in diabetic patients, although the numbers were small ($n = 102$).

The results to date have not settled the debate as to whether a low-protein diet is effective in slowing the loss of residual renal function in a large proportion of patients. However, these diets have been used effectively for more than 130 years to treat the symptoms resulting from CRF.[5] When properly applied, these diets do not lead to malnutrition, even in patients with advanced renal insufficiency.[3,4] For these reasons, we recommend instituting a low-protein diet in all patients that have symptoms attributable to uremia or to patients who exhibit progressive renal insufficiency despite the control of blood pressure and use of drugs to block angiotensin II. This requires education of the patient, interaction with a skilled dietitian, and proper monitoring of the quantity of protein eaten and the nutritional status.

References

1. Maroni BJ, Steinman T, Mitch WE: A method for estimating nitrogen intake of patients with chronic renal failure. Kidney Int 1985;27:58–65.
2. Hakim RM, Lazarus JM: Initiation of dialysis. J Am Soc Nephrol 1995;6:1319–1320.
3. Walser M, Hill S: Can renal replacement be deferred by a supplemented very-low-protein diet? J Am Soc Nephrol 1999;10:110–116.
4. Aparicio M, Chauveau P, de Precigout V, et al: Nutrition and outcome on renal replacement therapy of patients with chronic renal failure treated by a supplemented very-low-protein diet. J Am Soc Nephrol 2000;11:719–727.
5. Walser M, Mitch WE, Maroni BJ, et al: Should protein be restricted in predialysis patients? Kidney Int 1999;55:771–777.
6. Maroni BJ, Mitch WE: Role of nutrition in prevention of the progression of renal disease. Ann Rev Nutr 1997;17:435–455.
7. Mitch WE: Dietary requirements for protein and calories before dialysis. In Mitch WE, Klahr S (eds). Handbook of Nutrition and the Kidney, 4th edn. Philadelphia: Lippincott Williams and Wilkins, 2002, pp 135–156.
8. Mitch WE, Goldberg AL: Mechanisms of muscle wasting: The role of the ubiquitin-proteasome system. N Engl J Med 1996;335:1897–1905.
9. Goodship THJ, Mitch WE, Hoerr RA, et al: Adaptation to low-protein diets in renal failure: leucine turnover and nitrogen balance. J Am Soc Nephrol 1990;1:66–75.
10. Tom K, Young VR, Chapman T, et al: Long-term adaptive responses to dietary protein restriction in chronic renal failure. Am J Physiol 1995;268:E668–E677.
11. Kopple JD, Coburn JW: Metabolic studies of low-protein diets in uremia: I. Nitrogen and potassium. Medicine 1973;52:583–594.
12. Kopple JD, Greene T, Chumlea WC, et al: Relationship between nutritional status and the glomerular filtration rate: Results from the MDRD Study Group. Kidney Int 2000;57:1688–1703.
13. Maroni BJ, Staffeld C, Young VR, et al: Mechanisms permitting nephrotic patients to achieve nitrogen equilibrium with a protein-restricted diet. J Clin Invest 1997;99:2479–2487.
14. Kaysen GA: Biological basis of hypoalbuminemia in ESRD. J Am Soc Nephrol 1998;9:2368–2376.
15. Mitch WE, Price SR: Mechanisms activated by kidney disease and the loss of muscle mass. Am J Kidney Dis 2000;38:1337–1342.
16. Ikizler TA, Pupim LB, Brouillette JR, et al: Hemodialysis stimulates muscle and whole body protein loss and alters substrate oxidation in chronic hemodialysis patients. Am J Physiol Endocr Metab 2002;282:E107–E116.
17. Kaysen GA, Gambertoglio J, Felts J, et al: Albumin synthesis, albuminuria and hyperlipemia in nephrotic patients. Kidney Int 1987;31:1368–1376.
18. NKF-DOQI: Clinical practice guidelines for nutrition in chronic renal failure, National Kidney Foundation, Dialysis Outcomes Quality Initiative. Am J Kidney Dis 2000;35(Suppl 2):S1–S140.
19. Bergstrom J: Anorexia in dialysis patients. Sem Nephrol 1996;16:222–229.
20. Martin KJ: Requirements for calcium, phosphorus and vitamin D. In Mitch WE, Klahr S (eds). Nutrition and the Kidney, 3rd edn. Philadelphia: Lippincott-Raven, 1998, pp 87–106.
21. Block GA, Port FK: Re-evaluation of risks associated with hyperphosphatemia and hyperparathyoridism in dialysis patients: Recommendations for a change in management. Am J Kidney Dis 2000;35:1226–1237.
22. Brenner BM, Copper ME, de Zeeuw D, et al: Effects of losartan on renal and cardiovasular outcomes in patients with type 2 diabetes and nephropathy. N Engl J Med 2001;345:861–869.
23. Mitch WE, Wilcox CS: Disorders of body fluids, sodium and potassium in chronic renal failure. Am J Med 1982;72:536–550.
24. Masud T: Trace elements and vitamins in renal disease. In Mitch WE, Klahr S (eds). Nutrition and the Kidney, 4th edn. Philadelphia: Lippincott Williams & Wilkins, 2002, pp 233–252.
25. Yousuf S, Dagenais G, Pogue J, et al: Supplementation and cardiovascular events in high-risk patients. The Heart Outcome Prevention Evaluation Study Investigators. N Engl J Med 2000;342:154–160.
26. Brouhard BH, LaGrone L: Effect of dietary protein restriction on functional renal reserve in diabetic nephropathy. Am J Med 1990;89:427–431.
27. Zeller KR, Whittaker E, Sullivan L, et al: Effect of restricting dietary protein on the progression of renal failure in patients with insulin-dependent diabetes mellitus. N Engl J Med 1991;324:78–83.
28. Dullaart RP, Beusekamp BJ, Meijer S, et al: Long-term effects of protein-restricted diet on albuminuria and renal function in IDDM patients without clinical nephropathy and hypertension. Diabetes Care 1993;16:483–492.
29. Raal FJ, Kalk WJ, Lawson M, et al: Effect of moderate dietary protein restriction on the progression of overt diabetic nephropathy: A 6-month prospective study. Am J Clin Nutr 1994;60:579–585.
30. Mogensen CE: Dietary protein restriction and the progression of diabetic nephropathy. J Am Soc Nephrol 2002 (in press).
31. Fouque D, Laville M, Boissel JP, et al: Controlled low-protein diets in

chronic renal insufficiency: meta-analysis. Br Med J 1992;304:216–220.

32. Pedrini MT, Levey AS, Lau J, et al: The effect of dietary protein restriction on the progression of diabetic and nondiabetic renal diseases: A meta-analysis. Ann Intern Med 1996;124:627–632.

33. Fouque D, Wang P, Laville M, Boissel JP. Low-protein diets delay end-stage renal disease in nondiabetic adults with chronic renal failure. Nephrol Dial Transpl 2000;15:1986–1992.

34. Klahr S, Levey AS, Beck GJ, et al: The effects of dietary protein restriction and blood-pressure control on the progression of chronic renal failure. N Engl J Med 1994;330:878–884.

35. Levey AS, Adler S, Caggiula AW, et al: Effects of dietary protein restriction on the progression of advanced renal disease in the Modification of Diet in Renal Disease Study. Am J Kid Dis 1996;27:652–663.

36. Taal MW, Brenner BM: Renoprotective benefits of RAS inhibition: From ACEI to antiotensin II antagonists. Kidney Int 2000;57:1803–1817.

37. DCCT Research Group: Effect of intensive therapy on the development and progression of diabetic nephropathy in the Diabetes Control and Complications Trial. Kidney Int 1995;47:1703–1720.

38. Donadio JV, Bergstralh EJ, Offord KP, et al: A controlled trial of fish oil in IgA nephropathy. N Engl J Med 1994;331:1194–1199.

39. Kasiske BL, Lakatua JDA, Ma JZ, et al: A meta-analysis of the effects of dietary protein restriction on the rate of decline in renal function. Am J Kidney Dis 1998;31:954–961.

40. Junger P, Chauveau P, Ployard F, et al: Comparison of ketoacids and low-protein diet on advanced chronic renal failure progression. Kidney Int 1987;32(Suppl 22):S67–S71.

41. Bergstörm J, Alvestrand A, Bucht H, et al: Stockholm clinical study on progression of chronic renal failure – an interim report. Kidney Int 1989;36(Suppl 27):S110–S114.

42. Ihle BU, Becker GJ, Whitworth JA, et al: The effect of protein restriction on the progression of renal insufficiency. N Engl J Med 1989;321:1773–1777.

43. Rosman JB, Langer K, Brandl M, et al: Protein-restricted diets in chronic renal failure: A four year follow-up shows limited indications. Kidney Int 1989;27:S96–S102.

44. Locatelli F, Alberti D, Graziani G, et al: Prospective randomized, multicentre trial of effect of protein restriction on progression of chronic renal insufficiency. North Italian Cooperative Study Group. Lancet 1991;337:1299–1304.

45. Williams PS, Stevens ME, Fass G, et al: Failure of dietary protein and phosphate restriction to retard the rate of progression of chronic renal failure: A prospective, randomized, controlled trial. Q J Med 1991;81:837–855.

46. D'Amico G, Gentile MG, Fellin G, et al: Effect of dietary protein restriction on the progression of renal failure: A prospective randomized trial. Nephrol Dial Transplant 1994;9:1590–1594.

Iron and Erythropoietin-related Therapies

Ashraf I. Mikhail and Iain C. Macdougall

- Iron deficiency
- Serum ferritin
- Transferrin saturation
- Transferrin receptor
- Erythrocyte zinc protoporphyrin
- Hypochromic red cells

Iron therapy
- Oral iron
- Intravenous iron
- Monitoring intravenous iron therapy
- Reactions to intravenous iron
- Long-term toxicity

Erythropoietin therapy
- Novel erythropoiesis-stimulating protein
- Adverse effects of erythropoietin therapy
- Hyporesponsiveness to erythropoietin therapy
- Future strategies in the treatment of renal anemia

Anemia is present in the majority of patients with reduced renal function. The primary cause is insufficient production of erythropoietin. Additional factors that contribute to the pathogenesis of anemia in endstage renal disease (ESRD) are summarized in Table 71.1. If untreated, the anemia of ESRD is associated with reduced quality of life, limited opportunities for rehabilitation, and decreased survival (Table 71.2).

Iron deficiency

Iron deficiency is common in ESRD patients (Table 71.3). Erythropoietin therapy increases erythropoiesis and,

therefore, iron requirements. Normal body iron stores are 800–1200 mg.[1]

Serum ferritin

Ferritin is a metalloprotein that stores any iron in excess of needs. It is composed of a spherical protein shell enclosing a core of ferric oxide. Much of the body's iron is stored as ferritin in cells of the reticuloendothelial system. Serum ferritin levels, which correspond to total body iron stores, are normally 15–300 μg/L. Low serum ferritin (< 12 μg/L) is diagnostic of iron deficiency. The ferritin-to-storage iron ratio decreases with increasing iron load. At total iron stores below 500 mg, the average ratio is 15 mg storage iron per μg/L of ferritin. In patients with iron overload in whom the total storage iron level could be as high as 25 g, the ratio could be as low as 6 mg iron per 1 μg/L of ferritin.

Transferrin saturation

Transferrin saturation (TSAT) represents the percentage ratio of serum iron to total iron binding capacity. It is an indicator of the amount of iron that is readily available for erythropoiesis. A TSAT of 50% indicates that 50% of transferrin binding sites for iron transport are occupied by iron.

In chronic renal failure (CRF), TSAT levels < 20% are suggestive of iron deficiency. Functional iron deficiency results when a greater amount of iron is needed to support erythropoiesis than can be released from iron stores. In this condition TSAT decreases to levels consistent with iron deficiency despite a normal serum ferritin level.[2]

Table 71.1 Causes of anemia in patients with impaired renal function

Erythropoietin deficiency

Iron deficiency
  Repeated blood sampling
  Blood loss during dialysis
  Gastrointestinal bleeding
  Diminished oral intake (anorexia; diminished absorption)
Hyperparathyroidism
Inflammation or infection
Underdialysis
Aluminum toxicity
Vitamin B_{12} or folate deficiency
Shortened red-cell survival
Carnitine deficiency

Table 71.2 Effect of anemia on different physiological functions

General
  Fatigue
  Diminished exercise tolerance
  Drowsiness
Cardiovascular system
  Increased cardiac output
  Cardiac enlargement
  Left ventricular hypertrophy
  Angina
  Congestive heart failure
Endocrine system
  Altered menstrual cycles
  Reduced potency
Immune system
  Impaired immune responsiveness

Table 71.3 Tests used to evaluate iron status in patients with renal impairment

Test	Applications	Limitations
Ferritin	Low level is diagnostic of iron deficiency Extremely high level is diagnostic of iron overload	Acute-phase protein; high levels reflect infection or inflammation Reflects storage iron pool; not useful to detect functional iron deficiency
Transferrin saturation	Level below 20% suggests iron deficiency Level is usually low in functional iron deficiency	Low levels can be present in iron-replete persons High levels do not exclude functional iron deficiency Enormous diurnal variation due to variability of serum iron levels
Soluble transferrin receptor	Useful in detecting iron deficiency in patients with inflammatory conditions Low level may predict a good response to erythropoietin therapy	Expensive Serum level shows diurnal variation Not a useful marker of iron deficiency in patients receiving erythropoietin therapy Level does not drop below normal range until body iron stores are exhausted
Erythrocyte zinc protoporphyrin	High levels suggest iron deficiency Simple, inexpensive Requires small amount of blood (20 μl)	Long half-life: not ideal parameter to monitor response to parenteral iron supplementation Levels are elevated in uremia or inflammation
Hypochromic red cells	Useful in detecting functional iron deficiency Useful for monitoring the response to intravenous iron supplementation	Expensive: needs a special automated blood count analyzer False-negative results may be seen in patients not receiving erythropoietin Cannot reliably differentiate between absolute and functional iron deficiency

Transferrin receptor

Transferrin receptors are found on all cell membranes; they incorporate iron-bound transferrin into the cell. In conditions of iron deficiency, there is up-regulation of transferrin receptors to allow the cell to compete for maximum iron uptake. Soluble transferrin receptor (sTRF-R) is detectable in the peripheral blood. It is a truncated fragment of the receptor that lacks the cytoplasmic and transmembrane domains.

Estimation of sTRF-R can distinguish between iron deficiency anemia and the anemia of chronic disease. High sTRF-R is characteristic of iron deficiency while it remains unaffected in patients with chronic disease.[3] In anemia of chronic disease patients with CRF, sTRF-R can predict the response to erythropoietin therapy; the best response is achieved in patients with a low sTRF-R.[4]

Erythrocyte zinc protoporphyrin

Normally, ferrous iron is chelated to protoporphyrin IX to form heme. This reaction is catalyzed by ferrochelatase. In conditions of iron deficiency, the same enzyme chelates zinc to form zinc protoporphyrin.

Levels of zinc protoporphyrin of more than 90 μmol/mol heme indicate iron deficiency, although levels as low as 50 μmol per mole of heme can be seen in patients who respond adequately to iron therapy.

Levels of zinc protoporphyrin can be elevated in patients with CRF compared to the normal population. This could be due to interference with the assay in these patients. A high level in all CRF patients makes it unlikely that the test can identify patients who require iron supplementation during erythropoietin therapy.[5]

Hypochromic red cells

In patients with functional iron deficiency, iron deficient erythropoiesis occurs in the presence of normal body iron stores. Such patients have normal (or even elevated) serum ferritin levels. By measuring the percentage of hypochromic erythrocytes (defined as red blood cells with a hemoglobin concentration < 28 g/dL), it is possible to estimate bone marrow iron availability. When iron deficiency develops with erythropoietin therapy, the earliest change in indices is an increase in the percentage of hypochromic red cells.[6] Because of low erythropoiesis turnover in patients with CRF, red cell hypochromia may be normal in patients not receiving erythropoietin therapy. In the small subpopulation of patients who show hypochromia before commencing treatment, parenteral iron therapy usually leads to a rise in hemoglobin and improvement of hematological parameters.

Iron therapy

Oral iron

Several iron preparations are available (Table 71.4); all are simple and cheap. The most widely used is ferrous sulfate, which provides 65 mg of elemental iron per 200-mg tablet.

Several studies recommended primary oral iron therapy in peritoneal dialysis patients because it is more practical.[7,8] However, others have shown that in CAPD patients receiving oral iron therapy, there can be a progressive decline in serum ferritin levels once erythropoietin therapy is instituted, which necessitates switching to parenteral iron therapy.[9,10] Indeed, this form of therapy may be adequate only for patients not receiving erythropoietin.

For hemodialysis patients, intravenous iron supplementation should be used because the demands for iron frequently exceed the maximum quantity that can be supplied orally. For oral iron therapy to be effective, certain criteria should be fulfilled: at least 200 mg of elemental iron should be administered per day (usually two to three doses are required). Secondly, the tablets should be administered between meals to maximise absorption. Finally, enteric-coated formulation should *not* be used as most of the iron absorption occurs in the duodenum.

Gastrointestinal intolerance to oral iron is common (in about 20% of people) and dose-related. Intestinal absorption of iron is also severely impaired if functional iron deficiency develops in patients receiving erythropoietin when serum ferritin remains within the normal range.[11]

Intravenous iron

All intravenous iron preparations have in common a dense central core of ferric hydroxide, enveloped by a carbohydrate shell. After intravenous injection, the molecule is removed from the plasma by macrophages, and the iron is released where it binds to transferrin in plasma. There are four different iron preparations available for intravenous use (iron dextran, iron dextrin, iron sucrose, and iron sodium gluconate). They vary in molecular size, bioavailability, degradation kinetics, and side-effect profiles. The smaller the complex, the more rapidly the iron is released to bind to transferrin and to supply the bone marrow. After intravenous injection of low-molecular-weight complexes such as iron sodium gluconate, iron may be released too rapidly, thereby overloading the ability of transferrin to bind it, and leading to free iron reactions (see Reactions to intravenous iron, below). Thus, low doses of this preparation must be used (maximum 125 mg) compared, for example, with large complexes such as iron dextran where larger doses (1000 mg) can be administered safely.

There are four main indications to use parenteral iron in ESRD patients (Table 71.5). The aggressive use of intravenous iron is now known to enhance the response to erythropoietin therapy, even in patients who are iron-replete. A second advantage of this policy is a significant reduction in erythropoietin requirements (Table 71.6) because iron supply to developing red-cell precursors is a rate-limiting step for erythropoiesis. This can be overcome by supplying iron in a readily available form intravenously.

There are several ways of administering intravenous iron, either as a bolus or as an infusion (Table 71.7). For hemodialysis patients, low doses of iron (20–60 mg) can be administered with every dialysis session. Larger doses (100 mg) can be given weekly or monthly. Once optimal hemoglobin concentrations and iron stores are achieved, the required maintenance dose of parenteral iron for most patients ranges between 25 and 100 mg/week. For

Table 71.4 Available oral iron preparations

	Tablet size	Elemental iron
Ferrous sulfate	300 mg	65 mg
Ferrous fumarate	325 mg	108 mg
Ferrous gluconate	300 mg	35 mg
Ferrous succinate	100 mg	35 mg
Iron polysaccharide	10 mg/5 ml	?
Sodium iron edetate	190 mg/5 ml	27.5 mg

Table 71.5 Indications for parenteral iron therapy

Indication	Criteria
1. Iron deficiency	Serum ferritin < 100 µg/L Transferrin saturation < 20% Hypochromic red cells >10%
2. Preparation for erythropoietin therapy	Serum ferritin ≥ 100 µg/L
3. Functional iron deficiency	Serum ferritin ≥ 100 µg/L Transferrin saturation < 20% Hypochromic red cells > 10%
4. Adjuvant therapy to erythropoietin	See text

Table 71.6 Studies of aggressive intravenous iron supplementation in patients receiving erythropoietin

Reference	No of patients	Iron preparation	Duration of follow-up (months)	Erythropoietin dose reduction (%)
SunderPlassmann & Horl[12]	64	Sucrose	6	70
Fishbane et al[13]	52	Dextran	4	46
Macdougall et al[14]	37	Dextran	6	19
Silverberg et al[15]	41	Sucrose	6	61
Sepandj et al[16]	50	Dextran	6	35
Taylor et al[17]	46	Gluconate	6	33
Ahsan et al[18]	7	Dextran	12	26
Macdougall et al[19]	115	Sucrose	12	32
Besarab et al[20]	23	Dextran	6	40
Richardson et al[21]	386	Sucrose	24	30

Table 71.7 Regimens for administering intravenous iron[*]

Low dose	20–60 mg every dialysis session	Suitable for hemodialysis patients Any iron preparation can be used May be given as an intravenous "push"
Medium dose	100–400 mg	Usually intravenous infusions (100 mg may be given as a bolus injection) All iron preparations (maximum dose of iron gluconate 62.5–125 mg) Suitable for predialysis and patients on continuous ambulatory peritoneal dialysis
High dose	500–1000 mg	Must be given by intravenous infusion Only iron dextran or iron sucrose can be given at this dose Suitable for patients with large iron deficits

Adapted from Macdougall.[23]

predialysis and continuous ambulatory peritoneal dialysis (CAPD) patients, large intravenous iron doses can be given as infusions and repeated as needed.[22]

Monitoring intravenous iron therapy

Patients receiving intravenous iron should be monitored for signs of iron overload. Serum ferritin and TSAT should be measured 1 week after intravenous iron for small doses (< 200 mg) and at least two weeks after intravenous iron for large doses. It is recommended that intravenous iron therapy should be stopped whenever TSAT exceeds 50%, serum ferritin is ≥ 800 µg/L or whenever abnormal liver function tests develop. When serum ferritin has declined to < 800 µg/L (or TSAT to < 50%), parenteral iron can be resumed at a dose reduced by 30%–50%. Intravenous iron should also be stopped during any period of sepsis.

Reactions to intravenous iron

Two types of reaction are recognised. The first is IgE-mediated anaphylaxis, which is reported in 0.7% of people treated with iron dextran and is mediated by preformed dextran antibodies.[24] Anaphylactoid reactions (wheezing, myalgia, arthralgia, back pain, nausea, vomiting, and hypotension) are histamine mediated. They are caused by a transient overload of the transferrin molecule, resulting in release of free iron into the circulation.[25]

Long-term toxicity

It has been suggested that increased total body iron may increase the risk of cardiovascular disease[26] and cancer.[27] The relevance of these studies in ESRD patients has not been established.

Erythropoietin therapy

The introduction of erythropoietin has been critical to improving clinical management in patients with renal impairment. It is an essential in the management of anemia affecting the majority of hemodialysis patients, and a significant number of predialysis, CAPD, and renal transplant patients. Effective treatment of anemia with erythropoietin improves survival, decreases morbidity,[28] and improves quality of life.[29]

Subcutaneous administration of erythropoietin has a more favorable pharmacodynamic profile than intravenous administration (Table 71.8). When patients are switched from the intravenous to the subcutaneous route, hemoglobin is maintained with a 30% reduction in total weekly erythropoietin dose.[30] Thus, the erythropoietic response to a particular dose is greater with subcutaneous than with intravenous administration. The guidelines for erythropoietin therapy are summarised in Tables 71.9 and 71.10.

Novel erythropoiesis-stimulating protein

Novel erythropoiesis-stimulating protein (NESP) stimulates erythropoiesis by the same mechanism as erythropoietin. In contrast to erythropoietin (which contains three N-linked carbohydrate chains), NESP contains five N-linked carbohydrate chains, which allow it to be more stable in vivo with a two- to three-fold longer elimination half-life (Table 71.11).

Adverse effects of erythropoietin therapy

Adverse effects of erythropoietin therapy are listed in Table 71.12.

Hypertension, or an increase in antihypertensive therapy requirements, is found in 20–25% of patients receiving erythropoietin. This may be due to an increase in vascular endothelial reactivity, together with an increase in blood viscosity associated with an increase in red cell mass.

This hypertensive effect is exclusive to renal patients and is not observed in anemic patients without renal disease who are treated with erythropoietin.[32] Hypertensive encephalopathy mandates withholding erythropoietin therapy. Otherwise, antihypertensive therapy should be intensified when patients develop any rise in blood pressure.

Convulsions can occur secondary to hypertensive encephalopathy. Otherwise, erythropoietin therapy does not increase the risk of seizures when appropriate dosage recommendations are followed – even in those with a prior history of seizures.

There is equivocal evidence that erythropoietin therapy increases the risk of thrombosis in both native fistulae and

Table 71.8 Subcutaneous erythropoietin versus intravenous

	Subcutaneous	Intravenous
Half life	22–30 h	4–8 h
Bioavailability	20–34% of intravenous dose	
Dosage requirement	65–70% of intravenous dose	130–150% of subcutaneous dose per week
Frequency of administration	One to three times per week	Three times per week

Table 71.9 Initiation of erythropoietin therapy[31]

Subcutaneous route is preferable*
Encourage patients to self-administer the drug
Educate hemodialysis patients on the advantage of subcutaneous administration
Starting dose is 50–150 IU/kg/week, divided into two or three doses
For patients requiring intravenous administration the starting dose is 150–200 IU/kg/week
Higher starting doses may be needed in patients with severe anemia (hemaglobin < 8g/dL)
A single weekly injection can be used in patients receiving a small dose
A needle with the smallest possible gauge (29 G) should be used
Rotate injection sites (abdominal wall, thigh, arm)

*EPrex® is no longer licensed for subcutaneous administration.

Table 71.10 Titration of erythropoietin dosage[31]

Hb and reticulocyte count should be measured every 1–2 weeks after initiation of erythropoietin therapy or dose adjustment
Increase the weekly dose by 50% if Hb rise is < 2% of pretreatment Hb per month
After achieving target Hb
   Decrease the weekly dose by 25–30% if Hb exceeds the target level
   Decrease the weekly dose by 25–30% if the rate of Hb rise is > 2 g/dL/month

Hb, hemoglobin.

Table 71.11 Therapy guidelines for novel erythropoiesis-stimulating protein (NESP)

Starting dose 0.45 µg/kg per week or every other week
Patients receiving erythropoietin two or three times per week can be changed to NESP once weekly
Patients receiving erythropoietin once weekly can be changed to NESP once every other week
Increase the dose by 25% if the increase in Hb concentration is < 1 g/dL over a 4-week period
Decrease the dose by 25–50% if the increase in Hb concentration is > 2 g/dL over a 4-week period
Patients who are unable to tolerate subcutaneous NESP can be switched to the intravenous route using the
   same dosage without any reduction in therapeutic efficiency

Table 71.12 Possible side-effects of erythropoietin therapy

Skin irritation at injection site
Hypertension
? Convulsions and/or encephalopathy
Vascular acess thrombosis
Alopecia
Pure red cell aplasia
Myalgia and/or flu-like syndrome
? Hyperkalemia

Pure red cell aplasia develops in 1:10 000 patients treated with erythropoietin. It should be suspected whenever the patient's anemia becomes refractory to treatment (after exclusion of all other causes of hyporesponsiveness to treatment (Fig. 71.1). Bone marrow examination and the detection of antierythropoietin antibodies in serum confirms the diagnosis when erythropoietin therapy should be stopped. Other erythropoiesis-stimulating agents are equally ineffective and can exacerbate bone marrow suppression.

polytetrafluoroethylene (PTFE) grafts when patients are treated to normalize their hemoglobin.[33] However, the same study did not show any correlation between the dose of erythropoietin or hemoglobin level achieved, and the occurrence of vascular access thrombosis.

Hyporesponsiveness to erythropoietin therapy

This is defined as a failure to achieve and/or maintain the target hemoglobin levels at an erythropoietin dose of

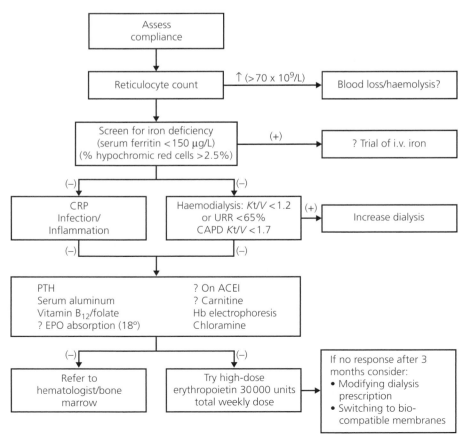

Figure 71.1 Algorithm for the management of poor responder patients to erythropoiesis-stimulating agents (ACEI, angiotensin-converting enzyme inhibitor; CAPD, continuous ambulatory peritoneal diaylsis; CRP, C-reactive protein; Dx, dialysis dose; EPO, erythropoietin; Hb, hemoglobin; HD, hemodialysis; PTH, parathyroid hormone; URR, urea reduction ratio). 18 h: check serum erythropoietin level 18 h post injection.

Table 71.13 Causes of inadequate response to erythropoietin

Chronic blood loss
Hemolysis
Hyperparathyroidism
Underdialysis
Iron deficiency
Folate, vitamin B_{12} deficiency
Aluminum toxicity
Malnutrition
Hemoglobinopathy
Autoimmune disease (e.g. systemic lupus erythematosus)
Malignancy (e.g. myeloma)
Infection
Uremic microinflammation
Angiotensin-converting enzyme inhibitor therapy
Primary bone-marrow disorder (e.g. myelodysplastic syndrome)
Antierythropoietin antibodies

450 IU/kg/week when administered intravenously, or 300 IU/kg/week when administered subcutaneously.[31] There are many different causes (Table 71.13), the commonest being iron deficiency. Concurrent infection and inflammation can impair the response to erythropoietin via the production of proinflammatory cytokines, which inhibit erythropoiesis. Parathyroidectomy can improve anemia in CRF patients with hyperparathyroidism.[34] In those receiving erythropoietin therapy, correction of hyperparathyroidism is often associated with a reduction in the total dose requirements of erythropoietin. Increasing dialysis adequacy, hemodiafiltration, water treatment, and the use of biocompatible hemodialysis membranes are all possible tools to improve erythropoietin responsiveness in dialysis patients (Fig. 71.1).

Future strategies in the treatment of renal anemia

Other erythropoietic substances are under development. The erythropoietic-mimetic peptides bind to the erythropoietin receptor and activate, causing identical intracellular signalling mechanisms to that of erythropoietin itself. The HCP inhibitors [Hematopoietic Cell Phosphatase] block the intracellular pathway that inhibits erythropoiesis. Fusing two intact erythropoietin molecules with a small peptide bridge produces an erythropoietin fusion protein with enhanced biological activity. Although short-term studies have shown erythropoietin gene therapy to be effective in animals, there are concerns over its safety and efficacy for use in people.

References

1. Council on Food and Nutrition, Committee on Iron Deficiency: Iron Deficiency in the United States. J Amer Med Assoc 1968;203:119–124.
2. Kaltwasser JP, Gottschalk R: Erythropoietin and iron. Kidney Int 1999;69:S49–S56.
3. Pettersson T, Kivivuori SM, Siimes MA: Is serum transferrin receptor useful for detecting iron-deficiency in anaemic patients with chronic inflammatory diseases? Br J Rheumatol 1994;33:740–744.
4. Beguin Y, Loo M, R'Zik S, et al: Early prediction of response to recombinant human erythropoietin in patients with the anemia of renal failure by serum transferrin receptor and fibrinogen. Blood 1993;82:2010–2016.
5. Braun J: Erythrocyte zinc protoporphyrin. Kidney Int 1999;69:S57–S60.
6. Schaefer RM, Schaefer L: The hypochromic red cell: a new parameter for monitoring of iron supplementation during r-huEPO therapy. J Perinat Med 1995;23:83–88.
7. Fishbane S, Maesaka JK: Iron management in end-stage renal disease. Am J Kidney Dis 1997;29:319–333.
8. Horl WH, Cavill I, Macdougall IC, et al: How to diagnose and correct iron deficiency during r-huEPO therapy – a consensus report. Nephrol Dial Transplant 1996;11:246–250.
9. Macdougall IC, Hutton RD, Cavill I, et al: Poor response to treatment of renal anaemia with erythropoietin corrected by iron given intravenously. BMJ 1989;299:157–158.
10. Wingard RL, Parker RA, Ismail N, et al:Efficacy of oral iron therapy in patients receiving recombinant human erythropoietin. Am J Kidney Dis 1995;25: 433–439.
11. Kooistra MP, Niemantsverdriet EC, van Es A, et al: Iron absorption in erythropoietin-treated haemodialysis patients: effects of iron availability, inflammation and aluminium. Nephrol Dial Transplant 1998;13:82–88.
12. SunderPlassmann G, Horl WH: Importance of iron supply for erythropoietin therapy. Nephrol Dial Transplant 1995;10:2070–2076.
13. Fishbane S, Frei GL, Maesaka J: Reduction in recombinant human erythropoietin doses by the use of chronic intravenous iron supplementation. Am J Kidney Dis 1995;26:41–46.
14. Macdougall IC, Tucker B, Thompson J, et al: A randomized controlled study of iron supplementation in patients treated with erythropoietin. Kidney Int 1996;50:1694–1699.
15. Silverberg DS, Blum M, Peer G, et al: Intravenous ferric saccharate as an iron supplement in dialysis patients. Nephron 1996;72:413–417.
16. Sepandj F, Jindal K, West M, et al: Economic appraisal of maintenance parenteral iron administration in treatment of anaemia in chronic haemodialysis patients. Nephrol Dial Transplant 1996;11:319–322.
17. Taylor JE, Peat N, Porter C, et al: Regular low-dose intravenous iron therapy improves response to erythropoietin in haemodialysis patients. Nephrol Dial Transplant 1996;11:1079–1083.
18. Ahsan N, Groff JA, Waybill MA: Efficacy of bolus intravenous iron dextran treatment in peritoneal dialysis patients receiving recombinant human erythropoietin. Adv Perit Dial 1996;12:161–166.
19. Macdougall IC, Chandler G, Elston O, et al: Beneficial effects of adopting an aggressive intravenous iron policy in a hemodialysis unit. Am J Kidney Dis 1999;34(Suppl 2):S40–S46.
20. Besarab A, Amin N, Ahsan M, et al: Optimization of epoetin therapy with intravenous iron therapy in hemodialysis patients. J Am Soc Nephrol 2000;11:530–538.
21. Richardson D, Bartlett C, Will EJ: Optimizing erythropoietin therapy in hemodialysis patients. Am J Kidney Dis 2001;38:109–117.
22. SunderPlassmann G, Horl WH: Erythropoietin and iron. Clin Nephrol 1997;47:141–157.
23. Macdougall IC: Strategies for iron supplementation: oral versus intravenous. Kidney Int Suppl 1999;69:S61–S66.
24. Fishbane S, Ungureanu VD, Maesaka JK, et al: The safety of intravenous iron dextran in hemodialysis patients. Am J Kidney Dis 1996;28:529–534.
25. Zanen AL, Adriaansen HJ, van Bommel EF, et al: 'Oversaturation' of transferrin after intravenous ferric gluconate (Ferrlecit) in haemodialysis patients. Nephrol Dial Transplant 1996;11:820–824.
26. Sullivan JL: Iron and the sex difference in heart disease risk. Lancet 198113;1(8233):1293–1294.
27. Weinberg ED: The role of iron in cancer. Eur J Cancer Prev 1996;5:19–36.
28. Eschbach JW, Abdulhadi MH, Browne JK, et al: Recombinant human erythropoietin in anemic patients with end-stage renal disease. Results of a phase III multicenter clinical trial. Ann Intern Med 1989;111:992–1000.

29. Grutzmacher P, Scheuermann E, Low I, et al: Correction of renal anaemia by recombinant human erythropoietin: effects on myocardial function. Contrib Nephrol 1988;66:176–184.

30. Bommer J, Barth HP, Zeier M, et al: Efficacy comparison of intravenous and subcutaneous recombinant human erythropoietin administration in hemodialysis patients. Contrib Nephrol 1991;88:136–143.

31. NKF-DOQI: Clinical practice guidelines for the treatment of anemia of chronic renal failure, National Kidney Foundation, Dialysis Outcomes Quality Initiative. Am J Kidney Dis 1997;30(Suppl 3):S192–S240.

32. Abels RI: Use of recombinant human erythropoietin in the treatment of anemia in patients who have cancer. Semin Oncol 1992;19(Suppl 8):29–35.

33. Besarab A, Bolton WK, Browne JK, et al: The effects of normal as compared with low hematocrit values in patients with cardiac disease who are receiving hemodialysis and epoetin. N Engl J Med 1998;339:584–590.

34. Mandolfo S, Malberti F, Farina M, et al: Parathyroidectomy and response to erythropoietin therapy in anaemic patients with chronic renal failure. Nephrol Dial Transplant 1998;13:2708–2709.

Anemia and Coagulopathy

Giuseppe Remuzzi, Arrigo Schieppati, and Luigi Minetti

Anemia

The correction of anemia by recombinant human erythropoietin (r-HuEpo) has shown that erythropoietin deficiency is the primary underlying defect in anemia of renal failure.[1] Erythropoiesis largely depends on the production of erythropoietin by the kidney, and in the progression to renal failure the hemoglobin (Hb) concentration has roughly the same clinical significance as the creatinine concentration. Prior to the introduction of r-HuEpo, about a quarter of chronic uremic patients were blood transfusion dependent. It has now become apparent that many symptoms previously attributed to uremia are in fact due to anemia. The most common cause of death among dialysis patients is cardiovascular disease, and anemia significantly contributes to the development of heart failure in chronic uremia.

Pathophysiology of anemia

The maintenance of red cell mass, and its adaptation to changes in oxygen need, is accomplished by erythropoietin, which acts as the mediator between the sensing mechanism for available oxygen, the regulation of erythropoietin production, and the erythroid marrow. Both the oxygen sensor and the site of synthesis of erythropoietin (peritubular capillary endothelial cells) are in the renal cortex.

Human erythropoietin was purified in 1977, and its molecular structure was characterized in 1986. It is a sialylglycoprotein composed of 165 amino acids. Its plasma level normally ranges between 15 and 25 mU/mL but may rise 100-fold in anemia. In chronic renal failure, erythropoietin production is much diminished, but the erythropoietin–hemoglobin feedback still operates, though at a lower setpoint. Erythropoietin is detectable in circulating blood after bilateral nephrectomy, consistent with experimental findings that about 10% is produced by the liver.

In autosomal dominant polycystic disease, anemia is less severe and serum erythropoietin is higher than is usually accounted for by increased serum creatinine concentrations, as if cystic kidneys retained better production of erythropoietin in spite of renal failure. When acquired polycystic kidney disease develops in hemodialysis patients there may be a significant spontaneous improvement in anemia. Cells containing mRNA for erythropoietin have been found in the walls of the cysts.

Anemia of renal failure is hypoproliferative, normochromic and normocytic, with a low reticulocyte count; however, a hemolytic component of varying importance is always associated with the decreased erythropoiesis. Red cell half-life is reduced to about a half to two-thirds of normal, but the defect is not intrinsic to the red cell, and could be due to uremic toxins.

Therapy for anemia
Dialysis

Renal anemia may improve once dialysis is started, and the improvement persists even at lower or unchanged serum erythropoietin levels, suggesting a role for circulating uremic toxins. Thus, both spontaneous and r-HuEpo-stimulated erythropoiesis[2] are improved by efficient dialysis. Apart from the specific effect of a better removal of toxins, dialysis relieves anemia by improving red cell survival, blood coagulation, nutritional status, and well-being.

Recombinant human erythropoietin (r-HuEpo)

The human gene for erythropoietin was cloned and expressed in 1984, and by the end of 1986 the efficacy of r-HuEpo in reversing the anemia of uremia was established. Large clinical trials were completed in USA and Europe so that less than 2 years later r-HuEpo was available for clinical use.

r-HuEpo contains the identical 165 amino-acid sequence of isolated natural erythropoietin. There are two forms of r-HuEpo – epoietin-α and epoietin-β – produced by genomic DNA (gDNA) and complementary DNA (cDNA) respectively. They differ in their oligosaccharidic component. Experimental and clinical findings suggest that their pharmacologic activity and all other biological effects are similar, though no direct comparison has been made. Epoietin-α has a mean half-life of 4–13 h after intravenous administration and around 24 h after subcutaneous injection. By the subcutaneous route, peaks are reached at 8–12 h and decline slowly thereafter; maximum levels are only about 10% of those achieved after the same intravenous dose.

The kinetics of epoietin-β seem to be a little different from epoietin-α. Both preparations appear to be eliminated primarily by nonrenal routes.

Besides erythropoiesis r-HuEpo therapy brings red cell survival back to normal; it increases erythrocyte elasticity and deformability and the antioxidant enzymatic system of red cells. Very likely all these improvements are achieved via rejuvenation of red cells. Treatment with r-HuEpo aims for the following: to make blood transfusions unnecessary; to prevent the consequences of severe anemia; to gain better improved rehabilitation and quality of life (Table 72.1).

Target hemoglobin

Some investigators and the DOQI work group[3] have suggested that the target of r-HuEpo therapy should be relying on hemoglobin level rather than hematocrit value. However many physicians still refer to hematocrit in evaluating the response to r-HuEpo therapy, so both indices are reported.

Anemic patients on dialysis have a shorter survival. Increase of hematocrit levels above 32% is associated with improved survival.[4]

The benefit of increased hemoglobin is mostly evident when cardiovascular morbidity and mortality is considered. In a clinical study the incidence of fatal and nonfatal myocardial infarction was significantly lower in hemodialysis patients who reached and maintained a normal hematocrit than in patients with hematocrit of 30%.

Significant relief of symptoms with a low risk of side-effects has been observed after r-HuEpo therapy in hemodialysis patients when the hemoglobin level is set between 9.5 and 11 g/dL[1] (roughly equivalent to hematocrit 28.5 and 33% respectively). The risk of development or worsening of hypertension and vascular thrombotic events, such as vascular access clotting and extracorporeal circuit thrombosis, as well as the decrease of plasma volume which reduces the efficiency of dialysis, have for some time kept clinicians from aiming for higher target hemoglobin. However, improvements in cardiac function, physical work capacity, quality of life, cognitive function, and sexual function have been reported after aiming for higher targets (11.5–13 g/dL).

The benefits and risks of complete correction of anemia and the optimal target hemoglobin have not yet been established. A study on more than 1200 hemodialysis patients with significant cardiac disease was discontinued June 1996 because of higher mortality in the group targeted toward a hematocrit of 42%, although the difference with the control group did not reach statistical significance. It is unclear why higher hematocrit was associated with enhanced mortality rate, and high hematocrit may not be the only explanation. However at the present it is not recommended to achieve the goal of hematocrit of 42% in hemodialysis patients with congestive heart failure.

In conclusion, according to investigators and current practice guidelines, elaborated in Europe[5] and the United States,[6] the target hemoglobin level should be greater than 11 g/dL. The upper limit for hemoglobin concentration has not been suggested by any of the available guidelines.

Dosage

The starting dose of r-HuEpo for most patients should be 50–150 IU/kg/week in two or three doses (typically 4000–8000 IU/week). Doses exceeding 300 IU/kg usually do not elicit further erythropoietic response.

Starting doses of 100 IU/kg three times a week by intravenous injection usually increase hemoglobin levels in 90% of patients. With this regimen hemoglobin usually increases by 1.5–2 g/dL in 4 weeks. Higher starting doses are employed when a faster rise is needed; however, a rise of more than 3 g/dL in 4 weeks should be avoided because of the possible exacerbation of hypertension.

Table 72.1 Treatment with recombinant human erythropoietin (r-HuEpo)

Route of administration	Intravenous for hemodialysis patients Subcutaneous for predialysis, hemodialysis, and CAPD patients
Optimal regimen	Thrice a week
Target hemoglobin	10–12 g/dL. Ht 30–36%
Starting dose	50–100 IU/kg i.v. thrice weekly or 30–60 IU/kg s.c. thrice weekly
Dose change	20–25 IU/kg thrice weekly
Interval to dose change	4-week for i.v. administration 6-week for s.c. administration
Optimal rate of rise in hemoglobin	2 g/dL or less every fourth week
Maintenance dose	Individually titrated

CAPD, continuous ambulatory peritoneal dialysis.

Several algorithms have been proposed to titrate r-HuEpo dose during the initial phase and for the maintenance of target hemoglobin levels, but none has been validated in a prospective fashion. Hemoglobin and hematocrit should be monitored every 1–2 weeks in the initial phase until target hemoglobin is reached, then every 2–4 weeks.

If the increase of hematocrit is less than 2% in 4 weeks, the r-HuEpo dose should be increased by 50%; if the rise of hematocrit is greater than 8%, the r-HuEpo should be decreased by 25%. It takes 4 weeks to fully assess the response to any change in dosage and any increase should not exceed 30 IU/kg three times per week each time.

When the target hemoglobin is about to be reached, the dosage should be reduced by about 25 IU/kg three times a week to avoid overshooting the target, and thereafter titrated down gradually.

By the subcutaneous route, the starting doses are lower, from 20–50 IU/kg three times a week. In a recent study on continuous ambulatory peritoneal dialysis (CAPD) patients the target hemoglobin was 10 g/dL. Therapy was started with subcutaneous doses of r-HuEpo 20 IU/kg three times a week and the dose increased by 20 IU/kg three times a week, every fourth week. The majority of patients reached the target hemoglobin within 6 months.[7]

In the maintenance phase, the minimal dosage of r-HuEpo needed to maintain target hemoglobin must be sought by adjusting the dose at intervals. The higher the target, the higher the maintenance dose: the median intravenous maintenance dose necessary to keep hemoglobin at about 12 g/dL is roughly 75 IU/kg three times a week, but the dispersion is wide as some patients need 25 IU/kg three times a week, and others more than 200 IU/kg three times a week. By the subcutaneous route, maintenance doses can be substantially lower; CAPD patients have been effectively managed with subcutaneous doses of r-HuEpo less than 40 IU/kg three times a week.

Frequency of dosing

The frequency of dosing depends on the route of administration.[1] Intravenous treatment must be given two or three times a week, while subcutaneous dosing can sometimes be given at larger intervals. For both routes, the thrice-weekly regimen is employed for the majority of patients, and twice weekly for a small part, while only a few patients find once a week is adequate.

Routes of administration

A number of studies have compared intravenous versus subcutaneous r-HuEpo administration in dialysis patients. Pooling together the results of these studies it could be concluded that on the average the dose of r-HuEpo needed to maintain a hematocrit of 33% was lower when administered subcutaneously than intravenously.

In a recent study,[8] subcutaneous administration was more cost-effective than intravenous injection. With the thrice-weekly dosage required to maintain the same target hemoglobin, 61% of the study patients could benefit from a lower weekly dose (from 18.5 to 26.5%) following the switch from intravenous to subcutaneous, while 39% required the same or higher doses. The maintenance dose for patients who received subcutaneous r-HuEpo diluted 1:2 with saline, to mitigate stinging at the injection site, was the same as the undiluted dose.[8] Besides some sparing effect, the subcutaneous route should also avoid the higher peaks of intravenous administration, with fewer side-effects.

For predialysis and peritoneal dialysis patients, subcutaneous administration should be always preferred, since it is easier to self-administer at home, and the arm veins are spared for possible future use as vascular access.

The intraperitoneal route has been tested in CAPD patients but is not cost-effective because absorption is poor (the bioavailability of intraperitoneally injected r-HuEpo is one-fifth to one-tenth of a subcutaneous dose).

Predialysis patients

Progression of renal insufficiency often goes in parallel with anemia. Low hemoglobin levels in the predialysis phase may have a determinant contributory role in left ventricular hypertrophy, which affects up to 75% of patients when dialysis is started.[9] Correction of anemia with r-HuEpo is associated with improved physical performance, although its efficacy in preventing cardiac disease has not yet been studied.

Concern that progression of renal disease could be accelerated by increasing hemoglobin with r-HuEpo therapy has been raised,[10] but no evidence of such an effect has been found in studies on people. In a study of 83 predialysis patients with anemia, randomly assigned to r-HuEpo treatment or a control group, anemia was corrected (hematocrit 36% or more) in 79% of the 43 treated patients and correlated with significant improvements in assessments of health-related quality of life.[11]

In conclusion r-HuEpo treatment in the predialysis phase is recommended, provided that high blood pressure is properly treated. Most studies have used subcutaneous r-HuEpo at doses of 50–60 IU/kg/week.[12] Iron deficiency should be corrected with oral iron to optimize the response.

Transplant patients

With immediate graft function, erythropoietin serum levels double within 7 days after transplantation from a mean baseline of about 18 mU/mL, and remain elevated until anemia is corrected (within 3 months). The majority of patients with adequate iron intake will develop iron deficiency by 6 months after transplantation and should receive iron supplementation.

The anemia in renal transplant recipients with chronic rejection can be effectively treated by r-HuEpo without significant effects on renal function.

Causes of inadequate response

More than 95% of patients will respond to r-HuEpo treatment, when iron stores are repleted, by attaining the target hemoglobin within 3–6 months after a prolonged correction phase and increments of dosage. When iron stores are adequate, the time to reach the target hemoglobin depends on the baseline hemoglobin concentration and the rate of hemoglobin increase. Inadequate response to r-HuEpo is defined as a failure to attain the target hemoglobin with maximum doses in the presence of adequate iron stores in 6 months. Maximum r-HuEpo doses are 300 U/kg/week subcutaneously and 450 U/kg/week intravenously.

Blunted response or lack of response may be due to a number of causes, the most common of which is iron deficiency. Other causes are: aluminum overload; underlying infectious, inflammatory or malignant diseases; gastrointestinal occult blood loss; underlying hematologic disease; severe hyperparathyroidism; folate or vitamin B_{12} deficiency; presence of circulating inhibitors of erythropoiesis; down-regulation of erythropoietin receptors on the surface of committed cells.

The iron deficiency may be primary to (preceding the r-HuEpo treatment) or secondary to consumption of iron deposits during the treatment. In the latter case, an initial good response then becomes subdued. Almost all patients become iron-deficient and require oral or parenteral iron replacement.[1,13] Iron stores can be assessed most accurately by staining the bone marrow for hemosiderin, but iron status must first be measured by serum iron ferritin and transferrin saturation. The protein ferritin is secreted into the plasma by the reticuloendothelial cells in response to the intracellular iron concentration, and is a good indicator of iron stores.[14] However, iron deficiency secondary to consumption of iron deposits by r-HuEpo-stimulated erythropoiesis may be concealed by apparently adequate ferritin levels, but disclosed by transferrin saturation less than 20%, and prompt erythropietic response to intravenous iron dextran.[13] During the correction phase serum iron fluctuates and transferrin iron is considered a superior marker of iron availability for heme synthesis.

The failure to supply enough iron despite oral iron supplementation and adequate iron stores as reflected by serum ferritin is called functional iron deficiency.[13] Mobilization of iron stores may be inadequate during rapid hemoglobin generation. The developing red cells will become hypochromic when insufficient iron is supplied to the erythron. Thus a quantitative assessment can be made of the amount of hemoglobin in newly released red cells by measuring the percentage of circulating red cells that are hypochromic; hypochromia is defined as a mean cell hemoglobin concentration (MCHC) less than 28 g/dL. More than 10% of hypochromic cells (normal range less than 2.5% of circulating red cells), in the absence of a hemoglobinopathy or inflammatory disease, should be diagnostic of functional iron deficiency.

Other more sophisticated tests for iron deficiency are the determination of serum transferrin receptor (STrR) concentrations and measurement of free erythrocytic protoporphyrin (FEP).[15] Serum transferrin receptor concentrations, measured with monoclonal antibodies, increase and correlate with the severity of iron store depletion, while serum ferritin is reaching its nadir. Free erythrocytic protoporphyrin levels measure the amount of protoporphyrin not incorporated into heme;[15] patients with a concentration of 90 μmol/mol heme, or more, were considered likely to be iron deficient. Free erythrocytic protoporphyrin and serum ferritin are similar as predictors of iron deficiency.[15]

Ascorbate supplementation may circumvent the resistance to r-HuEpo that is sometimes seen in iron-overloaded patients, particularly in the setting of functional iron deficiency.

In hemodialysis patients, aluminum overload may provoke microcytic anemia while iron deposits are normal. Aluminum and iron have common pathways for intestinal absorption, transport in the plasma, binding to transferrin, and uptake into the cell. Iron-depleted rats are more susceptible to aluminum accumulation.

In humans, aluminum overload may interfere with intestinal absorption of iron and its utilization in the erythropoietic response to r-HuEpo. In 11 hemodialysis patients, higher early levels of plasma aluminum were related to a smaller erythropoietic response to r-HuEpo and higher levels of protoporphyrin in red cells. Ferrochelatase activity and erythropoietic response were not correlated. This strengthens the suggestion that transferrin-bound aluminum may interfere with the insertion of iron into protoporphyrin to form heme.

Excess aluminum accumulation is becoming less common with increased use of deionizers and less use of aluminum-containing phosphate binders. Detection of aluminum in bone biopsies now has an incidence of less than 5%. Basal serum aluminum concentrations greater than 50 ng/mL and aluminum levels higher than 175 ng/mL after the deferoxamine (an aluminum-binding agent) challenge test (a single dose of 500–1000 mg intravenously) should indicate aluminum accumulation such as to interfere with the response to r-HuEpo. Chelation treatment with intravenous deferoxamine should improve aluminum-induced microcytic anemia and the form without microcytosis and, with questionable aluminum accumulation, it could also restore responsiveness to r-HuEpo.[16]

Erythropoiesis is negatively regulated by several macrophage-derived cytokines, including tumor necrosis factor α (TNFα), interleukin (IL) 1, IL-6, and tumor growth factor β (TGFβ), all of which are elevated in inflammatory processes. These cytokines have inhibitory effects on the erythroid progenitor cells that are targets for r-HuEpo. The cytokines may also impair iron metabolism by sequestering iron inside the macrophages. As a consequence the anemia observed with chronic infectious and inflammatory diseases has a low reticulocyte count for the degree of anemia, and may often be microcytic or hypochromic in spite of normal or raised serum ferritin.

Does this kind of anemia respond to r-HuEpo? There is now evidence that r-HuEpo overcomes the inhibition of erythropoiesis caused by inflammatory cytokines in chronic disease.[16] Unrecognized infection or subtle inflammation (possibly due to dialysis bioincompatibility) may contribute to the anemia of uremia. The association of chronic inflammatory disease with chronic renal failure constitutes a therapeutic challenge, as the anemia may be resistant to r-HuEpo at the usual dosage but may respond – at least partially – to high doses. Iron supplementation will be critical for erythropoietic response as the mobilization of iron deposits is hindered, and oral iron is unable to be enough for heme synthesis. In this kind of functional iron deficiency only intravenous iron will permit the erythropoietic response.

A clue to gastrointestinal occult blood loss is significant reticulocytosis in the absence of any rise in the hemoglobin concentration.[16] Hemodialysis patients with severe hyperparathyroidism need significantly more r-HuEpo. Vitamin B_{12}/folate deficiency is no longer considered a problem in r-HuEpo therapy. Some drugs too may influence erythropoiesis: for example angiotensin converting enzyme inhibitors can inhibit erythropoietin production, and adversely affect erythropoiesis.

Iron supplementation

Iron status should be monitored every month when r-HuEpo therapy is initiated and then every 2–3 months. Detection and correction of iron deficiency play a major role in the success of r-HuEpo. The total iron dose required can be calculated at any time by the hemoglobin iron deficit plus the amount needed to replenish iron stores. Ferritin levels lower than 100 ng/mL indicate iron deficiency (less than 50 or 30 ng/mL, absolute iron deficiency), and more than 600 ng/mL to reflect iron overload. With levels of more than 300 ng/mL, iron supplementation should, at least initially, be unnecessary.

During the correction phase the key factor is making iron available for heme synthesis, and the percentage of circulating hypochromic red cells is a better marker for assessing iron availability than transferrin saturation.[17] Iron supplementation should be aimed to keep serum ferritin higher than 100 ng/mL, transferrin saturation more than 20%, and hypochromic red cells less than 10%.[13]

In this phase the intravenous route is preferable (a loading dose of 100 mg iron dextran every dialysis session for 2–3 weeks, followed by 100 mg once a week or every 2 weeks) during the maintenance phase, and with a constant rate of erythropoiesis the assessment of iron stores is more reliable and gives a better basis for adjusting iron therapy.

A daily oral dose of about 200 mg of elemental iron (about one-sixth is absorbed) is appropriate in most patients.[11] Commercial oral iron preparations differ in their content of elemental iron, and a 325 mg tablet provides 107 mg ferrous fumarate, 65 mg ferrous sulfate, or 39 mg ferrous gluconate. In some patients the downward trend in ferritin in spite of oral iron supplementation indicates that intravenous iron dextran may be necessary. Iron dextran enhances the erythropoietic response even further, in spite of adequate iron stores and availability, and reduces r-HuEpo requirements by up to 47%.[13] New, well-tolerated, parenteral iron preparations (such as iron saccharate and iron gluconate) are leading to wider use of the intravenous route in the maintenance phase of r-HuEpo therapy, at different regimens: intermittent high doses (62.5–125 mg of ferric gluconate, once a week or every 2 weeks) or continuous low dose (10–20 mg per hemodialysis treatment).

Side-effects

The incidences (per patient-year) of some of the most frequently reported adverse events have been: hypertension (0.75); clotted vascular access (0.25); hyperkalemia (0.11); and seizures (0.048).

The relationship of seizures, not related to hypertension, and r-HuEpo therapy is questionable, since seizures are not infrequent in the untreated dialysis population (0.05–0.10). However, the rate of seizures appears to be higher during the first 90 days of r-HuEpo therapy than in the next 90 days. The incidence of seizures seems to be lower in epoietin-β patients than in those treated with epoietin-α. Strict control of the rate of hemoglobin rise (no more than 1.5 g/dL every 4 weeks) and close monitoring of blood pressure, appear warranted. (See Note added in proof.)

Hyperkalemia reflects less efficient dialysis (higher hematocrit means less plasma available for depuration) and poorer compliance with dietary prescriptions in patients experiencing improved well-being and quality of life.

The aggravation, or de novo appearance, of hypertension in patients during r-HuEpo therapy has been attributed to increased whole-blood viscosity, reversal of hypoxia-dependent peripheral vasodilatation, and activation of, or enhancement of vascular responsiveness to, vasoactive agents. Other mechanisms have been also suggested such as a functionally or structurally reduced cross-sectional area of the peripheral vascular bed, normalization of cardiac output, increase of red cell mass not perfectly balanced by a decrease of plasma volume.

Risk factors for the development or worsening of hypertension in dialysis patients include preexisting hypertension, rapid correction of anemia, high doses of r-HuEpo, whereas intravenous administration and 'nondipper' conditions are not. Increases in blood pressure are mostly reported during the first 90 days of therapy. In most cases, hypertension can be managed by reducing dry body weight, by starting or increasing antihypertensive therapy, and by reducing the dose of r-HuEpo. No patient should be excluded from r-HuEpo treatment because of increased risk of hypertension.

Future treatments of uremic anemia

Novel erythropoiesis stimulating protein (NESP) is a molecule that stimulates erythropoiesis by the same mechanisms as r-HuEpo.[18] Its chemical structure is such that the compound has an elimination half-life two or three times longer than r-HuEpo. Mean half-life of NESP (also called darbopoietin) is 49 h when given subcutaneously and 21 h for the intravenous route. This peculiar pharmacokinetic profile allows less frequent dosing. Clinical studies in more than 1500 patients have concluded that NESP is as effective and safe as r-HuEpo in correcting uremic anemia. The suggested initial dose of NESP is 0.45 µg/kg once a week either subcutaneously or intravenously. When the target hemoglobin level is reached, the maintenance dose of NESP is determined for the individual patient. To change from r-HuEpo to NESP, a rule of thumb is to divide the r-HuEpo dose by a factor of 200.

Recent data reported in an abstract showed that NESP maintained hemoglobin levels within the study target even when given once every 4 weeks.[19]

A new strategy that is being developed has targeted the erythropoietin receptor in search of a mimetic molecule. A family of peptides has been discovered and one member of the family, named erythropoietin mimetic peptide 1 (EMP1) is a promising new product.[20] This is a small compound with only 20 amino acids. Molecules of such small size might be delivered by inhalation or transdermally.

Coagulation disturbances of chronic renal failure

Uremic bleeding

An increased tendency to bleed has been known for centuries as a major feature of uremia. Ecchymoses, epistaxis, and gastrointestinal bleeding are most common; subdural hematoma occurs in 5–15% of people on hemodialysis, while hemopericardium and subcapsular hematoma of the liver are less frequent. Surgery or invasive procedures are always a risk for bleeding in uremic people.

Although the pathogenesis of uremic bleeding is multifactorial, platelet and endothelial dysfunction play major roles, while the platelet number is normal. Impaired platelet–platelet and platelet–vessel wall interactions result in a prolonged bleeding time, still the best predictor of clinical bleeding.[21] The evidence that several dialyzable 'toxins' (urea, creatinine, phenol, phenolic acids, or guanidinosuccinic acid) are involved in uremic platelet dysfunction is not compelling.

Quantitative and qualitative abnormalities of the von Willebrand factor (vWF) molecule, which promotes platelet adhesion and aggregation to subendothelial collagen, are also considered important in uremic bleeding. Interaction of vWF and platelet membrane glycoprotein GPIIb/IIIa is altered in uremia.[22]

Recent studies have emphasized the possibility that the bleeding tendency in uremia is a consequence of up-regulation of inducible nitric oxide(NO)-forming enzymes in the endothelium of systemic vessels, which reduces the platelets' capacity to interact with the vascular endothelial surface.

Platelet dysfunction is potentiated by the use of aspirin and other nonsteroidal anti-inflammatory drugs, which therefore should be employed with caution in uremic patients.

Other coagulation parameters are usually normal: partial thromboplastin time and prothrombin time are not altered in uremia.

Thrombosis of arteriovenous shunt

Paradoxically, uremic people may develop thromboembolism. The most frequent manifestation is vascular access thrombosis: about 0.5–0.8 episodes of fistula thrombosis occur per patient per year on hemodialysis.[23] The cause is still ill-defined: global coagulation screening tests showed a consistent increase of fibrinogen levels and decreased anticoagulant activity of protein C, but were otherwise normal. Alterations in the reactivity of platelets and leukocytes due to their continuous contact with artificial surfaces may also be relevant. About 75% of all cases of access thrombosis are associated with stenotic lesions in the venous system.

Raising the hematocrit with erythropoietin could further enhance the risk of clotting of dialyzers and vascular accesses. However a placebo-controlled study found that although it increased blood viscosity, erythropoietin did not enhance shunt thrombosis or heparin requirements.[24] In another study on 64 hemodialyzed patients with polytetrafluoroethylene (PTFE) grafts there were no significant differences in thrombectomies and mechanical problems per 1000 patient-days before and after erythropoietin.[25] Thus, erythropoietin (at low, medium, or high dosages) does not seem to promote graft thrombosis in uremics on hemodialysis.

Hypercoagulability in nephrotic patients

Nephrotic syndrome patients have a variety of hemostatic abnormalities that expose them to an enhanced risk of thromboembolism.[26] These include increased ability of platelets to aggregate, increased levels of coagulation cofactors (specifically V and VIII, vWf, factor VII, and fibrinogen) and reduced antithrombin III. In occasional patients, protein C and free protein S are also reduced. None of the above abnormalities however – except perhaps for reduced antithrombin III – are useful for defining individual patient risk for thromboembolic complications.

The main clinical manifestation of the hypercoagulability of nephrotics is renal vein thrombosis, which is particularly frequent in patients with membranous glomerulopathy. The literature indicates an average incidence of renal vein thrombosis in nephrotics of 35%, with individual studies reporting from 5–60%.[27] The incidence of thromboembolic complications other than renal vein thrombosis in nephrotic patients ranges from 10 to 40%. Most frequent clinical findings are pulmonary embolism and deep vein thrombosis of the extremities, but these patients may suffer thrombosis of the axillary and subclavian veins, and femoral, coronary, and mesenteric arteries.

Therapy in uremic bleeding

Dialysis

Hemodialysis shortens the prolonged bleeding time of uremics and partially corrects platelet and platelet–endothelial dysfunction. However, removal of uremic platelet toxins by hemodialysis is not enough to correct fully the hemostatic defects of uremia.[20]

Actually, the need for heparin administration to prevent clotting of the dialyzer speaks against the use of hemodialysis during active bleeding. It has been suggested that peritoneal dialysis is more effective than hemodialysis in removing uremic toxins, and studies on tests of platelet function show an improvement, but controlled studies about its clinical value are lacking. It has been suggested that peritoneal dialysis is more effective than hemodialysis in correcting platelet dysfunction, but again there is a lack of controlled studies. Several methods have been proposed to minimize blood loss during hemodialysis in bleeding patients, such as regional heparinization, low-molecular-weight heparins, prostacyclin, or no anticoagulation at all. The method of choice at our center (with satisfactory results) involves frequent flushes of saline through the dialyzer at intervals. This approach gave the best results when used in association with hemodiafiltration. This method is currently used after major surgery or trauma in hemodialysis patients.

Correction of anemia

Anemia is a major influence on the bleeding time and bleeding tendency of uremic people. A study on six uremic patients demonstrated for the first time that red cell transfusions shortened the bleeding time and controlled abnormal bleeding.[28] This was confirmed in a larger group of patients.[29] Relieving uremic anemia by erythropoietin also improved the hemostatic defects and normalized bleeding time[30] (Table 72.2). Therefore, correction of the anemia – either acutely by red blood cell transfusion or in the long term by the use of r-HuEpo – is currently a major part of the overall strategy for preventing and controlling abnormal bleeding in uremia.

Cryoprecipitate and desmopressin

Cryoprecipitate – which contains coagulation factor VIII, vWf, fibrinogen, and fibronectin – was used in uremics with very long bleeding times that did not improve with blood transfusions or hemodialysis or both.[31] In six uremic patients originally treated, the infusion of ten bags of cryoprecipitate was followed by normalization or significant shortening of the bleeding time, and allowed surgical procedures (in a few patients) without excessive blood loss. The effect, however, was delayed (nadir of bleeding time 4–6 h post infusion) and transient (lasting no longer than 24–36 h). Cryoprecipitate did not improve defects of platelet aggregation, whereas blood levels of factor VIII and vWf, which were normal or high before infusion, rose. The use of cryoprecipitate carries a small risk of transmitting viral diseases like hepatitis and AIDS.

Desmopressin, 1-deamino-8-D-arginine vasopressin (DDAVP), a synthetic derivative of antidiuretic hormone, was introduced in the late 1970s to control abnormal bleeding in patients with von Willebrand disease and mild hemophilia A.[32] DDAVP acts by increasing the release of vWf multimers from endothelial stores. DDAVP has been studied in uremics as a potentially safer alternative to cryoprecipitate. An open controlled trial showed that intravenous DDAVP at a dose of 0.4 µg/kg shortened the prolonged bleeding times of patients with chronic renal failure.[33]

This was confirmed in a randomized, placebo-controlled, double-blind crossover trial in 12 uremic people with a history of abnormal bleeding and prolonged bleeding times[34] infused intravenously with DDAVP, 0.3 µg/kg, added to 50 mL saline. Bleeding time was normalized in nine patients within 1 h of infusion, was less than 10 min at 2 h and 4 h, and had returned to baseline by 8 h (Table 72.2). While no significant changes were noted in platelet adhesion or aggregation, residual prothrombin, serum thromboxane B_2, or platelet cyclic AMP, levels of vWf in the blood increased above the already elevated baseline values.

Table 72.2 Therapeutic strategies for uremic bleeding

Treatment	Indication	Dosage	Effect		
			Start	Peak	End
Blood or RBC	Prophylaxis of bleeding in high-risk patients with anemia	According to the severity of anemia	PCV = 28–32 %		Related to RBC lifespan
Recombinant human erythropoietin	Prophylaxis of bleeding in high-risk patients with anemia	50–150 U/kg i.v.	PCV = 28–32%		
Cryoprecipitate*	Acute bleeding episodes	10 bags	1 h	4–12 h	24–36 h
Desmopressin†	Acute bleeding episodes	0.3 µg/kg i.v.‡ 0.3 µg/kg s.c. 3 µg/kg intranasal	1 h	2–4 h	6–8 h
Conjugated estrogens	Major surgery or when long-lasting effect is required	0.6 mg/kg/day i.v. infusion for 5 consecutive days	6 h	5–7 days	21–30 days

* Its use is not recommended, because there is no uniformly observed favorable effect.
†It loses efficacy when administered repeatedly.
‡Added to 50 mL saline and infused over 30 min.
RBC, red blood cells.

DDAVP was well tolerated with no changes in hematocrit and plasma osmolality. The effectiveness of DDAVP in shortening bleeding time and/or controlling the abnormal bleeding associated with invasive procedures (biopsies and major surgery) in chronic renal failure has been substantiated by additional studies in which the drug was given intravenously, subcutaneously, or intranasally. Repeated infusions, which may be required with major surgery, are associated with tachyphylaxis, probably due to depletion of vWf stores in endothelial cells. Although remarkably free of serious side-effects DDAVP is reported to cause a mild to moderate decrease in the platelet count, facial flushing, mild transient headache, nausea, abdominal cramps, mild tachycardia, water retention, and hyponatremia. There is a single report of a patient who suffered a stroke immediately after infusion of DDAVP.

From the data currently available it appears that DDAVP (0.3 µg/kg either intravenously or subcutaneously, or 3 µg/kg intranasally) is useful for treating acute bleeding in uremia and for preventing abnormal bleeding in connection with surgery or invasive procedures, and it is probably preferable to cryoprecipitate. In fact, because of variations in clinical response and the risk of transmitting viral disease, the authors do not use cryoprecipitate in their current clinical practice.

Conjugated estrogens

In a first study, six uremic people with bleeding tendency and prolonged bleeding time were given conjugated estrogens (orally in one patient, intravenously in the other five) for a total dose of 30–75 mg over 2–5 days. Bleeding times became shorter in all patients within 2–5 days of starting treatment, became normal in four patients, and remained normal for 3–10 days after discontinuation of the drug.

In a subsequent placebo-controlled, double-blind, crossover trial, conjugated estrogens were administered to six uremics with anemia and prolonged bleeding times (0.6 mg/kg added to 50 mL of saline solution and infused intravenously over a period of 40 min per day for 5 days) (Table 72.2). Bleeding time was already shortened hours after the first infusion, the effect lasting as long as 14 days, or 9 days after the last infusion.[35] No changes were noted in levels or multimeric structure of vWf. No serious side-effects were observed.

A dose-finding study showed that 0.3 mg/kg had no significant effect on bleeding time, but that the effect was clearly cumulative. The effect of a single infusion of 0.6 mg/kg disappeared within 72 h, while marked shortening of the bleeding time was achieved and maintained for 14 days with four or five infusions 24 h apart.[36] Studies confirmed the effects of oral estrogen in controlling abnormal bleeding using regimens of 0.6 mg/kg/day intravenously for 5 days, and 60 mg/day orally for 5 days.

There is also evidence from a small, placebo-controlled trial in four uremic patients that conjugated estrogen given orally at a dose of 50 mg/day may markedly shorten the prolonged bleeding time after an average of 7 days of treatment, and may be effective in controlling abnormal bleeding.[37] Besides transient hot flushes (rare), minor side-effects of conjugated estrogen include nausea, vomiting,

loss of libido, and gynecomastia, which may limit its prolonged use, particularly in men. The risks of malignancy and thromboembolic complications with intermittent high-dose, conjugated estrogen are unknown.

Avoidance of antiplatelet agents

In view of convincing evidence that uremic platelet function abnormalities are induced by toxins in plasma, transfusion of platelet concentrates is thought to be of little, if any, use for the control of abnormal bleeding, unless there is substantial thrombocytopenia.

Thrombosis of arteriovenous shunt
Acute thrombosis

The treatment of choice for acute arteriovenous shunt thrombosis is surgical thrombectomy. Pharmacological thrombolysis appears less effective although no study has formally compared the efficacy of surgical thrombectomy with pharmacological thrombolysis, and no comparative analysis has been done of the cost–benefit of the two techniques.

Intravenous infusion of streptokinase in one study – at a loading dose of 250 000 IU intravenously in 200 mL of 5% dextran over 30 min, followed by continuous intravenous infusion of 100 000 IU/h for 8–12 h – reported a success rate of about 60%[38] (Table 72.3). In another study of 79 patients, streptokinase was also injected directly into the clotted arteriovenous access – over 60 to 90 min for a maximum of 100 000 IU – and was successful in 68% of patients. Asymptomatic distal embolization (seen on angiogram) occurred in 7% of cases.[39]

In another study 14 consecutive hemodialysis access occlusions were treated with urokinase at a dose of 1–1.25 million IU infused at 20 000 IU/min by the crossed-catheter technique with the use of pediatric pumps after systemic heparin administration[40] (Table 72.2). This therapy restored patency within 1 h without significant complications in 11 of 14 occlusions. In 15 patients (14 arteriovenous grafts and one fistula) 10 mg tissue plasminogen activator (t-PA) was infused directly into the vascular access, at 2-h intervals, to a maximum of 30 mg. Angiography showed a decrease in clot volume in all cases and graft patency was restored in 10 of them. Three patients reclotted within 24 h and one had bleeding of the vascular access 5 days later. No bleeding occurred at remote sites[41] (Table 72.3).

Preventive measures

The efficacy of prophylaxis with antiplatelet drugs in prolonging the patency of vascular grafts has been assessed in few clinical trials, but the results are not conclusive (Table 72.3). In 1979 a randomized double-blind trial in 44 patients found that aspirin 160 mg/day was better than placebo in preventing shunt thrombosis in uremic patients,[42] reducing the incidence of thrombi from 0.46 to 0.16 per patient per month (P < 0.005). However, other studies have found that even low doses of aspirin further prolonged the bleeding time, and occasional patients given aspirin to prevent shunt thrombosis developed

Table 72.3   Pharmacological approaches to thrombosis of arteriovenous shunt

Treatment	Dosage	Indication	Reference
Streptokinase	Loading: 250 000 IU i.v. In 200 mnl of 5% dextran over 30 min Maintenance: 100 000 IU/h.i.v. for 8–12 h	Treatment	38
Streptokinase	Up to 100 000 IU i.v. Directly into the clotted arteriovenous access over 60–90 min	Treatment	39
Urokinase	1 000 000 to 1 250 000 IU i.v. At the rate of 20 000 IU/min with a pediatric micro- drif pump, after systemic heparin administration	Treatment	40
Tissue plasminogen activator	10 mg i.v. at 2 h intervals up to 30 mg As 10 ml each into the vascular access	Treatment	41
Antiplatelet agents*		Prophylaxis	
ASA[†]	160 mg/day orally		42
Dipyridamole	75 mg t.i.d. orally		44
ASA + dipyridamole[‡]	325 mg/day orally 75 mg t.i.d orally		44

* Results are not conclusive and are better in patients with arteriovenous shunt than in those with fistulas.
† Risk of severe gastrointestinal bleeding even with lower doses.
‡ Graft patency rate of 75% versus 79% with dipyridamole alone.

severe gastrointestinal bleeding. Recently, a metaanalysis of nine trials comprising 418 patients[43] indicated that antiplatelet treatment – essentially aspirin alone or aspirin plus dipyridamole – reduced the risk of vascular occlusions by 70%. The mean duration of these trials however was only 2 months. The absolute benefit of antiplatelet therapy appeared greater in patients with an arteriovenous shunt than in those with fistulas.

In a recent trial, dypiridamole alone 75 mg three times a day was superior to the same dose with aspirin 325 mg/day in maintaining patency of PTFE grafts after 1 year.[44] Thus patients on dipyiridamole alone had a graft patency rate of 79% at the end of the study, compared to 75% in the dipyridamole–aspirin combination group. However, the beneficial effect of dypiridamole was confined to the group of patients with a new graft, while those who already had a thrombosis of the PTFE graft did not benefit from the antiplatelet treatment. An intriguing finding of the above trial was that aspirin alone was no better than placebo, and actually increased the rate of graft thrombosis compared with dypiridamole or placebo.

Few clinical studies have tested the effect of the antiplatelet agent ticlopidine in preventing primary occlusion of native arteriovenous fistula and consistently reported a reduced incidence of thrombosis in the treated group.[45] All these studies however were small in size and short in duration. A new ticlopidine analog, clopidogrel, which seems devoid of the hematologic toxicity, is currently under investigation in a randomized controlled trial in the prevention of graft thrombosis.

There are few uncontrolled studies that have examined the effectiveness of systemic anticoagulation with warfarin in preventing occlusion of permanent central venous catheters, placed for other purposes than dialysis. These studies have suggested that low fixed-dose warfarin may reduce the risk of venous thrombosis. It is not known whether this indication can be extrapolated to hemodialysis permanent catheters.[46]

Therapy for hypercoagulability in nephrotic patients

Nephrotic syndrome patients with renal vein thrombosis or other thromboembolic complications need anticoagulation with heparin and warfarin (Table 72.4). There are not many data on doses and duration of treatment. The few published studies report ranges of treatment periods from 3–12 months, but in some patients anticoagulation was prolonged indefinitely. There is no evidence that thrombolytic therapy is superior to anticoagulant alone, despite some reports of promising results with streptokinase and urokinase (Table 72.4). In three cases published in 1984, systemic streptokinase[47] (50 000 IU loading dose over 30 min followed by 100 000 IU/h for 24 h, or 250 000 IU followed by a continuous infusion of 100 000 IU/h for 72 h)[48] was followed by lysis of thrombotic material documented by renal venography. In one case intraarterial thrombolytic therapy for isolated renal arterial and renal venous thrombosis was completed successfully within 24 h with urokinase infused through the renal artery (80 000 IU/h).[49] A review of the recent literature[50] includes 18 cases with repeated studies, in 14 of whom the renal veins were cleared by thrombolytic

Table 72.4 Prophylaxis and treament of thromboembolism in nephrotic patients

Treatment	Dosage	Indication	Reference
Low-molecular-weight heparin	4000 IU/day s.c. for 3–6 months. The dose should be reduced to 2000 IU/day s.c. if plasma creatinine > 200 μmol/L	Prophylaxis[¶]	52
Streptokinase	Loading: 50 000 IU i.v. administration over 30 min by peripheral vein Maintenance: 100 000 IU/h i.v. for 24 hours	Treatment[†]	47
Streptokinase	Loading: 250 000 IU i.v. by peripheral vein Maintenance: 100 000 IU/h i.v. for 72 h	Treatment[†]	48
Urokinase	80000 IU/h infused through the renal artery As 10 ml each into the vascular access	Treatment[‡]	49
Anticoagulants Heparin/warfarin	*	Treatment[§]	

* Little data available on doses and duration of treament (3–12 months).
[†]For renal vein thrombosis.
[‡]For simultaneous renal arterial and vein thrombosis
[§]For acute thrombosis start heparin followed by oral anticoagulants (warfarin) as long as the nephrotic state persists.
[¶]In patients with serum albumin < 2.5 g/dL.

therapy. However there are no studies so far that use a proper controlled design to compare thrombolytic therapy with heparin and oral anticoagulants. It appears from retrospective analysis that thrombolysis was used in more severe or bilateral cases. At present there is no basis for selecting which patients should be treated, especially when considering the additional risk of bleeding or embolic events.

Current recommendations are that patients with a diagnosis of acute thrombosis should start heparin (which usually leads to sudden improvement of renal function) followed by a regimen of oral anticoagulants (warfarin) that should probably be continued as long as the nephrotic state persists. Indeed, relapses of acute renal vein thrombosis have been reported after stopping oral anticoagulants. The use of warfarin in nephrotic syndrome must take into consideration the fact that this drug binds to a major extent to serum albumin, concentrations of which may vary rapidly in this condition. Whether purified antithrombin III should be added to heparin in cases of antithrombin III deficiency remains to be determined.

Patients with nephrotic syndrome are also at high risk for venous thromboembolism especially in connection with surgery, trauma, or prolonged bed rest, and therefore although anticoagulation has so far been considered mostly for acute thrombosis, the question of antithrombotic prophylaxis is of great importance (Table 72.4). A recent study, based on a decision analysis model, concluded that prophylactic oral anticoagulation while patients remain nephrotic enhances life expectancy by preventing pulmonary embolism,[51] and that the expected benefit is superior to the potential risk of bleeding induced by systemic anticoagulation. In patients with serum albumin lower then 2.5 g/dL prophylactic anticoagulation is strongly recommended since the risk of thrombo-

embolism increases steeply with more severe hypoalbuminemia. In a recent prospective uncontrolled trial[52] of 55 patients with nephrosis and severe hypoalbuminemia, low-molecular-weight heparin (40 mg enoxaparin, 4000 U/day) was given subcutaneously for 3 or 6 months or more to prevent thromboembolism. The data showed that the procedure was safe and heparin can be self-administered. During the treatment period no episodes of thrombosis were observed.

Aspirin and dipyridamole reverse the platelet hyperaggregability of nephrotic syndrome, but there are no studies to tell whether these drugs can actually prevent thromboembolism in patients with nephrotic syndrome.

Note added in proof

An alarming side effect of r-HuEpo is the development of antierythropoietin antibodies which is associated with transfusion dependent anemia, caused by a pure red cell bone marrow aplasia. Casadevall et al in early 2002[53] described and characterized 13 patients with pure red cell aplasia which had developed antibodies able to block the formation of erythroid colonies by normal bone marrow cells. Following this report, in July 2002, the European manufacturer of erythropoietin-α issued a "Dear Doctor Letter", warning that 141 suspected cases of pure red-cell aplasia had been reported world wide.[54] In 114 of the cases a bone marrow biopsy confirmed the erythroblastopenia. Anemia developed on average 10 months post therapy initiation, with a range of 1–92 months. Although the data are too scanty for a firm conclusion, it seems that the incidence of pure red-cell aplasia is higher in patients who are assuming r-HuEpo subcutaneously than in those who are assuming the drug intravenously. Therefore, the recommendation that a subcutaneous route should be preferred, should be waived until more data are available, and an intravenous route should be used. Moreover, the manufacturer of erythropoietin-α explicity recommends the use of intravenous r-HuEpo whenever possible.

When pure red-cell aplasia is suspected, r-HuEpo administration should be immediately interrupted. It is also recommended to avoid switching patients to other forms of r-HuEpo or to darbopoietin, since the antierythropoietin antibodies cross-react with all commercially available recombinant erythropoietic products.[53]

Immunosuppressive treatment was followed by disappearance of the antibodies in 16 of the cases described by Casadevall.[55]

References

1. Muirhead N, Bargman J, Burgess E, et al: Evidence based recommendations for the clinical use of recombinant human erythropoietin. Am J Kidney Dis 1995;26:S1–S24.
2. Ifudu O, Feldman J, Friedman EA: The intensity of hemodialysis and the response to erythropoietin in patients with end-stage renal disease. N Engl J Med 1996;334:420–425.
3. NKF-DOQI: Clinical practice guidelines for anemia in chronic kidney disease, 2000. National Kidney Foundation-Dialysis Outcomes Quality Initiative. I. Anemia work-up. Am J Kidney Dis 2001;37:S186–S189
4. Locatelli F, Conte F, Marcelli D: The impact of hematocrit levels and erythropoietin treatment on overall and cardiovascular mortality or morbidity: The experience of the Lombardy Dialysis Registry. Nephrol Dial Transplant 1998;13:1642–1644.
5. European Best Practice Guidelines for the Management of Anaemia in Patients with Chronic Renal Failure. Target Guideline 5: Target haemoglobin concentration for the treatment of the anaemia of chronic renal failure. Nephrol Dial Transplant 1999;14(Suppl 5):S11–S13.
6. National Kidney Foundation – Dialysis Outcomes Quality Initiative (NKF–DOQI). Clinical practice guidelines for anemia in chronic kidney disease, 2000. II. Target hemoglobin/hematocrit. Am J Kidney Dis 2001;37:S190–S193.
7. Barany P, Clyne N, Hylander B, et al: Subcutaneous epoietin beta in renal anemia: an open multicenter dose titration study of patients on continuous peritoneal dialysis. Perit Dial Int 1995;15:54–60.
8. Paganini EP, Eschbach JW, Lazarus JM, et al: Intravenous versus subcutaneous dosing of epoietin alpha in hemodialysis patients. Am J Kidney Dis 1995;26:331–340.
9. Harnett JD, Kent GM, Foley RN, Parfrey PS: Cardiac function and hematocrit level. Am J Kidney Dis 1995;25(Suppl 1):S3–S7.
10. Garcia DL, Anderson S, Rennke HG, Brenner BM. Anemia lessens and its prevention with recombinant human erythropoietin worsens glomerular injury and hypertension in rats with reduced renal mass. Proc Natl Acad Sci USA 1988;85:6142–6146.
11. Revicki DA, Brown RE, Feeny DH, et al: Health-related quality of life associated with recombinant human erythropoietin therapy for predialysis chronic renal disease patients. Am J Kidney Dis 1995;25:548–554.
12. Koch KM, Koene RAP, Messinger D, et al: The use of epoietin beta in anaemic predialysis patients with chronic renal failure. Clin Nephrol 1995;44:201–208.
13. Horl WH, Cavill I, Macdougall IC, et al: How to diagnose and correct iron deficiency during r-huEPO therapy: a consensus report. Nephrol Dial Transplant 1996;11:246–250.
14. Kalantar-Zadeh K, Hoffken B, Wunsch H, et al: Diagnosis of iron deficiency anemia in renal failure patients during the post-erythropoietin era. Am J Kidney Dis 1995;26:292–299.
15. Fishbane S, Lynn RI: The utility of zinc protoporphyrin for predicting the need for intravenous iron therapy in hemodialysis patients. Am J Kidney Dis 1995;25:426–432.
16. Macdougall IC: Poor response to erythropoietin; practical guidelines on investigation and management. Nephrol Dial Transplant 1995;10:607.
17. Wingard RL, Parker RA, Ismail N, et al: Efficacy of oral iron therapy in patients receiving recombinant human erythropoietin. Am J Kidney Dis 1995;25:433–439.
18. Macdougall IC: An overview of the efficacy and safety of novel erythropoiesis stimulating (NESP). Nephrol Dial Transplant 2001;16(Suppl 3):14–21.
19. Locatelli F, Olivares J, Walker R, et al: Novel erythropoiesis stimulating protein for treatment of anemia in chronic renal insufficiency. Kidney Int 2001; 60:741-747.
20. Barbone FP, Johnson DL, Farrel FX, et al: New epoietin molecules and novel therapeutic approaches. Nephrol Dial Transplant 1999;14(Suppl 2):80–84.
21. G. Remuzzi, E.C. Rossi. Hematological consequences of renal failure. In Brenner, BM (ed): Brenner and Rector's The Kidney, 5th edn, Vol. II. Philadelphia: WB Saunders Company, 1996, pp 2170–2186.
22. Escolar G, Cases A, Bastida E, et al: Uremic platelets have a functional defect affecting the interaction of von Willebrand factor with glycoprotein IIb–IIIa. Blood 1990;76:336–340.
23. Fan P, Schwab SJ: Hemodialysis vascular access. In Henrich WL (ed): The Principles and Practice and Dialysis. Baltimore: Williams & Wilkins, 1994, pp 22–37.
24. Shand BI, Buttimore AL, Hurrell MA, et al: Hemorheology and fistula function in home hemodialysis patients following erythropoietin treatment: a placebo-controlled study. Nephron 1993;64:53–57.
25. Standage BA, Schuman ES, Ackerman D, Gross GF, Rangsdale JW: Does the use of erythropoietin in hemodialysis patients increase dialysis graft thrombosis rates? Am J Surg1993;165:650–654.
26. Anderson S, Kennefick TM, Brenner BM. Renal and systemic manifestations of glomerular disease. In Brenner BM (ed): Brenner and Rector's The Kidney, 5th edn, Vol. II. Philadelphia: WB Saunders Company, 1996, pp 1981–2010.
27. Llach F: Hypercoagulability, renal vein thrombosis, and other thrombotic complications of nephrotic syndrome. Kidney Int 1985;28:429–439.
28. Fernandez F, Goudable C, Sie P, et al: Low haematocrit and prolonged bleeding time in uraemic patients: Effect of red cell transfusion. Br J Haematol 1985;59:139–148.
29. Livio M, Gotti E, Marchesi D, et al: Uraemic bleeding: Role of anemia and beneficial effect of red cell transfusions. Lancet 1982;2:1013–1015.
30. Viganò G, Benigni A, Mendogni D, et al: Recombinant human erythropoietin to correct uremic bleeding. Am J Kidney Dis 1991;18:44–49.
31. Janson PA, Jubelirer SJ, Weinstein MJ, et al: Treatment of the bleeding tendency in uremia with cryoprecipitate. N Engl J Med 1980;303:1318–1322.
32. Mannucci PM, Ruggeri ZM, Pareti FI, et al: 1-Deamino-8-D-arginine vasopressin: A new pharmacologic approach to the management of haemophilia and von Willebrand's diseases. Lancet 1977;1:869–872.
33. Watson AJ, Keogh JA: Effect of 1-deamino-8-D-arginine vasopressin on the prolonged bleeding time in chronic renal failure. Nephron 1982;32:49–52.
34. Mannucci PM, Remuzzi G, Pusineri F, et al: Deamino-8-D-arginine vasopressin shortens the bleeding time in uremia. N Engl J Med 1983;308:8–12.
35. Livio M, Mannucci PM, Viganò G, et al: Conjugated estrogens for the management of bleeding associated with renal failure. N Engl J Med 1986;315:731–715.
36. Viganò G, Gaspari F, Locatelli M, et al: Dose-effect and pharmacokinetics of estrogens given to correct bleeding time in uremia. Kidney Int 1988;34:853.
37. Shemin D, Elnour M, Amarantes B, et al: Oral estrogens decrease bleeding time and improve clinical bleeding in patients with renal failure. Am J Med 1990;89:436–440.
38. Matuszkiewicz-Rowinska J, Billip T, Omecka Z, et al: Systemic streptokinase infusion for declotting of hemodialysis arteriovenous fistulas. Nephron 1994;66:67–70.
39. Zeit RM: Arterial and venous embolization: declotting of dialysis shunts by direct injection of streptokinase. Radiology 1986;159:639–641.
40. Brunner MC, Matalon TA, Patel SK, McDonald V, Jensik SC: Ultrarapid urokinase in hemodialysis access occlusion. J Vasc Intervent Radiol 1991;2:503–506.
41. Ahmed A, Shapiro WB, Porush JG: The use of tissue plasminogen activator to declot arteriovenous accesses in hemodialysis patients. Am J Kidney Dis 1993;21:38–43.
42. Harter HR, Burch JW, Majerus PW, et al: Prevention of thrombosis in patients on hemodialysis by low dose aspirin. N Engl J Med 1979;301:577–579.

43. Antiplatelet Trialists' Collaboration. Collaborative overview of randomized trials of antiplatelet therapy. II: Maintenance of vascular graft of arterial patency by antiplatelet therapy. BR MED J 1994;308:159–168.

44. Sreedhara R, Himmelfarb J, Lazarus JM, et al: Anti-platelet therapy in graft thrombosis: results of a prospective, randomized, double-blind study. Kidney Int 1994;45:1477–1483.

45. Kaufman JS: Antithrombotic agents and the prevention of access thrombosis. Seminars Dial 2000;13:40–46.

46. Boraks P, Scale J, Price J, et al: Prevention of central venous catheter-associated thrombosis using minidose warfarin in patients with haematological malignancies. Br J Haemat 1998;101:483.

47. Rowe JM, Rasmussen RL, Mader SL, et al: Successful thrombolytic therapy in two patients with renal vein thrombosis. Am J Med 1984;77:1111–1114.

48. Burrow CR, Walker WG, Bell WR, et al: Streptokinase salvage of renal function after renal vein thrombosis. Ann Intern Med 1984;100:237–238.

49. Kennedy JS, Gerety BM, Silverman R, et al: Simultaneous renal arterial and venous thrombosis associated with idiopathic nephrotic syndrome: treatment with intra-arterial urokinase. Am J Med 1991;90:124–127.

50. Markowitz GS, Brignol F, Burns ER, et al: Renal vein thrombosis treated with thrombolytic therapy: case report and brief review. Am J Kidney Dis 1995;25:801–805.

51. Sarasin FP, Schifferli JA: Prophylactic oral anticoagulation in nephrotic patients with idiopathic membranous nephropathy. Kidney Int 1994;45:578–585.

52. Rostoker G, Durand-Zaleski I, Petit-Phar M, et al: Prevention of thrombotic complications of the nephrotic syndrome by the low-molecular-weight heparin enoxaparin. Nephron 1995;69:20–28.

53. Casadevall N, Nataf J, Viron B, et al: Pure red-cell aplasia and antierythropoietin antibodies in patients treated with recombinant erythropoietin. N Engl J Med 2002;346(7):469–475.

54. Agence française de sécurité sanitaire des produits de sante. Communique de presse. Available at http://agmed.sante.gouv.fr/htm/10/filcoprs/020704.htm as accessed September 2002.

55. Casadevall N. Antibodies against rHuEPO: native and recombinant. Nephrol Dial Transplant 2002;17(Suppl 5):42–47.

Calcium, Phosphorus, Renal Bone Disease, and Calciphylaxis

Francisco Llach and Francisco Velasquez-Forero

The term *renal osteodystrophy* was coined in 1943, 60 years after an association between bone disease and renal failure was discovered.[1] This term includes osteitis fibrosa, a reflection of secondary hyperparathyroidism (secondary HPT), osteomalacia (in the past often due to aluminum toxicity), adynamic bone disease (ABD) and mixed forms (mainly secondary HPT and osteomalacia). Additionally in children, rickets and skeletal deformities may also be present. Osteosclerosis and osteoporosis are less commonly observed. Of these lesions, osteitis fibrosa is characterized by a high bone turnover, whereas osteomalacia and ABD are characterized by low bone turnover. Here, we will analyze some pathogenetic clinical manifestations and diagnosis of the different forms of renal osteodystrophy but mostly discuss new therapeutics alternatives.

Pathogenetic considerations

High bone turnover disease

Several factors contribute to the high parathyroid hormone (PTH) levels characteristic of high bone turnover lesions. They include a decrease in calcitriol (calcitriol) synthesis by the failing kidney, the presence of hyperphosphatemia (via direct stimulation of PTH secretion) in endstage renal disease (ESRD), and an abnormality of the newly described calcium sensor receptor most likely due to uremia, calcitriol deficiency, and hyperphosphatemia.

Low bone turnover disease

In addition to osteomalacia (previously a common result of aluminum toxicity), a bone lesion named adynamic or aplastic bone disease (ABD) has been described with increasing frequency. The pathophysiology of low bone turnover states is not well known, except for aluminum-related bone disease. This bone lesion is characterized by low bone volume. Its frequency is steadily increasing in ESRD patients. The factors that may impair bone formation, mineralization, and bone turnover are given in Table 73.1.

Clinical signs and symptoms of osteodystrophy

Bone disease in patients with chronic renal failure (CRF) is usually asymptomatic. By the time symptoms are present, the patient usually has significant biochemical abnormalities and histologic evidence of bone disease. The usual symptoms of bone pain, muscular weakness, periarthritis, and pruritus are usually absent. However, two clinical syndromes have been increasing in frequency: coronary artery calcifications and calciphylaxis.

Recent evidence has revealed a high prevalence of *coronary artery calcifications* in the ESRD population. This probably plays a major role in the high cardiac morbidity and mortality. Indeed, strong relationships have been found between cardiac deaths and factors that favor metastatic calcification, i.e. hyperphosphatemia and increased calcium (Ca) × phosphorus (P) product.[2] In a large national study of data from more than 12 000 ESRD patients, higher mortality rates from coronary artery disease were found in patients with hyperphosphatemia (serum phosphorus > 6.5 mg/dL) than in patients with serum phosphorus of less than 6.5 mg/dL (relative risk 1.41; $P < 0.0005$). The risk for sudden death was also increased in patients with hyperphosphatemia as well as in patients with elevated Ca × P products (relative risk 1.07 per 10 mg^2/dL^2) and those with PTH levels > 495 pg/mL.[2] Factors predisposing to the development of metastatic calcifications are listed in Table 73.2. Calcifications of cardiac tissue have been reported in nearly 60% of dialysis patients.[3] These are most significant in the coronary arteries.

Table 73.1 Factors that may contribute to adynamic bone disease

Low serum PTH levels	Mechanism: PTx, diabetes mellitus, high calcium intake, high dialysate calcium, continuous ambulatory peritoneal dialysis, overtreatment with vitamin D, aluminum toxicity
Diabetes	Mechanism unknown: multifactorial? Low calcitriol levels? Abnormalities in PTH secretion?
Increasing age	Mechanism?
Increase calcium intake	Mechanism: oversuppression of PTH
Iron accumulation	
Fluoride therapy for osteoporosis	At toxic doses
Corticosteroid treatment	
Aluminum accumulation	Mechanism: aluminum on forming surface, aluminum in osteoblasts, increased serum Al
Acidosis	
Heparin therapy	

PTH, parathyroid hormone; PTx, parathyroidectomy.

Table 73.2 Factors predisposing to soft tissue calcifications

Hyperphosphatemia
Increase of Ca × P product
Increase in calcium intake
Adynamic bone disease
Secondary hyperparathyroidism
Age
Time on dialysis
Overuse of vitamin D derivatives

Coronary artery calcifications are much more common and severe in patients on hemodialysis.[4–6] Electron-beam computed tomography (EBCT) has high spatial and temporal resolution, and ultrafast (at subsecond intervals) imaging is triggered by the patient's ECG rhythm. Calcification of atherosclerotic plaques is found in the advanced stages of plaque transformation.[4] The extent of calcification noted by this technique correlates well with the severity of atherosclerotic lesions detected by coronary angiography.[6] When compared with coronary angiography as the reference standard, EBCT detected coronary artery disease with a sensitivity of 93% and a specificity of 73%.[6] Coronary artery calcifications detected by EBCT were found in the majority of patients on dialysis.[6] Braun et al[4] found that the incidence of coronary artery calcifications was 2.5–5 times greater in 49 patients on dialysis than in 102 non-dialysis patients of similar age. Furthermore, these calcifications worsened in the dialysis patients when EBCT studies were repeated 1 year later. Goodman et al[5] observed coronary artery calcifications to be highly prevalent (14 of 16 patients) in young adults, aged 20–30 years on dialysis, compared with healthy subjects of the same age (3 of 60 subjects). Calcium deposits in the mitral and aortic valves and of the myocardium are very common. This may contribute to conduction abnormalities and arrhythmias, left ventricular dysfunction, aortic and mitral stenosis, ischemia, congestive heart failure, and death. Most studies have found correlations of calcifications with uncontrolled hyperphoshatemia, an increased Ca × P product, and years on dialysis.[2–4] Patients with greater intakes of oral calcium had a higher incidence of coronary artery calcification.[5]

These data suggest that long-term imbalances in calcium and phosphorus underlie cardiac calcification. They raise the concern that long-term treatment with high doses of calcium-based phosphate binders with inappropriate vitamin D therapy may contribute to calcification. Vigilant monitoring of serum calcium and phosphorus and Ca × P product may reduce the incidence of cardiac calcification and its related morbidity and mortality. Control of serum calcium and phosphorus, and avoidance of excessive calcium intake should be part of a comprehensive approach to modify risk factors for coronary artery disease which are so prevalent in the ESRD population.

Calcific uremic arteriolopathy (CUA), also known as *calciphylaxis*, causes necrotic skin lesions which usually present as painful violaceous mottling similar to livedo reticularis, or as painful nodules, panniculitis. Seyle[7] first described a syndrome in an experimental animal in 1962 and postulated that two steps are required to produce ectopic systemic calcifications. The first step involves a systemic sensitization induced by agents such as parathyroid hormone (PTH), vitamin D, or a diet high in calcium and phosphorus. Second, after a time interval (known as the "critical period") exposure to appropriate challenging agents by subcutaneous injections resulted in macroscopic visible deposits of calcium salts (hydroxyapatite) at the site of injection and systematically and within 2–3 days. The challenging agents included local trauma, iron salt, egg albumin, polymyxin, and glucocorticoids; Selye named the syndrome "calciphylaxis." A few years later, a syndrome characterized by peripheral ischemic tissue necrosis, vascular calcifications, and cutaneous ulcerations was reported in uremic patients.[8] Because of its resemblance to Selye's animal model, it was named "calciphylaxis." However, there are significant differences between Selye's model and uremic calciphylaxis. The latter occurs primarily in the presence of uremia with abnormalities in divalent ions (PTH, hypercalcemia, and hyperphosphatemia) and vascular calcifications. It appears that uremic soft-tissue calcification (tumoral calcinosis) is the syndrome most analogous to Selye's.

It is important to review certain pathogenic factors. First, the presence of an uremic milieu together with a high $Ca \times P$ product is noted in the majority of reports.[8,9] Diffuse vascular calcifications were frequently noted in the early days of maintenance dialysis.[8] CUA was noted in 20% of dialysis patients with secondary hyperparathyroidism (HPT);[10] it increased to 58% in patients with clinical evidence of HPT and to 75% in patients with severe overt HPT.[16]

Second, the calcium content of the skin is increased in dialysis patients developing CUA.[11] It was provoked by a very high dialysate calcium concentration ([Ca]) of 4.0 mequiv./L.[11] A decrease in dialysate [Ca] dramatically improves CUA in some patients whereas a high dialysate [Ca] aggravates soft-tissue calcification.[11] Furthermore, CUA was associated with hypercalcemia induced by large oral doses of calcium carbonate ($CaCO_3$), and reversed by discontinuing it.[12] Many dialysis patients still ingest large doses of elemental calcium, but the long-term effects remain to be established. Almost all patients developing CUA were ingesting calcium-containing binders.

A third important pathogenic factor is a high PTH. Earlier, it appeared that HPT was an important risk factor in the development of CUA.[13] In this study Gipstein et al reported a series of patients with CUA, most with peripheral digital ulcers in whom parathyroidectomy (PTx) resulted in dramatic healing of the ulcers, and total disappearance of the syndrome in 61%. Marked hyperphosphatemia was present in each patient prior to CUA. Later, hyperphosphatemia was also associated with CUA[11] and was reversed by severe phosphorus restriction.

More recently, CUA has been reported in patients with PTH and divalent cation levels close to normal. We recently reported 14 patients with CUA, of whom only four had elevated PTH levels (870 ± 234 pg/mL).[14] In the remaining 10 patients, calcium, phosphorus, and PTH (< 250 pg/mL) all appeared to be well controlled. Coates et al[9] and Bleyer et al[15] report that obesity, especially in white women, is a predisposing factor. Morbid obesity was present in 11 of our 14 patients (79%) with CUA.[14] Coates et al[9] noticed a significant weight loss preceding the development of the skin lesion in 7 of 16 patients. In four patients, the lesions developed in areas that had obviously served as a site of insulin injection.[15] Patients with proximal calciphylaxis have poorer prognosis than those with acral CUA. Thus, Hafner et al[16] reported that 40 of 53 patients (75%) with distal location of necrosis survived, compared with 11 of 42 patients (26%) with proximal CUA ($P = 0.00001$).

Prevention and management of renal osteodystrophy

Important objectives include: (1) maintenance of normal serum calcium and phosphorus levels; (2) prevention of 2 HPT; (3) avoidance of toxic agents such as aluminum, iron, or fluoride and excessive calcium intake; (4) prevention and reversal of extraskeletal calcifications; and (5) avoidance of the hazards of treatment modalities (Table 73.3).

Table 73.3 Guidelines for management of renal osteodystrophy

General
Control of serum phosphorus (4.0–5.5 mg/dL)
Restrict dietary phosphorus within an adequate protein intake
Give phosphorus-binding agents: individual dosage should be proportional to size of the meals
Minimize the use of calcium-containing binders to 1 g/day
Do not use aluminum-containing phosphorus binders

Dietary calcium supplements
• Give oral calcium to supply 1 g/day in dialysis patients, but only if the serum phosphorus concentration is controlled and there is persistent hypocalcemia

Dialysate calcium concentration
• Use a 2.5 mequiv./L dialysate [Ca]
• Use a 2.0 mequiv./L dialysate [Ca] in individual patients with low bone turnover disease
• Do not use a dialysate [Ca] above 2.5 mequiv./l

Vitamin D metabolites
• Adequate control of serum phosphorus and any of the following:
• Hypocalcemia
• Secondary HPT (intact PTH > three times normal)
• Chronic renal failure in children
• Osteomalacia (with nutritional vitamin D deficiency or coexisting with secondary HPT)
• Concurrent anticonvulsant therapy
• Myopathy and muscle weakness

Dosing of vitamin D metabolites
• Calcitriol dose commensurate with PTH levels
  – Oral pulse therapy 2–8 g three times weekly
  – Intravenous calcitriol 0.5–8 g per HD three times weekly
• Paricalcitol dose commensurate with PTH levels PHH (μg/L)
  – 400–800, dose 4–2 μg with each dialysis
  – 800–1200, dose 8–12 μg with each dialysis
  – > 1200, dose 12–20 μg with each dialysis
• Doxercalciferol dose commensurate with PTH levels
  – Oral therapy 2.5–15 μg three times weekly
  – Intravenous 1–5 μg per HD three times weekly

Parathyroidectomy
• Ineffective medical treatment, evidence of severe secondary HPT, and any of the following:
• Persistent hypercalcemia (serum Ca^{2+} > 12 mg/dL)
• Progressive extraskeletal calcifications
• Persistent elevation of serum Ca^{2+} × phosphorus product
• Severe and intractable pruritus

Table 73.3 (cont'd)
- Symptomatic hypercalcemia after kidney transplantation (including secondary deterioration of renal function)
- Calciphylaxis (urgent PTx may be necessary)

Other factors
- Dialysate magnesium concentration of 0.6–1 mg/dL (0.5–0.7 mequiv./L); decrease if magnesium-containing phosphorus binders are used
- Water treatment: maintain aluminum < 5–10 μg/L and remove excess fluoride, calcium and magnesium in dialysate
- Infuse deferoxamine for aluminum chelation (1–5 mg/kg/week or every 10 days)
- Avoid concurrent treatment with barbiturates, phenytoin, glutethimide or corticosteroids

Prevention of phosphorus retention and hyperphosphatemia

Hyperphosphatemia is a silent killer in the dialysis population. A national study of two large, random samples of patients on hemodialysis showed that patients with elevated phosphorus or elevated Ca × P product had excessive mortality.[2,17] Those with serum phosphorus greater than 6.5 mg/dL had a 27% increase in mortality after adjustment for comorbid conditions. Some 39% of dialysis patients had hyperphosphatemia.[17] The goal should be to maintain predialysis serum phosphorus levels between 4.0 and 5.5 mg/dL. This requires a true commitment by the patient and the dialysis team in monitoring serum phosphorus, adjusting diets and phosphorus binders, and counseling.

The available options for reducing the phosphorus burden include (1) reducing dietary phosphorus intake; (2) preventing the absorption of phosphorus with phosphorus binders; and (3) enhancing the removal of phosphorus in dialysis. After these maneuvers, the control of hyperphosphatemia may become easier since the phosphorus efflux from bone decreases with lower PTH levels. Conversely, compliant patients have hyperphosphatemia from secondary HPT and/or increased individual susceptibility to phosphorus absorption.

Dietary phosphorus restriction

Dietary phosphorus restriction is the first step. The phosphorus intake of normal adults is 1–1.8 g/day. It depends primarily on consumption of meat and dairy products. Poultry, fish, liver, most soft drinks (especially cola), whole-grain breads, and some cereals, nuts and legumes are rich in phosphorus. With elimination of dairy products and limitation to 40 g of protein per day, the dietary intake of phosphorus is 650–1000 mg/day. Once a patient is on maintenance dialysis with a diet containing higher protein, phosphorus intake also rises. The National Cooperative Dialysis Study (NCDS) suggested that with commencement of dialytic therapy, patients should eat at least

0.8 g/kg/day protein. The average daily dietary intake of phosphorus in 162 hemodialysis patients who entered this study was 879 ± 248 mg.[18] With a more appropriate protein intake of 1 g/kg/day, the measured daily phosphorus intake ranged from 920 to 1200 mg, and when dietary protein was increased to 1.4 g/kg/day, the daily phosphorus intake was 1700–2400 mg. Thus, it may become difficult to achieve a balance between nutritional demands and limited phosphorus intake. Consequently, restriction of dietary phosphorus intake as the sole measure to avoid phosphorus retention is only feasible in patients with moderate CRF.

Phosphorus binders

Phosphorus binders are required for most patients with ESRD and for those with a glomerular filtration rate (GFR) of < 25–30 mL/min. The mass balance for phosphorus in dialysis patients is given in Table 73.4. Phosphorus binders decrease intestinal phosphorus absorption by creating poorly soluble phosphorus complexes in the intestinal tract. However, they do not exclude the need for restriction of phosphorus intake. Thus, 60–80% of ingested phosphorus is absorbed. Even with phosphorus binders, the net absorption of phosphorus can be greater than 50% especially if calcitriol is given. Phosphorus binders are more effective when phosphorus intake is lower than 1 g/day. With a greater intake (1.5–2 g/day), their binding capacity is markedly decreased. Binders should be taken immediately after meals. The dose should be "commensurate" with the size of the meal, and individualized for each patient according to serum phosphorus.

The available binders include sevelamer hydrochloride (Renagel), calcium acetate (Phoslo), $CaCO_3$, and calcium acetate, magnesium carbonate, and aluminum-based binders. Sevelamer is preferred over the calcium-based binders because it is calcium free. Patients can avoid problems related to calcium deposition and hypercalcemia. Most patients on dialysis are treated with vitamin D preparations that increase the hypercalcemia further. Aluminum-containing binders should be avoided because of the risk of bone disease and encephalopathy.

Sevelamer hydrochloride (Renagel) Sevelamer is a nonabsorbed hydrogel cross-linked polyallylamine hydrochloride, free of aluminum or calcium.[19] It is completely resistant

Table 73.4 Considerations regarding phosphorus removal and balance in dialysis patients with three different diets

	Phosphorus intake (mg/day)		
	900	1200	1500
Absorbed (60%)	540	720	900
Hemodialysis removal (mg/day) (700 mg/4 h) Dialysis three times a week			
Balance	+240	+420	+600

to digestive degradation. It is not absorbed. Partially protonated amines spaced one carbon from the polymer backbone interact with phosphorus anions by ionic and hydrogen bond. The in vivo efficacy of Renagel has been demonstrated in rats,[19] in normal volunteers[20] and in hyperphosphatemic ESRD patients.[21] In a randomized, placebo-controlled, double-blind trial of 36 maintenance hemodialysis patients followed over 8 weeks, it was found to be at least as effective as calcium carbonate or acetate. The reduction in serum phosphorus was significantly greater after 2 weeks of treatment with Renagel than with placebo. There was no significant change in serum calcium in either group. Furthermore, there was a significant decrease in phosphorus levels, which was associated with a decrease in PTH. Renagel also reduced serum total and low-density lipoprotein (LDL)-cholesterol.

The usual dose of Sevelamer is 2–8 g/day, given in divided 800-mg doses with a meal or large snack. A single supplemental oral calcium dose may be needed in some patients if hypocalcemia persists after hyperphosphatemia is controlled. This polymer offers advantages over traditional agents in the management of hyperphosphatemia. First, it abrogates the need for exposure to aluminum, magnesium, calcium overload, and potential hypercalcemia. Second, it allows the use of vitamin D and its analogs with minimal hypercalcemia. Ingestion of large amounts of calcium-containing binders and poor control of hyperphosphatemia may contribute to coronary artery disease. Sevelamer, being calcium free, may be preferable. A recent important randomized study in 202 hemodialysis patients contrasted the effect of Sevelamer with calcium-containing binders on biochemical parameters and on vascular calcifications over one year.[2] Both groups had similar control of hyperphosphatemia, but serum calcium concentration was significantly higher in those taking calcium binders, as was the incidence of hypercalcemic episodes. PTH levels remained below 150 pg/mL in patients ingesting calcium binders, despite reductions in vitamin D dosage and dialysate calcium concentration in some cases, while patients taking Sevelamer were more likely to reach target PTH levels (150–300 pg/mL). Furthermore, cholesterol levels were decreased by 50–60 mg/dL after Sevelamer. Finally, coronary, aortic, and valve calcification score (estimated by EBCT) increased significantly in patients on calcium binders but not those on sevelamer ($P = 0.009$).

Calcium-containing phosphorus binders Large doses of *calcium carbonate* (40% of elemental calcium) reduce phosphorus absorption.[25] Other calcium-based phosphorus binders include: *calcium acetate* (25% of elemental calcium), *calcium lactate* (12%) or *calcium gluconate* (8%). Calcium chloride should be avoided because it induces metabolic acidosis. The dose of calcium-containing phosphorus binders should be increased gradually until serum phosphorus is controlled. Hypercalcemia is the most common problem but constipation, changes in bowel habits, vague abdominal discomfort, and dyspepsia are often reported.

Hypercalcemia occurs in many patients on calcium binders; occasionally it requires withdrawal of the binder. A dialysate calcium concentration of 3.0–3.5 mequiv./L is often associated with hypercalcemic episodes.

Long-term side-effects of calcium-containing phosphorus binders are unknown. However, an excessive ingestion of calcium may contribute to the progression of coronary artery calcifications, increase adynamic bone disease, and contribute to tumoral calcinosis and calciphylaxis.

Aluminum-containing phosphorus binders Aluminum-containing phosphorus binders were standard before 1985. It has been suggested that there is little risk of aluminum intoxication with the ingestion of up to six capsules of aluminum hydroxide per day in the adult uremic patient, or at doses below *30 mg/kg* in children with ESRD. However, aluminum accumulation was noted in children undergoing peritoneal dialysis, although the dosage of aluminum gels did not exceed that amount. A progressive increase of plasma aluminum was noted, followed by a fall once the binder was discontinued. Consequently, no "safe" dose can be described. Moreover, larger doses are generally required to control serum phosphorus. We strongly recommend that aluminum binders should be abandoned in patients with CRF.

Other phosphorus binders *Magnesium carbonate* ($MgCO_3$) is an effective phosphorus binder. Hypermagnesemia does not occur provided the dialysate is magnesium free. The effect of magnesium supplementation in normal subjects after ingesting a meal supplemented with 5 mmol of magnesium acetate is to reduce the fractional gut absorption of phosphorus from 72% to 56%.[25] In general, $MgCO_3$ can be used together with a magnesium-free dialysate. Serum phosphorus came under control and remained unchanged over 2 years. Serum magnesium levels remained between 1.01 and 1.33 mmol/L. $MgCO_3$ was reported to be well tolerated by all patients. $MgCO_3$ binder with a low-magnesium dialysate is a good alternative to calcium binders.

Other binders include *calcium citrate* (21% elemental calcium), *ketovaline*, and *calcium ketoglutarate* or other calcium salts of ketoaminoacid and salts of polyuronic acid. Although calcium citrate is as effective as $CaCO_3$, its use should be limited because citrate salts markedly augment intestinal absorption of aluminum. Ketovaline is as effective as calcium acetate, but it is expensive. Calcium ketoglutarate is expensive. Some 30% has to be withdrawn due to gastrointestinal discomfort. The *polyuronic acid derivatives* are effective but there is not much experience with them.

A novel binder, *lanthanum carbonate*, has been evaluated recently in a randomized trial of 126 hemodialysis patients. Over 4 weeks it was well tolerated and reduced serum phosphorus and serum Ca × P product without hypercalcemia. In experimental animals, a dose of 1000–2000 mg/kg/day induced some decrease in bone formation and increase in osteoid tissue suggestive of osteomalacia. Current studies are evaluating the long-term effect of lanthanum carbonate in ESRD patients.

Dialysance of phosphorus

About 90% of patients on dialysis need further treatment to control hyperphosphatemia. The phosphorus removed during hemodialysis varies with the predialysis level of serum phosphorus and the efficiency of the dialyzer. In general, 500–600 mg phosphorus is removed during a 4-h conventional hemodialysis. The removal of phosphorus increased only to 600–700 mg per dialysis during 3 h of high-efficiency or high-flux dialysis. Others have described a phosphorus removal of 500–1000 mg. The amount removed declines steadily during treatment.

Several explanations account for the low mass transfer of phosphorus during hemodialysis. First, clearance by the dialyzers is 40–50% lower for phosphorus than for urea. The difference becomes greater at high blood flow rates. Second, the dialyzer clears only plasma phosphorus. Thus, excess of phosphorus, which accumulates between treatments, has a volume of distribution well beyond the extracellular space. The equilibration between the plasma and extravascular phosphorus is delayed. Consequently, serum phosphorus levels fall rapidly over the first 30–45 min of dialysis to values below 3.0 mg/100 mL. This reduces the phosphorus gradient between plasma and dialysate, resulting in a less efficient transfer. Furthermore, the initial decrease in serum phosphorus dictates an efflux of phosphorus from the intracellular space and bone, leading to a limited fall in phosphorus levels. *Postdialysis* serum phosphorus rebounds rapidly to predialysis values within 2–3 h after completion of dialysis. Finally, the increased hematocrit during erythropoietin reduces phosphorus removal during hemodialysis.

New dialyzer membranes have been used to improve phosphorus removal. The rates of clearance of phosphorus to urea with a cellulose or a polycarbonate membrane are 64% and 78% respectively. High-flux hemodialfiltration improves the ratio to only 30%. However, the mass removal rate of phosphorus is similar regardless of the membrane used. For example, the total phosphorus removed during 4 h of hemodialysis using a cuprophan membrane with a mean blood flow of 227 mL/min is 597 mg, while the removal with high-flux hemodialfiltration with a mean blood flow of 504 mL/min removes 721 mg. No differences in phosphorus transfer removal were noted in a preliminary comparison of dialysate solutions containing bicarbonate compared with acetate-based solutions. It is apparent that although dialysis removes substantial amounts of phosphorus, additional efforts to control hyperphosphatemia are required in 80–90% of patients.

The net removal of phosphorus may be slightly higher in continuous ambulatory peritoneal dialysis (CAPD) than in hemodialysis patients since CAPD is continuous and removes about 300 mg/day of phosphorus.

Treatment of hypocalcemia
Nutritional calcium supplements

Calcium carbonate or acetate can also be used to reverse a negative calcium balance. Patients with CRF have a normal or impaired intestinal calcium absorption. Patients with CRF are prescribed a diet with reduced dairy products and, consequently, low quantities of calcium. The dietary calcium intake in patients with advanced CRF is 400–700 mg/day. Generally, a neutral or positive balance for calcium can be achieved in uremic patients by increasing intake of calcium to 1.5 g/day. A positive calcium balance requires that calcium supplements be prescribed *between* meals. The amount prescribed should be ingested in several small doses.

$CaCO_3$ (4–10 g per day) administered to uremic patients reduced serum phosphorus and increased serum calcium and bicarbonate slightly. A daily oral dose of $CaCO_3$ 5–20 g given to hemodialysis patients improves bone biopsies and radiographs and reduces episodes of pseudogout and extraskeletal calcification, and reduces plasma alkaline phosphatase and serum PTH. However, patients with advanced CRF are more prone to develop hypercalcemia since urinary calcium is decreased. Calcium supplements should be used cautiously since the elevation of the Ca × P product predisposes to extraskeletal calcifications. Episodes of hypercalcemia are more frequent in patients with low serum phosphorus and, with ABD. Mild hypercalcemia (10.5–12 mg/dL) is usually asymptomatic, but patients may develop nausea, anorexia, vomiting, mental confusion, lethargy, pruritus, "red-eye syndrome," constipation, band keratopathy, and even sharp elevations in blood pressure.

The appropriate dialysate calcium concentration

Previously, the dialysate [Ca] was equivalent to diffusible calcium (e.g. 2.5 mequiv./L or 1.25 mmol/L); but because of hypocalcemia higher dialysate [Ca] (e.g. 3.5 mequiv./L) became preferable. Now, because of the high incidence of hypercalcemia from Ca^{2+}-containing binders, a return to a [Ca] of 2–5 mequiv./L dialysate has been promoted (Table 73.5).

The *ionized* blood [Ca] may fall during hemodialysis with a dialysate [Ca] of 2.5 mequiv./L. However, total blood calcium level may even increase because of an increase in serum albumin and correction of acidosis. A positive calcium balance occurs during hemodialysis with a dialysate [Ca] of 3.0–3.5 mequiv./L,[23] thereby delivering an inappropriate load of calcium with each dialysis. Dramatic increments in intradialytic serum ionized [Ca] occur with a dialysate [Ca] of 3.5 mequiv./L, whereas no significant changes occur with a dialysate [Ca] of 2.5 mequiv./L.[23] Flux of ionized calcium from dialysate to patient was observed with both 3.5 and 3.0 mequiv./L dialysate [Ca] but was not observed with 2.5 mequiv./L.[24] Thus, with a 3.5 mequiv./L dialysate [Ca], patients receive a large calcium

Table 73.5 Conditions associated with hypercalcemia in patients with renal failure

High dietary calcium uptake
Use of high-calcium dialysate (3–3.5 mequiv./L)
Treatment with vitamin D metabolites
Severe secondary HPT (tertiary HPT)
Aluminium-related bone disease
Phosphorus restriction and hypohosphatemia
Coexistence of other diseases causing hypercalcemia (e.g. multiple myeloma, sarcoidosis, tuberculosis, malignancy)
After successful kidney transplantation

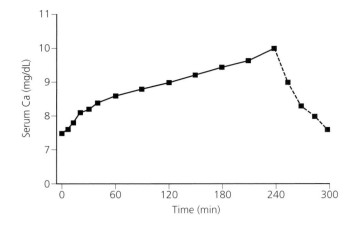

Figure 73.1 Intradialytic changes in serum calcium in five patients undergoing standard hemodialysis sessions of 4 h (dialysate calcium 3.5 mequiv./L). Note the increase in serum calcium and the fall to baseline values by 1 h after dialysis.

load during each dialysis, augmenting the risk of hypercalcemia; our own observations support this concern. By 1 h post dialysis the high serum [Ca] returns to predialysis values (Fig. 73.1) as calcium is deposited into soft tissue.[25] The intradialytic hypercalcemia is greater in patients with low bone turnover disease.

In two patients, massive tumoral shoulder calcifications marked a negative [Ca] gradient between dialysate and the patient blood, which induced the progressive disappearance of extraskeletal calcification.[26] Serum PTH was in the low-to-normal range and serum aluminum was consistently less than 20 µg/L. The patients were treated with *daily* hemodialysis using a dialysate [Ca] of 1 mequiv./L for a year. The *postdialysis* serum [Ca] steadily *decreased* with each dialysis; however, during the interdialytic period, plasma [Ca] actually became hypercalcemic for 8–12 weeks. During the 12 months of frequent dialysis therapy, the PTH level remained below 20 pg/mL, the tumoral calcification of the shoulder progressively disappeared and the patients' shoulders became functional.

There is little indication that a high dialysate [Ca] prevents bone disease. A dialysate [Ca] of 2.5 mequiv./L together with CaCO_3 may be effective in ameliorating secondary HPT. In addition, this dialysate [Ca] allows appropriate doses of calcium binders and vitamin D derivatives.[23]

Dialysate [Ca] of 3.5 mequiv./L in patients on CAPD provides higher [Ca] than those on hemodialysis[27] with a more prolonged PTH suppression. Peritoneal dialysate [Ca] of 2.5 mequiv./L is advisable in most patients treated with CAPD. In a randomized trial comparing 2.5 mequiv./L to 3.5 mequiv./L [Ca] dialysate, the 2.5 mequiv./L concentration reduced the frequency of severe hypercalcemia and allowed higher doses of calcitriol and CaCO_3. In a multi-center prospective randomized controlled trial, low dialysate [Ca] (2 mequiv./L) was compared with a standard dialysate (3.5 mequiv./L) concentration.[28] The lower [Ca] permitted an increase in the dose of CaCO_3 in patients who were maintained on a small dose of oral calcitriol (0.25 µg/day).

An increase in PTH may be corrected by appropriate dosing of calcitriol. In conclusion, dialysate [Ca] should be individualized. A dialysate [Ca] > 2.5 mequiv./L should be avoided whenever possible.

Use of calcitriol and its analogs

Despite appropriate intake of calcium and control of serum with phosphorus, with binders and a dialysate [Ca] of 3.5 mequiv./L, most patients develop overt secondary HPT. Appropriate use of calcitriol and its analogs has decreased the number of parathyroidectomies performed.[29] Patients should not be allowed to develop symptoms and signs of overt secondary HPT. Early therapy reduces PTH over 3–6 months, but requires a higher dose of calcitriol than for maintenance.

Two vitamin D_2 derivatives are available: 1-(OH)D_3 (alphacalcidol) and 1-(OH)D_2 (doxercalciferol), which is commercially available as Hecterol. Two nonhypercalcemic and nonhyperphosphatemic vitamin D analogs, 22-oxacalcitriol and 19-Nor-1,25(OH)_2D_2, have been developed, and the latter has been released as Zemplar.

Calcifidiol

The main disadvantages of calcifidiol are its lack of potency compared with calcitriol and its longer half-life. Several days are required for hypercalcemia to resolve. Deficiency of 25-(OH)D_3 is usually related to poor nutrition. Vitamin D supplementation in dialysis patients may be given at a dose of 1000–2000 U/day to induce "normal" 25-(OH)D_3 levels.

Calcitriol

Oral calcitriol (Rocaltrol) Oral calcitriol is highly efficacious in the treatment of patients with renal osteodystrophy. Doses of 0.25–2 µg/day to lower serum PTH, decrease bone resorption surface and marrow fibrosis, and improve symptoms in patients with secondary HPT, with a marked improvement in endosteal fibrosis and mineralization.

In a double-blind study of 31 dialysis patients, Berl et al gave either calcitriol, in an average dose of 0.82 µg/day, or regular vitamin D, in a small dose of 400 IU/day for 12 weeks; an increase in serum calcium, a decrease in serum PTH and improvement of osteitis fibrosa was noted only in those receiving calcitriol.[30] Two major problems with oral calcitriol are hypercalcemia and hyperphosphatemia. These usually occur late in therapy as PTH levels return to normal.

Prophylactic treatment in predialysis patients with calcitriol (0.125–0.50 µg) may prevent the development of secondary HPT. CRF may reverse and/or prevent secondary HPT but is associated with hypercalcemia, hyperphosphatemia, hypercalciuria, or impairment in renal function.[31] Children should always be treated to prevent growth retardation. Patients with slowly progressive CRF benefit from early therapy. Complications are usually reversible. Calcitriol impairs tubular creatinine secretion. Thus, serum creatinine may increase without change in true GFR.[32] Hypercalcemia may increase renal calcium–phosphorus deposition and impair renal function. In order to prevent secondary HPT, it is not yet clear whether it is better to administer calcitriol, to restrict phosphorus, or to add calcium supplements. Phosphorus restriction and calcium supplementation ameliorates secondary HPT in early CRF.[33]

Intravenous calcitriol (Calcijex) Calcitriol, given intravenously, directly inhibits the parathyroid gland. Thus, intravenous calcitriol administered three times weekly with dialysis suppresses PTH with less undesirable hypercalcemic episodes. The apparent additional benefit of intravenous calcitriol administration may be related to higher peak levels[34] and lack of direct contact of calcitriol with intestinal cell mucosa, which minimizes absorption of calcium and phosphorus. Oral administration of calcitriol, to maintain serum calcium at the upper limit of normal, did not alter PTH levels, but marked suppression of PTH levels (70.1 ± 3.2%) was observed in 20 patients receiving intravenous calcitriol.[35] A beneficial effect of intravenous calcitriol has been shown in patients intolerant to oral calcitriol, with persistent hypercalcemia and marked secondary HPT. Thus, hypercalcemia may not be an *absolute* contraindication to the use of intravenous calcitriol. Intravenous calcitriol improves osteitis fibrosa even in patients refractory to oral treatment.

Intravenous calcitriol has been used at an initial dose of 0.5–1 µg/dialysis. Depending on the PTH response, the maintenance doses are 0.5–4 µg/dialysis. Gallieni et al[36] used an average dose of 0.87 µg/dialysis in a large multicenter study. Cannella et al[37] used 30 ng/kg body weight per dialysis (2.1 µg/70 kg) with a dialysate [Ca] of 2.5 mequiv./L, calcium acetate as a phosphorus binder, and intermittent aluminum hydroxide as needed. They obtained control of PTH, improvement in bone histology, and a decrease in parathyroid gland size. Doses greater than 4 µg/dialysis may be effective in patients with severe HPT. Patients resistant to oral calcitriol may benefit from intravenous calcitriol. Cannella et al observed resistance to low intravenous doses calcitriol in some patients, but PTH responded to higher intravenous doses. Fernandez and Llach[38] found a sequential increase in calcitriol dose (2 µg–4 µg–6 µg) to be successful in patients with secondary HPT. Llach et al[39] reported the dose of intravenous calcitriol in patients with severe secondary HPT should be *commensurate* with the level of PTH. The mean initial maximum dose of calcitriol was 3.8 µg/dialysis. There was a dramatic decrease in PTH levels, and PTH decreased from 1826 ± 146 to 211 ± 48 pg/mL, whereas serum calcium and phosphorus remained unchanged in most patients.

In summary, intravenous calcitriol is effective in controlling secondary HPT in many patients, and the dose depends on its severity. The major problem with intravenous calcitriol is development of hypercalcemia and hyperphosphatemia which is more frequent as PTH approach normal levels.

Oral pulse therapy with calcitriol In patients with moderate secondary HPT a 4-µg pulse of oral calcitriol *twice weekly* reduced PTH and the size of the parathyroid glands. A controlled double-blind study by Quarles et al[40] compared oral pulse calcitriol (2–4 µg) versus equivalent doses of intravenous calcitriol in 19 hemodialysis patients. The initial effect of intravenous calcitriol on PTH was greater, but later PTH increased in both groups.[40] By the end of the study both intravenous and oral calcitriol doses were low because of hyperphosphatemia and hypercalcemia.

Other routes of administration *Intraperitoneal* calcitriol is effective in adult and pediatric CAPD patients. Calcitriol should be administered three times per week, in the peritoneal bag for the last dwelling of the day as the last 100 mL of the fluid is delivered to prevent absorption of calcitriol onto the bag. Intraperitoneal calcitriol achieves serum levels four- to fivefold higher than oral administration. Calcitriol given subcutaneously achieves higher serum levels than the oral route and similar levels to intraperitoneal.

Paricalcitol (Zemplar)

Hypercalcemia and hyperphosphatemia are common complications of calcitriol therapy. The structure of paricalcitol (Zemplar) is similar to calcitriol in the uremic rat.[41] Paricalcitol suppresses pre-pro-PTH mRNA in the uremic rat in a way similar to calcitriol, without inducing hypercalcemia or hyperphosphatemia.[42] Unlike calcitriol, its analog suppresses the intestinal vitamin D receptor resulting in a lack of calcemic activity. In a double-blind placebo-controlled, randomized multicenter study, 35 hemodialysis patients were treated three times weekly for 4 weeks with either intravenous paricalcitol (0.04–0.24 µq/kg) or placebo.[43] There was a significant reduction in PTH in patients treated with paricalcitol ($P = 0.006$). In phase III studies of 78 dialysis patients on intravenous paricalcitol or placebo for 12 weeks, PTH decreased from 785 ± 66 to 370 ± 73 pg/mL without significant changes in serum calcium or phosphorus (Fig. 73.2).[44] In a recent study, 37 patients with ESRD and severe HPT (PTH 901 ± 58 pg/mL) who were resistant to intravenous calcitriol were treated with paricalcitol for 16 months. PTH decreased from 901 pg/mL to 165 ± 24 pg/mL, while serum calcium and phosphorus did not change significantly. Thus, paricalcitol is safe and effective in dialysis patients with secondary HPT, and has less effect on serum calcium and phosphorus levels than calcitriol.

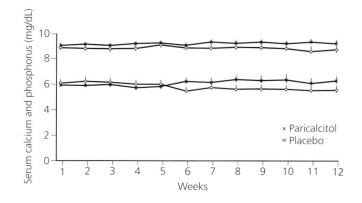

Figure 73.2 The values of serum calcium (Ca) (upper lines) and serum phosphorus (P) (lower lines) during the 12 weeks of study in placebo (O) and paricalcitol-treated (X) groups ($P < 0.05$).

Doxercalciferol (Hectorol)

Doxercalciferol (1α-OH-D$_2$) can suppress secondary HPT in ESRD.[46] Both doxercalciferol and alphacalcidol must undergo 25-hydroxylation in the liver to become the more biologically active form.

Rat studies showed similar effects of doxercalciferol and alphacalcidol in healing rachitic bone lesions, mobilizing calcium from bone, and enhancing intestinal calcium absorption, but much higher doses of doxercalciferol were required. However, doxercalciferol was less toxic than alphacalcidol. In women with postmenopausal osteoporosis, daily doxercalciferol doses as high as 5 μg were administered before hypercalciuria developed. In the uremic serum, calcium and phosphorus concentrations are unchanged after paricalcitol but increased with doxercalciferol. Thus, there is serious doubt about the selectivity (i.e. PTH suppression without inducing hypercalcemia or hyperphosphatemia) of this vitamin D analog in ESRD patients.

ESRD patients treated for 12 weeks with oral doses of doxercalciferol, either 4.0 μg/day or 4.0 μg three times a week, had PTH decreased from 672 ± 70 pg/mL to 289 ± 36 pg/mL, an increase in [Ca] from 8.8 mg/dL to 9.5 mg/dL, and episodes of hypercalcemia.

In a placebo-controlled study[47] (10 g three times weekly) 83% of the patients reached the target control for PTH (150–300 pg/mL), and the incidence of hypercalcemia was slight (3.26% for doxercalciferol, versus 0.46% for placebo, $P < 0.01$). Serum calcium rose during treatment, from 9.0 ± 0.1 mg/dL to 9.8 ± 0.1 mg/dL, and serum phosphorus remained unchanged. After 12 weeks of intravenous doxercalciferol treatment, PTH decreased below 50% of the initial value in 78% of patients, and the incidence of hypercalcemia was only 0.86%. Suppression of PTH levels was equivalent in the oral and the intravenous trials, but the incidence of hypercalcemia (> 11.2 mg/dL) was greater with oral administration. In both groups there was a substantial increase from baseline in serum calcium and phosphorus concentration. Thus doxercalciferol induces substantial hypercalcemia and hyperphosphatemia.

Alphacalcidol

Both short-term and long-term clinical trials in CRF have shown that 1-(OH)D$_3$ (alphacalcidol) is also effective in suppressing PTH. Treatment with phenobarbital, phenytoin, or glutethimide, or liver disease, impairs the hepatic 25-hydroxylation and results in impaired action of 1-α-(OH)D$_3$. The dose required to increase intestinal calcium absorption or to treat hyperparathyroid bone disease is one-and-a-half to two times that of calcitriol.

Calcimimetic agents

A new approach to decrease PTH uses calcimimetics, which stimulate the calcium-sensing receptor (CaSR) by minimizing the effect of blood ionized calcium.[48] High concentrations of the CaSR are found in the parathyroid cell membrane, in the kidney, in bone, the brain, and the lungs. Relatively small changes of extracellular ionized calcium activate the receptor. The CaSR is also sensitive to magnesium, trivalent elements, gadolinium and lanthanum, and polycationic compounds. Decreased secretion of PTH by parathyroid cells occurs within seconds of increasing blood ionized [Ca]. Stimulation of the receptors in the kidney leads to an increase in urinary calcium and magnesium.

Calcimimetic agents diminish release of PTH from the parathyroid glands across a wide range of blood-ionized calcium concentrations. Serum PTH levels fall within a few hours of oral administration, and serum calcium concentrations decline subsequently. The main calcimimetic studied is a phenylalkylamine (R)-N-(3-methoxy-alpha-phenylether)-3-(2-chlorophenyl)-2-propylamine (R-568).[49]

Experimental studies in uremic rats showed that R-568 acutely decreased proliferation of parathyroid cells[49] and reversed the histologic changes of osteitis fibrosa.

Short-term studies in patients on hemodialysis given single doses of R-568 showed an abrupt fall in PTH levels and, at higher doses, a fall in ionized [Ca]. Daily doses of R-568 100 mg administered to hemodialysis patients with secondary HPT reduced PTH levels by approximately 75% within 2 h and remained below pretreatment levels throughout the 15 days of the study. Blood ionized [Ca] decreased on the first day and 7 of the 16 patients dropped out of the study because of hypocalcemia.[50]

Thus calcimimetics are potent and rapid inhibitors of PTH secretion, but the development of hypocalcemia is a major concern. Unfortunately, the bioavailability of R-568 is low, and its metabolism is variable. Concomitant treatment with vitamin D may ameliorate the hypocalcemic effects.

Nonsurgical parathyroid gland intervention

Percutaneous fine-needle ethanol injection into enlarged parathyroid glands under ultrasonic guidance is successful in about 60% of people and in those who had relapsed after subtotal parathyroidectomy. The most common side-effect is transitory recurrent nerve palsy. *Selective* percutaneous ethanol injection in glands larger than 0.5 cm^3 renders patients responsive to medical therapy thereafter. Direct injection of calcitriol into enlarged parathyroid glands decreases PTH and restores the responsiveness to calcitriol.

Parathyroidectomy

The clinical indications for parathyroid surgery include the *unequivocal evidence of secondary HPT* (very high levels of serum PTH and/or the presence of osteitis fibrosa on bone biopsy), *together with any of the following:* (1) persistent hypercalcemia not attributable to other causes; (2) persistent hyperphosphatemia despite proper use of phosphorus binders; (3) serum Ca × P product that consistently exceeds 70–75 mg^2/dL^2; (4) progressive skeletal and articular pain, fractures or deformities due to secondary HPT; and (5) calciphylaxis. A 6–8-week trial with intravenous pulses of paricalcitol should be tried prior to parathyroidectomy.

The surgical procedures include (1) *subtotal* PTx; (2) *total* PTx *with autotransplantation*; and (3) *total* PTx *without* autotransplantation. Most important are the timing and a surgeon who is highly experienced. It is important to avoid spillage of abnormal cells, which may lead to recurrence. Some advocate PTx with autotransplantation, because this morbidity and mortality of a reoperation in the forearm is lower than in the neck. However, malignant degeneration of the autografted parathyroid tissue has been reported, as well as muscle invasion by recurrent parathyroid hyperplasia. Total PTx without autotransplantation still remains controversial. Parathyroid glands should be located *preoperatively* by sestamibi scan of the parathyroid glands, since the number and location of glands are highly variable. *During surgery*, the most suitable gland to retain is partially resected – usually the least hyperplastic one. Since the residual parathyroid tissue can undergo hyperplasia, a metal clip and/or a long, black silk suture should mark the remaining gland. Serum calcium concentration almost invariably falls after PTx. The degree of hypocalcemia is related to the severity of osteitis fibrosa. In the absence of PTH, calcium influx to the bone increases dramatically leading to hypocalcemia and the "hungry bone syndrome." To minimize the postoperative hypocalcemia, oral calcitriol 0.5–1.0 µg/day should be administered immediately after PTx with oral $CaCO_3$ (1–3 g of elemental calcium), and increased by 0.5–1.0 g/day at intervals of 3–7 days until serum calcium begins to increase. The goal is to maintain calcium levels above 8 mg/dL. If the serum calcium falls below 7.5 mg/dL, or if tetany appears, intravenous calcium should be given together with oral calcitriol. After PTx, careful monitoring of serum calcium is mandatory since tetany occurring in a uremic patient with severe bone disease may be catastrophic. In patients with marked skeletal disease, hypocalcemia may occasionally persist for 2–3 months after PTx. Normalization of elevated plasma alkaline phosphatase indicates that bone healing is largely completed. In the postoperative management of patients with marked periarticular calcifications, it may be wise to maintain a modest hypocalcemia – that is, a serum calcium level of 8.0–9.0 mg/dL – until the ectopic calcifications have resolved.

Failure of serum calcium concentration to decrease after surgery indicates either that too much residual parathyroid tissue was left, or that ectopic or supernumerary glands were missed, or that osteitis fibrosa was not responsible for the hypercalcemia.

Hypophosphatemia and *hypomagnesemia* are also frequent after PTx due to the "hungry bone syndrome." Phosphorus salts aggravate hypocalcemia and should not be given unless the serum phosphorus falls to < 1.5–2 mg/dL. Occasionally, the administration of *calcium-containing phosphorus binders* may be indicated to maintain serum phosphorus concentration in the range of 3.5–5.0 mg/dL. Calcium carbonate or acetate are the agents of choice, and aluminum salts must be avoided. If serum magnesium falls below 1.5 mg/dL, oral supplements of magnesium should be given. Hypomagnesemia may contribute to refractory hypocalcemia as it reduces PTH secretion and leads to skeletal resistance to the action of PTH. *Hyperkalemia* reflects the fact that PTH plays a role in potassium homeostasis. Even modest hyperkalemia in the immediate postoperative period may cause substantial electrocardiographic abnormalities associated with concomitant hypocalcemia.

Treatment of idiopathic adynamic bone disease

It seems advisable to *prevent* excessive suppression of PTH (less than one-and-a-half to three times the upper limit of normal) since mildly increased PTH is required for normal bone formation in dialysis patients. Most dialysis patients with PTH levels in the normal range may need to be treated with a dialysate [Ca] of 2.0 to 2.5 mequiv./L to increase PTH and improve the low-turnover bone state. The reversibility of parathyroid gland suppression in CAPD patients using a lower dialysate [Ca] has been confirmed.

Other treatments

Biphosphonates are analogs of pyrophosphate with a potent inhibitory effect on osteoclastic bone resorption. There are a few studies on bisphosphonates in CRF. Indications for these drugs may include hypercalcemic patients with increased bone turnover, and those with extraosseous calcifications due to high Ca × P product. Pamidronate has not been approved in CRF due to its potential nephrotoxicity. However, several reports suggest that pamidronate (60–90 mg) is safe and effective in the treatment of hypercalcemia induced by calcium-containing phosphorus binders, and/or calcitriol or alphacalcidol.

Patients undergoing regular dialysis receive periodic injections of *heparin* that is associated with decreased skeletal mineralization. A positive correlation has been shown between the rate of decrease in bone mass and the regular dosage of heparin in dialysis patients. Osteoporosis, multiple fractures and pseudoarthrosis have been reported in patients receiving 15 000–30 000 U/day of heparin over long periods of time. Dialysis patients may not receive sufficient heparin to cause problems. However, technetium-labeled heparin accumulates in the bones of the knees and shoulders in hemodialyzed patients.

Management of calciphylaxis

Patients with CUA can die of sepsis and ischemic events. The following therapy for CUA is recommended:

1. Stop oral calcium, use noncalcium-containing binders, and try to control serum phosphorus to less than 6.0 mg/dL.
2. If the patient has overt HPT (intact PTH above 600 pg/mL), emergency PTx should be performed.
3. If HPT is not present, daily dialysis (5–6 days per week) with a low dialysate [Ca] may be beneficial.
4. Debridement, local wound care, and treatment of sepsis are crucial.

Parathyroidectomy should be performed only in selected cases. Early reports recommending PTx were mostly patients with severe HPT,[13] whereas later reports showed that PTx was not successful.[16] Patients with low PTH levels can develop CUA that is unresponsive to PTx, and CUA occurs in patients after PTx. Thus, PTx should not be performed in patients with low PTH. In a review of 47 patients with CUA, Budisavijevic et al[51] described 31 patients who had PTx performed after developing CUA; 50% of those patients died in an average of 9 weeks from PTx.

Local injections in adipose areas (where the lesions usually develop), blood products, corticosteroids, and immuno-suppressants should be avoided. Hyperbaric oxygen therapy has improved CUA in CAPD patients.

References

1. Stanbury SW, Lumb GA: Metabolic studies of renal osteodystrophy: I. Calcium, phosphorus and nitrogen metabolism in rickets, osteomalacia and hyperparathyroidism complicating chronic uremia and the osteomalacia of the adult Franconi syndrome. Medicine 1962;41:1–31.
2. Ganesh SK, Stack AG, Levin NW, et al: Association of elevated serum PO_4, Ca × PO_4 product, and parathyroid hormone with cardiac mortality risk in chronic hemodialysis patients. J Am Soc Nephrol 2001;12:2131–2138.
3. Llach F: Cardiac calcifications: Dealing with another risk factor in patients with renal failure. Semin Dial 1999;12:293–295.
4. Braun J, Olendorf M, Moshage W, et al: Electron beam computed tomography in the evaluation of cardiac calcification in chronic dialysis patients. Am J Kidney Dis 1996;27:394–401.
5. Goodman WG, Goldin J, Kuzon BD, et al: Coronary artery calcification in young adults with ESRD who are undergoing dialysis. N Engl J Med 2000;342:1478–1483.
6. Achenback S, Moshage W, Rogers D, et al: Value of electron-beam computed tomography for the noninvasive detection of high-grade coronary artery stenoses and occlusions. N Engl J Med 1998;339:1964–1971.
7. Selye H: Calciphylaxis. Chicago, IL: University of Chicago Press, 1962.
8. Anderson DC, Stewart WK, Piercy DM: Calcifying panniculitis with fat and skin necrosis in a case of uremia with autonomous hyperparathyroidism. Lancet 1968;2:323–325.
9. Coates T, Kirkland GS, Dymock RB, et al: Ischemic tissue necrosis (calciphylaxis) in renal failure. Am J Kidney Dis 1998;32:384–391.
10. Katz AL, Hampers CL, Merrill JP: Secondary hyperparathyroidism and renal osteodystrophy in chronic renal failure: Analysis of 195 patients, with observations on the effects of chronic dialysis, kidney transplantation and subtotal parathyroidectomy. Medicine 1969;48:333–374.
11. Massry SG, Coburn JW, Hartenbower DL, et al: Mineral content of human skin in uremia. Effect of secondary hyperparathyroidism and hemodialysis. Proc Eur Dial Transplant Assoc 1970;7:146–148.
12. Campisol JM, Almirall J, Martin E, et al: Calcium-carbonate-induced calciphylaxis. Nephrology 1989;51:549–550.
13. Gipstein RM, Coburn JW, Adams DA, et al: Calciphylaxis in man. Arch Intern Med 1976;136:1273–1280.
14. Llach F, Goldblatt M, Freundlich RE, et al: The evolving pattern of calcific uremic arteriolopathy (calciphylaxis). J Am Soc Nephrol 2000; 11:567A.
15. Bleyer AJ, Choi M, Igwenezie B, et al: A case control study of proximal calciphylaxis. Am J Kidney Dis 1998;32:376–383.
16. Hafner J, Keusch G, Wahl C, et al: Uremic small artery disease with medical calcification and intimal hypertrophy (so-called calciphylaxis): A complication of chronic renal failure and benefit from parathyroidectomy. J Am Acad Dermatol 1995;33:954–962.
17. Block GA, Hulbert-Shearon TE, Levin NW, et al: Association of serum phosphorus and calcium × phosphate product with mortality risk in chronic hemodialysis patients: a national study. Am J Kidney Dis 1998;31:607–617.
18. Schoenfeld P, Henry R, Laird N: Assessment of nutritional status of the National Cooperative Dialysis Study population. Kidney Int 1980;23:580–588.
19. Rosenbaum DP, Holmes-Farley SR, Mandeville WH, et al: Effect of Renagel, a non-absorbable, cross-linked, polymeric phosphate binder on urinary phosphorus excretion in rats. Nephrol Dial Transplant 1997;12:961–964.
20. Burke SK, Slatopolsky EA, Goldberg DI: Renagel, a novel calcium- and aluminum-free phosphate binder, inhibits phosphate absorption in normal volunteers. Nephrol Dial Transplant 1997;12:1640–1644.
21. Chertow GM, Burke SK, Lazarus JM, et al: A phase II trial of poly(allylamine hydrochloride) (Renagel) in hemodialysis patients. Am J Kidney Dis 1997;1:66–71.
22. Raggi P, Burke SK, Dillon MA, et al: Sevelamer attenuates the progression of coronary artery and aortic calcifications compared with calcium-based phosphate binders. J Am Soc Nephrol 2001;12:239A.
23. Argiles A, Kerr PG, Canaud B, et al: Calcium kinetics and the long-term effects of lowering dialysate calcium concentration. Kidney Int 1993;43:630–640.
24. Hou SH, Zhao J, Ellman CF, et al: Calcium and phosphorus fluxes during hemodialysis with a low calcium dialysate. Am J Kidney Dis 1991;18:217–224.
25. Llach F, Coburn JW: Renal osteodystrophy and maintenance dialysis. In Maher JF (ed): Replacement of Renal Function by Dialysis. Dordrecht/Boston/Lancaster: Kluwer Academic Publishers, 1989, pp 911–952.
26. Fernandez E, Montoliu J: Successful treatment of massive uremic tumoral calcinosis with daily haemodialysis and very low calcium dialysate. Nephrol Dial Transplant 1994;9:1207–1209.
27. Bender FH, Bernardini J, Piraino B: Calcium mass transfer with dialysate containing 1.25 and 1.75 mmol/L calcium in peritoneal dialysis patients. Am J Kidney Dis 1992;20:367–371.
28. Weinreich T, Passlick-Deetjen J, Ritz E: Low dialysate calcium in continuous ambulatory peritoneal dialysis: a randomized controlled multicenter trial. The Peritoneal Dialysis Multicenter Study Group. Am J Kidney Dis 1995;25:452–460.
29. Cohen EP, Moulder JE: Parathyroidectomy in chronic renal failure: Has medical care reduced the need for surgery? Nephron 2001;89:271–273.
30. Berl T, Berns AS, Hufer WE, et al: 1,25 dihydroxycholecalciferol effects in chronic dialysis. A double blind-controlled study. Ann Intern Med 1978;88:774–780.
31. Ritz E, Kuster S, Schmidt-Gayk H, et al: Low dose calcitriol prevents the rise in 1,84 iPTH without affecting serum calcium and phosphate. Prospective placebo controlled multicenter trial (abstract). Nephrol Dial Transplant 1995;10:2228–2234.
32. Bertoli M, Luisetto G, Ruffatti A, et al: Renal function during calcitriol therapy in chronic renal failure. Clin Nephrol 1990;33:98–102.
33. Martinez I, Saracho R, Montenegro J, et al: The importance of dietary calcium and phosphorus in the secondary hyperparathyroidism of patients with early renal failure. Am J Kidney Dis 1997;29:496–502.
34. Reichel H, Szabo A, Uhl J, et al: Intermittent versus continuous administration of $1,25(OH)_2 D_3$ in experimental renal hyperparathyroidism. Kidney Int 1993;44:1259–1265.
35. Slatopolsky E, Weerts C, Thielan J, et al: Marked suppression of secondary hyperpararathyroidism by intravenous administration of 1,25 dihydroxycholecalciferol in uremic patients. J Clin Invest 1984;74:2136–2143.
36. Gallieni M, Brancaccio D, Padovese P, et al: Italian Group For The Study Of Intravenous Calcitriol: Low-dose intravenous calcitriol treatment of secondary hyperparathyroidism in hemodialysis patients. Kidney Int 1992;42:1191–1198.
37. Cannella G, Bonucci E, Rolla D, et al: Evidence of healing of secondary hyperparathyroidism in chronically hemodialyzed uremic patients treated with long-term intravenous calcitriol. Kidney Int 1994;46:1124–1132.
38. Fernandez E, Llach F: Guidelines for dosing of intravenous calcitriol in dialysis patients with hyperparathyroidism. Nephrol Dial 1996;11:96–101.
39. Llach F, Hervas J, Cerezo S: The importance of dosing intravenous calcitriol in dialysis patients with severe hyperparathyroidism. Am J Kidney Dis 1995;26:845–851.
40. Quarles LD, Yohay DA, Carroll BA, et al: Prospective trial of pulse oral versus intravenous calcitriol treatment of hyperparathyroidism in ESRD. Kidney Int 1994;45:1710–1721.
41. Brown AJ: Vitamin D analogues. Am J Kidney Dis 1998;32:S25–S39.
42. Slatopolsky EA, Finch J, Denda M, et al: A new analog of calcitriol, 19-Nor-$1,25(OH)_3D_2$ suppresses parathyroid hormone secretion in uremic rats in the absence of hypercalcemia. Am J Kidney Dis 1995;26:852–860.

43. Llach F, Keshav G, Goldblat MV, et al: Suppression of parathyroid hormone secretion in hemodialysis patients by a novel vitamin D analogue: 19-Nor-α-1,25–dihydroxyvitamin D_2. Am J Kidney Dis 1998;32:D48–D54.

44. Martin KJ, Gonzalez EA, Gellens M, et al: 19-Nor-α-1,25-dihydroxyvitamin D_2 (paricalcitol) safely and effectively reduces the levels of intact PTH in patients on hemodialysis. J Am Soc Nephrol 1998;9:1427–1432.

45. Llach F, Yudd M: Paricalcitol in dialysis patients with calcitriol-resistant secondary hyperparathyroidism. Am J of Kidney Dis. 2001;8:S45–S50.

46. Tan AUJ, Levine BS, Mazess RB, et al: Effective suppression of parathyroid hormone by 1 alpha-hydroxy-vitamin D2 in hemodialysis patients with moderate to severe secondary hyperparathyroidism. Kidney Int 1997;51:317–323.

47. Frazao JM, Chesney RW, Coburn JW: Intermittent oral 1-alpha-hydroxyvitamin D_2 is effective and safe for the suppression of secondary hyperparathyroidism in haemodialysis patients. 1-alpha-D2 Study Group. Nephrol Dial Transplant 1998;13:68–72.

48. Nemeth EF: Calcium receptors as novel drug targets. *In* Bikezikian JP, Raisz LG, Rodan GA (eds): Principles in Bone Biology. New York: Academic Press, 1996, pp 1019–1035.

49. Wada M, Furuya Y, Sakiyama J: The calcimimetic compound NPS R-568 suppresses parathyroid cell proliferation in rats with renal insufficiency: control of parathyroid cell growth via a calcium receptor. J Clin Invest 1997;100:2977–2983.

50. Antonsen JE, Sherrard, Andress DL: A calcimimetic agent acutely suppresses parathyroid hormone levels in patients with chronic renal failure. Kidney Int 1998;53:223–227.

51. Budisavijevic MN, Chiik D, Ploth DW: Calciphylaxis in chronic renal failure. J Am Soc Nephrol 1996;7:978–982.

Cardiovascular Complications of Endstage Renal Disease

Robert N. Foley and Patrick S. Parfrey

Background

Angina pectoris, myocardial infarction, dysrhythmia, cardiac failure, stroke, and peripheral vascular disease are common in endstage renal disease (ESRD). Treatment guidelines for hypertension and hypercholesterolemia are predicated on underlying risk levels. A cardiovascular event probability of 20% per decade defines high-risk status.[1,2] Incidence rates of approximately 10% per year are seen for both ischemic heart disease and cardiac failure in dialysis populations. These are orders of magnitude higher than in the general population.[3,4]

Treatment goals for uremic patients: risk factors and their management

The following are goals to minimize cardiovascular risk in patients with chronic kidney disease (Table 74.1): non-smoking; normal glycemia; blood pressure less than 130/85 mmHg; low-density lipoprotein (LDL)-cholesterol < 100 mm/dL; hemoglobin 11–12 g/dL; single pool variable volume $Kt/V > 1.2$ (or urea reduction ratio > 65%) in hemodialysis patients, and for CAPD (continuous ambulatory peritoneal dialysis) patients a total Kt/V_{urea} of at least 2.0 per week; total creatinine clearance of at least 60 L/week/1.73 m^2 for high and high-average transporters, and 50 L/week/1.73 m^2 in low and low-average transporters.

There have been very few controlled trials to define optimum management strategies in chronic kidney disease patients. The prescribing of potentially cardio-protective medications such as aspirin, statins, β-blockers, and angiotensin-converting enzyme inhibitors (ACEIs) to subjects with chronic kidney disease is typically far less than

50% even among those with cardiovascular disease.[5] The only solution to the therapeutic uncertainty created by lack of evidence is to create the evidence. It is our opinion that patients not entering trials should be treated as a "high-risk category" for management of classical risk factors.

Non-smoking, normal glycemia, and exercise

Healthy lifestyles should be advocated for renal patients. The evidence linking smoking to ESRD mortality is strongest in diabetic patients.[6] Smoking has been linked with death in hemodialysis patients in the US.[7] Diabetes accounts for half, or more, of new cases of ESRD. The natural history and risk factors for cardiac disease in diabetic ESRD need to be prioritized, given that both these factors clearly dominate outcome. There is evidence from the Diabetes Control and Complications Trial[8] that lower blood sugar levels reduce cardiovascular outcomes in diabetics without ESRD. Whether such an approach has an impact on survival in diabetic people with ESRD is unknown. High levels of glycosylated hemoglobin and advanced glycosylation endproducts have been associated with adverse outcomes in diabetic ESRD.[9,10]

Hypertension

Numerous trials in the 1970s and 1980s confirmed that treating blood pressure levels greater than 160/95 mmHg was beneficial. The reduction in the incidence of stroke, on average by 41%, was more dramatic than the reduction seen in coronary heart disease, which averaged 14%.[11] Treating hypertension is at least as beneficial in elderly subjects. Isolated systolic blood pressure should be treated in this patient group.[12] β-Blockers and diuretics formed the cornerstone of therapy in earlier studies. The dihydropyridine calcium channel antagonists, nifedipine and nitrendipine, were shown to be superior to placebo in reducing cardiovascular endpoints in elderly patients with systolic hypertension.[13,14]

It remains to be seen whether cardiovascular risk reaches a plateau, or even rises again, as blood pressure targets are lowered progressively in blood pressure trials. For example, in the HOT trial[15] felodipine was the primary antihypertensive; the trial failed to show that diastolic blood pressure targets below 80 mmHg were superior to targets below 85 mmHg or below 90 mmHg, when analyzed by group assignment with an intention-to-treat philosophy. When trying to generalize to renal patients, it should be borne in mind that the HOPE trial showed convincingly that ACEIs improve cardiovascular outcome

Table 74.1 Selected targets to minimize the risk of new cardiac disease and the progression of established cardiac disease in chronic kidney disease

Goal	Epidemiological evidence in CKD	RCT evidence in Non-CKD population	RCT evidence in CKD population	Comments
Nonsmoking	Yes	No	No	
Normal glycemia	Yes	Yes	No	
BP < 130/85	Yes and No ↑ BP associated with LVH, IHD, HF ↓ BP associated with death	Yes	No	Association between ↓ BP and death may reflect very high burden of endstage cardiomyopathy in ESRD patients
LDL < 100 mg/dl	Yes and No. Yes in transplant. No in dialysis. If anything ↓ cholesterol associated with death in dialysis	Yes	No	Association between ↓ cholesterol and mortality may be a reflection of malnutrition
Hemoglobin 11–12 g/dL	Yes	No	Yes	Clear benefits in terms of quality of life and LVH
$Kt/V > 1.2$ (or URR > 65%) in hemodialysis patients, total $Kt/V_{urea} > 2.0$ per week and a total creatinine clearance of at least 60 L/wk/1.73 m² for high high-average transporters and and 50 L/wk/1.73 m² in low and low-average transporters	Yes. Associated with CV and non-CV mortality	No	Awaited	

BP, blood pressure; CKD, chronic kidney disease; CV, cardiovascular; ESRD, endstage renal disease; HF, heart failure; IHD, ischemic heart disease; LDL, low-density lipoprotein; LVH, left ventricular hypertrophy; RCT, randomized controlled trial; URR, urea reduction ratio.

and survival in people at high cardiovascular risk. The age and comorbidity profile of participants in this study were broadly similar to current renal outpatient populations.[16]

Aggressive control of blood pressure reduces the rate of loss of renal function in chronic kidney diseases. Many trials with hard clinical endpoints have shown that ACEIs are superior to placebo.[17-19] Although these studies have usually aimed for equal blood pressure targets in both arms, the blood pressures achieved in the ACEI arms have tended to be lower, so that it has been difficult to quantify the extent to which renal protection reflects lower blood pressure or reduction of angiotensin II (Ang II) levels. Even in patients who become dependent on dialysis, an intervention that slows the rate of loss of residual renal function would be highly desirable. Whether ACEIs still have this effect after the onset of dialysis therapy is unknown. This class of agent has been shown to improve the outcome of patients with low ejection fractions and symptomatic cardiac failure, conditions that are very common in ESRD. We use ACEIs as preferred antihypertensive agents in chronic renal failure patients. There have been no randomised controlled trials in dialysis patients to support such a policy.

In the ongoing AASK trial,[20] after an interim analysis, in which only the relative effects of amlodipine and ramipril were compared, it was decided to stop the amlodipine arm because of superior renal outcomes in the ramipril arm. Although this study tells us that "ramipril is better than amlodipine" it cannot tell whether amlodipine per se has a neutral, beneficial, or harmful effect, because there was no placebo arm. Several recent studies have reported on the use of angiotensin II receptor antagonists (in type 2 diabetic patients with nephropathy).[21-23] The beneficial effect of these agents, and the lack of harm caused by calcium channel blockers are relevant because multiple antihypertensives are often needed to achieve recommended targets in renal failure populations.

An interesting epidemiological observation has been reported by several authors: the lower the blood pressure in the average dialysis patient the higher the mortality risk.[24,25] In our studies, cardiac enlargement, ischemic heart disease, and especially cardiac failure were major signs of impending death; high blood pressure (even within what is considered the "normal" range) was associated with progressive cardiac enlargement, and new-onset ischemic heart disease and cardiac failure. Admission to hospital for cardiac failure preceded two-thirds of all deaths; after admission for cardiac failure, low blood pressure was the single factor predictive of death. It is likely therefore, that the inverse association between blood pressure and mortality is a real phenomenon, and reflects the very high burden of endstage cardiomyopathy in dialysis patients. These observations strongly support aggressive treatment of hypertension to prevent endstage cardiomyopathy.[26]

Lipid abnormalities

Paradoxically, *low* serum cholesterol levels have been associated with mortality in large-scale epidemiological studies of ESRD[25]. It is likely that this reflects malnutrition and/or chronic inflammation, which are predictors of mortality. Certain lipoprotein types, which are not easily modifiable, most notably lipoprotein(a) (Lp(a)), are much higher in chronic renal failure and have been associated with adverse outcomes in some studies.[27,28] The evidence that lowering high cholesterol and LDL-cholesterol levels improves longevity is very compelling in nondialysis patients. Dietary intervention can have a significant impact on hyperlipidemia in patients who are highly motivated. Anorexia and malnutrition in dialysis patients appear to have very adverse effects on survival. Thus, adding further dietary restrictions may be hazardous. Our approach is to treat high cholesterol and LDL levels aggressively with a low threshold for using statins. A recent trial from the UK,[29] reported in the abstract that statin therapy is safe in patients with chronic kidney disease, in ESRD treated with dialysis, and in ESRD treated with transplantation. The CARE study[30] was a randomised trial that compared pravastatin to placebo in survivors of myocardial infarction, with total serum cholesterol less than 240 mg/mL. The abstract of another recent subgroup analysis, showed that 41% of the 4159 participants had glomerular filtration rates (GFR) below 75 mL/min. Pravastatin was equally effective in patients with and without chronic kidney disease in reducing the incidence of death or nonfatal myocardial infarction (the primary outcome), stroke, and coronary revascularization.[30]

Anemia

Anemia often accompanies chronic kidney disease. Chronic anemia leads to vasodilation, increased venous return, cardiac enlargement, and increased cardiac output.[31] In the long term, these compensatory mechanisms appear to be maladaptive. Several noninterventional studies have shown that anemia is associated with increased cardiac mass in uremic patients. The progressive cardiac enlargement starts relatively early in the course of chronic renal failure. Even moderate degrees of anemia are associated with progressive cardiac enlargement.[32] Several observational studies have suggested that anemia is an independent predictor of mortality in dialysis patients, within datasets where the vast majority of hemoglobin levels were between 6 and 12 g/dL.[33-35]

Several studies with small numbers have shown that partial correction of anemia partly corrects left ventricular (LV) hypertrophy in dialysis patients. The trade-offs are possibly lower cardiac mass, less cardiac failure, better quality of life, versus possibly more hypertension, increased thrombotic tendency, more expense. The trade-offs involved in adopting a policy of complete correction of anemia, as opposed to our current policy of partial correction, are addressed by several completed (and ongoing) randomised clinical trials worldwide. The studies completed to date have intervened late in the anemia–cardiac maladaptation endstage cardiomyopathy process. In the US Normal Hematocrit Trial[36] 1233 haemodialysis patients with ischemic heart disease or cardiac failure were randomly assigned to hematocrit targets of 30% or 42%. The primary outcome rates, death, or first nonfatal myocardial infarction, were similar in both groups, but patients assigned to the higher target had higher rates of vascular-access loss, and a decline in the adequacy of dialysis when compared with patients assigned to the lower hematocrit. Quality of life, however, was better in the group with normal hematocrit.

In the Canadian Normalization of Hemoglobin trial,[39] 146 hemodialysis patients with either concentric LV hypertrophy or LV dilation were randomly treated to hemoglobin levels of 10 g/dL or 13.5 g/dL. In patients with concentric LV hypertrophy, the changes in LV mass index were similar in both target groups. The changes in cavity volume index were similar in both targets in the LV dilation group. In the group with initially normal cavity volume there was an inverse correlation between the change in LV volume index and mean hemoglobin level. This hypothesis-generating result, that normal hemoglobin levels are better at preventing than regressing LV ventricular dilation, is attractive from a pathophysiological persepective;[37,38] it is the basis of an ongoing trial in patients new to hemodialysis. Normalization of hemoglobin led to clinically significant improvements in quality of life in terms of fatigue, depression, and personal relationships. Rates of loss and survival of vascular access were similar for both target groups.[39]

MacMahon et al[40,41] reported a randomized, double-blind crossover study in 14 hemodialysis patients. Performance was compared at rest and during a maximal incremental cycling exercise at a hemoglobin concentration of 10 and 14 g/dL, following an initial baseline test. Peak work rate and $V_{O_{2max}}$ were better at a hemoglobin level of 14 g/dL than at a hemoglobin of 10 g/dL. In addition, quality of life was improved, while LV dilation and systolic hyperfunction improved.

Uremia

Animal models show that characteristic features of uremia include: hypertrophy of ventricular myocytes; cardiac fibrosis; poor capillary blood supply relative to LV muscle mass; a limited ability to adjust cardiac output to alterations in preload and afterload; limited supplies of high-energy phosphate metabolites in cardiac myocytes; endothelial dysfunction; increased oxidative stress; and upregulation of procoagulation pathways.[42] In elegant experimental studies to prevent the morphological impact of uremia, parathyroid hormone (PTH) was a permissive factor, and some of the morphological changes were prevented with ACEIs, with blockade of central sympathetic outflow, and endothelin antagonists. Accelerated rates of ventricular myocyte apoptosis were seen in uremia. This provides key information that the morphological adaptations induced by uremia are maladaptive.

There is considerable clinical evidence to date to suggest that uremia exerts an independent impact on cardiac structure. LV hypertrophy, dilation, and systolic dysfunction improve for up to 2 years after renal transplantation.[43,44] This contrasts with observations on dialysis therapy, in which progressive cardiac enlargement and decompensation are common. There have been few large systematic studies to define sharp threshold levels of dialysis time and toxin removal. However, observational studies suggest that "more" is likely to be better than "less".[45]

Abnormalities of calcium–phosphate homeostasis are widespread in renal impairment. PTH is a calcium ionophore, and is likely to be a true uremic toxin at high levels. Experimental studies have shown deleterious effects on cardiac myocytes and all tissue types studied to date. Some studies have shown improvement in LV function and size after parathyroidectomy, while the inadequate hypertrophic response typical of uremic dilated cardiomyopathy has been related to high PTH levels in another study.[46] The role of calcium deposition remains contentious, because it is difficult to determine whether it has an innocent-bystander role, or is a true pathogenic factor. High calcium × phosphate product has been associated with shorter survival in hemodialysis patients.[47] In another study, hemodialysis patients underwent B-mode ultrasonography of the common carotid artery, aorta, and femoral arteries. Arterial and aortic stiffness were related to the degree of arterial calcification, which itself correlated with age, duration of hemodialysis, fibrinogen, and the prescribed dose of calcium-based phosphate binders.[48] Randomized controlled trials are needed to test cardiovascular outcomes using emerging phosphate reduction strategies that minimize calcium load, such as sevelamer, lanthanum, and calcimimetics.

Several recent observational studies suggest that low-grade inflammation is common in uremic patients, especially those with cardiovascular disease and malnutrition. This may partly explain the consistently strong association between hypoalbuminemia and cardiovascular events in renal impairment.[49,50] In one study, vitamin E and CRP (C-reactive protein) levels were associated with ultrasound carotid intima-media thickness, while the presence of plaques was associated with older age, oxidized LDL levels, and small Apo(a) isoform size.[51] Hyaluronan levels, which appear to be highest in subjects with malnutrition, inflammation, and cardiovascular disease, have been associated with short survival on dialysis.[52] Similar observations were seen when soluble adhesion molecules were studied.[53] Several pathways have been proposed that lead from inflammation to atherogenesis.[54] Increased expression of adhesion molecules on endothelial surfaces promotes the binding and activation of mononuclear cells and neutrophils, leading to oxidation of LDL. The acute phase reaction includes the hepatic release of atherogenic proteins like fibrinogen, Lp(a) and proteins that reduce the function of HDL. The overall pathobiology linking inflammation to atherosclerosis is not completely understood, but is susceptible to intervention at several levels.

Renal impairment is a state of endothelial dysfunction, with high levels of oxidative stress. These are features of chronic inflammatory states. A recent, noteworthy study examined the effect of high-dose vitamin E supplementation on cardiovascular outcomes in 196 hemodialysis patients with preexisting cardiovascular disease, randomly assigned to receive 800 IU/day of vitamin E or matching placebo. The primary endpoint was a composite of fatal or nonfatal myocardial infarction, ischemic stroke, peripheral vascular disease, or unstable angina. A primary endpoint ($P = 0.014$). was found in 16% patients assigned to vitamin E and 33% assigned to placebo. The beneficial impact of vitamin E was most marked for myocardial infarction, with a three-fold reduction in event rates.[55] These data are even more noteworthy because they have not been matched in much larger trials of antioxidant therapies in nonrenal populations. They point to the potential of novel, non-classical interventions in renal populations. Clearly, these data need confirmation in larger groups of patients with renal disease to enhance their generalizability.

Hyperhomocysteinemia

Homocysteine levels and renal function are inversely related.[56] Correction of folic acid deficiency reduces plasma homocysteine in patients with renal impairment. High doses of folic acid or methylated derivates can reduce homocysteine levels in subjects with renal failure, but full normalization of homocysteine levels has not been shown convincingly. The evidence that hyperhomocysteinemia is associated longitudinally with atherogenesis in renal impairment patients is inconclusive and no randomised trials with hard outcomes have been reported to date in patients with renal disease. Thus, there is a strong rationale to monitor folate levels, and to treat folate deficiency, but there is little evidence as yet to support super-supplementation. It is also true that supersupplementation is a low-risk strategy, and is unlikely to be harmful.

Diagnosis of cardiomyopathy

Chest radiography and electrocardiography are relatively insensitive tools for detecting cardiac enlargement. Echocardiography is easily performed and gives useful information about cardiac dimensions, valve function, systolic, and diastolic function. Cardiomyopathy often progresses rapidly in chronic uremia. We believe that echocardiography should be performed regularly in patients with chronic kidney disease.

Diagnosis of coronary artery disease

The questions "How to screen?" and "Who to screen?" have not been fully answered in people with chronic kidney disease. The role of noninvasive testing is still unclear. Exercise-based stress tests are usually inadequate in ESRD patients, because most are unable to reach a high enough level of exercise intensity. Of the other noninvasive screening tests available, adenosine thallium-201, dipyridamole thallium-201, and dobutamine stress echocardiography appear useful. Coronary arteriography remains the gold standard. In our opinion, ESRD patients with symptomatic ischemic heart disease should be investigated with coronary arteriography if the patient's physical state is such that revascularization would be seriously considered. The optimal approach to screening for coronary artery disease in asymptomatic renal transplant candidates has yet to be decided. Our current approach is to perform noninvasive screening on the following subgroups: patients over 45 years, diabetics over 25 years, smokers and those with ischemic changes on electrocardiography. Those who do not unequivocally have negative noninvasive screening tests should have arteriography.

Management of cardiomyopathy

The treatment goals of Table 74.1 apply to patients with concentric LV hypertrophy, LV dilation, and systolic dysfunction. ACEIs, CCBs, and β-blockers form the basis of antihypertensive therapy in concentric LV hypertrophy. Based on data from the nonuremic population, we use ACEIs as preferred therapy, and then β-blockers, in patients with LV dilation, systolic dysfunction, and symptomatic cardiac failure.

Management of coronary artery disease

Antiplatelet therapy, β-blockers, and ACE-inhibition are mainstays of preventive therapy, while calcium channel blockers and nitrates are useful additional components of symptomatic therapy. Dialysis patients fulfilling the anatomical criteria used in the general population are likely to benefit from coronary revascularization. Generally accepted criteria are: one-, two-, or three-vessel disease with angina refractory to medical management, where the intent is to relieve symptoms; left main coronary artery disease where the intent is to improve survival.

References

1. National Heart, Lung and Blood Institute. National Institutes of Health. http://www.nhlbi.nih.gov/guidelines/hypertension
2. National Heart, Lung and Blood Institute. National Institutes of Health. http://www.nhlbi.nih.gov/guidelines/hypercholesterolemia
3. Churchill DN, Taylor DW, Cook RJ, et al: Canadian hemodialysis morbidity study. Am J Kidney Dis 1992;19:214–234.
4. Foley RN, Parfrey PS, Sarnak MJ: Clinical epidemiology of cardiovascular disease in chronic renal disease. Am J Kidney Dis 1998;32(Suppl 3):S112–S119.
5. Tonelli M, Bohm C, Pandeya S, et al: Cardiac risk factors and the use of cardioprotective medications in patients with chronic renal insufficiency. Am J Kidney Dis 2001;37:484–489.
6. McMillan MA, Briggs JD, Junor BJ: Outcome of renal replacement therapy in patients with diabetes mellitus. Br Med J 1990;301:540–544.
7. Bloembergen WE, Stannard DC, Port FK, et al: Relationship of dose of hemodialysis and cause-specific mortality. Kidney Int 1996;50:557–565.
8. Effect of intensive diabetes management on macrovascular events and risk factors in the Diabetes Control and Complications Trial. Am J Cardiol 1995;75:894–903.
9. Manske CL, Wilson RF, Wang Y, et al: Prevalence of and risk factors for angiographically determined coronary artery disease in type I-diabetic patients with nephropathy. Arch Intern Med 1992;152:2450–2455.
10. Makita Z, Bucala R, Winston JA, et al: Reactive glycosylation endproducts in diabetic uremia and treatment of renal failure. Lancet 1994;343:1519–1522.
11. Collins R, Peto R, MacMahon S, et al: Blood pressure, stroke and coronary heart disease. Part 2. Short-term reductions in blood pressure: overview of randomised drug trials in their epidemiological context. Lancet 1990;335:827–838.

12. Lever AF, Ramsay LE: Treatment of hypertension in the elderly. J Hypertens 1995;13:571–579.
13. Gong L, Zhang W, Zhu Y, et al: Shanghai trial of nifedipine in the elderly (STONE).J Hypertens 1996;14:1237–1245.
14. Staessen JA, Fagard R, Thijs L, et al: Randomised double-blind comparison of placebo and active treatment for older patients with isolated systolic hypertension. The Systolic Hypertension in Europe (Syst-Eur) Trial Investigators. Lancet 1997;350:757–764.
15. Hansson L, Zanchetti A, Carruthers SG, et al: Effects of intensive blood-pressure lowering and low-dose aspirin in patients with hypertension: principal results of the Hypertension Optimal Treatment (HOT) randomised trial. HOT Study Group. Lancet 1998;351:1755–1762.
16. Yusuf S, Sleight P, Pogue J, et al: Effects of an angiotensin-converting-enzyme inhibitor, ramipril, on cardiovascular events in high-risk patients. The Heart Outcomes Prevention Evaluation Study Investigators. N Engl J Med 2000;342:145–153.
17. Lewis EJ, Hunsicker LG, Bain RP, et al: The effect of angiotensin-converting-enzyme inhibition on diabetic nephropathy. The Collaborative Study Group. N Engl J Med 1993;329:1456–1462.
18. Ruggenenti P, Perna A, Gherardi G, et al: Renal function and requirement for dialysis in chronic nephropathy patients on long-term ramipril: REIN follow-up trial. Gruppo Italiano di Studi Epidemiologici in Nefrologia (GISEN). Ramipril Efficacy in Nephropathy. Lancet 19998;352:1252–1256.
19. Maschio G, Alberti D, Janin G, et al: Effect of the angiotensin-converting-enzyme inhibitor benazepril on the progression of chronic renal insufficiency. The Angiotensin-Converting-Enzyme Inhibition in Progressive Renal Insufficiency Study Group. N Engl J Med 1996;334:939–945.
20. Agodoa LY, Appel L, Bakris GL, et al: African American Study of Kidney Disease and Hypertension (AASK) Study Group. Effect of ramipril vs amlodipine on renal outcomes in hypertensive nephrosclerosis: a randomized controlled trial. JAMA 2001;285:2719–2728.
21. Parving HH, Lehnert H, Brochner-Mortensen J, et al: Irbesartan in Patients with Type 2 Diabetes and Microalbuminuria Study Group. The effect of irbesartan on the development of diabetic nephropathy in patients with type 2 diabetes. N Engl J Med 2001;345:870–878.
22. Brenner BM, Cooper ME, de Zeeuw D, et al: RENAAL Study Investigators: Effects of losartan on renal and cardiovascular outcomes in patients with type 2 diabetes and nephropathy. N Engl J Med 2001;345:861–869.
23. Lewis EJ, Hunsicker LG, Clarke WR, et al: Collaborative Study Group: Renoprotective effect of the angiotensin-receptor antagonist irbesartan in patients with nephropathy due to type 2 diabetes. N Engl J Med 2001;345:851–860.
24. USRDS 1992: US Renal Data System Annual Report. IV: Comorbid conditions and correlations with mortality risk among 3,399 incident hemodialysis patients. Am J Kidney Dis 1992;5(Suppl 2):32–38.
25. Lowrie EG, Lew NL: Death risk in hemodialysis patients: the predictive value of commonly measured variables and an evaluation of death rate differences between facilities. Am J Kidney Dis 1990;15:458–482.
26. Foley RN, Parfrey PS, Harnett JD, et al: Impact of hypertension on cardiomyopathy, morbidity and mortality in end-stage renal disease. Kidney Int 1996;49:1379–1385.
27. Cressman MD, Heyka RJ, Paganini EP, et al: Lipoprotein(a) is an independent risk factor for cardiovascular disease in hemodialysis patients. Circulation 1992;86:475–482.
28. Goldwasser P, Michel MA, Collier J, et al: Prealbumin and lipoprotein(a) in hemodialysis: relationship with patients and vascular access survival. Am J Kidney Dis 1993;22:215–225.
29. Baigent C. The UK–Harp Steering Committee: Efficacy and safety of simvastatin and low-dose aspirin among patients with chronic renal disease: the UK Heart and Renal Protection (UK–HARP) pilot study (abstract). J Am Soc Nephrol 2001;12:190A.
30. Tonelli M, Moye L, Sacks F, et al: Pravastatin is effective for secondary prevention of cardiovascular events in patients with chronic renal insufficiency (abstract). J Am Soc Nephrol 2001;252A.
31. Muirhead N, Bargman J, Burgess E, et al: Evidence-based recommendations for the clinical use of human erythropoietin. Am J Kidney Dis 1995;26:S1–S24.
32. Levin A, Thompson CR, Ethier J, et al: Left ventricular mass index increase in early renal disease: impact of decline in hemoglobin. Am J Kidney Dis 1999;34:125–134.

33. Foley RN, Parfrey PS, Harnett JD, et al: The impact of anemia on cardiomyopathy, morbidity and mortality in end-stage renal disease. Am J Kidney Dis 1996;28:53–61.
34. Madore F, Lowrie EG, Brugnara C, et al: Anemia in hemodialysis patients: variables affecting this outcome predictor. J Am Soc Nephrol 1997;8:1921–1929.
35. Ma JZ, Ebben J, Xia H, et al: Hematocrit level and associated mortality in hemodialysis patients. J Am Soc Nephrol 1999;10:610–619.
36. Besarab A, Kline Bolton W, Browne JK, et al: The effects of normal as compared with low hematocrit in patients with cardiac disease who are receiving hemodialysis and epoetin. N Engl J Med 1998;339:584–590.
37. Katz AM: The cardiomyopathy of overload: an unnatural growth response in the hypertrophied heart. Ann Intern Med 1994;121:363–371.
38. Hunter JJ, Chien KR: Signaling pathways for cardiac hypertrophy and failure. N Engl J Med 1999;341:1276–1283.
39. Foley RN, Parfrey PS, Morgan J, et al: Effect of hemoglobin levels in hemodialysis patients with asymptomatic cardiomyopathy. Kidney Int 2000;58:1325–1335.
40. McMahon LP, McKenna MJ, Sangkabutra T, et al: Physical performance and associated electrolyte changes after haemoglobin normalization: a comparative study in haemodialysis patients. Nephrol Dial Transplant 1999;14:1182–1187.
41. McMahon LP, Mason K, Skinner SL, et al: Effects of haemoglobin normalization on quality of life and cardiovascular parameters in end-stage renal failure. Nephrol Dial Transplant 2000;15:1425–1430.
42. Middleton RJ, Parfrey PS, Foley RN: Left ventricular hypertrophy in the renal patient. J Am Soc Nephrol 2001;12:1079–1084.
43. Parfrey PS, Harnett JD, Foley RN, et al: Impact of renal transplantation on uremic cardiomyopathy. Transplantation 1995;60:908–914.
44. Rigatto C, Foley RN, Kent GM, et al: Long-term changes in LV hypertrophy after renal transplantation. Transplantation 2000;70:570–575.
45. Chan CT, Floras JS, Miller JA, et al: Improvements in LV systolic function with longterm nocturnal hemodialysis (abstract). J Am Soc Nephrol 2001;12:262A.
46. London GM, Fabiani F, Marchais SJ, et al: Uremic cardiomyopathy: an inadequate LV hypertrophy. Kidney Int 1987;31:973–980.
47. Block GA, Hulbert-Shearon TE, Levin NW, et al: Association of serum phosphorus and calcium × phosphate product with mortality risk in chronic hemodialysis patients: a national study. Am J Kidney Dis 1998;31:607–617.
48. Guerin AP, London GM, Marchais SJ, et al: Arterial stiffening and vascular calcifications in end-stage renal disease. Nephrol Dial Transplant 2001;15:1014–1021.
49. Yeun JY, Levine RA, Mantadilok V, et al: C-reactive protein predicts all-cause and cardiovascular mortality in hemodialysis patients. Am J Kidney Dis 2000;35:469–476.
50. Foley RN, Parfrey PS, Harnett JD, et al: Hypoalbuminemia, cardiac morbidity, and mortality in end-stage renal disease. J Am Soc Nephrol 1996;7:728–736.
51. Stenvinkel P, Heimburger O, Paultre F, et al: Strong association between malnutrition, inflammation, and atherosclerosis in chronic renal failure. Kidney Int 1999;55:1899–1911.
52. Stenvinkel P, Heimburger O, Wang T, et al: High serum hyaluronan indicates poor survival in renal replacement therapy. Am J Kidney Dis 1999;34:1083–1088.
53. Stenvinkel P, Lindholm B, Heimburger M, et al: Elevated serum levels of soluble adhesion molecules predict death in pre-dialysis patients: association with malnutrition, inflammation, and cardiovascular disease. Nephrol Dial Transplant 2000;15:1624–1630.
54. Kaysen GA: The microinflammatory state in uremia: causes and potential consequences. J Am Soc Nephrol 2001;12:1549–1557.
55. Boaz M, Smetana S, Weinstein T, et al: Secondary prevention with antioxidants of cardiovascular disease in endstage renal disease (SPACE): randomised placebo-controlled trial. Lancet 2000;356:1213–1218.
56. Bostom AG, Culleton BF: Hyperhomocysteinemia in chronic renal disease. J Am Soc Nephrol 1999;10:891–900.

Erectile Dysfunction as a Systemic Manifestation of Chronic Renal Failure

Manish P. Patel, J. Eric Derksen, and Culley C. Carson III

In men with chronic renal failure (CRF), quality of life is significantly impacted by erectile dysfunction (ED).[1] The etiology is often multifactorial. Uremia, medications, associated comorbid conditions and physiologic changes with dialysis, and the causative pathophysiology leading to the patient's CRF, should be considered prior to initiating treatment (Table 75.1).

Incidence

Is the incidence of ED greater than in normal men? Masters and Johnson[2] reported that the incidence of ED in normal men under the age of 50 years was less than 5%. The Massachusetts Male Aging Study reported that 5% of men at age 40 years have complete ED; and this rises to 50% among men aged 70.[3] Rodger et al[4] reported on 100 uremic men with a significantly higher prevalence. In a current study, Rosas et al[5] found that 82% of patients on hemodialysis had ED. ED was much more prevalent in the dialysis patients older than 50 years (63% in those younger than 50 compared with 90% in those older than 50).

Karacan[6] observed that rapid eye movement (REM) sleep was associated with penile tumescence, using a nocturnal penile tumescence (NPT) monitor. These studies showed that organic disturbances or pharmacological alteration of physiology correlated with altered NPT and impotency. If psychological factors predominate, the NPT results should

Table 75.1 Causes of erectile dysfunction in men with chronic renal failure

Anatomic (trauma, pelvic surgery renal transplant, vasculitis, penile surgery, arteriovenous malformations)

Structural
Tunica albuginea
Corpora cavernosa
Corpora spongiosum/glans penis

Vascular
Arterial compromise
Venoocclusive dysfunction

Neurologic
Autonomic innervation
Somatic innervation

Physiological
Endocrine
Abnormal testosterone metabolism and excretion
Stimulation of pituitary function
Elevated prolactin
Elevated parathyroid hormone
Diabetes mellitus

Neurogenic
Autonomic dysfunction
Supratentorial lesions (tumor, Alzheimer's disease, Parkinson's disease, trauma)
Infratentorial lesions
  Suprasacral
  Sacral
Peripheral somatic nervous system deterioration
Vascular
Arterial blood flow obstruction
Venous occlusive incompetence
Other
Pharmacologic causes
Hypoxia
Comorbid disease states (hypertension, diabetes mellitus, smoking, anemia, Paget's disease, Dupuytren's contracture, liver failure)
Pelvic radiation
Peyronie's disease
Psychosocial concerns

not be affected. Karacan reported that 50% of patients on hemodialysis had abnormal NPT.

Causes of erectile dysfunction in chronic renal failure: an overview

Physiologic factors in the evaluation of ED include: alterations in venous and arterial flow patterns, altered smooth muscle tone, hormonal aberrations, neurogenic abnormalities, and structural damage secondary to infection, trauma, or associated diseases. In addition, chronic fatigue, depression, and psychosocial stress may result from chronic, indolent illnesses that can contribute as psychological components of ED.[7]

Physiologic alterations in CRF predisposing to erectile dysfunction

In evaluation of a patient with CRF who presents with erectile problems, several physiologic processes must be considered: endocrine abnormalities, neurologic compromise, vascular insufficiency, venous incompetence, pharmacologic manipulations, psychological disturbances, and associated chronic diseases (such as hypertension, diabetes mellitus, anemia, and electrolyte abnormalities).

Endocrine abnormalities

CRF leads to abnormal hormonal balances throughout the hypothalamic–pituitary–gonadal axis. Semen quality is also affected and correlates with decreased testosterone levels.[8] The decrease in serum testosterone results from increased elimination, with maintained testicular hormone-binding capacity. Not all patients, however, have abnormal serum testosterone levels. Thus patients with CRF are likely to have a deficiency in hormone production and secretion as the primary mechanism for their hypogonadism, as well as an element of end-organ failure. Interestingly, giving exogenous testosterone to CRF patients with diminished levels of circulating testosterone does not improve erectile function or fertility.[9]

Men with CRF have abnormal secretion of luteinizing hormone, follicle-stimulating hormone, and prolactin. Luteinizing hormone levels are generally increased in response to low testosterone levels and because of a decrease in the metabolic clearance of luteinizing hormone.[10] Follicle-stimulating hormone is also elevated in those men with suboptimal spermatogenesis. The rise in serum luteinizing hormone and follicle-stimulating hormone correlates well with the pituitary response to hypothalamic stimulation by gonadotropin-releasing hormone (GnRH), which is preserved in the CRF patient. Thus, if the luteinizing hormone response to low testosterone levels is inadequate, a pituitary abnormality may be present.

The frequently elevated prolactin levels in men with CRF may cause sexual dysfunction. Medications that induce hyperprolactinemia include methyldopa, digoxin, cimetidine, and metoclopramide. Patients with hyperprolactinemia often have ED. Once the hyperprolactinemia is treated, erectile function improves, as does fertility.

Diabetes mellitus is a common cause of ED. The autonomic and sensory neuropathic dysfunction resulting in ED are not amenable to medical therapy. This is especially difficult for the young patient who has adequate vascular and venous function but insufficient neurologic ability to produce a sufficient erectile response.[10]

Neurogenic alterations

In the flaccid state and during detumescence, sympathetic neural activity predominates. Norepinephrine activates postsynaptic α_{1a}, α_{1b}, and α_{1b} receptors, and its activity is modulated by presynaptic α_2 receptors (Fig. 75.1).[11] Erections are mediated through the parasympathetic system via acetylcholine. Activation of muscarinic receptors liberates nitric oxide, which relaxes smooth muscle and causes erection. There are also nonadrenergic, noncholinergic (NANC) neurons that release nitric oxide (Fig. 75.2). Nitric oxide increases cyclic guanosine monophosphate (cGMP) production, which relaxes cavernous smooth muscle.[12]

In studies of 12 CRF patients with ED, an abnormal Valsalva maneuver correlated with abnormal NPT and diminished ability to achieve erections suitable for intercourse.[13] Peripheral neuropathy in CRF is frequent. Evaluation of patients with suspected neurogenic causes for impotency must rely on clinical judgment.[13]

Vascular compromise

Sexual stimulation releases nitric oxide, which relaxes smooth muscle and dilates the arterioles, thus increasing blood flow. Blood trapped in the expanding sinusoids

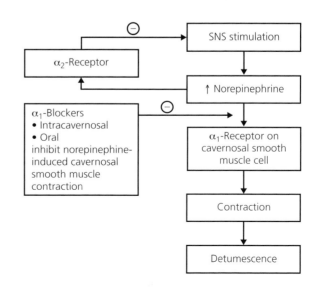

Figure 75.1 Sympathetic nervous system effect on cavernosal smooth muscle.

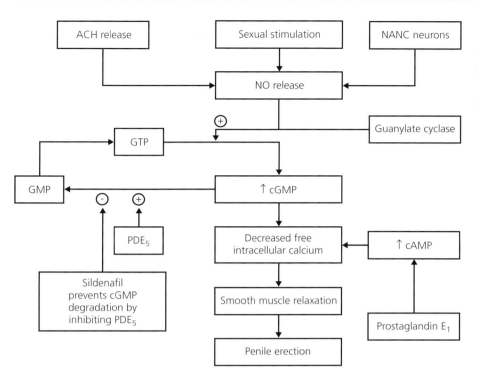

Figure 75.2 Nitric oxide-related (NO-related) neurogenic alterations. The primary pathway is cyclic GMP mediated while cyclic AMP acts secondarily. Both decrease intracellular calcium thus causing relaxation of smooth muscle. ACh, acetylcholine; GTP, guanosine triphosphate; NANC, nonadrenergic, noncholinergic.

compresses the venous system, increasing the pressure within the cavernosal bodies to approximately 100 mmHg. Contraction of the ischiocavernosus muscle further raises pressure in the penis leading to a rigid erection.

Acceleration of atherosclerosis leads to vasculogenic erectile dysfunction by occluding large vessels and their arterial tributaries. Therefore, regardless of age, vasculogenic ED occurs even in younger men with CRF. Kaufman et al[14] reported that 78% of impotent CRF patients had significant occlusive disease of the cavernosal artery.

Techniques to identify venous outflow abnormalities in ED include dynamic infusion studies, pharmacocavernosometry, and pharmacocavernosography.[15] In a series by Kaufman et al[16] 90% of CRF patients had venous occlusive incompetence.

Medicinal agents implicated in erectile dysfunction

Medications frequently associated with ED are listed in Table 75.2. Reductions in libido are seen with centrally acting agents like clonidine and reserpine, as well as drugs that increase prolactin levels. ED has been associated with virtually all antihypertensive agents. Calcium channel blockers (CCBs), angiotensin-converting enzyme inhibitors (ACEIs), angiotensin receptor blockers (ARBs), and α-adrenergic antagonists are least likely to cause iatrogenic ED. On the other hand, β-blockers, sympatholytics, and vasodilators are strongly associated.[17] These drugs, if causing ED, may be changed to α-adrenergic blocking agents such as terazosin, prazosin, or doxazosin, or ACEIs and CCBs.

Table 75.2 Medications associated with sexual dysfunction

Antihypertensive agents

Sympatholytics
Methyldopa
Clonidine
Reserpine
Guanethidine

β-Adrenergic antagonists
Propranolol
Pindolol
Atenolol
Metoprolol
Labetalol

Vasodilators
Hydralazine

Diuretics

Thiazides

Spironolactone

Other agents
Cimetidine
Digoxin

Clofibrate
Metoclopramide

Antidepressants
Tricyclics
Serotonin reuptake inhibitors

Anemia and diminished oxygen delivery

Low partial pressure of oxygen (Po_2) causes impotency by impairing cavernosal nitric oxide synthesis. Kim et al[18] found decreased nitric oxide synthesis and elevated smooth muscle tone in patients with low Po_2 at the corpora cavernosa. Luscher et al[19] found increased endothelium-derived contracting factors, which could further increase smooth muscle tone and inhibit erection. Finally, metabolites that inhibit nitric oxide synthase accumulation of CRF patients, possibly contributing to the ED.

Evaluation of erectile dysfunction in men with CRF

Erectile dysfunction in men with CRF should proceed systematically as outlined in Table 75.3. The use of NPT monitors can identify patients with a true organic cause for their ED whose vascular problems are suggested. Doppler screening studies, pharmacocavernosometry, pharmacocavernosography, dynamic infusion studies, and color Doppler response studies may be helpful. Finally, hormonal studies, including testosterone, luteinizing hormone, follicle stimulating hormone, and prolactin, should be obtained.

These may be supplemented by serum glucose, hemoglobin A_{1C}, lipid profile, and thyroid function studies.

Treatment options

Treatment options for ED are reviewed in Table 75.4.

Medical management of erectile dysfunction

Hormone regulation

Patients who have low testosterone levels may respond to replacement therapy which normally improves libido without a significant impact on potency or fertility. Effective replacements include injectable preparations, transdermal delivery systems, or sustained-release products. However, 100–200 mg of testosterone weekly by injection produces only small and variable responses in erectile function.[20] Clomifene citrate, which is a partial agonist of the estrogen receptor, increases secretion of gonadotropins and increases plasma testosterone in CRF.[21]

If hyperprolactinemia is found, chromophobic tumors of the anterior pituitary must be excluded, as men may present with ED or decreased libido. Methyldopa and reserpine interfere with dopamine secretion and therefore

Table 75.3 Evaluation of erectile dysfunction in men with chronic renal failure

History

Physical examination
General examination
GU examination: testicles, scrotum, phallus, meatus, prepuce, and glans
Digital rectal examination
Neurological examination: S2 to S4 sensation, bulbocavernosus reflex, anal wink, anal tone, and penoscrotal sensation

Laboratory evaluation to assess general and specific causes of erectile dysfunction
Serum testosterone
Luteinizing hormone
Follicle-stimulating hormone
Prolactin
Complete blood count
Serum glucose or hemoglobin A_{1C} and baseline electrolytes
Lipid profile
White men > 50 years and black men > 40 years should have a PSA test

Further referral to a urologist if considering
Doppler screening studies
Color Doppler ultrasound for flow
Pharmacocavernosography
Pharmacocavernosometry
Dynamic infusion studies
Nocturnal penile tumescence studies
Biothesiometry
Injection therapy
Surgical therapy

PSA, prostate-specific antigen.

Table 75.4 Treatment options in men with chronic renal failure and impotence

Medical
Medications
    Hormone replacement therapy
    Oral medications to improve arterial flow
    Intracavernosal injection therapy
    Transurethral therapy
    Dopaminergic agonists
    Erythropoietin
Devices
    Vacuum constriction device
    Constriction bands

Surgical
Revascularization techniques
Penile prosthetic devices

Psychiatric
Post-transplantation

Other issues
Adjust medications where appropriate
Control comorbid disease states
Evaluate for psychosocial stresses
Discuss expectations with patient
Routinely evaluate efficacy of therapy and patient satisfaction
Realize the changing patterns of erectile dysfunction and need to change therapy or modality
Consider early referral to a urologist

lead to hyperprolactinemia. If these causes are excluded, dopaminergic agonists may be of benefit.[22,23] Bromocriptine (1.25–5 mg daily) and lisuride hydrogen maleate (0.05–0.2 mg daily) decrease prolactin and elevate testosterone. Bromocriptine can induce hypotension, nausea, vertigo, and dizziness – side-effects that are intolerable to many patients. These side-effects are less prominent with lisuride hydrogen maleate.

Phosphodiesterase inhibitors

So far the Food and Drug Administration has approved only one selective type 5-phosphodiesterase inhibitor; sildenafil (Viagra, Pfizer) was introduced during 1998. Erectile function depends on the neuronal pathways (NANC neurons) and release of nitric oxide.[24,25] 5-Phosphodiesterase inhibitors inhibit the breakdown of cyclic GMP, thereby allowing continued relaxation of smooth muscle in the corpus cavernosum.[26] The best results in the initial human trials were obtained with 100 mg of sildenafil; however, up to 24% of men responded effectively on the 50-mg dosage schedule. Also significant was the increase in frequency of intercourse, with those receiving sildenafil making on average 5.9 successful attempts per month compared with 1.5 among those receiving placebo.[27] Sildenafil studies in patients on dialysis show a good response rate (66.7–80%). The majority of sildenafil responders had success with the 50-mg tablets.[28,29]

Sildenafil given to transplant patients does not perturb plasma levels and has a 60% satisfactory response rate.[30]

Most commonly reported side-effects are headache (16%), flushing (10%), and dyspepsia (7%).[31] Hypotensive side-effects occur particularly with concomitant nitrate administration. It is unclear how long the patient must wait until nitrates can be safely administered. Sildenafil decreases systolic and diastolic blood pressures by 10 and 7 mmHg respectively. Nitrate use leads to a synergistic increase in cyclic GMP levels, which can cause excessive hypotension and occasionally ischemic cardiac events or strokes.[32]

Sildenafil can be safely administered in CRF if there is no serious cardiac disease. Sildenafil is primarily metabolized in the liver but there is some renal excretion; lower doses are recommended initially (25 mg) in CRF patients.

Intracavernosal injection therapy

Alprostadil (Caverject; Edex), an exogenous form of prostaglandin E_1, administered by intracavernosal injection is the only approved agent. Alprostadil causes smooth muscle relaxation, vasodilation, and inhibition of platelet aggregation. Some 96% of alprostadil is locally metabolized within 60 min. No change in peripheral blood levels occurs[33] because of extensive pulmonary metabolism. Linet and Neff[34] concluded that alprostadil produced full erections in 70–80% of patients. Side-effects include pain (17%), hematoma or echymosis (1.5%), and priapism or prolonged erection (1.3%).

Other agents used alone or in combination with prostaglandin E_1 include papaverine and phentolamine mesylate (Regitine; CIBA Pharmaceuticals). Papaverine inhibits phosphodiesterase, leading to increases in cyclic AMP, elevated nitric oxide, and eventual relaxation of cavernosal smooth muscle and arterial dilation. Kapoor et al[35] reported on the use of papaverine in men with spinal cord injuries, who obtained satisfactory erections capable of successful penetration in 98%. Papaverine, however, causes priapism and fibrosis in up to 35% and 33% of men, respectively, with increased incidence in young and neurogenic patients.[36]

Phentolamine mesylate is a competitive nonselective alpha-adrenergic receptor antagonist. It has been used in combination with papaverine to increase blood flow. Side-effects include hypotension, reflex tachycardia, and nasal congestion.

These agents can be used successfully in CRF patients with vascular compromise, diabetic microangiopathy, moderate atherosclerosis, and partial arterial dysphasia, although higher doses may be necessary. Patients with venous occlusive disease may also benefit from increased engorgement of the corpora leading to increased compression of the tunica albuginea and therefore, occlusion of the emissary veins. It is interesting to note that patients with neurogenic and hormonal causes also do well with this therapy (as do older patients), without increased side-effects. Long-term use of these injection therapies is effective, with few complications in transplant patients.[37] No major complications on transplanted kidneys have been noted. The only contraindications to therapy are sickle cell anemia, severe psychiatric disorders, severe venous incompetence, and severe systemic disease.

Transurethral suppositories

The transurethral delivery system, Medicated Urethral System for Erection (MUSE), allows for delivery of alprostadril to the corpora by direct venous communication.[38] The mechanism of action of alprostadil has been discussed earlier. Success has been variable.

Erythropoietin, anemia, and erectile dysfunction

The treatment of anemia with recombinant human erythropoietin in men with CRF improves sexual performance[39] and elevates levels of follicle-stimulating hormone and testosterone.

Devices
Vacuum constriction devices and constriction bands

Vacuum constriction devices work by engorging the penis with blood by negative pressure. A constriction band is placed at the base of the penis for no longer than 30 min to avoid injury. These devices have local side-effects such as pain from the constriction band, entrapment of ejaculation by the constriction band, cold and dusky penis, numbness of the penis, and local irritation. Many men use these devices. Using the device can be difficult for men with a short penis or an extensive suprapubic fat pad. In those who need pharmacological manipulation for an adequate erection but who have evidence of venous incompetence, a constriction band alone may be used to sustain rigidity of the penis that is suitable for intercourse.

Surgical treatment of erectile dysfunction
Vascular procedures for erectile dysfunction

As most patients with renal failure have small-vessel disease, the use of revascularization techniques and venous occlusive surgery is not commonly employed. These judgments are best left to the urologist.

Penile prostheses

Implantation of a penile prosthesis is safe and usually successful, with low morbidity. Renal transplant patients commonly benefit from the device.[40] Such procedures should be performed after renal transplantation, if possible, because many men have improved sexual function, fertility, and potency after the operation. In immunocompromised patients, the risks of implanting an artificial device include prosthetic infection.[41]

Improvement in erectile dysfunction after renal transplantation

After renal transplantation, patients report improved erectile function and libido. Testosterone levels return to normal within 2–3 months, as do luteinizing hormone, follicle-stimulating hormone, and prolactin. Sperm counts normalize in 9–16 months. Patients who receive human chorionic gonadotropin (HCG) stimulation show improved responses with higher testosterone levels. Salvatierra et al[42] found pretransplant potency to be 22% while on dialysis; however, after renal transplant, 84% of men resumed levels of potency comparable to a time before the onset of uremia. Post-transplant psychological disturbances, except for anxiety, appear to diminish.

It is important to remember that a significant proportion of post-transplant men will continue to have erectile dysfunction despite normalization of hormone values and improved physiology.[43] Many of these patients suffer from vasculogenic ED. These patients should be evaluated in a way similar to pretransplant patients; treatment plans should be generated for their specific needs.

Conclusions

Erectile dysfunction includes a vast array of organic, anatomic and psychosocial elements, which make evaluation and treatment complex. However, a practitioner who observes a good history, physical examination, and laboratory evaluation can provide a great service to the quality of life of his patient with CRF. The physician must address the topic and make the patient feel comfortable with his changing physiology and anatomy. Renal transplantation has the potential to normalize hormone profiles and subdue some of the physiologic changes, although it may solve the problem in men because of associated comorbid conditions. Psychological, medical, and surgical therapies can be highly effective in correctly evaluated patients. A multidisciplinary approach to care should be employed that involves the primary-care physician, a nephrologist, urologist, psychiatrist, and psychologist.

References

1. Patel MP, Carson CC: The epidemiology, anatomy, physiology, and treatment of erectile dysfunction in chronic renal failure patients. Adv Ren Repl Ther 1999;6:296.
2. Masters WH, Johnson VF: Human sexual inadequacy. Boston, MA: Little, Brown and Co., 1990, pp 88–101.
3. Feldman HA, Goldstein I, Hatzichristou DG, et al: Impotence and its medical and psychosocial correlates: Results of the Massachusetts male aging study. Urology 1994;151:54–61.
4. Rodger KS, Fletcher K, Dewar JH, et al: Prevalence and pathogenesis of impotence in 100 uremic men. Uremia Invest 1984;8:89–96
5. Rosas SE, et al: Prevalence and determinants of erectile dysfunction in hemodialysis patients. Kidney Int 2001;59:2259–2266.
6. Karacan I: NPT/rigidometry. In Kirby RS, Carson CC, Webster GD (eds): Impotence: Diagnosis and Management of Erectile Dysfunction. Boston, MA: Butterworth Heinemann, 1991, pp 62–71.
7. Carson CC, Kirby R, Goldstein I: Textbook of Erectile Dysfunction. Oxford: Isis Medical Publishing. 1999, pp 551–562.
8. Copolla A, Cuomo C: Pituitary testicular evaluation in patients with chronic renal insufficiency in hemodialysis treatment. Minerva Med 1990;81:461–465.
9. Holdsworth S, Atkins RC, de Krettsker DM: The pituitary testicular axis in men with chronic renal failure. N Engl J Med 1977;296:1245–1251.
10. Brindley GS: Neurophysiology. In Kirby RS, Carson CC, Webster GD (eds): Impotence: Diagnosis and Management of Erectile Dysfunction. Boston, MA: Butterworth, Heinemann, 1991, p 27.
11. Traish AM, Netsuwan N, Daley J, et al: A heterogeneous population of alpha-1 receptors mediates contraction of human corpus cavernosum smooth muscle to norepinephrine. J Urol 1995;153:222–227.
12. Kim N, Vardi Y, Padma-Nathan H, et al: Oxygen tension regulates the nitric oxide pathway. Physiological role in penile erection. J Clin Invest 1993;91:437–442.
13. Campese VM, Procci WR, Levitan D, et al: Autonomic nervous system dysfunction impotence in uremia. Am J Nephrol 1982;2:140.
14. Kaufman J, Mutzichristou D, Mulhall J, et al: Impotence and chronic renal failure: A study of the hemodynamic pathophysiology. Urology 1994;151:612–618.
15. Carson CC: Impotence: New diagnostic modalities. Urol Annu 1992;6:229–311.
16. Kaufman J, Mutzichristou D, Mulhall J, et al: Impotence and chronic renal failure: A study of the hemodynamic pathophysiology. Urology 1994;151:612–618.
17. Brock GB, Lue TF: Drug-induced male sexual dysfunction. An update. Drug Safety 1993;8:414–426.
18. Kim N, Vardi Y, Padma-Nathan H, et al: Oxygen tension regulates the nitric oxide pathway. Physiological role in penile erection. J Clin Invest 1993;91:437–442.
19. Luscher TF, Borelungeri M, Duhi Y, et al: Endothelium-derived contracting factors. Hypertension 1992;14:117–126.
20. Lim VS: Reproductive function in patients with renal insufficiency. Am J Kidney Dis 1987;4:363–370.
21. Lim VS, Fang VS: Restoration of plasma testosterone levels in uremic men with clomiphene citrate. J Clin Endocrinol Metab 1976;43:1370–1374
22. Ruilope L, Garcia-Robles R, Paya C, et al: Influence of lisuride and dopaminergic agonist on the sexual function of male patients with chronic renal failure. Am J Kidney Dis 1985;3:182–187.
23. Muir JW, Besser GM, Edwards CW, et al: Bromocriptine improves reduced libido and potency in men receiving maintenance hemodialysis. Clin Nephrol 1983;20:308–314.
24. Zusman RM, Morales A, Classer DB, et al: Overall cardiovascular probable of sildenafil citrate. Am Cardiol 1999;83:35–44.
25. Chuang AT, Strauss ID, Murphy RA, et al: Sildenafil, a type 5 cyclic GMP-dependent relaxation in rabbit corpus cavernosum smooth muscle in vitro. J Urol 1998;160:257–261.
26. Boolell M, Allen MJ, Ballard SA, et al: Sildenafil: An orally active type 5 cyclic CMP-specific phosphodiesterase inhibitor for the treatment of penile erectile dysfunction. Int J Impot Res 1996;8:47–52.
27. Goldstein I, Lue TF, Padma-Nathan H, et al: Oral sildenafil in the treatment of erectile dysfunction. N Engl J Med 1998;338:1397–1404.
28. Chen J, et al: Clinical efficacy of sildenafil in patients on chronic dialysis. J Urol 2001;165:819–821.
29. Rosas SE, et al: Preliminary observations of sildenafil treatment for erectile dysfunction in dialysis patients. Amer J Kidney Dis 2001;37:134–137.
30. Prieto Castro R, Anglada Curado FJ. Regueiro Lopez JC, et al: Treatment with sildenafil citrate in renal transplant patients with erectile dysfunction. Br J Urol 2001;88:241–243.
31. Morales A, Gingell C, Collins M, et al: Clinical safety of oral sildenafil citrate (Viagra) in the treatment of erectile dysfunction. Int J Impot Res 1998;10:69–73.
32. Chuang AT, Strauss ID, Murphy RA, et al: Sildenafil, a type 5 cyclic GMP phosphodiesterase inhibitor, specifically amplifies endogenous cGMP- dependent relaxation in rabbit corpus cavernosum smooth muscle in vitro. J Urol 1998;160:257–261.
33. van Able H, Peskar BA, Sticht G, et al: Pharmacokinetics of vasoactive substances administered into the human corpus cavernosum. J Urol 1994;151:1227–1235.
34. Linet OI, Neff LL: Intracavernous prostaglandin E₁ in erectile dysfunction. Clin Invest 1994;72:139–143.
35. Kapoor VK, Chahal AS, Jyoti SP, et al: Intracavernous papaverine for impotence in spinal cord injured patients. Paraplegia 1993;31:6757–6764.
36. Barada JH, McKimmy RM: Vasoactive Pharmacotherapy. In Bennett AH (ed): Impotence. Philadelphia: WB Saunders, 1994, p 229.
37. Rodriguez Antolin A, Morales JM, Andres A, et al: Treatment of erectile impotence in renal transplant patients with intracavernosal vasoactive drugs. Transplant Proc 1992;24:105–112.
38. Padma-Nathan H, Bennett A, Gesundheit N, et al: Treatment of erectile dysfunction by the medicated urethral system for erection. J Urol 1995;153:975–984.
39. Imagawa A, Kawanish N, Numata A: Is erythropoietin effective for impotence in dialysis patients? Nephron 1990;54:95–109.
40. Kabalin JN, Kessler R: Successful implantation of penile prosthesis in organ transplant patients. Urology 1989;33:282–284.
41. Carson CC: Infections in genitourinary prostheses. Urol Clin North Am 1989;16:439–447.
42. Salvatierra O, Fortmann JL, Belzer FO: Sexual function in males before and after renal transplantation. Scand J Urol Nephrol 1992;26:181–186.
43. Reinberg N, Bumgardner CL, Aliabadi H: Urological aspects after renal transplantation. J Urol 1991;143:1087–1094.

Sleep Disorders and Renal Dysfunction

Elizabeth H. Nora, Eddie L. Greene, and Virend K. Somers

Introduction

Sleep disturbances and abnormal sleep patterns are common in people with chronic renal failure. Frequent sleep complaints include insomnia, hypersomnia, excessive snoring, and nocturnal limb movements. Specific clinical syndromes that are closely associated with sleep pathologies in patients with chronic renal failure include nocturnal myoclonus and the obstructive sleep apnea syndrome (OSA).

This very brief review will focus on OSA for several reasons. First, there are several potentially effective treatments for OSA. Second, OSA is associated with multiple quality-of-life issues, including daytime somnolence, irritability, impaired driving, fatigue, poor concentration, and decreased work performance, all of which may improve when OSA is treated effectively. These cognitive and functional characteristics of people with OSA overlap considerably with those that are manifest in people with chronic renal failure. Thus, in the patient with chronic renal failure who has obstructive sleep apnea, treatment of the sleep-related breathing disorder may help to improve symptoms previously thought to be secondary to renal dysfunction and uremia alone. Third, the pathophysiologic interactions between OSA and chronic renal failure may have important etiologic and therapeutic implications.

Obstructive sleep apnea

Sleep apnea syndrome is defined by an apnea–hypopnea index (AHI) of ≥ 15 apneic or hypopneic episodes per hour. More than five episodes per hour with a complaint of daytime sleepiness is also considered pathologic. An apneic episode is generally defined as ≥ 10-s interval without airflow, accompanied by desaturation or arousal. Hypopnea is defined by ≥ 10 s interval with less than 50% baseline airflow, accompanied by desaturation or arousal. Episodes of apnea or hypopnea can be caused by an obstructive mechanism, a central mechanism, or a mixture of both.

Prevalence and diagnosis of obstructive sleep apnea

In the general population of the USA, the prevalence of OSA is estimated at 2–4%[1]. However, among the population of patients with chronic renal failure, the estimated prevalence has ranged from as high as 66%[2] and 57%[3] to as low as 16.4%.[4] Even the lowest estimate of OSA is four times greater than that reported for the general population. Given the strong association of sleep disorders and chronic renal failure, a preliminary evaluation for OSA should be obtained when a patient is seen in the renal clinic. Screening can be performed by history or questionnaire. Routine questions include, "Do you snore?," "Has your bed partner noticed that you stop breathing when you sleep?," "Do you awake refreshed from sleep?," and "Do you fall asleep while driving?" When the clinician, spouse, or partner witnesses an apneic episode, this may also be an important sign of possible significant sleep apnea.

Observation of the patient during dialysis can also be useful. For example, if the patient regularly and promptly falls asleep during the dialysis treatment run, or if snoring or apnea/hypopnea are witnessed, the diagnosis is highly likely. Overnight pulse oximetry can provide a preliminary and inexpensive screening tool for the clinician to use in evaluating OSA. Multiple recurrent desaturations in the oxygen tracing are consistent with a clinical diagnosis of OSA. A primarily obstructive apnea mechanism often appears as a saw-tooth pattern on the oxygen saturation tracing. Nevertheless, the gold standard for diagnosing OSA is polysomnography. This is a comprehensive overnight study that uses an electrocardiogram and an electroencephalogram to monitor sleep stages, and also monitors oxygen saturation, limb movement, body position, airflow, and respiratory effort.

Pathophysiology

The classic risk factors for obstructive sleep apnea/hypopnea syndrome are obesity, male sex, and uvula–palatine–tracheal/craniofacial abnormalities.[5] However, people with chronic renal failure and OSA do not usually fit the expected profile. In particular, patients with ESRD and OSA are not consistently obese.[3,4] Thus many alternative mechanisms for the development of OSA in endstage renal disease (ESRD) have been hypothesized.[6] First, the build-up of uremic toxins may affect the central nervous system in a manner that reduces airway muscle tone and/or destabilizes respiratory drive.[6,7] Second, anemia is common in chronic renal failure and has been associated with changes in periodic breathing. Third, the chronic metabolic acidosis and hypocapnia that accompany ESRD can lower the apneic threshold. Fourth, neuropathies associated with the underlying cause of the renal failure (such as diabetes mellitus), or other metabolic abnormalities associated with chronic renal failure, can alter the respiratory drive and promote periodic breathing. A fifth possible mechanism is edema of the upper airway, resulting from sodium and water retention caused by activation of the renin–angiotensin–aldosterone system. As the radius of the airway decreases, the resistance to airflow increases exponentially (Poiseuille's law). If the resistance to airflow is high enough, or if other risk factors are also present, apnea or hypopnea can occur. This mechanism relates directly to the evidence that treatment of the renal failure and excessive volume retention by dialysis or ultrafiltration may help improve the severity of apnea.

Treatment of renal failure

If OSA is a consequence of chronic renal failure and uremia, does treatment of the renal disease improve the sleep apnea? Interestingly, a handful of case reports have demonstrated complete correction of the OSA after effective dialysis[7] or following a kidney transplant.[8] In these examples, severe untreated OSA confirmed by polysomnography was present prior to the initiation of dialysis or transplantation. In all these cases the symptoms associated with sleep apnea resolved and the quantitative estimate of sleep apnea severity was reduced. A small study of patients already on chronic hemodialysis did not corroborate these case studies.[2] Six of the 11 patients (55%) in this study had OSA as diagnosed by polysomnography. There was no difference in their apneic episodes on the nights after dialysis when compared to the nights during the interval between dialysis treatments. These data may not necessarily be contradictory given the differences in the populations studied.

Convincing data to support the supposition that the treatment of ESRD can improve sleep apnea arise from a recent study of 14 randomly selected patients on chronic hemodialysis.[3] Fifty-seven percent (8 of 14) had OSA. When those with OSA underwent an intensive program of daily, nocturnal hemodialysis there was a significant reduction in their apnea/hypopnea index from 46 ± 19 to 9 ± 9/h (see Fig. 76.1). This was accompanied by a significant decrease in serum creatinine levels and a significant increase in plasma bicarbonate concentrations. While multiple studies strongly support an association between ESRD and OSA, further work is needed to elucidate this relationship and the pathophysiology involved.

The compelling evidence for the increased prevalence of obstructive sleep apnea in patients with chronic renal disease, the decline in cognitive function arising from sleep deprivation and arousal during OSA, and the vascular and cardiac consequences associated with untreated sleep apnea all signify the importance of recognizing early sleep apnea in patients with chronic renal failure. It remains to be determined whether current specific

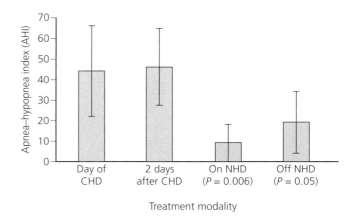

Figure 76.1 Graphical representation of data (adapted from Hanly and Pierratos)[3] depicting a significant reduction in the apnea–hypopnea index (AHI) with the use of nocturnal hemodialysis (NHD), compared with limited benefits from conventional hemodialysis (CHD). Study participants underwent 6–15 months of daily, nocturnal hemodialysis, which caused a significant reduction in their AHI ($P = 0.006$). On a night without NHD, participants still had a significant decrease in their AHI ($P = 0.05$).

treatments for chronic renal failure, uremia, and ESRD should be modified to emphasize the therapeutic strategies most likely to attenuate the severity of obstructive sleep apnea. This issue is especially important in the people with chronic renal failure who also have hypertension or severe ischemic heart disease.

Treatment of obstructive sleep apnea

Does treatment of OSA diminish the progression of renal dysfunction? The evidence suggesting an etiologic interaction between obstructive sleep apnea and hypertension,[6,9,10] and the very marked pressor and sympathetic responses to repetitive episodes of obstructive sleep apnea,[11] suggest that treatment of the sleep apnea may help decrease pressor stress on the kidney. Marked pressor responses to OSA, and the increased filtration, could cause maladaptive architectural changes leading to proteinuria and kidney damage. Proteinuria has been associated with sleep apnea independent of obesity, hypertension and diabetes.[12,13] Furthermore, in a small number of patients, the proteinuria disappeared with treatment of the OSA.[14]

Methods of treatment of obstructive sleep apnea

At minimum, treatment of OSA will improve quality of life. Therefore, treatment is important (see Fig. 76.2). Weight loss is always an option, although it is often difficult to achieve. Additionally, inclining the head of the bed, sleeping on one's side rather than back, and avoiding

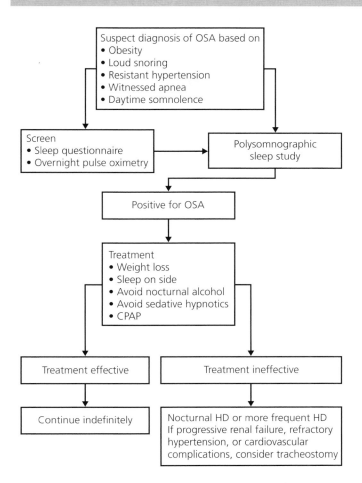

Suspect diagnosis of OSA based on
• Obesity
• Loud snoring
• Resistant hypertension
• Witnessed apnea
• Daytime somnolence

Screen
• Sleep questionnaire
• Overnight pulse oximetry

Polysomnographic sleep study

Positive for OSA

Treatment
• Weight loss
• Sleep on side
• Avoid nocturnal alcohol
• Avoid sedative hypnotics
• CPAP

Treatment effective

Treatment ineffective

Continue indefinitely

Nocturnal HD or more frequent HD
If progressive renal failure, refractory hypertension, or cardiovascular complications, consider tracheostomy

Figure 76.2 Algorithm depicting a suggested strategy for diagnosis and treatment of obstructive sleep apnea (OSA) in the setting of chronic renal failure (CPAP, continuous positive airway pressure; CV, cardiovascular; HD, hemodialysis).

alcohol, can all improve the symptoms of sleep apnea. After these measures, the preferred treatment of OSA is continuous positive airway pressure (CPAP). This device works in part by a direct application of Poiseuille's law. The CPAP effectively stents open the airway with positive pressure, which prevents the collapse or obstruction that occurs during inspiration. It is highly effective – if it is tolerated. Unfortunately there are less than ideal compliance rates with CPAP use due to the noise of the machine, discomfort from wearing the apparatus, nasal congestion, sensation of claustrophobia or suffocation from the mask, and drying of the mucous membranes. To ameliorate some of these complaints, nasal CPAP (nCPAP) is available. Instead of a full face-mask, this uses a small, triangular mask that covers only the nose. This has improved compliance in some patients. Alternatively an "Adam's circuit" can be used; this consists of two pressure prongs, one for each nostril, which some patients find more tolerable. The pressure setting on the CPAP machine can be adjusted individually for each patient, to provide the necessary positive pressure for stenting open the airways and to enhance comfort.

If CPAP is absolutely intolerable, there are a few less effective strategies, but some of these treatments do work well in renal failure patients because of their differing physiology and anatomy. One option is the anterior mandibular positioner (AMP). The device is most effective in people with a primary obstructive sleep apnea, but only in cases of mild-to-moderate obstruction (e.g. a raucous snorer who has few arousals).[15] Consequently, for people who have OSA associated with renal failure, and therefore likely a mixed central and obstructive pattern, this device is suboptimal. It is designed to displace the tongue and mandible anteriorly, thereby precluding upper airway collapse.[15] In direct comparison, both AMP and nCPAP reduce the AHI, though nCPAP reduces it more.[15] However, AMP is better tolerated than CPAP. The most common side effects attributed to AMP are sore teeth, tongue, and jaw, and trouble with chewing on the following morning. AMP is more convenient and portable compared toCPAP.

Several surgical procedures are also available as alternative strategies. These ENT (ear, nose and throat) procedures are most effective in strictly obstructive sleep apnea. Again, in the majority of cases of OSA that is associated with renal failure, these operations may not be successful since the apneas are both central and obstructive. The best-established surgery is the uvulopalatopharyngoplasty (UPPP). Newer versions of this procedure include laser-assisted uvulopalatoplasty (LAUP) or radiofrequency energy uvulopalatoplasty. The drawback of all of these procedures is their failure to reduce significantly the AHI over the long term, even in cases of pure obstructive sleep apnea,[16] although snoring may be ameliorated. Furthermore, there are no guidelines available yet to assess which patients are most likely to benefit.

If the above surgery is unsuccessful, there are several more salvage procedures. These include geniohyoid advancement with hyoid resuspension, maxillomandibular advancement, tongue suspension via Repose system, or base-of-tongue somnoplasty.[16] The group of patients for whom these procedures are beneficial is ill-defined, and the success rate is uncertain, depending greatly on the surgeon. These procedures are not widely available.

As a last resort for intractable sleep apnea, tracheostomy is a definitive treatment. This should only be considered in patients who are refractory to or noncompliant with CPAP and who have significant complications such as cor pulmonale, cardiac arrhythmias, or perhaps progressive renal failure. Interestingly, suggesting tracheostomy as the only remaining treatment option often increases the compliance with CPAP.

Many pharmacologic therapies have been tried for OSA but have shown little success except in specific situations.

The only other treatment modality available specifically for the renal failure patient with OSA is hemodialysis. Intriguing new evidence shows significant improvement in OSA with nocturnal hemodialysis.[3] Though there are many technical and financial limitations to using this treatment in all ESRD patients with OSA, the results are promising. Furthermore, the improvement in OSA with intensive hemodialysis suggests many possibilities for helping to clarify the pathophysiology of OSA in ESRD. Better understanding of the etiologic mechanisms will likely lead to novel and more effective therapeutic strategies.

References

1. Young T, Palta M, Dempsey J, et al: The occurrence of sleep-disordered breathing among middle-aged adults. N Engl J Med 1993;328:1230–1235.
2. Mendelson WB, Wadhwa NK, Greenberg HE, et al: Effects of hemodialysis on sleep apnea syndrome in end-stage renal disease. Clin Nephrol 1990;33:247–251.
3. Hanly PJ, Pierratos A: Improvement of sleep apnea in patients with chronic renal failure who undergo nocturnal hemodialysis. N Engl J Med 2001;344:102–107.
4. Kuhlmann U, Becker HF, Birkhahn M, et al: Sleep apnea in patients with end-stage renal disease and objective results. Clin Nephrol 2000;53:460–466.
5. Redline S, Strohl K: Recognition and consequences of obstructive sleep apnea hypopnea syndrome. Clin Chest Med 1998;19:1–19.
6. Fletcher EC: Obstructive sleep apnea and the kidney. J Am Soc Nephrol 1993;4:1111–1121.
7. Fein AM, Niederman MS, Imbriano L, et al: Reversal of sleep apnea in uremia by dialysis. Arch Intern Med 1987;147:1355–1356.
8. Auckely DH, Schmidt-Nowara W, Brown LK: Reversal of sleep apnea hypopnea syndrome in end-stage renal disease after kidney transplantation. Am J Kidney Dis 1999;34:739–744.
9. Peppard PE, Young T, Palta M, et al: Prospective study of the association between sleep-disordered breathing and hypertension. N Engl J Med 2000;342:1378–1384.
10. Brooks D, Homer RL, Kozar, LF, et al: Obstructive sleep apnea as a cause of systemic hypertension. Evidence from a canine model. J Clin Invest 1997;99:106–109.
11. Somers VK, Dyken ME, Clary MP, et al: Sympathetic neural mechanisms in obstructive sleep apnea. J Clin Invest 1995;96:1897–1904.
12. Chaudhary BA, Sklar AH, Chaudhary TK, et al: Sleep apnea, proteinuria, and nephrotic syndrome. Sleep 1988;11:69–74.
13. Sklar AH, Chaudhary BA, Harp R: Nocturnal urinary protein excretion rates in patients with sleep apnea. Nephron 1989;51:35–38.
14. Sklar AH, Chaundhary BA: Reversible proteinuria in obstructive sleep apnea syndrome. Arch Intern Med 1988;148:87–89.
15. Ferguson KA, Ono T, Lowe AA, et al: A short-term controlled trial of an adjustable oral appliance for the treatment of mild to moderate obstructive sleep apnea. Thorax 1997;52:362–368.
16. Loube DI: Technologic advances in the treatment of obstructive sleep apnea syndrome. Chest 1999;116:1426–1433.

CHAPTER 77

Neuropsychiatric Complications and Psychopharmacology of Endstage Renal Disease

Lewis M. Cohen, Michael J. Germain, and Edward G. Tessier

Neurological conditions
- Peripheral neuropathies
- Seizures
- Restless leg syndrome
- Insomnia
- Delirium
- Dementia

Psychiatric conditions
- Schizophrenia
- Adjustment disorders
- Anxiety disorders
- Depressive disorders
- Sexual disorders

Table 77.1 Etiology of organic brain syndrome in chronic renal disease

1. Common drugs leading to organic brain syndrome
   a. Psychotropic drugs
   b. Narcotics
   c. Illicit drugs
   d. Metoclopramide
   e. Antiseizure medications
   f. Cardiac medications, such as digoxin and amiodarone
   g. Transplant medications – calcineurin inhibitors, rapamycin, prednisone

2. Uremia
   a. Inadequate dialysis
   b. GFR of less than 12

3. Dialysis related
   a. Disequilibrium syndrome
   b. Dialysis dementia (secondary to aluminum intoxication)

4. Metabolic disturbance
   a. Hypoxemia
   b. Hypo- and hyperglycemia
   c. Sepsis
   d. Malignant hypertension

5. Structural neurological lesions
   a. Subdural hematoma
   b. Multiinfarct dementia
   c. Cerebral vascular accident

6. Electrolyte disturbances
   a. Hyper- and hypocalcemia
   b. Hypophosphatemia
   c. Hypermagnesemia
   d. Hyper- and hyponatremia

7. Anemia

8. Hyperparathyroidism

9. Heavy metal intoxications
   a. Lead
   b. Aluminum (dialysis dementia)
   c. Mercury
   d. Cadmium

10. Vitamin and mineral deficiencies
    a. Carnitine
    b. Zinc

11. Miscellaneous
    a. Hyper- and hypothyroidism
    b. Normal pressure hydrocephalus
    c. Sleep apnea
    d. Central pontine myelonolysis

Neuropsychiatric disorders are common in patients with endstage renal disease (ESRD). They include: the traditional 'organic brain' disorders (e.g. dementia and delirium), schizophrenia, a variety of stress and adjustment disorders, anxiety disorders, affective disorders, and miscellaneous other conditions. In a Medicare study involving 175 000 patients with ESRD, 9% were hospitalized for a mental condition during a one year period.[1] This chapter will briefly review the disorders and discuss recommended treatments as well as specific medications that are likely to produce neuropsychiatric symptoms. Several points are worth emphasizing:

1. Practically all psychotropic drugs can be used safely in people with ESRD. Most are fat soluble, easily pass the blood–brain barrier, are not dialyzable, are primarily detoxified by the liver, and are excreted in bile and not in urine. There are some notable exceptions which are detailed in the text and tables.
2. There is a paucity of research on the metabolism and efficacy of these agents. Future double-blind psychopharmacologic trials are greatly needed to assist nephrologists in management of this group of patients.
3. When individual patients cannot tolerate psychotropic medications, it is usually because of altered pharmacokinetics. The ESRD population is elderly, with multiple and severe comorbid disorders, often protein deficient, and prone to marked fluid and electrolyte shifts. Specific factors that influence the pharmacokinetics of psychotropic medications include: (a) excess gastric alkalinization that can affect drug absorption; (b) ascites and edema that influence drug distribution by increasing the apparent volume of distribution, requiring higher initial doses of medication; (c) dehydration and muscle wasting that decrease the volume of distribution, thereby requiring lower dosages of the drugs;

Table 77.2 Psychiatric and neurologic drugs used in renal failure

Drugs	Active metabolites	Reaction	Typical Adult dose	$t_{1/2}$	Adult dose in ESRD	$t_{1/2}$ in ESRD	Removed by dialysis?	Comment	Reference
Antidepressants – (SSRIs)									
Citalopram (Celexa®)	Desmethylcitalopram Didesmethylcitalopram Citalopram-N-oxide	Anxiety Agitation	20–60 mg daily	33–37 h	10–60 mg daily	43–49 h	H: no	ESRD has minimal impact on citalopram kinetics	27
Fluoxetine (Prozac®, Sarafem®)	Norfluoxetine: NF	Anxiety Agitation	20 mg daily	1–4 days NF 7–15 days	20 mg daily	1.8 days	H: no	No significant differences in fluoxetine and NF levels in renal failure	28
Fluvoxamine Luvox	No active metabolites	Anxiety Agitation	100–300 mg daily	15–22 h	100–300 mg daily	Similar to normal renal function	H: no	No significant differences in renal failure. Manufacture recommends lower initial doses	28, 29
Paroxetine (Paxil®)	No active metabolites	Anxiety Agitation	20–60 mg daily	17.3–25.1 h	10–30 mg daily	10.9–54.8 h		Increased AUC for paroxetine in ESRD (? related to metabolite that is inhibitor of CYP2D6). Reduced dosage recommended	28, 30
Sertraline (Zoloft®)	No active metabolites	Anxiety Agitation	50–200 mg daily	24 h	50–200 mg Daily	42–96 h	H: minimal	Minimal changes in kinetics in ESRD. Useful in sudden hemodialysis-related hypotension	31, 32

Table 77.2 (cont'd)

Drugs	Active metabolites	Reaction	Typical Adult dose	$t_{1/2}$	Adult dose in ESRD	$t_{1/2}$ in ESRD	Removed by dialysis?	Comment	Reference
Antidepressants (tricyclic)									
Amitriptyline (Elavil®)	Nortriptyline Hydroxyamitryptyline Hydroxynortriptyline	Sleep disturbance Confusion Delirium Hallucinations Paranoia Forgetfulness	25 mg q8h	32–40 h	25 mg q8h	32–40 h	H: no	Elevated conjugated metabolites observed in renal failure; probably no difference in dosing. Use of Therapeutic Drug Monitoring (TDM) with level of 75–175 µg/L may guide therapy if used for depression	28
Clomipramine (Anafranil)	Desmethylclopramine: DMC		100–250 mg daily	19–37 h DMC 54–77 h	No data	No data		Little data in ESRD	28
Desipramine (Norpramin®)	2-Hydroxydesipramine	Sleep disturbance Confusion Delirium Depression Forgetfulness Hallucinations Paranoia	100–200 mg daily	12–54 h	75–125 mg daily	No data	H: no CAPD: no	Effective in small trial for depression. Use of TDM with level of 100–160 µg/L may guide therapy if used for depression. Unconjugated amine and OH metabolites not removed by dialysis	28
Doxepin (Sinequan®)	Desmethyldoxepine		25 mg q8h	8–25 h	25 mg q8h	10–30 h	H: no CAPD: no		28
Imipramine (Tofranil®)	Desipramine	Sleep disturbance Confusion Delirium Hallucinations Paranoia Forgetfulness	25 mg q8h	6–20 h	25 mg q8h	No data	H: no CAPD: no		28
Nortriptyline (Aventil, Pamelor)	10-Hydroxynortriptyline E 10-hydroxynortriptyline Z 10-hydroxynortriptyline		25 mg q6-8h	18–93 h	25 mg q6-8h	15–66 h	H: no CAPD: no	Use of TDM with level of 50–150 µg/L may guide therapy if used for depression	28, 33

Table 77.2 (cont'd)

Drugs	Active metabolites	Reaction	Typical Adult dose	t$_{1/2}$	Adult dose in ESRD	t$_{1/2}$ in ESRD	Removed by dialysis?	Comment	Reference
Antidepressants (other)									
Amoxapine (Asendin®)	8-Hydroxyamoxapine: 8OHA 7-Hydroxyamoxapine: 7OHA		75–200 mg daily	8–30 h 8OHA 30 h 7OHA 4–6.5 h	75–200 mg daily	No data		Little data in ESRD	28
Bupropion (Wellbutrin, Zyban®)	Hydroxybupropion: HB Threobupropion: TB	Hallucinations Insomnia Agitation	100 mg q8h	10–21 h	100 mg q8h	No data		Risk for seizures with elevated levels of bupropion or metabolites. Use of TDM of bupropion (level 10–50 µg/L), HB (<1200 µg/L) and TB <400 µg/L) may guide therapy to avoid toxicity	28
Maprotiline (Ludiomil®)	Desmethylmaprotiline Maprotiline-N-oxide		75–150 mg daily	48–51 h	37.5–100 mg daily				
Mirtazapine (Remeron®)	Demethylmirtazapine: DMM		15–45 mg daily	20–40 h DMM 25 h	7.5–22.5 mg daily			Clearance reduced by about 50%. No clear role for TDM	34
Nefazodone (Serzone®)	Multiple including Hydroxynefazodone: NOH		50–150 mg daily	3–5 h NOH 2.5 h	50–150 mg b.i.d.	3–5.8 h NOH 4.4	H: minimal	Primarily nonrenal elimination. No clear role for TDM	35
Trazodone (Desyrel®)	Metachlorophenylpiperazine	Hypomania	150–400 mg daily	4–11 h	No data	No data		Predialysis levels of 50 mg: 85–89 ng/mL; postdialysis level 29–40 ng/mL. No clear role for TDM	36
Venlafaxine (Effexor®)	O-Desmethylvenlafaxine: ODV		37.5–225 mg XR daily	4 h ODV 4 h	37.5 mg to 112.5 XR daily	6–11 h ODV 9 h	H: no	No clear role for TDM	37

Drugs	Active metabolites	Reaction	Typical Adult dose	$t_{1/2}$	Adult dose in ESRD	$t_{1/2}$ in ESRD	Removed by dialysis?	Comment	Reference
Antimanic agents									
Lithium (Eskalith, Lithobid, Lithonate®)	None		900–1200 mg daily	14–28 h	200–600 mg daily	40 h	H: considerable CAPD: variable reports	Single dose after dialysis	38
Valproic acid/ Divalproex (Depakene®, Depakote®)	Unclear if active metabolites		15–60 mg/kg daily	6–17 h	15–60 mg/kg daily		H: modest	? Increased risk of pancreatitis with ESRD. Increased free levels in ESRD. Utilize free VPA levels with TDM	39
Antipsychotics (typical)									
Chlorpromazine (Thorazine®)	Chlorpromazine-N-oxide CPA sulf 7-OH-CPZ Nor-1-CPZ Nor-2-CPZ Nor-2-CPZ sulf 3-OH-CPZ		50–400 mg daily	11–42 h		11–42 h			40
Haloperidol (Haldol®)	Hydroxyhaloperidol plus other metabolites (activity not clear)		1–2 mg q8–12h	14–26 h	1–2 mg q8–12h	Similar		<1% excreted in urine	41
Perphenazine (Trilafon®)	Metabolite activity unknown		4–16 mg b.i.d. or q.i.d.	9.5 h					
Thioridazine (Mellaril®)	Mesoridazine (potency 2 × thioridazine) Sulforidazine	Prolonged QT interval	50–800 mg daily	21–24 h	No data	No data		Contraindicated in patients with prolonged QTc interval, concurrent fluoxetine, paroxetine, fluvoxamine therapy. Best avoided due to prolonged QT interval and risk for life-threatening arrhythmias may be higher with electrolyte shifts	

Table 77.2 (cont'd)

Drugs	Active metabolites	Reaction	Typical Adult dose	$t_{1/2}$	Adult dose in ESRD	$t_{1/2}$ in ESRD	Removed by dialysis?	Comment	Reference
Antipsychotics (atypical)									
Clozapine (Clozaril®)	N-Desmethylclozapine: NDC	Delirium and psychosis on withdrawal	12.5–450 mg slowly titrated	8–12 h NDC 13.2 h	Titrate to response and utilize TDM			Titrate dose to response Therapeutic drug monitoring may assist dosing in unclear circumstances. Avoid levels > 400 µg/L	42
Olanzepine (Zyprexa®)	N-Desmethylolanzapine Olanzapine-10-N-glucuronide		5–20 mg daily	32–38 h	5–20 mg	32–38 h		Dose adjustment not necessary in renal failure per manufacturer	43
Quetiapine (Seroquel®)	7-Hydroxyquetiapine N-Dealkylated quetiapine		150–750 mg b.i.d. or t.i.d.	6 h	150–750 mg b.i.d. or t.i.d.			Dosage adjustment not necessary in renal failure per manufacturer	
Risperidone (Risperdal®)	9-Hydroxyrisperidone		1–3 mg b.i.d	3–30 h 9ROH 19 h	0.5–1.5 mg b.i.d.	9ROH: 25 h		Wide variation in clearance noted between poor and extensive metabolizers. Clearance of sum of risperidone and 9ROH are reduced by 60% renal failure	44
Ziprasidone (Geodon®)	Inactive metabolites		20–80 mg b.i.d.	7 h	10–80 mg b.i.d.			No adjustment required for CrCl 10–60 mL/min per manufacturer. Some clinicians recommend avoiding in ESRD due to prolonged QT interval and risk for life-threatening arrhythmias that may be higher with electrolyte shifts	45

Table 77.2 (cont'd)

Drugs	Active metabolites	Reaction	Typical Adult dose	$t_{1/2}$	Adult dose in ESRD	$t_{1/2}$ in ESRD	Removed by dialysis?	Comment	Reference
Anxiolytics/hypnotics									
Alprazolam (Xanax®)	α-Hydroxyalprazolam < 15% of alprazolam	Hallucinations	0.25–5 mg t.i.d.	9–19 h	0.25–5 mg t.i.d.	9–19 h	H: minimal	Increased free fraction in ESRD. Minimal differences in dialysis-dependant patients	28, 46
Buspirone (Buspar®)	1-Pyrimidinylpiperazine: 1-PP		5 mg q8h	0.5–2.5 h 1-PP 6.3 h	5 mg q8h	1–5 h 1-PP 9 h	H: no	Considerable interindividual and intraindividual variability in kinetics in ESRD. Patients with renal failure may benefit from a 25–50%dose reduction	47
Clorazepate (Tranxene®)	Desmethyldiazepam: DMD		15–60 mg daily p.o.	DMD 57.3 h	15–60 mg daily p.o.	DMD 36.1 h		Increased free fraction DMD resulting in similar free levels in normal and renal insufficiency	48
Chlordiazepoxide (Librium®)	Multiple		15–100 mg daily	5–30 h	7.5–50 mg daily	? Similar		Decreased protein binding, increased clearance	57
Clonazepam (Klonopin®)	No active metabolites		0.5 mg t.i.d.	18–80 h	0.5 mg t.i.d.	? Same	H: no	Useful in restless leg syndrome	49
Diazepam (Valium®)	Desmethyldiazepam Oxazepam	Delusions Hallucinations	5–40 mg daily	92 h DMD 57.3 h	5–40 mg daily	37 h DMD 36.1 h	H: no	Elevated free levels of diazepam in ESRD. Increased free fraction DMD resulting in similar free levels in normal and renal insufficiency	28, 50
Lorazepam (Ativan®)	No active metabolites		1–2 mg b.i.d. or t.i.d.	9–16 h	0.5–2 mg b.i.d.	32–70 h	H: no	Manufacturer does not recommend in ESRD	28
Midazolam (Versed®)	α-Hydroxymidazolam conjugate: AHM-C	Prolonged sedation	1.25 mg i.v. titrate to response	1.2–12.3 h	1.25 mg i.v. titrate to response	1.2 – 12.3 h AMH-C: 50.4–76.8 h		? increased effect due to reduced protein binding?	28, 51

737

Table 77.2 *(cont'd)*

Drugs	Active metabolites	Reaction	Typical Adult dose	$t_{1/2}$	Adult dose in ESRD	$t_{1/2}$ in ESRD	Removed by dialysis?	Comment	Reference
Oxazepam (Serax®)	No active metabolites		30–120 mg daily usually in divided dose	6–25 h	30–120 mg daily usually in divided dose	25–90 h	H: no		28
Temazepam (Restoril®)	No active metabolites		15–30 mg hs prn	4–10 h	15–30 mg hs prn		H: no CAPD: no		28
Triazolam (Halcion®)	α-Hydroxytriazolam	Hallucinations Paranoia	0.125–0.5 mg hs prn	2–4 h	0.125–0.5 mg hs prn	2.3 h	H: no CAPD: no		28
Zaleplon (Sonata®)	No active metabolites		5–20 mg hs prn	1 h	? 5–10 mg hs prn			No dose adjustment needed per manufacturer for mild to moderate renal impairment. Not studied in ESRD	
Zolpidem (Ambien®)	No active metabolites		10 mg hs prn	2–3 h	Reduce dose by 50%	4–6 h		Increased free fraction	
Anticonvulsants									
Carbamazepine Tegretol®	Carbamazepine-10-11-epoxide 9-Hydroxymethyl-10-carbamoylacridan		100 mg b.i.d. to 400 mg q.i.d.	12–17 h (chronic dosing)	100 mg b.i.d. to 400 mg q.i.d	Similar to normal renal function	H: no CAPD: no		28
Gabapentin (Neurontin®)	Confusion Lethargy Hypoxia Coma		300–600 mg t.i.d.	5–7 h	300 mg every other day or 200–300 mg after each 4-h hemodialysis	132 h	H: yes CAPD: partial	Significant accumulation has occurred with typical dosing or interruption in hemodialysis	52, 58

Table 77.2 *(cont'd)*

Drugs	Active metabolites	Reaction	Typical Adult dose	$t_{1/2}$	Adult dose in ESRD	$t_{1/2}$ in ESRD	Removed by dialysis?	Comment	Reference
Phenytoin (Dilantin®)	Conjugated and unconjugated 5-(4-hydroxyphenyl)-5-phenylhydantoin: 4-OH-DPH (? activity)	Loose associations Psychosis Ataxia	200–400 mg daily	24 h (at low to moderate levels)	200–400 mg daily	24 h (at low to moderate levels) 4-OH-DPH levels ? (? significance)	H: no CAPD: no	Increased free levels secondary to uremia Monitor free phenytoin levels 1–2 mg/L	28, 53
Phenobarbital (Luminal®)	Inactive metabolite		60–250 mg daily	1.5–4.9 days	Unknown	Unknown	H: yes CAPD: conflicting reports	Partial renal clearance 15% for patients with normal renal function	59
Primidone (Mysoline®)	Phenobarbital: PB Phenylethyl-malonide: PEMA		125 mg t.i.d. titrated to 250–500 mg t.i.d.-q.i.d.	5–15 h PB: 1.5–4.9 days PEMA: 29–36 h	250–500 mg q12–24 h	? ↑ Primid one, PB, and PEMA levels	H: Modest	Report of flapping flapping tremor and CNS depression in patient with modest renal insufficiency and concurrent cimetidine therapy	27

CAPD, chronic ambulatory peritoneal dialysis; H, hemodialysis.

and (d) the high protein-binding affinity of these medications that in renal failure may leave a larger proportion of a given dose of medicine unbound and more available for efficacy, toxicity, or elimination.

4. Given these multiple and interacting factors it is no surprise that the *Physician's Desk Reference* generally recommends that patients with ESRD are administered no more than two-thirds the ordinary or maximum dose of most psychotropic medications. However, in our clinical experience and examination of the literature, we find that the majority of patients maintained with dialysis both tolerate and require ordinary dosages of many psychotropic medications. On the other hand, when the factors influencing pharmacokinetics are severe, it is logical to start with modest dosages and to increase cautiously.

5. It is fortunate that dialysis programs are legally mandated to provide access to renal social workers. Medications only help in certain situations. They do not substitute for the skilled provision of psychotherapy and counseling. They cannot replace clarification of complex individual and family matters. Ideally, a close working relationship ought to be established with community psychiatrists and mental health facilities.

Table 77.1 summarizes the many factors that can produce an organic brain syndrome in this population. Table 77.2 lists commonly used psychotropic medications, including a number of atypical antipsychotics and the new generation of antidepressant medications. Table 77.3 lists other medications that are widely used in this population, and which can produce neuropsychiatric symptoms as side effects. Alertness is needed to avoid misdiagnosis and mistreatment.

Neurological conditions

Patients with chronic kidney disease frequently manifest neurological symptoms. For patients over age 65 years who are maintained with dialysis, organic brain syndromes are a leading cause of hospitalization.[2] As renal function worsens, it is increasingly likely that a subtle or overt neurological symptom will occur.[3] Etiologic factors include medication side-effects that are worsened by diminished renal drug clearance, effects of the uremic milieu, dialysis and transplantation treatment effects, other comorbid conditions, and electrolyte disturbances.

Subtle subclinical deficits in cognitive function on neuropsychological testing are apparent in patients with uremia, as well as those with moderate renal insufficiency, and those who are considered to be adequately dialyzed. As renal function worsens, overt encephalopathy becomes apparent with confusion, delirium, stupor, and progression to coma.[4] Seizures can occur in advanced stages. If the alteration in mental status is due to uremia, dialysis will result in rapid improvement of mental status.

Peripheral neuropathies

The uremic state has an effect on the peripheral nervous system in virtually all patients.[5] Abnormal autonomic function occurs regularly. Delayed nerve conduction can frequently be measured. At a later stage, there may be sensory or motor peripheral neuropathy.

A steal syndrome from an arteriovenous (AV) fistula needs to be ruled out as a cause of peripheral neuropathy. The neurological deficit may be partially reversed if the fistula is banded or tied off. In the case of carpal tunnel syndrome where accumulation of β_2-microglobulin is suspected, dialysis can be intensified with large-surface-area dialyzers. Although wrist splints may relieve symptoms, surgery is often required. Polyneuropathy can be pharmacologically treated with low doses of tricylic antidepressants, gabapentin, or carbamazepine.

Postural hypotension can be effectively managed with thigh-high, moderate-graded compression stockings, and/or midodrine. Sudden intradialytic hypotension can be prevented by administering sertraline (50 mg) before dialysis. Gastroparesis and esophageal motility disorders may respond to a course of metoclopramide.

Seizures

Seizures are common in patients with chronic kidney disease, especially those undergoing hemodialysis.[6] Approximately 7% of patients may develop new-onset seizures as a consequence of a severe uremic state before dialysis is started, or secondary to hemodynamic and electrolyte shifts (disequilibrium syndrome) that occur during or shortly after dialysis sessions.[7] Medication-induced seizures can be due to an inadvertent effect of the drug (such as a rapidly increasing hematocrit with epoetin-alfa), toxic drug levels secondary to diminished renal clearance (such as penicillins, cephalosporins, acyclovir, amantidine, and high-dose intravenous contrast agents), accumulation of toxic metabolites (such as normeperidine), and subtherapeutic levels of maintenance antiseizure medication as a result of dialysis clearance. Other causes of seizure include: hemodynamic instability with hypotension and hypertension, dialysis dementia, alcohol withdrawal, electrolyte disturbances (involving calcium, sodium, glucose), and air emboli from hemodialysis.

The seizures of uremic encephalopathy can be prevented if dialysis is initiated early. Preventing seizures secondary to the dialysis disequilibrium syndrome that can occur when dialysis is started involves the gradual reduction of blood urea nitrogen (BUN) by low blood flows (200 mL/min), short dialysis (2–3 h), a small surface dialyzer, and diminished dialysate flow rates. Dialysis is performed on a daily basis initially. Dialysis disequilibrium can be prevented by giving intravenous mannitol (12.5 g of 25% solution) midway through sessions. Serum levels of antiepileptic drugs must be monitored in people with epilepsy, who may require additional medication immediately after dialysis.

In order to prevent seizures related to epoetin-alfa, initial doses should be low and adjusted to prevent a rapid increase in hematocrit. Patients with uncontrolled hypertension should first have their blood pressure controlled.

If a seizure occurs during dialysis, dialysis treatment should be stopped, the airway secured and – if hypoglycemia is suspected – intravenous glucose given. If the seizure persists, intravenous diazepam (5–10 mg) can be administered every 5 min. If respiratory depression occurs, flumazenil will reverse the effect of benzodiazapines, but may worsen control of the underlying seizure and render benzodiazepine therapy ineffective. A dose of dilantin (10–15 mg/kg) given at a rate no greater than 50 mg/min can be started. If the seizure was thought to be secondary to the uremic state, or a complication of the dialysis treatment, maintenance antiseizure medication may not be needed. If phenytoin is used chronically, a serum level of 1–2.5 mg/L of free phenytoin is recommended.

Restless leg syndrome

This is a common symptom found in over 50% of patients on chronic dialysis. This syndrome refers to a persistent and uncomfortable sensation in the lower extremities, which can only be relieved by movement of the legs. The symptoms occur more prominently at night and interfere with sleep. It is often confused with the burning foot syndrome, which is caused by vitamin B_6 deficiency or asymptomatic fasciculations, myoclonus, and painful muscle cramps. Treatment with heat packs and exercise can be effective, as can clonazepam, carbidopa/levodopa, dopamine agonists (pergolide), gabapentin, clonidine, and narcotics. Rotating these drug classes can be helpful in cases where tolerance occurs.

Insomnia

Insomnia is a common problem for patients with chronic kidney disease. Insomnia also occurs secondary to sleep apnea, restless leg syndrome, cramps, and the pain of peripheral neuropathy. Identification and treatment of these individual conditions will correct many cases of insomnia. Otherwise, nonpharmacological treatments (behavioral management and instruction in sleep hygiene practices) should be tried, and if not effective, a hypnotic such as temazepam, zolpidem, or zaleplon can be used on a short-term basis. Zaleplon is a new nonbenzodiazepine hypnotic agent, indicated for short-term treatment of insomnia. The manufacturer maintains that its pharmacokinetics are not altered in patients with renal insufficiency since less than 1% of the drug is excreted by the kidneys; however, there are substantial increases in the plasma concentrations of zaleplon metabolites in people with renal impairment, and the medication has been inadequately studied in hemodialysis populations.

Delirium

Attempts should be made to identify and correct the underlying causes of delirium in ESRD patients. There are several commonly used medications that may produce neuropsychiatric symptoms; these should be prescribed with caution. For example, acyclovir and meperidine are associated with delirium.[8,9] Clarithromycin has been reported to cause visual hallucinations in conjunction with peritoneal dialysis.[10]

Many cases are more etiologically complex, and require rapid treatment of symptoms, especially agitation. Pharmacological symptom management usually entails administration of the traditional neuroleptics, primarily haloperidol. In agitated, acutely delirious patients, this medication is commonly administered intravenously, through a slow push. The method is not formally approved, however, and there have been rare cases of torsade-de-pointes-type arrhythmias. There are several commonly used regimens for severe symptoms; a recent guideline merely lists the occasional use of 5–10 mg of haloperidol;[11] a more aggressive protocol calls for 5 mg to begin with and a doubling of the dose every 20 min until the patient is tranquilized, but arousable to painful stimuli.[12] Many psychiatric units medicate agitated patients with alternating doses of haloperidol and a benzodiazepine (e.g. lorazepam 1 mg or 2 mg) every 30 min to 1 h. Newer atypical neuroleptic agents such as clozapine, risperidone, and olanzapine hold promise for the future, but have not been systematically investigated.[13]

Dementia

Dialysis dementia, or dialysis encephalopathy, is a distinct, progressive, neurologic disorder whose etiology remains controversial.[7] It has been divided into three categories including an epidemic form that is often associated with aluminum, sporadic cases in which aluminum is not a factor, and a type that is associated with congenital or early-childhood renal disease. Dialysis dementia caused by aluminum toxicity can be treated with deferoxamine, large-surface-areas dialyzers, or charcoal hemoperfusion (see Chapter 84).

As the ESRD population ages, senile dementias are becoming more prevalent. Alzheimer's type of dementia has become a common comorbidity.

Psychiatric conditions

Schizophrenia

Pharmacological treatment of schizophrenia has been revolutionized by use of the atypical neuroleptics, including clozapine, risperidone, and olanzapine. Unlike traditional neuroleptics, this new generation of major tranquilizers effectively treats the negative symptoms of the disease, such as emotional blunting and apathy. Little is known about their properties in people with ESRD, and considerable caution is necessary. Olanzapine, for example, is largely metabolized by the liver but its metabolites are excreted in urine. Single-dose studies in patients with renal impairment indicate that special dosing is not required. However, multiple dose studies have not been conducted.

The traditional neuroleptics continue to be commonly employed in the management of schizophrenia. Recently, the Food and Drug Administration review of thioridazine, a widely used antipsychotic, resulted in a warning about prolongation of the ECG QTc interval, and association with torsade-de-pointes-type arrhythmias and sudden death. Thioridazine is now contraindicated with certain other drugs, including fluvoxamine, propranolol, paroxetine, and fluoxetine. An alternative tranquilizer should certainly be considered for patients with renal impairment.

Adjustment disorders

All renal replacement therapies and procedures force patients to be unusually dependent on technology and on medical staff.[14] Emotional difficulties can occur when highly independent individuals are compelled to behave passively. Dependency issues are especially accentuated by hemodialysis. Personality needs to be strongly considered when arranging therapy. People with renal disease should ideally be provided with information about each option by their nephrologist, and should be allowed to choose the treatment that is best suited to their situation, social circumstances, and personality characteristics. Decisions must be flexible, and staff must be aware of the possibility of a poor "fit", and the need to shift to a different modality.

Most chronic illnesses afford their victims some respite from continued awareness of the disease. For example, patients with heart conditions often have long asymptomatic periods, and those with cancer may have substantial periods of remission during which they have no pain and need no therapy. In contrast, patients with ESRD are constantly reminded of their illness. These patients must take multiple medications throughout the day, restrict fluids, and schedule their week around repetitive dialysis sessions. Furthermore, patients maintained with hemodialysis often require vascular access revisions and other procedures. The treatment has unfortunate effects on skin coloration and overall appearance, and on the surgical sites for access grafts. Peritoneal dialysis distorts the patient's body by distending the abdomen, and although most patients tolerate the cosmetic alterations, people who are greatly concerned with their appearance may have considerable difficulty accepting a change in abdominal girth. This therapy is all too often punctuated by episodes of peritonitis.

For most people, work is not merely a source of income, but also self-esteem. Unfortunately, many dialysis patients are retired, unemployed, or only able to maintain part-time jobs. The drop in income, the absence of employment benefits, and the additional costs of medication, transport, and special diets and equipment may have destructive effects on the individual and the family. When men or women lose their jobs because of ESRD, this places an added burden on the healthy spouse or partner. It is not unusual for roles to be reversed or expanded to manage daily responsibilities.[15]

Treatment for an adjustment disorder involves supportive and educational therapy by the nephrologist and social worker. Support by fellow patients and peer counselors can be beneficial in assisting patients and their families to accept the limitations of treatment. The more complex clinical situations should be identified, appropriate psychotherapy provided by the renal social workers, and referral made to the local mental health facilities. Pastoral counseling may be beneficial. Preparation and advanced warning about the possible stresses are ideal. Lastly, tincture of time is often a crucial factor in coping.

Anxiety disorders

Anxiety is one of the most common psychological symptoms seen in the physically ill. It may be particularly severe during or immediately preceding dialysis treatments. Rapid removal of fluid and electrolytes can produce hypotension, nausea, vomiting, and muscular cramps, and may result in considerable anxiety. Generalized anxiety about the future, fear about sexual performance, and apprehension over the ability to adjust to the ongoing demands of dialysis and the expectations of staff and family are frequent concerns for patients.

Pharmacological management is either directed at acute episodes of anxiety and panic, or at more generalized nervousness (Table 77.2). Since benzodiazepines are metabolized in the liver, dosage reduction is generally not necessary in ESRD. Exceptions included midazolam and chlordiazepoxide. It is not unusual to give ordinary doses of diazepam, ativan, alprazolam, and clonazepam before or during dialysis sessions. Selective serotonin reuptake inhibitors (SSRIs) are being used increasingly to treat panic and generalized anxiety disorders.

Depressive disorders

Examination of the ESRD literature suggests that subsyndromal depressive syndromes are likely in about 25% of patients, and major depression in 5%–22% of patients.[16] In dialysis facilities major depression is often unrecognized and untreated.

We would recommend a diagnostic approach that entails describing the criteria for major depression, eliciting patients' opinion as to whether they believe themselves to be depressed, and documenting the existence of associated factors, such as depressive episodes prior to the onset of renal failure, a family history of depression, and past suicide attempts.[17]

The association of depression and mortality in ESRD has been supported by several studies,[18] but not by others.[19] In one investigation,[20] the 2-year survival of patients with Beck Depression Inventory scores < 14 was 85%, while the survival rate for those with scores ≥ 25 was 25%. The most recent and comprehensive study used time-varying covariate survival analysis and found that depressive indices predicted survival at 1 year, and that higher levels of depressive affect were associated with increased mortality.[18]

Reviews of antidepressant management of ESRD have consistently found both SSRIs and tricyclic antidepressants to be beneficial.[21] Future double-blind psychopharmacologic trials are greatly needed to assist nephrologists in the management of these patients. Although the greatest body of experience is on the tricyclics, these have largely been supplanted by a newer generation of antidepressants. Tricyclics ought to be reserved for treatment-resistant depression (or other indications, such as peripheral neuropathy). The hydroxylated metabolites contribute to both the therapeutic and toxic effects of these medications in ESRD. Nortriptyline is a particularly useful tricyclic because of its meaningful serum levels. Imipramine and amitriptyline continue to be used for analgesia of neuropathic pain, while trazodone is commonly used as a sedative–hypnotic for insomnia.

SSRIs are often beneficial in ESRD, but have not been systematically or adequately researched. Fluoxetine is the best studied medication in this class, and appears to be both nontoxic and efficacious.[22] The kinetic profile of single doses of fluoxetine is unchanged even in anephric patients. A study of multiple doses concludes that renal function does not significantly alter either fluoxetine or norfluoxetine serum levels.

Sertraline has not been as intensively studied in this population, but it is also widely prescribed. Like fluoxetine, it is metabolized hepatically and excretion of the unchanged drug in urine is an insignificant route of elimination. Pharmacokinetic investigations in people with mild-to-severe renal impairment and matched controls show no significant differences. Sertraline has been used to help prevent sudden hemodialysis-related hypotension.[23]

Like sertraline and fluoxetine, citalopram kinetics are minimally changed in patients with ESRD and dose adjustment is probably not necessary. Interestingly, plasma concentrations of paroxetine hydrochloride are increased in people with renal impairment with the recommended initial dose for patients with severe renal insufficiency (10 mg) being half that of normal adults.

There are several non-SSRI antidepressant medications that should be used with caution or avoided with ESRD. For example, little is known about the pharmacokinetics of nefazodone hydrochloride in patients who have chronically impaired renal function. Careful dose adjustment is also necessary with venlafaxine, which is chiefly eliminated in urine along with its metabolites.[3] The elimination half-life of venlafaxine is prolonged and clearance is reduced in people who have chronic renal insufficiency or ESRD. Regular monitoring of blood pressure is recommended for those taking this drug. Bupropion hydrochloride has active metabolites, which are almost completely excreted through the kidney; these metabolites may accumulate in dialysis patients and predispose to seizures.

Care must be taken with patients receiving concurrent drugs metabolized by cytochrome P450 3A4 (e.g. tacrolimus, cyclosporin, sildenafil) when using antidepressants which are inhibitors of this isoenzyme. Inhibitors of cytochrome p450 3A4 include nefazodone, fluoxetine/norfluoxetine, fluvoxamine, paroxetine (a weak inhibitor), sertraline and valproic acid (a weak inhibitor). For many years, lithium has been the primary pharmacologic treatment of bipolar affective disorder. It has efficacy in acute episodes and in prevention of relapses. It is being replaced by classic anticonvulsant medications, such as depakote, carbamazepine, and gabapentine, which also significantly help these patients. For the relatively few bipolar patients with ESRD who require lithium (and do not respond to the anticonvulsants), treatment involves administration of a single dose (usually 600 mg) after each dialysis run. Because it is a small molecule that is readily dialyzed, lithium is eliminated by dialysis. A single dose will result in a steady serum level.[24] Serum lithium levels obtained before and after dialysis sessions are used to establish the proper dose. Ideally, lithium levels should be obtained immediately before dialysis and 2 h after completion of dialysis; the level obtained immediately after dialysis will often be lower than that observed later due to a postdialysis redistribution effect. A smaller dose (300 mg) may be given to augment the therapeutic effects of antidepressants in treatment-resistant unipolar depression.

Lithium can be nephrotoxic. Efforts should be made to substitute other drugs in patients with renal insufficiency. A long-term follow-up study has found that when the drug is discontinued, renal function will often improve.[25]

Sexual disorders

A majority of patients on dialysis experience diminished frequency of or interest in sex. Levy has observed that approximately 70% of men have partial or total impotence, and the majority of women are amennorheic or infertile.[21] He has also reported that even a successful kidney transplant does not always restore the patients' sexual function to that experienced before renal failure. Diminished libido and impaired sexual functioning are side effects of SSRIs. Behavioral psychotherapies may be helpful. Most men need surgical intervention for continued sexual functioning. Recent anecdotal reports suggest that sildenafil (Viagra) may hold promise for many patients. Double-blind crossover studies have been performed in over 3000 men with normal renal function, showing that irrespective of the cause of sexual dysfunction sildenafil is significantly more effective than placebo at inducing erections. Improvement in erectile function is associated with marked improvement of depressive symptoms and the patient's assessment of quality of life.[26] Sildenafil is contraindicated in people taking nitrates for coronary artery disease, as it can cause fatal hypotension. However, it has been shown to be safe and efficacious in patients with diabetes, spinal cord injury, and prostate cancer. For patients with ESRD who have not experienced significant hypotension during dialysis and are not receiving drugs known to be inhibitors of cytochrome p450 3A4 (see Depressive Disorders above), a low dose of sildenafil (25 mg) may be considered.

Table 77.3 Drugs producing neuropsychiatric toxicity in the general population with comments on likely effects for patients with renal failure

Drugs	Active metabolites	Reaction	Typical Adult dose	$t_{1/2}$	Adult dose in ESRD	$t_{1/2}$ in ESRD	Removed by dialysis?	Comment	Reference
Antiparkinsonian									
Amantadine (Symmetrel®)	Active metabolites	Hallucinations Agitation	100 mg q8–12 h	12 h	100 mg q7d	500 h	H variable reports	Accumulation in renal failure	28, 54
Anticholinergics									
Trihexyphenidyl (Artane®)		Hallucinations							
Benztropine (Cogentin®)		Confusion							31
Bromocriptine (Parlodel®)	Metabolites ? activity	Visual hallucinations							
Carbidopa/ Levodopa (Sinemet®)	Active metabolites	Hallucinations Agitation	25/100 mg t.i.d.	Carbidopa 2 h L-dopa 0.8–1.6 h	50% dose reduction	↑ Active metabolites			28
Analgesics									
Aspirin	Metabolites ? activity	Psychosis with toxic levels	650 mg q4h	2–3 h	Avoid full dose in ESRD	2–3 h	H negligible CAPD negligible		28
Codeine	Codeine 6-glucoronide Morphine	Hypotension Sedation CNS depression	30–60 mg q4–6h	2.5–4h	15–30 mg q4–6h	18 h		Hypotension; sedation has been reported in ESRD	28, 55
Ibuprofen (Motrin, Advil®)	Metabolites ? activity	Aseptic meningitis with lethargy Coma	200–800 mg t.i.d.	2–3.2 h	200–800 mg t.i.d.	2–3.2 h	H no CAPD no	Prostaglandin inhibition may result in renal dysfunction, uremic bleeding, and gastrointestinal bleeding, nephrotic syndrome, interstitial nephritis, hyperkalemia	28, 56
Indomethacin (Indocin®)	Inactive metabolites	Visual hallucinations Paranoid delusions	25–50 mg t.i.d.	4–12 h	25–50 mg t.i.d.	4–12 h	H no CAPD no	Prostaglandin inhibition may result in renal dysfunction, uremic bleeding, and gastrointestinal bleeding, nephrotic syndrome, interstitial nephritis, hyperkalemia	28

References

1. Kimmel PL, Tharner M, Richard CM, et al: Psychiatric illness in patients with end-stage renal disease. Am J Med 1998; 105:214–221.
2. USRDS. Excerpts from the United States Renal Data System 2000 Annual Data Report. National Institutes of Health NIDDK/DKUHD. Am J Kidney Dis 2000;36(suppl 2):S1–S239.
3. Fraser CL, Arieff AI: Neuropsychiatric complications of renal failure. In Brady HR, Wilcox CS (eds): Therapy in Nephrology and Hypertension: A Companion to Brenner and Rector's The Kidney. Philadelphia: WB Saunders Company, 2001, pp 488–490.
4. Fraser CL, Arieff AI: Metabolic encephalopathy as a complication of renal failure: mechanisms and mediators. New Horiz 1994;2:518–526.
5. Palmer, BF, Henrich, WL: Uremic mononeuropathy. In Rose, BD (ed): UpToDate. Wellesley, MA: UpToDate, 2001. http://www.uptodate.com
6. Barri YM, Golper TA: Seizures in patients undergoing hemodialysis polyneuropathy. In Rose, BD (ed): UpToDate. Wellesley, MA: UpToDate, 2001. http://www.uptodate.com
7. Arieff AI: Dialysis disequilibrium syndrome: Current concepts on pathogenesis and prevention. Kidney Int 1994;45:629–635.
8. Revenkar SG, Applegate AL, Markovitz DM: Delirium associated with acyclovir treatment in a patient with renal failure. Clin Infect Dis 1995;21: 435–436.
9. Stock SL, Catalono G, Catallano MC: Meperidine associated mental status changes in a patient with chronic renal failure. J Fla Med Assoc 1996;83:315–319.
10. Steinman MA, Steinman TI: Clarithromycin-associated visual hallucinations in a patient with chronic renal failure on continuous ambulatory peritoneal dialysis. Am J Kidney Dis 1996;27:143–146.
11. Schmidt RJ, Holley JL. Psychiatric illness in dialysis patients. In Rose BL (ed): UpToDate. Wellesley, MA: UpToDate, 2001. http://www.uptodate.com
12. Cassem NH, Hackett TP: The setting of intensive care. In Hackett TP, Cassem NH (eds): Massachusetts General Hospital Handbook of General Hospital Psychiatry. Saint Louis: The CV Mosby Co, 1978, pp 326–327.
13. Schwartz TL, Masand PS: The role of atypical antipsychotics in the treatment of delirium. Psychosomatics 2002;43:171–174.
14. Levy NB: Psychiatric consideration in the primary medical care of the patient with renal failure. Adv Ren Replace Ther 2000;7:231–238.
15. Reiss D: Patient, family and staff responses to end-stage renal disease. Am J Kidney Dis 1990;15:194–200.
16. O'Donnell K, Chung Y: The diagnosis of major depression in end-stage renal disease. Psychother Psychosom 1997;66:38–43.
17. Cohen LM, Steinberg MD, Hails KC, et al: The psychiatric evaluation of death-hastening requests: Lessons from dialysis discontinuation. Psychosomatics 2000;41:195–203.
18. Kimmel PL, Peterson RA, Weihs KL, et al: Multiple measurements of depression predict mortality in a longitudinal study of chronic hemodialysis outpatients. Kidney Int 2000;57:2093–2098.
19. Culp K, Flanigan M, Lowrie EG, et al: Modeling mortality risk in hemodialysis patients using laboratory values as time dependent covariates. Am J Kidney Dis 1996;28:741–746.
20. Shulman R, Price JDE, Spinelli J: Biopsychosocial aspects of lone-term survival on end-stage renal failure therapy. Psychol Med 1989;19:945–954.
21. Levy NB, Cohen LM: Central and peripheral nervous systems in uremia. In Massry SG, Glassock R (eds): Textbook of Nephrology, 4th edn. Philadelphia: Williams and Wilkins, 2001, pp 1279–1282.
22. Blumenfield, M, Levy NB, Spinowitz B, et al: Fluoxetine in depressed patients on dialysis. Int J Psychiatry Med 1997;27:71–80.
23. Dheenan S, Venketesan J, Grubb BP, Henrich WL: Effect of sertraline hydrochloride on dialysis hypotension. Am J Kidney Diseases 1998;31:624–630.
24. Port FK, Kroll PD, Rosenzweig J: Lithium therapy during maintenance hemodialysis. Psychosomatics 1979;20:130–132.
25. Braden GL: Lithium-induced renal disease. Primer on Kidney Disease, 3rd edn, San Diego, CA: Academic Press, 2001, pp 322–324.
26. Seidman SN, Roose SP, Menza MA, et al: Treatment of erectile dysfunction in men with depressive symptoms: Results of a placebo-controlled trial with sildenafil citrate. Am J Psychiatry 2001;158:1623–1630.
27. Joffe P, Larsen FS, Pedersen V, et al: Single-dose pharmacokinetics of citalopram in patients with moderate renal insufficiency or hepatic cirrhosis compared with health subjects. Eur J Clin Pharmacol 1998;54:237–242.
28. Aronoff GR, Berns JS, Brier ME, et al: Drug Prescribing in Renal Failure. Dosing Guidelines for Adults, 4th edn. Philadelphia, PA: American College of Physicians–American Society for Internal Medicine, 1999.
29. Perucca E, Gatti G, Spina E: Clinical pharmacokinetics of fluvoxamine. Clin Pharmacokinet 1994:27:175–190.
30. Doyle CD, Laher M, Kelly JG, et al: The pharmacokinetics of paroxetine in renal impairment. Acta Psychiatr Scand:80 (Suppl 350):89–90.
31. Wood KA, Harris MJ, Morreale A, et al: Drug-induced psychosis and depression in the elderly. Psych Clinics of North Amer 1988;11:167–193.
32. Brater DC: Drug Dosing in Renal Failure in Therapy in Nephrology and Hypertension. A Companion to Brenner and Rector's The Kidney. Philadelphia: WB Saunders Company, 2001, pp 641–653.
33. Nordin C, Betilsson L: Active hydroxymetabolites of antidepressants: emphasis on E-10-hydroxy-nortriptyline. Clin Pharmacokinet 1995;28:26–40.
34. Timmer CJ, Ad Sitsen JM, Delbressine LP: Clinical pharmacokinetics of mirtazapine. Clin Pharmacokinet 2000;38(6): 461–474.
35. Seabolt JL, DeLeon OA: Response to nefzaodone in a depressed patient with end-stage renal disease. Gen Hosp Psychiatr 2001;23:45–46.
36. Otani K, Tybring G, Mihara K, et al: Correlation between steady-state plasma concentration of mianserin and trazodone in depressed patients. Eur J Clin Pharmacol 1998;53:347–349.
37. Troy SM, Schultz RW, Parker VD: The effect of renal disease on the disposition of venlafaxine. Clin Pharmacol Ther 1994;56:14–21.
38. Lam YWF, Banerji S, Hatfield C, et al: Principles of drug administration in renal insufficiency. Clin Pharmacokinet 1997;32:30–57.
39. Lapierre O: Valproic acid intoxication in a patient with bipolar disorder and chronic uremia (letter). Can J Psychiatry, 1999;44:188.
40. Chetty M, Moodley SV, Mikller R: Important metabolites to measure in pharmacodynamic studies of chlorpromazine. Ther Drug Monit 1994;16:30–36.
41. Kudo S, Ishizaki T. Pharmacokinetics of haloperidol – an update. Clin Pharmacokinet 1999;37:435–456.
42. Guitton C, Abbar M, Kinowski JM, et al: Multiple-dose pharmacokinetics of clozapine in patients with chronic schizophrenia. J Clin Psychopharmacol 1998;18:470–476.
43. Callaghan JT, Bergstrom RF, Ptak LR, et al: Olanzapine – pharmacokinetic and pharmacodynamic profile. Clin Pharmacokinet 1999;37:177–193.
44. Heykants J, Haung ML, Mannens G: The pharmacokinetics of risperidone in humans: a summary. J Clin Psychiatry 1994; 55(5 Suppl):13–17.
45. Ereshefsky L. Pharmacokinetics and drug interactions: update for new antipsychotics. J Clin Psychiatry 1996;57(suppl):12–15
46. Schmith VD, Piraino B, Smith RB, et al: Alprazolam in end stage renal disease. J Clin Pharmacol 1991;31:571–579.
47. Caccia S, Vigano GL, Mingardi G, et al: Clinical pharmacokinetics of oral buspirone in patients with impaired renal function. Clin Pharmacokinet 1988:14:171–177.
48. Ochs HR, Rauh HW, Greenblatt DJ, et al: Clorazepate dipotassium and diazepam in renal insufficiency: serum concentrations and protein binding of diazepam and desmethyldiazepam. Nephron 1984;37:100–104.
49. Amiel M, Bryan S, Herjanic M: Clonazepam in the treatment of bipolar disorder in patients with non-lithium-induced renal insufficiency. J Clin Psychiatry 1987;48:424.
50. Ochs HR, Greenblatt DJ, Kaschell HJ, et al: Diazepam kinetics in patients with renal insufficiency or hypothyroidism. Br J Clin Pharm 1981;12:829–832.
51. Bauer TM, Ritz R, Huberthur C, et al: Prolonged sedation due to accumulation of conjugated metabolites of midazolam. Lancet 1995;346:145–147.
52. Wong MO, Eldon MA, Keane WF, et al: Disposition of gapapentin in anuric subjects on hemodialysis. J Clin Pharmacol 1995;35:622–626.

53. Borga O, Hoppel C, Odar-Cederlof I, et al: Plasma levels and renal excretion of phenytoin and its metabolites in patients with renal failure. Clin Phamacol Ther 1979;26:306–314.

54. Borison RL: Amantadine-induced psychosis in a geriatric patient with renal disease. Am J Psychiatry 1979;136:111–112.

55. Davies G, Kingswood C, Street M: Pharmacokinetics of opioids in renal dysfunction. Clin Pharmacokinet 1996;31:410–422

56. Hoppmann RA, Peden JG, Ober SK: Central nervous system side effects of non-steroidal anti-inflammatory drugs. Arch Intern Med 1991;151:1309–1313.

57. Wagner BKJ, O'Hara DA: Pharmacokinetics and pharmacodynamics of sedatives and analgesics in the treatment of agitated critically ill patients. Clin Pharmacokinet 1997;33:426–453.

58. Jones H, Agula E, Farber H: Gabapentin toxicity requiring intubation in a patient receiving long term Hemodialysis (letter). Ann Intern Med 2002;137:74–75.

59. Parto I, John EG, Heilliczer J: Removal of Phenobarbital during continuous cycling peritoneal dialysis in a child. Pharmacotherapy 1997;17:832–835.

78 Measures to Improve Quality of Life in Endstage Renal Disease Patients

Catherine Blake and William D. Plant

Background

Treatment outcomes in endstage renal disease (ESRD) have traditionally been measured in terms of morbidity and mortality. Increasing take-on rates (particularly of older patients), coupled with advances in renal replacement therapies, have led to greater focus on the measurement, maintenance, and improvement of health-related quality of life (QoL).[1–3] This is based upon the premise that health is "a state of complete physical, mental and social well-being and not merely the absence of disease and infirmity".[4] The concept of 'health' is therefore personal and abstract; both medical and nonmedical factors have an impact. It is difficult to capture its essence by direct measurement and certainly not by using single variables such as physiological measures of organ function.[5–7] Multi-dimensional assessment is required; the patient's own perception of well-being and QoL is a vital component.[5,8,9]

Defining quality of life

QoL is a difficult concept to describe, with no clear operational definition. This causes difficulties when interpreting results and comparing studies.[6,10] The terms *functional status*, *health status* and *QoL* are often used interchangeably and are (incorrectly) considered by many sources to define similar constructs.[11] Measures of *functional status* are largely concerned with physical health, based upon measurement of disability. *Health status* and *QoL* are broader concepts, encompassing both the physical and psychosocial dimensions of health.[12,13] *QoL* includes the personal responses, values and perceptions that are unique to each individual.[6] The term *health-related quality of life (HRQoL)* is also used to refer specifically to the physical, psychological, and social *dimensions* of health.[14] Throughout this text the following definition of *QoL* will be used: "a concept that takes account of the multidimensional nature of a person's well-being, reflecting the physical, psychological and social dimensions of health described by the World Health Organization, and which is influenced by personal beliefs, experiences and expectations as well as social and cultural factors".

Measurement of quality of life

Personal subjective perceptions are key to QoL assessments, which should evaluate daily-life performance in physical, psychological, and social dimensions.[8,14–17] Numerous QoL scales exist. Selection (generic/specific, self-report/interview, single item/battery) should reflect the objective of a study, and the validity, reliability and responsiveness of the instrument should already be established. *Disease-specific instruments* are generally more sensitive to changes in their target population; *generic instruments* are of greater value when comparing groups of patients with different conditions and when relating patients to the general population.[13] A *single index score* may be useful for economic and multivariate analyses, but a multi-item *profile* emphasizes the diverse aspects of QoL and allows a more clinical perspective.[7,13] QoL instruments are useful for discriminating between groups at one point in time, for monitoring change over time, and for predicting outcomes.[5]

Quality of life in endstage renal disease

Studies reporting QoL in renal patients were first published in the 1980s[18–20] and interest in QoL outcome measurement has grown dramatically since then.[16,21,22] The variation in the type and number of instruments used is notable; some studies have focused on one dimension only, whilst others consider global QoL. Commonly reported multidimensional measures include the Sickness Impact Profile (SIP)[23], the Short Form 36 (SF-36) health survey,[24] and the Kidney Disease Quality of Life Questionnaire (KDQoL).[25]

There is unequivocal evidence that QoL is impaired in dialysis patients when compared with the general population.[26–33] Transplant recipients also demonstrate impaired QoL although this is not as marked as in dialysis groups.[34–36] Limitations are reported mainly in the physical and social dimensions, while mental health scores tend to remain comparable to healthy individuals.[37] The maintenance of high psychological well-being in the majority of ESRD patients may result from an alteration in health values and expectations with chronic disease.[38,39] Up to 25% of ESRD patients report significant psychological distress.[28]

Factors affecting quality of life in endstage renal disease

Factors affecting QoL in ESRD have been identified mainly by cross-sectional studies, which allow comparisons between groups based on existing clinical and socio-demographic characteristics. Many of these report uni-variate relationships only, while others have used multivariate analysis to identify independent associations with QoL. Some prospective single-group and case-control studies using QoL indices as outcome measures have been conducted, but relatively few randomized controlled trials exist. Problems arise when comparing studies because of the considerable diversity in methodology, definition of QoL, choice of measurement instrument, and sample characteristics. Direct relationships between measures of clinical status and QoL may not always exist and variables affecting QoL are often interrelated. Broadly speaking, these may be divided into sociodemographic variables, clinical variables, and comorbid medical variables.

Relationships between these characteristics and the multidimensional SF-36, SIP and KDQoL questionnaires are summarized in Table 78.1, while clinical trials using these QoL scales as outcome measures are illustrated in Table 78.2. The main sociodemographic factors affecting QoL are age, gender, socioeconomic status, and educational level. Renal transplantation is associated with improved QoL, but this in part reflects patient selection. There are conflicting reports regarding the benefits of peritoneal dialysis (PD) over haemodialysis (HD). A recent critical review concluded that there was not enough evidence to support any significant difference in QoL between dialysis modalities.[63] Early referral for specialist treatment, adequacy of dialysis, maintenance of nutritional levels, and correction of anaemia are the main clinical factors associated with better QoL. Severity of comorbid illness is a strong predictor of less good QoL. Other factors affecting QoL are perceived burden of illness and the degree of social support.

Table 78.1 Factors affecting quality of life in endstage renal disease

Sociodemographic variables		
Age of patient	Older	Less good physical status[30,31,39]
	Younger	Less good mental health status[30,31,33,40,41]
Sex	Women	Less good global QoL scores[40–42,44,49,50]
Socioeconomic group	Lower group	Less good global QoL scores[40–42]
Educational level	Lower level	Less good global QoL scores[30,36,40,41]
Employment	Unemployed	Less good global QoL scores[31]
Social support	Living alone	Less good mental health status[33]
Race	White	Better global QoL scores[42,43]
Clinical variables		
Treatment modality	Transplant	Better global QoL scores than dialysis[26,29,36,41,44–47]
	Home HD and PD	Better global QoL scores than in-centre HD[27,29]
	HD and PD	same global QoL scores[63]
	PD	Better mental health status[27,48]
Preparation for dialysis	Early referral	Better global QoL scores[50]
Time since transplantation	Longer duration	Less good global QoL scores[36]
Serum albumin	Low	Less good global QoL scores[30,33,40]
Anemia	Low	Less good global QoL[27,36]
Kt/V urea	Better clearance	Better global QoL scores[33,51,52]
Serum creatinine	Low	Better global QoL scores[44]
Comorbidity		
	Complex	Less good global QoL scores[26,27,29,36,41,42]
	Diabetes mellitus	Less good global QoL scores[30]
	Cardiovascular disease	Less good global QoL scores[33,40]
	COPD	Less good global QoL scores[33]
	Musculoskeletal disease	Less good physical status[31]
Other		
Symptoms	Severe physical symptoms	Less good global QoL scores[53]
	Dialysis symptoms	Less good global QoL scores[32]
Sleep	Unsatisfactory	Less good global QoL scores[32]
Burden of disease	High burden	Less good global QoL scores[32]

COPD, chronic obstructive pulmonary disease; HD, hemodialysis; PD, peritoneal dialysis.

Table 78.2 Treatment interventions that improve quality of life

Intervention	Outcome in Intervention Group	Sample	Study type	Outcome measure	Reference
Correction of anaemia with erythropoeitin	Improved QoL	HD	RCT	SIP, KDQ	Canadian EPO Study[54]
		HD	RCT	SIP	McMahon et al[55]
		HD	CT	SIP	Moreno et al[56]
Exercise/counselling	Improved QoL	HD	CT	KI	Fitts et al[57]
Exercise	Improved QoL	CAPD	CT	KDQoL	Lo et al[58]
Exercise training	Improved physical QoL and objective physical function tests	HD	CT	SF-36	Painter et al[59]
	Low function patients improved significantly more in physical QoL than high function patients	HD	CT	SF-36	Painter et al[60]
Physical rehabilitation	Improved physical function and fewer problems with work and daily function due to emotional problems	HD	RCT	KDQoL	Tawney et al[61]
Predialysis education	Improved QoL	HD	CT	SIP	Klang et al[62]

CAPD, continuous ambulatory peritoneal dialysis; CT, controlled trial; HD, hemodialysis; KDQoL, Kidney Disease Quality of Life Questionnaire; PD, peritoneal diaylsis; RCT, randomized controlled trial; SIP, Sickness Impact Profile; SF-36, Short Form 36.

Recommendations

QoL measurement may be a valuable adjunct to objective clinical assessment in ESRD. Close relationships exist between self-reported QoL and morbidity and mortality outcomes.[28,40,64,65] These subjective measures may even be better predictors of outcome than clinical parameters.[28,53] There is also growing evidence that self-assessed physical and psychosocial well-being influences compliance and survival.[66,67] The inclusion of QoL assessment in the routine management of ESRD patients offers several advantages. Specific patient problems may be identified, thus directing clinical intervention. Nonmedical factors that affect QoL may be highlighted, and ways of improving quality of care identified. QoL assessment fosters more patient-centred treatment, enhancing communication between the patient and the healthcare team. Serial QoL measurement is valuable for patient surveillance over time and QoL assessment may direct healthcare planning and quality assurance initiatives.

Measures which may improve QoL are summarized in Table 78.3 and these reflect the five Es of renal rehabilitation identified by the Life Options Rehabilitation Council: education, encouragement, employment, exercise and evaluation.[68] Evaluation and regular reassessment are central to any initiative aimed at improving QoL. Adequacy of dialysis, correction of anaemia, careful management of comorbidity, maintenance of nutritional status, and exercise programs designed to enhance physical fitness are key factors in physical management. Education, patient involvement in decision-making, counselling, motivation, and the promotion of a positive ethos of rehabilitation are necessary components of psychological management and compliance. Vocational rehabilitation is an important consideration in social well-being, and every effort should be made to keep patients in work, or allow them to return to work. Efforts to enhance QoL therefore require a multidisciplinary approach, and this process should be started in the predialysis phase.

Table 78.3 Measures to improve quality of life

Physical
Correction of anemia
Maintenance of nutritional status
Adequacy of dialysis
Management of comorbidity
Exercise programs

Psychological
Education and choice of treatment
Psychological support/counselling

Social
Employment
  – Education and counseling
  – Retraining schemes
  – Flexibility of dialysis schedules
  – Physical fitness
Social supports
Patient support groups
Family education

Other
Early referral
Assessment and regular re-evaluation
Motivation and encouragement
Optimize compliance

References

1. Apolone G, Mosconi P: Review of the concept of quality of life assessment and discussion of the present trend in clinical research. Nephrol Dial Transplant 1998;13 (Suppl 1):65–69.

2. Reitig RA, Sadler JH, Mayer KB, et al: Assessing health and quality of life outcomes in dialysis: A report on an Institute of Medicine workshop. Am J Kidney Dis 1997;30:140–155.

3. Schrier RW, Burrows-Hudson S, Diamond L, et al: Measuring, managing and improving quality in the end-stage renal disease treatment setting: committee statement. Am J Kidney Dis 1994;24:383–388.

4. World Health Organization: The first ten years of the World Health Organization. Geneva, WHO, 1958;10:459.

5. Guyatt GH, Feeney DH, Patrick DL: Measuring quality of life. Ann Intern Med 1993;118:622–629.

6. Leplege A, Hunt S: The problem of quality of life in medicine. JAMA 1997;278:47–50.

7. Woodend AK, Nair RC, Tang AS: Definition of quality from a patient versus health care professional perspective. Int J Rehabil Res 1997;20:71–80.

8. Muldoon MF, Barger SD, Flory JD, Manuck SB: What are quality of life measurements measuring? BMJ 1998;316:542–545.

9. Slevin ML, Plant H, Lynch D, et al: Who should measure quality of life, the doctor or the patient? Br J Cancer 1988;57:109–112.

10. Gill TM, Feinstein AR: A critical appraisal of the quality of life measures. JAMA 1994; 272:619–626.

11. Dijkers MPJM, Whiteneck G, El-Jaroudi R: Measures of social outcomes in disability research. Arch Phys Med Rehabil 2000;81(Suppl 2):S46–S52.

12. Keith RA: Functional status and health status. Arch Phys Med Rehabil 1994;75:478–483.

13. McDowell I, Newell C: Measuring Health: A Guide to Rating Scales and Questionnaires, 2nd edn. New York: Oxford University Press, 1996, pp 381–383.

14. Testa MA, Simonson DC: Assessment of quality of life outcomes. N Engl J Med 1996;334:835–840.

15. Bergner M: Quality of life, health status, and clinical research. Med Care 1989;27(Suppl 3):S148–S156.

16. Gokal R: Quality of life in patients undergoing renal replacement therapy. Kidney Int 1993;40(Suppl 1):S23–S27.

17. Kimmel PL: Just whose quality of life is it anyway? Controversies and consistencies in measurement of quality of life. Kidney Int 2000;57(Suppl 74):S113–S120.

18. Simmons RG, Anderson C, Kamstra L: Comparison of quality of life of patients on continuous ambulatory peritoneal dialysis, hemodialysis, and after transplantation. Am J Kidney Dis 1984;4:253–255.

19. Evans RW, Manninen DL, Garrison LP Jr, et al: The quality of life of patients with end stage renal disease. N Engl J Med 1985;312:553–559.

20. Kutner NG, Brogan D, Kutner MH: End-stage renal disease treatment modality and patients' quality of life. Longitudinal assessment. Am J Nephrol 1986;6:396–402.

21. Edgell ET, Coons SJ, Carter WB et al: A review of health-related quality-of-life measures used in end-stage renal disease. Clin Ther 1996;18:887–938.

22. Cagney KA, Wu AW, Fink NE, et al: Formal literature review of quality-of-life instruments used in end-stage renal disease. Am J Kidney Dis 2000;36:327–336.

23. Bergner M, Bobbitt RA, Carter WB, et al: The sickness impact profile: Development of a final revision of a health status measure. Med Care 1981;19:789–805.

24. Ware JE, Snow KK, Kosinski M, Gandek B: SF-36 Health Survey Manual and Interpretation Guide. Boston, MA: Nimrod Press, 1993.

25. Hays RD, Kallich JD, Mapes DL, et al: Development of the kidney disease quality of life (KDQOL) instrument. Qual Life Res 1994;3:329–338.

26. Khan IH, Garratt AM, Kumar A, et al: Patients' perception of health on renal replacement therapy: evaluation using a new instrument. Nephrol Dial Transplant 1995;10:684–689.

27. Merkus MP, Jager KJ, Dekker FW, et al: Quality of life in patients on chronic dialysis: self-assessment 3 months after the start of treatment. The Necosad Study Group. Am J Kidney Dis 1997;29:584–592.

28. DeOreo PB: Hemodialysis patients assessed functional health status predicts continued survival, hospitalisation and dialysis attendance compliance. Am J Kidney Dis 1997;30:204–212.

29. Merkus MP, Jager KJ, Dekker FW, et al: Quality of life over time in dialysis: the Netherlands Cooperative Study on the Adequacy of Dialysis. NECOSAD Study Group. Kidney Int 1999;56:720–728.

30. Mingardi G, Cornalba L, Cortinovis E, et al: Health-related quality of life in dialysis patients. A report from an Italian study using the SF-36 Health Survey. DIA-QOL Group. Nephrol Dial Transplant 1999;14:1503–1510.

31. Blake C, Codd MB, Cassidy A, et al: Physical function, employment and quality of life in end-stage renal disease. J Nephrol 2000;13:142–149.

32. Carmichael P, Popoola J, John I, et al: Assessment of quality of life in a single centre dialysis population using the KDQOL-SF questionnaire. Qual Life Res 2000;9:195–205.

33. Mittal SK, Ahern L, Flaster E, et al: Self-assessed physical and mental function of haemodialysis patients. Nephrol Dial Transplant 2001;16:1387–1394.

34. Shield CF III, McGrath MM, Goss TF: Assessment of health-related quality of life in kidney transplant patients receiving tacrolimus (FK560)-based versus cyclosporine-base immunosuppression. FK560 Kidney Transplant Study Group. Transplantation 1997;64:1738–1743.

35. Tsuji-Hayashi Y, Fukuhara S, Green J, et al: Health-related quality of life among renal-transplant recipients in Japan. Transplantation 1999;68:1331–1335.

36. Rebollo P, Ortega F, Baltar JM, et al: Health related quality of life (HRQOL) of kidney transplant patients: Variables that influence it. Clin Transplant 2000;14:199–207.

37. Kutner NG: Renal Rehabilitation: where are the data? A progress report. Semin Dialysis 1996;9:387–389.

38. Dolan P: The effect of experience of illness on health status valuations. J Clin Epidemiol 1996;49:551–564.

39. Singer MA, Hopman WA, MacKenzie TA: Physical functioning and mental health in patients with chronic medical conditions. Qual Life Res 1999;8:687–691.

40. Harris LE, Luft FC, Rudy DW, et al: Clinical correlates of functional status in patients with chronic renal insuffficiency. Am J Kidney Dis 1993;21:161–166.

41. Rebollo P, Ortega F, Baltar JM, et al: Health-related quality of life (HRQOL) in end stage renal disease (ESRD) patients over 65 years. Geriatr Nephrol Urol 1998;8:85–94.

42. Bakewell AB, Higgins RM, Edmunds ME: Does ethnicity influence perceived quality of life of patients on dialysis and following renal transplant? Nephrol Dial Transplant 2001;16:1395–1401.

43. Julius M, Hawthorne VM, Carpentier-Alting P, et al: Independence in activities of daily living for end-stage renal disease patients: biomedical and demographic correlates. Am J Kidney Dis 1989;13:61–69.

44. Fujisawa M, Ichikawa Y, Yoshiya K, et al: Assessment of health-related quality of life in renal transplant and hemodialysis patients using the SF-36 health survey. Urology 2000;56:201–206.

45. Gross CR, Limwattananon C, Matthees B, et al: Impact of transplantation on quality of life in patients with diabetes and renal dysfunction. Transplantation 2000;70:1736–1746.

46. Jofre R, Lopez-Gomez JM, Moreno F, et al: Changes in quality of life after renal transplantation. Am J Kidney Dis 1998;32:93–100.

47. Wight JP, Edwards L, Brazier J, et al: The SF-36 as an outcome measure of services for end stage renal failure. Qual Health Care 1998;7:209–221.

48. Diaz-Buxo JA, Lowrie EG, Lew NL, et al: Quality of life evaluation using short form 36: comparison of hemodialysis and peritoneal dialysis patients. Am J Kidney Dis 2000;35:293–300.

49. Bro S, Bjorner JB, Tofte-Jensen P, et al: A prospective randomized multicenter study comparing APD and CAPD treatment. Perit Dial Int 1999;19:526–533.

50. Sesso R, Yoshihiro MM: Time of diagnosis of chronic renal failure and assessment of quality of life in hemodialysis patients. Nephrol Dial Transplant 1997;12:2111–2116.

51. Chen YC, Hung KY, Kao TW, et al: Relationship between dialysis adequacy and quality of life in long-term peritoneal dialysis patients. Perit Dial Int 2000;20:534–540.

52. Martin CR, Thompson DR: Prediction of quality of life in patients with end-stage renal disease. Br J Health Psychol 2000;5:41–55.

53. Merkus MP, Jager KJ, Dekker FW, et al: Predictors of poor outcome in chronic dialysis patients: The Netherlands Cooperative Study on the Adequacy of Dialysis. The NECOSAD Study Group. Am J Kidney Dis 2000;35:69–79.

54. Canadian Erythropoeitin Study: Association between recombinant erythropoietin and quality of life and exercise capacity of patients receiving haemodialysis. BMJ 1990;300:573–578.

55. McMahon LP, Mason K, Skinner SL, et al: Effects of haemoglobin normalisation on quality of life and cardiovascular parameters in end-stage renal failure. Nephrol Dial Transplant 2000;15(9):1425–1430.

56. Moreno F, Aracil FJ, Perez R, et al: Controlled study on the improvement of quality of life in elderly hemodialysis patients after correcting end-stage renal disease-related anaemia with erythropoietin. Am J Kidney Dis 1996;27:548–556.

57. Fitts SS, Guthrie MR, Blagg CR: Exercise coaching and rehabilitation counseling improve quality of life for predialysis and dialysis patients. Nephron 1999;82:115–121.

58. Lo C, Li L, Lo W, et al: Benefits of exercise training in patients on continuous ambulatory peritoneal dialysis. Am J Kidney Dis 1998;32:1011–1018.

59. Painter P, Carlson L, Carey S, et al: Physical functioning and health-related quality-of-life changes with exercise training in hemodialysis patients. Am J Kidney Dis 2000;35:482–492.

60. Painter P, Carlson L, Carey S, et al: Low-functioning hemodialysis patients improve with exercise training. Am J Kidney Dis 2000;36:600–608.

61. Tawney KW, Tawney PJW, Hladik G, et al: The Life Readiness Program: A physical rehabilitation program for patients on hemodialysis. Am J Kidney Dis 2000;36:581–591.

62. Klang B, Bjorvell H, Berglund J, et al: Predialysis patient education: effects on functioning and well-being in uraemic patients. J Adv Nurs 1998;28:360–344.

63. Gokal R, Figueras M, Ollé A, et al: Outcomes in peritoneal dialysis and haemodialysis—a comparative assessment of survival and quality of life. Nephrol Dial Transplant 1999;14(Suppl 6):S24–S30.

64. Ifudu O, Paul HR, Homel P, et al: Predictive value of functional status for mortality in patients on maintenance hemodialysis. Am J Nephrol 1998;18:109–116.

65. McClellan WM, Anson C, Birkeli K, et al: Functional status and quality of life: predictors of early mortality among patients entering treatment for end stage renal disease. J Clin Epidemiol 1991;44:83–89.

66. Kimmel PL, Peterson RA, Weihs KL, et al: Multiple measures of depression predict mortality in a longitudinal study of chronic hemodialysis outpatients. Kidney Int 2000;57:2093–2098.

67. DiMatteo MR, Lepper HS, Croghan TW: Depression is a risk factor for non-compliance with medical treatment: meta-analysis of the effects of anxiety and depression on patient adherence. Arch Intern Med 2000;160:2101–2107.

68. Life Options Rehabilitation Advisory Council: Renal Rehabilitation: Bridging the Barriers. Madison: Medical Education Institute, Inc, 1994, pp 1–144.

CHAPTER 79

Palliative and Supportive Care

Lewis M. Cohen and Michael J. Germain

This is the first edition of the textbook to include a chapter on palliative treatments for patients with endstage renal disease (ESRD). For most of the twentieth century, medicine focused almost single-mindedly on prolonging life and thwarting death; dialysis has certainly been one of the most successful life-supporting treatments to be developed. However, a paradigm shift is taking place. Medical disciplines are becoming increasingly attentive to the inevitability of death and the suffering that can sometimes accompany it.[1,2]

In 1991, the Institute of Medicine produced a report that directed the nephrology community to determine at what point the burden of dialysis outweighs the benefit.[3] The Renal Physician Association (RPA) and the American Society of Nephrology (ASN) jointly developed a clinical practice guideline: *Shared Decision Making in the Appropriate Initiation and Withdrawal of Dialysis*.[4] It concluded that familiarity with modern palliative medicine is required by nephrologists. This is necessary because: (1) there is a large symptom burden among ESRD patients; (2) there continues to be a high annual mortality rate (about 23%); (3) substantial numbers of deaths are preceded by the decision to terminate treatment (28% in New England); (4) quality of dying has not been previously emphasized and has not been the target of quality improvement efforts; and (5) advanced care planning is still the exception, rather than the rule.

Dialysis may support life, but not necessarily in a way that attends to quality of life. In a survey involving 80 patients receiving hemodialysis, the majority complained of being fatigued, while more than a third reported insomnia, cramping, and pruritis.[5] Neuropathic symptoms were endorsed by 29%, while 24% reported being of 'poor spirits'. We are unaware of any ongoing, systematically tested symptom treatment protocols for these problems.

If there is a subgroup of dying patients that ought to be receiving both maximal and ideal palliative care, it is those whose dialysis treatment has been terminated and who have on average only 8 days to live.[6] The majority of these patients are white, elderly, and diabetic. Three-quarters of the sample from our multicenter, prospective study had between three and seven comorbid illnesses, over half had inanition or failure-to-thrive syndromes, and on their last day of life caregivers reported that 30% of them had some agitation and 42% experienced pain.[7] A quality-of-dying instrument was used to examine three dimensions: time until death; pain and suffering; and psychosocial aspects. It showed that one in eight of the deaths were "bad" deaths.[8,9] In another study that examined all types of ESRD deaths from the perspective of the family and loved-ones, 57% of the respondents were unsure about or believed that the patient died with some pain, 24%

thought that the death was not peaceful, and 43% expressed regrets that the patient had not fulfilled his or her final wishes during the last days of life.[10]

Research shows that ongoing discussions about terminal care are rare; written advanced directives are completed by only 7–35% of chronic dialysis patients.[11,12] Patients often do not know that they have the option of withdrawal from dialysis; they frequently believe their physicians would not support such a choice.[13] Advanced care directives, such as The Five Wishes document (Aging with Dignity)[14] are extremely valuable educational tools, acting as focal points for such discussions and a means to document their wishes in patients' records.

"Do not resuscitate" (DNR) orders require written documentation, and the nephrology community has not been effective in providing patients with this option. In 1992, a seminal study demonstrated that over 8 years, 34% of 221 dialysis patients experienced cardiopulmonary arrest compared with 21% of a control (hospitalized) nondialysis population.[15] Of the successfully resuscitated dialysis patients, 78% died an average of 4.4 days later, and 95% of these people were on mechanical ventilation at the time of death. Six months after cardiopulmonary resuscitation (CPR), only 3% of ESRD patients were alive, compared with 9% of the control population ($P = 0.044$). This difference was not explained by age or comorbid conditions. As ESRD patients strongly support autonomy of decision-making, they ought to be informed about the extremely poor chance of survival with CPR.[16]

A successful palliative care program requires good patient–doctor communication (Fig. 79.1).[17] The doctor needs many skills, such as active listening, finding out how much a patient knows and wants to know, sharing information without "medispeak", reflecting back the patient's feelings, planning, and following through. Such skills will help patients to accept their prognosis and to engage in realistic advanced care planning. Involvement of the family is essential, as patients like to discuss advanced care planning with their loved-ones more than with the healthcare team.[18]

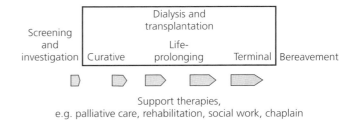

Figure 79.1 Supportive care model for renal disease.

Having conducted a demonstration project to integrate palliative care into the dialysis and renal transplant settings, we would suggest that (1) palliation should address both end-of-life care and general symptom management that starts with the beginning of the illness; (2) interdisciplinary cooperation is a necessity; (3) information about the circumstances surrounding deaths is often not known by the dialysis staff, but needs to be revealed if the practice of nephrology is to become more sensitive to these issues; and (4) contact with the families and loved-ones should not cease when the patient dies.

Several interventions can be incorporated, including: initiation of a didactic program to educate the healthcare team on the principles of modern palliative care (Table 79.1); regular assessment of patient symptoms; and treatment protocols or guidelines that are made available at the clinic nursing stations. We have found it useful to create renal morbidity and mortality conferences. These allow staff to review summaries from the hospital, nursing home, and clinic records of recently deceased patients. This information can be contrasted with data obtained from families through postal questionnaires, which elicits their perspective of the circumstances of the terminal care and death. Advanced care planning ought to be actively encouraged at clinics. Closer contact should be established with local hospice programs to facilitate referral of all patients who discontinue dialysis, as well as others who are clearly on the downward slope. Annual memorial services can be organized at dialysis clinics, and invitations provided to families, loved-ones, and staff who wish to celebrate the memories of patients who died in the

previous year. Such services are ecumenical events, which include inspirational readings, poetry, music, and a candle-lighting ceremony during which patient names are recited. After the formalities, family members are given refreshments, and have a chance to talk each about their loved-ones' last days and to share in the memories.

Figure 79.2 shows some of the results of a survey conducted with the demonstration project staff. A total of 16 physicians were sampled, including 3 private nephrologists, 10 nephrologists from a group practice, and 3 transplant surgeons. The series of didactic lectures, including several renal rounds, received the highest score and reflected the general interest in the subject. This was followed by the memorial service, which was rated very highly by almost all attendees. Although several of the physicians intentionally did not participate in the service, those who took part were extremely moved and commented that it had markedly influenced their practice.

Other interventions that should be developed include evidence-based palliative treatment protocols that can be made accessible to staff at the dialysis facility. Staff have different interests, clinical backgrounds, and expertise. Such guidelines can serve as a common, valuable resource. There could be one protocol for patients who terminate dialysis, another that could deal with patients who have cardiopulmonary arrest at the dialysis facility, and another for families of patients who are critically ill or dying. This last protocol would provide guidance on pain management, and address issues for families who chose to have a bedside vigil, which is not uncommon. It might also facilitate referral to a hospice, a valuable but rarely used

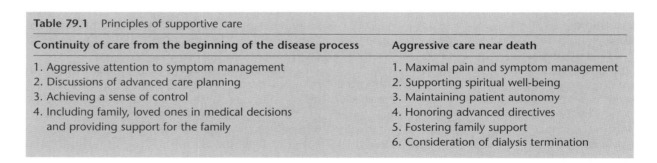

Table 79.1 Principles of supportive care

Continuity of care from the beginning of the disease process	Aggressive care near death
1. Aggressive attention to symptom management	1. Maximal pain and symptom management
2. Discussions of advanced care planning	2. Supporting spiritual well-being
3. Achieving a sense of control	3. Maintaining patient autonomy
4. Including family, loved ones in medical decisions and providing support for the family	4. Honoring advanced directives
	5. Fostering family support
	6. Consideration of dialysis termination

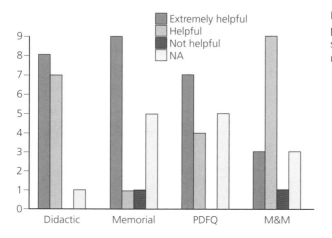

Figure 79.2 Renal palliative care interventions. Data from a survey of 16 participating nephrologists. Didactic, lecture series; memorial, memorial service; PDFQ, post death family questionnaire; M&M, morbidity and mortality conference; NA, no answer or did not participate.

resource. In 1996, for example, there were 14 253 people in North Carolina who received hospice care, but only 71 (0.5%) had ESRD.[19]

Pain is the most common and distressing physical problem for the dying patient with ESRD. Management is complicated because it also generally involves a geriatric subgroup. Over 90% of most opioid drugs are excreted via the kidneys, and many have active metabolites that may accumulate and cause distressing symptoms. This difficult situation is worsened by a paucity of hard data on the use of analgesics in ESRD.

Several drugs are best avoided altogether.[20] Meperidine results in accumulation of normeperidine, which is only half as potent an analgesic as the parent compound, but two to three time more likely to cause seizures. Elderly renal patients are especially likely to have CNS toxicity (agitation, myoclonus, and seizures). Use of propoxyphene or pentazocine is also undesirable. Levels of both the parent compounds and the active metabolites rise in renal failure, and can lead to increased risk of cardiac and neurologic sequelae. Adverse reactions can be further reduced by minimizing the use of mixed angonist/antagonist agents with strong psychotomimetic propensities, such as nalbuphine and butorphanol.

Morphine, often given intravenously, is the mainstay of pain control.[21] However, morphine 6-glucuronide is a more potent analgesic than morphine itself and equilibrates very slowly across the blood–brain barrier. Thus, patients may remain sedated for days after the drug is stopped. This may be beneficial if the patient is agitated or in intractable pain, but it could also deny that person the level of alertness necessary to achieve spiritual and interpersonal goals.

Fentanyl and hydromorphone are metabolized by the liver and therefore are good choices for severe pain in people with chronic kidney disease. The World Health Organization suggests a ladder approach, using non-narcotic analgesia first, then less potent narcotics such as codeine.[22] Oxycodone, hydromorphone, or morphine is used next if the pain is not controlled. Long-acting narcotics, such as extended-release morphine, oxycodone, and fentanyl patches can be used for constant pain, and should be supplemented with short-acting narcotics for breakthrough pain. Conversion formulas are available.

Table 79.2 Symptom guidelines

Symptom	Treatment	Dosage	Comments
Cramps	Quinine	260–325 mg p.o. prn	Give prior to symptoms. Limit to three doses daily
	Carnitine	1000–2000 mg i.v. during dialysis	Also used for cardiomyopathy, myopathy, refractory anemia
Restless leg syndrome	Clonazepam	0.5–2 mg hs prn	
	Carbidopa–levodopa	25/100 mg hs prn	
	Pergolide	0.05–0.2 mg q.i.d.	
	Pramipexole	0.3 mg q.i.d.	
Puritus	H₁ antagonists Clemastine	2.68 mg b.i.d. prn	Try any H₁ antagonist
	Skin moisturizer Hydrourea cream		
	Activated charcoal	6 g q.i.d. × 8 weeks	
	UVB light		
	Lidocaine i.v.	100 mg i.v. during dialysis	Potential seizures
	Ketotifen		Mast cell stabilizer
	Ondanstron	4 mg b.i.d.	High cost
	Plasmapheresis	3–4 exchanges	
Hypotension (intradialytic or persistent)	Alterations to the dialysis bath, temperature, sodium, ultrafiltration		
	Midadrine	1–10 mg t.i.d. prn or predialysis	Oral alpha-adrenergic agonist
	Sertraline	25–50 mg predialysis	
Anorexia	Megestrol	40–400 mg	Has been used in ESRD
	Dronabinol	2.5–5 mg b.i.d./t.i.d.	
Lethargy and fatigue	Methylphenidate	5–10 mg am and noon	Psychostimulant

hs, at bedtime; prn, as needed.

We believe in the traditional medical approach that treats the patients and their symptoms as the first priority. Table 79.2 lists some common ESRD symptoms and our recent guidelines. We would caution that these particular protocols have not been validated or tested with sufficient numbers of patients. They should be considered rough guides. Clinical recommendations are given in logical order, and begin with the need for patients to be well dialyzed.

In conclusion, the nephrology community has the opportunity to incorporate elements of modern palliative/ supportive care into the continuous quality improvement programs of their facilities. A renal palliative care module is being developed for the Education for Physicians on End-of-Life Care (EPEC) training program,[23] and should be available soon for nephrologists who are interested in mastering this subject. We predict that the practice of nephrology will become even more satisfying when it evolves beyond extending life as far as possible to also providing the best possible quality of life and the best possible end to patients lives.

References

1. Emanuel JE: Care for dying patients. Lancet 1997;349:1714.
2. Cohen LM: Suicide, hastening death, and psychiatry. Arch Intern Med 1998;158:1973–1976.
3. Levinsky N, Rettig R: Special report: The Medicare ESRD program. N Engl J Med 1991;324:1143–1148.
4. Moss AH. RPA and ASN Working Group: A new clinical practice guideline on initiation and withdrawal of dialysis that makes explicit the role of palliative medicine. J Palliative Med 2000;3:253–260.
5. Levy NB, Cohen LM: Central and peripheral nervous systems in uremia. In Massry SG, Glassock R (eds): Textbook of Nephrology, 4th edn. Philadelphia: Williams and Wilkins, 2001, pp 1279–1282.
6. Neu S, Kjellstrand CM: Stopping long-term dialysis: An empirical study of withdrawal of life-supporting treatment. N Engl J Med 1986;314:14–20.
7. Cohen LM, Germain M, Poppel DM, et al: Dialysis discontinuation and palliative care. Am J Kidney Dis 2000;36:140–144.
8. Cohen LM, McCue J, Germain M, et al: Dialysis discontinuation: A "good" death? Arch Intern Med 1995;155:42–47.
9. Cohen LM, Germain M, Poppel DM, et al: Dying well after discontinuing the life-support treatment of dialysis. Arch Intern Med 2000;160:2513–2518.
10. Woods A, Berzoff J, Cohen LM, et al: The family perspective of end-of-life care in end-stage renal disease: The role of the social worker. J Nephrol Social Work 1999;19:9–21.
11. Holly JL, Nespor S, Rault R: Chronic in-center hemodialysis patients' attitudes, knowledge, and behavior towards advance directives. J Am Soc Nephrol 1993;3:1405–1408.
12. Cohen LM, McCue JD, Germain MJ, et al: Denying the dying: Advance directives and dialysis discontinuation. Psychosomatics 1997;38:27–34.
13. Cohen LM, Germain M, Woods A, et al: Patient attitudes and psychological considerations in dialysis discontinuation. Psychosomatics 1993;34:395–401.
14. Aging with Dignity: The Five Wishes Document. http://www.agingwithdignity.org
15. Moss A, Holley J, Upton M: Outcome of cardiopulmonary resuscitation in dialysis patients. J Am Soc Nephrol 1992;3:1238–1243.
16. Moss AH, Hozayen O, King K, et al: Attitudes of patients towards cardiopulmonary resuscitation in the dialysis unit. Am J Kidney Dis 2001;38:847–851.
17. Germain M, Cohen L: Supportive care for patients with renal disease: Time for action. Am J Kidney Dis 2001;38:884–886.
18. Davison SN: Quality end-of-life care in dialysis units. Semin in Dialysis 2001;15:41–44.
19. Soltys FG, Brookins M, Seney J: Why hospice? The case for ESRD patients and their families. ANNA Journal 1998;25:619–624.
20. American Pain Society: Principles of Analgesic Use in the Treatment of Acute Pain and Cancer Pain, 4th edn. Glenview, IL: American Pain Society, 1999.
21. Levy M: Pharmacologic treatment of cancer pain. New Engl J Ped 1996;335:1124–1132.
22. Foley KM: The World Health Organization's Program in Cancer Pain Relief and Palliative Care. In Gebhardt G, Hammond DL, Jensen TS (eds): Proceedings of the 7th World Congress on Pain Progress in Pain Research and Management, Vol 2. Seattle, IL: IASP Press, 1994, pp 59–74.
23. Education for Physicians on End-of-Life Care. http://www.epec.net/content/about.html.

Health Economics of Endstage Renal Disease Treatment

Robert J. Rubin and Caitlin Carroll Oppenheimer

In 1999 about $18 billion was spent on endstage renal disease (ESRD) care in the USA.[1] The US government, under the Medicare program, paid about 70% ($12.7 billion), and private insurers and patients paid the rest. Although the expenditure per patient year at risk (YAR) has remained relatively stable (even declining in some instances), the Medicare program has continued to grow in absolute terms (slightly over 5% or $650 million from 1998 to 1999).[1] There is a belief that care can be delivered for a lower cost while offering higher quality to ESRD patients. In the USA, physicians are paid a monthly fee to care for dialysis patients (monthly capitation payment) and dialysis providers are paid a fixed amount per dialysis treatment per month (composite rate). As this amount has remained relatively stable over time, its value has decreased relative to inflation. Physicians and dialysis providers have had to find ways to increase their productivity by delivering the same or better quality care at a lower cost. In order to evaluate various measures to improve patient care, as well as maintain the economic viability of a practice or dialysis unit, it is useful to understand the economic tools available and how they can be used.

Methodologies

There are several ways to evaluate the economic and clinical effects of changes in the treatment of ESRD patients.

Cost–benefit analysis

This technique compares the costs of an intervention or treatment protocol with the benefits, identified in terms of monetary units. The benefits are typically measured as the change in medical expenditure and productivity. By converting the outcome to a monetary unit, interventions with a variety of outcomes can be compared. Key drawbacks are that changes in quality of life are not reflected in the analysis and it is difficult to measure the impact on "productivity" among nonworking people (such as the very old or young). While it is difficult to assign a value to a year of life that is free of disease, a standard benchmark is $100 000.[2] Multiple interventions can be ranked by their cost–benefit ratios. Clearly, as the cost–benefit ratio approaches a value of 1 the intervention becomes less desirable.

Cost-effectiveness analysis

This technique compares the costs of an intervention or treatment protocol with a measure of effectiveness. It identifies the trade-offs involved in making decisions about care. The costs are monetary and the effectiveness measure is reported in outcomes (life years gained or episodes averted) that are adjusted to reflect a measure of quality of life. The results are reported as cost per "quality adjusted life years" or QALYs. The advantage is that it avoids placing a value on a year of life. A recent example is the cost-effectiveness of retransplantation, which was determined as $9656 per QALY saved.[3] Table 80.1 shows the cost per QALY of some treatments for ESRD.

Cost minimization analysis

This technique analyzes two or more interventions or treatment protocols that are believed to be equal clinically, so that the only difference is the economic cost. An example of this type of study would be the cost consequences of using generic versus branded drugs.

Cost identification analysis

This technique identifies and totals all the costs of a particular intervention or treatment protocol. It is useful when comparing a new treatment protocol to an existing one. An example would be the effect of increasing Kt/V to 1.2 for all Medicare patients who have a Kt/V of less than 1. This intervention would increase dialysis costs by about $2340 per patient YAR but would decrease nondialysis spending by about $4670, a saving per patient YAR of $2330.[4] "Year at risk" is a technique used to standardize reporting of data on patients with varying follow-up times. The expenditures for all patients are summed and all patients receiving therapy during a given year contribute to the denominator based on the days during that year that they were in the program; thus a patient who was alive and on hemodialysis for 30 days in 1999

Table 80.1 Estimated cost per quality adjusted life year (QALY) gained by investing in different treatments

Treatment	Cost per QALY (US dollars)
Kidney transplant	9099
Home hemodialysis	33 345
Continuous ambulatory peritoneal dialysis	38 387
Hospital hemodialysis	42 444
Erythropoietin for dialysis anemia (with 10% reduction in mortality)	105 057
Erythropoietin for dialysis anemia (with no increase in survival)	243 978

Adapted from Maynard A. The Economic Journal 1991;101:1277–1286 with permission from the publisher.

contributes to the cost (numerator) and the time (denominator) for those 30 days.

These economic studies are frequently lumped together under the heading of "cost-effectiveness." However, it is important to understand a few methodological characteristics of these studies.

Perspective

Economic studies consider one or more perspectives (such as patient, provider, or payer). For example, per patient spending for a transplant in 1996 was $148 959 but Medicare spending per patient was $141 968. The difference between Medicare spending and total spending is relatively small for transplantation (5%), and substantially larger for hemodialysis (17%).[4] The difference is accounted for by payments that patients make, such as those relating to Part A (deductible, outpatient pharmaceuticals), and Part B (copayments). Therefore, an analysis that examines only the costs to Medicare, but which ignores outpatient pharmaceutical costs, would be appropriate from the perspective of the government but not from the perspective of the patient, as Medicare does not generally cover outpatient pharmaceutical costs.

In the example of cost identification cited above, increasing Kt/V to 1.2 would increase costs to the providers of dialysis care, but would decrease total costs from the government's perspective. Therefore, it would be cost-effective for Medicare but not for providers. However, if providers were responsible for all the costs (as they would be under a capitated system), then it would become cost-effective for the provider as well.

The societal perspective measures the net effect of all these perspectives. Generally, health economic studies analyze interventions for their effect on the healthcare system and the benefits to patients. A truly societal view should also value the effect of interventions on the nonhealth-related aspects of society, referred to as indirect costs. For example, if daily hemodialysis allowed patients to continue to work and be productive members of society then, from a societal perspective, the increased productivity of those patients might well offset any increased costs.

To better understand how these economic tools can be used, we describe the economics of renal replacement therapies.

Hemodialysis

Hemodialysis (HD) is the renal replacement treatment of choice for the majority of ESRD patients in the US. Direct comparison of cost-effectiveness between hemodialysis and peritoneal dialysis is not possible as no prospective study has satisfactorily determined differences in effectiveness between the two modalities. Differences in costs, as determined by Medicare payments, between the two modalities are well documented. In 1999, Medicare paid $48 370 per patient (year at risk) for diabetic hemodialysis patients and $37 911 per patient (year at risk) for diabetic peritoneal dialysis patients.[1]

There is widespread expectation that some or all of ESRD care will move towards capitation in the near future. Currently, routine payment for HD patients is comprised of three main components: the monthly capitation payment (MCP) made to physicians on a per patient basis, the dialysis facility reimbursement, and payment for ancillary services. The MCP includes all routine dialysis treatment in a given month. Services not covered include: surgical services, interpretation of tests, training of patients to encourage self-treatment, services not related to patients' renal disease, evaluation for renal transplantation, and physician services covered during a hospital stay as an inpatient. The dialysis facility reimbursement is a composite rate payment for all necessary dialysis services, equipment, and supplies. The composite rate has declined substantially on an inflation-adjusted basis. Some dialysis-related pharmaceuticals and supplies are paid as an add-on to the composite rate. These include erythropoietin, vitamin D injections, iron dextran, antibiotics, and some laboratory tests. Payments for ancillary services are an important component of dialysis facility revenues.

Under the current payment scheme, the incentives to reduce use of high-cost healthcare may not rest with the individuals who have the greatest opportunity to affect change. For example, in 1999 40% of total ESRD payments were for hospitalizations.[1] Reducing hospitalizations would benefit both the Medicare program and the individual patient, but the cost of providing additional services to the patient would likely be borne by the facility. Dialysis adequacy provides a useful illustration of such costs. Increasing Kt/V from 0.82 to 1.33 is associated with a 32% decrease in hospital days, which translates to an average saving of $5400 per patient.[5] A recent study found that a 0.1 lower Kt/V was associated with an 11% increase in number of hospitalizations, and $940 higher amount for Medicare inpatient reimbursement.[6] Figure 80.1 presents the strong linear relationship between Kt/V and hospitalizations.

Thus a strategy to deliver an improved level of dialysis should decrease costs. This would require increasing treatment times or increasing the size of the dialyzer used.[7] At the present time, however, most ESRD providers have

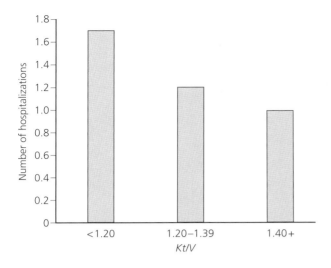

Figure 80.1 Relationship between Kt/V and number of hospitalizations ($n = 674$). With permission from the publisher Sehgal et al.[6]

Table 80.2 Estimated increase in dialysis spending to achieve 1.2 Kt/V threshold for all patients based on 1997 levels

	Kt/V value			
	≤ 1.0	1.0–1.1	≥ 1.2	Total
Percentage of adult hemodialysis patients	7%	15%	78%	100%
Increase in monthly capitation payment spending	$34	$0	$0	$2
Increase in dialysis facility/supplier spending	$393	$0	$0	$28
Total increase in dialysis-related spending	$427	$0	$0	$30

With permission from the Renal Physicians Association.[4]

Table 80.3 Cost estimates using three methods of increasing dialysis dose based on 1997 data

	Increase in Kt/V	Increase in cost (%)
Increase in dialysis time (10 min)	0.05	1.4
Switch to synthetic membrane	0.05	5.3
Switch to modified cellulose membrane	0.05	20.7

With permission from the Renal Physicians Association.[4]

little incentive to do so. An increase in spending by the dialysis facility or supplier of $393 should increase the Kt/V value of all patients from below 1.0–1.2 (Table 80.2).[7]

An increase in dialysis treatment time is a much less expensive means to increase Kt/V than a change in dialysis membrane (Table 80.3).

Vascular access

The average cost of morbidity related to vascular access is $7871 per patient YAR resulting in a cost to the Medicare program of between 14% and 17% of dialysis patient costs.[8] Feldman et al[9] identified trends in access-related morbidity suggesting that this high-cost aspect of care may be increasing. Vascular access morbidity also contributes to a reduction in the delivered dose of dialysis. Maintaining vascular access is another example of a high cost related aspect of therapy that has trade-offs for quality and cost of care.

The failure rate of arteriovenous (AV) grafts is higher than for AV fistulas.[10] The cost components of AV fistula placements have been discussed elsewhere.[11] McCarely et al[12] studied prospectively the effects of vascular access blood-flow monitoring, using the ultrasound dilution method, to identify and treat stenosis prior to thrombosis in patients using fistula or grafts. By the end of 33 months of monitoring of stenosis in 132 patients, the adjusted annual billed amount for vascular-access related events was 49% for grafts and 41% for fistula. Clearly, there are financial incentives to reduce morbidity from vascular access from the societal perspective, but not necessarily from the provider's perspective.

Current payment policy may not be structured to optimize the cost-effectiveness of available treatments or provide appropriate economic incentives to use them. The experience of erythropoietin provides evidence that changes in payment policy can affect provider behavior, and consequently clinical outcomes. In 1999, Medicare spent more than $1 billion on erythropoietin[1] whose widespread use has resulted in higher hematocrit levels and improved quality of life for many patients. When erythropoietin was first introduced in 1989, payment was made on a "per administration" basis rather than per unit. The average dose of erythropoietin remained low and stable into 1991 when Medicare began paying on a per unit basis. The average dose of erythropoietin subsequently increased and, by 1997, it had more than doubled. Approximately 70% of ESRD patients had a hematocrit of at least 31.[13] While causality cannot be proven from trend data, it is likely that the policy change affected behavior.

Peritoneal dialysis

Peritoneal dialysis (PD) is the choice of only 12% of dialysis patients in the USA.[1] Interestingly, its use has declined in recent years despite evidence that outcomes are generally similar, and costs are lower than HD.[14,15] However, there are no prospective randomized trials that conclusively determine whether equivalent outcomes exist for morbidity and mortality.

For PD patients, peritonitis is financially and clinically significant. A recent effort that identified spending for ESRD care (including Medicare payments as well as co-pays and deductibles) determined that average spending per year at risk on peritonitis for adult PD patients was $4635 in 1996, with over three-quarters of this spent on inpatient hospital services.[4] Reducing the incidence of

Table 80.4 Risk adjuster model results for within-year transplant patients

	Estimated coefficient (spending per YAR US$)	Patients in sample with characteristic (%)
Demographic factors		
Years of age (reference case 20–34)		
0–1	13 939	0
2–6	9517	1
7–12	14 050	1
13–15	3940	1
16–19	−3622	2
35–44	7668†	23
45–54	6243†	24
55–64	13 280‡	17
65+	21 191‡	7
Race (reference case white)		
Black	13 106‡	25
Sex (reference case female)		
Male	−3168	60
Years since onset of ESRD (reference case < 1)		
1–2	−17 215‡	40
3–4	−21 965‡	18
5+	−22 768‡	20
Wage Index (reference case mid 85 < index < 1.10)		
High index > 1.10	6042*	27
Low index < 0.85	−3793	23
Geographic region (reference case midwest)		
Northeast	10 273‡	20
West	−342	20
South	−2717	36
US Territories	7876	0.4
Disease-specific factors		
Diagnosis causing ESRD (reference case diabetes)		
Cystic kidney disease	−12 053‡	7
Other causes	−11 569‡	14
Hypertension	−13 685‡	20
Glomerulonephritis	−14 548‡	26
Other urologic	−8902	2
Number of transplants (reference case 1 Tx)		
Two transplants	−85 624‡	1
Transplant donor (reference case living-related donor)		
Cadaver transplant	−10 333‡	81
Intercept‡	−152 268	

$*P < 0.1$; $†P < 0.05$; $‡P < 0.01$.
Variables indicating missing or unknown data were included in the regression analysis, but are not given here. Reproduced with permission from the Renal Physicians Association.[4]

peritonitis would reduce costs and further strengthen the favorable economic position of PD relative to HD.

However, even if we assume equivalent efficacy between the two modalities and thus propose that PD is the least expensive (cost minimization) modality, it may still lag behind HD as the modality of choice. Traditional cost-effectiveness analysis reflects patient preferences and the perceived impact on quality of life. For PD patients it is possible that the impact of assuming responsibility for one's treatment reduces quality of life and thus diminishes the benefits of the lower cost therapy.

Transplantation

Transplantation is the most cost-effective renal replacement therapy (Table 80.1). The high cost of surgery is offset by a "long" period in which the patient requires little medical care. It is the only therapy that, if successful, is curative.

However, the number of people eligible for receiving a kidney transplant far exceeds the current supply of kidneys. One way to increase the supply of available kidneys is to use "expanded criteria" cadaver kidneys (EDK). The use of these donors is significantly more expensive than either cadaver or living-related transplants, although graft survival is similar.[16] Are the costs of EDK transplants greater, lesser, or equal to alternate renal replacement therapies, assuming roughly similar clinical outcomes? Modeling data show that after 6.6 years hemodialysis costs would be expected to exceed EDK transplant costs.[17] Therefore, it would be reasonable to proceed with the use of EDK transplants – assuming a graft survival, on average, of at least 6.6 years – while collecting economic data to verify the modeling results.

Given the scarcity of kidneys available for transplantation, it is useful to understand the cost-effectiveness of offering retransplantation to patients with failed grafts. The question to be answered is whether improvement in QALY from a second transplant is greater than the loss of QALY from someone else having to wait longer for their first transplant. The answer is that this policy has a cost per QALY of $9656.[3] However, the policy is, not unexpectedly, better for younger patients, lowering costs while increasing QALY, although it remains cost-effective for older patients. Costs are lower because the patients would be on dialysis less often and would be healthier following a transplant (on average).

All payers would like to be able to predict and therefore manage their financial risks. A risk adjustor model allows the payer to measure the degree to which its patient population may differ from a reference population. The risk adjustor may use demographic information (e.g. age or sex) or clinical information (e.g. cause of renal failure). In patients receiving a transplant one can construct a risk adjustor model using both demographic and clinical data (Table 80.4).[4] The base or reference case is a 20–34-year-old white woman who has had ESRD for less than 1 year and who lives in average-cost city in the midwestern United States; she has ESRD as a result of diabetes and she will

Table 80.5 Percentage difference between actual and predicted spending-within-year transplant patients

Group size	Mean predicted as % of actual spending*	90% of the time predicted $ are within (of actual spending)	98% of the time predicted $ are within (of actual spending)
10 patients	101%	16% to −13%	29% to −16%
20 patients	100%	11% to −9%	17% to −11%
40 patients	100%	7% to −7%	11% to −8%
60 patients	100%	6% to −5%	9% to −7%
100 patients	100%	5% to −4%	8% to −6%
500 patients	100%	2% to −2%	3% to −3%
600 patients	100%	2% to −2%	3% to −3%

*Rounded to nearest whole number.
Reproduced with permission from the Renal Physicians Association.[4]

receive a living-related donor kidney for her first transplant. As can be seen in Table 80.4, various demographic factors can dramatically affect the cost. For example, if she were 45–54, as are almost a quarter of transplant recipients, costs would be expected to increase by $6243. The cost would rise by an additional $10 333 if she received a cadaver transplant rather than a living-related donor transplant.

It is necessary to understand how good the model is in predicting actual costs. Table 80.5 shows that the model's ability to predict cost is a function of the number of patients (sample size). Thus, for groups of 100 patients the model would be ± 4–5% of actual spending 90% of the time and 6–8% for 98% of the time. These models are generally useful for predicting costs for larger groups of patients but they are based on historical costs and treatment protocols. When new treatment protocols are used both costs and outcomes change and the "old paradigms" are no longer valid. Newer immunosuppressive agents demonstrate this well.

The cost of immunosuppressive drugs is an important post-transplant cost. In the USA, patients who are not old or disabled have to pay for these drugs beginning 3 years after their transplant. The FDA approved mycophenolate mofetil in 1995, 12 years after the approval of cyclosporine. Tacrolimus and sirolimus have also been recently approved. Economic analyses will be important in determining whether these newer drugs alone or in combination with older therapies provide better clinical outcomes at equal or lower cost.[18] In performing the analyses, the perspective will be especially important as outpatient drug costs three years following a successful transplant place a real burden on patients.

Conclusion

Applying the tools of economics to ESRD enhances the decision-making powers of patients, providers, and payers. This chapter has identified a variety of analyses and healthcare scenarios that show that proper use of economic analysis can result in changes in practice and policy that might achieve more efficient use of resources as well as better patient outcomes.

References

1. USRDS 2001. US Renal Data System Annual Data Report: Atlas of End-Stage Renal Disease in the United States. National Institute of Diabetes and Digestive and Kidney Diseases. Bethesda, MD: National Institutes of Health, 2001.
2. Cutler DM, McClellan M: Is technological change in medicine worth it? Health Affairs 2001;20:11–29.
3. Hornberger JC, Best JH, Garrison LP Jr: Cost-effectiveness of repeat medical procedures: kidney transplantation as an example. Med Decis Making 1997;17:363–372.
4. The Lewin Group: Capitation Models for ESRD. Methodology and results. Renal Physicians Association, and American Society of Nephrology. Rockville MD and Washington DC: RPA–ASN, 2000.
5. Hakim RM, Breyer J, Ismail N, et al: Effects of dose of dialysis on morbidity and mortality. Am J Kid Dis 1996;23:661–669.
6. Sehgal AR, Dor A, Tsai AC: Morbidity and cost implications of inadequate hemodialysis. Am J Kid Dis 2001;37:1223–1231.
7. Daugridas JT, Ing T: Handbook of Dialysis. Boston, MA: Little and Brown, 1994.
8. USRDS 1997. US Renal Data System Annual Data Report. NIH and National Institute of Diabetes and Digestive and Kidney Diseases. Bethesda, MD: National Institutes of Health, 2001.
9. Feldman HI, Kobrin S, Wasserstein A: Hemodialysis vascular access morbidity. J Am Soc Nephrol 1996;7:523–535.
10. Woods JD, Turenne MN, Strawderman RL, et al: Vascular access survival among incident hemodialysis patients in the US. Am J Kidney Dis 1997;30:50–57.
11. Hakim R, Himmelfarb J: Hemodialysis access failure: A call to action. Kidney Int 1998;54:1029–1040.
12. McCarely P, Wingard RL, Shyr Y, et al: Vascular access blood flow monitoring reduces access morbidity and costs. Kidney Int 2001;60:1164–1172.
13. Greer JW, Milam RA, Eggers PW: Trends in use, cost and outcomes of human recombinant erythropoietin, 1989–98. Health Care Financ Rev, 1999;20:55–62.
14. Held PJ, Port FK, Turenne MN, et al: Continuous ambulatory peritoneal dialysis and hemodialysis: Comparison of patient mortality with adjustment for comorbid conditions. Kidney Int 1994;45:1163–1169.
15. Goeree R, Manalich J, Grootendorst P, et al: Cost analysis of dialysis treatments for end-stage renal disease. Clin Invest Med 1995;18:455–464.
16. Whiting, JF, Golconda , M, Smith, R, et al: Economic costs of expanded criteria donors in renal transplantation. Transplantation 1998;65:204–207.
17. Whiting, JF, Zavala, JW: The cost-effectiveness of transplantation with expanded donor kidneys. Transplant Proc 1999;31:1320–1321.
18. Gonin, JM: Maintenance immunosuppression: new agents and persistent dilemmas. Adv Renal Replace Ther 2000;7:95–116.

PART XIII
Maintenance Dialysis

HUGH R. BRADY

Technical Aspects of Hemodialysis

Bryan N. Becker and Gerald Schulman

General principles

Hemodialysis is a complex process performed with apparent simplicity. By attaching an extracorporeal circuit to a patient, the procedure of hemodialysis effectively removes uremic toxins and corrects acid–base disturbances in a manner approximating some of the functions of a natural kidney. This chapter presents a synopsis of dialyzers, dialysate composition, water treatment systems, and some of the technical aspects of hemodialysis.

Dialysis relies on the mass transfer across semipermeable membranes. The hemodialysis membranes separate the blood and dialysate compartments. Diffusion, convection, and ultrafiltration (UF) across the membrane are properties that are integral to the dialysis procedure. Diffusion describes the movement of solutes from one compartment to another, relying on a concentration gradient between the two compartments. This is the principal mechanism for toxin removal during hemodialysis. Convective transport involves the movement of solutes by bulk flow in association with fluid removal. Convective clearance is the mechanism of toxin removal by the depurative process known as hemofiltration. It is not dependent on concentration gradients and the magnitude of its contribution to clearance is directly related to the ultrafiltration rate. Mass solute removal across the dialyzer is a function of effective blood flow (Q_B) and differences between the afferent and efferent concentrations of solute, traditionally labeled as "arterial" and "venous" (C_A and C_V). Thus, the definition of diffusive dialyzer clearance (K), similar to creatinine clearance in the normal kidney, is calculated as:

$$K = (Q_B)(C_A - C_V)/C_A$$

where $(Q_B)(C_A - C_V)$ represents the amount of solute removal and C_A is the driving force.

The equation, however, neglects the contribution of convection. This phenomenon is directly related to ultrafiltration and involves the bulk movement of fluid across dialyzer membranes. The driving force for ultrafiltration is the hydrostatic pressure gradient across the membrane, the transmembrane pressure (TMP). With ultrafiltration, blood flow leaving the dialyzer (Q_{Bo}) is less than blood flow entering the dialyzer (Q_{Bi}). The difference between these values represents ultrafiltration (Q_{uf}). This can be incorporated into the above equation to yield a more precise definition of clearance:

$$(Q_{Bo}) = (Q_{Bi}) - (Q_{uf})$$

$$K = [Q_{Bi}(C_A) - (Q_{Bo} - Q_{uf})(C_V)]/C_A$$
$$= [Q_{Bi}(C_A - C_V) + (Q_{uf})(C_V)]/C_A$$

True clearance should be calculated by using the concentration in the aqueous compartment of blood and the concentration of solute in that compartment. Since solutes diffusing out of blood will appear in the dialysate, it is possible to calculate clearance for solutes not present in the incoming dialysate (e.g. urea) as:

$$K = Q_{Do}(C_{Do})/C_A$$

where C_{Do} and Q_{Do} are the concentrations of solute in the dialysate outlet and the effluent dialysate flow respectively. Although this equation provides a simple concept for determining clearance, the necessity of measuring low concentrations of any substance in the dialysate increases the error of measurement. Indeed, the most accurate measurement of dialyzer clearance is achieved when both "blood-side" and "dialysate-side" clearances are obtained, thus assuring mass balance.

The hemodialysis procedure

Blood circuit

Blood in the extracorporeal circuit is contained within tubing that is connected to the venous and arterial sides of a patient's access (Fig. 81.1). Needles are inserted into the patient's blood access and blood tubing is connected to the needle hubs. Blood is withdrawn from the arterial segment by the blood pump and pumped through the dialyzer back to the patient via the venous segment of tubing. Inadvertent entry of air into the dialysis circuit, air embolism, is a potentially lethal complication and is likeliest to occur between the vascular access site and the blood pump. Air can enter the dialysis circuit from areas around the arterial needle, through leaky or broken tubing or tubing connections, and through the saline infusion set. Air traps are located in the blood tubing to trap air and prevent air from entering the patient's circulation. Air detectors are linked to a relay switch that automatically clamps the venous blood line and shuts off the blood pump if air is detected.

Blood pumps used for hemodialysis (HD) are roller pumps that use the principles of peristaltic pumping to move blood through tubing. A compressible part of the tubing (the pump segment) is occluded between rollers and a curved rigid track. Elastic recoil refills the pump tubing after the roller has passed over it. The flow rate of the blood pump is dependent on the stroke volume, the speed of rotation of the rollers, and the volume of the pump segment. The blood flow rate displayed on the the dialysis machine is based on these three parameters, rather than an actual value from a blood flow probe. This can lead to significantly higher values for the displayed blood flow compared to the true blood flow rate. Incomplete occlusion of the pump segment due to a pump maladjustment leads to a reduced volume of blood with each pump rotation. This is a common cause of overestimation of blood flow and hence clearance. Careful maintenance of the pump is essential to insure that the prescribed dialysis dose is actually delivered to the patient.

Pressure monitors are usually located proximal to the blood pump and immediately distal to the dialyzer. The proximal monitor, the "arterial monitor," guards against excessive suction on the vascular access site by the blood pump and the distal monitor, the "venous monitor," gauges the resistance to blood return to the venous side of the vascular access. Some machines place the "arterial monitor" distal to the blood pump and proximal to the dialyzer to detect clotting in the dialyzer and more precisely estimate pressure in the dialyzer blood compartment. To prevent blood clotting in the dialyzer, an anticoagulant such as heparin is often infused into the circuit. A peristaltic pump or syringe pump delivers the anticoagulant into blood in the circuit via a T-tube or T-fitting usually located between the blood pump and the dialyzer.

A blood leak detector is usually placed in the dialysis circuit in the dialysate outflow line. If a blood leak develops

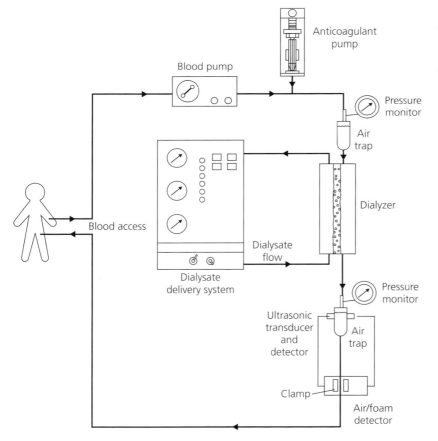

Figure 81.1 Blood circuit for hemodialysis procedure demonstrating the location of pressure monitors, air traps, air detectors, heparin pump, blood pump, and dialyzer. (From Feldman HI, Kinosian M, Bilker WB, et al: Effect of dialyzer reuse on survival of patients treated with hemodialysis. JAMA 1996;276:620–625. Copyright 1996, American Medical Association.)

Anticoagulant pump

Blood pump

Pressure monitor

Air trap

Blood access

Dialyzer

Dialysate flow

Dialysate delivery system

Ultrasonic transducer and detector

Pressure monitor

Air trap

Clamp

Air/foam detector

through the dialysis membrane, then blood leaking into the dialysate is sensed by the blood leak detector and the appropriate alarm is activated.

Dialysis solution circuit

Two properties of the dialysis solution that require constant monitoring are conductivity and temperature. A proportioning system dilutes a concentrated dialysis solution with water. If this system malfunctions, patient blood can be exposed to a hyperosmolar dialysis solution resulting in hypernatremia, or a hypoosmolar dialysis solution leading to hyponatremia and hemolysis. The primary solutes in the dialysis solution are electrolytes. Therefore, the concentration of the dialysis solution is reflected by the concentration of electrolytes and their electrical conductivity. Appropriate proportioning of water and the dialysis solution is monitored by a meter measuring conductivity of the product dialysis solution fed into the dialyzer.

A temperature monitor prevents complications related to a warm dialysis solution. A cool dialysis solution can be uncomfortable for the patient and is dangerous when the patient is unconscious, but otherwise may have therapeutic value in preventing hypotension. A warm dialysis solution (> 42 °C), however, can lead to hemolysis. If the conductivity or the temperature are outside of the normal range then a bypass valve diverts the dialysis solution around the dialyzer and directly to a drain.

On-line monitoring

Dialysis machines function as more than just dialysis delivery systems. Built-in monitors assess the physical characteristics of the dialysis solution as noted above and accrue data ranging from patient blood pressure and heart rate to treatment parameters, medication data, measures of delivered dialysis dose, plasma volume, thermal energy loss, and even dialysis access recirculation. Computerized medical information systems have been linked with dialysis delivery systems to provide information networks that can control treatments at individual patient stations while maintaining information and treatment records for future use. Some of these systems include the Smart Connection from Baxter Healthcare Corporation, the Althin Drake Willock System 1000, and a similar system designed by Fresenius. Real-time information regarding treatment parameters and patient information also can be visualized during dialysis treatments with the Cobe Centry 3 System, the Althin Drake Willock System 1000, and the Fresenius 2008H system. It is now possible to integrate data, such as comparing present and past dialysis treatments, into a real-time display to help gauge therapy, change prescription and ultrafiltration goals, and generate better immediate assessment of a patient's and unit's overall status.[1,2] Such on-line monitoring that allows sensors from the machine to change treatment parameters has been termed a biofeedback system (Fig. 81.2). Automatic biofeedback systems have the potential to reduce adverse events such as hypotension, to monitor the state of the hemodialysis access and to increase the efficiency of the hemodialysis treatment (Table 81.1).

A great deal of effort has been devoted to applying technological advances to improving measures of dialysis adequacy. Data from numerous studies during the last decade emphasize that the dose of dialysis greatly

Table 81.1 On-line features of the hemodialysis machine

Parameter	Consequence
Blood pressure	Changes in ultrafiltration rate, sodium modeling
Plasma volume by hemoglobin	Changes in ultrafiltration rate, sodium modeling
Thermal energy loss/gain	Change in dialysate temperature
Transient change in dialysate sodium	Measurement of Kt/V
Transient change in hemoglobin	Access blood flow, recirculation, cardiac output
Transient change in temperature	Access recirculation

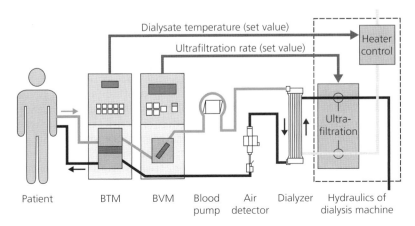

Figure 81.2 Elements of a hemodialysis biofeedback system. Patient input variables include blood pressure, plasma volume, sodium concentration, and plasma temperature. These inputs are measured by an online blood pressure monitor, a blood volume monitor (BVM), and a blood temperature monitor (BTM). The inputs lead to automatic adjustments by the hemodialysis machine of the ultrafiltration rate, dialysate temperature, and dialysate sodium concentration.

influences mortality and morbidity in ESRD patients. A standard measure of the dose of dialysis is the Kt/V urea index, where K = urea clearance, t = treatment time, and V = volume of urea distribution. When Gotch and Sargent reanalyzed data from the National Cooperative Dialysis Study,[3] they determined that values < 0.8 were associated with increased rates of patient morbidity. Additional studies have suggested that increasing Kt/V to values > 1.2–1.4 may improve patient survival.[4,5] Urea kinetic modeling is therefore an easy tool for assessing the adequacy of dialysis.

Traditionally, this technique has required multiple blood samples, accurate assessment of blood and dialysate flows and treatment times, and mathematical calculations, simplified somewhat by custom-designed software. On-line systems that accurately measure urea kinetics are now feasible (Biostat 1000, Baxter Healthcare Corporation), measuring urea concentration in dialysate effluent and determining urea kinetic parameters from concentration and time-dependent profile.[6,7] This does not require blood sampling and has the additional advantage of providing a Kt/V based on whole body urea clearance (2-pool model of urea kinetics) rather than traditional single-pool kinetics. Efforts to enhance the accuracy and simplicity of this system and other on-line urea monitoring devices are ongoing.

A recent variation employs sodium clearance in place of changes in urea concentration to simplify the measurement of on-line Kt/V. Sodium clearance across the dialyzer is almost identical to urea clearance. Thus, sodium concentration or dialysate conductivity can be used as a surrogate for urea. Sodium concentration, as a function of dialysate conductivity, is measured by sensors located pre- and post-dialyzer. Dialysis time, prescrbed Kt/V and the patient's urea volume, determined from a kinetic modeling session and not from anthropometrics, are entered into the machine. Clearance is measured by increasing the dialysate sodium concentration for a short period. This causes sodium to move from dialysate into the blood. By measuring the change in conductivity of the dialysate associated with its passage through the dialyzer, sodium clearance is determined and Kt/V can be calculated. Multiple measurements of Kt/V during the treatment allow one to determine if the prescribed goal will be reached. Common problems that prevent the goal from being reached include reduced actual blood flow or dialysate flow, reduced dialyzer performance, and access recirculation.

Other monitoring systems have been developed and used to monitor access flow and function during dialysis and to make accurate determinations of circulating blood volume during the dialytic procedure. Single- and dual-sensor systems using saline injections and sound velocity dilution calibration have been investigated as a method for accurately determining access flow during hemodialysis.[8] Similar efforts have led to noninvasive optical hematocrit monitoring to continually measure hematocrit during dialysis to better determine circulating blood volume.[9] As blood volume deceases, hematocrit increases. It is often possible to define a hematocrit in a patient above which hypotension is likely to occur.

The measurement of on-line blood volume with these devices can identify patients who are not near their estimated dry weight. In 18% of hemodialysis patients, a less than 5% decrease in blood volume was noted during routine hemodialysis sessions. In subsequent treatments, increased volume was successfully removed without hypotensive episodes.[10] The patients were able to have intradialytic fluid removal intentionally increased by 47% (average 0.8 L). The change in blood volume can be determined noninvasively during hemodialysis with these devices.[11] A critical hematocrit can be determined with these devices above which hypotension can be reliably predicted in 75% of patients.[12] Thus, these devices provide an added on-line safety measure to the treatment.

Characteristics of dialyzers

The classical view of membranes as inert structures providing solely fluid, ion, and molecular transport is now obsolete. Modern dialysis membranes display numerous physical, and adsorptive properties that contribute to the degree to which blood components are activated by the membranes. Membranes that produce little interaction with blood components such as white blood cells and the humoral components of plasma are described as being biocompatible. The structural compounds comprising the dialysis membranes may be their simplest distinguishing feature, dividing dialyzers into cellulosic, semisynthetic, and synthetic membranes. Although in decline, cellulose and its derivatives, cuprophane and cellulose acetate, continue to be the most commonly used membranes for dialysis worldwide. Cellulose extracted from cotton lint is dissolved in sodium hydroxide, and regenerated, and the membrane is then formed in an acid bath. Cuprophane is generated with an ammonium solution of copper hydroxide. Copper–ammonia–cellulose complexes are extruded into an acid bath producing a membrane with cuprammonium radicals. This modification yields greater diffusion and UF capabilities for cuprophane membranes compared to straight cellulose. Increasing glycerine content in membranes (average content for cuprophane = 5%) also affects these characteristics, as does membrane acetylation yielding greater solute and flux capacities to the membrane.

Synthetic membranes differ from cellulose-based dialyzers in several ways. All cellulose membranes have hydroxyl radicals at the surface that increase their hydrophilicity (membrane wettability). Techniques that mask hydroxyl radicals enhance hydrophobicity and increase protein adsorption.[13] Most synthetic membranes are thicker than less permeable cellulosic membranes. Membrane permeability is inversely proportional to membrane thickness and directly proportional to the membrane's intrinsic diffusion coefficient. However, synthetic membranes also display greater intrinsic diffusion coefficients and maintain their thickness when wet. Cuprophane and cellulose acetate membranes swell when wet.[14,15] A number of synthetic membranes also strongly bind blood proteins, causing decreases in their filtration efficiency.

Membranes can be symmetric or asymmetric. The smooth "skin" side interacts with blood for asymmetric membranes. Asymmetry, obtained by altering membrane precipitation during manufacturing,[16] allows for greater diffusive permeability. Hence, asymmetric membranes are very useful for hemofiltration. Polyacrylonitrile (PAN) and polysulfone (PS) membranes are commonly used asymmetric membranes. Polymethylmethacrylate (PMMA) membranes also manifest many of these characteristics. PAN, polyamide (PA), and PMMA membranes have low hydrophilicity and appreciable protein adsorption. Cellulose-based membranes have greater hydrophilicity and less adsorptive capacity.[16] Surface charge of the membranes also differs, which affects the sieving of charged solutes.[17]

Type of dialyzer

Three forms of dialyzers have been used for hemodialysis. Plate dialyzers, used in the early days of dialysis, consist of sheets of membranes separated by a spacer in rectangular compartments that are placed in parallel. This arrangement allows for low blood flow resistance and controlled UF.

Coil dialyzers are constructed from one or several pieces of membrane tubing wound around a central core. A support screen maintains the tubing in position. Blood flows through the tubing while dialysate flows through the supporting screen. Coil dialyzers are of historical interest only as they are rarely used. They are highly compliant with high blood flow resistance and variable UF rates.

Hollow-fiber dialyzers are the most common dialyzers in use today (Table 81.2). They consist of 10 000–15 000 hollow fibers wrapped in a bundle inside a plastic jacket. Each fiber has a diameter of 200–300 μm. Blood flows through the fibers while dialysate flows outside the fibers, typically in a countercurrent fashion. Hollow-fiber dialyzers are easy to use and provide low blood flow resistance, excellent mass transfer, low compliance, and controllable UF. Thus, the extracorporeal blood volume is constant and remains independent of transmembrane pressures. They require low (100–200 mL) priming volumes and are easier to re-use than the other types of dialyzers. Problems associated with early hollow-fiber dialyzers include increased blood clotting, blood loss, and residual ethylene oxide or formaldehyde in the potting compound that anchors the fibers to the dialyzer. These problems have largely been overcome with newer hollow-fiber dialyzers.[18]

A subset of hollow-fiber dialyzers are large-surface-area dialyzers (of high efficiency and high flux). These dialyzers have greater surface area than their conventional hollow-fiber counterparts and provide increased clearance for low molecular weight solutes as Q_b and Q_d are increased. High-flux dialyzers have surface areas as large as the high-efficiency dialyzers, with comparable clearance of substances with low molecular weights. In addition, they also significantly remove substances of higher molecular weight (> 10 000 Da) but also allow a high degree of hydraulic permeability. These dialyzers have low priming volumes; however, their marked hydraulic permeability requires constant UF monitoring.

Each dialyzer includes a specification sheet that gives operating information for the dialyzer. The K_{uf} is a function of the hydraulic permeability of the membrane and is expressed as the number of mL per hour ultrafiltration achieved for every mmHg of TMP. For example, if the K_{uf} is 4.0, the TMP required to remove 1000 mL/h is 250 mmHg. This pressure is assessed at the midpoint of the fibers. The values for K_{uf} supplied by manufacturers are derived from in vitro data and usually underestimate the actual clinical K_{uf} by 5–30%.[19] As most hollow-fiber dialyzers have pressure drops across the fibers, as blood is pushed by the blood pump at high pressures (generally 300–350 mmHg) and exits the dialyzers at lower pressures ≈ 100 mmHg, a "natural" TMP of 100–150 mmHg is possible. Thus, with a K_{uf} exceeding 5 mL/mmHg/h there is an obligate loss of 500 mL/h. Patients on these dialyzers may require fluid replacement if their UF requirements are < 500 mL/h. Because of this, with most synthetic membranes that have a $K_{uf} > 6.0$, monitoring is necessary to prevent hemodynamically significant errors in UF.

Solute clearance values for urea, creatinine, and vitamin B_{12} are also often supplied on the specification sheet. Clearance of these substances varies directly with hydraulic permeability, and the normal K_{uf} of many

Table 81.2 Representative list of commonly used hollow-fiber dialyzers

Model	Membrane	K_{uf}	KoA urea	Surface area (m^2)	Urea clearance (mL/min) Q_b = 200	Vitamin B$_{12}$ clearance (mL/min) Q_b = 200
Cobe 400-HG	Hemophan	5.3	570	0.9	177	57
Terumo C-101	Cellulose	3.5	520	1.0	171	54
Fresenius F-50	PS	30	700	0.9	176	95
Fresenius F-80	PS	60	945	1.8	192	139
Toray B1-1.6-H	PMMA	12	720	1.6	186	94
Gambro polyflux 160	PA	55	690	1.6	183	122
Gambro/Hospal Biospan 2400-S	AN-69	25	400	0.8	161	62

*From Daugirdas et al Handbook of Dialysis, 2nd edn. Boston: Little Brown, 1994, pp 30–52.
For a more extensive list of commonly used dialyzers and their specifications, refer to reference 14.
PA, polyamide; PMMA, polymethylmethacrylate; PS, polysulfone.

synthetic dialyzers can be altered by the manufacturer without requiring relabelling of the dialyzer. Dialyzer urea clearance is usually reported at various blood flow rates (e.g. 200, 300, and 400 mL/min) but at a specific dialysate flow rate (e.g. 500 mL/min). Creatinine clearance approximates 80% of urea clearance. Vitamin B_{12} clearance denotes the ability of the membrane to allow passage of solutes of larger molecular weight. High-flux and high-efficiency dialyzers significantly increase vitamin B_{12} clearance (> 100 mL/min at 200 mL/min blood flow) compared to conventional dialyzers (30–60 mL/min at 200 mL/min blood flow). For most dialyzers, in vivo clearance is 20–25% less than in vitro clearance.

Each dialyzer also has a mass transfer coefficient (*KoA*) for urea that provides a gauge of dialyzer efficiency. *KoA* determines the interrelationship between urea clearance and the flow rates of blood and dialysate, and therefore it can be used to estimate clearance at any given flow rate of blood and dialysate. *KoA* values of 200–300 mL/min are sufficient for small patients whereas *KoA* values near or > 700 mL/min are standard for high-efficiency dialyzers. Under any particular flow conditions there is a relationship between dialysance and *KoA*. Conversely, it is possible to determine the clinical performance of a dialyzer when blood or dialysate flow rates change or when a dialyzer membrane dysfunctions (e.g. by clotting). As such:

$$KoA = \frac{Q_B}{(1 - Q_B/Q_D)} \times \ln\left[(1 - D/Q_D)/1 - D/Q_B\right]$$

This equation can be rearranged to equate *D* (dialysance) as a function of *KoA* and flow rate:

$$D = \frac{e^{-[KoA\,(1 - Q_B/Q_D)/Q_B]} - 1}{e^{-[KoA\,(1 - Q_B/Q_D)/Q_B]} - 1/Q_D}$$

These equations are for coutercurrent flow. Similar expressions can be calculated for *KoA* during cocurrent flow:

$$KoA = \frac{Q_B}{(1 + Q_B/Q_D)} \times \log\left[Q_B/Q_D - D\,(1 + Q_B/Q_D)\right]$$

and when rearranged for D:

$$D = Q_B[1 - e^{-KoA\,(1 + Q_B/Q_D)/Q_B}/1 + Q_B/Q_D}$$

KoA can increase by as much as 10% as dialysate flow increases from 500 to 800 mL/min, perhaps due to changes in channeling of dialysate at different flow rates.

KoA has been thought to be a constant associated with a particular membrane, that can be used to calculate clearance as a function of any given blood flow and dialysate rates. It has recently been determined that *KoA* itself increases as dialysate flow increases.[20] This increase in *KoA* is thought to be due to changes in dialysate channeling through the hollow-fiber dialyzer. The implication of this finding is that the simple expedient of increasing dialysate flow from 500 to 800 mL/min can increase the *KoA* by as much as 10%. The delivered dose of the hemodialysis treatment can be increased by increasing dialysate flow without an increase in dialysis time or blood flow.

Biocompatibility

During hemodialysis, patients may experience a number of reactions that are a direct consequence of establishing the extracorporeal circuit. The number and severity of these reactions define the degree of dialysis biocompatibility. In the broadest sense, all aspects of the treatment such as dialysate composition and temperature, the nature of the anticoagulant or whether clearance is achieved predominantly by diffusion or convection, impact upon biocompatibility. However, it is the biocompatibility of the membrane surface itself that is most important and has been most closely studied. It is also important to remember that because hemodialysis is a repetitive process, even low-grade or minor membrane-induced reactions at each treatment can eventually lead to important clinical manifestations (Table 81.3).

The initial observation that transient neutropenia occurred during hemodialysis was made a quarter of a century ago.[21] It was later determined that complement activation via the alternative pathway, with generation of the anaphylatoxins C3a and C5a, was responsible for the decline in neutrophils shortly after initiation of hemodialysis.[22]

In this context, cellulosic hemodialysis membranes react with blood coursing through them. Free hydroxyl groups on cellulosic membranes activate complement via the alternative pathway. Membrane modifications that favor binding of factor H and inhibit binding of factor B (such as replacing hydroxyl groups with acetate side groups or diethylaminoethyl radicals) may ameliorate complement activation.[23,24] Further, complement activation is reduced as membrane hydrophobicity increases.[25] Surface charge further influences biocompatibility. Surfaces with a negative charge may interact with the Hageman factor and the contact pathway (kallikrein–kinin),[26] activating the contact pathway and generating bradykinin.[27,28] This may lead to severe adverse reactions in patients dialyzed against PAN membranes (specifically AN-69) while concomitantly receiving angiotensin-converting enzyme inhibitors (ACEIs).[29] ACEIs prevent bradykinin degradation. It should be noted that reused cellulosic membranes have also been implicated in these acute reactions.[30] Conceivably, reuse alters membrane characteristics, favoring bradykinin generation, although this has not yet been proved.

Table 81.3 Clinical manifestations of membrane biocompatibility/incompatibility

Anaphylactoid reactions

First-use syndrome

β_2-Microglobulin amyloidosis

Recovery from acute renal failure

Bacterial infection

Nutritional status

Loss of renal function

Response to vaccines

From Schulman and Levin.[25]

The effect of the format of the membrane is also significant. Format refers to the structure of the dialyzer rather than the nature of membrane. Dialyzers may be formatted as hollow-fiber or parallel-plate devices. The same membrane type may produce alterations in neutrophils (e.g. release of proteolytic enzymes) which differ depending on whether the membrane in the artificial kidney is formatted as hollow fibers or parallel plates.[31]

Finally, the adsorptive capacity of a membrane can affect its biocompatibility. PAN membranes bind vasoactive materials including C3a, C5a, and bradykinin to a greater extent than cuprophane.[32,33] The ability to adsorb potentially harmful substances may confer distinct advantages to certain membranes. On the other hand, beneficial substances may be removed and protein adsorption may alter the characteristics of the membrane.

Blood–membrane interaction

All humoral and cellular components in blood can potentially interact with the dialysis membrane. Interactions involving cellulosic membranes are associated with the greatest degree of complement activation. Generation of C3a and C5a is ultimately responsible for the clinical sequelae of blood–membrane interactions including contraction of vascular smooth muscle, increased vascular permeability, and formation of the membrane attack complex (C5b–C9). Complement generation also results in neutrophil activation. Release of enzymes such as lactoferrin, production of reactive oxygen species, synthesis of arachidonic metabolites, expression of adhesion receptors, and increases in monocyte cytokine gene transcription are all consequences of complement activation.[34]

The coagulation pathway is activated to a varying degree by dialyzer membrane surfaces. Anticoagulation during dialysis blunts this response. Cellular components of blood are also affected by hemodialysis membranes. Abnormal leukocyte function has been reported in chronic hemodialysis patients,[35,36] with complement-activating membranes inducing a greater degree of leukocyte dysfunction, defects in chemotaxis, and alterations in oxidative metabolism.[37] Peripheral blood mononuclear cells and monocytes harvested from patients chronically exposed to cuprophane membranes produce decreased concentrations of interleukin 1 (IL-1)[38] and tumor necrosis factor (TNF)[39] and exhibit reduced levels of interleukin 2 (IL-2) receptor expression[40] and variable degrees of natural killer cell activity dysfunction.[41]

Cytokines such as IL-1, IL-2, and TNF are thought to mediate some of the adverse reactions that are seen following hemodialysis with cuprophane membranes.[42] The paradox associated with this conclusion is that the performance index of in vitro cytokine generation by cells after they have been exposed to cellulosic membranes and then harvested from the peripheral circulation is downgraded at baseline and following endotoxin stimulation. It may be that repetitive insults are sufficient to produce adverse effects or that neutrophils and mononuclear cells produce tissue-level downregulation of cytokine production.[39]

Platelets also react with dialysis-membrane surfaces, but less information is available as to whether platelet function is affected by complement activation or other parameters of biocompatibility. Survival of red blood cells is significantly decreased in hemodialysis patients, although the cause for this is multifactorial. Red blood cells from hemodialysis patients appear to be more susceptible to the membrane attack complex (C5b–C9) than red blood cells from normal individuals.[43] The significance of these reactions is only partially understood at present. The extent to which any given membrane has been examined with respect to activation of each of the blood components differs (Table 81.4). Operationally, the lack of complement activation and early neutropenia during hemodialysis should serve as useful indices of biocompatible membranes.

Reuse of dialyzer

Reuse of dialyzer can impose its own direct effects on reactions during the hemodialysis treatment as well as indirectly via the production of alterations in membrane biocompatibility. During repetitive use, plasma proteins can coat dialysis membranes. The use of formaldehyde or glutaraldehyde without a bleach cycle fixes protein to the surface. This attenuates cuprophane-induced complement activation. However, many reuse procedures with these sterilants also include a bleach-containing cleansing cycle. This tends to restore the original surface of the membrane. Reuse with a mixture of peracetic acid and hydrogen peroxide also allows the surface of the membrane to become coated with protein, improving biocompatibility after reuse.

The increasing use of the newer synthetic membranes raises new issues with respect to reuse. Dialyzers manufactured with synthetic membranes have a favorable biocompatibility profile, even on first use. Therefore, there is no direct clinical benefit associated with reuse. However, the substantial cost of these dialyzers often means that reusing them saves costs. Reuse in this setting permits the introduction of these membranes into situations where

Table 81.4 Comparative bioincompatibility

Parameter	Relative order
Heparin consumption	Cuprophane > PS = PMMA
Complement activation	Cuprophane > cellulose acetate > PC > PAN
Leukopenia	Cuprophane > cellulose acetate > PC > PAN = PMMA
Granulocyte elastase	Cuprophane = PMMA > PS = PAN
Granulocyte adherence	Cuprophane > PS = PAN

Adapted from Mujaijsk R, Ivanovich P: Membranes fro extracorporeal therapy. *In* Maher JF (ed): Replacement of Renal Function by Dialysis. Dordrecht: Kluwer Academic Publishers, 1989, pp 181–188. With kind permission from Kluwer Academic Publishers.
PAN, polyacrylonitrile; PC, polyetherpolycarbonate; PMMA, polymethylmethacrylate; PS, polysulfone.

the cost would otherwise be prohibitive. A second issue relating to re-use of high-flux synthetic membranes involves changes in the fundamental characteristics of the membrane that are induced by the reuse procedure. A procedure using bleach increases porosity and makes the membrane more permeable to substances of larger molecular weight. This is obviously advantageous for removing injurious substances such as β_2-microglobulin. However, if the membrane opens too much, losses of albumin can be substantial. If hydrogen peroxide or peracetic acid is used as the sterilant, an opposite phenomenon occurs. The permeability of the membrane declines. This is clearly disadvantageous if removal of high-molecular-weight substances is deemed important.

Permeability and porosity

Synthetic high-flux membranes are being used increasingly in the USA. Advantages (or disadvantages) related to their use may result from improved biocompatibility, enhanced clearance and/or adsorption of large-molecular-weight substances, or both of these features. Even cellulose-triacetate membranes, cellulose-based high-efficiency membranes, have a relatively good biocompatibility profile. The majority of membranes used for conventional or high-efficiency hemodialysis are cellulose based or PMMA based. Polysulfone (PS) membranes, when configured as low-flux membranes for use without UF control (i.e. "biocompatibility" dissociated from "flux"), cause intermediate degrees of neutropenia and complement activation. The use of polyvinylpyrrolidone to accomplish this dissociation restores some hydrophilicity to the membrane and, thus, a tendency for complement activation.[44]

No large prospective long-term studies have attempted to differentiate effects related to high-flux and effects related to biocompatibility. Potential benefits of high-flux include enhanced middle-molecule clearance, removal of activated substances such as complement, clearance of β_2-microglobulin, and better lipid control due to the removal of a circulating inhibitor of lipoprotein lipase.[45] Potential disadvantages include albumin loss into the dialysate and the risk of introducing endotoxins or similar substances into the blood.

It is also apparent that reuse procedures may affect membrane properties. As mentioned, bleach may increase high-flux membrane permeability to substances with large molecular weights, while hydrogen peroxide or peracetic acid may decrease the permeability of the membrane. This alteration in permeability affects the membrane only when the membrane is configured as a high-flux membrane (e.g. PS or PMMA) but it is unimportant when the membrane is configured as a low-flux membrane. Reuse procedures may also alter the surface charge, potentially resulting in elaboration of bradykinin.

Clinical issues

Preliminary data from the US Renal USRDS registry,[46] as well as other studies, suggest that changing to newer membranes results in decreased mortality. Although these data are retrospective, they are consistent with other evidence suggesting chronic blood–membrane interactions with cellulosic membranes have long-term clinical consequences. Improvement in other aspects of hemodialysis treatment, such as increasing the delivered dose of dialysis, or improving blood pressure control, may mask or override adverse reactions to cellulosic membranes. Thus, superb survival has been reported with very long treatment times (high Kt/V) despite the use of cuprophane membranes, although meticulous control of hypertension and favorable demographics are also evident in this population.[47] Nevertheless, amyloidosis remains a problem in this setting.

Acute reactions

Anaphylactoid reactions associated with the use of new cuprophane membranes are well-established occurrences, although rare. The "first use" syndrome is characterized by signs and symptoms that include urticaria, cough, chest and back pain, dyspnea, and hypotension. It is usually seen within the first 15 min of hemodialysis. It has been suggested that some of these reactions are mediated by IgE antibodies directed against ethylene oxide which is used as a sterilant for cellulosic membranes. However, it should be noted that patients manifesting this reaction generate significantly higher levels of activated complement products than symptom-free patients.[48]

PAN membranes, specifically AN-69 (Hospal), can cause a similar syndrome in hemodialysis patients who are simultaneously receiving ACEIs. ACE is also a potent kinase that degrades bradykinin. PAN membranes generate high levels of bradykinin. Therefore, concomitant use of PAN membranes and an ACEI may lead to high levels of circulating bradykinin and adverse hemodynamic events.[29] The anaphylactoid reactions associated with ACEIs have also been reported with dialysis membranes other than PAN.[30] The common denominator in this instance may be that the most episodes occurred with reused dialyzers. The implication is that the reuse procedure affected the membrane surface in some way, perhaps altering the surface charge, increasing its negativity and potentiating bradykinin generation through the contact pathway.

Chronic reactions

Animal studies suggest that repeated activation of complement by cuprophane or zymosan delays recovery from ischemia-induced acute renal failure.[49] Residual renal function following a 5/6 nephrectomy also declines faster in animals exposed to cuprophane compared to control animals or animals exposed to PAN membranes.[50] Histology of animal kidneys shows neutrophil infiltration into the glomeruli of the those exposed to cuprophane or zymosan. Complement generation during the blood–membrane interaction of blood activated the leukocytes with potential detrimental consequences on organ function. A recent study in people with acute renal failure in intensive care units, matched for APACHE scores, showed more rapid recovery of renal function in those dialyzed with PMMA than those dialyzed using cuprophane membranes.[51]

There is evidence that the frequency and severity of β_2-microglobulin-induced amyloidosis also may be reduced by use of biocompatible membranes.[52] Peripheral blood mononuclear cells harvested from patients dialyzed against new cuprophane membranes produce greater amounts of β_2-microglobulin.[53] Proteases from complement-activated leukocytes potentially enhance polymerization of this protein into amyloid fibrils.[54] Moreover, cuprophane membranes do not significantly adsorb this protein nor permit significant passage of it.

Other potential chronic effects of bioincompatibility include a higher infection rate due to functional defects in peripheral blood leukocytes, a higher rate of graft infection,[37] and detrimental nutritional consequences.[55] Hypoalbuminemia, low cholesterol levels, low predialysis urea levels, and low creatinine levels (reflecting low muscle mass) have all been shown to correlate with increased mortality in the hemodialysis population.[56] While increasing the dose of dialysis may favorably influence these indices,[57] it is also true that the cytokine production may affect catabolism. Interestingly, an equivalent dose of hemodialysis (determined by Kt/V) leads to greater protein intake when PAN membranes are used than when cuprophane membranes are used. In such studies, the beneficial effects of increased permeability of the former membranes cannot be easily differentiated from their favorable biocompatibility profile.[44] Experiments employing sham dialysis also suggest that cuprophane causes skeletal muscle catabolism.[58]

Membrane choice for optimal dialysis

Membrane selection influences the frequency and number of adverse events related to hemodialysis therapy (Table 81.5). The membrane may also influence the response to vaccines or erythropoietin, and injury to various organs which may be mediated by inflammatory substances generated during blood–membrane interactions. Some recommendations have been suggested regarding membrane choice for optimal dialysis; they include:

1. Newer synthetic membranes offer established and theoretical advantages over cellulosic membranes.

Table 81.5 Factors influencing membrane choice

Biocompatibility of the membrane structure
    Composition and format
    Blood–membrane interactions
    Adsorptive properties
    Effect of reuse
Porosity/permeability
Diffusive and convective clearance

From Schulman G, Levin NW: Membranes for hemodialysis. Semin Dialysis 1994;7:251–256.

2. Synthetic membranes are beneficial when used in acute renal failure.
3. There is not enough information about the superiority of one synthetic membrane over another (one reasonable approach is to use the specific membrane found in a given study to ameliorate the particular adverse reaction of concern to the nephrologist); currently, the expense of the membrane should also factor in the decision.
4. Avoid the use of ACEIs when PAN membranes are selected – specifically AN-69. Caution must also be applied with reused membranes.
5. In most cases, the absence of complement activation and of neutropenia is a useful marker of biocompatibility.

Future developments in dialyzers

Advances in membrane manufacturing techniques are likely to yield dialyzers better able to remove substances of larger molecular weight (middle molecules). There have been advances in regulating pore-size dimensions, distribution, and geometry, that allow for increased sieving coefficients for molecules such as β_2-microglobulin, but not larger substances such as albumin.[59,60] Reducing the inner diameter of the hollow fibers has been shown to increase resistance in the blood compartment, which permits greater filtration of substances in the middle molecule range.[61] A sorbent system is being developed that also enhances the removal of larger substances; it will be placed in series with the dialyzer in the extracorporeal circuit.[62] The results of the HEMO study[63] will certainly impact on the importance of this technology. One arm of the prospective, randomized, multicenter trial compares the impact of high-flux versus low-flux membranes on morbidity and mortality in hemodialysis patients. If survival is improved with high-flux membranes in this trial, performance based on improved filtration of middle molecules will be a key feature of dialyzer evaluations.

Dialysate composition

One of the major aims of hemodialysis is the restoration of normal ion concentrations. As such, the levels of individual ions in the dialysate can be set to their desired plasma levels; however, in some instances dialysate levels are set for the *diffusible* fraction of the ion found in plasma. Dialysis solutions have undergone substantial changes since the inception of hemodialysis.

Dialysate glucose

In the early 1960s, high glucose concentrations in dialysis fluid were used to provide osmotic pressure for water removal. However, advances in hydraulic UF and the demonstration that high dialysate glucose (> 320 mg/dL) increased the risk for hyperosmolar syndrome, postdialysis hyperglycemia and hyponatremia[64] rendered the use of high dialysate glucose obsolete. Contemporary dialysis fluids range from glucose-free to slightly hyperglycemic (up to 200 mg/dL).[65] Most noninsulin dependent-diabetic patients tolerate well dialysis with glucose-free dialysate, despite losing 25–30 g of glucose across the dialyzer. However, this glucose loss may potentiate hypoglycemia[66–68] and adversely affect hemodialysis catabolism, raising levels of free amino acids during dialysis,[69] and increasing the intradialytic protein catabolic rate.[70] Ketogenesis and gluconeogenesis are usually sufficient to maintain serum glucose in the physiologic range despite reductions in plasma insulin, lactate, and pyruvate. By contrast, physiologic dialysate glucose (200 mg/dL) has few adverse effects,[71] aside from aggravating hypertriglyceridemia. Dialysate glucose can affect potassium removal, the risk of dialysis disequilibrium syndrome, and postdialysis fatigue. In general, an optimal dialysate glucose concentration is 100–200 mg/dL for most patients. However, in diabetic patients, insulin doses may require adjustment to account for this dialysis-imposed "glucose clamp" in which levels of plasma glucose may be kept constant during dialysis as a result of the concentration in the dialysate.

Dialysate sodium

Investigators comparing hemodynamic changes induced by conventional dialysis, UF, and sequential UF-dialysis found that plasma osmolality plays a pivotal role in maintaining hemodynamic stability during hemodialysis.[72–74] Isoosmolar fluid removal improved hemodynamic stability. During hemodialysis, the fall in extracellular osmolality is more rapid than corresponding changes in intracellular osmolality, resulting in extracellular to intracellular (ECF–ICF) fluid shifts, exacerbating volume depletion. This decline in plasma osmolality (P_{osm}) is more apparent with rapid solute removal that is not counteracted by sodium diffusing from dialysate into the blood. A low-sodium dialysate (< 135 mequiv./L) favors this ICF shift as plasma becomes more hypoosmolar following sodium movement from plasma to dialysate.

The reduction in plasma volume (PV) with UF and HD also increases plasma oncotic pressure and decreases capillary hydrostatic pressure. Both forces mobilize extravascular fluid. The degree to which PV decreases depends on the UF rate, fluid shifts, and the plasma refilling rate (PRR) from the ICF and interstitial fluid compartments. By maintaining a constant P_{osm}, a high-sodium dialysate minimizes intracellular water movement during dialysis, preserving PV.[72,73] A stable P_{osm} during dialysis enhances blood pressure stability,[74,75] especially when the dialysate sodium concentration is increased to ≥ 135 mequiv./L.[76–78] Hypo-osmolality impairs peripheral vasoconstriction during volume removal and exacerbates autonomic insufficiency. Hence, high-sodium dialysate, by maintaining stable P_{osm}, favorably influences compensatory mechanisms during volume removal.[70,79] Improved hemodynamic stability is paralleled by a reduction in cramping, nausea, vomiting, and headache during dialysis.[78–80] Furthermore, patients given higher dialysate sodium concentrations (144 mequiv./L) appear to have fewer hypotensive episodes.[80] Thus, a dialysate sodium

concentration of 140–145 mequiv./L is reasonable, gauging the optimal concentration to the patient's blood pressure, weight gain, and symptoms on dialysis.

The use of dialysate with higher sodium concentrations may lead to higher interdialytic weight gain because of increased thirst stimulated by an elevated serum tonicity. There was concern that hypertension or volume overload would be a consequence of this practice. Although there is an increase in interdialytic weight gain associated with higher dialysate sodium concentration, the excess volume is able to be removed successfully by increasing ultrafiltration rate. Adverse symptoms such as hypotension are mitigated by the greater hemodynamic stability associated with the higher sodium concentration. Indeed, it can be argued that the greatest improvement in intradialytic symptoms, such as hypotension, was due to the introduction of dialysate with a higher sodium concentration.

Sodium modeling

A strategy combining high and low levels of dialysate sodium is sodium-gradient hemodialysis. A high-sodium dialysate of 150 mequiv./L is used initially, which is then reduced automatically and progressively toward isotonic levels in one of three patterns. A linear, ramp pattern lowers sodium at a constant rate throughout the treatment. A step pattern maintains the high sodium for three-quarters of the treatment time and decreases the sodium to 135–140 mequiv./L for the rest. Finally, sodium is reduced from 150 to 140 mequiv./L in an exponential pattern. Sodium modeling can be incorporated into the biofeedback system described above. Sodium modeling allows the greatest sodium influx to the patient when urea and solute flux from the body is greatest. Theoretically, this technique is associated with fewer symptomatic hypotensive episodes although, in reality, it may not be any more advantageous than fixed high-sodium dialysate.[81–84] However, a recent prospective, crossover study in hypotension-prone hemodialysis patients (used as their own controls) compared standard dialysis (138 mequiv./L sodium) to step-sodium modeling, isolated ultrafiltration, cool dialysate, and constant high-sodium dialysate (144 mequiv./L). The volume removed was similar throughout the study. Sodium modeling and cool dialysate were found to be of greatest benefit in reducing hypotensive events and preserving postdialysis blood pressure. High-sodium dialysate was also shown to reduce hypotensive events as well. The authors conclude that sodium modeling should be the first approaching patients with intradialytic hypotension.[85] Sodium gradient dialysis may be beneficial in the initial dialysis of patients with advanced renal insufficiency and urea concentrations > 200 mg/dL, to decrease the risk of dialysis disequilibrium syndrome. Modeling may also be useful in patients with a low urea mass transfer coefficient, who have delayed urea equilibration between ICF and ECF.[72,86,87]

The concepts of sodium modeling can also be applied to UF, resulting in volume to be removed early in the dialytic session when the patient's intravascular volume is greatest. The UF rate can be gauged to decrease during dialysis as the intravascular volume declines: 50% UF during the first hour;

25% UF during the second hour; 15% UF during the third hour; and 10% UF during the fourth hour. Such a protocol, especially in combination with concurrent sodium modeling, may minimize cramping and symptomatic hypotension in patients prone to these complications.[88]

Dialysate buffer

Bicarbonate dialysis is the dialytic treatment of choice, conferring benefits over acetate dialysis, including a lower incidence of hypotension, hypoxemia, and improved left ventricular stroke work.[89-93] Metabolism of acetate occurs predominantly in the liver and skeletal muscle. Healthy people can metabolize acetate at a rate of up to 300 mM/h, whereas for elderly people and those on chronic hemodialysis the rate is about 3–3.5 mM/h.[94,95] Thus, older patients, especially those with underlying myocardial dysfunction and low muscle mass, may benefit from bicarbonate dialysate. Dialyzers with a large surface area, and increased blood flow rates enhance acetate transfer to the patient thereby increasing the acetate load for patients to metabolize.[91]

The hemodynamic instability associated with acetate dialysate buffer may be related to a number of factors including adenosine production,[72] IL-1 release,[96] and hypoxemia as a result of myocardial hypoperfusion and dysfunction.[97-100] Dialysate delivery systems also may play a role, as a change from a single-pass system to recirculation with cellulosic membranes can reduce hypoxemia during acetate dialysis.[101] In acetate dialysis, the transfer of carbon dioxide (CO_2) from blood to dialysate, results in reflex hypoventilation and hypoxemia with a decrease in the respiratory quotient: (CO_2 produced)/(O_2 consumed), producing hypocapnia and hypoventilation. Bicarbonate dialysate solutions with elevated $P\text{CO}_2$ levels reduce reflex hypoventilation and hypoxemia. However, when the dialysate bicarbonate concentration is > 35 mequiv./L hypoventilation may result from metabolic alkalosis.

Higher dialysate concentrations of sodium may improve hemodynamic instability related to acetate dialysis.[76,101-103] Nonetheless, bicarbonate is the dialysate buffer of choice in critically ill patients. In chronic hemodialysis patients, bicarbonate buffer may not offer added hemodynamic benefit when the sodium dialysate is higher than 140 mequiv./L. However, patients who metabolize acetate poorly tolerate bicarbonate dialysate better.[104]

Dialysate calcium

Because dialysate calcium equilibrates with the diffusible (ionized) fraction of plasma calcium, a dialysate calcium of 2.5 mequiv./L is equivalent to a serum calcium of 10 mg/dL. High dialysate calcium (3.5 mequiv./L) or low dialysate calcium (< 2.5 mequiv./L) has certain risks and advantages. Serum calcium is often reduced in advanced renal failure as a result of depressed production of 1,25-dihydroxyvitamin D and decreased absorption of calcium from the gastrointestinal tract. High dialysate calcium can improve indices of metabolic bone disease and reduce parathyroid hormone (PTH) levels.[105,106] High dialysate calcium can also improve hemodynamic stability during dialysis[107-109] as well as echocardiographic measures of left ventricular function.[110,111]

The main disadvantage of high dialysate calcium is hypercalcemia. Calcium-based phosphate binders, used preferentially over aluminum-containing antacids and oral or intravenous 1,25-dihydroxyvitamin D_3 are presently used in the management of hyperphosphatemia and to prevent uncontrolled secondary hyperparathyroidism.[112-114] High dialysate calcium can limit the effectiveness of this therapy by inducing hypercalcemia. To obviate hypercalcemia, lower dialysate calcium concentrations (2.5 mequiv./L) have been combined with high doses of oral calcium-containing phosphate binders and vitamin D sterols to control hyperphosphatemia[115] and secondary hyperparathyroidism.[116] Mild hypotension was the only major side effect associated with such dialysate calcium concentrations.[110,115] Thus, a dialysate calcium concentration of 2.5–2.7 mequiv./L is recommended for hemodynamically stable patients, particularly for those prone to hypercalcemia during treatment with vitamin D and calcium salts.

Dialysate potassium

Dialysis is the primary route of potassium elimination for hemodialysis patients[117,118] although the gastrointestinal tract also contributes to potassium excretion in individuals with ESRD. Typically, 50–80 mequiv. of potassium are removed with each dialysis treatment.[119] The rate of potassium removal during dialysis is largely a function of the concentration gradient between blood and dialysate. Blood and dialysate flow rates, dialyzer efficiency, and factors affecting transcellular potassium distribution such as pH, insulin and catecholamines, are also important.

The majority of dialyzed potassium originates intracellularly and must cross cell membranes before crossing the dialyzer membrane. Plasma potassium concentrations tend to "rebound" 4–5 h after dialysis, averaging 30% greater potassium values than immediately postdialysis.[120-122] This postdialysis rebound is important as an immediate postdialysis potassium value of > 5.5 mequiv./L is not considered "safe," and supplementation for postdialysis hypokalemia is not warranted.

The potassium rebound following hemodialysis reflects a two-compartment model. Potassium transit across cell membranes is believed to be the limiting factor in its removal during dialysis. As a result, potassium dysequilibrium is established, with transfer from ICF to ECF compartments during dialysis failing to replenish external potassium transfer to the dialysate. Net internal transfer continues following the termination of dialysis until a new steady-state potassium gradient is established. Potassium transfer is affected by many factors. Acidosis promotes potassium efflux from cells while alkalosis causes cellular potassium uptake; this is particularly important in hypokalemic patients with metabolic acidosis. Dialyzing patients with depletion of total body potassium can worsen hypokalemia when concurrent metabolic acidosis is corrected with parenteral bicarbonate during dialysis. Also, plasma tonicity can affect potassium distribution because tonicity favors movement of potassium into extracellular spaces and, consequently, its removal during dialysis. Hypertonic saline or mannitol, used for the treatment of hypotension or muscle cramps during dialysis, thus favors potassium removal during dialysis. Glucose-free dialysate, by lowering plasma insulin concentrations, also promotes the dialytic removal of potassium.

Low dialysate potassium can precipitate atrial and ventricular ectopic beats especially in patients with left ventricular hypertrophy, impaired left ventricular function, or in patients taking digoxin.[123] The frequency of arrhythmias is greatest during the first 2 h of dialysis, when potassium flux is greatest. Therefore, in some arrhythmia-prone patients, a "sequential" reduction in dialysate potassium may be safer for potassium removal.

Water treatment

Hemodialysis patients are exposed to as much as 600 liters of dialysis water a week, and to all its potential contaminants. Although water treatment systems (WTS) used by dialysis centers produce high-quality water for safe dialysis, WTS are susceptible to malfunction or to user error. Technical advances such as high-flux (HF) and high-efficiency (HE) dialysis, reuse, and bicarbonate dialysate have heightened awareness about water safety.

Hazards associated with dialysis water

Numerous reports of patient injury or death have been linked to improperly treated or inadequately monitored water used for hemodialysis. High levels of aluminum sulfate in dialysate water have been linked to bone disease (osteomalacia and aplastic bone disease) and dialysis-associated encephalopathy (dialysis dementia).[124–126] Limiting aluminum levels in dialysate water to 10 µg/L has resulted in a continued decline in the incidence and case fatality rate of dialysis dementia.[127,128]

Chloramines, used as bactericidal agents in treatment of municipal water, denature hemoglobin by oxidation and inhibition of the hexose monophosphate shunt. Chloramine exposure during dialysis has been associated with hemolysis, Heinz body hemolytic anemia, and methemoglobinemia.[129–131] There are other compounds with adverse effects in dialysis patients. Sodium azide, used frequently with glycerine as a preservative for WTS ultrafilters, has been associated with hypotension.[132] Fluoride, even at the recommended level of 1 mg/L, can cause osteomalacia and bone disease[133] as well as cardiac death.[134] Excess calcium and magnesium in dialysate water have been linked to the "hard water syndrome" – a constellation of symptoms including nausea, vomiting, weakness, flushing, and fluctuations in blood pressure.[135,136] Untoward effects have also been reported with nitrates (methemoglobinemia with cyanosis and hypertension),[137] copper (hemolytic anemia),[138,139] and zinc[140] in excess concentrations in dialysate water. Formaldehyde toxicity, secondary to improper disinfectant use and leaching from sediment filters, has caused hemolytic anemia and death.[141,142]

Essential components of water purification

The efficiency of a WTS depends on the capacity of the system, the nature of the water supply, variations in quality of municipal water, and the quality of product water. Figure 81.3 represents a WTS with temperature-blending valves, filters, water softening, carbon filters, reverse osmosis (RO), and deionizing stations. *Temperature-blending valves* mix incoming hot and cold water to provide an optimum water temperature for downstream components. Most RO membranes work with greatest efficacy at 77 °F (26 °C). Water temperature < 77 °F reduce the flow rate of the RO system and water > 100 °F (38 °C) may damage RO membranes. *Filters* remove particulate matter from the water. Sand filters remove particles of 25–100 µm; cartridge filters extract particles of 1–100 µm; and submicron filters remove

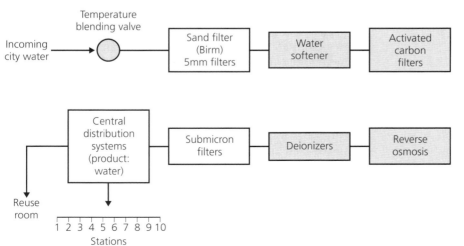

Figure 81.3 Components of a water treatment system. Deionizers are optional if reverse osmosis (RO) produces water of adequate quality. Granular activated carbon filters are always placed before the RO system to reduce water hardness and prevent scaling of the RO membranes. Deionization does not remove bacteria or endotoxins and should always be followed by ultrafiltration or submicron filters (From Ismail N, Becker BN, Hakim RM: Water treatment for hemodialysis. Am J Nephrol 1996;16:60–72. Reproduced with permission of S Karger AG, Basel.)

particles as small as 0.25 μm. In general, 5-μm filters are generally accepted as adequate protection for equipment and water treatment.

Water softeners, often sodium-containing cation-exchange resins, can remove calcium, magnesium, and other polyvalent cations from the feedwater. Because calcium and magnesium are removed from water in exchange for sodium, the amount of sodium released can be problematic. Removing calcium and magnesium prevents these ions from depositing on the RO system with resulting malfunction. *Granular activated-carbon filters* (GAC) absorb chlorine, chloramines, and other organic substances from the water. Carbon filters are porous with a high affinity for organic material. GAC can be contaminated with bacteria if they are not serviced properly or exchanged frequently. The size of the activated carbon bed depends on the empty bed contact time (EBCT). The EBCT calculation is:

$$EBCT = V \times 7.48 \text{ (gallons/cu.ft)}/Q$$

where V = carbon volume required in cubic feet and Q = water flow rate in gallons/min. EBCT differs for different substances. Recommended EBCT values are 6 min for chlorine removal and 10 min for chloramine removal. The Food and Drug Administration recommends that two GAC-filled tanks are used in series, with each tank having an EBCT of 3–5 min.

Reverse osmosis (RO) applies high hydrostatic pressure to a solution across a semipermeable membrane to prepare a purified solvent. RO rejects 90–99% of monovalent and divalent ions, and microbiologic contaminants, producing water safe for dialysis. An RO device is often used as pretreatment to deionization (DI), as an economic measure to provide longer service life for the DI system. Subsequent deionization of permeate (product) RO water is usually unnecessary. Deionization removes all types of cations and anions. The cation exchange resin exchanges hydrogen ions (H^+) for other cations; the anion exchange resin exchanges hydroxyl ions (OH^-) for other anions. DI efficacy is determined by measuring the resistivity of the effluent. Resistivity varies with temperature, therefore resistivity monitors must be temperature-compensated. When the DI system is exhausted, previously adsorbed ions can elute into the effluent, causing ion-related toxicities.[138,143]

Microbiology of hemodialysis systems

Water used by HD centers is usually obtained from the community water supply. Community water treatment can reduce bacteria and the concentration of endotoxins in the water; yet the dialysis WTS (apart from ultraviolet light) can still become contaminated with bacteria and endotoxins.[144,145] The primary microbial contaminants in dialysis fluids are water bacteria, Gram-negative bacteria and nontuberculous mycobacteria (Table 81.6). Nontuberculous mycobacteria in particular are problematic. They do not produce endotoxins, but they are more resistant to germicides than Gram-negative bacteria and they are infectious, especially in the setting of

inadequately disinfected dialyzers.[146–149] They can survive and multiply in RO-treated water or DI water that contains little organic matter.[144] Indeed, the CDC documented that nontuberculous mycobacteria were present in the water of 83% of dialysis centers surveyed in 1984.[146]

Sterilization destroys microorganisms, including highly resistant bacterial spores. Disinfection, in contrast, eliminates all but the highly resistant microorganisms.[150,151] Disinfection can be high level, intermediate, or low level, depending on the germicidal activity. High-level disinfection inactivates all microorganisms except bacterial spores. Low-level disinfection reduces the bacterial population to a "safe" level. WTS disinfection generally utilizes low-level disinfection. High-level disinfection is more often used for dialyzer reprocessing.

Pyrogenic reactions during hemodialysis

Pyrogenic reactions (PRs) often develop during or after dialysis treatment, with an incident rate of 0.5–12%.[151,152] A PR can be defined as chills (or rigors) and/or fever (oral temperature > 37.8 °C/100 °F) in a previously afebrile patient with no recorded signs or symptoms of infection before dialysis.[151,152] Hypotension is sometimes also included in the definition. Other signs of a PR are headache, myalgia, nausea, and vomiting. The symptoms usually begin 30–60 min into the dialysis treatment and stop shortly after, unless they are extreme. There appears to be little difference in PR rates between different hemodialysis modalities.[152]

Three lines of evidence implicate endotoxin in the pathogenesis of PR: (1) antiendotoxin antibodies in dialysis patients;[153,154] (2) *Limulus* lysate reactivity in plasma from patients experiencing PR;[155,156] and (3) an association of PR with fluids contaminated with Gram-negative bacteria.[156,157] It is unlikely that microorganisms cross intact dialyzer membranes because of their diameter of the pores. Rather, it is the endotoxins or other pyrogenic substances that probably gain access to the patient's bloodstream across the dialysis membrane.[156,158] Some of these substances are bacterial pyrogens released

Table 81.6 Naturally occurring water bacteria commonly found in hemodialysis systems

Gram-negative bacteria	Nontuberculous mycobacteria
Pseudomonas	*Mycobacterium chelonae*
Flavobacterium	*M. fortuitum*
Actinobacillos	*M. gordonae*
Alcaligenes	*M. scrofulaceum*
Xanthomonas	*M. avium*
Serratia	*M. abscessus*
Achromobacter	*M. intracellulare*
Aeromonas	

From Ismail N, Becker BN, Hakin RM: Water treatment for hemodialysis. Am J Nephrol 1996;16:60–72. Reproduced with permission of S. Karger AG, Basel.

by Gram-negative bacteria (Table 81.6),[159] including lipopolysaccharides (LPS), its subunit, layer A, other LPS fragments, peptidoglycans, muramylpeptides, exotoxins, and exotoxin fragments.

Assays for determining the permeability of pyrogens include the *Limulus* amoebocyte lysate (LAL) assay, the mononuclear cell (MNC) assay, radiolabeled LPS fragments, and neutrophil activation. Many bacterial substances, like endotoxin fragments, are small enough to penetrate tight cellulosic membranes. These fragments go undetected in the LAL assay. Thus, measuring in vitro cytokine production by mononuclear cells (MNCs) may be more sensitive and specific, allowing detection of these low-molecular-weight substances.[160–162]

The inability to detect passage of endotoxin across intact dialyzer membranes during conventional or HF dialysis[163–165] suggests that additional factors are probably involved in PR. Bacterial products such as endotoxins induce human MNC production of IL-1 and tumor necrosis factor alpha (TNFα).[159] Experimental data suggest that cultured MNCs increase IL-1 production in response to LPS, LPS fragments, or plasma proteins in the dialysate.[162,165,166] Moreover, LPS-like fragments can cross dialyzer membranes.[166] Interestingly, plasma must be present on the blood side for cytokine induction. LPS-binding proteins, complement, and other plasma proteins can be activated by regenerated cellulosic membranes[166] and amplify MNC cytokine production.[166–169] Evidence also suggests that endotoxin fragments can cross intact hemodialysis membranes and induce MNC cytokine production, particularly in the presence of plasma.

Additionally, severe PR in hemodialysis patients appear to correlate with the extent of bacterial contamination in the dialysate.[157] Recent studies have suggested that up to 35% of all water samples and 19% of all dialysate samples in the USA do not comply with AAMI standards (< 200 colony-forming units (CFU)/mL water, 2000 CFU/mL in dialysate). Presumably, bacteria adhere to and grow in the dialysis tubing, releasing endotoxin and endotoxin fragments into the dialysate.

Changing dialysis practices have had an impact on PRs. PRs have been reported with higher frequency in association with dialyzer reuse. Theoretically, use of RO and membrane integrity monitoring should lead to a decrease in the incidence of PRs.[170] The use of bicarbonate and HF dialysis have been linked with a higher risk of PR.[128] In dialysis units that used bicarbonate dialysis, a higher frequency of PR occurred only in centers that also performed HF dialysis. Centers that prepared their own bicarbonate dialysate also were more likely to report PRs than centers that used commercially prepared bicarbonate dialysate. The method for preparing bicarbonate dialysate entails potential contamination.[169] Acetate dialysate is prepared from a single concentrate at a concentration that prohibits bacterial growth (4.8 mol/L). However, bicarbonate dialysate must be prepared from two concentrates: an acid concentrate with a pH of 2.8 that is not conducive to bacterial growth and a 1.2 mol/L bicarbonate concentrate with a neutral pH. Bicarbonate concentrates can support halotolerant endotoxin-

producing, Gram-negative organisms. As many as 10^5–10^6 CFU/mL can develop in liquid bicarbonate in as few as 10 days following dialysate preparation. Because of this, active quality assurance should be exercised to use liquid bicarbonate concentrate (LBC) as soon as possible after manufacture or receipt by the dialysis center. Tanks and distribution lines containing stored LBC should be disinfected at least twice weekly.

Finally, dialyzer reuse practices has been associated with PR independent of HF dialyzer use.[128] Manual dialyzer reprocessing has been associated with higher incidence of PR compared to automated reprocessing.[150] Manual reprocessing can allow defects in dialyzer membranes to go undetected because testing for integrity of the membrane is generally not performed with this technique.

Several outbreaks of patient infection and PR have been reported in HD patients.[171–174] Many of these involved substandard reprocessing or poor water quality.[151] Inadequate mixing of germicide, or the use of a new germicide (chlorine dioxide, for example) have been implicated in several of these outbreaks.[152,175,176] Errors in the design and maintenance of a WTS were responsible for PR and Gram-negative bacteremia in another center.[176] Damage to RO membranes contributed to this outbreak, leading to the recommendation of a thorough inspection for RO damage whenever the RO system removes < 90–95% of total dissolved solids. Finally, though HD has been safely conducted outside the hospital or dialysis center setting, fatal endotoxemia occurred in dialysis patients at summer camp,[177] illustrating the importance of dialysis WTS in different environmental conditions.

The formaldehyde content used for disinfection also may be important for PRF. Formaldehyde 2% does not effectively or reproducibly eradicate mycobacterial organisms within 36 h.[172,178] If the concentration of formaldehyde is increased to 4%, mycobacteria cannot survive at room temperature beyond 24 h.[179] However, there is increasing evidence that lower concentrations of formaldehyde (e.g. 1%) can be effective if the dialyzers are kept at a temperature of 37–40 °C.[180]

Water quality standards for hemodialysis

A summary of the Association for the Advancement of Medical Instrumentation (AAMI) recommendations for safe and proper water treatment and the use of WTS components is listed in Table 81.7. Microbiologic samples should be assayed by the spread-plate or membrane-filtration technique. Internal fluid pathways should be disinfected weekly – the RO unit monthly. Aqueous formaldehyde 1–2%, glutaraldehyde, or chlorine-based disinfectants should be used to disinfect internal fluid pathways. Hot water (> 80 °C, 176 °F) is an alternative that avoids hazards associated with chemical germicides.

Low-level disinfection is adequate for WTS components. High-level disinfection is mandatory for dialyzer reprocessing. When reprocessing hemodialyzers, monitoring of water requires more stringent criteria; the water used for

Table 81.7 AMMI hemodialysis water quality standards

Microbiologic and endotoxin standards		
Type of fluid	Microbial count (CFU/mL)	Endotoxin (EU/mL)*
Water to prepare dialysate	≤ 200	No standard
Dialysate	≤ 2000	No standard
Water for reprocessing and rinsing	≤ 200	≤ 5
Water for dialyzer disinfectant	≤ 200	≤ 5

Chemical contaminants monitoring	
Contaminant	Suggested maximum level (mg/L)
Calcium	2
Magnesium	4
Sodium	70
Potassium	8
Fluoride	0.2
Chlorine	0.5
Chloramines	0.1
Nitrates	2
Sulfate	100
Copper, barium, zinc	0.1 each
Aluminum	0.01
Arsenic, lead, silver	0.005 each
Cadmium	0.001
Chromium	0.014
Selenium	0.09
Mercury	0.002

Adapted with permission from the AAMI, Association for the Advancement of Medical Instrumentation: AAMI Standard and Recommended Practices, Vol 3: Dialysis. Arlington: AAMI, 1993.
*5 EU = 1 ng; 230 mg/L where sodium concentration of the concentrates has been reduced to compensate for excess sodium in the water as long as conductivity of the water is being monitored continuously.

dialysate, for rinsing, reprocessing, and disinfecting the dialyzers should contain < 5 endotoxin units/mL (1 ng/mL).

Dialyzers can be treated with reverse ultrafiltration and sodium hypochlorite bleach < 1%, or cleaned with hydrogen peroxide 3% and peracetic acid 2%, then tested for leaks. Dialyzers can then undergo disinfection or sterilization with instillation of germicides into the blood and dialysate compartments for at least 24 h. Three commonly used agents are formaldehyde 4%, peracetic acid–hydrogen peroxide–acetic acid mixture (Renalin) and glutaraldehyde (Diacide). However, even 1% solutions of formaldehyde may have excellent germicidal efficacy when dialyzers are incubated at 40 °C for 24 h.[181] Heat sterilization at 105 °F for 20 h for reprocessing certain PS membranes has been successful.[182]

There are other clinical concerns about reprocessing of dialyzers. High residual formaldehyde levels in the dialyzer previously predisposed to anti-N-like antibody formation,[183] with resulting episodes of hemolysis and early transplant failure. However, no such reports have appeared since the use of more sensitive methods to detect residual formaldehyde. As mentioned, potential anaphylactoid reactions have also been noted in patients taking ACEIs who undergo HD with dialyzers that were reprocessed with Renalin or bleach.[184] These reactions probably reflect the characteristic of the membrane rather than the sterilant. Finally, increased mortality associated with manual dialyzer reprocessing using Renalin and glutaraldehyde has been reported.[185,186] A direct causative link between these germicides and increased patient mortality remains to be established.

References

1. Ronco C, Brendolan A, Milan M, et al: Impact of biofeedback-induced cardiovascular stability on hemodialysis tolerance and efficiency. Kidney Int 2000;58:800–808.
2. Ronco C, Ghezzi PM, La Greca G. The role of technology in hemodialysis. J Nephrol 1999;12(Suppl 2):S68–S81.
3. Gotch F, Sargent J: A mechanistic analysis of the National Cooperative Dialysis Study (NCDS). Kidney Int 1985;28:526–534.
4. Parker TF III: Role of dialysis on morbidity and mortality in maintenance hemodialysis patients. Am J Kidney Dis 1994;24:981–989.
5. Parker TF III, Husni L, Huang W, et al: Survival of hemodialysis patients is improved with a greater quantity of dialysis. Am J Kidney Dis 1994;23:670–680.
6. Keshaviah PR, Ebben JP, Emerson PF: On-line monitoring of the delivery of the hemodialysis prescription. Ped Nephrol 1995;Suppl:S2–S8.
7. Chauveau P, Naret C, Puget J, Zins B, et al: Adequacy of hemodialysis and nutrition in maintenance hemodialysis patients: clinical evaluation of a new on-line urea monitor. Nephrol Dial Transplant 1996;11:1568–1573.
8. Krivitski NM: Theory and validation of access flow measurement by dilution technique during hemodialysis. Kidney Int 1995;48:245–250.
9. Leypoldt JK, Cheung AK, Steuer RR, et al: Determination of circulating blood volume by continuously monitoring hematocrit during hemodialysis. J Am Soc Nephrol 1995;6:214–219.
10. Steuer RR, Germain MJ, Leypoldt JK, Cheung AK: Enhanced fluid removal guided by blood volume monitoring during chronic hemodialysis. Artif Organ 1998;22:627–632.
11. Steuer RR, Leypoldt JK, Cheung AK, Senekjian HO, Conis JM: Reducing symptoms during hemodialysis by continuously monitoring the hematocrit. Am J Kidney Dis 1996;27:525–532.
12. Steuer RR, Leypoldt JK, Cheung AK, Harris DH, Conis JM: Hematocrit as an indicator of blood volume and a predictor of intradialytic morbid events. ASAIO Journal 1994;40:M691–M696.
13. Mujais S, Schmidt B: Operating characteristics of hollow-fiber dialyzers. In Nissenson AR, Fine RN, Gentile DE (eds): Clinical Dialysis, 3rd edn. Norwalk, CT: Appleton and Lange, 1995, p 82.
14. Konstantin P, Bailey RM: Polycarbonate-polyether (PC-PE) flat sheet membrane: manufacture, structure and performance. Blood Purif 1985;4:6–12.
15. Gohl H, Raff M, Harttig D, et al: PC-PE hollow-fiber membrane. structure, performance characteristics, and manufacturing. Blood Purif 1985;4:23–31.
16. Gohl H, Konstantin P: Membrane and filters for hemofiltration. In Henderson LW, Quellhorst EA, Baldamus CA, Lysaght MJ (eds): Hemofiltration. Berlin: Springer-Verlag, 1986, p 41.
17. Leypoldt JK, Frigon RP, Henderson LW: Macromolecular charge affects hemofilter solute sieving. Trans Am Soc. Artif Intern Organs 1986;32:384–387.
18. Kaufman AM, Frinak S, Godmere RO, Levin NW: Clinical experience with heat sterilization for reprocessing dialyzers. ASAIO Journal 1992;38:M338–M340.
19. Sigdell JE: Operating characteristics of hollow-fiber dialyzers. In Nissenson AR, Fine RN, Gentile DE (eds): Clinical Dialysis, 2nd edn. San Mateo: Appleton and Lange, 1990, pp 106–107.
20. Leypoldt JK, Cheung AK. Increases in mass transfer-area coefficients and urea Kt/V with increasing dialysate flow rate are greater for high-flux dialyzers. Am J Kidney Dis 2001;38:575–579.

21. Kakplow LS, Goffinet JA: Profound neutropenia during the early phase of hemodialysis. J Amer Med Assoc 1968;203:1135–1137.

22. Akizawa T, Kitaoka T, Koshikawa S, et al: Development of a regenerated cellulose, non-complement activating membrane for hemodialysis. ASAIO Journal 1986;32:76–84.

23. Gohl H, Konstantin P: Membranes and filters for hemofiltration in hemofiltration. In Henderson LW, Quellhorst EA, Baldamus CA, Lysaght MJ (eds): Hemofiltration. Berlin: Springer-Verlag, 1986, pp 41–56.

24. Cheung AK: Interactions between plasma proteins and hemodialysis membranes, In Grunfeld JP, Back JF, Kreis H, Maxwell MH (eds): Advances in Nephrology, 22nd edn. Boston: Mosby Year Book, 1993, pp 417–434.

25. Schulman G, Levin NW: Membranes for hemodialyzers. Seminars Dial 1994;7:251–256.

26. Arbeit LA, Schulman G, Holmes T, et al: The bindery of vasoactive substances to dialysis membranes is proportional to the negativity of the surface potential (abstract). Proceedings of the Xth International Congress in Nephrology 1987;122.

27. Lemke HD, Fink E: Accumulation of bradykinin formed by the AN69 or PAN 17 DX-membrane is due to the presence of an ACE-inhibitor in vitro (abstract). J Am Soc Nephrol 1992;3:376.

28. Schulman G, Hakim RM, Arias R, et al: Bradykinin generation by dialysis membranes: Possible role in anaphylactic reaction. J Am Soc Nephrol 1993;3:1563–1569.

29. Parnes EL, Shapiro WB: Anaphylactoid reactions in hemodialysis patients treated with the AN69 dialyzer. Kidney Int 1991;40:1148–1152.

30. Pegues DA, Beck-Sagui M, Wooller SW: Anaphylactoid reactions associated with reuse of hollow fiber hemodialyzers and ACE inhibitors. Kidney Int 1992;42:1232–1237.

31. Hor WH, Schaefer RM, Heidland A: Effect of different dialyzers on proteinases and proteinase inhibitors during hemodialysis. Am J Nephrol 1985;5:332–326.

32. Sawada K, Malchesky PS, Guidubaldi JM, et al: In vitro evaluation of a relationship between human serum– or plasma–material interaction and polymer bulk hydroxyl and surface oxygen content. ASAIO Journal 1993;39:910–917.

33. Cheung AK, Chenoweth DE, Otsuka D, et al: Compartmental distribution of complement activation products in artificial kidneys. Kidney Int 1984;30:74–80.

34. Schindler R, Linnenweber S, Schulze M, et al: Gene expression of interleukin 1B during hemodialysis. Kidney Int 1993;43:712–721.

35. Greene WH, Ray C, Mauer SM: The effect of neutrophil chemotactic responsiveness. J Lab Clin Med 1976;88:971–974.

36. Bjorksten B, Mauer SM, Mills EL: The effect of hemodialysis on neutrophil chemotactic responsiveness. Acta Med Scand 1978;203:67–70.

37. Vanholder R, Ringoir S, Dhondt A, et al: Phagocytosis in uremic and hemodialysis patients: A prospective and cross-sectional study. Kidney Int 1991;39:320–327.

38. Friedlander MA, Hilbert CM, Wu YC, et al: Role of dialysis modality in responses of blood monocytes and peritoneal macrophages to endotoxin stimulation. Am J Kidney Dis 1993;22:11–23.

39. Pereira BJG, King AJ, Poutsiaka DD, et al: Comparison of first use and reuse of cuprophane membranes on interleukin-1 receptor antagonist and interleukin-1B production by blood mononuclear cells. Am J Kidney Dis 1993;22:288–295.

40. Zaoui P, Green W, Hakim RM: Hemodialysis with cuprophane membrane modulates interleukin-2 receptor expression. Kidney Int 1991;39:1020–1026.

41. Zaoui P, Hakim RM: Natural killer-cell function in hemodialysis patients: Effects of the dialysis membrane. Kidney Int 1993;43:1298–1305.

42. Dinarello CA, Koch DM, Shaldon S: IL-1 and its relevance in patients treated with hemodialysis. Kidney Int 1988;33:521–526.

43. Hakim RM: Personal communication.

44. Deppisch R, Betz M, Hansch GM, et al: Biocompatibility of the polyamide membranes in polyamide – the evaluation of a synthetic membrane for renal therapy. In Shaldon S, Koch KM (eds): Contribution to Nephrology. Basel: Karger, 1992, pp 26–46.

45. Seres DS, Strain GW, Hashim SA, et al: Improvement of plasma lipoprotein profiles during high-flux dialysis. J Am Soc Nephrol 1993;3:1409–1415.

46. Hornberger JC, Chernow M. Petersen J, Garber AM: A multivariate analysis of mortality and hospital admissions with high-flux dialysis. J Am Soc Nephrol 1993;3:1227–1237.

47. Charra B, Colemard E, Ruffet M, et al: Survival as an index of adequacy of dialysis. Kidney Int 1992;41:1286–1291.

48. Hakim RM, Breillatt J, Lazarus JM, et al: Complement activation and hypersensitivity reactions to dialysis membranes. N Engl J Med 1984;311:878–882.

49. Schulman G, Fogo A, Gung A, et al: Complement activation retards resolution of acute ischemic renal failure in the rat. Kidney Int 1991;40:1069–1074.

50. Gung A, Schulman G, Hakim R: Hemodialysis membrane choice influences maintenance of residual renal function (RRF) in an animal model (abstract). J Am Soc Nephrol 1991;2:237.

51. Hakim RM, Wingard RL, Parker RA: Effect of the dialysis membrane in the treatment of patients with acute renal failure. N Engl J Med 1994;331:1338–1342.

52. van Ypersele de Strihou C, Jadoul M, Malghem J, et al: Effect of dialysis membrane and patient's age on signs of dialysis-related amyloidosis. Kidney Int 1991;39:1012–1019.

53. Zaoui P, Stone WJ, Hakim RM: Effects of dialysis membranes on β_2-microglobulin production and cellular expression. Kidney Int 1990;38:962–968.

54. Hakim RM: Clinical implications of hemodialysis membrane biocompatibility. Kidney Int 1993;44:484–494.

55. Ikizler TA, Wingard RL, Hakim RM: Interventions to treat malnutrition in dialysis patients: the role of the dose of dialysis, intradialytic parenteral nutrition, and growth hormone. Am J Kidney Dis 1995;26:256–265.

56. Lowrie EG, Lew NL: Death risk in hemodialysis patients: The predictive value of commonly measured variables and an evaluation of death rate differences between facilities. Am J Kidney Dis 1990;15:458–482.

57. Lindsay RM, Spanner EA, Heidenheim P, et al: PCR, Kt/V and membrane. Kidney Int 1993;43(Suppl 41):S268–S273.

58. Guiterrez A, Alvestrand A, Wahren J, et al: Effect of in vivo contact between blood and dialysis membranes on protein catabolism in humans. Kidney Int 1990;38:487–494.

59. Bowry SK, Ronco C: Surface topography and surface elemectal composition analysis of Helixone, new high-flux polysulfone dialysis membrane. Int J Artif Organs 2001 24:757–64.

60. Ronco C, Brendolan A, Crepaldi C, Rodighiero M, Scabardi M: Blood and dialysate flow distributions in hollow-fiber hemodialyzers analyzed by computerized helical scanning technique. J Am Soc Nephrol 2002;13(Suppl l):S53–S61.

61. Ronco C, Brendolan A, Lupi A, Metry G, Levin NW: Effects of a reduced inner diameter of hollow fibers in hemodialyzers. Kidney Int 2000;58:809–817.

62. Winchester JF, Ronco C, Brady JA, et al: The next step from high-flux dialysis: appliction of sorbent technology. Blood Purif 2002;20:81–86.

63. Eknoyan G, Levey A, Beck G, et al: The hemodialysis (HEMO) study: Rationale for selection of interventions. Semin Dialysis 1996;9:24–33.

64. Mendelssohn S, Swartz CD, Yudis M, et al: High glucose concentration dialysate in chronic hemodialysis. ASAIO Journal 1967;13:249–253.

65. Rosborough DC, Van Stone JC: Dialysate glucose. Semin Dialysis 1993;6:260–263.

66. Ward RA, Wathen RL, Williams TE, et al: Hemodialysate composition and intradialytic metabolic, acid-base, and potassium changes. Kidney Int 1987;32:129–135.

67. Wathen RA, Keshaviah P, Hommeyer P, et al: The metabolic effects of hemodialysis with and without glucose in the dialysate. Am J Clin Nutr 1978;31:1870–1875.

68. Grajower MM, Walter L, Albin J: Hypoglycemia in chronic hemodialysis patients: Association with progranolol use. Nephron 1980;26:126–129.

69. Kopple JD, Swendseid ME, Shinaberger JH, et al: The free and bound amino acids removed by hemodialysis. ASAIO Journal 1973;19:309–303.

70. Ward RA, Shirlow MJ, Hayes JM, et al: Protein catabolism during hemodialysis. Am J Clin Nutr 1979;32:2443–2449.

71. Ramirez G, Butcher DE, Morrison AO: Glucose concentration in the dialysate and lipid abnormalities in chronic hemodialysis patients. Int J Artif Organs 1987;10:31–36.

72. Daugirdas JT: Dialysis hypotension: A hemodynamic analysis. Kidney Int 1991;39:233–246.

73. de Vries PMJM: Plasma volume changes during hemodialysis. Semin Dialysis 1992;5:42–47.

74. Palmer BF: The effect of dialysate composition on systemic hemodynamics. Semin Dialysis 1992;5:54–60.

75. Rosansky SJ, Rhinehart R, Shade R: Effect of osmolar changes on plasma arginine vasopressin (PAVP) in dialysis patients. Clin Nephrol 1991;35:158–164.

76. Wehle B, Asaba H, Castenfors J, et al: Hemodynamic changes during sequential ultrafiltration and dialysis. Kidney Int 1979;15:411–418.

77. Baldamus CA, Ernst W, Frei U, et al: Sympathetic and hemodynamic response to volume removal during different forms of renal replacement therapy. Nephron 1982;31:324–332.

78. Petitclerc T, Drueke T, Man N. Funck-Brentano JL: Cardiovascular stability on hemodialysis. Adv Nephrol 1987;16:351–370.

79. Raja R, Henriquez M, Kramer M, et al: Intradialytic hypotension – role of osmolar changes and acetate influx. Artif Organs 1985;9:17–21.

80. Henrich WL, Woodard TD, Blachley JD, et al: Role of osmolality in blood pressure stability after dialysis and ultrafiltration. Kidney Int 1980;18:480–488.

81. Dumler F, Grondin G, Levin NW: Sequential high/low sodium hemodialysis: An alternative to ultrafiltration. ASAIO Journal 1979;25:351–353.

82. Daugirdas JT, Al-Kudsi RR, Ing TS, et al: A double-blind evaluation of sodium gradient hemodialysis. Am J Nephrol 1985;5:163–168.

83. Raja R, Kramer M, Barber K, et al: Sequential changes in dialysate sodium (D_{Na}) during hemodialysis. ASAIO Journal 1983;24:649–651.

84. Bedichek E, Kirschbaum B, Sica D: Comparison of the hemodynamic and hormonal effects of hemodialysis using programmable vs constant sodium dialysate (abstract). J Am Soc Nephrol 1992;3:354.

85. Dheenan S, Henrich WL: Preventing dialysis hypotension: a comparison of usual protective maneuvers. Kidney Int 2001;59:1175–1181

86. Heineken FS, Evans MC, Keen ML: Intercompartmental fluid shifts in hemodialysis patients. Biotechnol Prog 1987;3:69.

87. Star RA, Hootkins R, Thompson JR, et al: Variability and stability of two pool urea mass transfer coefficient (abstract). J Am Soc Nephrol 1992;3:395.

88. Prospert FL, Ruffenach P: Ramped sodium dialysis (RSD) versus combined ramped sodium and ultrafiltration dialysis (RSD + RUD) compared to standard sodium dialysis (SD) (abstract). J Am Soc Nephrol 1996;7:1524.

89. Leunissen KML, Hoorntje SJ, Fiers HA, et al: Acetate versus bicarbonate hemodialysis in critically ill patients. Nephron 1986;42:146–151.

90. Graefe U, Milutenovich J, Follette WC, et al: Less dialysis induced morbidity and vascular instability with bicarbonate in dialysate. Ann Intern Med 1978;88:332–336.

91. Vincent JL, Vanherweghem JL, Degante JP, et al: Acetate induced myocardial depression during hemodialysis for acute renal failure. Kidney Int 1982;22:653–657.

92. Novello A, Kelsch RC, Easterling RE: Acetate intolerance during hemodialysis. Clin Nephrol 1976;5:29–32.

93. Hakim RM, Ponzer M-A, Tilton D, et al: Effects of acetate and bicarbonate dialysate in stable chronic dialysis patients. Kidney Int 1985;28:535–540.

94. Tolchin N, Roberts JL, Hayashi J, et al: Metabolic consequences of high mass-transfer hemodialysis. Kidney Int 1977;11:306.

95. Henrich WL: Hemodynamic instability during hemodialysis. Kidney Int 1986;30:605–612.

96. Lonnemann G, Bingel M, Koch KM, et al: Plasma interleukin-1 activity in humans undergoing hemodialysis with regenerated cellulosic membranes. Lymph Res 1987;6:63–70.

97. Garella S, Chang BS: Hemodialysis-associated hypoxemia. Am J Nephrol 1984;4:273–279.

98. Ross EA, Nissenson AR: Dialysis-associated hypoxemia: Insights into pathophysiology and prevention. Semin Dialysis 1988;1:33–39.

99. Wolff J, Pendersen T, Rossen M, et al: Effects of acetate and bicarbonate dialysis on cardiac performance, transmural myocardial perfusion and acid-base balance. Int J Artif Organs 1986;9:105–110.

100. Henrich WL, Woodard TD, Meyer BD, et al: High sodium bicarbonate and acetate hemodialysis: Double-blind crossover comparison of hemodynamic and ventilatory effects. Kidney Int 1983;24:240–245.

101. Vaziri ND, Wilson A, Mukai D, et al: Dialysis hypoxemia – role for dialyzer membrane and dialysate delivery system. Am J Med 1984;77:828–834.

102. Henrich WL, Woodard TD, Meyer BD, et al: High sodium bicarbonate and acetate hemodialysis: Double-blind crossover comparison of hemodynamic and ventilatory effects. Kidney Int 1983;24:240–245.

103. Mehta BR, Fischer D, Ahmad M, et al: Effects of acetate and bicarbonate hemodialysis on cardiac function in chronic dialysis patients. Kidney Int 1983;24:782–787.

104. Vinay P, Prud'homme, Vinet B: Acetate metabolism and bicarbonate generation during hemodialysis:10 years of observation. Kidney Int 1987;31:1194–1204.

105. Wing AJ: Optimum calcium concentration of dialysis fluid for maintenance haemodialysis. Br Med J 1968;4:145.

106. Johnson WJ, Goldsmith RS, Beabout JW: Prevention and reversal of secondary hyperparathyroidism in patients maintained by hemodialysis. Am J Med 1974;56:827–833.

107. Maynard JC, Cruz C, Kleerekoper M, et al: Blood pressure response to changes in serum ionized calcium during hemodialysis. Ann Intern Med 1986;104:358–361.

108. Sherman RA, Bialy GB, Gazinski B, et al: The effect of dialysate calcium levels on blood pressure during hemodialysis. Am J Kidney Dis 1986;8:244–247.

109. Fellner SK, Lang RM, Neumann A, et al: Physiological mechanisms for calcium-induced changes in systemic arterial pressure in stable dialysis patients. Hypertension 1989;13:213–218.

110. Henrich WL, Hunt JM, Nixon JV: Increased ionized calcium and left ventricular contractility during hemodialysis. N Engl J Med 1984;310:19–23.

111. Lang RB, Fellner SK, Neuman A, et al: Left ventricular contractility varies directly with blood ionized calcium. Ann Intern Med 1988;108:524–529.

112. Morton AR, Hercz G, Coburn JW: Control of hyperphosphatemia in chronic renal failure. Semin Dialysis 1990;3:219–223.

113. Mai ML, Emmett M, Shelkh MS, et al: Calcium acetate, an effective phosphorus binder in patients with renal failure. Kidney Int 1989;36:690–695.

114. Coburn JW: Use of oral and parenteral calcitriol in the treatment of renal osteodystrophy. Kidney Int 1990;38(Suppl 29):S54–S61.

115. Slatopolsky E, Weerts C, Norwood K, et al: Long-term effects of calcium carbonate and 2.5 mEq/L calcium dialysate on mineral metabolism. Kidney Int 1989;36:897–903.

116. Van der Merwe WM, Rodger RSC, Grant AC: Low calcium dialysate and high-dose oral calcetriol in the treatment of secondary hyperparathyroidism in haemodialysis patients. Nephrol Dial Transpl 1990;5:874–877.

117. Ketchersid TL, Van Stone JC: Dialysate potassium. Semin Dialysis 1991;4:46–51.

118. Spital A, Sterns RH: Potassium homeostasis in dialysis patients. Semin Dialysis 1988;1:14–20.

119. Sherman RA, Hwang ER, Bernholc AS, et al: Variability in potassium removal by hemodialysis. Am J Nephrol 1986;6:284–288.

120. Feig PU, Shook A, Sterns RH: Effect of potassium removal during hemodialysis on the plasma potassium concentration. Nephron 1981;27:25–30.

121. Hou S, McElroy PA, Nootens J, et al: Safety and efficacy of low-potassium dialysate. Am J Kidney Dis 1989;13:137–143.

122. Morgan AG, Burkinshaw L, Robinson PJA, et al: Potassium balance and acid-base changes in patients undergoing regular hemodialysis therapy. Br Med J 1970;I:779–783.

123. Morrison G, Michelson EL, Brown S, et al: Mechanism and prevention of cardiac arrhythmias in chronic hemodialysis patients. Kidney Int 1980;17:811–819.

124. Dunea G, Mahurkas SD, Mamdani B, et al: Role of aluminum in dialysis dementia.

125. Coburn JW, Norros KC, Sherrard DJ, et al: Toxic effects of aluminum in end-stage renal disease: Discussion of a case. Am J Kidney Dis 1988;12:171–184.

126. Llach F, Felsenfeld AJ, Coleman MD, et al: The natural course of dialysis osteomalacia. Kidney Int 1986;29(Suppl 18):S74–S79.

127. Tokars JI, Alter MJ, Favero MS, et al: National surveillance of hemodialysis-associated diseases in the United States, 1990. ASAIO Journal 1993;39:71–80.

128. Alter MJ, Favero MS, Moyer LA, et al: National surveillance of dialysis-associated diseases in the United States, 1989. Trans ASAIO, 1991;37:97–109.

129. Topple MA, Bland LA, Favero MS, et al: Investigation of hemolytic anemia after chloramine exposure in a dialysis center (letter). Trans ASAIO 1988;34:1060.

130. Yawata Y, Kjillstrand C, Buselmeier T, et al: Hemolysis in dialyzed patients: tap water-induced red blood cell metabolic deficiency. Trans ASAIO 1972;18:301–304.

131. Neilan BA, Ehlers SM, Kolpin CF, et al: Prevention of chloramine-induced hemolysis in dialyzed patients. Clin Nephrol 1978;10:105–108.

132. Gordon SM, Drachman J, Bland LA, et al: Epidemic hypotension in a dialysis center caused by sodium azide. Kidney Int 1990;37:110–115

133. Lough J, Noonan R, Gagnon R, et al: Effects of fluoride on bone in chronic renal failure. Arch Pathol 1975;99:484–487.

134. National News. Dialysis patients in Chicago die from fluoride poisoning; FDA issues safety alert. Contemp Dialysis Nephrol 1993;10–11.

135. Freeman RM, Lawton RL, Chamberlain MA: Hard-water syndrome. N Engl J Med 1967;276:1113–1118.

136. Evans DB, Slapak M: Pancreatitis in the hard water syndrome. Br Med J 1975;3:748.

137. Carlson DJ, Shapiro FL: Methemoglobinemia from well water nitrates: A complication of home dialysis. Ann Intern Med 1970;73:757–759.

138. Manzler AD, Schreiner CW: Copper-induced acute hemolytic anemia. A new complication of hemodialysis. Ann Intern Med 1970, 73:409–412.

139. Matter BJ, Pederson J, Psimenos G, et al: Lethal copper intoxication in hemodialysis. Trans ASAIO 1969;15:309–315.

140. Gallery EDM, Blomfield J, Dixon SR: Acute zinc toxicity in haemodialysis. Br Med J 1973;4:33.

141. Centers for Disease Control: Formaldehyde intoxication associated with hemodialysis – California. Epidemic Investigation Report EPI 81-73-2, May 7, 1984. Atlanta: Centers for Disease Control, 1984.

142. Orringer EP, Mattern WD: Formaldehyde-induced hemolysis during chronic hemodialysis. N Engl J Med 1976;294:1416–1420.

143. Johnson WJ, Taves DR: Exposure to excessive fluoride during hemodialysis. Kidney Int 1974;5:451–454.

144. Favero MS, Petersen NJ, Carson LA, et al: Gram negative water bacteria in hemodialysis systems. Health Lab Sci 1975;12:321–334.

145. Bland LA, Favero MS: Microbiologic aspects of hemodialysis systems. In Association for the Advancement of Medical Instrumentation, Vol. 3: Dialysis. Arlington, VA: American National Standards Inc., 1993, pp 257–265.

146. Carson LA, Bland LA, Cusick LB, et al: Prevalence of non-tuberculous mycobacterial in water supplies of hemodialysis centers. Appl Environ Microbiol 1988;54:3122–3125.

147. Lowry P, Beck-Sague CM, Bland LE, et al: Mycobacterium chelonae infections among patients receiving high-flux dialysis in a hemodialysis unit in California. J Infect Dis 1990;161:85–90.

148. Bolan G, Reingold AL, Carson LA, et al: Infestious with Mycobacterium chelonae in patients receiving dialysis and using processed hemodialyzers. J Infect Dis 1985;152:1013–1019.

149. Carson La, Petersen NJ, Favero MS, et al: Growth characteristics of atypical mycobacteria in water and their comparative resistance to disinfectants. Appl Environ Microbiol 1978;36:839–846.

150. Favero MS: Distinguishing between high-level disinfection, reprocessing, and sterilization. In Association for the Advancement of Medical Instrumentation: Technical Assessment Report No. 6. Reuse of Disposables: Implications for Quality Health Care and Cost Containment. Arlington, VA: American National Standards Inc., 1983, pp 19–20.

151. Favero MS, Bland LA: Microbiologic principles applied to reprocessing hemodialyzers. In Deane N, Wineman RJ, and Bemis JA (eds): Guide to Reprocessing of Hemodialyzers. Boston, MA: Martinus Nijhoff, 1986, pp 63–73.

152. Gordon SM, Oettinger CW, Bland LA, et al: Pyrogenic reactions in patients receiving conventional, high-efficiency, or high-flux hemodialysis treatments with bicarbonate dialysate containing high concentrations of bacteria and endotoxin. J Am Soc Nephrol 1992;2:1436–1444.

153. Jones DM, Tobin BM, Harlow GR, et al: Antibody production in patients on regular hemodialysis to organisms present in dialysate. Proc Eur Dial Transpl Assoc 1972;9:575–576.

154. Hindman SH, Favero MS, Carson LA, et al: Pyrogenic reactions during haemodialysis caused by entramural endotoxin. Lancet 1975;2:732–734.

155. Raij L, Shapiro FL, Michael AF: Endotoxemia in febrile reactions during hemodialysis. Kidney Int 1973;4:57–60.

156. Passavanti G, Buongiorno E, De Fino G, et al: The permeability of dialytic membranes to endotoxins: Clinical and experimental findings. Int J Artif Organs 1989;12:505–508.

157. Laurence RA, Lapierre ST: Quality of hemodialysis water: a 7-year multicenter study. Am J Kidney Dis 1995;25:738–750.

158. Dinarello CA: Interleukin-1 and its biologically related cytokines. Adv Immunol 1989;44:153–205.

159. Loppnon H, Brade H, Durbaum I, et al: IL-1 induction-capacity of defined lipopolysaccharide partial structures. J Immunol 1989;142:3229–3238.

160. Duff GW, Atkins E: The detection of endotoxin by in-vitro production of endogenous pyrogen: Comparison with limulus amebocyte lysate gelation. J Immunol Methods 1982;52:323–331.

161. Lonnemann G, Bingel M, Floege J, et al: Detection of endotoxin-like interleukin-1-inducing activity during in vitro dialysis. Kidney Int 1988; 33:29–35.

162. Evans RC, Holmes CJ: In vitro study of the transfer of cytokine inducing substances across selected high-flux hemodialysis membranes. Blood Purif 1991;9:92–101.

163. Favero MS, Port FK, Bernick JJ: In vivo studies of dialysis related endotoxemia and bacteremia. Nephron 1981;27:307–312.

164. Klinkman H, Falkenhagen D, Smollich BP: Investigation of permeability of highly permeable polysulfone membranes for pyrogens. Contrib Nephrol 1985;46:174–181.

165. Bingel M, Lonnemann G, Sheldon S, et al: Human interleukin-1 production during hemodialysis. Nephron 1986;43:161–163.

166. Hakim RM, Breillat J, Lazarus JM, et al: Complement activation and hypersensitivity reactions to dialysis membranes. N Engl J Med 1984;311:878–882.

167. Cavallon J-M, Fitting C, Haeffner-Cavaillon N: Recombinant C5a enhances interleukin-1 and. Eur J Immunol 1990;20:253–257.

168. Schindler R, Gelfand JA, Dinarello CA: Recombinant C5a stimulates transcription rather than translation of interleukin-1 (IL-1) and tumor necrosis factor: Translational signal provided by lipopolysaccharide or IL-1 itself. Blood 1990;76:1631–1638.

169. Urena P, Herbelin A, Zingraff J, et al: Permeability of cellulosic and non-cellulosic membranes to endotoxins subunits and cytokine production during in-vitro haemodialysis. Nephrol Dial Transplant 1992;7:16–28.

170. Gault MH, Duffett AL, Murphy JF, et al: In search of sterile, endotoxin-free dialysate. ASAIO J 1992;38:M431–M435.

171. Centers for Disease Control Clusters of bacteremia and pyrogenic reactions in hemodialysis patients. Georgia. Epidemic Investigation Report EPI 86-65-2, April 22, 1987. Atlanta: Centers for Disease Control, 1987.

172. Centers for Disease Control: Bacteremia associated with reuse of disposble hollow-fiber hemodialyzers. MMWR 1986;35:417–418.

173. Centers for Disease Control: Pyrogenic reactions in patients undergoing high-flux hemodialysis. California. Epidemic Investigation Report EPI 86-80-2, June 1, 1987. Atlanta: Centers for Disease Control, 1987,48.

174. Alter MJ, Favero MS, Miller JK, et al: Reuse of hemodialyzers. Results of nationwide surveillance for adverse effects. J Amer Med Assoc 1988;260:2073–2076.

175. Bland LA, Favero MS, Oxborrow GS, et al: Effect of chemical germicides on the integrity of hemodialyzer membranes. Trans ASAIO 1988;34:172–175.

176. Jenkins SR, Lin FUC, Lin RS, et al: Pyrogenic reactions and pseudomonas bacteremias in a hemodialysis center. Dialysis Transplant 1987;16:192–197.

177. Oberle MW, Favero MS, Carson LA, et al: Fatal endotoxemia in dialysis patients at a summer camp. Dialysis Transplant 1980;9:549–550.

178. Bolan G, Reingold AL, Carson LA, et al: Infections with Mycobacterium chelonae in patients receiving dialysis and using processed hemodialyzers. J Infect Dis 1985;152:1013–1019.

179. Bland LA, Favero MS. Microbiologic and endotoxin considerations in hemodialyzer reprocessing. In Association for the Advancement of Medical Instrumentation Vol. 3: Dialysis. Arlington, VA: American National Standards Inc., 1993, pp 45–52.

180. Gazenfield-Grazit E, Eliabou HE: Endotoxin antibodies in patients on maintenance hemodialysis. Israel J Med Sci 1969;5:1032–1035.

181. Hakim RM, Friedrich RA, Lowrie EG: Formaldehyde kinetics in reused dialyzers. Kidney Int 1985;28:936–943.

182. Kaufman AM, Frinak S, Godmere RO, et al: Clinical experience with heat sterilization for reprocessing dialyzers. ASAIO J 1992;38:M338–M340.
183. Vanholder R, NoensL, Eng RDS, Ringoior S: Development of anti-N-like antibodies during formaldehyde reuse in spite of adequate predialysis rinsing. Am J Kidney Dis 1988;11:477–480.
184. Pegues DA, Beck-Sague CM, Woollen SW, et al: Anaphylactoid reactions associated with reuse of hollow-fiber hemodialyzer and ACE inhibitor. Kidney Int 1992;42:1232–1237.
185. US Department of Health and Human Services, Food and Drug Administration: Tlk Paper T92–46, October 13, 1992.
186. Feldman HI, Kinosian M, Bilker WB, et al: Effect of dialyzer reuse on survival of patients treated with hemodialysis. J Amer Med Assoc 1996;276:620–625.
187. Daugirdas JT, Blake PG, Ing TS: Handbook of Dialysis, 3rd edn. Boston, MA: Little Brown Company, 2001, pp 46–66.
188. Ismail N, Becker BN, Hakim RM: Water treatment for hemodialysis. Am J Nephrol 1996;16:60–72.

Choice and Maintenance of Vascular Access

Eugene C. Kovalik and Steve J. Schwab

Hemodialysis is employed in three situations: (1) for chronic maintenance hemodialysis; (2) for acute renal failure; and (3) for the acute elimination of toxins or poisons from the body. Vascular access for chronic maintenance hemodialysis differs from the requirements for acute hemodialysis and acute poisonings in that long-term use is more important than ease of insertion and immediacy of function. During the 1960s, the Scribner shunt served for the provision of both acute and chronic hemodialysis. Since 2000, the provision of vascular access has focused more on the needs of the individual patient with multiple means of access to the circulation available.

Vascular access for acute hemodialysis

Requirements for vascular access in acute hemodialysis are best served by the use of dual-lumen, noncuffed temporary catheters (termed acute catheters), made of various materials including polyurethane, polyethylene, or polytetrafluoroethylene (PTFE). These materials have the useful property that at room temperature they are rigid, thus aiding insertion, but are pliable when they achieve body temperature after insertion. Acute vascular access should be easy to insert and be suitable for immediate use. The duration of use is of secondary importance.

Acute dialysis catheters may be placed in one of three anatomic locations: (1) the femoral vein; (2) the external jugular vein; or (3) the subclavian vein.

In most patients, the femoral vein is the easiest site to insert a catheter and is associated with the lowest risk of life-threatening complications. The major disadvantage of the femoral vein is that the patient must lie down while the catheter is in place, and there is a high rate of infection if the catheter is left in place for more than 5 days. A femoral catheter is particularly useful for acute renal failure or for acute toxin removal when the patient will only need one or two dialysis treatments. It is preferable to use femoral catheters 19–20 cm long, because recirculation in the femoral position is considerably lower than when shorter catheters are used (13–15 cm).

For patients who require longer periods of renal replacement therapy, the jugular approach is preferable. Catheters placed under aseptic conditions in either jugular vein may be left in place for up to 3 weeks. The complication rate associated with insertion into the jugular is considerably higher than that associated with femoral-line insertion; complications include pneumothorax and arterial or great vein puncture with associated mediastinal, pleural, or pericardial hemorrhage. There is also the risk of introducing an air embolism when inserting these catheters, and patients should be maintain the Trendelenburg position while the catheter is being inserted, until the caps have been placed on the end of the catheter. The risk of perforation of the great vein is probably greatest in patients who have previously had many line insertions and have developed central vein stenosis. It is imperative that a chest radiograph is taken before the initiation of hemodialysis after either jugular or subclavian lines are inserted, both to exclude the development of a pneumothorax, and to confirm that the position of the catheter is appropriate. If there is any doubt that the tip of the catheter is not within a great vein, a vascular study should be performed by injecting a small amount of contrast into the catheter under fluoroscopic control. Subclavian vein cannulation can also be performed, with a rate of immediate complications and catheter-life similar to jugular insertions. However, central vein stenosis – a late complication – occurs more often than with jugular insertions. Thus, cannulation of the subclavian vein for hemodialysis should be avoided when possible. It should especially be avoided in patients with chronic renal failure who will need future arteriovenous (AV) access placement.

There are two techniques that can be employed, when available, to reduce the complication rate of catheter insertion. The first uses ultrasound guidance to locate the position of the desired vein. Portable ultrasound devices are now used routinely to identify vessels for cannulation and for real-time cannulation. The number of serious and minor insertion complications are substantially reduced when ultrasound insertion techniques are used.

All temporary catheters carry the risk of bacterial infection due to contamination of the insertion tract or lumen. At the first sign of systemic infection or the development of fever, the catheter should be removed. The most common offending organism with jugular lines is *Staphylococcus aureus* or *Staphylococcus epidermidis*. Any signs of systemic infection should be treated with antibiotics following appropriate cultures. We routinely use a loading dose of vancomycin initially (10–20 mg/kg; our usual maximum dose is 2 g), pending bacteriologic identification of the organism and sensitivities. Patients with femoral catheters are also likely to become bacteremic from gram-negative organisms, and should be treated with vancomycin and either a third-generation cephalosporin, quinolone, or an aminoglycoside, pending the results of blood cultures. The culture results should guide antibiotic therapy after the initial dose. Combinations of vancomycin with an aminoglycoside must be used with caution because of the risk of ototoxicity. It is important to treat these patients for 2–3 weeks when cultures are positive and to confirm adequate antibiotic levels. We keep the trough level of vancomycin above 10–15 mg/mL. Patients who have only recently started hemodialysis may have moderate amounts of residual renal function, and hence the half-life of vancomycin may be as short as 48 h.

Uremic patients who develop *S. aureus* bacteremia have a relatively high incidence of metastatic complications; these patients may develop infectious endocarditis, septic arthritis, or epidural abscess. Patients who develop a metastatic focus of infection should have any accumulation of pus drained, and should be treated for up to 6 weeks with parenteral antibiotics.

Permanent vascular access

The nephrologist caring for patients with chronic renal failure and endstage renal disease (ESRD) has many important issues to deal with, but none is more important than the predialysis planning for vascular access. Without adequate access to the circulation, dialysis will be difficult and complications will be excessive. It is important for physicians who care for people with renal insufficiency to begin making plans at an early stage for the provision of renal replacement therapy, usually when the creatinine clearance is less than 25 mL/min or the serum creatinine is greater than 4 mg/dL. Early planning for the provision of vascular access is certainly cost-effective and saves the patient much discomfort because the need for emergency placement of central-vein dialysis catheters can be avoided.

A working group was established by the National Kidney Foundation (Dialysis Outcome Quality Initiative; DOQI) to develop clinical practice guidelines for establishing and maintaining vascular access in hemodialysis patients in the USA. This committee reviewed 1040 published articles on the provision of vascular access in hemodialysis patients. From their review of these papers, 40 guidelines were established in 1997[1] and were revised in 2001.[2] Because the work of this committee is the most authoritative review completed so far on the provision of vascular access for patients with renal failure, we shall make frequent reference to these guidelines throughout this chapter.

Types of permanent vascular access

Prior to creation of a new vascular access, it is important to evaluate the patient for possible central vein stenosis if risk factors exist. This is particularly important for patients who have undergone multiple previous vascular access procedures, or have had previous central line insertions on the side of the proposed access. Clinical clues that should raise suspicion for proximal venous stenosis include edema in the extremity, colateral vein development, differences in size of the extremities, and a current or previous pacemaker. If patients have any of these they should undergo venography; if there is still residual renal function and the patient is not on hemodialysis, magnetic resonance imaging (MRI) or ultrasound can be used to evaluate for central vein stenosis. If venous stenosis is identified, it is preferable to plan access for the contralateral side, if possible, although we have had success in performing angioplasty on central veins and then proceeding with fistula or PTFE insertion. Doppler ultrasound and MRI are valuable in patients with residual renal function in whom intravenous contrast should be avoided.

Primary fistula

In 1962 Cimino and Brescia[3] described the technique of anastomosis of the radial artery to adjacent veins. This technique allowed the repeated puncturing of veins for dialysis access. To date, the Cimino–Brescia AV fistula remains unrivaled when compared with any other form of long-term vascular access for either complication-free function or patency. Cumulative patency rates of primary fistula vary considerably between dialysis centers. The differences probably reflect multiple factors, such as the demographics of the local dialysis population, the expertise of the dialysis staff, and the skill and preferences of the vascular surgeons. The most frequent problem associated with AV fistulas is failure to mature, manifested by early thrombosis or inadequate blood flow rates. The reported incidence of a primary AV fistula failing to mature to a functional hemodialysis vascular access is 9–70%. In patients in whom it is not possible to create a primary radiocephalic AV fistula, an upper arm brachiocephalic fistula is a very reasonable alternative, and in our opinion it is preferable to the use of a PTFE graft. The upper arm brachiocephalic fistula can mature in most patients, even in those who have failed radiocephalic placement. Transposed brachiobasilic fistulas have been recently shown to have a patency similar to brachiocephalic and upper arm grafts, with a lower risk of infection and thrombosis than grafts. Thus, aggressive attempts at creating upper arm AV fistula are frequently rewarding in terms of avoiding the long-term complications of prosthetic grafts. Once the AV fistula has matured and begun to be used successfully, long-term function is excellent. Winsett and Wolma[4] reported that after 2 years of dialysis 90% of primary fistulas were functioning, and 80% were still functioning at 3 years. At our center the 3-year cumulative patency for native AV fistulas is 80% (excluding fistulas that never mature). The DOQI recommends that the creation of a primary AV fistula is, in most cases, the optimal form of vascular access for all hemodialysis patients.[1,2] There are only a few exceptions to this, notably in patients with severe congestive heart failure or angina, whom it is felt would not tolerate the increased cardiac output associated with such a procedure. A primary AV fistula should be constructed in at least 50% of all new patients with ESRD.

The DOQI also recommends that use of a primary AV fistula within 1 month of its creation is usually contra-indicated, as premature needling carries a considerable risk of causing a large hematoma in the arm, and risks sacrificing a lifetime of fistula access.[1] If dialysis is needed during the first 2 months after fistula creation, it is usually preferable to use a cuffed, tunneled catheter.

Polytetrafluoroethylene grafts

PTFE was introduced as material for vascular bypass grafts in 1976. Since then, this material has become the mainstay for dialysis vascular access when an autologous AV fistula is either believed to be technically impossible or has failed to mature. Using PTFE as a conduit, a fistula is created between an artery and vein in an upper limb. Such a graft accounts for more than 80% of the vascular procedures performed in the USA.[4] In other parts of the world the reverse is the case, with more that 80% of patients receiving a primary AV fistula. This difference probably relates to the increased proportion of aged patients in the USA who have diabetes and poor-quality veins, and the surgical practices that have evolved. Unfortunately, more than 40% of patients who present with ESRD in the USA have not had a vascular access created before the initiation of hemodialysis. One of the goals of the DOQI is to reverse this trend by increasing the percentage of primary AV fistulas in the US. Studies looking at the survival of grafts have noted cumulative patency rates for PTFE grafts of 63–90% at 1 year, and 50–77% at 2 years with fewer than 50% of synthetic fistulas surviving for more than 3 years. Most of these studies defined patency as persistent graft function regardless of whether the graft had undergone revision or thrombectomy or not. Unassisted graft patency (graft patency without graft revision, thrombectomy or angioplasty) has been reported by several authors to be 50–70% at 1 year. The successful use of PTFE grafts for long-term vascular access requires a vigorous prospective intervention plan. Details of this prospective treatment plan are discussed later in the chapter. Nonetheless, compared to native AV fistulas, the intervention rate to maintain this patency rate for PTFE grafts is five times greater than for native AV fistulas. At our center we have a 78% 3-year cumulative patency rate for PTFE grafts. The DOQI suggests that the cumulative patency rate for all dialysis grafts should not be less than the 70% at 1 year, 60% at 2 years, and 50% at 3 years.[1]

Newly inserted PTFE grafts should generally not be cannulated for at least 14–21 days, because adhesion of the subcutaneous tunnel and graft will not have occurred. Potential bleeding into the graft tunnel and hematoma of the graft tunnel may ruin the access site. Dialysis AV grafts should be considered mature when swelling of the access site has reduced to the point where its course is easily palpable. Attempts to cannulate a new PTFE dialysis AV graft in an edematous arm may lead to hematoma formation and graft laceration from inaccurate needle placement.

Dual-lumen cuffed tunneled catheters

Although an inferior choice for vascular access compared to either a primary AV fistula or PTFE grafts, dual-lumen or two single-lumen cuffed catheters have become important for providing vascular access for ESRD patients in the USA.[1,5] These catheters may be used in a number of circumstances, as initial vascular access while waiting for access to mature, or as a bridge between one access that has failed acutely and the establishment of another access. In addition, there is a subgroup of patients in whom all alternative sites have been exhausted. These catheters are commonly placed in jugular veins, but they can be placed for varying periods of time (under extreme circumstances) in the femoral veins, transhepatically, or by a translumbar route into the inferior vena cava. In addition, dual-lumen cuffed catheters may be used for patients with severe coronary artery disease or congestive heart failure who cannot tolerate the increase in cardiac output of about 10% that is induced by AV fistula. Dual-lumen cuffed catheters can provide adequate blood flows in order to achieve what is now the recommended dose of dialysis with a Kt/V of > 1.3. However, blood flows are inferior to those of either a PTFE graft or a primary AV fistula. In general, patients with dual-lumen catheter vascular access require longer treatment times.

The two major reasons for failure of dual-lumen cuffed catheters are thrombosis and infection.[5] There are some simple strategies to prolong the life of the catheter when it presents with poor flow. The first approach is to instil thrombolytic agents, made up to the volume of the internal lumen of the catheter and allowed to sit for up to 30 min.[1] This technique should successfully restore flow to the catheter in 75% of cases. Urokinase has been withdrawn from the US market, but tissue plasminogen activator (TPA) can be used by placing enough volume of a 1 mg/mL concentration to fill the catheter lumen and allowing it to dwell for 4–24 h prior to removal. If these techniques are unsuccessful, flow can almost always be restored with the assistance of interventional radiology. A gooseneck snare can be introduced through the femoral vein, and fibrin sheaths can be stripped off the tip of the catheter with restoration of flow in 95% of cases (Fig. 82.1).[6] Alternatively the catheter can exchanged over a guidewire, taking care to obliterate any fibrin sheath present so that the new catheter is not placed back into an existing fibrin sheath.

The main reason for permanent catheter failure is the high rate of infection (three or four episodes of catheter-related bacteremia per 1000 catheter days). In general, when patients become bacteremic as a result of a catheter-related infection, the catheter should be removed at the earliest opportunity. Patients should receive 2–4 weeks of appropriate antibiotic therapy after the catheter is removed. Although some authors report good success treating catheter-related bacteremia without removing the catheter, at our institution attempts to "salvage" the catheter by treating the patient for prolonged periods with antibiotics was successful in only 22% of cases.[7] Catheter exchange over a guidewire combined with antibiotic therapy has been reported to be successful in some studies when the tunnel tract was not infected (as outlined in Fig. 82.2).[8] Although cuffed catheters provide excellent intermediate access, they have a limited role in permanent access. Most catheters are

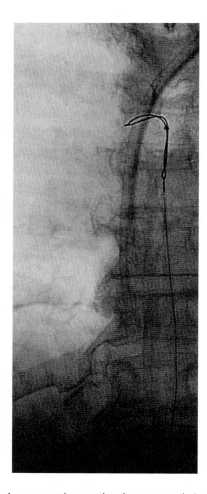

Figure 82.1 A gooseneck snare has been passed via the common femoral vein access and encircles the dual-lumen catheter. The catheter is shown here in the open position; in the closed position it may strip the fibrin sheath from the catheter as it is retracted. Reproduced with permission from Suhocki et al.[6]

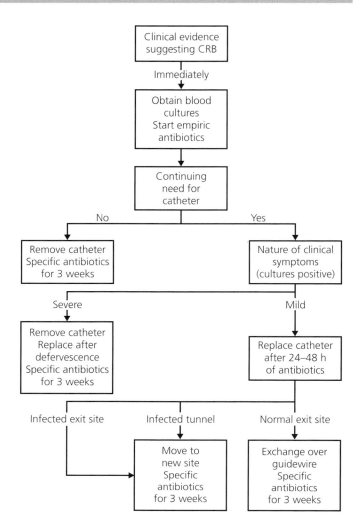

Figure 82.2 Management of catheter-related bacteremia (CRB). Reproduced with permission from Schwab and Beathard.[8]

removed secondary to tunnel tract infections or catheter-mediated bacteremia.

We believe that for patients with a survival prognosis of more than 6 months, some form of vascular access other than a cuffed catheter should be sought whenever possible. The role of the cuffed catheter, in our opinion, is to act as a "bridge" between other permanent AV access and to allow patients with ESRD to have adequate time for an AV fistula to mature. The DOQI recommends that tunneled cuffed catheters are the method of choice for temporary vascular access of more than 3 weeks.[1]

Catheters have been developed with subcutaneously implanted ports, which may make long-term use possible (Lifesite System, Vasca, Topsfield MA; Dialock System, Biolink, Boston, MA, USA). Although dialysis blood flow rates are marginally superior with these catheters the overwhelming reason to foster use of ports is the reduced rate of infection. Preliminary results with the Lifesite Access Port seem to support this, provided the appropriate germicide is used to sterilize the port pocket.

Reasons for access failure

Arteriovenous access thrombosis

Thrombosis is the leading cause of loss of AV access. Thrombosis occurring within a month of vascular access placement is due to technical errors in fistula construction or to premature use of the access.[5] After the first month, the unassisted thrombosis rate is approximately 0.5–0.8 episodes per patient per year. Access type greatly affects the rate of thrombosis: synthetic grafts clot more frequently than native fistulas. The major predisposing factor to graft thrombosis is anatomic venous stenosis, responsible for 80–85% of thromboses (Table 82.1).[1] Most cases of venous stenosis develop at or within 2–3 cm of the vein graft anastomosis and are due to hyperplasia of the fibromuscular intima and perivenous fibrosis. The remainder are located in more proximal veins, including central veins that may account for up to 16–20% of venous stenoses.[9] Previous prolonged cannulation of the subclavian vein, particularly if the catheter became infected, is the major risk factor associated with subclavian vein stenosis. Arterial stenosis accounts for fewer than 2% of graft failures.

About 10–15% of late-access thromboses occur in the absence of an identifiable anatomic lesion. Hypotension, intravascular volume depletion, hypercoagulable states, and prolonged compression of the fistula during sleep or by inexperienced nursing staff may lead to greatly decreased fistula flow and subsequent thrombosis. One of the chief causes of fistula thrombosis, in the absence of identifiable anatomical stenosis, is the use of excessive compression by the patient or dialysis staff on the vascular access when trying to achieve rapid hemostasis after hemodialysis.

An important complication of creating either a synthetic or primary AV fistula is the development of arterial steal. If not recognized and treated early, this may cause severe ischemia of the hand and complete loss of function of the limb. The patient with arterial steal will frequently have severe pain. On examination, there will be decreased capillary refilling and the radial pulse may be absent. In these circumstances it is important to either band or ligate the fistula or graft to decrease flow. It is also important to

distinguish arterial steal from nerve compression injury sustained during surgery. The symptoms are similar but the hand is usually warm with good capillary refill in compression injury. Nerve conduction studies are often needed to make the diagnosis. Treatment is supportive, as occlusion or banding do not usually improve symptoms.

Several risk factors are associated with an increased risk of vascular access thrombosis; these include: female sex, African-American race, advanced age, and diabetes mellitus. In addition, the use of erythropoietin may be related to an increased risk of graft thrombosis. In the Canadian Erythropoietin Study,[11] 14% of patients treated with erythropoietin developed graft thrombosis by 28 weeks of treatment compared with 2.5% of placebo-treated control subjects.[4] The presence of hypercoagulable states such as antiphospholipid antibody syndrome, or protein S or protein C deficiency, can also be associated with increased rates of graft thrombosis. In general, however, these are uncommon causes and should probably only be considered in patients who develop recurrent graft thrombosis in the absence of an identifiable anatomic lesion on fistulography.

Vascular access infection

Access infection is the most common reason for access failure when cuffed catheters are used for long-term access, and access infection is the second most common cause of graft failure when PTFE grafts are used. Failure of a primary AV fistula due to infection is extremely unusual. The successful use of prosthetic material as a form of vascular access depends critically on meticulous attention to aseptic techniques by the staff caring for ESRD patients. Before access cannulation, the relevent arm should be washed thoroughly with water and antibacterial soap. The limb should be further cleaned with 70% alcohol or 10% providone-iodine using a circular rubbing motion. Infection rates for each dialysis unit should be prospectively tracked in order to identify the source of infections, thus allowing corrective action to be taken.

Prophylaxis for vascular access infection with a variety of topical and intravenous antibiotics has been attempted in the past and has been aimed primarily at staphylococci.[11] Unfortunately, most agents have minimal or transient effects on skin or nasal carriage of the bacteria. Even effective antistaphylococcal agents such as rifampicin have limited clinical value because of resistant strains. Indeed, because of the emergence of vancomycin-resistant enterococci and staphylococci, nephrologists must be extremely cautious about liberal use of this agent. It is unlikely that newer antibiotic agents will be as effective for prophylaxis of bacterial infections in prosthetic grafts or catheters.

Pseudoaneurysm formation

An AV access that functions for a long time can often fail due to formation of an aneurysm or pseudoaneurysm. The reported incidence of aneurysm formation is 0.16 per 100 access months. The average hemodialysis patient will have two dialysis needles inserted per treatment, three treatments per week. For each year on hemodialysis, the graft or fistula

Table 82.1 Causes of prosthetic PTFE graft loss

Thrombosis
Anatomic lesions
Anastomotic stenosis
Central venous stenosis
Intragraft thrombosis
Nonanatomic etiologies
Low-flow state
Hypercoagulable state
Prolonged hemostasis
Infection
Pseudoaneurysm
Perigraft hematoma or seroma
Graft attrition

will undergo 312 needle cannulations. After 5 years this number will have reached 1570 needle insertions, which is more than most PTFE grafts can stand before they physically "wear out."

Strategies to prolong the life of polytetrafluoroethylene and primary arteriovenous fistulas

As we previously pointed out, stenosis of the graft vein anastomosis accounts for more than 80% of PTFE graft failures. It is sensible, therefore, to develop strategies for prospectively predicting the occurrence of graft thrombosis; then either surgical intervention or an endoluminal technique such as angioplasty can be used to dilate access stenosis. Four techniques are currently useful for detecting high-grade venous stenosis: (1) venous dialysis pressure measurement; (2) urea recirculation; (3) color Doppler evaluation; and (4) access flow measurement. Clinical features such as edema of the arm, pain over the access, and prolonged bleeding after hemodialysis, are relatively nonspecific but may signal impending graft thrombosis.

Early correction of venous stenosis with angioplasty or fistula revision reduces thrombosis rates and prolongs access viability. Early correction of venous stenosis with angioplasty or fistula revision reduces thrombosis rates and prolongs access viability.[1,10,12] In a prospective study at our institution, the rate of graft thrombosis among patients who underwent prospective monitoring for venous stenosis and treatment of venous stenosis when detected was reduced from 1.4 episodes per year to 0.15 episodes per year, when compared with patients who refused such intervention.[14] Other data from our institution and some larger studies are not as optimistic, but most studies show substantial improvement in access patency and decreased thrombosis rates in AV access when prospective surveillance and corrective interventions are used.

Venuos dialysis pressure

Venous dialysis pressure (VDP) can be an effective way to monitor AV grafts for venous stenosis. VDP can be measured either with blood flow (dynamic venous pressure) or without blood flow (static venous pressure). Both are useful, but static pressures have been shown to be more predictive of stenosis, largely because they eliminate many variables associated with erroneous values.

It is important to measure dynamic (VDP) pressure according to established protocols because many factors (the rate of extracorporeal blood flow, the compliance characteristics of the tubing, or needle size) can affect the result. We therefore adopted a protocol for measuring VDP in every patient at the initiation of dialysis for 2–5 min using a 15-gauge needle, before increasing to maximum blood flow (Table 82.2).[2] Such a protocol costs nothing and may be performed at every dialysis treatment. At our institution, using Cobe Century 3 dialysis machines, we consider three consecutive venous VDPs of more than

Table 82.2 Dynamic venous dialysis pressure monitoring protocol

To establish a baseline and establish trends, initiate measurement when the access is first used

Measure venous dialysis pressure from the hemodialysis machine at blood flow of 200 mL/min during the first 2–5 min of every hemodialysis session

Use 15-gauge needles (or establish protocol for different sizes of needle); ensure that the venous needle is in the lumen of the vessel and is not partially occluded by the vessel wall

Pressure must exceed the threshold three times in succession to be significant

At our institution, using Cobe Century 3 machines, three consecutive venous dialysis pressures of > 125 mmHg are an indication for fistulography; centers using different machines and variations of this technique need to define their own thresholds for fistulography

125 mmHg to be an indication for fistulography. The threshold for other machines has not been defined. It is important, however, to watch for trends in VDP rather than focus on individual readings. Trends in VDP are more predictive than absolute pressure values.

Static VDPs measured at zero blood flow are even more predictive but require specialized machinery. The technique of Besarab[2] is both predictive and relatively inexpensive (Table 82.3 and Fig. 82.3). For these reasons, the 2001 DOQI prefers static VDP.[2] VDP measurements are indirect measures of access flow. In either case, the techniques described apply only to AV grafts, and not fistulas, because colateral venous outflow in fistulas make VDP pressures unreliable.

Urea recirculation

Hemodialysis access recirculation occurs when dialyzed blood returning through the venous needle re-enters the extracorporeal circuit through the arterial needle. Recirculation is usually caused by a venous stenosis proximal to the venous needle that produces retrograde blood flow into the arterial needle. Recirculation can be quantified using the formula (where BUN is blood urea nitrogen):

$$\frac{(systemic\ BUN - dialyzer\ arterial\ BUN)}{(systemic\ BUN - dialyzer\ venous\ BUN)}$$

Prospective screening for abnormally elevated urea recirculation will allow the detection of venous stenosis. As with dialysis pressure, many factors influence recirculation. Urea recirculation depends on factors such as needle position, extracorporeal blood flow, cardiac output, intravascular volume, and venous and arterial stenosis. When performed in a standardized fashion, urea recirculation prospectively detects venous stenosis. It is crucial that each detail of this protocol is meticulously followed if consistent and clinically useful results are to be obtained, because even short delays in drawing blood samples can cause wide variations in calculated urea recirculation. Recirculation exceeding 10%

Table 82.3 Static intra-access pressure (IAP) monitoring protocol

1. Establish a baseline when the access has matured and shortly after the access is first used; trend analysis is more useful than any single measurement.
2. Assure that the zero setting on the pressure transducers of the dialysis delivery system has been calibrated to be accurate within ± 5 mmHg; if uncertain check the calibration (step 8).
3. Measure the mean arterial blood pressure (MAP) in the arm contralateral to the access.
4. Enter the appropriate output or display screen where venous and arterial pressures can be visualized (this varies for each dialysis delivery system); if a gauge is used to display pressures, the pressure can be read from the gauge
5. Stop the blood pump and cross clamp the venous line just proximal to the venous drip chamber with a hemostat (this avoids having to stop ultrafiltration for the brief period needed for the measurement); on the arterial line, no hemostat is needed since the occlusive roller pump serves as a clamp.
6. Wait 30 s until the venous pressure is stable, then record the arterial and venous intra-access pressure (IAP) values; the arterial segment pressure can only be obtained if a pre-pump drip chamber is available and the dialysis system is capable of measuring absolute pressures greater than 40 mmHg.
7. Unclamp the venous return line and restore the blood pump to its previous value.
8. If uncertain about the accuracy of the zero value on the pressure transducers, clamp the tubing from the drip chamber(s) to the pressure transducer protector(s). Pull off the pressure protector(s) from their nipples and record the zero value(s), P_0 (these are usually close to zero, but may deviate by 10 mmHg or more below or above zero). Replace the pressure transducers and protectors and unclamp the lines.
9. Determine the offset pressure(s), P_{offset}, between the access and the drip chamber(s) either by direct measurement (A) or using formula (B) based on the difference in height between the top of the drip chamber and the top of the arm-rest of the dialysis chair (Δ).
   (A) Measure the height from the venous or arterial needle to the top of the blood in the venous drip chamber in cm. The offset in mmHg = height (cm) × 0.76. For practical purposes the same value can be used for both if the drip chambers are at the same height.
   (B) Use the formula, offset in mmHg = 3.6 + 0.35 × Δ. The same value can be used for both if the drip chambers are the same height. If the drip chambers are not at equal heights, the arterial and venous height offsets must be determined individually. In a given patient with a given access the height offsets need to be measured only once and then used until the access location is altered by construction of a new access.
10. Calculate the normalized arterial and venous segment static intra-access pressure ratios, P_{IA}.
    Arterial P_{IA} = (arterial IAP + arterial P_{offset} − arterial P_0)/MAP
    Venous P_{IA} = (venous IAP + venous P_{offset} − venous P_0)/MAP
    Note: If the pressure is less than zero, algebraic subtraction of a negative number is equivalent to adding the absolute number.

Interpretation: Venous outlet stenosis can be detected with venous P_{IA} alone. Trend analysis is more useful than any single measurement. The higher the degree of stenosis at the outlet, the greater the venous P_{IA} pressure ratio. Strictures between the area of arterial and needle cannulation cannot be detected by measuring venous P_{IA}. Detection of these lesions requires the simultaneous measurement of pressures from both the arterial and venous needles. Central stenoses that have colateral circulation may have "normal pressures," but these usually present with significant ipsilateral edema. Accesses can be classified into the categories listed in the table below using the equivalent P_{IA} ratios from the arterial or venous needles; *the criteria must be met in each of two consecutive weeks to have a high likelihood of a 50% diameter lesion.* The criteria in bold type is the primary criterion for the location of the stenosis, the other is supportive.

Access type	Graft	Graft	Native	Native
Normalized P_{IA}	Arterial ratio	Venous ratio	Arterial ratio	Venous ratio
Normal	0.35–0.74	0.15–0.49	0.13–0.43	0.08–0.34
Stenosis				
Venous outlet	≥ 0.75	**≥ 0.5**	> 0.43 or	**≥ 0.35**
Intra-access	**≥ 0.75 and**	< 0.5	**> 0.43 and**	≥ 0.35
Arterial Inflow	**< 0.3**	NA	**< 0.13 +** clinical findings	NA

Patients who develop a progressive and reproducible increase in venous or arterial segment > 0.25 above their previous baseline irrespective of access type are also likely to have a hemodynamically significant lesion. Intra-access strictures are usually characterized by development of a difference between the arterial and venous pressure ratios > 0.5 in grafts or > 0.3 in native fistulas.

Reprinted with permission from National Kidney Foundation: DOQI Clinical Practice Guidelines 2000 Update for Vascular Access.

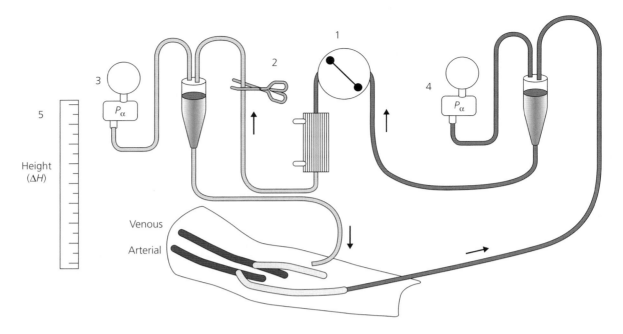

Figure 82.3   Arterial and venous pressure monitoring.

using the recommended two-needle method should prompt fistulography. Recirculation is the least predictive and the least sensitive method of using surveillance for venous stenoses. The DOQI no longer recommends it as a surveillance tool for detecting AV access stenoses.[2]

The measurement of access recirculation has been revolutionized with the development of sophisticated devices for the measuring access recirculation without the need to draw blood. Such devices will undoubtedly prove more reproducible and predictive of venous stenosis than the BUN method of detecting dialysis recirculation.[13] However, it is likely that any recirculation technique will detect impending access failure later rather than earlier because of the critical decrease in flow that must occur to develop recirculation.

Color flow Doppler evaluation

Doppler ultrasound may also be useful for detecting stenosis in vascular access grafts. The major drawbacks of this technique are the degree of variability between operators and its expense.[5] To date, no study has prospectively assessed its value in preventing fistula thrombosis. A potential application that avoids many of the pitfalls involves the sequential measurement of fistula blood flow velocity. When fistula blood flow velocity decreases significantly below a previously established baseline, venous stenosis may be present. The effects of prophylactic correction of these lesions on thrombosis rates has not been tested.

Access blood flow

Several new techniques have been developed to measure access blood flow. These include ultrasound and hemoglobin dilution techniques using a modified "Fick" principle. With current technology these observations of access flow are more reproducible than Doppler flow. Depner has reported that access flows lower than 600 mL/min were associated with access thrombosis, whereas access flows greater than 600 mL/min were unlikely to lead to thrombosis. One study of access flow monitoring showed significant cost savings in terms of missed treatments and hospitalizations.[14] Access survival for grafts improved significantly and that for native fistulas also showed a trend to improvement. The results for native fistulas were important because, as previously mentioned, venous pressure monitoring techniques do not work for AVFs and there is no other reliable method to follow native fistulas prospectively.[15] Figure 82.4 outlines the flow monitoring protocol.[14] In their 2001 update, The National Kidney Foundation DOQI favored either flow monitoring or static venous dialysis pressure monitoring protocols as the primary means for detecting vascular access stenosis.[2]

Venography and fistulography

A fistulogram is the "gold standard" for assessing vascular access patency because it gives detailed visualization of the fistula lumen, venous anastomosis, and proximal veins (Table 82.4). A fistulogram has limited value as a screening test because of its expense and because the overall prevalence of venous stenosis is relatively low. Screening techniques such as VDP and access flow and recirculation are used to select cases for fistulography.

Treatment of venous stenosis

Treatment of venous stenosis with at least short-term maintenance of vascular access patency is important clinically because it preserves other potential sites for future use.

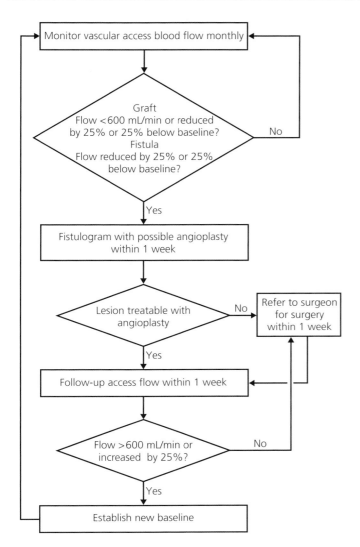

Figure 82.4 Access blood flow monitoring protocol. Reproduced with permission from McCarley et al.[14]

Table 82.4 Indications for fistulography
Graft thrombosis
Prolonged bleeding
Fistula arm edema
Pain in the arm during dialysis
Elevated venous pressures
Elevated fistula recirculation
Unexplained decrease in delivered dialysis dose
Decreased access flow

Percutaneous transluminal angioplasty (PTA), which is an outpatient procedure, corrects more than 80% of stenoses in both native and synthetic fistulas and in both venous outflow and arterial inflow tracts.[1,5,10] Prospective angioplasty of all venous stenoses that narrow the lumen by more than 50% improves fistula function and prolongs access survival. Angioplasty can be performed on both anastomotic and more proximal lesions, including central venous stenosis. The success of angioplasty in terms of preventing stenosis is best determined by the restoration of access flow back to near baseline values.[15] Failure to restore access flow indicates unsuccessful treatment.

The use of angioplasty requires continued monitoring because of the high restenosis rate (55–70% at 12 months). Recurrent lesions can be corrected by repeat angioplasty. The complication rate of each angioplasty procedure averages < 5%.

Lesions unsuitable for PTA can be surgically revised. Surgical revision of stenotic venous and arterial lesions remains the gold standard. It has the lowest recurrence rate but has generally been replaced (in the case of venous lesions) by angioplasty because of the disadvantages of extending the fistula site further up the involved extremity.

Insertion of endovascular stents has been advocated as a method to prevent recurrent stenosis after angioplasty. However, some controlled trials have been unable to show this benefit in most patients.[16] On the contrary, use of a Gianturco stent at the vein–graft anastomosis is associated with a faster recurrence rate than with angioplasty alone.[16] Similar findings have been noted with central vein stenoses, with improved patency seen only in elastic stenoses (which compromised 23% of lesions).[17] Thus, stents usually accelerate endothelial hyperplasia when placed into an abnormal endothelial bed. The role of fabric-covered and coated and irradiated stents remains to be determined.

Pharmacologic and other strategies to prolong access survival

A number of early trials showed that antiplatelet agents can prevent graft thrombosis in external shunts. Sreedhara et al. and others studied the effect of aspirin and dipyridamole in prolonging time to first thrombosis in PTFE grafts. These authors demonstrated a significant reduction in the number of graft thromboses in patients with newly created grafts who were treated with dipyridamole, compared with those treated with placebo.[18] However, there was no benefit in grafts that had previously thrombosed. Patients who have repeated thrombosis of AV access, but no significant anatomic stenosis on fistulography, may benefit from low-dose warfarin sodium (coumadin; 1–2 mg/day). In general, treatment of patients with coumadin anticoagulation has been unsuccessful in preventing AV access thrombosis (a Canadian multicenter trial was terminated). Unfortunately, long-term anticoagulation in hemodialysis patients clearly carries significant risk. In patients with AV access, the risks include bleeding, hematoma, and infection associated with periaccess hematoma, as well as gastrointestinal, uterine, and central nervous system bleeding. The DOQI does not currently recommend routine use of antiplatelet or anticoagulant preparations to prevent graft thrombosis.[1] The NIH has funded a multicenter clinical trial in the US to evaluate the role of pharmacologic agents in preventing AV access stenosis.

Treatment of thrombosed vascular access

Once thrombosis has developed in a PTFE graft, the therapeutic options include surgical thrombectomy, thrombolytic and mechanical dissolution. Available data do not indicate a clearcut preference between surgical thrombectomy and revision as compared to percutaneous mechanical or pharmacomechanical thrombolysis.[1] Since thrombosis is associated with underlying venous stenosis in more than 85% of cases, fistulography must be performed rapidly and the underlying stenosis corrected. Failure to do so will result in rapid repeat thrombosis. Thrombotic episodes in AV fistulas are difficult to resolve, neither percutaneous nor surgical techniques offer good results, but some studies suggest that radiological intervention can restore function to thrombosed native fistulas.[19]

Surgical thrombectomy using a Fogarty embolectomy catheter requires a small incision in the hemodialysis fistula. The clot is then removed by expansion of the catheter. This outpatient procedure is quick and has a very low complication rate.

Initial attempts to treat fistula thrombosis with thrombolytic agents, such as urokinase and streptokinase, yield disappointing results. Access patency could be reestablished in fewer than 60% of patients, almost all of whom required hospitalization and ran the risk of significant bleeding complications. However, dosing adjustments and technical advances have improved the success rate and reduced the incidence of bleeding in patients in whom there is no contraindication to thrombolytic therapy (e.g. a bleeding disorder, a recent bleeding episode, or severe hypertension).[20,21] As an example, use of the pulse-spray technique, which combines thrombolytic therapy with mechanical disruption of clots, rapidly established access patency in more than 90% of cases with minimal complications.[20] Fifty percent of these fistulas remained patent at 1 year. Underlying venous stenoses should be corrected during the same procedure.

Beathard[22] and Trerotola et al[23] have reported on the mechanical disruption of the clot in the graft without the use of any lytic agents. These investigators found a similar rate of success in opening the thrombosed grafts when comparing mechanical thrombolysis and surgical thrombectomy; however, grafts that had undergone mechanical thrombectomy achieved considerably higher longer-term patency.[22] In our view, however, the safety aspects of allowing the disrupted thrombus from the interior of the graft to embolize to the lungs have not yet been settled, and we do not currently practice these techniques.

Thrombolytic therapy is also useful in central venous thrombosis, where it is the only available choice. Advancing an infusion catheter into the clot with progressive dissolution is the preferred technique in this setting.

Nontraditional vascular access

In general, the principle when planning vascular access should be "as distal as possible for as long as possible."

Once both upper arms have been exhausted for both upper and lower arm PTFE grafts there are some more difficult options. These include axillary–axillary or axillary–jugular grafts, femoral grafts, or less commonly axillary–femoral grafts. If all these procedures are exhausted, the option of conversion to peritoneal dialysis should seriously be considered.

For patients who have truly run out of all sites on their upper limbs for vascular access, our preference is to create a graft from the axillary artery to the axillary vein on the opposite side.[24] Problems associated with this approach include difficulties in securing needles to the chest wall, and problems with hemostasis after removal of dialysis needles. Further, the graft may produce unwanted cosmetic results. At our institution these grafts are typically placed after a mean of nine previous access procedures, and 60% continue to function 3 years after creation. The axillary–axillary AV graft may also be positioned on one side of the chest.

The groin is clearly not a preferred site for AV grafts because of the increased infection risk, as well as patient discomfort and inconvenience. In extreme cases of vascular or infectious complications of the upper limbs, a loop thigh PTFE or saphenous vein AV graft may be constructed. Although sporadic good results with autologous saphenous vein grafts for hemodialysis have been noted, the consensus is that this autologous conduit is not recommended for hemodialysis access because of risks of stricture, pseudoaneurysm formation, infection and thrombosis, and because preservation of the saphenous vein is preferred for peripheral and coronary revascularization. When other options will not suffice, it is acceptable to use AV grafts in the lower limbs.

Long-term complications of vascular access

Overt vascular access-related cardiac decompensation occurs rarely, even in patients with underlying cardiac dysfunction. However, cardiac hypertrophy is a very frequent complication of long-term dialysis even with hypertension control, and the optimal correction of anemia with the use of recombinant erythropoietin. It is probable that part of the cardiac hypertrophy associated with ESRD is related to increased cardiac output related to the vascular access AV fistulas. In patients on dialysis for long periods of time, a primary AV fistula may become greatly dilated and aneurysmal, with large fractions of cardiac output passing through the fistula. Patients with cardiomyopathy can develop high-output heart failure with lower blood flows through the fistula. Limiting fistula flow by banding, or tying off some of the draining veins, may be attempted but often results in access thrombosis. Some of these patients may tolerate creation of a new smaller fistula on the contralateral arm. However, patients unable to tolerate a hemodialysis fistula should be converted to peritoneal dialysis or hemodialyzed by use of a permanent indwelling cuffed catheter.

References

1. NKF–DOQI: Dialysis Outcomes Quality Initiative: Clinical Practice Guidelines for Vascular Access, 1997. New York: National Kidney Foundation, 1997.

2. NKF–DOQI: Dialysis Outcomes Quality Initiative: Clinical Practice Guidelines for Vascular Access, 2001. New York: National Kidney Foundation, 2001.

3. Brescia M, Cimino J, Appel K, Harwich B: Chronic hemodialysis using venipuncture and a surgically created arteriovenous fistula. N Engl J Med 1966;275:1089–1092.

4. Winsett O, Wolma F: Complications of vascular access for hemodialysis. Southern Medical Journal 1985;78:513-517.

5. Fan P-Y, Schwab SJ: Vascular access: Concepts for the 1990s. J Amer Soc Nephrol 1992;3:1–11.

6. Suhocki PV, Conlon P, Knelson MH, Harland R, Schwab SJ: Silastic cuffed catheters for hemodialysis vascular access: Thrombolytic and mechanical correction of malfunction. Amer J Kidney Dis 1996;28:379–386.

7. Marr K, Sexton D, Conlon P, Corey G, Schwab S, Kirkland K: Catheter-related bacteremia and outcome of attempted catheter salvage in patients undergoing hemodialysis. Ann Intern Med 1997;127(4):275–280.

8. Schwab S, Beathard G: The hemodialysis catheter conundrum: Hate living with them, but can't live without them. Kidney Int 1999;56:1–17.

9. Barrett N, Spencer S, Melvor J, Brown E: Subclavian stenosis: A major complication of subclavian dialysis catheters. Nephrol Dialys Transpl 1988;4:423–425.

10. Lazarus J, Denker B, Owen W: Hemodialysis. In Brenner B (ed). Brenner's The Kidney, 5th edn. Philadelphia: WB Saunders, 1996, pp 2424–2506.

11. Boelaert JR, DeSmedt R, De Baere Y, Godard CA. Matthys EG: The influence of calcium mupirocin nasal ointment on the incidence of staphylococcus aureus infections in hemodialysis patients. Nephrol Dialys Transpl 1989;4:278–281.

12. Windus D, Audrain J, Vanderson R, Jendrisak MD, Picus D, Delmez JA: Optimization of high-efficiency hemodialysis by detection and correction of fistula dysfunction. Kidney Int 1990;38:337–341.

13. Lindsay RM, Burbank J, Brugger J. Bradfield E, Kram R: A device and a method for rapid and accurate measurement of access recirculation during hemodialysis. Kidney Int 1996;49:1152–1160.

14. McCarley P, Wingard R, Yu W,Petus W, Hakim R, Ikizler TA: Vascular access flow monitoring reduces access morbidity and costs. Kidney Int 2001;60:1164–1172.

15. Schwab S, Oliver M, Suhocki P, McCann R: Hemodialysis arteriovenous access: detection of stenosis and response to treatment as measured by vascular access blood flow. Kidney Int 2001;59:358–362.

16. Beathard GA: Gianturco self-expanding stents in the treatment of stenosis in dialysis access grafts. Kidney Int 1993;43:872–877.

17. Kovalik EC, Newman GE, Suhocki P, Knelson M, Schwab SJ: Correction of central venous stenoses: Use of angioplasty and vascular wallstents. Kidney Int 1994;45:1177–1181.

18. Sreedhara R, Himmelfarb J, Lazarus J, Hakim R: Antiplatelet therapy in graft thrombosis: results of a prospective randomized double blinded study. Kidney Int 1994;45:1477–1483.

19. Haage P, Vorwerk D, Wildberger J, Piroth W, Schurmann K, Gunther R: Percutaneous treatment of thrombosed primary arteriovenous hemodialysis access fistulae. Kidney Int 2000;57:1169–1175.

20. Valji K, Bookstein JJ, Roberts AC, Davis GB: Pharmacomechanical thrombolysis and angioplasty in the management of clotted hemodialysis grafts: early and late clinical results. Intervent Radiol 1991;178:243–247.

21. Ahmed A, Shapiro WB, Porush JG: The use of tissue plasminogen activator to declot arteriovenous accesses in hemodialysis patients. Amer J Kidney Dis 1993;21:38–43.

22. Beathard G: Comparison of mechanical thrombolysis and surgical thrombectomy for the treatment of thrombosed dialysis access grafts (abstract). J Amer Soc Nephrol 1994;5:407.

23. Trerotola SO, Lund GB, Scheel PJ Jr, Savader SJ, Venbrux AC, Osterman FA Jr: Thrombosed dialysis access grafts: percutaneous mechanical declotting without urokinase. Radiology 1994;191:615–617.

24. McCann R. Axillary Grafts for difficult hemodialysis access. J Vasc Surg 1996;24:457–462.

Hemodialysis Adequacy

Todd F. Griffith, Donal Reddan, and William F. Owen Jr

Historical beginnings of the measurement of hemodialysis adequacy

For more than 30 years, dialysis has provided successful "long term" life-sustaining replacement for absent renal function. Many patients have been dialyzed for longer than 10 years; and some have survived over 25 years.[1,2] In its 2001 Annual Data Report, the US Renal Data System counted approximately 340 000 Americans with endstage renal disease (ESRD), of whom 62% were being treated by maintenance hemodialysis.[3] However, despite our success in treating ESRD with dialysis, our knowledge of what constitutes the uremic toxins remains incomplete.[4] At its most fundamental level, the uremic syndrome is the result of the overall accumulation of multiple substances that interfere with physiological and biochemical functions. More than 40 different organic solutes are retained in renal failure,[5] and there are likely to be more. Retained substances range in size from molecular weights of less than 300 Da (e.g. urea, phosphorus, and purines) to ≥ 12 000 Da (e.g. β2-microglobulin, leptin,[6] and cystatin C).[7] Middle molecules are substances of 300–12 000 Da or more. The relative importance of these groups of uremic toxins (namely, the small and "middle" molecules) has been subject to significant unresolved controversy.[4,8] In many cases, which substance or substances should be removed, and in what quantity, remains unresolved. Furthermore, it is clear that the uremic syndrome is not only defined by retention of solutes/toxins, but also by deficiencies of other critical compounds, e.g. erythropoietin,[9] 1,25-dihydroxyvitamin cholecalciferol,[10] and micronutrients such as zinc and carnitine.[11–13]

The fragmented and incomplete understanding of uremia pathophysiology makes it difficult to define precisely an "adequate" amount of dialysis, and consequently compromises interpretation of the measure of dialysis adequacy. Ideally, definition of an adequate amount of dialysis should be based on removing the optimum amount of the uremic toxin to minimize short- and long-term patient morbidity and mortality. In the absence of such a definition, the appropriate amount of dialysis must be based on selection of a surrogate outcome measure and monitoring of its removal. In recent years within the USA, interest in defining adequate hemodialysis and its measurement has been intensified by the high annual gross mortality rate of Americans with ESRD. The mortality rate of US dialysis patients is greater than that of other comparably developed countries.[14–17] Both patient-dependent and dialysis-related factors have been proposed to account for these differences in outcome. Patient-dependent factors include older age and a higher occurrence of diabetes mellitus in the US ESRD population.[18–20] Other possible dialysis-related factors are the failure to achieve adequate solute clearance during hemodialysis, and dialyzer reuse.[21–25] It is clear that the global comparisons of ESRD patient outcomes rely on retrospective multivariable analyses that cannot completely adjust for population differences.[26] Regardless of the cause of the relatively higher mortality in the USA, it is indisputable that amount of dialysis matters.[22,27–38]

Interest in defining an appropriate dose of dialysis arose in the early 1970s, at which time mathematical models and formulations were being developed to assess the adequacy of hemodialysis. Interest in such mathematical models arose because of the clinical paradox that patients treated by peritoneal dialysis do not appear to develop uremic neuropathy, in spite of higher blood urea nitrogen (BUN) levels and creatinine concentrations than patients on hemodialysis.[39,40] Thus, it was proposed that the peritoneal membrane was able to remove selected uremic toxins of a higher molecular weight than urea with much greater efficiency than standard hemodialysis procedures. This theory led to the "square meter hour" hypothesis,[41] which related the efficiency of dialysis to the hours of treatment provided per week and the surface area of the dialysis membrane. The hypothesis seemed intellectually sound in view of the governing biophysical parameters for the clearance of middle molecular weight solutes (discussed later). Thereafter the same investigators devised the "dialysis index," which is the ratio of the calculated removal of a given molecular species to the minimal clearance of that molecular species necessary to maintain health.[42] In the absence of a pathologic and readily measurable molecular species to incriminate, insufficient dialysis was discerned historically by measuring the motor-nerve conduction velocity, electroencephalogram, and hematocrit. These clinical and laboratory studies were combined with assessments of patient activity, performance level, and dietary intake. However, clinical signs and symptoms are late clinical findings and are often unreliable for predicting hemodialysis adequacy.[43,44]

A body of evidence suggests that middle molecular weight solutes may be important in the pathophysiology of a number of comorbid conditions observed in-patients with ESRD[45-48] as well as hemodialysis patient survival.[49] For example, dialysis-associated amyloidosis is characterized by the accumulation of β_2-microglobulin modified by advanced glycation end products. Some evidence suggests that the occurrence of the disease may be attenuated by selective removal through an absorption column[50] or by certain dialysis membrane materials, some of which may have higher clearances for β_2-microglobulin (molecular weight of 12 500 Da).[51-53] The characteristic acquired lipoprotein lipase deficiency of chronic kidney disease may be attenuated by the use of high-flux hemodialysis membranes, and thereby decrease the severity of observed lipid perturbations.[55] Unfortunately, these provocative solutes lack adequate definitions and, subsequently, knowledge regarding their use as markers of dialysis adequacy is incomplete. Furthermore, most outcome studies for ESRD patients treated by hemodialysis have used the small molecular weight solute, urea, as a surrogate uremic toxin to determine hemodialysis adequacy.[22,28-38] Therefore, the discussion provided herein will focus on small molecular weight solutes like urea alone. The Hemodialysis (HEMO)[56] study of the National Institute of Diabetes, Digestive, and Kidney Disease, is a prospective, randomized trial of two dialysis doses delivered by high-flux or low-flux dialyzers. The study aims to evaluate the independent and combined effects of both membrane flux of larger molecular weight solutes and dialysis dose on patient mortality and morbidity.

The benchmark prospective study of hemodialysis adequacy is the National Cooperative Dialysis Study (NCDS).[38] Pending the full presentation of the results of the HEMO study[56] the NCDS is the only large-scale, prospective, randomized trial of hemodialysis dose and patient outcome (morbidity). This intervention trial was designed to evaluate two parameters thought to be critical outcome determinants related to hemodialysis adequacy. The first was the use of the change in the blood urea nitrogen (BUN) concentration as a marker of small molecular solute clearance, and the second was the length of each hemodialysis session as a surrogate for the clearance of middle molecular weight solutes. The latter was appropriate since removal of larger and/or less diffusive solutes is a function of the duration of hemodialysis as well as the membrane surface area. As for urea clearance, the time-averaged BUN concentration (TAC_{urea}) over a full weekly dialysis cycle was the measurement selected for quantifying and targeting urea clearance during hemodialysis, instead of the more conventional and easily quantified midweek predialysis BUN. Arguably, the long-term toxicity of ESRD is more likely a function of average "toxin" exposure (TAC_{urea}), rather than the peak plasma concentrations (midweek predialysis BUN). This issue is important for the clinician as well, in that the midweek predialysis BUN can vary substantially depending on the patient's dietary protein intake, as well as the amount of hemodialysis. All patients in the NCDS underwent rigorous and repeated kinetic modeling to achieve the specified TAC_{urea} for their assigned group.[57-59] The final study population consisted of 165 patients, randomized into four different intervention groups (2×2 factorial analysis). All patient groups were dialyzed three times per week. Groups I and III were modeled and dialyzed to TAC_{urea} 50 mg/dL, whereas groups II and IV were treated to TAC_{urea} of 100 mg/dL. Groups I and II were assigned the longer duration of hemodialysis, 4.5–5.0 h; groups III and IV had dialysis sessions of 2.5–3.5 h. The designated TAC_{urea} was achieved by varying the blood and dialysate flow rates and directions, and dialyzer surface area. All patients were followed for a minimum of 24 weeks.

The TAC_{urea} proved to be the most important determinant of patient morbidity and/or withdrawal from the study.[38,57-61] The proportion of patients not withdrawn for medical reasons or death by 9 months were 89% (group I: long dialysis time) and 94% (group III: short dialysis time) versus 55% and 54%, respectively, for groups II and IV. The duration of dialysis treatment had no effect on patient withdrawal. The TAC_{urea} was also a highly significant determinant of the rate of hospitalization, with fewer hospital admissions occurring in the low TAC_{urea} groups. Also, it was noted that group I had fewer hospitalizations than group III, and similarly group II had fewer hospitalizations than group IV. However, the effect of the length of hemodialysis was only statistically significant in the high TAC_{urea} groups (groups II and IV).[59,60] A stepwise logistic regression analysis of the data from the NCDS was performed to determine the effect of multiple treatment variables on the probability of an adverse outcome.[61] Death, withdrawal from the study, and/or hospitalization during the first 24 weeks of follow-up were again predicted by the TAC_{urea}. The second best outcome predictor was the protein catabolic rate (PCR),[38,60,61] equivalent to the dietary protein intake for hemodialysis patients in a steady state.[62] However, it was argued in a subsequent mechanistic analysis of the data from the NCDS that this statistical association was a consequence of the protocol design, namely that PCR was not an independent variable due to its interaction with TAC_{urea}.[63] Therefore, to achieve a predetermined TAC_{urea}, the amount of hemodialysis prescribed must be a function of the PCR. In other words, a greater PCR will require a greater amount of dialysis to achieve the same TAC_{urea}, and vice versa. Hence, any statistical correlation between TAC_{urea} and morbidity will be mirrored similarly by PCR. It should also be noted that the design of the NCDS did not set the PCR as a study variable. For all study groups, the PCR was permitted to fluctuate between the ranges of 0.8–1.4 g/kg/day (a range representing a grossly inadequate to perhaps a moderately excessive intake of dietary protein).

The NCDS supported the use of urea as an appropriate surrogate marker of small molecule clearance during hemodialysis and suggested that the degree of urea removal may predict patient outcome. However, the NCDS had a number of design limitations that compromise its external validity for a contemporary ESRD patient population and prevalent treatment practices. For example, the NCDS excluded older patients (> 60 years old) and diabetics, a patient profile that would exclude the preponderance of Americans with ESRD.[3] Furthermore, the participants in the NCDS were treated exclusively with cellulosic hemodialysis membranes that were not reused and acetate-buffered dialysis solutions; it may not be appropriate to generalize these findings to other increasingly prevalent biocompatible membrane materials and bicarbonate-based dialysis.[24,64] The follow-up period for the NCDS was ≤ 48 weeks and therefore did not adequately study mortality, a more fundamental long-term outcome. Despite these limitations, the NCDS is the foundation for subsequent analyses linking hemodialysis adequacy to patient morbidity and mortality. The NCDS firmly established the use of urea as a surrogate uremic toxin in the measurement of hemodialysis adequacy.

Principles and methods for quantifying the dose of hemodialysis

Many putative uremic toxins are products of protein metabolism.[8] Because it is impractical to measure the ever-increasing number of possible uremic toxins in routine practice, urea, a derivative of protein catabolism is the substance most often measured in clinical practice as a surrogate for the clearance of small molecules. Urea, which is small, is readily dialyzed and is the major catabolite of protein nitrogen[65] and constitutes 90% of waste nitrogen accumulated in body water between hemodialysis treatments.[62] Measurement of urea is simple, inexpensive, and universally available. Most importantly, its utility as a surrogate for hemodialysis treatment and outcomes has been validated, not the least by the NCDS,[38] and subsequently by other reports.[22,28-38] The Kt/V, the most

widely accepted measurement of hemodialysis dosing, was validated by a posthoc analysis of the NCDS data.[62,63] This expression of the dose of hemodialysis is best described as the fractional clearance of urea (Kt) as a function of its distribution volume (V), which approximates total body water. In turn, K is the dialyzer clearance of urea and is a function of the dialyzer clearance per surface area (KoA), and blood and dialysate flows (Q_b and Q_d respectively). The K is reported in L/min, dialysis treatment time (t) in minutes, and V in liters. Therefore, the Kt/V is a unit-less expression of solute clearance, adjusted for the patient's volume of urea distribution. Urea kinetic modeling is the clinical application of mathematical terms like Kt/V to describe the removal of urea during hemodialysis. Nearly all urea kinetic models that apply to hemodialysis are based on the law of conservation of mass, which means that the accumulation of any substance in the system is equal to the difference between the input and output. Hence, given adequate knowledge of its rate of accumulation, metabolism, excretion, and/or removal from the body, virtually any substance can be kinetically modeled. Finally it must be said that the accuracy of the model is only as good as the assumptions made to produce it. Adapting these principles to urea, we have:

systemic accumulation of urea =
urea input/generation – urea output/clearance

or expressed in the form of a differential equation:

$$d(V \times C)/dt = G - [(K_d + K_r) \times C]$$

where the change in urea content in the body [$d(V \times C)/dt$] is the result of the difference between net urea generation (G) and total body clearance by the dialyzer (K_d) and clearance by residual renal function (K_r). C is the concentration of urea, and V is the volume of distribution of urea.[62] For patients with ESRD, the values of C and V change during and between dialysis treatments. From this simple concept, the variable-volume, single-pool model[62] for urea kinetics has been derived and has been used clinically most often. This model assumes that: (1) urea accumulates in a single pool roughly equivalent to total body water during the interdialytic interval; (2) during a dialysis treatment, urea removal is equivalent from all body compartments; and (3) this single urea compartment expands in size between hemodialysis treatments (secondary to fluid retention) and diminishes in size with ultrafiltration during hemodialysis. As discussed in greater detail later, the second assumption has been challenged recently, giving rise to the use of clearance models of urea that assume at least two compartments.[56]

Use of formal urea kinetic modeling

When rigorously performed, formal urea kinetic modeling is a reproducible, quantitative method for measuring urea removal during hemodialysis. It has several advantages for assessing the adequacy of hemodialysis over alternative methods to measure the delivered dose of hemodialysis.

Assuming a single urea pool of variable volume, formal urea kinetic modeling is the recommended principle method for measuring hemodialysis dose. The three main strengths of formal urea kinetic modeling are given here.

1. Formal urea kinetic modeling can be utilized as a tool to prescribe individualized hemodialysis treatments to achieve the desired amount of hemodialysis (Kt/V) based on patient-specific parameters, such as residual renal function and the normalized protein catabolic rate (NPCR). To develop a hemodialysis prescription, it is necessary to obtain a dialyzer's urea clearance (K) for a variety of blood and dialysate flows in blood/water. To provide this information, the computational software for urea kinetic modeling uses the manufacturer's KoA to extrapolate a K value for that dialyzer that can be applied to different blood and dialysate flow rates. Furthermore, using computational software, formal urea kinetic modeling calculates the volume of distribution of urea by reiteration of two formulae that share common terms. The kinetic determination of V is based on the assumption of a single pool of urea that is coextensive with total body water and that expands during the interdialytic interval from fluid retention and contracts during hemodialysis by ultrafiltration. Assuming a thrice-weekly hemodialysis schedule, the computational software reiterates the following two formulae having shared terms, until unique values are found to satisfy both expressions.

$$V_t = Q_f \times t \left\{ \left[1 - \left(\frac{G - C_t (K + K_r - Qf)}{G - C_0 (K + K_r - Qf)} \right)^{\frac{Qf}{K + Kr - Qf}} \right]^{-1} - 1 \right\} \tag{83.1}$$

$$G = \frac{(K_r + \alpha) \left[C_0 - C_t \left(\frac{V_t + \alpha\theta}{V_t} \right)^{-\frac{K_r + \alpha}{\alpha}} \right]}{\left[1 - \left(\frac{V_t + \alpha\theta}{V_t} \right)^{-\frac{K_r + \alpha}{\alpha}} \right]} \tag{83.2}$$

In equation 83.1, V_t is the end-dialysis volume; Q_f is the rate of volume contraction during dialysis, which is calculated from total weight loss during dialysis divided by the length of dialysis, t; G is the interdialytic urea generation rate; K and K_r are the dialyzer and renal urea clearances, respectively; and C_t and C_0 are the BUN concentrations at the end and beginning of a dialysis treatment. In equation 83.2, α is the rate of interdialytic volume expansion and is calculated by the total interdialytic weight gain divided by the length of the interdialytic interval, θ.[62] With K and V apparent, the treatment time t can be determined easily to achieve the desired Kt/V. Formal urea kinetic modeling supports the derivation of various treatment time and blood flow combinations to achieve a target Kt/V. Thus, the use of formal urea kinetic modeling provides the hemodialysis care team with guidance about which specific parameters of the prescription to modify to achieve the desired hemodialysis dose based on individual patient parameters.

2. Formal urea kinetic modeling provides a means to readily check for errors in the delivered dose of hemodialysis, thereby offering a necessary mechanism for quality control. Formal urea kinetic modeling requires the measurement of pre- and postdialysis BUN concentrations, delivered hemodialysis treatment time, and dialyzer clearance of urea (at the blood and dialysate flow rates used). The formal urea kinetic modeling computer software assumes that all input data are accurate, and will use these values to calculate the volume of distribution of urea. In addition, most formal urea kinetic modeling programs will also calculate a volume of distribution based on anthropometric formulae.[66-68] The anthropometric volume of distribution of urea may be calculated by one of several formulae derived from sex-specific estimates of total body water (TBW) in healthy subjects. These are known as the Watson formulae[67] (equations 83.3–83.6) and the Hume–Weyer formulae[66] (equations 83.6 and 83.7). Equations 83.3 and 83.5 are for women, and equations 83.4 and 83.6 are for women:

$$TBW = 2.447 - (0.09156 \times age) + (0.1074 \times height) + (0.3362 \times weight) \tag{83.3}$$

$$TBW = -2.097 + (0.1069 \times height) + (0.2466 \times weight) \tag{83.4}$$

$$TBW = (0.194786 \times height) + (0.296785 \times weight) - 14.012934 \tag{83.5}$$

$$TBW = (0.34454 \times height) + (0.183809 \times weight) - 35.270121 \tag{83.6}$$

where TBW is the total body water.

Because these formulae were derived from analyses performed in healthy individuals, their general applicability to ESRD patients has been questioned. Based on measurements of total body water using bioelectrical impedance (BEI) in ESRD patients, a population-specific equation for calculating total body water has been derived:[68]

$$TBW = -0.07493713 \times age - 1.01767992 \times male + 0.12703384 \times ht - 0.04012056 \times wt + 0.57894981 \times diabetes - 0.00067247 \times wt^2 - 0.03486146 \times (age \times male) + 0.11262857 \times (male \times wt) + 0.00104135 \times (age \times wt) + 0.0186104 \times (ht \times wt) \tag{83.7}$$

Wt and ht are the patient's weight and height. Men and diabetic patients are assigned input values of 1.0 and women and nondiabetic subjects are assigned values of 0. In comparison with equations 83.3–83.6, this BEI-derived formula for ESRD patients correlates better with TBW as measured by BEI. Both the Watson and the Hume–Weyer formulae underestimate TBW by approximately 7.5%, and so may significantly overestimate the delivered dose of hemodialysis.[68]

By comparing the V derived from formal urea kinetic modeling with that from anthropometric data, possible errors related to the hemodialysis procedure may be

Table 83.1 Common reasons for a discrepancy between the kinetically derived and anthropometrically derived *V*

Kinetically derived V is larger than the anthropometric V
- Low blood flow from the angioaccess
- Inadequate dialyzer performance
- Dialysate flows less than prescribed
- Dialysis machine programmed incorrectly
- Premature completion of treatment
- Predialysis BUN sample was drawn after initiation of hemodialysis

Kinetically derived V is smaller than the anthropometric V
- Postdialysis BUN sample drawn from the venous blood line
- Postdialysis BUN sample drawn in the setting of significant fistula recirculation
- Postdialysis BUN sample drawn following a very efficient hemodialysis in a patient with a small *V* (high *K/V*)
- Postdialysis BUN sample inadvertently diluted with saline

Table 83.2 Common reasons for the delivered dose of hemodialysis falling below the prescribed dose

Compromised urea clearance
- Access recirculation
- Inadequate blood flow from the vascular access
- Inaccurate estimation of dialyzer performance
- Inadequate dialyzer reprocessing
- Dialyzer clotting during dialysis
- Blood pump/dialysate flow calibration errors
- Errors in prescribed blood and dialysate flow rates due to variability in blood pump tubing
- Dialysate flow rate that is inappropriately set too low
- Dialysate flow miscalibration
- Dialyzer leaks

Reductions in treatment time
- Inaccurate assessment of effective dialysis time using wristwatches
- Incorrect assumption of continuous treatment time because of failure to account for interruptions
- Premature discontinuation of hemodialysis for staff or unit convenience
- Premature discontinuation of hemodialysis to honor patient request/adherence
- Delay in starting dialysis session due to patient tardiness
- Wrong patient taken off dialysis
- Time on dialysis calculated incorrectly
- Time read incorrectly for initiation or completion of hemodialysis
- Clerical deficiencies

Laboratory or blood sampling errors
- Dilution of predialysis BUN blood sample with saline
- Drawing predialysis BUN blood sample after the start of dialysis
- Drawing postdialysis BUN blood sample before the end of dialysis
- Laboratory error due to calibration or equipment problems
- Drawing postdialysis BUN blood sample more than 5 min after dialysis completed

BUN, blood urea nitrogen.

detected. This is the principal benefit of formal urea kinetic modeling. A discrepancy between these two values for *V* should alert the dialysis care team to errors in dialysis delivery (see Table 83.1). In the case where the kinetically-derived *V* is larger than the anthropometrically derived *V*, the delivered dose of hemodialysis will be less than the prescribed dose. Alternatively, in instances where the kinetically-derived *V* is less than the expected anthropometrically-derived *V* (used for the initial hemodialysis prescription), the *Kt/V* may seem inappropriately high. If this erroneous *Kt/V* is interpreted without consideration of the urea distribution volume, a reduction in the dose of hemodialysis may appear appropriate. In this case, a reduction in hemodialysis dose may reduce the delivered hemodialysis dose to an unsafe level and so compromise the patient's well-being. This course of events would be observed when the hemodialysis dose was appropriate but an unappreciated error occurred in calculating *V*. Because of the enhanced rigor in ascertaining that the delivered dose of hemodialysis is correct, and the greater ease with which dosing deficiencies are detected, formal urea kinetic modeling provides the greatest support for continuous quality improvement efforts in the delivery of hemodialysis. Optimal quality improvement efforts require that the processes of care affecting patient outcome are routinely measured, that individual deficiencies are defined, and corrective steps implemented. Furthermore, formal urea kinetic modeling helps to identify one or more components in the hemodialysis treatment that were problematic, if the delivered dose did not mirror the prescribed dose (see Table 83.2).

3. Formal urea kinetic modeling accounts for the contribution of residual renal function to the sum total of the delivered hemodialysis dose. Some ESRD patients have significant residual renal function (K_r). Failure to account for substantial K_r will underestimate the actual total urea clearance and the NPCR. Because of the short duration of individual treatments, the impact of

residual renal function on total urea clearance during hemodialysis will be small. However, in the relatively long interdialytic period, residual renal function will significantly lower the predialysis BUN concentration. Graphically, when K_r is zero, the interdialytic rise in BUN concentration is linear. However, if $K_r > 0$, the rise in BUN concentration will be more shallow and curvilinear as a result of continuous renal excretion. Thus, when $K_r > 0$, less hemodialysis is required to achieve the same predialysis BUN level as when $K_r = 0$. The quantitative relationship that relates hemodialysis dose with and without residual renal function can be defined as:

$$kK_r = K_t - K'_t$$

where *K* and *K'* are the dialyzer urea clearances in the absence and presence of residual renal clearance,

Table 83.3   Error analysis*

Initial assessments
Elements of hemodialysis treatment to evaluate/correct immediately. These elements can be assessed noninvasively, using available data, and/or without incurring significant additional costs.

Clearance (K) less than assumed
Elements of the hemodialysis procedure affecting clearance include: dialyzer permeability (KoA), effective dialyzer surface area, blood flow and dialysate flow.
1. Assess fistula integrity to determine if there may be recirculation
   - Review arterial and venous needle placement, proximity, and orientation with patient care staff and patient
   - Verify direction of blood flow through angioaccess
2. Review written documentation of hemodialysis treatment, when *Kt/V* or URR was measured
   - Review hemodialyzer reuse log to evaluate total cell volume (TCV) of dialyzer
   - Review maintenance log for dialysis machine to check last calibration date and results
   - Review hemodialysis log to evaluate execution of prescribed versus actual treatment parameters, including:
     a blood flow rate (Q_b)
     b dialysate flow rate (Q_d)
     c type of hemodialyzer
     d extracorporeal pressures compared to previous sessions at prescribed Q_b
        i. Were prepump arterial pressures ≥ 200 mmHg?
        ii. Were prepump arterial or venous pressures close to upper limit per dialysis unit policy?
   - Review hemodialysis log for clinical events that may have resulted in a change in treatment parameters like the Q_b, such as hypotension, muscle cramps, chest pain, or problems with needle placement
3. Review for pattern of dialyzer clotting
   - May warrant review of patient's anticoagulation
4. Determine if dialyzer clearance is overestimated by reviewing formal urea kinetic modeling results on other patients using same model of dialyzer with same prescribed *Kt/V*
5. For delivery systems with computers, review the total liters of blood processed

Effective hemodialysis treatment time (T) less than prescribed
Hemodialysis treatment time is the total time at the prescribed blood and dialysate flow rates with the prescribed dialyzer, or is the dialysis time determined to provide an equivalent *Kt/V* at the prevailing blood and dialysate flow rates for a particular hemodialyzer.
1. Review written documentation of total duration of the dialysis treatment for determination of any of the following
   - Review patient arrival time in unit and transportation needs
   - Staff started hemodialysis late without a compensatory extension of the time on dialysis
   - Staff honored inappropriate patient request for early termination of hemodialysis treatment
     a Review understanding of dialysis treatment components with patient and direct patient care staff
   - Clinical events that may have caused premature discontinuation or interruption of hemodialysis, such as hypotension, muscle cramps, chest pain, etc.
   - Hemodialyzer blood leak
   - Problems with needle placement that required recannulation of angioaccess
   - Pressures in the extracorporeal circuit close to alarm limits

Errors in blood sampling or processing for calculating the delivered dialysis dose
Blood samples to support urea kinetic modeling must be performed in an operationally consistent manner that prevents the samples from being diluted with saline or heparin, collected without contamination by recirculated blood, and obtained at a time appropriate to support the measurement of hemodialysis adequacy. Review sampling procedure with patient care staff with focus on the following areas:
1. Low predialysis blood urea nitrogen (BUN) concentration
   - Review blood sampling procedure with patient's care provider
     a Were dialysis needles saline-filled?
     b Was blood sample drawn after the initiation of hemodialysis?
   - If available, consider having laboratory reassay sample
2. High postdialysis BUN concentration
   - Review blood sampling procedure with patient's care provider
     a Was blood sample drawn too late after the discontinuation of hemodialysis?
   - If available, consider having laboratory reassay sample

Table 83.3 *(cont'd)*

3. Low postdialysis BUN concentration
   - Review blood sampling procedure with patient's care provider
     a Was blood sample drawn before the discontinuation of hemodialysis?
     b Was blood sample drawn from the venous line?
     c Was blood sample drawn without flushing the dialysis lines and needle to eliminate recirculated blood?
     d Was the blood sample contaminated with saline from reinfusion?
   - If available, consider having laboratory reassay sample
4. Consider repeating pre- and postdialysis BUN sampling to determine *Kt/V* or URR, again.

*To help identify the problematic component(s) in hemodialysis delivery when the delivered dose does not mirror the prescribed dose, an error analysis algorithm should be used.[69,70]

†The hemodialysis care team should note that this list is not all-inclusive. However, the elements provided are the most common sources of error. If other components of the analysis are not revealing, perform a measurement of recirculation in the angioaccess using "two needles."[69]

respectively, and t is the treatment time. Here, k relates K_r to the difference between K and K', or the decrease in dialysis dose that is possible in the presence of residual renal function to achieve the same predialysis BUN. Therefore, the relationship between the total dialysis dose (KT), the dose provided by the dialyzer (K_t), and the contribution of the residual renal clearance (kK_r), are expressed by:

$$KT/V_t = K_t/V_t + kK_r/V_t$$

Computational software for formal urea kinetic modeling provides solutions for these equations. Formal urea kinetic modeling permits calculation of NPCR. The derivative formulae for PCR and NPCR are:

$$PCR = 9.35G + 0.29V_t$$

Because urea distribution volumes vary between 30–65% of body weight, it is improper to index the PCR simply be dividing PCR by the patient's body weight. The PCR must be presented in relation to the normalized body weight. Presuming the average volume of urea distribution is 58% of body weight, the patient's weight is converted to a normalized body weight (NBWt) by the following:

$$NBWt = V_t/0.58$$

and NPCR is thus expressed as:

$$NPCR = PCR/(V_t/0.58)$$

In patients who are not markedly catabolic or anabolic, the net protein catabolism will correlate closely with the dietary protein intake.[69–72] Since dietary records and histories are confounded by underreporting,[73,74] protein catabolic rate (calculated as part of formal urea kinetic modeling) will provide a more reliable estimate of dietary protein intake. Hence, use of the NPCR enables the dialysis care team to perform longitudinal analysis of the patient's nutritional status and to more soundly guide dietary counseling about protein intake.

Although the NCDS provided evidence that a high NPCR (presumably reflective of a better dietary protein intake) was associated with lower morbidity or lesser likelihood of treatment failure,[63] the design of the study was not ideal to prove conclusively that NPCR was an independent risk factor. However, several subsequent reports have statistically linked laboratory surrogates of nutrition to outcomes in chronic hemodialysis patients.[22,33,36,71,72,75–77] For example, a low serum albumin concentration (< 3.5 g/dL), which may be a laboratory surrogate of visceral malnutrition, was associated with a relative risk of death of 1.83 and 2.07 for diabetic and nondiabetic ESRD patients, respectively, although this difference was less when adjusted for Kt/V.[18] In a separate analysis of 13 473 ESRD patients, the serum albumin concentration was 21 times more powerful a predictor of death than was the dose of hemodialysis. Furthermore, the serum albumin concentration was an independent risk factor, apart from the dose of hemodialysis.[22] This finding is provocative because the serum albumin concentration has been linked to the adequacy of hemodialysis. Although not uniformly observed,[22] some investigators have reported a highly significant positive correlation between the serum albumin concentration and the dose of hemodialysis (Kt/V).[75,78] Arguably, patients who are inadequately dialyzed have a depressed appetite and a diminished protein-caloric intake. Thus, maintaining an adequate dose of hemodialysis may improve nutrition and patient survival.

The disadvantages of formal urea kinetic modeling are logistic. The complexity of the calculations requires the use of computational devices and software. The cost of computer devices and software may remain a consideration for some smaller hemodialysis units. Physical parameters, such as the K and V, are burdensome to measure and to monitor, and the actual treatment time can be difficult to determine. In addition, the time required for the dialysis unit staff to accurately collect and process all patient data to support these calculations may be significant in larger hemodialysis centers. Despite these relative limitations, both the National Kidney Foundation's Kidney Disease Outcomes Quality Initiative (KDOQI)[70] and the Renal Physicians Association's[69] evidence-based clinical practice guidelines agree that formal urea kinetic modeling is "the most rigorous method for prescribing dialysis treatment and evaluating the consistency with which the prescribed treatment is delivered to the patient..."[69]

Alternative methods of hemodialysis dose quantification

Recent literature suggests that only one alternative method of calculating Kt/V (Kt/V natural logarithm formula),[79] and one other measurement of the delivered dialysis dose (urea reduction ratio),[22,80] should be considered for routine use in clinical dialytic practice.

Kt/V natural logarithm formula

This second generation logarithm formula,[79] which was proposed based on the variable-volume single-pool urea kinetic model, accounts for the urea removed by both diffusive and convective clearance, the latter secondary to ultrafiltration.[70] Urea removal accomplished by convective transport is not associated with a change in the post- or predialysis BUN concentrations. Over a wide range of single-pool, variable volume Kt/V values derived by formal urea kinetic modeling (range 0.7–2.1), the second-generation logarithm formula for calculating Kt/V is accurate.[79,81,82] The original second generation logarithm formula for calculating Kt/V is:

$$Kt/V = -\ln(R - 0.008 \times t) + (4 - 3.5 \times R) \times UF/W$$

where ln is the natural logarithm, R is the post/predialysis BUN ratio, t is the dialysis session length in hours, UF is the ultrafiltration volume in liters, and W is the patient's postdialysis weight in kilograms. Using the aforementioned criteria of accuracy and completeness, the second generation logarithm formula for calculating Kt/V is the best alternative for dialysis care teams to use if they are not able to perform formal urea kinetic modeling. Although this simplified formula is convenient, its use alone will deprive the dialysis care team of the error check function for the delivered hemodialysis dose, as opposed to formal urea kinetic modeling. The logarithm calculation of Kt/V does not permit the rigorous, preemptive, quantitative analysis of the hemodialysis prescription possible with formal urea kinetic modeling. Furthermore, this formula does not support calculation of the NPCR. However, an approximation of the NPCR can be derived from a nomogram that uses patient-specific parameters and the Kt/V natural log formula.[83]

Urea reduction ratio (URR)

The URR is calculated simply from the fractional end-dialysis BUN concentration, which equals C_t/C_0 where C_t is the postdialysis BUN and C_0 the predialysis BUN.[22,80] Hence:

$$URR (\%) = 100 \times (1 - C_t/C_0)$$

which represents the fractional clearance of urea during a single hemodialysis treatment. Owing to the ease of calculation, this simple mode of measuring the dose of hemodialysis is immediately accessible. More importantly, the utility of URR as a measure that correlates with patient mortality has been validated in several clinical studies using different patient databases.[22,27,30] Therefore, URR may be no worse than Kt/V in defining mortality risk for hemodialysis patients. However, despite its ease of use, it

should be noted that there are limitations with URR as a measure of hemodialysis adequacy. URR does not account for the contribution of ultrafiltration to the final delivered dose of hemodialysis, in contrast to formal urea kinetic modeling or the Kt/V natural logarithm formula.[84–86] Recall that although urea is removed via convective clearance with ultrafiltration, this has no bearing on its plasma concentration. The failure to account for this additional urea removal limits the accuracy of the estimate of hemodialysis dose, depending on the volume of ultrafiltrate formed.[70] For example, a patient with a large ultrafiltration requirement will have a much higher dialytic dose when measured by formal UKM or the natural logarithm formula than will the same patient if no ultrafiltration is needed. However, the URR will be the same in both these circumstances, if all other parameters for the hemodialysis prescription are equal. This discrepancy between the dose of hemodialysis delivered in the presence and absence of ultrafiltration and its relationship to URR is illustrated in Fig. 83.1. Assuming a 3-h dialysis session, no residual renal function, and a volume of distribution of urea of 58% of body weight, the Kt/V derived using formal urea kinetic modeling is contrasted with the URR.[85] As illustrated in Fig. 83.1, a URR of 65% may correspond to a single-pool Kt/V of as low as 1.1 in the absence of ultrafiltration, or can be as great as approximately 1.35 when ultrafiltration of 10% of body weight occurs. Furthermore, because the relation between URR and Kt/V is curvilinear (see Fig. 83.1), modest decreases in the URR can result in a substantial decline in the Kt/V, especially in the target range of URR of $\geq$ 65%.

Using the URR alone, errors in the delivered dose of hemodialysis may be particularly difficult to ascertain. This limitation is a consequence of the inability of URR to support the calculation of V, for comparison with anthropometric-derived values. Also, similarly to the Kt/V calculated by the natural logarithm formula, achieving a target delivered dose of hemodialysis is an empirical exercise involving modification of the various components of the treatment prescription. Likewise, the URR does not support calculations of the NPCR and effectively ignores the contribution of residual renal function to urea clearance. Thus, although the URR is a useful tool to measure the delivered dose of hemodialysis for statistical outcome analyses,[22,23,30] it lacks sufficient accuracy and detail to routinely provide insight into problems with the dialysis prescription.

Percent reduction of urea

The percent reduction of urea, which is the fractional decline in the BUN concentration in a single hemodialysis session (not converted to a percent like the URR) can be used to calculate a Kt/V.[87,88] These formulae were derived by the linear correlation of the percent reduction of urea to the Kt/V derived from total dialysate collection and from formal urea kinetic modeling. However, because of the curvilinear relationship between the percent reduction of urea and Kt/V derived by formal urea kinetic modeling, the Kt/V extrapolated from the percent reduction of urea

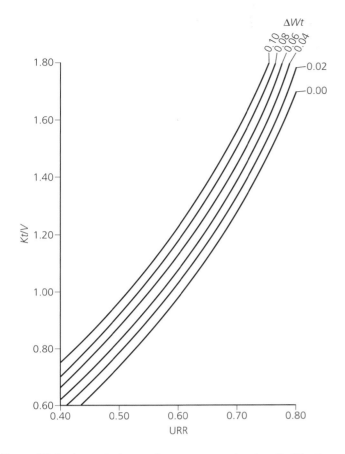

Figure 83.1 Impact of urea clearance secondary to ultrafiltration on the Kt/V. The family of curves is based on the assumption of a 3 h hemodialysis treatment and the absence of residual renal function. ΔWt is the volume ultrafiltered in liters divided by the patient's estimated dry weight in liters. The greater the ΔWt, the higher the Kt/V for any given URR value.[70]

can be incorrect by at least 20%. Setting an acceptable threshold for error of $\leq$ 5%, in comparison to formal urea kinetic modeling, the formula developed by Basile et al[88] is acceptable for the Kt/V range of 0.6–1.3. The formula developed by Jindal et al[87] is only acceptable over a very narrow Kt/V range of 0.9–1.1.[86] Although the formula by Basile et al was more accurate, it systematically overestimates the actual Kt/V in the critical range of $Kt/V < 1.0$. Because of their variability and unpredictability over the full range of Kt/V values, these formulae are not adequate for routine clinical use in measuring the delivered dose of hemodialysis.

Total dialysate collection

The clearance of urea as a surrogate for the clearance of small molecules during hemodialysis can also be quantified by collection of the dialysate.[89] Dialysate-based urea kinetic modeling has been considered by some to be the "gold standard" for dose quantification.[82,87,88,90] In the total dialysate collection technique, sometimes referred to as direct dialysis quantification, all the dialysate that passes through the dialyzer is collected. The total mass of urea removed can then be calculated as the product of the urea concentration of a representative sample of the dialysate collected and the collected volume. The obvious drawback to total dialysate technique is the impracticality of routinely collecting $\geq$ 90–150 L of spent dialysate that is usually generated during a single hemodialysis treatment. A more convenient technique is to collect only a small representative fraction of the total spent dialysate, sufficient to permit measurement of dialysate urea concentration.[91] The volume of spent dialysate can be calculated from the product of the dialysate flow rate and the total treatment time. The advent and application of built-in urea sensors in hemodialysis machines will permit the automation of dialysate urea quantification and make this method more feasible.[92,93] Although the total collection of dialysate may be the most accurate quantification of urea removed, there is no predetermined level of urea removal that defines an adequate dose of hemodialysis. Additionally, the accuracy of dialysate-based measurement of hemodialysis dose with an automated instrument has recently been questioned.[94,95] It is only through outcome correlation that a clinical measure can be declared useful,[95–97] and evidence for this has been lacking with the dialysate-based methods of urea quantification.

Duration of treatment

It has been suggested that the duration of the hemodialysis session is an independent measure of hemodialysis adequacy, segregated from Kt/V or URR. Dialysis treatment duration is longer in Europe and Japan compared to the USA, and this has been proposed as a contributing factor to the differential survival rates among these dialysis populations.[25,26,98] The proponents of dialysis duration as a unique measure of hemodialysis adequacy propose that extending the length of hemodialysis disproportionately increases the clearance of molecular weight solutes larger than urea (e.g. middle molecules). Because of their size, these molecules depend less on diffusive clearance than urea, if a conventional low flux dialyzer is used. Acknowledging that urea is only a marker solute for the uremic toxin(s) (it would not behave in the same biophysical manner as a middle molecular weight solute) treatment time becomes a crude surrogate for the clearance of these larger molecules. Therefore, a longer duration for hemodialysis may enhance patient survival,[26,36,99] and so offer an alternative measure not accounted for by urea-based kinetic modeling alone.

A second potential advantage of a longer time for hemodialysis treatments is the greater ease of establishing intravascular euvolemia. If the estimated dry weight is defined as the postdialysis weight that correlates with intravascular euvolemia, routinely achieving this weight may reduce the risk of cardiovascular complications, especially from hypervolemia and hypertension.[100] Both the ultrafiltration volume and the rate of ultrafiltration may affect blood pressure,[101–103] such that large ultrafiltration volumes or rapid ultrafiltration can result in hypotension and/or cramps. These symptoms are a frequent cause of the premature discontinuation of hemodialysis,[43,104,105] which in turn may result in the patient leaving dialysis above their true estimated dry weight. With a typical interdialytic weight gain, the cycle is repeated at the next dialysis, such that the patient is chronically hypervolemic. This cycle may be further exaggerated by the physiologically incorrect clinical practice of routinely relying upon hypotension and/or cramps to define estimated dry weight.[106–110] All of this may be confounded further by the deleterious effect of antihypertensive medications on the patient's intradialytic blood pressure.[111] Because some investigators have reported improved patient survival in the setting of greatly augmented blood pressure control associated with increased dialysis treatment times,[100] it has been argued that this is a causal relationship. Therefore, extending the duration of hemodialysis has been advocated as a means of minimizing intradialytic hypotension and improving the likelihood of achieving the patient's dry weight.[70]

Despite these clinically sound arguments, there are no clinical data to support a minimum time for hemodialysis treatment. The few studies that have attempted to statistically examine this issue are compromised by reliance on the prescribed hemodialysis time alone, instead of the delivered dialysis time.[22,38] The independent effects of time of treatment are inherently difficult to separate from dose of dialysis, defined by Kt/V.[112] Finally, as discussed in greater detail in a later section, the accuracy of the single-pool variable-volume model of urea kinetics becomes increasingly compromised with shorter dialysis times, such that the delivered dose of hemodialysis becomes increasingly overestimated.[70,113] On this basis there has been debate regarding whether dialysis treatment times should ever be less than 2.5 h.[70]

$K \times t$

Kt/V is derived by dividing one outcome measure ($K \times t$, a proxy for solute clearance) by another (V, a proxy of lean body mass and nutritive state). $K \times t$, V, total body water, body weight, and body mass index, all independently predict mortality risk in hemodialysis patients.[114] For each parameter, higher values correlate directly with patient outcome. Not surprisingly, paradoxical relationships result. For example, increasing V, a reflection of better nutritional health, may be associated with lower hemodialysis doses. This is unsurprising as many dialysis providers prescribe uniform dialysis doses regardless of variability in patient weight.[115] Increasing V without any alteration in $K \times t$ necessarily reduces the calculated dose of dialysis, Kt/V, and suggests an increased risk of death. In this case, this effect is abrogated by the reduced likelihood of death associated with an increased V. Therefore, some authors have advocated uncoupling $K \times t$ and V and measuring dose of hemodialysis with $K \times t$ alone.[116] Based on cross-sectional data, these authors proposed $K \times t$ thresholds of 40–45 L per treatment and 45–50 L per treatment for women and men, respectively.[116] Alternative theories exist which explain the complex and, occasionally, counterintuitive interactions described.[115] As yet, there are no prospective data supporting the substitution of $K \times t$ for Kt/V. The longitudinal nature of the HEMO study will facilitate the understanding of these complex interactions.[56]

Urea rebound—double-pool effects and recirculation
Double-pool models

As described earlier, the simplest model of urea distribution and concentration changes in anuric hemodialysis patients is the single-pool or single-compartment model which assumes that: (1) urea is distributed in a single compartment coextensive with total body water; (2) concentration equilibrium of urea prevails throughout this volume of distribution; and (3) the compartment will contract and expand uniformly during and between hemodialysis. This elementary model yielding the single-pool Kt/V has proven to be clinically useful in population studies and has received wide clinical acceptance. However, the actual anatomical distribution of urea comprises plasma, erythrocyte, interstitial, and intracellular water. Functionally, transfer between these compartments behaves as a diffusive process and can be described by the product of a volumetric mass transfer coefficient and the difference in concentration between the compartments.[62] However, this model omits another physiological consideration for urea kinetics during and between hemodialysis treatments – the variable distribution of blood flows to various vascular beds and organs. For example, in the anephric patient, approximately 80% of cardiac output is distributed to visceral organs (liver, gut, heart, and brain), which contain only 30% of total body water. In contrast, only 20% of the cardiac output is distributed to muscle, bone, and skin (primarily muscle), which account for 70% of total body water.[117]

During hemodialysis, the clearance of solutes is dependent on dialyzer clearance and the rate at which solutes can be conveyed from all body compartments into the dialyzer. The transfer of urea from the plasma water compartment into the dialysate may easily exceed its rate of transfer from other compartments into plasma water, functionally resulting in multiple compartments. This is a fundamental biophysical and practical basis for double-pool urea kinetic models, which are a more accurate and rigorous description of urea kinetics during hemodialysis. Specifically, one level of impedance of urea movement is from the intracellular compartment to the extracellular compartment, which is estimated to be approximately 800 mL/min.[117] This relative impedance of urea movement from the cells across the interstitium and into the blood compartment effectively renders the distribution of urea into two pools, one of which may become an unequilibrated reservoir. This biophysical reality obviously undermines a key assumption made in the formulation of the single-pool model.[118] In addition, the effect of differential organ perfusion will further contribute to this "disequilibrium" of urea removal.[119] Because of the preferential removal of urea from well-perfused, but relatively urea-depleted vascular beds during the course of hemodialysis, a single-pool, variable volume model for urea kinetics does not account for the different rates of urea transfer between these compartments.

The term "double-pool effects" describes the effect of this combination of biophysical phenomena on urea

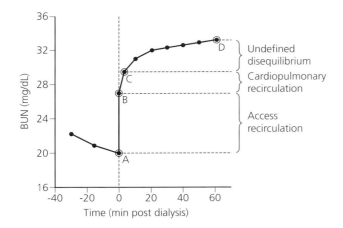

Figure 83.2 Biophysical and kinetic segregation of the components of urea rebound. After the completion of hemodialysis, the blood urea nitrogen (BUN) concentration increases. The increment from point A to point B is secondary to access recirculation; from point B to point C is secondary to cardiopulmonary recirculation; and point C to point D is secondary to flow–volume disequilibrium and/or diffusive impedance of urea (undefined disequilibrium).[70]

kinetics, namely diffusive impedance and flow–volume disequilibrium. As a consequence of this effect, release of sequestered urea begins at the cessation of a hemodialysis treatment and continues for 30–60 min (postdialysis urea rebound). The impedance of urea movement into plasma water and variation in organ perfusion are thought to be the major contributors to postdialysis urea rebound.[120–124] The postdialysis BUN concentrations measured before and after the occurrence of urea rebound will vary significantly, such that a much lower BUN concentration is observed before rebound than after (see Fig. 83.2). Thus, the effective delivered dose of dialysis will be overestimated, if this sequestered urea pool is large and not taken into consideration.

The extent of urea rebound varies greatly among patients, being influenced by variables such as the size and the efficiency of the dialyzer. In a study, the mean amount of urea rebound, measured as the percent increase in postdialysis BUN concentration immediately after dialysis versus 30 min post dialysis, was 17%.[122] However, in some patients, the extent of urea rebound was observed to be as great as 45%.[90] The use of dialyzers with high K (efficient, high-flux dialyzers), especially in a patient with a small V, increases the risk of significant double-pool effects.[122,125] Expressed mathematically, the severity of urea rebound is a function of K/V.[120,122,123] Therefore, the degree of rebound may be exaggerated in ESRD patients who are small-statured, have severely compromised cardiac output, or are subject to intradialytic hypotension.[120,122] On average, the equilibrated Kt/V (which is the Kt/V calculated using the 30 min postdialysis BUN sample) is approximately 0.2 less than the single-pool Kt/V.[122,126] For most patients, urea rebound is almost complete 15 min after discontinuation of hemodialysis but, for a minority, it may require up to 60 min.

Because of the inability to routinely predict which patients will have significant urea rebound, and in view of the potential deleterious impact of urea rebound on the delivered hemodialysis dose, the double-pool model seems to offer a better estimate of the true dose of hemodialysis. However, although this model better quantifies intradialytic urea removal, and so results in a more precise Kt/V and NPCR,[123,127] the need to obtain a 30–60 min postdialysis BUN sample makes it impractical in routine clinical practice. To overcome this limitation, several investigators have proposed different formulae to estimate the double-pool or equilibrated Kt/V (Kt/V_{eq}). Two of the most widely accepted formulae were derived by Smye et al[120,128] and Daugirdas et al.[83,119,125] The formula of Smye et al:

$$C_{eq} = C_0 e^{-\lambda T} \text{ and } \lambda = [1/(T - T_s)] \ln (C_s/C_t)$$

where C_{eq} is the equilibrated postdialysis BUN concentration, C_0 is the predialysis BUN concentration, C_s is the BUN concentration at a time T_s following the start of dialysis, C_t is the BUN concentration at the end of hemodialysis, T is the duration of hemodialysis (in minutes), and T_s is the time at which C_s is drawn (in minutes). The resultant C_{eq} is used to calculate an equilibrated Kt/V. The Kt/V_{eq} formulae of Daugirdas et al vary depending upon whether the patient received hemodialysis through an arteriovenous angioaccess (art Kt/V_{sp}) or a venous catheter (ven Kt/V_{sp}):

Arterial $Kt/V_{eq} =$
art Kt/V_{sp} – (0.60 × [art Kt/V_{sp} ÷ t]) + 0.03
Venous $Kt/V_{eq} =$
ven Kt/V_{sp} – (0.47 × [ven Kt/V_{sp} ÷ t]) + 0.02

where Kt/V_{sp} is the value of calculated Kt/V from the single-pool urea kinetic modeling. This group derived two formulae based on the assumption that if all other variables in the hemodialysis prescription are equal, the urea rebound from a venovenous access is less than with an arteriovenous access.[83,125] As discussed in greater detail in a later section, cardiopulmonary recirculation is lessened with venovenous sampling. Hence, the two formulae for KT/V_{eq} calculation depending on the blood sampling site. Indifferent of the location of the angioaccess, the shorter the treatment time, the larger the overestimation of Kt/V_{sp} in contrast to the equilibrated dialysis dose, Kt/V_{eq}. The Daugirdas formula for arteriovenous access has been validated against measurement of equilibrated Kt/V in patients enrolled in a HEMO pilot study.[129]

Although it is increasingly recognized that conversion to a double-pool model can enhance the accuracy of the measurement of the delivered hemodialysis dose, routine substitution of Kt/V_{eq} for Kt/V_{sp} may be problematic, and so is not recommended.[70] Reasons for this position include the: (1) impracticality of obtaining a 30–60 min BUN sample after the completion of hemodialysis; (2) uncertainty about the longitudinal validity of the above formulae for estimation of equilibrated Kt/V for an individual patient, particularly in light of changes in cardiac and nutritional status; and (3) absence of studies characterizing the dose–response relationship between Kt/V_{eq} and patient outcomes. Furthermore, it has been argued that rigorous monitoring of the Kt/V_{sp} and application of the hemodialysis dose recommendations from stringently evidence-based practice guidelines,[69,70] will assure patient safety equally as well as the use of double pool models.[70] Virtually all patient outcome studies have relied upon single-pool Kt/V determinations. Although there are no completed prospective outcome studies in adult ESRD population using the Kt/V_{eq}, the HEMO study that uses both Kt/V_{sp} and Kt/V_{eq} as measures of the delivered dialysis dose[56,129] will provide guidance for the utility of the double-pool model.

Recirculation

An additional biophysical variable confounding measurements of the delivered dose of hemodialysis is the occurrence of recirculation. During the process of hemodialysis, some of the blood that enters the dialyzer inlet may have flowed from the outlet, without first passing through the peripheral capillaries. This flow of previously dialyzed blood from the dialyzer outlet to the inlet is termed recirculation,[124,130–132] and if present, represents a separate component of urea rebound. Urea rebound is separable into two temporal phases, an early and late phase, before and after 3 min postdialysis, respectively. In turn, early urea rebound may be segregated into two components, both occurring as a consequence of different types of recirculation. The first component is secondary to blood recirculation within the angioaccess and is termed access recirculation. The second component of early urea rebound is a consequence of cardiopulmonary recirculation.[132]

Access recirculation occurs when a proportion of the blood returning to the patient through the venous needle/port is immediately drawn back into the arterial needle/port and dialyzed again. Common reasons for the occurrence of access recirculation are when the: (1) arterial needle is incorrectly placed downstream of the venous needle; (2) venous limb of the angioaccess is used for the arterial flow into the dialyzer and vice versa; or (3) when the blood pump speed exceeds the flow rate through the fistula (see Fig. 83.3).[132] The latter usually is a result of a critical stenosis in the angioaccess. Without a stenosis, fistula flow rates easily exceed 700 mL/min and are unlikely to be superseded by the extracorporeal blood flow rate (Q_b). Access recirculation begins to resolve immediately upon the completion of hemodialysis and its effects are completely abolished in less than a minute (usually about 20 s). Therefore, in the setting of access recirculation, a postdialysis BUN sample obtained either without flushing recirculated blood from the arterial line, or within the first 30 s post hemodialysis, will result in an erroneously low BUN concentration and an excessively large Kt/V, URR, and NPCR. The second component of early urea rebound, cardiopulmonary recirculation, is inevitable when hemodialysis is performed using an arteriovenous angioaccess.[83,133,134] Cardiopulmonary recirculation arises because of the routing of just-dialyzed blood through the veins to the heart, pulmonary circuit, and back to the angioaccess without the passage of this blood through any urea rich peripheral tissues.[130,135] Like access recirculation, cardiopulmonary recirculation causes urea rebound that

begins approximately 20 s after completion of the hemodialysis treatment. This effect dissipates in 2–3 min. Cardiopulmonary recirculation is observed only in cases of arteriovenous access since with a venous access, all blood returning from the dialyzer passes through peripheral tissues before being returned to the dialyzer. Similar to access recirculation, improper timing for sampling of the blood for measurement of the postdialysis BUN concentration will result in erroneous results from urea kinetic modeling.[70,136]

Uniformity of dose quantification and blood sampling

As implied from earlier discussions, the method for drawing the pre- and postdialysis BUN samples can greatly impact the results of the KT/V or URR measurement independent of the hemodialysis dose. Therefore, adoption of the same method of hemodialysis dose quantification (either Kt/V or URR) for all patients in a given facility will enhance consistency and enable meaningful comparison of data for a given patient over time, between different patients in the same center,

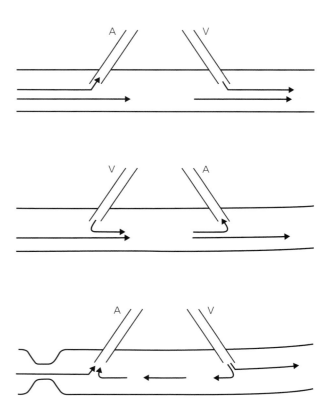

Figure 83.3 Schematic representation of angioaccess recirculation. A and V refer to the arterial and venous paths of blood flow, respectively. The uppermost panel illustrates the ideal situation of no access recirculation. The middle panel illustrates access recirculation secondary to reversal of the needle placement, so that the blood path is from the venous limb to the arterial limb of the access. The lower panel demonstrates access recirculation secondary to stenosis of the arterial limb of the access with resultant blood flow that is inadequate to meet the pump speed.[132]

and among different hemodialysis facilities.[136] In the absence of uniformity in measurement, meaningful longitudinal comparisons of delivered hemodialysis doses cannot be made. However, the adoption of one method of hemodialysis dose quantification does not preclude the use of another method as a supplementary measurement for some or all patients. Nevertheless, the dialysis facility must adopt a single, consistent, reproducible, and comparable measurement of the dose of hemodialysis. For example, if a center principally uses URR as the measurement of the delivered dose of hemodialysis, this can be supplemented episodically by the more precise measure of Kt/V derived from formal urea kinetic modeling. Similarly, a dialysis facility that uses single pool model Kt/V can supplement this with a measurement of the equilibrated Kt/V.

Blood sampling for the measurement of hemodialysis dose

Formal urea kinetic modeling To calculate Kt/V using formal urea kinetic modeling requires accurate measures of:

- pre- and postdialysis BUN concentration drawn at the first dialysis treatment of the week, and the predialysis BUN concentration at the following treatment in a thrice weekly hemodialysis schedule. Urea kinetic modeling based on two BUN samples (obtained on the pre- and postdialysis midweek BUN) has been described and validated for accuracy in comparison with classical three-sample urea kinetic modeling;[134]
- pre- and postdialysis weights at the time of the first dialysis treatment of the week;
- the actual treatment time (delivered time and not the prescribed time);
- the effective clearance of the dialyzer as calculated from the hemodialysis unit (not the in vitro value provided by the manufacturer that often overestimates the true in vivo value in plasma water).[137]

Daugirdas' second-generation natural logarithm formula To calculate Kt/V using the simplified Daugirdas formula requires:

- pre- and postdialysis BUN concentration drawn at the same hemodialysis session;
- the actual treatment time (delivered time);
- the patient's pre- and postdialysis weights.

Urea reduction ratio (URR) To calculate the URR requires:

- That pre- and postdialysis BUN concentrations are drawn at the same hemodialysis session. The accuracy of the calculated Kt/V or URR is highly dependent on proper blood sampling techniques for the pre- and postdialysis BUN concentrations.[136] Pre- and postdialysis blood sampling techniques must control for the site of the blood draw, needle or catheter preparation, blood and dialysate flow rates, ultrafiltration rate, and the timing of the blood sampling with respect to the initiation and termination of the hemodialysis treatment.[138] The ideal and accurate measurement of the Kt/V, URR, and NPCR requires:

- That predialysis BUN concentration is measured before hemodialysis begins and be obtained without dilution of the blood sample.[138]
- That postdialysis BUN concentration is measured after hemodialysis ends and angioaccess recirculation has resolved.[139,140]
- That laboratory processing of BUN samples is accurate.

Predialysis blood sampling procedures

The predialysis BUN must be drawn before dialysis begins to prevent this sample from being affected by the hemodialysis process. Sample dilution by heparin or saline must be avoided, or the predialysis BUN sample will register an artificially low concentration. A recent, evidence-based clinical practice guideline described a best clinical practice for blood sampling.[70]

Sampling technique when utilizing a fistula or graft

1. Obtain the blood specimen from the arterial needle prior to connecting the arterial blood tubing or flushing the needle. Ensure that no saline and/or heparin is in the arterial needle.
2. Do not draw sample if the hemodialysis treatment has commenced.

Sampling technique when utilizing a venous catheter

1. Withdraw any heparin and/or saline from the arterial port to prevent dilution of sample.
2. Using sterile technique, withdraw 10 mL of blood from the arterial port of the catheter. Do not discard this specimen if reinfusion is intended.
3. Connect a new syringe or collection device and draw the sample for BUN measurement.
4. Optional: reinfuse the 10 mL of blood withdrawn earlier. Initiate hemodialysis as per the dialysis unit's protocol.

Postdialysis blood sampling procedures

The timing of the acquisition of the postdialysis sample is even more critical.[136,138] Immediately upon completion of the hemodialysis treatment, if access recirculation is present, there will be some recirculated blood present in the angioaccess. If postdialysis blood sampling is performed in the presence of recirculated blood, it will dilute the blood sample and give a falsely reduced BUN concentration. This will result in an overestimation of the delivered dose of hemodialysis and the NPCR. Subsequently, cardiopulmonary recirculation and the double-pool effects will take place to complete the postdialysis urea rebound. As described earlier, although the most accurate method to account for these biophysical effects is to wait 30 min after the completion of dialysis, few patients will agree to waiting. An alternative, clinically applicable method that best supports the use of formal urea kinetic modeling is the "Slow Flow/Stop Pump Sampling Technique".[70]

Sampling technique for the postdialysis BUN concentration

1. At the completion of hemodialysis, turn off the dialysate flow (to terminate the hemodialysis process), and decrease the ultrafiltration rate to 50 mL/h (or to the lowest transmembrane pressure setting, or off).
2. Decrease the blood flow rate to 50–100 mL/min for 15 s. This step is performed to fill the arterial needle and blood tubing with nonrecirculated blood (to avoid the effect of access recirculation that may be present).
3. Proceed next with either of the two techniques: (a) slow flow or (b) stop pump.
   a. Slow-flow technique:
      i Immediately draw the blood sample for measurement of the postdialysis BUN concentration from the arterial needle/port.
      ii Stop the blood pump and complete the patient disconnection procedure as per dialysis unit protocol.
   b. Stop-pump technique:
      i After running the blood flow rate at 50–100 mL/min for 15 s to flush any recirculated blood from the angioaccess, immediately stop the pump.
      ii Clamp the arterial line and venous blood lines. Clamp the arterial needle tubing.
      iii The blood sample can be taken from the arterial port or the arterial needle tubing after disconnecting from the arterial blood line.
      iv Blood is then returned to the patient, and the disconnection procedure is continued and completed as per dialysis unit protocol.

Uniformity of blood sampling methods has several advantages. Firstly, as technical variability in blood sampling is minimized, the delivered doses of hemodialysis reported are comparable. Alternatively, a similar dose of hemodialysis reported by dialysis centers using different blood sampling methods may have varied "actual" dialysis doses, so are not comparable.[136] Secondly, the single-pool urea kinetic model mandates that the postdialysis BUN sample be measured without the effects of access recirculation and before significant urea rebound has occurred. The precise timing of the method of blood sampling advocated by the Kidney Disease Dialysis Outcomes Quality Initiative (KDOQI) meets this requirement.[70] Thirdly, the two recommended formulae for converting the single-pool Kt/V to a double-pool or equilibrated Kt/V value requires that the postdialysis BUN sample be obtained before urea rebound is completed. Therefore, the reproducibility and accuracy of these two blood sampling techniques outweigh the potential operational difficulties that may be encountered.

An alternative and widespread method of postdialysis BUN sampling is the Blood Reinfusion technique.[70] This involves blood sampling after the patient's blood has been completely reinfused. Its relative simplicity has made it a very popular technique, arguably with a lower likelihood of operational errors (the slow-flow/stop-pump techniques are more demanding technically).

For blood sampling by the blood reinfusion technique:

1. Return the patient's blood until the system is clear using a minimum volume of saline. The amount of saline used should be minimized, so that the postdialysis BUN concentration is not decreased because of systemic dilution from administered saline. This is a particular concern for patients with a small V. Tapping the dialyzer during blood return, or pinching the lines and releasing to flush the tubing may permit the use of less saline.
2. Clamp the blood and needle lines. Completely disconnect the patient from the extracorporeal circuit, as per the dialysis unit protocol.
3. Attach a 10-mL syringe to the arterial needle tubing using aseptic technique.
4. Unclamp arterial needle tubing/catheter. Withdraw and reinfuse 5–7 mL of blood several times to clear any remaining saline that could dilute the sample.
5. Clamp the arterial needle tubing/catheter after the line is filled with blood.
6. Utilizing a sterile technique, detach the syringe and set it aside.
7. Attach a multiple-sample luer adapter or a second syringe to vacutainer needle holder. Attach whichever of these devices is used to the end of the arterial fistula needle or catheter. Push the tube onto the holder.
8. Open the clamp on arterial needle tubing or catheter line to collect the postdialysis BUN sample. Clamp the line when the tube is full. Remove the adapter and needle holder or syringe.
9. Clamp the blood line, and complete the termination procedure as per dialysis unit protocol.

It is critical that the dialysis care team appreciate that the doses of hemodialysis measured by this blood sampling method will be systematically lower than those obtained using the slow-flow/stop-pump sampling techniques, even when the actual delivered dose of hemodialysis is the same.[136,139] This observed phenomenon is a consequence of variability in urea rebound that occurs in the time required for the sample to be obtained by the reinfusion technique. Therefore, continuous quality improvement initiatives that contrast the delivered dose of hemodialysis and NPCR between patients and facilities as clinical performance measurements, must not trivialize the potential for apparent differences arising from the blood sampling method alone.[136]

Frequency of the measurement of dialysis dose

Numerous outcome studies have correlated the dose of hemodialysis with patient morbidity and mortality.[22,27,28,30-32,34–38] As such, it is critical that the dose of hemodialysis be measured on a regular basis to ensure dialysis adequacy. Clinical signs and symptoms alone are not reliable indicators of hemodialysis adequacy. Measurement of the dose of hemodialysis should be performed monthly. This recommendation is based on the observation that most hemodialysis outcome studies relied upon monthly measurements.[21,30,35] Measurements performed less frequently may compromise the timeliness with which deficiencies in the delivered hemodialysis dose are detected, and hence may delay implementation of corrective steps. As in most dialysis facilities patients undergo monthly blood-based biochemical evaluations with monthly reporting of the institutional results, monthly measurement of the delivered hemodialysis dose is pragmatic. The frequency of dose measurement should be increased when patients are noncompliant and frequently miss treatments or have been "signed off" prematurely, for example when frequent problems are noted in the delivery of hemodialysis, such as poor blood flow, treatment interruptions, or clotting of the dialyzer; when wide variation in the delivered dose is observed in the absence of prescription changes; and/or when the hemodialysis prescription has been modified.

Defining and delivering an adequate dose of hemodialysis

Aggregate population recommendations

In 1996, the Renal Physician Association (RPA) released the first evidence-based, clinical practice guidelines on the adequacy of hemodialysis.[69] This document defined adequate hemodialysis as the "recommended quantity of hemodialysis delivered which is required for adequate treatment of ESRD such that patients receive full benefit of hemodialysis therapy."[69] At the time of its release, the only randomized, prospective, controlled trial that provided evidence for the required dose of hemodialysis was the National Cooperative Dialysis Trial (NCDS).[38] As previously discussed, reanalysis of the primary data from this trial showed that Kt/V values < 0.8 were associated with a relatively high rate of morbidity, whereas Kt/V between 1.0 and 1.2 were associated with a relatively lower rate of morbidity.[63] As described earlier, extrapolating from the NCDS to current dialysis practice is problematic, because of significant differences in patient mix and dialysis practice since the performance of the trial. Because of the paucity of definitive literature at the time of the RPA's Clinical Guidelines on Adequacy of Hemodialysis, a supplementary clinical decision analysis was performed using available data.[141] The initial analysis used a probabilistic model to assess how variables in the dialysis prescription effect a patient's quality-adjusted life expectancy (QALE). In a complementary analysis, lifetime costs and QALE were modeled to determine the "marginal cost-effectiveness of the components of the dialysis prescription."[142] On the basis of these analyses, the RPA recommended that "the delivered dose (Kt/V) should be at least 1.2."[69] For those using URR as a measure, the minimal dose (URR) should be at least 65%.[69] It should be noted that in the analysis by Hornberger,[142] the QALE continue to increase to a tested Kt/V level of 2.0. However, at Kt/V values of 1.4 and greater, a rapid increase in cost was noted secondary to the increased costs of the delivery of hemodialysis. This offset the savings achieved by fewer

hospitalizations. Thus, the RPA made a final recommendation that balanced the patient's quality-adjusted life expectancy and marginal cost-effectiveness of the dialysis dose.

Several published reports have suggested additional mortality benefit associated with a higher minimum dose of hemodialysis than advocated for in the RPA's Clinical Practice Guideline.[27,28,30-32,34,99] However, most of these reports were observational, retrospective analyses from self-selected dialysis centers. Some of their limitations include the comparison of patient outcomes to uncontrolled historical standards,[34,99] lack of randomization,[28,30,31] lack of standardization in the blood sampling method,[28,30,31] use of relatively broad categories of Kt/V or URR for analysis,[28,30,31] or major differences in clinical practice and patient behaviors compared to patients in the US.[99] Not all study results suggest an improved survival with delivered hemodialysis doses higher than Kt/V of 1.2 or URR of 65%.[22,29] A retrospective analysis of data from the Case Mix Adequacy Database, which used both single-pool (sp) and double-pool (dp) urea kinetic models, found no improvement in survival for a categorical Kt/V_{sp} of 1.2–1.4 or a Kt/V_{dp} of 1.0–1.2.[143] The NIH HEMO study will offer definitive guidance about the benefits of greater hemodialysis doses.

Based upon a review of the literature in this area of hemodialysis care since the publication of the RPA's Clinical Practice Guidelines, the DOQI Hemodialysis Adequacy Work Group recommended: (1) in the absence of definite and consistent evidence, the minimum dose of delivered hemodialysis as recommended should remain unchanged; and (2) the present literature does not support the definition of an optimal dose of hemodialysis.[70] Specifically, "the dialysis care team should deliver a Kt/V of at least 1.2 (single-pool, variable volume) for both adult and pediatric hemodialysis patients. For those using the URR, the delivered dose should be equivalent to a Kt/V of 1.2, i.e., an average URR of 65%. However, URR can vary substantially as a function of fluid removal".[70] In determining the minimum dose of hemodialysis as measured by the URR, it should be noted that the relationship between URR and Kt/V is greatly affected by the extent of the ultrafiltration.[84,85] Thus, the required URR to achieve the minimum adequate Kt/V of 1.2 can vary substantially as a function of fluid removal (see Fig. 83.1).

It is clear that many ESRD patients do not receive their prescribed dose of hemodialysis. Some previous studies reported that only 50% of the ESRD patients in the USA actually received their prescribed hemodialysis dose.[35,43] URR cannot be prescriptive, but it does offer a valid one-time analysis of the delivered dose of hemodialysis. Using the URR, a representative national survey of 6000 ESRD patients in the US revealed that in 1998 less than 75% of the patients surveyed received a URR ≥ 65%.[144] Although improvements in hemodialysis doses in the US have been achieved, a variety of factors can compromise the delivery of the prescribed hemodialysis dose.[35,43,105,145] These factors may be categorized into those that compromise urea clearance, reduce the hemodialysis treatment time, and/or result in errors in blood sampling. Again, it is emphasized that these problems in the delivered dose of hemodialysis will result in a discrepancy between the *V* derived from urea kinetic modeling and the *V* derived from anthropometric values (see Tables 83.1 and 83.2). A continuous quality improvement initiative that uses formal urea kinetic modeling will readily detect these problems in the delivered hemodialysis dose. In an effort to prevent the delivered dose of hemodialysis from declining to values below the recommended minimum dose, practitioners should prescribe doses of dialysis that are above these minimum values. In the NIH's HEMO study, where rigorous implementation and measurements of the hemodialysis prescription are executed, the 90% confidence interval for the single-pool *Kt/V* of 1.3 is 0.1 unit (personal communication, T. Greene, April 1995).[70] As such, KDOQI Practice Guidelines suggest that the prescribed minimum *Kt/V* should be 1.3.[70] For the URR, the HEMO study observed a 90% confidence interval of 4% (personal communication, T. Greene, April 1995).[70] Therefore, for those using URR, a minimum target URR of 70% should be set.[70] To achieve a desired *Kt/V*, *K* and *V* can be derived by various means and the treatment time *t* then determined. As such, *Kt/V* is prescriptive, but URR is not. In contrast to the *Kt/V*, strategies to increase the URR are subject to the preferences of the dialysis physician and are executed by trial and error. Specifically, an arbitrary estimate of the blood and/or dialysate flow rates, or the duration of treatment needed to achieve the target URR is prescribed and a follow-up URR is obtained. However, by using a series of nomograms, the URR can be correlated to an extrapolated *Kt/V*, and this value used to guide modification of the appropriate components of the hemodialysis prescription.[83]

Support for the current recommendation of a minimum *Kt/V* of 1.2 seems likely from the preliminary analysis of the results of the newly completed HEMO study. This prospective, randomized trial of two dialysis doses (equilibrated *Kt/V* of 1.05 versus 1.40) delivered by high-flux (β_2-microglobulin clearance > 20 mL/min) or low-flux dialyzers (β_2-microglobulin clearance < 10 mL/min) evaluated the independent and combined effects of both membrane flux of larger molecular weight solutes and dialysis dose on patient mortality and morbidity. Preliminary data analysis reveals no improvement in survival or decrease in hospitalization for all patients if they received a higher dialysis dose or greater membrane flux. Analysis of subgroups of patients is ongoing to determine if the absence of benefit is uniform.

Hemodialysis adequacy for selected patient subgroups

Diabetic patients

Collins et al[31] suggest that diabetics with ESRD may experience an approximately 40% reduction in their odds risk of death, if the minimum delivered Kt/V_{sp} is increased from 1.0–1.2 to ≥ 1.4. However, this finding has not been

observed uniformly in other studies of diabetics with ESRD.[30,143] Therefore, this discrepancy makes it difficult to routinely recommend a higher minimum dose of hemodialysis for diabetic patients.

Race and sex

Several observational analyses have reported that African-Americans with ESRD are more likely to receive less than the minimum appropriate dose of hemodialysis (as recommended by the RPA and DOQI).[144,146,147] However, this patient subgroup enjoys an improved survival rate in comparison to whites,[22,147,148] Despite knowledge of the cause of death, the basis of the improved survival for African-Americans is unclear. Potential explanations include: (1) the selective selection of healthier African-Americans for maintenance dialysis; (2) misdiagnosis or misclassification of the cause of ESRD among African-Americans; (3) improved nutrition among African-Americans; (4) African-Americans have better quality of life on dialysis and therefore adopt fewer deleterious health-related behaviors; and (5) a relatively lower susceptibility of African-Americans to the deleterious effects of inadequate hemodialysis.[147] A small body of evidence supports each of these conclusions. However, of relevance to the issue of appropriate hemodialysis dose by racial subgroups is a recent analysis using the patient database of Fresenius Medical Care (formerly National Medical Care, Lexington, MA, USA).[29] It is important to realize that all previous analyses of the relationship between the dose of hemodialysis and mortal risk were derived by statistically aggregating all patient subgroups (race, sex, diabetes), based on the assumption that their sensitivity is equivalent. Using a database of 18 144 representative ESRD patients, the analysis suggests that the previous clinical assumption of no difference in the odds risk of death among different racial groups and sex by URR is incorrect.[29] White patients (particularly white women) seem to be much more affected by the mortal risk of lower URR values than African-Americans (see Fig. 83.4). This differential racial sensitivity to lower hemodialysis doses, as measured by the URR, is not explained by differences in ages of patients. However, using a second-order equation to analyze death risk as a function of the URR, the death risk is minimized for all patient subgroups at a URR ≥ 65%, indifferent of the original discrepancy in death risk at lower URR values (see Fig. 83.5). This finding highlights the limitation of such subgroup analyses and suggests that efforts should be directed towards achieving this level of URR for all patients, regardless of the patient's race and sex (as recommended by the KDOQI Guidelines).[70] These findings underscore the limitation of URR and *Kt/V* as measures of the adequacy of hemodialysis, and support the contention that quality assurance efforts in this domain of care must be dynamic and reiterative to reflect the rapidly evolving knowledge base in dialysis care.

Twice-weekly hemodialysis

Twice-weekly hemodialysis is usually inadequate unless there is a significant amount of residual renal function (GFR > 5 mL/min). Because residual renal function

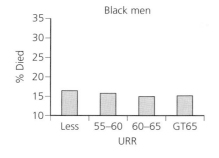

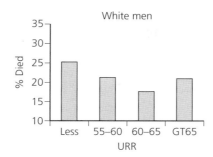

Figure 83.4 ESRD patient mortality as a function of urea reduction ratio (URR) categories for 1994. The patients have been partitioned by race and sex, and annual death rates determined.[29] GT means "greater than". In comparison to black men, white women were especially sensitive to URR values < 60%.[7]

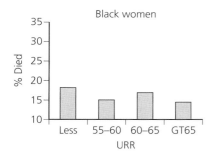

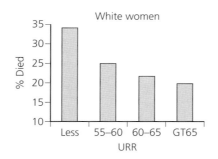

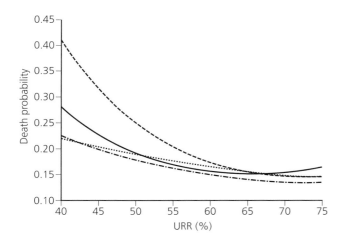

Figure 83.5 Age adjusted death probability for endstage renal disease patients as a function of urea reduction ratio (URR). The curve code is ······ black men; –·–·–·– black women; —— white men; –––––– white women. The URR is expressed as a second order variable.[29] Again, white women and men showed greater sensitivity to the mortality effects of URR values less than those recommended by the Renal Physician Association and DOQI Clinical Practice Guidelines on hemodialysis adequacy.[7]

declines with time, the presence of a significant amount of residual renal function at the initiation of maintenance hemodialysis mandates serial monitoring of renal function if the patient is undergoing twice-weekly hemodialysis. Such diligence will guide the appropriate addition of a third weekly hemodialysis treatment if renal function declines further. Unless the patients' residual renal function can be monitored serially and regularly, it is recommended that they are initiated on a thrice-weekly hemodialysis schedule from the onset.[70]

Inadequate delivery of hemodialysis – troubleshooting

Every effort should be made to ensure that ESRD patients receive their prescribed dose of hemodialysis. Whenever the prescribed dose falls below the minimum acceptable level, a systematic investigation should be initiated promptly to identify the cause of the deficiency. Because of the complexity and technical requirements of the hemodialysis procedure, deviations from the prescription may occur unintentionally. The dialysis care team must evaluate possible deviations that may significantly compromise the dose of hemodialysis. For this purpose, a clinical algorithm can be implemented in a dialysis facility to assist in the elucidation of potential technical problems (see Tables 83.2 and 83.3). Four treatment variables primarily affect the delivered dose of hemodialysis (as measured by Kt/V or URR). These variables are the clearance of the hemodialyzer, treatment duration, blood flow rate, and dialysate flow rates. Any of these components may vary for a given treatment. Therefore, small deviations in delivered dose are common and should be evaluated within the constraints of staff time and manpower. Significant underdelivery of the prescribed dose of hemodialysis (threshold of ≥ 20% decrement) should prompt further investigations. Errors that contribute to an apparent delivery of hemodialysis dose that is greater than that prescribed should also be investigated. Since the usual response to apparent overdelivery of the hemodialysis dose is by prescribing less dialysis, erroneous reports of overdelivery may lead to underdialysis with the anticipated consequences to morbidity and mortality. If the delivered dose of hemodialysis falls below a Kt/V of 1.2 or URR of 65% on a single determination, the dialysis care team is urged to consider the following interventions:

- Repeat the measurements and/or perform more frequent measurements of *Kt/V* or URR.
- Investigate potential errors using the clinical algorithm (see Table 83.3); in the interim, empirically increase the prescribed dose of hemodialysis.
- Suspend the use of the patient's reprocessed hemodialyzer (if dialyzer reuse is the practice of the unit).

References

1. Avram MM, Bonomini LV, Sreedhara R, Mittman N: Predictive value of nutritional markers (albumin, creatinine, cholesterol, and hematocrit) for patients on dialysis for up to 30 years. Am J Kidney Dis 1996;28:910–917.
2. Owen WF, Madore F, Brenner BM: An observational study of cardiovascular characteristics of long-term end-stage renal disease survivors. Am J Kidney Dis 1996;28:931–936.
3. USRDS/NIH-NIDDK 2001Annual Data Report: Atlas of End-Stage Renal Disease in the United States. Bethesda, MD: National Institutes of Health, National Institute of Diabetes and Digestive and Kidney Diseases, 2001.
4. Cheung AK: Quantitation of dialysis. The importance of membrane and middle molecules. Blood Purif 1994;12:42–53.
5. Vanholder R, De Smet R, Bogeleere P, Hsu C, Ringoir S: The uremic syndrome. *In* Jacobs C, Kjellstrand C, Koch K, Winchester J (eds): Replacement of Renal Function by Dialysis. Dordrecht: Kluwer Academic Publishers, 1996, pp 1–34.
6. Sharma K, Considine RV, Michael B, et al: Plasma leptin is partly cleared by the kidney and is elevated in hemodialysis patients. Kidney Int 1997;51:1980–1985.
7. Kabanda A, Jadoul M, Pochet JM, Lauwerys R, van Ypersele de Strihou C, Bernard A: Determinants of the serum concentrations of low molecular weight proteins in patients on maintenance hemodialysis. Kidney Int 1994;45:1689–1696.
8. Vanholder R, van Loo A, Dhondt AM, Glorieux G, De Smet R, Ringoir S: Second symposium on uraemic toxicity. Summary of a symposium held in Gent, Belgium, 22–24 September 1994. Nephrol Dialysis Transplant 1995;10:414–418.
9. Eschbach JW, Adamson JW: Anemia of end-stage renal disease (ESRD). Kidney Int 1985;28:1–5.
10. Mawer EB, Taylor CM, Backhouse J, Lumb GA, Stanbury SW: Failure of formation of 1,25-dihydroxycholecalciferol in chronic renal insufficiency. Lancet 1973;1(7804):626–628.
11. Cornelis R, Mees L, Ringoir S, Hoste J: Serum and red blood cell Zn, Se, Cs, and Rb in dialysis patients. Mineral Electrolyte Metab 1979;2:88.
12. Mahajan SK: Zinc metabolism in uremia. Int J Artif Organs 1988;11:223–228.
13. Golper TA, Ahmad S: L-carnitine administration to hemodialysis patients: has its time come? Semin Dialysis 1992;5:94–98.
14. Marcelli D, Stannard D, Conte F, Held PJ, Locatelli F, Port FK: ESRD patient mortality with adjustment for comorbid conditions in Lombardy (Italy) versus the United States. Kidney Int 1996;50:1013–1018.
15. Shinzato T, Nakai S, Akiba T, et al: Survival in long-term haemodialysis patients: results from the annual survey of the Japanese Society for Dialysis Therapy. Nephrol Dial Transplant 1996;11:2139–2142.
16. Held PJ, Brunner F, Odaka M, Garcia JR, Port FK, Gaylin DS: Five-year survival for end-stage renal disease patients in the United States, Europe, and Japan, 1982 to 1987. Am J Kidney Dis 1990;15:451–457.
17. Hull AR, Parker TF: Introduction and summary. Proceedings from the Morbidity, Mortality and Prescription of Dialysis Symposium, Dallas, TX, September 15 to 17, 1989. Amer J Kidney Dis 1990;15:375–383.
18. Keane WF, Collins AJ: Influence of co-morbidity on mortality and morbidity in patients treated with hemodialysis. Am J Kidney Dis 1994;24:1010–1018.
19. Hull AR: Predictors of the excessive mortality rates of dialysis patients in the United States. Curr Opin Nephrol Hypertens 1994;3:286–291.
20. Collins AJ, Hanson G, Umen A, Kjellstrand C, Keshaviah P: Changing risk factor demographics in end-stage renal disease patients entering hemodialysis and the impact on long-term mortality. Am J Kidney Dis 1990;15:422–432.
21. Owen WF Jr, Lew NL, Liu Y, Lowrie EG, Lazarus JM: The urea reduction ratio and serum albumin concentration as predictors of mortality in patients undergoing hemodialysis. N Engl J Med 1993;329:1001–1006.
22. Shaldon S. Unanswered questions pertaining to dialysis adequacy in 1992. Kidney Int Suppl 1993;41:S274–S277.
23. Tokars JI, Alter MJ, Favero MS, Moyer LA, Bland LA: National surveillance of dialysis associated diseases in the United States, 1991. ASAIO J 1993;39:966–975.
24. Held PJ, Blagg CR, Liska DW, Port FK, Hakim R, Levin N: The dose of hemodialysis according to dialysis prescription in Europe and the United States. Kidney Int Suppl 1992;38:S16–S21.
25. Held PJ, Levin NW, Bovbjerg RR, Pauly MV, Diamond LH: Mortality and duration of hemodialysis treatment. J Am Med Assoc 1991;265:871–875.
26. Reddan D, Szczech LA, Conlon PJ, Owen WF Jr: Contextual issues in comparing outcomes and care processes for ESRD patients around the world. Blood Purif 2001;19:152–156.
27. Szczech LA, Lowrie EG, Li Z, Lew NL, Lazarus JM, Owen WF Jr: Changing hemodialysis thresholds for optimal survival. Kidney Int 2001;59:738–745.
28. McClellan WM, Soucie JM, Flanders WD: Mortality in end-stage renal disease is associated with facility-to-facility differences in adequacy of hemodialysis. J Am Soc Nephrol 1998;9:1940–1947.
29. Owen WF Jr, Chertow GM, Lazarus JM, Lowrie EG: Dose of hemodialysis and survival: differences by race and sex. J Am Med Assoc 1998;280:1764–1768.
30. Held PJ, Port FK, Wolfe RA, et al: The dose of hemodialysis and patient mortality. Kidney Int 1996;50:550–556.
31. Collins AJ, Ma JZ, Umen A, Keshaviah P: Urea index and other predictors of hemodialysis patient survival. Am J Kidney Dis 1994;23:272–282.
32. Hakim RM, Breyer J, Ismail N, Schulman G: Effects of dose of dialysis on morbidity and mortality. Am J Kidney Dis 1994;23:661–669.
33. Lowrie EG: Chronic dialysis treatment: clinical outcome and related processes of care. Am J Kidney Dis 1994;24:255–266.
34. Parker TF 3rd, Husni L, Huang W, Lew N, Lowrie EG: Survival of hemodialysis patients in the United States is improved with a greater quantity of dialysis. Am J Kidney Dis 1994;23:670–680.
35. Acchiardo SR, Hatten KW, Ruvinsky MJ, Dyson B, Fuller J, Moore LW: Inadequate dialysis increases gross mortality rate. ASAIO J 1992;38:M282–M285.
36. Lowrie EG, Lew NL: Death risk in hemodialysis patients: the predictive value of commonly measured variables and an evaluation of death rate differences between facilities. Am J Kidney Dis 1990;15:458–482.
37. The National Cooperative Dialysis Study. Kidney Int Suppl 1983;13:S1–S122.
38. Lowrie EG, Laird NM, Parker TF, Sargent JA: Effect of the hemodialysis prescription of patient morbidity: report from the National Cooperative Dialysis Study. N Engl J Med 1981;305:1176–1181.
39. Tenckhoff H, Curtis FK: Experience with maintenance peritoneal dialysis in the home. Trans ASAIO 1970;16:90–95.
40. Tenckhoff H, Shilipetar G, Boen ST: One year's experience with home peritoneal dialysis. Trans ASAIO 1965;11:11–14.
41. Babb AL, Popovich RP, Christopher TG, Scribner BH: The genesis of the square meter-hour hypothesis. Trans ASAIO 1971;17:81–91.
42. Babb AL, Strand MJ, Uvelli DA, Milutinovic J, Scribner BH: Quantitative description of dialysis treatment: a dialysis index. Kidney Int Suppl 1975:23–29.
43. Delmez JA, Windus DW: Hemodialysis prescription and delivery in a metropolitan community. The St. Louis Nephrology Study Group. Kidney Int 1992;41:1023–1028.
44. Lindsay RM, Heidenheim AP, Spanner E, Baird J, Simpson K, Allison ME: Urea monitoring during dialysis: the wave of the future. A tale of two cities. Trans ASAIO 1991;37:49–53.
45. Djukanovic LJ, Mimic-Oka JI, Potic JB. The effects of hemodialysis with different membranes on middle molecules and uremic neuropathy. Int J Artific Organs 1989;12:11–19.

46. Asaba H, Alvestrand A, Furst P, Bergstrom J: Clinical implications of uremic middle molecules in regular hemodialysis patients. Clin Nephrol 1983;19:179–187.

47. Lowrie EG, Steinberg SM, Galen MA, et al: Factors in the dialysis regimen which contribute to alterations in the abnormalities of uremia. Kidney Int 1976;10:409–422.

48. Gotch FA, Sargent JA, Peters JH: Studies on the molecular etiology of uremia. Kidney Int Suppl 1975:276–279.

49. Leypoldt JK, Cheung AK, Carroll CE, et al: Effect of dialysis membranes and middle molecule removal on chronic hemodialysis patient survival. Am J Kidney Dis 1999;33:349–355.

50. Kazama JJ, Maruyama H, Gejyo F: Reduction of circulating beta$_2$-microglobulin level for the treatment of dialysis-related amyloidosis. Nephrol Dialysis Transplant 2001;16(Suppl 4):31–35.

51. Kay J: Beta$_2$-microglobulin amyloidosis. Amyloid: Int J Exp Clin Invest 1997;4:187–211.

52. Koch KM: Dialysis-related amyloidosis. Kidney Int 1992;41:1416–1429.

53. van Ypersele de Strihou C, Jadoul M, Malghem J, Maldague B, Jamart J: Effect of dialysis membrane and patient's age on signs of dialysis-related amyloidosis. The Working Party on Dialysis Amyloidosis. Kidney Int 1991;39:1012–1019.

54. Attman PO, Alaupovic P: Lipid abnormalities in chronic renal insufficiency. Kidney Int Suppl 1991;31:S16–S23.

55. Seres DS, Strain GW, Hashim SA, Goldberg IJ, Levin NW: Improvement of plasma lipoprotein profiles during high-flux dialysis. J Am Soc Nephrol 1993;3:1409–1415.

56. Eknoyan G, Levey AS, Beck GJ, et al: The Hemodialysis (HEMO) Study: rationale for selection of interventions. Sem Dialysis 1996;9:24–33.

57. Lowrie EG, Laird NM, Henry RR: Protocol for the National Cooperative Dialysis Study. Kidney Int Suppl 1983;13:S11–S18.

58. Sargent JA: Control of dialysis by a single-pool urea model: the National Cooperative Dialysis Study. Kidney Int Suppl 1983;13:S19–S25.

59. Parker TF, Laird NM, Lowrie EG: Comparison of the study groups in the National Cooperative Dialysis Study and a description of morbidity, mortality, and patient withdrawal. Kidney Int Suppl 1983;13:S42–S49.

60. Harter HR: Review of significant findings from the National Cooperative Dialysis Study and recommendations. Kidney Int Suppl 1983;13:S107–S112.

61. Laird NM, Berkey CS, Lowrie EG: Modeling success or failure of dialysis therapy: the National Cooperative Dialysis Study. Kidney Int Suppl 1983;13:S101–S106.

62. Gotch FA: Kinetic modeling in hemodialysis. In Nissenson AR, Fine RN, Gentile DE (eds): Clinical Dialysis, 3rd edn. East Norwalk, CT: Appleton & Lange; 1995, pp 156–188.

63. Gotch FA, Sargent JA: A mechanistic analysis of the National Cooperative Dialysis Study (NCDS). Kidney Int 1985;28:526–534.

64. Port FK, Orzol SM, Held PJ, Wolfe RA: Trends in treatment and survival for hemodialysis patients in the United States. Am J Kidney Dis 1998;32(Suppl 6:4):S34–S38.

65. Yeun JY, Depner TA: Principles of hemodialysis. In Owen WF, Pereira BJG, Sayegh MH (eds): Dialysis and Transplantation, 1st edn. Philadelphia: WB Saunders Co, 2000, pp 1–31.

66. Hume R, Weyers E: Relationship between total body water and surface area in normal and obese subjects. J Clin Pathol 1971;24:234–238.

67. Watson PE, Watson ID, Batt RD: Total body water volumes for adult males and females estimated from simple anthropometric measurements. Am J Clin Nutr 1980;33:27–39.

68. Chertow GM, Lazarus JM, Lew NL, Ma L, Lowrie EG: Development of a population-specific regression equation to estimate total body water in hemodialysis patients. Kidney Int 1997;51:1578–1582.

69. Committee of the Renal Physicians Association. Clinical Practice Guideline on Adequacy of Hemodialysis. Dubuque, IA: Kendall/Hunt Publishing, 1996.

70. NKFK/DOQI: Clinical Practice Guidelines for Hemodialysis Adequacy. Am J Kidney Dis 2001;37(Suppl 1):S7–S64.

71. Sargent JA, Gotch FA: Mathematic modeling of dialysis therapy. Kidney Int Suppl 1980; 10:S2–S10.

72. Sargent J, Gotch F, Borah M, et al: Urea kinetics: a guide to nutritional management of renal failure. Am J Clin Nutr 1978;31:1696–1702.

73. Little P, Barnett J, Margetts B, et al: The validity of dietary assessment in general practice. J Epidemiol Comm Health 1999;53:165–172.

74. Kortzinger I, Bierwag A, Mast M, Muller MJ: Dietary underreporting: validity of dietary measurements of energy intake using a 7-day dietary record and a diet history in non-obese subjects. Ann Nutrition Metab 1997;41:37–44.

75. Flanigan MJ, Lim VS, Redlin J: The significance of protein intake and catabolism. Adv Ren Replace Ther 1995;2:330–240.

76. Owen WF: Nutritional status and survival in end-stage renal disease patients. Mineral Electrolyte Metab 1998;24:72–81.

77. Leavey SF, Strawderman RL, Jones CA, Port FK, Held PJ: Simple nutritional indicators as independent predictors of mortality in hemodialysis patients. Am J Kidney Dis 1998;31:997–1006.

78. Yang CS, Chen SW, Chiang CH, Wang M, Peng SJ, Kan YT: Effects of increasing dialysis dose on serum albumin and mortality in hemodialysis patients. Am J Kidney Dis 1996;27:380–386.

79. Daugirdas JT: Second generation logarithmic estimates of single-pool variable volume Kt/V: an analysis of error. J Am Soc Nephrol 1993;4:1205–1213.

80. Lowrie EG, Lew NL: The urea reduction ratio (URR): a simple method for evaluating hemodialysis treatment. Contemp Dial Nephrol 1991;12:11–20.

81. Daugirdas JT: Rapid methods of estimating Kt/V: three formulas compared. Trans ASAIO 1990;36:M362–M364.

82. Flanigan MJ, Fangman J, Lim VS: Quantitating hemodialysis: a comparison of three kinetic models. Am J Kidney Dis 1991;17:295–302.

83. Daugirdas JT: Simplified equations for monitoring Kt/V, PCRn, eKt/V, and ePCRn. Adv Ren Replace Ther 1995;2:295–304.

84. Sherman RA, Cody RP, Rogers ME, Solanchick JC: Accuracy of the urea reduction ratio in predicting dialysis delivery. Kidney Int 1995;47:319–321.

85. Depner TA: Estimation of Kt/V from the URR for varying levels of dialytic weight loss: a bedside graphic aid. Sem Dialysis 1993;6:242.

86. Daugirdas JT: Linear estimates of variable-volume, single-pool Kt/V: an analysis of error. Am J Kidney Dis 1993;22:267–270.

87. Jindal KK, Manuel A, Goldstein MB: Percent reduction in blood urea concentration during hemodialysis (PRU). A simple and accurate method to estimate Kt/V urea. Trans ASAIO 1987;33:286–288.

88. Basile C, Casino F, Lopez T: Percent reduction in blood urea concentration during dialysis estimates Kt/V in a simple and accurate way. Am J Kidney Dis 1990;15:40–45.

89. Garred LJ: Dialysate-based kinetic modeling. Adv Ren Replace Ther 1995;2:305–218.

90. Bankhead MM, Toto RD, Star RA: Accuracy of urea removal estimated by kinetic models. Kidney Int 1995;48:785–793.

91. Ing TS, Yu AW, Wong FK, Rafiq M, Zhou FQ, Daugirdas JT: Collection of a representative fraction of total spent hemodialysate. Am J Kidney Dis 1995;25:810–812.

92. Keshaviah PR, Ebben JP, Emerson PF: On-line monitoring of the delivery of the hemodialysis prescription. Pediatr Nephrol 1995;9(Suppl):S2–S8.

93. Depner TA, Keshaviah PR, Ebben JP, et al: Multicenter clinical validation of an on-line monitor of dialysis adequacy. J Am Soc Nephrol 1996;7:464–471.

94. Depner TA, Greene T, Gotch FA, Daugirdas JT, Keshaviah PR, Star RA: Imprecision of the hemodialysis dose when measured directly from urea removal. Hemodialysis Study Group. Kidney Int 1999;55:635–647.

95. Depner TA: Assessing adequacy of hemodialysis: urea modeling. Kidney Int 1994;45:1522–1535.

96. Gabriel JP, Fellay G, Descombes E: Urea kinetic modeling: an in vitro and in vivo comparative study. Kidney Int 1994;46:789–796.

97. Lindsay RM, Henderson LW: Adequacy of dialysis. Kidney Int Suppl 1988;24:S92–S99.

98. Shinzato T, Nakai S, Akiba T, et al: Current status of renal replacement therapy in Japan: results of the annual survey of the Japanese Society for Dialysis Therapy. Nephrol Dial Transplant 1997;12:889–898.

99. Charra B, Calemard E, Ruffet M, et al: Survival as an index of adequacy of dialysis. Kidney Int 1992;41:1286–1291.

100. Charra B, Laurent G, Calemard E, et al: Survival in dialysis and blood pressure control. Contrib Nephrol 1994;106:179–185.

101. Rozich JD, Smith B, Thomas JD, Zile MR, Kaiser J, Mann DL: Dialysis-induced alterations in left ventricular filling: mechanisms and clinical significance. Am J Kidney Dis 1991;17:277–285.

102. Skroeder NR, Jacobson SH, Lins LE, Kjellstrand CM: Acute symptoms during and between hemodialysis: the relative role of speed, duration, and biocompatibility of dialysis. Artif Organs 1994;18:880–887.
103. Satoh Y, Iida T, Yamashita M, et al: Nature of refractory hypertension and its role in left ventricular function in patients on long-term hemodialysis. Nihon Univ J Med 1988;30:147–156.
104. Rocco MV, Burkart JM: Prevalence of missed treatments and early sign-offs in hemodialysis patients. J Am Soc Nephrol 1993;4:1178–1183.
105. LeFebvre JM, Spanner E, Heidenheim AP, Lindsay RM: Kt/V: Patients do not get what the physician prescribes. Trans ASAIO 1991;37:M132–M133.
106. Kinet JP, Soyeur D, Balland N, Saint-Remy M, Collignon P, Godon JP: Hemodynamic study of hypotension during hemodialysis. Kidney Int 1982;21:868–876.
107. de Vries JP, Kouw PM, van der Meer NJ, et al: Non-invasive monitoring of blood volume during hemodialysis: its relation with post-dialytic dry weight. Kidney Int 1993;44:851–844.
108. de Vries JP, Bogaard HJ, Kouw PM, Oe LP, Stevens P, De Vries PM: The adjustment of post dialytic dry weight based on non-invasive measurement of extracellular fluid and blood volumes. ASAIO J 1993;39:M368–M372.
109. Jahn H, Schohn D, Schmitt R: Hemodynamic modifications induced by fluid removal and treatment modalities in chronic hemodialysis patients. Blood Purif 1983;1:80–89.
110. Fishbane S, Natke E, Maesaka JK: Role of volume overload in dialysis-refractory hypertension. Am J Kidney Dis 1996;28:257–261.
111. Sulkova S, Valek A: Role of antihypertensive drugs in the therapy of patients on regular dialysis treatment. Kidney Int Suppl 1988;25:S198–S200.
112. Gotch FA, Sargent JA, Keen ML: Whither goest Kt/V? Kidney Int Suppl 2000;76:S3–S18.
113. Tattersall JE, DeTakats D, Chamney P, Greenwood RN, Farrington K: The post-hemodialysis rebound: predicting and quantifying its effect on Kt/V. Kidney Int 1996;50:2094–2102.
114. Lowrie EG, Chertow GM, Lew NL, Lazarus JM, Owen WF: The urea [clearance × dialysis time] product (Kt) as an outcome-based measure of hemodialysis dose. Kidney Int 1999;56:729–737.
115. Gotch FA: Kt/V is the best dialysis dose parameter. Blood Purif 2000;18:276–285.
116. Li Z, Lew NL, Lazarus JM, Lowrie EG: Comparing the urea reduction ratio and the urea product as outcome-based measures of hemodialysis dose. Am J Kidney Dis 2000;35:598–605.
117. Heineken FG, Evans MC, Keen ML, Gotch FA: Intercompartmental fluid shifts in hemodialysis patients. Biotechnol Progr 1987;3:69–73.
118. Cappello A, Grandi F, Lamberti C, Santoro A: Comparative evaluation of different methods to estimate urea distribution volume and generation rate. Int J Artif Organs 1994;17:322–330.
119. Daugirdas JT, Schneditz D: Overestimation of hemodialysis dose depends on dialysis efficiency by regional blood flow but not by conventional two pool urea kinetic analysis. ASAIO J 1995;41:M719–M724.
120. Smye SW, Evans JH, Will E, Brocklebank JT: Paediatric haemodialysis: estimation of treatment efficiency in the presence of urea rebound. Clin Phys Physiol Meas 1992;13:51–62.
121. Daugirdas JT: Bedside formulas for urea kinetic modeling. Contemp Dial Nephrol 1989;2:23–25.
122. Leblanc M, Charbonneau R, Lalumiere G, Cartier P, Deziel C: Postdialysis urea rebound: determinants and influence on dialysis delivery in chronic hemodialysis patients. Am J Kidney Dis 1996;27:253–261.
123. Abramson F, Gibson S, Barlee V, Bosch JP: Urea kinetic modeling at high urea clearances: implications for clinical practice. Adv Ren Replace Ther 1994;1:5–14.
124. Kaufman AM, Schneditz D, Smye S, Polaschegg HD, Levin NW: Solute disequilibrium and multicompartment modeling. Adv Ren Replace Ther 1995;2:319–329.
125. Daugirdas JT: Estimation of the equilibrated Kt/V using the unequilibrated post dialysis BUN. Semin Dialysis 1995;8:283–284.
126. Spiegel DM, Baker PL, Babcock S, Contiguglia R, Klein M: Hemodialysis urea rebound: the effect of increasing dialysis efficiency. Am J Kidney Dis 1995;25:26–29.
127. Stegeman CA, Huisman RM, de Rouw B, Joostema A, de Jong PE: Determination of protein catabolic rate in patients on chronic intermittent hemodialysis: urea output measurements compared with dietary protein intake and with calculation of urea generation rate. Am J Kidney Dis 1995;25:887–895.
128. Smye SW, Dunderdale E, Brownridge G, Will E: Estimation of treatment dose in high-efficiency haemodialysis. Nephron 1994;67:24–29.
129. Daugirdas JT, Depner TA, Gotch FA, et al: Comparison of methods to predict equilibrated Kt/V in the HEMO Pilot Study. Kidney Int 1997;52:1395–1405.
130. Sherman RA: Recirculation revisited. Semin Dialysis 1991;4:221–223.
131. Sherman RA, Levy SS: Rate-related recirculation: the effect of altering blood flow on dialyzer recirculation. Am J Kidney Dis 1991;17:170–173.
132. Tattersall JE, Chamney P, Aldridge C, Greenwood RN: Recirculation and the postdialysis rebound. Nephrol Dial Transplant 1996;11(Suppl 2):75–80.
133. Schneditz D, Kaufman AM, Polaschegg HD, Levin NW, Daugirdas JT: Cardiopulmonary recirculation during hemodialysis. Kidney Int 1992;42:1450–1456.
134. Depner TA, Cheer A: Modeling urea kinetics with two vs. three BUN measurements. A critical comparison. Trans ASAIO 1989;35:499–502.
135. Depner TA, Rizwan S, Cheer AY, Wagner JM, Eder LA: High venous urea concentrations in the opposite arm. A consequence of hemodialysis-induced compartment disequilibrium. Trans ASAIO 1991;37:M141–M143.
136. Owen WF Jr, Meyer KB, Schmidt G, Alfred H: Methodological limitations of the ESRD Core Indicators Project: an ESRD network's experience with implementing an ESRD quality survey. Am J Kidney Dis 1997;30:349–355.
137. Saha LK, van Stone JC: Differences between KT/V measured during dialysis and KT/V predicted from manufacturer clearance data. Int J Artif Organs 1992;15:465–469.
138. Lai YH, Guh JY, Chen HC, Tsai JH: Effects of different sampling methods for measurement of post dialysis blood urea nitrogen on urea kinetic modeling derived parameters in patients undergoing long-term hemodialysis. ASAIO J 1995;41:211–215.
139. Sherman RA, Matera JJ, Novik L, Cody RP: Recirculation reassessed: the impact of blood flow rate and the low-flow method reevaluated. Am J Kidney Dis 1994;23:846–848.
140. Daugirdas JT, Burke MS, Balter P, Priester-Coary A, Majka T: Screening for extreme postdialysis urea rebound using the Smye method: patients with access recirculation identified when a slow flow method is not used to draw the postdialysis blood. Am J Kidney Dis 1996;28:727–731.
141. Hornberger JC: The hemodialysis prescription and quality-adjusted life expectancy. Renal Physicians Association Working Committee on Clinical Guidelines. J Am Soc Nephrol 1993;4:1004–1020.
142. Hornberger JC: The hemodialysis prescription and cost effectiveness. Renal Physicians Association Working Committee on Clinical Guidelines. J Am Soc Nephrol 1993;4:1021–1027.
143. Levin NW, Stannard DC, Gotch FA: Comparison of mortality risk by Kt/V single-pool versus double-pool analysis in diabetic and non-diabetic hemodialysis patients (abstract). J Amer Soc Nephrol 1995;6:626.
144. Health Care Financing Administration, 1999 Annual Report. End-Stage Renal Disease Clinical Performance Measures Project. Baltimore: Department of Health and Human Services, Office of Clinical Standards and Quality, 1999.
145. Sargent JA: Shortfalls in the delivery of dialysis. Am J Kidney Dis 1990;15:500–510.
146. Sherman RA, Cody RP, Solanchick JC: Racial differences in the delivery of hemodialysis. Am J Kidney Dis 1993;21:632–634.
147. Price DA, Owen WF Jr: African-Americans on maintenance dialysis: a review of racial differences in incidence, treatment, and survival. Adv Ren Replace Ther 1997;4:3–12.
148. Bloembergen WE, Port FK, Mauger EA, Wolfe RA: Causes of death in dialysis patients: racial and gender differences. J Am Soc Nephrol 1994;5:1231–1242.

Complications Associated with Hemodialysis

Bertrand L. Jaber and Brian J. G. Pereira

Introduction

Since its experimental introduction in 1960, hemodialysis (HD) has become a widely performed and relatively safe procedure. Despite significant technological improvements in HD equipment and closer monitoring of patients by dialysis unit personnel, acute problems frequently occur during HD and can range from mild and transient, to catastrophic and fatal. This chapter will review the acute complications that are encountered during or directly related to HD therapy. The chronic organ system changes secondary to chronic renal failure and/or dialysis have been extensively reviewed elsewhere.[1]

Dialysis reactions

During HD, large volumes of blood are exposed to surface components of the extracorporeal circuit including the dialyzer, tubing, and other foreign substances related to the manufacturing and sterilization processes. This inter-action between the patient's blood and the extracorporeal system can lead to various adverse reactions (Table 84.1). These events represent a continuum of reactions that may range from mild to life-threatening anaphylactic/anaphylactoid reactions.[2]

Life-threatening anaphylactic and anaphylactoid reactions

Anaphylaxis is the result of an immunoglobulin E (IgE)-mediated acute allergic reaction in a sensitized patient, whereas anaphylactoid reactions result from the direct release of mediators by host cells. The onset of symptoms is usually immediate or within the first 5 min of initiation of dialysis, although a delay of up to 20 min may occur. Symptoms vary from subtle to quite severe and include burning/heat throughout the body or at the access site; dyspnea; chest tightness; angioedema; laryngeal edema; paresthesias involving the fingers, toes, lips or tongue; rhinorrhea; lacrimation; sneezing or coughing; skin

Table 84.1 Development, management, and prevention of dialysis reactions

Dialysis reaction	Onset during hemodialysis	Etiology	Course of action	Prevention
Life-threatening anaphylactic or anaphylactoid reaction	5–20 min	Ethylene oxide (first use dialyzer syndrome) Germicide (reuse dialyzer syndrome) AN69 dialyzer and ACE inhibitor interaction Renalin dialyzer reuse and ACE inhibitor interaction Medications (parenteral iron, heparin)	Stop hemodialysis Do not return blood to patient Epinephrine Corticosteroids Anti-histamines	Rinse dialyzer before use Use gamma/steam sterilized dialyzer Discontinue reuse with Avoid AN69 dialyzer wtih ACE inhibitor Discontinue reuse with renalin Use test dose for parenteral iron
Nonlife-threatening reaction	20–40 min	Complement activation	Continue hemodialysis	Use noncellulosic dialyzer membrane
Pyrogen reaction	Anytime	Endotoxin/bacterial contamination	Stop hemodialysis if hypotension present Blood cultures Antibiotics Antipyretics	Preventive strategies (Table 84.3)

flushing; pruritus; nausea or vomiting; abdominal cramps; and diarrhea. Predisposing factors include a history of atopy, elevated total serum IgE, eosinophilia and the use of angiotensin-converting enzyme inhibitors (ACEIs). The etiology of dialysis reactions (DR) is diverse and requires prompt investigation to help prevent further reactions.

Leachable substances

Allergy to ethylene oxide: "first use syndrome" The majority of severe DRs were initially ascribed to ethylene oxide (ETO) sterilized, complement-activating cellulosic membranes. Using a radioallergosorbent test (RAST), specific IgE antibodies against ETO conjugated to human serum albumin (HSA) were detected in patients with DR.[2] Indeed, when conjugated to human serum albumin, ETO acts as an allergen. While two-thirds of patients with such reactions have circulating IgE antibodies against ETO–HSA, one-third have a nonreactive RAST, possibly due to the adherence of ETO to a protein other than albumin, or due to non-ETO mediated mechanisms. Furthermore, 10% of patients with no prior history of DR have circulating levels of anti-ETO–HSA IgE antibodies.[2] ETO allergy became prominent with the introduction of hollow-fiber dialyzers. The potting compound used to anchor the hollow fibers in the dialyzer housing, acts as a reservoir for ETO and may impede its washout from the dialyzer. Indeed, even after prolonged periods of degassing and rinsing, the potting material may still contain significant amounts of ETO, leading to sensitization. Furthermore, delayed entry of ETO into the priming fluid has also been observed, and processing dialyzers before first use has reduced the incidence of these reactions.[2] If ETO allergy is suspected, changing to a gamma-sterilized or steam-sterilized dialyzer is appropriate.

Dialyzer reuse reactions: "reuse syndrome" As most residual ETO is washed out of the dialyzer during first use

and subsequent reprocessing, reuse reactions are likely to be due to other agents, such as the disinfectants used for dialyzer reprocessing. Commonly used disinfectants include formaldehyde, glutaraldehyde, and peracetic acid/hydrogen peroxide. Formaldehyde is a known allergen, and life-threatening reactions have been observed in HD patients in whom the RAST to formaldehyde was positive.[2]

Other leachable substances Other leachable substances suspected to cause DR include isopropyl myristate (used in the solution spinning process of hollow-fiber fabrication), isocyanates (found in the potting compound), and nonendotoxin *Limulus* amebocyte lysate (LAL)-reactive material (believed to be cellulose in nature and found during rinsing of cellulose hollow-fiber dialyzers).[2]

Membrane bioincompatibility

Evidence to support the hypothesis that life-threatening reactions follow complement activation during dialysis with unsubstituted cellulose membrane has been disputed.[2] Indeed, although DR have been observed during dialysis with complement-activating dialyzers, causality cannot be established as severe anaphylaxis itself causes C3a generation.[2] However, it is possible that secondary or concomitant release of complement fragments may amplify an IgE-mediated ETO reaction, for instance, by enhancing release of histamine or other mediators.[2]

Bradykinin-mediated reactions

Polyacrylonitrile (PAN) is a negatively charged synthetic membrane, which is composed of a copolymer of acrylonitrile and an aryl sulfonate. In recent years, severe anaphylactoid reactions have been reported in patients dialyzed with PAN membranes who were also on ACEIs.[2] Binding of Hageman factor XII to a negatively charged membrane leads to formation of kallikrein from prekallikrein, and the subsequent release of kinins (bradykinin) from kininogen. Although cuprophan and polymethylmethacrylate (PMMA) membranes display an ability to activate factor XII, PAN activates it to a greater extent.[2] Bradykinin is a molecule with a very short half-life that, in turn, activates production of prostaglandin and histamine release, with subsequent vasodilatation and increased vascular permeability. ACE inactivates bradykinin, and therefore, ACEIs can prolong the biological activities of bradykinin, which are highly calcium-dependent.[2]

Several anaphylactoid reactions have also been reported in patients dialyzed with bleach reprocessed polysulfone (PS) membranes and treated with ACEIs.[2] These reactions ceased once the use of bleach was discontinued. Furthermore, a cluster of anaphylactoid reactions was observed in patients dialyzed with different membranes and on ACEIs.[2] Hydrogen peroxide/peracetic acid was the reprocessing agent used, and the reactions abated once reprocessing was discontinued, despite continued use of ACEIs.

Dialysate factors

The use of acetate dialysate has been implicated in DR, and proposed mechanisms include interleukin-1 (IL-1) production by monocytes and prostaglandin/adenosine-mediated mechanisms.[2] Conversely, bicarbonate dialysate is highly susceptible to bacterial contamination, and bacterial products present in the dialysate can diffuse across both high-flux and low-flux membranes (see Bacterial contamination, below). Further, reprocessing of dialyzers, particularly with bleach, can increase the likelihood of reverse transfer of bacterial products from the dialysate to blood. These bacterial products can induce cytokine release by monocytes and consequently pyrogen reactions (PRs). Although PRs during dialysis are reported with a high frequency in dialysis units that use high-flux or reprocessed dialyzers, some authors suggest that they do not cause life-threatening reactions.[2]

Drug toxicity

Iron dextran Dextran, a mixture of synthetic glucose polymers, has been associated with systemic reactions. Anaphylactic reactions to iron dextran are due to this compound and occur in 0.6–1% of patient recipients.[2] The incidence of anaphylactic reactions is expected to rise, in view of the increasing need for parenteral iron dextran in erythropoietin-treated HD patients with absolute or functional iron deficiency. The precise mechanisms responsible for dextran-induced anaphylactoid reactions are elusive, but there seems to be dose-dependent histamine release from basophils that may account for the cardiovascular collapse.[2] Indeed, iron dextran at a dose >250 mg, is associated with hypotension and a serum sickness-like syndrome consisting of fever, headache, myalgia, arthralgia, and lymphadenopathy. Owing to this dose-related toxicity, iron dextran should always be initiated as a 25-mg test dose, with staff available to respond to reactions. If the test dose is uneventful, a course of therapy can then be given safely (100 mg/dialysis session for 10 doses).[3] Intravenous iron gluconate or sucrose may be an alternative for patients with severe iron deficiency anemia who are allergic to iron dextran.

Heparin Patients rarely exhibit hypersensitivity to heparin formulations but usually respond by substituting beef with pork heparin, or vice versa.[2] Heparin reduces aldosterone secretion by a direct action on the adrenal gland, leading to hypekalemia. It is not clear, however, whether this effect is due to heparin or its preservative, chlorbutol. The resultant hyperkalemia may be clinically significant in patients with underlying renal insufficiency.[2] However, this phenomenon has not been studied in the dialysis population, and heparin-associated complications are mainly related to bleeding (see Hemorrhage, below).

Deferoxamine Deferoxamine therapy for aluminum or iron chelation can produce hypotension during dialysis and rarely, allergic reactions, gastrointestinal disturbances, loss of vision, auditory toxicity, bone pain, or exacerbation of aluminum encephalopathy.[2]

Treatment and prevention

The treatment of severe anaphylactic and anaphylactoid reactions is similar; it requires immediate cessation of HD without returning the extracorporeal blood to the patient's circulation. Antihistamines (H_1 and H_2 antagonists), epinephrine, corticosteroids, and respiratory support should be provided if needed.[2] Specific preventive measures include rinsing the dialyzer immediately before first use, substituting ETO dialyzers with gamma- or steam-sterilized dialyzers, avoiding PAN membranes in patients on ACEIs, and possibly using angiotensin II receptor blockers instead of ACEIs in patients with dialyzer reuse reactions.

Mild reactions

Mild reactions consisting of chest or back pain often occur 20–40 min after initiation of HD with unsubstituted cellulose dialyzers. They are not characterized by anaphylactic or allergic reactions, and dialysis can usually be continued. Symptoms usually abate after the first hour, suggesting a relation to the degree of complement activation. Indeed, these reactions decrease with the use of substituted and reprocessed unsubstituted cellulose membranes, particularly when bleach has been omitted from the reuse procedure.[2] Some studies suggest that the incidence of chest and back pain parallels the degree of complement activation and increases with larger surface-area dialyzers.[2] However, a randomized crossover study comparing two similarly sized unsubstituted cellulose and PAN dialyzers showed no difference in these reactions between the two membranes, in spite of differences in complement activation.[2] Treatment with oxygen and analgesics is usually sufficient, and preventive measures include automated cleansing of new dialyzers or using noncellulose membranes.

Microbial contamination

Naturally occurring water bacteria commonly found in HD water systems include Gram-negative bacteria (GNB) such as *Pseudomonas* species and nontuberculous mycobacteria. GNB release endotoxin/lipopolysaccharide

(LPS) or other bacterial products, and nontuberculous mycobacteria are highly resistant to germicides.[2] Several factors during dialysis put patients at risk for exposure to bacteria and/or bacterial products, including contaminated water or bicarbonate dialysate, improperly sterilized dialyzers, and cannulation of infected grafts or fistulas.

Bicarbonate-containing solutions are highly susceptible to bacterial contamination.[2] If stored for too long, sodium bicarbonate breaks down to sodium carbonate that, along with glucose contained in the dialysate, is a growth medium for bacteria. When GNB reach excessively high concentrations in the dialysate, serious health risks to patients can occur, including PR with or without bacteremia. Indeed, outbreaks of clusters of infection in HD patients have been ascribed to bacterial contamination (Table 84.2). The passage of endotoxin from the dialysate into the blood can occur by diffusion or convection. The use of high-flux dialyzers, especially those reprocessed with bleach (which increases the permeability), increase the risk of passage of endotoxin from dialysate into blood – particularly of lipid A (~ 2000 Da), the active moiety of LPS. LPS interacts with plasma LPS-binding protein (LBP) and mediates cytokine production by interacting with the monocyte CD14 receptor.[2] Subsequent release of pyrogenic cytokines such as IL-1 and tumor necrosis factor produce a transient febrile reaction.[1]

Reprocessing of dialyzers has become a common practice in the USA because of decreased cost, improved biocompatibility, and fewer patient symptoms.[2] However, despite the general safety of this procedure, PR and bacteremia may supervene. Reprocessing involves rinsing, cleaning, testing, and sterilizing hollow-fiber dialyzers. PRs due to reprocessing have been attributed to improper disinfection procedures, inadequate potency of the solution used to disinfect the dialyzer, and inadequate measures to disinfect the O rings of dialyzers with removable headers.[2] In a survey by the Centers for Disease Control and Prevention in the US, the occurrence of PR in the absence of septicemia was reported by 21% of US dialysis centers.[4] Furthermore, the use of high-flux dialyzers (especially in conjunction with bicarbonate dialysate) and reprocessed dialyzers was associated with an increased incidence of PR.[4] Finally, intradialytic hypotension can also cause transient mesenteric ischemia that may be sufficient to damage the gastrointestinal mucosa, and lead to bacterial and/or LPS translocation.[2] Of note is an outbreak of bloodstream infection that was ascribed to repeated puncturing of single-use vials of epoetin-alfa.[5]

PR is a diagnosis of exclusion, as early septicemia should first be ruled out. Careful examination of the dialysis access is warranted, and blood cultures should be obtained. Treatment of PR includes antipyretics, empiric broad-spectrum antibiotics, cessation of ultrafiltration (UF) whenever hypotension is present, and selective hospitalization. An outbreak of bacteremia among several patients, involving a similar organism, should prompt a thorough search of the dialysis equipment for bacterial contamination.

Strategies for the prevention of PR are summarized in Table 84.3 and start with strict adherence to the standards of the Association for the Advancement of Medical

Table 84.2 Reactions and infections related to microbial contamination of dialysis fluids

Causative agents	Identifiable sources of contamination	Manifestations
Bacterial products		
Lipopolysaccharide	Back-filtration from enriched bicarbonate/glucose dialysate	Pyrogen reaction without bacteremia
	High-flux dialysis	
	Highly reprocessed dialyzers	
Microcystis aeruginosa exotoxin	Gut translocation following intradialytic hypotension	
(Microcystin-LR)	Carbon filters contaminated by blue–green algae	Acute hepatic necrosis
Bacteria		
Klebsiella pneumoniae	O-rings	Pyrogen reaction with bacteremia
Pseudomonas species	Hose connected to water spray device	
Xanthomonas maltophilia	Cross-contamination by technician's gloves	
Citrobacter freundii,	Cross-contamination of blood tubing by ultrafiltrate waste bag	
Acinetobacter species	Low levels of disinfectant	
Enterobacter species	Inadequate mixing of disinfectant with tap water	
Bacillus species	Inadequate potency of disinfectant despite standard measures	
Achromobacter		
Mycobacteria		
Mycobacterium chelonae abscessus	Inadequate potency of disinfectant despite standard measures	Pyrogen reaction with mycobacteremia
		Soft tissue infection
		Arteriovenous graft infection
Yeast		
Rhodotorula glutinis	Drain of hemodialysis machines	Unknown

Table 84.3 Strategies for prevention of bacterial contamination

Strict adherence to AAMI standards	Type of fluid	Microbial count	Endotoxin
	Water products	< 200 CFU/mL	< 2 EU
	Dialysate	< 2000 CFU/mL	No standard
	Reprocessed dialyzers	No growth	
Appropriate germicide	4% Formaldehyde*		
	1% Formaldehyde heated to 40°C*†		
	Glutaraldehyde†		
	Hydrogen peroxide/peracetic acid mixture (Renalin)*†		
	Heat sterilization (105°C for 20 h) for reprocessing of polysulfone membranes‡		
Wash and rinse the vascular access arm with soap and water			
Prior to cannulation, inspect vascular access for local signs of inflammation			
Scrub the skin with povidone iodine or chlorhexidine, allow to dry out for 5 min before cannulation			
Record temperature before and at the end of dialysis			
When central delivery systems are used	Clean and disinfect connecting pipes regularly		
	Remove residual bacteria or endotoxin by additional filtration		
When single-patient proportioning dialysis machines are used	Freshly prepare bicarbonate dialysate on a daily basis		
	Discard unused solutions at the end of each day		
	Containers should be rinsed and disinfected with fluids that meet AAMI standards, and should be air-dried before dialysate preparation		

*Minimum exposure of 11 h or 24 h to peracetic acid or formaldehyde, respectively, is required.
†These germicides are all equivalent or superior to 4% formaldehyde.
AAMI, Association for the Advancement of Medical Instrumentation; CFU, colony-forming units; EU, endotoxin unit.

Instrumentation (AAMI). In an era of high-flux dialysis and reuse, some authors believe that these recommendations are too liberal, and that sterile, pyrogen-free dialysis fluids should be used. Although this approach may offer clear advantages to patients, skepticism exists about the costs involved, and there is a lack of data to support its benefits.

Bloodline toxicity

Particle spallation

Bloodline components may enter the circulation by spallation, which is the release of silicone or polyvinyl chloride (PVC) particles induced by the roller pump.[6] Studies of the bioengineering aspects of spallation indicate these particles originate from cracks in the pump insert material, near the point of flexing; the cracks are caused by the repeated compression and relaxation of the tubing by the rollers.[6] With current high-flux technology demanding high pump speeds, spallation is more likely to occur. Quantitative studies indicate that the majority of particles released are < 5 μm in diameter and that the greatest release of particles occurs during the first hour of pumping. Although silicone has largely been replaced by PVC, the problem of spallation persists. Loading of animals with PVC or silicone particles induces IL-1 and prostanoid secretion by macrophages, and ascribed clinicopathologic effects include hepatomegaly, granulomatous hepatitis, and hypersplenism.[6] Future goals of bioengineering should include improving bloodline biocompatibility, with new designs of roller and pump segments, and internal coatings of the PVC tubing.

Leachable substances

The flexibility of PVC is achieved by the addition of a plasticizer, di(2-ethylhexyl)phthalate (DEHP). Phthalates are physically linked but not bound to PVC and hence may leach from the tubing matrix into the circulation. DEHP has been recovered from plasma and erythrocytes that were stored in plastic tubes.[6] While there is no clear evidence to confirm its toxicity, DEHP can bind to plasma lipids and lipoproteins, and significant tissue levels have been recovered at autopsy.[6] Furthermore, a hepatitis-like syndrome and necrotizing dermatitis have been reported in association with PVC exposure.[6] At present, bloodline reuse is practiced in 25% of dialysis units in the USA and may lead to biocoating of PVC tubing, giving a potential clinical advantage by reducing exposure to plasticizers.[6] Leachability studies of another plasticizer, trimellitate, from blood tubing show a lower release when compared with DEHP.[6]

Cardiovascular complications

Hypotension

Intradialytic hypotension requiring medical intervention occurs in 10–30% of treatments. The severity of hypotension in dialysis patients ranges from asymptomatic episodes to marked compromise of organ perfusion resulting in myocardial ischemia, cardiac arrhythmias, vascular thrombosis, loss of consciousness, seizures, and death. Any associated vomiting may be complicated by aspiration into the airways. Further, in patients with acute renal failure, intradialytic hypotension may induce further renal ischemia and retard recovery from acute renal failure.

The pathogenesis of intradialytic hypotension is complex.[7] UF rate and the volume of fluid removed are the primary causes for hypotension during dialysis. Indeed, a reduced plasma-refilling rate, coupled with impaired compensatory physiologic responses to hypovolemia, plays a major role. While UF rates of > 0.35 mL/min/kg will produce hypotension in most patients, slower UF rates with up to a 20% decrease in plasma volume are generally tolerated well. Analysis of the normal compensatory responses to hypovolemia suggests that central redistribution of the blood volume due to changes in peripheral vascular resistance are important for maintaining cardiac output. In dialysis patients, however, several factors impair the intradialytic increase in vascular resistance, and are due to patient-related and dialysis-related factors.[7] Patient-related factors include autonomic dysfunction (baroreflex impairment and alteration of heart rate responses) particularly in elderly and diabetic patients, use of antihypertensive medications, structural heart disease, cardiac arrhythmias, bacterial sepsis, hemorrhage, intradialytic venous pooling, increase in core body temperature, ingestion of food during dialysis, and anemia. Adenosine-mediated vasodilation due to acetate dialysate, low dialysate concentrations of sodium and/or ionized calcium, complement activation, or cytokine generation, may all contribute to intradialytic hypotension.[7] Indeed, IL-1 induces nitric oxide, which has been shown to correlate with intradialytic hypotension.[8] However, because cytokine generation may take several hours to occur, these contributing factors may account for prolonged postdialysis rather than intradialytic hypotension.[7] In addition, "sympathetic failure" has been well documented; this is due to the lack of an appropriate rise in plasma norepinephrine concentration during HD, and it may be a manifestation of baroreflex dysfunction and/or dialysis-related factors such as acetate dialysate.[7] The decreased sensitivity of the renin–angiotensin, adrenergic, and arginine vasopressin systems may also contribute to inadequate vasoactive responses to HD-induced hypovolemia.[7]

The immediate treatment of intradialytic hypotension is the restoration of the circulating blood volume by placing the patient in a Trendelenburg position while preventing aspiration, infusion of isotonic normal saline, infusion of hypertonic agents to enhance mobilization of extravascular fluid, and reduction/cessation of UF. With the advent of improved dialysis engineering principles, better preventive strategies have emerged. Indeed, cardiovascular instability and intradialytic hypotension have been minimized by the use of bicarbonate dialysate, volumetric control of UF, increased dialysate sodium concentrations, better assessment of the patient's "dry weight" (using bioelectric impedance or vena cava ultrasound), and the use of midodrine (an alpha-1 agonist), or cool dialysate (which increases catecholamines and vascular resistance).[9] The use of sodium modeling in a linear, step-drop or exponential program similarly reduces the incidence of hypotensive episodes. The use of salt-poor albumin offers no advantage to normal saline, but it costs more.

Other preventive strategies include: correction of anemia and hypoalbuminemia; withdrawal of antihypertensive drugs before dialysis; avoiding food before and during dialysis; counseling patients about weight gain; treating congestive heart failure and arrhythmias; and searching for other causes such as pericardial effusion.

Hypertension

Although less frequent than hypotension, hypertension occurring during or immediately after dialysis is an important risk factor for cardiovascular mortality. Indeed, cardiovascular disease is the leading cause of mortality in HD patients. Time-averaged blood pressure measurement correlates better with postdialysis blood pressure than with predialysis blood pressure, and dialysis patients often fail to show the normal "nocturnal dip" in blood pressure.

In two-thirds of patients, the mechanisms are partly volume-dependent. However, in up to half of patients, blood pressure control is not achieved despite fluid removal – a syndrome called "dialysis-refractory hypertension". In such patients, preexisting hypertension, volume depletion, hypokalemia-induced increased renin–angiotensin secretion, hypercalcemia-induced increased inotropism and vascular tone, and increased sympathetic tone during rapid UF in young patients with kidneys in situ, may play a role.[10,11] Intradialytic hypertension can also be precipitated by the use of hypernatric dialysate during sodium modeling.[12] Further, recombinant human erythropoietin (r-HuEpo) has been associated with a 20–30% incidence of new onset hypertension or exacerbation of hypertension, and transfusing HD patients to hematocrits of 40% is associated with increased blood viscosity and peripheral vascular resistance, and decreased cardiac output.[11] The higher vascular resistance in this situation is probably due to increased blood viscosity, which increases exponentially with the hematocrit, and the reversal of hypoxemic vasodilatation with correction of anemia.[11] Further, endothelial cell responses to various rheological and hormonal factors have been implicated partly in the pathogenesis of dialysis hypertension. Indeed, erythropoietin receptors are present on endothelial cells and elevated levels of endothelin-1, a potent vasoconstrictor, have been shown to correlate with increased blood pressure in patients receiving r-HuEpo intravenously (but not subcutaneously).[13] In addition, erythropoietin can cause a rise in resting cytosolic calcium concentration, which may increase vascular smooth muscle tone and vascular resistance.[14] Finally, in vitro studies also suggest a direct inhibitory effect of free hemoglobin on nitric oxide.

Although in practice an estimate of "dry weight" is determined clinically, treatment of intradialytic hypertension requires accurate determination of the patient's "dry weight."

It is reasonable to reduce the "dry weight" by 0.5 kg, observe the clinical response, and reevaluate periodically. A recent study using atrial natriuretic peptide measurements, suggests that a substantial number of patients with dialysis-refractory hypertension are not at their "true dry weight."[15]

Cardiac arrhythmias

Intradialytic atrial and ventricular arrhythmias are common in HD patients and the etiology is often multifactorial. Ischemic or hypertensive heart disease associated with left ventricular hypertrophy or congestive cardiomyopathy, uremic pericarditis, and conduction system calcification, are frequently encountered in adult patients with sustained or recurrent arrhythmias.[16,17] Silent myocardial ischemia is also common in dialysis patients. In addition, digitalis preparations, antiarrhythmic drugs, and other drugs, coupled with the constant acute and chronic alterations in fluid, electrolyte, and acid–base homeostasis, may precipitate arrhythmias during HD.[16] Indeed, hypocalcemia and hypomagnesemia may have additive effects on hypokalemia, whereas hypercalcemia, alkalosis and hypokalemia have additive effects on digitalis-related arrhythmias. Finally, myocardial ischemia from decreased myocardial oxygen delivery (due to intradialytic hypotension) or increased myocardial oxygen consumption (due to volume overload) can trigger arrhythmias in patients with underlying ischemic heart disease.

Measures to prevent arrhythmias include the use of bicarbonate dialysate and careful attention to dialysate concentrations of potassium and calcium. Use of zero potassium dialysate should be discouraged due to arrhythmogenic potential, and potassium modeling may be useful. In patients on digitalis, intracellular potassium shifts during dialysis should be minimized by ensuring that serum potassium does not fall below 3.5 mequiv./L, and by reducing both dialysate glucose and bicarbonate concentrations, when acid–base status permits. Serum digoxin levels should be regularly monitored and the need for the drug regularly reassessed. Dialysate calcium levels of 3.5 mequiv./L have been associated with cardiac ectopy in patients not taking digoxin.[17] Finally, maintenance of an adequate hemoglobin level, treatment of hypertension and congestive heart failure, and antianginal prophylaxis, offer additional precautions against cardiac arrhythmias. Whereas UF may improve myocardial oxygen consumption and reduce the likelihood of arrhythmias, intradialytic decrease in coronary blood flow has been demonstrated in adult HD patients,[18] and consequently may increase the risk of arrhythmias. Recognition and pharmacotherapy of acute and chronic arrhythmias in dialysis patients are beyond the scope of this chapter and have been reviewed elsewhere.[19]

Sudden death

Eighty percent of sudden deaths during dialysis are due to ventricular fibrillation and they are more frequently observed in the beginning of the week.[20,21] Although HD patients with ischemic heart disease are at increased risk for sudden death, other catastrophic intradialytic events need to be ruled out. The prompt recognition and treatment of life-threatening hyperkalemia, often encountered in young noncompliant patients, is imperative. When cardiopulmonary arrest occurs during dialysis, an immediate decision must be made as to whether the collapse is due to an intrinsic disease or whether technical errors have occurred, such as air embolism, unsafe dialysate composition, overheated dialysate, line disconnection, or sterilant in the dialyzer. Air in the dialysate, grossly hemolyzed blood, and hemorrhage due to line disconnection may be detected immediately. However, if no obvious cause is found, blood should not be returned to the patient, particularly if the arrest occurred immediately upon initiation of dialysis. A patient exposed to formaldehyde may have complained earlier of burning at the access site. If the event occurred during dialysis and a problem with dialysate composition is unlikely, blood may be returned to the patient; blood and dialysate samples should be sent immediately for electrolyte analysis, the dialyzer and blood lines saved for later analysis, and the dialysis machine replaced until all of its safety features are thoroughly evaluated for possible malfunction. While the management of cardiopulmonary arrest during dialysis should follow the standard principles of cardiopulmonary resuscitation, the diagnosis and management of technical errors are discussed later in this chapter.

Dialysis-associated steal syndrome (DASS)

Construction of an arteriovenous fistula or graft for HD access frequently results in reduction of blood flow to the hand. Although clinically significant ischemia does not usually result, symptomatic ischemia is by no means rare, particularly in patients with peripheral vascular disease and/or diabetes mellitus. Fistulas or grafts are classified as small if their diameter is < 75% of the diameter of the feeding artery, and large if > 75% of the diameter. Blood flow in the artery located distal to small fistulae or grafts remains orthodirectional, whereas larger fistulae or grafts cause retrograde flow in the distal artery, uniformly leading to "steal syndrome."[22] DASS has been reported in 6.4% and 1% of patients with radiocephalic fistulae or grafts, respectively.[23] Vascular steal can be exacerbated during HD. Symptoms of numbness, pain, and weakness of the hand may appear or worsen during HD, and clinical findings include coolness of the distal arm, diminished pulses, acrocyanosis, and (rarely) gangrene. Symptomatic DASS should be differentiated from other causes of painful limbs, including dialysis-associated muscle cramps, coexistent polyneuropathies due to diabetes mellitus or uremia, reflex sympathetic dystrophy, and entrapment mononeuropathies such as carpal tunnel syndrome associated with dialysis-related amyloidosis. Furthermore, acute ischemic monomelic mononeuropathy following the creation of an arm access is also known to occur,[24] and rapidly progressing acral gangrene may indicate calciphylaxis.

The evaluation of a painful hand includes pulse oximetry, plethysmography, Doppler flows, and arteriography. The treatment of DASS depends on its clinical severity and the anatomy of the access. Mild ischemia is common, manifest subjectively by coldness and paresthesias, and objectively by reduction in skin temperature, but with no loss of sensation or motion, and it generally improves with time.[25] The simplest way to improve distal perfusion is by ligation of the venous outflow of the fistula or graft. This procedure provides immediate improvement in perfusion but causes the elimination of a site for vascular access and the immediate need to form another one. There are other techniques that do not sacrifice the vascular access and yet improve distal perfusion. One is ligation of the artery distal to the origin of the fistula or graft, with or without establishing an arterial bypass from a point proximal to the fistula or graft to a point distal to the ligature. Alternatively, flow can be reduced by narrowing or "banding" the fistula or graft,[26] a method which has been refined by performing intraoperative digital plethysmography to assess the degree of luminal narrowing that is required.[23] Percutaneous transluminal angioplasty or laser recanalization is reserved for patients with inflow or outflow arterial disease.[27] Persistence of symptoms after an apparently successful correction of the vascular access flow should alert the clinician to other unrelated causes.

Neurologic complications

Muscle cramps

Prolonged involuntary muscle contractions or cramps are the most common acute neuromuscular complications observed during dialysis, and occur in 5–20% of patients.[28] Cramps are more frequently seen in anxious nondiabetic patients aged 30–50 years. They occur late during dialysis and frequently involve the legs. The discomfort typically takes 3 min to develop and 7 min to dissipate. Cramps lead to premature discontinuation of dialysis, accounting for about 15% of premature "sign-offs."[28] Electromyography performed during HD has shown tonic electrical activity in the muscles, which steadily increases throughout dialysis in those who develop cramps, as opposed to a steady decline in those who do not.[28] Furthermore, a subset of patients has an elevated predialysis level of serum creatinine phosphokinase during periods of cramps.[28]

The pathogenesis of intradialytic cramps is unknown. Plasma volume contraction and progressive hypoosmolality induced by HD are the two most important predisposing factors.[28] Hypomagnesemia and carnitine deficiency have also been incriminated.

The acute management of cramps is directed at increasing the plasma osmolality. Parenteral infusion of 23.5% hypertonic saline (15–20 mL), 25% mannitol (50–100 mL) or 50% dextrose in water (25–50 mL) has been shown to be equally effective.[29] However, hypertonic saline may result in postdialytic thirst, and both hypertonic saline and mannitol cause transient warmth or flushing during the infusion. Furthermore, large and repetitive infusions of mannitol may result in its retention, leading to increased thirst, interdialytic weight gain, and fluid overload.

Dextrose in water is preferred, particularly in nondiabetics, but causes transient hyperglycemia. A sublingual capsule of 10 mg nifedipine has been reported to provide relief of cramps without causing significant hypotension, and may be related to minimization of hypoosmolality-related changes in cellular ionized calcium levels.[28]

Preventive measures include dietary counseling to reduce excessive interdialytic weight gains. In patients without clinical signs of fluid overload, it is reasonable to increase the "dry weight" by 0.5 kg and observe the clinical response. In those patients who do not respond to the above measures, 5 mg of enalapril twice weekly has been shown to be effective, presumably by inhibiting angiotensin II-mediated thirst.[28] Oral quinine sulfate (325 mg) at the initiation of HD has been shown to reduce significantly the incidence of muscle cramps. Oxazepam at a dose of 5–10 mg, given 2 h before dialysis may also be effective in preventing cramps.[30] However, quinine sulfate is currently not approved as an over-the-counter product for the prevention of cramps and is only available by prescription; the Food and Drug Administration (FDA) in the US also regards it as both unsafe and ineffective except for its antimalarial properties. The use of sodium gradient HD is effective in minimizing intradialytic hypoosmolality and preventing hypotension. Proposed strategies include starting with a dialysate sodium concentration of 145–155 mequiv./L and a linear decrease to 135–140 mequiv./L by the completion of the treatment.[28,30] A comparison of sodium modeling using an exponential, linear, or step program has yielded similar results in decreasing intradialytic muscle cramping in young adults.[31] Finally, the affected muscle groups may benefit from stretching exercises during dialysis,[30] and carnitine supplementation has been shown to decrease the frequency of muscle cramps.[32]

Headache

Headache during dialysis is common and occurs in about 60% of HD patients.[33] The pain begins as a bifrontal discomfort 3–7 h into the dialysis session, and may become intense and throbbing, accompanied by nausea or vomiting. The headache is aggravated by the supine position and is not accompanied by visual disturbances.

The etiology of dialysis headache is unknown. It may be a subtle manifestation of the dialysis disequilibrium syndrome (DDS), or may be related to the use of acetate dialysate. The incidence of headaches may be lowered in several situations: with reused rather than new dialyzers; with dialysis sessions of 4 h rather than 2 h; with glucose-containing rather than glucose-free dialysate. It is not improved by the use of biocompatible membranes.[34] Furthermore, headache may be a manifestation of caffeine withdrawal, particularly in coffee-drinkers in whom an acute intradialytic drop in blood caffeine levels may be a precipitating factor.[30]

The treatment of dialysis headache consists of oral analgesics (acetaminophen). Preventive measures include a reduction in the blood flow rate during the early part of dialysis and a change to bicarbonate dialysate. Coffee ingestion during dialysis may also work.

Restless legs syndrome

The symptoms of restless legs syndrome (RLS) include deep paresthesias, and drawing and crawling sensations in the calves and legs that occur exclusively during rest and inactive seated or recumbent wakefulness, such as during HD.[35] Although the tendency to move can be momentarily suppressed, it is ultimately irresistible and movement of the legs yields prompt relief. Some patients also complain of discomfort bordering on pain at the same site. As a consequence, most patients have insomnia, and some suffer from anxiety or mild depression. The results of neurologic and electromyographic examinations are generally unremarkable.

Although the exact cause of RLS is unknown, iron deficiency anemia, vascular insufficiency, chronic lung disease, and abuse of caffeine have been implicated.[35] RLS is differentiated from peripheral neuropathy in which the paresthesias are constant and unrelieved by activity. The RLS may accompany early uremic neuropathy and disappear as the neuropathy progresses. Furthermore, RLS and insomnia are frequently encountered in severely uremic patients and are relieved within a few weeks of initiating dialysis therapy.[35] When symptoms develop in a stable HD patient, anxiety, progressive lower extremity vascular insufficiency, and inadequate dialysis need to be considered. Clonazepam taken before bedtime is temporarily effective but may result in unacceptable daytime drowsiness, whereas the shorter half-life benzodiazepines, such as temazepam, may preclude this effect.[35] Opiates are remarkably effective but have the potential for abuse and development of tolerance. Carbamazepine and levodopa have also been advocated but tolerance may develop rapidly.[35] Hence, a reasonable approach is to alternate chemically unrelated agents on a weekly or biweekly basis. These agents should be given early enough before dialysis to allow for absorption. Notably, in a nondialysis population the dopamine receptor agonist pramipexole has been shown to markedly ameliorate RLS.[36] A nonpharmacologic approach with transcutaneous electric nerve stimulation (TENS) is reserved for refractory cases, but experience of this is limited.[35] Once established, RLS is essentially a lifelong condition that may vary considerably in severity.

Dialysis disequilibrium syndrome (DDS)

Although DSS is no longer a frequent complication of maintenance dialysis, it is still a potential problem for patients with acute renal failure and patients with endstage renal disease (ESRD) who are starting HD, particularly with large surface area, high-flux dialyzers and shorter dialysis times. Risk factors include young age, severe azotemia, low dialysate sodium concentration, and preexisting neurologic disorders, such as recent stroke, head trauma, subdural hematoma, or malignant hypertension.[37] The incidence of DDS has decreased in recent years because of improvements in dialysis delivery technology, such as volumetric controlled machines, bicarbonate dialysate, sodium modeling, earlier recognition of uremic states, and earlier initiation of renal replacement therapy.

DDS commonly presents with restlessness, headache, nausea, vomiting, blurred vision, muscle twitching, disorientation, tremor, and hypertension. Major symptoms such as obtundation, seizures, coma, cardiac arrhythmias, or death occur occasionally. DDS usually occurs towards the end of dialysis and may be delayed up to 24 h. This syndrome is usually self-limited, but full recovery may take several days. Although cerebral edema is a consistent finding on computed tomographic scanning (CT scan), DDS remains a clinical diagnosis as laboratory tests, including electroencephalography (EEG), are nonspecific.

The pathogenesis of DDS is not fully known but it is largely due to cerebral edema. In early reports, DDS was attributed to transient osmotic disequilibrium due to more rapid removal of urea from blood than from cerebrospinal fluid (CSF), leading to an osmotic disequilibrium and subsequent cerebral edema. This "reverse urea effect" has been disputed.[37] Indeed, the development of paradoxical CSF acidosis during HD has been observed, with a resultant increase in osmotic activity, and it is aborted by slower dialysis.[37] Other factors that have been implicated include intracerebral accumulation of other osmotic solutes such as inositol, glutamine, and glutamate.[38]

Since DDS occurs during rapid HD, preventive measures include shorter and more frequent dialysis using small surface area dialyzers, high-sodium dialysate, and reduction in blood flow, especially in patients at risk for DDS. The use of a continuous infusion of mannitol during dialysis or the prophylactic use of anticonvulsants is not recommended, despite anecdotal reports of their efficacy.

Seizures

HD-associated seizures occur in < 10% of chronically dialyzed patients, but in a larger proportion of acutely dialyzed patients.[39] Seizures tend to be generalized and easily controlled. The presence of focal or refractory seizures, however, warrants evaluation for focal neurological disease, particularly intracranial hemorrhage. Other causes for seizures include DDS, uremic encephalopathy, acute aluminum intoxication, hypertensive encephalopathy, hypoglycemia, alcohol withdrawal, cerebral anoxia due to sustained intradialytic hypotension (i.e. from cardiac arrhythmias, hypersensitivity reaction, sepsis or hemorrhage), hyperosmolality due to hypernatremia, hypocalcemia, and use of epileptogenic drugs (i.e. theophylline, meperidine, β-lactamins). r-HuEpo therapy has also been implicated as a cause for seizures during dialysis. While this may be the case in hypertensive patients, where a rapid rise in hematocrit and subsequent rise in blood pressure may provoke hypertensive encephalopathy due to loss of autoregulation of the cerebral circulation, there is little evidence to suggest that seizures occur in normotensive patients on r-HuEpo.[40]

Treatment of established seizures requires cessation of dialysis, maintenance of airway patency, and investigation for metabolic abnormalities. Intravenous diazepam or clonazepam, and phenytoin may be required. Intravenous administration of 50% dextrose in water should be administered if hypoglycemia is suspected.

Acute aluminum neurotoxicity

Two distinct neurologic syndromes are associated with aluminum intoxication. The classic aluminum intoxication syndrome resulting from chronic exposure to oral or parenteral aluminum presents with insidious onset of "dialysis dementia," osteomalacia, microcytic anemia, and elevated plasma aluminum levels.[1] However, acute aluminum neurotoxicity occurs when the dialysate is contaminated with aluminum after administration of deferoxamine, resulting in higher aluminum levels, or following the concomitant oral intake of aluminum-based phosphate binders and citrate compounds. Citrate facilitates aluminum absorption in the small intestine, increases its solubility and promotes uptake by the central nervous system.[41] The acute onset of this syndrome consists of agitation, confusion, seizures, myoclonic jerks, coma, and death. Plasma aluminum levels are typically $> 500 \, \mu g/L$, and highly suggestive EEG findings include multifocal bursts of slow- or delta-wave activity and frequent spikes. The CT scan is usually normal and, in contrast to chronic aluminum toxicity, acute aluminum neurotoxicity in adults is fatal despite chelation therapy.

Hematologic complications

Complement activation and defective neutrophil and monocyte functions

HD patients are afflicted by several defects in cellular and humoral mechanisms including abnormal chemotaxis, adherence, phagocytosis, and release of mediators by neutrophils (PMN), impaired function of macrophage Fc receptors, and defective T-lymphocyte function.[1] Furthermore, during HD, blood is exposed to the dialyzer membrane and tubing, to soluble membrane constituents, bacterial products or solutes in the dialysate, and to the mechanical effects of being pumped through the HD circuit. These interactions can lead to activation of the complement, kinin, coagulation and fibrinolytic pathways, as well as cellular elements such as neutrophils, monocytes and lymphocytes.[33] Indeed, the magnitude of the activation of plasma and cellular elements of blood have been used as an index of "biocompatibility."[42] The definition of "biocompatibility" is frequently subject to the bias of the investigator or dialyzer manufacturer. The first dialyzers were made of cellulose ("unsubstituted cellulose"). However, high complement activation by hydroxyl groups on cellulose membranes (cellulose, cuprophan) and consequent activation of several plasma and cellular elements led to the development of newer membranes with lower complement-activating potential. These membranes have been loosely defined as "biocompatible".[42] Currently, the "biocompatible" membranes fall into two broad categories – the group of "substituted cellulose" dialyzers, wherein hydroxyl groups are substituted by tertiary amino groups (hemophan) or acetate (cellulose acetate and cellulose triacetate), and "synthetic" dialyzers, including PS, polyamide, PAN, PMMA, and polyvinyl alcohol. In general, biocompatible membranes activate less complement, have a higher β_2-microglobulin clearance, and greater hydraulic permeability. However, there is a considerable overlap between groups of dialyzers with respect to each of these properties.[42] Nonetheless, several reports have suggested that mortality in dialyzed patients with acute or chronic renal failure may be influenced by the selection of dialyzer membranes.

In the past decade, a number of clinical trials have compared the effects of cellulose-derived or synthetic dialyzer membranes on the clinical outcomes of patients with acute renal failure (ARF).[43] Table 84.4 summarizes the characteristics of these reports.[44] Limitations of these studies include quality differences, inconsistent randomization processes, absence of blinded dialyzer allocation, and the absence of power analyses. In some studies the comparison of synthetic to substituted rather than unsubstituted cellulose

Table 84.4 Summary of chronological trials assessing the impact of dialysis membrane biocompatibility on clinical outcomes in acute renal failure

Authors	Year	Trial type	Dialysis membrane		Patients (*n*)		APACHE II score		Survival (%)	
			BCM	BICM	BCM	BICM	BCM	BICM	BCM	BICM
Schiffl et al	1994	RCT	AN69	CU	26	26	24	24	62	35[†]
Hakim et al	1994	CT	PMMA	CU	37	35	29	29	57	37
Schiffl et al	1995	RCT	AN69, PAN	CU	38	38	23	24	63	34[†]
Kurtal et al	1995	CT	PA	CU	25	32	21	23	64	72
Assouad et al	1996	RCT	PMMA	CA	26	25	NR	NR	58	64
Himmelfarb et al	1998	CT	PMMA, PS	CU, HF	72	81	28	26	57	46[†]
Jörres et al	1999	RCT	PMMA	CU	84	76	24	23	60	58
Gastaldello et al	2000	RCT	PS	CA	89[*]	45	24	23[‡]	40	51
Albright et al	2000	CT	PS	CA	33	33	NR	NR	73	76

[*]Patients were randomized to either a low- (*n* = 41) or high-flux (*n* = 48) PS dialyzer.
[†]$P \leq 0.05$.
[‡]Survival was 37% and 42% in the low- and high-flux PS dialyzer groups respectively.
AN69, acrylonitrile 69; CA, cellulose acetate; CT, controlled trial; CU, cuprophan; HF, hemophan; NR, not reported; PA, polyamide; PAN, polyacrylonitrile; PMMA, polymethylmethacrylate PS, polysulfone; RCT, randomized controlled trial.

membranes may have confounded the results, as these dialyzers are not as bioincompatible. Further, the range of expected mortality among patients with ARF was very wide, rendering comparison between the studies even more difficult. None of the statistical analyses adjusted for dialysis dose, which may be an important determinant of outcomes.

An historical prospective study was based on a population drawn from the United States Renal Data System (USRDS) in collaboration with the ESRD networks in the USA; it studied 2410 randomly selected patients on chronic dialysis.[45] Compared to patients dialyzed with unsubstituted cellulose dialyzers, the adjusted relative mortality risk for patients dialyzed with either modified cellulose or synthetic dialyzers was 25–26% lower.[45] These data suggest that use of less biocompatible unsubstituted cellulose dialyzers was associated with an increased mortality in patients on chronic HD. More recently, similar data demonstrated a 31% lower adjusted relative infection risk among patients dialyzed with modified cellulose or synthetic dialyzers compared with unsubstituted cellulose dialzyers.[46]

The biological basis of the survival advantage in patients dialyzed with biocompatible membranes is speculative. Unsubstituted cellulose dialyzers are by far the most potent complement activators, resulting in activation of neutrophils, monocytes, and endothelial cells. Consequently, it is conceivable that the cells that are activated during dialysis may be less efficient in responding to subsequent challenges. Indeed, several cross-sectional studies and small short-term longitudinal studies have demonstrated multiple derangements in PMN function among patients on HD, particularly among those dialyzed with cellulose dialyzers.[1] In addition, several abnormalities in cytokine production by peripheral blood mononuclear cells (PBMCs) have also been reported.[47] However, to date, no definitive link has been established between the dialyzer membrane, immune cell dysfunction, and clinical outcome. Meanwhile, these observational studies should be interpreted as a demonstration of an association between the use of unsubstituted cellulose dialyzers and an increased mortality in patients on chronic HD. While these studies are "hypothesis-generating", a cause-and-effect relationship remains to be established between the use of unsubstituted cellulose dialyzers and increased mortality in patients on acute or chronic HD.

Intradialytic hemolysis

The causes of intradialytic hemolysis are shown in Table 84.5. Red blood cell (RBC) survival is decreased to around 66 days in HD patients despite good control of uremia, reflecting increased cell membrane fragility. During the early years of HD, dialyzer roller pumps caused traumatic RBC fragmentation,[48] and newer design technology has effectively eliminated this cause. Contamination of city water with chloramine, added to decrease bacterial contamination, or copper causes oxidative injury to RBC, leading to methemoglobinemia and acute hemolysis.[48] Deionization of the water supply or neutralization of the dialysis fluid with ascorbic acid, a reducing compound, can prevent complications from chloramine. Nitrate/nitrite

Table 84.5 Causes of intradialytic hemolysis

Mechanisms of injury	Etiologies
Traumatic fragmentation	Dialyzer roller pump
	Excessive suction at arterial access site
	Single needle dialysis
	High blood flow through a small needle
	Kinked dialysis catheter/tubing
	Right atrial subclavian catheter
Thermal	Overheated dialysate > 47°C
	Dialysate < 35°C, activation of anti-N cold agglutinin (formaldehyde)
Osmolar	Hypoosmolar dialysate
	Hyperosmolar dialysate
Oxidative injury	Chloramines
	Nitrite/nitrate
	Copper
	Drugs (quinine sulfate)
Reducing injury	Formaldehyde
Interference with cellular thiols	Copper
Interference with iron uptake	Aluminum
Inhibition of red blood cell glycolysis	Formaldehyde
G-6-PD* deficiency	Exacerbated by oxidants (quinine sulfate)
2,3-DPG† deficiency	Hypophosphatemia
Drug-induced microangiopathy	Quinine sulfate
Unknown	Zinc

*Glucose-6-phosphate dehydrogenase.
†2,3-Diphosphoglycerate.

intoxication can occur during home-HD of patients using well-water that is contaminated with urine from domestic animals, causing hemolysis via methemeglobinemia.

The retention of formaldehyde and hydrogen peroxide during dialyzer reprocessing has been associated with hemolysis.[48,49] Formaldehyde is a potent reducing agent that impairs RBC metabolism by inhibiting glycolysis, and may act as a hapten that induces hemolysis by formaldehyde-induced anti-N-like cold agglutinins.[48] Finally, rare causes that need to be considered include drug-induced hemolysis particularly in patients with glucose-6-phosphate dehydrogenase (G6PD) deficiency, microangiopathic hemolytic anemia (i.e., quinine sulfate), hypophosphatemia, hypersplenism, and insufficient dialysis.[48]

Patients with methemoglobinemia usually complain of nausea, vomiting, hypotension, and cyanosis, and oxygen therapy does not improve black-colored blood present in the extracorporeal circuit. Copper contamination should be suspected in the presence of skin flushing and abdominal pain or diarrhea. The diagnosis of acute hemolysis is self-evident when grossly translucent hemolyzed blood is observed in the tubing. Evaluation should include reticulocyte count, haptoglobin, lactodehydrogenase level, blood smear for schistocytes or Heinz bodies, Coombs test, and measurement of methemoglobin.[51] Survival of chromium-labeled RBC and examination of bone marrow may occasionally be indicated. More importantly, analysis of tap water for chloramines and metal contaminants, and thorough analysis of the dialysis procedure for clues of increased blood turbulence and mechanical RBC injury are recommended.

Thrombocytopenia

Heparin-induced thrombocytopenia is usually associated with heparin derived from bovine lung rather than bovine intestinal mucosa. The incidence of clinically suspected heparin-induced thrombocytopenia of 4% is probably an overestimate.[50] Pathophysiologic mechanisms have implicated an IgG-heparin immune complex disorder. Further, a delayed reaction that is associated with arterial and venous thrombosis may cause paradoxic clotting of the vascular access, and can be treated with low-molecular-weight heparin.[51] Transient thrombocytopenia may follow blood–membrane interactions and is maximum 1 h after starting dialysis, with platelet counts declining to < 100 000 per mm^3.[1] Further, thrombocytopenia may be secondary to other drugs commonly used during dialysis such as deferoxamine, vancomycin, or quinine sulfate.

Hemorrhage

Bleeding complications are commonly related to anticoagulation. Heparin confounds the uremic bleeding tendency, which is due to platelet dysfunction, abnormal platelet–vessel wall interaction, alteration of blood rheology and platelet adhesion due to anemia, and abnormal production of nitric oxide.[52] An increased incidence of spontaneous bleeding episodes has been reported in HD patients, particularly bleeding at specific sites such as gastrointestinal arteriovenous malformations, subdural hematoma, retroperitoneal bleeding, uremic hemopericardium, hemorrhagic pleural effusion, subcapsular hepatic hematoma, ocular anterior chamber hemorrhage, and skin hemorrhages including petechiae, ecchymosis, and subungual splinter hemorrhages.[53] Despite its limitations, the bleeding time is the best indicator of hemorrhagic tendency in dialysis patients. Specific treatment should be directed to the site of hemorrhage, and management of the bleeding propensity including treatment or reversal of uremic platelet dysfunction. Strategies to achieve improvement in platelet function include: an increase in r-HuEpo dose or transfusion of RBC to achieve a hematocrit > 30% in order to improve rheological platelets–vessel wall interactions; intravenous conjugated estrogens at 0.6 mg/kg/day for five consecutive days; intravenous or subcutaneous 1-deamino-8-D-arginine vasopressin (DDAVP) at 0.3 μg/kg over 15–30 min; and/or intravenous infusion of cryoprecipitate. For patients experiencing severe bleeding, particularly when related to anticoagulation, it is advisable to consider heparin-free dialysis, using normal saline flushes every 15–30 min with UF adjustments, regional heparin or citrate anticoagulation, low-molecular-weight heparin, heparin modeling, or prostacyclin.[1,54] In patients scheduled to undergo elective surgery or invasive procedures, it is recommended that aspirin is stopped a week earlier, the dose of anticoagulant is reduced to a minimum, and hematocrit is maintained above 30%. In some cases, DDAVP and/or estrogens may also be required.

Pulmonary complications

Hypoxemia

Upon exposure to bioincompatible dialyzers, in nearly 90% of patients, the arterial PaO_2 drops by 5–30 mmHg during HD, reaching a nadir between 30 and 60 min, and resolves within 60–120 min following discontinuation of dialysis.[1] This transient hypoxemia is commonly seen in patients dialyzed with unsubstituted cellulose dialyzers and with use of acetate dialysate.[55] The activation of the complement cascade following blood exposure to the free hydroxyl groups of cellulose membranes is believed to induce margination of leukocytes in the pulmonary vasculature, partly accounting for the observed ventilation/perfusion mismatch.[1] Other causes of this mismatch are related to impaired cardiac output due to a direct myocardial depressant effect of acetate.[55] However, the main factors implicated in the genesis of transient hypoxemia are due to hypoventilation that is itself of multifactorial origin.[55] Central hypoventilation occurs due to a decrease in carbon dioxide production following acetate metabolism (specific to acetate dialysate), loss of carbon dioxide in the dialyzer (with both acetate and bicarbonate dialysate), and rapid alkalinization of body fluids (specific to bicarbonate dialysate, particularly with large-surface-area dialyzers). The peripheral cause of hypoventilation has been ascribed to acetate-induced respiratory fatigue, especially in acutely ill patients. Finally, increased oxygen consumption in the order of 10% is observed during acetate dialysis and may contribute to hypoxemia.[55]

Transient dialysis-associated hypoxemia is usually of no clinical significance to patients unless preexisting chronic cardiopulmonary disease is present. Nevertheless, transient hypoxemia can be prevented by using biocompatible membranes, conventional bicarbonate dialysate and by increasing the fraction of oxygen in inspired air to 24–28% during dialysis.[55]

Sleep apnea

Sleep disturbances are reported in 67% of HD patients, compared to 14–42% in the general population.[56] Polysomnographic studies suggest a close correlation between sleep disturbances and blood urea nitrogen levels.[57] Sleep apnea (SA) affects 2–4% of the general adult population, and although unknown among HD patients, the prevalence may be as high as 30%.[57] Indeed, the prevalence of SA in the dialysis population is often underestimated since sleep during dialysis is often attributed to the long and boring nature of a HD session.

The pathogenesis of SA is unknown. Metabolic acidosis, chronic hypocarbia, and uremic toxins could result in central SA.[57] However, SA in HD patients is primarily obstructive in nature despite the fact that this population is not overweight, and has been ascribed to excessive reduction of muscle tone of the airway because of uremic myopathy or instability of respiratory control secondary to uremic neuropathy.[57] Furthermore, SA may be acutely worsened by HD due to removal of branch amino acids, or the use of acetate dialysate.[1] Elevated levels of circulating IL-1 and testosterone therapy have also been implicated.[57]

When present, snoring, nocturnal arousal, and excessive daytime sleepiness are highly suggestive of SA. The principal diagnostic test is a polysomnographic study performed in a sleep laboratory. In a cohort of patients who complained of daytime fatigue or sleepiness, polysomnographic studies demonstrated significant SA in up to 73% of those studied.[58] Careful detection of SA is important as nocturnal hypoxia may precipitate life-threatening cardiac arrhythmias, particularly in a population prone to metabolic abnormalities. The most useful and simplest treatment is the use of nasal continuous positive airway pressure (CPAP) which has significant pathophysiological consequences, including significant decrease in blood pressure, reduced arrhythmias, improved left ventricular function, and neuropsychological functions.[59] Clinical and polysomnographic improvement of SA has been documented following intensive HD and renal transplantation.[57,60] The regular use of screening questionnaires should be encouraged for early detection of SA in HD patients.[59] The effect of a high dose of dialysis or high-flux dialysis on SA has not been investigated.

Metabolic complications

Carbohydrate disturbances

Glucose intolerance encountered in uremia may result from an interplay between insulin resistance and decreased secretion. Insulin resistance has been attributed to altered receptor affinity that results in decreased specific binding of insulin along with increased level, and binding of glucagon to hepatic receptors.[1] Decreased secretion is due to decreased sensitivity of the β islet cells to glucose levels, and elevated parathyroid hormone (PTH) levels may interfere with insulin secretion.[61]

The initiation of HD usually improves glucose intolerance via several mechanisms, including the removal of uremic toxins that may contribute to insulin receptor alteration, positive calcium influx, and correction of total body potassium deficiency in patients previously on diuretics.[1] The use of glucose-free dialysate produces a net glucose loss of 30 g per dialysis treatment, whereas dialysate containing 200 mg/dL of glucose leads to a net glucose gain of 16–100 g per dialysis, a moderate caloric gain of up to 400 kcal per treatment. Diabetic HD patients do not develop volume contraction and hypersomolar coma despite significant hyperglycemia. However, hyperosmolality results in increased interdialytic weight gains due to increased thirst. Hyperkalemia and postdialysis hypokalemia can also occur. In some patients with type I diabetes mellitus, insulin requirement decreases significantly or even disappears, but the cause is unclear since residual endogenous insulin levels have not been reported.[1]

Hypoglycemia is rare, and usually a marker of multisystem failure. In uremic hypoglycemia, neuroglycopenic manifestations predominate because of coexistent autonomic dysfunction and lack of catecholamine response.[62] Use of insulin, oral hypoglycemic agents, propranolol (impairs glycogenolysis), salicylates, disopyramide (increases insulin secretion), or propoxyphene need to be investigated.[62] Additional triggering events are alcohol consumption, sepsis, chronic malnutrition, acute caloric deprivation, concomitant liver disease, congestive heart failure, or adrenal insufficiency.[62] Spontaneous hypoglycemia can occur and has been attributed to impaired glycogenolysis, diminished renal gluconeogenesis, impaired renal insulin degradation, and clearance.

Dialysate losses of alanine, a substrate for pyruvate synthesis may impair gluconeogenesis, and hypoglycemia associated with lactic acidosis can occur.[1] Postdialysis hypoglycemia is due to transient hyperinsulinemia that is induced by high dialysate glucose, and acetate that can suppress growth hormone secretion, a counterregulatory hormone.[1,62] Intradialytic parenteral nutrition (IDPN) can also result in postdialysis hypoglycemia which can be prevented by stopping IDPN 30–45 min before the end of dialysis. Finally, central pontine myelinolysis has been reported in diabetic dialysis patients, following frequent episodes of hyper/hypoglycemia.[63]

Lipid disturbances

Hyperlipidemia is common among HD patients, and the characteristic lipid abnormalities consist of elevated triglyceride levels, increased very low-density lipoprotein (VLDL) and decreased high-density lipoprotein (HDL) cholesterol.[1] HD patients usually have normal total cholesterol levels, and low levels are predictive of poor nutritional status and are associated with elevated mortality. Lipid disturbances in dialysis patients are primarily due to uremia and the etiologies include impaired lipolysis of VLDL due to a deficiency of lipoprotein lipase (LPL), presence of a poorly dialyzable LPL inhibitor, and disturbances in the apolipoprotein cofactors or lecithin-cholesterol-acyl transferase activity. Furthermore, hypertriglyceridemia may be exacerbated by the use of β-blockers, diuretics, androgens, or high carbohydrate diets. Associated abnormalities include increased chylomicron remnants and intermediate-density lipoprotein, and reduced levels of apolipoprotein A_1.[1]

Factors related to HD may also contribute to hyperlipidemia. Although acetate in the dialysate may be converted to long-chain fatty acids and cholesterol in the liver, careful studies suggest that < 5% is converted to lipids, and substitution of bicarbonate for acetate dialysate has no impact on lipid abnormalities.[1] Although absorption of glucose from peritoneal dialysate can lead to hyper-triglyceridemia, lower glucose concentrations present in dialysate do not contribute to hyperlipidemia in HD patients.[1] Heparin increases LPL activity and may transiently improve hypertriglyceridemia while increasing HDL cholesterol. Carnitine is necessary for oxidation of fatty acids and carnitine deficiency seen in HD patients could contribute to lipid abnormalities. However, dietary carnitine supplementation has had variable effects on lipid abnormalities.[1] Lipid peroxidation is increased in dialysis patients, due to decreased antioxidant activities such as ascorbic acid, tocopherol or selenium deficiency, and it is believed to accelerate atherosclerosis. Further, use of unsubstituted cellulose membranes intermittently activate neutrophil superoxide formation, and may result in increased lipid peroxidation.[64] Preliminary studies suggest that the use of high-flux dialysis may improve lipid abnormalities.[64] Finally, use of low-molecular-weight heparin instead of regular heparin has been shown to have beneficial effects on serum apolipoprotein levels.[65]

Treatment of hyperlipidemia includes dietary modifications that are usually difficult to institute due to preexisting dietary constraints imposed on HD patients. Drugs known to exacerbate hyperlipidemia should be avoided, and patients should be encouraged to exercise regularly. The use of lipid-lowering agents, such as gemfibrozil or a hydroxymethylglutaryl coenzyme A reductase (HMG CoA) inhibitor, increases LPL activity and cholesterol cell uptake, respectively. However, liver and muscle enzymes need to be closely monitored for the possibilities of drug-induced hepatitis or myositis. Finally, the use of eicosapentaenoic acid has also been suggested.[1]

Protein disturbances

Protein–calorie malnutrition is highly prevalent in HD patients and has been estimated to range between 20–70%. Increasing evidence links poor nutritional status to increased morbidity/mortality. Indeed, the National Cooperative Dialysis Study (NCDS) provides insights into the relation of urea and protein intake and suggests that dialysis adequacy is primordial in maintaining optimal protein intake. Furthermore, there is a significant correlation between low serum albumin and mortality.[66,67] Serum albumin concentration < 4 g/dL is a powerful predictor of mortality. The adjusted odds ratio of death is inversely related to serum albumin, and is about 1.48 for serum albumin concentration of 3.5–3.9 g/dL and 3.13 for concentrations of 3.0–3.4 g/dL.[66] The factors that affect the nutritional status of dialysis patients are decreased protein intake, anorexia due to uremic factors, gastrointestinal pathology, depression, comorbid illnesses, recurrent hospitalizations, multiple medications, and low socioeconomic status. Dialysis-related factors include the dose of dialysis, bioincompatible membranes, loss of amino acids into the dialysate, and the use of acetate, and high calcium dialysate.[67]

Compared to normal individuals, HD patients have significantly lower valine, serine, tyrosine, histidine and arginine levels, and significantly higher levels of taurine, aspartic acid, glycine, alanine, citrulline, proline and cystine,

reflecting a decreased essential amino acid/nonessential amino acid ratio.[1] Indeed, low valine levels correlate highly with established indices of malnutrition.[1] Recurrent losses of amino acids during HD are considerable and average 1.5–3 g per hour of dialysis. These losses are exacerbated by the use of glucose-free dialysate, reflecting increased gluconeogenesis due to mobilization of amino acids. In well-nourished patients, the dialysate losses of amino acids represent 3–4% of the weekly dietary intake of amino acids. Protein loss as high as 20 g in one HD session has been reported with PS dialyzers reprocessed with bleach. The negative nitrogen balance in patients on dialysis days, may be partly due to the loss of amino acids in the dialysate.[1] However, when protein intake is increased to 1.4 g/kg/day, the cumulative nitrogen balance (on dialysis and nondialysis days) becomes positive. Use of unsubstituted cellulose membranes has been linked to an increase in protein breakdown, due to release of prostaglandin (PGE$_2$) following blood–membrane interactions.[67]

Protein intake ≥ 1.2 g/kg/day and caloric intake ≥ 35 kcal/kg/day are usually sufficient to counteract lost amino acids. Glucose-containing dialysate should be used and protein intake of high biologic value should be emphasized. Recent studies promote the use of recombinant human growth hormone (r-hGH) as a potential strategy to promote anabolism in uremic patients.[67] IDPN is the most costly and least efficient nutritional supplement. Because of loss into the dialysate, only 70% of the nutrients are actually delivered to the patient. In a retrospective study, IDPN was beneficial in some patients with apparent improvement in serum albumin and survival.[68] IDPN should be considered in patients who cannot tolerate oral dietary supplements, but are able to ingest at least 50% of the prescribed caloric intake.[69]

Vitamin disturbances

Water-soluble vitamin supplements are recommended because of dietary restrictions, intradialytic losses and altered function of enzymatic systems.[1] The three water-soluble vitamins which are most likely to be deficient in the HD patient are folic acid, ascorbic acid (vitamin C), and pyridoxine (vitamin B$_6$). Folic acid deficiency may be due to inadequate intake, impaired absorption, interference with its activity by retained anions, or intradialytic losses, calculated at 100 μg/week.[70] Despite conflicting data on the need for folic acid supplementation, there is a consensus that discontinuation of folate supplementation does not result in deficiency for as long as 1 year.[70] Adequate folate levels promote RBC synthesis and may modulate homocysteine levels, a known cardiovascular risk factor. Recommended supplementation is 1 mg/day. Doses of ascorbic acid higher than 60 mg carry the risk of exacerbating hyperoxalemia/oxalosis.[1] Pyridoxine deficiency is caused by decreased intake or dialysate losses resulting in anemia, peripheral neuropathy, abnormal amino acid concentrations, and cell-mediated immune dysfunction.[1] The daily recommended dose of pyridoxine in HD patients is 10 mg. Intradialytic vitamin B$_{12}$ losses are insignificant with conventional dialyzers, but may be much larger with high-flux dialysis.[70] The recommended intake is 6 µg/day. Although several cases of Wernicke's encephalopathy have been reported in HD patients without a history of alcohol abuse, thiamine supplementation (vitamin B$_1$) is not routinely recommended unless malnutrition is present. Riboflavin, biotin and pantothenic acid levels are not usually decreased in HD patients, and no special supplementation appears to be required. However, biotin has been reported to improve several neurologic disorders in a small number of patients.[70]

Fat-soluble vitamins are usually not required except for vitamin D, which is discussed in the section on renal osteodystrophy. However, serum levels of vitamins A and E are usually elevated in HD patients and vitamin K deficiency does not occur unless the patient is receiving antibiotics.[1]

Electrolyte disturbances

Potassium removal during HD does not conform to single-pool kinetics.[71,72] The rate of removal of potassium from the extracellular space exceeds its rate of removal from the intracellular space. As serum potassium declines, the rate of removal decreases, but net potassium removal per treatment is around 100 mequiv., even with potassium-free dialysate. Potassium levels "rebound" within 5 h of finishing dialysis and may be 30% higher than immediate postdialysis values. Consequently, potassium supplementation in the postdialysis period, particularly before general anesthesia, should be avoided. The transfer of potassium from intracellular to extracellular compartments occurs at a slow rate and is affected by many factors, including pH, insulin, catecholamines, and membrane-bound Na$^+$,K$^+$-ATPase.

Potassium modeling and longer HD treatments have been suggested to avoid severe rebound.[71] The use of a zero-potassium dialysate bath should be avoided as it may precipitate rapid potassium fluxes, which may limit correction of acidosis, by impairing bicarbonate diffusion into the blood compartment.[72] Patients with marginal total body potassium stores (due to gastrointestinal losses) and metabolic acidosis are prone to life-threatening hypokalemia during HD, and intradialytic potassium losses combined with intracellular shifts due to correction of acidosis may acutely precipitate life-threatening muscle weakness or cardiac arrhythmias, particularly in patients on digoxin therapy.

Serum sodium disturbances in dialysis patients are usually due to incorrect dialysate concentration (see Technical malfunctions, below) and/or inadequate or excess consumption of free water.

Hypocalcemia is multifactorial and is usually secondary to hyperphosphatemia/dietary indiscretions, vitamin D deficiency, low calcium bath, or poor compliance, with calcium-containing phosphate binders or vitamin D therapy. Treatment includes a higher calcium bath, dietary counseling, and better compliance or timing of calcium-containing phosphate binders. Hypercalcemia is often associated with use of calcium-containing phosphate binders, with vitamin D therapy, malignancy and/or elevated calcium

dialysate. Treatment includes temporary discontinuation of vitamin D and calcium-containing phosphate binders, and HD using a low calcium bath may be necessary. The use of calcitonin or biphosphonate should be reserved for malignancy-associated hypercalcemia.

Hypophosphatemia can occur in dialysis patients, and when severe can cause respiratory arrest. Predisposing factors include poor nutritional intake, total parenteral nutrition (TPN), excessive phosphate binder therapy, or administration of frequent and intensive HD treatments. Although phosphorus levels can be increased by phosphorus-enriched dialysate, oral phosphorus supplementation usually suffices. Hyperphosphatemia usually reflects noncompliance with dietary restrictions, insufficient or inappropriate timing of phosphate binders to coincide with meals, use of phosphate-containing laxatives, or secondary hyperparathyroidism. Treatment includes reinforcing compliance with dietary restrictions, optimizing intake of binders, using large-surface-area dialyzers and longer HD treatment, and increasing phosphate clearance.

Hypomagnesemia is encountered in malnourished HD patients receiving TPN, whereas hypermagnesemia is caused by use of magnesium-containing laxatives, enemas, or antacids. Clinical manifestations include hypotension, weakness, and bradyarrhythmias, and HD is effective in lowering serum magnesium concentration.

Technical malfunctions

Air embolism

Improvements in dialysis machine safety monitors have reduced the incidence of air embolism. However, this catastrophic event can lead to death unless detected and treated early. The most vulnerable point of air entry into the extracorporeal circuit is the prepump tubing segment, where significant subatmospheric pressures of up to 250 mmHg prevail. Other points include other parts of the dialysis tubing, intravenous infusion circuits, especially with bottles, air bubbles from the dialysate, and central venous catheters. Furthermore, the use of high blood flows may allow rapid entry of large volumes of air despite small leaks.

Clinical manifestations depend on the volume of air, the site of introduction, the patient's position, and the speed at which air is introduced.[73] The volume of air required to produce clinical manifestations is unknown, and depends partly on preexisting cardiovascular or pulmonary disease. Microbubbles of air introduced at a slow rate dissolve slowly in the blood, and are better tolerated than macrobubbles, injected as a bolus. In the sitting position, air entry through a peripheral vein bypasses the heart and causes venous emboli in the cerebral circulation. The acute onset of seizures and coma, in the absence of precedent symptoms such as chest pain or dyspnea, is highly suggestive of air embolism. If the patient is supine, air introduced through a central venous line will be trapped in the right ventricle where it forms a foam and interferes with cardiac output and, if large enough, leads to obstructive shock. Further, dissemination of microemboli into the pulmonary vasculature occurs. In this event, dyspnea, dry cough, chest tightness, or respiratory arrest may occur. Further passage of air across the pulmonary capillary bed can lead to embolization to a major cerebral or coronary artery. Foam may be visible in the extracorporeal tubing and cardiac auscultation reveals a peculiar churning sound. In the Trendelenburg position, air emboli migrate to the venous circulation of the lower extremity, resulting in ischemia due to increased outflow resistance. Clinical manifestations include acrocyanosis, paresthesia and pain, and unless peripheral vascular disease coexists, the outcome is usually favorable.

Once the diagnosis is suspected, the first step is to clamp the venous blood line and stop the blood pump. For right heart air emboli, the patient is immediately placed in a recumbent position on the left side with the chest and head tilted downward. Cardiorespiratory support includes the administration of high-flow oxygen and endotracheal intubation and mechanical ventilation as needed. Aspiration of air from the ventricle by a percutaneously inserted needle or right atrial dialysis catheter can be attempted. If available, consideration should be given to hyperbaric oxygenation, where the patient undergoes decompression at a rate that allows the dissolved air to be expired through the lungs without coming out of solution[74].

Preventive measures depend primarily on dialysis machines that have venous air-bubble traps and foam detectors located just distal to the dialyzer, and a venous pressure monitor at the venous end. The detector is attached to a relay switch that simultaneously activates an alarm, shuts off the blood pump, and clamps the venous blood line if air is detected. Therefore, dialysis should never be performed with an inoperative air detection alarm system. Glass bottles containing intravenous solutions should be avoided since they create vacuum effects that can allow entry of air into the extracorporeal system. Further, dialysis catheters should be aspirated for blood return and flushed with saline before connection. When rinsing dialyzers with saline, all compartments should be filled up and air bubbles removed. Finally, in order to remove dissolved air, heating and degassing of dialysis water, particularly in the winter months, is accomplished by exposing heated water (34–39°C) to a high negative pressure during the purification process.[75]

Blood loss

Blood loss during HD can result from disengagement of the arterial or venous needle from the access, from separation of the venous or arterial line connections, from perforation or dislodging of the femoral or central line dialysis catheter, or from rupture of a dialysis membrane with or without malfunction of the blood leak detector. Clinical findings include hypotension, loss of consciousness, and cardiac arrest, sometimes within minutes of starting HD.[34] In addition, blood loss can occur following traumatic insertion of the dialysis catheter, leading to local pain from a rapidly expanding hematoma; to chest, shoulder, or neck pain from intrapericardial blood loss; to back,

flank, groin or lower abdominal quadrant pain or distention from retroperitoneal bleeding; or to hemoptysis from blood loss in the lungs.[34] Management of acute blood loss includes the immediate discontinuation of HD, pressure application for local hemostasis, hemodynamic support, and oxygen administration.

Incorrect dialysate composition

Incorrect dialysate composition occurs as a result of technical or human errors. There are two types of dialysate solution delivery systems. With central delivery, the solution used for the whole dialysis unit is produced by one machine by mixing liquid concentrate with purified water, and offers the advantage of reduced equipment and labor costs. With the individual system, each dialysis machine proportions its own dialysate liquid concentrate with purified water, permitting modification of the dialysate composition for a given patient. Because the primary solutes constituting the dialysate are electrolytes, the degree of dialysate concentration will be reflected by its electrical conductivity. Therefore, proper proportioning of concentrate to water can be achieved by a meter that continuously measures the conductivity of the dialysate solution as it is being fed to the dialyzer. Life-threatening electrolyte and acid–base abnormalities can be avoided if the conductivity alarm is functioning properly and the alarm limits are set correctly. However, in dialysis machines that are equipped with conductivity-controlled mixing systems, the system automatically changes the mixing ratio of the concentrates until the dialysate solution conductivity falls within the set limits. This may lead inadvertently to dialysate without any bicarbonate, with apparently acceptable conductivity. Therefore, if conductivity-controlled systems are used, it is safer to check also the dialysate pH before dialysis. Conductivity monitors can fail or can be improperly adjusted due to human error; nonetheless it is important for a person to monitor dialysate composition before every treatment, whenever a machine has been sterilized or moved about, or whenever a new concentrate is used. Furthermore, many nonstandardized solutions are available, some of which may be used with an inappropriate proportioning system. Therefore, it is essential that the supplies match the machine's proportioning ratio for which they were prepared to obtain the appropriate final dialysate composition.

Dysnatremias

Hypernatremia Hypernatremia occurs when concentrate or the ratio of concentrate to water is incorrect, and the conductivity monitors or the alarms are not functioning properly. The effects of hypernatremia are mainly caused by transcellular water shifts due to hyperosmolality, resulting in intracellular water depletion. Symptoms include profound thirst, headache, nausea and vomiting, seizures, coma, and death.[53] Aggressive treatment is essential, since mortality from acute severe hypernatremia (sodium > 160 mequiv./L) is greater than 70%.[76] Management includes cessation of dialysis, hospitalization, and infusion of 5% dextrose in water if the patient can tolerate a rapid increase in extracellular fluid volume. HD should be resumed using a different dialysis machine, particularly if a malfunction in conductivity monitoring is suspected. The dialysate sodium level should be 2 mequiv./L lower than the plasma level, and isotonic saline should be infused concurrently. Dialysis against a sodium level 3–5 mequiv./L lower than the plasma level may increase the risk of disequilibrium. UF with equal volume replacement with normal saline is another option.

Hyponatremia Failure to add concentrate, an inadequate ratio of concentrate:water, and malfunctions of the conductivity monitor or alarm can cause hyponatremia. Hyponatremia can also occur during the course of dialysis with a proportioning system, if the concentrate container runs dry and the conductivity set limits are inappropriate. Acute hypoosmolality causes hemolysis with hyperkalemia and hemodilution of all plasma constituents due to massive transfer of water from dialysate in the blood, leading to water intoxication.[53] Symptoms include restlessness, anxiety, pain in the vein injected with the hypotonic hemolyzed blood, chest pain, headache, nausea, and occasional severe abdominal or lumbar cramps. Pallor, vomiting, and seizures may be observed. Treatment of dialysis-induced hypoosmolality consists of clamping the blood lines and discarding the hemolyzed blood in the extracorporeal circuit. It is imperative to use high-flow oxygen and cardiac monitoring because of hyperkalemia and potential myocardial injury.[53] Dialysis should be restarted immediately, with a new batch of dialysate, a new dialyzer, and low-potassium dialysate, and a high transmembrane pressure should be applied to remove excess potassium and water.[53] Anticonvulsants are indicated for seizures, and blood transfusions may be needed for severe anemia. Finally, although acute (< 48 h) symptomatic hyponatremia has been corrected rapidly and safely with HD in nondialysis patients, there is no well-documented proof that HD against a high-sodium bath is safe in dialysis patients.[77] Even in the most acute symptomatic hyponatremic patient, a cautious approach is warranted, where a correction of sodium concentration by no more than 1–2 mequiv./L/h is the aim.[77]

Dyskalemias

The dialysate potassium concentration is usually 1–3 mequiv./L. Therefore, life-threatening hyperkalemia is uncommon in HD patients except in those who are markedly underdialyzed or following dietary indiscretion. Hyperkalemia can also develop following the use of single-needle dialysis.[53] Potassium-free dialysate should be discouraged, as it may precipitate cardiac arrhythmias, particularly in patients with left ventricular hypertrophy who are receiving digoxin, and may contribute to postdialysis fatigue. Intradialytic ECG monitoring should be reserved for problem patients on digitalis. Finally, with regards to the effects of packed RBC (PRBC) transfusion on potassium balance, various studies suggest that the potassium load per unit of transfused PRBC is 5–7 mequiv. for units stored for 14 and 21 days, respectively,[72] and,

therefore, intradialytic PRBC transfusion should not be discouraged.

Severe hypokalemia induced by HD can occur despite the use of a dialysate potassium concentration higher than that of the serum.[72] This is due to rapid correction of acidosis that leads to an intracellular shift of potassium. However, unless significant losses are due to vomiting, diarrhea, or nasogastric suction, hypokalemia is not generally considered a problem for HD patients.

Acid–base disturbances

HD patients have an alkali requirement of 240 mequiv. per treatment, taking into account daily acid generation and intradialytic losses of organic anions, which are bicarbonate precursors.[78] Detection and management of acid–base disorders in HD patients presents a challenge, because the serum bicarbonate is primarily regulated by dialysis.

Metabolic acidosis A downward trend in serum bicarbonate or an abrupt fall of more than 4 mequiv./L suggests the presence of a new metabolic acidosis.[78] Although acute intradialytic metabolic acidosis can occur due to improper mixing of concentrates or failure of pH monitors, other causes that need to be ruled out include diabetic or alcoholic ketoacidosis, lactic acidosis, toxic ingestions, increased protein catabolism, progressive loss of residual renal function, or dilutional acidosis.[78] When acetate dialysate is used, there is slight decrease in plasma bicarbonate during the first hour of dialysis because intradialytic bicarbonate losses have not yet been compensated for by the metabolism of acetate by muscle mitochondria. The diagnosis is usually suggested by the acute onset of hyperventilation during HD and confirmed by laboratory evaluation. Severe metabolic acidosis is treated by correcting the underlying cause, and HD with appropriate dialysate concentrate. In general, the use of acetate dialysate is not desirable because bicarbonate dialysate corrects acidosis in the most direct manner and provides better hemodynamic stability. Although dialysate bicarbonate levels of 35–38 mequiv./L are adequate in most circumstances, excessive correction of severe metabolic acidosis (bicarbonate < 10 mequiv./L), may lead to paradoxical acidification of the CSF and increased lactic acid formation by tissues.

Metabolic alkalosis The normal kidney can correct high plasma bicarbonate, whereas HD will maintain rather than repair metabolic alkalosis. Indeed, unless plasma bicarbonate is greater than 38–40 mequiv./L, no significant base is removed during HD with bicarbonate-based dialysate. However, with acetate dialysis, net alkali loss will occur when plasma bicarbonate is greater than 26–28 mequiv./L.[79] The presence of metabolic alkalosis is suggested by a rise in plasma bicarbonate by 4–5 mequiv./L from its usual value. Chronic respiratory acidosis usually does not need to be ruled out since plasma bicarbonate does not increase significantly in response to hypercapnia in anephric patients.[79] However, blood gas analysis is warranted to assess the respiratory response. Chloride-resistant alkalosis requires normal function for the maintenance of alkalosis and therefore, is unlikely to be observed in dialysis patients. The most common cause of metabolic alkalosis in HD patients is hydrochloric acid loss because of vomiting or nasogastric suction, and is usually seen in the setting of the intensive care unit (ICU). Attention should also be directed at identifying endogenous and exogenous sources of added alkali. Indeed, external sources of alkali or alkali precursors include sodium bicarbonate, calcium bicarbonate, citrate (blood products), lemon consumption, alkalinizing agents, lactate (Ringer solution), acetate (TPN solutions), and connection of the bicarbonate concentrate to the wrong port.[79] However, calcium bicarbonate supplementation, commonly used in dialysis patients, is minimally absorbed and, therefore, rarely produces elevation in plasma bicarbonate.[79] Finally, the combination of sodium polystyrene sulfonate (Kayexalate) and aluminum hydroxide can lead to absorption of alkali that is normally neutralized in the small intestine.[80] Acute treatment of metabolic alkalosis is rarely necessary as elevations to more than 40 mequiv./L are rarely seen because of bicarbonate removal by dialysis. Usually, removal of the alkali source is sufficient, and cimetidine (an H_2-receptor antagonist) or omeprazole (a gastric H^+,K^+-ATPase inhibitor) may be successful if loss of gastric acid is present. The administration of chloride salts to anephric patients with chloride-sensitive alkalosis will not repair the alkalosis, although reduction of plasma bicarbonate by dilution may be observed if large amounts are given. If a more rapid reduction in plasma bicarbonate is desired, modifying the dialysate bath (by replacing alkali with chloride, substituting bicarbonate with acetate dialysate, using acid dialysate, and hydrochloric acid infusion during citrate dialysis), is time-consuming, and these are often cumbersome therapeutic measures. Conventional bicarbonate dialysis or dialysis using lower dialysate bicarbonate levels (25–30 mequiv./L) is probably as effective and UF with saline replacement has been suggested.[79]

Severe metabolic alkalosis due to HD is rare and may be due to an error in the dialysate concentrates, reversed connection of bicarbonate and acid concentrate containers to the entry ports of the dialysis machine, or malfunction of the pH monitor. Furthermore, severe metabolic alkalosis can occur with regional citrate HD, and following continuous arteriovenous hemofiltration with dialysis.

Respiratory alkalosis The renal compensatory response to respiratory alkalosis or acidosis is absent in dialysis patients.[79] Acute respiratory acid–base disorders are, therefore, more likely to cause mixed acid–base disorders that may be life-threatening, due to extreme pH values.

During HD, despite losses of carbon dioxide into the dialysate, respiratory alkalosis does not occur. However, HD patients are more likely to suffer from anxiety, stroke and sepsis, which can cause respiratory alkalosis, and hepatic failure or pregnancy may be precipitating factors. Finally, an idiopathic hyperventilation syndrome has been described in a patient on CAPD, which disappeared once the patient was switched over to HD.[79]

Respiratory acidosis The concomitant presence of respiratory acidosis and renal failure is common in the ICU setting. REDY sorbent dialysis is a dialysate regenerating system, requiring only 6 L of dialysate compared to 120 L for a standard 4-h treatment.[81] The system comprises of a sorbent cartridge that has three different layers that participate in the epuration process. Although it offers some advantages over HD, REDY sorbent dialysis can cause acute hypercapnia.[81] Indeed, during dialysate regeneration, the breakdown of urea by urease that occurs in the second layer generates NH_4^+ and HCO_3^-. The third layer, consisting of zirconium phosphate, is a cation exchanger that exchanges Na^+ and H^+ for NH_4^+. Hence, carbonic acid is formed when HCO_3^- combines with H^+.

Fortunately, protons are partially buffered in the blood and carbon dioxide is eliminated by the lungs. However, the excess of carbon dioxide may be limited in patients with underlying pulmonary disease, resulting in hypercapnia and superimposed or worsening respiratory acidosis.[81] Moreover, blood returning from the patient is also hypercapnic and may contribute to furthering hypercapnia.

Mineral disturbances

In the early days of HD, dialysate was prepared using untreated tap water that contained high levels of calcium and magnesium. The "hard water syndrome" presents about an hour after the start of dialysis and symptoms include nausea, vomiting, hypertension, extreme weakness, lethargy (due to hypercalcemia), and a warm sensation in the skin (due to hypermagnesemia).[82] Acute pancreatitis may be observed. Currently, the water used for dialysate preparation is treated by deionization and reverse osmosis to control levels of divalent cations and to remove trace elements that may be present. However, in some rural areas the mineral content of the water is very high, and the syndrome can occur during home-HD despite seemingly adequate pretreatment of the water source. The diagnosis is confirmed by establishing elevated dialysate water calcium and magnesium levels. The first treatment is of the symptoms; dialysis should be stopped and restarted with properly treated water.

Metal contaminants that induce acute hemolysis include copper, zinc, and aluminum (see Intradialytic hemolysis, above). Intoxications with other metals such as lead and nickel may also occur.[53] Fluoride is a trace element that may accumulate in HD patients and deposit in bone.[83] Its contribution to renal osteodystrophy, however, is unclear.

Temperature monitor malfunctions

The heater raises the temperature of the incoming water to body temperature. Heating assists in the degassing of cold water and improves the mixing of water with dialysate concentrate. The internal controls of the thermostat are set up by the manufacturer to limit the dialysate temperature to 33–39°C. Malfunction of the thermostat in the dialysis machine can result in the production of excessively cool or hot dialysate. Accidental use of cool dialysate is not dangerous and has beneficial hemodynamic effects. However, a conscious patient will shiver, but hypothermia may occur in an unconscious patient. Overheated dialysate can cause immediate hemolysis and life-threatening hyperkalemia, particularly if the dialysate temperature rises above 51°C.[53] However, with temperatures of 47–51°C, the onset of hemolysis may be delayed for up to 48 h.[48]

If the dialysate temperature rises to 51°C, dialysis must be stopped immediately and blood in the system discarded. The patient should be monitored for hyperkalemia and transfused as necessary. Dialysis may be resumed to cool the patient by using dialysate temperature of 34°C, to treat hyperkalemia, and to allow blood transfusions. To prevent this potential catastrophic complication, visual and audible alarms are essential, as is a dialysate bypass for drainage, required with high-temperature alarms.

Miscellaneous complications

Postdialysis syndrome

An ill-defined "washed-out" feeling or malaise during or after HD is a common nonspecific symptom of about 33% of patients,[34] and has multifactorial origins. Reduced cardiac output, peripheral vascular disease, depression, poor conditioning, postdialysis hypokalemia or hypoglycemia, mild uremic encephalopathy, neuropathy, and myopathy may be contributing factors. Although this syndrome has been linked to membrane bioincompatibility via complement activation or cytokine production, a randomized, double-blind controlled study failed to show improvement by substituting cuprophan membranes with PS membranes.[84] Nonetheless, studies of amino acid balance suggest increased protein catabolism in the postdialysis period when unsubstituted cellulose membranes are used rather than cellulose acetate, PS or PAN membranes.[85] The use of glucose or bicarbonate dialysates has decreased the incidence of this syndrome, when compared to glucose-free, acetate-containing solutions. Malaise has also been ascribed to carnitine deficiency, which is important for muscle metabolism, and carnitine supplementation has been shown to improve patient well-being postdialysis.[32]

Pruritus

Pruritus is a common finding among dialysis patients, particularly in the summer. The etiology is often multi-factorial and includes xerosis, hypercalcemia, hyperphosphatemia from calcium phosphate crystal deposits in the skin, hyperparathyroidism, and inadequate dialysis.[86] Elevated plasma histamine and increased mast-cell proliferation in the skin have been reported in HD patients.[87]

In many cases, pruritus is more severe during or after dialysis and may be an allergic reaction to heparin, ethylene oxide, formaldehyde, or acetate. Indeed, in a subgroup of patients, use of gamma-sterilized dialyzers, cessation of use of formaldehyde as the germicide during reuse, and switching over to bicarbonate dialysate was associated with cessation of itching. Anecdotal reports suggest a likelihood of itching with cuprophan and new dialyzers compared to substituted cellulose and reused dialyzers.[34] Eczematous reactions to antiseptic solutions used to clean the vascular access site, rubber glove components (thiuram), nickel in the puncture needles, epoxy from glue in the tube-needle joint, or the collophane of glues used to maintain needles should be considered.[88]

Therapeutic strategies include the use of emollients and antihistamines, oral activated charcoal, ultraviolet therapy and sunbathing, ketotifen (a mast cell stabilizer), r-HuEpo therapy, or topical capsaicin.[87] Finally, dialysis prescription and adequacy should always be assessed.

Priapism

Priapism occurs in about 0.5% of male HD patients either during dialysis or 2–7 h after.[89] Although the majority of cases are idiopathic, a cause-and-effect relationship with HD has been suggested. Increased blood viscosity due to heparin, high hematocrit, r-HuEpo and androgen therapy, are the major incriminated factors.[90] Dialysis-induced hypoxemia, hypovolemia due to excessive UF, particularly in black men with sickle cell trait,[89] and the use of prazosin also play a role.[91] In the majority of patients, priapism is not related to sexual activity and occurs while on dialysis. The patient is usually awakened from sleep by a painful erection.

Prompt therapeutic interventions include corporal aspiration and irrigation. Dorsal penile block is achieved with 1% xylocaine without epinephrine, with intravenous sedation as necessary. Successful intracorporal irrigation with metaraminol has also been reported. Opiates are remarkably effective in controlling the pain but have the potential for abuse. Surgical procedures are designed to provide venous egress from the corpora cavernosa by way of a shunt. The prognosis is poor as secondary impotence is common despite bypass surgery. However, penile prostheses may be effective for the treatment of impotence.

Hearing and visual loss

The exact role of HD in hearing disturbances is unclear. Hearing impairment in HD patients has been reported[92] and may improve following transplantation.[93] In a recent audiometric study of HD patients, the incidence of hearing loss was 41% in the low, 15% in the middle, and 53% in the high frequency ranges, respectively.[93] Following a dialysis session, low frequency hearing improved in 38% of patients but worsened in 10%.[93] The low and high frequency losses, coupled with the spared middle frequency, result in a characteristic "dome-shaped" audiogram.[93] Advanced age, elevated plasma viscosity, and prior gentamicin administration are confounding factors of high frequency loss.[93] Improvement in low-tone frequencies after HD has been ascribed to the removal of uremic toxins, or fluctuations in fluid balance. Acute hearing loss during HD may be due to bleeding in the inner ear because of heparinization, or to hair cell injury of the cochlea from edema (endolymphatic hydrops).[53]

Visual loss is rare during HD, and is caused by occlusion of the central retinal vein, precipitation of acute glaucoma, anterior ischemic optic neuropathy associated with intradialytic hypotension, or Purtscher-like retinopathy due to leukoembolization.[94,95] Deferoxamine causes ocular toxicity and ototoxicity and serial audiovisual monitoring is required.[96] Finally, concomitant visual and hearing impairments can occur following the use of outdated cellulose acetate dialyzer membranes.[97]

Digoxin toxicity

HD patients are particularly prone to complications associated with the use of digoxin (see Cardiac arrhythmias, above). Coexistent metabolic alterations such as hypercalcemia, hypokalemia, and hypomagnesemia predispose to digoxin-induced arrhythmias, despite careful monitoring of drug levels. A syndrome consisting of recurrent abdominal pain associated with use of digoxin may occur shortly following dialysis, particularly after marked UF, and has been ascribed to digoxin-induced transient mesenteric ischemia.[53]

Acute fluoride poisoning

Fluoridation of municipal water is common, as is the reliance on reverse osmosis systems for dialysis water purification. Following exhaustion of deionizing columns, fluoride contamination of dialysate may cause acute fluoride poisoning. This manifests primarily by gastrointestinal symptoms and life-threatening hyperkalemia due to blockade of potassium channels, leading to significant extracellular potassium leakage.[98] This occurrence can be prevented by periodic testing of the dialysis water supply for fluoride content and maintenance of deionizing systems.

References

1. Lazarus JM, Denker BM, Owen WFJ: Hemodialysis. *In* Brenner BM, ed: The Kidney. Philadelphia: WB Saunders Company, 1996, pp 2424–2506.
2. Jaber BL, Pereira BJG: Dialysis reactions. Semin Dial 1997;10:158–165.
3. NKF–DOQI: Clinical practice guidelines for the treatment of anemia of chronic renal failure. National Kidney Foundation–Dialysis Outcomes Quality Initiative. Am J Kidney Dis 1997;30:192S-240S.
4. Tokars JI, Miller ER, Alter MJ, Arduino MJ: National surveillance of dialysis associated diseases in the United States, 1997. Semin Dial 2000;13:75–85.
5. Grohskopf LA, Roth VR, Feikin DR, et al: *Serratia liquefaciens* bloodstream infections from contamination of epoetin alfa at a hemodialysis center. N Engl J Med 2001;344:1491–1497.
6. Hoenich NA: Spallation and plasticizer release from hemodialysis blood tubing: a cause of concern? Semin Dial 1991;4:227–230.
7. Daugirdas JT: Dialysis hypotension: a hemodynamic analysis. Kidney Int 1991;39:233–246.
8. Beasley D, Brenner BM: Role of nitric oxide in hemodialysis hypotension. Kidney Int 1992;42:S96–S100.
9. Cruz DN, Mahnensmith RL, Brickel HM, Perazella MA: Midodrine and cool dialysate are effective therapies for symptomatic intradialytic hypotension. Am J Kidney Dis 1999;33:920–926.
10. Fellner SK: Intradialytic hypertension II. Semin Dial 1993;6:371–373.
11. Levin NW: Intradialytic hypertension I. Semin Dial 1993;6:370–371.
12. Sang GL, Kovithavongs C, Ulan R, Kjellstrand CM: Sodium ramping in hemodialysis: a study of beneficial and adverse effects. Am J Kidney Dis 1997;29:669–677.
13. Carlini R, Chamberlain I, Rothstein M: Intravenous erythropoietin (r-HuEPO) administration increases plasma endothelin and blood pressure in hemodialysis patients. Am J Hypertens 1993;6:103–107.
14. Vaziri ND: Cardiovascular effects of erythropoietin and anemia correction. Curr Opin Nephrol Hypertens 2001;10:633–638.
15. Fishbane S, Natke E, Maesaka JK: Role of volume overload in dialysis-refractory hypertension. Am J Kidney Dis 1996;28:257–261.
16. Bailey RA, Kaplan AA: Intradialytic cardiac arrhythmias I. Semin Dial 1994;7:57–58.
17. Kant KS: Intradialytic cardiac arrhythmias II. Semin Dial 1994;7:58–60.
18. Kenny A, Sutters M, Evans DB, Shapiro LM: Effects of hemodialysis on coronary blood flow. Am J Cardiol 1994;74:291–294.
19. Rutsky EA: Arrhythmias in hemodialysis patients. *In* Nissenson AR, Fine RN (eds). Dialysis Therapy. Philadelphia: Hanley & Belfus, Inc, 1993, pp 116–123.
20. Chazan J: Sudden deaths in patients with chronic renal failure on hemodialysis. Dial Transplant 1987;16:447–448.
21. Bleyer AJ, Russell GB, Satko SG: Sudden and cardiac death rates in hemodialysis patients. Kidney Int 1999;55:1553–1559.
22. Barnes RW: Hemodynamics for the vascular surgeon. Arch Surg 1980;115:216–223.
23. Odland MD, Kelly PH, Ney AL, Andersen RC, Bubrick MP: Management of dialysis-associated steal syndrome complicating upper extremity arteriovenous fistulas: use of intraoperative digital photoplethysmography. Surgery 1991;110:664–649 (Discussion 669–670).
24. Hye RJ, Wolf YG: Ischemic monomelic neuropathy: an under-recognized complication of hemodialysis access. Ann Vasc Surg 1994;8:578–582.
25. NKF–DOQI: Clinical practice guidelines for vascular access: Update 2000. National Kidney Foundation–Dialysis Outcomes Quality Initiative. Am J Kidney Dis 2001;37:137S–181S.
26. Schanzer H, Skladany M, Haimov M: Treatment of angioaccess-induced ischemia by revascularization. J Vasc Surg 1992;16:861–864.
27. Valji K, Hye RJ, Roberts AC, Oglevie SB, Ziegler T, Bookstein JJ: Hand ischemia in patients with hemodialysis access grafts: angiographic diagnosis and treatment. Radiology 1995;196:697–701.
28. Canzanello VJ, Burkart JM: Hemodialysis-associated muscle cramps. Semin Dialysis 1992;5:299–304.
29. Canzanello VJ, Hylander-Rossner B, Sands RE, Morgan TM, Jordan J, Burkart JM: Comparison of 50% dextrose water, 25% mannitol, and 23.5% saline for the treatment of hemodialysis-associated muscle cramps. ASAIO J 1991;37:649–652.
30. Bregman H, Daugirdas JT, Ing TS: Complications during hemodialysis. *In* Daugirdas JT, Ing TS (eds). Handbook of Dialysis. Boston: Little, Brown and Company, 1994, pp 149–168.
31. Sadowski RH, Allred EN, Jabs K: Sodium modeling ameliorates intradialytic and interdialytic symptoms in young hemodialysis patients. J Am Soc Nephrol 1993;4:1192–1198.
32. Ahmad S, Robertson HT, Golper TA, et al: Multicenter trial of L-carnitine in maintenance hemodialysis patients. II. Clinical and biochemical effects. Kidney Int 1990;38:912–918.
33. Bana DS, Yap AU, Graham JR: Headache during hemodialysis. Headache 1972;12:1–14.
34. Abuelo JG, Shemin D, Chazan JA: Acute symptoms produced by hemodialysis: a review of their causes and associations. Semin Dial 1993;6:59–69.
35. Krueger BR: Restless legs syndrome and periodic movements of sleep. Mayo Clin Proc 1990;65:999–1006.
36. Montplaisir J, Nicolas A, Denesle R, Gomez-Mancilla B: Restless legs syndrome improved by pramipexole: a double-blind randomized trial. Neurology 1999;23:938–943.
37. Arieff AI: Dialysis disequilibrium syndrome: current concepts on pathogenesis and prevention. Kidney Int 1994;45:629–635.
38. Silver SM, Sterns RH, Halperin ML: Brain swelling after dialysis: old urea or new osmoles? Am J Kidney Dis 1996;28:1–13.
39. Swartz RD: Hemodialysis-associated seizure activity. *In* Nissenson AR, Fine RN (eds). Dialysis Therapy. St Louis: Hanley & Belfus Inc, Mosby Year Book, 1993, pp 113–116.
40. Edmunds ME, Walls J: Pathogenesis of seizures during recombinant human erythropoeitin therapy. Semin Dial 1991;4:163–167.
41. Alfrey AC. Aluminum neurotoxicity. *In* Nissenson AR, Fine RN (eds). Dialysis Therapy. Philadelphia: Hanley & Belfus Inc, Mosby Year Book, 1993, pp 275–277.
42. Pereira BJG, Cheung AK: Biocompatibility of hemodialysis membranes. *In* Owen WF, Pereira BJG, Sayegh MH (eds). Dialysis and Transplantation: A Companion to Brenner and Rector's The Kidney. Philadelphia: WB Saunders Company, 1999, pp 32–56.
43. Karsou SA, Jaber BL, Pereira BJG: Impact of intermittent hemodialysis variables on clinical outcomes in acute renal failure: a critical review. Am J Kidney Dis 2000;35:980–991.

44. Modi GK, Pereira BJG, Jaber BLJ: Hemodialysis in acute renal failure: does the membrane matter? Semin Dial 2001;14:318–321.

45. Hakim RM, Held PJ, Stannard DC, et al: Effect of the dialysis membrane on mortality of chronic hemodialysis patients. Kidney Int 1996;50:566–570.

46. Bloembergen WE, Hakim RM, Stannard DC, et al: Relationship of dialysis membrane and cause-specific mortality. Am J Kidney Dis 1999;33:1–10.

47. Pereira BJ, Dinarello CA. Production of cytokines and cytokine inhibitory proteins in patients on dialysis. Nephrol Dial Transplant 1994;9:60–71.

48. Eaton JW, Leida MN: Hemolysis in chronic renal failure. Semin Nephrol 1985;5:133–139.

49. Gordon SM, Bland LA, Alexander SR, Newman HF, Arduino MJ, Jarvis WR: Hemolysis associated with hydrogen peroxide at a pediatric dialysis center. Am J Nephrol 1990;10:123–127.

50. Yamamoto S, Koide M, Matsuo M, et al: Heparin-induced thrombocytopenia in hemodialysis patients. Am J Kidney Dis 1996;28:82–85.

51. Pham PT, Miller JM, Demetrion G, Lew SQ: Clotting by heparin of hemoaccess for hemodialysis in an end-stage renal disease patient. Am J Kidney Dis 1995;25:642–647.

52. Remuzzi G, Rossi EC: Hematologic consequences of renal failure. In Brenner BM (ed). Brenner's The Kidney. Philadelphia: WB Saunders Company, 1996, pp 2170–2186.

53. Blagg C: Acute complications associated with hemodialysis. In Maher J (ed). Replacement of Renal Function by Diaysis: A Textbook of Dialysis. Dordrecht: Kluwer Academic, 1989, pp 750–771.

54. Caruana RJ, Smith MC, Clyne D, Crow JW, Zinn JM, Diehl JH: A controlled study of heparin versus epoprostenol sodium (prostacyclin) as the sole anticoagulant for chronic hemodialysis. Blood Purif 1991;9:296–304.

55. Cardoso M, Vinay P, Vinet B, et al: Hypoxemia during hemodialysis: a critical review of the facts. Am J Kidney Dis 1988;11:281–297.

56. Burmann-Urbanek M, Sanner B, Laschewski F, et al: Sleep disorders in patients with dialysis-dependent renal failure (in German). Pneumologie 1995;1:158–160.

57. Kimmel PL: Sleep apnea in end-stage renal disease. Semin Dial 1991;4:52–58.

58. Fletcher EC: Obstructive sleep apnea and the kidney. J Am Soc Nephrol 1993;4:1111–1121.

59. Man GCW: Obstructive sleep apnea. Med Clin North Am 1996;80:803–820.

60. Hanly PJ, Pierratos A: Improvement of sleep apnea in patients with chronic renal failure who undergo nocturnal hemodialysis. N Engl J Med 2001;344:102–107.

61. Fadda GZ, Hajjar SM, Perna AF, Zhou XJ, Lipson LG, Massry SG: On the mechanism of impaired insulin secretion in chronic renal failure. J Clin Invest 1991;87:255–261.

62. Arem R: Hypoglycemia associated with renal failure. Endocrin Metab Clin N Amer 1989;18:103–121.

63. Esforzado N, Poch E, Cases A, Cardenal C, Lopez-Pedret J, Revert L: Central pontine myelinolysis secondary to frequent and rapid shifts in plasma glucose in a diabetic haemodialysis patient. Nephrol Dial Transplant 1993;8:644–646.

64. Blankestijn PJ, Joles JA, Koomans HA: Does the modality of haemodialysis treatment affect lipoprotein composition? Nephrol Dial Transplant 1996;11:14–16.

65. Schneider H, Schmitt Y: Low-molecular-weight heparin – how does it modify lipid metabolism in chronic hemodialysis patients? (in German). Klin Wochenschr 1991;69:749–756.

66. Owen WFJ, Lew NL, Liu Y, Lowrie EG, Lazarus JM: The urea reduction ratio and serum albumin concentration as predictors of mortality in patients undergoing hemodialysis. New Engl J Med 1993;329:1001–1006.

67. Hakim RM, Levin N: Malnutrition in hemodialysis patients. Am J Kidney Dis 1993;21:125–137.

68. Capelli JP, Kushner H, Camiscioli TC, Chen SM, Torres MA: Effect of intradialytic parenteral nutrition on mortality rates in end-stage renal disease care. Am J Kidney Dis 1994;23:808–816.

69. Wolfson M: Use of intradialytic parenteral nutrition in hemodialysis patients. Am J Kidney Dis 1994;23:856–858.

70. Wolfson M: Use of water-soluble vitamins in patients with chronic renal failure. Semin Dial 1988;1:28–32.

71. Spital A, Sterns RH: Potassium homeostasis in dialysis patients. Semin Dial 1988;1:14–20.

72. Ketchersid TL, van Stone JC: Dialysate potassium. Semin Dial 1991;4:46–51.

73. O'Quin RJ, Lakshminarayan S: Venous air embolism. Arch Intern Med 1982;142:2173–2176.

74. Baskin SE, Wozniak RF: Hyperbaric oxygenation in the treatment of hemodialysis-associated air embolism. N Engl J Med 1975;293:184–185.

75. Butler BD: Biophysical aspects of gas bubbles and blood. Med Instrum 1985;19:59–62.

76. Covey CM, Arieff AI: Disorders of sodium and water metabolism and their effects on the central nervous system. In Brenner BM, Stein JH (eds). Contemporary Issues in Nephrology, Volume 1. New York: Churchill Livingstone, 1978, pp 212–241.

77. Sterns RH, Silver SM: Hemodialysis in hyponatremia: is there a risk? Semin Dial 1990;3:3–4.

78. Gennari FJ: Acid-base balance in dialysis patients. Semin Dial 2000;13:235–240.

79. Gennari HJ, Rimmer JM: Acid-base disorders in end-stage renal disease: part II. Semin Dial 1990;3:161–165.

80. Madias NE, Levey AS: Metabolic alkalosis due to absorption of "nonabsorbable" antacids. Am J Med 1983;74:155–158.

81. Shapiro WB: The current status of sorbent hemodialysis. Semin Dial 1990;3:40–45.

82. Freeman RM, Lawton RL, Chamberlain MA: Hard-water syndrome. N Engl J Med 1967;276:1113–1118.

83. Bello VA, Gitelman HJ: High fluoride exposure in hemodialysis patients. Am J Kidney Dis 1990;15:320–324.

84. Bergamo Collaborative Dialysis Study Group (BCDS): Acute intradialytic well-being: results of a clinical trial comparing polysulfone with cuprophan. Kidney Int 1991;40:714–719.

85. Salem M, Ivanovich PT, Ing TS, Daugirdas JT: Adverse effects of dialyzers manifesting during the dialysis session. Nephrol Dial Transplant 1994;9 (Suppl):127–137.

86. Osman Y, Poh-Fitzpatrick MB: Dermatologic disorders associated with chronic renal failure. Semin Dial 1988;1:86–90.

87. Weber M, Schmutz JL: Hemodialysis and the skin. Contr Nephrol 1988;62:75–85.

88. Feinstein EI: The skin. In Daugirdas JT, Ing TS (eds). Handbook of Dialysis. Boston: Little, Brown and Company, 1994, pp 583–589.

89. Singhal PC, Lynn RI, Scharschmidt LA: Priapism and dialysis. Am J Nephrol 1986;6:358–361.

90. Fassbinger W, Frei U, Issantier R, et al: Factors predisposing to priapism in haemodialysis patients. Proc Europ Dial Transplant 1977;12:380–386.

91. Nakamura N, Takaesu N, Arakaki Y: Priapism in haemodialysis patient due to prazosin? Brit J Urol 1991;68:551–552.

92. Rizvi SS, Holmes RA: Hearing loss from haemodialysis. Arch Otolaryngol 1980;106:751–756.

93. Gatland D, Tucker B, Chalstrey S, Keene M, Baker L: Hearing loss in chronic renal failure-hearing threshold changes following haemodialysis. J Roy Soc Med 1991;84:587–589.

94. Servilla KS, Groggel GC: Anterior ischemic optic neuropathy as a complication of hemodialysis. Am J Kidney Dis 1986;8:61–63.

95. Arora N, Lambrou FHJ, Stewart MW, Vidrine-Parks L, Sandroni S: Sudden blindness associated with central nervous symptoms in a hemodialysis patient. Nephron 1991;59:490–492.

96. Olivieri NF, Buncic JR, Chew E, et al: Visual and auditory neurotoxicity in patients receiving subcutaneous deferoxamine infusions. N Engl J Med 1986;314:869–873.

97. Hutter JC, Kuehnert MJ, Wallis RR, Lucas AD, Sen S, Jarvis WR: Acute onset of decreased vision and hearing traced to hemodialysis treatment with aged dialyzers. J Amer Med Assoc 2000;283:2128–2134.

98. McIvor M, Baltazar RF, Beltran J, et al: Hyperkalemia and cardiac arrest from fluoride exposure during hemodialysis. Am J Cardiol 1983;51:901–902.

Techniques in Peritoneal Dialysis

Sarbjit V. Jassal and Dimitrios G. Oreopoulos

The benefits of peritoneal dialysis lie in the simplicity and relatively low cost in comparison to in-center hemodialysis. The principles are simple and, together with the anatomy and physiology of the peritoneal membrane, these are discussed in detail elsewhere.[1] The peritoneal membrane behaves like a semipermeable, selective barrier for the diffusion of solutes and water from the capillary blood vessels into dialysate that is instilled during dialysis into the peritoneal space. To allow removal of nitrogenous wastes and other uremic toxins, a fixed volume of dialysate is filled into the intraabdominal peritoneal space and left in situ for a variable "dwell" time (during which solute equilibration occurs), and then the "spent" dialysate (effluent) is drained and discarded. This cycle is repeated at set intervals throughout the day. Adjustments can be made to the type and volume of dialysate, the period of dwell, and the frequency with which the cycles are repeated. Membrane permeability varies from one individual to another and may be influenced by peritonitis; physical factors, including vibration and physical activity; and drugs, such as β-adrenergic blockers, vasodilators, calcium channel blockers, and prostaglandin inhibitors. Alterations in the peritoneal solute transfer rates warrant dialysis to be tailored to the patient by altering the technique and dialysate prescriptions used.

To understand the techniques used in peritoneal dialysis it is important to discuss catheter types, the tubing and the connectology required, as well as the different dialysate solutions and systems in use currently. Because peritonitis and technique failures are the main problems encountered with peritoneal dialysis, numerous modifications have been produced.

Catheter types and connectology

Catheters

The sole purpose of the peritoneal dialysis catheter is to provide a quick, easily accessible route into the intraperitoneal space for dialysis, while minimizing risk of bacterial or fungal contamination. The inner end of the catheter is placed within the abdomen and lies adjacent to the parietal surface of the peritoneum. A middle portion lies in a subcutaneous tunnel. The outer end exits the abdomen and lies free on the abdominal surface. A sterile cap covers the outer tip of the catheter, allowing access for inflow and drainage of dialysate when necessary. The intraperitoneal portion is typically constructed from either silicone rubber or polyurethane and ranges in length from 12 to 16 cm. Most have multiple small 1-mm side holes to allow inflow and outflow of fluid. Some of the different types of catheter design are listed in Table 85.1. No single study has proved superiority of one type of catheter over the others, although the most favored catheters in use at present are the Tenckhoff catheter (with either a straight or coiled tip), the Missouri catheter, and the Oreopoulos Zellerman TWH catheter (Figs 85.1 and 85.2).

At the time of surgery, the catheter is fixed to the abdominal wall using either one or two Dacron cuffs, or a bead and flange. With the Dacron cuff, a fibrous mass develops around the cuff during a 5- to 6-week period. This helps to stabilize the catheter and acts as a physical barrier to bacteria that may be at the exit site (Fig. 85.1). The presence of a dual-cuffed subcutaneous portion of the catheter has not been proven to reduce exit site infections (although these studies are prone to type II errors); however, there does appear to be a more rapid response to treatment with antibiotics.[2,3] Catheters with a bead and flange at the internal fixation point often have an external Dacron cuff that can be secured to the anterior surface of the rectus sheath. By use of a purse-string suture, the bead is left on the intraperitoneal aspect of the peritoneum, and the flange on the external surface. This type of catheter can often prevent early-onset leakage and is beneficial if dialysis is to be started soon after catheter insertion. The subcutaneous and external portions are designed to reduce irritation of the subcutaneous tunnel and thus reduce exit-site and tunnel infections.

Angled or swan-neck catheters have a permanent bend in the subcutaneous portion allowing both the internal and external exits to point downward, with the subcutaneous catheter curvature lying convex upward.[4,5] The swan-necked peritoneal dialysis catheters are reported to have a longer 3-year survival probability, reduced peritonitis

Table 85.1 Selected catheter types

Catheter	Description
Standard Tenckhoff	Available with either one or two Dacron cuffs. Usually has a straight tip
Swan-Neck Arcuate	Features a permanent bend in the segment lying in the subcutaneous tunnel. Allows downwards direction of the exit site and intraperitoneal exit. Most catheters are available in this format. A modified version is also available with a pail handle appearance (two 90° bends on both sides of the deep cuff)
Missouri catheter	Similar to the Tenckhoff catheter except the straight intraperitoneal segment has a bead and flange. At insertion the slanted flange is positioned flat against the posterior rectus sheath and a purse-string suture tied between the flange and bead causing an almost leak-proof seal
Coil catheter	Similar to the Tenckhoff catheter but because of the curled tip it allows less "jet effect" and is potentially less prone to migration
Toronto Western catheter	As with the Missouri catheter it is secured with a bead and flange, but also has two discs perpendicular to the intraperitoneal portion of the catheter to help reduce catheter migration, omental wrapping, and reduce outflow obstruction
Presternal catheter	See text. This catheter is tracked subcutaneously to the chest wall and exits in the presternal area. Associated with fewer exit-site problems, the initial reports are favorable
Moncreif–Popovich	A modified Missouri catheter with an extra large external cuff, inserted up to 6 weeks before use and left completely buried until the surgical insertion wound is fully healed
Other types of catheters	Less favorable, including the LifeCath and Valli catheters. Intended to reduce catheter migration and omental wrapping
Cruz	Polyurethane catheter with two cuffs and a coiled intraabdominal segment. Bent permanently into a pail handle shape
Flex-Neck	A flexible catheter similar in appearance to regular catheters. Has a wider inside diameter to allow quicker fill and drain time
Ash Advantage	A T-shaped peritoneal dialysis catheter made of long grooves or flutes. Does not rely on side holes for drainage and is said to reduce occlusion due to omental wrapping and increase the speed of inflow and outflow

incidence, and fewer problems with catheter migration; however, the studies published have weak designs and contain few details about selection of patients and the type of dialysis systems used.[3,6–8]

The Moncrief–Popovich catheter and insertion technique uses a modified straight-tipped Missouri catheter that is inserted and maintained differently.[9] It is unique in that the whole catheter, including the portion that will eventually be left on the outer surface of the abdomen, is buried within the subcutaneous tissue at the time of insertion. After a variable period, ideally longer than 4–8 weeks, the outer portion of the catheter is exteriorized and dialysis is begun.[9] By burying the catheter completely, contamination of the wound and the catheter with bacteria is reduced. Wound healing occurs and stabilizing fibrous adhesions form around the Dacron cuffs during the next few weeks. Five-year results suggest that the catheter is associated with reduced episodes of peritonitis and a prolonged average catheter survival time.[10] Results are awaited from a randomized controlled trial comparing the Moncrief–Popovich catheter and insertion technique with standard techniques.

The presternal swan-necked catheter, described by Twardowski and colleagues,[12] is heralded as the catheter most suited for obese patients. This catheter follows the same principle as the swan-necked Missouri catheter but has an extra extension tubing, trimmed to the size of the patient, that is implanted in a subcutaneous track through the skin, allowing the exit site to lie on the chest wall. An extension is attached to the catheter by a titanium connector. Disconnection has not been reported, and in vitro studies suggest that more than three times the normal tension is required to cause separation of the catheters at this point.[11,12] The catheter is most useful in obese patients, those with abdominal stomas, patients with multiple exit-site infections, and patients who prefer to have the catheter exit from the chest site rather than the abdomen. Observational results appear excellent with a 2-year catheter survival of 95% compared with 75% 2-year survival of standard abdominal catheters in the same unit. The reported peritonitis rate is lower (one episode per 37.4 months compared with one per 20.5 months for abdominal catheters). The catheter has been used without problem in patients with malnutrition and severe cachexia, both conditions which preclude good wound healing.[13]

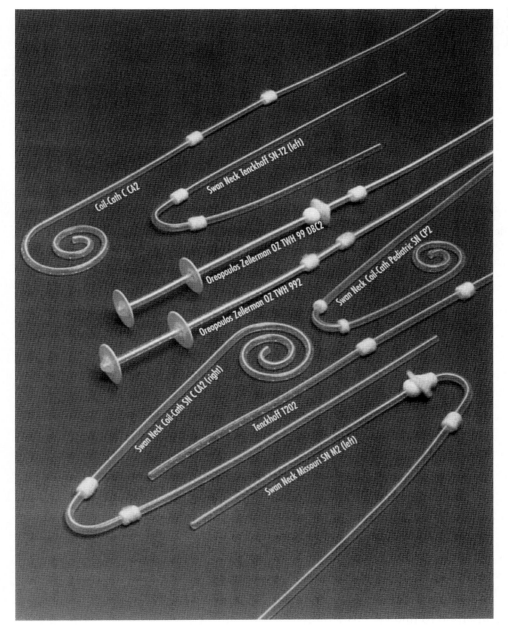

Figure 85.1 The most commonly used catheters. (Courtesy of Accurate Surgical Instruments, Toronto, Canada.)

Insertion techniques

Although catheters can be inserted at the bedside in an emergency, most are placed during a mini-laparotomy or with use of a laparoscope. Traditionally, those inserted acutely at the bedside using a blind technique are rigid, straight catheters used for a short period only. Acute catheters are prone to problems with catheter-tip migration, dialysate leaks, peritonitis, and bowel perforation, and therefore their use is not recommended. If an acute catheter must be used, removal and replacement with a tunnelled catheter is recommended after 3 days.

Surgical insertion of peritoneal catheters is well described elsewhere and involves dissection through the rectus muscle, into the peritoneal cavity.[14,15] The site should first be marked so as to avoid placing the exit site in a body fold or along the belt line. Catheters with curled or straight tips are inserted caudally into the pelvis by feel, avoiding adhesions, so that the tip lies between the visceral and parietal peritoneum. The internal cuff is usually fixed to the inner sheath of the rectus muscle; if present, the outer cuff can be fixed to the rectus sheath at least 2 cm from the exit site. Fixation closer to the exit site can result in problems with cuff extrusion at a later date. Sutures at the exit site should be avoided because this practice promotes exit-site infections. Placement of the catheter exit site on the left-hand side may reduce problems with slow drainage.[16]

Peritoneoscopic insertion is becoming increasingly popular. Insertion requires a peritoneoscope, steel cannula with internal trocar, and a spiral-wound Quill catheter

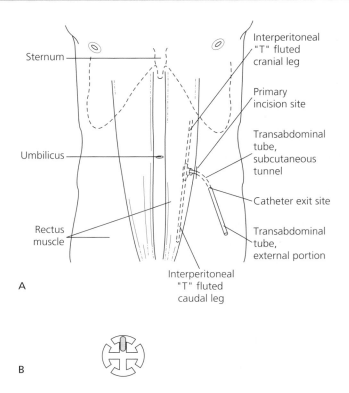

Figure 85.2 (A) The position of the Ash Advantage catheter after insertion. (B) The cross-sectional view of the flutes; the shaded area represents the radioopaque stripe. (Courtesy of Medigroup Inc., Division of Janin group, Inc., Naperville, IL, USA.)

guide surrounding the cannula. The peritoneoscope is inserted into the abdomen through a single small incision, air is insufflated, and the Quill and cannula are advanced into the optimal position. The scope and catheter are then removed, leaving the Quill catheter guide in place. The puncture site around the Quill is dilated, and the peritoneal dialysis catheter is advanced along the path of the Quill. After removal of the Quill, the position and function of the catheter are checked, and a subcutaneous path is created with use of a trocar.

In an unblinded randomized controlled trial, Gadallah et al have shown that peritoneoscopic insertion of the catheter is superior. Early complications like leakage and peritonitis were less common and the overall survival was longer with catheters inserted using the peritoneoscopic method.[17]

Care of the catheter

Although there is little evidence to suggest any benefit, antibacterial prophylaxis is advised, for all patients, at the time of insertion of a peritoneal dialysis catheter. Recommended practice guidelines suggest the intravenous (or intramuscular) administration of 1 g cephalosporin 1 h preoperatively and then again after 12 h. Alternatively, vancomycin 1 g as a single intravenous dose can be given preoperatively. With the emergence of vancomycin-resistant enterococci, this therapy is less favored at present.

Regular application of mupirocin at the catheter exit site has been shown to be effective in prevention of both exit-site infections and peritonitis.[18]

Because of the risks of leakage, wound dehiscence, and hernia formation, a "break-in period" of at least 2 weeks is recommended after catheter insertion. In practice, the time allocated for break-in varies because circumstances surrounding the need for peritoneal dialysis differ. Shorter break-in periods are associated with increased risks of leakage. Straining during defecation or coughing should be minimized if possible because both increase intra-abdominal pressure and therefore increase the chances of herniation and leakage. If difficulty with inflow is seen, simple interventions should be tried first, including bowel stimulation, clot dislodgement, and brisk ambulation. Catheter obstruction occurring soon after implantation is often due to a clot or fibrin plugs and may respond to flushing. If unsuccessful, streptokinase or alteplase can be used (see below, Difficulties encountered in the immediate postinsertion period).

In situations requiring acute dialysis, the patient is often already confined to bed rest and dialysis can be begun immediately. Initially, exchange volumes of 500 mL, with 1- to 2-h dwells, should be used, increasing to exchanges of 1000 mL after the first four exchanges. Unless leakage or discomfort occurs, the volume may be further increased after a day or two. Patients may experience diaphragmatic compromise and respiratory distress if the volume of exchanges is increased too rapidly, and respiratory function should be carefully assessed, especially in the intensive-care setting.

Patients requiring chronic dialysis can have dialysis planned over a period of a few weeks. If necessary, intermittent peritoneal dialysis may be started after the initial few days with use of low volumes (500–1000 mL). Exchange volumes may be increased in two to three dialysis sessions to 2000 mL. The patient should remain supine for most of the dialysis period, and activity during dialysis must be restricted. In practice, an intermittent peritoneal dialysis schedule of 20 h per session, two or three times a week, during a 2-week period, is sufficient to allow wound healing. Alternatively, symptoms can be managed with regular hemodialysis. In the ideal situation, the catheter should be inserted 4–6 weeks before use. Flushes with 1000 mL of 1.5% dextrose solution and 250 units of heparin should be done at the time of insertion, then on return to the nursing unit, and again at 24 h. Flushing should be continued at weekly intervals to maintain catheter patency until dialysis is commenced. Data from the Moncrief–Popovich technique, in which the catheter remains buried without flushing for some weeks, suggest that flushing at weekly intervals may not always be necessary, but no trials have addressed this issue to date. The exit site should be covered with a nonocclusive sterile gauze dressing and every attempt made to keep this site dry and free from any irritation. Dressing changes should be avoided if at all possible to allow optimal tissue repair around the catheter site. Chlorhexidine-based cleansing agents appear to be superior to iodine, with lower exit-site infections being identified.[19]

Difficulties encountered in the immediate postinsertion period

In the immediate postoperative period the patient should be assessed for pain or significant bleeding at the surgical site. The catheter can be flushed almost immediately. Leakage can develop any time after insertion but is most frequently seen early on. In most cases, leakage will stop if dialysis is discontinued for a time (from a few days to a few weeks). Dialysis leakage is more common in patients using steroids, in diabetics, obese patients, and in the elderly. Scrotal or labial swelling during peritoneal dialysis can be caused by a patent processus vaginalis or a subcutaneous leak in the anterior abdominal wall. The latter is often subtle and should be suspected when a patient has localized swelling or tenderness of the abdominal wall. The exact site of the leak can be determined with computed tomography after the infusion of 2000 mL of dialysis solution containing 100 mL of 50% diatrizoate. Patients should be encouraged to be mobile during the fill, to allow distribution of the dialysate throughout the abdomen, increasing the yield of the scan. Surgical repair is often required.

Inflow obstruction is often due to malposition of the catheter, or catheter-tip occlusion. Initial attempts with laxatives and ambulation may be successful, but repositioning is necessary in some cases. Occlusion due to omental stimulation appears to occur in response to peritoneal exposure to dialysate, although the degree to which this occurs is variable. Although it has been proposed that omental wrapping occurs in response to the unphysiologic nature of the dialysate (the pH ranges between 5.0 and 5.5) and the use of lactate in dialysate solutions, no study has addressed the issue of whether alteration of the composition of dialysate would reduce the frequency of omental wrapping.[20] Using a canine model, Moncrief et al[21] have shown that the intraabdominal presence of a catheter is insufficient to induce omental wrapping. In this study, catheter obstruction observed after the infusion of small volumes of dialysate suggesting that the dialysate itself, or the repeated inflow and outflow of fluid, is at least partly responsible. This observation has not yet been confirmed in human studies. There is weak evidence indicating that catheters placed on the left-hand side of the abdomen may have fewer problems with migration.[2] Catheter designs that reduce migration and omental wrapping include those with curled-tip, perpendicular disk-like structures (Oreopoulos Zellerman catheter; see Fig. 85.1), and a column disk (Lifecath). No single catheter has been clearly shown to be superior in this aspect.[20]

Outflow problems may be due to catheter migration, fibrin plugs, or clot formation within the catheter. Migration of the catheter appears to occur early in the course of its life. Migration is frequently seen on abdominal radiography, but radiologic findings do not always correlate with clinical evidence of obstruction or poor function. In a proportion of cases, surgical repositioning or peritoneoscopic manipulation can prolong catheter survival.[22] The latter is favored initially because it is less traumatic for the patient. During peritoneoscopy, air is insufflated into the abdomen, the catheter is clamped, and a curved metal rod is inserted through the catheter. With use of the rod as a support, the catheter tip is repositioned into the appropriate quadrant. The catheter position can be confirmed either radiologically or with use of the peritoneoscope. In some cases, the catheter will return to the same malposition shortly after manipulation – in these cases, surgical intervention is often required to remove adherent omentum or to release local adhesions.

Fibrin plugs or clots may be dissolved by a thrombolytic agent. One suggested protocol for administration of streptokinase is the reconstitution of 750 000 IU streptokinase in 30–100 mL of 0.9% saline and injection through the peritoneal catheter. Urokinase is preferable to streptokinase because of the lower incidence of allergic reactions, although it is no longer commercially available. As the withdrawal of urokinase, alteplase has been used as an alternative to streptokinase, albeit with lower success. A dose of alteplase (1 mg/mL) equal to the volume of the catheter plus transfer set is injected into the catheter and left for a minimum of a 2-h dwell.

Connectology

Connectology is the term used to describe the equipment and methods used to connect the dialysis system to the intraabdominal catheter. Numerous commercial preparations are available (Table 85.2). Connections are required between the catheter and the transfer set and between the transfer set and the dialysate container. Any system allowing the patient to be free of all tubing (except the intraperitoneal catheter) in between exchanges is referred to as a disconnect system. Because peritonitis rates correlate directly with the number of connections made, the connectology used can have a bearing on the incidence of peritonitis and thus on technique survival. Three basic techniques are available: the standard spike-and-port method, the Luer lock method, and assist devices.

The spike-and-port method of connection is the original and simplest method, involving the insertion of a plastic spike on the end of the tubing into a small sterile port on the dialysate bag. It requires fine control of both hands to prevent touch contamination of spike or port. Patients with visual impairment or poor hand coordination may have difficulty with this process. In a modified model (Inpersol system), a small rigid plastic sleeve covers the port, helping to guide the spike into the appropriate place. The spike is also partly protected with a clamshell-like structure, helping to prevent touch contamination and provide ease of insertion and removal.

The Luer lock system has an oversized Luer lock type of connection that involves a twisting action. The main advantage is that it does not require fine hand movements or good vision. Some transfer sets have the additional advantage of their Luer lock mechanisms being partially encased. The casing has a small reservoir that is prefilled at the time of manufacture with iodine or some other antiseptic solution (Fig. 85.3).

Assist devices are mechanized devices that use the spike-and-port principle but assist visually impaired or disabled patients to perform the connection. Unfortunately, the

Table 85.2 Currently available continuous ambulatory peritoneal dialysis systems

Commercial Name	Manufacturer	Comments	Number of connections per day*
Ultra set	Baxter Healthcare Inc, III	Y set with separate connection to dialysate bag Luer lock at patient catheter	12
Twin set	Baxter Healthcare Inc,	Y set with integrated disconnect system Luer lock at patient catheter	8
Freedom set	Fresenius, USA	Y set with separate connection to dialysate bag Luer lock at patient catheter 'Snap disconnect' lets the patient disconnect without exposing the end of the catheter	8
Fresenius double bag	Fresenius, USA	Y set with integrated disconnect system Luer lock at patient catheter 'Snap disconnect' allows the patient to disconnect without exposing the end of the catheter	4
NMC Dextrolyte II	NMC	Y set with separate connection to dialysate bag Luer lock at patient catheter 'Snap disconnect' allows the patient to disconnect without exposing the free end	8
T set		Y set with separate connection to dialysate bag Contains antiseptic in the system	8
		O set Y set with separate connection to dialysate reusable tubing	12

*Based on 4 exchanges per day

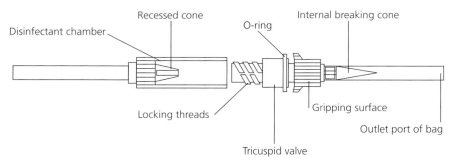

Figure 85.3 Diagrammatic representation of the Luer lock connector (Safe-Lock). (Courtesy of Fresenius Brent, Toronto, Canada.)

machines are often unpopular with patients because they require heavy portable batteries or an electric power outlet, and can be bulky. The main assist devices available use ultraviolet (UV) irradiation to sterilize the ends that will be connected.

Data derived from the US Renal Data System database suggest that the use of a UV flash system reduces peritonitis rates to 1/16.5 episodes per patient-month. When different bag systems were compared, however, the relative risk (by Cox analysis) of first peritonitis was still lower when a disconnect system or standard connect system was used.[23] In a nonrandomized series, technique survival and peritonitis-free time were higher in those using the prefilled Luer lock mechanism.[24] The highest peritonitis risk was seen in those using the spike-and-port system.

Dialysate solutions

Dialysate is supplied in disposable plastic bags, specially designed to allow administration of medication and easy connection. Dialysate bags are further sealed, and then sterilized, in a second envelope to avoid contamination of the ports during delivery. Most solutions are available in many volumes, from 1 to 5 L. Many patients use a 2.0-L fill volume, although recent recommendations are to increase to the maximal volume of dialysate tolerated by the patient. The introduction of a 2.5-L bag has increased the flexibility that can be offered to the individual patient. The potential volume of each bag exceeds that of the contained solution to allow for any ultrafiltrate at the end of the drain cycle. Solutions containing lower concentrations of calcium (1.25 versus 1.75 mmol/L) are available, allowing more patients with hyperphosphatemia to be treated with calcium-based phosphate binders.

Multiple dialysate solutions are now available, with different electrolyte concentrations, dextrose concentrations, buffers, and volumes. Recent work has shown that the use of heat-sterilized glucose solutions is associated with an increased amount of glucose degradation products (GDPs), hence stimulating glycosolation of both lipids and proteins. This is associated with increased morbidity and mortality. In an attempt to increase the biocompatibility of the dialysate solution new products containing polymerized glucose solutions, pH neutral solutions, and amino acid preparations are commercially available. The various products, the advantages and disadvantages and the indications for use are listed in Table 85.2. Gambro have developed a unique system (Gambrosol Trio Unica System) to reduce the GDPs produced during heat sterilization. They incorporate three separate solutions into one bag so that the compartments contain an isotonic component (Iso), a low glucose solution (LG) and a high glucose solution (HG). When the glucose contained in LG is mixed with the Iso, a glucose concentration of 1.5% is achieved; if HG and Iso are mixed the glucose solution is 2.5%. When all three compartments are mixed a glucose concentration of 3.9% is achieved allowing versatility in fluid management.

Systems used in peritoneal dialysis

Manual peritoneal dialysis

Continuous ambulatory peritoneal dialysis (CAPD) is the most common prescription of dialysis used throughout the world today. CAPD relies on long dwells with exchanges, performed periodically during a 24-hour period. CAPD is a manual system whereby the exchanges are performed four to five times a day by the patient at home, in school, or in any clean environment. Minimal equipment is required. Two different principles are used to design the transfer sets available today.

In the first, called the standard system (System II), dialysate fluid is run directly from the bag into the peritoneum. The connecting tubing is clamped during the dwell period; the tubing and empty bag are rolled up and stored in a little pouch by the patient's side, only to be opened when the dialysate effluent is to be drained back into the bag. This is then removed and discarded, and the cycle is repeated again.

The second system uses the 'flush before fill' principle (Fig. 85.4) and differs in that a small amount of fresh, sterile dialysate is flushed through the catheter and tubing system into the drain bag before any dialysate is instilled in the abdomen. Thus contaminating bacteria are flushed away with the dialysate effluent. The system has a Y-shaped piece of tubing (hence the name "Y set") that attaches at the stem to the patient's catheter. Because of the two arms of the tubing, two polyvinyl bags are required, one containing fresh dialysate, and another, which is empty at the start of the exchange, to collect

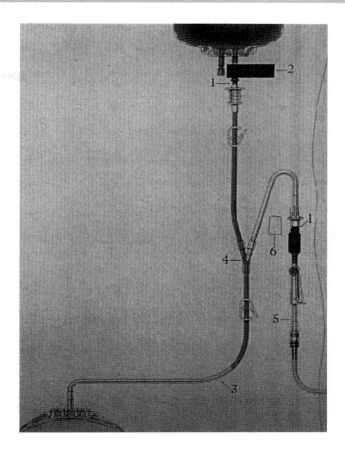

Figure 85.4 The Y set dialysis system and tubing. Features include the connection sites (1), the clip that prevents migration of organisms into the dialysate during spiking of the bag (2), and the flush before fill design (3). The Y set is so named because of the Y-shaped junction shown in the diagram (4). Short-length transfer sets and a prefilled disconnect cap increase the patient's comfort between exchanges (5 and 6). (Photograph provided by Baxter Healthcare Corporation, USA.)

dialysate effluent. At the end of a dwell period, the patient connects his or her catheter to the system being used and drains the dialysate effluent into an empty bag. The arm of the fresh dialysate bag is clamped shut throughout this period. Once draining is complete, the tubing between the patient and the Y piece is clamped, and a 100-mL aliquot of fresh dialysate is run from the fresh dialysate bag into the bag containing the effluent. The tubing to the effluent bag is then clamped, and the patient may proceed with instilling fresh dialysate into the peritoneal space. There are many variations of the flush-before-fill principle (Table 85.3), and the nomenclature can become confusing, but mainly these are limited to the Y-set principle. In most cases, the tubing comes attached to an empty but sterile drain bag, and the patient is left to make a connection between the dialysate bag and the tubing, and between the tubing and the catheter. In contrast, all the components of an "integrated disconnect system", including the dialysate bag, are preassembled and the whole system is sterilized as one unit. Only one connection is required, from the transfer set to the patient's catheter, reducing the chances

Table 85.3 Currently available dialysis solutions

Solution	Content	Indications	Comments
7.5% icodextrin (Extraneal)	Glucose polymer solution	Patients with ultrafiltration failure. Use once daily as a 8–12 h dwell	Absorption of glucose polymers is lower resulting in a prolonged osmotic effect. Also has lower GDP content. Associated with allergic rashes. May falsely elevate adequacy results[29]
1.1% amino acid solution (Nutrineal)	Mixture of 15 amino acids	Malnourished patients	Amino acids tend to be 80% absorbed therefore can supplement protein intake. May result in acidemia or inappropriate protein catabolism if high calorie foods are not consumed at the same time. In animal studies reduces mesothelial cell damage
Bicarbonate buffered solutions (Physioneal); awaiting data from Fresenius	Bicarbonate/lactate mixture or lactate free buffer	All/any patient population	Results in a more physiological pH in the dialysate. Believed to reduce mesothelial cell damage. Patient must be able to snap the connection and mix two solutions prior to administration
Dual or triple chamber lactate solutions (Stay-Safe and Gambrosol Trio)	Contain lactate in one section, with sterilized glucose contents in a separate chamber	All/any patient population	Results in a lower concentration of glucose degradation products during the process of heat sterilization. Believed to reduce mesothelial cell damage. Patient must be able to snap the connection and mix two solutions prior to administration

of touch contamination. At the end of the exchange, the transfer set, bag, and tubing are disconnected and discarded, leaving the patient free from all attachments. Another disconnect system, called the T-set system, allows reuse of the Y-shaped tubing. After the exchange, the tubing is filled with an antiseptic solution to minimize infection. This remains in situ until just before the next exchange, when the tubing is rinsed out with fresh dialysate and the stem is rinsed during the drainage of the spent dialysis. Unfortunately, although peritonitis rates are lower with the T set, the accidental instillation of antiseptic into the abdomen has made this a less popular technique. The O set system is so called because the two limbs of the Y tubing are joined to each other, forming an O shape when stored between exchanges.

Numerous studies have examined the benefits of the tubing and dialysis systems with reference to peritonitis rates, technique survival, and mortality of patients. Many are nonrandomized but still provide sufficient evidence to support the use of the integrated disconnect system (Table 85.4).

Automated peritoneal dialysis

Automated peritoneal dialysis is a generic term used to describe all peritoneal dialysis techniques where the dialysis exchanges are performed by a machine. Dialysis may be performed intermittently, for example for a period of 40 h twice a week (or 12 h three times a week), or on a daily basis. Intermittent therapies are rarely used because they provide inadequate dialysis clearances and should be restricted to use during the introductory period or postoperatively when short-term, low-volume dialysis therapy is needed.

Automated peritoneal dialysis (APD) is more usually used to describe all dialysis prescriptions administered by use of a cycler machine. The machine automatically cycles dialysis solution into and out of the abdomen at a predetermined volume and frequency. It can be used to supplement a normal CAPD day-exchange routine in cases in which adequacy is low; to provide a convenient mode of dialysis for patients returning to work, for example, or for those requiring help with their exchanges; or simply to optimize the dialysis prescription. In a small category of patients with fast-solute transfer, longer dwell periods lead to significant ultrafiltration failure, and a variation of APD called nocturnal intermittent peritoneal dialysis is used.

The machines used for home continuous dialysis have evolved from the original cyclers used for inpatient intermittent dialysis. The components of the systems include a dialysate holding station; a heater to warm the dialysate; a central control unit that monitors and controls the inflow, dwell, and drain of dialysate; and a method by which the dialysate effluent can be easily and safely disposed. For safety reasons, instillation and drainage depend on gravity, although a pump mechanism is used in some

Table 85.4 Summary of peritonitis rates in different peritoneal dialysis systems

Reference	Study design	Systems compared	Findings
Huang 2001[30]	C	Twin bag and APD	Lower peritonitis rates with APD (1/81.9 and 1/43.9 respectively)
Rodriquez-Carmona 1999[31]	C	CAPD versus APD	Lower peritonitis rates with APD compared with CAPD (1/38.4 and 1/18.7 respectively)
Kiernan 1995[32]	RCT	Y set (with no bag) versus 'twin bag'	Threefold decrease in peritonitis rates with fully connected (twin bag) system
Garcia-Lopez 1994[33]	CC	Disconnect (Y and O sets) versus standard	Lower peritonitis rates with disconnect (1/58 and 1/10 respectively)
Manili 1994[34]	D	T set	Low rates of peritonitis (1/50)
Teilens 1993[35]	C	Standard versus disconnect	Lower peritonitis rates with disconnect (1/34 and 1/10 respectively)
Viglino 1993[36]	RCT	T set versus Y set	No significant difference in peritonitis rates
Burkhart 1992[37]	C	Disconnect versus standard system	Lower peritonitis rates with disconnect (1/20 and 1/12 respectively)
Dasgupta 1992[38]	D	'Twin bag'	Twin bag peritonitis rates lower than previous rates for this unit
Dryden 1992[39]	RCT	Disconnect (Y set) versus standard	Lower peritonitis rates with Y set (1/25 and 1/9.7 respectively)
Port 1992[23]	C,Db	'Twin bag' versus standard versus UV + standard system	Twin bag system had the lowest peritonitis rates (1/21 versus 1/11 versus 1/16 respectively)

APD, automated peritoneal dialysis; C, cohort; CAPD, continuous ambulatory peritoneal dialysis; CC, case–control study; D, descriptive study design; Db, database; RCT, randomized controlled trial.
Peritonitis results are expressed as number of infections per patient-month.

cyclers to pump the dialysate onto a heating pad or to a raised container. With the aid of clamps, timers, weighing devices, and volume regulators, the cyclers can regulate the inflow, dwell, and outflow of dialysis solutions. Most machines can be programmed to allow a variable number of cycles, dialysate volumes, and dwell times, as well as to control the total time over which the whole cycle is completed. Recent advances have led to smaller, less intrusive machines and improved computerized controls that not only allow optimization of the prescription but also include superior database monitoring (Fig. 85.5). In some cases, the cycler can be linked to a modem and data can be directly transmitted to a central monitoring station, allowing easier follow-up of patients living in rural areas.

The different dialysate solutions used for APD are the same as for CAPD, the only difference being that 3-L and 5-L bags tend to be more convenient. Because larger volumes

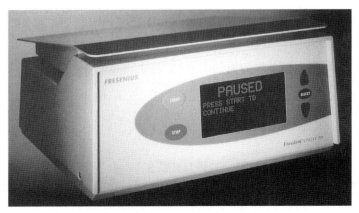

Figure 85.5 The IQ cycler, an example of a commercially available automated peritoneal dialysis system. (Courtesy of Fresenius Medical Care, USA.)

Table 85.5 Potential differences between peritoneal dialysis cycler machines and associated services

1. Can the same cycler can be used for both in-center dialysis (delivering up to 80 L over a 20-h period) and home patient use (delivering up to 18 L over a 10-h period)?
2. Should be quiet in operation
3. Portable (for patients who wish to travel), with traveling case available
4. Easily transported on carpet and hard floor while in operation
5. An additional midday exchange can be done with minimal number of connections and disconnections and the minimum number of additional tubing sets
6. Cycler tubing should be easily assembled; machine should be easy to prime and connect
7. Cycler stand should be available and included in the price
8. Tubing set is reusable, reducing the frequency with which connections need to be made
9. Cycler has the facility to finish with a 'day dwell' of different volume and/or concentration of dextrose
10. Sampling port should be specified
11. Dialysate should be supplied at regular intervals; arrangements for delivery to the patients home and pick up of unused materials should be made; if storage space is limited, the frequency of delivery is an important consideration
12. Installation, repair and exchange programs should be specified and maintained by the company; some companies will agree to provide a swap system so that no patient is left without a dialysis machine when technical repairs are required
13. A patient representative is often useful as a primary contact for difficulties encountered with the machine or dialysate deliveries
14. The company may provide on-site education for the nursing and technical staff in the use and maintenance of the cycler machines
15. Cost

of dialysate are required, the transfer sets often have a multipronged head, and multiple connections are required to set up the cycler. The principles of connectology are the same as in CAPD, and sets are available with both spike-and-port and Luer lock connections. In patients requiring administration of intraperitoneal medication, it is important to establish whether the cycler uses a mixture of dialysate from all bags at once, or uses dialysate from the bags in a sequential manner. If the dialysate is taken from each bag simultaneously, the drug can be injected into one bag only, and it will be mixed during the warming process; whereas a system that uses bags in a sequential manner needs to have the drug injected, in appropriate doses, into each bag. By mixing dialysate from all bags, the concentration of dextrose and thus the rate of ultrafiltration is stable. In addition, only one injection is required, reducing the chances of bacterial contamination. In contrast, the use of one bag at a time means that the concentration of drugs can be altered with time, an advantage for insulin administration, for example. Newer systems which control administration of medication, using a pump-like mechanism, are under development (Solumed, Newsol Technologies Inc., Toronto, Canada). Commercially available cyclers have the advantage of being more compact and more easily used by disabled patients. Some of the factors taken into consideration when purchasing APD machines are listed in Table 85.5.

Selection of patients

Peritoneal dialysis has the advantage of being cheaper, ideally suited for both home use and pediatric patients, and more easily performed than hemodialysis. In addition, it is associated with better preservation of renal reserve. With the advent of automated dialysis, sufficient dialysis can be offered to most patients regardless of body size. Although many data suggest that the survival on peritoneal dialysis is similar to that on hemodialysis, recent data from the US Renal Data System show a poorer survival on peritoneal dialysis in the older diabetic subgroup.[25,26] The equivalent data from database retrieval in Canada[27] do not confirm these findings, and controversy surrounds the role of peritoneal dialysis in older and diabetic patients.[21] With improved techniques in dialysis and increased target prescription levels, the available data may be obsolete, but this remains in question. Few absolute contraindications to peritoneal dialysis exist, particularly since the introduction of the Moncrief–Popovich and presternal catheters. Recent recommendations suggest that dialysis should be administered using an integrated approach, allowing the patient to transition from peritoneal dialysis, to hemodialysis and/or transplantation in a sequential, but timely manner.[28]

References

1. Burkhart JM, Nolph KD: Peritoneal dialysis. In Brenner BM, Rector FC (eds): The Kidney. Philadelphia: WB Saunders, 1996, pp 2507–2575.
2. Twardowski ZJ, Nolph KD, Khanna R, et al: The need for a "swan neck" permanently bent arcuate peritoneal dialysis catheter. Perit Dial Bull 1985;15:219–223.
3. Twardowski ZJ, Prowant BF, Khanna R, et al: Long-term experience with swan neck Missouri catheters. ASAIO Trans 1990;36:M491–M494.
4. Cruz C: Cruz catheter: implantation technique and clinical results. Perit Dial Int 1994;14(Suppl 3):S59–S61.
5. Cruz C: The Cruz catheter and its functional characteristics. Perit Dial Int 1997;17(Suppl 2):S146–S148.
6. Twardowski ZJ, Nichols WK, Nolph KD, et al: Swan neck presternal ("bath tub") catheter for peritoneal dialysis. Perit Dial Bull 1992;8:316.
7. Twardowski ZJ, Khanna R, Nolph KD, et al: Preliminary experience with the swan neck peritoneal dialysis catheter. ASAIO Trans 1986;32:64–67.

8. Hwang TL, Huang CC: Comparison of swan neck catheter with Tenckhoff catheter for CAPD. Adv Perit Dial 1994;10:203–205.

9. Moncrief JW, Popovich RP, Broadrick IJ, et al: A new peritoneal access technique for patients on peritoneal dialysis. ASAIO J 1992;39:62–65.

10. Moncrief JW, Popovich RP: Moncrief–Popovich catheter: implantation technique and clinical results. Perit Dial Int 1994;14(Suppl 3):S56–S58.

11. Moncrief JW, Popovich RP, Simmons E, et al: Peritoneal access technology. Perit Dial Int 1993;13:S121–S123.

12. Twardowski ZJ, Nichols WK, Nolph KD, et al: Swan neck presternal peritoneal dialysis catheter. Perit Dial Int 1993;13:S130–S132.

13. Twardowski ZJ, Prowant BF, Nichols WK, et al: Six-year experience with Swan neck presternal peritoneal dialysis catheter. Perit Dial Int 1998;18:598–602.

14. Gokal R, Ash SR, Helfrich GB: Peritoneal catheters and exit-site practices; towards, optimum peritoneal access. Perit Dial Int 1993;13:29–39.

15. Ash SR: Chronic peritoneal dialysis catheters: Effects of catheter design, materials and location. Semin Dial 1990;3:39–44.

16. Cuba de la Cruz M, Dimkovic N, Bargman J, et al: Is catheter function influenced by the side of the body in which the peritoneal dialysis catheter is placed? Perit Dial Int 2001;21:526.

17. Gadallah MF, Pervez A, El-Shahawy MA, et al: Peritoneoscopic versus surgical placement of peritoneal dialysis catheters: A prospective randomized study on outcome. Am J Kidney Dis 1999;33:118–122.

18. Casey M, Taylor J, Clinard P, et al: Application of mupirocin cream at the catheter exit site reduces exit-site infections and peritonitis in peritoneal dialysis patients. Perit Dial Int 2000;20:566–574.

19. Jones LL, Tweedy L, Warady BA: The impact of exit-site care and catheter design on the incidence of catheter-related infections. Adv Perit Dial 1995;11:302–305.

20. Ahmed MI, Rawal PA, Patel NM, et al: In vitro buffering capacity of residual peritoneal dialysate fluid: Implications for peritoneal dialysis therapy. Artif Organs 1992;16:416–418.

21. Moncrief JW, Popovich RP, Simmons E, et al: Catheter obstruction with omental wrap stimulated by dialysate exposure. Perit Dial Int 1993;13:S127–S129.

22. Simon ME, Pron G, Voros M, et al: Fluroscopically guided manipulation of malfunctioning peritoneal dialysis catheters. Perit Dial Int 1999;19:544–549.

23. Port FK, Held PJ, Nolph KD, et al: Risk of peritonitis and technique failure by CAPD connection technique: A national study. Kidney Int 1992;42:967–974.

24. Domrongkitchaiporn S, Karim M, Watson L, et al: The influence of continuous ambulatory peritoneal dialysis connection technique on peritonitis rate and technique survival. Am J Kidney Dis 1994;24:50–58.

25. Bloembergen WE, Port FK, Mauger EA, et al: A comparison of cause of death between patients treated with hemodialysis and peritoneal dialysis. J Am Soc Nephrol 1995;6:184–191.

26. Bloembergen WE, Port FK, Mauger EA, et al: A comparison of mortality between patients treated with hemodialysis and peritoneal dialysis. J Am Soc Nephrol 1995;6:177–183.

27. Fenton SS, Schaubel DE, Desmeules M, et al: Hemodialysis versus peritoneal dialysis: a comparison of adjusted mortality rates. Am J Kidney Dis 1997;30:334–342.

28. Blake PG: Integrated end-stage renal disease care: the role of peritoneal dialysis. Nephrol Dial Transplant 2001;16(Suppl 5):61–66.

29. Lilaj T, Dittrich E, Puttinger H, et al: A preceding exchange with polyglucose versus glucose solution modifies peritoneal equilibration test results. Am J Kidney Dis 2001;38:118–126.

30. Huang JW, Hung KU, Yen CJ, et al: Comparison of infectious complications in peritoneal dialysis patients using either a twin-bag system or automated peritoneal dialysis. Nephrol Dial Transplant 2001;16:604–607.

31. Rodriguez-Carmona A, Fontan PM, Fontan GT, et al: A comparative analysis on the incidence of peritonitis and exit-site infection in CAPD and automated peritoneal dialysis. Perit Dial Int 1999;19:253–258.

32. Kiernan L, Kliger A, Gorban-Brennan N, et al: Comparison of continuous ambulatory peritoneal dialysis related infections with different Y-tubing exchange systems. J Am Soc Nephrol 1995;5:1835–1838.

33. Garcia-Lopez E, Mendoza-Guevara L, Morales A, et al: Comparison of peritonitis rates in children on CAPD with spike connector versus two disconnect systems. Adv Perit Dial 1994;10:300–303.

34. Manili I, Brunori G, Camerini C, et al: Low incidence of peritonitis with the T set. Adv Perit Dial 1994;10:147–149.

35. Tielens E, Nube MJ, Vet JA, et al: Major reduction of CAPD peritonitis after the introduction of the twin-bag system. Nephrol Dial Transplant 1993;8:1237–1243.

36. Viglino G, Colombo A, Cantu P, et al: In vitro and in vivo efficacy of a new connector device for continuous ambulatory peritoneal dialysis. Perit Dial Int 1993;13:S148–S151.

37. Burkart JM, Jordan JR, Durnell TA, et al: Comparison of exit-site infections in disconnect versus nondisconnect systems for peritoneal dialysis. Perit Dial Int 1992;12:317–320.

38. Dasgupta MK, Fox S, Gagnon D, et al: Significant reduction of peritonitis rate by the use of twin-bag system in a Canadian regional CAPD program. Adv Perit Dial 1992;8:223–226.

39. Dryden MS, McCann M, Wing AJ, et al: Controlled trial of a Y set dialysis delivery system to prevent peritonitis in patients receiving continuous ambulatory peritoneal dialysis. J Hosp Infect 1992;20:185–192.

Complications of Peritoneal Dialysis

John D. Williams and Simon Davies

Infectious complications
- Peritonitis
  - Prevention
- Eosinophilic peritonitis
- Exit-site infection
- Tunnel infection

Noninfectious complications
- Inadequate ultrafiltration
- Catheter malfunction
  - Inflow failure
  - Outflow failure
  - Fibrin in dialysate
  - Fluid leaks
- Pain
  - Inflow
  - Backache
  - Generalized pain
  - Outflow pain
- Bleeding
  - After catheter insertion
  - Exit site
  - Blood-stained dialysate
- Chyloperitoneum
- Metabolic complications

Loss of peritoneal function is a major factor leading to treatment failure in peritoneal dialysis (PD) Although the precise biological mechanisms responsible for these changes have not been defined, it is widely assumed that alterations in peritoneal function are related to structural changes in the peritoneal membrane. There is accumulating, albeit indirect, evidence that continuous exposure to components of bioincompatible dialysis solution as well as repeated episodes of bacterial peritonitis play a major role in the long-term changes seen in peritoneal function (ultrafiltration loss and increased solute clearance). To date, however, the relationship between structure and function has not been fully defined. Although a number of studies have identified various mesothelial, vascular, and interstitial changes in peritoneal morphology during PD, the factors responsible for these have not been identified. These changes include loss or degeneration of mesothelial cells; thickening of the submesothelial compact collagenous zone (variously described as fibrosis or sclerosis); changes in the structure and number of blood vessels; and reduplication of vascular basement membrane.

Recent studies have quantified the changes within the submesothelial collagenous zone and demonstrated a progressive increase in thickness with time on PD

(Fig. 86.1). Changes within the peritoneal vascular bed have also been identified. These include progressive changes to the structure of small vessels ranging from subtle thickening of the subendothelial matrix through to complete obliteration of vessels (Fig. 86.2). There is thus accumulating evidence that changes occur in both the interstitial and vascular compartments of the dialysed peritoneal membrane.[1] Although it is likely that these changes are related to time on dialysis, to peritonitis, and perhaps to dialysis solution components, the exact relationships are poorly understood, as is the possible contribution of uremia.

In a small proportion of patients, there is extensive thickening and fibrosis of the peritoneal membrane (Fig. 86.3). This can occur after severe or recurrent peritonitis. It was originally described following exposure to acetate in the dialysate, the use of chlorhexidine as an antiseptic, and the administration of the β-blocker practolol. Clinically, it usually presents with poor ultrafiltration and reduced peritoneal transport.

Some patients develop an encapsulating, sclerotic reaction in which the bowel is enveloped in a thick cocoon of fibrous tissue, causing obstruction. Such individuals present with anorexia, nausea, malnutrition, and partial or complete intestinal obstruction. Whether this is a variant of extensive peritoneal fibrosis or a separate entity is unknown.

Infectious complications

Peritonitis

Although the introduction of disconnect systems has reduced the incidence of peritonitis it remains one of the most important complications of long-term PD. A single episode is rarely life-threatening, but repeated or prolonged inflammation remains a major cause of treatment failure and results in a forced switch to haemodialysis.

The diagnosis should be suspected in any patient who develops a cloudy bag or abdominal pain. Fever may also be present but is not a universal feature of peritonitis. Patients should be advised to contact their dialysis unit immediately if they have a cloudy bag or persistent abdominal pain. Samples of the dialysate should be taken for cell counting and microbiological examination. The diagnosis is confirmed by finding more than 100 white blood cells/mm³ of which at least 50% are polymorphonuclear leukocytes. A Gram stain of the spun deposit should also be performed to help identify the type of causative organism, although this will only reveal the pathogen in a minority of cases. For most patients,

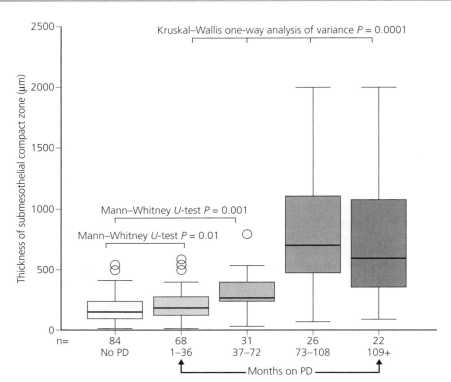

Figure 86.1 Changes in the thickness of the peritoneal membrane with origin of biopsy and time on PD. The submesothelial compact zone was measured in micrometers in samples taken from normal individuals, uremic predialysis patients, hemodialysis patients, and from patients undergoing PD, grouped according to duration of dialysis. Data are presented as box plots representing interquartile ranges.

treatment will have to be empirical, pending full results of culture and sensitivity tests. Various culture techniques have been proposed but white cell lysis is often helpful in increasing the yield of a positive growth.

There is no "gold standard" treatment for peritonitis in a PD patient. A number of regimens have been found reasonably effective, none of which give a 100% cure rate without relapse, and there has been no study that compares all the different schedules proposed. A further complicating factor is the recent emergence of vancomycin-resistant enterococci; and there is concern that large-scale use of this antibiotic selects for these organisms with the potential for transfer of the resistance to other species such as staphylococci – especially methicillin-resistant *Staphylococcus aureus* (MRSA). As a consequence, alternative regimens avoiding vancomycin have been proposed.

The Advisory Committee on Peritonitis Management of the International Society of Peritoneal Dialysis has published detailed guidelines and algorithms for the management of this condition.[2] The recommended initial empirical therapy is a first-generation cephalosporin, such as cephazolin or cephalothin, combined with an aminoglycoside (paying attention to residual renal function). Both types of antibiotic are administered as a loading dose in the first bag and then as a maintenance dose in subsequent bags. Suggested doses of cephalosporin are 500 mg/L for loading and 125 mg/L for maintenance. Once the culture result is available the regimen should be modified accordingly.

If an enterococcus is identified (Gram positive) the cephalosporin should be stopped and ampicillin added at a dose of 125 mg/L. *S. aureus* treatment includes adding oral rifampicin 600 mg daily. If the organism is not an MRSA, an alternative is to use a specific Gram-positive antibiotic such as flucloxacillin or rifampicin. If other Gram-positive organisms are identified then the cephalosporin should be continued. Though in vitro tests may suggest resistance of coagulase-negative staphylococci to cephalosporins, the in vivo concentration of the drug is usually sufficient to overcome this potential problem. If, however, clinical improvement is slow or fails to occur, then vancomycin may be given at a dose of 30 mg/kg intraperitoneally every 7 days. If the organism is an MRSA then vancomycin should be given using the same regimen.

Finally, for uncomplicated Gram-positive infections, an oral cephalosporin can be substituted for the intraperitoneal cephalosporin during the second week of therapy (summarized in Fig. 86.4).

If the culture is negative, combined therapy of cephalosporin and aminoglycoside should be continued for 2 weeks, assuming there is a clinical response (summarized in Fig. 86.5).

If a Gram-negative microorganism is identified, then the subsequent management will depend on the sensitivity (summarized in Fig. 86.6). If the bacteria are sensitive to the cephalosporin then it should be continued. On the other hand, the isolation of *Pseudomonas* requires the withdrawal of the cephalosporin and the addition of an alternative antibiotic with demonstrable activity against the organism, such as a quinolone.

The isolation of multiple organisms including anerobes strongly suggests major bowel pathology, including perforation or a diverticular abscess. Metronidazole should

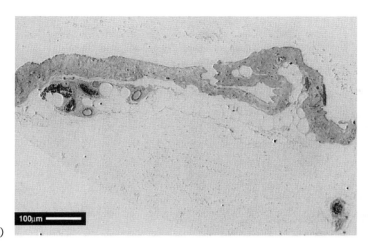
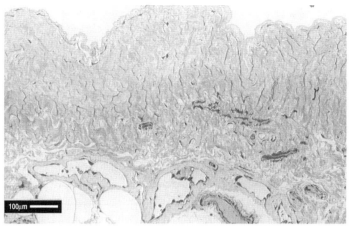

Figure 86.2 Morphological features of the parietal peritoneum. Biopsies from (A) a normal individual and (B) a patient who had been on peritoneal dialysis for 7 years. Toluidine blue.

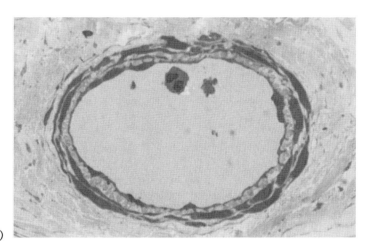
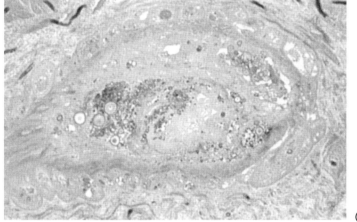

Figure 86.3 Morphological features of blood vessels in the parietal peritoneum. (A) A normal arteriole. (B) A venule with its vascular lumen occluded by connective tissue containing small calcific deposits.

be added to the regimen intravenously to begin with (the intravenous dose is 500 mg three times a day). In this situation, urgent surgical review is required pending a laparotomy.

The identification of yeasts on the Gram-stain and/or isolation of yeasts or fungi on culture are matters for serious concern. Many clinicians would recommend removing the peritoneal catheter as soon as possible because this type of infection can be difficult to eradicate in the presence of a foreign body. There is recent experience suggesting that a combination of an imidazole such as fluconazole and flucytosine may be of benefit. The recommendation for adults is daily fluconazole at an oral or intraperitoneal dose of 200 mg, and flucytosine at a loading dose of 2 g orally with a maintenance dose of 1 g/day. Amphotericin B is no longer recommended. Unfortunately oral flucytosine is not universally available.

The optimum duration of treatment has not been clearly defined by controlled trials. At present it is recommended that for Gram-positive organisms therapy should be for 14 days, except in the case of *S. aureus* when 21 days is suggested. For culture negative episodes 14 days should suffice. The same is true in the case of single organism Gram-negative peritonitis, but 21 days is recommended for *Pseudomonas*, *Stenotrophomonas*, or multiple organisms. Fungal or yeast infections require 4–6 weeks of therapy (or 7–10 days of therapy after catheter removal).

A wide variety of other antibiotics to those cited have been tried with success. In particular, a commonly used regimen is an oral quinolone such as ciprofloxacin instead of an aminoglycoside. The reader is referred to the Advisory Committee recommendations for details.[2]

If a patient is not systemically ill they can be treated successfully on an outpatient basis. It is extremely important, however, that they are followed-up either in the clinic or by telephone. In the majority of cases, clinical resolution, as judged by clearing of the bags, starts within 48 h. If there is no improvement within 96 h despite the

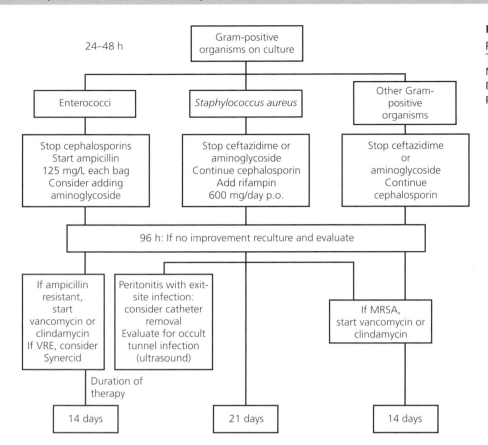

24–48 h

Figure 86.4 Management of Gram-positive peritonitis. (Reproduced with permission from The Advisory Committee on Peritonitis Management of The International Society of Peritoneal Dialysis-Related Peritonitis Treatment Recommendations: 2000 Update.)

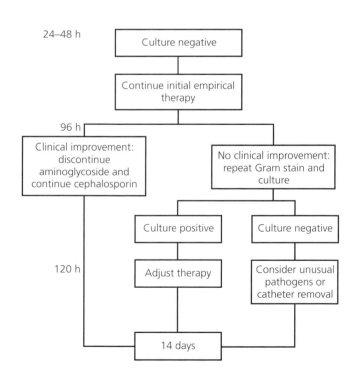

Figure 86.5 Management of culture-negative peritonitis. (Reproduced with permission from The Advisory Committee on Peritonitis Management of The International Society of Peritoneal Dialysis-Related Peritonitis Treatment Recommendations: 2000 Update.)

correct antibiotic, as judged by sensitivity tests, then the fluid must be retested for cell count, Gram-stain and culture. In the case of a persistent *S. aureus* infection, an underlying tunnel infection should be excluded (see section on Tunnel infection). In all other situations where there is a failure to improve, serious consideration should be given to removing the catheter. The possibility of intra-abdominal or gynecological disease, or the presence of unusual organisms such as mycobacterium, should also be considered.

For patients on automated peritoneal dialysis (APD), regimens similar to those outlined above are used but the dialysis should be modified so that it lasts a full 24 h, with 3- to 4-h dwells. Once there is clinical resolution, the usual APD regimen can be recommenced, but with a daytime bag containing the antibiotics, until completion of the treatment.

Relapsing peritonitis is defined as separate infective episodes caused by the same organism within 4 weeks of finishing the previous course of antibiotics. In Gram-positive infections a 4-week course of a cephalosporin together with oral rifampicin should be tried. The recurrence of *S. aureus* infection should trigger a search for a pericatheter infection or tunnel. Relapsing MRSA-related peritonitis will require a prolonged course (4 weeks) of vancomycin or clindamycin. If enterococci or Gram-negative organisms are the cause, then the possibility of intraabdominal disease or a diverticular abscess should be considered. Again a repeat course of antibiotics chosen by

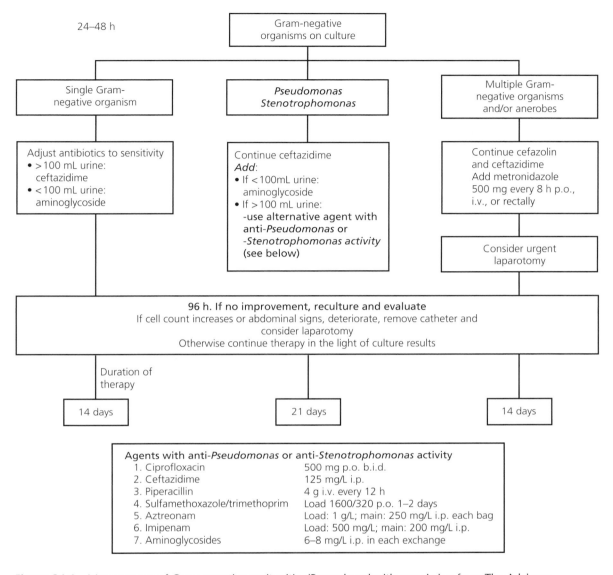

Figure 86.6 Management of Gram-negative peritonitis. (Reproduced with permission from The Advisory Committee on Peritonitis Management of The International Society of Peritoneal Dialysis-Related Peritonitis Treatment Recommendations: 2000 Update.)

sensitivity testing should last 4 weeks. As before, in the case of a relapse, removal of the catheter should be considered if there is no improvement within 4 days.

The best regimen for catheter replacement after removal for peritonitis has not been defined. There are theoretical benefits for the withdrawal of PD as replacement renal therapy for a brief period and avoiding the presence of an intraperitoneal foreign body, or altering host defences by instilling dialysate. Some centers, however, practice removal and replacement of the catheter at the same time under antibiotic cover.[3] Such an approach has, in fact, met with anecdotal success. Each patient should be judged individually to decide what is in his or her best interests.

Prevention

Because of the high rate of peritonitis experienced during the early years of continuous ambulatory peritoneal dialysis

(CAPD), considerable efforts have been made to prevent this serious complication.

A large number of studies have attempted to identify a cohort of patients who by virtue of altered host-defense mechanisms might be more susceptible to episodes of peritonitis. To date, however, there is no evidence that a correctable biological defect predisposes patients to an increased risk of peritonitis.

In contrast, significant advances have been made in the design of delivery systems in an attempt to reduce bacterial entry into the peritoneal cavity and thus reduce peritoneal infection. Buoncristiani and colleagues were the first to show that a Y-set system significantly reduced the rate of infection. This has been confirmed in several randomly allocated, prospective controlled trials.[4] An integrated twin-bag system, one bag for unused fluid and the other for drainage, is connected to a Y-shaped tube, which has a short stem to link it to the catheter. The principle of the system is that the drainage tube is flushed free of contaminating bacteria before fresh fluid is run in. In addition, there is a reduction in the number of times that the continuity of the tubing is broken. These Y systems act by greatly reducing the effects of touch contamination, thus reducing the rate of coagulase-negative staphylococcal infection. This system is now the standard for CAPD. The Y set does not, however, affect the incidence of *S. aureus* peritonitis.[5]

In contrast to *Staphylococcus epidermidis*, carriage of *S. aureus* appears to be confined to a minority of individuals. These patients are more likely to acquire peritonitis. Perez-Fontan and colleagues[6] reported that following the use of nasal mupirocin by nasal carriers of this organism, the rate of *S. aureus* infection was reduced. Unfortunately, they also observed a significant increase in Gram-negative peritonitis. However, the study was not randomly allocated but used historical control subjects. Bernardini and colleagues[7] reported that either oral rifampicin or mupirocin applied to the exit site reduced the rate of *S. aureus* peritonitis. However, the European trial of nasal mupirocin in carriers of this species of bacteria did not show a significant difference in the rate of peritonitis due to this organism (although it did reduce exit-site infections).[8] Thus, it is not certain that regular use of mupirocin will reduce the rate of peritoneal infection caused by *S. aureus*.

Unfortunately there is no proven method of decreasing the incidence of Gram-negative infections. Clearly one should avoid PD, if possible, in any patient with a stoma or fistula. Part of the difficulty is that Gram-negative organisms often cause problems in the elderly, probably as a result of diverticular disease. Other than keeping the bowels regular by judicious use of fibre, no other measures seem to reduce this type of infection.

Eosinophilic peritonitis

This condition is diagnosed when the patient presents with a cloudy bag of effluent, which is found to contain eosinophils on microscopy rather than neutrophils. The fluid is culture-negative. It is an uncommon event but tends to occur within the first few weeks of starting PD. The cause is unknown but is assumed to be some form of reaction to the cannula or to the dialysate. It is usually self-limiting and no treatment is required. Certain brands of vancomycin have also been reported to cause a chemical peritonitis, but withdrawal of the drug is usually followed by remission.

Exit-site infection

Exit-site infection has become an important complication of long-term PD. The actual incidence reported varies markedly from center to center, but a major difficulty appears to be the lack of a strict definition. A detailed review by Luzar[9] concluded that it occurred on average at a rate of 0.48 episodes per patient year. There does not appear to be a difference when CAPD is compared to continuous cycling PD. The most common infecting organism is *S. aureus*, either alone or in association with another species of bacteria.[10] A detailed photographic record of exit-site appearance (healthy, traumatized and infected) has been published.[11]

The diagnosis is suspected on clinical grounds usually by the presence of marked erythema of, or discharge from, the exit site. Increased scab formation also makes the diagnosis likely. There is often, but not invariably, local tenderness around the exit site and over the outer cuff. Although a positive culture is not essential to diagnose an exit-site infection, an attempt to determine the causative microorganism should be made. It is essential to culture any exudate rather than just to sample the surrounding skin. The latter procedure, even with a moistened swab, may grow only skin commensals, which are not the cause of the problem.

Unfortunately, there appear to be no satisfactory trials comparing different therapeutic regimens: thus, the following recommendations are based on anecdotal experiences from a variety of centers in different countries. Consensus guidelines have been published[11] (Table 86.1).

The main treatment options are systemic antibiotics and a local therapy. If there is any discharge or significant associated cellulitis it is essential to start with a systemic antibiotic. Because *S. aureus* is the common organism, an agent effective against this species should be prescribed. Unless there is prior evidence that the patient carries MRSA, flucloxacillin at a dose of 500 mg four times a day is appropriate. Alternatively, a cephalosporin can be used if the patient is allergic to penicillin. In most patients, the drug can be given orally but if the individual is systemically ill, then the antibiotics should be administered intravenously until clinical improvement occurs. Hospitalisation is not necessary for most patients. If the infection is resistant to methicillin, an alternative to flucloxacillin should be used. In a few cases, the organism may be sensitive to a cephalosporin. In the majority of resistant cases, however, vancomycin should be given as a 1-g intravenous dose (or intraperitoneally if the dwell time is at least 6 h). The dose is repeated once a week for up to 4 weeks. Vancomycin should not be used as the preferred therapy for exit-site infections in view of the emergence of vancomycin-resistant enterococci and the concern that this resistance could transfer to other bacteria.

Should the culture grow a Gram-negative organism, then ciprofloxacin in an oral dose of 500 mg twice daily will be effective in most cases. Other antibiotics should be substituted according to the in-vitro sensitivity results.

It is recommended that treatment should continue for a minimum of 2 weeks. In Gram-positive infections, if there is no improvement within 7 days, rifampicin 600 mg/day should be added. If complete healing does not take place after 4 weeks of therapy, then further measures should be considered. A number of centers have recommended exteriorizing and shaving the outer cuff. If this cuff is visible or even close to the exit site, it is likely to be involved in the infection. Under local anesthetic, the cuff

Table 86.1 Management of exit-site infection

1. Evaluate	Equivocal – stain or scabbing		Definite – purulent	Cuff or tunnel involvement
2. Investigate	Culture swab		Culture swab	Culture swab, ultrasound
3. Initial treatment		Cauterize exuberant granulation tissue		
	Tropical mupirocin		Appropriate antibiotic course	
4. 48 hours	Reassess in light of antibiotic sensitivities			
	Spread to tunnel, consider catheter removal			
5. Follow-up	Presistent *Staphylococcus aureus* infections, add rifampicin			
	Accompanying peritonitis, remove catheter			

Reproduced with permission from The Advisory Committee on Peritonitis Management of the International Society of Peritoneal Dialysis-related Peritonitis Treatment Recommendations: 2000 Update.

is exposed by an incision along the line of the catheter. The cuff is freed by blunt dissection and then carefully shaved off the catheter. There is often temporary resolution of infection after this procedure and it may prolong catheter life for 6–12 months.[12] If the infection persists or relapses then catheter removal must be considered, because there is a high risk that the exit-site infection will lead to peritonitis. It is important that the new exit site is located through a different part of the anterior abdominal wall. If the infection is controlled, and there is no evidence of sepsis along the tunnel, it is possible to insert a new catheter under antibiotic cover at the same time as the old one is removed. In a few individuals, it is possible to suppress the infection with a prolonged course of antibiotics, but again there is a risk of subsequent peritonitis. The exact regimen should be tailored to meet the clinical needs of each patient.

Whenever exit-site infection occurs, increased local measures are necessary. The site should be cleaned at least once and preferably twice daily with povidone–iodine. An alternative antiseptic, preferred by some centers, is hydrogen peroxide. If there is only erythema and no significant discharge, these measures may be effective on their own. Topical mupirocin has also been advocated for treatment, though experience is limited. This agent cannot be used with polyurethane catheters because it causes structural changes to the plastic and eventual catheter failure (it appears to be harmless to silicon cannulas). Where there is exuberant granulation tissue, Khanna and Twardowski[12] advocate the application of a silver-nitrate stick to the granulation tissue, taking care to avoid the surrounding skin. There is also anecdotal evidence for the beneficial use of hypertonic saline (3%).

In summary, however, failure of initial therapy and recurrence of infection should be considered as strong indications for catheter removal and replacement.

Because exit-site infection can be intractable, it is clearly important to avoid circumstances under which it might occur. Prophylaxis must start at the time of implantation. There are studies suggesting that the use of a single dose of parental antibiotic reduces the early infection rate. It is clear, however, that vancomycin should no longer be used

for this purpose. A cephalosporin is probably the best alternative although, because of the association between nasal carriage of *S. aureus* and exit-site infections, preoperative nasal mupirocin might prove effective. There are, in addition, several studies that look specifically at the prevention of *S. aureus* exit-site infections. Zimmerman and colleagues[13] showed that regular rifampicin reduced this complication but some resistance to the antibiotic did appear during the course of the study. Bernardini and colleagues[7] confirmed this result using historical control subjects and showed a similar benefit with daily topical mupirocin. Perez-Fontan et al[6] treated *S. aureus* nasal carriers with nasal mupirocin. They showed a significant fall in *S. aureus* exit-site infections but a rise in Gram-negative infections. Once again, the control subjects were historical, so exact interpretation is difficult. A large European randomly allocated prospective study showed that the regular use of nasal mupirocin by patients who were proven nasal carriers of *S. aureus* reduced the rate of exit-site infection with this organism by two-thirds.[8] There was no significant increase in other infections.

Thus, it is clear that regular mupirocin can prevent *S. aureus* exit-site infections, but the most appropriate, cost-effective regimen has not been determined. The choices are to treat all patients; to screen for carriage, then treat; or to use mupirocin only if infection occurs. All of these strategies have advantages and disadvantages. A pharmacoeconomic analysis is currently under way and its findings will be awaited with interest.

A controlled trial has suggested that the regular use of povidone–iodine was associated with reduced infection when compared to soap and water.[14]

One technique that appears promising is the use of silver ions. This inhibits bacterial growth. A silver ring placed at the exit site has been tried[15] and attempts are now being made to coat the catheter directly with silver. Controlled trials are awaited.

It has also been claimed that the type of catheter can influence the rate of exit-site infection. At least two trials, however, were unable to show any difference between the swan-neck and straight cannulas.[16,17] It remains possible that the caudal direction of the exit site with a swan neck may encourage drainage and thus reduce the severity of any infection, but this hypothesis remains unproven. The Moncrief–Popovich catheter, in a technique where it is buried subcutaneously for several weeks before use, was introduced in an attempt to reduce this complication. Their initial experience, however, gave a rate of 0.55 episodes per patient year,[18] which is no improvement over that reported for standard cannulas.

The next important preventive measure is the avoidance of dialysate leakage. This can be minimized by implanting the catheter through the rectus sheath or not commencing PD for at least 2 weeks after insertion. Should dialysis be necessary, small volumes (500 mL for adults) with no dwell should be used initially, slowly increasing over 10 days. In addition, catheter movements should be minimized by using tape and a dressing of gauze with a nonocclusive cover. This should not be changed for several days unless there is excess bleeding. It is unclear when daily dressing should start. Suggested times are between 2 and 8 weeks after implantation.

Tunnel infection

This is defined as an infection occurring between the two cuffs. This problem is a relatively rare occurrence. Diagnosis is suggested by the classical signs of inflammation appearing along the line of the catheter. Sometimes, but not always, there is an associated exit-site infection. The diagnosis may be aided by ultrasonography. If this shows a fluid collection around the cannula, a tunnel infection should be suspected. Treatment of tunnel infection is similar to that of the exit site and must involve systemic antibiotics, but the chances of resolution are much lower and thus serious consideration should be given to catheter removal in every case. This is mandatory if there is associated peritonitis.

Noninfectious complications

Inadequate ultrafiltration

Insufficient ultrafiltration leading to fluid overload is one of the most common problems associated with long term PD. The incidence of this problem increases with time on treatment, in part from changes in membrane function, but also from the loss of residual urine volume that contributes to satisfactory fluid balance. One study would suggest that up to 30.9% of patients have this problem by 6 years of treatment.[19]

In defining ultrafiltration failure it is possible to take either a patient- or a membrane-centered approach. The former is a relative definition: it is the inability to achieve sufficient peritoneal fluid removal to maintain adequate fluid balance; it is influenced by many factors including fluid intake, residual urine volume, and the acceptability of using hypertonic (4.25% dextrose) exchanges. The latter is based on the absolute measurement of the ultrafiltration capacity of the peritoneal membrane, using standardized methods (see below), and is influenced by the intrinsic

properties of the membrane, such as characteristics of solute transport and fluid reabsorption rates. The clinician needs to integrate these two approaches to identify and manage fluid balance in the PD patient.

Insufficient ultrafiltration should be suspected if there is clinical evidence of fluid overload (Fig. 86.7). This problem is more difficult to identify in PD than HD patients, partially because it can develop insidiously, but also because driving the weight down to an appropriate 'dry weight' using sequential ultrafiltration during dialysis sessions is not possible. Edema, hypertension, unexplained low plasma albumin, low daily ultrafiltration volumes in anuric patients (< 750 mL), excessive dependence on hypertonic exchanges (≥ 2 per day), or increases in weight disproportionate to changes in the mid-arm circumference all suggest that there is a problem. These findings should lead the clinician to evaluate peritoneal membrane function.

Membrane function should be assessed using a standardized 4-h dwell as in the peritoneal equilibration test (PET)[20,21] or the simplified standardized permeability analysis (SPA).[22] The only important difference between these methods is the concentration of dextrose used (2.5% for PET, 4.25% for SPA). Both tests measure two aspects of membrane function, the ultrafiltration capacity and the rate of transfer of creatinine – low molecular weight solute transport. The ultrafiltration capacity is the net volume of fluid removed during the dwell, and is a function of several aspects of the membrane. A value of < 200 mL using the PET or < 400 mL using the SPA have been taken as indicators of ultrafiltration failure.[21,22] Solute transport rates can be best thought of as a measure of the effective peritoneal surface area. High solute transport will be associated with rapid absorption of glucose during a dialysis dwell, so reducing the osmotic gradient and thus achieved ultrafiltration, and this is the single most important cause of ultrafiltration failure. It is also the only aspect of membrane function that has been shown to change with time on treatment.[23]

If membrane function is normal (see Fig. 86.8) and the total achieved ultrafiltration is reasonable (> 1000 mL/day), then it is likely that fluid balance problems can be addressed through patient education and ensuring good glycemic control in diabetics. If the ultrafiltration capacity of the membrane is poor, but solute transport normal, then it is important to exclude a reversible mechanical cause. This is especially the case if the loss of ultrafiltration appears to have developed rapidly. The reason may be obvious – a catheter malposition, or constipation (abdominal x-ray), or the development of a scrotal and subcutaneous leak – but deep cuff leaks are more difficult to identify and require a contrast CT scan. Once mechanical causes are excluded, patients with persistent poor ultrafiltration capacity and solute transport rates below average (dialysate/plasma, D/P, creatinine ratio < 0.64) will usually require switching to hemodialysis once residual urine volume, which can be augmented by diuretics,[24] has disappeared. This is, however, a relatively rare form of ultrafiltration failure.

Much more common is high-solute-transport ultrafiltration failure. Owing to the loss in osmotic gradient

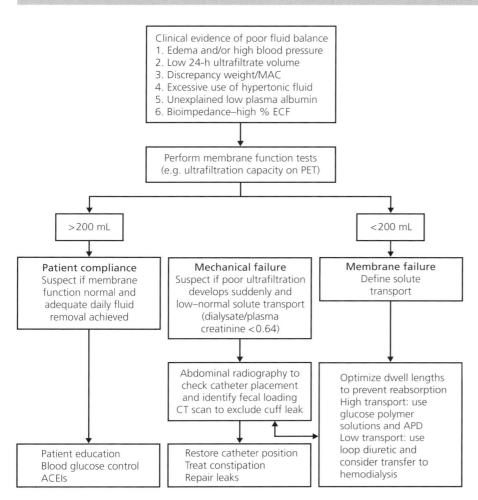

Figure 86.7 Algorithm for assessing and managing fluid balance and ultrafiltration failure.

Clinical evidence of poor fluid balance
1. Edema and/or high blood pressure
2. Low 24-h ultrafiltrate volume
3. Discrepancy weight/MAC
4. Excessive use of hypertonic fluid
5. Unexplained low plasma albumin
6. Bioimpedance–high % ECF

Perform membrane function tests
(e.g. ultrafiltration capacity on PET)

>200 mL

<200 mL

Patient compliance
Suspect if membrane function normal and adequate daily fluid removal achieved

Mechanical failure
Suspect if poor ultrafiltration develops suddenly and low–normal solute transport (dialysate/plasma creatinine <0.64)

Membrane failure
Define solute transport

Abdominal radiography to check catheter placement and identify fecal loading CT scan to exclude cuff leak

Optimize dwell lengths to prevent reabsorption
High transport: use glucose polymer solutions and APD
Low transport: use loop diuretic and consider transfer to hemodialysis

Patient education
Blood glucose control
ACEIs

Restore catheter position
Treat constipation
Repair leaks

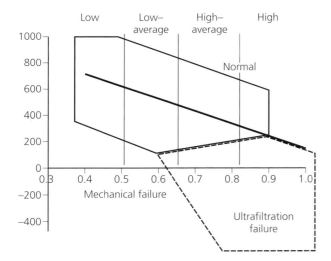

Figure 86.8 The relationship between solute transport (x axis) and ultrafiltration capacity observed in the peritoneal equilibration test (PET). The bold regression line reflects the inverse relationship between these measures (see text). This and the areas defined as normal or representing mechanical and ultrafiltration (UF) failure were established from 1800 consecutive measurements.[21,23]

described above, patients with this problem will frequently reabsorb from their longer dialysis exchanges. The solution to this problem is to use automated peritoneal dialysis (APD) to enable short exchanges to be performed during the night, combined with a glucose polymer to achieve maximum ultrafiltration during the long day dwell.[25]

Catheter malfunction
Inflow failure

A 2-L bag of dialysate should take 15 min or less to run into the peritoneal cavity. If inflow is significantly slowed or nonexistent, then mechanical causes should first be eliminated. The tubing and catheter should be checked for kinks, all clamps or rollers must be open for the inflow position, and all frangible seals fully broken. In the absence of such problems, the catheter should be flushed vigorously with 20 mL of heparinized saline. If the catheter now becomes patent, it is wise to add heparin at 500 U/L for the next few cycles. This is because the cause of blockage is usually a fibrin plug. If the catheter remains blocked, the abdomen must be radiographed. If the cannula is in a reasonable position in the pelvis, an attempt to restore patency should be made with the use of urokinase; 2 mL containing 25 000 units of urokinase should be infused into the lumen of the catheter and left in situ for 2–4 h. The catheter is then flushed and if inflow is restored, heparin should be added to the dialysate for the next few cycles. Should this procedure not be successful but fibrin is still thought to be the cause, an endoscopy brush may sometimes prove successful in unblocking the catheter.

If the radiographs show the catheter to be malpositioned, then an attempt should be made to reposition the catheter tip into the pelvis. This can be done using a sterile semirigid rod, shaped into a curve and slid down the lumen of the catheter under radiographic screening control. The rod is then rotated. Sometimes the catheter will then move easily and slide back into the pelvis. The technique is not practical when the cannula has a swan-neck configuration. Alternatively, the cannula can be repositioned at laparotomy or peritoneoscopy. It will often be found to be wrapped in omentum. Under these circumstances, current practice is to "hitch" the omentum out of the way in the upper abdomen. This avoids an omentectomy (preserving the omentum for future use if necessary) but prevents the omentum from blocking the catheter for a second time. An algorithm for managing inflow failure is shown in Fig. 86.9.

Outflow failure

The reasons for this problem are similar to those causing inflow failure. In addition, constipation is a well-recognized cause of outflow problems. Loading of the bowel with fecal material is often obvious on a plain film of the abdomen. If constipation is a likely cause of the problem, it should be treated by oral laxatives or an enema. Sometimes a strong laxative such as sodium picosulfate (Picolax) is necessary to ensure sufficient evacuation for drainage of the dialysate. Subsequently, bowel action should be kept regular by increasing the fibre in the diet and, if necessary, the addition of a mild laxative such as lactulose or senna.

Fibrin in dialysate

During peritonitis, it is common for fibrin to be present in the dialysate. If there is any restriction of dialysate flow, the bags should be heparinized to a concentration of 500 units/L. A few patients have fibrin formation in the absence of peritonitis. The bag may appear cloudy immediately on drainage, but the fibrin will aggregate on standing. The first time this happens a sample must be sent to the microbiology laboratory to exclude infection. If this proves negative, the patient can be reassured. If catheter plugging occurs, regular use of heparin is recommended. This can often be confined to the overnight bag for CAPD or the daytime dwell (if used) for those receiving APD.

Fluid leaks

External On occasions, fluid may leak from the exit site or even the incision site where the cannula was inserted into the peritoneal cavity. This is usually a problem that

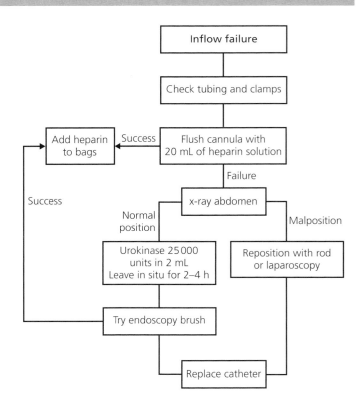

Figure 86.9 Algorithm for managing failure of dialysate inflow.

occurs early, particularly if dialysis is started soon after cannula insertion. Whenever possible, elective insertion of the catheter should be performed at least 2 weeks before dialysis is required. In addition, the use of the paramedian approach for the peritoneal entry site is thought to minimize the chances of this complication. If a leak occurs, then PD should be withheld for as long as possible. If dialysis is necessary then temporary use of hemodialysis should be used for 2 weeks. Alternatively, after at least 48 h of a "dry" abdomen, PD can be recommenced with the aid of a cycler using a low volume (500 mL for adults) and no dwell. Volumes are then progressively increased during 10 days. Should the leak recur despite either of these regimens, surgical repair of the peritoneal entry site will be required. It may be better to completely remove the first catheter and replace with a new one at a different site. Once again, if at all possible, the abdomen should be left dry for 2–4 weeks to allow full healing with sealing, particularly around the inner cuff.

Internal

Abdominal wall edema Edema of the anterior abdominal wall can occur as part of generalized fluid retention. In this situation there is almost invariably a significant amount of peripheral edema. Treatment involves restricting fluid intake and using more hypertonic bags to improve fluid removal.

Isolated edema of the abdominal wall suggests an internal leak from the peritoneal cavity. This is particularly likely to occur from the catheter insertion site or a previous incision. It also sometimes occurs in association with an overt hernia. The site of the leak can be visualized by computerized tomography after the intraperitoneal instillation of contrast media. It may be necessary for the patient to stand or perform other maneuvers to increase intraabdominal pressure before the leak can be seen. An alternative diagnostic test is to perform scintigraphy after injecting a compound labelled with technetium-99m, such as DTPA. If a major leak is visualized, then surgical repair will be required. Often, however, the patient can be managed conservatively by bed rest and using low-volume cycles with little or no dwell. Cessation of PD for 2 weeks with temporary hemodialysis may also allow the leak to seal permanently.

Genital edema This symptom can be caused by the same processes as abdominal wall edema and the management is identical. In addition, genital edema can also be caused by a patent processus vaginalis with or without an associated inguinal hernia. As before, the leak should be visualized by using computer tomography or scintigraphy. Any hernia requires surgical repair, but once again a small leak may seal off spontaneously if PD is suspended, or with continued use of bed rest, low volumes, and a scrotal support for affected men.

Vagina Leakage of dialysate through the vagina has been described, though relatively rarely. It is not clear whether this phenomenon occurs through the fallopian tubes or by tracking of fluid through fascial planes to the vaginal vault. There is often an associated peritonitis. Diagnosis is confirmed by the presence of fluid in the vagina with a glucose content much higher than that the patient's blood glucose level. If the fallopian tubes are the cause then tubal ligation should cure the problem. Otherwise, leaving the abdomen dry for 2 weeks may allow for spontaneous healing. A recurrence may mean that transfer to hemodialysis would be in the patient's best interest.

Hydrothorax A pleural effusion can occur because of generalized fluid overload or local lung disease, but occasionally it is due to a leak of dialysate through the diaphragm. This more commonly occurs on the right side. A leak is most simply confirmed by aspirating some of the effusion and finding that it has a glucose concentration that is higher than of the patient's blood glucose. Initially conservative measures should be tried. These include stopping PD, aspirating the effusion to dryness and leaving the abdomen dry for 2 weeks (using hemodialysis if necessary). This regimen is effective in a number of patients. If the condition recurs, then pleurodesis should be tried. Various agents have been advocated including tetracycline, talc, autologous blood, and fibrin glue (see Bargman[26] for details) but there are no comparative studies to indicate the best regimen.

Hernias

The inevitable increase in intraabdominal pressure due to the presence of a large volume of fluid in the abdomen will mean that any weakness in the abdominal wall may give way, creating a hernia. Hernias are relatively common in PD patients. The major risks are incarceration and strangulation of bowel. The commonest sites are inguinal, incisional, pericatheter, and periumbilical. Less common sites have been reviewed by Bargman.[26] Any patient commencing long-term PD with a hernia should have it repaired. This can be done at the same time as catheter insertion. Pericatheter hernias are less likely if the catheter is inserted in a paramedian position and PD is not started for at least 10 days after the procedure. If a hernia subsequently develops during PD treatment, it should be electively repaired. Postoperatively, the patient should be treated by low-volume (500 mL) cycles with no dwell using a cycler. The volume is progressively increased and CAPD can recommence after 10 days. Alternatively, the patient can be treated by temporary hemodialysis. Should hernias become a recurrent problem, a switch to nightly PD should seriously be considered because intraabdominal pressure is lower in the supine position. The only other option is a transfer to hemodialysis.

Prolapse One special form of hernia is uterine prolapse. Once again the increased abdominal pressure particularly during CAPD will exacerbate this problem. Though uncommon, it can be difficult to treat. Ring pessaries are sometimes helpful for controlling the uterine descent. If these are not successful then a repair should be considered. In the absence of published information, it is suggested that postoperatively the patient should receive low-volume cycles, or switch temporarily to hemodialysis (i.e. managed in the same way as for ordinary hernias).

Pain

Inflow

Soon after the commencement of PD, patients may experience pain during inflow of the fluid. This is particularly likely to occur if dialysis commences immediately or within a few days of catheter insertion. It is presumably related to blunt trauma of the peritoneum. This problem usually disappears with time but may require the temporary use of simple analgesics. Slowing the rate of inflow will often reduce the symptoms. Curled-tip catheters are thought to reduce the likelihood of this type of pain. The introduction of air can also produce discomfort. Care with the bag-exchange technique should eliminate this hazard.

Pain invariably occurs during peritonitis. The treatment is the same as for any case of peritonitis together with sufficient analgesia if clinically necessary.

A small number of individuals have persistent inflow pain. At least some of these can be treated successfully by increasing the pH of the fluid from the usual acidic level of 5.3 to neutral by using neutral pH bicarbonate-based solutions.[27]

Backache

In a minority of patients, particularly those undergoing CAPD or having a daytime dwell in association with APD, backache may occur. The presence of a large volume of fluid in the abdomen distorts the normal body balance and posture, exacerbating any tendency to lordosis of the spine. Patients with preexisting back problems are most likely to have an exacerbation of their backache although by no means will they all be affected. It is important to investigate the symptom so as to exclude treatable or serious disease. This includes plain views of the spine and if necessary magnetic resonance imagining. Renal osteodystrophy, if present, must be treated appropriately. If, however, the problem appears to be due to degenerative disease of the spine (spondylolisthesis or osteoporosis) adjusting the PD regimen can be beneficial. Reducing the volume of dialysate may help but may adversely affect adequacy (see Chapter 87). Avoidance of fluid in the abdomen while the patient is upright will often allow considerable improvement. This means transferring those on CAPD to nightly PD and avoiding a daytime dwell. If this is ineffective, a switch to hemodialysis should be tried. In addition to the above, exercises for the back are sometimes useful.

Generalized pain

If peritonitis occurs, some patients will develop generalized abdominal pain, particularly if treatment is delayed. This symptom usually disappears within a few days of controlling the infection. A fixed or strangulated hernia may also cause persistent abdominal pain. Local pain can occur in association with exit-site or tunnel infections. Specific treatment of the cause will eliminate the symptom.

Outflow pain

Some patients have discomfort or even pain when the dialysate runs out. This emptying sensation is abolished when the next cycle runs in. This commonly occurs during peritonitis but may be experienced in the absence of infection during the first few weeks of treatment. In the latter situation, the symptom usually disappears with time.

Bleeding
After catheter insertion

Immediately after the catheter is placed in the peritoneal cavity, a small amount of bleeding can occur from the operation wounds. If excessive, this will usually respond to firm pressure. Rarely, it may be necessary to reopen the wound and secure the bleeding point.

Exit site

The exit site can be a source of blood loss at any time while a peritoneal cannula is in place. A common cause is the removal of a crust before actual separation has occurred. The bleeding almost invariably stops with local pressure but a raw area remains which is liable to get infected. Regular cleansing of the exit site with povidone–iodine will reduce the chances of this complication. Patients must be instructed not to pull off the crust but await its natural separation. Severe infection of the exit site may, on occasion, be accompanied by secondary hemorrhage. This again will usually respond to firm pressure with gauze dressings. The subsequent management is the same as for any exit-site infection.

Blood-stained dialysate

This is an uncommon event, and although it is rarely serious it can cause considerable alarm to the patient. In some individuals, there is a clear history of trauma to the abdomen or of unexpected strain. Some women relate the episode to their menstrual cycle at the time of ovulation or menstruation. Other less common causes are listed in Table 57.8 of Brenner and Rector's The Kidney. The treatment is to flush the abdomen with a few cycles of dialysate containing heparin (500 units/L) to minimize the chances of clotting in the cannula. It has been suggested that ice-cold dialysis fluid will stop the bleeding more quickly. There is no controlled trial of this, and the procedure is uncomfortable. The problem usually resolves spontaneously and is often visible in only one outflow. It is unusual for the blood-stained dialysate to be associated with infection, although it is wise to have the fluid cultured. Routine use of antibiotics is not necessary. In the rare event of significant hemorrhage occurring, an urgent laparotomy is required.

Chyloperitoneum

An occasional patient may present with a milky effluent. The initial reaction is to suspect peritonitis, but closer inspection reveals that the fluid is not completely opaque and microscopy does not show excess white cells. This appearance is thought to be due to the presence of chylomicrons in the dialysate. There is no obvious cause in some patients but malignant neoplasm in the retroperitoneum, including lymphoma, can present this way. Reasonable steps should be taken to exclude such a diagnosis. In the absence of malignant disease there is no specific treatment.

Metabolic complications

The use of glucose-based hyperosmolar solutions for PD results in a significant increase in the glucose load experienced by the patient. A number of reports have measured the daily glucose absorption, which is estimated as between 100 and 200 g/day.

The resulting metabolic effect is a persistent tendency for patients on CAPD to develop hyperglycemia and hyperinsulinemia. In a number of individuals, frank diabetes may develop. This unused glucose load is also thought to contribute to an increased risk of atherogenesis.

Changes in lipid metabolism peculiar to CAPD are more difficult to define. Triglycerides and cholesterol increase during the first year on CAPD. This is due to an increase in very-low-density and low-density lipoproteins (LDL). The greater the degree of hyperlipidemia at the start of therapy, the worse will be the changes with time on CAPD. In addition, there was an indication that lipoprotein (a) levels may increase with time on CAPD (although these results are not universally confirmed). On the whole, however, proatherogenic lipid levels are more common in patients on CAPD than those on hemodialysis.

A number of studies have demonstrated the effectiveness of cholesterol-lowering agents in patients on CAPD. Both lovastatin and simvastatin (hydroxymethylglutaryl-coenzyme A reductase inhibitors) have been shown effective in reducing total cholesterol and LDL-cholesterol while increasing high-density lipoprotein cholesterol. The long-term effects of such intervention on cardiovascular morbidity and mortality, however, have yet to be established.

References

1. Williams JD, Craig KJ, Topley N, von Ruhland C, Fallon M, Newman GR, Mackenzie RK, Williams GT: Morphological changes in the peritoneal membrane of patients with renal disease. J Amer Soc Nephrol 2002;13:470–479.

2. Keane WF, Bailie GR, Boeschoten E, et al: Adult peritoneal dialysis-related peritonitis treatment recommendations: 2000 update. Perit Dial Int 2000;20:396–411.

3. Paterson AD, Bishop MC, Morgan AG, Burden RP. Removal and replacement of Tenckhoff catheter at a single operation. Lancet 1986;8518: 1245–1247.

4. MacLeod A, Grant A, Donaldson C, et al: Effectiveness and efficiency of methods of dialysis therapy for end-stage renal disease: systematic reviews. Health Technol Assess 1998;2:1–166.

5. Holley J L, Bernardini J, Piraino B: Infecting organisms in continuous ambulatory peritoneal dialysis on the Y set. Am J Kid Dis 1994;23:569–573.

6. Perez-Fontan M, Garcia-Falcon, Rosales M, et al: Treatment of Staphylococcus aureus nasal carriers in continuous ambulatory peritoneal dialysis with mupirocin. Am J Kid Dis 1993;22:708–712.

7. Bernardini J , Piraino B, Holley J, et al: A randomized trial of Staphylococcus aureus prophylaxis in peritoneal dialysis patients: Mupirocin calcium ointment 2% applied to the exit site versus cyclic oral rifampicin. Am J Kidney Dis 1996;27:695–700.

8. The Mupirocin Study Group: Nasal mupirocin prevents Staphylococcus aureus exit-site infection during peritoneal dialysis. J Am Soc Nephrol 1996;7:2403–2408.

9. Luzar MA: Exit-site infection in continuous ambulatory peritoneal dialysis: A review. Perit Dial Int 1991;11:333–340.

10. Twardowski ZJ, Prownant BF: Classification of normal and diseased exit sites. Perit Dial Int 1996;16(Suppl 3):S32–S50.

11. Gokal R, Alexander S, Ash S, et al: Peritoneal catheters and exit site practices toward optimum peritoneal access: 1998 update. Official report from the International Society for Peritoneal Dialysis. Perit Dial Int 1998;18:11–33.

12. Khanna R, Twardowski ZJ: Recommendations for treatment of exit site pathology. Perit Dial Int 1996;16(Suppl 3):S100–S104.

13. Zimmerman SW, Ahreus E, Johnson CA, et al: Randomized controlled trial of prophylactic rifampin for peritoneal dialysis-related infections. Am J Kidney Dis 1991;18:225–231.

14. Luzar MA, Brown C, Balf D, et al: Exit site care and exit-site infection in CAPD: Results of a randomised multicenter trial. Perit Dial Int 1990;10:25–29.

15. Kahl AA, Grosse-Siestrop C, Kahl KA, et al: Reduction of exit-site infections in peritoneal dialysis by local application of metallic silver: A preliminary report. Perit Dial Int 1994;14:177–180.

16. Hwang TL, Huang CC: Comparison of Swan neck catheter with Tenckhoff catheter for CAPD. Adv Perit Dial 1994;10:203–205.

17. Eklund BH, Honkanen EO, Kala AF, et al: Catheter configuration and outcome in patients on continuous ambulatory peritoneal dialysis: A prospective comparison of two catheters. Perit Dial Int 1994;14:70–74.

18. Moncreif JW, Popovich RP, Dasgupta M, et al: Reduction in peritonitis incidence in continuous ambulatory peritoneal dialysis with a new catheter and implantation technique. Perit Dial Int 1993;13(Suppl 2):S329–S331.

19. Heimburger O, Waniewski J, Werynski A, Tranaeus A, Lindholm B: Peritoneal transport in CAPD paients with permanent loss of ultrafiltration capacity. Kidney Int 1990;38:495–506.

20. Twardowski ZJ, Nolph KD, Khanna R, Prowant BF, Ryan LP, Moore HL, et al: Peritoneal equilibration test. Perit Dial Bull 1987;7:138–147.

21. Davies SJ, Brown B, Bryan J, Russell GI: Clinical evaluation of the peritoneal equilibration test: a population-based study. Nephrol Dial Transplant 1993;8:64–70.

22. Ho-dac-Pannekeet MM, Atasever B, Struijk DG, Krediet RT: Analysis of ultrafiltration failure in peritoneal dialysis patients by means of standard peritoneal permeability analysis. Perit Dial Int 1997;17:144–150.

23. Davies SJ: Montoring of long-term membrane function. Perit Dial Int 2001;21:225–230.

24. Medcalf JF, Harris KP, Walls J: Role of diuretics in the preservation of residual renal function in patients on continuous ambulatory peritoneal dialysis. Kidney Int 2001;59:1128–1133.

25. Posthuma N, ter Wee PM, Verbrugh HA, Oe PL, Peers E, Sayers J, et al: Icodextrin instead of glucose during the daytime dwell in CCPD increases ultrafiltration and 24-h dialysate creatinine clearance. Nephrol Dial Transplant 1997;12:550–553.

26. Bargman JM: Noninfectious complications of peritoneal dialysis. In Gokal R, Nolph KD (eds): The Textbook of Peritoneal Dialysis. Dordrecht: Kluwer, 1994, pp 555–562.

27. Mactier RA, Sprosen TS, Gokal R, et al: Bicarbonate and bicarbonate/lactate peritoneal dialysis solutions for the treatment of infusion pain. Kidney Int 1998;53:1061–1067.

Adequacy of Peritoneal Dialysis

Peter G. Blake

The term "adequacy of dialysis" has traditionally been used to refer to small-solute clearance in both hemodialysis (HD) and peritoneal dialysis (PD). There is, however, an increasing sense that it should take into account other elements of the dialysis prescription. In this review of adequacy of PD, emphasis will be given to small-solute clearance; however, attention will also be paid to the equally important areas of volume status and nutrition.

The issue of comparative outcomes on PD, relative to HD, is also a key measure of the adequacy of PD as a renal replacement therapy. It has been a controversial topic and will be reviewed here.

Small-solute clearance

In the late 1980s, the first attempts were made to extrapolate to PD the principles of quantification and prescription of dialytic dose established for HD in the aftermath of the National Cooperative Dialysis Study.[1] In the 1990s, numerous studies attempted to show that measurements of fractional urea clearance (Kt/V) and creatinine clearance corrected for body surface area (CrCl) correlated with, or were predictive of, patient well-being and survival. More recently, the first major randomized control trials in this area have been carried out.

Principles of quantification

Small-solute clearance in PD comprises a peritoneal and a residual renal component. The latter is particularly important in that it accounts for a greater proportion of overall clearance achieved than is the case in HD, and because it appears to persist longer in PD patients.

The peritoneal component is calculated by collecting dialysate effluent for 24 h and by measuring its urea and creatinine content. These are then divided by the serum urea and creatinine levels, respectively, to give peritoneal urea clearance (Kt) and creatinine clearance. Dialysate creatinine levels may need to be corrected for the high dialysate glucose content as this interferes with the assay used in some laboratories. The renal component is calculated in the same way with a 24-h urine collection. However, in the case of creatinine clearance, an average of residual renal urea and creatinine clearance is typically used because unmodified creatinine clearance substantially overestimates the true glomerular filtration rate. These clearances are then normalized to total body water (V) to give Kt/V, or to 1.73 m^2 body surface area to give CrCl. The value for V is estimated using anthropometric formulas, such as those of Watson, based on age, sex, height, and weight.[2] These estimates, compared with a "gold standard" such as deuterium oxide dilution, are, on average, reasonably accurate in nonobese patients but tend to give an overestimate of V in those who are overweight.[3] Nevertheless, because most of the clinical literature is based on a V calculated according to these equations and because they are relatively simple, they remain the method of choice. Body surface area is estimated by the Du Bois formula.[4] Kt/V and CrCl values are typically expressed as weekly, rather than daily, clearances (Tables 87.1 and 87.2).

Attempts to estimate Kt/V and CrCl using abbreviated methods based on the peritoneal equilibration test (PET) are not sufficiently accurate for clinical practice. Computer programs that calculate clearances are widely available. These can also be used to model patients and predict the clearances that a given prescription will achieve, but they are not accurate enough to replace the 24-h collection in clinical practice. Collections are more cumbersome in patients on automated PD (APD) than in those on continuous ambulatory PD (CAPD) because of the greater volumes involved, and many units train patients to record or measure effluent volumes and then to take a representative aliquot of dialysate for measurement of urea and creatinine.

Table 87.1 Formulas required to calculate Kt/V

Kt/V	= 7 (daily peritoneal Kt/V plus daily renal Kt/V)
Daily peritoneal Kt	= $\dfrac{\text{24-h dialysate urea content}}{\text{Serum urea}}$
Daily renal Kt	= $\dfrac{\text{24-h urine urea content}}{\text{Serum urea}}$
V (by Watson)	= 2.447–0.09516 A + 0.1704 H + 0.3362 W (in males) or
	= –2.097–0.1069 H + 0.02466 W (in females)

A, age (years); H, height (cm); W, weight (kg).

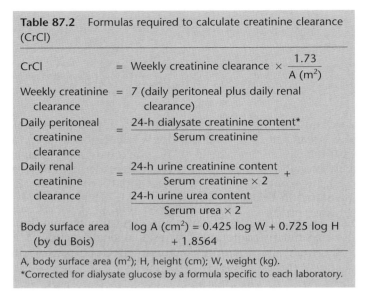

Table 87.2 Formulas required to calculate creatinine clearance (CrCl)

CrCl	$= \text{Weekly creatinine clearance} \times \dfrac{1.73}{A \ (m^2)}$
Weekly creatinine clearance	$= 7 \ (\text{daily peritoneal plus daily renal clearance})$
Daily peritoneal creatinine clearance	$= \dfrac{\text{24-h dialysate creatinine content}^*}{\text{Serum creatinine}}$
Daily renal creatinine clearance	$= \dfrac{\text{24-h urine creatinine content}}{\text{Serum creatinine} \times 2} + \dfrac{\text{24-h urine urea content}}{\text{Serum urea} \times 2}$
Body surface area (by du Bois)	$\log A \ (cm^2) = 0.425 \log W + 0.725 \log H + 1.8564$

A, body surface area (m^2); H, height (cm); W, weight (kg).
*Corrected for dialysate glucose by a formula specific to each laboratory.

Typically, residual renal function declines gradually towards zero over the first 2–3 years on PD, and so total clearance will also decrease if the dialysis prescription is not modified (Fig. 87.1).[5] In recent years, much effort has gone into making such modifications. In general, collections should be performed shortly after commencing PD and then every 4 months subsequently so as to allow timely detection of declines in residual function; collections should also be performed after any alteration in prescription or unexpected clinical event. There are data suggesting that daily collections are not very reproducible, mainly, but not only, because of major variations in the urinary component.[6] A 48-h urine collection might therefore be preferable in some patients. An unexpected result should certainly be confirmed with a repeat collection.

The urea and protein content of the same 24-h collections carried out to calculate clearance can be used to measure the normalized protein equivalent of nitrogen appearance (nPNA), which, in a stable patient, is an estimate of dietary protein intake. There are numerous formulas for calculating nPNA, but evidence suggests that those of Bergstrom are best (Table 87.3).[7,8] Also, these collections allow measurement of total creatinine excretion, which can, in turn, be used to estimate lean body mass (Table 87.4).[9] Similarly, measurement of total protein or albumin losses can be helpful in the evaluation of low serum albumin values.

Total *Kt/V* values achieved in PD are typically one-half to two-thirds of those in HD. This might suggest major underdialysis, but it must be remembered that the efficiency, in terms of solute removal, of clearance delivered intermittently is much less than that of the same amount of clearance delivered continuously.[10] Also, continuous modalities avoid the substantial disequilibria of intermittent ones. Furthermore, it has been suggested that continuous modalities are at an advantage because peak levels of uremic toxins are theoretically lower for a given quantity of clearance than is the case with intermittent modalities. It has been proposed that peak rather than mean levels of small solutes are proportional to uremic toxicity.[1]

Clinical studies on adequacy of peritoneal dialysis

Initial studies correlating small-solute clearance and patient outcomes gave varied results and tended to have multiple

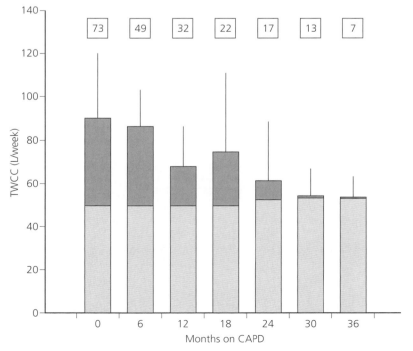

Figure 87.1 Change in CrCl with time and CAPD. The lighter areas indicate the proportion of CrCl accounted for by peritoneal and renal clearance respectively. Figures in the boxes refer to the number of patients at each 6-month interval. (From Blake PG, Balaskas EV, Izatt S, Oreopoulos DG: Is total creatinine clearance a good predictor of clinical outcomes in CAPD? Perit Dial Int 1992;12:353–358.)

Table 87.3 Bergstrom formulas for estimating protein equivalent of nitrogen appearance (PNA) in patients on peritoneal dialysis

PNA (g/day) =   20.1 + 7.50 (daily dialysate plus urine urea nitrogen content (g/day))

or

15.1 + 6.95 (daily dialysate plus urine urea nitrogen content (g/day)) + daily dialysate plus urine protein content (g/day)

The same formulas with urea concentrations expressed in SI units are as follows:

PNA (g/day) =   20.1 + 0.209 (daily dialysate plus urine urea content (mmol/day))

or

15.1 + 0.195 (daily dialysate plus urine urea content (mmol/day)) + daily dialysate plus urine protein content (g/day)

Modified from Bergstrom et al.[7]
In all cases, normalized PNA (nPNA) = PNA/desirable body weight.

Table 87.4 Formulas for calculating lean body mass by the method of Keshaviah et al[9]

Lean body mass (kg)	= 7.38 + 0.029 [creatinine production (mg/day)]
Creatinine production (mg)	= Creatinine excretion + creatinine degradation
Creatinine excretion (mg/day)	= 24-h dialysate creatinine* content (mg) + 24-h urine creatinine content (mg)
Creatinine degradation (mg/day)	= 0.38 [Serum creatinine (mg/dL)] × [Body weight (kg)]

*Corrected for dialysate glucose by a formula specific to each laboratory.

methodological flaws. The Canada/USA (CANUSA) study avoided some of these problems in that it was multicenter and prospective and in that it followed almost 600 incident CAPD patients for up to 3 years, giving it unprecedented statistical power.[12] It was, however, a cohort study with no mandated interventions. CANUSA demonstrated a predictive power for both Kt/V and CrCl, such that a 5 L/week lower CrCl was associated with a 7% greater relative risk of dying, and a 0.1 unit/week lower Kt/V was associated with a 5% greater relative risk of dying. Peritoneal dialysis prescriptions in CANUSA patients were mainly the standard 4×2 L/week and very few were altered with time, so that changes in clearance were mainly due to declines in residual function. CANUSA, on closer analysis, showed a correlation between residual renal clearance and subsequent mortality, but could not show one between peritoneal clearance alone and mortality (Table 87.5).[13] However, the design of the study did not really allow this issue to be addressed.

Subsequent to CANUSA, a variety of other prospective and retrospective studies showed similar correlations between small-solute clearance and clinical outcomes, but all were similarly confounded by residual renal function.[14–16] None could show an independent effect of peritoneal clearance on outcomes, even when there was significant variation in PD dose (Table 87.5).[16] Notwithstanding this, clinical practice guidelines from various bodies proposed target Kt/V and CrCl values in the middle to late 1990s.[17,18] Most notably, the US National Kidney Foundation Dialysis Outcomes Quality Initiative (DOQI) set a weekly Kt/V target of 2.0 for CAPD. For CrCl, the target was set at 60 L/week, although this was subsequently modified down to 50 L/week for low and low average transporters (see below and Table 87.6).[17,18,19] Slightly higher targets were set for APD, with and without day dwells, on the grounds that these are somewhat more intermittent modalities than CAPD (Table 87.5). These new clearance targets had a major impact on PD prescription and led to increased use of higher dwell volumes in CAPD and of multiple day dwells in APD.[20] The result was a notable increase in delivered clearances.

Randomized controlled trials

The first major randomized controlled trials addressing the effectiveness of raising peritoneal clearance have recently appeared. Mak et al[21] compared 4×2 L with 3×2 L in 82 prevalent CAPD patients in a single-center study in Hong Kong. Follow-up was for 12 months and, during this time, Kt/V fell in both groups owing to loss of residual renal function. By the end of 12 months, the weekly Kt/V values in the control and intervention groups were 1.67 and 2.02 respectively. No significant difference was seen in clinical outcomes. This study was, however, significantly underpowered in terms of patient numbers.

Table 87.5 Relative risks of mortality associated with peritoneal and residual clearance*

	CANUSA	Rocco et al	ADEMEX
Renal Kt/V (per 0.1/week increment)	Not reported	0.88 ($P = 0.003$)	0.94 ($P = 0.005$)
Peritoneal Kt/V (per 0.1/week increment)	Not reported	1.00 ($P = 0.81$)	1.00 ($P = 0.78$)
Renal CrCl (per 10 L/week increment)	0.88 ($P < 0.05$)†	0.60 ($P < 0.001$)	0.89 ($P = 0.01$)
Peritoneal CrCl (per 10 L/week increment)	1.00 (not significant)†	0.90 ($P = 0.41$)	1.03 ($P = 0.56$)

*Data taken from the CANUSA,[13] Rocco et al,[16] and ADEMEX[22] studies.
†Per 5 L/week increment in CrCl.

Table 87.6 US National Kidney Foundation "DOQI" weekly clearance targets for PD

	Kt/V	CrCl
CAPD	2.0	60 L*
APD with a day dwell	2.1	63 L
APD with no day dwell	2.2	66 L

*50 L for low and low–average peritoneal transporters.
Kt/V, fractional urea clearance; CrCl, creatinine clearance; CAPD, continuous ambulatory peritoneal dialysis; APD, ambulatory peritoneal dialysis.
Modified from Golper et al.[19]

The largest and most definitive randomized controlled trial on this topic, published in 2002. This was the Adequacy of Dialysis in Mexico (ADEMEX) study involving 960 incident and prevalent CAPD patients recruited from 25 centers in Mexico.[22] Participating patients were randomized to one of two groups. The control group was maintained on a standard 4 × 2 L CAPD prescription, whereas the intervention group had their prescription augmented in order to achieve a peritoneal creatinine clearance of 60 L/week. A very small number of patients who could achieve a peritoneal creatinine clearance of 60 L/week on the standard prescription were excluded from the study. The increases in clearance in the intervention group were made using a larger dwell volume or a fifth exchange, delivered with a night exchange device. Follow-up was for an average of 2 years and the primary endpoint was survival. A large variety of secondary endpoints were also examined. Unlike previous studies, ADEMEX had substantial statistical power to detect endpoint differences. The control group received, on average, a weekly peritoneal CrCl of 46 L and a weekly peritoneal *Kt/V* of 1.62, whereas the intervention group had values of 57 L and 2.13 respectively. Corresponding values for total *Kt/V* are 1.80 and 2.27 and for CrCl are 54 L and 63 L per week respectively (Table 87.7). There were no significant differences in either primary or secondary outcomes between the two groups. In particular, the relative risk of mortality for a patient included in the intervention group was 1.00 compared with a patient in the control group (Fig. 87.2 and Table 87.5). This result was surprising to many and, given the high quality of the study, has brought into question the appropriateness of the DOQI treatment recommendations.

In support of the ADEMEX findings are the results of another randomized control trial from Lo et al.[23] This study involved 322 incident CAPD patients recruited from six centers in Hong Kong between 1996 and 1999. These patients were randomized to three different *Kt/V* targets: 1.5–1.7/week, 1.7–2.0/week, and > 2.0/week. The three groups achieved the targeted *Kt/V* levels and no difference was found in 2-year survival rates. There was, however, a significantly greater study dropout rate of patients in the group with a *Kt/V* below 1.7/week, but the authors concluded that *Kt/V* should be maintained above 1.7/week. This study was somewhat underpowered to detect mortality differences but, in the light of the ADEMEX study, its findings are not so surprising.

These studies particularly show that residual renal function cannot be replaced on a one-to-one basis by peritoneal clearance. The whole notion of adding the two together may no longer be justifiable. Given that increasing peritoneal clearance is not a neutral intervention and may have lifestyle implications for the patient in terms of mechanical symptoms, time commitment, and cost, it is important to avoid an unnecessarily aggressive approach to PD prescription. However, these studies do not prove that there is no link between peritoneal clearance and outcome. Clearly, there is some relationship in that zero dialysis guarantees an adverse outcome. Thus, there is no evidence that doses below those recorded by the ADEMEX control group, for example, are safe. Furthermore, the Lo et al[23] study would suggest that total *Kt/V* values below 1.7 are problematic.

A possible conclusion from all this new evidence is to define a total *Kt/V* target in the region of 1.7–1.8/week, but it is perhaps more logical to set a purely peritoneal clearance target of 1.65–1.7/week and consider residual renal function as a bonus. A corresponding peritoneal clearance target might be 45–50 L/week, which is what the ADEMEX control group received.

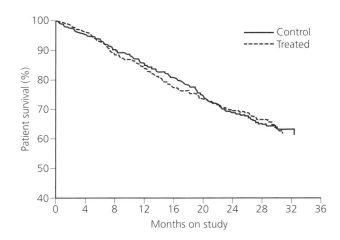

Figure 87.2 Life-table intent-to-treat analysis of patient survival in the intervention and control groups in the ADEMEX study. (Reproduced from Paniagua R, Amato, D, Vonesh E, et al: Effect of increased peritoneal clearances on mortality rates in peritoneal dialysis: ADEMEX, a prospective randomized controlled trial. J Am Soc Nephrol 2002;13:1307–1320.)

Table 87.7 Peritoneal and total clearances delivered in the ADEMEX study

	Control	Intervention
Peritoneal *Kt/V* (per week)	1.62	2.13
Total *Kt/V* (per week)	1.80	2.27
Peritoneal CrCl (L/week)	46.1	56.9
Total CrCl (L/week)	54.1	62.9

An alternative interpretation is that the whole *Kt/V* and CrCl model may be flawed. The normalization to body water and body surface area may not be appropriate, or peritoneal small-solute clearance may simply not be the best measure of the effectiveness of PD. A more holistic clinical approach with less attention to numbers and more to the patients' clinical status may be preferable.

Peritoneal transport status

Patients differ in the rapidity at which urea, creatinine, and other solutes equilibrate with dialysis solution across their peritoneal membrane. This is classically measured by the peritoneal equilibration test (PET) in which dialysate and plasma levels of urea and creatinine are measured during a 4-h, 2-L, 2.5% dextrose dwell carried out under standard conditions.[24] Equilibration curves are constructed for patients, who are defined as low, low average, high average, and high transporters (Fig. 87.3). It is generally believed that PET status is a measure of the "effective" or vascular surface area of the peritoneal membrane, but, interestingly, it does not correlate with body size. Patients who are high transporters equilibrate quickly and so, in that sense, dialyze well, but they ultrafilter poorly because their osmotic gradient for glucose dissipates rapidly. They might be expected to do better with short dwell times, as in APD, but they need to avoid prolonged day dwells with glucose-based PD solutions. They also have higher dialysate protein losses and are prone to more marked hypoalbuminemia. Conversely, low transporters ultrafilter well, lose less protein in their dialysate, and have higher serum albumin levels, but they equilibrate slowly. Thus, in low transporters large-volume dwells with longer treatment times are best for achieving good clearance. In practice, even low transporters achieve reasonable urea equilibration, typically exceeding 85% in standard CAPD. However, creatinine equilibration is significantly reduced, especially with the short duration dwells of APD, and CrCl targets are difficult to achieve once residual renal function is lost. Despite this, results from the CANUSA study and other studies suggest that low, rather than high,

transporters have substantially superior long-term outcomes on CAPD.[25] This again supports the notion that peritoneal small-solute clearance alone is not a good predictor of patient outcome on PD. Rather, it suggests that volume status may be more important as high transporters have more problems in this regard. These findings have led to the suggestion that high transporters might preferentially be directed to APD and to the use of alternative osmotic agents to dextrose, especially when residual renal function is lost (see below).[18] These findings have also resulted in the target CrCl values for low transporters being set at a lower level of 50 L/week in the 2001 revised DOQI guidelines.[19]

Increasing peritoneal dialysis dose

Despite the controversy about target clearances in PD, it is important to understand how delivered clearance can be increased in PD patients. In CAPD, the best strategy to raise dialytic dose is to increase dwell volumes to 2.5 L. This is usually well tolerated and minimally disruptive of lifestyle. Larger patients may require and tolerate 3-L volumes. The alternative approach of increasing the frequency of daytime manual exchanges to more than four will tend to lead to inadequate spacing of the exchanges so that equilibration is less complete and is also likely to increase the risk of patient noncompliance. A fifth exchange, however, can be carried out with a nighttime exchange device and, as two of the dwells will now be in the supine position, scope for larger volume dwells increases.

APD offers alternative strategies, although it should not be viewed as a panacea for inadequate PD. If carelessly prescribed, it can lead to clearances that are actually less than those on standard CAPD. Daytime dwells are required to achieve clearance targets in APD patients unless residual renal function is very good or unless the patient is very small or is a high transporter. In heavier patients and in low transporters, especially when residual renal function is poor, 2-day dwells are frequently required. The cost of this approach can be reduced by using the cycler solutions and tubing to perform the daytime exchange. If two daytime

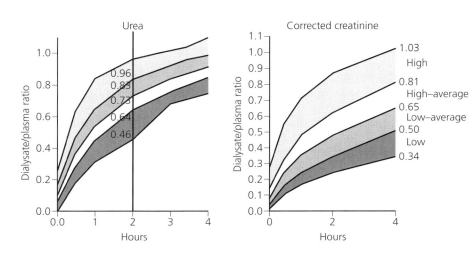

Figure 87.3 Peritoneal equilibration test results. Ranges of values for D/P urea and D/P creatinine (corrected) in standard PET. (From Twardowski et al.[24]

exchanges are being carried out, the number of cycled exchanges can be limited to four or even three in order to minimize cost.

With regard to the actual cycler prescription, 2.5-L, or even higher, dwell volumes are usually well tolerated, given that APD is delivered in the supine position. Nine hours should be the standard time spent each night on the cycler. Increasing the frequency of cycler exchanges above six or seven over 9 h gives only modest increases in clearance, and so is generally not cost-effective.[26] The problem is that too much of the cycling time is spent on draining and filling and too little on actual dialysis. Tidal techniques, which maintain a constant residual volume throughout the cycling time, were devised to help with this problem but they are not effective in increasing clearance and are only useful when the final phase of drainage is slow or painful.

With both CAPD and APD, hypertonic solutions can be used to increase clearance by maximizing ultrafiltration, but this strategy increases the risk of dehydration as well as that of obesity, hyperglycemia, hyperlipidemia, and, perhaps, long-term peritoneal membrane damage. With all strategies, patient lifestyle and willingness to comply should be kept in mind. As stated already, dialysis dose should be remeasured soon after each prescription alteration.

In some cases, the CrCl target is achieved but that of the Kt/V is not. This is typically seen in patients with substantial residual renal function because of the disproportionate contribution of tubular creatinine secretion. The converse situation, in which the Kt/V target is achieved but the CrCl is not, is seen in patients who are low transporters because they have relatively poorer creatinine equilibration. It is also seen in patients with short dwell times, as in APD, in which creatinine equilibration is disproportionately affected.

Volume status in peritoneal dialysis

The favorable prognosis associated with low PET status gives support to the notion that volume status is an important determinant of outcome in PD patients.[25] There are no high-quality data to prove that good volume management improves outcome. However, cardiovascular disease is the biggest cause of morbidity and mortality in dialysis patients generally, and hypertension, a crucial risk factor, is very common in this population and very influenced by volume status.

Management of volume status has recently been the subject of International Society of Peritoneal Dialysis clinical practice guidelines.[27] Key factors that need to be taken into account in managing volume status in PD patients, in addition to PET findings, include salt and water intake, residual renal function, and adherence to the PD prescription. Useful strategies to control volume status include dietary salt and water restriction when required, the use of high-dose loop diuretics in patients who still have urine output, and education of patients in the significance of fluid overload and hypertension.

There are a number of key factors in the prescription, however, that can be modified. These are the dwell time, the tonicity of solution used, and the choice of osmotic agent. Prolonged dwell times are associated with greater peritoneal fluid absorption. This is particularly an issue with the nighttime dwell in CAPD and with the daytime dwell in APD. One approach is to break up these long dwells by introducing a nighttime exchange device in CAPD or a daytime exchange in APD. This intervention will increase not only net ultrafiltration but also clearance. Ultrafiltration can also be enhanced, in both short and long dwells, by increasing the tonicity of the glucose solution used. However, this strategy is limited by the adverse effects of increased glucose absorption. These include hyperglycemia, hyperlipidemia, obesity, and peritoneal membrane damage. A more attractive approach to avoid fluid absorption from long-duration dwells has become possible in recent years with the introduction of the alternative osmotic agent icodextrin.[28] This is a large-molecular-weight glucose polymer that induces ultrafiltration by colloid osmosis. Because the icodextrin molecule is too large to be absorbed across the peritoneal membrane, the osmotic gradient does not dissipate and there is sustained ultrafiltration throughout the duration of a long dwell. Icodextrin is now frequently used as the long daytime dwell in APD and as the nighttime dwell in CAPD. There is a modest amount of lymphatic absorption of icodextrin with subsequent metabolism to maltose, but no toxicity related to this has been identified after 10 years' experience. The only disadvantages of icodextrin are its higher cost and a small but significant rate of exfoliative skin rashes. Besides improving ultrafiltration, the reduced exposure to glucose of patients on icodextrin can lead to less weight gain and less hyperglycemia and hypertriglyceridemia. In general, average high and high transporters should be directed towards APD and/or icodextrin if problems arise with volume status.[18] This will often first occur when residual renal function falls off.

Patient compliance

Patient compliance with PD exchanges is an important issue. Methodology to detect noncompliance is limited. Ratios between actual and predicted creatinine excretion have not been found to be helpful, but sudden rises in creatinine excretion in a given patient are suggestive of noncompliance. These sudden rises suggest that patients, on the day of their collections, are dialyzing out creatinine that accumulated on previous noncompliant days. Questionnaires are likely to understate the prevalence of noncompliance and checks on home inventory are probably the nearest there is to a gold standard. Using the latter methodology, one US group found a 40% rate of significant noncompliance.[29] A large, multicenter, questionnaire-based study suggested that the problem was most likely to occur in patients who were young, employed, African-American, and on more than four CAPD exchanges daily.[30] There is a need to be aware of this problem.

Malnutrition in peritoneal dialysis

Malnutrition is prevalent in dialysis patients generally, and one international study found, using subjective nutritional assessment, that 8% of 224 CAPD patients had severe malnutrition and a further 33% had mild-to-moderate malnutrition.[31]

A number of nutritional indices have been shown to predict adverse outcomes. Lower serum albumin is associated with greater mortality, hospitalization rates, and technique failure.[12] In the CANUSA study, the relative risk of dying decreased by 6% for each 1 g/L rise in the serum albumin. In PD patients, however, serum albumin may not primarily be a nutritional marker. A number of studies have shown that high peritoneal transport status and the presence of inflammation, as indicated by a raised serum C-reactive protein level, are the major predictors of a low serum albumin.[32,33]

Lean body mass, estimated by creatinine excretion according to the method of Keshaviah et al,[11] and total body nitrogen, estimated by neutron activation analysis,[34] have also been shown to predict survival, as has the relatively simple clinical tool of subjective global assessment.[12] The predictive data for the nPNA are less consistent. Some of this discrepancy may be related to variation in the methods of measurement and normalization. Evidence suggests that the Bergstrom formula, which was specifically derived from PD patients, is most accurate in that it takes full account of the high nonurea, nonprotein nitrogen losses in these patients.[7,35] Normalization to desirable rather than actual weight is preferable. No clear target for nPNA has been validated. On theoretical grounds, 1.2 g/kg/day has been proposed but is rarely achieved, and neutral nitrogen balance may be possible at significantly lower values.[7,17] Caloric intake has been relatively poorly studied and, although it has been shown to be as important as protein intake for nitrogen balance, no clear studies correlating it with outcome have been published. The general recommendation is that patients receive 35 kcal/kg/day, although this should be reduced for obese pateints.[17] In many patients, 20% or more of calories will come from dialysate glucose absorption. Other nutritional indices such as serum prealbumin, insulin-like growth factor 1 (IGF-1) levels, anthropometrics, and bioelectric impedance are not widely used.

Malnutrition in dialysis patients is typically multifactorial. Food intake is often low owing to uremia per se, dietary restrictions, socioeconomic issues, possible dialysate-induced compression of viscera, and, often most significantly, comorbidity, including gastrointestinal disease, cardiovascular disease, and depression. Patients also have obligatory dialysate nitrogen and protein losses and may be catabolic from inadequate intake as well as from intercurrent illnesses, inflammation, and acidosis. The role of endocrine dysfunction, and in particular of the growth hormone IGF-1 axis in impairing the balance between anabolism and catabolism in uremia, has also been recognized.

Management of malnutrition

Interventions to treat malnutrition are not well validated. They include increases in dialytic dose, oral protein, and carbohydrate supplementation; intraperitoneal amino acids; and administration of anabolic hormones such as androgens and recombinant growth hormone and IGF-1.

A small number of studies, mostly uncontrolled, have looked at the effect of prospective increases in peritoneal clearance on nutrition.[36,37] In general, these studies have shown conflicting results with regard to protein intake, with some showing an increase and others no change. The methodology is often confounded by mathematical coupling between indices of dialysis dose and those of nutrition. In studies that have looked at serum albumin, there has been no clear beneficial effect. The ADEMEX study also failed to show a nutritional advantage for the high-clearance group.[22]

There have been numerous studies on intraperitoneal amino acids. Initially, these were confounded by associated increases in uremia and acidosis. However, more recently, the amino acid composition of the preparations has been favorably modified, and strategies for administering them have improved so that they are now given as one exchange in the daytime in association with oral caloric intake. Recent trials have confirmed an increase in nitrogen balance, a fall in phosphate consistent with an anabolic effect, favorable changes in IGF-1 levels, and an increase in serum albumin that appears to be significant only in more severely hypoalbuminemic patients.[38] There remain some questions, however, as to how sustained these beneficial effects are.

One small randomized controlled trial has shown a benefit for anabolic steroids in increasing lean body mass and functional performance in malnourished HD and PD patients, but concerns about side-effects have limited their use.[39] Studies on recombinant growth hormone and IGF-1 have been small and short term, but have shown impressive anabolic effects.[40] Effects on serum albumin have been less impressive. Cost and toxicity concerns limit the use of these recombinant agents to research studies at present.

The relative ineffectiveness of most of these nutritional interventions in PD patients raises questions about the nature of malnutrition in dialysis patients generally. Although many patients are malnourished, which is a predictor of adverse outcomes, it is not clear whether malnutrition is the proximate cause of those outcomes or whether its correction, when possible, will lead to an improvement in those outcomes. It is at least as plausible that malnutrition is a consequence of comorbidity or inflammation, which is the true proximate cause of the patients' morbidity and mortality. If the latter is the case, attempts to treat the malnutrition, without dealing with underlying causes, may be ineffective both in terms of nutritional status and in terms of ultimate clinical outcomes. Recent data linking malnutrition, inflammation, and cardiovascular disease may be pertinent in this regard.[41]

Comparative outcome studies

Interest in adequacy of dialysis has also focused attention on comparative outcomes between HD and PD. Most data come from national or renal registries and none is from randomized control trials. Patient mortality is the usual endpoint used in these studies. A controversial US Registry study published in 1995 suggested an excess mortality on PD, but the methodology was unusual in that the majority of the first year in dialysis was omitted from the analysis.[42] This leads to a systematic bias against PD, as outcomes on the modality are relatively better in the early years on dialysis.

Subsequent and more contemporary studies from the US, Canadian, Danish, and Lombardy Registries all show a similar picture.[43–46] PD has a survival advantage over HD during the first 2–3 years of dialysis. This advantage is most marked in younger patients and in nondiabetics (Fig. 87.4). In the USA, but not elsewhere, no significant early advantage for PD is seen in older diabetics; indeed, in older female diabetics, HD has a significant advantage.[43] After 2 years of dialysis, data are less detailed but PD appears to lose its advantage. The reason for the early survival benefit of PD is uncertain. One possibility is that it relates to better retention of residual renal function on PD. Another possibility is that it simply represents a baseline case mix advantage for PD that cannot be detected in registry studies. It is, however, found in countries with both high and low PD use.[43,44,46]

Technique failure is undoubtedly more common in PD than in HD. The most frequent causes are peritonitis, social reasons, and "inadequate dialysis." There is recent evidence that technique failure rates in PD are falling, principally because of better prevention and management of peritonitis.[47]

A reasonable conclusion from the above is that modality selection should not be significantly influenced by registry data. PD is at least as good, if not better, than HD in the early years for patients who choose that option. Given its cost advantage in most developed countries, this suggests that PD is a more cost-effective initial therapy. Subsequently, many patients will need to move to HD as a result of technique failure, and often loss of residual renal function may be associated with this. A dialysis delivery system based on early use of PD but easy availability of HD after 2–3 years might be maximally cost-effective. This concept has been described as "integrated dialysis care."

Specific management recommendations

As a result of the recent ADEMEX study, there is substantial confusion as to how best to prescribe PD. Clearance guidelines, in particular, will need to be revisited. In the mean time, clinicians need to define an approach that maximizes patient outcomes by avoiding interventions which are unproven and which may have significant negative cost and lifestyle implications.

A reasonable strategy is to monitor clearances shortly after the patient initiates PD, and routinely at 4- to 6-month intervals subsequently. Clearances should also be remeasured soon after any alteration in the prescription and in response to any unexplained clinical changes. Measurements should comprise Kt/V and CrCl and include both their renal and peritoneal components.

In light of the recent trials, a reasonable approach would be to ensure that each patient receives at least a peritoneal Kt/V of 1.7/week. Residual renal function should be considered a bonus. If, however, residual renal function is very substantial, i.e. in excess of 5 mL/min, it may be possible to manage with a peritoneal Kt/V of 1.5. If the patient is not doing well and appears to be manifesting uremic symptoms, an increase in the peritoneal clearance component above 1.7 can be attempted, but the ADEMEX study suggests that this is generally not effective.

There is no convincing evidence that CrCl is any more useful than Kt/V, but it would be wise to keep the peritoneal component above 45 L/week.

Careful attention should be paid to volume status, with the aim of keeping patients edema free and their blood pressure levels at or below 130/80 mmHg. Long-duration dextrose dwells should be avoided if volume status is a problem. In such settings, the use of APD and icodextrin for long dwells should be considered. PET status should be

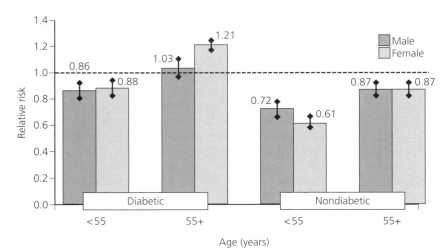

Figure 87.4 Relative mortality risk for PD compared with HD in incidents in US dialysis patients, 1994–1998. (Reproduced from Collins AJ, How W, Xia H, et al: Mortality risks of peritoneal dialysis and hemodialysis. Am J Kidney Dis 1999;34:1065–1074.)

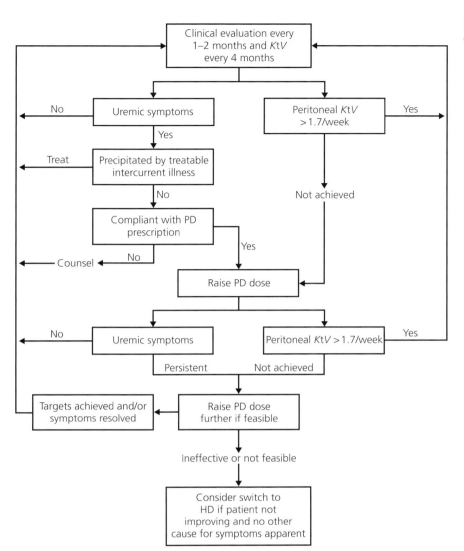

Figure 87.5 Algorithm for the management of clearances in peritoneal dialysis.

established in order to identify patients who are at risk of volume overload and who might require these interventions.

A multidisciplinary approach to malnutrition is recommended. Patients should be screened for this by a combination of tools, including clinical evaluation; assessment of dietary protein and calorie intake by a renal dietitian; subjective global assessment; measurements of serum urea, creatinine potassium, and albumin; serial 24-h creatinine excretion as an index of lean body mass; and nPNA. The limitations of each of these indices should be kept in mind, and no individual index should be emphasized to the exclusion of the others. Warning signs for malnutrition include decreasing body weight, low or declining subjective global assessment status, decreasing lean body mass or blood urea, and nPNA below 0.8 g/kg/day using the Bergstrom formula with normalization to desired or standard weight. Serum albumin below 30 g/L should be investigated, not only with nutrition in mind but also with regard to PET status and the presence of inflammation, which may frequently be subclinical.

Preventive strategies for malnutrition include a timely start on dialysis; targeting a dietary protein intake above 1 g/kg body weight per day and a dietary calorie intake above 35 kcal/kg/day; vitamin supplementation; and an "adequate" PD prescription.

Therapeutic strategies ideally involve a multidisciplinary approach with dietary counseling; diagnosis and treatment of comorbidity with special attention to upper gastrointestinal disease and depression; correction of poor dentition; awareness of cultural and socioeconomic issues; avoidance of excessive numbers of medications; and correction of acidosis and, where possible, inflammation. If this is unsuccessful, interventions to consider are oral calorie and protein supplementation and the use of intraperitoneal amino acids. Administration of anabolic steroids may sometimes have a role. A trial of HD may be appropriate if the nutritional status is not improving and if no clear cause for this can be identified.

References

1. Teehan BP, Schleifer CR, Sigler MH, et al: A quantitative approach to the CAPD prescription. Perit Dial Bull 1985;5:152–156.

2. Watson PR, Watson ID, Batt RD: Total body water volumes for adult males and females estimated from simple anthropometric measurements. Am J Clin Nutr 1980;23:27–39.
3. Wong K-C, Xiong D-W, Kerr PG, et al: Kt/V in CAPD by different estimations of V. Kidney Int 1995;48:563–569.
4. Du Bois D, Du Bois EF: A formula to estimate the approximate surface area of height and weight be known. Arch Intern Med 1916;17:863–871.
5. Blake PG, Balaskas EV, Izatt S, Oreopoulos DG: Is total creatinine clearance a good predictor of clinical outcomes in CAPD? Perit Dial Int 1992;12:353–358.
6. Rodby RA, Firanek CA, Cheng YG, et al: Reproducibility of studies of peritoneal dialysis adequacy. Kidney Int 1996;50:267–271.
7. Bergstrom J, Heimburger O, Lindholm B: Calculation of the protein equivalent of total nitrogen appearance from urea appearance. Which formulas should be used? Perit Dial Int 1998;18:467–473.
8. Kopple JD, Gao XL, Qing DP: Dietary protein, urea nitrogen appearance and total nitrogen appearance in chronic renal failure and CAPD patients. Kidney Int 1997;52:486–94.
9. Keshaviah PR, Nolph KD, Moore, HL, et al: Lean body mass estimation by creatinine kinetics. J Am Soc Nephrol 1994;4:1475–1485.
10. Depner TA: Quantifying hemodialysis and peritoneal dialysis: examination of the peak concentration hypothesis. Semin Dial 1994;7:315–317.
11. Keshaviah PR, Nolph KD, VanStone JC: The peak concentration hypothesis: a urea kinetic approach to comparing the adequacy of continuous ambulatory peritoneal dialysis and hemodialysis. Perit Dial Int 1989;9:257–260.
12. Churchill ND, Taylor DW, Keshaviah PR, and the CANUSA Peritoneal Dialysis Study Group: Adequacy of dialysis and nutrition in continuous peritoneal dialysis: association with clinical outcomes. J Am Soc Nephrol 1996;7:198–207.
13. Bargman JM, Thorpe KE, Churchill DN for the CANUSA Peritoneal Dialysis Study Group: Relative contribution of residual renal function and peritoneal clearance to adequacy of dialysis: a reanalysis of the CANUSA Study. J Am Soc Nephrol 2001;12:2158–2162.
14. Maiorca R, Brunori G, Zubani R, et al: Predicative value of dialysis adequacy and nutritional indices for mortality and morbidity in CAPD and HD patients: a longitudinal study. Nephrol Dial Transplant 1995;10:2295–2305.
15. Diaz-Buxo JA, Lowrie EG, Lew NL, et al: Associates of mortality among peritoneal dialysis patients with special reference to peritoneal transport states and solute clearance. Am J Kidney Dis 1999;33:523–534.
16. Rocco M, Souci JM, Pastan S, McClellan WM: Peritoneal dialysis adequacy and risk of death. Kidney Int 2000;58:446–457.
17. National Kidney Foundation. NKF-DOQI: clinical practice guidelines for peritoneal dialysis adequacy. Am J Kidney Dis 1997;30 (Suppl 2):S67–S136.
18. Blake PG, Bargman J, Bick J, et al: Clinical practice guidelines of the Canadian Society of Nephrology for Peritoneal Dialysis Adequacy and Nutrition. J Am Soc Nephrol 1999;10 (Suppl 13):S311–S321.
19. Golper TA, Churchill DN, Blake PG, et al: NKF-K/DOQI clinical practice guidelines for peritoneal dialysis adequacy: update 2000. Am J Kidney Dis 2001;37 (Suppl 1):S65–S136.
20. Perez RA, Blake PG, Jindal KA, et al: Changes in peritoneal dialysis practices in Canada 1996–1999. Perit Dial Int 2003;22:53–57.
21. Mak SK, Wong PN, Lo KT, et al: Randomized perspective study of the effect of increased dialytic dose on nutritional and clinical outcomes in continuous ambulatory peritoneal dialysis patients. Am J Kidney Dis 2000;36:105–114.
22. Paniagua R, Amato, D, Vonesh E, et al: Effect of increased peritoneal clearances on mortality rates in peritoneal dialysis: ADEMEX, a prospective randomized controlled trial. J Am Soc Nephrol 2002;13:1307–1320.
23. Lo WK, Cheng IKP, Ho YW, et al: Effect of Kt/V on CAPD survival in a prospective randomized study. Perit Dial Int 2001;21 (Suppl 2): S17.
24. Twardowski ZJ, Nolph KD, Khanna R, et al: Peritoneal equilibration test. Perit Dial Bull 1987;7:138–147.
25. Churchill DN, Thorpe KE, Nolph KD, Keshaviah PR, Oreopoulos DG, Page D: Increased peritoneal membrane transport is associated with decreased patient and technique survival for continuous peritoneal dialysis patients. J Am Soc Nephrol 1998;9:1285–1292.
26. Perez RA, Blake PG, McMurray S, Mupas L, Oreopoulos DG: What is the optimal frequency of cycling in automated peritoneal dialysis? Perit Dial Int 2000;20:548–556.
27. Mujais S, Nolph K, Gokal R, et al: Evaluation and management of ultrafiltration problems in peritoneal dialysis. Perit Dial Int 2000;20 (Suppl 4):S5–S21.
28. Mistry CD, Gokal R, Peers E: A randomized multicenter clinical trial comparing isosmolar icodextrin with hyperosmolar glucose solutions in CAPD. Kidney Int 1994;46:496–503.
29. Bernardini J, Piriano B: Compliance in CAPD and CCPD patients as measured by supply inventories during home visits. Am J Kidney Dis 1998;31:101–107.
30. Blake PG, Korbet SM, Blake R, et al: A multicenter study of non-compliance with continuous peritoneal dialysis exchanges in U.S. and Canadian patients. Am J Kidney Dis 2000;35:506–514.
31. Young GA, Kopple J, Lindholm B, et al: Nutritional assessment of CAPD patients: an international study. Am J Kidney Dis 1991;17:462–471.
32. Blake PG, Flowerdew G, Blake RM, et al: Serum albumin in patients on continuous ambulatory peritoneal dialysis — predictors and correlations with outcomes. J Am Soc Nephrol 1993;3:1501–1507.
33. Yeun JY, Kaysen GA: Acute phase proteins in peritoneal dialysate albumin loss are the main determinants of serum albumin in peritoneal dialysis patients. Am J Kidney Dis 1997;30:923–927.
34. Pollock CA, Ibels LS, Allen BJ, et al: Total body nitrogen as a prognostic marker in maintenance dialysis. J Am Soc Nephrol 1995;6:82–88.
35. Mandolfo S, Zucchi A, Cavalieri D'Oro L, Corradi B, Imbasciati E: Protein nitrogen appearance in CAPD patients: what is the best formula? Nephrol Dial Transplant 1996;11:1592–1596.
36. Blake PG, Oreopoulos DG: Answers to all your questions about peritoneal urea clearance and nutrition in CAPD patients. Perit Dial Int 1996;16:248–251.
37. Davies, SJ, Phillips L, Griffiths AM, Naish PF, Russell GI: Analysis of the effects of increasing delivered dialysis treatment to malnourished peritoneal dialysis patients. Kidney Int 2000;57:1743–1754.
38. Jones M, Hagen T, Vonesh E, et al: Use of a 1.1% amino acid dialysis solution to treat malnutrition in peritoneal dialysis patients. J Am Soc Nephrol 1995;10:1432–1437.
39. Johansen KL, Mulligan K, Schambelan M: Anabolic effects of nandrolone decanoate in patients receiving dialysis: a randomized controlled trial. JAMA 1999;281:1275–1281.
40. Fouque D, Peng SC, Shamir E, Kopple JD: Recombinant human insulin-like growth factor-one induces an anabolic response in malnourished CAPD patients. Kidney Int 2000;57:646–654.
41. Stenvinkel P, Heimburger O, Lindholm B, Kaysen GA, Bergstrom J: Are there two types of malnutrition in chronic renal failure? Evidence for relationships between malnutrition, inflammation, and atherosclerosis. Nephrol Dial Transplant 2000;15:953–960.
42. Bloembergen WE, Port FK, Mauger EA, et al: A comparison of mortality between patients treated with hemodialysis and peritoneal dialysis. J Am Soc Nephrol 1995;6:177–183.
43. Collins AJ, How W, Xia H, et al: Mortality risks of peritoneal dialysis and hemodialysis. Am J Kidney Dis 1999;34:1065–1074.
44. Fenton SSA, Schaubel DE, Desmeules M, et al: Hemodialysis versus peritoneal dialysis: a comparison of adjusted mortality rates. Am J Kidney Dis 1997;30:330–342.
45. Locatelli F, Marcelli D, Conte F, et al: Survival and development of cardiovascular disease by modality of treatment in patients with end-stage renal disease. J Am Soc Nephrol 2001;12:2411–2417.
46. Heaf JG, Lokkegaard H, Madsen M: Initial survival advantage of peritoneal dialysis relative to haemodialysis. Nephrol Dial Transplant 2002;17:112–117.
47. Schaubel DE, Blake PG, Fenton SS: Trends in CAPD technique failure: Canada 1981–1997. Perit Dial Int 2001;21:365–371.

Patient Selection for Dialysis, the Decision to Withdraw Dialysis, and Palliative Care

Alvin H. Moss

Background
Nephrologists' reported practices of withholding and withdrawing dialysis
Patient preferences for dialysis decision-making
Practice guidelines for selection of dialysis patients
• Rationale for practice guidelines
• Recommendation for practice guidelines
Deciding to withhold or withdraw dialysis in individual cases
• The process of informed consent as the paradigm for decision-making
• Deciding for the incompetent patient
• Resolving conflict between the surrogate and the nephrologist
• Ethical principles in decision-making
• Legal basis for deciding to withhold or withdraw dialysis
• The role of advance care planning
Caring for patients after the decision has been made to withhold or stop dialysis
• Response to a patient's refusal of dialysis
• Response to a patient's request to stop dialysis
Dialysis decision-making in acute renal failure
Conclusions

The consequences of these factors are twofold: the numbers of patients on chronic dialysis and the cost of the ESRD program to the federal government have exceeded all initial projections several times over; and observers of dialysis, including physicians and nurses actively providing it, have questioned the appropriateness of dialyzing 10–15% of the current patients because of their short life expectancy and limited quality of life. This chapter will examine the following topics: the reported practices of nephrologists and the perspectives of patients regarding dialysis decision-making; the data documenting significant variation in decisions to start patients on dialysis and supporting the establishment of practice guidelines for dialysis patient selection; the recommendations of the Renal Physicians Association and the American Society of Nephrology clinical practice guideline, *Shared Decision-Making in the Appropriate Initiation of and Withdrawal from Dialysis*; a process for dialysis decision-making in individual cases that is based on ethics and the law; and recommendations for caring for a patient after the decision has been made to withhold or stop dialysis. It will also describe briefly the medical and ethical issues in deciding whether or not to initiate dialysis in a patient with acute renal failure.

Background

In a span of just 30 years, the process of patient selection for dialysis has been transformed from an intensive one in which each candidate was carefully scrutinized by a multidisciplinary committee for acceptability to one in which almost any patient, or family of a patient, who requests dialysis receives it. Nephrologists, medical ethicists, and health-policy experts have identified many factors to explain this transformation, but most prominent among them are the following: (1) federal legislation that pays for dialysis for all patients with endstage renal disease (ESRD) who are eligible for Medicare; (2) improvements in medical science and technology that have made it possible to achieve long-term survival for some patients who were previously thought to be too sick to undergo dialysis (for example, the elderly and those with diabetes); (3) a changing ethical and legal environment in which respect for patient autonomy and the right of patient self-determination have become almost decisive in medical decision-making to start or stop a life-sustaining treatment like dialysis; (4) the financial self-interests of nephrologists who stand to increase their incomes by treating larger numbers of dialysis patients; and (5) the absence of any attempt prior to 2000 to define formally patients who would be inappropriate for dialysis.

Nephrologists' reported practices of withholding and withdrawing dialysis

In the 1990s, research studies of nephrologists' dialysis decision-making began to emerge.[1–4] These studies provided insight into what decisions nephrologists would typically make in a variety of circumstances and why they made the decisions that they did. These studies documented that deciding to withhold and withdraw patients from dialysis are frequent occurrences for the vast majority of nephrologists. Most withhold one to five patients and withdraw one to ten patients from dialysis each year. The findings of these studies agree with the 1994 Annual Report of the US Renal Data System in which withdrawal from dialysis was listed as the second most common cause of death after cardiac causes.[5] In one study, nine out of ten nephrologists would stop dialysis at the request of a competent patient, but only six out of ten would agree to stop dialysis for an irreversibly incompetent patient at the family's request if the patient's wishes were unknown. In this study, only one of 100 nephrologists would stop dialysis for an irreversibly incompetent patient for whom the nephrologist felt dialysis should be stopped if the family requested that dialysis be continued and the patient's wishes were unknown. The authors concluded that consensus exists among nephrologists regarding the right of competent patients to determine the course of their care, including stopping dialysis. They also concluded that nephrologists disagree about the management of incompetent patients with unclear prior wishes, and that they have difficulty making decisions for such patients.[1]

In a study of medical directors of dialysis units, nine out of ten indicated that they would agree to stop dialysis at the request of a competent patient, but only one-third would stop dialysis of a permanently and severely demented patient without advance directives. One-sixth of the medical directors would start dialysis for a permanently unconscious patient if requested, but the remainder would not. In this study, some respondents indicated that although they thought dialysis was inappropriate for the demented and permanently unconscious patients, they would not withdraw or withhold it unless they could "convince" the families to agree. Other respondents specifically noted that they would be afraid to stop dialysis for the patient with severe dementia if there was the potential for litigation from family members who wanted dialysis continued. In interpreting the results of their study, the authors suggested that some nephrologists may misunderstand the ethical and legal aspects of making decisions for such patients and may feel obligated to provide dialysis to all patients for whom it is requested.[2]

Similarly, in a study of dialysis decision-making by nephrologists in Canada, the UK, and the USA, more than nine out of ten nephrologists from all three countries would respect a competent patient's refusal to start dialysis. But, American nephrologists would offer dialysis significantly more often to demented patients, severely disabled diabetic patients, and patients in a persistent vegetative state, than would Canadian or British nephrologists.[3] The American nephrologists significantly more often gave "respect for the patient or family request" as the first reason to offer dialysis, and ranked "fear of law suit" higher as a reason to offer dialysis than their counterparts in the other countries. The British and Canadian nephrologists significantly more often cited "adequate quality of life" as a reason to offer dialysis than the Americans did. Despite these variations, there was never more than a 30% difference in the practice of offering dialysis among the three groups. The greatest agreement on offering dialysis was for the young competent patient with muscular dystrophy (more than 90% in each group). Fewer than 10% of each group thought that dialysis should be offered to patients in a persistent vegetative state.

Patient preferences for dialysis decision-making

In making decisions about which patients should be selected for dialysis, input from patients is important because they are, as a group, the best to judge under which circumstances dialysis would be viewed as beneficial and when it would be burdensome. Regrettably, there are few studies of patient preferences regarding dialysis, and only one examined the interaction between health state and treatment modalities.[6] In this study, 25% or fewer of the patients would want to continue dialysis in three health states: severe stroke, severe dementia, and permanent coma. These findings agree with another study in which 74% of dialysis patients said they would want to stop dialysis if they became permanently and severely demented.[7]

Practice guidelines for selection of dialysis patients

Rationale for practice guidelines

These cited studies point to significant variations in the decision-making of nephrologists in cases in which the patients lacked decision-making capacity and their wishes were not clear. On the other hand, there appeared to be a consensus among nephrologists to honor the wishes of competent patients who want to refuse or to stop dialysis, and there seemed to be general agreement among the nephrologists and patients that dialysis is not appropriate when there is profound neurologic impairment. In this setting, in which there is broad agreement on some issues and considerable variation on others, practice guidelines would appear to be beneficial. Five benefits of practice guidelines for patient selection for dialysis have been previously noted; such guidelines may:

1. Improve the understanding of physicians, nurses, and other dialysis healthcare providers of the ethical principles and processes involved in making decisions to withhold or withdraw dialysis.
2. Promote medically and ethically sound decisions in a more uniform fashion than has been the case up to now.
3. Assist dialysis facilities and hospitals in developing policies related to these issues.
4. Provide an acceptable moral framework for dialysis decision-making, that will increase the understanding of the general public and help to avoid outrage like that which occurred in the early 1960s when the criteria for patient selection used by the Seattle committee became known.
5. Establish a standard of care for dialysis patient selection, perhaps reducing the liability concerns of nephrologists who practice according to the guidelines.[8]

Recommendation for practice guidelines

The idea of practice guidelines for patient selection for dialysis is not new. By 1978, just 5 years after the passage of the federal legislation creating the Medicare ESRD program, Belding Scribner (one of the early nephrologists who pioneered dialysis) was concerned about "how not to dialyze" certain patients with poor prognoses. He recognized even then the need for a "deselection committee."[9] The Institute of Medicine Committee for the Study of the Medicare End-Stage Renal Disease Program (IOM Committee), which issued its report in 1991, acknowledged that the existence of the public entitlement for treatment of ESRD did not oblige physicians to treat all patients who have kidney failure with dialysis or transplantation.[10] This Committee noted that for some ESRD patients the burdens of dialysis might substantially outweigh the benefits. Specifically, the Committee questioned the appropriateness of providing dialysis to two groups of patients: those with a limited life expectancy despite the use of dialysis, and those with severe neurological disease. The first group included patients with kidney failure and other life-threatening illnesses, such as atherosclerotic cardiovascular disease, cancer, chronic pulmonary disease, and AIDS. The second group included patients whose neurologic disease rendered them unable to relate to others, such as those in a persistent vegetative state, or with severe dementia, or cerebral vascular disease. The IOM Committee recommended that guidelines be drafted to assist nephrologists in making these decisions so that dialysis would be used appropriately.

The Renal Physicians Association (RPA) and the American Society of Nephrology (ASN) heeded this call for a clinical practice guideline and published it in 2000 (the RPA/ASN guideline).[11] To draft this guideline, the RPA and ASN organized a working group that included representatives from multiple disciplines and organizations within the dialysis community, kidney patients, internal and family medicine physicians, and experts in bioethics and health policy. The working group developed *a priori* analytic frameworks regarding decisions to withhold or withdraw dialysis in patients with acute renal failure and endstage renal disease. Systematic literature reviews were conducted to address pre-specified questions derived from the frameworks. In most instances, the relevant evidence that was identified was contextual in nature and only provided indirect support to the recommendations. In formulating their nine recommendations, the working group used research evidence, case and statutory law, and ethical principles. They recommended shared decision-making as the basis for making decisions about starting and stopping dialysis. Shared decision-making is a process by which physicians and patients agree on a specific course of action based on a common understanding of the treatment goals and the risks and benefits of the chosen course, compared with the alternative courses. These recommendations appear in Table 88.1. Their recommendations for who should be dialyzed, though more systematically developed and justified, are consistent with those previously recommended.[8] This agreement suggests that there is now a real consensus in the nephrology community on this topic (Table 88.2).

Table 88.1 Renal Physicians Association and the American Society of Nephrology (RPA/ASN) recommendations for initiation and withdrawal of dialysis (with permission from the RPA[11])

Recommendation No. 1: Shared decision-making
A patient–physician relationship that promotes shared decision-making is recommended for all patients with either ARF or ESRD. Participants in shared decision-making should involve at a minimum the patient and the physician. If a patient lacks decision-making capacity, decisions should involve the legal agent. With the patient's consent, shared decision-making may include family members or friends and other members of the renal care team.

Recommendation No. 2: Informed consent or refusal
Physicians should fully inform patients about their diagnosis, prognosis, and all treatment options, including: 1) available dialysis modalities, 2) not starting dialysis and continuing conservative management which should include end-of-life care, 3) a time-limited trial of dialysis, and 4) stopping dialysis and receiving end-of-life care. Choices among options should be made by patients or, if patients lack decision-making capacity, their designated legal agents. Their decisions should be informed and voluntary. The renal care team, in conjunction with the primary care physician, should insure that the patient or legal agent understands the consequences of the decision.

Recommendation No. 3: Estimating prognosis
To facilitate informed decisions about starting dialysis for either ARF or ESRD, discussions should occur with the patient or legal agent about life expectancy and quality of life. Depending upon the circumstances (e.g. availability of nephrologists), a primary care physician or nephrologist who is familiar with prognostic data should conduct these discussions. These discussions should be documented and dated. All patients requiring dialysis should have their chances for survival estimated, with the realization that the ability to predict survival in the individual patient is difficult and imprecise. The estimates should be discussed with the patient or legal agent, patient's family, and among the medical team. For patients with ESRD, these discussions should occur as early as possible in the course of the patient's renal disease and continue as the renal disease progresses. For patients who experience major complications that may substantially reduce survival or quality of life, it is appropriate to discuss and/or reassess treatment goals, including consideration of withdrawing dialysis.

Recommendation No. 4: Conflict resolution
A systematic approach for conflict resolution is recommended if there is disagreement regarding the benefits of dialysis between the patient or legal agent (and those supporting the patient's position) and a member(s) of the renal care team. Conflicts may also occur within the renal care team or between the renal care team and other healthcare providers. This approach should review the shared decision-making process for the following potential sources of conflict: (1) miscommunication or misunderstanding about prognosis; (2) intrapersonal or interpersonal issues; or (3) values. If dialysis is indicated urgently, it should be provided while pursuing conflict resolution, provided the patient or legal agent requests it.

Table 88.1 (*cont'd*)

Recommendation No. 5: Advance directives
The renal care team should attempt to obtain written advance directives from all dialysis patients. These advance directives should be honored.

Recommendation No. 6: Withholding or withdrawing dialysis
It is appropriate to withhold or withdraw dialysis for patients with either ARF or ESRD in the following situations:
Patients with decision-making capacity who, being fully informed and making voluntary choices, refuse dialysis or request dialysis be discontinued.
Patients who no longer possess decision-making capacity who have previously indicated refusal of dialysis in an oral or written advance directive.
Patients who no longer possess decision-making capacity and whose properly appointed legal agents refuse dialysis or request that it be discontinued.
Patients with irreversible, profound neurological impairment such that they lack signs of thought, sensation, purposeful behavior, and awareness of self and environment.

Recommendation No. 7: Special patient groups
It is reasonable to consider not initiating or withdrawing dialysis for patients with ARF or ESRD who have a terminal illness from a nonrenal cause or whose medical condition precludes the technical process of dialysis.

Recommendation No. 8: Time-limited trials
For patients requiring dialysis, but who have an uncertain prognosis, or for whom a consensus cannot be reached about providing dialysis, nephrologists should consider offering a time-limited trial of dialysis.

Recommendation No. 9: Palliative care
All patients who decide to forgo dialysis or for whom such a decision is made should be treated with continued palliative care. With the patient's consent, persons with expertise in such care, such as hospice health care professionals, should be involved in managing the medical, psychosocial, and spiritual aspects of end-of-life care for these patients. Patients should be offered the option of dying where they prefer including at home with hospice care. Bereavement support should be offered to patients' families.

ARF, acute renal failure; ESRD; endstage renal disease.

Table 88.2 The consensus on patients for whom dialysis is inappropriate

1. Patients who refuse dialysis or who have previously indicated they did not want it
2. Patients who are terminally ill from a non-renal disease
3. Patients who are permanently unconscious
4. Patients who are unable to relate to others
5. Patients who are unable to cooperate with the dialysis process

Deciding to withhold or withdraw dialysis in individual cases

The process of informed consent as the paradigm for decision-making

The ethical and legal literature agree that medical decisions for individual patients (such as withholding or withdrawing dialysis) should be made according to the process of informed consent, in which there is active, shared decision-making.[12] This agreement formed the basis for the first two recommendations in the RPA/ASN guideline. Thus, if a physician determines that a patient has decision-making capacity, the patient is informed of his/her medical condition – in this case ESRD – and of all the benefits, risks, and consequences associated with each of the available treatment options, including the option not to undergo dialysis. After determining the patient's values and preferences, the physician recommends what might be best for the patient, based on those preferences. Through further conversations, in which there is mutual participation and respect, the patient reaches a decision about dialysis – whether to consent to it or to refuse it. For some patients, the balance of the benefits and the burdens of dialysis may not be clear, and the nephrologist may not know whether to recommend dialysis or not. In such situations, there is an ethical recommendation for a limited trial of dialysis, of about 30 days. During this time, the patient's responses to dialysis can be assessed, and afterwards both the patient and physician are in a better position to decide about continuation.

Deciding for the incompetent patient

If the patient lacks decision-making capacity, physicians make decisions with the patient's agent as designated in the patient's advance directive (e.g. durable power of attorney for healthcare or healthcare proxy). If the patient has not completed a written advance directive specifying an agent, physicians must make decisions with a surrogate who should be appointed according to the provisions of the state law in which the care is being provided. Surrogates should base their decisions on what the patient would choose if he or she were competent to do so; and if the patient's views about treatment are unknown, their decision should be based on the patient's best interests.

Resolving conflict between the surrogate and the nephrologist

Occasionally there are conflicts between the surrogate and the nephrologist in which the surrogate requests dialysis and the nephrologist does not believe it is appropriate. Based on the studies reviewed here, many nephrologists report that they would do as the surrogate requests, even if they thought it was wrong. In yielding to pressure from the surrogate, nephrologists potentially weaken the integrity of their specialty, and they shirk their responsibility to be good stewards of the federally funded ESRD program – a program to which every taxpayer, including every nephrologist, contributes. Recommendation 4 of the RPA/ASN guideline provides a systematic approach for resolving these conflicts.

Withholding or withdrawing dialysis of an incompetent patient, over the objections of the family or surrogate, may be both ethical and legal.[13] Such decisions should be made openly and should focus clearly on the patient's wishes or best interests. At a minimum, such decisions should be reached only after following Recommendation 4 of the RPA/ASN guideline, including extended conversation with the patient's surrogate about the diagnosis of ESRD, about options for treatment including palliative care without dialysis, the prognosis, and the reasons for not offering or for stopping dialysis; the agreement of other members of the dialysis team including at least one other nephrologist; the concurrence of an ethics committee (if available); a detailed note in the patient's medical record documenting all of the factors relevant to the decision; and an attempt to transfer the patient's care if the surrogate wishes it. If the patient is already receiving dialysis and if (after all of the above steps) the surrogate still requests dialysis, and no other nephrologist has been found who is willing to accept the patient in transfer for dialysis, then the surrogate is given some time (usually 72 h) to consider other options, including contacting a lawyer, before dialysis is stopped. Such a course of action by the nephrologist is justified for patients who are deemed inappropriate for dialysis (Table 88.2). In using such an approach, for example, a nephrologist might refuse to dialyze a patient who is permanently unconscious, basing his decision on Recommendation 6 of the RPA/ASN guideline. In taking such an approach, nephrologists should indicate that they understand the surrogate's request and should give an explanation along the lines of: "I am sorry, but we do not dialyze patients in your loved one's condition. Our profession is guided by ethical principles that require us to be of benefit and do no harm. In your loved one's case, dialysis cannot help her get better, and it may harm her." Nephrologists say this not because we lack respect or compassion for the surrogate but because our primary commitment is to the patient.[13]

Ethical principles in decision-making

Ethical justifications and general and specific principles to be used in making decisions about offering or not offering dialysis were articulated by the End-Stage Renal Disease Data Advisory Committee to the US Renal Data System in their 1993 annual report. This report included the deliberations of an ad hoc committee gathered to examine bioethical issues related to ESRD; the ad hoc committee was composed of nephrologists, ethicists, and health-policy experts. The Data Advisory Committee endorsed the recommendations of this ad hoc committee. The report described two ethical justifications for withholding or withdrawing dialysis: the right of patients to refuse dialysis based on the ethical principle of respect for autonomy and the legal right of self-determination; and a judgement that dialysis does not offer a reasonable expectation of medical benefit based on the ethical principles of beneficence and nonmaleficence.[14]

Legal basis for deciding to withhold or withdraw dialysis

The ethical principle of respect for patient autonomy is applied to care of the dialysis patient through the process of obtaining informed consent or refusal. In turn, the obtaining of consent or refusal is firmly grounded in the law – common law, constitutional law, and federal statute. The right of patients to accept or refuse dialysis is first based on common law dating back to the 1914 case of *Schloendorff v. Society of New York Hospital*. In this case, Justice Benjamin Cardozo wrote "Every human being of adult years and sound mind has a right to determine what shall be done with his body." In the 1990 US Supreme Court case of *Cruzan v. Director*, the legal doctrine of informed consent was determined to be a constitutionally protected right. The Supreme Court justices held "The doctrine of informed consent arose in recognition of the value society places on a person's autonomy and as the primary vehicle by which a person can protect the integrity of his body. If one can consent to treatment, one can also refuse it. Thus, as a necessary corollary to informed consent, the right to refuse treatment arose".[15] The Patient Self-Determination Act (included in the Congressional Omnibus Reconciliation Act of 1990, Public Law 101–508) became effective on December 1, 1991 and protected by federal statute the right of dialysis patients to consent to or to refuse dialysis. It is important for nephrologists to understand the law because if a nephrologist were to dialyze a competent patient against his/her will the nephrologist could be civilly liable for medical battery.

The role of advance care planning

Deciding to stop a life-sustaining treatment like dialysis for an incompetent patient is among the most difficult ethical problems faced by physicians.[13] Because there is a presumption in favor of continued dialysis for patients who cannot and have not expressed their wishes, patients' rights to forgo dialysis in certain situations are usually difficult to achieve unless patients have explicitly stated their preferences in advance or named a surrogate to speak on their behalf. The usual practice of nephrologists in treating patients who have become incompetent, and who have never provided either oral or written advance directives regarding their preferences for stopping dialysis, is to continue dialysis. These considerations underscore the importance of advance care planning with dialysis patients. Advance care planning is a process in which a patient's preferences for a healthcare proxy and for future medical care under a variety of circumstances are determined (sometimes in the form of a written advance directive), are updated, and then followed in a manner in which the patient intended once the patient loses decision-making capacity.

Advance care planning has been recognized as particularly important for dialysis patients for three reasons:[16] almost half of the dialysis population is elderly, and the elderly are the most likely to withdraw or be withdrawn from dialysis; prior discussion of advance directives has been shown to help dialysis patients and their families to approach death in a reconciled fashion;[17] and unless a specific directive to withhold cardiopulmonary resuscitation is obtained – which can be done in the framework of advance care planning – it will be automatically provided although it rarely leads to extended survival in dialysis patients. For these reasons, nephrologists have been encouraged to discuss the circumstances under which patients would want to discontinue dialysis and forgo cardiopulmonary resuscitation and to urge patients to complete written advance directives.

Caring for patients after the decision has been made to withhold or stop dialysis

Response to a patient's refusal of dialysis

Patients with ESRD may have encephalopathy or depression that renders them decisionally incapable. The first assessment of patients with ESRD who refuse dialysis is whether they have decision-making capacity. If they have decision-making capacity, then the nephrologist should determine whether the refusal of dialysis is valid. The nephrologist is obligated to determine why the refusal has been made, to ensure that the patient correctly under-stands the information that has been presented and the consequences of the decision. Patients and families should be informed that death from uremia may take a week or a month, depending on the circumstances, that death from uremia is usually a comfortable one in which the patient

becomes increasingly somnolent and then dies, and that if dialysis is not initiated it will be necessary to maintain salt and fluid restrictions so that pulmonary edema does not occur and mar the comfort of the dying process.[18]

If the refusal is judged to be valid, then the patient should be considered terminally ill, because a terminal illness is defined as one in which death is expected within 6 months or less. At this point, the dialysis team should refer the patient to a hospice or adopt a hospice-like approach to patient care.[19] Such an approach considers medical, emotional, social, and spiritual needs of the dying patient and the family. If the team remains involved in the patient's care – such continuity is desirable – they should take the following steps: (1) encourage the patient to participate with them in advance care planning, which may include completion of written advance directives and should include eliciting the patient's preferences for the site of death and for a surrogate decision maker once the patient loses decision-making capacity; (2) issue a do-not-resuscitate order that applies to the outpatient setting; (3) discuss with the patient and family contingencies for the final hours of the patient's life so that the family or caregivers do not panic and call emergency medical services when the patient experiences a cardiopulmonary arrest; and (4) address the needs of the family with regard to grieving while the patient is dying, and bereavement after the patient has died.

Response to a patient's request to stop dialysis

A patient's request to stop dialysis should trigger a systematic response on the part of the dialysis team, including the inquiry in Table 88.3.[16] Such an inquiry might uncover potentially reversible factors responsible for the patient's request, including difficulties with dialysis

---

Table 88.3 Questions to be answered in responding to a patient's request to stop dialysis

1. Does the patient have decision-making capacity or is the patient's cognitive capacity diminished by depression, encephalopathy, or other disorder?
2. Why does the patient want to stop dialysis?
3. Are the patient's perceptions about the technical or quality-of-life aspects of dialysis accurate?
4. Does the patient really mean what he/she says or is the decision to stop dialysis made to get attention, help, or control?
5. Can any changes be made that might improve life on dialysis for the patient?
6. Would the patient be willing to continue dialysis while the factors responsible for the patient's request are being addressed?
7. Has the patient discussed his/her desire to stop dialysis with significant others such as family, close friends, or spiritual advisors? What do they think about the patient's request?

treatments, concerns about the burdens that the patient is placing on family, undue influence or pressure from outside sources, conflict between the patient and others, and dissatisfaction with the dialysis modality, the time, or the setting. It is usual for most dialysis units to ask a patient who wishes to stop dialysis to be evaluated by a counseling professional, either a psychiatrist, psychologist, or social worker, or someone in pastoral care, to be sure that the patient has decision-making capacity and that reversible factors are identified. Dialysis units also usually try to persuade patients to stay on dialysis for a period of time to see if patient satisfaction is increased as reversible factors are addressed.

Dialysis decision-making in acute renal failure

The ethical principles for making dialysis decisions in the setting of acute renal failure have been described to be the same as those for chronic renal failure.[20,21] When confronted with a decision about whether to dialyze a patient with acute renal failure who satisfies the medical indications for dialysis, a nephrologist has basically three options: to initiate dialysis without any limitations; to start dialysis on a time-limited trial; or to refuse to offer dialysis. The justifications for offering dialysis are that the patient wants it (respect for patient autonomy) and that the patient is likely to benefit from it (beneficence). The justification for offering dialysis on a time-limited basis is that the patient wants it, but the balance of the benefits and burdens of dialysis is unclear. After a time-limited trial, dialysis for acute renal failure can be continued if the patient is benefiting from it (beneficence) or stopped if dialysis and the continued life it is sustaining are deemed burdensome (dialysis is stopped to refrain from harming the patient further – nonmaleficence). Nephrologists are not obliged to offer dialysis to patients with multiple organ system failure that includes acute renal failure, for whom dialysis can be reasonably predicted to be nonbeneficial because it cannot substantially affect their chance of survival or end their dependence on intensive care. For example, it seems to be well established that dialysis will not likely benefit acute renal failure patients who have five or more organs systems in failure.[20,21]

Conclusions

Since the inception of dialysis for chronic renal failure in the early 1960s, dialysis decision-making has undergone a dramatic transformation. Dialysis selection committees have disappeared, and decisions about whether to start or stop dialysis are made within the confines and privacy of the patient–physician relationship, governed by the process of informed consent.

The wide range of discretion afforded to patients and nephrologist in making decisions about dialysis has resulted in a large variation in the way these decisions are made. Commentators on the ESRD program, including nephrology physicians and nurses, are concerned that many patients

being dialyzed are not appropriate candidates. Research indicates that many nephrologists will dialyze incompetent patients at the request of patients' families, even if they think dialysis of such patients is inappropriate. Practice guidelines for patient selection for dialysis have been developed by the RPA and ASN as a means to improve dialysis decision-making and to reduce variation in the decisions that are made.

Excluding those patients who are identified as inappropriate dialysis candidates by the RPA/ASN guideline, the best approach for patient selection seems to be a liberal policy for accepting patients who might benefit from dialysis, combined with a readiness to withdraw patients from dialysis when the burdens of treatment outweigh the benefits. Successful implementation of such a policy requires good advance care planning at the start of dialysis and continuing dialogue between the physician, the patient, and the family, about the patient's values, wishes, and goals. Patients should be informed that they have the right to stop dialysis. However, the goal of the nephrologist and the dialysis team should be to optimize the care of each patient, so that each patient is satisfied with his/her quality of life, and chooses to continue dialysis until a catastrophic event occurs. When it does occur, good advance care planning will prove its worth, because then everyone will know that the patient would no longer wish to receive dialysis, and it may be withdrawn, with the patient, family, and dialysis team all reconciled to the patient's death. Renal palliative care (see Chapter 79) should have been begun at the start of dialysis with pain and symptom management and advance care planning; it will now become especially important for ensuring that the patient is comfortable and that the patient and the family receive psychosocial and spiritual support, including bereavement support when the patient dies.

References

1. Singer P: The End-State Renal Disease Network of New England: Nephrologists' experience with and attitudes towards decisions to forgo dialysis. J Am Soc Nephrol 1992;2:1235–1240.
2. Moss AH, Stocking CB, Sachs GA, et al: Variation in the attitudes of dialysis unit medical directors toward decisions to withhold and withdraw dialysis. J Am Soc Nephrol 1993;4:229–234.
3. McKenzie JK, Moss AH, Feest TG, et al: Dialysis decision-making in Canada, the United Kingdom, and the United States. Am J Kidney Dis 1998;31:12–18.
4. Sekkarie MA, Moss AH: Withholding and withdrawing dialysis: The role of physician specialty and education and patient functional status. Am J Kidney Dis 1998;31:464–472.
5. USRDS 1994. United States Renal Data System 1994 Annual Report. Bethesda, MD: The National Institutes of Health, 1994, D20.
6. Singer PA, Thiel EC, Naylor CD, et al: Life-sustaining treatment preferences of hemodialysis patients: implications for advance directives. J Am Soc Nephrol 1995;6:1410–1417.
7. Kaye M, Lella JW: Discontinuation of dialysis therapy in the demented patient. Am J Nephrol 1986;6:75–79.
8. Moss AH: To use dialysis appropriately: the emerging consensus on patient selection guidelines. Adv Renal Replacement Ther 1995;2:175–183.
9. Fox R, Swazey J: The Courage to Fail: A Social View of Organ Transplants and Dialysis, 2nd edn. Chicago, IL: University of Chicago Press, 1978, p 370.
10. Rettig RA, Levinsky NG (eds): Kidney Failure and the Federal Government. Washington, DC: National Academy Press, 1991, pp 51–61.

11. Renal Physicians Association and the American Society of Nephrology: Shared Decision-Making in the Appropriate Initiation of and Withdrawal from Dialysis. Washington, DC: RPA, 2000.

12. President's Commission for the Study of Ethical Problems in Medicine and Biomedical and Behavioral Research. Making Health Care Decisions. Washington, DC: US Government Printing Office, 1982, pp 27–39.

13. Keating RF, Moss AH, Sorkin MI, Paris JJ: Stopping dialysis of an incompetent patient over the family's objection: is it ever ethical and legal? J Am Soc Nephrol 1994;4:1879–1883.

14. ESRD Data Advisory Committee: 1993 Annual Report. Washington, DC: US Department of Health and Human Services, 1993, pp 29–33.

15. Meisel A: The Right to Die 1994 Cumulative Supplement 2. New York: John Wiley & Sons, 1994, p 17.

16. Moss AH: Dialysis decisions and the elderly. Clin Geriatr Med 1994;10:463–473.

17. Swartz RD, Perry E: Advance directives are associated with "good deaths" in chronic dialysis patients. J Am Soc Nephrol 1993;3:1623–1630.

18. Kjellstrand CM: Practical aspects of stopping dialysis and cultural differences. *In* Kjellstrand CM, Dossetor JB (eds): Ethical Problems in Dialysis and Transplantation. Dordrecht, The Netherlands: Kluwer Academic Publishers, 1992, pp 103–116.

19. Neely KJ, Roxe DM: Palliative care/hospice and the withdrawal of dialysis. J Pall Med 2000;3:57–67.

20. MacKay K, Moss AH: Acute dialysis of patients with multiple organ dysfunction syndrome: should it be done? Semin Dial 1996;5:412–416.

21. MacKay K, Moss AH: To dialyze or not to dialyze: An ethical and evidence-based approach to the patient with acute renal failure in the intensive care unit. Adv Renal Replace Ther 1997;4:288–296.

PART XIV
Transplantation

CHRISTOPHER S. WILCOX

The Evaluation and Preparation of Donors and Recipients for Renal Transplantation

V. Ram Peddi and M. Roy First

Living donor transplants
- Blood type and histocompatibility
- Medical and social evaluation of the potential living donors

Cadaver donor transplants
- Neurological evaluation of the potential cadaver kidney donor
- Medical evaluation of the potential cadaver kidney donor

Evaluation and preparation of the recipient
- Age
- Infections
- Gastrointestinal disease
- Lower urinary tract disease
- Malignancy
- Cardiovascular disease
- Special consideration for patients with type 1 diabetes mellitus
- Surgical preparation of the patient

Conclusion

To date, over 500 000 kidney transplants (living donor and cadaver) have been performed worldwide, more than 200 000 of which have been in the USA.[1] With the current therapeutic advances in solid organ transplantation, graft survival rates have reached unprecedented levels. According to the 2000 United Network for Organ Sharing (UNOS) kidney registry, the overall 1- and 5-year graft survival rates were 89.4% and 64.7%, respectively, for cadaveric kidney transplants and 94.5% and 78.4%, respectively, for recipients of living donor kidneys.[2] Patient survival rates after 1 and 5 years for cadaveric organ recipients are 95% and 82%, respectively, and for recipients of living donor transplants 98% and 91% respectively.[2] Further analysis of the UNOS data indicate that, from 1988 to 1996, the half-life for grafts from living donors increased steadily from 12.7 to 21.6 years, and that for cadaver donor allografts from 7.9 to 13.8 years. The average yearly reduction in the relative hazard of graft failure beyond 1 year was 4.2% for all recipients, 0.4% for those recipients who had an acute rejection episode, and 6.3% for those who did not have an acute rejection.[3]

This improvement in outcome after renal transplantation has resulted in a more liberal selection of patients.[4] The demand for kidney transplants far exceeds the supply of available organs. Although the number of patients on the waiting list for a kidney transplant has increased by 61.5%, from 17 883 in 1990 to 46 489 in 1999, during the same period organ donation increased at the much slower rate of 24.5%, from 9358 to 12 400.[2] As a result, the median

waiting time for a kidney transplant increased from 380 days in 1990 to 1099 days in 1997.[2] In addition to providing a better quality of life, renal transplantation is strikingly cost-effective. Theoretically, a successful transplant could save approximately $100 000 per patient over 5 years compared with maintenance dialysis.[5] Currently, there are more than 50 000 patients in the USA awaiting cadaver renal transplantation.[2]

Living donor transplants

Transplantation from living donors, especially human leukocyte antigen (HLA)-identical siblings, remains superior to cadaver renal transplantation.[1,2] Living donor transplantation can be elective, sparing the recipient a long waiting period on dialysis. It also eases the shortage of cadaver donor organs. With the more potent immunosuppression now available, living donation has been extended to less histocompatible intrafamilial donors and spouses. The results from a spousal donor transplant are superior to those of cadaver donor transplantation.[6] Currently, approximately 40% of renal transplants in the USA are from live donors, 22% of whom are emotionally related or not related to the recipient.[2] The frequency of living donor transplantation varies significantly from one country to the next: 3% in France, 5% in Germany, 8% in Australia, 12% in the UK, 27% in the USA, 25% in the Scandinavian countries, and 40% in Greece. In some countries, particularly India, Turkey, and other Middle East nations, kidney donation is almost exclusively from live donors. The risk of death related to kidney donation has been estimated to be 0.03–0.06%.[7-9] Serious complications in 0.23–2.5% of patients after donor nephrectomy[7-12] are mainly attributable to pneumothorax, pneumonia, wound infection, urinary tract infection, hemorrhage, and deep vein thrombosis.

An individual should be considered as a potential living donor only if the following basic requirements have been fulfilled:[4,6-12]

1. The donor and recipient are ABO blood group compatible.
2. The warm T-lymphocyte cross-match is negative.
3. The person is in excellent physical condition, emotionally stable, and well motivated.
4. The individual is willing to undergo donor nephrectomy, is fully informed about the procedure, and is not under pressure from family members to donate a kidney.

Laparoscopic donor nephrectomy, now routinely performed at several centers, has reduced the morbidity of kidney donation and thereby encouraged more potential living donors to donate. The laparoscopic procedure causes less postoperative pain, shorter hospitalization, and early resumption of functional activity for the donor.[13] Laparoscopic donor nephrectomy is technically more difficult and may be associated with longer warm ischemia time and delayed graft function, especially in the hands of inexperienced surgeons. However, technical complications are the same as for open nephrectomy in centers where this procedure is routinely performed. The short-term graft survival data are similar for patients receiving kidneys from open donor nephrectomy.[13] Long-term graft survival data are awaited.[14]

Blood type and histocompatibility

The potential donor and recipient must be ABO blood group compatible; however, Rh factor incompatibility is not a contraindication to transplantation. Transplantation of blood group A_2 and A_2B kidneys into selected B blood group recipients has been successfully performed in some centers.[15] As B blood group cadaveric transplant recipients wait longer before cadaver transplantation than other blood group recipients, this form of transplantation across the ABO barrier is generating increased interest.

HLA typing and the mixed lymphocyte culture (MLC) are performed on the recipient and potential donors.[16] Excellent long-term outcomes are associated with HLA-identical sibling transplants. Results of transplantation between one haplotype-matched (haploidentical) living related donor, completely mismatched living related donors, and living unrelated renal donors are superior to those obtained with cadaver organs. The MLC should be part of the selection procedure between potential related donors who share equivalent numbers of HLA antigens.

The cytotoxic T-cell cross-match must be negative immediately before transplantation in order to proceed with surgery. A positive high-titer B-cell cross-match is also a contraindication to live donor transplant; however, transplantation may proceed in the presence of a low-titer B-cell cross-match, provided that the T-cell cross-match and the flow cytometry cross-match are negative.[17]

Medical and social evaluation of the potential living donors

All potential donors must be emotionally stable and well motivated to donate a kidney. They must have the opportunity to meet in private with the physicians and social worker on the transplant team, so as to be sure that donation is voluntary and based on full awareness of relevant information. Coercion to donate kidneys is not acceptable. Under no circumstances is payment to a donor acceptable. Living unrelated kidney donors should be considered only if they have a close personal relationship with the recipient, such as a spouse or a lifelong friend. However, given the marked survival advantage with renal transplantation compared with dialysis, and the long waiting lists for cadaver kidneys, other sources of live donation that are being entertained include exchange of living donor kidneys between pairs of individuals with incompatible blood types (paired live donor kidney exchange program) and nondirected donation of kidney by a living donor ("good Samaritan" donor) to a recipient unknown to the potential donor.[18,19]

All potential donors who are willing to donate a kidney should be meticulously evaluated to ensure that they are in excellent general health and that there are no contraindications to the removal of one kidney.[4,9,12] The evaluation of potential donors is indicated in Table 89.1.

The potential donor undergoes thorough history-taking and physical examination with the aim of detecting unsuspected disease such as diabetes, hypertension, anemia, renal calculi, or malignancy. Blood tests should be carried out to detect infections that could be transmitted to the recipient: cytomegalovirus (CMV), Epstein–Barr virus (EBV), HIV, and hepatitis C virus (HCV).[4,8,12,20] The remainder of the studies assess whether renal function and structure are completely normal. The donor work-up is an outpatient process. The potential donor should preferably be a nonsmoker and should not be more than 25% above ideal body weight.[21] Cardiac stress testing is recommended

---

Table 89.1 Evaluation of potential living donors

Aims
  To detect unsuspected diseases such as diabetes, hypertension, hyperlipidemia, anemia, renal calculi, or malignancy in the donor
  To detect infections that may be transmitted from the donor to the recipient
  To assess whether renal function and structure are normal

Clinical assessment
  Complete history and physical examination with multiple blood pressure measurements in the supine and erect positions

Laboratory studies
  Complete blood count
  BUN, serum creatinine, electrolytes
  Fasting blood glucose (GTT if family history of diabetes)
  Serum calcium, phosphorus, uric acid
  Liver function tests
  Fasting lipids
  PT and PTT
  Urine analysis, microscopy, and culture
  24-h urine for creatinine, protein, calcium, and uric acid
  Hepatitis B and C serology
  Antibodies to CMV, EBV, HIV, *Treponema pallidum*
  HLA typing
  ECG
  Chest radiograph
  Intravenous pyelography
  Renal ultrasound or CT scan (only with family history of polycystic kidney disease)
  Renal arteriogram

BUN, blood urea nitrogen; GTT, glucose tolerance test; CMV, cytomegalovirus; EBV, Epstein–Barr virus; CT, computed tomography; HLA, human leukocyte antigen; PT, prothrombin time; PTT, partial thromboplastin time.

---

in potential donors over 40 years of age with known risk factors for coronary artery disease.[21] Minor health problems need not exclude an individual from being a potential donor.[21]

The age of the potential donor is obviously important, and different criteria are used by the various transplant centers.[8,12] Minors should not be considered for kidney donation except in special circumstances. In the USA, it is necessary to obtain permission from a court of law to use a kidney from a donor who has not attained the age of majority. Older donors must be evaluated very carefully. Donors up to age 70 years have been used provided that they were in excellent health. Following unilateral nephrectomy, kidney donors who have been followed as long as 30 years exhibit a slight reduction in glomerular filtration rate and a mild increase in urine protein excretion. The prevalence of hypertension in these donors is no different from that of their healthy siblings who did not donate a kidney.[7]

Cadaver donor transplants

Cadaver donors continue to be the main source of kidneys as the success rate of such transplants continues to improve. After harvesting, kidneys can be preserved by simple hypothermic storage for up to 36 h or by continuous perfusion for up to 72 h,[22] allowing ample time for histocompatibility testing on donor and recipient, evaluation and preparation of the potential recipient, and transportation of the kidney to the best potential recipient.

Neurological evaluation of the potential cadaver kidney donor

The procurement of cadaver organs for transplantation has raised unique legal and ethical issues. The criteria for brain death have been clearly established in recent years (Table 89.2). In general, a 24-h period of observation of the neurological status is necessary, but if the potential donor's condition is unstable and the neurologist or neurosurgeon has determined that brain death has occurred the kidneys may be harvested after consent is obtained from the patient's next of kin. To avoid a conflict of interest, it is important that the declaration of death be the responsibility of the potential donor's physician. It is appropriate to initiate discussion with family members about organ donation before death so that written permission can be obtained in advance from the family and, if necessary, from the medical examiner.

Medical evaluation of the potential cadaver kidney donor

The medical criteria for an ideal cadaver kidney donor are outlined in Table 89.3. Kidneys from infant donors have a higher incidence of technical problems when transplanted singly, therefore transplantation en bloc of both kidneys is

Table 89.2 Neurological evaluation of the potential cadaver donor

24-h observation of the neurological status is necessary, provided the potential donor is medically stable

To avoid conflict of interest, declaration of death is the responsibility of the potential donor's physician

Criteria for brain death
Cerebral unresponsiveness
Brainstem unresponsiveness
No activity on EEG for 30 min or absence of cerebral blood flow on radionuclide study or contrast angiography

Toxic screen free of depressant drugs (particularly barbiturates)

Table 89.3 Medical evaluation of potential cadaver donors

Age: infant to 70 years

Obtain thorough medical history

No evidence of
Long-standing or severe hypertension
Long-standing diabetes mellitus
Primary renal disease
Systemic disease affecting the kidneys
Systemic bacterial, viral, or fungal infection
HIV infection or hepatitis as indexed by negative serology for HIV, HBV, HCV
Perforated abdominal viscus
Malignancy other than primary brain tumor or treated squamous or basal cell skin cancer

Normal BUN, creatinine (minor terminal elevations are acceptable)

Normal urinalysis at the time of admission

Maintenance of good urine output is ideal

HBV/HCV, hepatitis B/C virus; BUN, blood urea nitrogen.

in order with donors younger than 3 years.[23] Single kidneys may be transplanted from donors aged between 4 and 70 years; however, donors older than 55 years of age must be carefully evaluated. Donors with mild hypertension or diabetes of short duration are not excluded from consideration, provided that blood urea nitrogen and serum creatinine levels are normal and there is no proteinuria. For these donors and for those older than 55 years, post-mortem renal biopsy is advisable for assessment of the viability of the kidney as a donor organ.[24] Frozen sections should be made after harvesting, and an assessment made of the extent of arteriolar nephrosclerosis, glomerular sclerosis, and interstitial fibrosis.

The serious shortage of donor kidneys has prompted many institutions to expand their donor criteria.[25,26] In an attempt to increase the utilization of suboptimal kidneys, transplantation of both marginal kidneys (dual transplant) into a single recipient has been performed at some centers. This has been found to offer good short-term results without exposing the recipient to delayed posttransplant renal recovery, acute allograft rejection, or major surgical complications.[27] There has been renewed interest in the use of "nonheart-beating donors," with good short-term results.[28,29] Ideally, renal perfusion should be maintained during the terminal phase of the patient's care by appropriate administration of intravenous fluids. Minor terminal elevations in blood urea nitrogen (BUN) and creatinine in the donor are not a contraindication to the use of the kidneys.

All donors should be carefully evaluated for signs of infection. Generalized or abdominal sepsis excludes a donor from further consideration; however, donors with terminal mild pulmonary infection or bacteriuria related to an indwelling catheter are often acceptable, provided that the infecting organism has been identified and appropriate antibiotics have been given. Evidence of HIV infection is a contraindication to donation. Kidneys from hepatitis B virus (HBV) surface antigen-positive donors should be used only in HBV-positive recipients. Every attempt should be made to obtain a medical history from the potential donor's family, physician, and medical records. High-risk behavior, such as male homosexual activity or intravenous drug use, excludes people from consideration as kidney donors, regardless of their HIV antibody status. Controversy exists about potential donors with antibodies to HCV.[20] Although the majority of centers reject such potential donors, other centers accept them. Currently, in our center, kidneys from these donors are considered for transplantation only into HCV RNA-PCR-positive recipients. The CMV antibody status of the potential donor is also determined. In the past, certain transplant centers regarded a kidney from a CMV-seropositive donor as a contraindication for a recipient who was seronegative. Given the current availability of potent prophylactic antiviral therapy, however, this is no longer a reason not to proceed with renal transplantation.

Evaluation and preparation of the recipient

The approach to the transplant evaluation process of the potential recipient is illustrated in Fig. 89.1. Early referral to the transplant center when the glomerular filtration rate (GFR) is in the 25 mL/min range is mandatory. Preemptive living donor transplantation without the previous initiation of dialysis has been found to be associated with a 52% reduction in the risk of allograft failure during the first year after transplantation and with better long-term allograft survival than transplantation after initiation of dialysis.[30] A similar correlation between better posttransplant outcome and shorter duration of dialysis has been reported with cadaver transplantation.[31]

Pretransplant evaluation must include a detailed medical and psychological evaluation of the potential recipient. Patients must be healthy enough to undergo the surgical procedure and to withstand the potential problems of immunosuppressive therapy. Potential recipients should meet with the transplant team so that their questions can be answered and to ensure that they understand the procedure and have realistic expectations. The pretransplant work-up, the side-effects of immunosuppressive agents, the complex and demanding medical regimen, the possibility of recurrence in the allograft of the patient's native kidney disease, and rehabilitation potential of the prospective recipient need to be discussed at this time.

The pretransplant evaluation of the recipient is described in Table 89.4. The aim is to detect any problem that might reduce the chances of success of the operation and to take corrective measures when necessary. Not all patients with endstage renal disease (ESRD) are candidates for transplantation. Patients of advanced age or those with significant systemic illness are generally not acceptable candidates. Contraindications to transplantation are listed in Table 89.5.

Age

The age range for transplantation has been broadened in recent years with the advent of more effective immunosuppressive therapy. Good results have been reported in children as young as 1 year. Growth retardation is an important aspect of childhood renal failure that improves after successful transplantation. At the other end of the age range, there is no well-defined cutoff point. In the past, patients older than 50 years were not accepted for transplantation because of a higher mortality rate, but currently patients up to 75 years are being accepted. In the older patients, a diligent pretransplant assessment must be performed. Currently, over 50% of patients on the UNOS kidney transplant waiting list are 50 years of age or older.[2]

Infections

Infection remains a significant cause of morbidity and mortality after transplantation. Treatable infections must be eradicated before transplantation. Infections of the sinuses, ears, chest, urinary tract, and the feet of diabetics and patients with peripheral vascular disease must be cleared up prior to transplantation. Dental caries should be treated to reduce the risk of dental abscess after transplantation. Chest radiography should be performed for signs of pulmonary tuberculosis or other pulmonary infection. Potential recipients who are seronegative for CMV are at high risk of developing serious CMV infection if given a seropositive donor organ and should be given prolonged prophylactic antiviral therapy after transplantation.[32] Seropositive recipients are also at risk for CMV infection, usually a milder variety, owing either to reactivation of the virus or to acquisition of a different strain of virus from a seropositive donor. Thus, prophylactic antiviral agents are usually administered to all combinations that include a CMV-seropositive donor or recipient.[32] Controversy exists with regard to patients who are HBV surface antigen positive or HCV antibody positive because of the risk of later developing progressive liver disease and death from liver failure.[33] In these patients, liver biopsy

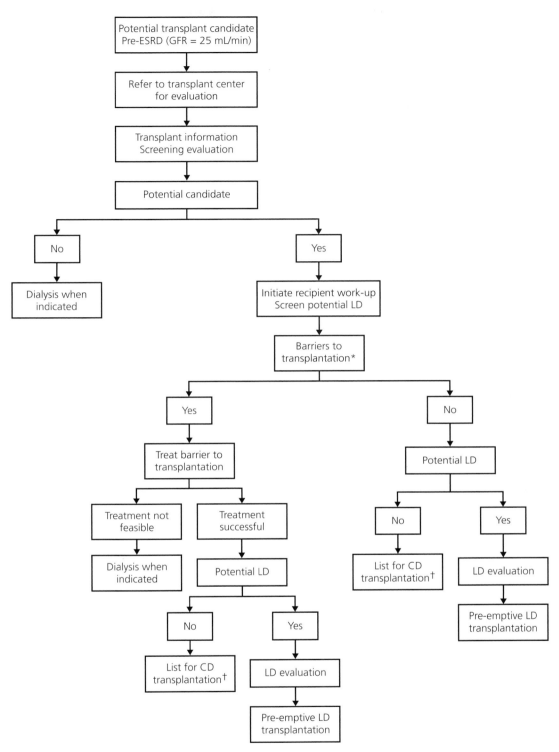

Figure 89.1 Approach to the transplant evaluation process of the potential renal transplant recipient. LD, living donor; CD, cadaver donor; GFR, glomerular filtration rate; ESRD, endstage renal disease. *Common barriers to transplantation include vascular disease, infection, carcinoma, smoking, alcohol or other substance use, obesity, and noncompliance to medical treatment. †Patients may not accrue waiting time on the United Network of Organ Sharing (UNOS) waiting list until GFR ≤ 20 mL/min or initiation of dialysis.

should be performed to assess the histological severity of the disease before transplantation.

A potential candidate for organ transplantation who is seropositive for HIV antibody but is asymptomatic should not necessarily be excluded from candidacy for organ transplantation, but should be advised that he or she may be at increased risk of morbidity and mortality because of immunosuppressive therapy.[2] The currently available highly active antiretroviral therapy has improved survival and decreased morbidity in HIV-positive patients. As such, there is now increased interest in transplantation in HIV-positive patients with undetectable viral loads and CD4+ cell counts of at least 200 cells/mm³.[34] However, a recent national random survey of 271 US nephrologists reported low rates of recommendation for renal transplantation in HIV-positive patients.[35]

Table 89.4 Pretransplant evaluation of kidney recipients

Complete history and physical examination

Dental evaluation

Gynecologic evaluation

Laboratory studies
  Liver function tests
  HBV and HBC screening
  Antibodies to CMV, HIV, EBV
  Urine culture
  PSA*

Radiology studies
  Chest radiograph
  Upper gastrointestinal series or endoscopy†
  Barium enema or colonoscopy‡
  Gallbladder ultrasonography
  Voiding cystourethrography§
  Mammography¶
  Bone densitometry

HBV/HCV, hepatitis B/C virus; CMV, cytomegalovirus; EBV, Epstein–Barr virus; PSA, prostate-specific antigen.
*Male patients > 50 years.
†In the presence of symptoms or history of peptic ulcer disease.
‡Age > 40 years and/or family history of colon cancer.
§In diabetic patients or in patients with a history of recurrent urinary tract infections.
¶Female patients > 40 years.

Table 89.5 Contraindications to renal transplantation

Age > 75 years
Active infection
Severe cardiovascular disease
Severe pulmonary disease
Severe chronic liver disease
Malignancy*
Active vasculitis or glomerulonephritis
Uncorrectable lower urinary tract disease†
Primary oxalosis‡
Morbid obesity
Severe psychosocial problems
Current drug or alcohol abuse
Positive current T-cell cross-match

*Cure from malignancy with no evidence of recurrence is not a contraindication.
†Patients unwilling to undergo creation of an ileal conduit or to perform frequent self-catheterizations.
‡Patients should undergo combined kidney and liver transplantation.

Gastrointestinal disease

Because of the serious consequences of bleeding from a peptic ulcer after transplantation, endoscopic examination should be performed in patients with symptoms or a history of peptic ulcer disease. If an ulcer is present, it should be treated medically for 6 weeks, followed by repeat endoscopy. If the ulcer has not healed, surgical therapy should be performed before transplantation. Some institutions perform a barium enema or colonoscopy in potential transplant recipients over age 40 years, so that the transplant team will be aware of the presence of diverticular disease or colonic polyps. Patients who have localized diverticular disease and a history of acute diverticulitis or perforation of a diverticulum should be considered for a pretransplant segmental colectomy, and colonic polyps should be removed and examined histologically. The value of this approach has been questioned.[36] Gallbladder ultrasonography is often included in the pretransplant evaluation. Our practice is to advise patients with gallstones to have a cholecystectomy, thus avoiding the danger of acute cholecystitis after transplantation.

Lower urinary tract disease

Patients with recurrent urinary tract infections should have a voiding cystourethrogram. If persistent high-grade reflux is demonstrated, bilateral nephrectomy and ureterectomy is indicated. Treatment causes of lower urinary tract obstruction, such as prostatic hypertrophy, should be corrected before transplantation. For patients with a neurogenic bladder, the transplant ureter can be anastomosed into an ileal conduit; alternatively, frequent self-catheterization should be considered after transplantation. Both of these maneuvers carry the risk of recurrent urinary tract infection after transplantation. Prostate-specific antigen (PSA) should be measured in male recipients older than 50 years.

Malignancy

Patients with an incurable malignancy should not be considered for transplantation. Except for localized basal or squamous cell carcinomas of the skin, patients who have undergone curative resection or treatment of malignancy should have a disease-free interval of 1–10 years before being considered for a transplant. The duration of the disease-free period should be determined by what is known about the natural history of the particular tumor. A thorough evaluation must be carried out before transplantation to ensure that the patient is indeed free of recurrence.

Cardiovascular disease

Vascular disease is present in a significant proportion of dialysis patients, especially older patients and those with diabetes mellitus. Occlusive arteriosclerotic vascular disease has become the major cause of death in patients with a functioning allograft.[33] If the severity of the vascular disease would preclude successful rehabilitation and longevity, transplantation is contraindicated. Patients with severe angina should be carefully evaluated for critical coronary artery disease amenable to angioplasty or bypass surgery. Similarly, patients with peripheral vascular disease or extracranial carotid artery disease should be evaluated for correctable lesions.

Special consideration for patients with type 1 diabetes mellitus

The risks and benefits of pancreas or islet cell transplantation should be discussed with patients with ESRD and type 1 diabetes mellitus. Transplant recommendations for such patients are listed in Table 89.6. Patients < 50 years of age and with minimal or no cardiovascular disease and left ventricular ejection fraction of > 50% are the best candidates for vascularized pancreas transplantation. The major benefits of pancreas transplantation include improved quality of life as a result of normalization of blood glucose levels, prevention of recurrent diabetic nephropathy in the allograft, and improvement or stabilization of the long-term complications of diabetes. When compared with kidney transplantation alone in patients with type 1 diabetes mellitus, kidney and pancreas transplantation has been shown to improve patient survival.[37] Patients with cardiovascular disease who are not candidates for vascularized pancreas transplantation should be considered for islet transplantation, which is a far less invasive procedure.[38]

Surgical preparation of the patient

Surgical procedures that should be performed to lessen the likelihood of serious consequences after transplantation were outlined earlier. Bilateral nephrectomy is indicated for the control of severe hypertension that is not controlled with drug therapy and effective fluid removal by dialysis, for high-grade vesicoureteral reflux, for recurrent episodes of acute pyelonephritis, and occasionally for massive enlargement of polycystic kidneys. Pretransplant parathyroidectomy should be considered for dialysis patients with severe secondary hyperparathyroidism and symptomatic bone disease.

Conclusion

The current success of renal transplantation has led to a more liberal selection policy. However, if success rates are to be maintained, all potential transplant recipients, especially those who fall into a high-risk category, need to be evaluated carefully before transplantation, and attempts must be made to eliminate conditions that might adversely affect short- and long-term outcomes.

References

1. Cecka JM: The UNOS Scientific Renal Transplant Registry-2000. In Terasaki PI, Cecka JM (eds): Clinical Transplants 2000. Los Angeles: UCLA Tissue Typing Laboratory, 2001, p 1.
2. United Network of Organ Sharing: 2000 Annual Report of The U.S. Scientific Registry of Transplant Recipients and the Organ Procurement and Transplant Network, Washington, DC. www.UNOS.org. Accessed on 10/29/2001.
3. Hariharan S, Johnson CP, Bresnahan BA, et al: Improved graft survival after renal transplantation in the United States, 1988 to 1996. N Engl J Med 2000;342:605–612.
4. First MR: Pretransplantation evaluation and preparation of donors and recipients. In Jacobson HR, Striker GF, Klahr S (eds): The Principles and Practice of Nephrology, 2nd edn. Philadelphia: BC Decker, 1995, p 805.
5. United States Renal Data System: USRDS 1996, Annual Data Report. Am J Kidney Dis 1996;28 (Suppl 2):1.
6. Terasaki PI, Cecka M, Gjertson DW, et al: High survival rates of kidney transplants from spousal and living unrelated donors. N Engl J Med 1995;333:333–336.
7. Najarian JS, Chavers BM, McHigh LE, et al: 20 years or more of follow-up and living kidney donors. Lancet 1992;340:807–810.
8. Bia MJ, Ramos EL, Danovitch GM, et al: Evaluation of living renal donors. The current practice of US transplant centers. Transplantation 1995;60:322–327.
9. Bay WH, Hebert LA: The living donor in kidney transplantation. Ann Intern Med 1987;106:719–727.
10. Weiland D, Sutherland DER, Chavers B, et al: Information on 628 living related kidney donors at a single institution with long-term follow-up in 472 cases. Transplant Proc 1984;16:5.
11. Blohme I, Fehrman I, Norden G: Living donor nephrectomy. Scand J Urol Nephrol 1992;26:149–153.
12. Kasiske BL, Ravenscraft M, Ramos EL, et al: The evaluation of living renal transplant donors: clinical practice guidelines. J Am Soc Nephrol 1996;7:2288–2313.
13. Ratner LE, Buell JF, Kuo PC: Laparoscopic donor nephrectomy: pro. Transplantation 2000;70:1544–1546.
14. Barry JM: Laparoscopic donor nephrectomy: con. Transplantation 2000;70:1546–1548.
15. Bryan CF, Shield CF III, Nelson PW, et al: Transplantation rate of the blood group B waiting list is increased by using A2 and A2B kidneys. Transplantation 1988;66:1714–1717.
16. Colombe BW, Garovoy MR: The major histocompatibility system of humans. In Jacobson HR, Stricker GF, Klahr S (eds): The Principles and Practice of Nephrology, 2nd edn. Philadelphia: BC Decker, 1995, p 798.

Table 89.6 Transplantation recommendations for patients with endstage renal disease (ESRD) and type 1 diabetes mellitus (DM)

Patient characteristic	Transplant recommendation
Patients with ESRD and stable type 1 DM	Living donor kidney transplant followed by cadaver pancreas transplantation or simultaneous pancreas–kidney transplantation if there is no suitable living donor
Patients with ESRD and labile type 1 DM or patients with DM-induced severe autonomic neuropathy	Consider simultaneous pancreas–kidney transplantation as the first option
ESRD patients who are candidates for cadaver kidney transplant and are high risk for vascularized pancreas transplant	Living donor kidney followed by islet cell transplantation or simultaneous cadaver kidney and islet cell transplantation
Type 1 DM patients with previous kidney transplant and stable GFR of > 50 mL/min	Pancreas or islet cell after kidney transplantation

GFR, glomerular filtration rate.

17. Ting A, Welsh K: HLA matching and crossmatching in renal transplantation. *In* Morris PJ (ed): Kidney Transplantation: Principles and Practice, 4th edn. Philadelphia: WB Saunders, 1994, p 109.
18. Gridelli B, Remuzzi G: Strategies for making more organs available for transplantation. N Engl J Med 2000;343:404–410.
19. Matas AJ, Garvey CA, Jacobs CL, et al: Nondirected donation of kidneys from living donors. N Engl J Med 2000;343:433–436.
20. Pereira BJG, Mildord EL, Kirkman RL, et al: Transmission of hepatitis C virus by organ transplantation. N Engl J Med 1991;325:454–460.
21. The Authors for the Live Organ Donor Consensus Group: Consensus statement on the live organ donor. JAMA 2000;284:2919–2926.
22. Marshall VC, Jablonski P, Scott DF: Renal preservation. *In* Morris PJ (ed): Kidney Transplantation: Principles and Practice, 4th edn. Philadelphia: WB Saunders, 1994, p 86.
23. Cosimi AB: The donor and donor nephrectomy. *In* Morris PJ (ed): Kidney Transplantation: Principles and Practice, 4th edn. Philadelphia: WB Saunders, 1994, p 56.
24. Lloveras L: The elderly donor. Transplant Proc 1991;23:2592–2595.
25. Alexander JW, Davies CB, First MR, et al: Single pretransplant donor-specific transfusion in cadaver and living related donor renal transplantation. Transplant Proc 1993;25:485–487.
26. Alexander JW, Zola JC: Expanding the donor and pool: use of marginal donors for solid organ transplantation. Clin Transplant 1996;10:1–19.
27. Remuzzi G, Grinyo J, Ruggenenti P, et al: Early experience with dual kidney transplantation in adults using expanded donor criteria. Double Kidney Transplant Group (DKG). J Am Soc Nephrol 1999;10:2591–2598.
28. Winjen RMH, Booster MH, Stubenitsky BM, et al: Outcome of transplantation of non-heart-beating donor kidneys. Lancet 1995;345:1067–1070.
29. Gonzalez C, Casstelao AM, Torras J, et al: Long-term function of transplanted non-heart-beating donor kidneys. Transplant Proc 1995;27:2948–2950.
30. Mange KC, Joffe MM, Feldman HI: Effect of the use or nonuse of long-term dialysis on the subsequent survival of renal transplants from living donors. N Engl J Med 2001;344:726–731.
31. Cacciarelli TV, Sumrani N, DiBenedetto A, et al: Influence of length of time on dialysis before transplantation on long-term renal allograft outcome. Transplant Proc 1993;25:2474–2476.
32. Patel R, Syndman DR, Ruben RH, et al: Cytomegalovirus prophylaxis in solid organ transplant recipients. Transplantation 1996;61:1279–1289.
33. First MR: Long-term complications after transplantation. Am J Kidney Dis 1993;22:477–486.
34. Stock PG, Roland M, Carlson L, et al: Renal transplantation in HIV+ patients. Am J Transplant 2001;2:164, Abstract 114.
35. Thamer M, Hwang W, Fink NE, et al: U.S. nephrologists' attitude towards renal transplantation: results from a national survey. Transplantation 2001;71:281–288.
36. McCune TR, Nylander WA, VanBuren DH, et al: Colonic screening prior to renal transplantation and its impact on post-transplant colonic complications. Clin Transplant 1992;6:91–96.
37. Becker BN, Brazy PC, Becker YT, et al: Simultaneous pancreas–kidney transplantation reduces excess mortality in type 1 diabetic patients with end-stage renal disease. Kidney Int 2000;57:2129–2135.
38. Shapiro AM, Lakey JR, Ryan EA, et al: Islet transplantation in seven patients with type 1 diabetes mellitus using a glucocorticoid-free immunosuppressive regimen. N Engl J Med 2000;343:230–238.

Technical Aspects of Renal Transplantation and Surgical Complications

Donald C. Dafoe

Recipient evaluation
Procurement
Transplant operation
Surgical complications
- Wound complications
- Bleeding
- Urine leak
- Vascular thrombosis
- Obstruction of the collecting system
- Lymphocele
- Vesicoureteral reflux
- Transplant renal artery stenosis
Miscellaneous complications

Renal transplantation is regarded by most physicians as the preferred treatment for chronic renal failure.[1] A successful renal transplant improves a patient's independence and rehabilitation. Transplantation is more cost-effective than other modalities. According to the United Network for Organ Sharing, the 1-year graft survival rate for 22 423 renal allografts (live and cadaver donor) placed into adult recipients during 1997–1998 in the USA was 91%. The recipient mortality in the first year was less than 5%.[2] Rejection and the donor shortage are the major obstacles to routine application of renal transplantation. As the proportion of grafts lost to rejection diminishes and the value of each donor graft increases, the importance of technical perfection is magnified. Surgical skills are best exercised in the context of judicious intra- and perioperative decision-making based on a thorough understanding of medicine and biology.

Recipient evaluation

The renal graft is usually transplanted heterotopically in the extraperitoneal iliac fossa of the pelvis. In most cases, the native kidneys are left intact. From the narrow yet important perspective of technical issues, the evaluation of the renal transplant candidate raises several questions:

- Is the domain of either iliac fossa or pelvis adequate?
- Will arterial inflow and venous outflow be sufficient?
- What is the condition of the urine-collecting system and bladder?

Most often, a careful medical history and physical examination of the candidate will provide the answers to these questions and no further anatomical studies are necessary. Examination of the abdomen may reveal surgical scars, masses, organomegaly, or abdominal wall defects that

dictate the site of the transplant. For example, a right subcostal incision implies that the superior epigastric artery has been sacrificed at prior surgery. Since the inferior epigastric artery is taken during the transplant surgery, placement of the graft on the right could result in a disastrous loss of abdominal wall tissue secondary to devascularization. In the patient with polycystic kidney disease, physical examination may find a large native kidney encroaching on the iliac fossa. A nephrectomy may be necessary either before or synchronous with the transplant. Palpation of weak or absent femoral pulses betrays serious vascular disease that may contraindicate renal transplantation. If the groin pulses are unequal, the graft should be placed on the side with the stronger pulse. Similarly, the graft should be placed on the side opposite to unilateral leg swelling or other stigmata of venous disease. Previous surgery in the lower abdomen (e.g. vascular reconstruction) may require additional studies (e.g. arteriography).

Routine cystoscopy or cystography is not indicated. These studies may be of value when there is a history of voiding problems, massive urinary reflux, recurrent infections, or prior urological procedures. A cystogram in a patient who has been anuric or oliguric for several years while on dialysis may demonstrate a small-capacity, noncompliant bladder. In the instance of an unsatisfactory urinary reservoir, an ileal loop or bladder augmentation may be needed in advance of the transplant.

Bilateral native nephrectomy is seldom necessary, but indications include symptomatic polycystic kidney disease (e.g. cyst rupture, bleeding), massive vesicoureteral reflux, heavy proteinuria, persistent upper tract infection, severe renovascular hypertension, and symptomatic stone disease.

Procurement

Brain death standards for cadaver donors are stringent.[3] There are accepted general donor criteria such as no extracranial malignancy or HIV infection. However, given the severe donor organ shortage, general criteria are expanding. For example, the upper age limit is now 70 years. Consideration is now given to kidneys from donors with diabetes or hypertension of short duration (e.g. less than 5 years). Nonheart-beating donors are more commonplace. Grafts may function after as long as 48 h of cold storage preservation, but the incidence of delayed graft function increases proportionately with prolonged preservation time.

The retrieval of cadaver donor kidney grafts is usually one component of a complex multiple organ procurement. A common technique employed is in situ perfusion using iced preservation solution and en bloc removal of both kidneys based on the aorta and inferior vena cava. Multiple arteries are found in approximately 20% of donors. During procurement, care is taken to leave multiple arteries intact. In a cadaver donor, renal arteries can be centered on a Carrel patch of donor aorta to facilitate the arterial anastomosis. The hilum of the renal graft is not disturbed to avoid arterial arborizations. Because the arterial blood supply to the kidney is segmental, inadvertent ligation of a polar artery, for example, creates a discrete infarct. If the vessel supplies the upper pole, a small scar of little consequence may result. On the other hand, a lower pole vessel is important because it supplies the ureter. A devascularized ureter will necrose and leak or fibrose and obstruct. Damage to a large accessory artery may result in slough of parenchyma manifesting as a caliceal cutaneous fistula. This problem usually requires transplant nephrectomy. To ensure good vascularization of the graft ureter, the procurement surgeon leaves a "fan" of investing periureteral tissue. Iliac vessels are routinely procured from the cadaver donor for possible bench reconstruction if any graft vessels are severed or damaged.

When the source of the renal graft is a live donor – a genetically or emotionally related individual – the technical issues are similar to those of the cadaver donor procurement. With a live donor, the surgeon has the advantage of preoperative imaging of the renal vasculature. Arteriography, spiral computed tomography, or magnetic resonance angiography will uncover multiple vessels or an early bifurcation of the renal artery off the aorta. If both kidneys have a single artery and vein, the left kidney is preferred because of the longer vein. A longer vein facilitates the sew-in and the donor nephrectomy, particularly if the surgery is performed laparoscopically. A guiding principle is: if there is a defect (e.g. a simple cyst), the live donor is left with the more perfect kidney.

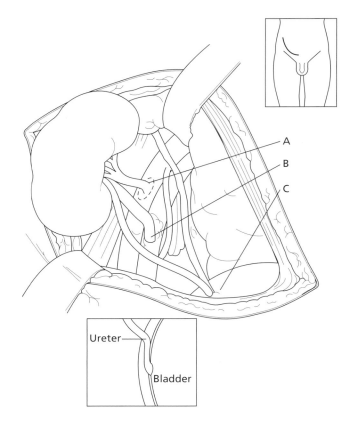

Figure 90.1 The renal allograft is implanted in the extraperitoneal iliac fossa. The arterial blood supply to the graft is from either the internal iliac artery or the external iliac artery (as shown, **A**) and venous drainage is into the external iliac vein (**B**). The ureteroneocystostomy is created between the graft ureter and the bladder (**C**). This mucosa-to-mucosa connection is covered by reapproximation of divided detrusor muscle, thus preventing reflux. (From Hardy JB: Hardy's Textbook of Surgery, 2nd edn. Philadelphia: JB Lippincott, 1988.)

Transplant operation

General endotracheal anesthesia is induced with the patient in the supine position on the operating table.[4] A urinary balloon catheter is inserted. Intraoperative monitoring may include a central venous pressure catheter, pulse oximetry, and arterial blood pressure line. A curvilinear incision is made in either the right or left lower abdomen (Fig. 90.1). (In theory, the renal graft can be transplanted anywhere that there is a suitable recipient artery, vein, and urine conduit or reservoir.) The extraperitoneal iliac fossa is used because of the presence of the iliac vessels and its proximity to the urinary bladder. The transplant is protected by the iliac bone posterolaterally and the abdominal musculature anteriorly; yet the graft is superficial enough for percutaneous biopsy. Three layers of the abdominal wall – the external oblique, internal oblique, and transverses abdominis – are divided to afford access to the iliac fossa. The diaphanous peritoneal membrane is rolled medially off the external iliac vessels. It is common practice to anastomose the transplant artery end-to-side on the external iliac artery. Alternatively, the distal internal iliac artery is ligated and

divided, and the proximal vessel is used for end-to-end anastomosis with the graft renal artery. Bilateral ligation of the distal internal iliac artery in the performance of serial bilateral renal allografts is discouraged to prevent vasculogenic impotence. Lymphatic channels that overlie the iliac vessels are divided to expose the artery and vein. These channels are ligated to prevent lymphatic leaks, lymphocele formation, and subsequent ureteral obstruction or iliac vein compression. The renal vein is routinely sewn to the side of the external iliac vein. The time that transpires between removing the graft from the iced slush and reperfusion with oxygenated blood is known as "the warm ischemia time." This period ranges from 25 to 45 min. Warm ischemia time longer than 45 min in cadaver renal transplantation is associated with increased incidence of delayed graft function; longer than 60 min may render the patient permanently dialysis dependent (primary nonfunction).

Urinary drainage from the renal graft is established by surgically connecting the graft ureter to the bladder. The ureteroneocystostomy is usually accomplished via the extravesical approach, whereby the spatulated end of the transplant ureter is sewn to the bladder, mucosa to mucosa, after incision through detrusor muscle. The detrusor muscle is then reunited to buttress the anastomosis and create an antireflux valve. Other techniques of ureteroneocystostomy include tunneling of the graft ureter via cystotomy (Leadbetter–Politano) and sewing of the native ureter to the transplant renal pelvis (ureteropyelostomy). After meticulous hemostasis is achieved, the wound is closed in two layers. At most centers, drains or ureteral stents are not used routinely. Depending on the patient's body habitus, the operation lasts for 2–4 h. In children, the relative size discrepancy between the graft and the recipient may dictate placement of the renal transplant intraperitoneally by anastomosis to the aorta and inferior vena cava.[5]

If the pretransplant evaluation reveals a contracted, noncompliant bladder, a urine reservoir can be established with an ileal loop – a segment of ileum with one end brought out as an ostomy – or bladder augmentation with a segment of intestine. Alternatively, the small bladder of disuse may be gradually expanded before transplantation by gradual filling over time with incrementally larger volumes to produce adequate bladder capacity. If bladder urodynamics are markedly abnormal, the bladder may be used as a passive reservoir coupled with intermittent self-catheterization after transplantation.

Surgical complications

Wound complications

Wound infection is the most common complication after renal transplantation. Contributory factors include obesity, diabetes, uremia with protein malnutrition, and exogenous immunosuppression. Typically, the characteristic findings of fever, local erythema, swelling, and drainage present 4–7 days after surgery. If the infection is confined to the subcutaneous space, treatment consists of opening the skin to allow drainage, followed by local wound care measures such as packing until the wound heals in. If there is significant cellulitis or systemic illness, antibiotics are warranted. The antibiotic selected depends on the Gram stain and culture. Gram-positive organisms are usually responsible. If there is a suspicion of a subfascial abscess, an ultrasound study may be helpful or the removal of fascial sutures will demonstrate deep involvement. Drainage of clear fluid from the wound is common, especially in obese patients. Placement of a collection bag over the wound will allow the determination of creatinine in the fluid to distinguish urine (from a urine leak) from serum (lymphatic leak or a draining seroma). A seroma, a subcutaneous collection of tissue fluid, can be left alone to resolve with time or can be drained either by repeated needle aspiration or by drain placement. The approach depends on the clinical circumstances. Dehiscence of the transplant wound is unusual. However, the inhibition of wound healing from the malnutrition of chronic renal failure and steroid immunosuppression may contribute to fascial disruption. Dehiscence requires emergent reoperation and reclosure.

Bleeding

Characteristically, "surgical" bleeding – requiring a return to the operating room – presents in the early postoperative period with tachycardia, hypotension, and, after volume resuscitation, a falling hematocrit. Bleeding is more likely in renal transplant recipients than normal patients because of decreased platelet adhesiveness secondary to uremia. This platelet defect may be reversed with vasopressin or intravenous estrogen. Some surgeons fully heparinize renal transplant recipients, and this practice may contribute to bleeding. Heparin effect can be countered with protamine. A falling hematocrit in the early postoperative period should not be ascribed to "medical" causes. Correction of clinically significant bleeding is amenable only to reexploration. A bleed at the vascular anastomosis or a vessel in the graft hilum is often the culprit. Mild hematuria that resolves without intervention is not uncommon.

Urine leak

The prevalence of urine leak is approximately 2%. A large urine leak at the ureter-to-bladder anastomosis due to a technical flaw results in a rapid fall-off in urine output in the early postoperative period. Later, ureteral necrosis and leak may be due to procurement errors (e.g. degloving) or ischemia from rejection-induced vasculitis and thrombosis of periureteral blood supply. Labial or scrotal edema may occur. Clear fluid from the wound may be distinguished from the more common finding of a draining seroma by a creatinine determination on the fluid: if the fluid is urine, the creatinine value will be much higher than the synchronous serum creatinine. There may be a sensation of fluid ballottability around the graft on examination. The patient may complain of pain from the inflammation of extravasated urine. Fever may occur from superimposed infection. The suspicion or a urine leak is confirmed by a radionuclide scan showing extravasation of "hot" tracer outside the confines of the collecting system.[6] If ultrasonography demonstrates a fluid collection, the collection is tapped and the fluid analyzed for creatinine to make the diagnosis of "urinoma." Emergent exploration is the treatment of choice for a urine leak. Treatment of a leak with interventional radiologic techniques such as percutaneous nephrostomy and drain placement is successful only for small leaks at the ureteroneocystostomy. Although these techniques are helpful for diagnosis or as a temporizing measure in patients who are unfit for surgery (e.g. untreated urinary infection), the definitive solution is surgery. Reconstruction of the ureter may involve reimplantation after cutting back to well-vascularized tissue. If the transplant ureter is too short to reach the bladder, the bladder may be extensively mobilized and fixed superiorly to the psoas muscle – a psoas "hitch;" the distal native ureter may be sewn to the transplant pelvis, or a tube can be fashioned from the bladder wall (Boari flap) to bridge the gap. After reconstruction, a ureteral stent is used to deter another leak and a drain is placed to allow egress of urine until the urinary mucosa heals watertight. The drain is removed when output ceases, and the stent is cystoscopically removed at 6 weeks.

Vascular thrombosis

The prevalence of thrombosis of the transplant artery or vein is 1%. Clinically, acute anuria raises the concern of graft thrombosis. Occasionally, loss of the renal transplant from thrombosis is masked by increased urine production from dormant native kidneys in response to diuretics and volume loading. Hyperacute rejection can result in thrombosis, but faulty technique is usually responsible. Technical problems include intimal dissection, especially in recipients with long-standing diabetes or hypertension; kinking of the artery or vein from malpositioning of the graft; torsion of the vessels; and narrowing of the anastomosis. Doppler ultrasonography or radionuclide scanning show greatly decreased or no flow to the graft.[4] If the index of suspicion for thrombosis is high – for example, an uneventful live donor graft that does not diurese postoperatively – the patient should be taken back for immediate exploration. Arteriography is seldom of value and delays surgical exploration. At exploration, arterial thrombosis is suggested by a small, pale kidney; with venous thrombosis, the kidney transplant is blue, swollen, and, sometimes, bleeding from a fracture. Thrombectomy and graft salvage have been reported, but warm ischemia that lasts more than 45–60 min results in irreversible injury. When the vascular compromise is incomplete (e.g. venous kinking), the chance of salvage is improved, but a prolonged delay in graft function can be expected. Protracted warm ischemia or primary nonfunction of a graft mandates transplant nephrectomy.

Obstruction of the collecting system

Obstruction occurs in about 2% of renal transplants. Blockage of urine flow in the early postoperative period may be the result of technical misadventure in the construction of the ureteroneocystostomy – such as a too-tight antireflux tunnel – or a problem with the graft ureter – such as a twist, entrapment by the spermatic cord, or an extrinsic compression by a urinoma. Weeks to months after the transplant surgery, an ultrasonographic investigation of an elevated serum creatinine value may uncover a dilated urine collecting system due to ureteral stricture, stone disease (either de novo, retained, or of donor origin), fungus balls, shed tissue from papillary necrosis, or lymphocele. A fungus ball is often superimposed on a partial obstruction or a retained foreign body. After percutaneous needle biopsy, hemorrhage can fill the pelvis with clot, but the thrombolytic effect of urokinase in urine makes obstruction of the collecting system unusual.

If the collecting system is massively dilated on ultrasonography, the patient should be scheduled for a definitive surgical repair. When a dilated transplant ureter with mild-to-moderate hydronephrosis is seen, the urodynamic significance of the findings may be uncertain. If renal transplant function is only mildly impaired, a

furosemide "washout" radionuclide study may be helpful. An antegrade pyelogram provides the best image and can be converted to a percutaneous nephrostomy (PCN) to decompress the obstructed system. If there is a clinically significant obstruction, there will be a postobstructive diuresis and a fall in the serum creatinine. In equivocal cases, a Whitaker test can be performed. This is a manometric study of urodynamics by saline infusion through the PCN. If there is an obstruction, the pressure in the manometer will rise steadily as saline is infused. The disadvantage of decompression of the collecting system is difficulty in localizing a full renal pelvis during the definitive surgical repair. Another disadvantage of an indwelling decompressing catheter is the introduction of infection. Balloon dilatation of a ureteral stricture and stenting have been reported, but disruption of the ureter and recurrent strictures are an issue. Furthermore, stenting introduces a foreign body that may be a nidus for encrustation, stone formation, or infection. The best approach is surgical correction. This is carried out either by graft ureter reimplantation or, more commonly, by rerouting of urine from the transplant renal pelvis into the native ureter. In constructing the ureteropyelostomy, the native kidney does not have to be removed; rather, the ureter is ligated and any residual function is shut down by the resultant hydrostasis.

Lymphocele

Transected lymphatic channels that course over the iliac vessels may leak lymph and develop into a lymphocele – a cyst-like collection of lymph that may impinge on the graft ureter. The standard treatment for lymphocele is surgical fenestration. A window is created in the lymphocele wall via the laparoscope or open surgery to allow lymph to drain into the peritoneal cavity, where it is absorbed. A lymphocele can also be treated by sclerosis with iodine or caustic antibiotic preparation (e.g. tetracycline) to obliterate the cavity.

Vesicoureteral reflux

Voiding cystography in transplant recipients demonstrates a reflux rate of 2–6%. Whether urine reflux, per se, damages a renal transplant is debatable; what is not debatable is the deleterious effect of reflux when infection is present. Antibiotic suppression of urinary tract infection will decrease the incidence of graft pyelonephritis, but if infections recur a revision of the ureteroneocystostomy is indicated to eliminate reflux.

Transplant renal artery stenosis

Typically, transplant renal artery stenosis (TRAS) usually occurs months after transplant surgery. TRAS has a prevalence of approximately 5–10%. The etiologic factors implicated include technical error with narrowing of the arterial anastomosis, torsion of the artery, and intimal hyperplasia or arteriosclerosis from rejection or altered hemodynamics. TRAS often has an insidious onset. The diagnosis is suggested by hypertension that is intractable to an escalating regimen of antihypertensive drugs. Such hypertension is associated with a gradual rise in serum creatinine. It was learned that the addition of an angiotensin-converting enzyme (ACE) inhibitor to the regimen abruptly increased the serum creatinine value in patients with TRAS; thus, ACE inhibitors are now used as a provocative diagnostic test for TRAS. On physical examination, a bruit may be heard over the transplant, but this finding is nonspecific. Radionuclide scintigraphy and Doppler ultrasonography miss the diagnosis unless the TRAS is extremely tight. If a screening study is desired because the diagnosis is in question, imaging options include spiral computed tomographic angiography, magnetic resonance angiography, and carbon dioxide angiography. These options limit dye load and the associated insult to the graft. Ultimately, direct angiography is the definitive study. With angiography, if TRAS is present, percutaneous transluminal angioplasty (PTA) can be carried out at that time. If PTA fails or sufficient radiologic expertise is not available, surgical correction by patch angioplasty (preferred over saphenous vein bypass) can be attempted. However, the surgical approach has a high rate of graft loss. PTA has been surprisingly durable; nevertheless, the clinician must be vigilant for recurrent TRAS after PTA.

The picture of TRAS can be mimicked by a stenotic proximal iliac artery ipsilateral to the renal transplant or an arteriovenous fistula (AVF) after needle biopsy. Both entities share the underlying pathophysiology of TRAS: underperfusion of the renal parenchyma distal to the lesion with activation of the renin–angiotensin mechanism. Careful auscultation over the graft may distinguish the two entities. AVF is suggested by a bruit during both systole and diastole. Iliac artery stenosis can be treated by PTA and stenting. An AVF may continue to grow until it is therapeutically interrupted or treated. Embolization to obliterate the AVF is definitive treatment, but the nephron mass beyond the fistula will be sacrificed.

Miscellaneous complications

Leg edema ipsilateral to the graft is common owing to ligation of lymphatics and/or compression of the external iliac vein by the graft. The diagnosis of deep venous thrombosis may be entertained, and, if the index of suspicion is high, a Doppler study or venography is indicated.

Femoral nerve injury is a rare complication. Neuropraxis of the femoral nerve may result from retractor trauma or ischemia. Patients with preexisting diabetic neuropathy are particularly susceptible. Femoral nerve injury is manifested by the inability of the supine patient to lift the leg off the bed. Restoration of function, assisted by physical therapy, takes several weeks.

References

1. Suthanthiran M, Strom TB: Renal transplantation. N Engl J Med 1994;331:365–376.
2. 2000 Annual Report of the U.S. Scientific Registry for Transplant Recipients and the Organ Procurement and Transplantation Network: Transplant Data: 1990–1999. U.S. Department of Health and Human Services, Health Resources and Services Administration, Office of Special Programs, Division of Transplantation, Rockville, MD. Richmond, VA: United Network for Organ Sharing.
3. Phillips MG (ed): Organ Procurement, Preservation and Distribution in Transplantation. United Network for Organ Sharing. Richmond, VA: William Byrd Press, 1991.
4. Dafoe DC, Alfrey EJ: Urologic aspects of renal transplantation. In Hanno PM, Wein AJ (eds): Clinical Manual of Urology, 2nd edn. New York: McGraw-Hill, 1994.
5. Tejani AH, Fine RN (eds): Pediatric Renal Transplantation. New York: Wiley Liss, 1994.
6. Becker JA, Choyke PL, Hill M, et al: Imaging the transplanted kidney. In Pollack HM (ed): Clinical Urography. Philadelphia: WB Saunders, 1990.

Diagnosis and Management of Renal Allograft Dysfunction

John P. Vella and Mohamed H. Sayegh

Immediately post transplantation
Early post transplantation
- Approach to diagnosis
- Acute renal allograft rejection
- Diagnosis
- Pathology
Late acute dysfunction
- Late chronic dysfunction
The approach to management: acute rejection
- Pulse corticosteroids
- Polyclonal antibody therapy
- OKT3
- Recurrent rejection
- Management of chronic allograft dysfunction
- Calcineurin inhibitor nephrotoxicity
  – Acute toxicity
  – Chronic calcineurin inhibitor nephrotoxicity
Trends for the future

The most common complication of renal transplantation is allograft dysfunction, which not infrequently leads to graft loss. The United Network of Organ Sharing (UNOS) registry data indicate that 1- and 3-year graft survival rates average 93% and 86%, respectively, for recipients of living related donor kidneys and 87% and 76%, respectively, for recipients of cadaveric donor kidneys.[1] A number of risk factors have been identified for lower cadaver renal allograft survival, which include retransplantation, prior sensitization with more than 50% panel reactivity, the presence of delayed graft function, the number of rejection episodes, donor age less than 5 and greater than 60 years, greater degrees of human leukocyte antigen (HLA) mismatching, and allograft dysfunction at discharge (plasma creatinine concentration above 2 mg/dL or 176 µmol/L).[2] During the 10 years between 1985 and 1995, the effects of factors such as transfusion and the duration of first grafts has disappeared, while the effects of factors such as cold ischemia time, regrafts, and original disease have diminished in magnitude. Other factors, including HLA matching, donor age, and race, continue to exert significant influence.[3]

As a result, the differential diagnosis is best approached by considering the time periods after transplantation (Table 91.1).

Immediately post transplantation

Delayed graft function (DGF) is defined as renal failure persisting after transplantation. Less than 5% of kidneys with DGF never function (primary nonfunction). The major cause for DGF is postischemic acute tubular necrosis (ATN),[4] the incidence of which increases when the cold ischemia time exceeds 24 h and when the dose of

Table 91.1 Rejection rescue protocol

Rejection (Banff 1997 classification)		Treatment options
Borderline change		Optimize immunosuppressive drug levels
Grade IA	Moderate tubulitis (> 4 mononuclear cells in > 25% of biopsy sample)	1. Optimize immunosuppressive drug levels
Grade IB	Severe tubulitis (> 10 mononuclear cells in > 25% of biopsy sample)	2. Consider switch to tacrolimus or MMF or sirolimus 3. Adjunctive therapy (statin) 4. Recycle oral steroids or pulse intravenous steroids
Grade IIA	Mild-to-moderate arteritis in at least one blood vessel	5. If unresponsive, polyclonal anti-T-cell antibody therapy or OKT3
Grade IIB	Severe arteritis (> 25% loss of luminal area)	
Grade III	Transmural arteritis with fibrinoid necrosis and perivascular inflammation	Optimize immunosuppressive drug levels Switch to tacrolimus OKT3
Antibody-mediated rejection		Optimize immunosuppressive drug levels Switch to tacrolimus OKT3 Therapeutic plasma exchange until donor-specific antibody is removed

MMF, mycophenolate mofetil.

cyclosporine (CsA) therapy exceeds 10 mg/kg/day. ATN is a feature of calcineurin inhibitor (CI) therapy. Tacrolimus may be less nephrotoxic than cyclosporine.[5] Renal ultrasonography should always be performed in order to exclude a vascular catastrophe such as thrombosis of the transplant renal artery or vein. Isotope renography may also detect functionally significant obstruction or a urine leak. Atheroembolism of the renal artery or renal vein thrombosis can occur, but are rare causes of DGF. The diagnosis of allograft rejection in patients with DGF who are maintained on dialysis can be made only by renal biopsy. The approach to such patients with DGF varies with patient risk (Fig. 91.1A). Factors connoting high risk include sensitization, retransplants (especially those who lost the previous graft within the first 3 months), and cold ischemia time exceeding 24 h. High-risk patients should have a renal biopsy performed during days 3–5 to rule out acute rejection. A repeat biopsy should be performed in 3–5 days if rejection is not seen and DGF persists. Low-risk patients (unsensitized patient, first transplant, and cold ischemic time < 24 h) should have a biopsy performed during days 7–10, which can be repeated a week later should DGF persist.

Prolongation of DGF by concurrent CI therapy has led to the use of sequential induction regimens with anti-lymphocyte antibody therapies in many centers (see below). Provision of adequate immunosuppression while avoiding "toxic" CI levels is desirable during DGF, as there is some evidence to suggest that the incidence of acute rejection is increased by DGF.[6] Initial studies suggested that DGF is associated with poorer long-term graft survival;[7] however, more recent reports indicate that graft survival is not significantly different when comparing DGF with no DGF for patients *without rejection*.[8] Immunological injury may play a role in some cases of DGF. Evidence to support this is provided by the observation that the incidence of DGF is increased in presensitized, retransplant patients.[7] Therapy of DGF includes supportive care (dialysis) and minimizing nephrotoxins (notably calcineurin inhibitors and some antibiotics). The use of vasodilators such as dopamine has been largely discredited. Early reports suggesting that diltiazem and/or iloprost – a prostacyclin analog – may prevent DGF have not been reproduced. As diltiazem can elevate CI levels, this drug should be used with caution in any transplant patient in whom there is a potential for CI toxicity. At present, no form of therapy is generally accepted as being superior to supportive care and maintenance of adequate immunosuppression to prevent intercurrent acute rejection.

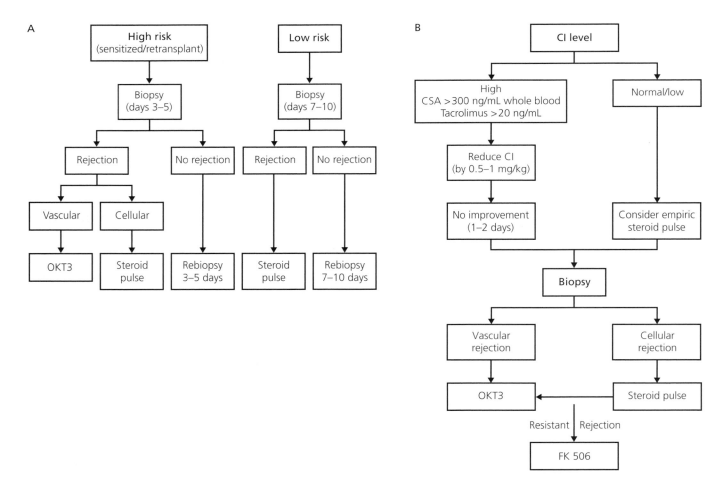

Figure 91.1 (A) The approach to patients with delayed graft function. (B) The approach to patients with rising creatinine levels after immediate graft function. CI, calcineurin inhibitor.

Hyperacute rejection is a rare and generally preventable cause of primary nonfunction.[9] There is no effective therapy and graft nephrectomy is necessary.

Accelerated rejection can occur in patients with or without DGF; it refers to rejection episodes occurring 2–5 days after transplantation.[9] The diagnosis of accelerated rejection is usually established by renal biopsy, which may show predominantly cellular rejection or predominantly vascular-type rejection. It is important to make this pathological distinction as the approach to therapy is different.

Early post transplantation

The differential diagnosis is substantially different in patients with initial graft function who then develop renal insufficiency within the first 3 months post transplantation. The major causes in this setting are: acute rejection, which is most common; CI nephrotoxicity; thrombotic angiopathy; and urinary tract obstruction or decreased renal perfusion due to effective circulating volume depletion, infection, and recurrent or de novo renal disease.

Approach to diagnosis

Early allograft dysfunction is characterized by a plasma creatinine concentration that is stable at an elevated level or is increasing.[10] Unless there is evidence to suggest infection or recurrent disease (such as heavy proteinuria or a nephritic urine sediment with red cells and red cell casts), the evaluation of such patients is commenced by measuring and adjusting the dose of CI (Fig. 91.1B). A renal biopsy is performed if no improvement is noted within 1–2 days or if the creatinine continues to rise. If, on the other hand, the plasma CsA concentration is normal or low, a biopsy is performed or empirical pulse steroid therapy is given with adjustment made of the CsA dose until levels are within the "therapeutic" range. Renal ultrasonography should be performed prior to renal biopsy to exclude a urinary leak or obstruction.

Acute renal allograft rejection

Acute renal allograft rejection is defined as an acute deterioration in allograft function that is associated with specific pathologic changes in the transplant that have been categorized by the Banff consortium (see below).[11] The incidence of acute rejection and when it occurs vary with the induction therapy used for immunosuppression. Registry data indicate that the incidence of acute rejection has greatly declined over the last 6 years and is now in the region of 10–20% depending on the source of the kidney as well as recipient characteristics.[1] Kidneys which recover function still have a 10% decrease in 1-year survival when compared with rejection-free kidneys.[12] Acute rejection episodes also have a negative impact on long-term graft survival, being the major clinical predictor of chronic rejection, which is responsible for most grafts lost after the first year post transplantation.

Diagnosis

The presence of acute renal allograft rejection should be suspected in every transplant patient in whom the creatinine fails to settle or is rising with decreased urine output and hypertension. Only 8% of patients with functioning grafts have a first episode of rejection after 1 year;[13] these episodes are often associated with noncompliance with medical therapy and/or low drug levels.[14] Acute vascular occlusion can be excluded by a radionuclide flow scan.[15]

Percutaneous renal allograft biopsy or fine needle kidney aspiration are frequently necessary (Fig. 91.1B).[16]

Pathology

An international standardization of criteria for the histologic diagnosis of renal allograft rejection has been recently performed that is of value to guide therapy and for the gradation of biopsy samples for research.[17] Semiquantitative lesion scoring focuses on tubulitis and arteritis and includes a minimum threshold for interstitial inflammation. Type I is tubulointerstitial rejection without arteritis; type II is vascular rejection with intimal arteritis; and type III is severe rejection with transmural arterial changes. Biopsies with only mild inflammation are graded as "borderline/suspicious for rejection." Chronic/sclerosing allograft changes are graded based on the severity of tubular atrophy and interstitial fibrosis. Antibody-mediated rejection, hyperacute or accelerated acute in presentation, is also categorized, as are other significant allograft findings (Table 91.1).

Late acute dysfunction

When acute allograft dysfunction develops more than 3 months after transplantation, the differential diagnosis should include prerenal azotemia due to volume depletion, CsA nephrotoxicity, urinary tract infection or obstruction, acute rejection possibly due to reduction in immunosuppression or noncompliance, recurrent or de novo renal disease, and renal artery stenosis.[18] The risk of late acute rejection is increased in patients who are tapered off CsA[14] or steroids.[19] Bearing in mind that renal transplant recipients rarely achieve a GFR exceeding 55–60 mL/min, a creatinine of less than 2 mg/dL represents good, although certainly not normal, renal function. Long-term transplant patients who miss several doses of steroids risk adrenal insufficiency.

Late chronic dysfunction

Many patients have slowly progressive renal disease over a period of years after renal transplantation. The major etiologic considerations in this setting are: chronic rejection, chronic CsA nephrotoxicity (discussed below), hypertensive nephrosclerosis from poorly controlled hypertension, chronic urinary tract obstruction, and recurrent or de novo renal disease.

The most common cause of allograft failure after the first year post transplant is the incompletely understood clinicopathological entity variously called chronic allograft dysfunction, transplant glomerulopathy, or chronic rejection.[20] This accounts for 25–30% of patients with endstage renal disease awaiting retransplantation. Up to one-third of patients who require kidney transplants currently have previously been engrafted.

The approach to management: acute rejection

(The pharmacology of the major classes of drugs used is reviewed in Chapter 12.)

Happily, the introduction of novel immunosuppressive agents such as mycophenolate, tacrolimus, and sirolimus as well as the availability of effective cytomegalovirus (CMV) prophylaxis have combined to greatly reduce the early risk of rejection to 10–20%.[21] In the event that rejection occurs, treatment should be started when the diagnosis is suspected and should not be delayed until the results of the allograft biopsy are available. The intensity of therapy will largely be dictated by the severity of the rejection episode as well as response to initial therapy (see Table 91.2 for one approach).

In this age of greatly reduced rejection risk, it is useful to investigate the root cause of a rejection episode (Table 91.2).

Pulse corticosteroids

Corticosteroids remain one of the cornerstones of most induction, maintenance, and rescue immunosuppressive regimens. Steroids are lympholytic when given in high dosage (methylprednisolone 0.5–1 g/day given over 3–5 days for example) and can reverse acute rejection in up to 75% of cases. After completing the steroid pulse, oral steroids are restarted using the same dosage the patient had been taking. The CI dose should be increased only if the serum levels are subtherapeutic. The urine output increases and the serum creatinine starts decreasing within 3–5 days. The major complication of pulse steroids is increased susceptibility to infection, especially oral candidiasis. Other potential problems include acute hyperglycemia, hypertension, peptic ulcer disease, and psychiatric disturbances including euphoria and depression. Prophylactic antacids/H_2 blockers as well as oral antifungal therapy are generally recommended.[22] Steroid resistance is defined as a lack of improvement in urine output or the plasma creatinine concentration within 5 days. Second-line therapy consists of antilymphocyte antibodies, either polyclonal antilymphocyte antibodies or monoclonal OKT3.

Polyclonal antibody therapy

Polyclonal anti-T-cell antibodies can be prepared in rabbits or horses. Antilymphocyte serum (ALS; Thymoglobulin, Sangstat, Menlo Park, CA, USA) is prepared by immunizing rabbits with human lymphoid cells derived from cultured B-cell lines. Antithymocyte globulin (ATG), a preparation commonly used in Europe, is an equine hyperimmune globulin. ALS has been used for prophylaxis and primary and second-line therapy of acute rejection. A typical recommended dose for acute rejection is 10–15 mg/kg daily for 7–10 days. The reversal rate is 75–100%, with the plasma creatinine concentration returning to baseline after several days. Fever and chills develop in a majority of patients during the initial ALS infusion. Anaphylactic reactions, including respiratory distress and hypotension, are exceedingly rare. To minimize the allergic manifestations, patients are usually pretreated with corticosteroids, antihistamines, and antipyretics. A pruritic skin rash (20%) and presumed antiplatelet antibody-induced thrombocytopenia of varying severity (50%) can occur late, but ALS does not generally induce a host antibody response to the rabbit or horse serum. As a result, there is a greater opportunity for successful readministration. ALS has also been used to reverse rebound rejection following OKT3 administration in patients with high titers of anti-mouse antibodies, which limit retreatment with OKT3 (see below).[22]

OKT3

OKT3 is a murine monoclonal antibody that is directed against the CD3 antigen complex that is closely associated with the T-cell receptor.[23] CD3 is involved in transducing signals from the T-cell receptor to the nucleus, leading to cytokine-mediated T-cell activation. The mechanism of action of OKT3 is related to inhibition of cell-mediated immunity via modulation/clearing of $CD3^+$ T cells. OKT3 has been used both as the primary treatment of acute rejection and as rescue therapy for resistant rejection.[24] The usual dose of OKT3 is 5 mg intravenously daily for 10–14 days. Up to 94% of steroid or ALS-resistant rejection can be expected to reverse with OKT3 treatment.[25] The plasma creatinine concentration typically increases for the first 2–3 days of OKT3 therapy and then declines. Rebound

Table 91.2	Preventable causes of rejection
	Preventable causes of rejection
Inadequate drug	Azathioprine
Inadequate dose	Failure to aggressively optimize CI or SRL levels in the early posttransplant period
Noncompliance	Failure to take medication Youth Side-effects (especially cosmetic such as weight gain, acne and hirsutism) Drug or alcohol abuse Financial
Drug interaction	Various drugs can reduce CI and SRL drug levels Dilantin Phenobarbital Rifampin St John's wort

CI, calcineurin inhibitor; SRL, sirolimus.

rejection occurs in approximately 50% of cases; roughly 75% of these episodes can be reversed by pulse steroids. OKT3 is also used as primary therapy in the minority of patients who have predominantly vascular rejection, a process that is generally resistant to steroids and ALS.[25]

In vitro, OKT3 acts as a T-cell mitogen. Many of the first-dose reactions commonly seen are generally thought to be due to initial binding to the CD3 complex, mediating T-cell release of cytokines. These reactions include: fever (70–100%), rigors (30%), nausea, vomiting, and diarrhea (15–20%), hypotension, chest pain, dyspnea, and wheezing (10–20%), and occasionally frank pulmonary edema. This last complication is rarely seen unless the patient is volume overloaded; therefore, patients should be dialyzed or diuresed prior to OKT3 therapy. Dyspnea may also be related to complement activation and subsequent pulmonary vascular neutrophil sequestration.[26] Antihistamines, antipyretics, and methylprednisolone (250 mg for two doses) are usually given prior to OKT3 to minimize these side-effects, all of which decrease with repeated exposure. Higher steroid doses should be avoided to prevent a potential increase in the procoagulant effect of OKT3.[27] Other serious complications that can occur after the administration of OKT3 include graft thrombosis,[28] infections, and aseptic meningitis. Rarely, patients receiving OKT3 develop arterial and venous thrombi within the graft, leading to loss of the graft.[28] In almost one-half of those cases reported, the characteristic feature is thrombosis within glomerular capillaries and veins suggestive of the thrombotic microangiopathy similar to hemolytic uremic syndrome. This complication is most likely to occur with high-dose OKT3 (10 mg/day) rather than with the current recommendation of 5 mg/day. The OKT3-induced increase in coagulation may be mediated by the release of tumor necrosis factor (TNF) (and perhaps other cytokines) from circulating mononuclear cells.[29] The development of this syndrome in the early postoperative period suggests that endothelial cell injury due to ischemia and/or surgery may contribute to intrarenal thrombus formation.[28] A similar pattern of injury may be seen as a result of other causes, which include cyclosporine therapy and de novo or recurrent hemolytic uremic syndrome post transplant.

OKT3 can predispose to potentially life-threatening infections, especially those due to cytomegalovirus.[30] Total exposure is an important determinant of risk with almost 100% of patients suffering an episode of infection after three courses.[31] Patients receiving multiple courses may develop Epstein–Barr virus-related lymphoproliferative disorders.[32] Aseptic meningitis characterized by lymphocytosis and elevated cerebrospinal fluid protein occurs in up to 5% of patients who receive OKT3 and is usually self-limiting, although differentiation from other causes of infectious meningitis is essential.

Recurrent rejection

Approximately 15–20% of renal transplant patients have recurrent episodes of acute rejection. The success rate of retreatment with OKT3 in this setting is related to its ability to modulate/clear CD3$^+$ T cells.[33] This in turn is determined by two important factors: circulating anti-mouse antibody titers and timing of the rejection episode. Roughly 50–60% of patients who receive OKT3 will produce human anti-mouse antibodies (HAMA), generally in low titers (< 1:100). Low antibody titers do not affect the response to retreatment (reversal rate almost 100%) if the rejection episode occurs within 90 days after transplantation. On the other hand, titers above 1:100 or recurrent rejection beyond 90 days is associated with a reversal rate of less than 25%. The reversal rate is essentially zero when both high HAMA titers and late rejection are present. It is hoped that the development of genetically engineered humanized monoclonal antibodies (OKT3) will largely eliminate the anti-antibody response, thereby increasing the utility of anti-T-cell antibodies in the treatment of recurrent rejection.

Our current protocol is to treat a first episode of acute, predominantly cellular rejection with a steroid pulse. A second pulse may be given before resorting to anti-lymphocyte therapy in patients who show a partial clinical and histological response. Although OKT3 and ALS are as, or perhaps more, effective as pulse steroids in reversing acute rejection, they are associated with a higher incidence of side-effects and there is no evidence that long-term graft survival is improved. We therefore reserve these agents for steroid-resistant or recurrent rejection. OKT3 is also indicated in primarily vascular rejection.[25] It is important to confirm the diagnosis of rejection by renal biopsy before starting antilymphocyte therapy. In some cases, the steroid pulse has reversed the rejection process, but renal failure persists because of acute tubular necrosis and/or CsA toxicity, both of which can accompany acute rejection. Patients who rebound after OKT3 or ALS are treated with a steroid pulse. In the absence of a response, we offer a second and, rarely, a third course of OKT3 provided that there is neither high titers of anti-mouse antibodies nor late acute rejection (beyond 90 days) and the patient is free of active infection.

Recent uncontrolled trials suggest that tacrolimus may be effective as rescue therapy for acute renal allograft rejection that is unresponsive to the above regimen. One report switched 77 patients with biopsy-proven ongoing acute rejection from CsA to tacrolimus.[34] The overall response rate was 74%, with responders having a mean plasma creatinine concentration of 2.35 mg/dL (207 μmol/L) at 14 months. Even dialysis-dependent patients had a 50% response rate. Preliminary data on the role of mycophenolic acid as rescue therapy for biopsy-proven acute rejection revealed a response rate of 69% in patients who failed standard pulse steroid or OKT3. More recently, attention has turned to sirolimus as rescue therapy for refractory rejection with early promising results.[35] There are no data available at present to ascertain whether tacrolimus, mycophenolate, or sirolimus is superior as rescue therapy for resistant rejection.

Management of chronic allograft dysfunction

The management of chronic renal allograft rejection remains one of the major challenges facing transplant physicians and surgeons.[36] Therapeutic strategies are summarized in Table 91.3. Immunosuppressive therapy is generally ineffective, except for those patients in whom the precipitating cause is inadequate immunosuppression because of noncompliance or aggressive drug tapering. There is currently a great deal of interest in the hypothesis that switching patients who are experiencing graft dysfunction from a nephrotoxic CI to sirolimus may abrogate the decline in GFR. Certainly, there are some interesting studies indicating that sirolimus is at least as effective as CsA in preventing rejection.[37,38]

Intravenous pulse or oral minipulse corticosteroid administration may be beneficial if there is evidence of active acute rejection on allograft biopsy. Nonimmunologic interventions should be focused primarily on aggressive control of blood pressure and possibly of hyperlipidemia.[36,39] It remains to be determined whether angiotensin-converting enzyme (ACE) inhibitors provide any special benefit. A recent short-term study showed that lisinopril decreased protein excretion in transplant recipients with hypertension and proteinuria without adversely affecting renal hemodynamics or causing significant hyperkalemia.[40] The long-term impact of such therapy on progression of allograft dysfunction is unknown. Other therapeutic modalities that have been considered but are not yet proven to be effective in controlled human trials include antiplatelet agents, thromboxane antagonists, fish oil, and a low protein diet.

Calcineurin inhibitor nephrotoxicity

The toxic effects of CIs can be divided temporally and pathogenically into two discrete categories. Acute

Table 91.3 Chronic allograft dysfunction (CAD): therapeutic strategies

Prophylactic interventions	
Alloantigen-dependent mechanisms	
Optimize HLA match	Long-term benefit greatest with matching for HLA-A > HLA-B > HLA-DR
Avoidance of sensitization to HLA	Up to 6% differential in 3-year graft survival in patients who are highly sensitized compared with nonsensitized (under CsA)

Blood transfusion effect
  1-DR matching
  Donor-specific transfusion
	Up to 10% improvement in 3-year graft survival in those who did not become sensitized to HLA

Avoidance of acute rejection
  MMF
  Neoral versus CsA (?)
  Tacrolimus
  Antibody induction therapy
	Impact of newer immunosuppressive agents and antibody induction protocols on chronic graft loss remains unproven. Tacrolimus can negate impact of sensitization on long-term graft loss

Alloantigen-independent mechanisms
  Nephron undersupply
  Donor–recipient age matching
  Donor–recipient weight matching
  Double kidney transplants
	Theoretical benefits from providing adequate nephron dose. Optimizing this variable may conflict with organ procurement

Renal injury
  Minimize cold ischemia time
  Preservation solution
	Risk of ATN is greatly increased when cold ischemia exceeds 24 h. Risk of CAD increases if ATN is complicated by acute rejection

Therapeutic interventions	
CMV	Potential benefits of antiviral chemotherapy
Hyperfiltration	Potential benefits of preventing/treating hyperfiltration
Hypertension	CCBs probably of maximal benefit early post transplant when calcineurin inhibitor dosage is highest
Proteinuria	Potential benefit of reducing proteinuria (unproven)
Hyperhomocysteinemia	Potential benefit of reducing homocysteine levels (unproven)
Hyperlipidemia	HMGCoA reductase inhibitors reduce risk of acute rejection. Unproven benefit in preventing CAD

HLA, human leukocyte antigen; CsA, cyclosporine A; MMF, mycophenolate mofetil; ATN, acute tubular necrosis; CAD, chronic allograft dysfunction; CMV, cytomegalovirus; CCBs, calcium channel blockers; HMGCoA, hydroxymethylglutaryl CoA reductase inhibitors.

nephrotoxicity manifests as azotemia, which is largely reversible after dose reduction and is due predominantly to vasoconstriction. Chronic CI toxicity manifests as irreversibly progressive renal disease and hypertension and is due to fibrogenesis.

Acute toxicity

Renal transplant patients treated with CsA or tacrolimus (calcineurin inhibitor, CI) may develop nephrotoxicity, which can manifest in many ways. In addition to azotemia, other renal effects of CsA include tubular dysfunction with concomitant electrolyte and acid–base disturbances and, rarely, thrombotic microangiopathy. A similar pattern of renal injury is associated with the use of tacrolimus. Attention must also be paid to drug dose and to drug interactions. In the earliest clinical renal transplant trials using CsA, a high incidence of oliguric ATN and primary nonfunction was observed; the risk was greatest with prolonged ischemia time of the donated kidney prior to transplantation. Subsequent trials using lower doses of CsA showed that these problems were dose related. Studies in experimental animals have demonstrated that CsA causes vasoconstriction of the afferent and efferent glomerular arterioles and reductions in renal blood flow and glomerular filtration rate (GFR). However, CsA is not a "direct" vasoconstrictor and the exact mechanism of vasoconstriction is unclear: there appears to be substantial impairment of endothelial cell function, leading to reduced production of vasodilators (prostaglandins and nitric oxide) and enhanced release of vasoconstrictors (endothelin and thromboxane). Increased sympathetic tone may also be present, although renal vasoconstriction occurs even in denervated kidneys. The increase in renal vascular resistance induced by CsA is not corrected with time. Maintenance CsA therapy is associated with transient reductions in renal plasma flow and glomerular filtration rate, which correlate both with dose and with peak CsA levels reached 2–4 h after the oral dose and which reverse when reasonable drug levels are attained. Administration of a calcium channel blocker can prevent the renal vasoconstriction. This observation constitutes part of the rationale for the use of calcium channel blockers to treat hypertension in CsA-treated transplant recipients. The increase in vascular resistance may be reflected clinically by an elevated plasma creatinine concentration and hypertension. Acute CsA nephrotoxicity is usually reversible with cessation of therapy. The important clinical problem is to differentiate CsA-induced renal dysfunction from acute rejection. The only definitive diagnostic test is biopsy of the renal allograft. Although there are no specific pathologic changes induced acutely by CsA, the absence of cellular or vascular rejection, coupled with tubular damage including vacuolization of the tubular epithelial cells, strongly suggests CI nephrotoxicity. In addition, the presence of rejection does not exclude concomitant CI toxicity. Rarely, vascular lesions similar to those seen in the thrombotic microangiopathies are seen. This lesion is idiosyncratic and is presumably initiated by CI-induced injury to the vascular endothelial cells. Affected patients present with acute renal failure that is usually irreversible

and usually leads to graft loss. However, some patients undergo partial recovery if CsA is discontinued.

Chronic calcineurin inhibitor nephrotoxicity

Chronic cyclosporine nephrotoxicity is manifested by renal insufficiency due to glomerular and vascular disease, abnormalities in tubular function, and an increase in blood pressure. The biopsy reveals an obliterative arteriolopathy, suggesting the cause is primary endothelial damage. Ischemic collapse or scarring of the glomeruli, vacuolization of the tubules, and focal areas of tubular atrophy and interstitial fibrosis also occur. These changes are typically seen with high-dose CsA therapy (> 6 mg/kg/day). The factors responsible for chronic CsA nephrotoxicity are not well understood. It has been proposed that the arterial lesions are the primary abnormality, with ischemia being responsible for the tubular and interstitial lesions. However, animal studies have shown that the vascular and interstitial findings can be dissociated. Recent data suggest that transforming growth factor β (TGF-β), a cytokine with both potent immunosuppressive and fibrogenic properties, is upregulated by CsA in an experimental model of chronic CsA nephropathy. The development of interstitial fibrosis is also associated with increased expression of osteopontin, a potent macrophage chemoattractant, by the tubular epithelial cells. Other evidence that supports an alternative mechanism for CsA toxicity is the observation that administration of either an endothelin A receptor antagonist or calcium channel blockers can prevent hypertension and reductions in renal plasma flow and yet have no impact on the development of arteriolopathy.

The best information available to support the hypothesis of chronic CsA nephrotoxicity comes from cardiac transplant patients and patients with autoimmune diseases in whom the nephrotoxic potential of CsA can be evaluated in the absence of coexisting acute or chronic renal allograft rejection. These patients have a 35–45% reduction in GFR. Early studies suggested that up to 10% of heart transplant recipients progressed to endstage renal disease after 8 years of continuous CsA therapy. More recent reports using low-dose CsA have noted a much lower risk of less than 3%. Whether there is a "safe" dose of CsA that is effective immunologically but does not cause progressive renal dysfunction is difficult to answer because of the lack of well-controlled prospective trials comparing different dose regimens. Short-term studies in patients receiving CsA for nonrenal autoimmune diseases suggest that a maintenance dose below 5 mg/kg/day may not lead to progressive chronic nephrotoxicity. However, trials in which 5 mg/kg/day were given for longer periods found elevations in the plasma creatinine concentration, a fall in glomerular filtration rate, and the development of hypertension in over 80% of patients. Longer observations in heart transplant recipients receiving low-dose maintenance CsA have demonstrated an acute fall in the glomerular filtration rate that then remains stable for at least 3–4 years. A similar pattern is seen after liver transplantation and in patients with rheumatoid arthritis. Furthermore, repeat renal biopsies in a small number of patients with rheumatoid arthritis receiving cyclosporine did not show progressive histologic changes at 3 years. The applicability of these findings to renal allografts is uncertain – it has been suggested, for example, that the denervated kidney may be less susceptible to CsA-induced renal injury. Retrospective longitudinal studies of cadaver renal transplant recipients suggest that most patients maintained on 3–5 mg/kg/day of CsA after the first year have stable plasma creatinine levels for up to 5–9 years. Long-term stabilization of the glomerular filtration rate has also been demonstrated in a prospective trial. However, the significance of these studies is somewhat uncertain in view of their often retrospective nature and lack of routine performance of repeat renal biopsies.

There are no studies to clearly define the optimal dose of CsA in renal transplantation. Typically, the induction dose is in the range of 8–10 mg/kg/day in the perioperative period. The dose is then tapered over 6 months to a maintenance dose of approximately 4 mg/kg/day. Plasma CsA levels are monitored to maintain 12-h trough plasma CsA levels between 50 and 150 ng/mL (or whole blood levels between 150 and 300 ng/mL) once the patient has passed the first few months post transplant without rejection episodes.

In view of the utility of CsA in transplantation and autoimmune diseases, there has been a great deal of interest in developing new therapeutic strategies to minimize its nephrotoxic potential. Animal data and preliminary observations in humans suggest that fish oil may be beneficial. Animal and human data also suggest that concurrent administration of calcium channel blockers may be protective against CsA nephrotoxicity, at least in part by minimizing renal vasoconstriction. However, there is at present no proof that these agents increase graft survival. A similar lack of benefit on long-term renal function has been noted with nifedipine in two studies of hypertensive transplant recipients receiving CsA. The likely explanation for the inability to demonstrate a long-term benefit with calcium channel blockers in patients treated with CsA is that reversal of renal vasoconstriction, although beneficial, does not affect the concurrent upregulation of TGF-β, therefore interstitial fibrosis can proceed uninterrupted.

Trends for the future

Given the current lack of consensus on the optimal regimen for immunosuppression of renal transplant recipients with our existing array of drugs, it is likely that new drugs, as they are approved, will initially cloud the issues further. The important properties to be sought in any new treatment protocol are greater specificity, decreased side-effects, and greater efficacy in the management of chronic rejection. The combination of effective antiproliferative activity, as exhibited by these newer agents and the well-established effect of CsA on T-cell activation, offers the potential for the development of new regimens which fulfill at least some of these criteria.

The holy grail of transplantation is the induction of tolerance, which is specific acceptance of allograft tissue without immunosuppression in the presence of an intact humoral and cell-mediated immune system.[41,42] Clinical strategies of tolerance have been investigated with the use of blood transfusion[43] or donor bone marrow infusion.[44] Currently, we and others are actively researching the implications of T-cell activation blockade by a variety of different mechanisms. One strategy is to interfere with T-cell recognition of alloantigen by blocking the peptide/T-cell receptor signal, thus abrogating the antigen-specific component of the immune response.[45] Another strategy is to interfere with various costimulatory pathways that are also necessary for full T-cell activation, and thus induce antigen-specific unresponsiveness.[46] Some of these strategies may undergo clinical evaluation in the near future.

References

1. Cecka JM: The UNOS Scientific Renal Transplant Registry. Clin Transplant 1999;1–21.
2. Cecka JM, Terasaki PI: The UNOS Scientific Renal Transplant Registry. Los Angeles: UCLA Tissue Typing Laboratory, 1995.
3. Terasaki PI, McClelland JD, Yuge J, et al: Advances in kidney transplantation. In Terasaki PI (ed): Clinical Transplants. Los Angeles: UCLA Tissue Typing Laboratory, 1995, p 487.
4. Lim EC, Terasaki PI: Early graft function. In Terasaki PE (ed): Clinical Transplants. Los Angeles: UCLA Tissue Typing Laboratory, 1991, p 401.
5. Ahsan N, Johnson C, Gonwa T, et al: Randomized trial of tacrolimus plus mycophenolate mofetil or azathioprine versus cyclosporine oral solution (modified) plus mycophenolate mofetil after cadaveric kidney transplantation: results at 2 years. Transplantation 2001;72:245–250.
6. Yokoyama I, Uchida K, Kobayashi T, et al: Effect of prolonged delayed graft function on long-term graft outcome in cadaveric kidney transplantation. Clin Transplant 1994;8:101–106.
7. Sanfilippo F, Vaughn WK, Spees EK, et al: The detrimental effects of delayed graft function in cadaver donor renal transplantation. Transplantation 1984;38:643–648.
8. Troppmann C, Gillingham KJ, Gruessner RW, et al: Delayed graft function in the absence of rejection has no long-term impact. A study of cadaver kidney recipients with good graft function at 1 year after transplantation. Transplantation 1996;61:1331–1337.
9. Braun WE: The immunobiology of different types of renal allograft rejection. In Milford EL (ed): Renal Transplantation: Contemporary Issues in Nephrology, Vol 19. New York: Churchill Livingstone, 1989, p 45.
10. Nickerson P, Jeffery J, Rush D: Long-term allograft surveillance: the role of protocol biopsies. Curr Opin Urol 2001;11:133–137.
11. Racusen LC, Solez K, Colvin RB, et al: The Banff 97 working classification of renal allograft pathology. Kidney Int 1999;55:713–723.
12. Cecka JM, Terasaki PI: Early rejection episodes. In Terasaki PE (ed): Clinical Transplants. Los Angeles: UCLA Tissue Typing Laboratory, 1989, p 425.
13. Burke JF, Pirsch JD, Ramos EL, et al: Long-term efficacy and safety of cyclosporine in renal-transplant recipients. N Engl J Med 1994;331:358–363.
14. Sanders CE, Curtis JJ, Julian BA, et al: Tapering or discontinuing cyclosporine for financial reasons: a single center experience. Am J Kidney Dis 1993;21:9–15.
15. Meyer M, Paushter D, Steinmuller DR: The use of duplex Doppler to evaluate renal allograft dysfunction. Transplantation 1990;50:974–978.
16. Helderman JH, Hernandez J, Sagalowski A, et al: Confirmation of the utility of fine needle biopsy of the renal allograft. Kidney Int 1988;34:376–381.
17. Solez K, Axelsen RA, Benediktsson H, et al: International standardization of criteria for the histologic diagnosis of renal allograft rejection: the Banff working classification on renal transplant pathology. Kidney Int 1993;44:411–422.

18. Frem GJ, Rennke HG, Sayegh MH: Late renal allograft failure secondary to thrombotic microangiopathy–human immunodeficiency virus nephropathy. J Am Soc Nephrol 1994;4:1643–1648.

19. Hricik DE, Whalen CC, Lautman J, et al: Withdrawal of steroids after renal transplantation: clinical predictors of outcome. Transplantation 1992;53:41–45.

20. Womer KL, Vella JP, Sayegh MH: Chronic allograft dysfunction: mechanisms and new approaches to therapy. Semin Nephrol 2000;20:126–147.

21. Denton MD, Magee CC, Sayegh MH: Immunosuppressive strategies in transplantation. Lancet 1999;353:1083–1091.

22. Delmonico FL, Tolkoff-Rubin N: Treatment of acute rejection. *In* Milford EL (ed): Renal Transplantation: Contemporary Issues in Nephrology, Vol 19. New York: Churchill Livingstone, 1989, p 129.

23. Schroeder TJ, First MR: Monoclonal antibodies in organ transplantation. Am J Kidney Dis 1994;23:138–147.

24. Norman DJ, Barry JM, Bennett WM, et al: The use of OKT3 in cadaveric renal transplantation for rejection that is unresponsive to conventional anti-rejection therapy. Am J Kidney Dis 1988;11:90–93.

25. Ortho Multicenter Transplant Study Group. A randomized trial of OKT3 monoclonal antibody for acute rejection of cadaveric renal transplants. N Engl J Med 1985;313:337–342.

26. Raasvekt MHM, Bemelman FJ, Schellekens P, et al: Complement activation during OKT3 treatment: a possible explanation for respiratory side effects. Kidney Int 1993;43:1140–1149.

27. Abramowicz D, Pradier O, De Pauw L, et al: High dose glucocorticoids increase the procoagulant effects of OKT3. Kidney Int 1994;46:1596–1602.

28. Abramowicz D, Pradier O, Marchant A, et al: Induction of thromboses within renal grafts by high-dose prophylactic OKT3. Lancet 1992;339:777–778.

29. Pradier O, Marchant A, Abramowicz D, et al: Procoagulant effect of the OKT3 monoclonal antibody: involvement of tumor necrosis factor. Kidney Int 1992;42:1124–1129.

30. Oh CS, Stratta J, Fox RJ: Increased infections associated with the use of OKT3 for the treatment of steroid resistant rejection in renal transplantation. Transplantation 1988;45:68–73.

31. Thistlethwaite JR Jr, Stuart JK, Mayes JT, et al: Complications and monitoring of OKT3 therapy. Am J Kidney Dis 1988;11:112–119.

32. Swinnen LJ, Costanza-Nordin MR, Fisher SG, et al: Increased incidence of lymphoproliferative disorders after immunosuppression with the monoclonal antibody OKT3 in cardiac transplant recipients. N Engl J Med 1990;323:1723–1728.

33. Norman DJ, Shield CF 3rd, Henell KR, et al: Effectiveness of a second course of OKT3 monoclonal anti-T cell antibody for treatment of renal allograft rejection. Transplantation 1988;46:523–529.

34. Jordan ML, Shapiro R, Vivas SA, et al: FK506 "rescue" for resistant rejection of renal allografts under primary cyclosporine immunosuppression. Transplantation 1994;57:860–865.

35. Hong JC, Kahan BD: Sirolimus rescue therapy for refractory rejection in renal transplantation. Transplantation 2001;71:1579–1584.

36. Hostetter TH: Chronic transplant rejection. Kidney Int 1994;46:266–279.

37. Kreis H, Cisterne JM, Land W, et al: Sirolimus in association with mycophenolate mofetil induction for the prevention of acute graft rejection in renal allograft recipients. Transplantation 2000;69:1252–1260.

38. Groth CG, Backman L, Morales JM, et al: Sirolimus (rapamycin)-based therapy in human renal transplantation: similar efficacy and different toxicity compared with cyclosporine. Sirolimus European Renal Transplant Study Group. Transplantation 1999;67:1036–1042.

39. Tullius SG, Tilney NL: Both alloantigen-dependent and -independent factors influence chronic allograft rejection. Transplantation 1995;59:313–318.

40. Traindl O, Falger S, Reading S, et al: The effects of lisinopril on renal function in proteinuric renal transplant recipients. Transplantation 1993;55:1309–1313.

41. Nickerson PW, Stenrer W, Steiger J, et al: In pursuit of the "Holy Grail;" allograft tolerance. Kidney Int 1994;45:s40–s49.

42. Turka LA, Sayegh MH: T-cell tolerance. *In* Tilney NL, Strom TB, Leendert LC (eds): Transplantation Biology. Philadelphia: Lipincott-Raven, 1996, pp 503–515.

43. Lagaaij EL, Hennemann IP, Ruigrok M, et al: Effect of one-HLA-DR-antigen-matched and completely HLA-DR-mismatched blood transfusions on survival of heart and kidney allografts. N Engl J Med 1989;321:701–705.

44. Brennan DC, Mohanakumar T, Flye MW: Donor-specific transfusion and donor bone marrow infusion in renal transplantation tolerance: a review of efficacy and mechanisms. Am J Kidney Dis 1995;26:701–715.

45. Sayegh MH, Krensky AM: Novel immunotherapeutic strategies using MHC derived peptides. Kidney Int 1996;49 (Suppl 53):S13–S20.

46. Sayegh MH, Turka LA: T cell costimulatory pathways: promising novel targets for immunosuppression and tolerance induction. J Am Soc Nephrol 1995;6:1143–1150.

CHAPTER 92

Cardiovascular and Other Noninfectious Complications after Renal Transplantation

William E. Braun

Introduction

The half-life for cadaver allografts that are still functioning at 1 year ($T_{1/2}$) has increased from approximately 7.5–8 years in the early 1990s to about 13 years currently. Consequently, there will be large numbers of successfully treated renal transplant recipients requiring long-term care in the context of chronic immunosuppression.

Recommendations for the outpatient surveillance of renal transplant recipients has been provided by the Clinical Practice Guidelines Committee of the American Society of Transplantation.[1] Because there are "virtually no scientific data on which to base decisions regarding the optimal frequency or type of contact between renal transplant recipients and transplant centers," an empirical set of guidelines is offered. Renal transplant recipients should have regular follow-up in a transplantation center. The purpose of such follow-up visits is not only to provide graft surveillance and optimization of immunosuppression but also to evaluate, treat, and anticipate complications and comorbid conditions as well as to provide education

and experienced counseling. In general, those patients with essentially an uncomplicated early post-transplant course and functioning allograft who are discharged within 1 week of receiving a graft will be monitored two or three times per week for the first month, with about two follow-up visits within that period of time if continuing improvement and a stable course is established. Between 1 and 3 months after transplantation, laboratory monitoring is performed usually on a weekly basis, with follow-up visits at 2- to 4-week intervals. If the clinical course remains uncomplicated, monitoring is carried out midway between, and with, follow-up visits that are at approximately monthly intervals up to 6 months, every 2–3 months from 6 months up to 1 year, every 3–4 months from 1 to 3 years, every 4–6 months for the first 3–5 years, and every 6 months to 1 year thereafter.

The usual laboratory tests include measuring serum creatinine, blood urea nitrogen, electrolytes, glucose, calcium, magnesium, phosphorus, and albumin levels, and usually blood levels of the immunosuppressants being used along with a complete blood count and urinalysis. Lipid studies, liver function tests, serum uric acid, and 24-h urine collection for protein and creatinine are carried out every 3–12 months, depending on the clinical problems and medications. Diabetic patients should have their hemoglobin A_1C levels monitored every 3 months, and those patients receiving HMG-CoA reductase inhibitors (statins) should have their serum alanine aminotransferase (ALT) and creatine kinase (CK) enzyme levels checked every 3 months.

For annual follow-up visits, additional studies are performed that include an expanded history and physical examination, chest radiograph, electrocardiogram, and examination of three stool specimens for occult blood. In addition, a pelvic examination and Papanicolaou smear for women aged 18 years and older and for sexually active teens should be carried out, along with a breast examination and mammogram for women aged 40 years and older. Men aged 40 years and older should have a digital rectal examination and their prostate-specific antigen (PSA) levels checked. A screening colonoscopy examination should be carried out in patients aged 50 years and at appropriate intervals thereafter. Because the serum creatinine level may overestimate renal function, a direct determination of glomerular filtration rate (GFR) may be indicated using [^{125}I]iothalamate or similar techniques. If the urinalysis suggests infection, a urine culture should be carried out even in asymptomatic individuals. Similarly, patients with leukopenia and no specific symptoms should have not only adjustment of the dose of azathioprine or mycophenolate mofetil but also cytomegalovirus (CMV) studies (CMV-DNA).

The major causes of mortality in renal allograft recipients in descending order of frequency are coronary heart disease (CHD), malignancies, sepsis, and liver failure. Factors causing allograft dysfunction (often associated with hypertension and proteinuria) include a variety of prerenal events, cyclosporine or tacrolimus nephrotoxicity, rejections (acute cellular, vascular, and chronic), recurrent or de novo glomerulonephritis and other nephropathies, renal artery stenosis, pyelonephritis, and obstruction.

Cardiovascular disease

Cardiovascular disease remains the leading cause of mortality in recipients of renal allografts, and its proportion of total deaths has increased. Moreover, cardiovascular disease accounts for 36% of patients dying with a functioning graft in the first 10 years after transplantation. By 15 years after renal transplantation, about 23% of patients develop ischemic or coronary heart disease (CHD), 15% develop cerebrovascular disease (CVD), and 15% of patients develop peripheral arterial disease (PAD).[1]

Coronary heart disease

Within 4 years after renal transplantation, the prevalence of CHD is 11%, a frequency that exceeds the 9.5% prevalence of CHD existing before transplantation and that is three to four times that expected.[2] However, when compared with renal transplant recipients prior to 1986, the relative risk of CHD deceased to 0.60 between 1986 and 1992, and even further to 0.27 after 1992.[3] Moreover, in patients who suffered an acute myocardial infarction (MI) between 1990 and 1996, compared with those who suffered an acute MI between 1977 and 1984, there has been a 51% reduction in the risk of cardiac mortality.[4]

The management of CHD can be directed at three levels: (1) medical treatment of CHD risk factors; (2) diagnosis and interventional treatment of established CHD; (3) consideration of agents for secondary prevention of cardiovascular events or having potentially important secondary benefits in the prevention of CHD.

Level I: medical treatment of CHD risk factors
(Table 92.1)

Post-transplantation risk factors for CHD may be classified as not modifiable, difficult to modify, in transition, and modifiable (Table 92.1). Interventional studies have not been reported in transplant recipients. In one major study, hypertension and low-density lipoprotein (LDL) cholesterol could no longer be identified as CHD risk factors, apparently because of intensive treatment.[5] CHD risk factors in renal transplant recipients, when compared with those in the nontransplant population, include risks specific to transplantation (acute rejections, prednisone and cyclosporine use, pretransplant splenectomy), risks disproportionately accentuated by transplantation (diabetes mellitus, age, cigarette smoking),[3] risks of similar magnitude (male sex, hypertension, low high-density lipoprotein (HDL) and high LDL cholesterol), risks that may reflect another process at work (hypoalbuminemia reflecting increased interleukin 1 (IL-1) and IL-6 inflammatory activity), and probable new risks that have been uncovered in different segments of the general population.[2,3,5] For example, in the Heart Outcomes Prevention Evaluation (HOPE) study, it was found that *any* degree of albuminuria, even below the threshold for microalbuminuria, was a risk factor for MI, stroke, or cardiovascular death in nondiabetics as well as diabetics.[6] Additionally, a serum creatinine level of $\geq$ 1.4 mg/dL was found to be a significant risk factor for cardiovascular death and was independent of known cardiovascular death risk factors

Table 92.1 Post-transplantation risk factors* for coronary heart disease

Not modifiable	Difficult to modify	In transition	Modifiable
Increasing age†‡	Smoking†	Each acute rejection†‡	Hypertension§
Male sex†‡	Excess weight	Prednisone dose‡	Elevated total cholesterol ‡
Pretransplantation CHD	Sedentary lifestyle	Cyclosporine dose	LDL ≥130 mg/dL§
Atherosclerotic disease	Lp (a)	Post-transplantation de	HDL (each 10 mg/dL)†
In carotid arteries†‡		novo diabetes mellitus	LVH
In peripheral vessels†‡			Elevated homocysteine level
Plaque burden in coronary arteries			
Pretransplantation diabetes mellitus†‡			
Family history of premature CHD			
Pretransplantation splenectomy†			

HDL, high-density lipoprotein; CHD, coronary heart disease; LDL, low-density lipoprotein; LVH, left ventricular hypertrophy.
*Not all risk factors have been subjected to analysis.
†Independent risk factor for post-transplantation CHD identified by multivariate analysis.
‡Risk factor for post-transplantation CHD identified by discriminate analysis.
§These traditional risk factors did not appear in some analyses presumably because they were aggressively treated.
Adapted from Braun WE: Noninfectious complications of renal transplantation. *In* Therapy in Nephrology and Hypertension: A Companion to Brenner & Rector's The Kidney. Philadelphia: WB Saunders, 1999, pp 625–633.

and treatment.[7] Elevation of C-reactive protein (CRP) identifies a population at increased risk for cardiovascular disease.[8]

Risk assessment The first step in risk management is risk assessment. The 10-year risk for developing CHD can be assessed by CHD risk scoring systems that were published in 1998[9] and 2001.[10] The former evaluates diabetes as a weighted risk factor and provides 10-year CHD risk estimates as absolute percentages in comparison with an age- and gender-matched population.[9] The latter establishes three risk categories: > 20%, ≤ 20%, and < 10% (Table 92.2).[10]

It has become clear that the risk factors for CHD are essentially the same as the risk factors for progression of renal disease and include hypertension, hyperlipidemia, hyperglycemia, aging, smoking, proteinuria, and renal insufficiency. Consequently, cardioprotective strategies are also renoprotective.

Hypertension Hypertension is a well-established risk factor (see Chapters 59 and 63).

Hyperlipidemia In the general population, elevated total and LDL cholesterol levels, low levels of HDL cholesterol, and hypertriglyceridemia are risk factors for CHD. It seems highly likely that the same type of lipid-associated cardiovascular risk will be found in renal transplant recipients. Hyperlipidemia occurs in 50–80% of renal transplant recipients treated with prednisone and calcineurin inhibitors, particularly cyclosporine. It usually consists of elevated LDL cholesterol, apolipoprotein B, triglycerides, and very low density lipoproteins (VLDL); and low, normal, or even slightly elevated serum HDL cholesterol levels.[11] This contrasts with chronic dialysis patients, who usually have high triglyceride and low HDL levels. Lipoprotein a (LP-a) levels that are elevated with chronic renal failure usually improve after renal transplantation.

Factors contributing to post-transplantation hyperlipidemia include a genetic basis, increasing age, male sex, postmenopausal state in women, excess body weight, impaired renal function, nephrotic-range proteinuria, diabetes mellitus, hypothyroidism, and certain immunosuppressants. Cyclosporine[12] and glucocorticoids promote hyperlipidemia. With sirolimus, severe hypercholesterolemia and hypertriglyceridemia were 3 to 4 times more frequent than with cyclosporine and were maximal after approximately 2 months of therapy.[13] It has been estimated, by use of the Framingham model, that sirolimus in doses of 2 or 5 mg/day would cause a small increased incidence of two or three new cases of CHD per thousand renal transplant recipients per year, respectively.[13]

The mechanisms of hyperlipidemia after renal transplantation are incompletely understood.[14] Hypercholesterolemia tends to improve within the first 6–12 months after transplantation when prednisone and cyclosporine doses are being tapered, as may hypertriglyceridemia and hypercholesterolemia when sirolimus doses are decreased. Nevertheless, significant hyperlipidemia warrants treatment if it persists afterwards (Table 92.3).

It is important to consider secondary causes of dyslipidemias: for hypercholesterolemia, these are hypothyroidism, obstructive liver disease, androgens, prednisone, cyclosporine, and sirolimus; and for hypertriglyceridemia, these are diabetes mellitus, chronic excessive alcohol consumption, progestins, and sirolimus.

There are three categories of risk that modify LDL cholesterol treatment goals in nontransplant patients and can serve as a basis for treating transplant recipients: (1) CHD and CHD risk equivalents that carry a 10-year risk > 20% for a major coronary event and have an LDL goal of less than 100 mg/dL; (2) multiple risk factors that carry a 10-year risk of 20% for a major coronary event and have an LDL cholesterol goal of less than 130 mg/dL; and (3) a 0–1 risk factor that carries a 10-year risk < 10% for a major

Table 92.2 LDL cholesterol goals and cutoff points for therapeutic lifestyle changes (TLC) and drug therapy in different risk categories

Risk category	LDL goal (mg/dL)	LDL level to initiate lifestyle changes (mg/dL)	LDL level to consider drug therapy (mg/dL)
CHD or CHD risk equivalents (10-year risk > 20%)	< 100	≥ 100	≥ 130 (100–129; drug optional)*
2+ risk factors (10-year risk ≤ 20%)	< 130	≥ 130	10-year risk 10–20%: ≥ 130 10-year risk < 10%; ≥ 160
0–1 risk factor †	< 160	≥ 160	≥ 190 (160–189: LDL-lowering drug optional)

LDL, low-density lipoprotein; CHD, coronary heart disease.
*Some authorities recommend the use of LDL-lowering drugs in this category if an LDL cholesterol level of < 100 mg/dL cannot be achieved by therapeutic lifestyle changes. Others prefer the use of drugs that primarily modify triglycerides and HDL, e.g. nicotinic acid or fibrate. Clinical judgement also may call for deferring drug therapy in this subcategory.
†Almost all people with 0–1 risk factor have a 10-year-risk < 10%; thus 10-year risk assessment in people with a risk factor of 0–1 is not necessary.
With permission from NCEP Adult Treatment Panel III Report. JAMA 2001;285:2486.

Table 92.3 Adult Treatment Panel III Classification of LDL, total, and HDL cholesterol, and triglyceride levels (mg/dL)

LDL cholesterol	< 100	Optimal
	100–129	Near or above optimal
	130–159	Borderline high
	160–189	High
	≥ 190	Very high
Total cholesterol	< 200	Desirable
	200–239	Borderline high
	≥ 240	High
HDL-cholesterol	< 40	Low
	≥ 60	High
Triglycerides	< 150	Normal
	151–199	Borderline high
	200–499	High
	≥ 500	Very high

With permission from The National Cholesterol Education Program (NCEP) Expert Panel on Detection, Evaluation, And Treatment of High Blood Cholesterol In Adults (Adult Treatment Panel III). JAMA 2001;285:2486.

coronary event and has an LDL goal of less than 160 mg/dL.

Lowering LDL cholesterol is achieved by therapeutic lifestyle changes (TLC) and drug therapy. The essential features of TLC include a reduced intake of saturated fats (less than 7% of total calories) and cholesterol (less than 200 mg/day), weight reduction, and increased physical activity.[10]

Drug therapy includes statins, bile acid sequestrants, nicotinic acid, and fibric acid derivatives (Table 92.4). Because post-transplant hyperlipidemia is most often dominated by an elevated LDL cholesterol level, statins will be the group of drugs most frequently used (e.g. atorvastatin, fluvastatin, lovastatin, pravastatin, and simvastatin). Because atorvastatin is the most potent, it is usually started first at a dose of 10 mg daily.[15] Pravastatin has been reported to have immunosuppressive effects, and is metabolized in the liver by sulfation; fluvastatin is metabolized by CYP2C9; the other statins are metabolized by the CYP3A4 system, which is also involved in the metabolism of cyclosporine, tacrolimus, and sirolimus.[15] Consequently, when these immunosuppressants are used in combination with a statin metabolized by CYP3A4, there is potential toxicity from increased statin levels. Patients should be monitored every 3–6 months, or as clinically indicated, with ALT levels being measured for hepatic toxicity and CK enzymes for muscle toxicity. Other statin side-effects include alopecia, insomnia, gastrointestinal symptoms, and drug interactions with warfarin, macrolide antibiotics (such as erythromycin), fibric acid analogs, niacin, nondihydropyridine calcium channel blockers, azole antifungal agents, histamine 2 blockers, and grapefruit juice.[15] Impaired renal function

may require lower doses of statins. Ingestion of food increases the bioavailability of lovastatin.[15]

When associated with sirolimus, hypertriglyceridemia may diminish as the dosage of sirolimus declines, but treatment may well be warranted for severe elevations. The use of fibric acid analogs (gemfibrozil, bezafibrate, fenofibrate, and ciprofibrate) or nicotinic acid may be indicated. The last three fibric acid drugs may increase serum creatinine in cyclosporine-treated patients, and fenofibrate and bezafibrate may increase plasma homocysteine.[11,16] Fibric acid analogs should be avoided in those with severe renal disease or severe hepatic disease, and the dose should be reduced in patients with impaired renal function.[11]

Combined lipid abnormalities characterized by both high LDL cholesterol and triglyceride levels are more difficult and riskier to treat. Atorvastatin at doses of 20 mg and higher at times may be effective monotherapy, but the addition of a second agent such as gemfribrozil or niacin may be appropriate. Under such circumstances, very close clinical and laboratory follow-up is warranted.

Additional benefits of statins include a reduction in the level of circulating endothelin 1 and decreases in systolic, diastolic, and pulse pressure,[17] reduced CRP, and reduction of acute primary coronary events[8] and antiproliferative effects.[18,19]

Post-transplant diabetes mellitus (PTDM) Post-transplant diabetes mellitus (PTDM) is usually detected within the first year, with a reported frequency of 4–20%.[20] A glucose tolerance test 1 year after transplantation may be worthwhile for those patients not exhibiting PTDM. A previous decline in PTDM, observed before 1995 when cyclosporine was used with lower doses of glucocorticoids, has been reversed, with an increase in PTDM now being attributed to older and heavier recipients as well as to better absorbed cyclosporine formulations.[21] Risk factors for PTDM include glucocorticoids and calcineurin inhibitors (tacrolimus being a greater risk than cyclosporine), age > 45 years, male sex, African-American and Hispanic race, family history of diabetes, excess body weight, cadaver-allograft recipient, acute rejection, and CMV and HCV infection. The purine antagonists do not appear to be diabetogenic; information on sirolimus is incomplete.

The complications of PTDM are likely to be the same as those seen in patients with pretransplant diabetes mellitus.[22] At least three cases of de novo diabetic nephropathy have been reported in PTDM patients. Patients with PTDM are usually best managed by collaborative care with an endocrinologist or diabetologist. Nevertheless, the transplant nephrologist needs to evaluate carefully the medications being used because of the potential for side-effects that include edema (the thiazolidinedione derivatives pioglitazone and rosiglitazone), higher blood levels of drugs because of decreased renal function (insulin, metformin, sulfonylurea derivatives), lactic acidosis (metformin), and competitive metabolism by CYP3A4 (short-acting insulin secretogogues such as repaglinide, and nateglinide to a lesser extent). The effect of hepatic

Table 92.4 Drugs affecting lipoprotein metabolism

Drug class, agents, and daily doses	Lipid/lipoprotein effects	Side-effects	Contraindications	Clinical trial results
HMG-CoA reductase inhibitors (statins)*	LDL ↓18–55% HDL ↑5–15% TG ↓7–30%	Myopathy; increased liver enzymes	*Absolute*: active or chronic liver disease *Relative*: concomitant use of certain drugs¶	Reduced major coronary events, CHD deaths, need for coronary procedures, stroke, and total mortality
Bile acid sequestrants†	LDL ↓15–30% HDL ↑3–5% TG no change or increase	Gastrointestinal distress; constipation; decreased absorption of other drugs	*Absolute*: dysbeta-lipoproteinemia; TG > 400 mg/dL *Relative*: TG > 200 mg/dL	Reduced major coronary events and CHD deaths
Nicotinic acid‡	LDL ↓5–25% HDL ↑15–35% TG ↓20–50%	Flushing; hyperglycemia; hyperuricemia (or gout); upper gastrointestinal distress; hepatotoxicity	*Absolute*: chronic liver disease; severe gout *Relative*: diabetes; hyperuricemia; peptic ulcer disease	Reduced major coronary events, and possibly total mortality
Fibric acids§	LDL ↓5–20% (may be increased in patients with high TG) HDL ↑10–20% TG ↓20–50%	Dyspepsia; gallstones; myopathy; unexplained non-CHD deaths in WHO study	*Absolute*: severe renal disease; severe hepatic disease (see text also)	Reduced major coronary events

HMG-CoA, 3-hydroxy-3-methylglutaryl coenzyme A; LDL, low-density lipoprotein; HDL, high-density lipoprotein; TG, triglycerides; ↓, decrease; ↑, increase; CHD, coronary heart disease.
*Lovastatin (20–80 mg), pravastatin (20–40 mg), simvastatin (20–80 mg), fluvastatin (20–80 mg), and atorvastatin (10–80 mg).
†Cholestyramine (4–16 g), colestipol (5–20 g), and colesevelam (2.6–3.8 g).
‡Immediate-release (crystalline) nicotinic acid (1.5–3 g), extended-release nicotinic acid (1–2 g), and sustained-release nicotinic acid (1–2 g).
§Gemfibrozil (600 mg twice daily), fenofibrate (200 mg), and clofibrate (1000 mg twice daily).
¶ Cyclosporine, tacrolimus, sirolimus, macrolide antibiotics, various antifungal agents, and other drugs metabolized by CYP3A4 (fibrates and niacin should be used with appropriate caution; see text).
With permission from NCEP Adult Treatment Panel III Report. JAMA 2001;285:2486.

insufficiency on drug metabolism should be considered. A 5-year, randomized, controlled clinical trial of kidney transplant recipients who had insulin-requiring diabetes mellitus as their original disease compared standard insulin therapy with optimized glycemic control.[23] The standard therapy group had more than a twofold increase in the volume of the mesangial matrix per glomerulus, a three-fold increase in arteriolar hyalinosis, and greater thickening of the glomerular basement membrane. However, severe hypoglycemic episodes were more frequent in the optimized group.

Patients with PTDM require diabetes education and diet instruction. They should monitor their glycemic control with a home glucose diary, have their hemoglobin A1c levels checked every 3 months, have regular ophthalmologic evaluations, regular foot care, regular evaluation of complications from a variety of neuropathies (autonomic neuropathy with orthostatic hypotension, peripheral neuropathy, gastroenteropathy, bladder dysfunction, neuropathic bone disease), and appropriate periodic cardiovascular evaluation of the coronary arteries, carotid arteries, and peripheral vascular system.

Because of the striking benefit of angiotensin-converting enzyme inhibitors (ACEIs) in slowing the progression of diabetic nephropathy in type 1 diabetics and of the angiotensin receptor blockers (ARBs) in type 2 diabetics,[24,25] these antihypertensives are preferred in patients with PTDM. Ramipril reduced the development of new diabetes in high-risk individuals in the HOPE trial.[26] ACEIs and ARBs can cause adverse effects including acute renal failure or hyperkalemia when used with high doses of cyclosporine, which cause afferent arteriolar vasoconstriction, or nonsteroidal anti-inflammatory agents, which block afferent arteriolar dilatation, or when used in volume contracted states or in the presence of transplant renal artery stenosis or compromised renal function.

Patients with renal insufficiency or those receiving an ACEI, an ARB, or spironolactone could experience life-threatening hyperkalemia.[27] Patients should be informed about the relatively frequent side-effect of cough with ACEIs and the uncommon but potentially severe side-effect of angioedema with ACEIs and even ARBs. The dose of diabetogenic immunosuppressants should be kept as low as possible.

Cigarette smoking In a study of 1334 transplant recipients, 24.7% of whom smoked, the relative risk for a major cardiovascular event was 1.56 for those smoking 11–25 pack–years at transplant and 2.14 for those smoking > 25 pack–years ($P < 0.001$).[28] The relative risk of invasive malignancy was 1.91 and of death with a functioning graft 1.42. The effects of smoking appeared to reduce 5 years after stopping. Adverse renal hemodynamic effects, coagulation alterations, and endothelial injury result from smoking and are particularly injurious in diabetics.[29,30] Cigarette smoking is an independent risk factor for type 2 diabetes mellitus.[31]

Nicotine causes arousal or sedation, dampens unpleasant emotions, and develops special psychological significance for users.[32] There are basically three ways in which smoking cessation may be achieved: (1) self-motivated spontaneous cessation; (2) counseling and behavioral therapies; and (3) pharmacotherapies.[33] One or more of these should be offered to every smoker.

It has been estimated that approximately 50 million Americans have stopped smoking, 95% of whom have stopped of their own accord.[32,33] Individuals who stop smoking typically experience physical withdrawal symptoms, which peak in 2–4 days and generally disappear in 10–14 days. Even years later, many individuals will continue to experience the periodic desire to smoke. Smoking even a single cigarette in response to these urges can frequently lead to an extended relapse. Persistent urging by a physician may motivate a patient to cease smoking. The next most effective methods are behaviorally oriented programs by an experienced psychologist or physician experienced in smoking-cessation therapy. There is a strong, dose–response relationship between the intensity of counseling and its effectiveness. The three types of counseling and behavior therapies that were found to be especially effective were providing practical counseling in problem-solving and skills training, development of a social support mechanism as part of the treatment (intra-treatment social support), and development of a social support network outside of treatment (extratreatment social support).[33]

Pharmacologic aids to smoking cessation include bupropion or nicotine replacement as gum, inhaler, nasal spray, or patch. Clonidine is an efficacious second-line pharmacotherapy. When only pharmacologic methods are used, 1-year cessation rates rarely exceed 20%. Multicomponent behaviorally oriented programs can improve the long-term cessation rate to approximately 30–40%.[34] The use of over-the-counter nicotine patches without concurrent psychosocial treatment resulted in low success rates of around 13% at 6 months.[34] Common nicotine skin patch side-effects include skin irritation, insomnia, vivid dreams, and nausea. Skin irritation can usually be reduced by changing the location of the skin site for patch application. Bupropion (Zyban, Wellbutrin), 150 mg each morning for 9 weeks, when compared with a nicotine patch alone, a combination of the nicotine patch and bupropion, or placebo resulted in abstinence rates after 1 year of 30.3%, 16.4%, 35.5%, and 15.6%, respectively, clearly indicating greater success with combination therapy including bupropion, or bupropion alone.[35] Sustained-release bupropion reduced the relapse rate and weight gain after smoking cessation.[36] Bupropion appears to be metabolized in the liver by enzyme systems other than CYP3A4 that are involved in the metabolism of cyclosporine, tacrolimus, and sirolimus. Bupropion has not been studied in patients with renal insufficiency, but dose reduction may be needed. Side-effects of bupropion include seizure and other neurologic symptoms (insomnia, headache, abnormal dreams, dizziness, disturbed concentration), dry mouth, nausea, constipation, arthralgia, and back pain. Contraindications include seizure disorder, prior or current bulimia or anorexia nervosa, and monoamine oxidase inhibitor use.

Hyperhomocysteinemia Hyperhomocysteinemia has been observed in 65–70% of renal transplant recipients.[37] Fasting plasma homocysteine (tHcy) levels greater than 10 μmol/L are generally considered to be abnormal.[1] In a metaanalysis of 27 studies, mild-to-moderate elevations of tHcy occurring either during fasting or after methionine loading were a significant and independent risk factor for coronary, cerebrovascular, and peripheral vascular disease in the general population.[38] However, the results of prospective studies have been inconclusive, and it has not yet been demonstrated that reduction of elevated tHcy levels results in any reduction of cardiovascular morbidity and mortality.[39] One study demonstrated that elevated tHcy causes atherosclerosis in a multi-step process.[40] Factors known to increase tHcy levels include deficiencies of folate, B_6 (pyridoxine), B_{12} (cyanocobalamin), impaired renal function, and certain drugs.[16]

Management of elevated tHcy should include measurements of blood levels of folate, B_6, and B_{12}. Hyperhomocysteinemia in renal transplant recipients responded to treatment with 2.4 mg/day of folic acid, 50 mg/day of vitamin B_6, and 0.4 mg/day of vitamin B_{12}.[37] In this study, 5 of the 10 renal transplant recipients achieved tHcy levels < 12 μmol/L, and overall there was a 28% reduction in tHcy levels. In 55 stable renal transplant recipients treated with cyclosporine, tHcy levels decreased from 36.9 ± 21.3 μmol/L to 27.7 ± 14.8 μmol/L by 6 months after transplantation, although the levels remained higher than controls (16.0 ± 5.3 μmol/L) and higher than those in a normal population.[41] It is currently unclear what constitutes optimum treatment. Certainly, if deficiencies of folate, B_6, and B_{12} are detected, they should be corrected. For those patients who have normal levels of these factors and stable renal function but elevated tHcy levels, an interim treatment designed to avoid adding three new pills to a transplant recipient's already large medication list is a single pill taken once per day, such as Nephrocap or Nephrovite Rx, containing 1.0 mg folic acid, 10 mg of pyridoxine, and 6 μg of cyanocobalamin among other components.[42]

Level II: diagnosis and interventional treatment of established CHD

Renal transplant recipients should be evaluated before, and annually after, transplantation in order to identify those who are at high risk for CHD. A formal coronary evaluation should identify newly symptomatic patients and profile their coronary risk.[9,10] For patients with angina pectoris, atypical chest pain, or a high-risk profile,[9,10] further study with stress testing or possibly coronary angiography may identify those needing intervention. Because of the duration and clustering of coronary risk factors in renal transplant recipients, it is appropriate to use imaging studies rather than the traditional exercise electrocardiography as the initial test.[43,44] Imaging stress testing is either nuclear-based (assessing perfusion) or echo-based (assessing myocardial function), and each of these may use either exercise or pharmacologic stressors (dipyridamole, adenosine, or dobutamine).

Screening for coronary disease by electron beam computed tomography (CT) scanning and coronary calcium scoring (CCS) remains unproved.[45,46] Although plaque burden is a coronary risk factor,[47] and CCS reflects plaque,[48] calcified plaques are relatively stable.[49]

Results of percutaneous transluminal angioplasty (PTCA) and coronary artery bypass grafting (CABG) have improved appreciably. Coronary artery stenting (CAS) may improve substantially in the near future by the use of sirolimus-coated stents to suppress neointimal proliferation.[50] In this study of 2989 renal transplant recipients, 83 required myocardial revascularization (PTCA or CABG) before or after renal transplantation.[51] None of the 45 patients revascularized after transplantation experienced allograft loss or significant change in function. Survival rates of the 45 patients were 93%, 78%, and 60% at 1, 3, and 5 years respectively.[51] Early-phase risk factors for death included hypertension and revascularization carried out before 1989. Late-phase risk factors for death included diabetes mellitus, a greater number of pre-CABG myocardial infarctions, renal transplantation before 1984, older age, and unstable angina before CABG. These authors concluded that coronary angiography, PTCA, and CABG are safe in patients with functioning renal allografts.[50] In another series of 31 patients who received CABG after renal transplantation, there was one early postoperative death and two episodes of transplant renal dysfunction occurred.[52] A retrospective United States Renal Data Systems (USRDS) database search from 1995 to 1998 identified 912 patients who were hospitalized for CABG, 613 hospitalized for PTCA, and 626 for PTCA/CAS.[53] In-hospital deaths were 4.9% for CABG, 4.2% for PTCA, and 2.2% for CAS. At 3 years event-free survival from combined cardiac endpoints (cardiac death and acute MI) was 88.9% for CABG, 84.8% for CAS, and 80.2% for PTCA.[53] These authors concluded that, after comorbidity adjustment, renal transplant patients in the USA have similar 3-year survival after PTCA, CAS, and CABG (75.8%, 78.9%, and 77.0%, respectively), but fewer serious cardiac events after CABG.

Level III: consideration of agents useful for primary/secondary prevention of cardiovascular events or having potentially important secondary benefits in the prevention of CHD

The use of aspirin or enteric-coated aspirin (65–325 mg/day) for those without aspirin sensitivity is recommended.[1] β-Adrenergic receptor blockers have a special role in the secondary prevention of cardiac morbidity and mortality.

Renal transplant recipients who either have established CHD or are at considerable risk for developing it should take certain "preferred" medications that have a primary indication in a transplant recipient and also have a secondary antiproliferative or antifibrotic effect. Most of these effects have been demonstrated only in experimental models and for only certain cell types. Examples include ACEIs to block transforming growth factor (TGF)-β-mediated extracellular matrix protein synthesis by fibroblasts[54] and ARBs that shunt angiotensin II to binding sites on AT_2 receptors with inhibition of endothelial cell proliferation.[55] Spironolactone (25 mg/day) reduced morbidity and mortality in patients with severe congestive heart failure who were also receiving ACEIs, probably because it reduced myocardial and vascular fibrosis.[56] Statins can block the proliferative effect of epidermal growth factor,[19] have an antihypertensive effect,[57] and may favorably affect osteoporosis.[58] Sirolimus inhibits vascular smooth muscle cell proliferation by blocking cell cycle progression at the G1–S stage.[13,50] One study found that coating coronary artery stents with sirolimus prevented neointimal proliferation.[50] However, there may be circumstances in which an antiproliferative state is undesirable (e.g. extensive wound healing or prolonged acute tubular necrosis).

Recent information indicates that combining an ACEI, an ARB, and a β-blocker has an adverse effect on the myocardium.[59] Consequently, there can be no presumption of additive beneficial effects of untested drug combinations.

New immunosuppression protocols that either avoid or rapidly eliminate glucocorticoids and/or calcineurin inhibitors should offer substantial promise in reducing the risk for CHD.

Cerebrovascular disease (CVD)

Duplex ultrasounds of the carotid arteries should be performed if there is a decreased carotid arterial pulse, a bruit over the carotid artery, or a neurologic syndrome consistent with carotid artery disease. Post-transplant CHD and CVD are strongly predictive of one another. In addition to traditional risk factors, elevated levels of tHcy are also associated with extracranial carotid artery stenosis,[60] as well as cerebral macro- and microangiopathy.[61]

In symptomatic patients with high-grade carotid artery stenosis by angiography, the benefit of carotid endarterectomy is well documented. In asymptomatic patients with carotid artery stenosis of ≥ 80%, intervention should be considered.[62] In the Asymptomatic Carotid Atherosclerosis Study (ACAS), the estimated incidence of ipsilateral strokes within 5 years and perioperative strokes or death within 30–42 days of randomization were reduced by 66% in men and by 17% in women.[62]

Patients with autosomal dominant polycystic kidney disease (ADPKD) require special attention for CVD. The overall prevalence of an asymptomatic intracranial aneurysm (ICA) determined by magnetic resonance angiography (MRA) is approximately 12%. The prevalence increases to 24% in those with a positive family history of an ICA or subarachnoid hemorrhage in conjunction with ADPKD, and is about 5% in those with a negative family history. In patients with ADPKD who have a family history of ICA or subarachnoid hemorrhage, or who have neurologic symptoms suggestive of an ICA, MRA is usually the initial study. Repeat screening with MRA every 5 years has been a general recommendation for ADPKD patients with no prior aneurysm.[63] If acute symptoms of an ICA rupture or sentinel bleed develop, or surgery is planned, usually for a larger aneurysm (generally 7 mm), cerebral angiography will often be performed. Control of hypertension and timely neurosurgical judgement and skill are the main elements of treatment.

Peripheral arterial disease (PAD)

Diabetic renal transplant recipients with pretransplant CHD have a sevenfold greater risk of amputation within 3 years of evaluation for transplantation.[64] Non-diabetics with renal allografts functioning for > 20 years also risk lower limb ischemia requiring amputation.[65] About one-third of patients in the general population with PAD have typical claudication that results in amputation in 5% of patients within 5 years.[66] About 5–10% of patients have critical leg ischemia. Their risk of limb loss is substantial. However, more than 50% of patients having PAD on the basis of abnormal ankle–brachial (A/B) index ratios do not have typical claudication or critical leg ischemia, but they do have reduced ambulatory activity and quality of life. Diminished femoral and/or pedal pulses, iliofemoral bruits, the presence of coronary, carotid, or renal arterial disease, or a high-risk CHD profile are indications to measure the A/B index. An A/B index value that is less than 0.90 at rest, or more than 0.90 at rest but that decreases by 20% after exercise, is diagnostic.[66]

Patients with PAD in the general population should have risk factor assessment and treatment, and should receive antiplatelet therapy with aspirin or clopidogrel in order to inhibit platelet aggregation.[66] Clopidogrel (75 mg once daily) is extensively metabolized by the liver and is said to not require dosage adjustment with impaired renal function. It is contraindicated with active bleeding or hypersensitivity. Side-effects include thrombotic thrombocytopenic purpura, longer time for cessation of bleeding, myelotoxicity, gastrointestinal symptoms, rash, and other skin disorders. Treatment of claudication begins with exercise therapy and possibly drugs such as cilostazol.[66] Cilostazol is metabolized primarily by CYP3A4, and consequently numerous drug interactions are a concern, particularly with cyclosporine, tacrolimus, and sirolimus (see also Hyperlipidemia). Because cilostazol and several of its metabolites inhibit phosphodiesterase III, and several drugs with this effect have caused decreased survival in patients with class III or IV congestive heart failure, it is contraindicated in patients with congestive heart failure of any severity. Other side-effects of cilostazol include headache, dizziness, palpitation, tachycardia, diarrhea, peripheral edema, pharyngitis, and rhinitis. If claudication does not improve, studies to determine the site of the occlusive lesion(s) should be undertaken with a view to endovascular or surgical intervention.[66]

Angiographic studies in renal transplant recipients will usually be performed using nonionic radiocontrast material or MRA in order to minimize the risk of renal dysfunction. Those patients having standard angiograms with radiocontrast material should be prehydrated intravenously and possibly receive acetylcysteine.[67]

Post-transplantation erythrocytosis (PTE)

PTE, defined as a persistently elevated hematocrit > 51%, occurs in about 15% of renal transplant patients (range 4–22%), usually within the first 2 years. The consequences of PTE are primarily thromboembolic events, which may be seen in up to 22% of patients.

The development of PTE does not correlate with serum erythropoietin levels.[68] Angiotensin II stimulates the proliferation of normal early erythroid precursors, having increased numbers of AT_1 receptors, which correlates with the hematocrit in patients with PTE.[69,70] Consequently, ACEIs and ARBs are the treatments of choice for PTE, although phlebotomy may be useful at times. Because some patients may have a rapid fall in hematocrit, or less commonly a spontaneous remission, careful monitoring is necessary. Intermittent therapy may be effective in some patients.

Malignant disease

The incidence of de novo malignant neoplasms is increased after renal transplantation. The most frequent malignant neoplasms encountered and their relative risks (RR) are skin cancers (RR 4–21); non-Hodgkin's lymphomas (RR 28–49); carcinomas of the uterus and cervix (RR 14), vulva-perineum (RR 100), hepatobiliary tree (RR 30), and Kaposi sarcoma (RR up to 400–500 in certain ethnic groups).[71] Several clinical profiles for individuals prone to developing certain malignancies are as follows: post-transplantation lymphoproliferative disease (PTLD) in those patients seronegative for the Epstein–Barr virus (EBV) who have been treated with antilymphocyte, antithymocyte, or OKT3 monoclonal antibodies and/or are receiving higher doses of cyclosporine and mycophenolate mofetil; Kaposi sarcoma in those of Arabic, Jewish, black, or Mediterranean ancestry or with evidence of human herpes virus 8 or human immunodeficiency virus infection; carcinoma of the cervix and vulva in those with papillomavirus, and possibly herpes genitalis infections, or multiple sexual partners; hepatocellular carcinomas in those with persistent hepatitis B antigenemia, cirrhosis, and/or hepatitis C of long duration; carcinomas of the skin in fair-skinned or older individuals with unprotected sun exposure and long-duration use of azathioprine with its metabolite thioguanine; recurrent malignant disease in those who before transplantation had a malignant neoplasm with a medium or high rate of recurrence[72] (Table 92.5). Recommendations of the American Cancer Society are used for cancer surveillance, but they may need to be applied with increased frequency or with invasive testing in high-risk individuals[73] (see above).

Two of the most frequently encountered malignant neoplasms after transplantation have clinical features worth noting. Non-Hodgkin's lymphoma (NHL) can develop in the first year. The average time after transplantation for PTLD is 32 months, with a range of 1–254 months. Three special characteristics of PTLD after transplantation are its extranodal involvement in 70% of patients compared with 35% of nontransplant controls, central nervous system involvement in 26% (with 63% confined to the brain), and microscopic or gross involvement of the allograft in 20% of patients, sometimes simulating rejection. Discon-

tinuation or massive reduction of purine antagonists and calcineurin inhibitors is usually the initial step in therapy for PTLD. Additional therapy is often necessary and includes chemotherapy, radiotherapy, surgical excision, acyclovir, ganciclovir, and anti-CD20 monoclonal antibody. Potential side-effects of anti-CD20 antibody now include fatal reactivation of CMV infection.[74] In a study of 435 patients, total remissions were achieved 29%; approximately one-fourth of remissions were induced by the decrease or elimination of nonsteroidal immunosuppressants[75] (Table 92.6). An increase in the prednisone dose is often necessary to protect the allograft when other immunosuppressants are withdrawn. Whether to resume lower doses of nonsteroidal immunosuppression after regression of PTLD is a difficult question. Some recipients with PTLD in full remission can maintain stable allograft function for years while on prednisone alone. Although reinstitution of lower dose nonsteroidal immunosuppression after PTLD regression has been recommended by some, the life-threatening risk of PTLD recurrence has led others to avoid restarting it.[73] Retransplantation in a small number of patients who had complete remission of PTLD has a 9% PTLD recurrence rate. At least 1 year of documented complete PTLD remission should elapse before retransplantation.[73]

Squamous cell carcinomas of the skin and lip constitute about one-third of all new malignant neoplasms after renal transplantation. In transplant recipients, post-transplantation squamous cell carcinomas tend to be

Table 92.5 Three groups of malignant neoplasms with different post-transplantation recurrence rates

Recurrence rate	Type of malignant neoplasm
Low: 0–10%	Incidental renal cell, testicular, cervical, and thyroid cancers and lymphoma
Medium: 11–25%	Carcinomas of the corpus uteri, colon, prostate (nonfocal), and breast, and Wilms tumor
High: > 25%	Invasive bladder cancers, sarcomas, melanomas, symptomatic renal cell carcinoma, nonmelanoma skin cancer, and multiple myeloma

Adapted from Penn I: The effect of immunosuppression on preexisting cancer. Transplantation 1993;55:742–747, © 1993, The Williams & Wilkins Company, Baltimore.

Table 92.6 Complete remissions of post-transplantation non-Hodgkin's lymphoma with different therapies*

Therapy	Number of patients†	
Decreased immunosuppression (purine antagonists or calcineurin inhibitors)	96	(34)
Excision	47	(15)
Chemotherapy	26	(7)
Acyclovir	31	(1)
Radiotherapy	17	(3)
Immunostimulation	5	(0)

*Complete remissions were achieved in 131 (29%) of 455 patients, some of whom received more than one form of therapy.
The remaining 324 patients either received no treatment, did not respond to treatment, or were currently being treated.
†The figures in parentheses are the numbers of patients having a complete remission when a particular treatment was the only therapy given.
Adapted from Penn I: Tumors after renal and cardiac transplantation. Hematol Oncol Clin North Am 1993;7:431–445.

multiple, have a more aggressive course, and are a more common cause of cancer death than in the general population. Transplant recipients developing skin cancers are about 30 years younger than their counterparts in the general population. Skin cancer risk can be lessened by wearing protective clothing, avoiding direct sun exposure, and using sun blocks. Thioguanine, the active metabolite of azathioprine, may be a chemical carcinogen for the skin. A dose reduction of azathioprine in patients with multiple or severe skin cancers may be indicated. Squamous cell carcinomas typically require frequent surgical treatment. A dermatologist should examine and treat the patient at intervals appropriate to the risks.[76] Other modes of therapy include episodic topical 5-fluorouracil, and topical or systemic retinoids.[76] Numerous side-effects have been reported with 0.5 to 2 mg/kg/day doses of retinoids, including hepatotoxicity, pancreatitis, pseudotumor cerebri, numerous ophthalmologic complications, inflammatory bowel disease, hypertriglyceridemia and decreased HDL-cholesterol, hyperglycemia, hyperostosis, osteoporosis, alopecia, mucocutaneous lesions, and elevated creatine kinase levels. Retinoids may need dose adjustment in renal insufficiency and should not be used by women who are, or intend to become, pregnant.

Liver disease

Liver disease occurs in 7–24% of patients early after transplantation, and contributes to later mortality in 8–28% of patients. The clinical presentation of liver disease has several forms: acute viral hepatitis (hepatitis A, B, and C, CMV, herpes simplex, human herpesvirus (HHV)-6, EBV); drugs (e.g. statins, azole antifungal medications, ACEIs, isoniazid, and high doses of acetaminophen); chronic hepatitis caused by hepatitis B or C; cholestasis caused by obstructive lesions as well as by azathioprine, cyclosporine, and tacrolimus; veno-occlusive disease associated with CMV and azathioprine; infiltrative disease that may be reversible (fat and iron deposition) or progressive (amyloid and malignancies); peliosis hepatis; and alcoholism, which can cause chronic hepatitis and cirrhosis and may often occur in conjunction with other causes. Because so many drugs, including alcohol, can affect liver function, all of the patient's medications and habits should be carefully evaluated.

The histopathology of post-transplantation liver disease has been evaluated by biopsies in 307 patients – 230 in a French study and 77 in an American study.[77,78] It includes fatty metamorphosis, chronic persistent hepatitis, chronic active hepatitis in various stages, cirrhosis, hemosiderosis, hepatic peliosis, and drug-related cholestasis. The levels of serum liver enzymes were not discriminating. In the American study, progression to cirrhosis was seen only in patients with early or advanced chronic active hepatitis or with untreated hemosiderosis.[78] Transition from early chronic active hepatitis to advanced chronic active hepatitis occurred in 60% of patients, with an annual rate of histologic progression of 13%. Older age and female sex

were risk factors for progression. In both studies, liver histopathology offered the best prediction of liver disease. Patients with liver disease usually die beyond the seventh year after transplantation, most often because of infection.

Hepatitis B infection has been dramatically reduced by hepatitis B vaccination in hemodialysis (HD) patients and by isolation of hepatitis B surface antigen (HB$_s$Ag)-positive HD patients. After transplantation, the spontaneous conversion rate from HB$_s$Ag positive to negative was 0–3% compared with 19% in HD patients. A clinical, virologic, and histopathologic study of 151 HB$_s$Ag-positive kidney transplant recipients observed for a median of 125 months documented high rates of persistent viral replication (50%) and reactivation (30%).[79] Histologic worsening occurred in 85% of patients and cirrhosis developed in 28%, with hepatocellular carcinoma occurring in 23% of those with cirrhosis. There were markedly worse histopathologic changes from hepatitis C (HCV) and B (HBV) coinfection. It was concluded that chronic hepatitis B infection is a definite risk, but not a contraindication, for renal transplantation in the absence of cirrhosis; the latter is best managed by continuation of dialysis or combined liver/kidney transplant. Factors associated with histologic deterioration were alcohol consumption, HCV coinfection, older age, female sex, and presence of chronic active hepatitis. The presence of HBV-DNA and/or hepatitis B e antigen (HBeAg) prior to transplantation was associated with an increased risk of progression of liver disease and death from liver failure. In a recent comprehensive study, 128 HB$_s$Ag-positive patients had significantly worse 10-year patient and graft survivals than either HCV-positive or noninfected patients (10-year patient survival: 55 ± 6%, 65 ± 5%, and 80 ± 3%, $P < 0.001$, for HB$_s$Ag-positive, HCV-positive, and noninfected patients respectively; 10-year graft survival: 36 ± 5%, 49 ± 5%, and 63 ± 3%, $P < 0.0001$, for HB$_s$Ag-positive, HCV-positive, and noninfected patients respectively).[80]

Active hepatitis B in renal transplant recipients has been treated with lamivudine, a reverse transcriptase inhibitor, in doses of 75–100 mg/day for more than 6 months. Lamivudine is mostly excreted in the urine. Therefore, dose reduction is necessary for impaired renal function.[81] The area under the curve (AUC) for lamivudine is increased by trimethoprim–sulfamethoxazole. Elevation of serum alanine aminotransferase (ALT) may be seen after initiation of treatment with lamivudine and may represent the development of lamivudine resistance that is accelerated after transplantation.[81] Consequently, HBV, DNA, and ALT should be monitored every 3 months in patients receiving lamivudine.[81] Side-effects include malaise, fatigue, nausea, vomiting, and neutropenia. Lactic acidosis, severe hepatomegaly with steatosis, and death have been reported with antiretroviral nucleoside analogs, alone or in combination with lamivudine.

Hepatitis C has become the most common cause of chronic liver disease in renal transplant recipients. The prevalence of anti-HCV antibody among renal transplant recipients has ranged from 11% to 49%, and 74–94% of these patients are viremic (positive for HCV-RNA). Post-transplant liver disease occurs in 19–64% of those with, compared with 2–19% of those recipients without, HCV antibody. Patient and graft survivals with HCV infection are reduced, although they remain somewhat better than in those positive for hepatitis B (see above). The most common causes of patient mortality are liver failure, sepsis, and CHD. Other complications of HCV infection include cryoglobulinemia, glomerular lesions (membranoproliferative, membranous, fibrillary, and immunotactoid glomerulonephritis, and thrombotic microangiopathy), and hepatocellular carcinoma (HCC). A few patients who have hepatitis C may fail to make antibody to hepatitis C; these patients can be detected only by testing for HCV-RNA. Treatment for hepatitis C involves the use of pegylated interferon-α, with or without ribavirin.[81] However, interferon-α often causes irreversible renal allograft rejection. Therefore, treatment of hepatitis C after transplantation with such a protocol is typically not undertaken. Treatment of such patients should be considered before transplantation. However, ribavirin can cause life-threatening hemolysis in patients with renal failure in whom it is contraindicated.

Patients who have hepatitis B, hepatitis C, or both should be monitored indefinitely for development of HCC with liver imaging (ultrasound, magnetic resonance imaging (MRI)), α-fetoprotein determinations, assessment of viral load, and liver function tests.

Immunization for hepatitis A and B should be considered for those at risk.

Abstinence from alcohol is recommended for those with hepatitis. Prolonged reduction of azathioprine in recipients with chronic hepatitis has been said neither to alter the course of the liver disease nor to predispose to graft failure, but complete cessation of azathioprine may be followed by decreased graft function or failure. The effect of reduced mycophenolate mofetil dosage on graft function in patients with hepatitis B or C has not been reported. However, because these purine antagonist immunosuppressants, and possibly calcineurin inhibitors also, may promote viral replication, conservative use of immunosuppressive drugs should be employed whenever possible.

Gastrointestinal diseases

Perforation of the colon can now be managed with low mortality and often maintenance of allograft function when there is a high clinical index of suspicion, prompt exteriorization of the perforated colon, reduction of immunosuppression to minimal levels, and appropriate antibiotic coverage. In a series of 1000 renal transplants, the incidence of colon perforations was 1.1%. More than one-half of the cases of perforation of the colon occur within 3 months of renal transplantation. Diverticulitis was the cause in approximately 70%, with smaller contributions from iatrogenic factors, ischemia, impaction, and colonic ulcers and colitis. The key factors for successful management are prompt surgical and antiobiotc therapy, minimization of immunosuppression, and support of the patient and allograft with the equivalent of about 15 mg/day of prednisone.

A variety of gastrointestinal symptoms occur with cyclosporine, mycophenolate mofetil, and sirolimus, particularly diarrhea with the last two. Early endoscopy of the upper and lower intestinal tract is often necessary to clarify the issue. If *Helicobacter pylori* is identified as the etiologic agent in a peptic ulcer, a 2-week course of two antibiotics (e.g. amoxicillin 1000 mg b.i.d. and clarithromycin 500 mg b.i.d.) and lansoprazole 30 mg b.i.d. is recommended. Clarithromycin can increase blood levels of immunosuppressants metabolized by CYP450.

Musculoskeletal disorders

Osteoporosis

Many renal transplant recipients have unrecognized osteopenia or osteoporosis at transplantation. Compounding that problem is the fact that "as many as 60% of renal transplant recipients treated with corticosteroids may lose sufficient bone mineral density to meet the definition of osteoporosis in the first 18 months after transplantation."[1] By 6 months after renal transplant, patients receiving therapy with cyclosporine, azathioprine, and low-dose prednisone had a 2.8% decrease in the bone mineral density (BMD) of the lumbar vertebrae (cancellous bone) and a 4.2% decrease in the BMD of the femoral neck.[82] Once the prednisone dose was < 7.5 mg/day, subsequent decreases in BMD appeared to parallel those for age-matched individuals.[83]

At a mean follow-up of 8.1 years after renal transplantation, annual BMD loss was 1.75% compared with normal annual bone loss of 0.5% per year for females before and 1% per year for females after menopause. Twenty years after transplantation, osteoporosis was present in 41%, severe osteopenia in 15%, moderate osteopenia in 15%, mild osteopenia in 8%, and normal BMD in 21%.[84] Subnormal testosterone levels were seen in nearly one-half of the males with significant BMD loss.

Cumulative steroid dose and female sex are independent risk factors for low vertebral BMD.[85] Hyperparathyroidism (HPT), hypogonadism in males, postmenopausal state in females, diabetes mellitus, and metabolic acidosis secondary to graft dysfunction, but not the cumulative dose of cyclosporine, are risk factors for osteoporosis.

Spontaneous fractures occur frequently in transplant recipients. Severe neuropathic bone and joint destruction (Charcot's joint), usually in the tarsal and metatarsal joints, may develop insidiously and present with ankle and pedal edema and unstable gait.

In addition to treating specific contributing factors, such as female or male hormone deficiencies, treatment begins with the appropriate use of calcium and vitamin D supplements; in the case of osteoporosis or possibly even severe osteopenia, oral bisphosphonates such as alendronate or risedronate, or calcitonin as a nasal spray, may be added to the treatment regimen. Alendronate and risedronate may reduce fracture rates by more than 40%.[86] Avoiding cigarette smoking, excessive alcohol and caffeine intake, treating hypocalcemia and vitamin D deficiency, and an exercise program are mainstays of therapy. Basic requirements for males are 1000 mg of elemental calcium and 400 international units (IU) of vitamin D daily; for those over 50 years of age, the supplemental dose of calcium is increased to 1200 mg; and for those over 70 years of age, vitamin D is increased to 600 IU. Women who are premenopausal and not pregnant require 1000 mg/day of elemental calcium, which increases to 1500 mg/day if they are postmenopausal and not taking estrogens.[87] Frank osteoporosis, and possibly severe osteopenia, are usually treated with one of the oral bisphosphonates: alendronate in doses of 10 mg/day, or 70 mg/week, or risedronate at doses of 5 mg/day, or 35 mg/week. Alendronate and risedronate should be taken while upright, with 170–230 mL water, at least 30 min before the first food or medication. The patient should not chew or suck on the tablet because of potential mucosal irritation and should not lie down for at least 30 min thereafter. Bisphosphonates should not be given in the presence of hypocalcemia or in patients with a creatinine clearance < 35 mL/min because of lack of study data. Oral bisphosphonates should be avoided in those with symptomatic upper gastrointestinal tract disease or delayed gastric emptying. Calcium-, magnesium-, and aluminum-containing medications interfere with the absorption of the bisphosphonates and should be taken several hours apart. Intravenous pamidronate 0.5 mg/kg at the time of transplant and 1 month later,[88] and intravenous ibandronate in four doses at 3-month intervals, have been used to prevent osteoporosis.[89] A short-term study of prophylactic intravenous pamidronate demonstrated protection against the reduction of BMD.[88] Among side-effects reported with alendronate and risedronate are dysphasia, esophagitis, and esophageal and gastric ulcers. Side-effects of pamidronate include hypocalcemia, febrile reactions, and collapsing focal segmental glomerulosclerosis reported in seven patients receiving high doses in the course of treatment for malignancy.[90] Bisphosphonates may aggravate preexisting low-turnover bone disease and hyperparathyroidism.[89] Etidronate, a nonnitrogen-containing bisphosphonate, must be used in a cyclical fashion in order to reduce the risk of bone demineralization. Calcitonin nasal spray (200 IU/day) reduced new vertebral fractures by 33% in 1255 postmenopausal osteoporotic women.[85] Side-effects of calcitonin include allergy and nasal irritation. Raloxifene, a selective estrogen receptor modifier for postmenopausal women (60 mg/day), reduces vertebral fractures by 30%.[86] Side-effects include flushing and hot flashes, leg cramps, and thromboembolic events.

Hyperparathyroidism (HPT)

HPT may contribute to osteoporosis, osteitis fibrosa, lytic lesions (Brown tumors), pathologic fractures, ectopic calcifications, and calciphylaxis. Parathyroid function may return to normal if the allograft functions well. Persistent secondary HPT may occur if the parathyroid glands had developed nodular hyperplasia and/or if renal allograft function is impaired.[91] After transplantation, improvement in HPT may be seen in about 50% of patients.

Indications for parathyroidectomy have generally been the occurrence of acute hypercalcemia > 12.5 mg/dL in the immediate post-transplant period, asymptomatic hypercalcemia > 12 mg/dL persisting for more than 1 year after transplantation, and symptomatic hypercalcemia.[92] During a 29-year period, only 38 of 4344 renal transplant recipients required parathyroidectomy for tertiary HPT, at a mean of 2.7 years after transplantation.[92] Calcimimetic agents that directly inhibit PTH secretion by activating calcium-sensing receptors in the parathyroid glands are currently being tested in hemodialysis patients.[93]

Avascular necrosis (AVN)

When glucocorticoids were the major immunosuppressant, the prevalence of AVN was 3–41%, but in the cyclosporine era it has generally been < 5%. Risk factors for AVN include cadaver transplants, repeat transplants, frequent acute rejections, alcohol consumption, glucocorticoids, and osteoporosis.

The weight-bearing long bones are the most frequently affected sites. Diagnosis is confirmed by MRI.

Initial conservative measures for the hip include avoidance of weight-bearing. Orthopedic surgical procedures for AVN include core decompression before collapse of the femoral head, and total hip replacement for more extensive disease. Once the disease has occurred, an abrupt decrease or discontinuation of glucocorticoids does not appear to be helpful and may jeopardize the allograft.

A syndrome of severe, episodic bone pain involving primarily both knees and ankles that is often worse at night and in recumbency has been associated with the use of cyclosporine.[94] The pain often responds to calcium channel blockers, but a small number of patients may develop AVN in the affected knee.

Gout

In patients receiving cyclosporine, the prevalence of hyperuricemia is 30–80%, and 2–28% develop symptomatic gout. In the precyclosporine era, hyperuricemia developed in 19–55%, and gout occurred in 0–8% within 10 years of transplantation but increased to 23% after 20 years.[84] The diagnosis of acute gout can be made with a good history, physical examination, and, in certain cases, joint aspiration and examination of the fluid for monosodium urate crystals in polymorphonuclear leukocytes. Glucocorticoids may mute the full expression of acute gout.

A modified protocol for the use of colchicine in the treatment of acute gout in stable renal transplant recipients is shown in Table 92.7[95] and tophaceous gout in Table 92.8.[95] Allopurinol alone over time may help to reduce the frequency of acute attacks. Colchicine may cause myoneuropathy with elevated serum creatine kinase particularly when used for long periods in patients with impaired renal function on receiving statins. Other treatments for acute gout include nonsteroidal anti-inflammatory drugs that have considerable risk in renal

Table 92.7 A modified protocol for colchicine in the treatment of acute gout in stable renal transplant recipients

Day 1	Colchicine 0.6 mg orally q1h × 2 maximum, but stop if any dose causes diarrhea
Day 2	Colchicine 0.6 mg orally q1h × 2 maximum, but stop if any dose causes diarrhea
Day 3–9	Colchicine 0.6 mg orally once daily, but stop if diarrhea occurs

Note: The objective is to terminate the acute painful inflammatory joint symptoms while minimizing the risk of toxicity. One should be thoroughly familiar with each patient's drug sensitivities and with other potential side-effects, including myopathy, neuropathy, alopecia, myelosuppression, and rarely fatality, and with drug interactions, especially with immunosuppressants. Lower doses or drug avoidance are necessary for those with a glomerular filtration rate (GFR) < 50 mL/min per1.73 m^2. The risks and benefits of treatment, alternative treatment, or nontreatment must be carefully evaluated for each patient. Prudent clinical judgment and careful monitoring are essential. Also adjust allopurinol, azathioprine, diuretics, and diet as needed.
(From reference 91, with permission from Elsevier Science.)

Table 92.8 A modified protocol for managing tophaceous gout in stable renal transplant recipients

For patients on azathioprine
  Allopurinol 50 mg/day; azathioprine reduced by 50–75% (no more than 50 mg/day)
  Monitor complete blood count, liver, and renal function
  Reduce or eliminate diuretic, if possible; diet as needed
For patients on mycophenolate mofetil
  Allopurinol 100 mg/day
  Monitor complete blood count, liver, and renal function
  Reduce or eliminate diuretic if possible; diet as needed
  Ultrasound of renal allograft for obstruction or stones; treat as indicated
Urine alkalinization to pH of ~ 6.5–7.0*
Appropriate hydration
If GFR is > 50 mL/min per 1.73 m^2, probenecid 250 mg twice per day may be initiated
If no side-effects or toxicity are encountered, one may cautiously increase allopurinol and continue close monitoring

Note: The objective is to decrease urate deposits while minimizing drug toxicity or damage to the allograft. One should be thoroughly familiar with each patient's drug sensitivities and with the potentially serious side-effects of each component of treatment, medications, and fluids, including the broad range that may be seen with allopurinol and probenecid. One should also be aware of any potential drug interactions, especially with immunosuppressants. With impaired renal function (GFR < 50 mL/min per 1.73 m^2), azathioprine doses are often reduced, and allopurinol and probenecid may need to be avoided entirely. The risks and benefits of treatment, alternative treatment, or nontreatment must be carefully evaluated for each patient. Prudent clinical judgement and careful monitoring are essential.
*Approaches to alkalinize the urine (and some of their risks) when clinically safe include the use of potassium citrate (hyperkalemia, alkalosis); sodium citrate, sodium bicarbonate (hypertension, fluid retention, possibly nephrolithiasis), and acetazolamide (paresthesiae, renal stone) may be more problematic.
(From reference 91, with permission from Elsevier Science.)

transplant recipients[58] by reducing the GFR, causing hyperkalemia, and at times interstitial nephritis, or proteinuria with minimal change in the disease. The new cyclooxygenase 2 inhibitors have not been reported as being safer. Glucocorticoids may be used for an acute gouty attack[58] at doses in the range 0.5–1.0 mg/kg of prednisone for 3–7 days with tapering to the maintenance dose within 14 days.[58] Adrenocorticotrophic hormone (ACTH) 40–80 IUs given intramuscularly has also been used.[58] It may be appropriate to substitute mycophenolate mofetil for azathioprine to permit higher doses of allopurinol. Similarly, a change from cyclosporine to another immunosuppressant not having adverse renal hemodynamic and hyperuricemic effects may be appropriate. Losartan has a uricosuric effect that is not extended to other members of its ARB class. Diuretics should be avoided or used in reduced doses.

Hypophosphatemia

Hypophosphatemia may be caused by massive diuresis immediately post transplantation, by persistence of secondary hyperparathyroidism early post transplantation, and later by defective renal phosphate reabsorption, glycosuria, glucocorticoid therapy inhibiting proximal tubular reabsorption of phosphate, and even the inadvertent use of phosphate binders as antacids. Complications of severe hypophosphatemia include rhabdomyolysis, impaired left ventricular function and possibly ventricular arrhythmias, impaired pulmonary function presumably related to respiratory muscle impairment, defects in erythrocyte metabolism with possible hemolysis, insulin resistance, osteomalacia, and renal tubular defects resembling Fanconi syndrome. Oral supplementation with phosphorus-containing compounds may be needed.

Hypomagnesemia

Cyclosporine, tacrolimus, and sirolimus may cause renal magnesium wasting and hypomagnesemia. Magnesium depletion is associated with intracellular calcium overload, cardiac arrhythmias, and changes in the coronary vasculature similar to those seen in accelerated atherosclerosis, neurologic, and gastrointestinal symptoms. The hypomagnesemia caused by cyclosporine is typically not accompanied by hypocalcemia or hypokalemia. Oral replacement is with magnesium oxide (400 mg) once or twice daily.

Ocular disease

The most common ocular complication in glucocorticoid-treated renal transplant recipients is posterior subcapsular cataracts, occurring in about 10%. Patients may require cataract surgery and lens implantation. It is important to inquire regularly about the state of the patient's vision in transplant follow-up visits, to evaluate the presence of a cataract with a standard ophthalmoscope at a +10-diopter setting, and to encourage regular ophthalmologic exams.

Regular ophthalmologic examinations are essential for diabetic recipients of renal transplants. Allograft recipients who develop CMV disease should have an ophthalmologic examination to detect CMV retinitis, which may require more extensive treatment (see Infectious complications after renal transplantation). Herpetic keratoconjunctivitis, toxoplasmosis retinitis, ophthalmic herpes zoster, and enophthalmitis are conditions requiring urgent treatment by an experienced ophthalmologist and infectious disease specialist.

Psychiatric illnesses

Depression after renal transplantation is common. Discussions with the patient's family may help to reveal problems with alcohol or substance abuse, sleep disturbances, and compliance with medication. Collaborative treatment with psychiatric care is indicated. Medications prescribed mostly by psychiatrists may (1) have side-effects that overlap with those of major immunosuppressants or resemble other disease states (e.g. selective serotonin uptake inhibitors causing tremor, diarrhea, weight gain and edema with prolonged use, and platelet dysfunction and bleeding; venlafaxine causing dose-dependent increases in blood pressure); (2) require dose adjustment because of impaired renal function (e.g. gabapentin, venlafaxine, and mirtazapine); or (3) be metabolized significantly by hepatic CYP3A4 and affect levels of cyclosporine, tacrolimus, and sirolimus as well as other drugs (see Hyperlipidemia) that share the same pathway (e.g. nephazodone) (see Chapter 67).[96]

References

1. Kasiske BL, Vazquez MA, Harmon WE, et al: Recommendations for the outpatient surveillance of renal transplant recipients. American Society of Transplantation. J Am Soc Nephrol 2000;11 (Suppl 15):S1–S86.
2. Kasiske BL: Risk factors for accelerated atherosclerosis in renal transplant recipients. Am J Med 1988;84:985–992.
3. Kasiske BL, Chakkera HA, Roel J: Explained and unexplained ischemic heart disease risk after renal transplantation. J Am Soc Nephrol 2000;11:1735–1743.
4. Herzog CA, Ma JZ, Collins AJ: Long-term survival of renal transplant recipients in the United States after acute myocardial infarction. Am J Kidney Dis 2000;36:145–152.
5. Kasiske BL, Guijarro C, Massy ZA, et al: Cardiovascular disease after renal transplantation. J Am Soc Nephrol 1996;7:158–165.
6. Gerstein HC, Mann JF, Yi Q, et al: Albuminuria and risk of cardiovascular events, death, and heart failure in diabetic and nondiabetic individuals. JAMA 2001;286:421–426.
7. Mann JF, Gerstein HC, Pogue J, et al: Renal insufficiency as a predictor of cardiovascular outcomes and the impact of ramipril: the HOPE randomized trial. Ann Intern Med 2001;134:629–636.
8. Ridker PM, Rifai N, Clearfield M, et al: Measurement of C-reactive protein for the targeting of statin therapy in the primary prevention of acute coronary events. N Engl J Med 2001;344:1959–1965.
9. Wilson PW, D'Agostino RB, Levy D, et al: Prediction of coronary heart disease using risk factor categories. Circulation 1998;97:1837–1847.
10. Executive Summary of The Third Report of The National Cholesterol Education Program (NCEP) Expert Panel on Detection, Evaluation, And Treatment of High Blood Cholesterol In Adults (Adult Treatment Panel III). JAMA 2001;285:2486–2497.
11. Massy ZA, Kasiske BL: Posttransplant hyperlipidemia: mechanisms and management. J Am Soc Nephrol 1996;7:971–977.
12. Ligtenberg G, Hene RJ, Blankestijn PJ, et al: Cardiovascular risk factors in renal transplant patients: cyclosporin A versus tacrolimus. J Am Soc Nephrol 2001;12:368–373.
13. Saunders RN, Metcalfe MS, Nicholson ML: Rapamycin in transplantation: a review of the evidence. Kidney Int 2001;59:3–16.
14. Podder H, Stepkowski SM, Napoli KL, et al: Pharmacokinetic interactions augment toxicities of sirolimus/cyclosporine combinations. J Am Soc Nephrol 2001;12:1059–1071.
15. Chong PH, Seeger JD, Franklin C: Clinically relevant differences between the statins: implications for therapeutic selection. Am J Med 2001;111:390–400.
16. Westphal S, Dierkes J, Luley C: Effects of fenofibrate and gemfibrozil on plasma homocysteine. Lancet 2001;358:39–40.
17. Glorioso N, Troffa C, Filigheddu F, et al: Effect of the HMG-CoA reductase inhibitors on blood pressure in patients with essential hypertension and primary hypercholesterolemia. Hypertension 1999;34:1281–1286.
18. Katznelson S: Immunosuppressive and antiproliferative effects of HMG-CoA reductase inhibitors. Transplant Proc 1999;31:22S–24S.
19. Vrtovsnik F, Couette S, Prie D, et al: Lovastatin-induced inhibitions of renal epithelial cell proliferation involves a p21 ras activated, AP-1-dependent pathway. Kidney Int 1997;52:1016–1027.
20. Jindal RM: Posttransplant diabetes mellitus: a review. Transplantation 1994;58:1289–1298.
21. Cosio FG, Pesavento TE, Osei K, et al: Post-transplant diabetes mellitus: increasing incidence in renal allograft recipients transplanted in recent years. Kidney Int 2001;59:732–737.
22. Williams ME: Management of the diabetic transplant recipient. Kidney Int 1995;48:1660–1674.
23. Barbosa J, Steffes MW, Sutherland DE, et al: Effect of glycemic control on early diabetic renal lesions. A 5-year randomized controlled clinical trial of insulin-dependent diabetic kidney transplant recipients. JAMA 1994;272:600–606.
24. Lewis EJ, Hunsicker LG, Clarke WR, et al: Renoprotective effect of the angiotensin-receptor antagonist irbesartan in patients with nephropathy due to type 2 diabetes. N Engl J Med 2001;345:851–860.

25. Brenner BM, Cooper ME, de Zeeuw D, et al: Effects of losartan on renal and cardiovascular outcomes in patients with type 2 diabetes and nephropathy. N Engl J Med 2001;345:861–869.

26. Yusuf S, Gerstein H, Hoogwerf B, et al: Ramipril and the development of diabetes. JAMA 2001;286:1882–1885.

27. Schepkens H, Vanholder R, Billiouw JM, et al: Life-threatening hyperkalemia during combined therapy with angiotensin-converting enzyme inhibitors and spironolactone: an analysis of 25 cases. Am J Med 2001;110:438–441.

28. Kasiske BL, Klinger D: Cigarette smoking in renal transplant recipients. J Am Soc Nephrol 2000;11:753–759.

29. Orth SR, Ritz E, Schrier RW: The renal risks of smoking. Kidney Int 1997;51:1669–1677.

30. Ritz E, Benck U, Franek E, et al: Effects of smoking on renal hemodynamics in healthy volunteers and in patients with glomerular disease. J Am Soc Nephrol 1998;9:1798–1804.

31. Manson JE, Ajani UA, Liu S, et al: A prospective study of cigarette smoking and the incidence of diabetes mellitus among US male physicians. Am J Med 2000;109:538–542.

32. DeNelsky GY, Bower ME: Smoking cessation in cardiac preventive health. In Robinson K (ed): Preventive Cardiology. Armonk, NY: Futura Publishing Co., 1998, pp 325–353.

33. Fiore MC, Bailey WC, Cohen SJ, et al: Treating tobacco use and dependence. In Quick Reference Guide for Clinicians. Rockville, MD: US Department of Health and Human Services, October, 2000.

34. Helge TD, Denelsky GY: Pharmacologic aids to smoking cessation. Cleve Clin J Med 2000;67:818, 821–818, 824.

35. Jorenby DE, Leischow SJ, Nides MA, et al: A controlled trial of sustained-release bupropion, a nicotine patch, or both for smoking cessation. N Engl J Med 1999;340:685–691.

36. Hays JT, Hurt RD, Rigotti NA, et al: Sustained-release bupropion for pharmacologic relapse prevention after smoking cessation. A randomized, controlled trial. Ann Intern Med 2001;135:423–433.

37. Bostom AG, Shemin D, Gohh RY, et al: Treatment of hyperhomocysteinemia in hemodialysis patients and renal transplant recipients. Kidney Int 2001;59 (Suppl 78):S246–S252.

38. Boushey CJ, Beresford SA, Omenn GS, et al: A quantitative assessment of plasma homocysteine as a risk factor for vascular disease. Probable benefits of increasing folic acid intakes. JAMA 1995;274:1049–1057.

39. Eikelboom JW, Lonn E, Genest J Jr, et al: Homocyst(e)ine and cardiovascular disease: a critical review of the epidemiologic evidence. Ann Intern Med 1999;131:363–375.

40. Welch GN, Loscalzo J: Homocysteine and atherothrombosis. N Engl J Med 1998;338:1042–1050.

41. Arnadottir M, Hultberg B, Wahlberg J, et al: Serum total homocysteine concentration before and after renal transplantation. Kidney Int 1998;54:1380–1384.

42. Friedman AN, Bostom AG, Selhub J, et al: The kidney and homocysteine metabolism. J Am Soc Nephrol 2001;12:2181–2189.

43. Lee TH, Boucher CA: Clinical practice. Noninvasive tests in patients with stable coronary artery disease. N Engl J Med 2001;344:1840–1845.

44. Braun WE, Marwick TH: Coronary artery disease in renal transplant recipients. Cleve Clin J Med 1994;61:370–385.

45. Detrano RC, Wong ND, Doherty TM, et al: Coronary calcium does not accurately predict near-term future coronary events in high-risk adults. Circulation 1999;99:2633–2638.

46. He ZX, Hedrick TD, Pratt CM, et al: Severity of coronary artery calcification by electron beam computed tomography predicts silent myocardial ischemia. Circulation 2000;101:244–251.

47. Grundy SM: Primary prevention of coronary heart disease: integrating risk assessment with intervention. Circulation 1999;100:988–998.

48. Block GA, Port FK: Re-evaluation of risks associated with hyperphosphatemia and hyperparathyroidism in dialysis patients: recommendations for a change in management. Am J Kidney Dis 2000;35:1226–1237.

49. Kullo IJ, Edwards WD, Schwartz RS: Vulnerable plaque: pathobiology and clinical implications. Ann Intern Med 1998;129:1050–1060.

50. Sousa JE, Costa MA, Abizaid A, et al: Lack of neointimal proliferation after implantation of sirolimus-coated stents in human coronary arteries: a quantitative coronary angiography and three-dimensional intravascular ultrasound study. Circulation 2001;103:192–195.

51. Ferguson ER, Hudson SL, Diethelm AG, et al: Outcome after myocardial revascularization and renal transplantation: a 25-year single-institution experience. Ann Surg 1999;230:232–241.

52. Dresler C, Uthoff K, Wahlers T, et al: Open heart operations after renal transplantation. Ann Thorac Surg 1997;63:143–146.

53. Herzog CA, Ma JZ, Collins A: Three-year survival of renal transplant recipients in the US after coronary artery bypass surgery, coronary angioplasty, and coronary stenting. J Am Soc Nephrol 2001;11:719A.

54. Kagami S, Border WA, Miller DE, et al: Angiotensin II stimulates extracellular matrix protein synthesis through induction of transforming growth factor-beta expression in rat glomerular mesangial cells. J Clin Invest 1994;93:2431–2437.

55. Monton M, Castilla MA, Alvarez Arroyo MV, et al: Effects of angiotensin II on endothelial cell growth: role of AT-1 and AT-2 receptors. J Am Soc Nephrol 1998;9:969–974.

56. Pitt B, Zannad F, Remme WJ, et al: The effect of spironolactone on morbidity and mortality in patients with severe heart failure. Randomized Aldactone Evaluation Study Investigators. N Engl J Med 1999;341:709–717.

57. Borghi C, Prandin MG, Costa FV, et al: Use of statins and blood pressure control in treated hypertensive patients with hypercholesterolemia. J Cardiovasc Pharmacol 2000;35:549–555.

58. Clive DM: Renal transplant-associated hyperuricemia and gout. J Am Soc Nephrol 2000;11:974–979.

59. Cohn JN, Tognoni G: A randomized trial of the angiotensin-receptor blocker valsartan in chronic heart failure. N Engl J Med 2001;345:1667–1675.

60. Selhub J, Jacques PF, Bostom AG, et al: Association between plasma homocysteine concentrations and extracranial carotid-artery stenosis. N Engl J Med 1995;332:286–291.

61. Fassbender K, Mielke O, Bertsch T, et al: Homocysteine in cerebral macroangiography and microangiopathy. Lancet 1999;353:1586–1587.

62. Executive Committee for the Asymptomatic Carotid Atherosclerosis Study. Endarterectomy for asymptomatic carotid artery stenosis. JAMA 1995;273:1421–1428.

63. Kasiske BL, Ramos EL, Gaston RS, et al: The evaluation of renal transplant candidates: clinical practice guidelines. Patient Care and Education Committee of the American Society of Transplant Physicians. J Am Soc Nephrol 1995;6:1–34.

64. Manske CL, Wilson RF, Wang Y, et al: Atherosclerotic vascular complications in diabetic transplant candidates. Am J Kidney Dis 1997;29:601–607.

65. Braun WE, Avery R, Gifford RW Jr, et al: Life after 20 years with a kidney transplant: redefined disease profiles and an emerging nondiabetic vasculopathy. Transplant Proc 1997;29:247–249.

66. Hiatt WR: Medical treatment of peripheral arterial disease and claudication. N Engl J Med 2001;344:1608–1621.

67. Tepel M, van der GM, Schwarzfeld C, et al: Prevention of radiographic-contrast-agent-induced reductions in renal function by acetylcysteine. N Engl J Med 2000;343:180–184.

68. Danovitch GM, Jamgotchian NJ, Eggena PH, et al: Angiotensin-converting enzyme inhibition in the treatment of renal transplant erythrocytosis. Clinical experience and observation of mechanism. Transplantation 1995;60:132–137.

69. Mrug M, Stopka T, Julian BA, et al: Angiotensin II stimulates proliferation of normal early erythroid progenitors. J Clin Invest 1997;100:2310–2314.

70. Gupta M, Miller BA, Ahsan N, et al: Expression of angiotensin II type I receptor on erythroid progenitors of patients with post transplant erythrocytosis. Transplantation 2000;70:1188–1194.

71. Penn I: Cancers in cyclosporine-treated vs azathioprine-treated patients. Transplant Proc 1996;28:876–878.

72. Penn I: The effect of immunosuppression on pre-existing cancers. Transplantation 1993;55:742–747.

73. Penn I: Neoplasm following transplantation. In Norman DJ, Turka LA (eds): Primer on Transplantation. Mt Laurel, NJ: American Society of Transplantation, 2001, pp 268–275.

74. Suzan F, Ammor M, Ribrag V: Fatal reactivation of cytomegalovirus infection after use of rituximab for a post-transplantation lymphoproliferative disorder. N Engl J Med 2001;345:1000.

75. Penn I: Tumors after renal and cardiac transplantation. Hematol Oncol Clin North Am 1993;7:431–445.

76. Berg D, Otley CC: Skin cancer in organ transplant recipients: epidemiology, pathogenesis, and management. J Am Acad Dermatol 2002;47:1–17.

77. Debure A, Degos F, Pol S, et al: Liver diseases and hepatic complications in renal transplant patients. Adv Nephrol 1988;17:375–400.

78. Rao KV, Anderson WR, Kasiske BL, et al: Value of liver biopsy in the evaluation and management of chronic liver disease in renal transplant recipients. Am J Med 1993;94:241–250.
79. Fornairon S, Pol S, Legendre C, et al: The long-term virologic and pathologic impact of renal transplantation on chronic hepatitis-B virus infection. Transplantation 1996;62:297–299.
80. Mathurin P, Mouquet C, Poynard T, et al: Impact of hepatitis B and C virus on kidney transplantation outcome. Hepatology 1999;29:257–263.
81. Gane E, Pilmore H: Management of chronic viral hepatitis before and after renal transplantation. Transplantation 2002;74:427–437.
82. Kwan JT, Almond MK, Evans K, et al: Changes in total body bone mineral content and regional bone mineral density in renal patients following renal transplantation. Miner Electrolyte Metab 1992;18:166–168.
83. Grotz WH, Mundinger FA, Gugel B, et al: Bone mineral density after kidney transplantation. A cross-sectional study in 190 graft recipients up to 20 years after transplantation. Transplantation 1995;59:982–986.
84. Braun WE, Richmond BJ: Osteoporosis and gout before and after 20 years with a functioning renal transplant. Graft Organ Cell Transplant 1999;2:S119.
85. Wolpaw T, Deal CL, Fleming-Brooks S, et al: Factors influencing vertebral bone density after renal transplantation. Transplantation 1994;58:1186–1189.
86. Maricic MJ, Gluck OS: Osteoporosis: therapeutic options for prevention and management. J Musculoskel Med 2001;18:415–425.
87. Scheiber LB, Torregrosa L: Early intervention for postmenopausal osteoporosis. J Musculoskeletal Med 1999;16:276–285.
88. Fan SL, Almond MK, Ball E, et al: Pamidronate therapy as prevention of bone loss following renal transplantation. Kidney Int 2000;57:684–690.
89. Grotz W, Nagel C, Poeschel D, et al: Effect of ibandronate on bone loss and renal function after kidney transplantation. J Am Soc Nephrol 2001;12:1530–1537.
90. Markowitz GS, Appel GB, Fine PL, et al: Collapsing focal segmental glomerulosclerosis following treatment with high-dose pamidronate. J Am Soc Nephrol 2001;12:1164–1172.
91. Massari PU: Disorders of bone and mineral metabolism after renal transplantation. Kidney Int 1997;52:1412–1421.
92. Kerby JD, Rue LW, Blair H, et al: Operative treatment of tertiary hyperparathyroidism: a single-center experience. Ann Surg 1998;227:878–886.
93. Goodman WG, Hladik GA, Turner SA, et al: The calcimimetic agent AMG073 lowers plasma parathyroid hormone levels in hemodialysis patients with secondary hyperparathyroidism. J Am Soc Nephrol 2002;13:1017–1024.
94. Barbosa LM, Gauthier VJ, Davis CL: Bone pain that responds to calcium channel blockers. A retrospective and prospective study of transplant recipients. Transplantation 1995;59:541–544.
95. Braun WE: Modification of the treatment of gout in renal transplant recipients. Transplant Proc 2000;32:199.
96. Abramowicz M (ed.): Drugs for depression and anxiety. Med Lett 1999;41:33–38.

CHAPTER

93
Prevention and Treatment of Infection in the Kidney Transplant Recipient

Nina E. Tolkoff-Rubin and Robert H. Rubin

Temporal sequence of infection following transplantation
- Infections in the first month post transplant
- One to six months post transplant
  - Viral infections in the kidney transplant recipient
  - The herpes group viruses
  - Cytomegalovirus
  - Epstein–Barr virus-associated lumphoproliferative disorder
  - Herpes simplex viral infection in the renal transplant patient
  - Varicella-zoster virus infection in the renal transplant patient
  - Human herpesvirus 6 infection in the renal transplant patient
  - Hepatitis in the renal transplant patient
  - Community-acquired respiratory viruses in the renal transplant patient
  - Papovaviruses in the renal transplant patient
  - Invasive aspergillosis
  - *Pneumocystis carinii* pneumonia
- More than 6 months post transplant
Summary

As a result of innovations in immunosuppression, increasing understanding of the immunologic mechanisms involved in the rejection process, and improved preventative and curative therapy for key infections, kidney transplantation has been transformed from an experiment in human immunobiology to the most practical means of rehabilitating patients with endstage renal disease of diverse etiologies. One-year graft survival from living donors exceeds 90%, with grafts from cadaveric donors exceeding 85% survival. The two barriers to long-term allograft function remain rejection and infection. What is new, however, is the recognition that these two processes are closely linked, with similar arrays of cytokines, chemokines, and growth factors – the mediators of inflammatory injury – being released by the recipient as a consequence of both rejection and infection. The therapeutic prescription for the transplant patient should always be thought of as having two components: (1) an immunosuppressive regimen to prevent and treat rejection and (2) an antimicrobial strategy, whose nature is determined by the intensity and components of the immunosuppressive approach taken, to make this safe. Certain general principles need to be delineated:[1–5]

1. Prevention of infection is the primary goal of the clinician. Failing that, early recognition and initiation of therapy are necessary if the patient is going to survive microbial invasion. This task is rendered more difficult by the impaired inflammatory response present in most transplant patients, which is a consequence of the anti-rejection approach that is used. As a consequence of immunosuppression, signs and symptoms of infection can be greatly attenuated, thus leading to later diagnosis, at which time the microbial burden can be far higher than that of the normal host. Thus, there is a need for the early utilization of such imaging approaches as chest computed tomographic (CT) studies as well as magnetic resonance imaging (MRI) and positron emission tomography (PET). Similarly, even innocuous-appearing skin lesions, if unexplained, merit biopsy and culture to recognize disseminated infection. In 20–30% of patients with nocardial or fungal infection, skin lesions are the earliest sign of disseminated infection.

2. Drug interactions between antimicrobial agents and the calcineurin inhibitors are of great clinical importance. The calcineurin inhibitors cyclosporine and tacrolimus are metabolized by hepatic cytochrome P450 enzymes and thereby lead to drug interactions:
   a. Upregulation of cyclosporine and tacrolimus metabolism will result in decreased blood levels and an increased risk of rejection unless dosage adjustment of the calcineurin inhibitor is accomplished. Antimicrobial agents having this effect include rifampicin, nafcillin, and isoniazid.
   b. Downregulation of cyclosporine and tacrolimus metabolism will result in increased blood levels, an increased risk of nephrotoxicity, and the possibility of over immunosuppression and an increased risk of infection. Antimicrobial drugs producing this effect are the macrolides (erythromycin > clarithromycin > azithromycin) and the azoles (ketoconazole > itraconazole > voriconazole > fluconazole).
   c. Synergistic nephrotoxicity is defined as the occurrence of nephrotoxicity in a patient with appropriate calcineurin inhibitor blood levels upon the initiation of therapy with one of several antimicrobial agents: amphotericin, aminoglycosides, vancomycin, and high doses of trimethoprim–sulfamethoxazole, fluroquinolones, and pentamadine.

   Whereas the first two of these interactions can be managed by close monitoring of calcineurin inhibitor blood levels and dosage adjustment, synergistic nephrotoxicity can only be prevented by attempting to avoid nephrotoxins and making sure that the patient is euvolemic. In addition, the choice of antimicrobial to be used favors the prescription of advanced spectrum β-lactams, azoles rather than amphotericin, and a renewed emphasis on preventing infection.

3. Antimicrobial therapy in transplantation can be used in four different modes. The first mode is the *prophylactic*,

in which the antimicrobial agent is administered to an entire population before a particular event. This requires an infection that is sufficiently common and/or important to justify such an intervention, and a nontoxic drug that can achieve the desired effect. By far the most effective prophylactic strategy in transplantation is the use of low-dose trimethoprim–sulfamethoxazole, which not only prevents urinary tract infection and urosepsis but also *Pneumocystis carinii* pneumonia, listeriosis, nocardiosis, and toxoplasmosis. The second mode is the *empiric* mode, in which broad-spectrum antimicrobial therapy is administered to patients with fever of unclear origin. There are two major indications for such therapy in febrile organ transplant patients: the presence of leukopenia (a neutrophil count < 500/mm^3) and/or the occurrence of rigors. The third mode is the *preemptive*, in which antimicrobial agents are administered to a subgroup of patients found to be at particularly high risk of clinically important infection due to the presence of certain clinical/epidemiologic or laboratory markers. The aim is to prevent the occurrence of symptomatic disease, and to focus antimicrobial interventions on patients who would most benefit from them. Finally, there is the *therapeutic* mode, in which antimicrobial agents are administered to patients with clinically important infections.

4. The risk of any infection, particularly opportunistic infection, in the transplant patient is determined primarily by the interaction of three factors: *technical/anatomic abnormalities* that lead to tissue infarction, fluid collections, and the requirement for indwelling drains, catheters, and vascular access devices; the *environmental exposures* that the patient encounters; and a complex function termed the *net state of immunosuppression*. If an exposure is great enough, even patients who have received minimal immunosuppression can develop life-threatening infection; witness outbreaks of *Aspergillus* during hospital construction and outbreaks of *Legionella* due to contaminated hospital water supplies. By contrast, if the net state of immunosuppression is sufficiently high, even minor exposure to agents present in the normal environment can cause major infections.

The net state of immunosuppression is determined by the interaction of several factors: any continuing host defense defects that were present prior to the transplant; the dose, duration, and nature of the immunosuppressive therapy (the single most important determinant of the net state of immunosuppression); leukopenia and thrombocytopenia; any process or foreign body that adversely affects the primary mucocutaneous barrier to infection; metabolic abnormalities such as protein–calorie malnutrition and, perhaps, diabetes and uremia; infection with one or more of the immunomodulating viruses, e.g. cytomegalovirus (CMV), Epstein–Barr virus (EBV), hepatitis B and/or C virus (HBV and HCV), and, perhaps, human herpesvirus 6 (HHV-6) and HIV.

The importance of the various contributors to the net state of immunosuppression is illustrated by the following statistics from the Massachusetts General Hospital: if one stratifies transplant patients on the basis of a serum albumin of less than or more than 2.5 g/dL, those who are hypoalbuminemic have a 10-fold increase in the incidence of life-threatening infection. Approximately 90% of patients with opportunistic infection are infected with one or more of the immunomodulating viruses; indeed, the 10% exceptions are usually due to an overwhelming environmental exposure. Table 93.1 provides an overview of the different infections that occur in the transplant population.

Temporal sequence of infection following transplantation

There is an expected temporal sequence (Fig. 93.1) that may then be used in three ways: in the differential diagnosis of a clinical syndrome possibly due to microbial invasion in the individual patient; as a tool for infection control – exceptions to the timetable almost invariably represent environmental contamination that needs to be identified and eliminated; and as a guide for the design and implementation of effective preventative strategies. For renal transplants, it is convenient to divide the post-transplant course into three time periods: the first month, the period 1–6 months post transplant, and the late period > 6 months post transplant.

Infections in the first month post transplant

There are three important categories of infection in the first month post transplant:

1. More than 95% of these infections are the same bacterial and candidal infections of the wound, lungs, urine, surgical drains, and vascular access devices that occur in nonimmunocompromised patients undergoing comparable surgery. The major factor in the pathogenesis of these infections is a technical/anatomic mishap during the transplant operation or peritransplant period that leads to devitalized tissue, a fluid collection (blood, lymph, or urine), and the need for devices (e.g. drainage catheters, vascular access devices, endotracheal tubes) that abridge or compromise the mucocutaneous surfaces of the body that constitute the primary barrier to infection. Although prophylactic antibiotics aimed at urinary tract infection and staphylococci (e.g. cefazolin when patients are called to the operating room and continuing for no more than 24 h) can decrease the incidence of these infections, the major determinant is the technical skill with which the operation is performed and the perioperative care is accomplished. Solid organ transplant recipients are the most unforgiving of all surgical patients when it comes to technical problems in their management, and the presence of these problems almost invariably leads to infection.

2. Uncommonly, the allograft itself is infected, either because of infection in the donor or because of contam-

Table 93.1 Categories of infection in renal transplant recipients

Infections related to the operation
Infections occurring in any surgical patient
  Bacterial or candidal line-associated bloodstream infection
  Bacterial wound infection
  Aspiration pneumonia related to intubation, sedation, etc.
  Urinary tract infections associated with external catheters
Infections related to technical complications of transplantation
  Anastomic leak or breakdown
  Wound or intraabdominal hematoma
  Urinary tract infections related to need for internal drainage devices or stents

Infections conveyed by the allograft
Bloodstream bacterial or fungal infection
Viral
  Hepatitis B and C
  HIV
  Epstein–Barr virus

Urinary tract infections

Opportunistic infections
Viral infections
  Herpesviruses (cytomegalovirus, herpes simplex virus, varicella-zoster virus, Epstein–Barr virus, human herpesvirus 6, Kaposi's sarcoma-associated herpesvirus, or human herpesvirus 8)
  Hepatitis viruses
  Human papillomaviruses
  HIV
Infections due to nosocomial exposure
  Aspergillus sp.
  Legionella sp.
  Resistant bacteria
    Pseudomonas aeruginosa and other Gram-negative rods
    Methicillin-resistant *Staphylococcus aureus*
    Vancomycin-resistant *Enterococcus*
Infections due to community exposure
  Endemic fungal infections
    Histoplasma capsulatum
    Coccidioides immitis
    Blastomyces dermatitidis
  Other environmental saprophytes
    Cryptococcus neoformans
    Aspergillus sp.
    Nocardia asteroides
    Pneumocystis carinii
  Infections acquired by ingestion of contaminated food or water
    Salmonella sp.
    Listeria monocytogenes
    Strongyloides stercoralis
  Mycobacterium tuberculosis and other mycobacteria

Community-acquired respiratory tract infections
Influenza, parainfluenza, adenovirus, and respiratory syncytial virus
Legionella sp.

ination from handling prior to organ implantation. There are three types of donor infection that have an impact on the recipient:
a. Chronic infection with hepatitis viruses and HIV and latent infection with *Mycobacterium tuberculosis*, the

endemic mycoses (blastomycosis, coccidioidomycosis, and histoplasmosis), and CMV. The efficiency of transmitting replicating virus (HBV, HCV, or HIV) from the donor via the allograft approaches 100%, so careful serologic screening of the donor for these infections

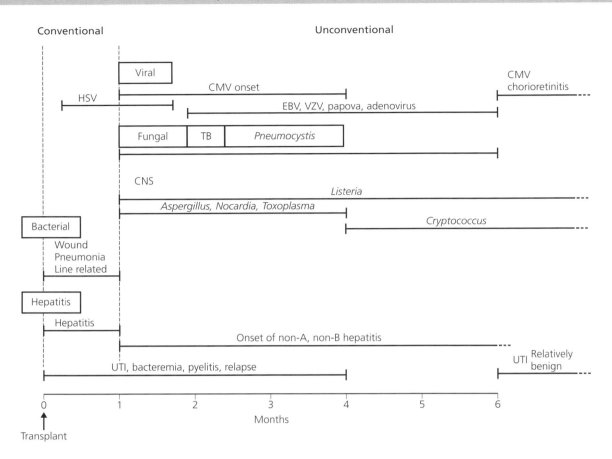

Figure 93.1 Temporal sequence of infection after renal transplantation. (From Rubin RH: Infection in the organ transplant recipient. *In* Rubin RH, Young LS (eds): Clinical Approach to Infection in the Compromised Host, 3rd edn. New York: Plenum Medical Book Co., 1994.)

is essential. Latent tuberculosis or mycotic infection within the allograft has been described. Latent CMV is a real issue, and knowing the serologic status of the donor and recipient will help to determine the preventative strategies that will be employed post transplant.[1–4]

b. Acute infection that was responsible for the patient's demise. The critical determination is whether this infection will be conveyed with the allograft. For example, it is now clear that such processes as meningococcal and pneumococcal meningitis may be lethal for an individual, but, provided that appropriate bactericidal antibiotic therapy has been administered for > 3 days, consideration of this individual as a possible donor is not unreasonable.[6]

c. The biggest concern regarding donor-related infection is acute infection associated with the intensive care unit exposure that many cadaveric donors receive before they are deemed potential donors. Thus, infection of vascular access devices and/or urinary catheter-related infection can contaminate the allograft. In particular, bacteremia and candidemia at the time of organ harvest can contaminate the allograft and threaten the vascular suture line, potentially leading to a mycotic aneurysm and catastrophic rupture.

Although a recent report suggested that donor bacteremia was not a major problem, it must be stressed that virulent organisms, such as *Pseudomonas aeruginosa* or *Staphylococcus aureus*, are a significant risk.[6–12]

3. Finally, infections that were present pretransplant, which may be made more serious by the surgery and posttransplant immunosuppression. Of particular concern are bacteremia and candidemia at the time of transplant (again threatening the vascular suture line), pneumonia or other forms of lung injury (chemical injury to aspiration or pulmonary infarction), and urinary tract infection. Lung injury of any type is at risk of Gram-negative or fungal superinfection, and should be allowed to heal before transplanting the patient. Patients with chronic viral infection (e.g. hepatitis) should undergo a full evaluation prior to transplant, including liver biopsy, since posttransplant immunosuppression will amplify the extent of these viral processes.[1–6,13]

From these basic principles, the approach to fever and possible infection in this first month can be derived. Diagnostically, a complete blood count (CBC) for neutropenia, urinalysis and urine culture, and two sets of blood cultures are drawn. If sputum is available, a Gram stain and culture are appropriate. A standard chest radiograph is indicated, particularly in patients who have been oversedated or who have been vomiting. Chest CT is appropriate in the face of symptoms referable to the lung or ongoing fevers that are not well explained by the conventional chest film. All vascular access devices should be removed and replaced with fresh sticks (i.e. not changed over a wire). Finally, an ultrasound of the allograft should be performed to look for a local leak or significant fluid collection. Even without a recognized technical complication, the presence of such a collection in someone without a convincing alternative explanation for fever should prompt aspiration for culture. Infected collections require percutaneous or surgical drainage and antimicrobial therapy. Since the advent of cyclosporine and tacrolimus, allograft rejection in adults has become an uncommon cause of fever; however, in children, fever may be the first sign of rejection.

The most common form of bacterial infection in the first few months post transplant has traditionally been a urinary tract infection (UTI). The need for bladder catheters in the first several days post transplant and the trauma to the kidney that occurs with harvesting, transport, and implantation, as well as possible immunologic trauma, account for a reported incidence of UTI of 35–79%. In addition, a UTI in the first few months after transplant is frequently associated with signs of pyelonephritis, bacteremia, and a high rate of relapse when treated with a standard course of antibiotics. Fortunately, UTI (and urosepsis) has been virtually eliminated by oral prophylaxis with either low-dose trimethoprim–sulfamethoxazole (TMP/SMX) at a dose of one single-strength tablet at bedtime or ciprofloxacin at a dose of 250 mg at bedtime for 6–12 months post transplant. TMP/SMX has the added advantage of providing effective prophylaxis against *P. carinii*, *Nocardia asteroides*, *Listeria monocytogenes*, *Toxoplasma gondii*, and *Salmonella* species. In a small percentage of patients, UTIs recur after the highest risk period and after routine prophylaxis has been completed. This should prompt a search for anatomic factors predisposing to infection, such as nephrolithiasis, prostatic hypertrophy, bladder outlet obstruction, or urodynamic problems. If no correctable problem is identified, long-term prophylaxis should be considered.[14–18]

Fungal infections in this period are typically caused by *Candida* species (especially *Candida albicans*). *Candida* species are found in the gastrointestinal tract, on the skin, and in the vagina, and both colonization and disease are increased in diabetics and patients on preoperative antibiotics or immunosuppressants. Candidal infections are sufficiently common to warrant prophylaxis. Topical therapy, such as clotrimazole troches 10 mg orally twice a day or nystatin suspension 3 mL swish and swallow orally twice a day, is recommended during the first 6 months after transplantation but also during times when increased immunosuppressants or antibiotics are used.

The most common manifestation of candidal infection is mucocutaneous overgrowth, such as thrush, vaginitis, or intertrigo. Topical therapy to the skin with ketoconazole or clotrimazole, or increased oral therapy with nonabsorbable agents such as clotrimazole troches five times a day, is usually sufficient. When topical treatment fails,

fluconazole (100–200 mg/day orally), adjusted for renal function, is highly effective.

Candidal UTI is often iatrogenic, through catheters. It may result in ascending infection, pyelonephritis, and fungemia. One mechanism for this is obstructive uropathy due to a "fungal ball" at the ureterovesical junction, seen particularly in diabetics with neurogenic bladders. We advocate removal of any catheters and treatment with systemic antifungal agents (not topical therapy to the bladder) of even asymptomatic candiduria. Placement of a three-way catheter to treat topically can produce bacterial superinfection. Fluconazole 200 mg/day orally or, if the organism is thought not to be susceptible (e.g. *Candida krusei* or *Candida glabrata*), low-dose (10 mg/day) amphotericin B combined with flucytosine are effective regimens.

Candidal bloodstream infection is particularly associated with indwelling central lines, ascending UTIs, or breaches of mucosal integrity. Even transient candidemia requires treatment. Fluconazole can be utilized if the candidal isolate is known to be *C. albicans* or other species that are susceptible to fluconazole; however, if there is a question about this, voriconazole, caspofungin, or a lipid amphotericin preparation provides broader coverage while toxicity is minimized. The vascular access catheter(s) must be removed, whichever drug is chosen. For critically ill patients, many centers are utilizing combination therapy with caspofungin and voriconazole or a lipid amphotericin preparation.

The classic opportunistic infections are not seen in the first month post transplant, when the daily dose of immunosuppressant is the highest, underlining the fact that it is the duration of immunosuppression, or the "area under the curve," rather than simply the daily dose that is the major determinant of the net state of immunosuppression. Thus, a single case of invasive aspergillosis in the first month post transplant should trigger an investigation for an environmental hazard.

One to six months post transplant

The dominant form of infection during this time is that caused by the immunomodulating viruses, particularly CMV and EBV. The combination of sustained immunosuppression and one or more of these viruses makes possible the occurrence of a variety of opportunistic infections. Specifically, the net state of immunosuppression is now great enough for opportunistic infections to occur without the requirement for an intensive environmental exposure; however, if such an exposure were to occur, its effects would be greatly amplified during this particularly vulnerable time. Thus, the approach to be taken to prevent infection during this time has three components: an effective strategy to prevent viral infection; low-dose trimethoprim–sulfamethoxazole prophylaxis; and assurances that the air supply and potable water supply are free of risk.

Viral infections in the kidney transplant recipient

Four groups of viruses are of special significance: the herpes group viruses, especially CMV, EBV, and, perhaps, human herpesvirus 6 (HHV-6); the hepatitis viruses HBV and HCV; the community-acquired respiratory viruses, most notably respiratory syncytial virus (RSV), influenza, and adenoviruses; and the papovaviruses, most notably JC and BK viruses.

The herpes group viruses

The herpes group viruses CMV, EBV, HHV-6, herpes simplex virus 1 and 2 (HSV-1 and HSV-2), varicella-zoster virus (VZV), and HHV-7 and -8 share several characteristics in common that make them particularly effective pathogens in renal transplant recipients:

1. *Latency.* Once infected with a herpes group virus, the individual is infected for life, with latent virus present in a variety of cells once replication has ceased. The laboratory marker for latent infection is the presence of antibody to the particular virus (seropositivity) in the absence of viral replication. The stability of the latency varies with the different viruses. Thus, HSV-1 and -2, as well as EBV, are relatively unstable, with frequent reactivation; CMV, HHV-6, and probably HHV-7 and -8 are quite stable, requiring proinflammatory events for reactivation to occur.
2. *Cell association.* Herpes group viruses are highly cell associated, which results in limited routes of transmission: intimate contact, transplantation, transfusion of blood products containing viable leukocytes, and pregnancy. Such cell association renders humoral immunity relatively inefficient in the control of infection, while emphasizing the importance of major histocompatibility complex (MHC)-restricted, virus-specific cytotoxic, T cells in the control of these infections.
3. *Malignancy.* All herpes group viruses should be considered potentially oncogenic. However, thus far, only EBV (posttransplant lymphoproliferative disease (PTLD)) and HHV-8 (Kaposi's sarcoma) have been linked to malignancies. Cytokines, chemokines, and growth factors liberated as part of the recipient's inflammatory response to a virus can increase the occurrence of PTLD, with, for example, CMV increasing the risk of PTLD approximately 10-fold.

Cytomegalovirus

In addition to the syndromes directly attributable to viral infection, CMV is associated with immune dysregulation, an increased incidence of bacterial and fungal infections, a higher rate of both acute and chronic allograft injury, and a 10-fold rise in the occurrence of EBV-associated PTLD. Antimicrobial strategies during this period are centered on the prevention and treatment of CMV infection. The most common clinical manifestation of CMV is a nonspecific febrile illness, often with leukopenia, thrombocytopenia, and liver function test abnormalities. However, fever may be seen in concert with many other clinical syndromes, ulcers anywhere in the gastrointestinal tract, hepatitis or pancreatitis, pneumonitis, and, as a later complication, chorioretinitis. There are three major patterns of CMV infection in organ transplantation. Each carries a different risk of clinical disease, and thus may warrant a different preventive strategy.

1. *Primary infection (R–/D+).* Here, a CMV-seronegative recipient (R–) receives cells latently infected with CMV from a seropositive donor (D+). In most instances, these latently infected cells are within the allograft, although viable leukocyte-containing blood products can also transmit latent virus. More than 60% of patients who are primarily infected experience symptomatic disease.
2. *Reactivation infection (R+/D–).* Here, seropositive recipients reactivate their own endogenous latent virus. The recipient has some preexisting immunity, and the rate of symptomatic disease is approximately 10–15%.
3. *Superinfection (R+/D+).* Here, a seropositive recipient receives an organ from a seropositive donor. In more than half of these patients, some or all of the virus that reactivates can be shown to be of donor origin. This group has a higher rate of symptomatic infection than the reactivation group mentioned previously, ranging from 20% to 30%.

For all three of these forms of CMV there are three pathways by which CMV can be reactivated. The most important is triggered by tumor necrosis factor (TNF) in the circulation. Thus, the reason that other infections, allograft rejection, antilymphocyte antibody administration, and sepsis of diverse etiologies can trigger CMV reactivation is that all result in the elaboration of TNF. The other two pathways are through cyclic AMP, with epinephrine and norepinephrine having this effect, as do certain proinflammatory prostaglandins.[19–24]

Seropositive patients treated with antilymphocyte antibodies (e.g. antithymocyte globulin or the monoclonal antibody OKT3) have an increased incidence of symptomatic disease (e.g. when these antibodies are used as antirejection therapy, the incidence of symptomatic disease rises from 15% to 65%).[24]

Given the protean effects of CMV on the transplant recipient, it is not surprising that much effort has been expended in the development of preventative strategies. Two general strategies can be employed: prophylaxis and preemptive therapy. Prophylaxis is recommended in dealing with R–/D+ patients, who are at risk of primary infection. Three to six months of oral valganciclovir, with or without an induction course of intravenous ganciclovir, is quite effective in preventing CMV disease. (This has largely replaced less effective regimens, such as acyclovir, hyperimmune globulin, and oral ganciclovir, which has a poor bioavailability profile.) The dose of ganciclovir used for prophylaxis is 5 mg/kg/day; for valganciclovir, 900 mg/day is utilized. All doses of ganciclovir and valganciclovir must be decreased in the face of renal dysfunction. Although such a prophylactic program would work for the R+ recipient, many centers prefer one of two preemptive approaches. The first requires regular monitoring for evidence of presymptomatic viremia as tested by polymerase chain reaction (PCR) or the pp65 antigenemia assay. If monitoring is carried out appropriately, preemptive therapy can be as effective as prophylaxis, with fewer patients exposed to the antiviral drugs. The second approach is the initiation of ganciclovir (or valganciclovir) concomitant with antilymphocyte therapy, continuing for 3 months, which reduces symptomatic disease from 65% to essentially 0%.[25–27]

Treatment of clinical CMV disease is with intravenous ganciclovir, 5 mg/kg twice daily (or oral valganciclovir in doses designed to mimic the pharmacokinetics of the intravenous drug, 900 mg twice daily). Dosages are decreased in the face of renal dysfunction. We advocate treatment with full doses until viremia is cleared, and then oral therapy for 3 months to prevent relapse. Relapse, with the risk of ganciclovir resistance arising, is particularly common in patients with primary infection, in those with an allograft that is a six-antigen mismatch, and in those who have received inadequate doses or durations of therapy. The major toxicity of ganciclovir is myelosuppression; however, most patients can tolerate a treatment course, although some may require support with granulocyte colony-stimulating factor or erythropoietin/red blood cell transfusions. Foscarnet, a nucleotide analog, has excellent CMV activity; however, because it is a very nephrotoxic drug, with loss of prodigious amounts of magnesium and calcium in the urine, its use is restricted to patients with ganciclovir-resistant infection.[1]

The diagnosis of CMV rests on the demonstration of replicating virus in the bloodstream or in tissues. Traditional cell culture on a fibroblast cell monolayer, with the development of a characteristic cytopathic effect in tissue culture, may take 1–3 weeks. In patients without an apparent or accessible end organ to biopsy, demonstration of virus in the bloodstream by other techniques is necessary. Although the so-called shell viral culture, or early antigen culture, is rapid because it uses antibody to detect an antigen made by the virus in the early phase of replication, it is less sensitive than traditional cell culture.[8] Direct staining of the buffy coat produced from a patient's blood sample with an antibody to a particular CMV antigen (the pp65 antigen) is rapid, sensitive, and appears to have excellent predictive value for clinical disease and relapse. This currently is the preferred method of diagnosis at many centers.[9] Molecular methods such as the polymerase chain reaction, particularly if quantitative, offer similar results. It is important to emphasize that these two methods provide a useful measurement of viral load, which is the key consideration in predicting the gravity of the clinical situation and the intensity of therapy that will be required.[25–33]

Epstein–Barr virus-associated lymphoproliferative disorder

Infection with EBV in normal hosts may be asymptomatic or may result in the self-limited lymphoproliferative disease known as infectious mononucleosis. The virus is transmitted through saliva and initiates lytic infection in the epithelial cells of the oropharynx. Subsequently, B lymphocytes trafficking through this lymphoid-rich tissue become infected, and B-cell proliferation, activation, and immortalization ensue. In nonimmunocompromised hosts, this B-cell proliferation is controlled by potent T-cell responses. However, immunosuppression markedly impairs these responses, and EBV may be associated with the progressive and often fatal syndrome of PTLD.[12] The overall risk of PTLD in kidney transplantation is estimated to be 1–3%. The highest risk occurs with primary EBV infection;

because most adults are already seropositive before transplantation, the highest incidence is found in children. The incidence of PTLD has risen in recent years, coincident with the use of more potent immunosuppressive regimens, particularly cyclosporine, tacrolimus, and antilymphocyte antibodies.[1]

PTLD often presents with fever and leukopenia. The organ systems most commonly involved are the gastrointestinal tract (pain, bleeding, obstruction, perforation) and the central nervous system (mental status changes, focal cranial nerve or motor abnormalities, or meningitis). Unlike lymphoma in the general population, it is not uncommon for the lymph nodes to be totally free of disease (with negative CT scans) in the face of active PTLD at other sites. The allograft is a favored site of PTLD, and biopsies should be carefully reviewed. The pathology of B-cell tumors causing disease may simply show polyclonal aggregates of B cells or, because the B-cell proliferation and activation favor mutational events, it may show a frank, monoclonal lymphoma.[1,34,35]

Because the mortality of established PTLD in these patients is more than 50% and because some tumors (particularly in primary infection) respond to decreasing or stopping immunosuppression, it is recommended that kidney transplant patients cease taking immunosuppression drugs, even if this means losing the allograft as a result of rejection. At present, the additional treatment of choice is the administration of an anti-B-cell antibody. For further therapy, a wide assortment of remedies has been employed: antivirals (which work on the lytic, not the mostly latent, B-cell infection induced by EBV), immunoglobulin plus interferon, radiation, and chemotherapy. Perhaps most interesting is the report of success in the treatment of patients with PTLD, in whom other therapies had failed, with a monoclonal antibody to interleukin 6. Another innovative form of therapy involves the infusion of donor leukocytes that are likely to contain cytotoxic T cells presensitized to EBV or the infusion of patient-derived, expanded EBV-specific cytotoxic T cells.[1,35–38]

There is a particularly urgent need to focus on prevention. EBV can be isolated from the pharyngeal secretions of 10–20% of normal hosts who are seropositive, from up to 50% of transplant patients, and from up to 80% of transplant patients receiving antilymphocyte antibodies. Investigators have asked whether there is a relationship between the amount of EBV shed in the pharynx, the number of infected B cells, and the subsequent risk of PTLD. Although patients with higher levels of EBV DNA in the oropharynx were more likely to develop PTLD, they were also taking higher doses of immunosuppressants and were more likely to have primary infection.[13] This study could not prove a causal relationship, however it is tempting to postulate that increased EBV replication in the oropharynx might result in an increased number of infected B cells and therefore confer a higher risk for PTLD. If such a relationship did exist, a preventive antiviral strategy similar to that employed for CMV – using ganciclovir, the drug with best activity – might decrease the risk of PTLD.

Finally, it has been shown that symptomatic disease with CMV is a significant independent risk factor for the development of subsequent PTLD.[14] This could relate to the profound immune dysregulation seen during symptomatic CMV infection, including alterations in cytotoxic and helper T cells as well as in cytokines. Thus, strategies aimed at prevention of CMV could conceivably also decrease the incidence of PTLD both by altering the cytokine milieu produced in response to CMV replication and by direct antiviral effects against EBV.[1-37]

Herpes simplex viral infection in the renal transplant patient

HSV infection is probably the second most common symptomatic viral infection affecting the transplant recipient after CMV. Approximately one-half of HSV-seropositive patients and two-thirds of those who excrete the virus will develop visible mucocutaneous lesions ~ 2 weeks post transplant. The lesions peak in severity 4–6 weeks post transplant, with increases in immunosuppression prolonging the process. The lesions themselves are usually more severe in immunosuppressed patients than in immunologically normal individuals, with large, painful, crusted ulcerations being common. Intraoral and esophageal infection may occur in association with herpes labialis, particularly if the mucosa has been traumatized by endotracheal or nasogastric tubes. The great majority of cases of oral HSV infection are due to HSV-1. Although herpetic orolabial infection in the transplant patient can cause heaped up, verrucous lesions of the lips, patients who fail to respond to acyclovir therapy should be biopsied to rule out a squamous cell carcinoma.[39-41]

Anogenital infection, usually due to HSV-2, in transplant patients can be quite severe, with large coalescing ulcerations that often do not have clear-cut vesicles. Tzanck preparations are typically negative. Specific diagnosis can be accomplished by viral cultures or direct detection by immunofluorescence of material taken on a swab of the lesion.[42]

Virtually all of the HSV infection observed in transplant patients is due to reactivation of endogenous latent virus. Primary infection conveyed by the allograft is quite rare, as is disseminated infection and encephalitis.[1,39-41]

The antiviral era has totally changed the occurrence of HSV infection, as acyclovir and ganciclovir are quite effective in both preventing and treating clinical episodes due to this virus. Most transplant centers either prescribe prophylaxis with oral acyclovir (400 mg three times daily) or rely on their CMV preventative programs to prevent HSV disease. If symptomatic infection develops, it is easily treated with oral acyclovir or valacyclovir for 7–10 days, with longer courses being used if immunosuppression is being increased.[43,44]

Varicella-zoster virus infection in the renal transplant patient

Primary VZV infection results in disseminated visceral disease that includes hemorrhagic pneumonia and skin lesions, encephalitis, pancreatitis, hepatitis, and disseminated intravascular coagulation. If diagnosed early, intravenous acyclovir (10 mg/kg three times daily) can be life-saving. Because of the gravity of the illness, it is essen-

tial that the serologic status of transplant patients and candidates be known. Seronegative individuals should receive the varicella vaccine with documentation of seroconversion. If the vaccine is given post transplant, then close observation of the recipient as an outpatient post vaccination is indicated because this is a live, attenuated vaccine that could conceivably cause serious disease. In our experience, this has not occurred – we have seen only with a few cutaneous vesicles. A bigger problem in immunosuppressed patients is a failure to seroconvert, which should trigger a booster dose. It is unclear whether an individual who fails to seroconvert is at all protected. Our policy is to give the vaccine and, if no seroconversion occurs, to give prophylactic treatment with zoster immune globulin and/or antiviral therapy.

Reactivation of the VZV infection produces cutaneous zoster in transplant patients, usually without visceral involvement but not uncommonly with some cutaneous spread beyond the affected dermatome. In the preantiviral era, zoster occurred in ~ 10% of transplant recipients, but with the widespread use of preventive antiviral therapies the incidence of zoster has decreased significantly. Treatment of zoster with oral fanciclovir or valacyclovir will hasten the healing of the skin lesions.[1,45-46]

Human herpesvirus 6 infection in the renal transplant patient

HHV-6 is a β-herpesvirus that is closely related to CMV. Primary infection with HHV-6 usually occurs in the first year of life, causing a febrile exanthem – roseola (also called exanthem subitum). HHV-6 viremia, almost always because of endogenous reactivation, can be documented by PCR in 30–50% of transplant recipients, often in association with active CMV disease. It is more difficult to define what HHV-6 is doing in the transplant patient. At present, it would appear that HHV-6 can cause fever with or without mononucleosis, interstitial pneumonitis, hepatitis, bone marrow suppression, and encephalitis. In addition, some investigators have postulated that this virus has indirect effects similar to those linked to CMV. Finally, there is evidence that the combination of HHV-6 and CMV causes a more severe clinical syndrome than either virus by itself. At present, it appears that HHV-6 is similar to CMV in being sensitive to ganciclovir.[47-49] Clearly, there is much more to be learned about this virus, and presumably HHV-7.[50-54]

Hepatitis in the renal transplant patient

Chronic hepatitis is present in 10–15% of renal transplant patients. It is now apparent that both HBV and HCV infection are responsible for this. The course of these viruses is exacerbated by immunosuppression, and over a 10-year period a significant proportion of patients who do not respond to antiviral therapy progress to endstage liver disease and/or hepatocellular carcinoma. Because of this risk, we advocate liver biopsy prior to transplant in patients who have serologic markers of active viral replication. HBV infection is well managed with lamivudine therapy; however, 1–3 years after initiating such therapy resistant mutants appear. Liver transplant patients benefit from the combination of HBV immune globulin and lamivudine, and the question of whether such combination therapy would be useful in kidney transplant patients is currently under study. Fortunately, there are additional anti-HBV drugs undergoing clinical trials that appear to be quite promising as it is likely that a therapeutic strategy akin to that used against HIV will be necessary, namely multiple drugs to overcome the appearance of resistance.[1,3,4]

HBV is far more virulent than HCV in terms of progression to endstage liver disease or cancer. However, therapy is becoming available, and the prognosis is reasonably good because of this. In contrast, HCV is more desultory, but the therapy currently available (ribavirin plus interferon) is far less effective, with no other drugs on the horizon.[1]

Both HBV and HCV are easily transmitted with an allograft from a donor with replicating virus. Because of the slow course of HCV, some transplant groups have advocated transplanting kidneys (and other organs) from HCV-positive donors, particularly to those who are HCV positive. Our approach is to accept this policy for patients in extremis in their need for a heart or a liver, but as life can be maintained on dialysis we have not accepted this approach for kidneys.[1]

Community-acquired respiratory viruses in the renal transplant patient

Transplant patients are particularly susceptible to infection by the respiratory viruses that circulate in the community. The severity of these illnesses is greater than in the general population, with viral pneumonia being far more common in transplant patients than in the immunologically normal. Of at least equal importance, superinfection with such bacteria as *Streptococcus pneumoniae*, *Haemophilus influenzae*, *Staphylococcus aureus*, and Gram-negative bacilli is also far more common. Trials of influenza vaccine in renal transplant patients have shown a lack of toxicity or adverse effects, but a disappointing level of efficacy. Unfortunately, there is little information on the efficacy of amantadine or the neuraminidase inhibitors in this setting. Thus, avoidance of influenza exposures is exceedingly important in preventing this infection and its consequences.

A particularly virulent respiratory syncytial virus (RSV) that causes an increased rate of pneumonia and mortality has been observed in both pediatric and adult transplant patients with acute respiratory failure. Because there are some anecdotal reports suggesting that aerosolized ribavirin therapy may have therapeutic efficacy for this infection, an aggressive approach to diagnosis is appropriate.[1,4]

Other respiratory viruses noted to cause serious disease in transplant patients include adenoviruses, parainfluenza, and rhinovirus. Because our therapies are relatively primitive for this class of infection, and because transplant patients have a significantly higher rate of complications than the general population, it is worth a special effort to isolate them from such exposures throughout their posttransplant course.

Papovaviruses in the renal transplant patient

The papovaviruses are divided into two genera – the polyomaviruses and the papillomaviruses. The human polyomaviruses, JC virus and BK virus (JCV and BKV), cause significant disease in the transplant recipient. JCV is the causative agent of progressive multifocal leukoencephalopathy – a subacute, progressive demyelinating disease of the central nervous system. BKV is an important cause of tubulointerstitial nephritis in the kidney transplant patient, which can mimic rejection. At present, there is no treatment for either of these processes except to decrease immunosuppressive therapy.[1,4]

Progressive multifocal leukoencephalopathy is a demyelinating disease of the white matter of the brain, which is characterized clinically by the development of progressive motor and sensory deficits, dementia, and death, usually within 6 months. This is an uncommon process, which is virtually always due to reactivation of latent JCV that was acquired in childhood.[55-57]

BKV has been linked to ureteral strictures for more than 30 years. Far more important, however, has been the increasing incidence of progressive interstitial nephritis due to this virus that has been linked to excessive immunosuppression, especially regimens that include tacrolimus with or without mycophenolate, and significant rejection episodes. It has been suggested that damage to the tubular epithelium by rejection plays an important role in the severe tubulointerstitial nephritis that develops. BKV nephritis has a poor prognosis, with progressive renal dysfunction being the rule.[1,58,59] Papillomavirus infection in transplant patients causes warts, which can be so numerous as to be disfiguring. The level of immunosuppression is the prime factor which determines the severity of the warts in the individual patient. Malignant transformation, particularly in sun-exposed areas, has been well documented. A particular subgroup of papillomaviruses, the epidermodysplasia verruciformis-associated types, has been linked to the pathogenesis of cutaneous and anogenital squamous cell carcinomas in these patients. Cervical papillomavirus is similarly more extensive in transplant recipients, is also modulated by the intensity of immunosuppression, and has been linked to the pathogenesis of cervical cancer in both the general population and among transplant patients.[56,57,60,61]

Invasive aspergillosis

Aspergillus species are ubiquitous in the soil and thus in the hospital environment. Invasive aspergillosis of the lungs and sinuses occurs after an intense environmental exposure, such as construction, in the face of excessive immunosuppression or following CMV infection. Avoidance of exposure in the hospital, for example masks while traveling off the unit, may help prevent some cases. In addition, if *Aspergillus* colonization of the respiratory tract is detected, given the increased risk of invasion in immunosuppressed patients, preemptive antifungal therapy should be considered, with careful monitoring of cyclosporine or tacrolimus levels.[62-65]

The most common clinical manifestation is pulmonary disease, which is the primary portal of entry for this organism (the sinuses and damaged skin being the other sites of interest). Invasive aspergillosis at any site should be thought of as being angioinvasive, with the three basic characteristics of invasive aspergillosis stemming from this event: tissue infarction, hemorrhage, and metastasis. Common presenting symptoms of invasive aspergillosis include cough, pleuritic chest pain, and fever with radiographic evidence of nodules or infiltrates progressing to infarcts or cavitary disease, although others also occur. Dissemination to the central nervous system is common, is often not detected premortem, and is nearly universally fatal by the time it is detected. All patients with pulmonary aspergillosis should have imaging of the central nervous system even in the absence of symptoms, and central nervous system aspergillosis should be considered in all patients with kidney transplants and neurologic disease. Early diagnosis and treatment are necessary for successful treatment of this entity. Thus, early biopsy is indicated to permit adequate diagnosis of the disease. The therapy of invasive aspergillosis is currently in a state of flux. Traditionally, high-dose intravenous amphotericin B (1.0–1.25 mg/kg/day for the deoxycholate product or 5–12.5 mg/kg/day of the lipid amphotericin preparation) has been the standard of care. Recently, a study comparing the efficacy of voriconazole with amphotericin in the treatment of invasive aspergillosis has demonstrated that voriconazole (initial dose 6 mg/kg twice daily to load the patient, then 4 mg/kg twice daily) is far better than amphotericin in terms of both efficacy and side-effect profile. Another newly licensed drug is the echinocandin preparation caspofungin. This agent was tested in compassionate trials of patients with unacceptable toxicity and/or failure to respond to therapy, with a 41% significant response noted. At the moment, there is a lack of information on this drug, although it is postulated that its major use for invasive aspergillosis will be as part of a two- or even three-drug combination to treat disease, especially metastatic or disseminated disease.[1,62–68]

Pneumocystis carinii pneumonia

There is at least a 10% incidence of *P. carinii* pneumonia (PCP) in kidney transplant patients who receive no prophylaxis. Although most infection can be treated successfully, the first-line therapies have significant toxicities. A minimum of 6 months' prophylaxis should therefore be given to all kidney transplant patients, especially to those groups of patients who have poor transplant results (too much acute and chronic rejection, excessive amounts of immunosuppression, and, often, recurrent herpes group viral infection). One tablet of single-strength (80/400 mg) TMP/SMX daily is nearly universally effective and provides prophylaxis against other infections, as previously mentioned. Treatment-limiting toxicity is rare at the prophylactic dose, the most common side-effects being rash and fever. Other options for prophylaxis appear to be less effective, but include daily dapsone, monthly intravenous or aerosolized pentamidine, and daily atovaquone.[1,4]

PCP typically manifests with cough, fever, and dyspnea. Chest radiographs may show the typical bilateral interstitial infiltrates but may also appear normal, particularly in the early phase of disease. So-called induced sputum, a deep specimen obtained after breathing nebulized saline, has a very high sensitivity in patients with AIDS (80–95%), especially when monoclonal antibody staining of the specimen

is used.[16] Although this has not been studied prospectively in organ transplant patients, experience suggests that the sensitivity is much less, possibly owing to the lower organism burden in the lungs of these patients. In patients who are severely ill, treatment should be started and bronchoalveolar lavage should be the first diagnostic procedure. If the lavage result is negative, transbronchial biopsy will not provide much additional information; therefore, open lung biopsy – by thoracoscopic means to decrease the morbidity of the procedure, if possible – should be the next procedure.[1,4]

There are several treatment regimens for PCP.[17] First-line treatment for severe PCP is intravenous TMP/SMX at doses of 15 mg/kg/day, given as one-fourth of this dose every 6 h, if the creatinine clearance is greater than 50 mL/min. The total daily dose is reduced by 50% and the interval increased to 12 h for creatinine clearances of 30–50 mL/min; the drug is not recommended if the creatinine clearance is below 30 mL/min. Sulfamethoxazole levels should be measured after five doses, aiming for levels between 10 and 15 mg/dL but no higher. TMP/SMX at these doses has the following toxicities: fever and rash, renal dysfunction, hyperkalemia, bone marrow suppression, hepatitis, and pancreatitis. Intravenous pentamidine, 4 mg/kg/day, is effective therapy for PCP, but may be associated with hypotension and hypoglycemia during the infusion and renal and electrolyte abnormalities during the treatment course. Unfortunately, toxicities requiring a change in treatment from one of these drugs to the other are common in this patient population. If both drugs cause serious toxicity in a patient, or after the patient responds, therapies that appear to be effective for mild-to-moderate PCP are clindamycin plus primaquine or atovaquone alone. PCP may worsen for 3–5 days after institution of therapy, presumably owing to the host's immune response to the killing of organisms. Experience in AIDS patients suggests that high-dose corticosteroids may ameliorate this response and may improve outcome in patients with severe PCP ($Po_2 < 60$ or A–a gradient > 35).[17] An increase in corticosteroid dose followed by tapering the dose as tolerated appears to have similar effects in patients with kidney transplants.[1,4]

More than 6 months post transplant

Patients who are alive with a functioning allograft, and thus requiring continuous immunosuppression, can be divided into three groups. Approximately 75% of them have good allograft function, are on decreased doses of immunosuppressants, and are free of chronic viral infections. These patients develop infections that are similar to those observed in the community, particularly respiratory viral infection (e.g. influenza, respiratory syncytial virus, adenovirus, rhinovirus, and parainfluenza). Although the epidemiology is similar in both populations, in the transplant patient there is a far higher incidence of both viral and bacterial pneumonia.[1,4]

About 10–15% of patients who survive into this period have chronic viral infections with CMV, EBV, HBV, HCV, or, much less commonly, HIV. Because immunosuppressive therapy renders the host's defenses unable to clear these infections effectively, patients not only develop complications as a result of these infections but do so with a decreased latency period. These complications include organ failure (hepatic failure and cirrhosis with HBV or HCV), malignancy (hepatocellular carcinoma or EBV-associated lymphoproliferative disease), or AIDS.

Finally, 5–15% of these patients, whom we call the chronic n'er-do-wells, are characterized by relatively poor allograft function and one or more episodes of acute or chronic rejection, requiring excessive immunosuppression. These patients are at highest risk of late opportunistic infections such as *P. carinii*, *Cryptococcus neoformans*, *L. monocytogenes*, or *N. asteroides*. This group may warrant long-term or lifetime antimicrobial prophylaxis with low-dose TMP/SMX, clotrimazole, and acyclovir.[1,4]

Summary

Infection has always been a major threat to kidney transplant patients on immunosuppressive therapy. Improvements in the prevention and treatment of infections have contributed greatly to the improved outcome in these patients. However, it is obvious that the available information is still incomplete, and further well-designed studies are needed to delineate patients at high risk for infection as well as the optimal types, doses, and durations of preventive or therapeutic regimens in these patients. It is hoped that the development of new, effective, and less toxic antimicrobial agents will assist in this effort. The underlying principle remains that infection and rejection are always closely linked and that the immunosuppression required to optimize allograft function requires an optimal antimicrobial program to render it as safe as possible. Two principles need to be united in developing such a program. First, the intensity of antimicrobial therapy, both pharmacologic and environmental, must be matched to the intensity of the immunosuppressive program being employed. Second, different time points in the posttransplant course carry a higher risk of different forms of infection, thus necessitating the use of different antimicrobial strategies and different diagnostic and empiric treatment regimens.

References

1. Rubin RH: Infection in the organ transplant patient. *In* Rubin RH, Young LS (eds): Clinical Approach to Infection in the Compromised Host, 4th edn. New York, Kluwer/Academic Press, 2002.
2. Hariharan S, Johnson CP, Bresnahan BA, et al: Improved graft survival after renal transplantation in the United States, 1988 to 1996. N Engl J Med 2000;342:605–612.
3. Rubin R, Ikonen T, Gummert J, et al: The therapeutic prescription for the organ transplant recipient: the linkage of immunosuppression and antimicrobial strategies. Trans Infect Dis 1999;1:29–39.
4. Fishman JA, Rubin RH: Infection in organ-transplant recipients. N Engl J Med 1998;338:1741–1751.
5. Rubin RH, Wolfson JS, Cosimi AB, et al: Infection in the renal transplant recipient. Am J Med 1981;70:405–411.
6. Gottesdiener KM: Transplanted infections: donor-to-host transmission with the allograft. Ann Intern Med 1989;110:1001–1016.
7. Rubin R, Fishman J: A consideration of potential donors with active infection: is this a way to expand the donor pool? Transpl Int 1998;11:333–335.
8. Johnston L, Chui L, Chang N, et al: Cross-Canada spread of methicillin-resistant *Staphylococcus aureus* via transplant organs. Clin Infect Dis 1999;29:819–823.
9. Nelson PW, Delmonico FL, Tolkoff-Rubin NE, et al: Unsuspected donor pseudomonas infection causing arterial disruption after renal transplantation. Transplantation 1984;37:313–314.
10. McCoy GC, Loening S, Braun WE, et al: The fate of cadaver renal allografts contaminated before transplantation. Transplantation 1975;20:467–472.
11. Spees EK, Light JA, Oakes DD, et al: Experiences with cadaver renal allograft contamination before transplantation. Br J Surg 1982;69:482–485.
12. Freeman RB, Giatras I, Falagas ME, et al: Outcome of transplantation of organs procured from bacteremic donors. Transplantation 1999;68:1107–1111.
13. van der Vliet JA, Tidow G, Kootstra G, et al: Transplantation of contaminated organs. Br J Surg 1980;67:596–598.
14. Rubin RH, Fang LS, Cosimi AB, et al: Usefulness of the antibody-coated bacteria assay in the management of urinary tract infection in the renal transplant patient. Transplantation 1979;27:18–20.
15. Tolkoff-Rubin N, Cosimi A, Russell P, et al: A controlled study of trimethoprim–sulfamethoxazole prophylaxis of urinary tract infections in renal transplant recipients. Rev Infect Dis 1982;4:614–618.
16. Fox BC, Sollinger HW, Belzer FO, et al: A prospective, randomized, double-blind study of trimethoprim–sulfamethoxazole for prophylaxis of infection in renal transplantation: clinical efficacy, absorption of trimethoprim–sulfamethoxazole, effects on the microflora, and the cost–benefit of prophylaxis. Am J Med 1990;89:255–274.
17. Maki DG, Fox BC, Kuntz J, et al: A prospective, randomized, double-blind study of trimethoprim–sulfamethoxazole for prophylaxis of infection in renal transplantation. Side effects of trimethoprim–sulfamethoxazole, interaction with cyclosporine. J Lab Clin Med 1992;119:11–24.
18. Hibberd P, Tolkoff-Rubin N, Doran M, et al: Trimethoprim–sulfamethoxazole compared with ciprofloxacin for the prevention of urinary tract infection in renal transplant recipients. Online J Curr Clin Trials 1992;document 15.
19. Reinke P, Prosch S, Kern F, et al: Mechanisms of human cytomegalovirus (HCMV) (re)activation and its impact on organ transplant patients. Trans Infect Dis 1999;1:157–164.
20. Fietze E, Prosch S, Reinke P, et al: Cytomegalovirus infection in transplant recipients. The role of tumor necrosis factor. Transplantation 1994;58:675–680.
21. Stein J, Volk HD, Liebenthal C, et al: Tumour necrosis factor alpha stimulates the activity of the human cytomegalovirus major immediate early enhancer/promoter in immature monocytic cells. J Gen Virol 1993;74:2333–2338.
22. Prosch S, Staak K, Stein J, et al: Stimulation of the human cytomegalovirus IE enhancer/promoter in HL-60 cells by TNF-alpha is mediated via induction of NFkB. Virology 1995;208:107–116.
23. Docke WD, Prosch S, Fietze E, et al: Cytomegalovirus reactivation and tumour necrosis factor. Lancet 1994;343:268–269.
24. Hibberd PL, Tolkoff-Rubin NE, Cosimi AB, et al: Symptomatic cytomegalovirus disease in the cytomegalovirus antibody seropositive renal transplant recipient treated with OKT3. Transplantation 1992;53:68–72.
25. Chou S: Newer methods for diagnosis of cytomegalovirus infection. Rev Infect Dis 1990;12 (Suppl 7): S727–S736.
26. Paya CV, Wold AD, Smith TF: Detection of cytomegalovirus infections in specimens other than urine by the shell vial assay and conventional tube cell cultures. J Clin Microbiol 1987;25:755–757.
27. van den Berg AP, van der Bij W, van Son WJ, et al: Cytomegalovirus antigenemia as a useful marker of symptomatic cytomegalovirus infection after renal transplantation – a report of 130 consecutive patients. Transplantation 1989;48:991–995.
28. Cope AV, Sweny P, Sabin C, et al: Quantity of cytomegalovirus viruria is a major risk factor for cytomegalovirus disease after renal transplantation. J Med Virol 1997;52:200–205.
29. Cope AV, Sabin C, Burroughs A, et al: Interrelationships among quantity of human cytomegalovirus (HCMV) DNA in blood, donor–recipient serostatus, and administration of

methylprednisolone as risk factors for HCMV disease following liver transplantation. J Infect Dis 1997;176:1484–1490.

30. Hassan-Walker AF, Kidd IM, et al: Quantity of human cytomegalovirus (CMV) DNAemia as a risk factor for CMV disease in renal allograft recipients: relationship with donor/recipient CMV serostatus, receipt of augmented methylprednisolone and antithymocyte globulin (ATG). J Med Virol 1999;58:182–187.

31. Tong CY, Cuevas LE, Williams H, et al: Prediction and diagnosis of cytomegalovirus disease in renal transplant recipients using qualitative and quantitative polymerase chain reaction. Transplantation 2000;69:985–991.

32. Emery VC, Sabin CA, Cope AV, et al: Application of viral-load kinetics to identify patients who develop cytomegalovirus disease after transplantation. Lancet 2000;355:2032–2036.

33. Griffiths P, Cope A, Hassan-Walker A, et al: Diagnostic approach to cytomegalovirus infection in bone marrow and organ transplantation. Trans Infect Dis 1999;1:179–186.

34. Cheeseman SH, Henle W, Rubin RH, et al: Epstein–Barr virus infection in renal transplant recipients. Effects of antithymocyte globulin and interferon. Ann Intern Med 1980;93:39–42.

35. Harris NL, Ferry JA, Swerdlow SH: Posttransplant lymphoproliferative disorders: summary of Society for Hematopathology Workshop. Semin Diagn Pathol 1997;14:8–14.

36. Oertel SH, Anagnostopoulos I, Bechstein WO, Liehr H, Riess HB: Treatment of posttransplant lymphoproliferative disorder with the anti-CD20 monoclonal antibody rituximab alone in an adult after liver transplantation: a new drug in therapy of patients with posttransplant lymphoproliferative disorder after solid organ transplantation? Transplantation 2000;69:430–432.

37. Durandy A: Anti-B cell and anti-cytokine therapy for the treatment of PTLD: past, present, and future. Trans Infect Dis 2001;3:104–107.

38. Fischer A, Blanche S, Le Bidois J, et al: Anti-B-cell monoclonal antibodies in the treatment of severe B-cell lymphoproliferative syndrome following bone marrow and organ transplantation. N Engl J Med 1991;324:1451–1456.

39. Cheeseman SH, Rubin RH, Stewart JA, et al: Controlled clinical trial of prophylactic human-leukocyte interferon in renal transplantation. Effects on cytomegalovirus and herpes simplex virus infections. N Engl J Med 1979;300:1345–1349.

40. Rubin RH, Tolkoff-Rubin NE: Viral infection in the renal transplant patient. Proc Eur Dial Transplant Assoc 1983;19:513–526.

41. Ho M: Virus infections after transplantation in man. Brief review. Arch Virol 1977;55:1–24.

42. Stone WJ, Scowden EB, Spannuth CL, et al: Atypical herpesvirus hominis type 2 infection in uremic patients receiving immunosuppressive therapy. Am J Med 1977;63:511–516.

43. Griffin P, Colbert J, Williamson E, et al: Oral acyclovir prophylaxis of herpes infection in renal transplant recipients. Transplant Proc 1985;17:84–85.

44. Pettersson E, Hovi T, Ahonen J, et al: Prophylactic oral acyclovir after renal transplantation. Transplantation 1985;39:279–281.

45. Rifkind D: The activation of varicella-zoster virus infections by immunosuppressive therapy. J Lab Clin Med 1966;68:463–474.

46. Luby JP, Ramirez-Ronda C, Rinner S, et al: A longitudinal study of varicella-zoster virus infections in renal transplant recipients. J Infect Dis 1977;135:659–663.

47. Sing N: Human herpesviruses-6, -7, and -8 in organ transplant recipients. Clin Microb Infect 2000;6:453–459.

48. Okuno T, Higashi K, Shiraki K, et al: Human herpesvirus 6 infection in renal transplantation. Transplantation 1990;49:519–522.

49. Gudnason T, Dunn D, Brown N, et al: Human herpesvirus 6 infections in hospitalized renal transplant recipients. Clin Transplant 1991;5:359–364.

50. Yoshikawa T, Suga S, Asano Y, et al: A prospective study of human herpesvirus-6 infection in renal transplantation. Transplantation 1992;54:879–883.

51. Yoshikawa T, Suga S, Asano Y, et al: A prospective study of human herpesvirus-6 infection in renal transplantation. Transplantation 1992; 54:879–83.716.

52. Dockrell DH, Smith TF, Paya CV: Human herpesvirus 6. Mayo Clin Proc 1999;74:163–170.

53. Garner S: Prevalence in England of antibody to polyomavirus (B.K.). Br Med J 1973;1:77–78.

54. Shah KV, Daniel RW, Warszawski RM: High prevalence of antibodies to BK virus, an SV40-related papovavirus, in residents of Maryland. J Infect Dis 1973;128:784–787.

55. Brown P, Tsai T, Gajdusek DC: Seroepidemiology of human papovaviruses. Discovery of virgin populations and some unusual patterns of antibody prevalence among remote peoples of the world. Am J Epidemiol 1975;102:331–340.

56. Boubenider S, Hiesse C, Marchand S, et al: Post-transplantation polyomavirus infections. J Nephrol 1999;12:24–29.

57. Howell DN, Smith SR, Butterly DW, et al: Diagnosis and management of BK polyomavirus interstitial nephritis in renal transplant recipients. Transplantation 1999;68:1279–1288.

58. Binet I, Nickeleit V, Hirsch HH, et al: Polyomavirus disease under new immunosuppressive drugs: a cause of renal graft dysfunction and graft loss. Transplantation 1999;67:918–922.

59. Leventhal B, Soave R, Mouradian J, et al: Renal dysfunction and hyperglycemia in a renal transplant recipient. Transplant Infect Dis 1999;1:288–294.

60. Boubenider S, Hiesse C, Marchand S, et al: Post-transplantation polyomavirus infections. J Nephrol 1999;12:24–29.

61. Howell DN, Smith SR, Butterly DW, et al: Diagnosis and management of BK polyomavirus interstitial nephritis in renal transplant recipients. Transplantation 1999;68:1279–1288.

62. Mullen D, Silverberg S, Penn I, et al: Squamous cell carcinoma of the skin and lip in renal homograft recipients. JAMA 1976;229:729–734.

63. Savin JA, Noble WC: Immunosuppression and skin infection. Br J Dermatol 1975;93:115–120.

64. Tolkoff-Rubin N, Hovingh G, Rubin R: Central nervous system infections. In Wijdecks E (ed) Neurologic Complications in Organ Transplant Recipients. Boston: Butterworth Heinemann, 1999, pp 141–168.

65. Britt RH, Enzmann DR, Remington JS: Intracranial infection in cardiac transplant recipients. Ann Neurol 1981;9:107–119.

66. Weiland D, Ferguson RM, Peterson PK, et al: Aspergillosis in 25 renal transplant patients. Epidemiology, clinical presentation, diagnosis, and management. Ann Surg 1983;198:622–629.

67. Montero CG, Martinez AJ: Neuropathology of heart transplantation: 23 cases. Neurology 1986;36:1149–1154.

68. Tolkoff-Rubin N, Hovingh G, Rubin R: Central nervous system infections. In Wijdecks E (ed) Neurologic Complications in Organ Transplant Recipients. Boston: Butterworth Heinemann, 1999, pp 141–168.

69. Nielsen HE, Korsager B: Bacteremia after renal transplantation. Scand J Infect Dis 1977;9:111–117.

PART XV
Drugs and the Kidney

CHRISTOPHER S. WILCOX

Drug Dosing in Renal Failure

D. Craig Brater

Numerous drugs are eliminated by the kidney and thereby require dose adjustment in patients with renal insufficiency.[1-4] In addition, some drugs that themselves are not dependent upon the kidney for excretion are converted in the liver to active metabolites that accumulate in patients with diminished renal function.[5,6] To avoid toxicity from either parent drug or active metabolites, doses of many drugs must be adjusted downward in patients with decreased renal function. The precision required in this dose adjustment is not always great and depends upon the therapeutic index of individual drugs. For example, penicillins and cephalosporin antibiotics have wide margins of safety. Many antibiotics in these classes are administered in smaller doses to patients with severe renal insufficiency, but doing so does not require the same degree of precision as dose adjustment with drugs having narrow therapeutic indices such as aminoglycoside antibiotics. With the latter, serum concentrations are measured to assure attainment of therapeutic yet nontoxic levels.

In addition to drug accumulation because of compromised elimination pathways, the patient treated with any of the several methods of hemodialysis, hemofiltration, or peritoneal dialysis presents an additional challenge. Drug may be removed by the procedure itself, thereby requiring compensatory dose supplementation, the extent of which is a function of the amount of drug removed.[1] The ability of dialysis to remove drugs is influenced by factors such as binding of drug to protein, which limits dialyzability, molecular size, etc. These factors are highly variable among drugs, even those in the same chemical class, rendering a priori predictions impossible. One must rely on published data from appropriate patient populations to guide therapy. In addition, for drugs with narrow therapeutic indices, drug serum concentrations can be measured.

This chapter will discuss principles of drug dosing that will serve as a framework for dosing regimen adjustment in patients with renal insufficiency. Dosing guidelines for patients with various degrees of renal dysfunction,

including dialysis, are offered in the appendix (Tables A94.1–A94.3).

It is possible to predict and anticipate some of the effects that renal disease and dialysis will have on drug disposition. Renal insufficiency will cause drugs eliminated by the kidney to accumulate. In general, accumulation sufficient to be of clinical concern occurs if 30% or more of the drug is eliminated in the urine unchanged. A characteristic of renal insufficiency is accumulation of endogenous organic acids in plasma. Predictably, these acids can compete with acidic xenobiotics for binding to albumin and thereby diminish protein binding. Similarly, any cause of hypoalbuminemia results in diminished binding of drugs bound to albumin. As will be discussed, changes in protein binding can influence the concentration of unbound, pharmacologically active drug in plasma.

All forms of dialysis require the passage of the removed substance across a membrane. For a drug, certain characteristics predict its ability to be removed by a dialytic procedure. Avid binding to circulating proteins prevents dialytic removal. Theoretically, large size also restricts removal, but most xenobiotics are small enough that this factor is only rarely important. A drug that is widely distributed in tissues with only a small component of the total body burden circulating in plasma may readily cross a dialysis membrane. However, the amount removed during dialysis is trivial and clinically unimportant.

Understanding the pharmacokinetic characteristics of a drug is the framework upon which the following discussion is based. In turn, such an understanding allows predictions that can be helpful for clinicians when dealing with a clinical situation in which insufficient clinical information is available.

Principles of dose adjustment

Loading dose

Use of some drugs entails administration of a loading dose in order to rapidly attain therapeutic drug concentrations.[7-9] This approach is usually employed in therapeutic settings in which an effective drug concentration is needed quickly. The thought process that is undertaken in deciding whether to give a loading dose entails weighting the urgency of the clinical setting and, thereby, the rapidity with which a pharmacologic effect is needed against the half-life of the drug. If a loading dose is not given, the time needed to reach plateau drug concentrations is four times the half-life. If this time is long relative to the clinical need, a loading dose strategy should be employed. The loading dose needed is a function of the volume of distribution (V_d) of the drug and the target blood concentration to initially be attained ($C_{initial}$):

Loading dose = ($C_{initial}$) (V_d)

For example, if the V_d for a drug such as an aminoglycoside antibiotic is 0.25 L/kg and the desired peak serum concentration is 8 mg/L, the necessary loading dose can be calculated as follows:

Loading dose = (8 mg/L) (0.25 L/kg)
= 2 mg/kg

It is customary for clinicians to think in terms of the loading dose itself as opposed to calculating it from values for V_d and the desired concentration. This habit can be hazardous, particularly in settings where the patient's disease may influence V_d and thereby mandate a change in the loading dose. For example, if the V_d of a drug in a patient with renal insufficiency is one-half that in a patient with normal renal function, and the patient with renal disease received a "standard" loading dose, the resulting initial concentration would be twice that expected, with a consequent risk of toxicity. To illustrate using the previous example, if the "normal" loading dose of 2 mg/kg were administered to a patient whose V_d was 0.125 L/kg (i.e. one-half the usual value), then a concentration of 16 mg/L would result:

2 mg/kg = ($C_{initial}$) (0.125 L/kg)
$C_{initial}$ = 2 mg/kg ÷ 0.125 L/kg
= 16 mg/L

It should be clear from this example that clinicians need to be alert to changes that occur in the V_d of drugs. Such data are provided in the appendix (Table A94.1) for patients with renal disorders. The loading dose can be calculated as shown previously if the desired concentration is known. Alternatively, if the clinician knows the usual loading dose, the data in Table A94.1 can be used to calculate a modified dose:

Usual loading dose/Modified loading dose
= Normal V_d/Patient's V_d

or,

Modified loading dose
= (Patient's V_d/Normal V_d) × Usual loading dose

The direct proportionality between loading dose and V_d should make such dose adjustments easy and routine.

A caution that needs emphasis concerning loading doses and V_d is the influence of changes in drug protein binding. In patients with renal insufficiency, the protein binding of many drugs is decreased.[10,11] This is particularly true for acidic drugs bound to serum albumin, wherein accumulated endogenous organic acids can displace drug from binding sites.[12]

For drugs such as phenytoin, valproate, and warfarin, all of which are highly protein bound, a decrease in binding to albumin might be expected to cause an increase in the unbound concentration and thereby result in increased effect. However, the increased free drug is also readily available for metabolism of these drugs by the liver such that the unbound concentration is no different from that in patients with normal renal function.[10,11,13,14] In other words, in patients with normal renal function, a total serum concentration of phenytoin of 10 mg/L yields 1 mg/L of free drug; in contrast, in a patient with endstage renal disease (ESRD), the same dose results in a lower total concentration of 5 mg/L but the same free, pharmacologically active phenytoin concentration (Table 94.1).

The lesson here is that for phenytoin (and valproate) the same pharmacologically active unbound serum concentration occurs at a lower total concentration. Clinical laboratories usually measure total drug concentration. Hence, in a patient with renal insufficiency or with hypoalbuminemia (which also results in decreased protein binding), the "therapeutic" serum concentration expressed as total drug is less than in patients with normal renal function. If the clinician is not cognizant of this fact, he or she may inappropriately administer larger doses to increase the total drug concentration. The result is a concomitant increase in the unbound concentration to potentially toxic levels.

Maintenance dose

A maintenance dose maintains desired steady-state drug concentrations.[7–9] This dose is determined by the desired average drug concentration, $C_{average}$, and the clearance (Cl) of the drug from the body:

Maintenance dose = ($C_{average}$) (Cl)

If a drug is administered as a continuous intravenous infusion, the maintenance dosing rate is the infusion rate of the drug. If a drug is administered as separate, intermittent intravenous doses, the dosing rate is expressed as:

Dosing rate = Individual dose/Dosing interval

Lastly, if a drug is administered by mouth, one must incorporate a term that accounts for incomplete bioavailability, the fraction of dose absorbed (F). In this circumstance, the maintenance dosing rate becomes:

Table 94.1 Phenytoin concentration in patients with normal renal function and those with endstage renal disease (ESRD)

Concentration	Bound	+	Free	=	Total	Percentage bound
Normal renal function	9	+	1	=	10 mg/L	90
ESRD	4	+	1	=	5 mg/L	80

Dosing rate $= (F)$ (Individual dose)/Dosing interval

Hence, depending on the route of administration, any of the following relationships may apply:

Infusion rate	$= (C_{average})$ (Cl)
Dose/Dosing interval	$= (C_{average})$ (Cl)
$F \times$ Dose/Dosing interval	$= (C_{average})$ (Cl)

It should be apparent from these relationships that a change in clearance mandates a proportional change in the rate of drug administration if the average drug concentration is to remain the same. In patients with renal insufficiency, the clearance of drugs or their metabolite(s) is often diminished and, consequently, maintenance doses must be adjusted. Guidelines for doing so are offered in the appendix (Table A94.3).

Half-life

The half-life ($T_{1/2}$) of a drug refers to the time required for the serum concentration to decrease by 50%. The rate of elimination of most drugs (exceptions being phenytoin and salicylate) is independent of drug serum concentration and is referred to as being linear. This means that the $T_{1/2}$ is independent of serum concentration; as such, the time for a drug's concentration to decrease from 100 to 50 units of concentration is the same as it takes to decrease from 10 to 5 units.

Many clinicians use $T_{1/2}$ synonymously with clearance of a drug. In so doing, they presume that an increase in $T_{1/2}$ indicates a decrease in clearance that thereby requires a compensatory decrease in the maintenance dose. This misconception can lead to errors in dose adjustment in patients with renal insufficiency. As opposed to solely being a reflection of the clearance of a drug, $T_{1/2}$ is a function of both V_d and Cl:

$$T_{1/2} = 0.693 \; V_d/Cl$$

Hence, a change in $T_{1/2}$ can reflect either a change in V_d, a change in Cl, or a change in both. The correct dosing regimen adjustment that must be made depends on whether an alteration in V_d or in Cl is responsible for the change in $T_{1/2}$. If $T_{1/2}$ increases solely because of an increase in V_d, the loading dose should be increased while the maintenance dose should remain unchanged. If one incorrectly assumed that $T_{1/2}$ increased because Cl decreased, a "normal" loading dose and a diminished maintenance dose would be administered. Doing so would result in a loading dose that is too small, which thereby would not attain the desired initial concentration, and an inappropriately diminished maintenance dose, which would maintain a lower drug concentration than desired. The result could be lack of efficacy.

A good example of this potential scenario is the use of digoxin in patients with renal insufficiency. In patients with mild-to-moderate renal insufficiency, the V_d of digoxin is approximately the same as in patients with normal renal function whereas Cl may be about one-half to two-thirds of normal.[15] In such patients, the $T_{1/2}$ rises in proportion to the diminished Cl. In patients with severe renal insufficiency, however, V_d is decreased to one-half to two-thirds of normal, and Cl is decreased even more to about one-third of normal.[15,16] In this setting $T_{1/2}$ is influenced by both parameters, and though half-life is prolonged compared with patients with normal renal function, it is little different from that in the patient with mild-to-moderate renal insufficiency. In the patient with severe renal insufficiency, if the change in $T_{1/2}$ were erroneously presumed to only reflect the decrease in digoxin clearance and thereby impact only on the maintenance dose, a serious dosing error would occur. Since no downward adjustment in loading dose would be made, the initial concentration would be higher than desired; in addition, the decrease in maintenance dose would be underestimated so that the patient's steady-state serum concentration would be maintained at a higher concentration than desired. The hazards of such an error are obvious.

One must realize the limitations of using $T_{1/2}$ to predict dosing adjustments; instead, one must dissect it into its component parts of V_d and Cl. Of what use, then, is $T_{1/2}$? Knowing $T_{1/2}$ allows one to determine the time necessary for serum drug concentrations to reach steady state. Steady state is reached after administering drug for four to five times the $T_{1/2}$. As discussed previously, this delay in attaining plateau drug concentrations can be avoided by giving a loading dose designed to attain the desired drug concentration quickly.

It is important to remember that the concept of attainment of steady state applies to any change in dose, not just starting therapy. For example, if a maintenance dose is doubled, four to five times the $T_{1/2}$ is required for the serum concentration to reach the new plateau. Similarly, if the maintenance dose is decreased, four to five times the $T_{1/2}$ must elapse for the new, lower steady-state concentration to be reached. Lastly, if drug is stopped altogether, four to five times the $T_{1/2}$ is needed for concentrations to become negligible.

In summary, the half-life should be used to predict the time necessary for a drug to reach steady-state concentrations. It is a hybrid value influenced by both V_d and Cl and as such provides no direct information about loading or maintenance dose.

Dosing regimens

When renal dysfunction dictates a need to modify the dosing regimen, several options are available. Changes in loading dose simply entail giving a larger or smaller dose depending on whether V_d is increased or decreased. Whether to modify a loading dose may be unknown. In such cases, one should first decide whether or not a loading dose strategy is actually necessary. If so, one should err on the side of caution and administer a smaller loading dose than usual. If monitoring of clinical endpoints and/or serum drug concentrations shows the dose to have been too low, a supplementary dose can be given. In contrast, if too large a dose is administered, the clinician may be faced with iatrogenic drug toxicity and the need for remedial measures until the drug concentration diminishes, the time of which is dependent on half-life.

For adjusting maintenance doses of a drug, several strategies can be employed. The primary objective is to maintain the same average drug concentration as would occur if the patient did not have renal disease. Because the majority of drugs obey linear or first-order elimination kinetics, change in clearance can be compensated by a proportional change in the dosing rate:

Usual maintenance dose/Modified maintenance dose
= Usual clearance/Patient's clearance

or,

Modified maintenance dose
= (Patient's clearance/Usual clearance) × Usual maintenance dose

Hence, if the clearance of a drug in a patient with renal insufficiency is one-half the "normal" value, then the patient's maintenance dose should be one-half that usually administered. Such dose modifications will maintain the average steady-state drug concentration to be the same in the patient with renal disease as in those with normal renal function.

If a patient is receiving drug by continuous intravenous infusion, maintenance dose modification simply requires a modified infusion rate. If, however, the patient is receiving intermittent doses, reduction of the total dose being administered can be accomplished in three different ways:

1. Decreasing each individual dose and maintaining the same dosing frequency; this approach is often referred to as the variable dose method.
2. Maintaining the same individual dose but administering each dose less frequently; this approach is called the variable frequency (or interval) method.
3. Modifying both individual doses and the frequency of their administration, which is a combination method.

All three methods attain the same average drug concentration. For example, if 1200 mg of a drug is administered to a patient with normal renal function as 400 mg every 8 h, and one wished to administer one-half as much drug to a patient with renal insufficiency, viable options include:

1. 200 mg every 8 h;
2. 600 mg every 24 h;
3. 300 mg every 12 h.

Over a course of therapy, the total amount of drug administered with each of these regimens is the same, and it is half that in the patient with normal renal function. These regimens differ, however, in the profile of serum drug concentrations. Regimens with closer dosing frequencies and smaller individual doses result in less difference between peak and trough drug concentrations. Which of these options is best to employ is a function of the drug and disease being treated. For example, for an antibiotic with a long postantibiotic effect, having a considerable period of time with low serum concentrations may not be worrisome. In contrast, for a drug that must be maintained within a narrow concentration range to maximize efficacy (e.g. an antiarrhythmic or anticonvulsant), a regimen would be needed that minimizes fluctuations in serum concentrations.

There is no general rule that can be applied in terms of maximum length of a dosing interval – 24 h seems a reasonable rule of thumb. Clinicians should realize the different options available and try to collate these options with individual therapeutic settings. For example, if a patient is not responding to a drug, the clinician should realize that a possible explanation is an inappropriate dosing regimen. Similarly, signs of toxicity shortly after administration of an individual dose may indicate a need to give drug more frequently in smaller doses to optimize the dosing regimen in an individual patient.

Dialysis

Patients with ESRD treated with dialysis (including hemofiltration) have an additional mechanism by which drugs can be eliminated.[17–20] If substantial elimination by these routes occurs, supplemental dosing must be given. In patients maintained on hemodialysis, this is most easily accomplished by administering a supplemental dose of drug at the completion of the dialysis session. The dose given is the amount of drug removed during the procedure.

With continuous ambulatory peritoneal dialysis (CAPD), there is essentially a continual process of drug removal. In this setting, the patient's total clearance of a drug equals clearance relative to the patient's residual level of renal function plus clearance via CAPD. One simply adjusts the dosing regimen (either individual dose, dosing interval, or both) upwards in proportion to the added increment in clearance from CAPD.

It is not infrequent for clinicians to encounter a setting where they are administering a drug to a patient receiving dialysis and are unable to find any information about dialytic removal of the agent. In this setting, one can often gain insight into the dialyzability of a drug by examining some of its pharmacokinetic parameters. One limitation to removal by dialysis is molecular size. If a drug is too large to pass across the dialysis membrane (including the peritoneum), it will not be removed by dialysis. This applies, for example, to vancomycin and amphotericin. Drugs that are highly bound to serum proteins have restricted access to the dialysis membrane since only free, unbound drug can cross this barrier. Hence, if a drug is bound in excess of 90%, it is unlikely that dialysis will contribute appreciably to its elimination. Drugs that are water soluble are more readily dialyzed; in turn, a clue that a drug is water soluble is the fact that these drugs are usually eliminated predominantly by the kidney as unchanged drug. Lastly, drugs with large volumes of distribution have minimal dialyzability. Conceptually, one can think with such drugs that of the total amount of drug in the body only a small portion resides in the vascular space with the dominant portion being in peripheral tissues. The drug in the vascular space can be removed but, once dialysis ends, the large amount of drug in the tissues can refill the vascular compartment; the dialysis procedure thereby removes only an insignificant quantity of the total amount of drug in the body.

Specific examples can be used to illustrate these principles. Aminoglycoside antibiotics are water soluble and eliminated primarily by the kidney (100% of the dose is normally excreted unchanged in the urine), they have negligible protein binding, and they have small volumes of distribution (0.25 L/kg). These drugs are removed by dialysis procedures in sufficient quantities to require dose supplementation. In contrast, cefonicid has a small V_d (0.10 L/kg), but is highly bound to serum proteins (98%) and thereby is not removed by hemodialysis or CAPD. Cefadroxil, on the other hand, despite having a somewhat larger V_d than cefonicid (0.30 L/kg) is only 16% bound to serum proteins. Dialytic removal is sufficient with this cephalosporin to require supplemental dosing. Lastly, drugs such as phenothiazines and tricyclic antidepressants that have very large V_d values (> 10 L/kg) are not eliminated by dialysis even if they are negligibly bound to serum proteins.

Table A94.2 in the appendix lists the amount of a drug removed by dialysis (as a percentage of a "normal" dose in a patient with normal renal function). This value allows calculation of the increment in dosing that must be given to compensate for removal by dialysis. The table does not include removal of drugs by hemoperfusion, hemofiltration, or hemodiafiltration. Hemoperfusion is applicable to toxicologic settings and is discussed in the chapter on poisoning (Chapter 96).

For hemofiltration, one should remember that this procedure removes unbound drug in the serum. The amount removed (and thereby the dose increment needed) can be calculated as:

Amount removed (mg)
= Serum concentration (mg/L) × Unbound
   fraction × Ultrafiltration rate (L/min) × Time of
   procedure (min)

The ultrafiltration rate and the duration of the hemofiltration procedure are known. The unbound fraction can be found in the published literature.[1] Serum concentration can be directly measured for many drugs. Alternatively, the average concentration at steady state can be reasonably estimated as:

Average concentration (mg/L)
= Dosing rate (mg/min)/Clearance (mL/min)

Active metabolites

As noted in the introductory comments, even though many drugs are not themselves eliminated by renal routes, they are converted by the liver to active metabolites that depend on the kidney for excretion. Hence, in patients with renal disease, the metabolite can accumulate, causing its own pharmacologic effect(s).[5,6] For example, meperidine is converted to normeperidine, which is not an analgesic like the parent drug but rather is a central nervous system stimulant. It is excreted by the kidney and accumulates in patients with renal insufficiency. Even in elderly patients with mild decrements in renal function, this metabolite can reach sufficient concentrations to cause seizures. Its use in patients with renal compromise requires lower doses of meperidine (which may limit its efficacy). A better alternative is to use another analgesic such as morphine for which the parent drug and metabolite(s) do not depend on the kidney for elimination. For many drugs, whether there are active metabolites is unknown, much less whether they accumulate in patients with renal disease. Clinicians should be aware that metabolites may cause problems. Unanticipated responses to drugs should raise this thought and may often prompt discontinuation of a drug in the hope that an adverse response dissipates.

Dosing recommendations

When renal insufficiency affects the volume of distribution of a drug (see Table A94.3 in the appendix), the loading dose must be modified. More commonly, one needs to compensate for decreased clearance of drugs by adjusting the maintenance dose. Principles for doing so have been discussed previously, the most important of which is the proportionality that exists between clearance, dose, and steady-state serum drug concentration. Hence, a clearance that is one-half that of normal can be compensated for by decreasing the dose to one-half of normal. Different strategies for dose adjustment have also been discussed; the clinician can change each individual dose, the interval between them, or both. Which strategy to use depends on the drug and the individual patient, but a reasonable starting point for most drugs is to first lengthen the interval until a maximum of 24 h is reached, after which further modification of the individual dose is appropriate.

Table A94.3 in the appendix offers recommendations for modification of the maintenance dose in patients with various degrees of renal insufficiency. These guidelines should serve only as starting points of therapy. Subsequent dosing requires tailoring the regimen to each individual patient, which in turn must be based on clinical endpoints and/or measurement of serum concentrations of drugs.

References

1. UpToDate, Wellesly, MA, 2001.
2. Brater DC: The pharmacological role of the kidney. Drugs 1980;19:31–48.
3. Tucker G: Measurement of the renal clearance of drugs. Br J Clin Pharmacol 1981;12:761–770.
4. Lam YWF, Banerji S, Hatfield C, et al: Principles of drug administration in renal insufficiency. Clin Pharmacokinet 1997;32:30–57.
5. Drayer DE: Pharmacologically active drug metabolites: therapeutic and toxic activities, plasma and urine data in man, accumulation in renal failure. Clin Pharmacokinet 1976;1:426–443.
6. Verbeeck RK, Branch RA, Wilkinson GR: Drug metabolites in renal failure: pharmacokinetic and clinical implications. Clin Pharmacokinet 1981;6:329–345.
7. Holford NHG, Sheiner LB: Kinetics of pharmacologic response.

Pharm Ther 1982;16:143–166.

8. Gibaldi M, Levy G: Pharmacokinetics in clinical practice. I. Concepts. J Am Med Assoc 1976;235:1864–1867.

9. Gibaldi M, Levy G: Pharmacokinetics in clinical practice. 2. Applications. J Am Med Assoc 1976;235:1987–1992.

10. Oie S: Drug distribution and binding. J Clin Pharmacol 1986;26:583–586.

11. Reidenberg MM, Drayer DE: Alteration of drug–protein binding in renal disease. Clin Pharmacokinet 1984;9:18–26.

12. Gulyassy PF, Bottini AT, Stanfel IA, et al: Isolation and chemical identification of inhibitors of plasma ligand binding. Kidney Int 1986;30:391–398.

13. MacKichan JJ: Protein binding drug displacement interactions. Fact or fiction? Clin Pharmacokinet 1989;16:65–73.

14. Greenblatt DJ, Sellers EM, Koch-Weser J: Importance of protein binding for the interpretation of serum or plasma drug concentrations. J Clin Pharmacol 1982;22:259–263.

15. Sheiner LB, Rosenberg BG, Marathe VV: Estimation of population characteristics of pharmacokinetic parameters from routine clinical data. J Pharmacokinet Biopharm 1977;5:445–479.

16. Gault MH, Churchill DN, Kalra J: Loading dose of digoxin in renal failure. Br J Clin Pharmacol 1980;9:593–597.

17. Gibson TP, Nelson HA: Drug kinetics and artificial kidneys. Clin Pharmacokinet 1977;2:403–426.

18. Keller E, Reetz P, Schollmeyer P: Drug therapy in patients undergoing continuous ambulatory peritoneal dialysis. Clinical pharmacokinetic considerations. Clin Pharmacokinet 1990;18:104–117.

19. Reetz-Bonorden P, Böhler J, Keller E: Drug dosage in patients during continuous renal replacement therapy. Pharmacokinetic and therapeutic considerations. Clin Pharmacokinet 1993;24:362–379.

20. Bressolle F, Kinowski J-M, de la Coussaye JE, et al: Clinical pharmacokinetics during continuous haemofiltration. Clin Pharmacokinet 1994;26:457–471.

Appendix

Table A94.1 Effect of renal disease on volume of distribution*

Drug	V_d (L/kg)	
	Normal renal function	**ESRD**
Analgesics		
Codeine	3.5–6.0	7.3
Nalmefene	8.2	17.1
Salicylate	0.15	Increase (no change)[†]
Anesthetics and drugs used during anesthesia		
Thiopental	1.9 (12)	3.0 (12)
Antianxiety agents		
Abecarnil	14	19 (no change)
Oxazepam	1.0	Increase (no change)
Anticoagulants, antifibrinolytics, and antiplatelet agents		
Sulfinpyrazone	0.06	Increase (no change)
Warfarin	0.11–0.20	Increase (no change)
Anticonvulsants		
Phenytoin	0.5–1.0	Increase (no change)
Valproate	0.2–0.4	Increase (no change)
Antihistamines		
Roxatidine	3.2	2.0
Anti-inflammatory agents		
Azapropazone	0.15–0.25	No change (decrease)
Diflunisal	0.10–0.13	0.27 (no change)
Oxaprozin	0.07–0.25	(decrease)
Antimicrobial agents/antibacterials		
Cephalosporins		
Cefazolin	0.11–0.14	0.17
Cefoxitin	0.27	Increase
Macrolide antibiotics		
Erythromycin	0.6–0.8	1.2
Penicillins		
Azlocillin	0.18	0.3
Timocillin	0.15–0.24	Increase (no change)
Quinolones		
Norfloxacin	3.2	1.7
Antifungals		
Miconazole	2–3	Decrease
Bronchodilators		
Albuterol	2.0–2.5	0.8
Cardiovascular agents		
Blood lipid-lowering agents		
Acifran	0.5	(Decrease to 1/3 normal)
Clofibrate	0.14	Increase (no change)
Cardiac inotropes		
Digitoxin	0.73	Increase (no change)
Digoxin	$V_d = 3.84 + 0.0446\ CrCl$	
Hormonal agents		
Insulin-like growth factor	0.15	0.07–0.09
Miscellaneous		
Bendazac	0.18	Increase (no change)

*V_d, volume of distribution; ESRD, endstage renal disease; CrCl, creatinine clearance.
[†]Values in parentheses indicate data for unbound drug.

Table A94.2 Percentage of a dose removed by one session of hemodialysis or 24 h of continuous ambulatory peritoneal dialysis (CAPD)

Drug	Hemodialysis	CAPD
Analgesics		
Meperidine	Negligible	Negligible
Methadone	Negligible (< 1%)	Negligible (< 1%)
Nalmefene	Negligible	Negligible
Propoxyphene	Negligible	Negligible
Salicylates	Negligible	Negligible
Tilidine	Negligible (< 1%)	
Tramadol	Negligible (7%)	
Anesthetics and drugs used during anesthesia		
Gallamine	Considerable	Considerable
Antianxiety agents, sedatives, and hypnotics		
Buspirone	Negligible	
Chloral hydrate	Negligible	
Ethchlorvynol	Negligible	
Glutethimide	Negligible	
Meprobamate	Negligible	
Methaqualone	Negligible	
Oxazepam	Negligible	
Phenobarbital	Negligible	
Zopiclone	Negligible	
Anticholinergics and cholinergics		
Cisapride	Negligible	
Metoclopramide	Negligible	
Pirenzipine	11–15%	
Anticoagulants, antifibrinolytics, and antiplatelet agents		
Warfarin	Negligible	Negligible
Low-molecular-weight heparins	Negligible	
Anticonvulsants		
Gabapentin	50%	
Ethosuximide	45%	
Levetiracetam	25–50%	
Phenytoin	Negligible	Negligible
Primidone	30%	
Topiramate	50%	
Valproic acid	Negligible (1%)	Negligible
Antihistamines		
Cetirizine		Negligible (9%)
Cimetidine	10–20%	Negligible (1.6%)
Famotidine	Negligible (6–16%)	Negligible (4.5%)
Fexofenadine	Negligible (< 1.7%)	
Levocabastine	Negligible (11%)	
Loratadine	Negligible	
Nizatidine	Negligible (10%)	
Ranitidine	50–60%	Negligible (< 1%)
Anti-inflammatory agents		
Azapropazone	Negligible	Negligible
Bromfenac	Negligible	
Leflunomide	Negligible	Negligible
Lornoxicam	Negligible	
Nabumetone	Negligible	
Oxaprozin	Negligible	Negligible

Table A94.2 (*cont'd*)

Drug	Hemodialysis	CAPD
Penicillamine	30%	
Sulindac	Negligible	
Antimicrobial agents		
Aminoglycosides		
Aminoglycosides	50%	20–25%
Spectinomycin	50%	
Carbapenems		
Imipenem	80–90%	Negligible
Meropenem	50–70%	
Cephalosporins		
Cefaclor	33%	
Cefadroxil	50%	
Cefamandole	50%	Negligible (5%)
Cefazolin	50%	20%
Cefdinir		Negligible (1.4–7.2%)
Cefipime	40–70%	26%
Cefixime	Negligible (1.6%)	Negligible
Cefmenoxime	16–51%	Negligible (< 10%)
Cefmetazole	60%	
Cefodizime	50%	Negligible (15%)
Cefonicid	Negligible	Negligible (6.5%)
Cefoperazone	Negligible	Negligible
Ceforanide	20–50%	
Cefotaxime	60%	Negligible (5%)
Cefotetan	Negligible (5–9%)	
Cefotiam	30–40%	
Cefoxitin	50%	Negligible
Cefpirome	32–48%	Negligible (12%)
Cefpodoxime	50%	
Cefprozil	55%	
Cefroxadine	50%	
Cefsulodin	60%	
Ceftazidime	50%	Negligible
Ceftibuten	39%	
Ceftizoxime	50%	Negligible (16%)
Ceftriaxone	40%	Negligible (4.5%)
Cefuroxime		20%
Cephacetrile	50%	
Cephalexin	50–75%	30%
Cephalothin	50%	
Cephapirin	20%	
Macrolide antibiotics		
Clindamycin	Negligible	Negligible
Dirithromycin	Negligible	
Lincomycin	Negligible	Negligible
Monobactams		
Aztreonam	40%	Negligible
Carumonam	51%	
Moxalactam	30–50%	Negligible (15–20%)
Nitroimidazoles		
Metronidazole	45%	Negligible (10%)
Ornidazole	42%	Negligible (6%)
Tinidazole	40%	
Oxazolindiones		
Linezolid	33%	

Table A94.2 *(cont'd)*

Drug	Hemodialysis	CAPD
Penicillins		
Amdinocillin	32–70%	Negligible (< 4%)
Amoxicillin	30%	
Ampicillin	40%	
Azlocillin	30–45%	
Carbenicillin	50%	
Cloxacillin	Negligible	
Dicloxacillin	Negligible	
Methicillin	Negligible	
Mezlocillin	20–25%	24%
Nafcillin	Negligible	
Oxacillin	Negligible	
Penicillin	50%	
Piperacillin	30–50%	Negligible (6%)
Temocillin	50%	Negligible
Ticarcillin	50%	Negligible
Polymyxins		
Colistin	Negligible	Negligible
Quinolones		
Ciprofloxacin	Negligible (2%)	Negligible (0.4–1.6%)
Enoxacin	Negligible	
Fleroxacin	Negligible (3–7%)	Negligible (< 10%)
Levofloxacin	Negligible	Negligible
Lomefloxacin	Negligible	
Norfloxacin	Negligible	
Ofloxacin	Negligible (15–25%)	Negligible (4–6%)
Pefloxacin	Negligible	
Temafloxacin	Negligible (9.4%)	
Streptogramins		
Quinupristin–dalfopristin	Negligible	
Sulfonamides		
Sulfamethoxazole	50%	Negligible (8%)
Trimethoprim	50%	Negligible (7%)
Tetracyclines		
Doxycycline	Negligible	Negligible
Minocycline	Negligible	Negligible
Vancomycin	Negligible	Negligible (15–20%)
Teicoplanin	Negligible	Negligible (5%)
Antifungals		
Amphotericin B	Negligible	
Fluconazole	40%	Negligible (18%)
Flucytosine	50%	
Itraconazole	Negligible	Negligible
Ketoconazole	Negligible	Negligible
Miconazole	Negligible	Negligible
Antimalarials		
Chloroquine	Negligible	
Mefloquine	Negligible	
Quinine	Negligible	
Antituberculous agents		
Para-aminosalicylic acid	50%	
Ethambutol	Negligible (12%)	
Isoniazid	75%	

Table A94.2   (cont'd)

Drug	Hemodialysis	CAPD
Antiviral agents		
Acyclovir	60%	Negligible (< 10%)
Amantadine	Negligible	
Cidofovir	50%	Negligible
Didanosine	20–67%	Negligible
Foscarnet	27–58%	
Ganciclovir	Negligible	
Lamivudine	Negligible	
Ribavirin	Negligible (8%)	
Vidarabine	50%	
Zidovudine	Negligible	Negligible
Antineoplastics and antimetabolites		
Cyclophosphamide	30–60%	
Etoposide	Negligible	
Methotrexate	Negligible	
Paclitaxel	Negligible	
Antiulcer agents		
Lansoprazole	Negligible	
Omeprazole	Negligible	
Pantoprazole	Negligible	
Rabeprazole	Negligible	
Bronchodilators		
Dyphylline	28%	
Theophylline	40%	
Zileuton	Negligible (0.5%)	
Cardiovascular agents		
Antianginal agents		
Amlodipine	Negligible	Negligible
Bepridil	Negligible	
Diltiazem		Negligible (< 0.1%)
Felodipine	Negligible	
Isradipine	Negligible	
Nifedipine	Negligible (< 1%)	Negligible
Antiarrhythmics		
N-Acetylprocainamide	50%	Negligible
Amiodarone	Negligible	
Bretylium	Negligible	
Cibenzoline	Negligible	
Disopyramide	Negligible (2–4%)	
Flecainide	Negligible (1%)	Negligible
Lorcainide	Negligible (8–12%)	
Mexiletine	Negligible	Negligible
Procainamide	Negligible	Negligible (< 5%)
Propafenone	Negligible	
Quinidine	Negligible (<?)	
Recainam	Negligible (9%)	
Sematilide	20–25%	
Sotalol	40–57%	
Tocainide	25%	Negligible (2%)
Antihypertensives		
α_1-Adrenergic antagonists		
Doxazosin	Negligible	
Urapadil	Negligible (6.5%)	

Table A94.2   (cont'd)

Drug	Hemodialysis	CAPD
Angiotensin antagonists		
Candesartan	Negligible	
Erbesartan	Negligible	
Irbesartan	Negligible	
Losartan	Negligible	Negligible
β-Adrenergic antagonists		
Acebutolol	Negligible	
Atenolol	50%	
Carvedilol	Negligible	
Esmolol	Negligible	Negligible
Labetalol	Negligible (2–5%)	Negligible (0.14%)
Metoprolol	Negligible	
Nadolol	50%	
Centrally acting α$_2$-stimulants		
Clonidine	Negligible	
Guanfacine	Negligible	
Converting enzyme inhibitors		
Captopril	35–40%	Negligible (< 1%)
Cilazapril	Negligible (14%)	
Enalapril	50%	
Fosinopril		Negligible (2%)
Lisinopril	50–60%	
Omapatrilat	Negligible	
Perindopril	55%	
Quinapril		Negligible (2.6%)
Vasodilators		
Buflomedil	Negligible (3.4–6.7%)	
Diazoxide	Negligible	
Ketansirin	Negligible	
Minoxidil	24–43%	
Blood lipid-lowering agents		
Bezafibrate	Negligible	Negligible (1.6%)
Clofibrate	Negligible	
Fenofibrate	Negligible	
Gemfibrozil	Negligible	
Pravastatin	Negligible	
Cardiac inotropes		
Digoxin	Negligible	Negligible (8%)
Fab	Negligible	Negligible

Hormonal agents		
Epoetin		Negligible (2.3%)

Hypoglycemic agents		
Repaglinide	Negligible	
Rosiglitazone	Negligible	

Hypouricemic agents		
Allopurinol	40%	

Psychotherapeutic agents		
Citalopram	Negligible (< 1%)	
Lithium	Considerable	Considerable
Olanzapine	Negligible	
Sertindole	Negligible (< 0.1%)	
Sertraline	Negligible	
Tianeptine	Negligible	

Table A94.2 (cont'd)

Drug	Hemodialysis	CAPD
Steroids		
Prednisone	Negligible	
Miscellaneous		
Cyclosporine	Negligible	
Mycophenolate	Negligible	
Sulbactam		Negligible
Tazobactam	30–50%	Negligible (11–13%)

Table A94.3 Dosing recommendations in patients with renal insufficiency (relative to normal dose)

Drug	>50	20–50	< 20	Drug	>50	20–50	< 20
Analgesics				Levetiracetam		1/2	1/3
Butorphanol			1/2	Oxcarbazepine			1/2
Codeine			1/2	Toperamate			1/2
Meperidine		Avoid		Vigabatrin		1/2	1/4
Metamizol			1/3	*Antihistamines*			
Nalmefene			1/2	Cetirizine			1/3
Propoxyphene		Avoid		Cimetidine		1/2	1/6
Tramadol			1/2	Ebastine			1/2
Anesthetics and drugs used during anesthesia				Famotidine	1/2	1/3	1/5
Alcuronium			1/3	Fexofenadine			1/2
Doxacurium			1/2	Levocabastine			1/3
Gallamine			1/8	Nizatidine	1/2	1/4	1/4
Metocurine			1/2	Ranitidine	1/2	1/3	1/4
Pancuronium			1/5	Roxatidine	3/4	1/2	1/4
Pipecuronium			1/2	*Anti-inflammatory agents*			
Rapacuronium			2/3	Azapropazone	1/2	1/5	1/10
D-Tubocurarine			1/2	Diflunisal			1/2
Vecuronium		Avoid		Indobufen		1/2	1/3
Antianxiety agents				Ketoprofen			1/2
Acamprosate			1/3	Ketorolac		Avoid	
Buspirone		1/2	1/4	Oxaprozin			1/2
Anticholinergics and cholinergics				Penicillamine		!Avoid	
Metoclopramide		1/2	1/4	Tiaprofenic acid			1/2
Neostigmine		1/2	1/3	Ximoprofen			1/3
Pirenzipine			1/2	*Antimicrobial agents/antibacterials*			
Pyridostigmine	1/2	1/3	1/5	Aminoglycosides	1/3	1/2	1/4
Anticoagulants, antifibrinolytics, and antiplatelet agents				Carbapenems			
Desirudin			1/6	Biapenem			1/4
Iloprost			1/2	Imipenem		1/2	1/4
Lamifiban			1/10	Meropenem		1/2	1/3
Lotrafiban			1/2	Cephalosporins			
Low-molecular-weight heparins			1/2	Cefaclor		1/2	1/4
Sulotroban	1/2	1/5	1/20	Cefadroxil	1/2	1/4	1/8
Tirofiban			1/2	Cefamandole	1/2	1/3	1/4
Tranexamic acid	1/2	1/4	1/8	Cefazolin	1/2	1/4	1/6
Anticonvulsants				Cefdinir			1/10
Gabapentin	1/2	1/4	1/8	Cefepime	2/3	1/5	1/8
				Cefetamet	1/2	1/4	1/8

Table A94.3 *(cont'd)*

Drug	Creatinine clearance (mL/min)			Drug	Creatinine clearance (mL/min)		
	>50	20–50	< 20		>50	20–50	< 20
Cefixime		1/2	1/3	Gatifloxacin			1/4
Cefmenoxime	1/2	1/4	1/6	Levofloxacin			1/6
Cefmetazole	2/3	1/2	1/3	Lomefloxacin			1/6
Cefodizime			1/2	Norfloxacin			1/2
Cefonicid	1/2	1/5	1/10	Ofloxacin			1/2
Ceforanide	1/2	1/3	1/5	Rufloxacin			2/3
Cefotaxime		1/2	1/4	Sparfloxacin			1/2
Cefotetan	1/2	1/4	1/10	Temafloxacin	3/4	1/2	1/4
Cefotiam		3/4	1/2	Sulfonamides			
Cefoxitin	1/2	1/4	1/6	Sulfamethoxazole			1/2
Cefpirome		1/2	1/4	Sulfisoxazole	3/4	1/2	1/4
Cefpodoxime		1/4	1/8	Trimethoprim			1/2
Cefprodoxime	1/2	1/3	1/5	Tetracyclines			
Cefprozil			1/2	Tetracycline		1/3	1/10
Cefroxadine		1/2	1/4	Urinary bacteriostatics			
Cefsulodin	1/2	1/4	1/10	Cinoxacin			1/10
Ceftazidime	1/2	1/5	1/10	Fosfomycin			1/4
Ceftibuten		1/2	1/6	Vancomycin-like agents			
Ceftizoxime	1/2	1/4	1/10	Teicoplanin		1/2	1/3
Cefuroxime		1/2	1/4	Vancomycin	2/3	1/2	1/10
Cephacetrile	1/2	1/4	1/10				
Cephalexin		1/3	1/10	*Antifungals*			
Cephalothin	2/3	1/2	1/6	Fluconazole		1/2	1/3
Cephapirin		1/2	1/3	Flucytosine	1/2	1/3	1/4
Cephradine		1/3	1/10	Miconazole			1/3
Loracarbef	1/2	1/4	1/10	Terbinafine			1/2
Chloramphenicol and thiamphenicol							
Thiamphenicol	1/2	1/3	1/10	*Antimalarials*			
Macrolide antibiotics				Chloroquine	1/2	1/5	1/10
Clarithromycin			1/3	Quinine		1/2	1/3
Lincomycin		1/2	1/3				
Roxithromycin			1/2	*Antituberculous agents*			
Monobactams				Ethambutol		1/2	1/3
Aztreonam	1/2	1/3	1/4	Isoniazid			1/2
Carumonam	2/3	1/3	1/6				
Moxalactam	1/2	1/3	1/10	*Antiviral agents*			
Penicillins				Acyclovir		1/2	1/5
Amdinocillin		1/2	1/4	Amantadine	1/2	1/5	1/10
Amoxicillin		1/2	1/6	Cidofovir	1/2	1/5	1/10
Ampicillin	1/2	1/4	1/10	Didanosine			1/3
Azlocillin		1/2	1/4	Ganciclovir	1/2	1/5	1/10
Carbenicillin	1/3	1/5	1/10	Lamivudine		1/3	1/10
Methicilin		1/2	1/4	Oseltamivir		Avoid	
Mezlocillin	1/2	1/4	1/8	Penciclovir		1/2	1/4
Penicillin		1/5	1/8	Rimantadine			1/2
Piperacillin		1/2	1/3	Stavudine		1/5	1/10
Ticarcillin	1/2	1/3	1/4	Zalcitabine		1/2	1/4
Timocillin		1/2	1/4	Zanamivir			1/2
Polymyxins				Zidovudine			1/2
Colistin	1/2	1/3	1/6				
Quinolones				*Antineoplastic agents*			
Ciprofloxacin			1/2	Bleomycin			1/2
Enoxacin	1/2	1/3	1/4	Carboplatin		1/2	1/3
Fleroxacin	3/4	1/2	1/3	Etoposide		1/2	1/3
				Exemestane			1/3
				Methotrexate		Undefined	
				Oxaliplatin			1/2

Table A94.3 (cont'd)

Drug	Creatinine clearance (mL/min) >50	20–50	< 20
Pentostatin			1/2
Ralitrexed		1/2	Avoid
Topotecan			1/2
Antispasticity agent			
Tizanidine			1/4
Bronchodilators			
Albuterol			1/3
Dyphylline		Avoid	
Enprofylline		Avoid	
Cardiovascular agents			
Antianginal agents			
Isradipine			1/4
Lercanidipine			1/2
Antiarrhythmics			
Acecainide		1/2	1/4
(N-acetylprocainamide; NAPA)			
Bretylium			1/5
Cibenzoline		1/2	1/3
Disopyramide		1/2	1/5
Dofetilide		1/2	Avoid
Encainide		1/2	1/4
Flecainide			1/3
Procainamide (see NAPA)			
Recainam		1/2	1/4
Sematilide	1/2	1/4	1/4
Sotalol		1/3	1/8
Tocainide		3/4	1/2
Antihypertensives			
Acebutolol		1/2	1/3
Atenolol		1/2	1/4
Betaxolol			1/2
Benazepril			1/4
Bisoprolol		1/2	1/3
Buflomedil			1/2
Candesartan			1/2
Captopril	1/2	1/6	1/12
Carteolol		1/2	1/4
Cetamolol			1/3
Cilazapril	3/4	1/2	1/4
Clonidine		1/2	1/3
Delapril			1/3
Diazoxide		2/3	1/2
Enalapril		1/3	1/5
Eposartan			2/3
Fosinopril			1/2
Guanadrel	1/2	1/5	1/10
Imidapril			1/2
Lisinopril		1/2	1/4
Methyldopa			1/2
Metoprolol			1/2
Minoxidil			1/2

Drug	Creatinine clearance (mL/min) >50	20–50	< 20
Moezipril			1/4
Moxonidine			1/3
Nebivolol			1/2
Nadolol	3/4	1/2	1/4
Pentopril		Avoid	
Perindopril			1/10
Pinacidil			1/2
Quinapril	1/2	1/4	1/8
Ramipril		2/3	1/3
Rilmenidine	2/3	1/3	1/5
Spirapril			1/3
Temocapril			1/2
Trandolapril			1/3
Blood lipid-lowering agents			
Acifran		1/4	Avoid
Bezafibrate	2/3	1/3	1/6
Ciprofibrate			1/2
Clofibrate	1/2	1/4	1/10
Fenofibrate			1/6
Lovastatin			1/2
Cardiac inotropes			
Digoxin	1/2	1/3	1/5
Flosequinan			1/3
Milrinone			1/10
Piroximone			1/2
Diuretics			
Acetazolamide (for glaucoma)	1/2	1/2	1/3
Triamterene	1/2	1/3	1/4
Hormonal agents			
Goserelin			1/4
Lanreotide			1/2
Octreotide			1/2
Triptorelin			1/2
Hypoglycemic agents			
Chlorpropamide		Avoid	
Metformin		Avoid	
Repaglinide			1/2
Tolrestat			1/2
Hypouricemic agents			
Allopurinol	2/3	1/3	1/6
Colchicine			1/2
Psychotherapeutic agents			
Acamprosate		Avoid	
Milnacipran		1/2	1/4
Mirtazapine			2/3
Quetiapine			1/4
Reboxetine			2/3
Remoxipride			1/2
Resperidone			2/3
Sulpiride	2/3	1/2	1/4
Tianeptine			1/3
Venlafaxine			1/2

Table A94.3 *(cont'd)*

Drug	Creatinine clearance (mL/min)		
	>50	20–50	< 20
Sympathomimetics			
Dolasetron			1/2
Miscellaneous			
Dextran 40			1/4
EDTA		1/2	1/4
Sildenafil			1/2
Sulbactam			1/5
Tazobactam			1/4

EDTA, ethylene diamine tetraacetic acid.

CHAPTER 95

Diuretics: Use in Edema and the Problem of Resistance

David H. Ellison and Christopher S. Wilcox

Sites and mechanisms of action
- Proximal tubule diuretics
- Loop diuretics
- Distal convoluted tubule diuretics
- Collecting duct diuretics

Pharmacokinetics

Clinical use of diuretics
- Acute renal failure
  - Prevention
  - Treatment
- Chronic renal insufficiency
- Nephrotic syndrome
- Heart failure
- Cirrhosis and ascites
- Idiopathic edema

Toxicity and use in special circumstances
- Azotemia and extracellular fluid volume depletion
- Hypokalemia
- Hyponatremia
- Glucose intolerance
- Hyperlipidemia
- Metabolic alkalosis
- Ototoxicity
- Impotence
- Hyperuricemia and gout

Diuretic resistance
- General causes
- Therapeutic approaches
  - High-dose and intravenous diuretic therapy
  - Combined diuretic therapy
  - Continuous diuretic infusion
- Additional measures in specific circumstances
  - Endopeptidase inhibitors and atrial peptides
  - Vasopressin V_2 receptor antagonists
  - Albumin
  - Circulatory support and inotropic agents
  - Ultrafiltration
- General approach to patients with diuretic resistance

The problem of edema was noted in the earliest days of recorded history. "Flooding of the heart" was described by the ancient Egyptians, and cures were often heroic.[1] Diuretics, from the Greek "diouretikos" (promoting urine), have been employed for hundreds of years. Paracelsus recognized the diuretic properties of mercury, which remained in common use until the twentieth century.[1] The modern era of diuretics began during the 1950s and 1960s with the development of thiazides and loop diuretics. These drugs were developed empirically, without prior knowledge of ion transport mechanisms. Although few new diuretics have become available during the past 10 years, our understanding of diuretic-sensitive transport pathways has exploded, and progress in rational therapeutic approaches to edematous conditions has continued. This chapter will review uses of diuretic drugs to treat edematous conditions. Where data from controlled trials support particular approaches, or where consensus recommendations on therapy are available, they will be emphasized. The reader is referred elsewhere for a discussion of diuretic treatment of hypertension and nonedematous disorders (Chapters 4, 35, 37, 38, and 54).

Sites and mechanisms of action

Diuretics are usually classified according to their sites and mechanisms of action. The sites and mechanisms of action of the most commonly used diuretics are shown in Fig. 95.1. Recommended doses are summarized in Table 95.1.

All of the diuretic drugs in clinical use act primarily on the renal tubules to inhibit Na reabsorption and increase fractional Na excretion. Active NaCl reabsorption is driven by the Na,K-ATPase pump, which is expressed at the basolateral membrane (the blood side) of epithelial cells along the nephron, keeping intracellular Na concentration low. Each nephron segment possesses unique apical mechanisms that permit Na to move across the luminal membrane; these specific transport pathways at the luminal membrane form the molecular bases of diuretic action. Together, active Na extrusion from the basolateral membrane and passive Na entry across the luminal membrane permit vectoral Na transport in the absorptive direction.[2]

Proximal tubule diuretics

An important pathway by which Na crosses the luminal membrane of proximal tubule cells involves electroneutral exchange of Na for H. Protons then titrate filtered bicarbonate, forming carbonic acid, which dehydrates to CO_2 and H_2O, a reaction catalyzed by carbonic anhydrase. Carbonic anhydrase inhibitors interfere with enzyme activity both inside the cell and within the brush border. The net result is impaired Na, HCO_3, Cl, and water reabsorption by the proximal tubule and increased renal Na, Cl, HCO_3 and water excretion (for more details, see reference 3). Because carbonic anhydrase inhibitors are relatively weak diuretics, their use as diuretic drugs is limited.

Loop diuretics

Approximately 25% of the filtered NaCl is reabsorbed along the loop of Henle. An electroneutral Na/K/2Cl transport pathway generates net NaCl reabsorption because much of

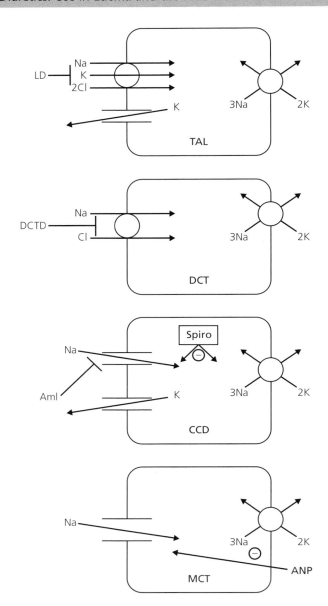

Figure 95.1 Principal cellular sites and mechanisms of action of the most commonly used classes of diuretics. TAL, thick ascending limb; DCT, distal convoluted tubule; CCD, cortical collecting duct; MCT, medullary collecting tubule; LD, loop diuretics; DCTD, distal convoluted tubule diuretics; Aml, amiloride; Spiro, spironolactone; ANP, atrial natriuretic peptide.

the absorbed K is recycled. Loop diuretics such as furosemide, bumetanide, and torsemide inhibit the action of the Na/K/2Cl pathway directly (see Fig. 95.1 and reference 3). Loop diuretics are potent ("high ceiling") drugs that promote the excretion of Na and Cl, together with K. Although they inhibit K reabsorption along the thick ascending limb, their effects on K excretion reflect predominantly their tendency to increase K secretion along the distal nephron. Loop diuretics increase magnesium and calcium excretion. Loop diuretics also impair the ability of the kidney to elaborate urine that is either very concentrated or very dilute and have important hemodynamic effects, both within the kidney and systemically.

They increase secretion of vasodilatory prostaglandins and often reduce cardiac preload, when administered acutely. Loop diuretics block the tubuloglomerular feedback mechanism and tend to preserve glomerular filtration rate.

Distal convoluted tubule diuretics

Distal convoluted tubule (DCT) diuretics (thiazides and thiazide-like drugs) bind to the Na/Cl transporter expressed at the apical membrane of cells along the distal tubule (see Fig. 95.1 and reference 4). DCT diuretics impair urinary diluting capacity, but they have no effect on urinary concentrating ability. Most DCT diuretics become less effective when the glomerular filtration rate drops below 40 mL/min. DCT diuretics increase magnesium excretion but, in contrast to loop diuretics, reduce urinary calcium excretion.

Collecting duct diuretics

Sodium reabsorption by the collecting duct system, which amounts to only 3% of the filtered NaCl load, is primarily electrogenic (current generating), unlike transport along more proximal segments. Three major groups of diuretics act predominantly in the collecting duct. *Sodium channel blockers* (see Fig. 95.1), such as triamterene and amiloride,[5,6] act from the lumen to inhibit Na movement through Na channels in collecting duct cells. Because these drugs impair Na movement along the cortical collecting duct, the lumen-negative transepithelial voltage declines, inhibiting K secretion secondarily. This effect accounts for their K-sparing action. The second class of collecting duct diuretics is represented by *spironolactone*, a competitive antagonist of aldosterone. Aldosterone stimulates Na reabsorption and K secretion along the collecting duct. It also increases the magnitude of the lumen-negative transepithelial voltage. By inhibiting the action of aldosterone, spironolactone causes mild natriuresis and potassium retention. Spironolactone has troubling estrogenic side-effects;[7] a new more selective aldosterone antagonist, eplerenone, is currently under development and may be available shortly.[8]

Atrial natriuretic peptide (ANP) and congeners act at many sites both in the kidney and elsewhere to reduce left atrial pressure, decrease blood pressure, and increase renal salt excretion. As shown in Fig. 95.1, a major site of ANP action in the kidney is along the medullary collecting tubule. Natriuretic peptides are metabolized by endopeptidases. Drugs that inhibit neutral endopeptidase increase plasma ANP concentrations. In hypertensive patients, this reduces blood pressure, increases glomerular filtration rate (GFR) and renal Na excretion, and decreases the plasma renin activity.[9] Nesiritide is a recombinant brain natriuretic peptide that was recently approved for use in decompensated heart failure.[10]

Osmotic diuretics, such as mannitol, do not interfere directly with specific transport proteins but rather act as osmotic particles in tubule fluid. This inhibits both fluid and NaCl reabsorption (for more details, please see reference 3). Thus, these drugs tend to increase the excretion not only of fluid but also of Na, K, Cl, bicarbonate, and other

Table 95.1 Commonly prescribed classes of diuretic and recommended dose range

Class of diuretic	Available dose sizes	Daily dose range (starting dose to maximum recommended* dose)
Carbonic anhydrase inhibitors		
Acetazolamine	125 mg, 250 mg, 500 mg	125–375 mg
Loop diuretics		
Furosemide	20 mg, 40 mg, 500 mg; 1 mg/mL (pediatric); 10 mg/mL (injection)	20–1000 mg
Bumetanide	1 mg, 5 mg; 1 mg/5 mL (liquid); 0.5 mg/mL (injection)	0.5–10 mg
Torsemide	5 mg, 10 mg, 20 mg, 100 mg; 5 mg/mL (injection)	5–200 mg
Ethacrynic acid	50 mg; 50 mg (powder for injection)	25–400 mg
Distal convoluted tubule diuretics		
Bendrofluazide	2.5 mg, 5 mg	2.5–10 mg
Chlorothiazide	250 mg, 500 mg, 0.5 mg	250–2000 mg
Cyclopenthiazide	25 mg, 50 mg	25–100 mg
Hydrochlorothiazide	12.5 mg, 25 mg, 50 mg	12.5–200 mg
Hydroflumethiazide	25 mg, 2.5 mg	25–200 mg
Indapamide	1.25 mg, 2.5 mg	1.25–5 mg
Methychlorthiazide	2.5 mg, 5 mg	2.5–10 mg
Polythiazide	1 mg, 0.5 mg	0.5–4 mg
Chlorthalidone	50 mg	25–200 mg
Mefruside	25 mg	12.5–100 mg
Metolazone	0.5 mg, 5 mg	0.5–10 mg (up to 150 mg has been used in renal failure)
Collecting duct diuretics		
Na channel blockers		
Amiloride	5 mg	5–20 mg
Triamterene	50 mg, 100 mg	50–250 mg
Spironolactone	25 mg, 50 mg, 100 mg	50–400 mg
Brain natriuretic peptide		
Osmotic diuretics		
Mannitol	5%, 10%, 15%, 20%, 25%	25–200 g

*The maximum safe dose of most diuretics is rarely indicated or advantageous.

solutes. The urinary osmolality during osmotic diuresis tends to approach that of plasma, regardless of the state of hydration. Osmotic diuretics increase renal blood flow and wash out the medullary solute gradient – effects which contribute to the diuretic-induced impairment in urinary concentrating capacity.

Pharmacokinetics

All diuretics in clinical use, except spironolactone and nesiritide, have their predominant site of action on the luminal membrane of the nephron. Therefore, to be effective, they must reach the systemic circulation in active form, and be concentrated in tubular fluid.

Loop diuretics are generally well absorbed. The bioavailability of furosemide is 50–69%.[3] Some 95–99% is bound to albumin. Therefore, glomerular filtration is negligible. However, approximately one-half of an oral dose of furosemide is eliminated unchanged by the kidneys, where it is secreted avidly by a probenecid-sensitive proximal mechanism (Fig. 95.2). Carbonic anhydrase inhibitors, loop diuretics, and thiazides are weak organic anions (OA⁻). They are taken up across the basolateral membrane of the proximal tubule by an organic anion transporter (OAT).[11] Presently, four OAT genes have been identified and are expressed in the kidney.[11] OAT-1 and OAT-3 have been shown to have high affinity for loop, thiazide, and carbonic anhydrase diuretics.[12,13] The OAT is a tertiary active countertransport system in which organic

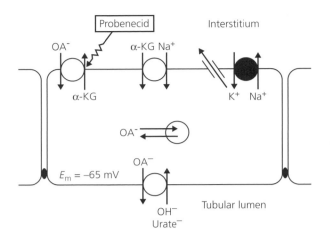

Figure 95.2 Cell model for secretion of organic anions (OA⁻) by proximal tubule cells. For description, see text. Carbonic anhydrase, loop, and thiazide diuretics can all be transported by the organic anion transporter (OAT) in exchange for α-ketoglutarate (αKG).

anions are exchanged for intracellular alpha-ketoglutarate (αKG⁻). The intracellular levels of αKG⁻ are kept high by a parallel cotransporter of Na⁺/αKG⁻. This utilizes the favorable electrochemical gradient for Na⁺ created by the operation of the basolateral Na⁺,K⁺-ATPase and a negative membrane potential (E_m) created by a basolateral K⁺ conductase. Other organic anions can compete with substrates such as diuretics for transport by OAT. These include β-lactam and sulfonamide antibiotics, nonsteroidal anti-inflammatory agents, antiviral agents such as adefovir, p-aminohippurate, methotrexate, uric acid, and a number of endogenous organic anions. Within the cytoplasm, OA⁻ can be taken up and released from intracellular vesicles.

The luminal brush border secretory pathway for OA⁻ and diuretics is less well defined. Two mechanisms have been identified. One is a voltage-driven OA⁻ transporter that derives energy from the E_m. This process can transport loop diuretics and thiazides in addition to p-aminohippurate and urate.[14] There is also an organic anion: urate/hydroxyl anion countertransport mechanism that could provide an exit route for diuretics from the proximal tubule cells.[11]

The uptake of loop diuretics into the proximal tubule is stimulated by alkalosis.[15] Uptake is strongly enhanced by albumin across the range found in plasma.[16] Therefore, the accumulation of organic anions and urate, and the acidosis and reduction in serum albumin concentration that frequently accompany chronic renal disease, may limit nephron secretion of active furosemide and other loop diuretics, thiazides, and carbonic anhydrase inhibitors.

A parallel process also located within the proximal tubule serves to bioinactivate furosemide specifically.[17,18] Studies in experimental animals have shown that, following peritubular uptake into the early segment of the proximal tubule, furosemide is metabolized by uridine diphosphate–glucuronyl transferase (UDTG) to the inactive glucuronide, which is secreted into the proximal lumen.[19] This uptake process is *inhibited* by serum albumin,[19] in contrast to the uptake process that transports active furosemide into the tubular lumen. Therefore, a reduction in serum albumin concentration may reduce the secretion of active furosemide, but increases the renal uptake and metabolism to the inactive glucuronide. These studies in animals have yet to be confirmed by clinical investigation. Approximately one-half of an oral dose of furosemide is eliminated unchanged by the kidney, whereas one-half is eliminated as the inactive glucuronide. In contrast, other loop diuretics such as bumetanide and torsemide are not subjected to major glucuronidation. They are metabolized by a cytochrome P450 process in the liver to inactive metabolites.[20,21] Thiazide diuretics are mostly excreted in active form.

There is normally a sigmoidal relationship between the log of the rate of renal excretion of loop diuretics and the increase in natriuresis (see Fig. 95.3). This is analogous to a dose–response curve. Inhibition of proximal secretion with probenecid increases the plasma diuretic concentration and reduces the natriuresis, but does not perturb this relationship between natriuresis and diuretic excretion. This is consistent with the effect of probenecid whereby it inhibits the uptake of loop diuretics rather than blocks their action on the nephron.[22] A similar interaction occurs with indomethacin.[23] However, the main effect of non-steroidal anti-inflammatory drugs is to reduce the responsiveness of the tubule to furosemide.[22] This is predominantly the result of reduced generation of prostaglandin E_2 because the natriuretic response to furosemide can be restored in indomethacin-treated rats by microperfusion of prostaglandin E_2 into the nephron.[24] A reduced dietary salt intake and repeated administration of furosemide during salt restriction cause a shift in the natriuresis–drug concentration curve to the right, and thereby diminish the natriuretic responsiveness to a unit delivery of diuretic to the tubule lumen.[25]

There are some pharmacokinetic differences between loop diuretics. Bumetanide is more extensively metabolized than furosemide, which accounts for its shorter half-life.[21] Torsemide is less extensively metabolized and more bioavailable than other loop diuretics and has a rather longer half-life.[20,26,27] DCT diuretics are handled at the kidney similarly to loop diuretics. The more lipid-soluble drugs (e.g. bendroflumethiazide and polythiazide) are more potent, have a more prolonged action, and are more extensively metabolized.[28]

Of the distal, potassium-sparing agents, triamterene is well absorbed. It is rapidly hydroxylated to metabolites that retain some diuretic activity.[29] The drug and its metabolite are excreted by the kidney, with a half-life of approximately 3–5 h. Amiloride is incompletely absorbed. It is secreted in active form into tubular fluid.[30] It has a longer duration of action – approximately 18 h. Spironolactone is an aldosterone antagonist. It is metabolized to active compounds (canrenones).[31] It is readily absorbed and bound to plasma proteins. It has an elimination half-life of approximately 20 h, and takes up to 48 h to become fully effective.

Nesiritide (brain natriuretic peptide; BNP) is approved only for intravenous use. It exhibits biphasic disposition

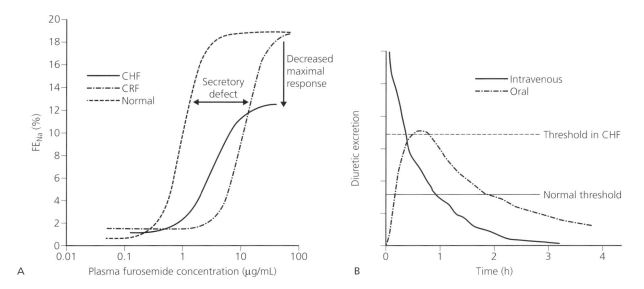

Figure 95.3 Dose–response curve for loop diuretics. A, the fractional Na excretion (FE_{Na}) as a function of plasma loop diuretic concentration. Compared with normal subjects, patients with chronic renal failure (CRF) show a rightward shift in the curve owing to impaired diuretic secretion. The maximal response is preserved when expressed as FE_{Na} (but not when expressed as absolute Na excretion). Patients with congestive heart failure (CHF) demonstrate a rightward and downward shift, even when expressed as FE_{Na}, and thus are relatively diuretic resistant. B, comparison of the response to intravenous and oral doses of loop diuretics. In a normal individual (Normal), an oral dose may be as effective as an intravenous dose because the time above the natriuretic threshold (indicated by the 'Normal threshold' line) is approximately equal. If the natriuretic threshold increases (as indicated by the 'Threshold in CHF' line), then the oral dose may not provide a high enough serum level to elicit natriuresis.

from the plasma. The mean terminal half-life is approximately 18 min. The mean initial half-life is approximately 2 min.

Clinical use of diuretics

A general approach to diuretic treatment of edema is presented in Fig. 95.4. Use of diuretics to treat specific disorders is discussed below.

Acute renal failure

Acute renal failure is frequently associated with a decline in urine output. Obstruction of kidney tubules by casts and sloughed cells may contribute to renal dysfunction in some cases. Patients who develop oliguria in the setting of acute renal failure have mortality rates that are higher than those in whom oliguria does not develop. For all these reasons, diuretic drugs have been used commonly in attempts to prevent or treat acute renal failure (see also Chapter 4).

Prevention

Several studies have examined the ability of diuretics, including mannitol, to prevent renal failure in high-risk situations. Mannitol reduces the risk of postkidney transplant acute renal failure.[32] Mannitol is also commonly employed as prophylaxis for patients undergoing vascular surgery, although data in support of its efficacy are mixed.[33] Mannitol may also be effective as part of a regimen of

forced alkaline diuresis in the setting of crush injuries and rhabdomyolysis,[34] although controlled studies are not available. In a subset of patients with diabetic kidney disease, mannitol was found to reduce the likelihood of acute renal failure after cardiac catheterization, but the number of patients studied was small.[35] On the other hand, in several situations, mannitol provides no prophylactic benefit. In a well-controlled study of radiocontrast-induced acute renal failure, both mannitol and furosemide were inferior to 0.45% NaCl as prophylaxis.[36] Further, mannitol itself may induce acute renal failure.[37] In reviewing data concerning mannitol and acute renal failure, Conger[33] concluded that mannitol has an established role only in preventing primary transplant dysfunction. Most clinicians would also use mannitol (12.5 g initial dose followed by 50–100 g/24–48 h) to prevent myoglobinuric acute renal failure.

Fewer data are available concerning loop diuretics as prophylaxis for acute renal failure. As discussed above, furosemide does not appear to have a role in prophylaxis from radiocontrast-induced acute renal failure.[36] Lassnigg and colleagues[38] reported that neither dopamine nor furosemide was superior to saline to prevent renal failure following cardiac surgery. Thus, loop diuretics are not indicated for prophylaxis against acute renal failure.

Treatment

High doses of loop diuretics (2–15 mg/kg) can effectively restore urine output in some patients with oliguric acute renal failure.[39,40] This may be a useful effect because increasing water and electrolyte excretion makes

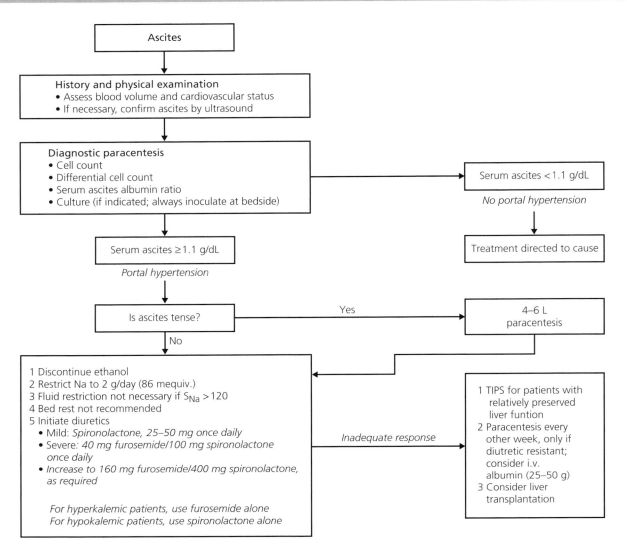

Figure 95.4 Algorithm for treating patients with ascites. TIPS, transjugular intrahepatic portosystemic shunting; CV, cardiovascular; EtOH, ethanol. Based in part on recommendations of Runyon.[71]

controlling extracellular fluid volume easier. Patients who respond to diuretic infusion with an increased urine output also demonstrate reduced mortality. This is not believed to indicate that diuretic drugs improve overall prognosis in acute renal failure. Shilliday and colleagues[41] randomized patients with acute renal failure to either loop diuretics or placebo. All patients received dopamine and mannitol. The results showed that loop diuretics significantly increased urine output, but they did not affect the requirement for dialysis or the time until renal recovery. These data suggest that a positive response to diuretics identifies a less severely affected subgroup of patients. Further, high-dose loop diuretic infusion in the setting of acute renal failure is not necessarily benign. In one study, deafness occurred in 3.4% of patients treated with high doses of furosemide (3 g/day in addition to an initial bolus).[40] Renal failure impairs metabolic clearance of loop diuretics, especially furosemide. Thus, renal failure is a risk factor for loop diuretic-induced ototoxicity. To

summarize, several studies indicate that loop diuretics can increase urine output in the setting of oliguric acute renal failure. Continuous infusion may be especially effective in this regard. Despite increasing urine output, there is no convincing evidence that loop diuretics (or mannitol) improve prognosis, reduce the need for dialysis, or speed recovery from acute renal failure. Many investigators recommend a trial of loop diuretics for patients with oliguric acute renal failure to attempt to increase urine output. If diuresis does not ensue or if excessive doses are required, diuretic treatment can be stopped without jeopardizing prognosis.

In experimental renal failure, atrial natriuretic peptide was shown to speed recovery from a renal insult.[42] Unfortunately, this effect could not be replicated in human acute renal failure,[43] although a subgroup analysis suggested a beneficial effect in oliguric patients. At this time, atrial natriuretic peptide cannot be recommended routinely to treat patients with acute renal failure.

Chronic renal insufficiency

Sodium and water retention occurs very commonly in the setting of chronic renal failure. Dietary NaCl restriction is an important method of controlling hypertension and edema, but when this is not sufficient diuretic therapy is necessary. Loop diuretics are preferred because DCT diuretics alone are usually ineffective when the GFR is less than 30 mL/min.

The ability of loop diuretics to increase *fractional Na excretion* (FE_{Na}) is preserved as the GFR declines (see Fig. 95.3).[27,44,45] This indicates that the *absolute* increase in renal Na excretion elicited by a ceiling dose of loop diuretic *declines* in proportion to the decline in GFR. In addition, the dose of drug required to achieve a given increment in NaCl excretion in chronic renal failure increases because accumulated organic acids compete with diuretics for proximal tubule secretion, as shown in Fig. 95.3. When the GFR is 15 mL/min, only one-fifth to one-tenth as much loop diuretic is secreted as in a normal individual.[27]

Patients with *chronic* renal insufficiency, however, usually do remain responsive to loop diuretics, even when the GFR is as low as 10–15 mL/min, providing they are prescribed at a higher dose. DCT diuretics, on the other hand, are relatively ineffective for patients whose GFRs are below 30 mL/min, when they are administered by themselves. Although DCT diuretics (thiazides and others) lose their effectiveness as sole agents as the GFR declines, these drugs remain effective in renal failure when added to a regimen that includes a loop diuretic, as discussed below.[46]

Nephrotic syndrome

Nephrotic syndrome is the combination of proteinuria ≥ 3.5 g/24 h, hypoalbuminemia, and edema. Hypoalbuminemia may contribute to edema by reducing plasma oncotic pressure and permitting a shift of fluid out of the capillaries and into the interstitium. In this case, one would anticipate that the plasma volume would be lower than normal. Although this mechanism may be of central importance for patients with minimal change nephropathy or severe hypoalbuminemia,[47] many nephrotic patients do not show evidence of plasma volume depletion. This has led to an alternative "overflow hypothesis," which posits that primary renal salt retention underlies the edema of nephrotic syndrome.[48] Evidence in support of this hypothesis includes observations that the sympathetic nervous system and the renin–angiotensin–aldosterone axis are often not strongly stimulated in nephrotic patients, that many such patients are hypertensive, and that natriuresis during treatment often begins before plasma oncotic pressure rises. Yet, primary renal salt retention alone does not cause edema because escape occurs.[49] Thus, it seems likely that some component of fluid shift out of the vascular tree is a necessary component of nephrotic edema.[50] In many patients, and especially in diabetic nephrosis, primary renal salt retention does occur and plays an important role.

Regardless of mechanism, diuretics are important for treating nephrotic edema. As with other causes of edema, dietary salt restriction plays a central and facilitating role in treatment. Because most nephrotic patients are significantly diuretic resistant,[27] distal convoluted tubule diuretics are generally not employed even as first-line agents. Loop diuretics, such as furosemide 40–60 mg/day, can be administered orally and increased to a maximum of 240 mg/day as single or divided doses.

Intravenous albumin has been utilized to treat nephrotic edema for more than 50 years. Early work showed that some nephrotic patients achieve natriuresis with albumin alone, presumably because plasma volume increases.[51] After loop diuretics were introduced into clinical practice, albumin was no longer used by itself because diuretic drugs were found to be more effective. Nevertheless, despite concerns about efficacy and safety, the combination of albumin and loop diuretics continues to be used commonly to treat nephrotic edema, especially in pediatric patients. Controlled studies in adults suggest that albumin may potentiate diuresis or natriuresis when combined with a loop diuretic, but only modestly.[52–54] Studies in children, in whom the diagnosis is often minimal change nephropathy, suggest that combined loop diuretics and albumin infusion effectively reduces extracellular fluid volume.[55,56] This effect is transient, unless remission is achieved, and complications are common. Several concepts for rational albumin use can be advanced. first, the therapeutic approach should be based on a careful assessment of the vascular volume. As discussed above, some patients – especially adult patients, patients with diabetic nephropathy, or patients with focal and segmental glomerulosclerosis – have extracellular fluid volume expansion. In this setting, albumin use should be discouraged because it can increase blood pressure in up to 46% of cases.[56] In contrast, for patients who appear to be volume depleted, especially patients with minimal change disease and profound hypoalbuminemia, albumin may be indicated. For children, albumin is generally administered as a 25% solution (1 g/kg body weight for 1–4 h) together with furosemide 1.5 mg/kg. Such treatment has been reported to induce a 0.4-kg weight loss per infusion and can be repeated five or more times.[55,57]

First, although diuretic resistance in nephrotic patients can result from impairments in diuretic delivery into tubular fluid, patients with nephrotic syndrome usually demonstrate normal diuretic clearance,[58] suggesting that other mechanisms predominate. Another cause might be diuretic binding to albumin in the tubule lumen. In normal individuals, tubule fluid is nearly protein free. Patients with nephrotic syndrome, however, filter albumin into tubule fluid. Kirchner and coworkers[59] showed that albumin in tubule fluid blunts the ability of loop diuretics to inhibit Na and Cl transport. In animal models, inhibiting diuretic binding restores a normal response, but a recent study in human nephrotic syndrome suggests that this is not a predominant mechanism; thus, binding inhibitors should not be considered as therapeutic options.[58]

Heart failure

Heart failure is a common disorder that affects as many as 4.8 million people in the USA, leading to as many as

250 000 deaths per year. General aspects of heart failure diagnosis and treatment are beyond the scope of this chapter, and the interested reader is referred elsewhere.[60] The discussion below will focus instead on the role of diuretics in treating heart failure. Systolic dysfunction (left ventricular ejection fraction $\leq$ 40%) is the best-understood form of heart failure and the most morbid. When left ventricular function is impaired, cardiac output declines. This leads to a drop in mean arterial pressure and activation of neurohumoral systems, including the renin–angiotensin–aldosterone (RAA) axis. Activation of the RAA system, together with other factors, leads to salt and fluid retention, with resulting symptoms of dyspnea, exercise intolerance, and edema.

Diuretic drugs have been used to treat congestive heart failure for more than 500 years, and they continue to play a central role in heart failure treatment today. During the past 20 years, several forms of heart failure treatment have been shown not only to improve symptoms but also to prolong life, at least in the subset of patients with systolic dysfunction. Except for the aldosterone antagonist spironolactone, which will be considered separately below, no diuretic drug has been shown to prolong life. Yet it is very clear that, except in mild cases, most patients suffering from congestive heart failure require diuretic treatment to control symptoms of fluid overload, and it is probably impossible to conduct placebo-controlled trials to determine whether diuretics reduce mortality. Early attempts to withdraw diuretics and treat congestive heart failure (CHF) patients with angiotensin-converting enzyme inhibitors alone frequently led to recrudescence of volume overload.[61] However, because diuretics have not been shown to affect mortality, these drugs should never be employed as monotherapy for patients with systolic dysfunction. Instead, they should be employed for symptomatic control as supplementary but essential agents. They should always be combined with moderate restriction of dietary Na (approximately 2 g Na/day).

During the past 25 years, the goal of diuretic treatment of heart failure has changed. Consensus panels now suggest that the goal is to *eliminate symptoms and signs of fluid retention*.[60] While rapid diuresis may lead to azotemia or symptomatic hypotension, the appearance of these complications should prompt a slowing or a temporary cessation of diuretic treatment. Once the patient has stabilized, additional attempts to control extracellular fluid volume expansion should be made. The "dry weight" can be estimated as the weight at which symptoms of orthopnea and paroxysmal nocturnal dyspnea disappear, the jugular venous pressure returns to normal, and edema disappears. Once this weight is determined, successful diuretic therapy is adjusted based on daily weight measurement. The renal function may be modestly depressed compared with baseline when the patient achieves "dry weight."

When a diuretic is indicated for symptoms and signs of extracellular fluid volume expansion, either thiazides or loop diuretics can be employed. Although some texts suggest that thiazide diuretics should be used as initial therapy for patients with mild disease,[27] others indicate that loop diuretics are employed preferentially.[62] There are few objective data supporting one or the other approach. In general, the efficacy and safety of loop and distal convoluted tubule diuretics appear to be similar.[63–65] A lower incidence of postural hypotension has been reported when treating elderly patients with loop rather than distal convoluted tubule diuretics,[66] but other studies suggest that distal convoluted tubule diuretics are tolerated better.[65]

A dose of 25–50 mg/day of hydrochlorothiazide is commonly employed to treat patients with mild heart failure. When the disease process is more advanced, a loop diuretic is commonly employed. A typical regimen is initiated with 20 mg of furosemide once daily for patients with normal renal function.[27] Because the dose–response curve for loop diuretics is steep, it is important to ensure that the chosen dose exceeds the diuretic threshold. This is often obtained by doubling the diuretic dose until a clear natriuretic and diuretic response ensues or until a safe maximal dose is obtained. Most ambulatory patients can detect such an effect within 4 h and can identify the effective dose in this manner. Once a satisfactory dose is reached, it can be administered up to twice daily or more to ensure adequate contraction of the extracellular fluid volume. A higher dietary salt intake requires more frequent dosing. When intake is high enough, even a potentially effective diuretic dose does not contract the extracellular fluid volume, because postdiuretic NaCl retention overcomes initial natriuresis.[25]

Patients with congestive heart failure may develop diuretic resistance owing to impaired diuretic absorption across the gastrointestinal tract (see Fig. 95.3). Brater and coworkers[67] showed that absorption of furosemide and bumetanide is slowed in congestive heart failure, leading to a 50% decrease in peak urinary diuretic concentrations. In contrast, the *bioavailability* (which is the percentage of total dose absorbed in active form) of the two drugs is unchanged.[68] Inasmuch as loop diuretics must achieve a critical "threshold" concentration to inhibit salt transport effectively, slowed gastrointestinal absorption may lead to diuretic resistance and may explain the observation that intravenous diuretic therapy is often effective for a patient who has become resistant to oral agents. In some patients, the speed of absorption improves with clearance of edema.[69] Bowel wall edema, impaired gastrointestinal motility, and altered bowel wall perfusion may all participate in delayed diuretic absorption.

Cirrhosis and ascites

First, ascites is a common complication of hepatic cirrhosis. It results primarily from three mutually reinforcing processes. First, systemic and splanchnic vasodilation reduce the "effective" arterial pressure (predominantly determined by the mean arterial pressure), leading to renal salt retention. Second, fluid transudes from plasma to the interstitium owing to hypoalbuminemia. Third, increased blood volume and portal resistance lead to portal hypertension. Together, these processes lead to extracellular fluid volume expansion, with a predominance of fluid in the peritoneal cavity (ascites).

Most patients with ascites have cirrhosis, but nonhepatic causes may be responsible in as many as 20%. Many causes of nonhepatic ascites (such as peritoneal carcinomatosis) do not respond to diuretic treatment, thus accurate diagnosis is essential. All patients should be questioned about risk factors for cirrhosis and examined carefully. Approximately 1500 mL of fluid must be present to detect flank dullness. An abdominal ultrasound can be used to confirm ascites. Diagnostic paracentesis should include a cell count and a differential and serum–ascites albumin gradient. If the gradient is ≥ 1.1 g/dL, the patient has portal hypertension (positive predictive value = 97%).[70]

An algorithm for treating cirrhotic ascites is shown in Fig. 95.4. The first component is abstinence from alcohol. Abstinence can improve portal pressure in some patients.[71] The second factor is to restrict the dietary Na intake to 2 g/day (86 mequiv./day). A more severe Na restriction will promote more rapid reduction in extracellular fluid volume, but is considerably less palatable. Restricting water intake is usually not necessary, unless the serum Na level is < 120 mmol/L; bed-rest is not generally recommended.

For patients with tense ascites, a large-volume (4–6 L) paracentesis is usually indicated. This treatment is usually tolerated well, improves well-being, and leads to rapid resolution of ascites,[72] although not to improved prognosis. The use of colloid during or after paracentesis remains a subject of debate.[73–75] Many investigators suggest that a single paracentesis of 4–6 L can be tolerated without administering albumin, especially if edema is present. If there is no edema and if paracentesis is repeated, then albumin (25–50 g) can be administered.[71] Following paracentesis, diuretics must be initiated or continued to reduce the rate or likelihood of recurrence.[76]

While large-volume paracentesis has assumed an important role in treating patients with tense ascites, approximately 90% of ascitic patients can be controlled with diuretics and salt restriction.[77] Thus, practice guidelines approved by the American Association for the Study of Liver Disease emphasize the primary role of diuretics to treat cirrhotic ascites. Spironolactone has traditionally been the drug of choice. Concerns about hyperkalemia, slow onset of action, half-life, and side-effects have prompted investigation of other agents for these patients. Amiloride does not induce painful gynecomastia, as does spironolactone, but amiloride appears to be less effective.[78] In randomized controlled trials, spironolactone was also shown to be more effective than furosemide, when given alone, and had a lower incidence of side-effects.[79,80] When ascites is mild, spironolactone may be administered at 25–50 mg/day. There is no pharmacokinetic justification for the common practice of administering spironolactone more than once daily.[81] When ascites is more pronounced, spironolactone is usually initiated together with furosemide. A regimen of 100 mg spironolactone and 40 mg furosemide has been found empirically to lead to the highest ratio of efficacy to side-effects.[71] The rapid onset of furosemide action initiates diuresis before the onset of spironolactone action (at approximately 2 weeks[79]). Further, spironolactone attenuates furosemide-induced hypokalemia and furosemide attenuates spironolactone-induced hyperkalemia. Doses can be increased to a maximum of 400 mg spironolactone/

160 mg furosemide. Furosemide can be withheld initially from hypokalemic patients. Conversely, spironolactone must be used carefully for patients with intrinsic renal disease, especially diabetic nephropathy. Eplerenone, a more selective aldosterone antagonist with fewer antiestrogenic side-effects, is likely to be available in the near future.

As for other edematous conditions, treatment is best documented by daily weight loss. For patients who have peripheral edema, there is no clear maximal rate of weight loss. For patients without edema, daily weight losses should not exceed 0.5 kg.[82] Severe hyponatremia (< 120 mmol/L), prerenal azotemia (creatinine > 2.0 mg/dL), or encephalopathy should prompt cessation of diuretics.

Patients who are refractory to diuretic treatment or who require repeated paracenteses should be considered for alternative approaches. A recent report compared paracentesis with transjugular intrahepatic portosystemic shunting (TIPS) for patients with either refractory or recurrent ascites.[83] In that study, TIPS was associated with better survival and less ascites at 3 and 6 months than large-volume paracentesis. In addition, TIPS increased GFR and urinary sodium excretion. While these impressive results suggest an important role for TIPS in treating patients with cirrhotic ascites, this approach is best reserved for patients with refractory ascites who have only mild hepatic encephalopathy, mild elevations in bilirubin, and relatively normal renal function.[84] Definitive therapy of cirrhotic ascites often involves liver transplantation.

Idiopathic edema

Idiopathic edema is diagnosed by excluding other systemic and local (venous, lymphatic, and neural) causes.[85] The classic features of idiopathic edema include periodic swelling of the legs, hands, and face in addition to abdominal bloating, occurring almost exclusively in women. Idiopathic edema is frequently associated with eating disorders; when present in obese individuals, it often disappears or improves if weight is lost. Many patients who suffer from idiopathic edema are already taking diuretics when first evaluated, and diuretic abuse may be a component of the disorder. Thus, it is not clear whether diuretics should be used as treatment. A low-salt diet should be prescribed, and adherence to the prescribed regimen can be confirmed by measuring urine sodium excretion. If diuretics are used, they may be given at night, when they may be more effective. Spironolactone is a good choice because its action is prolonged, making rebound edema less of a problem, and because it prevents the effects of secondary hyperaldosteronism. Potassium-sparing diuretics such as amiloride will also help to address the hypokalemia that frequently accompanies idiopathic edema. Unfortunately, diuretics usually fail to control the edema.[85]

Toxicity and use in special circumstances

The main metabolic adverse effects of diuretics are listed in Table 95.2; these and other adverse side-effects are

Table 95.2 Adverse and clinically useful metabolic effects of diuretics

DCT diuretics	Loop diuretics	CCD diuretics
Hypokalemia	Hypokalemia	Hyperkalemia
Hyponatremia		
Hypocalciuria and	Hypercalciuria	Hypocalciuria
hypercalcemia	Hypermagnesuria	Hypermagnesuria
Hypomagnesuria		
Hyperuricemia		
Hyperglycemia	Hyperglycemia	
Hyperlipidemia	Hyperlipidemia	

DCT, distal convoluted tubule; CCD, cortical collecting duct.

discussed elsewhere in more detail.[3] Toxic effects can be divided into metabolic effects, which are often dose related, and idiosyncratic effects, which are dose independent. The latter usually manifest as allergic sulfonamide-like skin reactions that can occasionally develop into severe and life-threatening Stevens–Johnson syndrome.

Azotemia and extracellular fluid volume depletion

Diuretics are frequently administered to treat edematous expansion of the extracellular fluid volume. Edema usually results from a decrease in the "effective" arterial blood volume. Overzealous diuretic usage or intercurrent complicating illnesses can lead to excessive contraction of the intravascular volume, orthostatic hypotension, renal dysfunction, and sympathetic overactivity. Although patients suffering from congestive heart failure usually require diuretic therapy, the combination of diuretics and angiotensin-converting enzyme inhibitors is especially likely to cause renal dysfunction. High diuretic doses or extreme dietary NaCl restriction may predispose to renal dysfunction during therapy with diuretics and angiotensin-converting enzyme (ACE) inhibitors for congestive heart failure.[86,87] In such cases, it is important to attempt to continue ACE inhibitors, in view of their effects on mortality. Functional renal failure in such patients often responds to a reduction in diuretic dose or a liberalization in dietary NaCl intake, permitting continued administration of the ACE inhibitor. Other patients at increased risk for relative contraction of the intravascular volume during loop diuretic therapy include the elderly,[88] patients with preexisting renal insufficiency,[89] patients with right-sided heart failure or pericardial disease, and patients taking nonsteroidal anti-inflammatory drugs.

Hypokalemia

Hypokalemia occurs commonly during therapy with both loop and DCT diuretics. A measurable decline in serum K concentration is nearly universal in patients given DCT diuretics, but most patients do not become frankly hypokalemic.[90] The clinical significance of diuretic-induced hypokalemia continues to be debated.[91–97] Hypokalemia may be more common during treatment with long-acting DCT diuretics, such as chlorthalidone, than with shorter-acting DCT diuretics, such as hydrochlorothiazide, or with the very short-acting loop diuretics.[98] DCT diuretics also increase urinary magnesium excretion and can lead to hypomagnesemia, which may cause or contribute to the hypokalemia observed under these conditions.[99,100] Some studies suggest that maintenance magnesium therapy can prevent or attenuate the development of hypokalemia,[101] but this has not been supported universally. Hypokalemia also occurs commonly during therapy with loop diuretics, although the magnitude is smaller than that induced by distal convoluted tubule diuretic (loop diuretics 0.3 mmol/L compared with distal convoluted tubule diuretics 0.5–0.9 mmol/L[98,102]). During chronic diuretic therapy with loop diuretics, the degree of potassium wasting correlates best with volume contraction and serum aldosterone levels.[103]

Hyponatremia

Diuretics have been reported to contribute to more than one-half of all hospitalizations for serious hyponatremia. Hyponatremia is especially common during treatment with DCT diuretics, compared with other classes of diuretics, and the disorder is potentially life-threatening.[104] Several factors contribute to DCT diuretic-induced hyponatremia. DCT diuretics inhibit solute transport in the "diluting segment" of the kidney, they can reduce the glomerular filtration rate, they contract the extracellular fluid volume, and they lead to hypokalemia.[105] All of these factors, plus their ability to stimulate water consumption in some patients, may contribute to potentially life-threatening hyponatremia. Hyponatremia is less common with loop diuretics because these drugs block the concentrating mechanism. In fact, loop diuretics are commonly used to treat hyponatremia, when combined with hypertonic saline, for the syndrome of inappropriate antidiuretic hormone (ADH) secretion.[106,107] The combination of loop diuretics and angiotensin I-converting enzyme inhibitors has been reported to correct hyponatremia in the setting of congestive heart failure.[108]

Glucose intolerance

Glucose intolerance is a dose-related complication of DCT diuretic use.[109,110] The pathogenesis remains unclear, but several contributory factors have been suggested. First, diuretic-induced hypokalemia may decrease insulin secretion by the pancreas, via effects on the membrane voltage of pancreatic β cells. When hypokalemia was prevented by oral potassium supplementation, the insulin response to hyperglycemia normalized, suggesting an important role for hypokalemia.[111] Hypokalemia may also interfere with insulin-mediated glucose uptake by muscle, but most patients demonstrate relatively normal insulin sensitivity.[112] Other factors may also contribute to glucose intolerance. Volume depletion may stimulate catecholamine secretion, but volume depletion during therapy with DCT diuretics is usually very mild. Recently, it has been suggested that DCT diuretics directly activate calcium-activated potassium channels that are expressed by pancreatic β cells.[113] Activation of these channels is known to inhibit insulin secretion.

Hyperlipidemia

DCT diuretics increase levels of total cholesterol, total triglyceride, and low-density lipoprotein (LDL) cholesterol and reduce the level of high-density lipoprotein (HDL).[112] Definitive information about the mechanisms by which DCT diuretics alter lipid metabolism is not available, but many of the mechanisms that affect glucose homeostasis have been suggested to contribute. Hyperlipidemia, like hyperglycemia, is a dose-related side-effect, and one that wanes with chronic diuretic use. In recent large clinical studies, the effect of *low-dose* DCT diuretic treatment on serum LDL was not significantly different from placebo.[114] Further, hypertension treatment with DCT diuretics has now been shown clearly to reduce the risk of stroke, coronary heart disease, congestive heart failure, and cardiovascular mortality.[115]

Metabolic alkalosis

DCT and loop diuretics frequently cause metabolic alkalosis. Diuretics cause metabolic alkalosis via several mechanisms. They increase the excretion of bicarbonate-free acidic urine and they stimulate the renin–angiotensin–aldosterone pathway. Aldosterone directly stimulates H secretion by the medullary collecting tubule[116] and increases the magnitude of the transepithelial voltage in the cortical collecting duct. Hypokalemia also contributes to metabolic alkalosis by increasing ammonium production,[117] stimulating bicarbonate reabsorption by proximal tubules,[118,119] and increasing the activity of the H/K ATPase in the distal nephron.[120] Finally, contraction of the extracellular fluid volume stimulates Na/H exchange in the proximal tubule and may reduce the filtered load of bicarbonate. All of these factors may contribute to the metabolic alkalosis observed during chronic loop diuretic treatment.

Ototoxicity

Ototoxicity is the most common toxic effect of loop diuretics that is unrelated to their effects on the kidney. Deafness, which is usually temporary, can be permanent.[121,122] It appears likely that all loop diuretics cause ototoxicity because it can occur with chemically dissimilar drugs such as furosemide and ethacrynic acid.[121,122] The mechanism of ototoxicity involves expression of the secretory isoform of the Na/K/2Cl in the stria vascularis.[123–126] Ototoxicity appears to be related to the peak serum concentration of loop diuretic and therefore tends to occur during rapid drug infusion of high doses. For this reason, this complication is most common in patients with uremia.[127] It has been recommended that furosemide infusion be no more rapid than 240 mg/h.[128] In addition to renal failure, infants, patients with cirrhosis, and patients receiving aminoglycosides or *cis*-platinum may be at increased risk for ototoxicity.[127]

Impotence

Impotence is a common side-effect of thiazide diuretics and should be elicited by direct questioning.[129]

Hyperuricemia and gout

Thiazide and loop diuretics raise plasma uric acid concentration because they reduce the ECF (extracellular fluid) volume and increase the proximal tubule fluid reabsorption; they also compete with the urate secretory mechanism. Thus, they can aggravate or precipitate gout.

Diuretic resistance

General causes

Resistance to a diuretic implies an inadequate reduction in extracellular fluid volume during treatment with moderate to high diuretic doses (Table 95.4). The evaluation and management of diuretic resistance is summarized in Table 95.3 and Fig. 95.4.

The first step is to ensure that the patient has renal edema. This must be differentiated from lymphatic or venous obstruction, from idiopathic edema, or from a complication of therapy, such as with a calcium entry blocker (CEB) that redistributes fluid from the plasma to the interstitial compartment.

The second step is to assess compliance. Therapy with a loop diuretic or thiazide is almost invariably accompanied by a fall in serum potassium concentration and increase in plasma bicarbonate and urate concentrations. Therefore, failure to detect these changes from pretreatment values suggests noncompliance. Noncompliance with the diuretic prescription often results from adverse effects, including impotence. However, the commonest cause of resistance to diuretics is failure to comply with restriction of NaCl intake. For patients with mild edema, a diet with no added salt, using a KCl substitute, and abstinence from salted or canned foods is usually sufficient to reduce Na intake to a target of 100 mmol/24 h (2.3 g Na/24 h). For patients with diuretic resistance or severe edema, the help of a dietitian is necessary to reduce daily Na intake to levels of 80 mmol or below. Dietary Na compliance can be assessed by a 24-h urine collection for Na excretion (with concurrent estimation of creatinine to judge the adequacy of the collection). Providing a patient is stable and has not just started or stopped diuretic therapy, renal Na excretion is a valid approximation to Na intake.

The third step is to search for pharmacokinetic or pharmacodynamic limitations of diuretic action. Diuretic absorption in patients with severe edema may be

Table 95.3 Identification and management of general causes of diuretic resistance

Cause or example	Identification	Management
1 Nonrenal edema		
Lymphatic or venous obstruction	Diagnose from clinical history and examination	Institute appropriate nondiuretic therapy
Cyclic edema	Ask about periodicity (women)	Institute appropriate therapy
CEB therapy	Obtain drug history	Reduce dose of CEB or substitute another agent
2 Noncompliance		
With diuretic prescription	Check for fall in S_K, rise in plasma HCO_3 and urate levels with loop or thiazide therapy; urinary diuretic screen	Counsel patient and ask direct questions concerning adverse effects and problems with impotence
With diet	Measure 24-h Na excretion, corrected for creatinine excretion. Goal (mmol Na/24 h) is: mild hypertension or edema, < 100; severe hypertension or edema, < 80	Obtain dietary consultation; repeat 24-h urine to ensure problem is corrected
3 Pharmacokinetic alterations		
Incomplete or delayed absorption Increase dose or use i.v.	Measure plasma levels	Change to more bioavailable drug
Decreased renal function	Quantify GFR	Increase dose in proportion to decline in GFR
4 Pharmacodynamic alterations		
Edematous states	Clinical examination	Increase diuretic dose
Activation of RAA axis	Measure PRA	Consider ACEI, AT_1 antagonist, or spironolactone
Intranephronal adaptation to primary diuretic		Consider concurrent use of second diuretic
5 Adverse drug interactions		
NSAIAs	Obtain drug history	Reduce dose or discontinue NSAIA

CEB, calcium entry blockers; NSAIAs: nonsteroidal anti-inflammatory agents; AT_1, angiotensin 1 receptor blocker; PRA, plasma renin activity; RAA, renin–angiotensin axis; GFR, glomerular filtration rate; ACEI, angiotensin-converting enzyme inhibitor.

incomplete or delayed because of edema or poor blood flow to the intestines. A decrease in renal function that limits GFR decreases the fraction of diuretic eliminated in active form via the tubular lumen. Doses of loop diuretics should be increased in proportion to the decline in GFR (or creatinine clearance). Patients with severe edema typically exhibit diuretic resistance because of salt-retaining mechanisms in nephron segments whose reabsorptive processes are not blocked by the diuretic. There may be pronounced activation of the renin–angiotensin–aldosterone (RAA) axis that can be assessed by measurement of plasma renin activity (PRA) and which is caused by the combined actions of the underlying disease state and the diuretic. Intranephronal adaptations occur during diuretic therapy that enhance reabsorption at other sites. This can be addressed rationally by adding a second diuretic, as described below. Finally, nonsteroidal anti-inflammatory agents (NSAIAs) can limit both the natriuretic and antihypertensive action of diuretics.

Therapeutic approaches
High-dose and intravenous diuretic therapy

High doses of loop diuretics are frequently employed to treat severe volume overload, especially when treatment is urgent. Ceiling doses of furosemide, bumetanide, and torsemide have been estimated (see Table 95.4). When given as a bolus, ceiling doses of furosemide range from 80 mg intravenously (i.v.) in hepatic cirrhosis to 500 mg i.v. in severe acute renal failure. The ceiling dose is that which provides maximal inhibition of the Na/K/2Cl cotransporter, thereby reaching the plateau of the loop diuretic dose–response curve. Administering doses that are higher than the ceiling frequently do increase 24-h urinary NaCl excretion further because the time during which the urinary diuretic concentration is above the natriuretic threshold is prolonged, but the effects of higher doses are often only marginally more effective. It is almost always better to increase the frequency of administration rather than administer extremely large doses.

High doses of loop diuretics given intravenously lead to peripheral vasodilation that may be clinically useful in patients suffering from congestive heart failure who experience symptomatic relief before significant volume and NaCl losses have occurred. In one study,[130] patients with extracellular fluid volume expansion following an acute myocardial infarction experienced a decline in left ventricular filling pressure and an improvement in dyspnea within 5–15 min of receiving 0.5–1 mg/kg of intravenous furosemide. The early decline in left ventricular filling

Table 95.4 Ceiling doses of loop diuretics

	Furosemide		Bumetanide		Torsemide	
	i.v.	p.o.	i.v.	p.o.	i.v.	p.o.
Renal insufficiency						
GFR 20–50 mL/min	80–160	160	4–8	4–8	50	50
GFR < 20 mL/min	200	240	8–10	8–10	8–10	100
Severe acute renal failure	500	NA	12	NA	200	NA
Nephrotic syndrome	120	240	3	3	20–50	20–50
Cirrhosis	40–80	80–160	1	1–2	10–20	20
Congestive heart failure	40–80	80–160	1–2	1–2	10–20	20

Ceiling dose indicates the dose that produces the maximal increase in FE_{Na}. Larger doses may increase net daily natriuresis by increasing the *duration* of natriuresis without increasing the maximal rate. All doses in milligrams. (Based on Brater DC: Diuretic therapy. N Engl J Med 1998;339:387–395.)
NA, not available.

pressure resulted from increased venous capacitance rather than diuresis. Pretreatment of animals with indomethacin greatly attenuates furosemide-induced venodilation, suggesting that prostaglandin secretion contributes importantly to the effects of loop diuretics on vascular tone.[131]

Although venodilation and improvements in cardiac hemodynamics frequently result from intravenous loop diuretic therapy in acute left ventricular failure, other reports indicate that the hemodynamic response may be more complex. Loop diuretics stimulate renin secretion by activating the macula densa mechanism as well as by reducing extracellular fluid volume. In two series, 1–1.5 mg/kg furosemide boluses, administered to patients with chronic congestive heart failure, resulted in transient *deterioration* in hemodynamics (during the first hour), with a decline in stroke volume index, an increase in left ventricular filling pressure, and exacerbation of congestive heart failure symptoms.[132,133] These changes were attributed primarily to activation of the renin–angiotensin system; angiotensin-converting enzyme inhibitors (ACEIs) attenuated the pressor response. Johnston et al[134] reported that low-dose intravenous furosemide increased venous capacitance but that higher doses did not, suggesting that high-dose furosemide stimulates sufficient renin secretion and angiotensin II generation to overwhelm the prostaglandin-mediated vasodilatory effects.

While these data concerning potentially deleterious effects of loop diuretics provide cautionary information, it should be emphasized that intravenous loop diuretics remain the primary therapy for patients in acute pulmonary edema because they usually do improve symptoms before natriuresis, suggesting that, even when cardiac output falls, most patients experience a rapid *decline* in left ventricular filling pressure. Further symptomatic improvement occurs later with natriuresis.

The major limitation of high doses of loop diuretics is drug toxicity. Fluid and electrolyte complications result directly from the diuresis and natriuresis. For diuretic-*resistant* patients, however, direct drug toxicity, most commonly ototoxicity, may also occur and is an important consideration during high-dose or prolonged therapy. All loop diuretics cause ototoxicity in experimental animals, and clinical ototoxicity has been reported following ethacrynic acid, furosemide, and bumetanide administration. Ototoxicity is usually reversible, but has been irreversible occasionally; its incidence may be increased in patients exposed to other ototoxic agents, such as the aminoglycosides.[135] Ototoxicity may be especially common following ethacrynic acid administration and appears to be related to the serum concentration of the drug. Furosemide toxicity has been reported when serum levels exceed 100 µg/mL and can be minimized by administering the diuretic < 10 mg/min.[135,136] Myalgias may occur following high doses of bumetanide. Continuous infusion of diuretics avoids high peak levels and the concomitant toxicity (see Continuous diuretic infusion, below) in diuretic-resistant patients.

Another complication of high-dose furosemide treatment may be thiamine deficiency. Chronic furosemide administration has been reported to lead to thiamine deficiency in animals and, in some reports, in humans. In one study,[137] patients with congestive heart failure who had received 80 mg daily of furosemide for at least 3 months were randomized to receive intravenous thiamine or placebo. Intravenous thiamine led to improved hemodynamics, natriuresis, and an improvement in indices of thiamine status. This work must be confirmed before thiamine can be recommended routinely for patients using prolonged high-dose loop diuretic treatment, but it raises the possibility that loop diuretics may predispose to nutritional deficiencies.

Combined diuretic therapy

Diuretic resistance can often be treated with two classes of diuretic used simultaneously. Controlled trials[138] suggest little or no benefit from giving two agents of the same class (e.g. ethacrynic acid and furosemide). In contrast, adding a proximal tubule diuretic or a distal convoluted tubule diuretic to a loop diuretic is often dramatically effective. Distal convoluted tubule diuretics added to loop diuretics are synergistic (the combination is more effective than the sum of the effects of each drug alone) (see Table 95.5 for regimens).

Distal convoluted tubule diuretics do not alter the pharmacokinetics or the bioavailability of loop diuretics. The addition of a distal convoluted tubule diuretic to a loop diuretic enhances NaCl excretion via several mechanisms (for a review, see Ellison[2]). The most important mechanism is probably by inhibiting NaCl transport along the distal tubule where tubular Na and Cl uptake is stimulated by the loop diuretic. During prolonged use of loop diuretics for resistant edema, distal nephron cells become hypertrophic and hyperplastic and there is an increase in the density of Na/K ATPase pump sites, in the density of Na/Cl cotransporters, and in the intrinsic capacity to reabsorb Na and Cl. Thus, when microperfused with a standard NaCl load, distal tubules from animals treated chronically with loop diuretics reabsorb Na and Cl up to three times more rapidly than those of control animals.[139] Because distal convoluted tubule diuretics can inhibit apical Na/Cl cotransport by the distal tubule even under these stimulated conditions, the effects of these diuretics will be greatly magnified in patients in whom high doses of loop diuretics have led to hypertrophy and hyperplasia. Wilcox and coworkers[140] showed that the natriuretic effect of chlorothiazide in humans was enhanced following treatment with furosemide for 1 month. These data suggest that daily oral furosemide treatment, even in modest doses, may be sufficient to induce adaptive changes along the distal nephron and that these may be treated with combination drug therapy.

When a second class of diuretic is added, the dose of loop diuretic should not be altered because the shape of the loop diuretic dose–response curve is not affected by addition of other classes of diuretic. Thus, the loop diuretic should be given in an effective or ceiling dose (Table 95.4). The choice of distal convoluted tubule diuretic is arbitrary. Many clinicians choose metolazone because its half-life is longer than some classic thiazide diuretics and because

metolazone has been reported to remain effective even when the glomerular filtration rate is low. Yet, direct comparisons between metolazone and classic thiazides have shown little difference in natriuretic potency when combined with loop diuretics in patients with nephrotic edema, congestive heart failure, or azotemia.[46,141,142]

Distal convoluted tubule diuretics may be added in full doses (see Table 95.5) when a rapid and robust response is needed, but this is likely to lead to complications and an extremely close follow-up is mandatory. We advocate hospitalizing patients when initiating aggressive combination therapy. Fluid and electrolyte depletion, sometimes massive, occurs commonly during combination diuretic therapy. Serious side-effects are noted in up to two-thirds of published reports describing combination therapy.[143] One reasonable approach is to establish a therapeutic target weight and achieve control of the expanded extracellular fluid volume by adding escalating daily doses of a distal convoluted tubule diuretic. When the target weight is attained, the distal convoluted tubule diuretic can be prescribed three times weekly and the dose adjusted on the basis of the patient's weight.

Another approach to combination therapy may be a short fixed course. Comparison was made of adding a thiazide-type diuretic to furosemide for either a fixed 3-day period or adjusting the dose to achieve targeted volume losses during 5–7 days. Both regimens were equally effective in reducing extracellular fluid volume and symptoms; surprisingly, natriuresis and diuresis continued even after the thiazide-type diuretic was discontinued during the fixed regimen.[141] For the outpatient requiring combined therapy, one approach is to add a modest dose of distal convoluted tubule diuretic, such as 2.5–5 mg/day of metolazone, for 3 days only. Higher doses or longer time periods are effective but probably too dangerous for routine outpatient usage. Because distal convoluted tubule diuretics are absorbed more slowly than loop diuretics (peak levels at 1.5–4.0 h for distal convoluted tubule diuretics compared with 0.5–2.0 h for loop diuretics), it is rational to administer the distal convoluted tubule diuretic 0.5–1 h prior to the loop diuretic.

Drugs that act on the collecting duct, such as amiloride and spironolactone, can be added to a regimen of loop diuretics, but their effects are generally less dramatic than those of distal convoluted tubule diuretics. The combination of spironolactone and loop diuretics has not been shown to be synergistic, but can prevent hypokalemia while maintaining renal Na excretion. Collecting duct diuretics are used commonly to treat patients with cirrhosis of the liver in whom hypokalemia must be avoided because it predisposes to hepatic encephalopathy. As discussed above, the combination of furosemide and spironolactone is now considered the preferred regimen for cirrhotic ascites.[71] Cortical collecting duct diuretics also reduce magnesium excretion, making hypomagnesemia less likely than when combined with loop diuretics.

In the setting of congestive heart failure, spironolactone was shown recently to reduce mortality.[144] Aldosterone antagonists may also have a role for symptomatic treatment of resistant edema in congestive heart failure patients. Barr

---

Table 95.5 Combination diuretic therapy

To a ceiling dose of a loop diuretic (Table 95.1) add:

Distal convoluted tubule diuretics
    Metolazone 2.5–10 mg p.o. daily*
    Hydrochlorothiazide (or equivalent) 25–100 mg p.o. daily
    Chlorothiazide 500–1000 mg intravenously

Proximal tubule diuretics
    Acetazolamide 250–375 mg daily or up to 500 mg i.v.

Collecting duct diuretics
    Spironolactone 100–200 mg daily
    Amiloride 5–10 mg daily

*Metolazone is generally best given for a limited period of time (3–5 days) or should be reduced in frequency to three times per week once extracellular fluid volume has declined to the target level. Only in patients who remain volume expanded should full doses be continued indefinitely, based on the target weight.

et al[145] randomized 42 patients with New York Heart Association class II–III congestive heart failure to either 50–100 mg/day of spironolactone or placebo added to a regimen of loop diuretics and ACEIs. Spironolactone increased urinary Na excretion, increased the urinary Na/K ratio, increased the serum magnesium concentration, and reduced ventricular arrhythmias. Others have reported similar results.[146,147] Nevertheless, hyperkalemia is a concern when adding spironolactone to ACEI therapy, especially in those patients with renal insufficiency.[148] In one study, potentially life-threatening hyperkalemia during spironolactone treatment was found to be predicted by renal insufficiency, diabetes, older age, a risk for dehydration, and concomitant use of other medications that may cause hyperkalemia.[149]

Combination diuretic therapy is often indicated for hospitalized patients in an intensive care unit who need urgent diuresis because of diuretic resistance in the setting of obligate fluid and solute loads. Two intravenous drugs are available to supplement loop diuretics for combination therapy: chlorothiazide (500–1000 mg once or twice daily) and acetazolamide (250–375 mg up to four times daily). Chlorothiazide has relatively potent carbonic anhydrase-inhibiting capacity in the proximal tubule. It also blocks the thiazide-sensitive Na/Cl cotransporter in the distal convoluted tubule and has a longer half-life than some other thiazides. Both chlorothiazide and acetazolamide can act synergistically with loop diuretics. Acetazolamide is especially useful when metabolic alkalosis complicates the treatment of edema since this may make it difficult to correct hypokalemia or to wean a patient from a ventilator.[150] The use of acetazolamide can correct alkalosis without the need to administer saline. In other situations, combination diuretic therapy may be targeted at the underlying disease process. Theophylline is a very mild diuretic, but acts synergistically with loop diuretics and may be useful when bronchospasm and edema are present together. For patients with left ventricular dysfunction, afterload reduction may enhance diuresis, both acutely and over the longer term, although the effects of ACEIs on diuretic efficacy are complex.

Continuous diuretic infusion

For hospitalized patients who are resistant to diuretic therapy, continuous diuretic infusions can be considered (see Table 95.6). These have several potential advantages. first, because they avoid troughs of diuretic concentration, they prevent the postdiuretic NaCl retention that normally follows the natriuresis. Second, constant infusion yields a greater acute natriuresis than bolus therapy. In one study of patients with chronic renal failure, a continuous infusion of bumetanide was 32% more efficient than a bolus of the same dose.[152] In another study of patients with severe congestive heart failure, 60–80 mg/day of furosemide was more effective when given as a continuous infusion following a loading dose (30–40 mg) than when given as bolus doses three times daily. Bumetanide has a short half-life; torsemide has a longer half-life; and furosemide is intermediate. Therefore, one may anticipate

that the ratio of the efficiency of continuous infusion to bolus would be greatest for bumetanide and least for torsemide. Bolus torsemide may prove to be an alternative approach to continuous bumetanide infusion. Third, poorly documented observations suggest that some patients who are resistant to large doses of diuretics given by bolus may respond to continuous infusion.[153,154] These studies have failed to compare equivalent doses or to randomize the treatments, but Van Meyel et al[154] showed natriuresis during constant infusion in patients who had failed to respond to 250 mg of furosemide given as a bolus. Fractional Na excretion varied in a linear manner with total daily furosemide dose between 480 and 3840 mg/day. Fourth, the diuretic response can be more easily titrated and is smoother with continuous diuretic infusion. Magovern and Magovern[155] reported successful diuresis of hemo-dynamically compromised patients after cardiac surgery by continuous furosemide infusion. Infusing loop diuretics continuously may reduce the sympathetic discharge and activation of the renin–angiotensin system and may moderate the abrupt solute and fluid losses that occur following a large intravenous bolus. Finally, drug toxicity from loop diuretics, such as ototoxicity (observed with all loop diuretics) and myopathies (with bumetanide), appear to be less common when the drugs are administered as continuous infusions. Total daily furosemide doses exceeding 2 g have been well tolerated when administered over 24 h (see Table 95.6), but these high infusion rates may lead to toxic serum concentrations if continued for prolonged periods in patients with renal failure. Torsemide, which has a relatively greater clearance by hepatic metabolism, may be preferred for prolonged high-dose therapy.

Additional measures in specific circumstances
Endopeptidase inhibitors and atrial peptides

Atrial natriuretic peptide (ANP) and other biologically active peptides are degraded by neutral endopeptidases. Therefore, drugs that inhibit these enzymes increase

Table 95.6	Continuous infusion of loop diuretics	
	Starting bolus	**Infusion rate**
Furosemide	20–80 mg	2–80 mg/h (20)*
Bumetanide	1 mg	0.2–2 mg/h (1)
Torsemide	25 mg	1–50 mg/h (10)

*A recommended starting dose is given in parentheses for each drug. In general, the lowest dose range for continuous infusion will be effective in patients with well preserved renal function who have not previously been treated with loop diuretics. The highest doses should be reserved for patients with severe renal insufficiency and profound diuretic resistance. At high continuous doses, toxicity may develop, especially during furosemide infusion in patients with impaired renal function. (Doses derived from Martin SJ, Danziger LH: Continuous infusion of loop diuretics in the critically ill: a review of the literature. Crit Care Med 1994;22:1323–1329.)

plasma ANP levels and cause natriuresis. Indeed, neutral endopeptidase inhibitors given to hypertensive subjects do increase plasma ANP concentrations, lower blood pressure,[156] and, when given to normotensive subjects, increase glomerular filtration and renal Na excretion and decrease the plasma renin activity.[9] Therefore, such therapy might potentiate diuretic-induced Na and fluid loss. This hypothesis was tested in a dog model of acute congestive heart failure. Furosemide alone leads to natriuresis, but this was accompanied by a decrease in GFR and marked activation of the renin–angiotensin axis. During low-dose ANP infusion, the furosemide-induced natriuresis was potentiated and the GFR was now stabilized without activation of the RAA axis.[157] Therefore, endopeptidase inhibition or ANP infusion might be effective in treating loop diuretic resistance, but this requires validation in human subjects. As discussed above, brain natriuretic peptide has recently been approved for use in decompensated congestive heart failure.[10]

Vasopressin V$_2$ receptor antagonists

Arginine vasopressin (AVP) acts on specific vasopressin V$_2$ receptors in the kidney to promote free-water reabsorption. Specific, nonpeptide, orally active V$_2$ receptor antagonists are available for experimental use. A V$_2$ antagonist has been shown to be an effective diuretic in hydropenic human subjects, in whom it increased urine flow and decreased urine osmolality.[158] In a rat model of cirrhosis, a V$_2$ antagonist enhanced free-water excretion and urinary dilution.[159] V$_2$ antagonists may be of considerable utility in promoting free-water excretion and normalizing serum sodium concentration in patients with diuretic-induced hyponatremia. However, they will have to be used with care, since, in these circumstances, the hyponatremia can represent renal free-water retention, which is a final line of volume defense during forced diuretic-induced natriuresis.

Albumin

The use of albumin to treat nephrotic edema and in the setting of therapeutic paracentesis was discussed above. Hypoalbuminemia may contribute to diuretic resistance in other situations and albumin infusion may be considered. Hypoalbuminemia can lead to diuretic resistance by increasing the diuretic's volume of distribution, thereby reducing diuretic delivery to the renal tubules. In rats born without the ability to synthesize albumin, the volume of distribution of furosemide increased nearly 10-fold, an effect largely corrected by albumin. Further, premixing of albumin with furosemide increased the percentage of diuretic recovered in the urine from 7% to 18%, reduced furosemide's volume of distribution, and increased its renal delivery.[160] In four hypoalbuminemic furosemide-resistant patients, administering 30 mg furosemide mixed with 6 g albumin increased urine volume, whereas neither furosemide nor albumin alone had any effect. In contrast, a recent study compared the effects of furosemide with or without albumin for hypoalbuminemic patients (mean albumin 3 g/dL) who were not diuretic resistant.[161] Albumin did not potentiate the effect of furosemide in this study. This study indicates that albumin does not increase

efficacy of loop diuretics in patients whose albumin levels are near 3 g/dL. Most investigators believe that albumin should only be considered for diuretic-resistant patients whose serum albumin concentration is less than 2 g/dL. In this situation, consideration should be given to premixing 5 mg furosemide per gram of albumin for infusion.

Circulatory support and inotropic agents

Acute dopamine infusion increases renal plasma flow, urinary sodium excretion, GFR, and the functional status of patients with moderate to severe congestive heart failure. Beregovich and coworkers[162] showed that cardiac output and urinary sodium excretion rose progressively as dopamine infusion was increased from 1 to 5 and 10 μg/kg/min in patients with classes III and IV congestive heart failure. However, stroke volume and urinary flow rate peaked at 5 μg/kg/min, and several patients developed sinus tachycardia or striking increases in systemic vascular resistance at doses ≥ 5 μg/kg/min. Although acute effects of dopamine infusion on renal sodium excretion and cardiac hemodynamics are often dramatic, natriuretic effects typically wane after 12–24 h.[163]

Dobutamine is a dopamine derivative that is a potent inotrope without significant effects on mesenteric or systemic vascular tone or blood pressure. Both dopamine and dobutamine have been reported to improve cardiac output, renal perfusion, and, in some situations, urinary Na excretion. Hilberman et al[164] compared the effects of dopamine and dobutamine in 12 patients who had undergone open heart surgery and developed depressed left ventricular performance postoperatively. The drugs were administered in random order in doses that increased cardiac output equally (dopamine 5.0 ± 1.8 and dobutamine 3.5 ± 1.8 μg/kg/min). While they had similar effects on renal plasma flow, renal vascular resistance, and glomerular filtration rate, dopamine increased urinary flow rate by 2.8-fold and Na excretion by 4.6-fold more than dobutamine. Since dopamine can increase urinary Na and water excretion during treatment with dobutamine in patients with congestive heart failure, it appears to have unique natriuretic properties. These studies provide a rationale for combining low doses (2–5 μg/kg/min) of dopamine and dobutamine in critically ill patients.

Two other studies limit the enthusiasm for dopamine when added to a loop diuretic to treat congestive heart failure. In one study of six patients with chronic stable congestive heart failure, neither dopamine nor dobutamine was more effective than placebo in increasing urine volume.[165] In a randomized crossover study,[166] dopamine (1–3 μg/kg/min) did not increase urinary solute and water excretion when added to a maximally effective dose of furosemide given to patients with stable heart failure, but did lead to potentially serious tachyarrhythmias in several patients. Although this study does not provide evidence supporting the use of low-dose dopamine in patients with congestive heart failure, the patients studied were stable and *did* respond to furosemide alone. Whether dopamine might elicit diuresis in patients who become *refractory* to furosemide alone was not addressed.

Some data do support dopamine use in critically ill

patients with mild-to-moderate renal dysfunction. In two uncontrolled studies of critically ill patients, dopamine (1.5–2.5 µg/kg/min) increased urine output by 42–50% in patients with baseline urinary outputs <0.5–1 mL/kg/h.[167,168] In a controlled, crossover study of critically ill patients comparing dopamine (200 µg/min) with dobutamine (175 µg/min) or placebo, dopamine increased urine output significantly without affecting creatinine clearance, whereas dobutamine increased creatinine clearance significantly without affecting urine output.[169] Taken together, these data suggest that dopamine may increase renal Na and water excretion in some patients with mild-to-moderate renal dysfunction.

Dopamine has also been recommended in acute renal failure to enhance renal perfusion, increase urinary NaCl excretion, and enhance recovery. Small uncontrolled studies suggested that low doses of dopamine increase urine output in postoperative renal failure and reported that dopamine (4 µg/kg/min) improved urine output in a small group of patients with postoperative acute renal failure. A study of 328 critically ill patients at risk for renal failure showed that low doses of dopamine did not protect against renal failure.[170] Similarly, in a study of cardiac surgery patients, dopamine did not protect against acute renal failure.[38] Thus, there is little support for a role for dopamine in protecting against renal dysfunction.

In summary, dopamine and dobutamine are clearly effective inotropes that increase cardiac output and can improve renal perfusion and Na and water excretion when administered to patients with systolic dysfunction. In contrast, data supporting a role for low ("renal")-dose dopamine to protect against acute renal failure, to treat stable congestive heart failure, or to treat diuretic resistance are lacking.

Ultrafiltration

Most patients who appear to be resistant to diuretics respond to one of the approaches outlined (Table 95.3 and Fig. 95.4). Side-effects of diuretic therapy such as prerenal azotemia and metabolic alkalosis, rather than diuretic resistance, usually limit the ability to reduce extracellular fluid volume further. When pharmacological therapy fails, plasma ultrafiltration, with or without accompanying hemodialysis, may be used to remove extracellular fluid. Agostoni et al[171] randomized patients with congestive heart failure to equal volume removal by ultrafiltration or furosemide. The extracellular fluid volume remained contracted following ultrafiltration but rebounded to baseline after the intravenous diuretic treatment was discontinued. The extracellular fluid volume rebound following loop diuretic usage was associated with a brisk rise in plasma renin and angiotensin II levels. ECF volume contraction induced by diuretics or ultrafiltration stimulates renin secretion via effects on vascular fullness, but loop diuretics additionally stimulate renin secretion directly via the macula densa. This loop diuretic-induced counter-regulatory hormonal response may contribute to more rapid fluid reaccumulation. These interesting results suggest a role for ultrafiltration in the rare patient with extracellular fluid volume overload that cannot be controlled using conventional therapy.

General approach to patients with diuretic resistance

A general approach to diuretic resistance is given in Figs 95.4 and 95.5 and Table 95.3. It is important to establish a

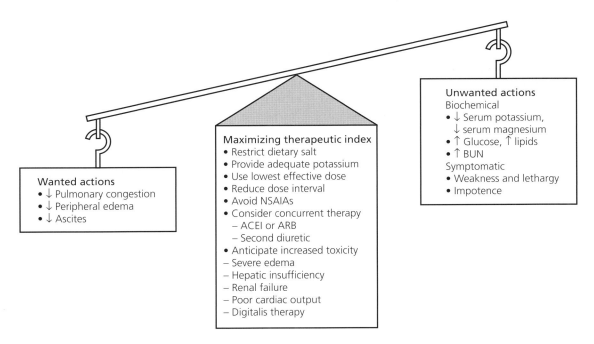

Figure 95.5 Balancing the desirable and undesirable actions of diuretics. NSAIAs, nonsteroidal anti-inflammatory agents; P, plasma concentration; BUN, blood urea nitrogen; Cr, creatinine; ARB, angiotensin receptor blocker.

target response. This can be defined by a set weight, by clearance of peripheral edema, or by improvement in respiratory or other symptoms. Some patients require modest edema to maintain renal perfusion and general well-being, but recent recommendations for treating heart failure recommended keeping patients quite dry.

Noncompliance with dietary prescription can be determined by measuring the sodium excretion rate over 24 h. If excretion exceeds 100 mmol (43 mmol Na = 1 g Na; 100 mmol = 2.3 g), then excessive dietary NaCl intake is likely contributing to the apparent resistance.

If diuretic resistance persists despite effective NaCl restriction, the dose of loop diuretic should be doubled until a response is obtained or until the ceiling dose (Table 95.4) is attained. A distinct increase in urinary output should be noted within 4 h of an oral diuretic dose if a clinical response has been attained. If the response is still inadequate, poor gastrointestinal absorption should be considered and a drug with a higher and more consistent bioavailability, such as torsemide, should be selected, or the diuretic should be given intravenously.

If the response remains inadequate, combination diuretic therapy should be considered (Table 95.5). This is best initiated under observation in hospital. The most potent combination is metolazone or a thiazide added to a loop diuretic, but this approach carries a significant risk of hypokalemia, azotemia, and severe volume depletion. For patients whose serum potassium concentration or blood pressure is low, adding a collecting duct diuretic such as spironolactone or amiloride is preferable. These patients must be followed for the potential development of *hyperkalemia*, especially those who are on concomitant ACEI therapy.

For those patients who remain unresponsive, more aggressive therapy in hospital is indicated with intravenous loop diuretic infusions that can be combined, if necessary, with intravenous or oral distal convoluted tubule diuretics or carbonic anhydrase inhibitors. While the role of ultrafiltration remains unclear, it should be considered in selected unresponsive patients with intractable congestive cardiac failure.

References

1. Eknoyan G: A history of diuretics. *In* Seldin DW, Giebisch G (eds): Diuretic Agents: Clinical Physiology and Pharmacology. San Diego: Academic Press, 1997, pp 3–28.
2. Ellison DH: Diuretic resistance: physiology and therapeutics. Semin Nephrol 1999;19:581–597.
3. Wilcox CS: Diuretics. *In* Brenner BM (ed): The Kidney. Philadelphia, 2000, pp 2219–2252.
4. Okusa MD, Ellison DH: Physiology and pathophysiology of diuretic action. *In* Seldin DW, Giebisch G (eds): The Kidney: Physiology & Pathophysiology. Philadelphia, 2000, pp 2877–2922.
5. Busch AE, Suessbrich H, Kunzelmann K, et al: Blockade of epithelial Na$^+$ channels by triamterene-underlying mechanisms and molecular basis. Pflügers Arch 1996;432:760–766.
6. Velázquez H, Wright FS: Effects of diuretic drugs on Na, Cl, and K transport by rat renal distal tubule. Am J Physiol 1986;250:F1013–F1023.
7. Rose LI, Underwood RH, Newmark SR, et al: Pathophysiology of spironolactone-induced gynecomastia. Ann Intern Med 1977;87:398–403.
8. Delyani JA, Rocha R, Cook CS, et al: Eplerenone: a selective aldosterone receptor antagonist (sara). Cardiovasc Drug Rev 2001;19:185–200.
9. Wilkins MR, Unwin RJ, Kenny AJ: Endopeptidase-24.11 and its inhibitors: potential therapeutic agents for edematous disorders. Kidney Int 1993;43:273–285.
10. Colucci WS, Elkayam U, Horton DP, et al: Intravenous nesiritide, a natriuretic peptide, in the treatment of decompensated congestive heart failure. Nesiritide Study Group. N Engl J Med 2000;343:246–253.
11. Sweet DH, Bush KT, Nigam SK: The organic anion transporter family: from physiology to ontogeny and the clinic. Am J Physiol Renal Physiol 2001;281:F197–F205.
12. Cha SH, Sekine T, Fukushima JI, et al: Identification and characterization of human organic anion transporter 3 expressing predominantly in the kidney. Mol Pharmacol 2001;59:1277–1286.
13. Uwai Y, Saito H, Hashimoto Y, et al: Interaction and transport of thiazide diuretics, loop diuretics, and acetazolamide via rat renal organic anion transporter rOAT1. J Pharmacol Exp Ther 2000;295:261–265.
14. Krick W, Wolff NA, Burckhardt G: Voltage-driven *p*-aminohippurate, chloride, and urate transport in porcine renal brush-border membrane vesicles. Pflügers Arch 2000;441:125–132.
15. Loon NR, Wilcox CS: Mild metabolic alkalosis impairs the natriuretic response to bumetanide in normal human subjects. Clin Sci (Colch) 1998;94:287–292.
16. Pichette V, Geadah D, du Souich P: The influence of moderate hypoalbuminaemia on the renal metabolism and dynamics of furosemide in the rabbit. Br J Pharmacol 1996;119:885–890.
17. Sear JW: Drug biotransformation by the kidney: how important is it, and how much do we really know? Br J Anaesth 1991;67:369–372.
18. Sommers DK, Meyer EC, Moncrieff J: The influence of co-administered organic acids on the kinetics and dynamics of frusemide. Br J Clin Pharmacol 1991;32:489–493.
19. Pichette V, du Souich P: Role of the kidneys in the metabolism of furosemide: its inhibition by probenecid. J Am Soc Nephrol 1996;7:345–349.
20. Blose JS, Adams KF Jr, Patterson JH: Torsemide: a pyridine-sulfonylurea loop diuretics. Ann Pharmacother 1995;29:396–402.
21. Brater DC: Disposition and response to bumetanide and furosemide. Am J Cardiol 1986;57:20A–25A.
22. Chennavasin P, Seiwell R, Brater DC: Pharmacokinetic dynamic analysis of the indomethacin–furosemide interaction in man. J Pharmacol Exp Ther 1980;215:77–81.
23. Chennavasin P, Seiwell R, Brater DC, et al: Pharmacodynamic analysis of the furosemide–probenecid interaction in man. Kidney Int 1979;16:187–195.
24. Kirchner KA, Martin CJ, Bower JD: Prostaglandin E2 but not I2 restores furosemide response in indomethacin-treated rats. Am J Physiol 1986;250:F980–F985.
25. Wilcox CS, Mitch WE, Kelly RA, et al: Response of the kidney to furosemide. I. Effects of salt intake and renal compensation. J Lab Clin Med 1983;102:450–458.
26. Brater DC: Clinical pharmacology of loop diuretics. Drugs 1991;41 (Suppl 3):14–22.
27. Brater DC: Diuretic therapy. N Engl J Med 1998;339:387–395.
28. Welling PG: Pharmacokinetics of the thiazide diuretics. Biopharm Drug Dispos 1986;7:501–535.
29. Mutschler E, Gilfrich HJ, Knauf H, et al: Pharmacokinetics of triamterene. Clin Exp Hypertens 1983;A5:249–269.
30. Somogyi AA, Hovens CM, Muirhead MR, et al: Renal tubular secretion of amiloride and its inhibition by cimetidine in humans and in an animal model. Drug Metab Dispos 1989;17:190–196.
31. Andriulli A, Arrigoni A, Gindro T, et al: Canrenone and androgen receptor-active materials in plasma of cirrhotic patients during long-term K-canrenoate or spironolactone therapy. Digestion 1989;44:155–162.
32. Bonventre JV, Weinberg JM: Kidney preservation ex vivo for transplantation. Annu Rev Med 1992;43:523–553.
33. Conger JD: Interventions in clinical acute renal failure: What are the data? Am J Kidney Dis 1995;26:565–576.
34. Better OS, Stein JH: Early management of shock and prophylaxis of acute renal failure in traumatic rhabdomyolysis. N Engl J Med 1990;322:825–829.
35. Weisberg LS, Kurnik PB, Kurnik BR: Risk of radiocontrast in

patients with and without diabetes mellitus. Kidney Int 1994;45:259–265.

36. Solomon R, Werner C, Mann D, et al: Effects of saline, mannitol, and furosemide on acute decreases in renal function induced by radiocontrast agents. N Engl J Med 1994;331:1416–1420.

37. Dorman HR, Sondheimer JH, Cadnapaphornchai P: Mannitol-induced acute renal failure. Medicine (Baltimore) 1990;69:153–190.

38. Lassnigg A, Donner E, Grubhofer G, et al: Lack of renoprotective effects of dopamine and furosemide during cardiac surgery. J Am Soc Nephrol 2000;11:97–104.

39. Anderson RJ, Linas S, Berns AS, et al: Nonoliguric acute renal failure. N Engl J Med 1977;296:1134–1138.

40. Brown CB, Ogg CS, Cameron JS: High dose frusemide in acute renal failure: a controlled trial. Clin Nephrol 1981;15:90–96.

41. Shilliday IR, Quinn KJ, Allison ME: Loop diuretics in the management of acute renal failure: a prospective, double-blind, placebo-controlled, randomized study. Nephrol Dial Transplant 1997;12:2592–2596.

42. Conger JD, Falk SA, Hammond WS: Atrial natriuretic peptide and dopamine in established acute renal failure in the rat. Kidney Int 1991;40:21–28.

43. Allgren RL, Marbury TC, Rahman SN, et al: Anaritide in acute tubular necrosis. Auriculin Anaritide Acute Renal Failure Study Group. N Engl J Med 1997;336:828–834.

44. Van Olden RW, Van Meyel JJM, Gerlag PGG: Sensitivity of residual nephrons to high dose furosemide described by diuretic efficiency. Eur J Clin Pharmacol 1995;47:483–488.

45. Voelker JR, Cartwright-Brown D, Anderson S, et al: Comparison of loop diuretics in patients with chronic renal insufficiency. Kidney Int 1987;32:572–578.

46. Fliser D, Schröter M, Neubeck M, et al: Coadministration of thiazides increases the efficacy of loop diuretics even in patients with advanced renal failure. Kidney Int 1994;46:482–488.

47. Oliver WJ, Owings CL: Sodium excretion in the nephrotic syndrome: relation to serum albumin concentration, glomerular filtration rate, and aldosterone secretion rate. Am J Dis Child 1967;113:352–362.

48. Ichikawa I, Rennke HG, Hoyer JR, et al: Role for intrarenal mechanisms in the impaired salt excretion of experimental nephrotic syndrome. J Clin Invest 1983;71:91–103.

49. Reinhardt HW, Boemke W, Palm Ü, et al: What causes escape from sodium retaining hormones? Acta Physiol Scand 1990;139 (Suppl 591):12–17.

50. Schrier RW, Fassett RG: A critique of the overfill hypothesis of sodium and water retention in the nephrotic syndrome. Kidney Int 1998;53:1111–1117.

51. Luetscher JA Jr, Hall AD, Kremer VL: Treatment of nephrosis with concentrated human serum albumin. I. Effects on the proteins of body fluids. J Clin Invest 1949;28:700–712.

52. Akcicek F, Yalniz T, Basci A, et al: Diuretic effect of frusemide in patients with nephrotic syndrome: is it potentiated by albumin? Br Med J 1995;310:162–163.

53. Fliser D, Zurbruggen I, Mutschler E, et al: Coadministration of albumin and furosemide in patients with the nephrotic syndrome. Kidney Int 1999;55:629–634.

54. Sjöström PA, Odlind BG: Effect of albumin on diuretic treatment in the nephrotic syndrome. Br Med J 1995; 310:1537.

55. Baum M: Ask the expert. Pediatr Nephrol 2000;14:184–185.

56. Haws RM, Baum M: Efficacy of albumin and diuretic therapy in children with nephrotic syndrome. Pediatrics 1993;91:1142–1146.

57. Weiss RA, Schoeneman M, Greifer I: Treatment of severe nephrotic edema with albumin and furosemide. NY State J Med 1984;84:384–386.

58. Agarwal R, Gorski JC, Sundblad K, et al: Urinary protein binding does not affect response to furosemide in patients with nephrotic syndrome. J Am Soc Nephrol 2000;11:1100–1105.

59. Kirchner KA, Voelker JR, Brater DC: Binding inhibitors restore furosemide potency in tubule fluid containing albumin. Kidney Int 1991;40:418–424.

60. Advisory Council to Improve Outcomes Nationwide in Heart Failure: Consensus recommendations for the management of chronic heart failure. On behalf of the membership of the Advisory Council to Improve Outcomes Nationwide in Heart Failure. Am J Cardiol 1999;83:1A–38A.

61. Richardson A, Scriven AJ, Poole-Wilson PA, et al: Double-blind comparison of captopril alone against frusemide plus amiloride in mild heart failure. Lancet 1987;2:709–711.

62. Gomberg-Maitland M, Baran DA, Fuster V: Treatment of congestive heart failure: guidelines for the primary care physician and the heart failure specialist. Arch Intern Med 2001;161:342–352.

63. Gillies A, Morgan T, Myers J: Comparison of piretanide and chlorothiazide in the treatment of cardiac failure. Med J Aust 1980;1:170–172.

64. Levy B: The efficacy and safety of furosemide and a combination of spironolactone and hydrochlorothiazide in congestive heart failure. J Clin Pharmacol 1977;17:420–430.

65. Viherkoski M, Huikko M, Varjoranta K: The effect of amiloride/hydrochlorothiazide combination vs furosemide plus potassium supplementation in the treatment of oedema of cardiac origin. Ann Clin Res 1981;13:11–15.

66. Heseltine D, Bramble MG: Loop diuretics cause less postural hypotension than thiazide diuretics in the frail elderly. Curr Med Res Opin 1988;11:232–235.

67. Brater DC: Pharmacokinetics of loop diuretics in congestive heart failure. Br Heart J 1994;72 (Suppl):40–43.

68. Brater DC, Day B, Burdette A, et al: Bumetanide and furosemide in heart failure. Kidney Int 1984;26:183–189.

69. Vasko MR, Brown-Cartwright D, Knochel JP, et al: Furosemide absorption altered in decompensated congestive heart failure. Ann Intern Med 1985;102:314–318.

70. Runyon BA, Montano AA, Akriviadis EA, et al: The serum–ascites albumin gradient is superior to the exudate–transudate concept in the differential diagnosis of ascites. Ann Intern Med 1992;117:215–220.

71. Runyon BA: Management of adult patients with ascites caused by cirrhosis. Hepatology 1998;27:264–272.

72. Gines P, Arroyo V, Quintero E: Comparison of paracentesis and diuretics in the treatment of cirrhotics with tense ascites: results of a randomized study. Gastroenterology 1987;93:234–241.

73. Luca A, Garcia-Pagán JC, Bosch J, et al: Beneficial effects of intravenous albumin infusion on the hemodynamic and humoral changes after total paracentesis. Hepatology 1995;22:753–758.

74. Peltekian KM, Wong F, Liu PP, et al: Cardiovascular, renal, and neurohumoral responses to single large-volume paracentesis in patients with cirrhosis and diuretic-resistant ascites. Am J Gastroenterol 1997;92:394–399.

75. Tito L, Gines P, Arroyo V, et al: Total paracentesis associated with intravenous albumin management of patients with cirrhosis and ascites. Gastroenterology 1990;88:146–151.

76. Fernandez-Esparrach G, Guevara M, Sort P, et al: Diuretic requirements after therapeutic paracentesis in non-azotemic patients with cirrhosis. A randomized double-blind trial of spironolactone versus placebo. J Hepatol 1997;26:614–620.

77. Stanley MM, Ochi S, Lee KK, et al: Peritoneovenous shunting as compared with medical treatment in patients with alcoholic cirrhosis and massive ascites. Veterans Administration Cooperative Study on Treatment of Alcoholic Cirrhosis with Ascites. N Engl J Med 1989;321:1632–1638.

78. Angeli P, Dalla Pria M, De Bei E, et al: Randomized clinical study of the efficacy of amiloride and potassium canrenoate in nonazotemic cirrhotic patients with ascites. Hepatology 1994;19:72–79.

79. Fogel MR, Sawhney VK, Neal EA, et al: Diuresis in the ascitic patient: a randomized controlled trial of three regimens. J Clin Gastroenterol 1981;3(Suppl 1):73–80.

80. Perez-Ayuso RM, Arroyo V, Planas R, et al: Randomized comparative study of efficacy of furosemide versus spironolactone in nonazotemic cirrhosis with ascites. Relationship between the diuretic response an the activity of the renin–aldosterone system. Gastroenterology 1983;84:961–968.

81. Sungaila I, Bartle WR, Walker SE, et al: Spironolactone pharmacokinetics and pharmacodynamics in patients with cirrhotic ascites. Gastroenterology 1992;102:1680–1685.

82. Pockros PJ, Reynolds TB: Rapid diuresis in patients with ascites from chronic liver disease: the importance of peripheral edema. Gastroenterology 1986;90:1827–1833.

83. Rossle M, Ochs A, Gulberg V, et al: A comparison of paracentesis and transjugular intrahepatic portosystemic shunting in patients with ascites. N Engl J Med 2000;342:1701–1707.

84. Lake JR: The role of transjugular shunting in patients with ascites. N Engl J Med 2000;342:1745–1747.

85. Kay A, Davis CL: Idiopathic edema. Am J Kidney Dis 1999;34:405–423

86. Packer M: Identification of risk factors predisposing to the development of functional renal insufficiency during treatment with converting-enzyme inhibitors in chronic heart failure. Cardiology 1989;76(Suppl. 2):50–55.

87. Packer M, Lee WH, Medina N, Yushak M, Kessler PD: Functional renal insufficiency during long-term therapy with captopril and enalapril in severe congestive heart failure. Ann Intern Med 1987;106:346–354.

88. Smith WE, Steele TH: Avoiding diuretic related complications in older patients. Geriatrics 1983;38:117–119.

89. Kaufman AM, Levitt MF: The effect of diuretics on systemic and renal hemodynamics in patients with renal insufficiency. Am J Kidney Dis 1985;5:A71–A78.

90. Siegel D, Hulley SB, Black DM, et al: Diuretics, serum and intracellular electrolyte levels, and ventricular arrhythmias in hypertensive men. JAMA 1992;267:1083–1089.

91. Flaker G, Villarreal D, Chapman D: Is hypokalemia a cause of ventricular arrhythmias. J Crit Illness 1986;2:66–74.

92. Freis ED: Critique of the clinical importance of diuretic-induced hypokalemia and elevated cholesterol level. Arch Intern Med 1989;149:2640–2648.

93. Harrington JT, Isner JM, Kassirer JP: Our national obsession with potassium. Am J Med 1982;73:155–159.

94. Kaplan NM: Our appropriate concern about hypokalemia. Am J Med 1984;77:1–4.

95. Kaplan NM: How bad are diuretic-induced hypokalemia and hypercholesterolemia? Arch Intern Med 1989;149:2649.

96. Kassirer JP, Harrinton JT: Diuretics and potassium metabolism: a reassessment of the need, effectiveness and safety of potassium therapy. Kidney Int 1977;11:505–515.

97. Myers MG: Diuretic therapy and ventricular arrhythmias in persons 65 years of age and older. Am J Cardiol 1990;65:599–603.

98. Ram CVS, Garrett BN, Kaplan NM: Moderate sodium restriction and various diuretics in the treatment of hypertension: effects of potassium wastage and blood pressure control. Arch Intern Med 1981;141:1015–1019.

99. Dorup I: Magnesium and potassium deficiency. Its diagnosis, occurrence and treatment in diuretic therapy and its consequences for growth, protein synthesis and growth factors. Acta Physiol Scand 1994;150(Suppl 618):7–55.

100. Rude RK: Physiology of magnesium metabolism and the important role of magnesium in potassium deficiency. Am J Cardiol 1989;63:31G–34G.

101. Dorup I, Skajaa K, Thybo NK: Oral magnesium supplementation restores the concentrations of magnesium, potassium and sodium–potassium pumps in skeletal muscle of patients receiving diuretic treatment. J Intern Med 1993;233:117–123.

102. Palmer BF: Potassium disturbances associated with the use of diuretics. In Seldin DW, Giebisch G (eds): Diuretic Agents: Clinical Physiology and Pharmacology. San Diego: Academic Press, 1997, pp 571–583.

103. Wilcox CS, Mitch WE, Kelly RA, et al: Factors affecting potassium balance during frusemide administration. Clin Sci 1984;67:195–203.

104. Ashraf N, Locksley R, Arieff A: Thiazide-induced hyponatremia associated with death or neurologic damage in outpatients. Am J Med 1981;70:1163–1168.

105. fichman MP, Vorherr H, Kleeman CR, et al: Diuretic-induced hyponatremia. Ann Intern Med 1971;75:853–863.

106. Hantman D, Rossier B, Zohlman R, et al: Rapid correction of hyponatremia in the syndrome of inappropriate secretion of antidiuretic hormone: an alternative treatment to hypertonic saline. Ann Intern Med 1973;78:870–875.

107. Schrier RW: New treatments for hyponatremia. N Engl J Med 1978;298:214–215.

108. Dzau VJ, Hollenberg NK: Renal response to captopril in severe heart failure: role of furosemide in natriuresis and reversal of hyponatremia. Ann Intern Med 1984;100:777–782.

109. Carlsen JE, Kober L, Torp-Pedersen C, et al: Relation between dose of bendrofluazide, antihypertensive effect, and adverse biochemical effects. Br Med J 1990;300:975–978.

110. Shalev H, Ohali M, Abramson O: Nephrocalcinosis in pseudohypoaldosteronism and the effect of indomethacin therapy. J Pediatr 1994;125:246–248.

111. Helderman JH, Elahi D, Andersen DK, et al: Prevention of the glucose intolerance of thiazide diuretics by maintenance of body potassium. Diabetes 1983;32:106–111.

112. Toto RA: Metabolic derangements associated with diuretic use: insulin resistance, dyslipidemia, hyperuricemia, and anti-adrenergic effects. In Seldin DW, Giebisch G (eds): Diuretic Agents: Clinical Physiology and Pharmacology. San Diego: Academic Press, 1997, pp 621–636.

113. Pickkers P, Schachter M, Hughes AD, et al: Thiazide-induced hyperglycaemia: a role for calcium-activated potassium channels? Diabetologia 1996;39:861–864.

114. Grimm RH Jr, Flack JM, Granditis GA: Treatment of Mild Hypertension Study (TOMHS) Research Group. Long-term effects on plasma lipids of diet and drugs to treat hypertension. JAMA 1996;275:1549–1556.

115. Psaty BM, Smith NL, Siscovick DS, et al: Health outcomes associated with antihypertensive therapies used as first-line agents. JAMA 1997;277:739–745.

116. Stone DK, Seldin DW, Kokko JP, et al: Mineralocorticoid modulation of rabbit medullary collecting duct acidification. J Clin Invest 1983;72:77–83.

117. Tannen RL: The effect of uncomplicated potassium depletion on urine acidification. J Clin Invest 1970;49:813–827.

118. Soleimani M, Aronson PS: Ionic mechanism of Na^+-HCO_3^- cotransport in rabbit renal basolateral membrane vesicles. J Biol Chem 1989;264:18302–18308.

119. Soleimani M, Grassl SM, Aronson PS: Stoichiometry of Na^+-HCO_3^- cotransport in basolateral membrane vesicles isolated from rabbit renal cortex. J Clin Invest 1987;79:1276–1280.

120. Wingo CS, Straub SG: Active proton secretion and potassium absorption in the rabbit outer medullary collecting duct. Functional evidence for proton-potassium-activated adenosine triphosphatase. J Clin Invest 1989;84:361–365.

121. Maher JF, Schreiner GF: Studies on ethacrynic acid in patients with refractory edema. Ann Intern Med 1965;62:15–29.

122. Nochy D, Callard P, Bellon B, et al: Association of overt glomerulonephritis and liver disease: a study of 34 patients. Clin Nephrol 1976;6:422–427.

123. Bosher SK: The nature of ototoxicity actions of ethacrynic acid upon the mammalian endolymph system. I. Functional aspects. Acta Otolaryngol 1980;89:407–418.

124. Hidaka H, Oshima T, Ikeda K, et al: The Na–K–Cl cotransporters in the rat cochlea: RT-PCR and partial sequence analysis. Biochem Biophys Res Commun 1996;220:425–430.

125. Ikeda K, Oshima T, Hidaka H, et al: Molecular and clinical implications of loop diuretic ototoxicity. Hear Res 1997;107:1–8.

126. Mizuta T, Adachi M, Iwasa KH: Ultrastructural localization of the Na–K–Cl cotransporter in the lateral wall of the rabbit cochlear duct. Hear Res 1997;106:154–162.

127. Star RA: Ototoxicity. In Seldin DW, Giebisch G (eds): Diuretic Agents: Clinical Physiology and Pharmacology. San Diego: Academic Press, 1997, pp 637–642.

128. Wigand ME, Heidland A: Ototoxic side effects of high doses of furosemide in patients with uremia. Postgrad Med J 1971;47:54–56.

129. Chang SW, fine R, Siegel D, et al: The impact of diuretic therapy on reported sexual function. Arch Intern Med 1991;151:2402–2408.

130. Dikshit K, Vyden JK, Forrester JS, et al: Renal and extrarenal hemodynamic effects of furosemide in congestive heart failure after acute myocardial infarction. N Engl J Med 1973;288:1087–1090.

131. Wilcox CS: Diuretics. In Brenner BM (ed): The Kidney. Philadelphia, 1996, pp 2299–2330.

132. Curran KA, Hebert MJ, Cain BD, et al: Evidence for the presence of a K-dependent acidifying adenosine triphosphatase in the rabbit renal medulla. Kidney Int 1992;42:1093–1098.

133. Francis GS, Siegel RM, Goldsmith SR, et al: Acute vasoconstrictor response to intravenous furosemide in patients with chronic congestive heart failure. Ann Intern Med 1985;103:1–6.

134. Johnston GD, Nicholls DP, Leahey WJ: The dose–response characteristics of the acute non-diuretic peripheral vascular effects of frusemide in normal subjects. Br J Clin Pharmacol 1984;18:75–81.

135. Ryback LP: Ototoxicity of loop diuretics. Otolaryngol Clin N Am 1993;26:829–844.

136. Nierenberg DW: Furosemide and ethacrynic acid in acute tubular necrosis. West J Med 1980;133:163–170.

137. Shimon I, Almog S, Vered Z, et al: Improved left ventricular function after thiamine supplementation in patients with congestive heart failure receiving long-term furosemide therapy. Am J Med 1995;98:485–490.

138. Chemtob S, Doray J-L, Laudignon N, et al: Alternating sequential dosing with furosemide and ethacrynic acid in drug tolerance in the newborn. Am J Dis Child 1989;143:850–854.

139. Ellison DH, Velázquez H, Wright FS: Adaptation of the distal convoluted tubule of the rat: structural and functional effects of dietary salt intake and chronic diuretic infusion. J Clin Invest 1989;83:113–126.

140. Loon NR, Wilcox CS, Unwin RJ: Mechanism of impaired natriuretic response to furosemide during prolonged therapy. Kidney Int 1989;36:682–689.

141. Channer KS, McLean KA, Lawson-Matthew P, et al: Combination diuretic treatment in severe heart failure: a randomised controlled trial. Br Heart J 1994;71:146–150.

142. Garin EH: A comparison of combinations of diuretics in nephrotic edema. Am J Dis Child 1987;141:769–771.

143. Oster JR, Epstein M, Smoler S: Combined therapy with thiazide-type and loop diuretic agents for resistant sodium retention. Ann Intern Med 1983;99:405–406.

144. The Randomized Aldactone Evaluation Study (RALES): Effectiveness of spironolactone added to an angiotensin-converting enzyme inhibitor and a loop diuretic for severe chronic congestive heart failure. Am J Cardiol 1996;78:902–907.

145. Barr CS, Lang CC, Hanson J, et al: Effects of adding spironolactone to an angiotensin-converting enzyme inhibitor in chronic congestive heart failure secondary to coronary artery disease. Am J Cardiol 1995;76:1259–1265.

146. Dehlström U, Karlsson E: Captopril and spironolactone therapy for refractory congestive heart failure. Am J Cardiol 1993;71:29A–33A.

147. Van Vliet AA, Donker AJM, Nauta JJP, et al: Spironolactone in congestive heart failure refractory to high-dose loop diuretic and low-dose angiotensin-converting enzyme inhibitor. Am J Cardiol 1993;71:21A–28A.

148. Zannad F: Angiotensin-converting enzyme inhibitor and spironolactone combination therapy: new objectives in congestive heart failure treatment. Am J Cardiol 1993;71:34A–39A.

149. Schepkens H, Vanholder R, Billiouw JM, et al: Life-threatening hyperkalemia during combined therapy with angiotensin-converting enzyme inhibitors and spironolactone: an analysis of 25 cases. Am J Med 2001;110:438–441.

150. Miller PD, Berns AS: Acute metabolic alkalosis perpetuating hypercarbia: a role for acetazolamide in chronic obstructive pulmonary disease. JAMA 1977;238:2400–2401.

151. Martin SJ, Danziger LH: Continuous infusion of loop diuretics in the critically ill: a review of the literature. Crit Care Med 1994;22:1323–1329.

152. Rudy DW, Voelker JR, Greene PK, et al: Loop diuretics for chronic renal insufficiency: a continuous infusion is more efficacious than bolus therapy. Ann Intern Med 1991;115:360–366.

153. Gerlag PGG, van Meijel JJM: High-dose furosemide in the treatment of refractory congestive heart failure. Arch Intern Med 1988;148:286–291.

154. Van Meyel JJM, Smits P, Dormans T, et al: Continuous infusion of furosemide in the treatment of patients with congestive heart failure and diuretic resistance. J Intern Med 1994;235:329–334.

155. Magovern JA, Magovern GJ Jr: Diuresis in hemodynamically compromised patients: continuous furosemide infusion. Ann Thorac Surg 1990;50:482–484.

156. Ogihara T, Rakugi H, Masuo K, et al: Antihypertensive effects of the neutral endopeptidase inhibitor SCH 42495 in essential hypertension. Am J Hypertens 1994;7:943–947.

157. Fett DL, Cavero PG, Burnett JR: Low-dose atrial natriuretic factor and furosemide in experimental acute congestive heart failure. J Am Soc Nephrol 1993;4:162–167.

158. Shimizu K: Aquaretic effects of the nonpeptide V_2 antagonist OPC-31260 in hydropenic humans. Kidney Int 1995;48:220–226.

159. Tsuboi Y, Ishikawa SE, Fujisawa G, et al: Therapeutic efficacy of the non-peptide avp antagonist OPC-31260 in cirrhotic rats. Kidney Int 1994;46:237–244.

160. Inoue M, Okajima K, Itoh K, et al: Mechanism of furosemide resistance in analbuminemic rats and hypoalbuminemic patients. Kidney Int 1987;32:198–203.

161. Chalasani N, Gorski JC, Horlander JC Sr, et al: Effects of albumin/furosemide mixtures on responses to furosemide in hypoalbuminemic patients. J Am Soc Nephrol 2001;12:1010–1016.

162. Beregovich J, Cianchi C, Rubler S, et al: Dose-related hemodynamic and renal effects of dopamine in congestive heart failure. Am Heart J 1974;87:550–557.

163. Braun GG, Bahlmann F, Brandl M, et al: Long term administration of dopamine: is there development of tolerance? Prog Clin Biol Res 1989;308:1097–1099.

164. Hilberman M, Maseda J, Stinson EB, et al: The diuretic properties of dopamine in patients after open-heart operation. Anesthesiology 1984;61:489–494.

165. Good J, Frost G, Oakley CM, et al: The renal effects of dopamine and dobutamine in stable chronic heart failure. Postgrad Med J 1992;68 (Suppl 2):S7–S11.

166. Vargo DL, Brater DC, Rudy DW, et al: Dopamine does not enhance furosemide-induced natriuresis in patients with congestive heart failure. J Am Soc Nephrol 1996;7:1032–1037.

167. Flancbaum L, Choban PS, Dasta JF: Quantitative effects of low-dose dopamine on urine output in oliguric surgical intensive care unit patients. Crit Care Med 1994;22:61–66.

168. Parker S, Carlon GC, Isaacs M, et al: Dopamine administration in oliguria and oliguric renal failure. Crit Care Med 1981;9:630–632.

169. Duke GJ, Briedis JH, Weaver RA: Renal support in critically ill patients: low-dose dopamine or low-dose dobutamine? Crit Care Med 1994;22:1919–1925.

170. Bellomo R, Chapman M, finfer S, et al: Low-dose dopamine in patients with early renal dysfunction: a placebo-controlled randomised trial. Australian and New Zealand Intensive Care Society (ANZICS) Clinical Trials Group. Lancet 2000;356:2139–2143.

171. Agostoni P, Marenzi G, Lauri G, et al: Sustained improvement in functional capacity after removal of body fluid with isolated ultrafiltration in chronic cardiac insufficiency: failure of furosemide to provide the same result. Am J Med 1994;96:191–199.

96 Dialysis and Hemoperfusion in the Treatment of Poisoning and Drug Overdose

James F. Winchester

Poisoning is a major public health concern. Although mortality is low in patients managed at home or hospital, the volume of patients is enormous. Approximately 2 million patients in 2000 were reported to the American Association of Poison Control Centers (AAPCC);[1] 1074 patients (116 of whom were aged < 6 years; 153 aged between 6 and 19; and 805 aged > 19 years of age) succumbed to their toxic exposure. The AAPCC covers approximately 96.2% of the US population, and similar poison centers are spread throughout Europe and other countries. The nephrologist is often consulted in poisoning cases, particularly for drug removal. In the 2000 AAPCC report, 6680 patients were treated with alkalinization of the urine, 1207 received hemodialysis, and 82 received hemoperfusion or other extracorporeal intervention. The purpose of this chapter is to outline the initial approach to the poisoned subject, briefly discuss initial management, and then to discuss areas where the nephrologist may assist in management of the patient with forced diuresis, recent advances in dialysis, and related techniques.[2] Additionally, the criteria for clinical judgement as to when these techniques should be used in the management of poisoning will be given. For treatment of specific poisons, the reader is referred to a recent comprehensive textbook.[3]

Initial approach

The algorithm in Fig. 96.1 gives a reasonable approach to all poisoned patients, and allows triage of patients to intensive care, hyperbaric chambers, etc. Rapid assessment and stabilization of the airway, of ventilation, and of hemodynamic status are required. To achieve this, airway intubation, supplemental oxygen, assisted ventilation, and intravenous fluid infusion may be needed. The temperature and respiratory rate should be measured frequently. Hypoglycemia should be ruled out without delay. Unconscious patients, and those suffering convulsions, should receive oxygen, naloxone, and dextrose. In alcoholics, thiamine should also be given, ideally before the dextrose infusion. In general, the management of seizures due to poisoning is similar to that of seizures due to other causes. Rectal diazepam may be used if intravenous access is difficult. Seizures induced by overdoses of isoniazid and anticholinergic agents may respond to pyridoxine and physostigmine respectively. The benzodiazepine antagonist flumazenil has been incriminated in seizure induction, and is less widely used now than previously.[4]

Theophylline-induced seizures are often difficult to control and may require general anesthesia. Alterations in body temperature may be treated by passive external warming and cooling, or by peritoneal lavage. Details of the medication, dose, quantity, and time of ingestion should be elicited. Other informants such as family, the patient's physician's and pharmacist's previous records, and empty medicine bottles may provide crucial information. Frequently, more than one medication, including alcohol, may be involved. Physical examination of pupil appearance, breath odors, unusual vital signs, and respiratory pattern may define further the nature of the ingestion.

The anion gap is increased in poisoning with salicylate, ethylene glycol, and methanol, and is decreased with lithium. In contrast, an osmolal gap (between measured and calculated osmolality) may aid in the identification of an alcohol poisoning (ethylene glycol, methanol, isopropyl alcohol). If the patient has already received therapy, or if the poisoning is well advanced, the anion and osmolal gap calculations may be misleading.

Gastric lavage, emetics, cathartics, and oral sorbents

Gastric lavage and syrup of ipecacuanha are not as effective as once thought. They are now recommended only up to 1 h after ingestion, unless drugs with a known delaying effect on gastric emptying have been ingested (tricyclics or massive doses of aspirin or barbiturate poisoning).[5] Polyethylene glycol solutions, used for gut preparation for endoscopy, are useful in clearing the bowel of poisons, particularly if the drug ingested is a slow-release preparation (lithium, iron, theophylline). Caution must be used with lavage, emesis, cathartics, and oral charcoal in unconscious patients; such procedures should

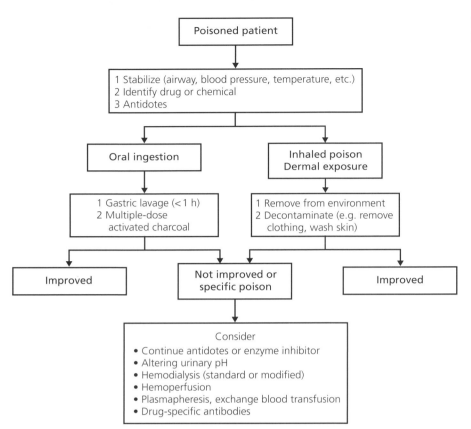

Figure 96.1 Simplified management of the poisoned patient.

be preceded by airway intubation with a cuffed tube to prevent aspiration of gastric contents. Gastric lavage and emesis are contraindicated in petroleum distillate or caustic ingestions because of the risk of hydrocarbon aspiration in the former and gastrointestinal rupture in the latter. Multiple doses of activated charcoal have been shown to be effective (50 g every 2–6 h) in patients with a wide range of drug ingestions.[6] This is particularly recommended for barbiturate, anticonvulsant, theophylline, aspirin, quinine, or dapsone ingestion.[7] Oral charcoal significantly shortens drug half-life through interruption of the enterohepatic circulation of some agents, e.g. barbiturates, digitalis preparations, and theophylline.

Altering urinary pH

Drugs that are weak acids or bases exist in solution as nonionized or ionized species. Nonionized molecules are usually lipid soluble and diffuse across cell membranes, whereas ionized forms are unable to penetrate lipid membranes.

Excretion of drugs by the kidney involves three main processes: glomerular filtration, tubule secretion at the proximal convoluted tubule, and passive tubule reabsorption. Increasing the pH of tubular fluid increases the degree of ionization of weak acids. This reduces drug reabsorption by lowering its nonionic diffusion. The reverse applies to weak bases. The dissociation of a weak acid or base is determined by its dissociation constant

(pK_a) and the pH gradient across the tubule membrane. At a pK_a equal to the pH, the concentrations of nonionized drug and ionized drug are equal. Elimination of weak acids by the kidney is increased by alkaline urine for drugs having pK_a values in the range 3.0–7.5, whereas for weak bases elimination is increased in acid urine if their pK_a is 7.5–10.5. Drugs that respond to urinary pH manipulation have the following characteristics: predominantly renally eliminated in the unchanged form; the drug is a weak electrolyte with a pK_a in the appropriate acidic or basic range; the drug is confined to the extracellular fluid compartment; and the drug is minimally protein bound. Phenobarbital (pK_a 7.2) and thiopental (pK_a 7.6) have similar dissociation constants; however, because of different lipid partition coefficients (phenobarbital coefficient 3, thiopental coefficient 80), 25–50% of phenobarbital is excreted unmetabolized in the urine compared with < 1% of thiopental, rendering alteration of urinary pH of no value in the latter. Forced diuresis (300–500 mL/h) may be complicated by the development of hyponatremia and water intoxication, pulmonary edema, cerebral edema, hypokalemia, and either alkalinemia or acidemia secondary to the use of alkaline or acidic agents respectively. For these reasons, forced diuresis must be accompanied by close vigilance and measurement of urinary pH, at least hourly, and of electrolytes, every 1–2 h initially and frequently thereafter. In salicylate intoxication, acidemia also increases the amount of nonionized and diffusible salicylic acid in the blood, and thereby enhances its accumulation within cerebral tissue.[8]

Correction of acidemia may also induce potassium shifts – cellular and renal – and serum potassium should be measured frequently.[9]

Attention has also been given to the administration of alkali without the copious quantities of fluid accompanying "forced" diuresis, demonstrating that similar quantities of salicylate can be recovered in urine over the same time period without the inherent dangers of fluid administration.[10]

In moderate-to-severe salicylate poisoning, examination of the Done nomogram for estimating the severity of poisoning in relation to time of ingestion assists in the decision of whether to employ forced alkaline diuresis.[11] It may be necessary to resort to dialysis or hemoperfusion when the levels of salicylate exceed 130 mg/dL at 6 h after ingestion or exceed the (extrapolated) initial level of 160 mg/dL, or when there is an unresponsive acidosis or the development of renal failure. Dialysis should be used when other measures have failed and persistent manifestations of salicylate poisoning, with progressive deterioration, are seen.[12]

For alkaline diuresis, the urinary pH should be maintained within the range 7.5–8.5 by adjustment of the amount of bicarbonate administered. Diuresis can be initiated by using furosemide or osmotic diuretic agents such as mannitol or urea. Mannitol may cause hyponatremia and hyperosmolality. In salicylate poisoning, frequently some degree of dehydration is present before initiation of treatment; therefore, 1 L of 5% dextrose containing 25 mequiv./L bicarbonate and 75 mequiv./L sodium and appropriate levels of potassium (judged on the initial serum potassium level) should be given. The goal of treatment is to maintain a urine flow of 300–500 mL/h, and either mannitol or bolus doses of furosemide, 20 mg, may be required to maintain the diuresis; 10–20 mequiv./L of potassium in infused fluid may also be required. The following drugs are amenable to alkaline diuresis: phenobarbital, when the plasma level exceeds 10 mg/dL; barbital, when the plasma level exceeds 10 mg/dL; and salicylates, when the plasma level exceeds 50 mg/dL (relative to time of ingestion). Forced alkaline diuresis has also been shown to be of benefit in the treatment of 2,4-dichlorophenoxyacetic acid (2,4-D) poisoning.[13]

In acid diuresis, 1 L of 5% dextrose in normal saline per hour is given in the first 1–2 h, with added arginine or lysine hydrochloride (10 g i.v. over 30 min). Thereafter, 5% dextrose in normal saline is given every 2 h. Ammonium chloride, 4 g every 2 h, should be administered orally. In those patients who cannot tolerate a nasogastric or duodenal tube, a 1–2% solution of ammonium chloride in normal saline should be given intravenously. With either technique, the dose is adjusted to maintain a urinary pH of 5.5–6.5. Plasma potassium should be monitored. Urinary pH should be measured at least hourly. Forced acid diuresis can increase the excretion of amphetamines, fenfluramine, phencyclidine, and quinine. Acid diuresis may or may not be indicated in the management of poisoning with these agents. Ascorbic acid (1 g every 6 h in adults) can also be administered orally to acidify the urine.

Chloride loading (especially ammonium chloride) increases the excretion of bromide; bromide excretion can be further increased with administration of mannitol, loop diuretics, or dialysis.[14] In contrast, lithium excretion is not further enhanced by ammonium chloride, water, saline, or loop diuretics.

Dialysis techniques for removing poisons

Many substances can be removed by hemodialysis and peritoneal dialysis. Exhaustive reviews of state-of-the-art dialysis in poisoning have been published. Prior to discussion of dialysis in drug poisoning, it is worthwhile considering the basic principles of dialysis, factors favoring drug removal with dialysis, and the potential problems associated with dialysis in poisoned patients.

Principles of dialysis

Many dialysis techniques are available: peritoneal dialysis and hemodialysis utilize natural and artificial semipermeable membranes respectively. Hemodialysis uses either aqueous dialysate or sorbent-containing dialysate.[15] Direct extensions of hemodialysis have used the principle of ultrafiltration, whereby drug removal accompanies the ultrafiltrate. Drug removal may also be increased by continuous arteriovenous hemofiltration (CAVH), CAVHD, CVVH, and CVVHD – modifications of hemodialysis that process continuous (C), arterial (A), or venous (V) blood, or hydrostatically ultrafiltered (H) or dialysed and ultrafiltered (D) blood. Blood may be subjected to these techniques at high or low rates through membranes that have pores larger than conventional dialysis membranes[16] over a continuous 24-h period.[17]

Factors governing drug removal are: solute (or drug) size; the lipid–water partition coefficient; the degree of protein binding; the volume of distribution; and the maintenance of a concentration gradient.[18] Other factors include blood flow rate through the dialyzer, dialysate flow rate, dialyzer surface area, and the characteristics of the specific membrane chosen. For example, lithium exists in whole body water and is not protein bound; in contrast, amitriptyline is 96.4% bound to serum albumin, but is also bound more avidly in muscle to produce a large apparent volume of distribution (8.3 L/kg of body weight). Consequently, lithium is eminently dialyzable and amitriptyline is not.

Drug clearances reach a plateau above a blood flow rate of 200–300 mL/min. Therefore, for larger molecule drugs, the rate of removal can be increased by increasing the surface area.

Factors governing drug removal with dialysis

Drug removal rates with dialysis are best calculated from in vitro experiments, using protein-containing solutions with the drug added to mimic the clinical situation. It is also important to consider the intercompartmental transfer of drugs from tissues into plasma;[19] however, the influence of this factor on removal of most drugs is unknown.

Plasma protein binding is an important factor limiting the dialysis of drugs. However, with some drugs, for example salicylate, the bound salicylate is highly ultrafilterable, thus making salicylate an ideal dialyzable drug. Lipid solubility of drugs also governs their removal by dialysis. Ethchlorvynol and glutethimide are examples of highly lipid-soluble drugs. Their removal is low with aqueous dialysis but increases with lipid dialysis, which allows partitioning in lipid globules within the dialysate. However, with modern dialysis and with large surface area dialyzers,[20,21] "lipid" dialysis has fallen into disuse. Additional techniques, such as the use of activated charcoal or resin hemoperfusion, are more appropriate.

Ultrafiltration dialysis (e.g. CAVH) increases the solvent drag of the solute. Therefore, it has been evaluated for treating poisoning with agents such as paraquat.[22] However, with conventional hemodialyzer membranes, the degree of increase in clearance is rather small.[1] The clearance of solutes by the process of ultrafiltration, however, is greatly enhanced if the membrane has larger pores.[23] Although these large-pore membranes are not specifically used for poisoning therapy, it is known that removal of solutes ranging from 64 Da (urea) up to 1500 Da (vitamin B_{12}) is identical; this type of treatment allows higher clearance rates for large-molecular-weight drugs. With CAVH and other methods that use low blood flow rates without dialysis, drug removal is modest. For example, the clearances of creatinine and matching drugs are about 5 mL/min over a 24-h period. Therefore, other techniques are usually employed.

Peritoneal dialysis is the least effective method for removing drugs in view of the slower dialysate transit times within the abdominal cavity. It can be used as a temporizing measure until other techniques are established. Operant conditions for hemodialysis include the use of maximal blood flow rates (including pressor support of the circulation) and use of bicarbonate dialysis at high flow rates. For the continuous therapies, continuous heparinization and inspection of the apparatus for clots along with restoration of ultrafiltered fluid are necessary. Prolonged, or repeated, dialysis may be required in treating poisoning by lithium, ethchlorvynol, glutethimide, and midazolam to avoid large rebounds in drug concentration after the procedure, which might cause a relapse of intoxication. Table 96.1 lists the reported dialyzable drugs.[24]

Sorbent hemoperfusion

Hemoperfusion refers to the passage of blood through a column containing sorbent particles. It was introduced in the 1940s,[25] refined during 1950–1970,[26–28] and adopted for clinical use in poisoning in the 1970s and 1980s.[29–31] Hemoperfusion relies on the physical process of drug adsorption. In many instances, drug removal is far better than with hemodialysis, peritoneal dialysis, or forced diuresis. Activated charcoal hemoperfusion and resin hemoperfusion devices are available. In addition, antibody- or antigen-coated charcoal hemoperfusion is available for specific autoimmune states,[32] removal of cytotoxic antibody prior to renal transplantation,[33] or endotoxin binding to fibers.[34] Washing, and coating the particles with a polymer solution, decreases platelet aggregation without losing efficiency of adsorption.

Certain resins have been shown to be most effective in the removal of lipid-soluble drugs, with drug clearance rates exceeding those achieved by charcoal hemoperfusion. Available hemoperfusion devices and the contained sorbents are shown in Table 96.2.

Hemoperfusion is instituted with a column that contains between 100 and 300 g of activated charcoal, or 650 g (wet weight) of polystyrene resin, in a circuit resembling hemodialysis. Hemoperfusion can be combined with hemodialysis to increase core temperature, to increase drug-removing efficiency, or to correct acidosis. Blood flow rates should be the highest achievable. Pressure devices can detect interior rises in pressure, which serve as an index of thrombosis occurring inside the device.

Removal of lipid-soluble drugs, such as glutethimide and methaqualone, is far more efficient with XAD-4 resin hemoperfusion than with activated charcoal.

Table 96.3 lists representative drugs that have been reported to be removed by various types of hemoperfusion.

Complications of hemoperfusion

Transient platelet depletion (average loss 30%) occurs with coated or uncoated charcoal or resin preparations. Greater falls in platelet counts were previously observed with the resin preparations; however, with the newly developed highly biocompatible resins, this is no longer the case.[35] Reductions in serum calcium and serum glucose, transient falls in white blood cell counts, and a reduction of 1–2°F in body temperature may also be seen. Hypotension is not a complication of the circulation of blood in the extracorporeal circuit, but pressor agents used to maintain the blood pressure are removed. Hence, it is recommended that such agents should be infused distal to the devices.

Criteria for consideration of hemodialysis or hemoperfusion in poisoning

The decision about whether a patient should undergo active drug removal is not always easily made. It is based on the clinical features of poisoning. Hemodialysis or hemoperfusion should be considered if the patient's condition progressively deteriorates despite intensive supportive therapy with appropriate fluid balance, correction of acid–base abnormalities, pressor infusion, and forced diuresis.

Table 96.1   Drugs and chemicals removed with dialysis*

Antimicrobials/anticancer	Ticarcillin	5-Fluorouracil	(Encainide)	Amanitin
Cefaclor	(Clindamycin)	(Methotrexate)	(Flecainide)	Demeton sulfoxide
Cefadroxil	(Erythromycin)		(Lidocaine)	Dimethoate
Cefamandole	(Azithromycin)	*Barbiturates*	Metoprolol	Diquat
Cefazolin	(Clarithromycin)	Amobarbital	Methyldopa	Glufosinate
Cefixime	Metronidazole	Aprobarbital	(Ouabain)	Methylmercury
Cefmenoxime	Nitrofurantoin	Barbital	N-Acetylprocainamide	complex
Cefmetazole	Ornidazole	Butabarbital	Nadolol	(Organophosphates)
(Cefonicid)	Sulfisoxazole	Cyclobarbital	(Pindolol)	Paraquat
(Cefoperazone)	Sulfonamides	Pentobarbital	Practolol	Snake bite
Ceforamide	Tetracycline	Phenobarbital	Procainamide	Sodium chlorate
(Cefotaxime)	(Doxycycline)	Quinalbital	Propranolol	Potassium chlorate
Cefotetan	(Minocycline)	(Secobarbital)	(Quinidine)	
Cefotiam	Tinidazole		(Timolol)	*Miscellaneous*
Cefoxitin	Trimethoprim	*Nonbarbiturate hypnotics,*	Sotatol	Acipimox
Cefpirome	Aztreonam	*sedatives, tranquilizers,*	Tocainide	Allopurinol
Cefroxadine	Cilastatin	*anticonvulsants*		Aminophylline
Cefsulodin	Imipenem	Carbamazepine	*Alcohols*	Aniline
Ceftazidime	(Chloramphenicol)	Atenolol	Ethanol	Borates
(Ceftriaxone)	(Amphotericin)	Betaxolol	Ethylene glycol	Boric acid
Cefuroxime	Ciprofloxacin	(Bretylium)	Isopropanol	(Chlorpropamide)
Cephacetrile	(Enoxacin)	Clonidine	Methanol	Chromic acid
Cephalexin	Fluroxacin	(Calcium channel blockers)	*Analgesics, antirheumatics*	(Cimetidine)
Cephalothin	(Norfloxacin)	Captopril	Acetaminophen	Dinitro-o-cresol
(Cephapirin)	Ofloxacin	(Diazoxide)	Acetophenetidin	Folic acid
Cephradine	Isoniazid	Carbromal	Acetylsalicylic acid	Mannitol
Moxalactam	(Vancomycin)	Chloral hydrate	Colchicine	Methylprednisolone
Amikacin	Capreomycin	(Chlordiazepoxide)	Methylsalicylate	4-Methylpyrazole
Dibekacin	PAS	(Diazepam)	(D-Propoxyphene)	Sodium citrate
Fosfomycin	Pyrizinamide	(Diphenylhydantoin)	Salicylic acid	Theophylline
Gentamicin	(Rifampin)	(Diphenylhydramine)		Thiocyanate
Kanamycin	(Cycloserine)	Ethiamate	*Antidepressants*	Ranitidine
Neomycin	Ethambutol	Ethchlorvynol	(Amitriptyline)	
Netilmicin	5-Fluorocytosine	Ethosuximide	Amphetamines	*Metals, inorganics*
Sisomicin	Acyclovir	Gallamine	(Imipramine)	(Aluminum)†
Streptomycin	(Amantadine)	Glutethimide	Isocarboxazid	Arsenic
Tobramycin	Didanosine	(Heroin)	Monoamine oxidase inhibitors	Barium
Bacitracin	Foscarnet	Meprobamate	Moclobemide	Bromide
Colistin	Ganciclovir	(Methaqualone)	(Pargylline)	(Copper)†
Amoxicillin	(Ribavirin)	Methsuximide	(Phenelzine)	(Iron)†
Ampicillin	Vidarabine	Methyprylon	Tranylcypromine	(Lead)†
Azlocillin	Zidovudine	Paraldehyde	(Tricyclics)	Lithium
Carbenicillin	(Pentamidine)	Primidone		(Magnesium)
Clavulinic acid	(Praziquantel)	Valproic acid	*Solvents, gases*	(Mercury)†
(Cloxacillin)	(Fluconazole)		Acetone	Potassium
(Dicloxacillin)	(Itraconazole)	*Cardiovascular agents*	Camphor	(Potassium dichromate)†
(Floxacillin)	(Ketoconazole)	Acebutolol	Carbon monoxide	Phosphate
Mecillinam	(Miconazole)	(Amiodarone)	(Carbon tetrachloride)	Sodium
(Mezlocillin)	(Chloroquine)	Amrinone	(Eucalyptus oil)	Strontium
(Methicillin)	(Quinine)	(Digoxin)	Thiols	(Thallium)†
(Nafcillin)	(Azathioprine)	Enalapril	Toluene	(Tin)
Penicillin	Bredinin	Fosinopril	Trichloroethylene	(Zinc)
Piperacillin	Busulfan	Lisinopril		
Temocillin	Cyclophosphamide	Quinapril	*Plants, animals, herbicides,*	
		Ramipril	*insecticides*	
			Alkyl phosphate	

This table will be updated periodically at http://www.arrtjournal.org.[48]
( ), poor removal; ( )†, removed with chelating agent; PAS, p-aminosalicylic acid.

Table 96.2 Some available hemoperfusion devices

Manufacturer	Device	Sorbent type	Amount of sorbent	Polymer coating
Clark*	Biocompatible system	Carbon	50, 100, 250 mL	Heparinized polymer
Gambro*	Adsorba	Norit Carbon	100 or 300 g	Cellulose acetate
Nextron Medical	Hemosorba Ch-350	Petroleum bead carbon	170 g	PolyHema

*Smaller devices for use in children.

Table 96.3 Drugs and chemicals removed with hemoperfusion*

Barbiturates
Amobarbital
Butabarbital
Hexabarbital
Pentobarbital
Phenobarbital
Quinalbital
Secobarbital
Thiopental
Vinalbital

Nonbarbiturate hypnotics, sedatives and tranquilizers
Carbamazepine
Carbromal
Chloral hydrate
Chlorpromazine
(Diazepam)
Diphenhydramine
Ethchlorvynol
Glutethimide
Meprobamate
Methaqualone
Methsuximide
Methyprylon
Phenytoin
Promazine

Promethazine
Valproic acid

Analgesics, antirheumatics
Acetaminophen
Acetylsalicylic acid
Colchicine
d-Propoxyphene
Methylsalicylate
Phenylbutazone
Salicylic acid

Antimicrobials/anticancer
(Doxorubicin)
Ampicillin
Carmustine
Chloramphenicol
Chloroquine
Clindamycin
Dapsone
Doxorubicin
Gentamicin
Ifosfamide
Isoniazid
(Methotrexate)
Pentamidine
Thiabendazole

(5-Fluorouracil)
Vancomycin

Antidepressants
(Amitriptyline)
(Imipramine)
(Tricyclics)

Plant and animal toxins, herbicides, insecticides
Amanitin
Chlordane
Demeton sulfoxide
Dimethoate
Diquat
Endosulfan
Glufosinate
Methylparathion
Nitrostigmine
(Organophosphates)
Phalloidin
Polychlorinated biphenyls
Paraquat
Parathion

Cardiovascular
Atenolol
Cibenzoline succinate

Clonidine
Digoxin
(Diltiazem)
(Disopyramide)
Flecainide
Metoprolol
N-Acetylprocainamide
Procainamide
Quinidine

Miscellaneous
Aminophylline
Cimetidine
(Fluoroacetamide)
(Phencyclidine)
Phenols
(Podophyllin)
Theophylline

Solvents, gases
Carbon tetrachloride
Ethylene oxide
Trichloroethane
Xylene

Metals
(Aluminum)†
(Iron)†

*This table will be updated periodically at http://www.arrtjournal.org.[48]
( ), poor removal; ( )†, removed with chelating agent.
Reproduced from Winchester JF: Dialysis and hemoperfusion in poisoning. Adv Renal Replacement Ther 2002;9:26–30.[48]

Suggested clinical criteria are: progressive deterioration despite intensive supportive therapy; severe intoxication with depression of midbrain function; development of the complications of coma, such as pneumonia or septicemia, and underlying conditions predisposing to such complications (e.g. obstructive airway disease); impairment of normal drug excretory function in the presence of hepatic, cardiac, or renal insufficiency; intoxication with agents with metabolic and/or delayed effects, e.g. methanol, ethylene glycol, and paraquat; and intoxication with an extractable drug or poison that can be removed at a rate exceeding endogenous elimination by liver or kidney. These criteria should be considered with information about plasma concentrations of drugs. However, drug concentration may be misleading since most patients take more than one drug. For further discussion on the effect of dialysis/hemoperfusion on specific agents, see a recent review.[36]

Plasma exchange and exchange blood transfusion

Both of these techniques have been used infrequently in the treatment of poisoning.[37] With a 3- to 4-L plasma exchange, the maximal quantity of drug removed is its plasma concentration times the volume of plasma removed. Therefore, this is used for removal of highly protein-bound drugs. Chromic acid and chromate poisoning have been treated with mixed success,[38] but otherwise its role is unclear. Plasma exchange with subsequent plasma perfusion over sorbents has been used for a variety of poisons. Exchange blood transfusion has been used especially when hemolysis and methemoglobinemia have complicated the poisoning (e.g. sodium chlorate poisonings).

Hemoperfusion and hemodialysis with chelation

Aluminum and iron intoxication in dialysis patients can be treated with deferoxamine in conjunction with dialysis (continuous ambulatory peritoneal dialysis or hemodialysis) or hemoperfusion for removal of the deferoxamine–aluminum complex. Clinical improvement in the osteomalacia component of renal osteodystrophy, encephalopathy, iron overload, and anemia have been reported.[39,40] Heavy metals and their salts are not removed efficiently by dialysis or hemoperfusion alone. During hemodialysis, metal removal may be enhanced with certain chelating agents, such as N-acetylcysteine or cysteine. In contrast, removal of mercury and thallium by hemoperfusion appears to be modest at best. Chelating microspheres or chelate–metal groups for adsorption may eventually prove useful for heavy metal removal.[41,42]

Immunopharmacology

Immunopharmacology is limited to digoxin poisoning[43] and snakebite.[44] When injected, Fab fragments of antibodies to drugs or venom combine with a high degree of specificity to their antigenic targets. In potentially fatal cases of glycoside poisoning, Fab fragment administration has resulted in a response far greater than that obtained with conventional therapy. In the presence of renal failure, however, for drugs that depend on renal elimination, the effectiveness of Fab fragment administration may be reduced. Potentially fatal cases of digoxin poisoning have been treated successfully by Fab antibody fragments, but failures have also been reported, and the cost of treatment is high. Immobilized antibody on hemoperfusion devices may offer an alternative.[45] In dialysis patients (in whom vascular access facilitates interventional therapy), a judgement to use either hemoperfusion or Fab antibody fragments is required, especially since the elimination half-time of digoxin in anephric patients can be substantially reduced with the addition of hemoperfusion. Newer resin hemoperfusion devices have been used for removing digoxin (C. Ronco, personal communication).[46] Recurrent digoxin poisoning in renal failure patients has been reported 24–48 h after receiving Fab antibodies.[47]

References

1. Litovitz TL, Klein-Schwartz W, White S, et al: 2000 Annual report of the American Association of Poison Control Centers Toxic Exposure Surveillance System. Am J Emerg Med 2000; 19: 337–395.
2. Jacobs C, Kjellstrand CM, Koch KM, Winchester JF (eds): Replacement of Renal Function by Dialysis, 4th edn. Dordrecht: Kluwer Academic Publishers, 1996
3. Haddad LM, Shannon MW, Winchester JF (eds): Clinical Management of Poisoning and Drug Overdose, 3rd edn. Philadelphia: WB Saunders Co, 1997.
4. Doyon S, Roberts JR: Reappraisal of the "coma cocktail." Dextrose, flumazenil, naloxone and thiamine. Emerg Med Clin North Am 1994;12:301–316.
5. Kulig K: Initial management of ingestions of toxic substances. N Engl J Med 1992;326:1677–1681.
6. Chyka PA: Multiple-dose activated charcoal and enhancement of systemic drug clearance: summary of studies in animals and human volunteers. J Toxicol Clin Toxicol 1995;33:399–405.
7. American Academy of Clinical Toxicology; European Association of Poisons Centres and Clinical Toxicologists: Position statement and practice guidelines on the use of multi-dose activated charcoal in the treatment of acute poisoning. J Toxicol Clin Toxicol 1999;37:731–751.
8. Mayer SE, Melmon KL, Gilman AG: Introduction: the dynamics of drug absorption, distribution and elimination. In Gilman AG, Goodman LS, Gilman A (eds): The Pharmacological Basis of Therapeutics, 6th edn. New York: Macmillan, 1981, p 1.
9. Gabow PA, Peterson LN: Disorders of potassium metabolism. In Schrier RW (ed): Renal and Electrolyte Disorders, 2nd edn. Boston: Little, Brown & Co, 1980, p 183.
10. Prescott LF, Balali-Mood M, Critchley JA, et al: Diuresis or urinary alkalinization in salicylate poisoning? Br Med J 1982;285:1383–1386.
11. Done AK: Salicylate intoxication: significance of measurements of salicylate in blood in cases of acute ingestion. Pediatrics 1960;26:800–807.
12. Schreiner GE: Dialysis of poison and drugs: annual review. Trans Am Soc Artif Intern Organs 1970;16:544–568.
13. Vale JA, Rees AJ, Widdop B, et al: Use of charcoal haemoperfusion in the management of severely poisoned patients. Br Med J 1975;1:5–9.
14. Horowitz BZ: Bromism from excessive cola consumption. J Toxicol Clin Toxicol 1997;35:315–320
15. Ash SR, Carr DJ, Blake DE, et al: Effect of sorbent-based dialytic therapy with the Biologic-DT on an experimental model of hepatic failure. Trans Am Soc Artif Intern Organs 1993;39:M675–M680.
16. Henderson LW, Silverstein MAE, Ford CA, et al: Clinical response to maintenance hemodiafiltration. Kidney Int 1975;7:S58–63.
17. Kaplan AA: Continuous arteriovenous hemofiltration and related therapies. In Jacobs C, Kjellstrand CM, Koch KM, et al (eds): Replacement of Renal Function by Dialysis, 4th edn. Dordrecht: Kluwer Academic Publishers, 1996, p 390.
18. Maher JF: Principles of dialysis and dialysis of drugs. Am J Med 1977;62:475–481.
19. Gibson TP, Atkinson AI: Effect of changes in intercompartment rate constants on drug removal during hemoperfusion. J Pharm Sci 1978;67:1178–1179.
20. Kane SL, Constantiner M, Staubus AE, et al: High-flux hemodialysis without hemoperfusion is effective in acute valproic acid overdose. Ann Pharmacother 2000;34:1146–1151.
21. Palmer BF: Effectiveness of hemodialysis in the extracorporeal therapy of phenobarbital overdose. Am J Kidney Dis 2000;36:640–643.
22. Pond SM, Johnston SC, Schoof DD, et al: Repeated hemoperfusion and continuous arteriovenous hemofiltration in a paraquat poisoned patient. J Toxicol Clin Toxicol 1987;25:305–316.
23. Henderson LW: Biophysics of ultrafiltration and hemofiltration. In Jacobs C, Kjellstrand CM, Koch KM, Winchester JF (eds): Replacement of Renal Function by Dialysis, 4th edn. Dordrecht: Kluwer Academic Publishers, 1996, p 146.
24. Winchester JF: Active methods for detoxification. In Haddad LM, Shannon MW, Winchester JF (eds): Clinical Management of Poisoning and Drug Overdose, 3rd edn. Philadelphia: WB Saunders Co, 1997.
25. Muirhead EE, Reid AF: Resin artificial kidney. J Lab Clin Med 1948;33:841–844.
26. Schreiner GE: The role of hemodialysis (artificial kidney) in acute poisoning. Arch Intern Med 1958;102:896–904.
27. Yatzidis IT, Voudiclari S, Oreopoulos D, et al: Treatment of severe barbiturate poisoning. Lancet 1965;2:216–217.
28. Chang TMS: Artificial Cells. Springfield, IL: Charles C Thomas, 1972.
29. Hampel G, Crome P, Widdop B, et al: Experience with fixed-bed charcoal haemoperfusion in the treatment of severe drug intoxication. Arch Toxicol 1980;45:133–141.
30. Gelfand MC, Winchester JF, Knepshield JH, et al: Charcoal

hemoperfusion in severe drug overdosage. Trans Am Soc Artif Intern Organs 1977;23:599–605.

31. Verpooten GA, De Broe ME: Combined hemoperfusion–hemodialysis in severe poisoning: kinetics of drug extraction. Resuscitation 1984;11:275–289.

32. Terman DS, Buffaloe G, Mattioli C, et al: Extracorporeal immunoadsorption: initial experience in human systemic lupus erythematosis. Lancet 1979;2:824–827.

33. Hakim RM, Milford E, Himmelfarb J, et al: Extracorporeal removal of anti-HLA antibodies in transplant candidates. Am J Kidney Dis 1990:16:423–431.

34. Ronco C, Brendolan A, Scabardi M, et al: Blood flow distribution in a polymyxin coated fibrous bed for endotoxin removal. Effect of a new blood path design. Int J Artif Organs. 2001;24:167–172.

35. Ronco C, Brendolan A, Winchester JF, et al: First clinical experience with an adjunctive hemoperfusion device designed specifically to remove beta 2-microglobulin in hemodialysis. Contrib Nephrol 2001;133:166–173.

36. Golper TA, Marx MA, Shuler C, et al: Drug dosage in dialysis patients. In Jacobs C, Kjellstrand CM, Koch KM, Winchester JF (eds): Replacement of Renal Function by Dialysis, 4th edn. Dordrecht: Kluwer Academic Publishers, 1996, p 750.

37. Gurland HJ, Samtleben W, Lysaght MJ, et al: Extracorporeal blood purification techniques: plasmapheresis and hemoperfusion. In Jacobs C, Kjellstrand CM, Koch KM, Winchester JF (eds): Replacement of Renal Function by Dialysis, 4th edn. Dordrecht: Kluwer Academic Publishers, 1996, p 472.

38. Meert KL, Ellis J, Aronow R, et al: Acute ammonium dichromate poisoning. Ann Emerg Med 1994;24:748–750.

39. Winchester JF: Management of iron overload. Semin Nephrol 1986;4

40. Chang TMS, Barre P: Effect of desferrioxamine on removal of aluminum and iron by coated charcoal haemoperfusion and haemodialysis. Lancet 1983;2:1051–1053.

41. Margel S: A novel approach for heavy metal poisoning treatment, a model. Mercury poisoning by means of chelating microspheres; hemoperfusion and oral administration. J Med Chem 1981;24:1263–1266.

42. De Groot G, van Heijst AN, van Kesteren RG, et al: An evaluation of the efficacy of charcoal haemoperfusion in the treatment of three cases of acute thallium poisoning. Arch Toxicol 1985;57:61–66.

43. Martiny SS, Phelps SJ, Massey KL: Treatment of severe digitalis intoxication with digoxin-specific antibody fragments: a clinical review. Crit Care Med 1988;16:629–635.

44. Dart RC, Seifert SA, Boyer LV, et al: A randomized multicenter trial of crotalinae polyvalent immune Fab (ovine) antivenom for the treatment for crotaline snakebite in the United States. Arch Intern Med 2001;161:2030–2036.

45. Savin H, Marcus L, Margel S, et al: Treatment of adverse digitalis effects by hemoperfusion through columns containing antidigoxin antibodies bound to agarose polyacrolein microsphere beads. Am Heart J 1987;113:1078–1084.

46. Tsuruoka S, Osono E, Nishiki K, et al: Removal of digoxin by column for specific adsorption of beta(2)-microglobulin: a potential use for digoxin intoxication. Clin Pharmacol Ther 2001;69:422–430

47. Ujhelyi MR, Robert S, Cummings DM, et al: Disposition of digoxin immune Fab in patients with kidney failure. Clin Pharmacol Ther 1993;54:388–394.

48. Winchester JF: Dialysis and hemoperfusion in poisoning. Adv Renal Replacement Ther 2002;9:26–30.

(Suppl 1):22.

PART XVI
Use of the Internet

HUGH R. BRADY

Internet Resources for Nephrologists
Robert O. Stuart

History of the Internet
• The World Wide Web and medicine
thekidney.org

There is a growing mountain of research. But there is increased evidence that we are being bogged down today as specialization extends. The investigator is staggered by the findings and conclusions of thousands of other workers – conclusions which he cannot find time to grasp, much less to remember, as they appear. Yet specialization becomes increasingly necessary for progress, and the effort to bridge between disciplines is correspondingly superficial.

The difficulty seems to be, not so much that we publish unduly in view of the extent and variety of present-day interests, but rather that publication has been extended far beyond our present ability to make real use of the record. The summation of human experience is being expanded at a prodigious rate, and the means we use for threading through the consequent maze to the momentarily important item is the same as was used in the days of square-rigged ships.

Wholly new forms of encyclopedias will appear, ready-made with a mesh of associative trails running through them, ready to be dropped into the memex (computer with hyperlinks) and there amplified. The lawyer has at his touch the associated opinions and decisions of his whole experience, and of the experience of friends and authorities. The patent attorney has on call the millions of issued patents, with familiar trails to every point of his client's interest. The physician, puzzled by his patient's reactions, strikes the trail established in studying an earlier similar case, and runs rapidly through analogous case histories, with side references to the classics for the pertinent anatomy and histology.

This extended quote by Vannevar Bush from the July 1945 issue of *The Atlantic Monthly* presciently identified not only the problems of information overload and accessibility but also pointed a way toward their solution.[1] More than 50 years later, the absolute quantity of information and its rate of accumulation have grown by several orders of magnitude (Fig. 97.1).[2] The acceleration of data accumulation and increasingly digital nature of information suggests that in the very near future information will be virtually synonymous with what is available through the Internet. The essential challenge for

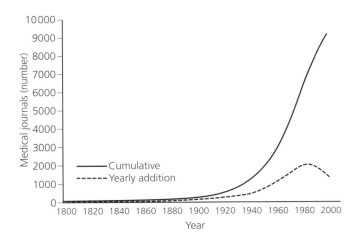

Figure 97.1 Growth in medical periodicals with time. Data are derived from a list of MEDLINE-indexed journals (ftp://ncbi.nlm.nih.gov/pubmed). The dates reflect the individual journal's date of founding publication and not date of initial MEDLINE or Index Medicus index inclusion. Currently, almost 10 000 biomedical periodicals are indexed in MEDLINE, although the rate of growth appears to be decreasing.

the future becomes, then, to ensure that the growth of actual knowledge keeps pace with that of mere facts.

History of the Internet

After the Soviet launch of Sputnik in 1957, the USA established the Defense Advanced Research Projects Agency (DARPA), which was tasked with the development of military science and technology. A critical concern at the time was maintaining a functional communications infrastructure in the event of nuclear war. Traditional modes of communication such as the telephone were considered unreliable in this circumstance owing to their highly centralized nature. Building on then recent advances in information technology theory, the concept of a decentralized network of communications nodes trading discrete packets of data was put forward in the early 1960s and first put into practice in 1969 as the ARPANET (Advanced Research Projects Agency Network). This earliest version of what became the Internet at first connected a mere four computers at the University of California (Los Angeles, Santa Barbara), University of Stanford, and the University of Utah.[3,4]

The next few years saw incremental growth of the network and rapid expansion of capabilities to include early versions of most current functionality, including the first transcontinental link from UCLA to BBN Inc. in Cambridge, MA (1970), application of e-mail to the

ARPANET (1972), the first realtime chat application (1972), the first international connections (to University College of London via Norway (1973)), and the still-current foundations of network protocols such as TCP/IP (Transmission Control Protocol/Internet Protocol) (1974–1975).

By the late 1970s, the vast majority of universities had no network connectivity. In 1979, many such institutions not directly connected to ARPANET were connected via a nonmilitary network termed CSNET (Computer Science Network). The creation of CSNET significantly expanded the net, connecting about 150 institutions and tens of thousands of new users. Although practically restricted to a very technically oriented population, in 1983 this "Net" made its first entrée into the popular culture with the publication of William Gibson's *Neuromancer*, in which the term cyberspace (among others) was coined. In 1986, the NSFNET (National Science Foundation Network) was established to provide high-speed links between six supercomputing centers. By 1990, this network had taken over the older ARPANET, thus forming the next generation of the Internet. The complexity of the current network of networks composing the Internet is almost beyond imagination.

The World Wide Web and medicine

However, the real explosion in networking functionality and popularity awaited realization of Vannevar Bush's original vision in the form the World Wide Web (WWW), a term and technology developed at CERN (European Organization for Nuclear Research) by Tim Berners Lee between 1991 and 1993. Although the original entity was purely text based and devoted to physics research, the essential ingredient – hyperlinks connecting myriad pages of related information – was present. Shortly thereafter, in 1993, the first graphical browser, Mosaic, developed at the National Center for Super Computing Applications led to an explosion in the growth of the WWW. By popular demand, in 1995 online services such as Compuserve, Prodigy, and AOL began offering internet access in addition to proprietary content. Subsequent developments in the size and ability of the WWW to carry an almost limitless variety of multimedia content are quite familiar to all (Fig. 97.2).

The explosion in the growth of the WWW makes it almost synonymous with the "Internet." However, the older components still operate: Telnet (access and control of a remote computer), FTP (file transfer protocol used for data exchange), Gopher (an early attempt at hierarchically organizing network content), and of course e-mail and chat. The massive growth of resources present on the Internet and especially the WWW present considerable opportunities as well as challenges for the sharing of biomedical information. Physicians are generally familiar with online sources of information such as MEDLINE or perhaps GenBank (ncbi.nlm.nih.gov). Current technology makes it entirely possible to make the sum total of the medical literature available to everyone. Increasingly, the thorny problem of copyright restrictions is dealt with by a variety of means, including institutional subscriptions

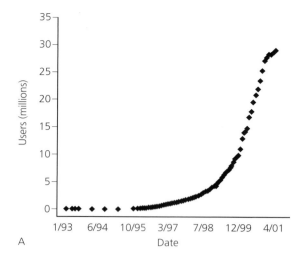

A

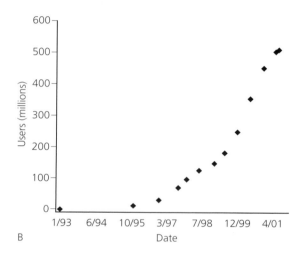

B

Figure 97.2 Internet growth. **A**, Growth of the WWW. Data reflect the number of WWW servers as a function of time. As would be expected, growth of the WWW awaited widespread adoption of graphical browser software. Note also that, like the growth in medical journals (Fig. 97.1), growth in the number of WWW servers may be decelerating somewhat, indicating a (perhaps temporary) saturation of the market. **B**, Increase in Internet users. Data from www.nua.ie/surveys/. Note the fairly consistent, and surprisingly low, ratio of ~ 20:1 server computers to individual users.

and making slightly older (~ 6 months) literature freely available.[5]

Nevertheless, two vexing problems remain: the accessibility and validity of information. There are essentially two commonly used methods of making sense of the jumble of information available on the Internet: search engines and specialized WWW sites containing curated links and annotations. Search engines vary considerably in the results obtained (Table 97.1). Despite their power, search engines still leave something to be desired in that they are unable to group together pages that are superficially unrelated and they tend not to prioritize results. A few search utilities monitor users' responses in order to prioritize pages based on popularity – the utility becomes "smarter" the more people use it.

Table 97.1 Nephrology search engine results

Search engine	2001	1998
Yahoo (yahoo.com)	41	14
AltaVista (altavista.digital.com)	158 383	12 755
Excite (excite.com)	3920	6898
Google (google.com)	187 000	NA

NA, not available.

Table 97.2 Nephrology categories in thekidney.org

General nephrology sites
Professional societies
Online journals
Continuing medical education
Academic renal divisions
Medical schools
Endstage renal disease
National Institutes of Health
Resources for research

Fortunately, in the case of nephrology (and medicine generally), there are excellent "list pages" and "portals" with many links organized and annotated according to the needs of the target audience. It is a simple matter to use such a page as a home base from which one explores. Another, perhaps less acute, problem lies in the ephemeral nature of some information on the Internet. One novel approach to the problem is the Internet archive (web.archive.org), which seeks to capture periodic snapshots of the entire WWW for later retrieval. It is said to be the largest database in existence with over 100 terabytes of data.

Physician Internet use is as high as 100% in some studies.[6] In addition, as a matter of course, physicians are able to distinguish medical fact from fiction on the Internet. Patients, too, make use of the Internet, although probably to a lesser extent than physicians.[6] In many cases, the medical information sources available via the WWW are the first line of patient inquiry. Although many reputable sources of medical information geared toward the general public can be found, a great many more range from the dubious to the frankly fraudulent. It stretches the limits of physician responsibility to demand a thorough knowledge of Internet-derived medical nonsense. Nevertheless, it is important to realize that patients have easy access to unreviewed medical concepts and even drugs via online pharmacies that may be located in other countries. Questions directed in this area may become a standard part of the medical history.

thekidney.org

The electronic resource accompanying this chapter is available at www.thekidney.org and is organized into several logical categories (Table 97.2). Included in the WWW site are nearly 400 links to nephrology resources on the Internet. The links were compiled through use of search engines and other nephrology sites. The link list is not nearly as exhaustive as the 187 000 possibilities suggested by one search utility, but it does represent the most popular and stable sites. Most of the current links were continuously functional in the 3 years between editions of this text.

Included here are several general nephrology sites. Particularly useful are: MedNets/nephrology (www. mednets.com/nephrol.htm); NephrologyLinx (www. nephrologylinx.com/index.cfm), which has an easily accessible synopsis of current clinical literature; and RenalNet (www.renalnet.org/). As of 2001, it is possible that almost all scholarly journals and professional societies have a presence on the WWW (to include even The Flat Earth Society (www.flat-earth.org) and the Luddites (www.Luddite.com)). Medical education via the WWW is an ever-expanding enterprise. Most medical school curricula incorporate WWW-based resources, and quite a few textbooks are available, in part or total, on the WWW. Notable here are: *Harrison's Principles of Internal Medicine*,[7] *UpToDate*,[8] and *Scientific American Medicine*.[9] Most online textbooks require a subscription. In addition, most academic renal divisions, dialysis companies, and essentially all medical schools have a presence on the WWW.

Technology giveth and technology taketh away, and not always in equal measure. A new technology sometimes creates more than it destroys. Sometimes, it destroys more than it creates. But, it is never one-sided.[10] The Internet represents an astounding opportunity for paradigm-shattering leaps in medical education, remote diagnosis and treatment, medical record-keeping, and business management. At the same time, the very same technology will threaten physician and patient alike with loss of privacy and independence, and drowning by a vast sea of facts. Computer science and the Internet roll forward quite independently of physicians, who, nevertheless, recognize that the basic human condition remains the same despite the superficial changes.

References

1. Bush V: How we may think. Atlantic Monthly 1945;July.
2. National Center for Biotechnology Information: PubMed Interim Report 2001. *Online* ftp://ncbi.nlm.nih.gov/pubmed/
3. Zakon RH: Hobbes Internet Timeline, 2001. *Online* http://www.zakon.org/robert/internet/timeline/
4. Cerf V: A brief history of the Internet and related networks. *In* Aboba B (ed): The Online User's Encyclopedia. New York: Addison Wesley, 1993.
5. Lipman D: PubMed Central decentralized. Nature 2001;410:740.
6. Jadad AR, Sigouin C, Cocking L, Booker L, Whelan T, Browman G: Internet use among physicians, nurses, and their patients. JAMA 2001;286:1451–1452.
7. Braunwald E, Fauci AS, Isselbacher KJ, et al: Harrison's Principles of Internal Medicine, 15th edn. New York: McGraw Hill. *Online* http://www.harrisonsonline.com/
8. Rose BD (ed): UptoDate. Wellesley, MA: UpToDate Inc. *Online* http://uptodate.com

9. Dale DC (ed): Scient ific American Medicine. New York: Scientific
American Inc. *Online* http://www.samed.com/
10. Postman N: Speech to the German Informatics Society, Oct 11, 1990.
Online http://www.eff.org/Net_culture/Criticisms/

Index

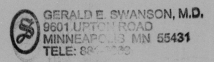